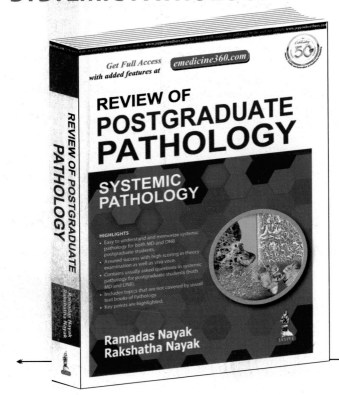

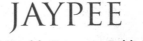

REVIEW OF
POSTGRADUATE PATHOLOGY
GENERAL PATHOLOGY

Authors

Ramadas Nayak MBBS MD
Professor (former Head), Department of Pathology
Yenepoya Medical College, Yenepoya (Deemed to be University)
Mangaluru, Karnataka, India
Formerly, Head, Department of Pathology, Kasturba Medical College
Mangaluru, Manipal Academy of Higher Education, Manipal
Karnataka, Mangaluru, India
askdr.nayak@gmail.com

Rakshatha Nayak MBBS MD DNB
Assistant Professor, Department of Pathology
Kasturba Medical College, Mangaluru, Affiliated to Manipal Academy of Higher Education, Manipal
Karnataka, Mangaluru, India

Foreword

Lt Gen Dr MD Venkatesh, VSM (Retd)

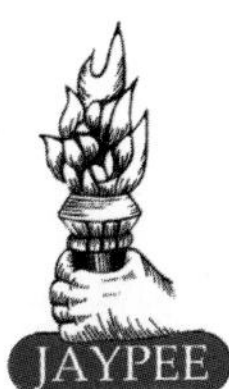

JAYPEE BROTHERS MEDICAL PUBLISHERS
The Health Sciences Publisher
New Delhi | London

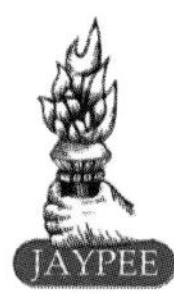

Jaypee Brothers Medical Publishers (P) Ltd

Headquarters
EMCA House
23/23-B, Ansari Road, Daryaganj
New Delhi 110 002, India
Landline: +91-11-23272143, +91-11-23272703
+91-11-23282021, +91-11-23245672
E-mail: jaypee@jaypeebrothers.com

Corporate Office
Jaypee Brothers Medical Publishers (P) Ltd.
4838/24, Ansari Road, Daryaganj
New Delhi 110 002, India
Phone: +91-11-43574357
Fax: +91-11-43574314
E-mail: jaypee@jaypeebrothers.com

Overseas Office
JP Medical Ltd.
83, Victoria Street, London
SW1H 0HW (UK)
Phone: +44-20 3170 8910
Fax: +44(0)20 3008 6180
E-mail: info@jpmedpub.com

Website: www.jaypeebrothers.com
Website: www.jaypeedigital.com

Inquiries for bulk sales may be solicited at: jaypee@jaypeebrothers.com

Review of Postgraduate Pathology: General Pathology */ Ramadas Nayak, Rakshatha Nayak*

First Edition: **2022**

ISBN: 978-93-90595-56-3

Printed at: Sanat Printers

Dedication

Students who inspired us,
Patients who provided the knowledge,
Our teachers, friends, parents, and family members,
who encouraged and supported us.

FOREWORD

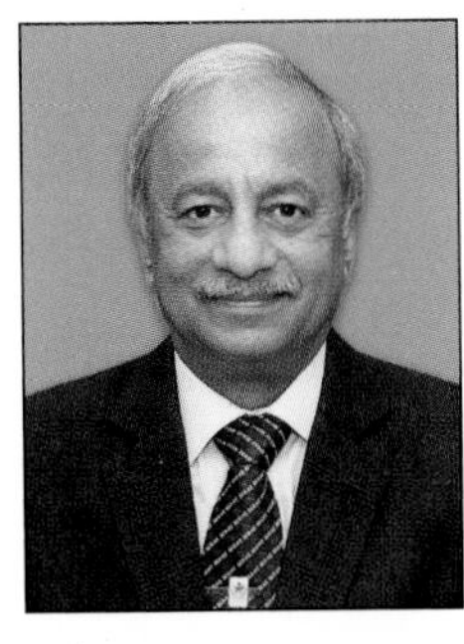

Lt Gen Dr MD Venkatesh, VSM (Retd)
Vice Chancellor
Manipal Academy of Higher Education
Manipal, Karnataka, India

It gives me great pleasure to be writing the foreword for the book titled "Review of Postgraduate Pathology General Pathology" authored by my dear friend Dr Ramadas Nayak, Professor of Pathology at Yenepoya University, Mangaluru and co-authored by Dr Rakshatha Nayak, Assistant Professor of Pathology at Kasturba Medical College, Mangaluru. Dr Ramadas Nayak has used his over 4 decades of professional and teaching experience to the fullest in authoring this remarkable book. The book has been written in a very lucid and simple language. The book has been structured in 17 chapters under the headings of "Basics of Pathology", "General Pathology", and "Immunopathology" and contents of the book are current, up-to-date, and well-researched. The illustrations and tables have been very judiciously used to emphasize important points for easy understanding and retention. I am sure that this easy-to-read book will be very helpful for the postgraduate students of pathology in their understanding of "pathology" and will help as a quick reference book in "pathology". It will serve them well in their preparation for their examinations. I congratulate my friend Dr Ramadas Nayak for his committed efforts toward authoring quality books for the benefit of undergraduate and postgraduate medical students. This present book is one more in the long list of popular books in "pathology" that he has authored. I congratulate the authors and publishers for this remarkable effort and I am sure that this book will be a welcome addition as study material for students of "pathology" and should find a place in the library of all medical colleges.

PREFACE

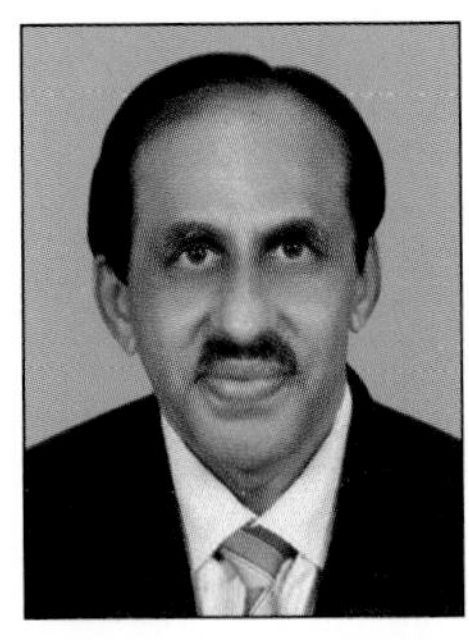

Ramadas Nayak

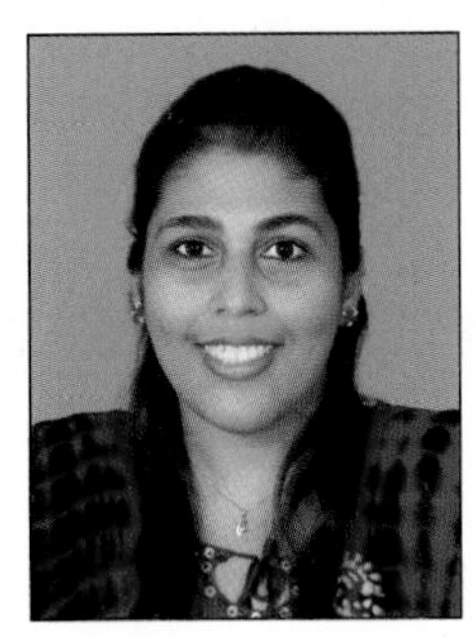

Rakshatha Nayak

The knowledge of pathology is a constantly evolving and emerging speciality. To reflect this, there is a great need to constantly educate oneself, besides reviewing frequently, recent developments and evolving molecular techniques to support the morphological assessment of diagnosis, prognosis, and response to treatment. Pathology is a rapidly expanding, ever-changing, and interesting field in medicine.

Our experience in teaching made us aware of difficulties faced by the postgraduate student of pathology to cope with the basics, advances, routine laboratory work, and interpretation of routine slides. This enthused us to help them by providing a book with "basics of pathology" and "general pathology" in a lucid manner. Most of the students struggle to get the basics in pathology right, which are usually not provided by the standard textbooks in "pathology". The motivation and inspiration for writing the book were the struggles faced by our postgraduate students. The main aim of this book is to provide a sound knowledge of pathology by understanding the disease mechanisms which lay the foundation for basic science. We hope that the reader can learn by construing material given in the book. Writing a postgraduate book was a marathon task which took almost 2.5 years to complete. The challenges we encountered included new information being available online, by the time writing of the entire book was completed.

Every attempt has been made to present information in a simplified text augmented with the use of colored images and illustrations, tables, text boxes, and flowcharts. There was a tremendous increase in the understanding of molecular pathology and same is highlighted in all the relevant chapters.

ORGANIZATION

This book consists of 17 chapters and is organized into three sections namely "Basics of Pathology", "General Pathology", and "Immunopathology".

Section 1—Basics of Pathology: It provides an overview of the basic knowledge and consists of chapters namely cell as a structural unit, cellular activation, maintaining cell populations, extracellular matrix, and basics of genetics.

Section 2—General Pathology: It consists of introduction to pathology; cellular responses to injury, adaptation and cell death; inflammation and healing; hemodynamic disorders, thromboembolism and shock; neoplasia; infections and infestations; genetic disorders and molecular pathology; diseases of infancy and childhood; and environmental and nutritional diseases.

Section 3—Immunopathology: It deals with normal immune response and hypersensitivity; autoimmune diseases and rejection of tissue transplants; and immunodeficiency diseases and amyloidosis.

We realized that postgraduate students find it difficult to understand, remember, and answer the questions during examinations in a satisfying manner. Though many pathology textbooks are available, postgraduates face difficulty in refreshing their knowledge during examinations. This book fills the niche to provide basic information to a postgraduate in a nutshell. Majority of questions that may appear in Paper I of postgraduate examination is also provided. Keywords are shown in bold words so that the student can rapidly go through the book the previous day or just before the examination. Most students are fundamentally "visually oriented". As the saying "a picture is worth a thousand words", this further encouraged us to provide many illustrations.

This book can serve as a source of "general pathology" for postgraduates in pathology. Numerous illustrations, gross photographs, photomicrographs, tables, text boxes, flowcharts, and X-rays have been incorporated for easy understanding of the subject.

ACKNOWLEDGMENT

- Our sincere thanks to all our family members, especially Smt Rekha Nayak, Ms Rashmitha Nayak, Mr Ramnath Kini, Master Rishab Kini, and Mr Ramnath Nayak (Chartered Accountant), who have patiently accepted our long preoccupation with this work.
- We are grateful to Lt Gen (Dr) MD Venkatesh, Vice-Chancellor, Manipal Academy of Higher Education, Manipal, Karnataka (India) for writing the "Foreword" and support.
- We are indebted to Dr Ramdas M Pai (Chancellor), Dr HS Ballal (Pro-Chancellor), and Dr Dilip G Naik (Pro Vice-Chancellor) of Manipal Academy of Higher Education, Manipal, Karnataka (India) for their support. We are grateful to our beloved Dean, Dr M Venkatraya Prabhu, Kasturba Medical College, Mangaluru, Karnataka (India) for his constant support and encouragement.
- We wish to express our gratitude to Mr Yenepoya Abdulla Kunhi (Honorable Chancellor), Mr Mohammed Farhaad Yenepoya (Hon Pro-Chancellor), Dr M Vijaya Kumar (Vice-Chancellor) and Dr KS Gangadhara Somayaji (Registrar), Yenepoya (Deemed to be University), Mangaluru, Karnataka, India.
- We are thankful to all our friends who contributed fantastic images for this book. Our sincere thanks to Dr Sharada Rai (Professor and Head), Department of Pathology, Kasturba Medical College (Mangaluru), Manipal Academy of Higher Education, Manipal.
- We would like to express our gratitude to all our friends, colleagues, undergraduate and postgraduate students (Department of Pathology, Yenepoya Medical College and Kasturba Medical College, Mangaluru) who helped us in the different stages of preparing the manuscript; to all those who provided support, talked things over, read, offered comments and assisted in the editing, proofreading, and graphic designing.
- A special thanks to Shri Jitendar P Vij (Group Chairman), Mr Ankit Vij (Managing Director), Mr MS Mani (Group President) of M/s Jaypee Brothers Medical Publishers (P) Ltd, New Delhi (India) for publishing the book in the same format as wanted, well in time. We are grateful to Shri Jitendar P Vij for unmasking our talent as authors.
- We would like to offer a huge appreciation to the wonderful work done by Dr Richa Saxena (Associate Director-Professional Publishing), Ms Pooja Bhandari (Production Head), Ms Sunita Katla (Executive Assistant to Group Chairman and Publishing Manager), Ms Nedup Denka Bhutia (Development Editor), Dr Ravindra Pandey (Editor), Mr Ajay Kumar Sharma (Production Senior Manager), Ms Seema Dogra (Cover Visualizer), Mr Manoj Kumar (Typesetter), Mr Keshav Kumar (Proofreader), Mr Rajesh Gurugundi (Image Designer) of M/s Jaypee Brothers Medical Publishers (P) Ltd, New Delhi, India.
- We thank Mr Venugopal V Regional Head–Business Development (Digital) and Mr Gajanana Prabhu of M/s Jaypee Brothers Medical Publishers (P) Ltd for taking this book to every corner of Karnataka.
- Last but definitely not least, a thank you to our postgraduate students. Without you, we would not write. You make all our books possible.
- There are many more people we could thank, but space and modesty compel us to stop here.

IMAGES CONTRIBUTION

We are extremely grateful to all my friends who willingly provided required images for this book:

- Dr Anuradha CK Rao (Professor); Dr Krishnaraj Upadhyaya (Professor); Dr Indra Puthran (Professor); Dr Supriya P (Assistant Professor); Dr Renuka Patil (Assistant Professor); Dr Subha Sudhakar (Assistant Professor); Dr Vidya Rekha Kamath (Assistant Professor); Dr Divya A (Associate Professor); Dr Deepa Mary Thomas (Assistant Professor); Dr Prema Saldhana (Professor and Head), Department of Pathology, Yenepoya Medical College. Dr Vidya Pai (Professor); Dr Neha Haswani (Assistant Professor); and Dr Rouchelle G Tellis (Addl Professor and HOD) of Department of Microbiology, Yenepoya Medical College. Dr Yashodhar Bhandary (Associate Professor), Yenepoya Research Centre, Yenepoya (Deemed to be University), Deralakatte, Mangaluru, Karnataka, India.
- Dr Sharada Rai, Professor and Head, Department of Pathology; Dr Jagadish Rao PP, MBBS, MD, Diplomate NB, PGDCFS, Dip Cyber Law, PGCTM, MNAMS, District Medicolegal Consultant (Government Wenlock District Hospital), and Associate Professor, Forensic Medicine and Toxicology; Dr Archith Boloor, Associate Professor, Department of Medicine; Dr Sonali Ullal, Associate Professor, Department of Radiodiagnosis; and Dr Suresh Kumar Shetty, Honorary State Medicolegal Consultant, Government of Karnataka and Professor, Department of Forensic Medicine and Toxicology, Kasturba Medical College, Affiliated to Manipal Academy of Higher Education (Manipal), Mangaluru, Karnataka, India.
- Dr Seethalakshmi NV (Professor); Dr Annie Jojo (Professor); Dr Ajit Nambiar (Professor and Head); Dr Indu R Nair (Additional Professor); and Dr Meera Subramanian (Senior Lecturer), Department of Pathology, Amrita Institute of Medical Sciences, Ponekkara PO, Kochi, Kerala, India.
- Dr Jayaram N Iyengar, Managing Director; and Dr Ananth Vikas, Anand Diagnostic Laboratory (A Neuberg Associate) — Neuberg Anand Reference Laboratory, Bengaluru, India.
- Dr Sriram Bhat M, Professor and Head, Department of Surgery, Kasturba Medical College, a constituent of Manipal Academy of Higher Education, Manipal, Mangaluru, Karnataka, India.
- Dr T Reba Philipose (Professor and Head); Dr Muktha R Pai (former Professor and HOD); and Dr Arvind P (Associate Professor), Department of Pathology, AJ Institute of Medical Sciences and Research, Mangaluru, Karnataka, India.
- Dr Ramesh Chavan (Professor); Dr Ashwini Ratnakar (Assistant Professor), Department of Pathology, Jawaharlal Nehru Medical College, Belagavi, KLE (Deemed to be University), Karnataka, India.
- Dr Prasanna Shetty B (Professor and Head) and Dr Sulatha Kamath (Professor), Department of Pathology, MS Ramaiah Medical College, Bengaluru, India.
- Dr Jayashree K (Professor and Head) and Dr Rekha A Nair (Professor), Department of Pathology, Regional Cancer Institute, Thiruvananthapuram, Kerala, India.
- Dr Veena Shenoy, MD, Associate Professor, and Residency Program Director, Department of Pathology, The University of Mississipi Medical Center, Mississippi, USA.
- Dr Surendra Nayak Kapadi, MD, Department of Histopathology, Ministry of Health, Maternity Hospital, Sabha Area, Kuwait.
- Dr Kanthilatha Pai, Professor and Head, Department of Pathology, Kasturba Medical College, Manipal Academy of Higher Education, Manipal, Karnataka, India.
- Dr S Sankar, MBBS, MD, Professor and Head, Department of Pathology, Dean, Faculty of Allied Health Sciences, KUHS, Government Medical College, Kottayam, Kerala, India.
- Dr Vandana Kamath, Associate Professor of Pathology, Christian Medical College, Vellore, Tamil Nadu, Chennai, India.
- Dr Nandeesh BN and Dr Anita Mahadevan (Professor and Head of Department), Department of Neuropathology, National Institute of Mental Health and Neuro-Sciences (NIMHANS), Bengaluru, Karnataka, India.
- Dr Jayaprakash Shetty, Vice-Dean, Professor and Head of Department Pathology, KS Hegde Medical Academy Mangaluru, affiliated to Nitte University Mangaluru, Karnataka, India.

- Dr Jayaprakash CS, Professor and Head of Department Pathology, Father Muller Medical College, Kankanady, Mangalore, Karnataka, India.
- Dr Dayananda S Biligi, Professor and HOD, Department of Pathology, Bangalore Medical College and Research Institute, Bengaluru, Karnataka, India.
- Dr Narayana Murthy C, Professor and Head, Department of Pathology, Basaveshwara Medical College and Hospital, Chitradurga, Karnataka, India.
- Dr Malathi, Kidwai Memorial Institute of Oncology, Bengaluru, Karnataka, India.
- Dr Tanuj Kanchan, Professor, Department of Forensic Medicine and Toxicology, All India Institute of Medical Sciences, Jodhpur, Rajasthan, India.
- Dr Niranjana Murthy B, Professor and Head of Department Pathology, Sri Siddartha Medical College, Tumkur, affiliated to Siddartha (deemed to be University) Tumkur, Karnataka, India.
- Dr Vinit Anand (Professor and Head of Department); Dr Vaibhav Nayak (Professor); Dr Indudhara PB (Professor); Dr Ganga H (Associate Professor); and Dr Harshitha KS (Senior resident) of Subbaiah Institute of Medical Sciences, Shivamogga, Karnataka, India.
- Dr Francisco Couto, Director, Professor of Pathology; Dr RGW Pinto (Professor and Head); Dr Premila de Sousa Rocha (Associate Professor); Dr Suresh RS Mandrekar; Dr Shruti U Shetye (Tutor); Dr Merline Augustine (Tutor); and Dr Priyanka Raghuvir Mashelkar (Tutor), Department of Pathology, Goa Medical College, Bambolim, Goa, India.

CONTENTS

SECTION 1: BASICS OF PATHOLOGY

SECTION 2: GENERAL PATHOLOGY

SECTION 3: IMMUNOPATHOLOGY

SECTION

1

BASICS OF PATHOLOGY

CHAPTER 1

Cell as a Structural Unit

CHAPTER OUTLINE

CELL

Pathology (Greek, *pathos* = suffering, *logos* = study) literally means the study of *suffering* and it deals with the study of *disease*. Rudolf Virchow (Father of Cellular Pathology) stated that the disease originates at the cellular level. With the present advances in medicine, we realize that cellular disturbances occur as a result of alterations in molecules (genes, proteins, and others) which influence the survival and behavior of cells. Thus, the modern pathology deals with the *cellular* and molecular abnormalities that produce diseases. Hence, it is necessary to know the *normal* cellular structure and function.

NORMAL CELL STRUCTURE AND FUNCTIONS

- A cell is the fundamental unit of life.
- All cells are tridimensional, although when viewed under the light microscope on a glass slide, they appear to be flat.

Components of the Cell (Fig. 1)

All cells share the fundamental structural components. Each cell has three essential components—(1) cell membrane, (2) cytoplasm, and (3) nucleus.

Cell Membrane/Unit Membrane

- It is the outer boundary of the cell.
- **Light microscopy:** The membrane appears at the periphery as a thin condensation.

Function of Cell Membrane

Cell membrane plays a critical role in virtually every aspect of cell function. These include:

- **Compartmentalization:** The plasma membrane is a continuous, unbroken sheet that encloses the contents of the entire cell, whereas the nuclear and cytoplasmic membranes enclose diverse intracellular spaces. Membrane compartmentalization allows to perform specialized activities without external interference and allows to regulate the cellular activities independently.
- **Scaffold for biochemical activities:** Membranes are also a distinct compartment themselves and provide the cell with an extensive framework or scaffolding. This helps in orderly effective interaction.
- **Providing a selectively permeable barrier:** Membranes prevent the unrestricted exchange of molecules from one to the other. However, they provide the means of communication between the compartments they separate.

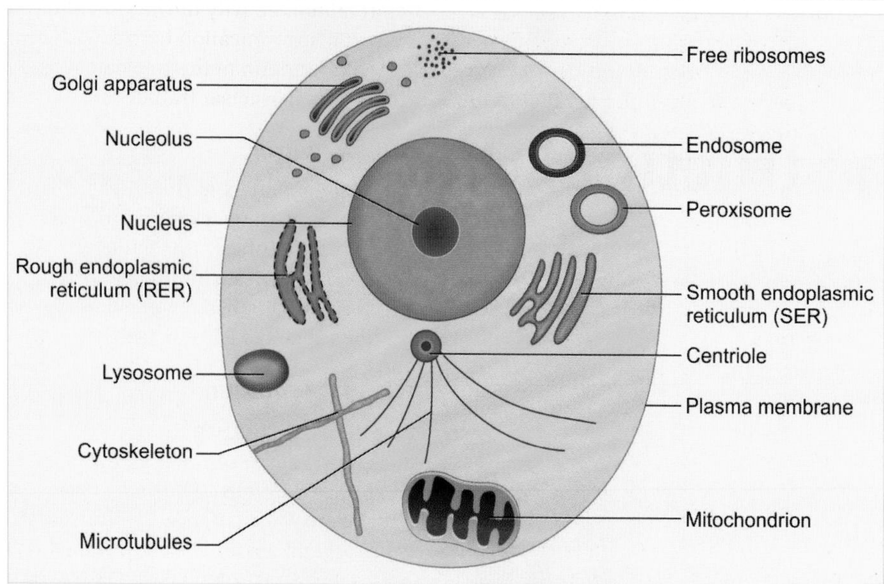

FIG. 1: Various constituents of cell.

- **Transporting solutes:** The plasma membrane contains the machinery for transporting substances from one side of the membrane to another. This allows a cell to accumulate substances (e.g., sugars and amino acids), that are necessary to fuel its metabolism and build its macromolecules. The plasma membrane is also capable of transporting specific ions. This establishes ionic gradients across itself. This is especially important in nerve and muscle cells.
- **Responding to external signals:** The plasma membrane plays an important role in the response of a cell to external stimuli, a process called as **signal transduction**. Membranes have receptors **which** combine with specific complementary structure/molecules (or **ligands**). Different types of cells have membranes with different receptors and can recognize and respond to different ligands. The interaction of a plasma membrane receptor with an external ligand generates a signal that stimulates or inhibits internal activities. For example, signals at the plasma membrane prepare the cell for division.
- **Intercellular interaction:** The plasma membrane mediates the interactions between a cell and its surrounding. For example, it allows cells to recognize and signal one another, to adhere to each other, and to exchange materials and information.
- **Energy transduction:** Membranes are involved in the processes of conversion of one type of energy to another type (energy transduction). Membranes are also involved in the transfer of chemical energy from carbohydrates and fats to adenosine triphosphate (ATP).

Cytoplasm

- Cytoplasm or cytosol is the component of the cell, located between the nucleus and the cell membrane.
- **Light microscopy:** Various products of cell metabolism may be seen in the cytoplasm, and appear as granules or vacuoles.

Cytoplasmic Organelles

Ultrastructurally, the cytoplasm is composed of—(1) organized cell components, or organelles; (2) the cytoskeleton (discussed on pages 15–22), and (3) cytoplasmic matrix.

Organized components of the cytoplasm

They mainly consists of—(1) membranous systems, (2) ribosomes, (3) mitochondria, (4) lysosomes, and (5) centrioles.

- **Membranous system:** It is composed of—(1) the endoplasmic reticulum, and (2) the Golgi complex.
  - **Endoplasmic reticulum:**
    - **Appearance:** It is a closed system of unit membranes forming tubular canals and flattened sacs or cisternae. It subdivides the cytoplasm into a series of compartments.
    - **Types:** The membranes of the endoplasmic reticulum may be "rough", i.e., rough endoplasmic reticulum (RER) (i.e., covered with numerous attached granules), or "smooth", i.e., smooth endoplasmic reticulum (SER) (i.e., free of any particles).
    - **Function:** RER is abundant in metabolically active cells.
  - **Golgi complex:**
    - **Appearance:** It consists of a series of parallel, doughnut-shaped flat spaces or cisternae and spherical or egg-shaped vesicles demarcated by smooth membranes.
    - **Function:** They synthesize and package cell products for the cell's own use and for export.
- **Ribosomes**
  - They are found in all cells.
  - Two types of ribosomes namely free and attached.
  - **Functions:**
    - Free ribosomes produce proteins for the cell's own use.
    - Attached ribosomes produce proteins for export.

- **Mitochondria:** They are present in all eukaryotic cells.
  - **Appearance:** Each mitochondrion is composed of two membranes. The outer membrane is a continuous, closed-unit membrane. Running parallel to the outer membrane is the inner membrane that forms numerous crests or invaginations.
  - **Function:** Most important function is the formation of energy-producing ATP from phosphorus and adenosine diphosphate (ADP). ATP is exported into the cytoplasm and is an essential source of energy for the cell.
- **Lysosomes:** Lysosomes are intracellular organelles that contain degradative enzymes.
  - **Appearance:** Electron microscopically, appears as spherical or oval structures.
  - **Function:**
    - Lysosomal enzymes perform the digestion of a wide range of macromolecules, including proteins, polysaccharides, lipids, and nucleic acids.
    - They participate in the removal of phagocytized foreign material.
- **Centrioles**
  - **Appearance:** They are short tubular structures, usually located in the vicinity of the concave face of the Golgi complex.
  - **Function:** Play a key role during cell division.

Cytoplasmic matrix

The space within the cytoplasm, not occupied by the membranous system, the cell skeleton, or by the organelles, is called as the cytoplasmic matrix. It is composed of proteins and free ribosomes.

Nucleus

Nucleus is the central processing unit of the cell and is the controlling center of the cell. It contains mainly deoxyribonucleic acid (DNA) that governs the genetic and functional aspects of cell activity. It is present within the cytoplasm. The important components of the nucleus are—(1) nuclear envelope (nuclear membrane, pore, and lamina), (2) nuclear matrix, (3) nuclear chromatin, and (4) nucleoli.

Nuclear Envelope

Nuclear envelope separates the nucleus from the cytoplasm. It consists of three parts—(1) nuclear membrane, (2) nuclear pore, and (3) nuclear lamina.

Nuclear membrane

The nuclear membrane is subdivided into outer nuclear membrane (ONM), inner nuclear membrane (INM), and perinuclear space. ONM is continuous with the endoplasmic reticulum. It contains multiple ribosomes on its cytoplasmic side. The INM is parallel to ONM and is directly attached to the nuclear lamina. The space in between ONM and INM is called as perinuclear space. Nuclear membrane acts as a physical barrier between cytoplasm and nucleus and helps in chromatin remodeling and gene expression.

Nuclear pore

In positions, where INM and ONM fuse with each other, they make the hole on the nuclear membrane. There are multiple nuclear pores in both ONM and INM. The number of nuclear pores varies from few hundreds to thousands depending on the metabolic activity of the cell. The nuclear pore is the site of direct communication between the nucleus and cytoplasm. The main function of the nuclear pore is the facilitation of the cytoplasmic to nuclear traffic and *vice versa*.

Nuclear Matrix

The nuclear matrix is the internal skeleton of the nucleus. It consists of network of ribonucleic acid (RNA), protein complexes, peripheral nuclear lamin, and residual nucleoli. Its composition varies with nuclear activities. The nuclear matrix protein (NMP) is tissue specific and involved in many vital functions of cell (e.g., gene transcription and translation).

Nuclear Chromatin

Chromatin structure

Chromatin represents the uncoiled chromosome of the interphase nucleus. The individual chromosomes occupy specific position of the nucleus which is referred to as chromosomal territories. Chromatin consists of DNA, histone, and nonhistone proteins.

Classification of chromatin

Chromatin can be classified as heterochromatin and euchromatin. The heterochromatin consists of condensed portion of chromatin where genes are usually inactive. Euchromatin is less condensed and consists of actively transcribed genes. Heterochromatin and euchromatin (refer Fig. 2 in Chapter 5) are seen in the cells/tissues under light microscope.

Nucleolus

Nucleolus is the subnuclear, round to oval, small structure seen within the nucleus. In normal resting nuclei, the nucleoli are seen as round or oval structures occupying a small area within the nucleus. It is not attached to the nuclear membrane and is usually situated in the center of the nucleus; however, their position may vary. They vary in number from 1–3. The size of the nucleolus depends upon the requirement of ribosome and protein synthesis. Hence, in a metabolically active cell with more amount of protein synthesis, the cells will show larger nucleoli. Nucleolus can be easily detectable by light microscope. In histological section stained by routine hematoxylin and eosin (H&E), the nucleoli appear as deep eosinophilic round structures. In cytology smears stained by May Grunwald Giemsa stain, the nucleoli appear as light-blue colored structures.

Nucleosome is the basic unit of chromatin and discussed in detail in Chapter 5.

Relative volumes, numbers, and role of intracellular organelles in a hepatocyte are presented in **Table 1.**

CELLULAR HOUSEKEEPING

Introduction

Q. Write a short essay on cellular housekeeping.

The viability, normal activity and intracellular homeostasis of cells depend on housekeeping functions that all differentiated cells must perform. The **normal housekeeping functions are usually compartmentalized within membrane-bound intracellular organelles (Fig. 1**).

Table 1: Relative volumes, numbers, and role of intracellular organelles* in a hepatocyte.

Compartment/intracellular organelle	*Percentage (%) of total volume*	*Number/cell*	*Role*
Cytosol (cytoplasm) has a plasma membrane	54	1	Metabolism, transport, and protein translation
• Mitochondria	22	1,700	Generation of energy, apoptosis
• Endoplasmic reticulum			
○ Rough endoplasmic reticulum (RER)	9	1	Membrane synthesis and synthesis of secreted proteins
○ Smooth endoplasmic reticulum (SER), Golgi apparatus	6	1	Modification, sorting, and catabolism of proteins
• Endosomes	1	200	Intracellular transport and export, ingestion of extracellular substances
• Lysosomes	1	300	Cellular catabolism
• Peroxisomes	1	400	Metabolism of very long-chain fatty acids
Nucleus It consists of • Nuclear membrane • Nucleoli • Chromatin, and • Nuclear matrix	6	1	Cell regulation, proliferation, deoxyribonucleic acid (DNA) transcription

**Note*: Ribosome, cytoskeleton, centrioles, and cytoplasmic vacuoles are not mentioned in the above table.

Box 1: Housekeeping functions.

- Protection from the environment
- To get nutrients
- Metabolism
- Communication
- Movement
- Renewal of senescent molecules
- Molecular catabolism
- Generation of energy

Housekeeping Functions

These are listed in **Box 1**.

Advantages of compartmentalization

The advantages of isolating certain cellular functions within membrane-bound distinct compartments are as follows:

- Potentially injurious degradative enzymes or reactive metabolites can be concentrated or stored at high concentrations in these specific organelles.
- Helps to prevent damage to other cellular constituents.
- Compartmentalization helps in creation of unique intracellular environments (e.g., low pH or high calcium) that are needed for certain enzymes or metabolic pathways.

Synthesis of Proteins

- New proteins needed for the plasma membrane or secretions are synthesized in the RER. These are physically assembled in the Golgi apparatus.
- Proteins needed for the cytosol are synthesized on free ribosomes.
- **Smooth endoplasmic reticulum:** These are the site of synthesis of steroid hormone and lipoprotein. They are abundant in certain cell types such as gonads and liver. SER also modifies hydrophobic compounds such as drugs into water-soluble molecules for export.

Molecular Catabolism

Q. Write a short essay on peroxisomes.

When the proteins and organelles get damaged, they must be broken down. These are taken up into the cell by endocytosis. They are catabolized in the cells. These molecules are constantly being degraded and renewed. Their breakdown takes place at three different sites and serves different functions.

1. **Proteasomes** (refer pages 184–185): These are "disposal" complexes which degrade denatured or "tagged" cytosolic proteins and release short peptides. In few cases, these released short peptides are presented to class I or class II major histocompatibility molecules which will produce an adaptive immune response (refer Chapter 15). In other cases, proteasomal degradation of regulatory proteins or transcription factors can shut down cellular signaling pathways.
2. **Lysosomes:** These are intracellular organelles containing powerful enzymes that can digest a wide range of macromolecules (e.g., proteins, polysaccharides, lipids, and nucleic acids). The phagocytosed microbes and damaged or unwanted cellular organelles are also destroyed or degraded in lysosomes. This process is called as autophagy (refer pages 156–159).
3. **Peroxisomes:** These are specialized organelles in the cell which contain catalase, peroxidase, and other oxidative enzymes. They breakdown very long-chain fatty acids, and during this process, they generate hydrogen peroxide.

Regulation of Contents and Position of Cellular Organelles

The contents and location of cellular organelles are very well regulated.

- **Endosomal vesicles:** They transfer the internalized material to the appropriate intracellular sites. The newly synthesized materials are directed to the cell surface or targeted organelle by endosomal vesicle.
- **Cytoskeleton:** It controls the movement of both organelles and proteins within the cell and its environment. Cytoskeletal proteins also regulate cellular shape and intracellular organization. They are needed for maintaining *cell polarity*. This is very important in epithelia, in which the apical (top of the cell) and the basolateral (bottom and side of the cell) are exposed to different environments and have distinct functions (discussed in details on pages 15–22).
- **Mitochondria:** Its functions include:
    - **Major source of energy** for the cell is the ATP. It is generated through oxidative phosphorylation in the mitochondria.
    - Mitochondrion is also an important **source of metabolic intermediates** which are necessary for anabolic metabolism.
    - **Synthesis of certain macromolecules** (e.g., heme)
    - **Initiation and regulation of apoptosis:** Through its sensors of cell damage.

Generation of Energy

Cell growth and maintenance need a constant supply of both energy and the building blocks required for synthesis of macromolecules. In growing and dividing cells, all of the organelles need to be replicated (organellar biogenesis) and also to be present in all daughter cells following mitosis. The macromolecules and organelles have limited span of life (e.g., life span of mitochondria is about 10 days). Hence, it is necessary to have mechanisms for the recognition and degradation of "worn out" cellular components. The final catabolism occurs in lysosomes.

Housekeeping Genes

Q. Write a short essay on housekeeping genes.

A small percentage of genes, called as housekeeping genes, and their gene products are necessary for the function and maintenance of all cells. They are named so because they keep cells running. These genes are expressed, transcribed, and translated in all cells at a relatively constant rate and not known to be subject to regulation. They remain unaffected by environmental conditions. Housekeeping genes often lack the CCAAT and TATA boxes.

The cytosine bases in the CpG islands of housekeeping genes escape the methylation process (they are unmethylated). Therefore, these genes tend to be expressed and remain transcriptionally active in most cell types.

Q. Describe the cell ultrastructure and its role in health and disease (for answer refer individual chapters)

Plasma Membrane

All cells are bounded by an external membrane, called the **plasma membrane** (cell membrane). **It protects the cell and through this nutrient is obtained.** It is the outermost component of the cell and forms closed compartments around the cytoplasm to define cell boundaries. It separates cytoplasm from its external or extracellular environment namely **extracellular matrix (ECM) and** the **intercellular space**. Plasma membrane (and all other organellar membranes) of cells is a thin, fragile, dynamic fluid structure static lipid sheaths measuring about 5–10 nm in width. It encloses the contents of the entire cell.

Composition of Plasma Membrane

The membrane is a bimolecular (lipid–protein) layer composed of approximately equal amounts (by weight) of lipids and proteins. The lipid bilayer acts as a structural backbone and sheet of lipids form the backbone of cell membrane. Most of the chemical reactions of cells take place in aqueous polarized solution. Since **lipids are immiscible with water, the lipid of the cell membrane effectively prevents random movements of water-soluble materials into and out of the cell**. Thus, the contents of different compartments are kept separate and ion gradients between different compartments are maintained. Proteins embedded within the lipid bilayer (of phospholipids, cholesterol), carry out most of the specific functions. They act as channels which allow selective passage of particular ions and molecules. Some type of cell signaling is also mediated by membrane proteins. The plasma membrane functions as a selective barrier that regulates the passage of materials into and out of the cell and facilitates the transport of specific molecules.

Membrane lipids (Fig. 2)

The lipid bilayer consists of two distinct leaflets namely, inner and outer. Membranes contain a variety of lipids, all of which are **amphipathic**; that is, they **contain both hydrophilic (water-loving/polar) and hydrophobic (water-fearing/nonpolar) regions**. The amphipathic phospholipids with hydrophilic head groups face the aqueous environment. The hydrophobic lipid tails interact with each other to form a barrier to passive diffusion of large or charged molecules.

The lipid bilayer is composed of a heterogeneous collection of different phospholipids. The main phospholipids in the cell membrane are phosphoglycerides. The distribution of phospholipids in each half of the bilayer is different or asymmetric. Examples of asymmetry include:

- Certain membrane lipids (e.g., *phosphatidylcholine* and *sphingomyelin*) are more abundant in the outer half.
- Certain membrane lipids [e.g., *phosphatidylserine* (negative charge) and *phosphatidylethanolamine*] are more concentrated in the inner layer/leaflet (cytosolic face).
- Some of the outer lipids are known as glycolipids, include oligosaccharide chains. They extend outward from the cell surface (outer face) to the extracellular region. There they contribute to a delicate coating on the cell surface area called the glycocalyx.

  Composition of cell membrane is summarized in **Box 2**.

Cellular processes involved with asymmetric partitioning of phospholipids

The asymmetric partitioning of phospholipids plays an important role in several cellular processes:

- **Phosphatidylinositol:** It is present on the inner membrane leaflet. It can be phosphorylated and serves as an electrostatic scaffold for intracellular proteins. Alternatively, polyphosphoinositides can be hydrolyzed by phospholipase C. These can produce intracellular second signals such as diacylglycerol and inositol trisphosphate.

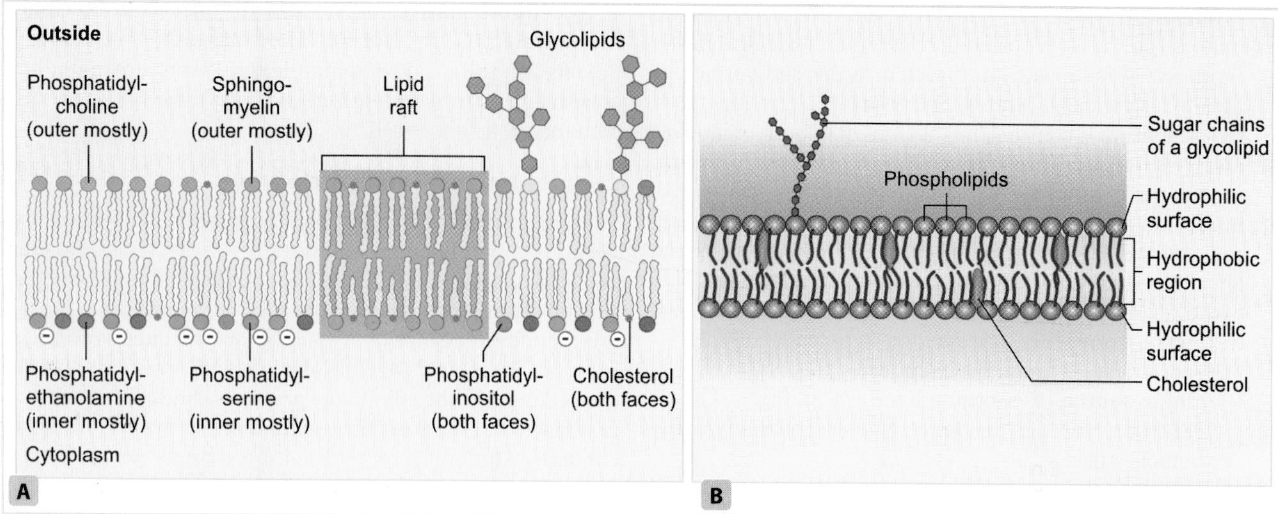

FIGS. 2A AND B: Organization of plasma membrane. (A) The plasma membrane is a bilayer of phospholipids, cholesterol, and associated proteins. The distribution of phospholipid within the plasma membrane is asymmetric. The phosphatidylcholine and sphingomyelin are present in the outer leaflet, and phosphatidylserine (negative charge) and *phosphatidylethanolamine* are mainly seen on the inner leaflet. The glycolipids are found on the outer face where they contribute to the extracellular glycocalyx. Nonrandom partitioning of certain membrane components such as cholesterol creates membrane domains termed as lipid rafts. (B) Structure of plasma membrane depicting hydrophobic and hydrophilic surfaces.

Box 2: Composition of cell membrane.

- Lipids: Phospholipids, cholesterol, and glycolipids
  - Double layer, hydrophilic ends outer side and hydrophobics ends facing each other
- Proteins:
  - Integral protein incorporated within the membrane
  - Transmembrane protein present through complete breadth
  - Peripheral membrane protein is present on the inner and outer surface of the membrane
- Carbohydrates: Glycoproteins and glycolipids

- **Phosphatidylserine:** It is normally restricted to the inner face. It has a negative charge and is involved in electrostatic interactions with proteins. However, when it flips to the extracellular face, it helps in apoptosis. In platelets, it serves as a cofactor in the clotting of blood.
- **Glycolipids and sphingomyelin:** They are mainly expressed on the extracellular face. Glycolipids (and particularly gangliosides, with complex sugar linkages and terminal sialic acids give them negative charges) are important in cell-cell and cell-matrix interactions, including inflammatory cell recruitment and sperm-egg interactions.

Lipid rafts

The lipid structure of plasma membranes is not homogeneous. This creates nonrandom partitioning of certain membrane components along with patches in the plasma membrane. These specialized membrane patches or areas in the **outer leaflet** of the lipid bilayer are termed as **lipid rafts** (**Fig. 2A**). Membrane proteins move laterally within the lipid bilayer, with less movement in **lipid raft** areas. These lipid rafts have higher concentrations of cholesterol and saturated fatty acids (glycosphingolipids, sphingolipids) and certain proteins which reduce lipid fluidity.

Membrane Proteins

Various ways of association of membrane proteins with the lipid bilayer

The protein component inserted into the cell membrane has different intrinsic solubilities in various lipid domains. They tend to accumulate in certain regions of the membrane (e.g., rafts) and become depleted from others. These nonrandom distributions of lipids and proteins in the cell membrane have impact on cell-cell and cell-matrix interactions, intracellular signaling and the generation of specialized membrane regions involved in secretory or endocytic pathways. **The plasma membrane has a variety of proteins and glycoproteins.** Membrane proteins can be grouped into four distinct classes depending on the intimacy of their relationship to the lipid bilayer. Protein interaction with the lipid bilayer of cell membrane is arranged in one of four general patterns (**Fig. 3**):

- **Integral and transmembrane proteins (1 and 2 in Fig. 3):** Most protein molecules are embedded (directly incorporated) within the lipid bilayer (intrinsic or integral proteins) itself. Many membrane proteins traverse the entire thickness of the lipid bilayer membrane. They extend and protrude from both the extracellular and cytoplasmic sides of the membrane (i.e., they form part of their mass on either side namely, from one side to the other). Hence, are called transmembrane proteins. When these transport proteins traverse the lipid layer many times, they are called ***multipass transmembrane proteins (2 in Fig. 3)***. Peripheral proteins show a looser association (embedded within) with one of the two membrane surfaces (inner or outer lipid leaflet), particularly the inner. Membrane-associated proteins may traverse the membrane (singly or multiply) via one or more relatively hydrophobic α-helical amino acid sequences. Depending on the sequence and hydrophobicity of these amino acid sequences, such proteins may be enriched or excluded from lipid rafts and other membrane domain. Integral membrane protein molecules usually contain

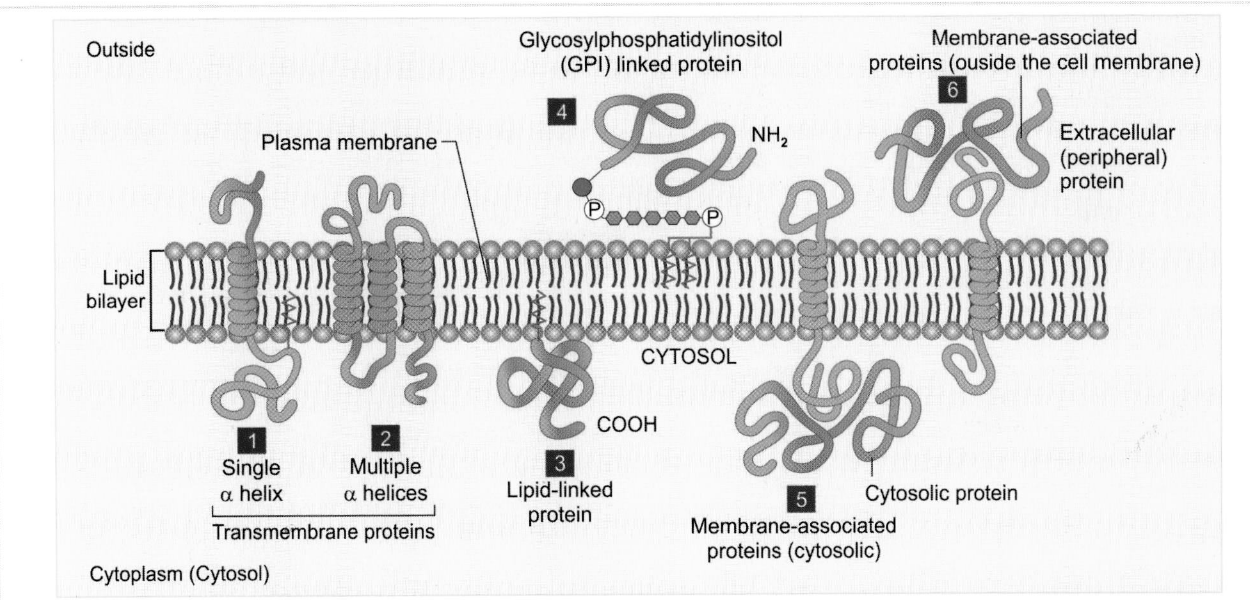

(COOH: carboxy terminal; NH_2: amino terminal)

FIG. 3: Various type of membrane protein interaction with lipid layer.

positively charged amino acids in their cytoplasmic domains which are attached to the negatively charged head groups of membrane phospholipids. Parts of many integral proteins protrude from both the outer or inner membrane surface. Similar to glycolipids (described previously), the carbohydrate moieties of glycoproteins project from the external surface of the plasma membrane and contribute to the glycocalyx. This glycocalyx forms the important components of proteins acting as receptors. These receptors participate in important interactions such as cell adhesion, cell recognition, and the response to protein hormones. Similar to lipids, the distribution of membrane polypeptides (proteins) is different in the two surfaces of the cell membranes. Hence, all membranes in the cell are asymmetric. Membrane proteins functioning as components of large enzyme complexes are less mobile, particularly those involved in the transduction of signals from outside the cell. Such protein complexes are located in lipid rafts (refer page 8).

- **Extracytosolic proteins: Proteins on the extracytoplasmic** (extracellular) **face** may anchor or get attached to the membrane via glycosyl phosphatidyl inositol linkages (GPI) on the face of the membrane (**4 in Fig. 3**).
- **Interaction with extracellular and/or intracytoplasmic proteins:** Apart from protein-protein interactions within the membrane, membrane proteins can also associate or **interact with extracellular and/or intracytoplasmic proteins**. This creates large, relatively stable complexes (e.g., the *focal adhesion complex*). Extracellular proteins can noncovalently associate with transmembrane proteins and help to attach or anchor them to the cell.
- **Membrane-associated proteins (5 and 6 in Fig. 3):** They do not extend into the interior of the lipid bilayer at all and are located entirely outside of the lipid bilayer, on either the cytoplasmic (**5 of Fig. 3**) or extracellular side (**6 of Fig. 3**). These proteins are often known as **peripheral proteins.** They are attached to the surface of the membrane by noncovalent bonds. **Lipid-anchored proteins (3 of Fig. 3)** are located outside the lipid bilayer, on either the extracellular or cytoplasmic surface. They are covalently linked to a lipid molecule that is situated within the bilayer.
    - **Cytosolic proteins:** Proteins may be synthesized in the cytosol. These **proteins on the cytosolic face** may associate with or get inserted into the cytosolic side of the plasma membrane through post-translational modifications. Examples are:
        - **Farnesyl anchor:** Farnesylation (i.e., attachment to prenyl groups such as farnesyl, related to cholesterol)
        - Addition of fatty acids
            - Palmitoyl anchor: Attachment by palmitic acid or
            - Myristoyl anchor: Attachment by myristic acid
        - Some membrane proteins are anchored to cytoplasmic structures by the cytoskeleton (**Fig. 4**).

Structure of membrane and its contents are summarized in **Figure 4**.

Cell Polarity

Most of the cells in the body are polarized or have certain orientation. For example, the epithelial cells have distinct polar distribution, such as luminal surface and basolateral surface facing toward the basement membrane and side of the cell. This polarity of the epithelial cells is due to various membrane protein complexes. Three types of polarity complex proteins are observed in the membrane of the epithelial cells:

- PAR (CDC42-PAR3-PAR6-aPKC) are involved in the apical polarization.
- Crumbs (Crb-PALS-PATJ) are involved in the apical polarization.

- Scribbles (Scrib-Dlg-Lgl) responsible for basolateral polarization.

They are also involved in the asymmetric cell division, cell proliferation, and cell migration. Loss of epithelial cell polarity complexes is related with tumor progression and invasion.

Salient features of cell polarity are presented in **Box 3**.

Cilia and Flagella

Cilia and flagella (**Box 4**) represent the mobile extensions from the surface of the cytoplasm. Cilia are small, regular, and multiple in number, whereas, flagellum is a single slender structure. Cilia are seen on the epithelial lining of the upper respiratory tract and fallopian tube. Cilia are usually lost in the malignant tumors arising from the bronchial epithelium. Hence, in the presence of cilia on the cell it is justifiable to safely exclude the possibility of malignancy. Cilia help in the movement of the particles or organism in one direction.

Brush Border

The surface of few specialized epithelial cells shows multiple microvilli termed as brush border (**Box 4**). They are regular finger-like projections on the cell surface about 1 μ in length. Microvilli are seen on the luminal surface of the intestinal epithelium and the proximal tubular epithelial cells of kidney. On light microscopy, they give a fuzzy appearance to the surface of epithelium. The brush border increases the surface area of the cell and helps in better absorption of the substances from the lumen (e.g., intestinal lumen or tubular lumen).

Salient features of cilia and brush border are presented in **Box 4**.

Functions of Membrane Proteins

Transmembrane proteins can translate mechanical forces (e.g., from the cytoskeleton or ECM) and chemical signals across the membrane. These features are also observed within the various organellar membranes. Transmembrane proteins are involved in:

- **Ion and metabolite transport:** The plasma/cell membrane functions as a selective barrier regulating the passage of materials into and out of the cell. Thus, it facilitates the transport of specific molecules. It keeps the ion content

Box 3: Salient features of cell polarity.

- Major polarity complex protiens: PAR (CDC42–PAR3–PAR6–aPKC), Crumbs (Crb–PALS–PATJ), and Scribbles (Scrib–Dlg–Lgl). They are also involved in asymmetric cell division, cell proliferation, and migration
  - PAR and Crumbs: Apical polarity
  - Scribbles: Basolateral polarity
- Many polarity complex proteins may be mutated in cancer
- Cell polarity protein complexes are involved in epithelial mesenchymal transition (EMT), tumor progression, and invasion

Box 4: Salient features of cilia and brush border.

Cilia and flagella
- Extensions from the surface of cytoplasm
- Cilia are present on the lining epithelium of the upper respiratory tract and fallopian tube
- Function: Movement of the particles or organism in one direction

Brush border
- Regular finger-like projections on the cell surface seen in few specialized epithelial cells (e.g., intestinal epithelium and proximal tubular epithelial cells of kidney)
- Function: Helps in better absorption of the substances from the large surface area

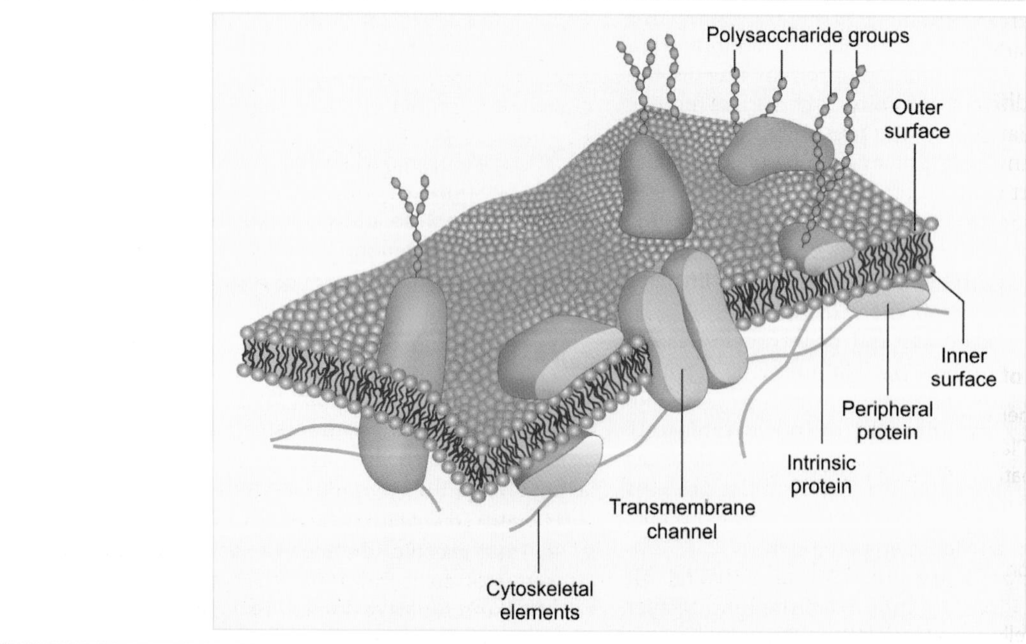

FIG. 4: Structure of membrane and its contents.

of cytoplasm constant, which differs from that of the extracellular fluid. The plasma membrane has **selective permeabilities** and acts as a barrier. It maintains differences in composition between the inside and outside of the cell. Selective membrane molecular permeability is brought out by the action of specific **transporters** and **ion channels.**

- **Fluid-phase and receptor-mediated uptake of macromolecules:** The plasma membrane exchanges molecules with the extracellular environment by **exocytosis** and **endocytosis.**
- **Cell-ligand, cell-matrix, and cell-cell interactions:** Membrane plays key roles in **cell-cell interactions,** cell to its environment interaction, and in **transmembrane signaling**.

Changes in plasma membrane components can affect water balance, ion flux, and many processes within the cell. Specific deficiencies or changes in any components of membrane (e.g., caused by mutations in genes encoding membrane proteins) can produce a variety of **diseases.**

Functions of plasma membrane are listed in **Box 5**.

Many of plasma membrane proteins function together as larger complexes. These proteins may form complexes under the control of chaperone molecules in the RER or by lateral diffusion in the plasma membrane. Lateral diffusion refers to the lateral movement of lipids and proteins in the membrane. Usually, membrane lipids and proteins are free to move laterally**,** if they are no restrictions by certain interactions. The lateral diffusion is characteristic mechanism of many protein receptors (e.g., cytokine receptors). These receptors dimerize or trimerize in the presence of ligand to form functional signaling units.

Transport across the cell membrane may be brought out by one of the mechanisms:

- **Simple diffusion:** Passive, down an ionic or concentration gradient, or
- **Facilitated diffusion** via ion channel or carrier proteins (which does not require energy), or
- **Active:** Only via carrier proteins which need energy and usually against a gradient.

Passive membrane diffusion (Fig. 5)

The lipid bilayer is relatively impermeable to all molecules except the smallest and/or most hydrophobic molecules. So, to import or export charged molecules, it needs specific transmembrane transporter proteins; the internalization or externalization of large proteins, complex particles, or even cells requires to encircle the molecules with segments of the plasma membrane.

- **Small nonpolar molecules: A molecule** is termed **nonpolar** when there is an **equal sharing of electrons between the two atoms of a diatomic molecule** or because of the symmetrical arrangement of polar bonds in a more complex molecule. Small, nonpolar molecules such as O_2 and CO_2 **easily dissolve in lipid bilayers** of cell membrane. Hence, they rapidly diffuse across the membrane, similar to hydrophobic molecules (e.g., steroid-based molecules such as estradiol or vitamin D).
- **Polar molecules:** A polar molecule has a net **dipole** as a result of the opposing charges (i.e., having partial positive and partial negative charges) from polar bonds arranged asymmetrically (e.g., water is a polar molecule since it has a slight positive charge on one side and a slight negative charge on the other).
    - **Small polar molecules** (<75 daltons in mass, such as water, ethanol, and urea) can **easily cross cell membranes.** Dalton is a unit used in expressing the molecular weight of proteins.
    - **Larger polar molecules:** The lipid bilayer forms an **effective barrier** for the passage of larger polar molecules, even those only slightly >75 daltons (e.g., glucose).
- **Ions:** They **cannot pass through the lipid bilayers** though small, because of their charge and high degree of hydration.

Carriers (Transporters) and Channels

Small charged solutes can move across the membrane using either carriers or channels. Unique plasma membrane protein complexes are required for crossing the membranes by the larger polar molecules which support normal cellular functions (e.g., uptake of nutrients and disposal of waste). Carriers and channels are the two main classes of membrane transport proteins. C*hannel proteins* and *carrier proteins* are used for crossing of low-molecular-weight species (ions and small molecules up to approximately 1,000 daltons). Note that similar pores and channels are also needed for transport across organellar membranes. Each transported molecule (e.g., ion, sugar, nucleotide) needs a highly specific carrier protein/transporter (e.g., glucose but not galactose):

- **Channel proteins (2 of Fig. 5A):** Plasma membranes contain transmembrane channels which are narrow pore-like structures (hydrophilic pores) composed of proteins that constitute selective ion channels. They interact with the solute to be transported. When open, they allow rapid passive movement of solutes across the membrane. They are usually restricted by size and charge. Examples include water and small inorganic ions. *Channels* are used when concentration gradients can drive the solute movement. Ion channels are very **selective** and, in most cases, allow the passage of only one type of ion (Na^+, Ca^{2+}, etc.). Ion channels are open transiently and thus are "**gated.**" Gates can be controlled by opening or closing.
- **Carrier (transporters) proteins (4 of Fig. 5A):** They bind to their specific solute to be transported and undergo a series of conformational changes to transport specific small molecules or sometimes a class of molecules (such as ions, sugars, or amino acids) across the lipid bilayer of membranes. The conformational changes alternately expose the solute-binding site on one side of the membrane

Box 5: Functions of plasma membrane.

- Transport: Selective permeability of various substances
- Signal transduction: Plasma membrane has many receptors that transport information from external surface via intracellular signaling molecules
- Maintenance of cell polarity
- Cell-to-cell recognition
- Intercellular joining
- Attachment of intracellular cytoskeleton to the extracellular matrix
- Cell identification

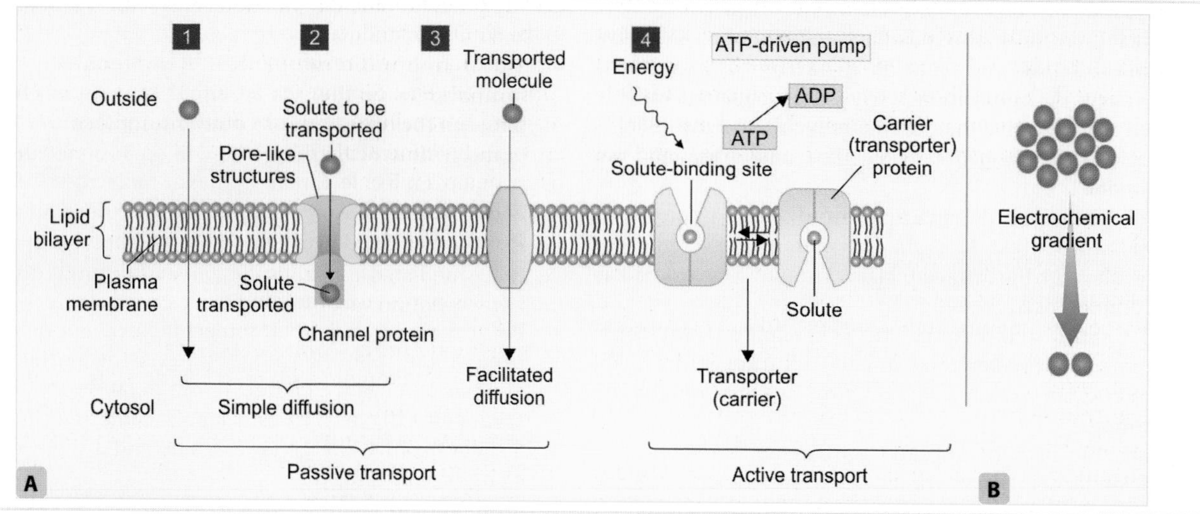

FIGS 5A AND B: (A) Mechanism of active and passive transport through cell membrane. Channel protein (2) forms a pore across the membrane through which specific solutes can passively diffuse. A transporter (4) alternates between two conformations, so that the solute-binding site is sequentially accessible on one side of the membrane and then on the other. (B) Mechanism of transport by electrochemical gradient.

and then on the other. Their transport is relatively a slow process. *Carriers* are required when solute is moved *against* a concentration gradient.

Mechanism of Transport (Figs. 5 and 6, Table 2)

- **Passive transport (1 to 3 of Fig. 5):** Molecules can **passively** traverse the membrane by **simple diffusion** or by **facilitated diffusion.** It does not require energy. Simple diffusion may occur with or without channel proteins. **Facilitated diffusion** involves either certain transporters or ion channels. All channels and many carriers (transporters) permit solutes to cross the membrane only passively ("downhill"). This process is called passive transport. In these situations, there is a concentration and/or electrical gradient between the inside and outside of the cell (**Fig. 5B**). This *passive transport* drives spontaneous movement of solute against an electrochemical gradient toward equilibrium. Almost all plasma membranes have an electrical potential difference across them, with the inside being negative relative to the outside. This contrasts with **active transport**, which **requires energy** because it constitutes movement. **Hormones** can regulate facilitated diffusion by changing the number of transporters available. For example, insulin via a complex signaling pathway can recruit **glucose transporters (GLUT)** from an intracellular reservoir. This increases glucose transport in fat and muscle.
- **Active transport (4 of Fig. 5A):** The process of active transport differs from diffusion, in active transport, that the molecules are transported against concentration (electrochemical) gradient; hence, requires energy. In contrast, passive transport does not need energy. The energy for active transport can come from (i) the hydrolysis of ATP, (ii) electron movement, or (iii) light. Usually energy is released by ATP hydrolysis (ATP-driven pumps) or a coupled ion-concentration gradient. Example for transporter ATPases is the notorious *multidrug resistance (MDR) protein* also called P-glycoprotein. MDR is present

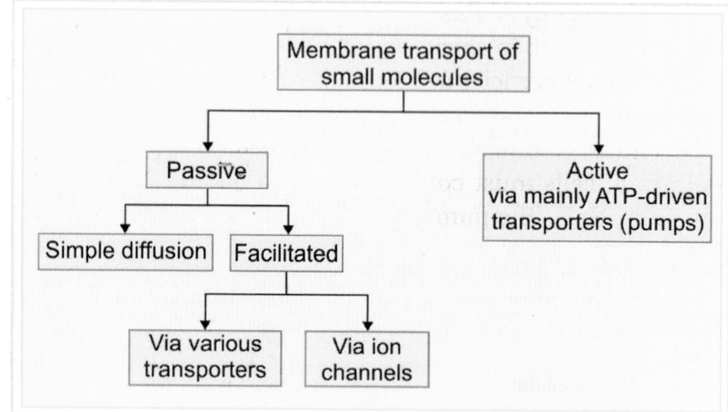

FIG. 6: Two types of membrane transport of small molecules.

Table 2: Various methods of transfer of material and information across membranes.

Cross-membrane movement of small molecules	***Cross-membrane movement of large molecules***
• Diffusion (passive and facilitated) • Active transport	• Endocytosis • Exocytosis
Signal transmission across membrane	***Intracellular contact and communication***
Cell surface receptors • Signal transduction [e.g., glucagon→ cyclic adenosine monophosphate (cAMP)] • Signal internalization coupled with endocytosis [e.g., low density lipoprotein (LDL) receptor]	• Passive (simple) diffusion of solute from higher to lower concentration • Facilitated diffusion is passive transport of solute from higher to lower concentration mediated by specific protein transporter • Active transport • Extracellular microvesicle and exosome secretion and uptake

at elevated levels in many human cancer cells and they pump polar compounds (e.g., chemotherapeutic drugs) out of cells and may render cancer cells resistant to treatment to a variety of chemically unrelated cytotoxic drugs that are widely used in cancer chemotherapy. This active transport is mediated by transporters (carrier molecules and not channels).

Osmosis

Water spontaneously moves "downhill" across a membrane from a solution of lower solute concentration (relatively high-water concentration) to one of higher solute concentration (relatively low-water concentration). This process is called **osmosis**, or *osmotic flow*. Membranes allow free passage of water. Water moves into and out of cells by osmosis, depending on relative solute concentrations.

- **Hypertonicity:** When salt in the extracellular space is more than in the cytosol, it is termed hypertonicity. It causes a net movement of water out of cells into the extracellular region.
- **Hypotonicity:** When salt in the extracellular is less than in the cytosol, it is termed hypotonicity. It causes a net movement of water into cells.

Ion-exchanging ATPases

The cytosol is rich in charged metabolites and protein species. These charged particles attract a large number of counter ions (oppositely charged counterparts) that tend to increase the intracellular osmolarity. As a consequence, to prevent over hydration, cells must constantly pump out small inorganic ions (e.g., Na^+). The pumping out usually occurs through the activity of membrane ion-exchanging ATPases. If there is loss of the ability to produce energy (e.g., in a cell injured by toxins or ischemia), it will result in osmotic swelling and eventual rupture of cells. Similar transport mechanisms operate to regulate intracellular and intraorganellar pH. Most cytosolic enzymes function at pH 7.4, whereas lysosomal enzymes work best when pH is 5 or less.

Receptor-mediated and Fluid-phase uptake

Receptor-mediated and fluid-phase uptake of material involves membrane-bound vacuoles (**Fig. 7**).

Endocytosis (1 in Fig. 7 and 1 in Fig. 18) The process of uptake of fluids or macromolecules (large molecules) by the cell is termed *endocytosis*. It occurs by two fundamental mechanisms:

- **Endocytosis through caveolae:** Caveolae ("little cavities or caves") are **noncoated** invaginations of the plasma membrane. **Caveolae** may be derived from lipid rafts. Caveolin is the major structural protein of caveolae. *Caveolae* endocytose extracellular fluid, membrane proteins, and some receptor-bound molecules (e.g., folate) in a process driven by caveolin proteins, concentrated within lipid rafts. Certain small molecules (including some vitamins) are taken up by forming invaginations. Endocytotic vesicles are formed when part of the plasma membrane invaginates. They enclose a small volume of extracellular fluid and its contents. Then these vesicles get pinched off from the plasma membranes. The bilayer lipid membrane or **vesicle** then fuses with other membrane structures. Thus, endocytosis transports its contents to other cellular compartments or also back to

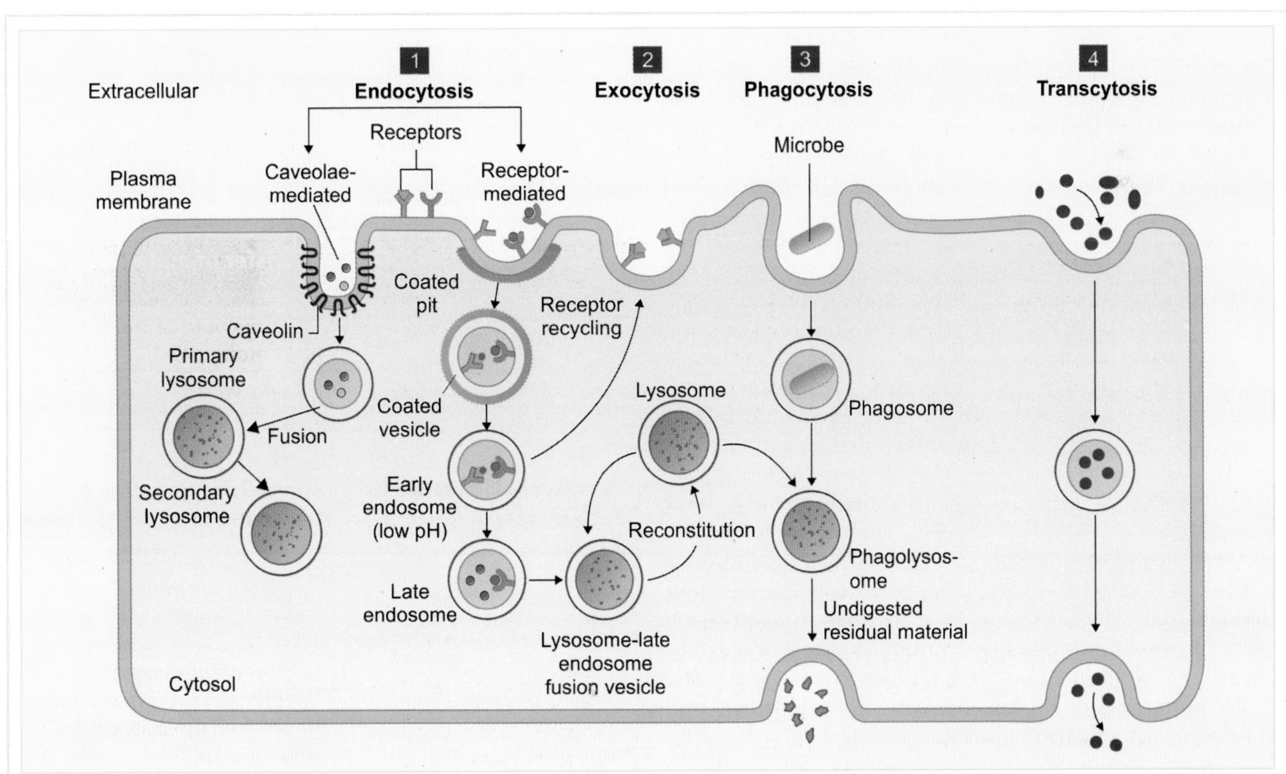

FIG. 7: Movement of small molecules and larger structures across membranes. The lipid bilayer is relatively impermeable to all molecules except the smallest and/or most hydrophobic molecules. For the import or export of charged species needs specific transmembrane transporter proteins, vesicular traffic, or membrane deformations (for details refer text).

the exterior of the cell. Majority of endocytotic vesicles fuse with **primary lysosomes in the cytoplasm and** form **secondary lysosomes.** The hydrolytic enzymes present in the lysosomes digest the macromolecular contents and release amino acids, simple sugars, or nucleotides. These are carried out of the vesicles to be (re)used by the cell. Endocytosis is associated with GPI-linked molecules, cyclic adenosine monophosphate (cAMP)-binding proteins, SRC-family kinases, and the folate receptor.

- ○ **Potocytosis** (literally "cellular sipping") is a type of receptor-mediated endocytosis in which small molecules are transported across the plasma membrane of a cell. In potocytosis, there is internalization of caveolae with any bound molecules and associated extracellular fluid. The caveolae operate in the transmembrane delivery of some molecules (e.g., folate). They also contribute to the regulation of transmembrane signaling and/or cellular adhesion via the internalization of receptors and integrins. Mutations in caveolin may be observed in muscular dystrophy and electrical abnormalities of the heart.

- **Pinocytosis: Pinocytosis** ("cellular drinking") of extracellular fluid is a fluid-phase process that virtually occurs in all cells. This is discussed in detail on page 29.
- **Receptor-mediated endocytosis (refer 1 in Fig. 7):** It is the major uptake mechanism for certain larger molecules (macromolecules) such as transferrin and low-density lipoprotein (LDL). These macromolecules bind to specific cell-surface receptors and molecules get internalized through a membrane invagination process driven by an intracellular matrix of clathrin proteins. It involves *clathrin coated pits and vesicles.* Clathrin is a hexamer of proteins that spontaneously assembles into a basket-like framework and forms clathrin-coated pits (buds) on the cytosolic surface of membrane. It drives to form the invagination and a vesicle. The macromolecule or ligand to be internalized (by itself as in pinocytosis or by binding to the receptor), rapidly invaginates and pinches off to form a *clathrin-coated vesicle.* After internalization, clathrin-coated vesicles transport molecules from the plasma membrane to internal compartments. The vesicles then rapidly uncoat and fuse with an acidic intracellular structure called the *early endosome.* It progressively matures to late endosome. The clathrin dissociates and can be reused/recycled to the same or different regions of the plasma membrane or may fuse with lysosomes and ultimately degraded. Defects in receptor-mediated transport of LDL are responsible for familial hypercholesterolemia.

Exocytosis (refer 2 in Fig. 7) It is the process by which large molecules (e.g., cell-surface proteins, such as receptors, ion channels, and transporters) are exported or released from cells to the exterior. In exocytosis, proteins synthesized and packaged in membrane-bound vesicles fuse with the plasma membrane and discharge their contents to the extracellular space.

A comparison of the mechanisms of endocytosis and exocytosis is presented in **Figure 8**.

Phagocytosis (3 in Fig. 7 and 2 of Fig. 18) In this process, there is formation of a nonclathrin-mediated membrane invagination of large particles by specialized phagocytes (e.g., macrophages or neutrophils). The resulting phagosomes fuse with lysosomes and degrade the internalized material.

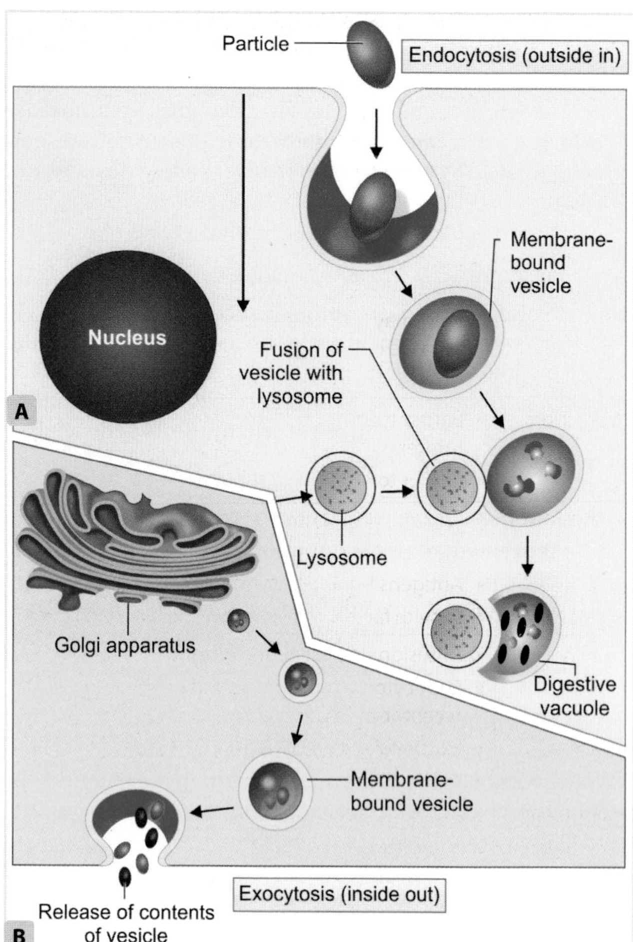

FIGS. 8A AND B: A comparison of the mechanisms of endocytosis and exocytosis. (A) Endocytosisl; and (B) Exocytosis.

Transcytosis (4 in Fig. 7): Transcytosis is the process in which there is movement of endocytosed vesicles between the apical and basolateral compartments (i.e., to a different surface of plasma membrane from where it originated) of cells. This mechanism is used for transferring large amounts of solute and/or bound ligand from one face of a cell to another (across epithelial barriers such as ingested antibodies in maternal milk across intestinal epithelia) or for the rapid movement of large volumes of solute. Increased transcytosis may play a role in the increased vascular permeability seen in inflammation and tumors.

Three pathways by which materials are moved to lysosomes are presented in **Figure 18**.

Summary of functions of plasma membrane is presented in **Table 3**.

Channelopathies

Q. Short essay on channelopathies.

Normal functions of ion channels

Ion channels are transmembrane pore-forming proteins. They allow ions (e.g., Na^+, K^+, Ca^{2+} and Cl^-), to enter or exit cells. This ion traffic is important for control of several physiological functions. These include heartbeat, muscle contraction and relaxation, regulation of insulin secretion in pancreatic β cells, etc. For example, activation and inactivation of Na^+ and K^+ channels determine the action potential in neurons, and

Table 3: Summary of functions of plasma membrane.

Cellular mechanism	*Membrane functions*
Structure	• Usually thicker than the membranes of intracellular organelles • Contains all cellular organelles • Maintains relationship with cytoskeleton, endoplasmic reticulum, and other organelles • Outer surfaces in many cells are not smooth. They may have cilia or even microvilli; both are capable of movement • Maintenance of fluid and electrolyte balance
Protection	• Barrier to toxic molecules and macromolecules (proteins, nucleic acid, and polysaccharides) • Barrier to foreign microbes and cells
Activation of cell	• Hormones (regulation of cellular activity) • Mitogens (cellular division) • Antigens (antibody synthesis) • Growth factors (proliferation and differentiation)
Transport	• Diffusion and exchange diffusion • Endocytosis (pinocytosis and phagocytosis); receptor-mediated endocytosis • Exocytosis (secretion) • Active transport
Cell-to-cell interaction	• Communication and attachment at junctional complexes • Symbiotic nutritive relationships • Release of enzymes and antibodies to extracellular environment • Relationships with extracellular matrix

Ca^{2+} channels are important in contraction and relaxation of cardiac and skeletal muscle.

Channelopathies are inherited or acquired disorders of ion channels. Ion channel myopathies are group of inherited or acquired disorders due to mutations of ion channels. They are characterized by myotonia, relapsing episodes of hypotonic paralysis associated with abnormal serum potassium levels, or both.

Inherited channelopathies

Mutations in ion channel genes cause a variety of diseases.

- Cardiac arrhythmias (e.g., short and long QT syndromes)
- Neuromuscular syndromes (e.g., myotonias, familial periodic paralysis)
- Inherited disorders affecting skeletal muscle contraction, heart rhythm and nervous system function. These are due to mutations in genes that encode voltage-gated Na^+ channels.
- Certain pediatric epilepsy syndromes
- **Cystic fibrosis:** It is due to a mutation in a chloride channel and affects mucus and sweat-secreting cells of various organs.
- **Diabetes mellitus:** In pancreatic β cells, ATP-sensitive K^+ channels regulate insulin secretion. Mutations in these channel genes can lead to certain forms of diabetes.
- **Retinitis pigmentosa:** Some types of retinitis pigmentosa may be due to mutations in ion channels.
- Mutations in gap junctions, channels that provide direct communication between cells, may also be associated with a variety of inherited diseases.
- Channelopathies may reflect gains (epilepsy, myotonia) or losses (weakness) of ion channel function.
- Different mutations of the same ion channel may result in different disorders. For example, inherited mutations in a single Na^+ channel in skeletal muscle can produce either hyperkalemic or hypokalemic periodic paralysis. However, mutations in different genes may give rise to the same phenotype. For example, mutations in different skeletal muscle Na^+ channels may cause hyperkalemic periodic paralysis.

Acquired channelopathies

These include evolution of some cancers and autoimmune neurologic conditions.

- **Autoantibodies** may cause disorders of both ligand-gated ion channels (receptors) and voltage-gated ones. For example, **myasthenia gravis** and **autoimmune neuropathy** are due to autoantibodies versus nicotinic acetylcholine receptors, which control ion channels.
- **Neuromuscular disorders:** Autoantibodies against voltage-gated Ca^{2+} and K^+ channels may produce diverse neuromuscular disorders.
- **Tumor development:** Ion channels are involved in cell cycle progression and may play a role in tumor development.
- **May cause death:** Up to 20% of sudden unexplained deaths and 10% of sudden infant death syndrome (SIDS) are due to cardiac arrhythmias. These are associated with mutations in the Na^+ channel and are responsible for long QT syndrome.
- Majority of patients with mucolipidosis type IV and autosomal dominant polycystic kidney disease have mutations in cell membrane Ca^{2+} channels.

CYTOSKELETON

Q. Describe cytoskeletal abnormalities.
Q. Describe the cytoskeleton in health and disease.
Q. Describe in detail pathology of cytoskeletal abnormalities.

The skeletal system of a human consists of hard elements (e.g., bone, cartilage) that support the soft tissues of the body and play main role in mediating bodily movements. Similarly, the cells also have a "skeletal system" termed as a **cytoskeleton** which has similar functions as skeleton. The cytoskeleton acts like the "bones" and "muscles" of a cell. The **cytoskeleton** is an **intracellular scaffolding of proteins,** rods, and tubules. The cytoskeleton network of protein filaments extends throughout the cell, giving the cell structure and keeping the organelles in place.

Functions

Cytoskeleton forms an elaborate interactive network. It is responsible for the cell's architecture with and positioning the various organelles (e.g., epithelial in which certain organelles are arranged in a defined order from the apical to the basal end of the cell) within the interior of the cell. It maintains the three-dimensional physical shape of cells and resists forces that tend to deform the shape. It provides structural support to all cell functions. Thus, cytoskeleton is responsible for the **ability of cells to adopt a particular shape, maintain polarity, organize the intracellular organelles, and movement.**

- Some cytoskeletal elements transport cellular contents and some are involved in motion of the cells (motor molecules) which convert chemical energy into mechanical energy.
- It forms a network of tracks that direct the **movement of materials and organelles within cells.** For example, delivery of mRNA molecules to specific parts of a cell, the movement of membranous carriers from the endoplasmic reticulum to the Golgi complex.
- The force-generating apparatus which moves cells from one place to another (e.g., cilia that protrude from the cell's surface). For example, locomotion of sperm, white blood cells, and fibroblasts.
- An essential component of the **cell's division machinery.** Cytoskeletal elements make up the apparatus which separate the chromosomes during mitosis and meiosis and for splitting the parent cell into two daughter cells during cytokinesis.

Types (Fig. 9)

The cytoskeleton of the cells is mainly composed of three major well-defined classes or types of fibrillar proteins (filamentous structures), **namely—(1) microfilaments (actin filaments), (2) intermediate filaments, and (3) microtubules.** Each of these cytoskeletal filaments is a polymer of protein subunits held together by weak, noncovalent bonds. This type of construction helps in rapid assembly and disassembly and they undergo continuous break down and built up as a cell performs specific activities. These types are distinguished by protein type, diameter, and way in which they aggregate into larger structures. Each cytoskeletal element has distinct properties.

Diagrammatic appearance of three major components of the cytoskeleton namely—(1) microtubules, (2) intermediate filaments, and (3) microfilaments is presented in **Figure 9.**

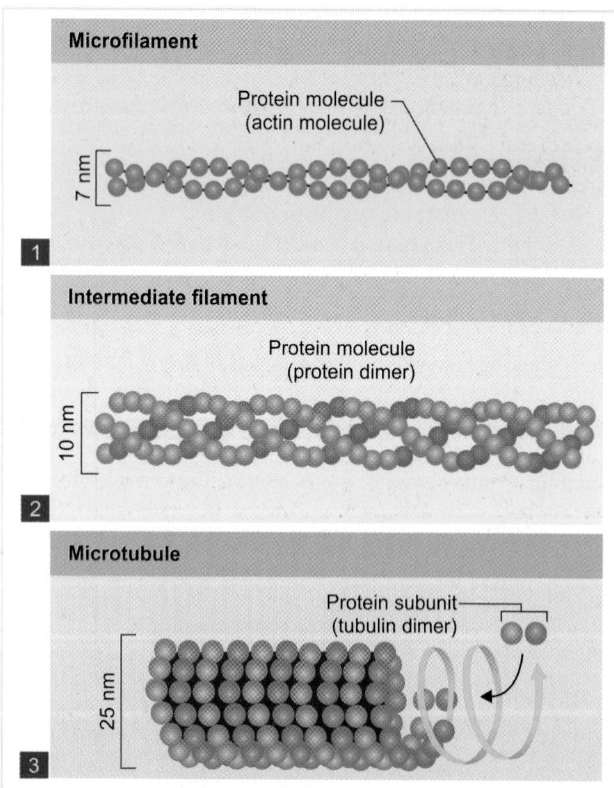

FIG. 9: Diagrammatic appearance of three major components of the cytoskeleton, namely—(1) microfilaments, (2) intermediate filaments, and (3) microtubules.

Microfilaments (Actin Filaments)

Q. Short essay on microfilaments.

Structure of Microfilaments (1 in Fig. 9)

Microfilaments are **extremely fine strands** (fibrils measuring 5–9 nm in diameter), polymers of the protein **actin.** They are part of a cell's cytoskeleton. Microfilaments are the **smallest filaments of the cytoskeleton** and are composed of two strands of subunits of the protein actin (hence also called actin filaments) wound in a spiral. **Each actin filament (F-actin) consists of two protofilaments** twisted together to form a helix. The **terms actin filament, F-actin, and microfilament are basically synonyms for this type of filament.** The **protofilaments** are made up of multiple globular actin monomers (G-actin) joined together head to tail and associated with ATP molecules to provide energy for contraction. Microfilaments are the most abundant cytosolic proteins in cells. Like microtubules, microfilaments are polar. Their positively charged (+) end is jagged (barbed) and their negatively charged (-) end is pointed. The plus end grows faster than the minus end. Histologically, actin filaments can be well-demonstrated in skeletal muscle cells. In muscle cells, the actin filaments form a stable arrangement of bundles with the motor protein myosin. Contraction occurs when the actin and myosin filaments slide relative to each other driven by the release of energy from hydrolysis of ATP molecules. It is the basis of muscle contraction. In nonmuscle cells, F-actin assembles via an assortment of actin binding proteins into well-organized bundles and networks that control cell shape and movement.

Function of Microfilaments (Box 6)

- Protection of cells against deformation and are responsible for the cells to **withstand stretching and compression.**
- Maintain shape of cell and help in **attachment of one cell to another.**
- **Cell movement:** Actin plays a central role in cell movement (especially unicellular organisms like amoebae), pinocytosis, and phagocytosis. During movement, one end of a microfilament elongates while the other end shortens, and myosin acts as a motor in the process. Microfilaments

Box 6: Functions of microfilaments.

- Withstand stretching and compression
- Maintain shape of the cell
- Movement of cell: Actin can shorten its length and helps in the movement of the cell as in phagocytosis or pinocytosis
- Help in contraction of muscle fibers by binding to the myosin
- Cell division (cytokinesis)
- Help in the transport of various vesicles within the cytoplasm

also play a role in cytoplasmic streaming. Cytoplasmic streaming is the process of flow of cytoplasm (the contents of the cell, including the fluid part called cytosol) throughout the cell. It helps nutrients, waste products, and cell organelles to travel from one part of the cell to another. Microfilaments can attach to a cell organelle and undergo contraction, thereby pulling the organelle to a different area of the cell.

- **Muscle contraction:** One of the main roles of microfilaments is to contact muscles. Their concentration is greater in muscle cells, where they form myofibrils (the basic unit of the muscle cell). In muscle cells, actin along with the protein myosin forms a complex called actomyosin. This actomyosin causes contraction and relaxation of the muscles. The sarcomeres are the basic unit of muscle tissue and consist of groups of actomyosin.
- **Cell division:** Microfilaments help in cell division (during mitosis). Microfilaments help in the process of cytoplasmic division of a cell (cytokinesis) and physically separating the cell into two daughter cells. During cytokinesis, first there is formation of a ring of actin around the cell that is separating, and then myosin proteins pull on the actin and cause it to contract. The ring gets narrower around the cell, dragging the cell membrane with it, till it splits into two daughter cells. Once the cells are separated, the microfilaments depolymerize, or break down, into actin molecules causing the ring to disassemble.
- Actin may also bind to intrinsic plasma membrane proteins to anchor them in position.
- Microfilaments also serve other functions in the cell through proteins that interact with actin.

Absence or abnormalities in any of these proteins results in a genetic disease.

Intermediate Filaments

Q. Short essay on intermediate filaments.
Q. Short essay on intermediate filaments in health and disease.

Intermediate filaments have great strength, and they make the cells capable to withstand the mechanical stress that occurs when cells are stretched. They are strong and rope-like. They are found mainly in the cytoplasm of most cells and lamin intermediate filament is also found within the nucleus.

Structure (2 in Fig. 9)

They are tough, solid, flexible, unbranched, rope-like fibers composed of a variety of related proteins. Intermediate filaments are larger than microfilaments. They have a diameter of 8–10 nm, intermediate between those of microtubules (thick) and microfilaments (thin). They provide structural support and mechanical strength to cells that are subjected to physical stress, including neurons, muscle cells, and the epithelial cells that line the body's cavities. They are present in the cytoplasm as well as nucleus of the cell. All intermediate filaments consist of paired proteins nested as coiled rods. Unlike microtubules and microfilaments, intermediate filaments are chemically heterogeneous group of structures. Thus, they are composed of different proteins in different cell types. Intermediate filaments are very few in many cell types but are most abundant in nerve cells and skin cells. Most types of intermediate filaments are cytoplasmic except one type called laminins which are nuclear. Intermediate filaments bear tension in the cell, give the cell structure, and organize cell organelles and tether them in place.

Q. Classify intermediate filament proteins and discuss diseases related to their mutations.

Types

There are about six biochemically and immunologically distinct types.

Depending on the polypeptide subunits, on the type of cell in which they are found, biochemical, genetic, and immunologic criteria; intermediate filaments can be divided into six major classes (**Box 6**). These include—(1) cytokeratin, (2) vimentin, (3) desmin, (4) glial fibrillary acidic protein (GFAP), (5) neurofilaments (NFs), (6) lamins and nestin. Cytokeratins (CKs) are a complex group of about 20 polypeptides, whereas other four types consist of a single polypeptide unit. Individual types of intermediate filaments have characteristic tissue-specific patterns of expression. Hence, they are used for identifying the cellular origin of poorly differentiated tumors.

Based on the molecular structure of proteins, intermediate filaments can be **divided into six main groups/types** (**Box 7**).

Filensin is an unclassified intermediate filament expressed during the differentiation of the vertebrate lens epithelial cells.

Keratins (Cytokeratins)

Q. Write short essay on cytokeratins.
Q. Explain cytokeratin immunostaining profile in diagnostic pathology.

Cytokeratins or better named as keratins are a family of **water-insoluble, intracellular** (intracytoplasmic) **fibrous intermediate filament proteins** present in almost all epithelia as well as in some nonepithelial cell types. They help the cells to resist stress. The epithelial keratin intermediate filaments

Box 7: Classification of intermediate filaments according to molecular structure.

Types I (acidic) and II (basic): Present in epithelial and hair (trichocytic) keratins

Type III: It consists of four varieties namely—
- Vimentin: It is expressed mainly in mesenchymal cells and also in leukocytes, vascular endothelial cells and some epithelial cells
- Desmin: Present in the skeletal and cardiac muscle fibers
- Glial fibrillary acidic protein (GFAP): Present in astrocytes and other glial cells
- Peripherin: Seen in the peripheral neurons and cranial nerves

Type IV: It contains of neurofilaments expressed in mature neurons
- Alpha (α) internexin: These are expressed in developing central nervous system

Type V is mainly nuclear lamins. These are seen underneath the nuclear membrane (such as Lamin A, Lamin B, and Lamin C). It also helps in chromatin organization and gene expression

Type VI: It consists of only nestin and is present in stem cells of the central nervous system and in developing skeletal muscle

comprise about 20 distinct type of keratin polypeptides. The polypeptides are numbered 1 through 20 (**Table 4**). They are classified depending on the basis of their molecular weight (MW) (ranging from 40,000 to 68,000). According to isoelectric pH value (ranging from 5 to 8), they are classified as the type II (basic) keratins and the type I (acidic) keratins. In each category, CKs are numbered in order of decreasing size from low molecular weight (LMWCKs) to high molecular weight (HMWCKs). This combination constitutes keratin catalog, which shows a tissue specific distribution throughout the epithelia. Keratin filaments constitute the primary structural proteins of epithelial cells (e.g., epidermal cells, liver cells, and pancreatic acinar cells). Keratins are an excellent marker for epithelial differentiation in tumors irrespective of whether the tumor is of endodermal, neuroectodermal, mesenchymal, or germ cell derivation. These are used as histochemical markers for various epithelia. This family of keratins is important in diagnostic immunohistochemistry (IHC) for the identification of carcinomatous differentiation as well as for identification of specific carcinoma subtypes. Common keratins and their distribution are presented in **Table 4**.

Though there are several keratins, those that are functionally useful in determining site of origin remain limited (namely keratins 5, 7, 8, 14, 17, 18, 19, and 20). Keratin antigens and their significance are presented in **Table 5**.

The CK5/6 may be useful in the differential diagnosis of metastatic carcinoma in the pleura versus epithelial mesothelioma. Usefulness of CK5 and CK5/6 is listed in **Box 8**.

Usefulness of CK7/CK20 immunoprofiles in select neoplasms is presented in **Table 6**.

Key diagnostic usefulness of CKs is presented in **Table 7**.

Table 4: Common keratins and their distribution.

Type II (basic) keratin	*Distribution in normal tissue*	*Type I (acidic) keratin*
Cytokeratin (CK) 1	Epidermis of palms and soles	CK9 and CK 10
CK 2	Epithelia in all locations	CK 11
CK 3	Cornea	CK12
CK 4	Nonkeratinizing squamous epithelia	CK13
CK 5	Basal cells of squamous and glandular epithelia, myoepithelial, mesothelium	CK 14 and CK 15
CK 6	Squamous epithelia, especially hyperproliferative	CK16
CK 7*	Simple epithelia	CK17
CK 8*	Basal cells of glandular epithelia, myoepithelial	CK18*
	Simple epithelia, most glandular and squamous epithelia (basal)	CK19*
	Simple epithelia of intestines and stomach, Merkel cells	CK20*

* Low molecular weight (LMWCKs) and remaining are high molecular weight (HMWCKs).

Keratins in nonepithelial tumors (Box 9)

The keratins may give positive results in nonepithelial mesenchymal tissues or melanocytic lesions especially with keratins 8 and 18 and, less commonly, keratin 19.

Vimentin

This is one of the cytoplasmic intermediate filaments (MW 57,000/57 kD) that was initially isolated from a mouse fibroblast culture. Vimentin is characteristic of mesenchymal cells, such as endothelial cells, fibroblasts, and vascular smooth muscle cells. In mesenchymal tumor pathology, it has to be noted that vimentin shows a greater amino acid homology to desmin, neurofilament proteins (NFPs), and glial fibrillary acidic protein (GFAP) than to the keratins. Though vimentin is considered as restricted to mesenchymal cells, vimentin has been found in many other neoplasms including a variety of carcinomas. Thus, pathologists rarely use vimentin as a diagnostic marker in soft tissue tumors. However, it can be used as a useful control marker to make sure that the tissue has been properly fixed and processed. If vimentin cannot be easily detected in nonneoplastic endothelial cells, fibroblasts, and

Table 5: Keratin antigens and their significance.

Cytokeratin/CK antigen (antibody)	*Significance*
CK8 (35BH11 and CAM5.2)	Carcinomas of simple epithelium
Pankeratin (AE1/AE3)	Carcinomas of simple and complex epithelium
CK1/10 (34B4)	Squamous cell carcinoma
CK7 (OV-TL 12/30)	Nongastrointestinally-derived carcinomas
CK20 (K20)	Most gastrointestinal carcinomas; mucinous ovarian, biliary, transitional, and Merkel cell carcinoma
CK19 (RCK 108) —good screening marker for epithelial neoplasms	Most carcinomas; many carcinomas with squamous component; myoepithelial cells
CK1/5/10/14 (34betaE12)	Basal cells of prostate; most duct-derived carcinomas
CK18/19 (PKK1)	Most carcinomas
CK10/11/13/14/15/16/19 (AE1)	Most squamous lesions and many carcinomas
CK8/14/15/16/18/19 (MAK-6)	Most carcinomas

Box 8: Usefulness of cytokeratin (CK) 5 and CK5/6.

- Good marker for demonstration of squamous and transitional cell differentiation
- Useful for differential diagnosis of mesothelial differentiation versus adenocarcinoma in lung
- Give positive reaction with myoepithelial cells of breast and basal cells of prostate
- Sensitive and specific markers of basal-like phenotype of breast carcinoma

Table 6: Cytokeratin (CK) 7/CK20 immunoprofiles in select neoplasms.

CK7+/CK20+	CK7+/CK20–
• Transitional cell carcinoma • Pancreatic carcinoma • Ovarian mucinous carcinoma • Gastric adenocarcinoma **CK7–/CK20–** • Squamous cell carcinoma, lung • Prostate adenocarcinoma • Renal cell carcinoma • Hepatocellular carcinoma • Adrenocortical carcinoma • Few thymic carcinoma	• Non-small cell carcinoma of lung • Small cell carcinoma of lung • Breast carcinoma (ductal and lobular) • Non-mucinous ovarian carcinoma • Endometrial adenocarcinoma • Gastric adenocarcinoma • Pancreatic ductal adenocarcinoma • Cholangiocarcinoma • Mesothelioma • Squamous cell carcinoma of cervix **CK7–/CK20+** • Colorectal adenocarcinoma • Merkel cell carcinoma

Table 7: Key diagnostic usefulness of cytokeratins immunomarkers.

Immunomarker	*Significance*
CAM5.2 and AE1/AE3	These are broad coverage antibodies used for detection of carcinomatous differentiation. For screening, both of them should be used together
CK7 (+)	Tumors include adenocarcinomas of breast, lung, ovary, endometrium, and pancreas; mesothelioma, urothelial carcinomas, thymic carcinomas; squamous cell carcinoma of uterine cervix; and fibrolamellar variant of hepatocellular carcinomas
CK7 (negative/ rare positive)	Renal, prostate, adrenocortical, squamous (except uterine cervix), small cell carcinomas, and hepatocellular carcinomas
CK20 (+)	Colorectal, pancreas (~60%), gastric (~50%), cholangiocarcinoma (~40%), mucinous ovarian, Merkel cell, and urothelial carcinomas (~30%)
CK20 (negative/rare positive)	Most breast, lung, and salivary gland carcinomas, hepatocellular, renal, prostate, adrenocortical, squamous, and small cell carcinomas
CK7/CK20	Refer **Table 6**

other mesenchymal elements routinely present in any tissue section, then this section should not be used for interpretation.

Key features of vimentin coexpression in carcinomas are presented in **Table 8**.

Desmin

This is a muscle-type intermediate filament (MW 53,000/53 kD) found in cells of smooth and striated muscle and in a lesser amount in myofibroblasts. It is abundant in parenchymal (compared to vascular) smooth muscle cells. It forms the scaffold on which actin and myosin contract. It is seen in the majority of rhabdomyoma, leiomyoma, rhabdomyosarcoma (RMS), and leiomyosarcoma (LMS).

Box 9: Keratin in nonepithelial tumors.

- Focal presence in several sarcomas
- Focal rare presence (with CAM5.2) in melanoma
- Common in plasma cells (plasmacytoma) and rare in other lymphoid neoplasms (anaplastic large cell lymphoma)
- Common in dendritic cells of lymph nodes (CAM5.2)
- Antibody AE1/AE3 may give spurious positive keratin in astrocytic neoplasms
- "Secretory variant" of meningiomas may express keratin in (~30%)

Table 8: Vimentin coexpression in carcinomas.

Significance of vimentin immunomarkers	*Tumors*
Commonly positive	Renal, endometrioid endometrial, salivary gland, follicular thyroid, and sarcomatoid (spindle cell) carcinomas, "basal-like" breast carcinomas, and stromal components of malignant mixed Müllerian tumors
May be seen in few cells in 10–20% of tumors	Colorectal, lung, breast, prostate, and ovarian adenocarcinomas
Not diagnostically useful	Body cavity effusion specimens
Vimentin positive (usually)	Epithelial and sarcomatoid mesotheliomas
Internal quality control	Mesenchymal and endothelial cells regularly immunostain with vimentin, and this is used as an internal quality control for the quality of immunoreactivity in any tissue

Glial Fibrillary Acidic Protein

It has a MW 48,000–52,000 (48 to 52kD). It is present in astrocytes (normal, reactive, and neoplastic), ependymal cells (developing, reactive, and neoplastic) and oligodendrocytes (developing and neoplastic but not expressed by mature oligodendroglia) that support neurons. Nonglial tissues which may stain positive with GFAP include Schwann cells, myoepithelial cells, Kupffer cells, and some chondrocytes. GFAP can be used as a second-line marker (positive ~30%) for malignant peripheral nerve sheath tumor (MPNST).

Neurofilaments

They are loosely packed intermediate filaments present in the cytoplasm of mature and developing neurons and their processes, paraganglionic cells, and certain normal neuroendocrine (NE) cells. They are protein triplets composed of three major subunits [low (L), medium (M), and high (H) MW subunits]—NF-L, NF-M, and NF-H (MW 68,000, 150,000, and 200,000, respectively). They impart strength and rigidity.

Lamins A, B, and C

Lamin intermediate filaments form a structural layer on the inner side of the nuclear membrane and provide attachment sites for the chromosomes. Diagrammatic cross section through the nuclear envelope with relation to nuclear lamins is presented in **Figure 10**.

Nestin (Neuroectodermal Stem Cell Marker)

Nestin is defined as a class VI intermediate filament protein. It is present in dividing cells only during the early stages of development (transient expression) in the central nervous system (CNS), peripheral nervous system and in myogenic and other tissues. Nestin is needed for survival, renewal, and mitogen-stimulated proliferation of neural progenitor cells. Nestin expression in the cytoplasm identifies neuroepithelial stem cells, myoblasts, and myotubes (during early stages of skeletal myogenesis). Nestin is used as a marker of multipotent neural stem cells (NSCs). Once the tissue differentiates, nestin becomes downregulated and is replaced by tissue-specific intermediate filament proteins.

Unclassified Intermediate Filament

Filensin is seen in the epithelial cells of the lens at the time of differentiation

Intermediate filaments and their expression is presented in **Figure 11**.

Tissue distribution of the major intermediate filament proteins is presented in **Table 9**.

Organization of the cytoskeleton in polarized epithelial cells of small intestine is shown in **Figure 12**.

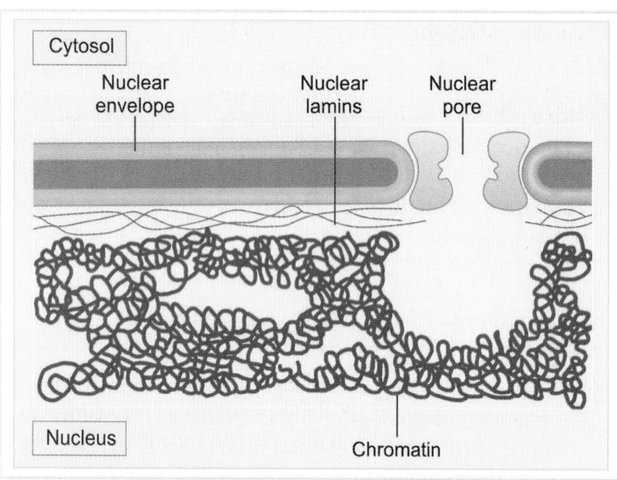

FIG. 10: Diagrammatic cross section through the nuclear envelope. The intermediate filaments of the nucleus namely lamin, line the inner face of the nuclear envelope and provide attachment sites for the chromosomes.

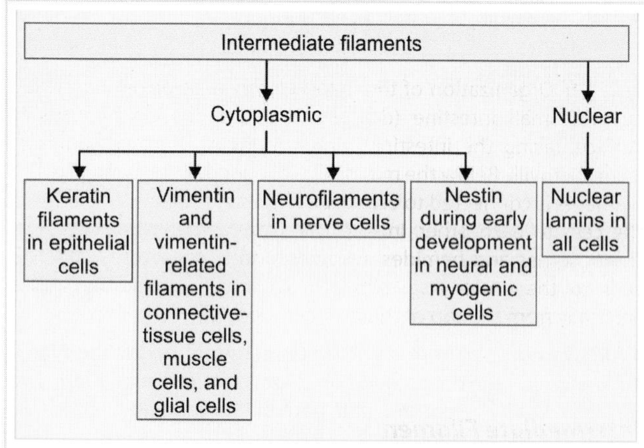

FIG. 11: Intermediate filaments and their expression.

Table 9: Tissue distribution of the major intermediate filament proteins.

Sequence type	*Intermediate filament protein*	*Primary tissue distribution*	*Function*
I	Keratin (acidic) (11 epithelial and 4 hair keratin)	Epithelial cells	Tensile strength
II	Keratin (basic) (8 epithelial and 4 hair keratin)	Epithelial cells of the hair and nail	Tensile strength
III	Vimentin	Mesenchymal cells, leukocytes, endothelial cells, and some epithelial cells	Supports the cytoplasmic membrane and helps in proper positioning of organelles
III	Desmin	Sarcomeres in skeletal and cardiac muscle cells	Helps in stabilizing sarcomere of the contracting muscle fibers
III	Glial fibrillary acidic protein (GFAP)	Astrocytes and other glial cells	Support glial cells
III	Peripherin	Neurons of the dorsal root ganglia, sympathetic ganglia, and cranial nerves	Supports neurons
IV	Neurofilament (NF)-light, NF-medium, and NF-high	Mature neurons	Form the cytoskeleton of the dendrites and axons
V	Lamin A, B, and C	Nuclear envelopes of all cell types	Control of assembly of the nuclear envelope during mitotic event and chromatin organization
VI	Nestin	Stem cells in the central nervous system	Survival, renewal and mitogen-stimulated proliferation of neural progenitor cells

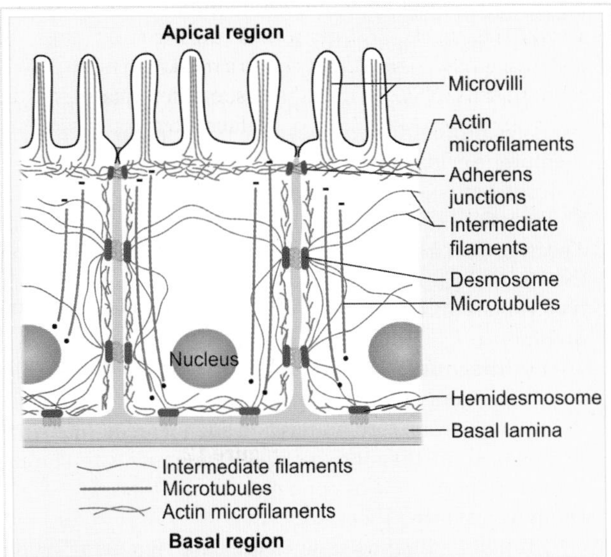

FIG. 12: Organization of the cytoskeleton in polarized epithelial cells of small intestine (diagrammatic). At the apical (upper) surface, facing the intestinal lumen, bundles of actin filaments form microvilli. Below the microvilli, a circumferential band of actin filaments is connected to cell–cell adherens junctions that anchor the cells to each other. Intermediate filaments are anchored to desmosomes and hemidesmosomes, and connect the epithelial cells to the underlying extracellular matrix. Microtubules run vertically from the top of the cell to the bottom.

Intermediate Filaments in Diseases

Used for categorization of tumors

Antibodies specific to intermediate filaments are useful in categorization of undifferentiated solid tumor cells. For example, the presence of CKs, detected by IHC, points to an epithelial origin (carcinoma).

Rhabdoid tumor of the kidney (RTK)

Microscopically, it consists of sheets of discohesive tumor cells with large vesicular nuclei, prominent nucleoli, and abundant eccentric cytoplasm containing large eosinophilic inclusions. Ultrastructurally, these eosinophilic inclusions in the cytoplasm of tumor cells consist of whorls of intermediate filaments that are characteristic but not specific for the tumor.

Merkle cell carcinoma

Ultrastructurally, the tumor cells show dense-core neurosecretory granules (sometimes arranged immediately beneath the cell membrane) and tightly packed perinuclear intermediate filaments.

Embryonal rhabdomyosarcoma

A morphological variant which shows tumor cells containing cytoplasmic globular inclusions composed of intermediate filaments and produce a rhabdoid appearance.

Gemistocytes in diffuse astrocytomas

Gemistocytes (gemistos meaning laden or full), these reflect an accumulation of glial-type intermediate filaments (GFAPs) that form compacted paranuclear whorls and extend into stout cytoplasmic processes.

Atypical teratoid/rhabdoid tumors of CNS

The cytoplasm of the rhabdoid cell contains intermediate filaments and is immunoreactive for epithelial membrane antigen and vimentin.

Rhabdoid meningioma

It consists of sheets of tumor cells with hyaline eosinophilic cytoplasm containing intermediate filaments.

Tuberous sclerosis

Cortical hamartomas in tuberous sclerosis may show some large cells with appearances intermediate between glia and neurons (large vesicular nuclei with nucleoli resembling neurons, and abundant eosinophilic cytoplasm resembling gemistocytic astrocytes). They may express intermediate filaments of both neuronal (NF) and glial (GFAP) types.

Fibrillary astrocytoma

Composed of GFAP.

Mallory–Denk bodies

These appear as clumped, amorphous, eosinophilic material in ballooned hepatocytes. They consist of tangled skeins of intermediate filaments such as keratins 8 and 18 in complex with other proteins such as ubiquitin. These inclusions are a characteristic but not specific feature of alcoholic liver disease.

Diseases due to Mutations in Genes Coding Intermediate Filaments

- Epidermolysis bullosa simplex; K5 or K14 mutation. K5 and K14 genes code for keratin 5 and keratin 14, respectively.
- Laminopathies are a group of rare genetic disorders caused by mutations in the genes coding nuclear laminins. These include Hutchinson-Gilford progeria syndrome, dystrophies of skeletal and/or cardiac muscles, and various lipodystrophies.

Microtubules

Structure (3 in Fig. 9)

Microtubules are bigger than intermediate filaments, at 23 nm. They are long, hollow, unbranched, relatively rigid tubes, composed of subunits of the protein called tubulin. Each microtubule consists of pairs of (dimers of α- and β-) tubulin, assembled into a hollow tube. The dimers of α- and β-tubulin are arranged in constantly elongating or shrinking hollow tubes with a defined polarity. The ends of tubes are designated "+" or "–." The "–" end is usually embedded in a *microtubule organizing center (MTOC* or *centrosome)* near the nucleus where it is associated with paired *centrioles*. The "+" end elongates or recedes in response to various stimuli by the addition or subtraction of tubulin dimmers. This addition or deletion of molecules changes the length of the microtubule. Microtubules are involved in several important cellular functions. Long, hollow microtubules provide many cellular movements. Cells contain both individual tubulin molecules as well as formed microtubules. They have guanosine triphosphatase (GTPase) enzyme activity. They are present in the cytoplasm of almost all cells and support intracellular transport and cell organization. Microtubules are components of a diverse array of structures, including the mitotic spindle of dividing cells and the core of cilia. When the cell needs microtubules to carry out a specific function (e.g., cell division), free tubulin dimers self-assemble to form more microtubules. After the cell division, some of the microtubules separate into individual tubulin dimers, thereby replenishing the cell's supply of building blocks. Thus, there is building up as well as break down of microtubules.

Functions (Box 10)

- **Transporting organelles within the cell:** Act as support cables for "molecular motor" proteins. Thus, it allows the movement of vesicles and organelles around cells. The anterograde (– to +) transport is brought by kinesins motors, whereas retrograde (+ to –) motion is brought out by dyneins motors.
- **Provides mechanical support** for separating sister chromatid (mitotic spindle) during mitosis/cell division.
- **Cilia:** Microtubules are also components of hair-like structures called **cilia** and flagella. There are two types of cilia namely—(1) motile cilia and (2) primary cilia.
  - **Motile cilia** have one more pair of microtubules than primary cilia and they can move. Coordinated movement of motile cilia is responsible for the movement of the cell or propelling the substances along the cell surface. For example, motile cilia cause expulsion of particles along the respiratory tract (e.g., in bronchial epithelium), movement of egg cells in the female reproductive tract and flagella in sperm.
  - **Primary cilia:** Many types of cells have primary cilia—single, nonmotile projections on nucleated cells. They serve a sensory function and act like an antenna, sensing signals from outside the cell and pass them to particular locations inside cells. For example, primary cilia sense light entering the eyes, urine leaving the tubules of kidney. Though these cilia do not move, they stimulate some cells to move (e.g., cells that help in wound healing). Absence of primary cilia is observed in some diseases (e.g., polycystic kidney disease). Cells may have many motile cilia but usually have only one primary cilium that does not move. The core of *primary* cilia helps to regulate proliferation and differentiation.

Microtubules prepared from living tissue contain additional proteins, called **microtubule-associated proteins** (or **MAPs**). MAPs consist of a heterogeneous collection of proteins.

Cytoskeleton in Disease

Q. Write short note on cytoskeleton in disease.

Molecular disturbances of the cytoskeleton are best seen on freely movable cells in body fluids. In blood, change of red blood cells (RBCs) shape can lead to elliptic or spherical RBCs.

- **Disorders of RBC shape**
  - Hereditary spherocytosis
  - Hereditary elliptocytosis
- **Parasitic disease:** The process of entry of the malaria parasites probably involves active participation of the cell membrane cytoskeleton.
- **Role of cytoskeleton in carcinogenesis:** Cytoskeleton filaments are present in many tumors. Examples include: Keratins in carcinomas (tumors of epithelial origin), the glial-fibrillary acid protein in gliomas, vimentin in lymphomas and nonmuscle sarcomas, and protein of NFs in tumors originating in the sympathetic nervous system.
  - **For diagnosis:** For example, the presence of characteristic keratin variants in particular carcinomas (e.g., squamous cell carcinomas and adenocarcinomas) may be used for diagnosis of these carcinomas, including early lymph node or bone marrow metastases.
- **Diagnosis of other diseases**:
  - **Prenatal diagnosis:** Intermediate filament typing can be used for prenatal diagnosis. For example, the presence of amniotic fluid cells containing glial filaments or NFs may suggest a malformation of the central neural system.
  - Abnormal intermediate filaments may be present in muscle cells in various muscle diseases and brain cells (e.g., in Alzheimer's disease and others).

Box 10: Main functions of microtubules.

- Intracellular transport of vesicles containing proteins from the Golgi apparatus to plasma membrane
- Mitotic spindle movement: The mitotic spindles are formed by microtubules. The chromatids are separated and pulled to each daughter cell nucleus by the mitotic spindles formed by microtubules
- Movements of cilia and flagella
- Mechanical support

CELL-CELL INTERACTIONS

There are many different types of cells in the body that dynamically interact with each other by diverse structures and in different ways. **Cells interact and communicate with one another by forming junctions and junctional complexes. These junctions provide mechanical links and facilitates surface receptors ligand. Similar junctional complexes also mediate interaction of cells with the ECM.** These interactions must be precisely and carefully controlled to correctly determine the structures and functions of tissues.

Q. Describe the role of cell adhesion molecules in health and disease (for role of adhesion molecules in inflammation and other diseases refer pages 284–290.

Types of Cell Junctions

Classification of cell junctions is presented in **Box 11**.

Cell junctions are organized into three basic types. Various cell junctions in an epithelial cell of the small intestine are presented in **Figure 13**.

Box 11: Classification of cell junctions.

- Occluding (tight) junctions between the cell-to-cell
- Anchoring junctions
  - Cell-to-cell: Adherens junction and desmosomes
  - Cell-to-matrix: Hemidesmosomes
- Communicating (gap) junction

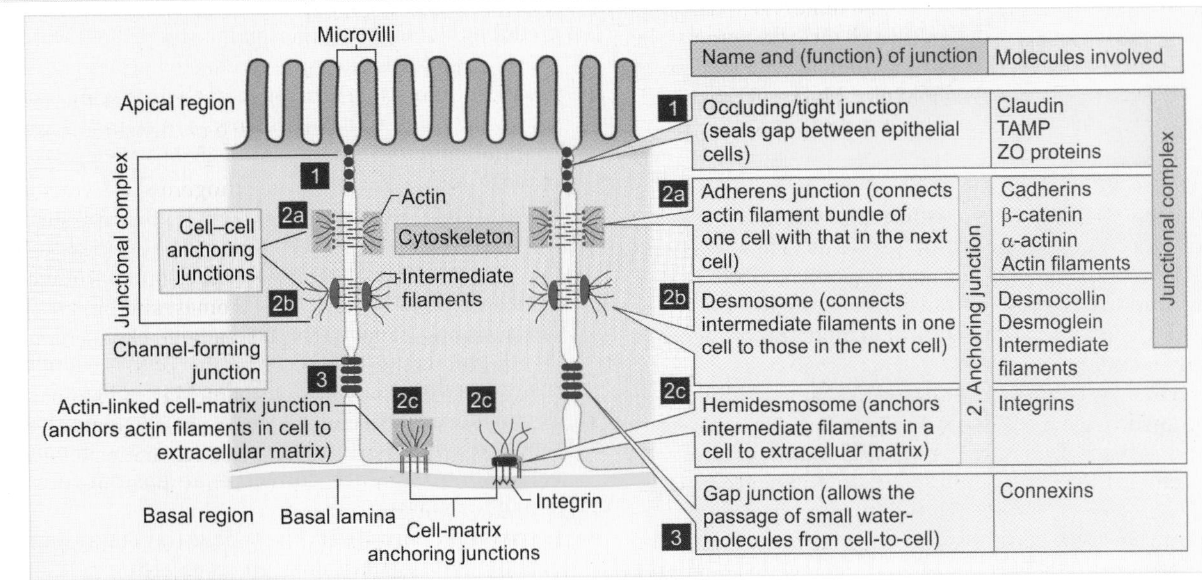

(TAMP: tight junction-associated MARVEL protein; ZO: zonula occludens)

FIG. 13: Various cell junctions in an epithelial cell of the small intestine. The tight junctions are peculiar to epithelia and the other types also occur (in modified forms) in various nonepithelial tissues.

Occluding Junctions (Tight junctions)

They hold or seal adjacent epithelial cells closely together (**1 in Fig. 13**). They create a continuous barrier that block or seal the gap between the cells. When viewed en face by freeze-fracture electron microscopy, occluding junctions appear to form a tight mesh like network of macromolecular contacts between neighboring cells. The complexes that mediate these cell–cell interactions are composed of multiple transmembrane proteins. These include tetraspanning claudin and tight junction-associated MARVEL protein (TAMP) families (e.g., occludin and claudin). They connect to many intracellular adaptor and scaffolding proteins, including the three members of the zonula occludens protein family (ZO-1, ZO-2, ZO-3) and cingulin.

Functions

- Occluding junctions create a high-resistance continuous selectively permeable barrier that seals the space between cells, thereby prevents or restricts the paracellular (between cells) movement of ions and other molecules.
- Maintain cellular polarity by forming the boundary between apical and basolateral domains of cells.
- These junctions (along with desmosomes) are dynamic structures. They can dissociate and reform as and when required to facilitate epithelial proliferation or migration of inflammatory cells.

Q. Write essay on cellular interaction with extracellular matrix.

Anchoring Junctions

Anchoring junctions mechanically attach cells and their intracellular cytoskeletons to other adjacent cells or to the ECM. These are two types of anchoring junctions namely: Adherens junctions and desmosomes.

Adherens junctions

They transmembrane adhesion molecules that connect actin microfilament bundle in one cell with that in the next cell. Adherens junctions are usually closely associated with and beneath occluding/tight junctions (**2A in Fig. 13**). Both adherens junctions and desmosomes (see below) are formed by homotypic (similar structures) extracellular interactions between transmembrane glycoproteins on adjacent cells. These glycoproteins are called as cadherins. They can influence cell shape and/or motility. Loss of the epithelial adherens junction proteinE-cadherin is responsible for the discohesive invasion pattern observed in some gastric carcinomas and lobular carcinomas of the breast.

Desmosomes

Q. Short essay on tonofilaments.

Desmosomes are disk-shaped structures at the surface of cell. They are more basal and form many types of junctions. They are matched with identical structures at an adjacent cell surface (**Fig. 14** and **2B of Fig. 13**). Desmosomes contain larger members of the cadherin family. Epithelial desmosomes attach to cable-like filaments of cytokeratin, sometimes called as tonofilaments. Such intermediate filaments are very strong and desmosomes cause firm cellular adhesion and provide strength throughout the epithelium. Desmosomes connect intermediate filaments in one cell to those in the next cell or cell to ECM.

Cell-to-cell desmosomal junctions Attachment of cell-to-cell are formed by the homotypic association of transmembrane glycoproteins called cadherins (**Figs. 13** and **14**).

- **Spot desmosome** or **macula adherens** (*macula* = Latin for **spot**): When the adhesion focus between cells is small and circular or **spot**-like (snap-like or rivet like) in outline, it is termed as spot desmosome. In spot desmosomes,

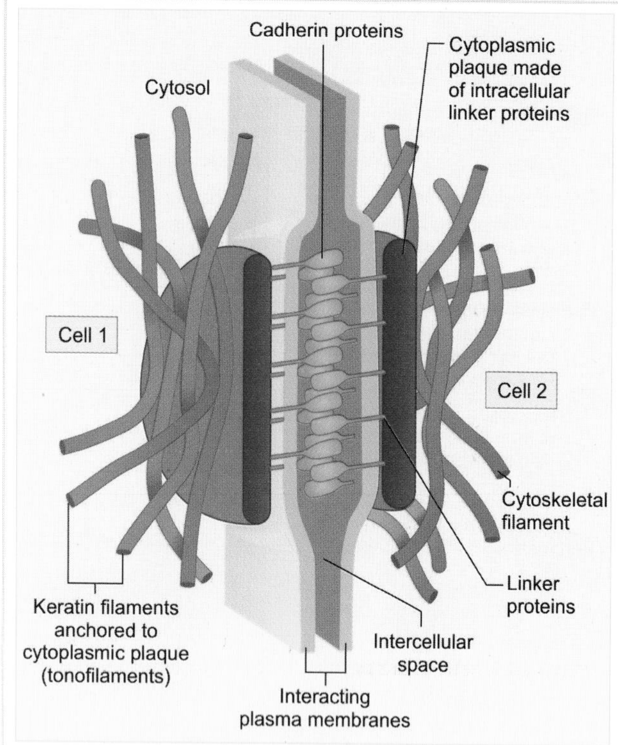

FIG. 14: Diagrammatic representation of desmosomes. Desmosomes link the keratin intermediate filaments of one epithelial cell (cell 1) to those of another (cell 2). On the cytoplasmic surface of each interacting plasma membrane is a dense plaque made up of a mixture of intracellular linker proteins. A bundle of keratin filaments (tonofilaments) is attached to the surface of each plaque. The cytoplasmic tails of transmembrane cadherin proteins bind to the outer face of each plaque whereas their extracellular domains interact to hold the neighboring cells to each other. Cadherin proteins attach one cell to another. Identical cadherin molecules present in the plasma membranes of adjacent cells bind to each other extracellularly. Inside the cell, cadherins are attached, via linker proteins, to cytoskeletal filaments—either actin filaments or keratin intermediate filaments.

the cadherins are linked to intracellular intermediate filaments (**keratin intermediate filaments** also known as **tonofilaments**) and allow extracellular forces to be mechanically communicated (and dissipated) over multiple cells. Intracellular **cytokeratin intermediate filaments (tonofilaments)** of the **cytoskeleton** are anchored in the attachment plaques on the two cytoplasmic surfaces of each **desmosome.** Tonofilament is made up of keratins and is found in all epithelial cells, but is particularly well developed in the epidermis. The tonofilaments, in the cells of the stratum basale of epidermis, consist of **keratin 5** and **keratin 14, and in** spinosum, **keratin 1** and **keratin 10**.

- **Belt desmosome:** In this, there are broad bands of adhesion between cells. The transmembrane adhesion molecules associated with belt desmosomes are intracellular actin microfilaments. They can influence cell shape and/or motility.

Cell to ECM (extracellular matrix)

- **Hemidesmosome (Figs. 2C in Fig. 13** and **15):** When an adhesive focus attaches the cell to the sECM, it is called a hemidesmosome (half of a desmosome). This is because the other half of the desmosome is not present within the ECM. The transmembrane connector proteins involved are called integrins. Similar to cadherins, they attach to intracellular intermediate filaments (also called **keratins** or **tonofilaments**), and functionally link the cytoskeleton to the ECM.
- **Focal adhesion complexes** (refer page 35) are large macromolecular complexes which are found at hemidesmosomes. They are composed of more than 100 proteins and are localize hemidesmosomes. These include proteins that can generate intracellular signals when cells are subjected to increased stress. For example, endothelium in the bloodstream or cardiac myocytes in a heart failure.
- Tonofilaments are keratin intermediate filaments that form tonofibrils in the cytosol of epithelial tissue. In epithelial cells, tonofilaments converge at desmosomes and hemidesmosomes.
- **Junctional complex:** The occluding/tight junction occupies the most apical position of the cell. This is followed by the adherens junction and then by a parallel row of desmosomes. All these three (**1, 2A** and **2B in Fig. 13**) together form a structure called a junctional complex.

Integrins

Focal adhesions attach cells to the ECM and important molecules involved are integrins. Integrins are the most important large family of transmembrane two-chain glycoproteins. They are composed of α- and β-subunits. Integrins consist of a heterodimeric combination of one of 18 different α-subunits and 8 different β-subunits. There are about 24 different combinations found and, depending on the combination, the integrins act as receptors for a variety of different ECM proteins. Integrin molecules are attached to the actin cytoskeleton inside the cytosol. This attachment is mediated by a network of proteins grouped together on the cytoplasmic side of the focal adhesions. These proteins mediate a physical connection from the cell interior to exterior, as well as serve role in signaling and regulating cell adhesion. This network of proteins includes kinases, phosphatases, and adaptor molecules.

Functions

- Integrins attach cell's intracellular cytoskeleton to a diverse type of molecules (ligands) present in ECM such as laminin and fibronectin. They functionally and structurally link the intracellular cytoskeleton with the outside world.
- Integrins also mediate cell–cell adhesive interactions. For example, integrins on the surface of leukocytes are necessary for its firm adhesion to endothelium and transmigration across the endothelium at sites of inflammation. They mediate the adhesion of leukocytes to endothelium and of various cells to the ECM. They are normally expressed in a low-affinity form on leukocyte plasma membranes and do not adhere to their specific ligands. However, when the leukocytes are activated by chemokines, they cause firm adhesion.
- They play a critical role in platelet aggregation.
- In addition to its property of focal attachment to underlying substrates, by binding through the integrin receptors, it can trigger signaling cascades. These may influence cell locomotion, proliferation, shape, and differentiation.

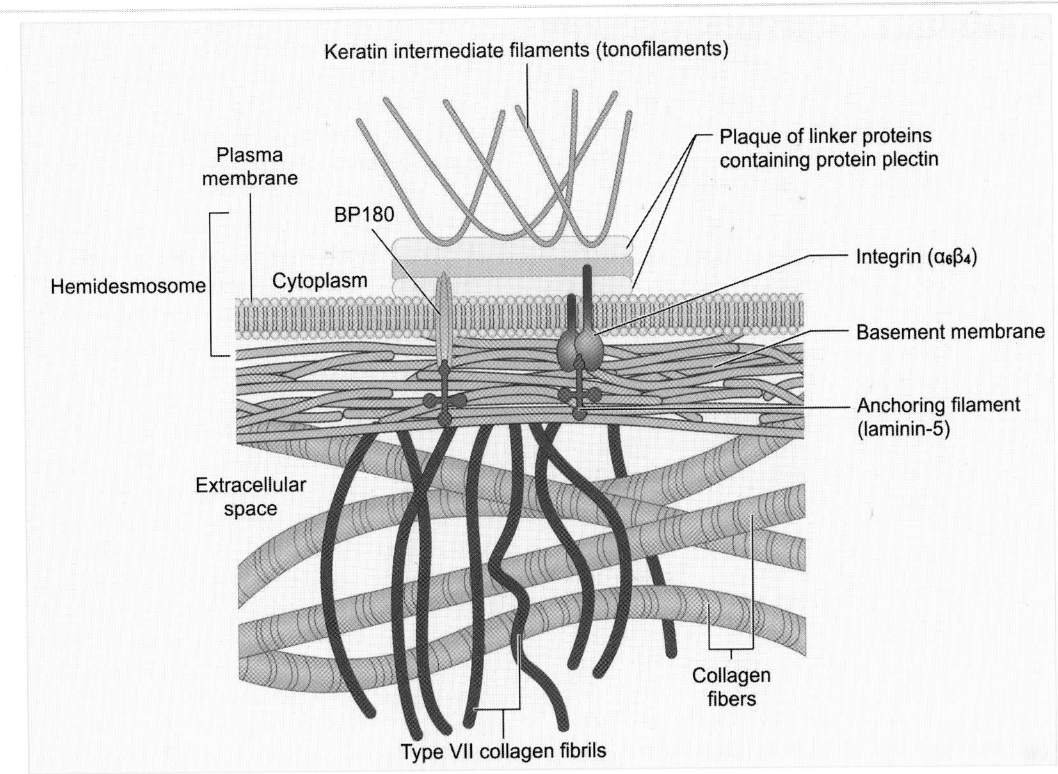

FIG. 15: Schematic diagram showing the major components of a hemidesmosome in epidermal cells. Hemidesmosomes are differentiated sites at the basal surfaces of epithelial cells where the cells attach the keratin intermediate filaments (tonofilaments) in an epithelial cell to underlying basal lamina/basement membrane. This linkage is mediated by a transmembrane attachment complex containing integrins and not by cadherins. Electron micrograph of hemidesmosomes shows the dense plaque of linker proteins on the inner surface of the plasma membrane and the intermediate filaments projecting into the cytoplasm. The $\alpha_6\beta_4$ integrin molecules of the epidermal cells are linked to cytoplasmic intermediate filaments by a protein called plectin. This protein plectin is present in the dark-staining plaque of linker proteins. The basement membrane is anchored by anchoring filaments of a particular type of laminin through integrin. A second transmembrane glycoprotein (BP180) maintains the linkage between the intracellular and the extracellular structural elements involved in epidermal adhesion. The collagen fibers are part of the underlying dermis.

Functions

They provide cell-to-cell adhesion and mechanical strength. Hemidesmosomes attach the cell with ECM namely basal lamina.

Communicating Junctions (Gap Junctions)

Gap junctions (**3 of Fig. 13**) are channels (channel-forming junctions) which bridge the gaps between adjacent cells. It creates direct channels which link the cytoplasm of one to that of the other adjacent cell. They are found near the basal end of the cells. The junction consists of a dense planar array of 1.5–2 nm narrow gaps or pores (called *connexons*). They are formed by hexamers of transmembrane protein *connexins*. These pores permit or mediate the passage of chemicals, electrical signals, ions, nucleotides, sugars, amino acids, vitamins, and other small molecules from one cell to another. The permeability of the gap junction is rapidly reduced when there is lowering of intracellular pH or increase in the intracellular calcium. Gap junctions play important role in cell–cell communication. For example, in cardiac myocytes, cell-to-cell calcium movement occurs through gap junctions. This allows the myocardium to behave as a functional syncytium capable of coordinated waves of contraction responsible for heartbeat.

Functions

Gap junctions are continuous channels between the two adjacent cells and therefore, the cells can rapidly share small molecules and ions.

Summary of various cell-to-cell interactions is presented in **Table 10**.

BIOSYNTHETIC MACHINERY: ENDOPLASMIC RETICULUM AND GOLGI APPARATUS

Endoplasmic Reticulum

The cytoplasm of most cells contains a convoluted membranous network (reticulum) called as ER. This network extends throughout the cytosol, from the surface of the nucleus to the cell membrane. It encloses a series of intercommunicating branching tubules (channels) and flattened sacs or lumens called cisternae. The tubules and sacs interconnect and their membranes are continuous with the outer nuclear membrane (ONM). The compartment enclosed by ER is also continuous with the space between the inner and ONMs. Thus, the ER and nuclear membranes form a continuous sheet enclosing a single internal space,

Table 10: Summary of various cell-to-cell interactions.

Name	Function
Occluding (tight) junction	Seals the adjacent/neighboring cells together in an epithelial sheet. It prevents leakage of extracellular molecules between them and also helps to polarize the cells
Anchoring junctions	
• Cell-to-cell: Adherent junction and desmosome	Joins the intermediate filaments in one cell to those of neighboring cells
• Cell-to-matrix: Hemidesmosome	It anchors intermediate filaments in a cell to the basal lamina
Communicating (gap) junction	They form channels that permit small, intracellular, water-soluble molecules, including inorganic ions and metabolites, to pass from cell-to-cell

called the ER lumen or the *ER cisternal space.* The membrane surface of ER is up to 30 times than that of the cell membrane.

Functions

Endoplasmic reticulum is a major site for vital cellular activities. **There is a constant renewal of all cellular constituents. These include structural proteins, enzymes transcription factors, and the phospholipid membranes of the cell. This is kept in balance by synthesis and intracellular degradation.**

- **Synthesis of proteins and lipids:** The proteins synthesized in RER include:
  - **All transmembrane proteins and lipids:** Required for the plasma membrane.
  - **Soluble proteins:** Found within cell's organelles, including the ER itself, Golgi complex/apparatus, lysosomes, endosomes, secretory vesicles.
  - **Secreted proteins:** Almost all of the proteins that will be secreted to the cell exterior, plus those destined for the lumen of the ER, Golgi apparatus, or lysosomes are initially delivered to the ER lumen.
- **Synthesis of other molecules:** ER is also the initial site of synthesis of all molecules destined for export out of the cell.

The various functions of the ER are essential to every cell. The relative importance of ER varies greatly between individual cell types. The **endoplasmic reticulum (ER)** is divided into two subcompartments, the **RER** and the **SER**. They are distinguished by the presence or absence of ribosomes. Most cells have scanty regions of smooth ER, and the ER is often partly smooth and partly rough.

The rough ER has ribosomes bound to its cytosolic surface, whereas the smooth ER lacks associated ribosomes.

Rough Endoplasmic Reticulum

In RER, there are **membrane-bound ribosomes** on the cytosolic surface.

Synthesis of Proteins

Polypeptides/proteins are synthesized at two distinct locations within the cell namely:

1. **Within membrane-bound ribosomes (RER):** Certain polypeptides are synthesized on ribosomes attached to the cytosolic surface of the RER membranes. Ribosomes are organelles that are not membrane-enclosed. Ribosomes synthesize both soluble and integral membrane proteins. Most of these proteins are destined either for secretion to the exterior of cell or for other organelles in the interior of cell. The proteins are transported into other membrane-enclosed organelles only after their synthesis is complete. The proteins are transported into the ER as they are synthesized.
2. **In free ribosomes:** Free ribosomes are ribosomes that are not attached to the RER. They synthesize all other proteins/polypeptides encoded by the nuclear genome. These are subsequently released into the cytosol. The RER is the starting point of the biosynthetic pathway.

Synthesis of Proteins in RER (Fig. 16)

Rough endoplasmic reticulum is the site of **synthesis of the proteins** but also produces **carbohydrate chains**, most of the **lipid** for the rest of the cell (e.g., phospholipids) and functions as a **store for Ca^{2+} ions** (used in many cell signaling responses). RER synthesizes and segregates proteins not destined for the cytosol. Many ribosomes can bind to a single mRNA molecule; hence a polyribosome is usually formed. If the mRNA encodes a protein with an ER signal sequence, the polyribosome becomes attached to the ER membrane. This directs the signal sequences on multiple growing polypeptide chains. The individual ribosomes associated with such an mRNA molecule can return to the cytosol after the completion of translation. In the cytosol, these can intermix with the pool of free ribosomes. The steps in synthesis of protein RER are as follows:

- Synthesis of the polypeptide begins on a free ribosome. A newly translated signal sequence emerges from the ribosome. This process is directed by the newly translated N-amino terminus of a secretory nascent protein contains 15–40 amino acids. It includes a specific sequence of hydrophobic residues comprising the **signal sequence or signal peptide**.
- As the newly translated signal sequence emerges from the ribosome, signal sequence or peptide binds to protein complex called the signal-recognition particle (SRP). SRPs stop further translation (polypeptide elongation) until the SRP–ribosome nascent chain complex can contact the ER membrane.
- SRP–ribosome complex then binds to an SRP receptor (SR) present within the ER membrane. SRP then releases the **signal sequence or signal peptide**, allowing translation to continue with the nascent polypeptide chain transferred to a translocator complex (also called a translocon or protein-conducting channel) through the ER membrane. This leads to more firm attachment of the ribosome to the ER. It is followed by release of the SRP.
- The nascent polypeptide passes into the lumen of the ER. This is followed by the cleavage of **signal sequence or signal peptide** inside the lumen of the RER by an enzyme called as the signal peptidase.
- Translation continues and the growing polypeptide pushes itself toward lumen of ER. Simultaneously, chaperones and other proteins serve to "pull" the nascent polypeptide through the translocator complex.
- After the release of polypeptides from the ribosome, post-translational modifications and proper folding of the polypeptides continue. The proper folding occurs with the help of ER chaperones, such as **binding immunoglobulin**

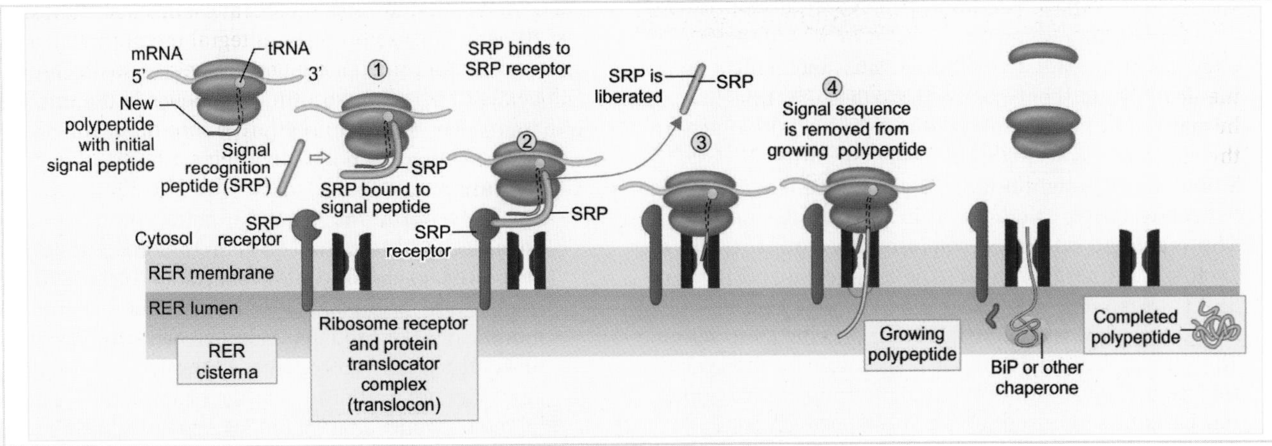

FIG. 16: Steps in synthesis of protein in rough endoplasmic reticulum (RER).

protein (BiP). BiP is an HSP70_molecular chaperone located in the lumen of ER. Chaperone molecules retain proteins in the ER till proper folding and conformation is achieved. If a protein fails to fold and assemble properly, it is retained and degraded within the ER. Excess accumulation of misfolded proteins, either due to accumulation beyond the capacity of the ER to edit and degrade them, leads to the ER stress response (also called the unfolded protein response or the UPR). This stimulates cell death through apoptosis.

- Proteins will be either extruded into the lumen of ER or get integrated into the membrane of ER. Proteins to be integrated into the ER must fold properly to perform its function and assemble into higher order complexes. Proper folding of the extracellular domains of many proteins involves the formation of disulfide bonds. Mutations which disrupt disulfide bond formation may be inherited and cause several disorders (e.g., familial hypercholesterolemia).

Importance of the ER Editing Function

For example, *cystic fibrosis* is most commonly associated with misfolding of the CFTR membrane transporter protein. This is due to the most common mutation in the *CFTR* gene with loss of a single amino acid residue (phenylalanine 508). This leads to misfolding, ER retention, and degradation of the CFTR protein. The loss of CFTR function also leads to abnormal epithelial chloride transport, hyperviscous bronchial secretions and recurrent infections of airway.

Salient features of endoplasmic reticulum are presented in **Box 12**.

Salient features of ribosomes are presented in **Box 13**.

Box 12: Salient features of endoplasmic reticulum.

Ultrastructurally, appear as tubular and cistern-like spaces and vesicular structures folded in the cytoplasm.

Rough endoplasmic reticulum (RER)
- Membrane of RER is continuous with nuclear membrane
- Beaded in appearance due to ribosome particles attached to the surface
- Function: Synthesis of secretory proteins and lysosomal enzymes

Smooth endoplasmic reticulum (SER)
- Connected to Golgi apparatus and plasma membrane
- Function: Synthesis of lipids

Box 13: Salient features of ribosomes.

Structure
- Present as free ribosomes in cytosol and membrane bound form attached to the endoplasmic reticulum
- Made up of rRNA (ribosomal RNA) and proteins
- Consists of 2 units—(1) smaller 40s and (2) larger 60s
- Small subunits have the binding site for mRNA (messenger RNA) and tRNA (transfer RNA)
- rRNA of the larger subunit has enzymatic activity to catalyze the peptide bond

Function
- Sites of protein synthesis, decode the information from mRNA, and help the molecules of tRNA to assemble the particular amino acids to make a protein

Smooth Endoplasmic Reticulum

Smooth endoplasmic reticulums lack bound ribosomes. The SER in most cells is relatively sparse. However, they are extensively developed in a number of cell types, including those of skeletal muscle, kidney tubules, and steroid-producing endocrine glands. They form the transition zone from RER to transport vesicles moving to the Golgi.

Functions

- **Synthesis of steroid hormones** in the endocrine cells of the gonad and adrenal cortex
- **Detoxification:** In the liver, chronic use or repeated exposure of a wide variety of organic compounds that are metabolized by the SER (including barbiturates and ethanol) can lead to reactive hyperplasia of the SER in liver cells. Detoxification is performed by a system of oxygen transferring enzymes (oxygenases), including the *cytochrome P450* family. These enzymes do not have substrate specificity, hence, capable of oxidizing numerous different hydrophobic compounds and convert them into more hydrophilic compounds that can be easily excreted. The effects are not always beneficial. For example, the

relatively harmless compound benzo[*a*]pyrene can be converted into a potent carcinogen by the "detoxifying" enzymes of the SER. Cytochrome P450s metabolize many medications, and genetic variation in these enzymes among humans, may be responsible for individual differences in the effectiveness and side effects of many drugs.

- **Sequestering calcium ions:** The SER also is responsible for sequestering calcium within the cytoplasm of cells. The regulated release of calcium ions from the SER of skeletal and cardiac muscle cells (specialized form of SER known as the *sarcoplasmic reticulum* in muscle cells) into the cytosol is responsible for triggering contraction. The sarcoplasmic reticulum is responsible for the cyclical release and sequestration of calcium ions that regulate muscle contraction and relaxation, respectively.

Salient features of Golgi complex are presented in **Box 14**.

Golgi Apparatus

Golgi apparatus or Golgi complex is a dynamic organelle that consists of organized stacks of disk like, membrane-enclosed compartments called *Golgi cisternae.* Golgi complex is primarily a "processing plant" and is not uniform in composition from one end to the other. Each Golgi stack is divided into cis, ***medial***, and ***trans*** **cisternae;** the cis face is entry face near the ER and the trans face is the exit face near the plasma membrane. The composition of the membrane compartments from the *cis* to the *trans* face is different. Each compartment is composed of a network of interconnected tubular and cisternal structures: The cis Golgi network (CGN) and the trans Golgi network (TGN), respectively. Newly synthesized membrane proteins, secretory, and lysosomal proteins, leave the ER and enter The Golgi complex at its *cis* face (cis end). Then they progress along the Golgi apparatus where proteins that were originally synthesized in the rough ER are sequentially modified in specific ways. The TGN is a sorting station where proteins are segregated into different types of vesicles heading either to the plasma membrane or to various intracellular destinations.

The RER sends many of its proteins and lipids destined for other organelles or for extracellular export to the *cis* face of Golgi apparatus.

- The Golgi apparatus progressively modifies and completes post-translational **modification of proteins** in an orderly fashion. The macromolecules move from *cis* to *trans* face and during this, they are shuttled between the various cisternae within membrane-bound vesicles.
- In ER, *N-linked oligosaccharide* is attached *en bloc* to many proteins and then trimmed while the protein is still in the ER. As macromolecules move in the Golgi apparatus, these **N-linked oligosaccharides are trimmed** and further modified in a stepwise fashion. This trimming helps the proteins to fold and to transport misfolded proteins to the cytosol for degradation in proteasomes. Thus, Golgi apparatus play an important role in controlling the quality of proteins exiting from the ER.
- **Glycosylation**
    - The **glycoproteins** are proteins that contain oligosaccharide chains (glycans), bound to amino acids. **Glycosylation** is the enzymatic attachment of sugars, and is the most common post-translational modification of proteins. Many proteins also undergo reversible glycosylation with a single sugar (*N*-acetyl glucosamine) bound to a serine or threonine residue. (Nonenzymatic attachment of sugars to proteins is referred to as **glycation**. This process can have serious pathologic consequences as in in poorly controlled diabetes mellitus).
    - The Golgi complex plays a key role in the assembly of the carbohydrate component of glycoproteins and glycolipids. Glycosylation occurs in Golgi apparatus by adding O-linked oligosaccharides (sugar moieties linked to serine or threonine) to proteins and lipids. The glycosylation helps in directing molecules to lysosomes (via the mannose-6-phosphate receptor) and some glycosylation adducts may be important for cell–cell or cell–matrix interactions, or for clearing senescent cells (e.g., platelets and red cells).
- The Golgi apparatus **packages, addresses and dispatches lipids and proteins to various proper destinations**. In the *CGN*, proteins are recycled back to the ER. In the *TGN*, proteins and lipids are dispatched to other organelles (including the plasma membrane) or to secretory vesicles destined for extracellular release.
- Golgi apparatus initiates packing, concentration, and storage of secretory products.

Cells with prominent Golgi complex: These are found in cells specialized for secretion. These include goblet cells of the intestine, bronchial epithelium (secreting large amounts of polysaccharide-rich mucus), and plasma cells (secreting large quantities of antibodies).

Diagrammatic appearance of a portion of a Golgi complex is shown in **Figure 17**.

Box 14: Salient features of Golgi complex.

Membrane bound cistern-like spaces arranged in polarized fashion

Functions:

- Processing of protein received from rough endoplasmic reticulum. N-linked and O-linked glycosylation of proteins and lipids
- Storage of calcium
- Platform for various cell signaling

WASTE DISPOSAL: LYSOSOMES AND PROTEASOMES

Three routes available for degradation of intracellular macromolecules. These include (i) lysosomes, (ii) proteasomes and (iii) peroxisomes. Cells mainly depends on lysosomes to digest internalized material and accumulated internal waste.

Lysosomes

Q. Describe the function (analyze the role) of lysosome in health, cell injury (refer Chapter 7) and disease (refer pages 834–845).

Lysosomal Function in Health

Lysosomes are small (0.2–0.4 µm) membrane-bound vesicles found in the cytosol of the cell. They are the cell's digestive

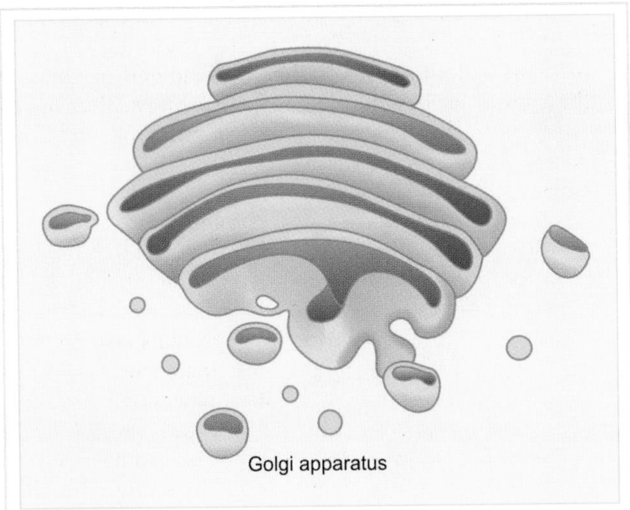

FIG. 17: Diagrammatic appearance of a portion of a Golgi complex. The elements of the *cis* and *trans* compartments are often discontinuous and appear as tubular networks.

organelles containing many (bag of) degradative enzymes produced in the RER and carried over in Golgi apparatus.

Contents

There are at least 50 different hydrolytic enzymes (**Table 11**). These include acid hydrolases (i.e., enzymes that function best in acidic pH ≤5), proteases, nucleases, lipases, glycosidases, phosphatases, and sulfatases (**Table 11**). All the enzymes of a lysosome have their optimal activity at an acid pH and thus are **acid hydrolases**. The pH optimum of these enzymes is suited to the low pH of the lysosomal compartment, which are about 4.6. These enzymes are less active at the neutral pH of cells and most extracellular fluids. Thus, if a lysosomal enzyme is released into the cytosol (where the pH is between 7.0 and 7.3), they cause little degradation of cytosolic components. Cytosolic and nuclear proteins usually not degraded in lysosomes, but degraded in the large multiprotein complexes in the cytosol are called as proteasomes.

Table 11: List of various enzymes present in lysosome.

Enzyme	*Substrate*
Phosphatases	
• Acid phosphatase	Phosphomonoesters
• Acid phosphodiesterase	Phosphodiesters
Nucleases	
• Acid ribonuclease	Ribonucleic acid (RNA)
• Acid deoxyribonuclease	Deoxyribonucleic acid (DNA)
Proteases	
• Cathepsin	Proteins
• Collagenase	Collagen
Glycosaminoglycan (GAG)-hydrolyzing enzymes	
• Iduronate sulfatase	Dermatan sulfate
• β-galactosidase	Keratan sulfate
• Heparan N-sulfatase	Heparan sulfate
• α-N-acetyl glucosaminidase	Heparan sulfate
Polysaccharidases and oligosaccharidases	
• α-glucosidase	Glycogen
• Fucosidase	Fucosyloligosaccharides
• α-mannosidase	Mannosyloligosaccharides
• Sialidase	Sialyloligosaccharides
Sphingolipid hydrolyzing enzymes	
• Ceramidase	Ceramide
• Glucocerebrosidase	Glucosylceramide
• β-hexosaminidase	GM_2 ganglioside
• Arylsulfatase A	Galactosylsulfatide
Lipid hydrolyzing enzymes	
• Acid lipase	Triacylglycerols
• Phospholipase	Phospholipids

Synthesis of lysosomal enzymes

Lysosomal enzymes are initially synthesized in the ER lumen. They move from ER to the Golgi apparatus in which they are tagged with a mannose-6-phosphate (M6P) residue. Such M6P-modified proteins are then delivered to lysosomes through trans-Golgi vesicles that express M6P receptors.

Functions of lysosomes

Lysosomes form closed compartments in which the composition of the lumen (the aqueous interior of the compartment) differs substantially from that of the surrounding cytosol.

Breakdown of material (Fig. 18) The lysosomal enzymes can hydrolyze virtually every type of macromolecule. The macromolecules destined for catabolism in the lysosomes arrive by one of the three pathways:

- **Pinocytosis or receptor-mediated endocytosis:** Lysosomes are the site of degradation/breakdown of material brought into the cell from the extracellular environment. These **materials may be taken up** into the cells **by** fluid-phase **pinocytosis or** receptor-mediated **endocytosis.** These materials pass from plasma membrane to early endosome to late endosome, and ultimately into the lysosome. In the process of passage of the material from plasma membrane to lysosome, they become progressively more acidic. The first acidic compartment encountered by the material is early endosome, and in late endosome, proteolytic enzymes begin significant digestion. The late endosomes mature into lysosomes.
- **Phagocytosis:** Phagocytosis of microorganisms or large fragments of matrix or debris occur primarily in phagocytic cells (macrophages and neutrophils). In phagocytic cells, lysosomes function as scavengers. In phagocytosis, large, insoluble particles/materials (e.g., bacteria) are enveloped by the plasma membrane and internalized to form a *phagosome*. This phagosome subsequently fuses with a lysosome to form phagolysosome. Ingested microorganisms are usually inactivated by the low pH of the lysosome and then digested enzymatically.
- **Autophagy** (refer pages 156–159): Lysosomes also play an important role in organelle turnover, that is, the regulated destruction of the cell's own organelles and their replacement. Lysosomes are responsible for degradation

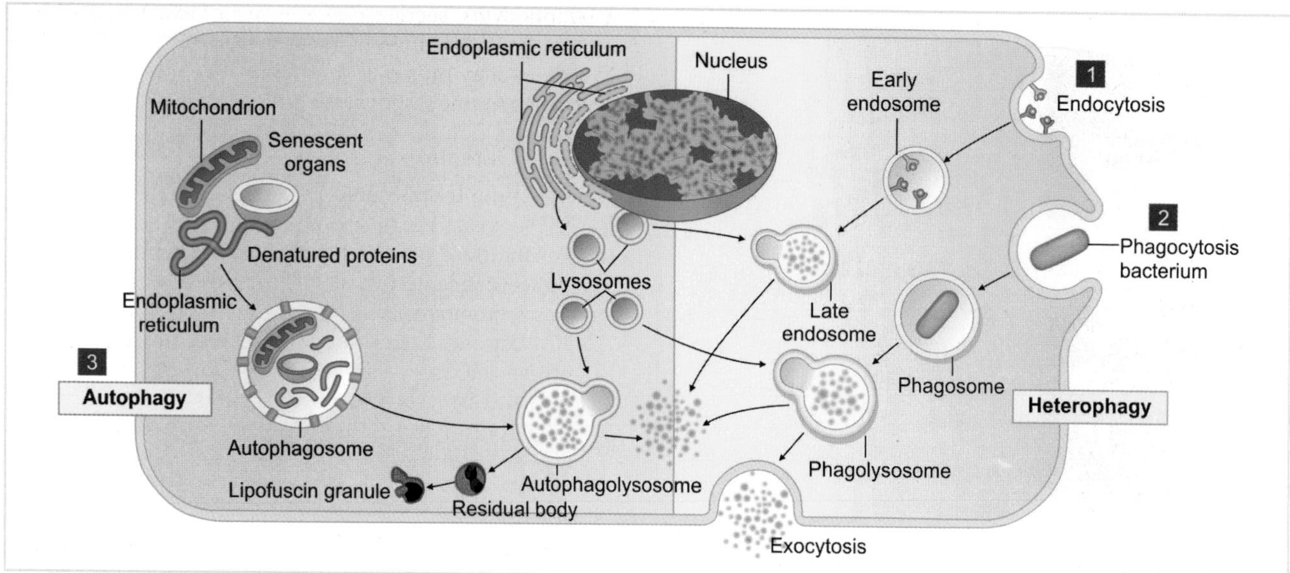

FIG. 18: Pathways of degradation and removal of materials by lysosomes. Heterophagy is digestion within a cell of a substance taken in by endocytosis of phagocytosis from the cell's environment. (1) Pinocytosis and endocytosis: Soluble macromolecules and molecules bound to proteins on the cell surface are taken into the cell by invagination of segments of the plasma membrane and form endosomes. Then, they are delivered to lysosomes. (2) Phagocytosis: Whole cells and other large, insoluble particles are phagocytosed and move from the cell surface to lysosomes. (3) Autophagy: Worn-out organelles and bulk cytoplasmic components form autophagosome and are delivered to lysosomes through the autophagic pathway. Within the acidic lumen of a lysosome, hydrolytic enzymes degrade proteins, nucleic acids, lipids, and other large molecules.

of many old (senescent organelles) or unnecessary cellular constituents (components) or large protein complexes that have become obsolete for the cell or organism. The process by which an old/aged organelle is degraded in a lysosome is termed as autophagy ("eating oneself"). In 2016, Nobel Prize was awarded to Yoshinori Ohsumi for his discoveries of mechanism of autophagy. During autophagy, an obsolete organelle (e.g., mitochondrion) is surrounded by a double membrane derived from the ER. The double membrane progressively expands to encircle a collection of structures and forms an *autophagosome.* The outer membrane of this *autophagosome* then fuses with a lysosome to produce an *autophagolysosome.* Inside these *autophagolysosomes,* the enclosed organelle is degraded and the breakdown products are made available to the cell. Apart from facilitating the turnover of aged and defunct cellular constituents, autophagy also is used to preserve viability of cell during depletion of nutrients. After the completion of the digestive process in the autophagolysosome, the organelle is termed as a *residual body.* Depending on the type of cell, the contents of the residual body may be completely removed from the cell by exocytosis, or they may remain within the cytoplasm indefinitely as a *lipofuscin granule (wear and tear pigment).* Lipofuscin granules increase in number as an individual becomes older. These granules are considered a major characteristic of the aging process.

Pathways of degradation and removal of materials by lysosomes are presented in **Figure 18.**

Proteasomes

Discussed under protein misfolding further on pages 184 and 185.

Peroxisome

It is a membrane-bound organelle (formerly known as a microbody), found in the cytoplasm of almost all cells. They also degrade intracellular macromolecules. Peroxisomes contain about 50 different enzymes and these are involved in a variety of biochemical pathways in different types of cells. Peroxisomes originally were defined as organelles that carry out oxidation reactions and leads to the production of hydrogen peroxide. Peroxisomes also contain the enzyme catalase, which decomposes hydrogen peroxide. A variety of substrates are broken down by such oxidative reactions in peroxisomes.

Exosomes

Q. Write a short essay on exosomes.

Definition

Exosomes are defined as small extracellular membrane vesicles of endocytic origin.

Formation

The exact mechanism of generation of endosomes is not fully understood. Exosomes may be released either:

- From cells upon fusion of a multivesicular body (MVB, which is an intermediate endocytic compartment in the cytoplasm of cell) with the plasma membrane (**Fig. 19**) or
- Released directly from the plasma membrane.

Multivesicular bodies can either deliver its content to lysosomes for degradation or can fuse with the cell surface to release intraluminal vesicles as exosomes.

A subtype of exosomes is also present in ECM bio scaffolds (nonfluid).

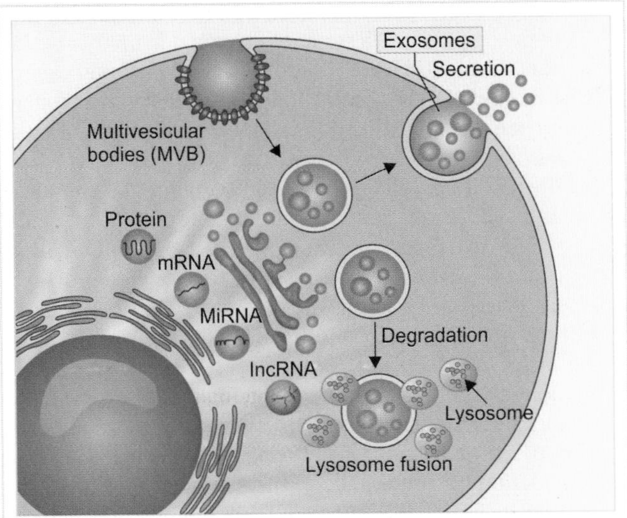

FIG. 19: Exosome formation from multivesicular body (MVB).

Cardinal Features

- Exosomes are vesicles having a saucer shape and measure about 30–150 nm in diameter. These vesicles are bound by a lipid bilayer.
- Released by almost all types of cells.
- Present in all body fluids.
- They are loaded with microRNAs (miRNAs) and other bioactive contents.
- Payload very cell specific.

Composition of the exosomes secreted by various cells reveals the presence of some common proteins as well as some cell-type specific proteins. This indicates that exosomes are secreted subcellular components and are produced by different cell types. Exosomes can transfer proteins, lipids, mRNA, and microRNA into acceptor or recipient cells. These RNAs may have functional effects in recipient cells.

Functions of Exosomes

Exosomes have specialized functions and play a key role in some processes.

- **Intracellular signaling:** Exosomes probably provide a means of intercellular communication and of transmission of macromolecules between cells.
- **Waste management:** Exosomes eliminate undegraded endosomal or lysosomal proteins and membranes.
- **Disease:** Exosomes play a role in the spread of proteins, lipids, mRNA, miRNA, and DNA. Thus, they may act as a contributing factor in the development of several diseases. Exosomes provide a means of intercellular communication. They may also act as vehicles for "bad" communication or spread. Exosomes may propagate spread of neurodegenerative protein. Examples include Aβ (in Alzheimer's disease), tau (in numerous neurodegenerative diseases), prions (in transmissible spongiform encephalopathies), alpha-synuclein (in Parkinson's disease), and superoxide dismutase 1 (in amyotrophic lateral sclerosis).
- Coagulation
- **Immune system:** B cells, dendritic cells, and mast cells of the immune system appear to release exosomes constitutively. Dendritic cells are specialized to activate T lymphocytes, secrete higher levels of exosomes upon interaction with antigen-specific CD4+ T lymphocytes. Exosomes may thus play a functional role in mediating adaptive immune responses to pathogens and tumors.

Methods of Detection

- **Nanoparticle tracking analysis:** It is a highly sensitive method for visualization and analysis of exosomes.
- Exosomal surface markers-based exosome characterization
    - **Fluorescence-activated cell sorting (FACS):** It is the most common method used to analyze the different physical and chemical characteristics of exosome in suspension. This method uses light scattering properties of vesicles to analyze and sort individual exosomes using specific fluorescently labeled antibodies.
    - **Western blotting:** This technique is used for detecting specific proteins and semiquantitative estimation of protein.
    - **Enzyme-linked immunosorbent assay (ELISA):** It uses a solid-phase enzyme immunoassay (EIA) to detect the presence of a specific single protein on the surface of exosomes using a single or a pair of antibodies.
- **Flow cytometry:** It is an optical method to detect exosomes in suspension. However, it cannot detect single exosomes due to limited sensitivity and potential measurement artifacts as exosomes.
- **Tunable Resistive Pulse Sensing (TRPS)-based exosome characterization**: TRPS is a technique that detects even single exosomes and can be used to measure the size of exosomes.
- **Other methods:** These include transmission electron microscopy, atomic force microscopy, Raman microscopy, etc.

Applications

Exosomes have altered characteristics in many diseases, such as cancer and autoimmune diseases. Hence, they have potential for diagnostic and therapeutic applications.

- **Therapeutics:** Exosomes may have a potential therapeutic application as they have the ability to elicit potent cellular responses in vitro and in vivo.
- Exosomes mediate regenerative outcomes to injury and disease. This is similar to bioactivity of stem cell populations.
- Exosomes secreted by human circulating fibrocytes (a population of mesenchymal progenitors) are involved in normal wound healing via paracrine signaling.
- **Drug delivery:** Exosomes may be used as vectors for drug delivery. The exosomes are composed of cell membranes, rather than synthetic polymers. Thus, they do not elicit immune response and are better tolerated by the host. Thus, exosomes may be used as a vehicle for the delivery of cancer drugs.
- Exosomes can be used for prognosis and as a biomarker in health and disease.

CELLULAR METABOLISM AND MITOCHONDRIAL FUNCTION

Mitochondria

Mitochondria contain their own DNA genome (circularized, about 1% of the total cellular DNA). These DNAs encode about

1% of the total cellular proteins and about 20% of the proteins involved in *oxidative phosphorylation*. Though their genomes are small, mitochondria can perform all the steps of DNA replication, transcription, and translation.

Features

Depending on the cell structure, mitochondria vary considerably in size and shape. They change shape over time but are most often elongated, sausage-shaped organelles. Mitochondria are dynamic, can constantly fuse (fusion) with one another, or split (fission) in two. Mitochondria are very mobile, moving around the cell by using microtubules. They tend to localize at intracellular sites where there is maximum requirement of energy. The number of mitochondria in cells is highly variable and the number of mitochondria in a cell depends on the balance between fusion by mitochondrial fission (division) and fusion, and by autophagy.

Appearance (Fig. 20)

Each mitochondrion has four compartments:

- ***Outer mitochondrial membrane***: Each mitochondrion has two separate and specialized membranes namely outer and inner. The outer mitochondrial membrane completely encloses the mitochondrion and serves as its outer boundary. It is relatively permeable because of its pore-forming protein known as ***porin***. The porin proteins form aqueous channels and allow free passage of small (<5,000 daltons) molecules. Larger molecules (and even some smaller polar species) need specific transporters. The outer membrane contains enzymes which convert certain lipid substrates into a form that can be metabolized within the mitochondrion.
- ***Inner mitochondrial membrane:*** It is thinner than the outer and is subdivided into two interconnected domains.
    - **Inner boundary:** It lies just inside the outer mitochondrial membrane, forming a double-membrane outer envelope. It is particularly rich in the proteins needed for the import of mitochondrial proteins. The inner membrane contains the cytochromes, the carrier molecules of the electron transport chain, and the enzymes involved in ATP production.
    - **Cristae:** The other domain is present within the interior of the organelle as a series of invaginated membranous sheets, called **cristae.** They project into the inner cavity. In some cell types, mitochondria typically have tubular cristae. The cristae contain a large amount of membrane surface, which contain the machinery (the enzymes of the respiratory chain) required for aerobic respiration and ATP formation. Aerobic respiration takes place within the matrix and on the inner membrane. This process is enhanced by the large surface area provided by the cristae.
- ***Mitochondrial matrix***: The ***inner cavity*** is filled by the ***mitochondrial matrix***. The matrix is the site of the mitochondrial DNA and ribosomes (of considerably smaller size than those found in the cytosol). It contains the most of metabolic enzymes, such as the enzymes involved in oxidation of fatty acids and the Krebs cycle of the citric acid cycle. The matrix also contains many ***dense matrix granules***, the function of which is not known.
- ***Intermembranous space***: It is the space between the two membranes namely outer and inner. It also contains a variety of enzymes.

Energy Generation

Cellular respiration

All functions of cells require a continuous supply of energy. The energy is derived from the sequential breakdown of organic molecules during the process called ***cellular respiration***. Mitochondria are the main organelles involved in cellular respiration. The energy generated during cellular respiration is ultimately stored in the form of ATP molecules. In all cells, ATP forms a pool of readily available energy for all the metabolic functions of the cell. The main substrates for cellular respiration are simple sugars (glucose) and lipids (fatty acids).

- ***Glycolysis* (Fig. 21):** Glycolysis is the main pathway of glucose (and other carbohydrate) metabolism. It consists of a series of reactions that extract energy from the breakdown of glucose to form two molecules of pyruvate. Glycolysis starts in the cytosol of all cells. It can function either aerobically or anaerobically, depending on the availability of oxygen and the electron transport chain. The

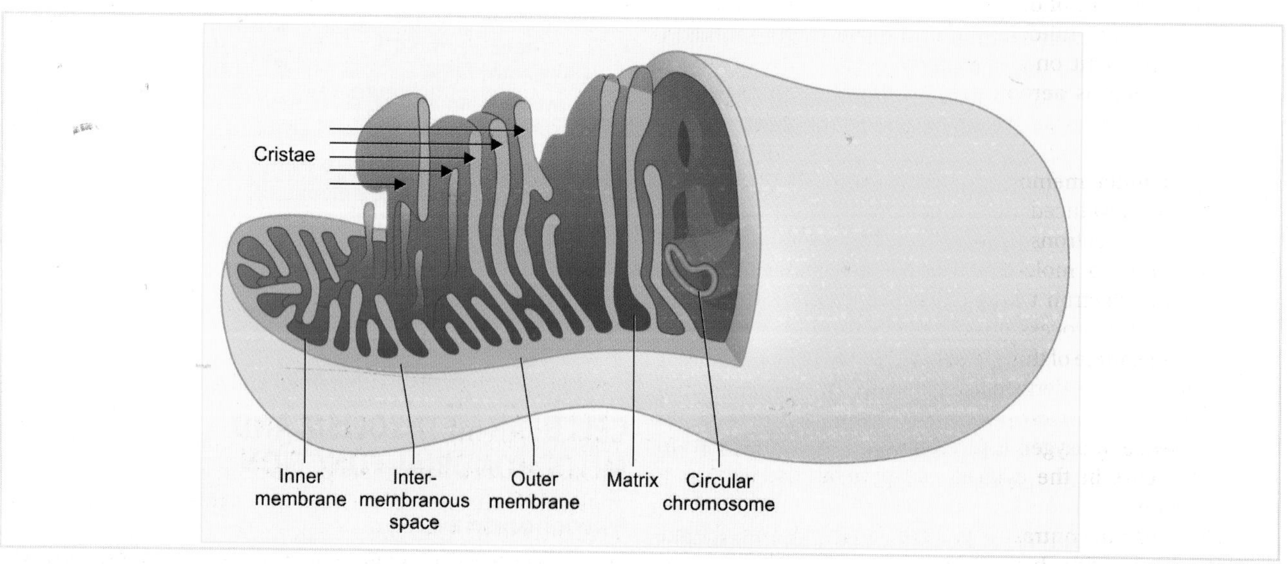

FIG. 20: Diagrammatic appearance of mitochondria.

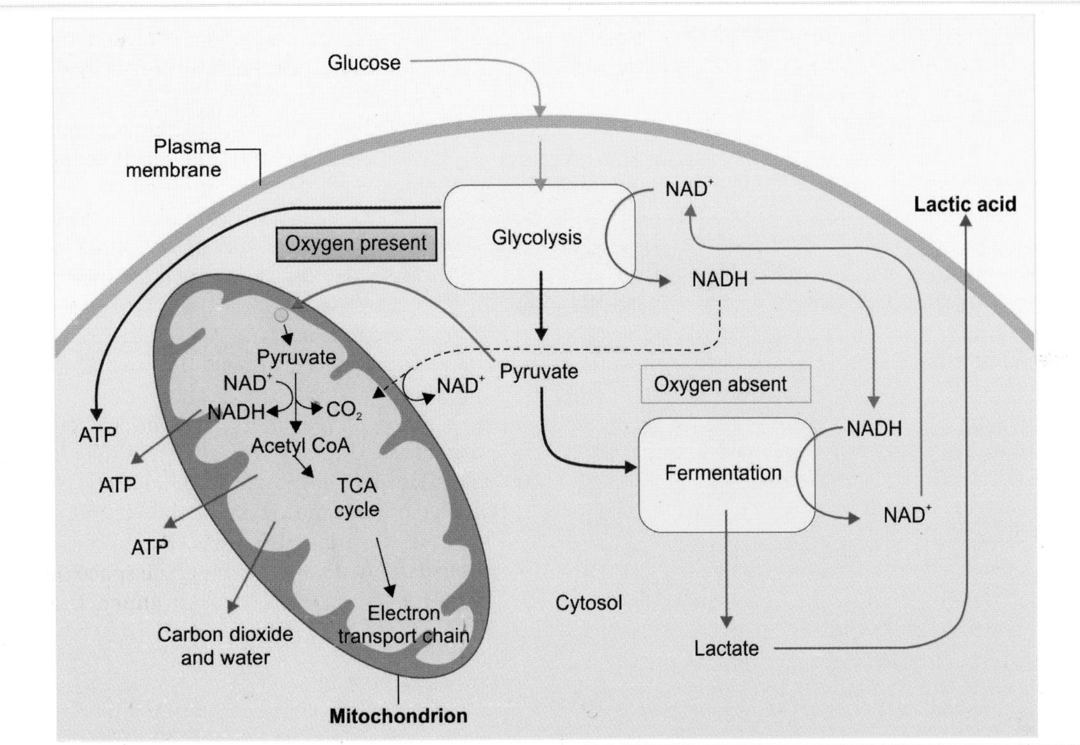

[ATP: adenosine triphosphate; NAD: nicotinamide adenine dinucleotide oxidized form; NADH: nicotinamide adenine dinucleotide reduced form; TCA cycle: tricarboxylic acid cycle, also known as Krebs cycle or citric acid cycle (CAC)]

FIG. 21: Carbohydrate metabolism in cells. The glycolysis produces pyruvate. In the presence of O_2, the pyruvate moves into the matrix (aided by a membrane transporter) and is degraded to carbon dioxide and water. This process forms a large quantity of ATP. In the absence of O_2, the pyruvate reduced NADH to lactate.

two products of glycolysis are pyruvate (pyruvate is the salt of pyruvic acid), and nicotinamide adenine dinucleotide reduced form (NADH). During this process a small amount of ATP is formed. The products of glycolysis (pyruvate and NADH) can be metabolized in two different ways, depending on the type of cell in which they are formed and the presence or absence of oxygen (i.e., aerobic or anaerobic).

- ○ ***Aerobic respiration:*** Under aerobic conditions (in the presence of oxygen), pyruvate is transported from cytosol into mitochondria. Mitochondrial respiration is dependent on a continuous supply of oxygen and is termed as aerobic respiration. In the presence of oxygen, pyruvate is degraded to carbon dioxide and water. Mitochondria utilize an ionic gradient across their inner membrane for the synthesis of ATP. The NADH produced during glycolysis donates its high-energy electrons from the original molecule (e.g., glucose) to molecular oxygen. The energy released during electron transport is used in the formation of ATP. This process gives a large quantity of ATP. The major source of the energy required for all basic cellular functions are derived from oxidative metabolism.
- ○ ***Anaerobic respiration:*** Glycolysis occurring in the absence of oxygen is termed as anaerobic respiration. It occurs in the cytosol and pyruvate is reduced to lactate.

- ***Fatty acids:*** In contrast to glucose, fatty acids pass directly into mitochondria. In the mitochondria, fatty acids are also degraded to carbon dioxide and water. This generates a large amount of ATP.

They are found in large numbers in metabolically active cells (e.g., liver and skeletal muscle). When there is excess availability of fuel, most cells convert glucose and fatty acids into glycogen and triglycerides, respectively, for storage.

Reactive Oxygen Species

The mitochondrion is also an important source of reactive oxygen species (e.g., oxygen free radicals, hydrogen peroxide) produced as a natural (usually low-level) byproduct of substrate oxidation and electron transport. Hypoxia, toxic injury, or even mitochondrial aging can lead to increased levels of intracellular oxidative stress.

Intermediate Metabolism

The abundant generation of high-energy ATP by pure **oxidative phosphorylation** also "burns" glucose to CO_2 and H_2O. This leads to non-availability of carbon moieties needed for synthesis of lipids or proteins.

Warburg effect

Rapidly growing cells (both benign and malignant) need more carbon moieties for synthesis of lipids or proteins. For this reason, rapidly growing cells increase glucose and glutamine uptake but decrease their production of ATP per glucose molecule in the presence of adequate oxygen. They form lactic acid instead of ATP. This will provide more carbon moieties for the synthesis of lipids or protein. In 1924, the biochemist

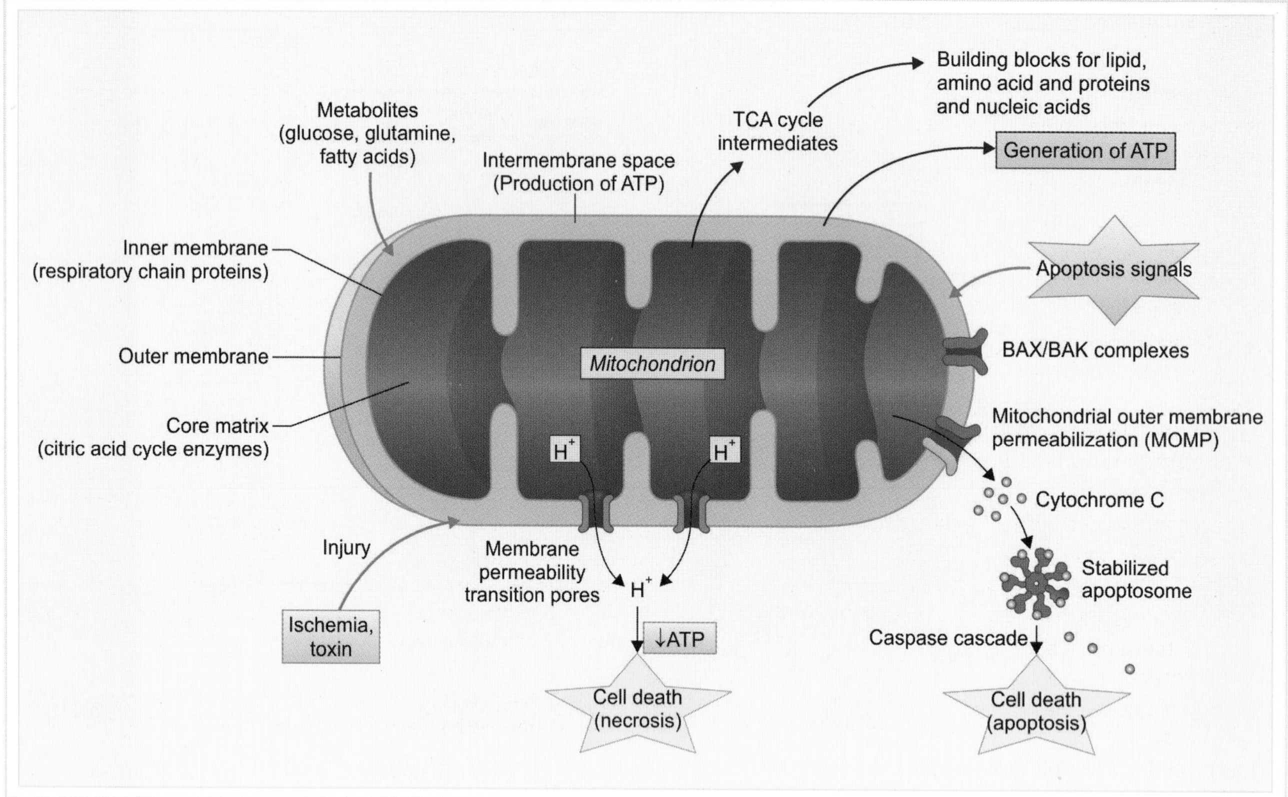

[ATP: adenosine triphosphate; TCA cycle: tricarboxylic acid cycle, also known as Krebs cycle or citric acid cycle (CAC)]

FIG. 22: Various roles of the mitochondria. Apart from the efficient generation of ATP from carbohydrate and fatty acid substrates, mitochondria play an important role in intermediary metabolism and cell death (necrosis and apoptosis).

Otto Warburg and his colleagues discovered that cancer cells take up large amounts of glucose and metabolize it via glycolysis to lactic acid, even in the presence of oxygen (or aerobic glycolysis). This observation was termed the **Warburg effect.** Both glucose and glutamine provide carbon moieties needed for the mitochondrial tricarboxylic acid (TCA) cycle. Instead of generating ATP, intermediates of TCA cycle are used for the synthesis of lipids, nucleic acids, and proteins. Thus, mitochondrial metabolism can be modified depending on the growth state of the cell either to support cellular maintenance or cellular growth. Finally, growth factors, supply of nutrients, and availability of oxygen, as well as cellular signaling pathways and sensors that respond to these exogenous factors, control these metabolic decisions (refer pages 487–491).

Cell Death by Necrosis or Apoptosis

On the one hand, mitochondria are factories which produce energy in the form of ATP which allow the cells to survive; on the other hand, they are involved in causing death (necrosis and apoptosis) of the cells when they are exposed to severe injurious agents. It also regulates the balance of cell survival and death. Mitochondria play central roles in the regulation of "apoptosis".

Mitochondria can be damaged or undergo degenerative changes by genetic disorders or oxygen free radicals. Mitochondria undergo regular renewal and their turnover is rapid. Probably, their half-lives range from 1 to 10 days, depending on the tissue, nutritional status, metabolic demands, and intercurrent injury. During fertilization, the ovum contributes to the majority of cytoplasmic organelles to the fertilized zygote. Hence, mitochondrial DNA is entirely *maternally inherited.* The protein constituents of mitochondria can be derived from both nuclear and mitochondrial genetic transcription. Thus, inheritance of mitochondrial disorders may be X-linked, autosomal, or maternal.

Various roles of the mitochondria are summarized in **Figure 22**.

Salient features of mitochondria are presented in **Box 15.**

TENSINS

Q. Write a short essay on tensins in health and disease.

Introduction

Organs have special designed functions and consist of complex three-dimensional structure composed of cells embedded in ECM (extracellular matrix). During organogenesis, cells migrate to the appropriate location and stay in the location in order to maintain tissue integrity. Following injury, it may be necessary for cells to migrate to damaged areas and then undergo remodeling into the normal structure as part of tissue repair. The processes of organogenesis, organ homeostasis, and repair require controlling of cell adhesion so that it is possible to have cell motility and maintain cell stasis.

Cell adhesion is mainly of two types—(1) intercellular adhesion (i.e., adhesions between cells) or (2) cell-to-matrix adhesion (page 22 and Fig. 13 of Chapter 1).

Box 15: Salient features of mitochondria.

Structure
- Double membrane bound structure
- Parts: Outer and inner membrane, intermembranous space, cristae, and mitochondrial matrix
- Outer membrane
  - Rich in porin
  - Allows small ions and proteins to pass through
  - Connected with endoplasmic reticulum
- Inner membrane
  - Rich in cardiolipin
  - Impermeable to protein, ion, and electrons
  - Rich in ATP synthase, respiratory chain protein complexes (e.g., NADH dehydrogenase complexes, cytochrome b, c1 and cytochrome oxidase) and transport protein complexes
- Mitochondrial matrix
  - Rich in enzymes of citric acid cycle and mitochondrial DNA
- Functions: Power house of the cell. Mainly involved in energy production in the form of ATP synthesis
  - Citric acid cycle: Its main reactions occur in mitochondria
  - Electron transport: It occurs during oxidative phosphorylation
  - Storage of calcium: Play a important role in calcium homeostasis
  - Cell cycle: Signalling platform for progression of cell cycle
  - Apoptosis: Involved in intrinsic pathway of activation of apoptosis and activation of proapoptotic enzymes.

The intercellular adhesion is maintained through intercellular junctions, whereas cell-to-matrix adhesion is maintained mainly through focal adhesions. In both types of adhesions, they represent the points of contact between cells or between the cell and the ECM. The cell adhesion consists of many molecular complexes seen at the cell membrane and are linked internally to the cytoskeleton in the cytosol. In response to environmental factors, these complexes can be either assembled or disassembled. This will allow the cells to become attached or detached from each other and the ECM and thereby regulate the cell motility.

The Structure and Function of Focal Adhesions

These are discussed on page 24. Focal adhesion complexes are large macromolecular complexes which are found at hemidesmosomes. Focal adhesions attach cells to the ECM and important molecules involved are integrins. Integrin molecules are attached to the actin cytoskeleton inside the cytosol. These include proteins that can generate intracellular signals when cells are subjected to increased stress. This attachment is mediated by a network of proteins grouped together on the cytoplasmic side of the focal adhesions. These proteins have mediated a physical connection from the cell interior to exterior, as well as serve a role in signaling and regulating cell adhesion. This network of proteins includes kinases, phosphatases, and adaptor molecules and one of these molecules is called tensin (**Fig. 23**). Other molecules include talin, paxillin, vinculin, focal adhesion kinase (FAK), p130 cas, a-actinin, and zyxin.

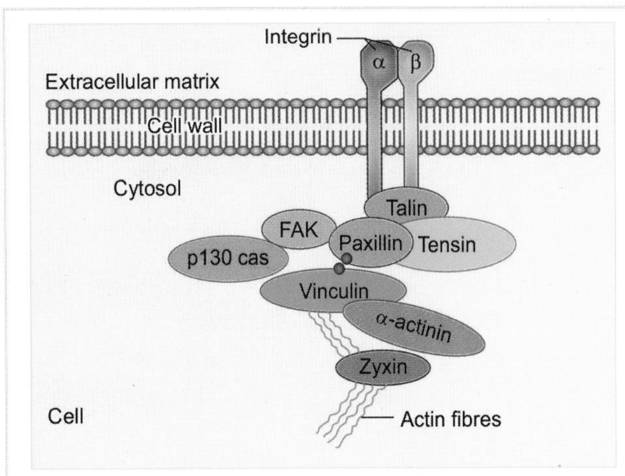

FIG. 23: Diagrammatic representation of typical focal adhesion complexes. It consists of α- and β-heterodimeric integrin molecules externally attached to the extracellular matrix (ECM) and intracellular, cytoplasmic tails connect to a network of proteins and the actin cytoskeleton in the cytosol. It is also associated with a complex of linking molecules (e.g., vinculin and talin).

Table 12: Tensin gene family.

Name of the gene	*Location in the chromosome*	*Sites**
Tensin 1 (*TNS1*, OMIM 600076),	Chromosome 2q 35-36	Tensin 1 is present in most tissues. Tensins 1, 2, 3 are found in highest levels in the human heart, skeletal muscles, kidney, and lung. Tensin 3 is also found in placenta
Tensin 2 (*TENC1*, OMIM 607717),	Chromosome 12q13	
Tensin 3 (*TNS3*, OMIM 606825)	Chromosome 7p12.3	
Tensin 4, commonly called C-terminal Tensin-like, Cten (*TNS4*, OMIM 608385)	Chromosome 17q21.2	Placenta and prostate

*Very low or no expression of tensin is observed in brain, thymus, and circulating leukocytes

Tensin Proteins

Tensin proteins are located at the specialized regions of plasma membrane called focal adhesions. The focal adhesions are formed around a transmembrane core of an αβ integrin heterodimer. Tensins are one of the molecules involved in molecular bridges between integrins and the actin cytoskeleton. The Tensin family members play crucial roles in main cellular processes including adhesion, migration, proliferation, differentiation, and apoptosis.

Tensin Gene Family

The Tensin gene family consists of four members. The four genes and their location in the chromosomes are presented in **Table 12**.

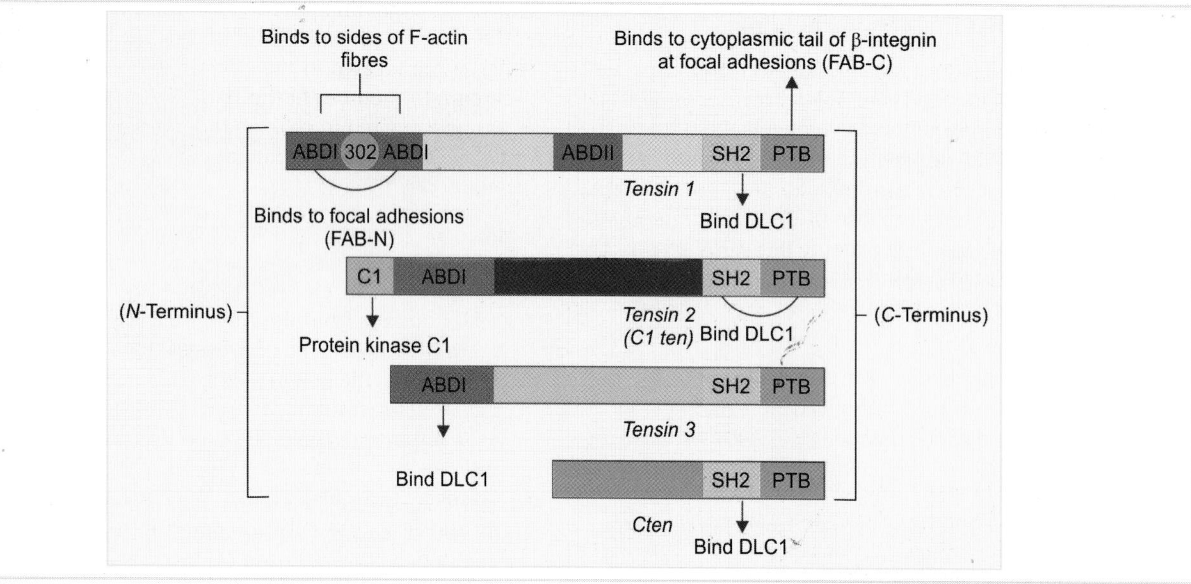

(C-terminus: carboxy terminus; DLC1: deleted in liver cancer 1; N-terminus: amino terminus; PTB: phosphotyrosine-binding domain; SH2: Src-homology 2)

FIG. 24: Diagrammatic representation of the structure of Tensin family protein. Tensins 1, 2 and 3 have both domains for binding to cytoskeletal proteins (ABD) and signal transduction components (SH2). Cten does not have the N-terminal.

Structure of Tensin Proteins (Fig. 24)

Tensin is a multidomain protein and can bind to several structural and signaling molecules. Tensins 1, 2 and 3 have highly homologous N- and C-terminal ends but structure of central regions are different. In general, the N-terminus consists of actin-binding domains (ABD), where as the C-terminus contains an Src-homolgy 2 (SH2) domain and a phosphotyrosine-binding domain (PTB) (**Fig. 24**). Thus tensins have both domains for binding to cytoskeletal proteins (ABD) and signal transduction components (SH2).

Tensin 1

- It contains SH2 and ABD regions similar to the tumor suppressor phosphatase and Tensin homolog (PTEN).
- Tensin 1 has **two actin-binding sites** in the ABDs and one in the central region.
- **Phosphotyrosine-binding (PTB) domains** are known for binding phosphorylated tyrosines. Through this PTB domain, Tensin 1 (and the other Tensins) **binds to the cytoplasmic tail of β-integrins** independently of phosphorylation.
- The **SH2 domain** at the C terminus can **bind to phosphorylated tyrosine residues on proteins** [e.g., FAK, deleted in liver cancer (DLC) 1 and phosphoinositide 3 (PI3) kinase]. Tensin 1 also contains phosphorylated tyrosine residues and can link an SH2 containing cytoskeletal protein with signal transduction to the actin cytoskeleton.
- At both the N- and C-termini, there are **focal adhesion-binding** (FAB) **domains** which are needed for localization to focal adhesions.

Tensin 2

- The structure of Tensin 2 is similar to that of Tensin 1. The central region of Tensin 2 is rich in proline and can **act as a binding site for proteins containing Src homology 3** (SH3) or WW domains.
- It is the **only tensin having protein kinase C domain** at the N-terminus.

Tensin 3

- The structure of Tensin 3 is similar to that of Tensin 1.
- Contains tyrosine residues and are potential sites of phosphorylation and can bring out signal transduction.

Cten

- C-terminus of tensin (Tensin 4, commonly called C-terminal Tensin-like, Cten) shows a high degree of homology. Hence, included in the Tensin family of proteins. However, it does not have the N-terminus ABD domains of Tensins 1, 2 and 3.
- Cten still contains the signaling component of other Tensins but does not have the actin binding capability. They may play a unique role in cellular processes.
- It is also localized to focal adhesion region of cytosol similar to other Tensins, it is also found in the nucleus.

The Tensins are linked to multiple upstream and downstream signaling factors and interact differentially with such components to bring out their response.

Functional Activity of Tensins

Cell Adhesion and Motility

Tensins are important for stabilizing cell adhesion and regulating cell motility. Recruitment of Tensins to the focal adhesions depends on the state of maturation of the focal adhesions.

- Tensin 2 is recruited to focal complexes during early stage focal adhesions.
- In contrast, Tensin 1 and Tensin 3 are found in the mature form of focal adhesions known as "fibrillar adhesions".
- In contrast to other Tensins 1 and 3, Cten stimulates cell motility and this is performed through two mechanisms:
  1. Following activation of epidermal growth factor receptor (EGFR) signaling, Tensin 3 levels decrease while cellular Cten levels simultaneously increase (without affecting the other Tensin proteins). The raised levels of Cten displace Tensin 3 from the focal adhesions. This process is called as the "**Tensin Switch**". Since

Cten does not have the N-terminus ABD, it cannot bind the actin stress fibres. This causes detachment of focal adhesions from the actin cytoskeleton. This gives rise to actin remodeling and cytoskeletal rearrangements and allow for migration of cell.

2. Secondly, SH2 domain of **Cten** can bind to DLC1 and replace Tensin 3 to **form a complex with DLC1**. This results in an inhibition of DLC1 which no longer promotes Rho family guanosine triphosphatase (GTP)-activating protein (Rho-GAP activity). This in turn leads to increased RhoA-GTP-mediated signal transduction via ROCK and subsequent motility (**Figs. 25A** and **B**).

Other Functional Activity

Tensin proteins can activate and are targets of other signaling molecules.

- Focal adhesion kinase forms complex with Tensin 1 and vinculin and mediate signal transduction.
- Growth hormone stimulation can cause FAK-mediated tyrosine phosphorylation of Tensin 1.
- Forced expression of Cten in epithelial cell lines can upregulate and stabilize both FAK and integrin-linked kinase (ILK). This may be associated with induction of cell motility. This may be involved in epithelial–mesenchymal transition. These can downregulate E-cadherin. It is noted that there is a possible crosstalk between adherens junctions and focal adhesions.

Cell Survival and Apoptosis

Cell survival: Tensins are involved in signaling pathways, many of which involve the regulation of multiple biological processes including cell adhesion and survival. For example, the PI3 kinase/Akt signaling pathways support cell survival through activation of phosphatidylinositol-(3,4,5)-trisphosphate (PIP3). Cten located in the nucleus can form a complex with β-catenin (a member of the Wnt signaling pathway). Forced expression of Cten in colonic and pancreatic cancer cell lines has been found to stimulate anchorage-independent colony formation.

Apoptosis: Tensins can be targeted by caspases during apoptosis.

- **Caspase 3 can cleave Tensin 1** and separate the SH2/PTB domains from the ABD. The loss of the SH2 domain results in loss of a PI3 kinase-mediated cell survival signal. Also, the integrins become detached from the actin cytoskeleton resulting in disruption of focal adhesions. This is an important step in the cellular change characteristic of apoptosis.
- Caspase 3 can **also cleave Cten** and release a fragment, containing only the phosphotyrosine-binding (PTB) domain. This detached fragment can induce apoptosis by competing for binding sites in the cytoplasmic tails of β-integrin and disrupting the links between integrins and actin fibres.

Regulation of Tensin Proteins

The upstream pathways regulating Tensin protein expression are completely known. There are two main pathways that may be involved, namely—(i) the EGFR signaling pathway and (ii) the signal transducer and activator of transcription 3 (Stat3) signaling pathway.

- **EGFR signaling pathway:** Activation of EGFR signaling through EGF stimulation or c-ErbB2 activity leads to the

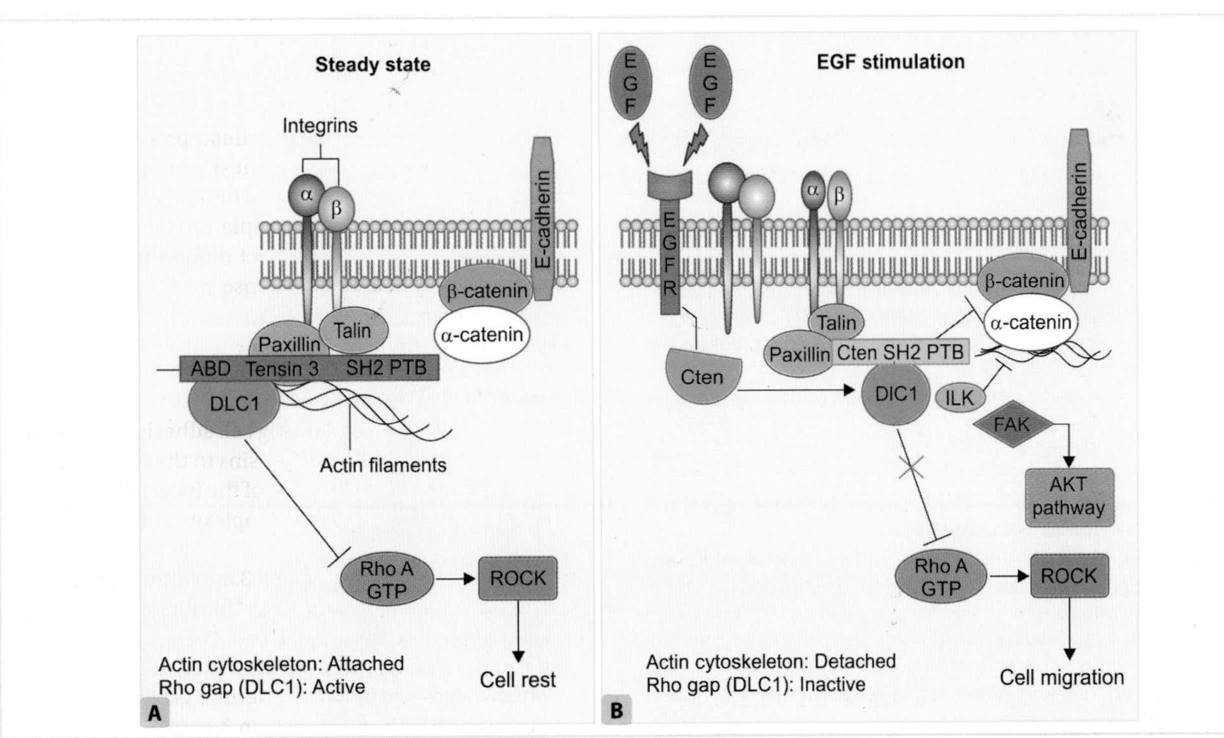

(DLC1: deleted in liver cancer 1; FAK: focal adhesion kinase; GTP: guanosine triphosphate; ILK: integrin-linked kinase; ROCK: Rho-associated protein kinase; SH2: Src-homology 2)

FIGS. 25A AND B: Diagrammatic representation of the structure of Tensin family protein. Tensins 1, 2 and 3 have both domains for binding to cytoskeletal proteins (ABD) and signal transduction components (SH2). Cten does not have the N-terminal.

Tensin switch (refer page 36). This is characterized by a decrease in levels of Tensin 3 and an increase in Cten (**Fig. 25B**). However, the other Tensins remain unaffected. The signaling pathway probably involves the *KRAS/BRAF/* mitogen activated protein kinase (MAPK) pathway.
- **Stat3 signaling:** This pathway may be involved in regulating expression of Cten. Stat3-dependent overexpression of Cten can disrupt cell adhesion and induce motility. This disruption of cell adhesion and motility can be abolished by inhibition of Cten.

Apart from the EGFR and Stat3 signaling, other factors may also regulate the Tensin proteins. These include the ECM, platelet-derived growth factor, thrombin, angiotensin, *Bcr/Abl*, etc.

Role of Tensins in Carcinogenesis

Tensins are concerned with cell motility. Hence, they can be involved in carcinogenesis, particularly the promotion of metastasis. Role of Tensins in carcinogenesis is complex.
- Investigations on Tensin 3 and Cten reveal that Tensins are involved in disease progression. Tensin 1 was found to be downregulated in tumors of the prostate, breast, kidney, and skin. Tensin 2 has been reported to be downregulated in cancers of the kidney and lung. This suggests that they may have tumor suppressor activity.
- In contrast, in hepatocellular carcinoma, Tensin 2 was found to be overexpressed in 46% of tumors in comparison to normal liver tissue.
- Tensins 1, 2, and 3 generally have a tumor suppressive activity. Reduced expression of these Tensins has been observed in tumors of the thyroid, kidney, and breast. In contrast, other studies in breast, melanoma, and non-small cell lung carcinoma indicate that they have oncogenic effect.
- Cten is not normally present in most tissues and raised levels have been observed in tumors of the lung, thymus, colon, breast, and pancreas, suggesting that it has an oncogene role. It was also found that greater levels of expression are associated with advanced disease stage and metastasis.
- Breast carcinoma: Cten expression has been shown to stimulate cell motility. Immunohistochemical analysis found no correlation between Cten expression and tumor size. However, there was a significant association with HER2/ErbB2 positive tumors, reduction in estrogen receptor expression, lymph node metastasis, tumor size, grade, and poor Nottingham prognostic index. Patients with high tumor expression of Cten had a poorer prognosis than those with low level of expression and also had increased risk of developing metastasis.
- Colorectal cancer: Cten expression was found to correlate with advanced stage, poor prognosis, and distant metastasis. Studies support an oncogenic role of Cten in colorectal tumors.
- Target for therapy: Though there are conflicting reports regarding the role of Tensins in carcinogenesis, they are still considered to have potential as targets for therapeutic agents.
  - Tensin 1 induction is associated with anticancer properties in epithelioid cancers and leukemia cells.
  - Tensin 2 has been considered as a novel therapeutic target in myleproliferative disorders.
  - Cten being under the regulation of the EGFR signaling pathway, it may be a molecular target in those colorectal tumors resistant to anti-EGFR therapies due to downstream BRAF and KRAS mutations.

Conclusion

Tensins are important in regulating cell adhesion and cell migration and they are regulators of cell migration. They bind to the actin cytoskeleton and mediate signal transduction events at focal adhesion regions. Since they play a role in regulation of cell migration, they may be involved in cancer metastasis. Cten is generally a marker of poor prognosis and may be involved in the development of metastasis. The targeting of the cell migratory machinery by using the Tensin family of genes may be used as therapeutic target for anticancer therapies.

BIBLIOGRAPHY

1. Andersson ER. The role of endocytosis in activating and regulating signal transduction. *Cell Mol Life Sci*. 2011;69:1755.
2. Andersen JL, Kornbluth S. The tangled circuitry of metabolism and apoptosis. *Mol Cell*. 2013;49:399.
3. Banasik JL, Copstead LC. Pathophysiology,6th edition. Philadelphia: Saunders Elsevier; 2019.
4. Burke PJ. Mitochondria, bioenergetics and apoptosis in cancer. *Trends Cancer*. 2017;3:857.
5. Choi AM, Ryter SW, Levine B. Autophagy in human health and disease. *N Engl J Med*. 2013;368:651.
6. English AR, Zurek N, Voeltz GK. Peripheral ER structure and function. *Curr Opin Cell Biol*. 2009;21:596.
7. Exosomal biomarkers for cancer diagnosis and patient monitoring https://www.tandfonline.com/doi/abs/10.1080/14737159.2020. [Last accessed on 2021 January 14].
8. Friedman JR, Nunnari J. Mitochondrial form and function. *Nature*. 2014;505:335.
9. Guillot C, Lecuit T. Mechanics of epithelial tissue homeostasis and morphogenesis. *Science*. 2013;340:1185.
10. Hetz C, Chevet E, Oakes SA: Proteostasis control by the unfolded protein response. *Nat Cell Biol*. 2015;17:829.
11. Johnson DS. Establishing and transducing cell polarity: common themes and variations. *Curr Opin Cell Biol*. 2017;51:33.
12. Kaur J, Debnath J. Autophagy at the crossroads of catabolism and anabolism. *Nat Rev Mol Cell Biol*. 2015;16:461.
13. Kumar V, Abbas AK, Aster JC. Robbins basic pathology, 10th edition. Philadelphia: Saunders Elsevier; 2018.
14. Kumar V, Abbas AK, Fausto N, et al. Robbins and Cotran pathologic basis of disease, 10th edition. Philadelphia: WB Saunders; 2021.
15. Pignatelli M, Gallagher P. Recent Advances in Histopathology- 23. New Delhi: JP Medical; 2014.
16. Simons K, Sampaio JL. Membrane organization and lipid rafts. *Cold Spring Harb Perspect Biol*. 2013;3:1.
17. Strayer DS, Saffitz JE. Rubin's Pathology: Mechanism of Human Disease, 8th edition. Philadelphia: Wolters Kluwer; 2020.
18. Tait SW, Green DR. Mitochondria and cell death: outer membrane permeabilization and beyond. *Nat Rev Mol Cell Biol*. 2010;11:621.
19. Wong E, Cuervo AM. Integration of clearance mechanisms: the proteasome and autophagy. *Cold Spring Harb Perspect Biol*. 2010;2:1.
20. Xie L, Zeng X, Hu J, Chen Q. Characterization of nestin, a selective marker for bone marrow derived mesenchymal stem cells. *Stem Cells Int*. 2015.

CHAPTER 2

Cellular Activation

CHAPTER OUTLINE

The English poet John Donne expressed his belief in the interdependence of humans and phrased that—"**No man is an island**". The same can be said of the cells that—"**No cell lives in isolation".** Cells are specialized to carry out one or more specific functions. Many biological processes need various cells to work together and to coordinate their activities. For this, cells should communicate with each other. Cell communication is an important aspect of any tissue, and heart of all these communication systems are regulatory proteins that produce signals, which are sent from one place to another in the body or within a cell. The signals are processed to provide clear and effective communication. This cell communication is brought out by a process called **cell signaling**. The molecules which initiates this communication are called *signal molecules.* Communication between cells is mediated mainly by extracellular signal molecules. Cell signaling makes the cells to respond in an appropriate manner to a specific environmental stimulus. Cell signaling affects almost every aspect of cell structure and function. Cell signaling is also involved in the regulation of cell growth, division, and differentiation during development, as well as their behavior in adult tissues. Loss of cellular communication and the controls that maintain normal relationships of cells can lead to unregulated growth (cancer) or an ineffective response to an extrinsic stress (as in shock). If the cell signaling involved in cell division loses control, it can produce a malignant tumor.

CELL SIGNALING

Cell signaling is a vital and integral part of modern cell biology. It controls the inner workings of cells and allows them to respond, adapt and survive. Each cell is constantly exposed to various types of signals. These signals must be "interpreted" and integrated into responses so that they benefit the organism as a whole.

Main events for cell signaling mechanisms: (1) Arrival of signaling molecule at the cell, (2) perception of the signal, usually by dedicated proteins referred to as receptors, (3) transmission of the signal by the receptor into the cell, (4) passing on of the "message" to a series of cell signaling components, often referred to as a cell signaling cascade, and (5) carrying the "message" to its final destination, perhaps the cytoplasm or the nucleus.

Source of Signals

The sources of the signals can be classified as:

- **Extracellular signals:** They determine whether a cell lives or dies, whether it remains quiescent, or whether it is stimulated to perform a specific function.
  - **Pathogens and damage to neighboring cells:** Many cells have the capacity to sense and respond to damaged cells (*danger signals*) and foreign invaders such as microbes (refer pages 221–224).

- **Cell-cell contacts:** These are mediated through adhesion molecules and/or gap junctions. Gap junction signaling between adjacent cells is through hydrophilic connecting channels. These junctions allow the movement of small ions (e.g., calcium), metabolites, and second messenger molecules (e.g., cAMP) through them (refer pages 22 to 25 of Chapter 1).
- **Cell-extracellular matrix (ECM) contacts:** These are mediated through integrins (refer page 24 and pages 233 and 234).
- **Secreted molecules:** The most important secreted molecules include *growth factors* (refer Table 2), *cytokines* (pages 291–304), and *hormones* (which are secreted by endocrine organs and they act on different cell types away from the cell).

- **Intercellular signals:** They are important in the developing embryo, to maintain tissue organization, and to ensure that tissues respond in an adaptive and effective fashion to various threats (e.g., local tissue trauma or a systemic infection).

Types of Signaling Molecules

There are several varieties or kinds of extracellular signal molecules. These include:

- **Amino acids and amino acid derivatives: Example, glutamate, glycine, acetylcholine, epinephrine, dopamine, and thyroid hormone**. These molecules act as neurotransmitters and hormones.
- Dissolved gases, e.g., NO and CO
- Retinoids
- **Steroids derived from cholesterol:** Steroid hormones regulate sexual differentiation, pregnancy, carbohydrate metabolism, and excretion of sodium and potassium ions.
- **Eicosanoids:** They are derived from a fatty acid named arachidonic acid. Eicosanoids regulate a variety of processes such as pain, inflammation, blood pressure, and blood clotting.
- **Variety of small polypeptides and proteins:** Some of these are present as transmembrane proteins on the surface and others are part of, or associate with, the ECM. Finally, a large number of proteins are excreted into the extracellular environment where they are involved in regulating processes such as cell division, differentiation, the immune response, or cell death and cell survival.
- Nucleotides

Most of these signal molecules are released into the extracellular space by exocytosis from the signaling cell. Signals may cause differentiation of cells, stimulate proliferation, or may direct the cell to perform a specialized function. Many cells need certain signals to survive and in the absence of these exogenous signals, cells may die by apoptosis. The signal molecules may be mainly divided into two types (**Fig. 1**) namely: (i) Hydrophobic (bind directly to receptors on cytosol) or (ii) hydrophilic (binds to receptor on extracellular surface).

- **Hydrophobic signaling molecules:** These molecules spontaneously diffuse through the plasma membrane and bind to target receptors present in the cytosol **Figure 1**. In most of the cases, the receptor-hormone complex moves into the nucleus and binds to specific regulatory sequences in deoxyribonucleic acid (DNA). Then, it either activates or represses expression of specific target genes.

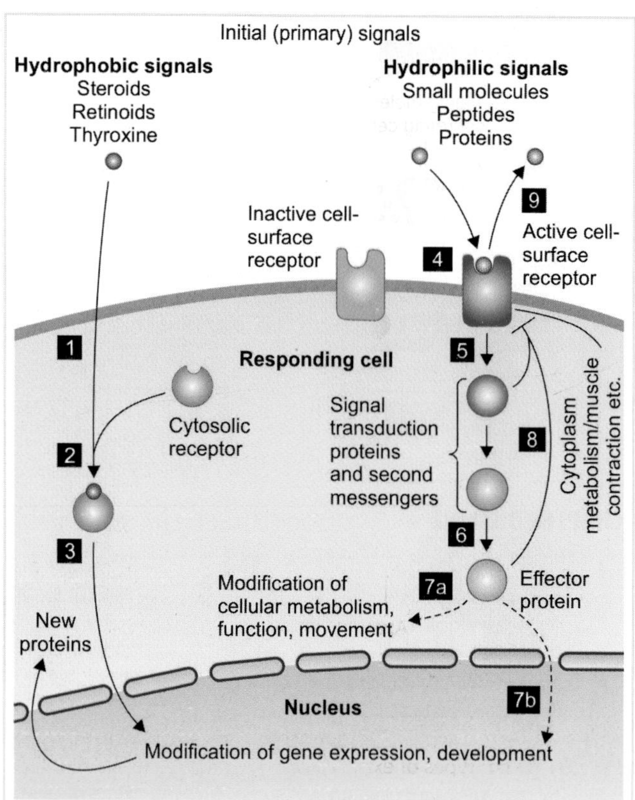

FIG. 1: Overview of cell signaling. Hydrophobic signaling molecules diffuse through the plasma membrane (Step 1) and bind to receptors in the cytosol (Step 2). The receptor–signal complex then moves into the nucleus (Step 3) and binds to transcription-control regions in deoxyribonucleic acid (DNA). This may activate or repress gene expression. The hydrophilic molecules cannot diffuse across the cell membrane. They bind to specific cell-surface receptor proteins and trigger a conformational change in the receptor, thus activate it (Step 4). The activated receptor in turn activates one or more downstream signal transduction proteins or small-molecule second messengers (Step 5). This activates one or more effector proteins (Step 6). The end result of a signaling cascade varies depending on the signal.

Examples for hydrophobic signals include steroids, retinoids, and thyroxine.

- **Hydrophilic signaling molecules:** They **constitute majority of signaling molecules**. These signaling molecules are too large and too hydrophilic to diffuse through the plasma membrane. These signaling molecules bind to **cell-surface receptors** that are integral membrane proteins embedded in the plasma membrane. Examples include small molecules (adrenaline, acetylcholine), peptides (glucagon), and proteins (insulin, growth hormone).

Downstream and upstream: Often in signaling pathways terms such as downstream and upstream are used. Downstream means later on in the pathway, whereas upstream means coming before. Such terms are also used in genetics.

Types of Signaling (Fig. 2)

Cells usually communicate with each other through **messenger molecules or signals**. Signaling pathways can be classified into

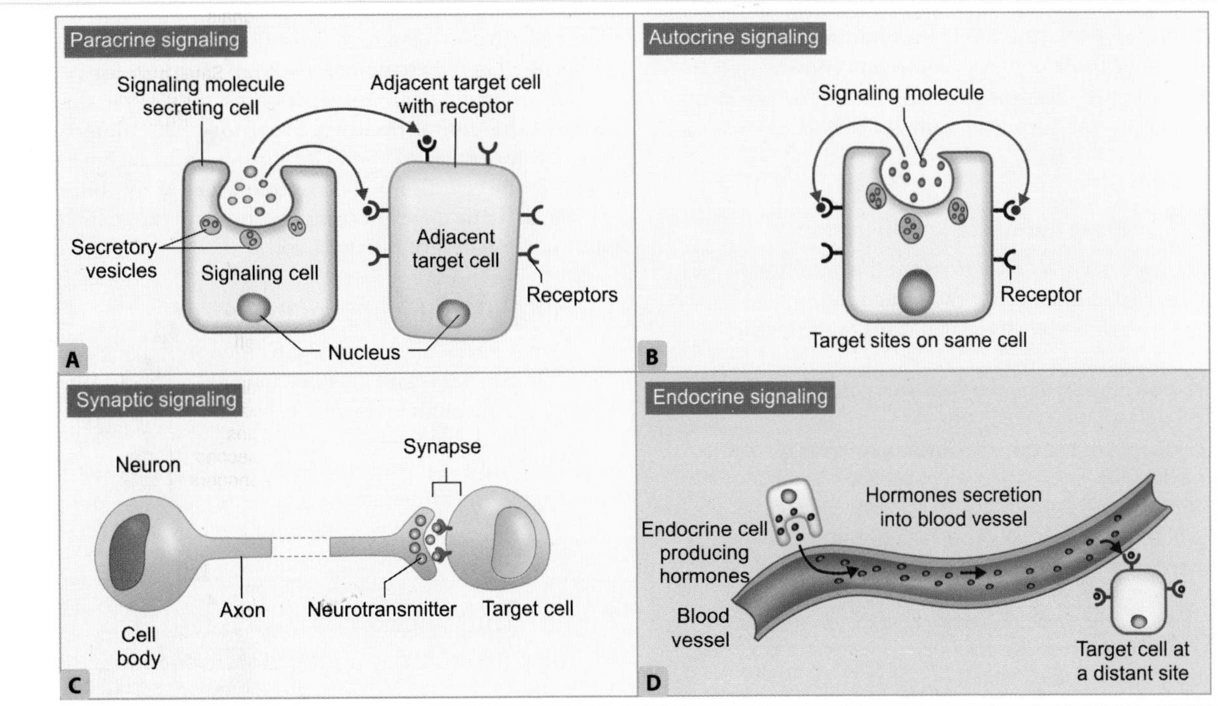

FIGS. 2A TO D: Types of extracellular signaling (A) Paracrine (B) Autocrine (C) Synaptic and (D) Endocrine signaling.

different types based on the relationships between the cells which send signals and those which receive it. Depending on the source of the ligand and the location of its corresponding receptors (i.e., in the same, adjacent, or distant cells), the modes of signaling can be divided four types.

1. **Paracrine signaling:** In this, signaling molecule or secrete factor is produced by one cell type (signaling cell) and signals travel or diffuse a short distance. It acts on the appropriate receptors present on the adjacent target cells or cells that are in close proximity (or immediate vicinity) of the cell from which the message molecule originated. The target cell activated by signal is usually of a different type. For example, in healing by repair, growth factor produced by macrophage (one cell type) has growth effect on fibroblast (adjacent target cells of different type). After the signaling, the secreted signal is rapidly degraded, taken up by other cells, or trapped in the ECM.
2. **Autocrine signaling:** In this type, the cell that is secreting or producing a signal molecule itself expresses receptors on its surface that can respond to signal. Consequently, cells releasing the signals will stimulate (or inhibit) the cells which secretes them. Thus both signaling cell and responding cell is same. Examples for autocrine signaling includes liver regeneration, proliferation of antigen-stimulated lymphocytes, and tumors. Autocrine signaling can be a means to adjust groups of cells undergoing synchronous differentiation during development. It can be used to amplify (positive feedback) or dampen (negative feedback) to a particular response.
3. **Synaptic signaling:** This type of signaling is performed by neurons that transmit signals electrically along their axons and release neurotransmitters at specialized cell junctions (synapses), which are often located far away from the neuronal cell body. Thus, activated neurons secrete neurotransmitters at specialized cell junctions (i.e., synapses) onto target cells. Synaptic signaling only occurs between cells with the synapse, between a neuron and the muscle and it is controlled by neural activity. Example acetylcholine is a neuromuscular transmitter produced at the nerve endings that cats on acetylcholine (ACh) receptor on skeletal muscle cells.
4. **Endocrine signaling:** In this type, signals are usually carried by the blood and travel throughout the body and act on target cells that are typically located far away (at a distant) from the source (signaling cell) or site of its synthesis in the body. Endocrine messengers are produced by cells of endocrine organs and are called hormones.

   For example, a insulin is and hormone released into the blood circulation from β cells of the islets of Langerhan in the pancreas and acts on many target cells at a distance. Thyroid-stimulating hormone secreted by pituitary (endocrine) gland acts on (TSH) receptor and activate thyroid (another endocrine gland) cells to produce thyroid hormones.

OVERVIEW OF CELLULAR SIGNALING

Various steps in normal cell proliferation are presented in **Box 1**.

Signal Molecules

Cells receive and transmit hundreds of different signaling molecules collectively called the growth factor signals. Cell signaling is initiated with the release of a signaling or messenger molecule called growth factors and these are termed *ligands* (ions or neutral molecules) produced by a signaling cell. It has to be received by the target/responding cell. **The signal irrespective of their** nature or **source is transmitted to the cell via a specific *receptor* protein.** The signal can produce an effect or specific response, only if target cells express (or have) a receptor. This should be a complimentary **receptor** that specifically recognizes and binds that particular signal molecule. **Ligands usually have high affinities for receptors** and at physiological concentrations they have **specificity to bind the complimentary receptors.** The molecules can be soluble, bound to the ECM, or bound to the surface of a neighboring cell. They may be **stimulatory or inhibitory.** They can act in many different combinations and they can influence almost any aspect of cell behavior.

Box 1: Steps in normal cell proliferation.

- **Binding of a growth factor to its specific receptor** on the plasma/cell membrane
- Transient and limited **activation of the growth factor receptor**
- **Activation** of many **signal transducing proteins** on the inner leaflet of the plasma membrane
- **Transmission of the transduced signal across the cytosol to the nucleus.** This is achieved by second messengers or a cascade of signal transduction molecules
- Induction and **activation of nuclear regulatory (transcription) factors.** They initiate and regulate deoxyribonucleic acid (DNA) transcription. There will be synthesis of other cellular components that are required for cell division. These include organelles, membrane components, and ribosomes
- **Entry and progression** of the cell **into the cell cycle.** This ultimately leads to division of cell

Binding of Molecules to Receptor

The signal binds the receptor and then initiates a cascade of intracellular events and produce the necessary response in the target cell. The binding site of the receptor recognizes the signal molecule with high specificity. This ensures that the receptor responds only to the appropriate signal and not to the many other signaling molecules surrounding the cell. Many signal molecules act at very low concentrations. Types of recptors are discussed on page 43–51.

Signal Transduction Pathways (Fig. 3)

Q. Write a short essay on signal transduction pathways.

The binding or interaction activates the receptor. This causes relay of signal across the plasma membrane (in case of

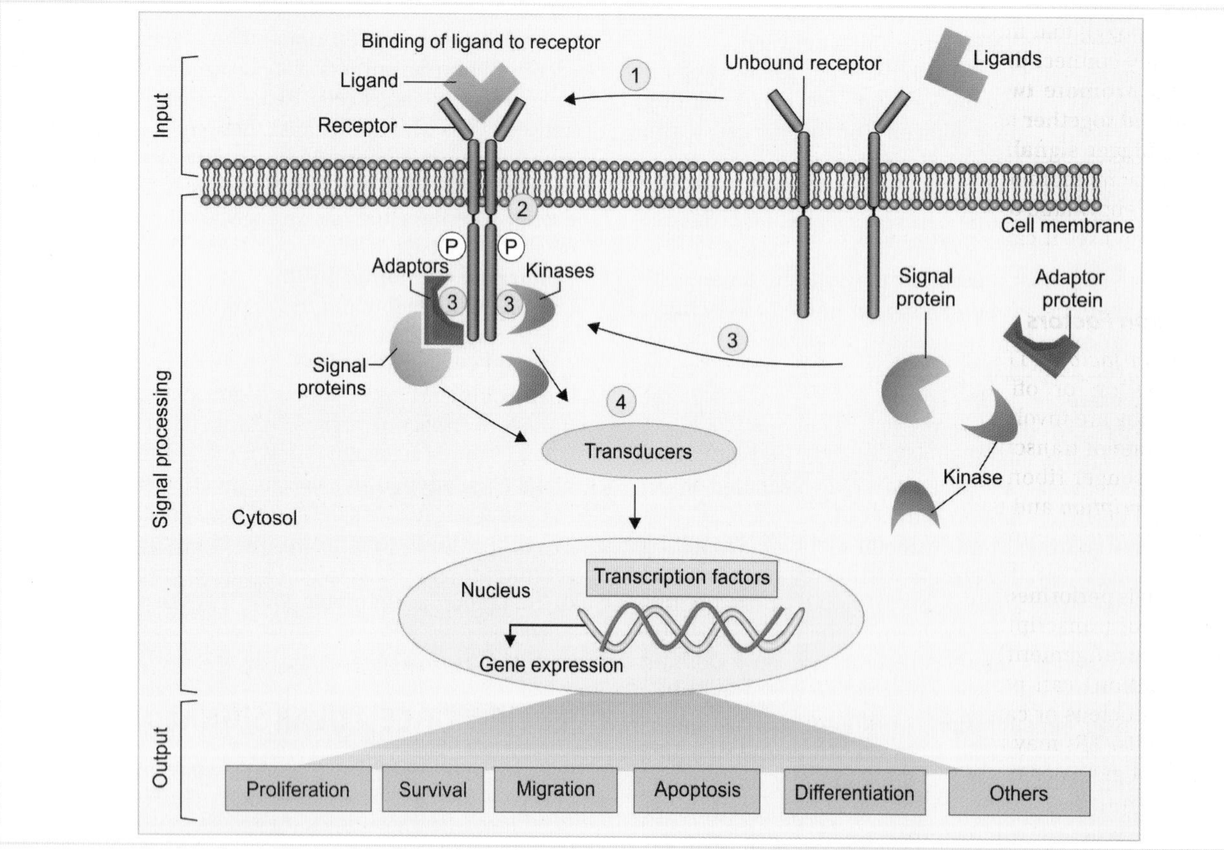

FIG. 3: Features of growth factor signal transduction. The basic process involved in growth factor signaling pathway: (1) Binding of growth factor; (2) Ligand-induced receptor dimerization, activation of intrinsic kinase activity, and autophosphorylation at specific tyrosine residues or serine/threonine residues [in transforming growth factor-beta (TGF-β)]; (3) The phosphorylated receptors act as docking sites for adaptor proteins or directly bind to a wide range of molecules; (4) Activate downstream signaling pathways that regulate a variety of cellular processes. Most of these signaling pathways, the signals from the membrane pass through the cytoplasm into the nucleus [except for interleukin (IL)-6 which via signal transducing adaptor proteins (STAPs) transmit signals directly from the membrane to the nucleus].

receptor on surface of cell) to the receptor's cytoplasmic domain. Once the signal has reached the inner surface of the plasma membrane, it is transmitted into the cell interior. This in turn activates one or more *intracellular signaling pathways* or *systems*. These systems depend on *intracellular signaling proteins*, which process the signal inside the receiving cell and deliver it to the concerned intracellular targets. The **overall process of converting or translating information carried by extracellular signals into intracellular responses**/changes inside a cell, as well as the individual steps in this process, is called **signal transduction.** The chain of intermediates is termed a **signal transduction pathway** because it transduces, or converts, information from one form into another as a signal is relayed from a receptor to its targets. Some signal transduction pathways may have two or three intermediates, others can involve more than a dozen. The targets at the end of signaling pathways are called *effector proteins*, which are altered in some way by the incoming signal and elicit the appropriate response/change in cell behavior. The signals transduced by cell surface receptors are often deranged in developmental disorders and in cancers.

Adaptor Proteins

Signal transducing adaptor proteins (STAPs) are essential *protein* molecules that are accessory to main **proteins** in a signal transduction pathway. They play a key role in organizing intracellular signaling pathways. These proteins may contain a few specific domains [e.g., SH2 or SH3 (SH=Src family kinases homology)] that mediate protein-protein interactions that physically connect different enzymes. They **function as linkers** that **promote two or more signaling proteins to become joined together as part of a signaling complex and generate a bigger signaling complex.** The adaptors can be integral cellular membrane proteins or cytosolic proteins. They lack intrinsic enzymatic activity. By recruiting the protein to signaling complexes it can determine downstream signaling events.

Transcription Factors

Transcription factors (TFs) are proteins that help to turn specific genes "on" or "off" by binding to nearby specific DNA sequence. They are involved in the process of converting, or controlling rate of transcription of genetic information from DNA to messenger ribonucleic acid (RNA). This process is termed t*ranscription* and is the first step of gene expression. Most signal transduction pathways ultimately influence cellular function by modulating gene transcription. The gene transcription is performed through the activation and nuclear localization of transcription factors (TFs). Conformational (structural arrangement) changes of TFs (e.g., following phosphorylation) can permit translocation/movement of TF into the nucleus or can expose specific DNA or protein-binding motifs. TFs may result in the expression of either a limited set of genes or may produce widespread effects on gene expression. The most important TFs that regulate the expression of gene needed for growth are *MYC* and *JUN*, and a TF that leads to growth arrest is triggered by the expression of genes is TP53. TFs have a modular design, they usually have domains that bind DNA and others that interact with other proteins (e.g., components of the RNA polymerase complex) required for transcription.

- **Deoxyribonucleic acid (DNA)-binding domains:** They allow the specific binding of transcription factore (TFs) to short DNA sequences. Some TFs **may bind to binding sites in the promoter region of the gene,** close to the site where transcription starts. However, **most TFs bind widely throughout genomes** which include long-range regulatory elements such as enhancers. Enhancers are spatially located close to the genes they regulate and act by looping back to gene promoters. These enhancers may appear to be far away in terms of genomic sequence. Thus, chromatin organization appears to be important in regulating gene expression in both normal physiological and pathological situations.
- **Interaction with other proteins:** To induce transcription, a transcription factor (TF) must also have protein-protein interaction domains. This will directly or indirectly recruit histone-modifying enzymes, chromatin-remodeling complexes, and most importantly, RNA polymerase—the large multiprotein enzymatic complex that is required for RNA synthesis.

Termination of Signaling

Finally, signaling has to be terminated. This is important because cells have to be responsive to additional messages that they may receive. First process in termination is to eliminate the extracellular messenger molecule.

- **Producing extracellular enzymes:** Certain cells perform this by producing extracellular enzymes that destroy specific extracellular messengers.
- **Internalization of activated receptors:** In other cases, activated receptors are internalized. Once inside the cell, the receptor may be degraded together with its ligand. This can decrease the sensitivity of cell to subsequent stimuli.
- **Within endosomes:** The receptor and ligand may be separated within an endosome. Then the ligand is degraded and the receptor is returned to the cell surface mainly into five classes (see **Fig. 4**):
    i. G protein-coupled (GPCRs).
    ii. Ion channel linked.
    iii. Containing intrinsic enzymatic activity.
    iv. Tyrosine kinase linked.
    v. Intracellular.

SIGNALING RECEPTORS

Receptors are proteins (usually present on cell surface), which bind to ligands (signaling molecules known as first messengers) and cause responses.

Types of Signaling Receptors (Fig. 4 and Box 2)

Cellular receptors are grouped into different types depending on the signaling mechanisms and their activation of intra-cellular biochemical pathways. Receptors may be present on the surface of a cell (cell-surface or transmembrane) or present within the cell (intracellular or cytosol) in the cytoplasm or nucleus (**Fig. 4**).

Intracellular Receptors (Refer 4 of Fig. 4)

Receptors on cytosol: These receptor proteins are inside the target cell (either cytoplasm or nucleus). The signal molecule

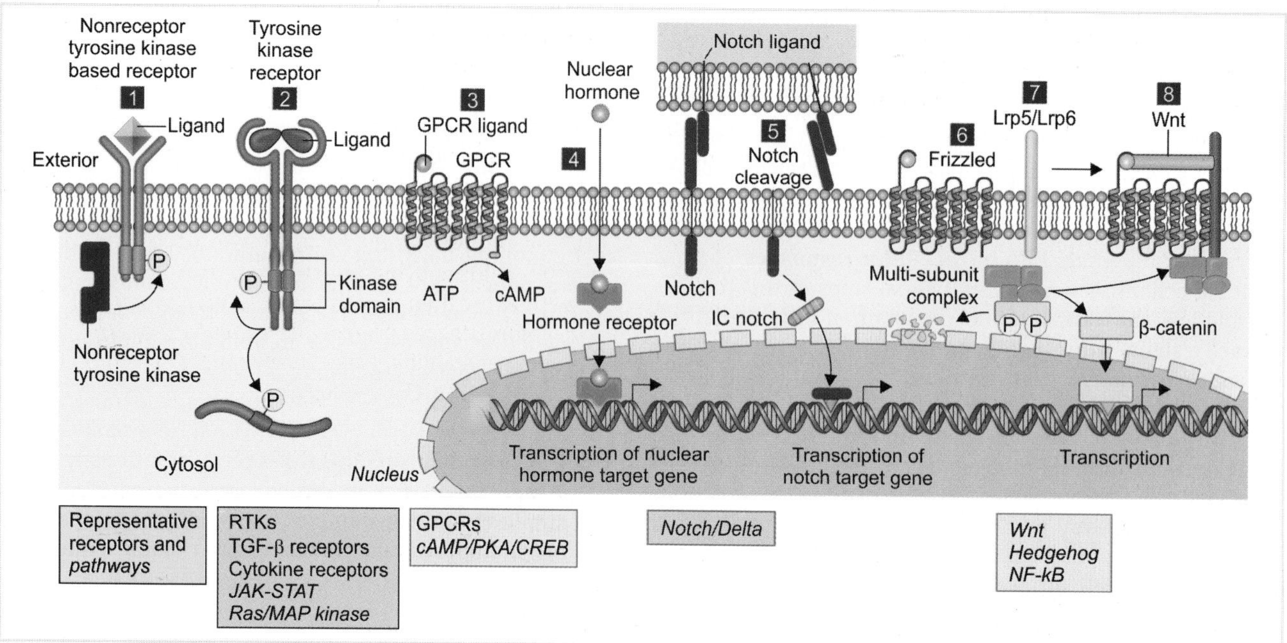

(ATP: Adenosine triphosphate; cAMP: cyclic adenosine monophosphate; CREB: cAMP-response element binding protein; GPCR: G protein-coupled receptor; Lrp5/Lrp6: low-density lipoprotein receptor–related proteins 5 and 6; PKA: protein kinase A)

FIG. 4: Types of signaling receptors in receptor-mediated signaling. (1) Receptors using a nonreceptor tyrosine kinase (2) Receptor tyrosine kinase [these receptors are protein kinases or are associated with a cytosolic kinase]. These kinases are activated by ligand binding followed by receptor dimerization. Some of these kinases directly phosphorylate and activate transcription factors (TFs)]. (3) Seven-transmembrane receptor linked to heterotrimeric G proteins [activate the larger guanosine triphosphate (GTP) binding Gα proteins, which in turn activate specific kinases or other signaling proteins]. (4) A nuclear receptor that binds its ligand and influences transcription (5) Notch, which recognizes a ligand on another cell and can enter the nucleus and influence transcription of specific target genes. (6) and (8) Wnt/Frizzled pathway that releases intracellular β-catenin. The released β-catenin migrate to the nucleus and act as a TF(transcription factor). (7) Lrp5/Lrp6, low-density lipoprotein (LDL) receptor related proteins 5 and 6, act as coreceptors in Wnt/Frizzled signaling.

Box 2: Major receptor families with examples.

Major classes of cell-surface receptors

- **Enzyme-linked receptors:** They contain either intrinsic enzyme activity on their intracellular domain or associate directly with an intracellular enzyme. Ligand binding produces a conformational change and is transmitted via a transmembrane helix which activates the enzyme, initiating signaling cascades
  - **Receptor serine/threonine kinases (RSTKs):** Contains intrinsic serine/threonine kinase activity. e.g., TGFβ receptors
  - **Receptor tyrosine kinases (RTKs):** Contains intrinsic tyrosine kinase activity Examples are as follows:
    - Epidermal growth factor (EGF) receptor family (ErbB family)
    - Insulin receptor family
    - Platelet-derived growth factor (PDGF) receptor family
    - Vascular endothelial growth factor (VEGF) receptor family
    - Fibroblast growth factor (FGF) receptors family)
    - Nerve growth factor (NGF) receptor family
  - **Tyrosine-kinase associated receptors:** Receptors that associate with proteins that have tyrosine kinase activity (e.g., cytokine receptors, **TNF** receptors)
  - **Receptor guanylyl cyclases:** Contain intrinsic cyclase activity [e.g., atrial natriuretic peptide (ANP)]
  - **Receptor tyrosine phosphatases**
- **G protein-coupled receptors:** They bind a ligand and activate a membrane protein called a G-protein, which then interacts with either an ion channel or an enzyme in the membrane (e.g., acetylcholine, epinephrine, thrombin, vasopressin)
- **Ion channel linked receptors (channel-linked receptors also called ligand-gated ion channels):** They bind a ligand and open a channel through the membrane that allows specific ions to pass through (e.g., neurotransmitter receptors)

Intracellular receptors

E.g., receptors for vitamin D and steroid hormones

has to enter the cell cytosol to bind directly to them. The signal molecule in these, should be sufficiently small and hydrophobic to diffuse across the target cell's plasma membrane.

Intracellular receptors include receptors for transcription factors (TFs) that are activated by lipid-soluble ligands. The signals can easily pass across the plasma membranes. In the cytosol, they interact with intracellular proteins to form a receptor-ligand complex that directly binds to nuclear DNA. They can result in either activation or repression of gene transcription. For example, vitamin D and steroid hormones, which activate nuclear hormone receptors. A small and/or nonpolar signaling ligand can also diffuse into adjacent cells. For example, nitric oxide (NO) which passes through endothelial cells, regulates intravascular pressure. NO is produced in activated endothelial cell and diffuses into adjacent vascular smooth muscle cells. This activates the enzyme guanylyl cyclase to generate cyclic guanosine monophosphate (cGMP). This in turn causes relaxation of smooth muscle relaxation. This is the method by which endothelium can regulate vasomotor tone.

Cell-surface Receptors (Transmembrane Receptors) (Fig. 4)

Transmembrane receptors: In most cases, the cell-surface receptors are transmembrane proteins present at the extracellular surface of the responding (target) cell. They do not enter the cytosol or nucleus. When the extracellular signal molecule (a ligand), binds to these specific receptor proteins on the surface of the target cells , they become activated. This generates various intracellular signals that alter the behavior of the cell. They convert an extracellular ligand-binding event into intracellular signals that alter the behavior of the target cell. These cell-surface receptors act as *signal transducers.* Three general categories of cell-surface receptors include: ion-channel, G-protein, and enzyme-linked protein (e.g., receptors associated with kinases) receptors.

Major classes of cell-surface receptors

There are many receptors to fill the vital role of the detection of extracellular signals. However, in spite of the vast array of extracellular molecules that need to be detected by a single cell (includes hormones, cytokines and chemokines), most cell-surface receptors fall mainly into four major classes. Depending on the receptor, ligand binding , they are of the following types:

1. Open ion channels (**Ion channel linked**): They are usually present at the synapse between electrically excitable cells (refer 2 of Fig. 5 of Chapter 1) (e.g., Cystic fibrosis transmembrane conductance regulator).
2. **G protein-coupled receptors (GPCRs):** They activate an associated guanosine triphosphate (GTP)-binding regulatory protein *(G protein).* They are associated with growth factor signaling pathways involved in cell proliferation (refer Fig. 6 and pages 45–46).
3. **Receptors associated with kinase activity:** They belong to enzyme-linked receptor group. They activate an endogenous or associated enzyme, usually a tyrosine kinase. They are also associated with growth factor signaling pathways involved in cell proliferation (for details refer page 47).
   - **Receptor protein-tyrosine kinases** (**RTKs**) (for details refer page 48)
   - **Nonreceptor or cytoplasmic protein-tyrosine kinases** (for details refer page 47)
4. **Trigger a proteolytic event or change protein binding or stability to activate a latent transcription factor (Fig. 4):** Originally, these receptors were recognized as important for embryonic development and cell fate determination. However, they have been found to be a common feature of multiple pathways which regulate normal development. They participate in the functions of mature cells, especially within the immune system. These pathways rely on protein-protein interactions, rather than enzymatic activities, to transduce signals. These allow them to achieve very precise control. These receptors trigger a proteolytic event or a change in protein binding or stability. This in turn activates a latent TF (e.g., Notch, Wnt, and Hedgehog).

Ion Channel Linked Receptors

These receptors are often involved in the detection of neurotransmitter molecules. Hence, they are sometimes referred to as transmitter-gated ion channels. Binding of the ligand to the receptor changes the ion permeability of the plasma membrane. The receptor undergoes a conformational change and either opens or closes an ion channel. This permits the efflux or influx of specific ions. However, this is only a transient event and the receptor returns to its original state very rapidly. Example for ion channel receptor sis the acetylcholine receptor.

G Protein-coupled Receptors

Q. Write short essay on G-protein-coupled receptors.

These are polypeptides that characteristically traverse the plasma membrane seven times [hence designated as seven-transmembrane (7TM) or serpentine receptors] (**Figs. 5 and 3 in Fig. 4**). Many of them have a common mode of action, that is, they interact with G proteins, hence the name G protein-coupled receptors. But some of them control signal transduction pathways in different ways. There are >1,500

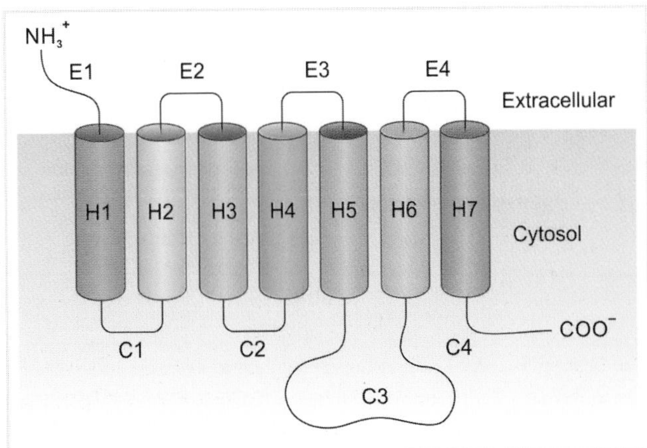

(COO^-: carboxy terminal; NH_3: amino terminal)

FIG. 5: General structure of G protein-coupled receptors. They contin seven transmembrane α-helical regions (H1–H7), four extracellular segments (E1–E4), and four cytosolic segments (C1–C4).

such receptors. They contain seven transmembrane α-helical regions (H1–H7), four extracellular segments (E1-E4), and four cytosolic segments (C1–C4). Its N-terminus is on the exoplasmic face and the C-terminus is on the cytosolic face of the plasma membrane.

Mechanism of Action (Fig. 6)

G protein-coupled receptors (GPCR) act indirectly (through GTP) to regulate the activity of target protein (which is usually either an enzyme or an ion channel). The interaction between the activated receptor and target protein is mediated by GTP. Different steps are:

- The ligand binds to the **GPCRs** (**Fig. 6A**). This increases the affinity of receptor with an intracellular GTP-binding protein (G protein). These are called as G proteins because they bind guanine nucleotides, either guanosine diphosphate (GDP) or GTP. G proteins are heterotrimeric because all of them consist of three different polypeptide subunits, called α, β, and γ. At baseline, G proteins contain GDP.
- Interaction of ligandin with the receptor induces a conformational change in receptor. It activates G protein through the exchange of GDP for GTP. The Gα subunit of G protein releases its GDP and GDP is replaced by GTP (**Fig. 6B**).
- The Gα subunit dissociates from the Gβγ complex and binds to an effector (e.g., adenylyl cyclase in **Fig. 6B**). This activates the effector target protein. This can change the concentration of one or more small intracellular signaling molecules (if the target protein is an enzyme), or it can change the ion permeability of the plasma membrane (if the target protein is an ion channel).
- Downstream signaling of the activated effector (e.g., adenylyl cyclase) generates cyclic adenosine monophosphate (cAMP) (**Fig. 6D**) and inositol-1,4,5-triphosphate (IP_3), the latter releasing calcium from the endoplasmic reticulum (ER).
- The GTPase activity of Gα hydrolyzes the bound GTP, deactivating Gα (**Fig. 6E**).
- The Gα reassociates with Gβγ and reforms the trimeric G protein. This brings to end of the activity of the effector.
- The receptor will be phosphorylated by a *G protein-coupled receptor kinase* (*GRK*) (**Fig. 6G**).
- The phosphorylated receptor binds to an arrestin molecule (**Fig. 6H**), which inhibits the ligand-bound receptor from activating additional G proteins. In unstimulated cell arrestin molecules are localized in the cytoplasm in this basal "inactive" conformation. Active phosphorylated GPCRs recruit arrestin to the plasma membrane. The receptor bound to arrestin is taken up by endocytosis.

Examples of some of the ligands that operate by means of this pathway are—bradykinin, calcitonin, dopamine, epinephrine (adrenaline), glucagon, histamine, leukotrenes, neurotensin, parathyroid hormone, prostaglandin, serotonin and somatostatin.

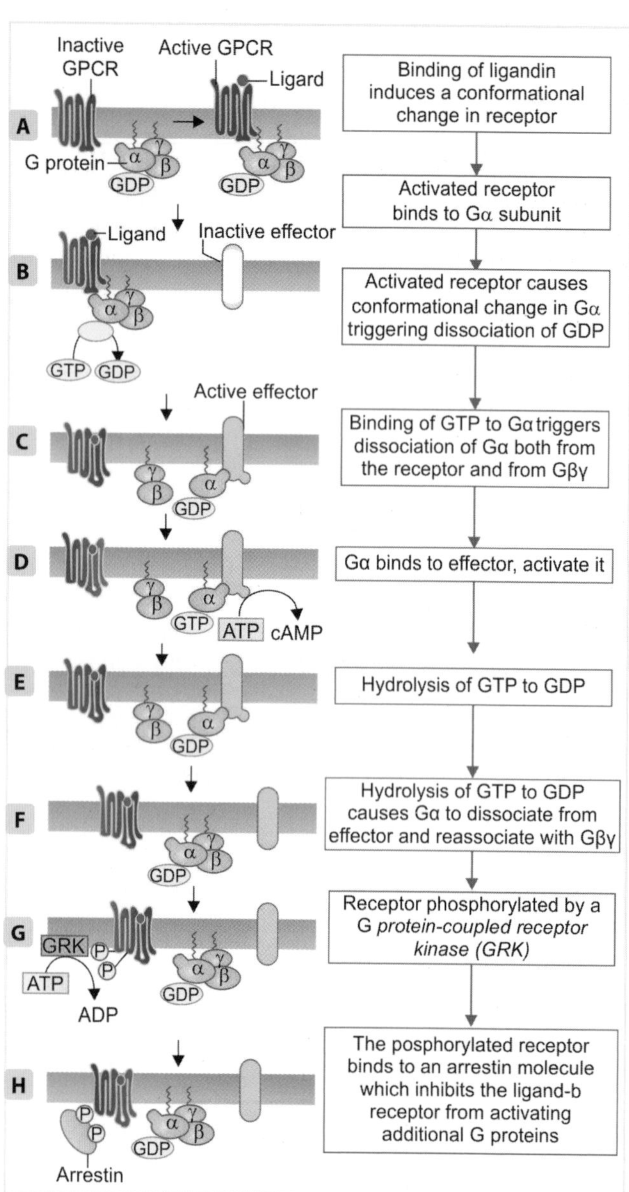

(ADP: adenosine diphosphate; ATP: adenosine triphosphate; GDP: guanosine diphosphate; G protein: guanine nucleotide-binding proteins; GPCR: protein-coupled receptors; GTP: guanosine triphosphate)

FIG. 6: The mechanism of receptor-mediated activation (or inhibition) of effectors by means of heterotrimeric G proteins (Parts A to H).

Disorders Associated with G Protein-coupled Receptors

Inherited disorders can occur due to defects in both GPCRs and heterotrimeric G proteins.

- **Defective G protein-coupled receptor:** Familial hypocalciuric hypercalcemia, neonatal severe hyperparathyroidism, hyperthyroidism (thyroid adenomas), familial male precocious puberty, X-linked nephrogenic diabetes insipidus, retinitis pigmentosa.
- **Defective G protein:** Albright's hereditary osteodystrophy and pseudohypoparathyroidisms, McCune-Albright syndrome, pituitary and thyroid tumors, adrenocortical and ovarian tumors.

G Proteins that Regulate the Production of Cyclic Adenosine Monophosphate

Cyclic adenosine monophosphate acts as a second messenger in some signaling pathways. An extracellular signal can rapidly increase the concentration of cAMP more than 20-fold within seconds. Such a rapid response needs a balance between rapid synthesis of the molecule and its rapid breakdown or removal. cAMP is produced from adenosine triphosphate (ATP) by an enzyme called adenylyl cyclase. cAMP is short-lived (unstable) in the cell because it is rapidly and continuously destroyed/hydrolyzed by specific cAMP phosphodiesterases to form 5′-AMP. Many extracellular signals act by increasing cAMP concentrations inside the cell and other extracellular signals act through different GPCRs and reduce cAMP levels.

Cyclic adenosine monophosphate produces its effects mainly by activating cAMP dependent protein kinase A (PKA). This PK phosphorylates specific serines or threonines on selected target proteins (both intracellular signaling proteins and effector proteins) and regulate their activity. Since the target proteins are different from one cell type to another, the effects of cAMP markedly vary depending on the cell type.

G Proteins Signal via Phospholipids (Fig. 7)

Many GPCRs and receptor protein-tyrosine kinases (RTKs) can also initiate signaling pathways by converting phospholipids of cell membranes into second messengers. One of the lipid-splitting enzymes involved is the plasma membrane-bound enzyme phospholipase C-β (PLC-β). There are several classes of PLC, these include—the β class, which is activated by GPCRs and the γ class is activated by a class of enzyme coupled receptors called RTKs. The PLC-β acts on a phosphorylated inositol phospholipid (a *phosphoinositide*) called phosphatidylinositol 4,5-bisphosphate [PI (4,5) P_2]. Phosphatidylinositol (PI) is a phospholipid present in small amount and bound to the inner half of the plasma membrane lipid bilayer. Receptors that activate this inositol phospholipid signaling pathway activate PLC-β in much the same way that G proteins activates adenylyl cyclase. The activated phospholipase then cleaves/hydrolyzes the PI (4,5) P_2 to produce two important so-called second messengers or products namely—1,2-diacylglycerol (DAG) and IP_3. Signaling via the *IP_3/DAG pathway* leads to an increase in cytosolic Ca^{2+} and to activation of PKC.

- **Inositol 1,4,5-trisphosphate (IP_3):** IP_3 is a sugar phosphate, small, water-soluble molecule formed at the membrane. It is capable of rapid diffusion from the plasma membrane into the interior of the cell. On reaching the ER, it binds to and opens specific IP_3-gated Ca^{2+}-release channels (also called IP_3 receptors) located at the surface of the ER membrane. Ca^{2+} stored in the ER is released through the open channels and quickly increases the Ca^{2+} concentration in the cytosol. This in turn propagates the signal by influencing the activity of Ca^{2+}-sensitive intracellular proteins (**Fig. 7**).
- **Diacylglycerol (DAG)** is a lipid molecule that remains in the plasma membrane after its formation by PLC-β. There it recruits and activates effector proteins of which best-studied is *PKC*, which phosphorylates serine and threonine residues on a wide variety of target proteins.

Examples of cell responses in which GPCRs activate plasma-membrane-bound enzyme PLC-β are presented in **Table 1**.

Receptors Associated with Kinase Activity

Protein-tyrosine kinases (PTKs) are enzymes that **phosphorylate** specific tyrosine residues present on **protein substrates**. Protein-tyrosine phosphorylation is a mechanism for signal transduction. These kinases are involved in the regulation of growth, division, differentiation, survival, attachment to the ECM, and migration of cells. Mutation of protein-tyrosine kinases can cause continual activity leading to uncontrolled cell division and the development of cancer. One type of unregulated version of the protein-tyrosine kinase ABL is observed in leukemia.

Downstream phosphorylation is a common pathway of signal transduction. Conformational changes in receptor can stimulate intrinsic receptor *PK* activity or promote the

Table 1: Examples of cell responses in which G protein-coupled receptors (GPCRs) activate plasma membrane-bound enzyme phospholipase C-β (PLC-β).

Target tissue	*Signal molecule*	*Major response*
Liver	Vasopressin	Breakdown of glycogen
Pancreas	Acetylcholine	Secretion of amylase
Smooth muscle	Acetylcholine	Contraction of muscle
Blood platelets	Thrombin	Aggregation of platelet

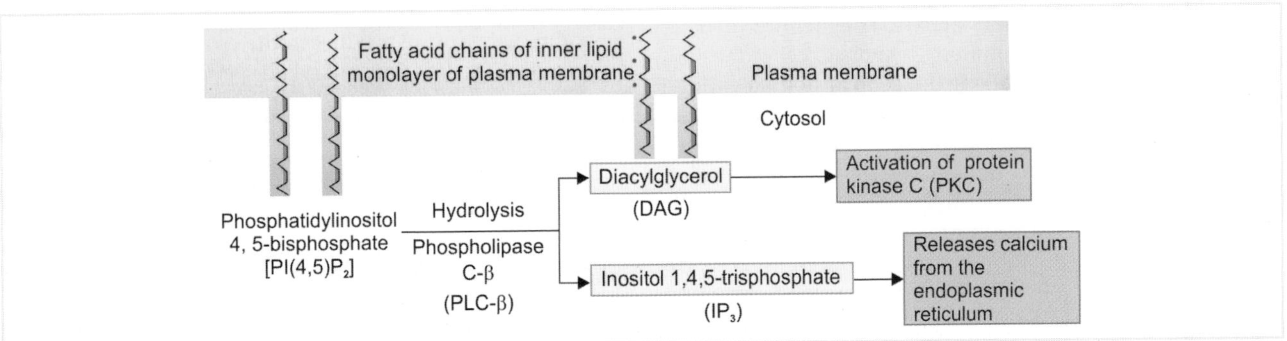

FIG. 7: Hydrolysis of phosphatidylinositol 4,5-bisphosphate [PI(4,5)P_2] by phospholipase C-β produces two second messengers namely—inositol 1,4,5-trisphosphate (IP_3) and diacylglycerol (DAG). IP_3 diffuses through the cytosol and releases Ca^{2+} from the endoplasmic reticulum. The DAG remains in the membrane and helps to activate protein kinase C (PKC).

enzymatic activity of recruited intracellular kinases. These kinases add charged phosphate residues to target molecules. *Tyrosine kinases* phosphorylate specific tyrosine residues. The *serine/threonine kinases* add phosphates to distinct serine or threonine residues. The *lipid kinases* phosphorylate lipid substrates. For each event of phosphorylation, there is also a potential counter-regulatory *phosphatase*, an enzyme which removes the phosphate residue. Thus, the signals are modulated where phosphatases act as inhibitors in signal transduction.

Classification

Protein-tyrosine kinases can be divided in two groups:

1. **Receptors containing intrinsic enzymatic activity:** These receptors constitute a quite heterogeneous class of receptors. They are integral membrane proteins that contain a single transmembrane helix and an extracellular ligand binding domain. They are characterized by the presence of a **catalytic activity integral within the receptor polypeptide**. This catalytic activity is controlled by the ligand binding event. The ligand (signal) binding domain of the receptor kinase is found on the cell surface (extracellular side of the membrane), while the kinase enzymatic activity resides in the cytoplasmic part of the protein. These receptors are mainly of two types:
   i. **Receptor serine/threonine kinases** with serine/threonine kinase activity or
   ii. **Receptor tyrosine kinases (RTKs) or receptor protein-tyrosine kinases** with tyrosine kinase activity.
2. **Receptors linked to separate tyrosine kinases (Nonreceptor or cytoplasmic protein-tyrosine kinases or tyrosine kinase linked receptors):** Several receptors do not themselves have intrinsic catalytic activity (e.g., immune receptors, some cytokine receptors, and integrins), that is they do not contain a tyrosine kinase domain. These receptors have **separate intracellular protein called *nonreceptor tyrosine kinase***. Such kinases are normally present in the cytoplasm of the cell. On activation of the receptors by ligand binding, the activated receptor adopts a new conformation. This new conformational change is recognized by these kinases in the cytoplasm. These enzyme interacts with receptors and phosphorylates specific motifs on the receptor or other proteins. This class of receptors is commonly referred to as the **cytokine receptor superfamily**, because they are commonly involved in the recognition of cytokines and growth factors.

   Nonreceptor protein-tyrosine kinases are regulated indirectly by extracellular signals. They control diverse processes such as the immune response, cell adhesion, and neuronal cell migration. The cellular homolog of the transforming protein of the Rous sarcoma virus is called SRC. SRC is an important family of non-RTKs *(Src-family kinases)*. SRC contains unique functional regions called *Src-homology (SH)* domains. The SH2 domains usually bind to receptors phosphorylated by another kinase and allow the aggregation of multiple enzymes. The SH3 domain is responsible for protein–protein interactions, and often involves proline-rich domains.

Receptor Protein-tyrosine Kinases

Receptor protein-tyrosine kinases are a class of receptors that translate the presence of extracellular messenger molecules into changes inside the cell. *RTKs* are integral membrane proteins.

Components of receptor tyrosine kinases

All RTKs have three components, namely:

- An extracellular domain containing a ligand-binding site.
- A single hydrophobic transmembrane α helix, and
- A cytosolic segment that has a domain with protein tyrosine kinase activity.

Examples

Many extracellular signal proteins act through RTKs. These include epidermal growth factor (EGF), insulin, insulin-like growth factor-1 (IGF-1), platelet-derived growth factor (PDGF), fibroblast growth factor (FGF), vascular endothelial growth factor (VEGF), and macrophage-colony-stimulating factor (M-CSF). Their receptors are RTKs.

Most RTKs are monomeric (monomer is a molecule and large numbers of monomers combine to form polymers by a process called polymerization), and ligand binding to the extracellular domain induces formation of receptor dimers. The formation of functional dimers is a step needed for activation of all RTKs.

Steps of Receptor Tyrosine Kinase Activation (Figs. 8A and B)

- The intrinsic kinase activity of an RTK is very low in the resting, unstimulated (no ligand bound) state (**Figs. 8A** and **B**).
- Receptor protein-tyrosine kinases contain a flexible domain termed the *activation loop* on the cytosolic side of the receptor. In the resting state, the activation loop is nonphosphorylated (unphosphorylated) and assumes a conformation that blocks or obstructs protein tyrosine kinase activity, thereby prevents ATP from entering it.
- Binding of ligand (signal protein) to the ligand-binding domain on the extracellular side of the receptor causes a conformational change that promotes dimerization of the extracellular domains (regions) of receptor. Two ways of dimerization are shown in **Figures 8A** and **B**. It brings transmembrane segments of receptor and their cytosolic domains (regions) close together. This activates the tyrosine kinase domain and leads to phosphorylation of tyrosine side chains on the cytosolic part of the receptor. The phosphorylation leads to a conformational change in the activation loop that unblocks kinase activity. The resulting enhanced activity of kinase can then phosphorylate additional tyrosine residues in the cytosolic domain of the receptor. The PKs phosphorylate specific tyrosine residues of cytoplasmic substrate proteins which bind to sites for various intracellular signaling proteins that relay the signal. The phosphorylation alters the activity, localization, or ability of these substrate proteins to interact with other proteins within the cell.

Mechanism of action of receptors associated with kinase activity are discussed in detail on pages 51–61.

Other Classes of Receptors

Receptor Proteins of the Notch Family

Notch is a single-pass transmembrane protein found on the cell surface and its ligand (signal protein) is called

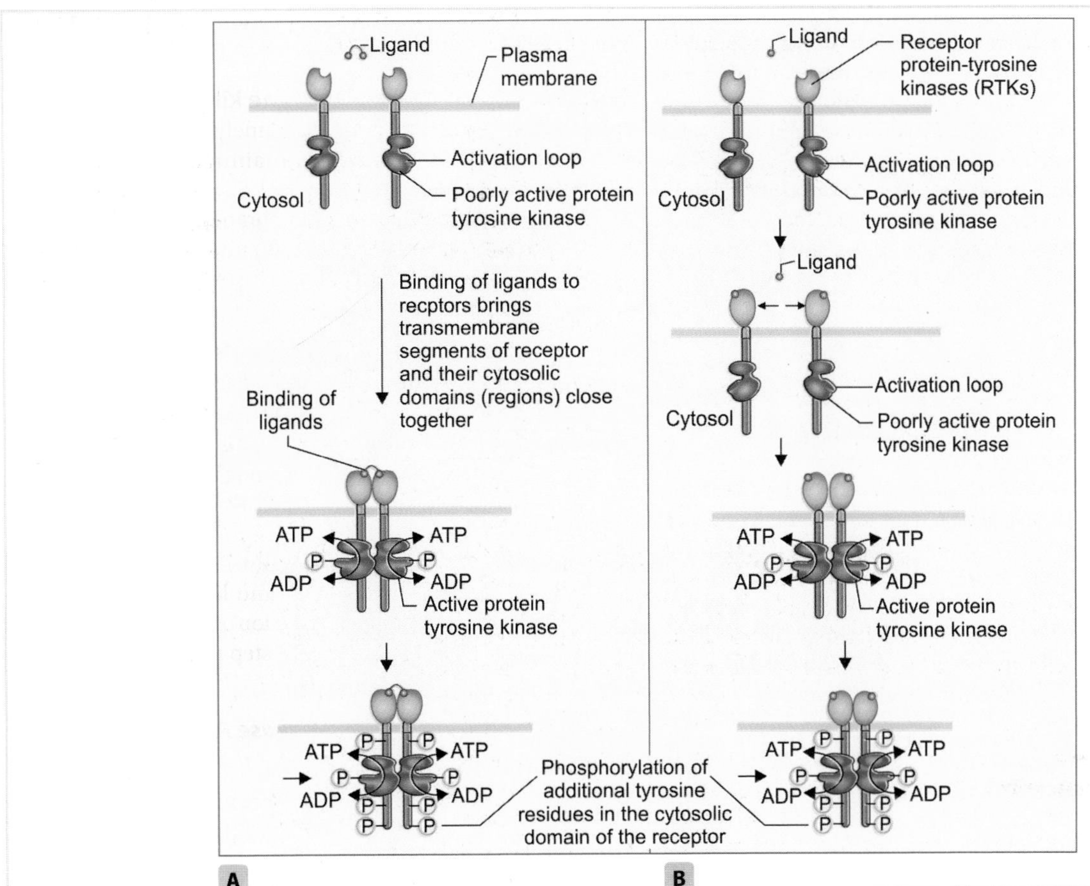

FIGS. 8A AND B: Steps in the activation of a receptor protein-tyrosine kinase (RTK). Two ways of dimerization are shown here. (A) Single ligandin binds 2 receptors. (B) Each ligandin binding receptors separately.

Delta. Notch acts as a latent transcription regulator and is the simplest and most direct signaling pathway from a cell-surface receptor to the nucleus. The extracellular domain of Delta on the signaling cell binds to Notch on an adjacent responding cell (immediate neighboring cell but not on the same cell) and signals to neighboring cell (**5** in **Fig. 4**). For example, during development when a precursor cell commits to become a neural cell, it signals to its immediate neighbor cell not to become neural, and the inhibited cells instead develop into epidermal cells. When this signaling process is defective, a huge excess of neural cells is produced at the expense of epidermal cells, which is lethal. This process is called *lateral inhibition.* Notch is activated when Delta ligand binds to Notch receptors on another cell and causes proteolytic cleavage of the cytoplasmic tail of Notch receptor by a plasma membrane-bound protease. Notch needs this cleavage to function. The released tail translocates into the nucleus and acts by binding to a DNA-binding protein. It converts transcriptional repressor into a transcriptional activator to activate the transcription of a set of Notch response genes.

Wnt Protein Ligands (Figs. 9A to C and See 6 and 8 in Fig. 4)

The word *Wnt* is an amalgamation of *wingless* (*Wg*), the corresponding fly gene of *Drosophila,* with *int* for the retrovirus integration site in mice. The principal signaling receptor for Wnt proteins is transmembrane *Frizzled (meaning shrivelled) (Fz).* They regulate the intracellular levels of transcription regulator β-catenin, hence called as *Wnt/β-catenin pathway.* The *β-catenin* is multi-talented protein that binds to E-cadherin. A portion of the cell's β-catenin is located at cell–cell junction and functions as membrane-cytoskeleton linker protein and controls cell–cell adhesion. In the absence of Wnt, remaining β-catenin molecules that are not attached to cell-adhesion molecules are bound in a cytosolic *destruction complex.* The complex has tumor suppressor gene called adenomatous polyposis coli (APC) protein as an integral part. APC is so named because its loss may result in colorectal cancer. *APC* encodes a cytoplasmic protein whose dominant function is to promote the degradation of β-catenin. This complex rapidly degrades β-catenin by ubiquitin directed proteasome in the cytoplasm. Wnts are soluble factors that bind WNT receptors. Wnt binding to Fz (and other coreceptors) prevent the APC-mediated degradation of β-catenin and frees the β-catenin. This allow it to translocate to the nucleus and it associates with a TF [*ternary complex factor (TCF)*]. It functions as a coactivator to induce expression of particular target genes, often promotes cell proliferation. If there is loss or mutation of APC (e.g., in colon cancers), β-catenin degradation is prevented. In such situation, the WNT signaling response is inappropriately activated even in the absence of WNT factors.

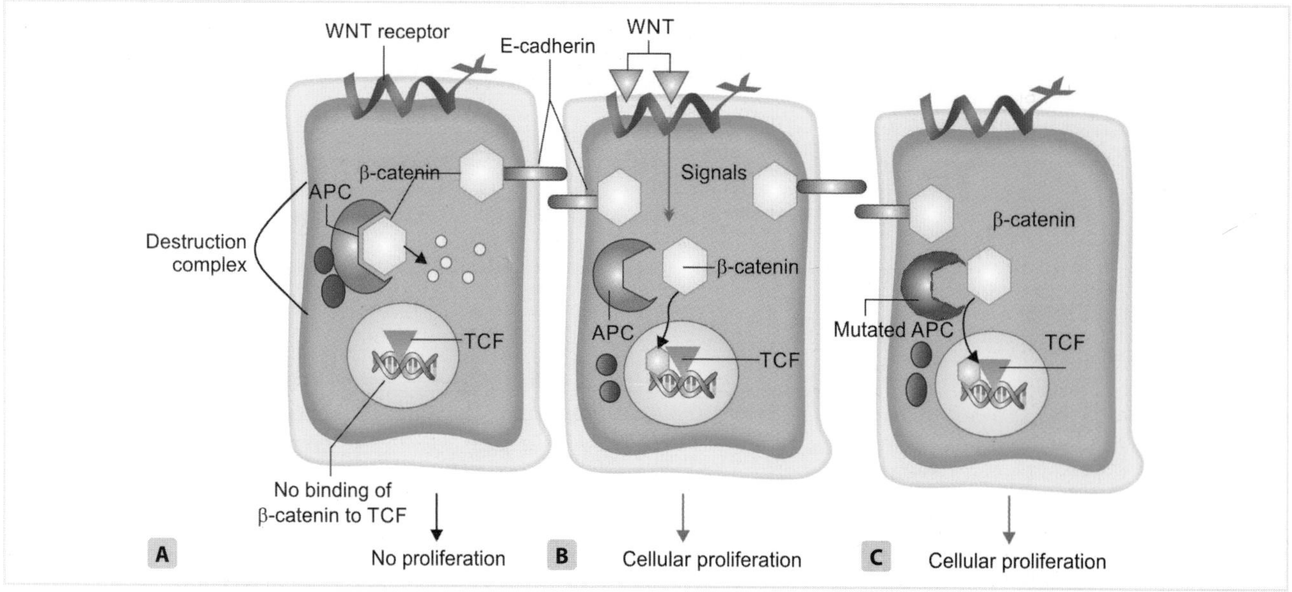

FIGS. 9A TO C: Role of adenomatous polyposis coli (APC) in regulating the β-catenin. APC and β-catenin are components of the WNT signaling pathway—(A) In resting cells, β-catenin forms a complex with APC protein. This complex destroys β-catenin and is associated with low intracellular levels of β-catenin. (B) When cells are stimulated by WNT molecules, the destruction complex is not formed. There is no destruction of β-catenin and leads to increase in their cytoplasmic levels. β-catenin translocates to the nucleus, where it binds to transcription factor called ternary complex factor (TCF). This activates several genes involved in the cell cycle and cell cycle progresses. (C) When *APC* is mutated or absent, the β-catenin cannot be destroyed and cell enters into the cell cycle. The cells behave as though they are under constant stimulation by the WNT pathway.

Hedgehog Signaling

Q. Write short note on Hedgehog signaling.

The Hedgehog (Hh) signaling pathway acts similar to the Wnt pathway. Both activate latent transcription regulators by inhibiting their degradation. They both trigger a switch from transcriptional repression to transcriptional activation. It relieves repression of target genes. The effects of Hh are mediated by a latent transcription regulator called Cubitus interruptus (Ci), the regulation of which is similar to the regulation of β-catenin by Wnts. Hh functions by blocking the proteolytic processing of Ci, thereby changing it into a transcriptional activator. This is achieved by a convoluted signaling process that depends on three transmembrane proteins—Patched, iHog, and Smoothened. Hh signaling can promote cell proliferation, and excessive Hh signaling can lead to cancer. Inactivating mutations in one of the *Patched* genes occur frequently in *basal cell carcinoma* of the skin.

Nuclear Factor Kappa-light-chain-enhancer of Activated B Cells-dependent Signaling Pathway (Fig. 10)

The nuclear factor kappa-light-chain-enhancer of activated B cells (NF-κB) proteins are transcription regulators that are central to many stressful, inflammatory, and innate immune responses. Various cell-surface receptors activate the NF-κB signaling pathway.

- ***Toll-like receptors*** recognize pathogens and activate this pathway in triggering innate immune responses.
- The receptors for ***tumor necrosis factor*-α (*TNF*-α) and *IL1***, which are cytokines that induce inflammatory responses, also activate this signaling pathway.

Mechanism

The toll-like and IL1 receptors belong to the same family of proteins whereas TNF receptors belong to a different family. However, all of them, act in similar ways to activate NF-κB.

- In the resting state of both the Wnt and Hedgehog (Hh) pathways, a key transcription factor (TF) is ubiquitinylated and undergoes proteolytic degradation. This generates a protein fragment that acts as a transcriptional repressor. Activation of the signaling pathway blocks ubiquitinylation and releases the TF in its active state.
- The NF-κB pathway (**Fig. 10**) works in the opposite manner. In the resting state (unstimulated cells), the NF-κB transcription factor (TF) is tightly bound to an inhibitor protein called IκB that holds NF-κB in an inactive state within the cytoplasm. When activated, two related kinases, IκB kinase α (IKKα) and IKKβ cause ubiquitinylation of the inhibitor IκB followed by its degradation and releases NF-κB from an inhibitor. The released NF-κB can translocate to the nucleus and turn on the transcription of hundreds of genes that participate in inflammatory and innate immune responses.
- Similar to the Wnt and Hh signaling, excessive NF-κB signaling is found in a number of human cancers.

Modular Signaling Proteins, Hubs, and Nodes

Traditional linear view of signaling consists of steps such as receptor activation, triggering of an orderly sequence of biochemical intermediates, changes in gene expression and the biological response. This looks as oversimplification of the process because, it is found that any initial signal results in multiple primary and secondary effects, each of which contributes in varying degrees to the final outcome. This is

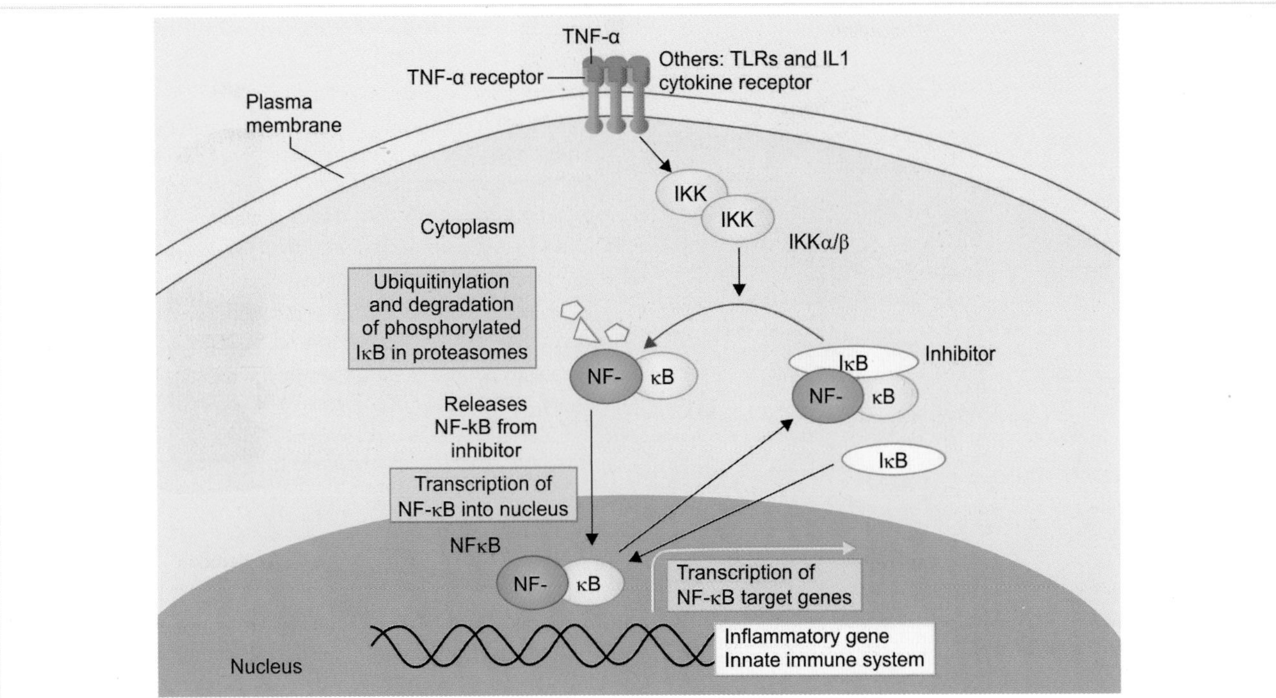

(IKK: IκB kinase)

FIG. 10: The activation of the nuclear factor kappa-light-chain-enhancer of activated B cells (NF-κB) pathway by tumor necrosis factor-alpha (TNF-α).

especially in case of signaling pathways that rely on enzymatic activities. For example, phosphorylation of protein can lead to association with a number of other molecules. This may result in multiple effects such as:

- Activation or inactivation of enzyme
- Localization of transcription factors (TFs) to nucleus or cytoplasm
- Activation or inactivation of TF
- Polymerization or depolymerization of actin
- Degradation or stabilization of protein
- Activation of feedback inhibitory or stimulatory loops

By comparing it with computer networks, signal transduction can be visualized as a kind of networking. The protein–protein complexes can be considered **nodes** and the biochemical events feeding into or originating from these nodes can be thought of as **hubs.**

SIGNALING TRANSDUCTION PATHWAYS (FIG. 11)

Q. Describe the signal transduction pathways.

Signal transduction is the process of transferring a signal across or through a cell.

Many extracellular signals can also affect gene expression, thereby inducing long-term changes in cell function. **The main signaling pathways that cells use to influence gene expression are listed in Box 3.**

Classification

Depending on the sequence of intracellular events, signal transduction pathways can be classified into several basic types. Though every signaling pathway has its own subtleties and distinctions, almost all signal transduction pathways can be grouped into one of these basic types.

1. **Receptor associated kinase:** It is a very common type of signal transduction pathway. Steps involved in signaling from a tyrosine kinase-based receptor are presented in **Figure 11**. In this type, the binding of a ligand to its complimentary receptor triggers activation of a receptor-associated kinase. These receptors usually have a single transmembrane domain and are activated by **ligand-induced receptor dimerization**. The kinase may be an intrinsic component of the cytosolic domain of the receptor protein or may be tightly attached to the cytosolic domain of the receptor. These kinases may act in one of the following ways:
   a. **Direct phosphorylation:** In this type, the kinases usually directly phosphorylate and activate a variety of signal-transducing proteins, including transcription factor (TFs) located in the cytosol, Lipid-soluble ligands can diffuse into cells. They interact with intracellular proteins to form a receptor-ligand complex. This can directly binds to nuclear DNA. It can either activate or repress gene transcription.
   b. **Activation through GTP-binding proteins:** In this, receptor kinases activate small GTP-binding "switch" proteins such as RAS. Steps involved in signaling from a tyrosine kinase-based receptor are presented in **Figure 11**. Many signal transduction pathways activated by RAS, involve several kinases (**Fig. 12**). In this pathway, one kinase phosphorylates and thus activates (or occasionally inhibits) the activity of another kinase. Eventually one or more of these kinases phosphorylate and activate TFs.

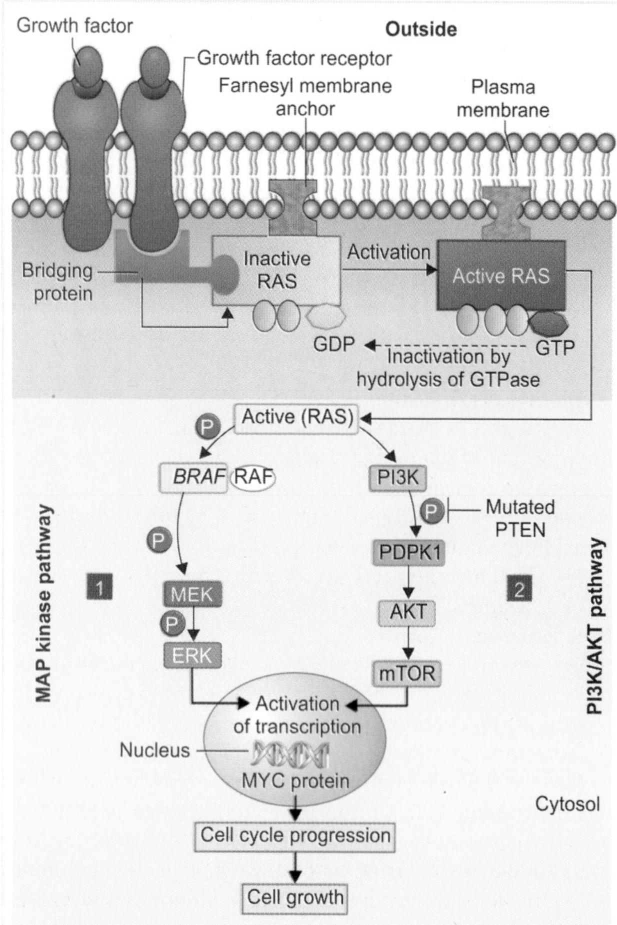

(mTOR: mammalian target of rapamycin)

FIG. 11: Steps involved in signaling from a tyrosine kinase-based receptor. RAS is anchored to the cell membrane by the farnesyl moiety and is essential for its action. Binding of the growth factor (ligand) to growth factor receptor causes dimerization of receptor and autophosphorylation of tyrosine residues. Attachment of adapter (or bridging) proteins couples the receptor to inactive, guanosine diphosphate (GDP)-bound RAS. GDP forms guanosine triphosphate (GTP) and produce activated RAS. The activated RAS stimulates downstream regulators of cell proliferation by two pathways—(1) RAF/ERK/MAP kinase pathway and (2) PI3K/AKT pathway, which in turn send the signal to the nucleus, resulting in cell proliferation. Activated RAS interacts with and activates RAF [also called as mitogen-activated protein *(MAP) kinase]*. RAF phosphorylates MAP kinase (MAPK), and activated MAPK phosphorylates other cytoplasmic proteins and nuclear transcription factors. This leads to cellular responses. Activated RAS can also activate phosphatidylinositol 3-kinase (PI3K), which in turn can activate other signaling systems. The active GTP state is short-lived because an enzyme GTPase hydrolyzes GTP to GDP. The cascade is turned off when the activated RAS hydrolyzes GTP to GDP and thereby converts active RAS to inactive RAS. Mutations in RAS that lead to delayed GTP hydrolysis can thus lead to augmented proliferative signaling. Growth factor receptors, RAS, PI3K, MYC and D cyclins are oncoproteins. These are activated by mutations in various cancers.

Box 3: Signaling pathways which influence gene expression.

- Receptor serine kinases (activate Smads)
- Cytokine receptors and the Janus kinase/signal transducer and activator of transcription protein (JAK/STAT) signaling pathway
- Receptor tyrosine kinases (**Fig. 11**)
- The RAS/mitogen-activated protein (MAP) kinase pathway
- Phosphoinositide signaling pathways
- Signaling pathways controlled by ubiquitinylation and protein degradation: Wnt, Hedgehog, and NF-κB
- Signaling pathways controlled by protein cleavage: Notch/Delta, sterol regulatory element-binding protein (SREBP), and Alzheimer's Disease
- Integration of cellular responses to multiple signaling pathways: Insulin action

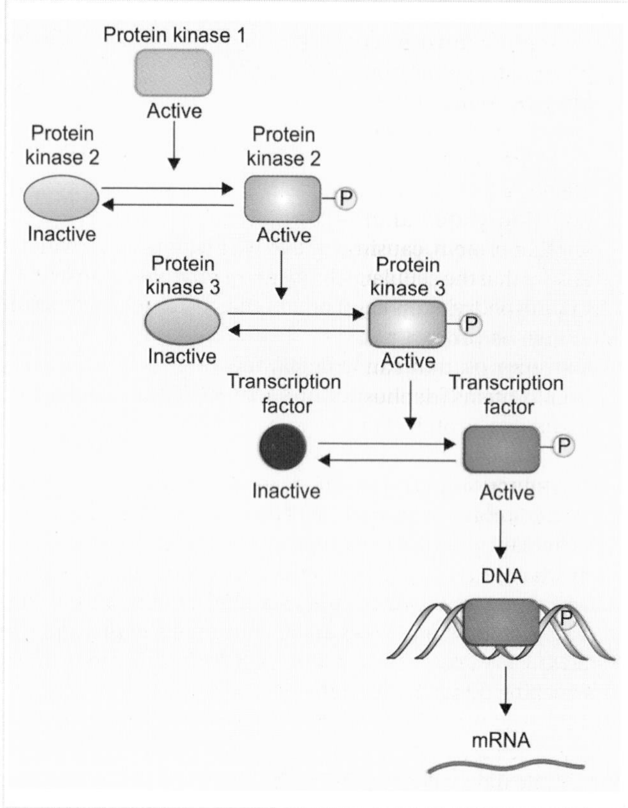

FIG. 12: Steps in signal transduction pathway involving several kinases. It consists of protein kinases and protein phosphatases whose catalytic actions change the conformations, and thus the activities, of the proteins they modify. In this example, protein kinase 1 activates protein kinase 2 and activated protein kinase 2 phosphorylates protein kinase 3, activating the enzyme. Protein kinase 3 then phosphorylates a transcription factor (TF), increases its affinity for a site on the deoxyribonucleic acid (DNA) and the transcription factor (TF) binds to the DNA.

2. **Cytosolic kinase:** In this type, receptors become activated by conformational changes induced by ligand binding. For example, the receptors with seven membrane-spanning segments, activate GTP-binding Gα proteins (**Fig. 6**). Their activation usually leads to activation of one or more PKs. These in turn phosphorylate and activate multiple target proteins, including transcription factors (TFs).
3. **Protein subunit dissociation:** In this signaling pathway, binding of a ligand to a receptor causes disassembly of a multiprotein complex in the cytosol. This in turn, releases a transcription factor (TF) which translocates into the nucleus and affects gene expression.
4. **Protein cleavage:** In this another common type, proteolytic cleavage of an inhibitor or of the receptor itself releases an active transcription factor (TF). Then the TF moves into the nucleus

Steps in the signal transduction pathway: The signal molecules or ligand that binds the receptor is called the first messenger. When they bind to receptors, they induce signal transduction pathways. These signal transduction pathways generally involve the addition or removal of phosphate groups and this leads to the activation of proteins.

- **Phosphorylation cascade:** Enzymes that transfer phosphate groups from ATP to a protein are called **protein kinases**. Many of the relay molecules involved in a signal transduction pathway are protein kinases and often act on other protein kinases in the pathway. Usually this creates a phosphorylation cascade, in which one enzyme phosphorylates another, which then phosphorylates another protein, causing a chain reaction. It is important to ensure that the cellular response is regulated appropriately. In phosphorylation cascade, there are a group of proteins known as protein phosphatases. **Protein phosphatases** are enzymes that can rapidly remove phosphate groups from proteins (dephosphorylation). Protein phosphatases, inactivate protein kinases and thus acts as "off switch" in the signal transduction pathway. Turning the signal transduction pathway off is essential when the signal is no longer present. Another importatnt aspect of dephosphorylation is that it makes protein kinases available for reuse and enables the cell to respond again when another signal is received.
- **Second messengers:** Kinases are not the only the molecules utilized by cells in signal transduction. **Second messengers** can also relay signals received by receptors on the cell surface to target molecules in the cytoplasm or the nucleus. These secondary molecules are small, nonprotein, water-soluble molecules or ions. Examples of second messengers include cyclic AMP (cAMP) and calcium ions.

Most important signal transduction pathways are discussed below.

Receptor Serine Kinases that Activate Smads

This family consists of receptor serine kinases [the **transforming growth factor-beta (TGF-β) receptor family**] and large family of their signaling molecules (the TGF-β family) that bind to them. These receptors phosphorylate, and thus trigger the activation of a class of TFs (the **Smads**). **Smads regulate several cell developments, growth, and differentiation pathways. Smads** (or **SMADs**) consist of a family of structurally similar transcription factors (TF) which are involved in receptors of the TGF-β superfamily. The abbreviation SMADS refers to the homologies to the *Caenorhabditis elegans* SMA ("small" worm phenotype) and *Drosophila* MAD ("Mothers against Decapentaplegic") family of genes. There are three types of Smad protein functions in the TGF-β signaling pathway namely—receptor-regulated Smads (R-Smads; Smads 2 and 3), common partner Smads (Co-Smads-Smad4), and inhibitory Smads (I-Smads)

In unstimulated cells, Smads are located in the cytosol. When cells are activated, they travel into the nucleus to regulate transcription. The TGF-β pathway has widely diverse effects in different types of cells. This is because different members of the TGF-β family activate different members of the TGF-β receptor family. This in turn activates different members of the Smad class of TFs. Also, same activated Smad protein partners with different TFs, and thus activates different sets of genes, in different types of cells.

The TGF-β family consists of a number of related extracellular signaling molecules. TGF-β is produced by many cells in the body and there are three human TGF-β isoforms, TGF-β 1, 2, and 3.

Main function of TGF-β:

- **To prevent the proliferation of cells.** This is performed by inducing the synthesis of proteins such as p15INK4B, which inhibit the cyclin-dependent kinases (CDKs). CDKs are necessary for progression into the S phase of the cell cycle (see Fig. 7 of Chapter 3). TGF-β inhibits the growth of both the secreting cells (autocrine signaling) and neighboring cells (paracrine signaling). Loss of TGF-β receptors, or of any of intracellular signal transducing proteins involved in the TGF-β pathway, releases cells from this growth inhibition and is seen frequently in the early development of human tumors.
- TGF-β proteins also **promote expression of cell-adhesion molecules and extracellular-matrix molecules**. This plays an important role in tissue organization.
- Other members of the TGF-β family:
    - **Activins and the inhibins:** They affect early development of the urogenital tract.
    - **Bone morphogenetic protein (BMP)**, now called BMP7 has the ability to induce bone formation in cultured cells. It is used clinically to strengthen bone after severe fractures. Other BMP proteins were recognized, most have nothing to do with bones. They are involved in development, formation of mesoderm, and of the earliest blood-forming cells. Some maintain the undifferentiated state in cultures of embryonic and adult stem cells.

Significance: Loss of TGF-β signaling plays an important role in the early development of many cancers. Many tumors contain inactivating mutations in either TGF-β receptors or Smad proteins and thus are resistant to growth inhibition by TGF-β.

- Most **pancreatic cancers** contain a deletion in the gene encoding Smad4 and thus cannot induce cell cycle inhibitors in response to TGF-β.
- Retinoblastoma (Rb), colon and gastric cancer, hepatocellular carcinoma, and some T and B-cell tumors are also unresponsive to TGF-β growth inhibition.
- Mutations in Smad2 also commonly occur in several types of tumors.

Tyrosine-kinase Associated Receptors

Protein tyrosine kinases phosphorylate specific tyrosine residues on target proteins. The phosphorylated target proteins can then activate one or more signaling pathways. These regulate most aspects of cell proliferation, differentiation, survival, and metabolism.

There are two large classes of receptors activate protein tyrosine kinases and both of them activate similar intracellular signal transduction pathways. These receptors are:

1. **Receptor tyrosine kinases (RTKs)**, in which the tyrosine kinase enzyme is an intrinsic part of the receptor's polypeptide chain.
2. **Cytokine receptors**, in which the receptor and kinase are separate polypeptides, encoded by different genes, yet are tightly bound together. The large family of cytokine receptors includes receptors for many kinds of local mediators (collectively known as *cytokines*), as well as receptors for some hormones (e.g., *growth hormone* and *prolactin*).

Cytokine Receptors and the JAK/STAT Signaling Pathway

In cytokine receptors, the tightly bound kinase is known as a *JAK kinase*. The cytokine receptors utilize a novel, short signal transduction pathway called the **JAK/STAT pathway**. The "JAK" portion of the name is an acronym for Janus kinases. (Janus is a two-faced Roman god who protected entrances and doorways.) "STAT" is an acronym for "signal transducers and activators of transcription". JAK/STAT pathway operates by more direct route without the involvement of second messengers. STAT TF binds to the activated receptor, becomes phosphorylated by the JAK kinase. STAT proteins are located in the cytosol and are called as *latent transcription regulators* because they migrate into the nucleus and regulate gene transcription only after they are activated. Once phosphorylated, STAT molecules move/translocate from the cytoplasm to the nucleus. In the nucleus, they bind to specific DNA sequences [e.g., interferon-stimulated response element (ISRE)] and directly activate transcription. Negative feedback regulates the responses mediated by the JAK–STAT pathway.

Janus kinases play an essential role regulating hematopoiesis and proliferation of blood cells. Point mutation JAK2V617F leads to activation of the JAK/STAT signaling pathways and leads to development of myeloproliferative diseases (MPDs) such as polycythemia vera (PV), essential thrombocythemia (ET), and primary myelofibrosis (PMF). JAK2V617F is a somatic mutation. Thus, it is present only in the hematopoietic cell compartment but not in germline DNA. This mutation is common in most MPD patients. JAK also activates the MAPK and phosphatidylinositol-3 kinase (PI3K) signaling pathway, resulting in increased proliferation and survival of cells harboring the JAK2V617F mutation.

Overview of signal transduction pathways triggered by receptors that activate protein tyrosine kinases is presented in **Figure 13**.

Examples of extracellular signal proteins that act through cytokine receptors and the JAK–STAT signaling pathway are listed in **Box 4**.

RAS Pathway (Refer Figs. 11 and 14)

Retroviruses are small viruses that carry their genetic information in the form of RNA. Some of these viruses contain genes, called oncogenes, which enable them to transform normal cells into tumor cells. RAS was originally discovered as the product of a retroviral oncogene. Later it was found that it was derived from its mammalian host. Thus, the name RAS refers to the discovery of the viral oncogene v-RAS (Rat Sarcoma). It was later discovered that about 30% of all human cancers contain mutant versions of *RAS* genes. RAS proteins are part of a superfamily of >150 small G proteins. Two main cellular pathways in which the RAS protein operates are **(i) RAS-MAP(mitogen-activated protein) kinase cascade and (ii) phosphoinositide-3 kinase (PI3K) pathways (phosphoinositide signaling pathway (Fig. 11)**. It is to be noted that apart from these two effectors, an increasing

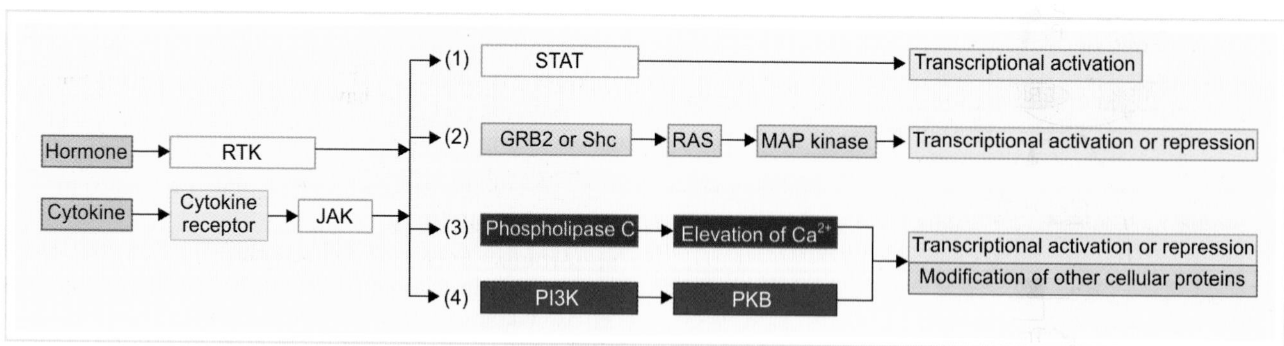

(GRB2: growth factor receptor-bound protein 2; JAK: Janus kinase)

FIG. 13: Overview of signal transduction pathways triggered by receptors that activate protein tyrosine kinases. Receptor tyrosine kinases (RTKs) as well as cytokine receptors activate multiple signal transduction pathways that regulate transcription of genes. (1) In the most direct pathway (mainly by cytokine receptors), a signal transducer and activator of transcription protein (STAT) transcription factor (TF) binds to the activated receptor, becomes phosphorylated, moves to the nucleus, and directly activates transcription. (2) Binding of adapter protein (GRB2 or Shc) to an activated receptor activates the RAS/mitogen-activated protein (MAP) kinase pathway. The Shc family of adaptor proteins is a group of proteins that lacks intrinsic enzymatic activity. (3) and (4) Two phosphoinositide pathways are triggered by recruitment of phospholipase C-γ and phosphatidylinositol-3 kinase (PI3K) to the membrane. Elevated levels of Ca^{2+} and activated protein kinase B (PKB) modulate the activity of TFs and also of cytosolic proteins that are involved in metabolic pathways or cell movement or shape.

Box 4: Examples of extracellular signal proteins that act through cytokine receptors and the Janus kinase/signal transducer and activator of transcription protein (JAK/STAT) signaling pathway.

- Interferon-γ
- Interferon-α
- Erythropoietin
- Prolactin
- Growth hormone
- Granulocyte–macrophage-colony-stimulating factor

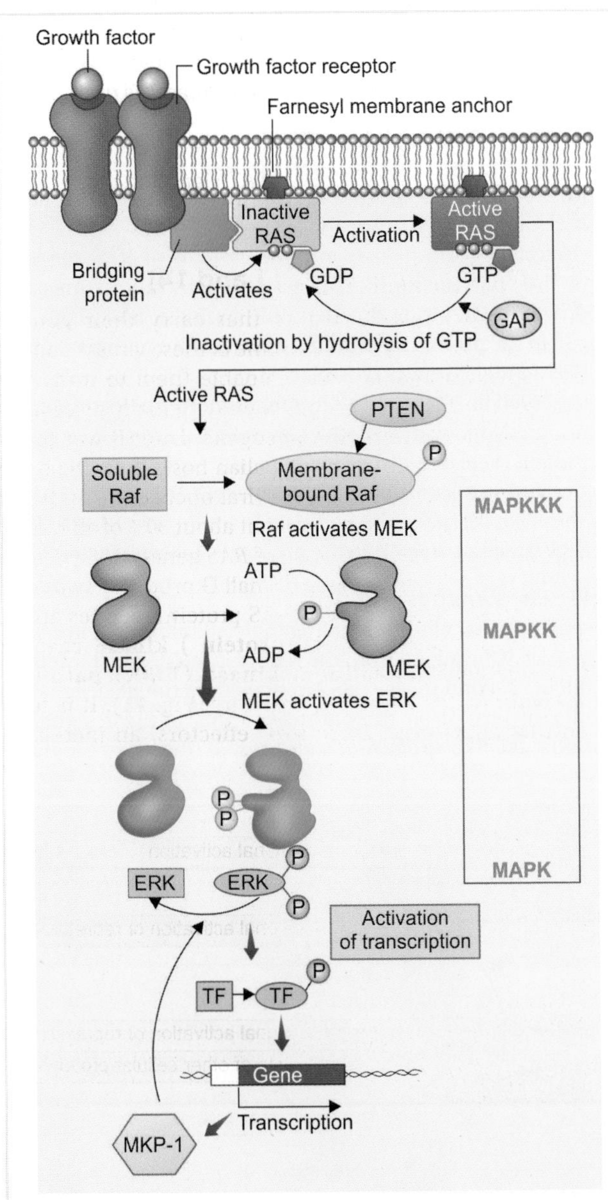

(Raf: MAPKKK; Mek: MAPKK; Erk: MAPK; TF: transcription factor).

FIG. 14: The steps of a RAS-mitogen-activated protein (MAP) kinase cascade

number of molecules that specifically interact with RAS have been identified. These proteins are involved in the regulation of numerous processes. These include cell division, differentiation, gene expression, cytoskeletal organization, vesicle trafficking, and nucleocytoplasmic transport. Almost all RTKs and cytokine receptors activate the *RAS/MAP kinase pathway.*

***Significance*:** RAS is an important protein that is subsequently activated by the signaling complexes on the receptor tyrosine kinases. These proteins are involved in the regulation of numerous processes. These include cell division, differentiation, gene expression, cytoskeletal organization, vesicle trafficking, and nucleocytoplasmic transport. Almost all RTKs and cytokine receptors activate the RAS/MAP kinase pathway.

The monomeric *RAS protein* belongs to a family of membrane-associated small G proteins called the *GTPase superfamily* of intracellular switch proteins. RAS proteins (product of *RAS* gene) are attached to the cytoplasmic aspect (inner surface) of the plasma membrane by a lipid group farnesyl membrane anchor. RAS is also anchored to the ER and Golgi membranes. This anchor is embedded in the inner leaflet of the lipid bilayer. RAS is functionally similar to the heterotrimeric G proteins. Like G proteins, RAS also acts as both a switch and a molecular timer. However, unlike heterotrimeric G proteins, RAS consists of only a single small subunit. RAS proteins are present in two different forms—(1) an active GTP-bound form; and (2) an inactive GDP-bound form (see **Fig. 11**). Normally, RAS proteins orderly flip back and forth (or cycle) between an active or excited signal-transmitting state (GTP bound-on state) and an inactive or quiescent state (GDP bound-off state). Stimulation of RTKs by growth factors activate RAS. This leads to exchange of GDP for GTP. The cycling between active and inactive states of RAS is aided by accessory proteins that bind to the G protein and regulate its activity. These accessory proteins include:

- ***GTPase-activating proteins* (*GAPs*):** RAS by itself has GTPase activity and some capability to hydrolyze a bound GTP to GDP (inactive GDP-bound form). But this capability of exchange of the nucleotide is greatly accelerated or catalyzed by interaction with specific GAPs. Mutations in one of the RAS-GAP genes cause neurofibromatosis 1 (NF1), a disease in which patients develop large numbers of neurofibromas.
- ***Guanine nucleotide-exchange factors* (*GEFs*).** An inactive RAS is converted to the active form when the bound GDP is replaced with a GTP. The activation of RAS is performed by protein called GEFs.
- ***Guanine nucleotide-dissociation inhibitors* (*GDIs*).** GDIs are proteins inhibit the release of a bound GDP and maintaining the inactive, GDP-bound state.

The subsequent conformational changes generate active RAS. The **active RAS-GTP binds and activates downstream signaling proteins namely the MAPK and PI3K/AKT**. The active GTP state is short-lived, by. However, hydrolysis of GTP is very slow in the absence of a GAP. The GAP has additional catalytic residues and can lead to inactive GTP to GDP-bound state.

RAS-MAP Kinase Cascade (Figs. 11 and 14)

The RAS-MAP kinase cascade is turned on by variety of extracellular signals. They play a key role in cell proliferation and differentiation. The pathway relays extracellular signals from the plasma membrane through the cytoplasm and into the nucleus. **MAPK pathway is a major signaling path that transmits membrane receptor signals to nuclear transcription factors (TFs).** The different steps of the pathway are as follows:

- This pathway is activated when a **growth factor,** such as EGF or PDGF **binds to the extracellular domain of growth factor receptor.** It leads to the **autophosphorylation of tyrosine residues of the receptor.** In order to activate RAS, **two cytosolic bridging proteins (GRB2 and Sos)** must first be recruited to link between the receptor and RAS. GRB2 is an *adapter protein* (it has no enzyme activity) and serves as a link between the activated receptor protein and Sos. Sos is a guanine nucleotide exchange protein (GEF) that catalyzes conversion of inactive GDP bound RAS to the active GTP-bound form. As a result, GDP is released and is replaced by GTP.
- The GTP-bound form of RAS has high affinity for the serine/threonine kinase c-RAF (RAF1). RAF has sequential kinase activity and causes **phosphorylation three times.** Hence, Raf is an important signaling protein and is known as a MAP kinase kinase kinase (MAPKKK)/MAP3Ks. These MAP3K function as the entry point for the MAPK pathway. MAP kinase kinases (MAPKKs) are dual specificity kinases, i.e., they can phosphorylate tyrosine as well as serine and threonine residues. The **three-step phosphorylation** mentioned below **is characteristic of all MAP kinase cascades.**
  - **First-step phosphorylation:** GTP-RAS recruits the protein Raf (Raf = MAPKKK) to the membrane, where it is phosphorylated and thus activated. This c-RAF is the proto-oncogene homologue to the viral v-RAF oncogene. Apart from c-RAF, there are two other RAF kinases (A-RAF and B-RAF). Mutations in B-RAF are found in many tumors.
  - **Second-step phosphorylation:** Activated c-RAF phosphorylates and activates another dual specificity kinase named MEK. MEK is a MAPKK (Mek = MAPKK).
  - **Third-step phosphorylation:** MEK in turn phosphorylates and activates still another kinase termed ERK. ERK is a MAPK (Erk = MAPK).
- Activated ERK (MAPK) translocates into the nucleus where it phosphorylates transcription factors (TFs) such as Elk-1.
- Phosphorylation of the TFs increases their affinity for regulatory sites on the DNA. This leads to an increase in the transcription of specific genes (e.g., *Fos, Myc,* and *Jun*) that are involved in the growth response and regulation of the cell cycle. One of the genes whose expression is stimulated encodes a MAPK phosphatase (MKP-1). Members of the MKP family can remove phosphate groups from both tyrosine and threonine residues of MAPK. This in turn inactivates MAPK and stops further signaling activity along the pathway.

Mutations affecting RAS pathway

- **Mutations in the human *RAS* gene** can lead to tumor formation. These mutated RAS prevent the protein from hydrolyzing the bound GTP (active) back to the GDP (inactive) form. Thus, mutant version of RAS remains in the "on" position. This sends a continuous message downstream along the signaling pathway and keeps the cell in the proliferative mode. Mutations in members of the RAS family namely, H-RAS, N-RAS, and K-RAS have been observed in 20–30% of all human tumors. For example, the mutated/oncogenic H-RAS can drive G0 arrested cells into the cell cycle in the absence of mitotic signals.
- **Activating mutations in the *Raf* gene:** They are observed in about 50% of melanomas. This mutant *Raf* stimulates MEK-ERK signaling in cells in the absence of growth factors.

Molecular switches (Fig. 15)

Most of the intracellular signaling molecules are proteins. They help to relay the signal from the receptor into the cell by either producing second messengers or activating the next signaling or effector protein in the pathway. Many of these signaling proteins act like *molecular switches.* When they receive a

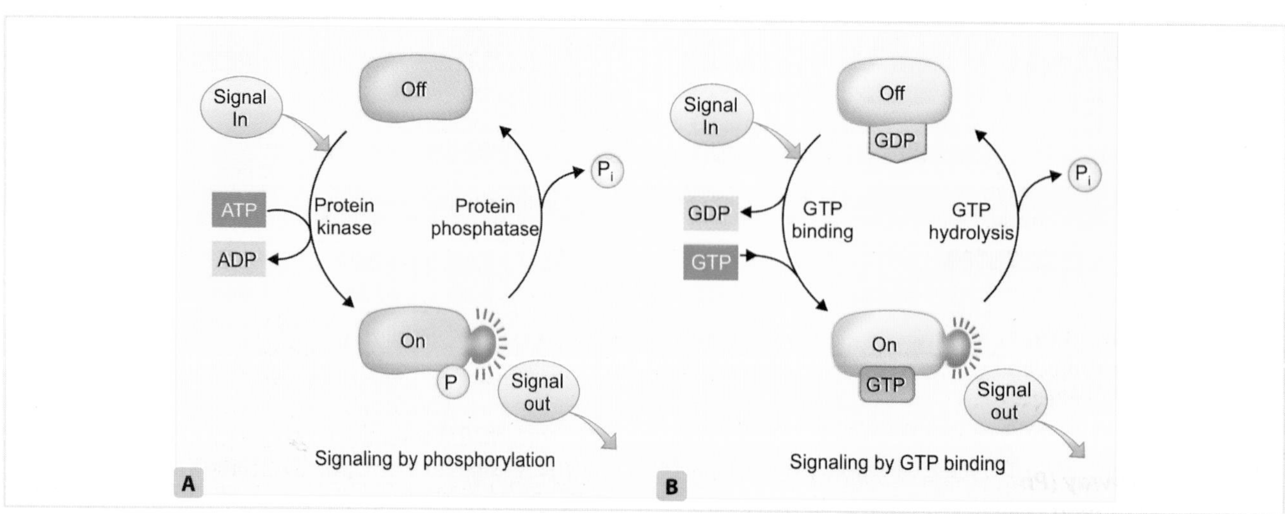

FIGS. 15A AND B: Two types of intracellular signaling proteins that act as molecular switches. (A) A protein kinase adds a phosphate from adenosine triphosphate (ATP) to the signaling protein, and a protein phosphatase removes the phosphate. (B) A guanosine triphosphate (GTP) binding protein is induced to exchange its bound GDP for GTP.

signal, they switch from an inactive to an active state. The active state is maintained only till another process switches them off. Then they return to their inactive state. The switching off is as important as the switching on. After transmitting a signal, every activated molecule in the pathway must return to its original, inactivated state by switch off mechanism. Then only it can be ready to transmit another signal. There are two main classes of molecular switches namely:

- **Phosphorylation (Fig. 15A):** In this type, proteins are activated or inactivated by phosphorylation.
  - Switch moves in **one direction by a protein kinase (PK)**. The protein kinase (PK) adds one or more phosphate groups to specific amino acids on the signaling protein. There are two main types of PK namely—(1) serine/threonine kinases (major group) which phosphorylate the serines and threonines in their targets, and (2) tyrosine kinases, which phosphorylate proteins on tyrosines.
  - The **other direction of switch is by a protein phosphatase**. This removes the phosphate groups.

  The activity of any protein in this phosphorylation pathway **depends on the balance between** the **activities of the kinases that phosphorylate** it and of the **phosphatases that dephosphorylate** it. Many intracellular signaling proteins controlled by phosphorylation are themselves PKs, and these are mostly organized into kinase cascades. Once into kinase cascades, one protein kinase (PK) activated by phosphorylation, phosphorylates the next PK in the sequence, and so on. Thus, it relays the signal onward and, in certain cases, they amplify it or spread it to other signaling pathways.
- **GTP-binding proteins (Fig. 15B):** The other important class of molecular switches consists of GTP-binding proteins. These proteins switch between an "on" (actively signaling) state when GTP is bound and an "off" state when GDP is bound. There are two major types of GTP-binding proteins.
  - **G proteins:** These are large **trimeric GTP-binding proteins.**
  - **Small monomeric GTPase:** They are also called **monomeric GTP-binding proteins**.
    Specific regulatory proteins control both types of GTP-binding proteins. One is GAPs which cause an "off" state by increasing the rate of hydrolysis of bound GTP. Other is GEFs which activate GTP-binding proteins and switches "on" state.
- **Others:** Apart from phosphorylation or GTP binding, there are some signaling proteins which are switched on or off other methods. These methods include—by the binding of another signaling protein or a second messenger (e.g., cAMP or Ca^{2+}), or by covalent modifications other than phosphorylation or dephosphorylation, such as ubiquitinylation.

It is to be born in mind that, most signaling pathways contain inhibitory steps, and a sequence of two inhibitory steps can have the same effect as one activating step. This *double-negative* activation is very common in signaling systems.

PI3K/AKT Pathway (Phosphoinositide Signaling Pathway)

Besides the IP_3/DAG pathway (refer **Fig. 7**), many activated RTKs and cytokine receptors initiate another phosphoinositide pathway by recruiting the enzyme *PI3K* to the membrane.

Phosphatidylinositol (PI) is a unique membrane lipid. It can undergo reversible phosphorylation at multiple sites on its inositol head group. Phosphorylation of PI produces a variety of lipids called phosphoinositides. PI3K is lipid kinase enzyme involved in the phosphorylation of PI. PI3K is a plasma membrane-bound enzyme and is recruited to the cytosolic surface of the plasma membrane by binding to phosphotyrosines. Both RTKs and GPCRs can activate it. PI3K can also be recruited to the cell membrane by means of RAS. When activated, PI3K can phosphorylate PI (**Fig. 16A**) at the 3, 4, and 5 positions of the inositol ring to produce several phosphoinositides such as PI 3-phosphate [PI(3)P], PI 3,4-bisphosphate [PI(3,4)P_2], and PI 3,4,5-trisphosphate [PI(3,4,5)P_3]. Of these, PI(3,4,5)P_3 is most significant because it can serve as a docking site for various intracellular signaling (signal-transducing) proteins and can form signaling complexes. This complex relays the signal into the cell from the cytosolic face of the plasma membrane. PI(3,4,5)P_3 transduce signals downstream in several important pathways. In some cells, this *PI3K pathway* can trigger cell division and prevent apoptosis, thereby ensuring cell survival and growth.

It is to be noted that there is a difference between this use of phosphoinositides and their use described earlier. Earlier it was mentioned that (refer page 57and **Figs. 7** and **16**), PI(4,5)P_2 is cleaved by PLC-β (in the case of GPCRs) or PLC-γ (in the case of RTKs) to produce soluble IP_3 and membrane-bound DAG. By contrast, PI(3,4,5)P_3 is not cleaved by either PLC. PI(3,4,5)P_3 is produced from PI(4,5)P_2.

Phosphatidylinositol-3,4,5-trisphosphate remains in the plasma membrane till it is dephosphorylated by specific *phosphoinositide phosphatases.* Important phosphatase is the *phosphatase and tensin homologue deleted on chromosome 10 (PTEN)* phosphatase, which dephosphorylates the 3 position of the inositol ring. Mutations in PTEN can be found in many advanced cancers. The cells lacking PTEN have elevated levels of PI(3,4,5)P_3 and PKB activity. Since, PKB exerts an antiapoptotic effect, loss of PTEN reduces apoptosis. These mutations prolong signaling by PI3K and promote uncontrolled cell growth. There are various types of PI3Ks. PI3Ks activated by RTKs and GPCRs belong to class I. RTKs activate *class Ia PI3Ks* whereas GPCRs activate *class Ib PI3 kinases.*

Activation of PI3K

It can occur by at least three independent pathways, all of which start with binding of a ligand to receptor tyrosine kinases (RTKs). It is not clear which of these pathways predominates in different physiological situations.

- Via RAS signaling pathway (described below).
- By direct binding of the regulatory subunit of PI3K, p85, to phospho-YXXM motifs (in which X indicates any amino acid) within the RTK. This triggers activation of the p110 catalytic subunit of PI3K.
- Depends on the adaptor protein GRB2. This binds preferentially to phospho-YXN motifs of the RTK.

PI3K–AKT signaling pathway (Fig. 16)

Phosphoinositides stimulate phosphorylation dependent signaling by interaction with pleckstrin homology (PH) domain. Intracellular signaling proteins bind to PI(3,4,5)P_3 produced by activated PI3K via a specific interaction domain. The PI(3,4,5)P_3 recruits two PKs to the plasma membrane via their PH domains namely Akt/AKT (also called *PKB*) and

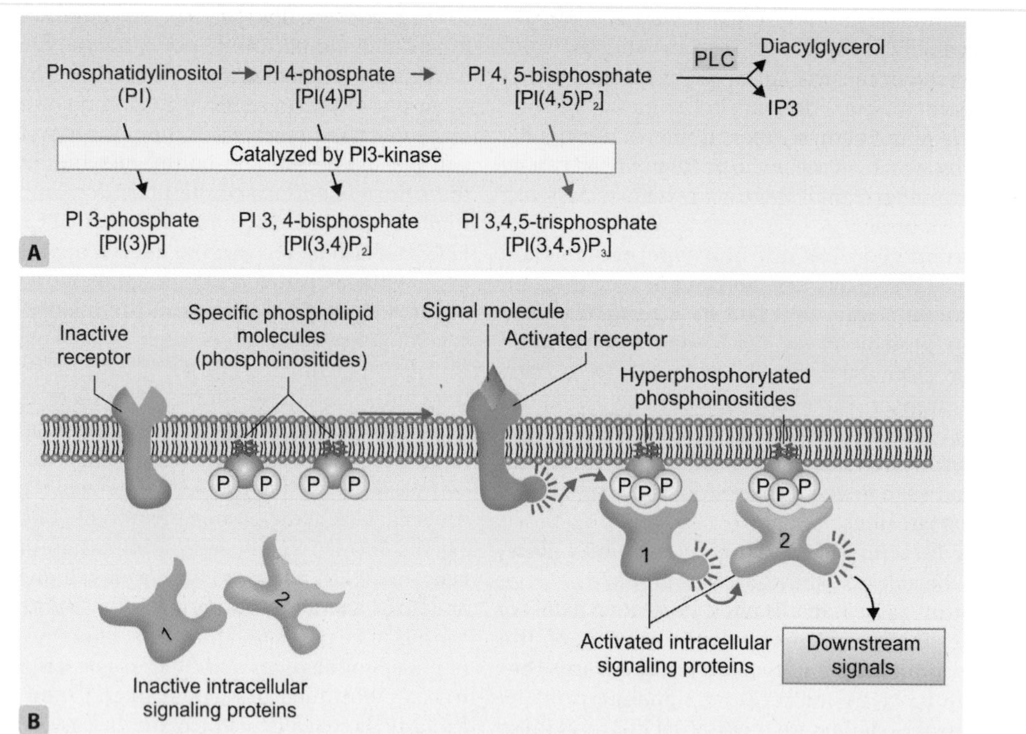

FIGS. 16A AND B: Production of molecules involved in phosphoinositide signaling pathways. (A). Activated PI3K can phosphorylate PI at the 3, 4, and 5 positions of the inositol ring to produce several phosphoinositides such as PI 3-phosphate [PI(3)P], PI 3,4-bisphosphate [PI(3,4) P2], and PI 3,4,5-trisphosphate [PI(3,4,5)P3]. PI(3,4,5)P3 can be converted into diacylglycerol or IP3,(B) Steps involved in phosphoinositide signaling pathways. PI(3,4,5)P3 can serve as a docking site for various intracellular signaling (signal-transducing) proteins and can form signaling complexes. This complex relays the signal into the cell from the cytosolic face of the plasma membrane. PI(3,4,5)P3 transduce signals downstream in several important pathways.

phosphoinositide-dependent PK 1 (*PDPK1*). Akt is serine/threonine PK which gets activated by this pathway. In the PK AKT (PKB), PI(3,4)P_2 binds to the PH domain of AKT, thereby releasing an autoinhibitory conformation. This results in partial kinase activation by the kinase PDPK1 (refer **Fig. 11**). Full activation of AKT is performed by a second phosphorylation by the mammalian target of rapamycin complex 2 (mTORC2). There are other kinases also involved as a secondary activator of AKT.

Target of Rapamycin

The control of cell growth by the PI3K-Akt pathway depends partly on a large PK called TOR (named as the target of *rapamycin).* It is a bacterial toxin which inactivates the kinase and is used as an immunosuppressant as well as anticancer drug). TOR was originally detected in yeasts and in mammalian cells, it is called mTOR. It is present in cells in two functionally distinct multiprotein complexes.

- **mTOR complex 1:** It contains the protein *raptor* and this complex is sensitive to rapamycin. Its functions are:
  - Stimulates cell growth by promoting ribosome production and protein synthesis as well as by inhibiting protein degradation.
  - Promotes both cell growth and cell survival by stimulating nutrient uptake and metabolism. The mTOR in complex 1 integrates inputs from various sources (including *growth factors* and nutrients such as amino acids), both of which help activate mTOR and promote cell growth. The growth factors activate mTOR mainly via the PI3K-Akt pathway. The net result is that Akt activates mTOR and thereby promotes cell growth.
- **mTOR complex 2:** It contains the protein *rictor* and is insensitive to rapamycin. Its functions are:
  - Help to activate Akt (see **Fig. 16**)
  - Regulates the actin cytoskeleton via Rho family GTPases

The *PI3K-Akt signaling pathway* is the major pathway activated by the hormone *insulin.* It also plays an important role in promoting the survival and growth of many cell types. Once activated Akt can phosphorylate various target proteins at the plasma membrane, in the cytosol, and nucleus. This inactivates most of the target proteins.

The transduction of signals from RTKs and cytokine receptors begins with the formation of multiprotein complexes associated with the plasma membrane. These complexes initiate the RAS/MAP kinase pathway (refer page 56)

Phosphorylation of these messenger molecules is regulated by PI3K family members. PTEN can antagonize the activity of lipid phosphatases.

Convergence, Divergence, and Crosstalk Among Different Signaling Pathways

All the signaling pathways described earlier were discussed as linear pathways leading directly from a receptor at the cell surface to an end target. In actual fact, these signaling pathways in the cell are much more complex than mentioned in the previous pages.

Examples of convergence, divergence, and crosstalk among signaling pathways:

- **Convergence:** Signals from a different unrelated receptor, each binding to its own complimentary ligand, can *converge* to activate a common effector, such as RAS or Raf (**Fig. 17**). Example, three types of receptors namely GPCRs, RTKs, and integrins may bind to very different ligands. But all of them can lead to the use of the same adaptor protein and activate RAS and transmit signals down the MAP kinase pathway. Thus, as a consequence of this convergence, signals from different types of receptors can lead to the transcription and translation of a similar set of growth promoting genes in each target cell.
- **Divergence:** Signals from the same ligand, such as EGF or insulin, can *diverge* to activate different effectors, thereby leading to diverse cellular responses. Signal divergence may be observed in virtually all the signal transduction that have been described in this chapter.
- **Crosstalk:** Signals can move back and forth between different pathways, a phenomenon termed as *crosstalk*. It was discussed earlier that number of signaling pathways work as if each operated as an independent, linear chain of events. However, it is the fact that the information circuits that operate in cells are more like an interconnected web in which components produced in one pathway can participate in events occurring in other pathways.

These characteristics of cell-signaling pathways are presented diagrammatically in **Figures 18** and **19**.

Signaling pathways provide a mechanism for routing information through a cell. The cell receives information about its environment through the activation of various surface receptors. These receptors act like sensors to detect extracellular stimuli. The cell-surface receptors can bind only to specific ligands and are not affected by the presence of any variety of unrelated molecules. A single cell may contain dozens of different receptors sending signals to the cell interior

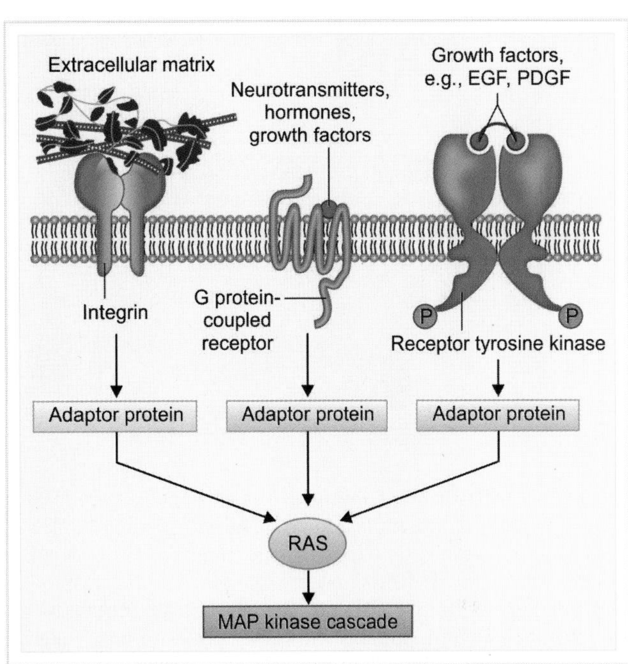

FIG. 18: Convergence of signals. Signals transmitted from a G protein-coupled receptor, an integrin, and a receptor tyrosine kinase all converge on RAS. Then they are transmitted along the mitogen-activated protein (MAP) kinase cascade.

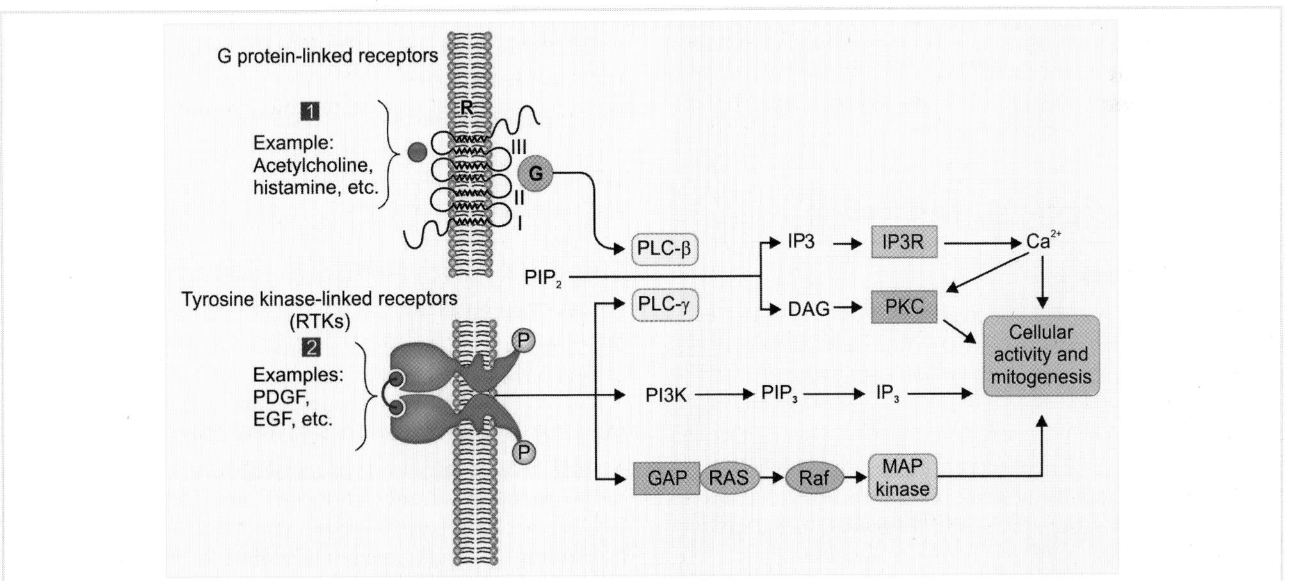

FIG. 17: Examples of convergence, divergence, and crosstalk among various signal transduction pathways. This outlines the two signal transduction pathways initiated by receptors that act by means of—(1) heterotrimeric G proteins lionked receptors, and (2) receptor protein-tyrosine kinases (RTKs). The two pathways converge by the activation of different phospholipase C (PLC) isoforms, both of which lead to the production of the same second messengers [inositol trisphosphate (IP_3) and diacylglycerol (DAG)]. Activation of the RTKs by either platelet-derived growth factor (PDGF) or epidermal growth factor (EGF) leads to the transmission of signals along three different pathways and this an example of divergence. Crosstalk between the two types of pathways by calcium ions by action of IP_3 can act on various proteins, including protein kinase C (PKC), whose activity is also stimulated by DAG.

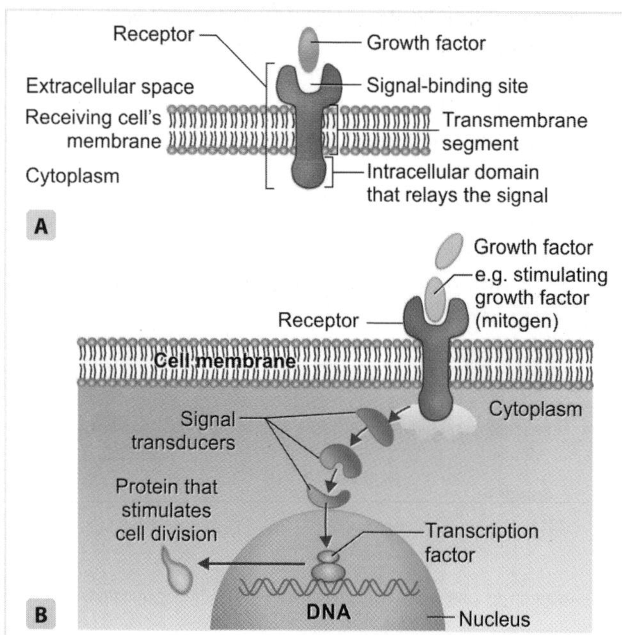

FIGS. 19A AND B: Steps involved in signaling through growth factors. Binding of growth factors to its receptors starts the signal transduction cascades. (A) A growth factor binds to the extracellular domain of a growth factor receptor in the cell membrane. (B) This binding transmits a signal to the intracellular domain of the receptor. This in turn interacts with other signaling molecules. At the end of the signal transduction cascade are transcription factors that can turn on or off the expression of genes. It finally stimulates cell division.

simultaneously. Once they are transmitted into the cell, signals from these receptors can selectively go through a number of different signaling pathways. These pathways may cause a cell to divide, change shape, activate a particular metabolic pathway, or even commit suicide. In this way, the cell integrates information received from different sources and elicits an appropriate and comprehensive response.

GROWTH FACTORS AND RECEPTORS

Growth Factors

Q. Write short essay on growth factors.

Q. Describe the role of growth factors in health and disease (for disease refer pages 444–447).

Definition

Growth factor is a molecule/substance which signals/stimulates the activity of proteins that are needed for cell survival, differentiation, proliferation/**growth and division** of living cells.

There are many growth factors. Though their protein structures have significant diversity, they have a remarkably similar overall mechanism of relaying signals. Growth factors produce their effects by interacting with **specific receptors** on cell surfaces. This initiates **various signaling events. Main role of growth factors is to stimulate the activity of genes that are needed for cell growth and cell division.** Growth factors can act in an **endocrine**, **paracrine**, or **autocrine** manner (refer **Fig. 2**). They affect a wide variety of cells to produce a **mitogenic response.**

Box 5: Consequences of gene expression by growth factor.

- Promote entry of cell into the cell cycle
- Relieve blocks on cell cycle progression, thereby promotes cell replication
- Inhibit apoptosis
- Enhance synthesis of components needed for division of cells(e.g., nucleic acids, proteins, lipids, carbohydrates)

Significance: Growth factors bind to specific receptors and influence expression of genes. Its consequences are summarized in **Box 5**. Apart from stimulation of cell proliferation and/or survival, growth factors can regulate nongrowth activities ssuch as migration, differentiation, and synthetic capacity of cells.

Growth factors regulate proliferation of cells at steady state and in response to injury, when there is need for replacing the irreversibly damaged cells. Uncontrolled cell proliferation can occur when there is dysregulation of growth factor activity or when there is alteration in growth factor signaling pathways that leads to constitutively activation of cell proliferation. Many growth factor pathway genes are proto-oncogenes. Because these genes have proliferative effects, gain-of-function mutations convert them into oncogenes. These oncogens lead to uncontrolled cell division and can be precursors to cancer. Growth factors can signal through any of the pathways shown in **Fig. 4**. Most growth factors mainly involve receptors with intrinsic kinase activity (**Fig. 11**).

Signaling Mechanisms of Growth Factor Receptors

The **receptor-mediated signal transduction** process is activated by the binding of ligands (e.g., growth factors and cytokines) to specific receptors. Receptor activation leads to expression of specific genes.

Steps in Growth Factors Mediated Cell Division (Figs. 19A and B)

Q. Write short essay on signaling mechanisms in cell growth.

Binding of Growth Factors to Receptors

Growth factors come into contact with proteins named **growth factor receptors** found on the surface of a cell (i.e., ligands bind to receptors). Most growth factors deliver their message by binding to specific receptors embedded in the membrane of the receiving cell (i.e., cell which will be prompted to grow or to stop growing). The growth factor receptors are proteins that have three parts namely—(1) a signal-binding site outside the cell, (2) a transmembrane segment that passes through the cell membrane, and (3) an intracellular domain that relays the signal (i.e., the binding of growth factor) to other proteins inside the cell's cytoplasm.

Signal Transduction Cascades

Series of biochemical reactions called as **signal transduction cascade** occurs within that cell. The cytoplasmic proteins that transmit the signal inside the cell is called as **signal transducers.** There are several different signal transducers and one of the examples of a signal transduction system is the RAS protein (refer **Fig. 11**). RAS is a molecular switch that exists in two forms:

1. **Inactive form:** In this form, RAS is bound to GDP (RAS–GDP).
2. **Active form:** In this form, RAS is bound to GTP (RAS–GTP).

When a growth factor activates a growth factor receptor, the intracellular domain of the receptor flips the RAS switch to on by exchanging GDP for GTP. Next, RAS–GTP activates a series of three enzymes called **protein kinases.** They add phosphate groups to other proteins. The first kinase in the chain activates the second kinase, which in turn activates the third kinase. The RAS–GTP turned on by three PKs is termed as a *MAP kinase cascade* (**Figs. 11, 14 and 20**).

Transcriptional Regulation of Cell-cycle Genes

The final components of most growth-factor-initiated signal transduction cascades are **activation of genes that encode transcription factors (TFs)** in the nucleus. These TFs either activate or repress the expression of specific genes. The products of these activated genes either promote or inhibit cell proliferation. In RAS-mediated signaling, the MAP kinase phosphorylates specific TFs in the nucleus. These TFs influence the expression of the cell-cycle genes. Important cell-cycle genes activated in response to growth factors are the *cyclins* and CDKs.

Simplified schematic representation steps involved in transduction and transcription from the surface of the cell to nucleus is presented in **Figure 21**.

Effects of Growth Factor Action

Growth factors induce cell proliferation by **binding to specific receptors**, and deliver positive growth signals to the target cells. These signals stimulate the **expression of genes** whose products have several functions which include:

- **Activation of cell cycle:** Promote entry of cells into the cell cycle. Growth factors are not only involved in the proliferation of cells at steady state but also needed for replacement of irreversibly damaged cells after injury.
- Relieve blocks which prevent cell cycle progression (thus promoting replication)
- Prevention of apoptosis
- Increases the synthesis of cellular components (nucleic acids, proteins, lipids, carbohydrates) needed for a mother cell to produce two daughter cells.

Growth factors are proteins that usually stimulate cell proliferation and/or survival. But they can also have nongrowth activities, including migration, differentiation, and synthetic capacity. Growth inhibitory factors also exist. For example, TGF-β inhibits the growth of certain cells. Thus, chronic exposure to either increased amounts of a growth factor, or to decreased amounts of a growth inhibitory factor, can change the balance of cellular growth.

Various Types of Growth Factors (Table 2)

Selected growth factors that are involved in two important proliferative processes (1) tissue repair, and (2) tumor development are summarized in **Table 2.**

Hepatocyte Growth Factor

Hepatocyte growth factor (HGF; also known as scatter factor) was originally recognized as a growth factor produced by platelets that stimulated DNA production in rat hepatocytes in primary culture. It was biochemically distinct from PDGF.

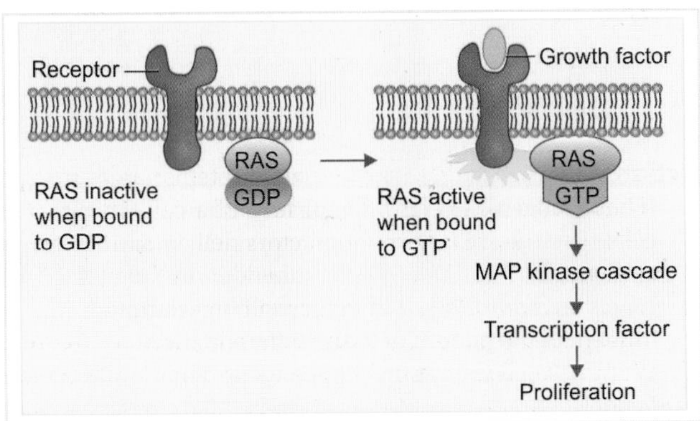

FIG. 20: RAS-mediated signal transduction cascade. The RAS protein is an intracellular signaling molecule. When a growth factor binds to the cellular receptor, inactive RAS bound to GDP becomes active by binding to GTP.

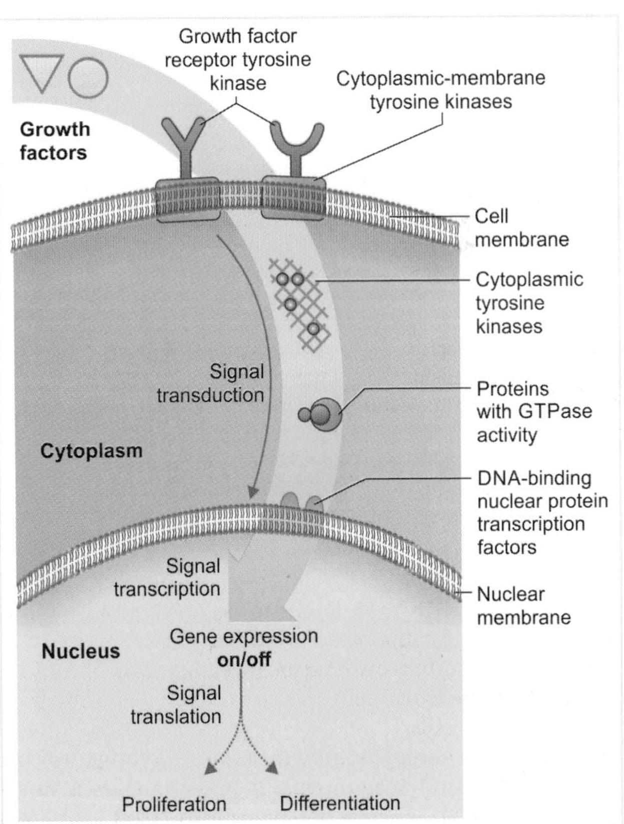

FIG. 21: Simplified schematic representation steps involved in transduction and transcription from the surface of the cell to nucleus.

Table 2: Growth factors involved in regeneration and repair.

Type of growth factor	*Receptor*	*Source*	*Functions*
Growth factor			
Epidermal growth factor (EGF) family EGF-α	EGF receptor (EGFR): • EGFR1 (ERBB1) • ERBB2 (HER-2 or HER2/Neu)	Activated macrophages, salivary glands, keratinocytes, etc.	• Mitogenic for epithelial cells, and fibroblasts • Stimulates migration of epithelial cell • Formation of granulation tissue
Hepatocyte growth factor (HGF) (scatter factor)	Mesenchymal epithelial transition factor (c-MET)	Fibroblasts, stromal cells in the liver, endothelial cells	• Increases proliferation of hepatocytes and other epithelial cells • Increases cell motility
Transforming growth factor-alpha (TGF-α)	EGFR	Activated macrophages, keratinocytes, etc.	Stimulates proliferation of hepatocytes and many other epithelial cells
Platelet-derived growth factor (PDGF) • Isoforms A, B, C, D	Platelet-derived growth factor receptor (PDGFR) α and β	Platelets, macrophages, endothelial cells, smooth muscle cells, keratinocytes	• Chemotactic for neutrophils, macrophages, fibroblasts, and smooth muscle cells • Activates and stimulates proliferation of fibroblasts, endothelial, neuroglial cells, and other cells • Stimulates production of extracellular matrix (ECM)
Vascular endothelial growth factor (VEGF) • Isoforms A, B, C, D	Vascular endothelial growth factor receptor (VEGFR)-1, VEGFR-2, and VEGFR-3	Mesenchymal cells	• Mediates functions of endothelial cells; proliferation, migration, invasion, survival of endothelial cells • Increases vascular permeability
Fibroblast growth factors (FGFs), [includes acidic (aFGF, or FGF-1) and basic (bFGF, or FGF-2)]	Fibroblast growth factor receptors (FGFRs) 1–4	Macrophages, mast cells, endothelial cells, etc.	• Chemotactic and mitogenic for fibroblasts, myoblasts • Stimulates endothelial cells,s angiogenesis and synthesis of ECM protein
Transforming growth factor beta (TGF-β) and related growth factors • TGF-β isoforms (TGF-β1, TGF-β2, TGF-β3)	TGF-β receptors (types I and II)	Platelets, T lymphocytes, macrophages, endothelial cells, keratinocytes, smooth muscle cells, fibroblasts	• Chemotactic for leukocytes and fibroblasts • Potent fibrogenic agent, stimulates ECM protein synthesis • Suppresses acute inflammation • Regulates differentiation of some cell types (e.g., cartilage)
Keratinocyte growth factor (KGF) (i.e., FGF-7)	Keratinocyte growth factor receptor (KGFR)	Fibroblasts	Stimulates migration, proliferation, and differentiation of keratinocyte
Cytokines			
Tumor necrosis factor (TNF) and interleukin (IL)-1 participate in wound healing • TNF and IL-6 are involved in liver regeneration	TNF receptor (TNFR), or death receptor, for TNF, IL-1 receptor (IL-1R) for IL-1 and IL-6 receptor (IL-6R) also known as CD126 (cluster of differentiation 126) for IL-6		TNF activates macrophages; regulates other cytokines and has multiple functions

Subsequently, HGF were found to be involved in various physiological and pathological processes.

Source: Hepatocyte growth factor is produced by fibroblasts and most mesenchymal cells, as well as endothelium and non-hepatocyte liver cells.

Synthesis: Hepatocyte growth factor belongs to the plasminogen family of proteins. It is secreted as a single polypeptide in an inactive precursor (pro-HGF) form. It is proteolytically activated by a thrombin-like soluble enzyme called HGF activator (HGFA) or by serine proteases released at sites of injury (site-specific).

Actions

- It has mitogenic effects on hepatocytes and most epithelial cells, such as biliary, pulmonary, renal, mammary, and epidermal.
- It acts as a *morphogen* in embryonic development (i.e., it influences the pattern of tissue differentiation).
- Promotes cell migration (hence its designation as *scatter factor*).
- Enhances hepatocyte survival.

Significance of MET receptor: MET is the receptor for HGF, it has intrinsic tyrosine kinase activity. MET is frequently overexpressed or mutated in tumors (e.g., renal and thyroid papillary carcinomas). Thus, MET inhibitors may be of value for cancer therapy.

Epidermal growth factor and transforming growth factor-α

Both of these factors belong to the EGF family and bind to the same receptors, which explain why they share many biologic activities.

Source: Epidermal growth factor and TGF-α are produced by macrophages and a variety of epithelial cells.

Action: They are mitogenic for hepatocytes, fibroblasts, and a host of epithelial cells.

Epidermal growth factor receptor family

Epidermal growth factor ligands signal through a group of membrane receptors with intrinsic tyrosine kinase activity known as epidermal growth factor receptors (EGFRs or ERBB receptors). Well known receptors in this group are four namely, EGFR1 (also known as ERB-B1, or simply EGFR) and *ERBB2 receptor* (also known as *HER2*); ERBB3, and ERBB4. These four receptors share similar structural features.

Significance

- EGFR1 mutations and/or amplification frequently seen cancers such as lung, head and neck, breast, and brain.
- *ERBB2 receptor* (*HER2*) is overexpressed in a subset of breast cancers.
- Tumors with these receptors have been successfully targeted by antibodies and small molecule antagonists.

Platelet-derived Growth Factor (PDGF)

Platelet-derived growth factor is a family of several closely related proteins. They are dimers consisting of two chains (designated by pairs of letters). Three isoforms of PDGF (AA, AB, and BB) are constitutively active whereas PDGF-CC and PDGF-DD need activation by proteolytic cleavage.

Source: Platelet-derived growth factor is stored in platelet granules and is released on activation of platelets. They were originally isolated from platelets (hence the name). It is also produced by many other cells such as activated macrophages, endothelium, smooth muscle cells, and a variety of tumors.

Action: All PDGF isoforms produce their effects by binding to two PDGF cell surface receptors namely, PDGFR-α and β. Both of these have intrinsic tyrosine kinase activity.

- Platelet-derived growth factor induces proliferation of fibroblast, endothelial, and smooth muscle cell; synthesis of matrix, and is chemotactic for these cells (and inflammatory cells). Thus, it promotes recruitment of the cells into areas of inflammation and tissue injury.

Vascular Endothelial Growth Factor (VEGF)

Vascular endothelial growth factors are a family of homodimeric proteins. These include VEGF-A, B, C, and D, and placental growth factor (PlGF) (**Fig. 22**).

Actions: Vascular endothelial growth factors bind to a family of RTKs [VEGF receptors (VEGFR)-1, 2, and 3]; VEGFR-2 is highly expressed in endothelium and is responsible for angiogenesis.

- VEGF-A is simply known as VEGF. It is the major *angiogenic* factor which stimulates the development of blood vessel after injury and in tumors.
- VEGF-B and placental growth factor (PlGF) are involved in development of embryonic vessel.
- VEGF-C and D stimulate both angiogenesis and lymphatic development (*lymphangiogenesis*).
- VEGFs are also involved in the maintenance of normal adult endothelium (i.e., not involved in angiogenesis). Their expression is high in epithelial cells adjacent to fenestrated epithelium such as podocytes in the kidney, pigment epithelium in the retina, and choroid plexus in the brain.
- VEGF induces angiogenesis by promoting endothelial cell migration, proliferation (capillary sprouting), and formation of the vascular lumen.
- VEGFs also induce vascular dilation and increased vascular permeability. VEGF was originally termed vascular permeability factor to indicate these vascular activities.

Inducers of vascular endothelial growth factor

- **Hypoxia:** It is the most important inducing factor for production of VEGF, through pathways that involve intracellular hypoxia-inducible factor (HIF-1).
- **Other VEGF inducers:** These include PDGF and TGF-α which are produced at sites of inflammation or wound healing.

Uses of Anti-vascular endothelial growth factor antibodies

VEGFs bind to a family of tyrosine kinase receptors. These include VEGFR-1, VEGFR-2, and VEGFR-3. VEGFR-2 is highly

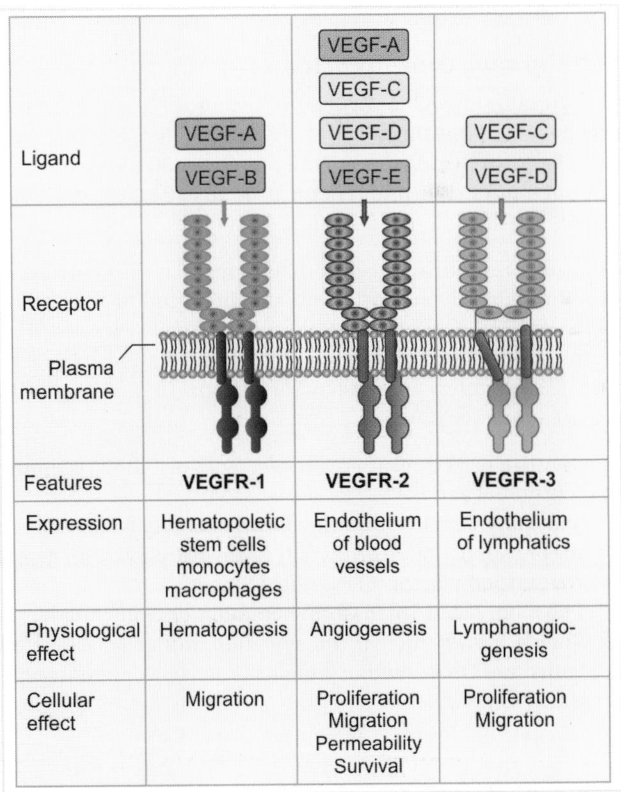

FIG. 22: Various vascular endothelial growth factors and its receptors.

expressed in endothelium and is the most important receptor involved in angiogenesis.

- **Cancers:** Antibodies against VEGF can be used for the treatment of several tumors (e.g., renal and colon cancers) which need angiogenesis for their spread and growth.
- **Ophthalmic diseases:** Used for diseases such as "wet" age-related macular degeneration (AMD is a disorder characterized by inappropriate angiogenesis and vascular permeability and causes adult-onset blindness), the angiogenesis associated with retinopathy of prematurity, and the leaky vessels that lead to diabetic macular edema.
    - Increased levels of soluble versions of VEGFR-1 (s-FLT-1) may cause pre-eclampsia (hypertension and proteinuria) in pregnant women. This is by "sequestering" the free VEGF required for maintaining normal endothelium.

Fibroblast Growth Factor (FDF)

Fibroblast growth factor is a family of growth factors consisting of >20 members. Most important being acidic FGF (aFGF, or FGF-1), basic FGF (bFGF, or FGF-2), and FGF-7 [also called keratinocyte growth factor (KGF)].

Mechanism of Action: Fibroblast growth factors, after release, associate with heparan sulfate in the ECM. This acts as a reservoir for inactive factors which can be subsequently released by proteolysis (e.g., at sites of wound healing). FGFs transduce signals through four tyrosine kinase receptors [fibroblast growth factor receptors (FGFRs 1–4)].

Actions: Fibroblast growth factors are involved in wound healing, hematopoiesis, and development. bFGF is also involved in angiogenesis.

Transforming Growth Factor-β (TGF-β)

Transforming growth factor-β is distinct from TGF-α (described previously). It has three isoforms (TGF-β1, TGF-β2, TGF-β3). Each isoform belongs to a family of about 30 members and includes bone morphogenetic proteins (BMPs), activins, inhibins, and Müllerian inhibiting substance.

Source: Transforming growth factor-β1 is homodimeric protein which is most widely distributed and is commonly called as TGF-β. It is produced by many cell types, such as platelets, endothelium, and mononuclear inflammatory cells. TGF-β is secreted as a precursor that needs proteolysis to release the active protein.

Mechanism of Action: There are two types of TGF-β receptors namely types I and II.

- They have **serine/threonine kinase activity** which induce the phosphorylation of a variety of downstream cytoplasmic transcription factors (TFs) called *Smads.*
- Phosphorylated Smads form heterodimers with Smad4.
- Smad4 allows nuclear translocation and gets associated with other DNA-binding proteins to activate or inhibit gene transcription.

Actions

- **Pleiotropic:** TGF-β has multiple and often opposing effects. Their actions depend on the tissue and concurrent signals. Agents with such diversity or multiplicity of effects are termed as "pleiotropic with a vengeance". It plays an important role in many physiological processes such as adhesion, migration, differentiation, apoptosis, and the determination of cell fate.
- **Scar formation:** TGF-β is mainly involved in scar formation after injury and checks the inflammation during wound healing. TGF-β stimulates the synthesis of collagen, fibronectin, and proteoglycans. It inhibits degradation of collagen by—(1) decreasing matrix metalloproteinase (MMP) activity, and (2) increasing the activity of tissue inhibitors of metalloproteinases (TIMPs).
- **Fibrosis:** TGF-β is also involved in fibrosis of lung, liver, and kidneys during chronic inflammation.
- **Anti-inflammatory:** TGF-β is an anti-inflammatory cytokine. It serves to limit and terminate inflammatory responses by inhibiting lymphocyte proliferation and the activity of other leukocytes.

Examples of other growth factors are presented in **Table 3**.

Table 3: Examples of other growth factors and their physiological actions.

Growth factor	Physiological actions
Insulin-like growth factor 1 (IGF-1)	• Collaborates with platelet-derived growth factor (PDGF) and epidermal growth factor (EGF) • Stimulates proliferation of fat cells and connective tissue cells
Insulin-like growth factor 2 (IGF-2)	• Collaborates with PDGF and EGF • Stimulates or inhibits response of most cells to other growth factors • Regulates differentiation of some cell types (e.g., cartilage)
Transforming growth factor-beta (TGF-β; multiple subtypes)	• Stimulates or inhibits response of most cells to other growth factors • Regulates differentiation of some cell types (e.g., cartilage)
Interleukin-2 (IL-2)	Stimulates proliferation of T lymphocytes
Nerve growth factor (NGF)	Promotes axon growth and survival of sympathetic and some sensory and central nervous system (CNS) neurons
Hematopoietic cell growth factors (IL-3, GM-CSF, G-CSF, M-CSF, erythropoietin)	Promote proliferation and growth of white and red blood cells

(G-CSF: granulocyte colony-stimulating factor; GM-CSF: granulocyte–macrophage colony-stimulating factor; M-CSF: macrophage colony-stimulating factor)

BIBLIOGRAPHY

1. Alberts B, Johnson A, Lewis J, Morgan D, Raff M, Roberts K, Walter P. Molecular Biology of the cell, 6th edition. New York: Taylor & Francis; 2015.
2. Bradshaw RA, Dennis EA. Functioning of Transmembrane Receptors in Cell Signaling, 1st edition. Academic Press: 2011
3. Duronio RJ, Xiong Y. Signaling pathways that control cell proliferation. *Cold Spring Harb Perspect Biol*. 2013;5:1.
4. Hancock: Cell signalling. 3rd edition. New York Oxford: Wiley; 2010.
5. Horst A. Molecular pathology, Sound Parkway: CRC Press; 2018.
6. Iwasa J, Marshall W. Karp's cell and molecular biology, 8th edition. Hoboken:John Wiley & Sons: 2016.
7. Karp G. Molecular and cell biology: Concepts and experiments. 6th edition. Hoboken: Taylor & Francis; 2010.
8. Kumar V, Abbas AK, Aster JC. Robbins basic pathology, 10th edition. Philadelphia: Saunders Elsevier; 2018
9. Kumar V, Abbas AK, Fausto N, et al. Robbins and Cotran pathologic basis of disease, 10th edition. Philadelphia: WB Saunders; 2021.
10. Morrison DK: MAP kinase pathways. *Cold Spring Harb Perspect Biol.* 2012;4:1.
11. Nusse R, Clevers H: Wnt/β-catenin signaling, disease, and emerging therapeutic modalities. *Cell.* 2017;169:985.
12. Perona R: Cell signalling: growth factors and tyrosine kinase receptors. *Clin Transl Oncol.* 2011;8:77.
13. Purves D, Augustine GJ, Fitzpatrick D, et al., Neuriscience, 2nd edition. Sunderland (MA): Sinauer Associates; 2001.
14. Ria R , Melaccio A, Racanelli V, Vacca A: Anti-VEGF Drugs in the treatment of multiple myeloma patients. *J Clin Med.* 2020;9:1765.
15. Shukla, Arun K: Methods in Cell Biology. Elsevier: 2016.
16. Strayer DS, Saffitz JE. Rubin's Pathology: Mechanism of Human Disease, 8th edition. Philadelphia: Wolters Kluwer; 2020.

CHAPTER 3

Maintaining Cell Populations

CHAPTER OUTLINE

PROLIFERATION AND CELL CYCLE

Q. Write a short essay on cell cycle.
Q. Discuss the molecular events in cell growth.

For growth or replacement of dead/damaged/normally lost cells, it requires additional cells. For this, new ones must be produced by **cell division,** or **proliferation.** Cell proliferation is essential for the development and maintenance of steady state tissue homeostasis (stable system maintenance).

Somatic cells are produced by the division of existing cells in an orderly sequence of events. For cellular proliferation/division to generate two daughter cells, first accurate, complete duplication/replication of deoxyribonucleic acid (DNA) should occur along with coordinated synthesis of all other constituents of cells (biosynthesis of other cellular components). This is followed by equal distribution of DNA and other cellular constituents (e.g., organelles) to produce two identical daughter cells through mitosis and cytokinesis (division of the cytoplasm, exclusive of nuclear division, that occurs during the final stages of mitosis and meiosis to form daughter cells). This sequence of duplication is called as the **cell cycle.** Proliferation of cells is characterized by DNA replication and mitosis. Cell division occurs throughout the life, although different cell types divide more or less often than others. Cells have variation in their proliferative capacity, depending on the cell type and the age of the individual.

Cell Cycle

Definition of Cell Cycle: The **sequence of events that control DNA replication and mitosis** and **results in cell division** is called the *cell cycle.*

Phases of Cell

Cells may be cycling or quiescent. Different phases of cell cycle are presented in **Box 1** and **Figure 1**. Cells that divide continuously (e.g., intestinal mucosa, hematopoietic progenitor cells) always undergo transition from mitosis (M phase) to G_1 (gap 1) and undergo continuous cell division. By contrast, cells that divide (replicate) infrequently (e.g., hepatocytes) are in a quiescent phase (G_0). These cells in G_0 may enter G_1 phase when they receive various stimuli. Cells in G_1 phase then synthesize their DNA in S phase and proceed to G_2 and ultimately to M phase (**Fig. 1**). Following mitosis, cells again enter G_1, if they are in an actively dividing mode or to G_0 phase.

Box 1: Different phases of cell cycle.

- G_1 (presynthetic) phase
- S (DNA synthesis) phase
- G_2 (premitotic) phase
- M (mitotic) phase

(DNA: deoxyribonucleic acid)

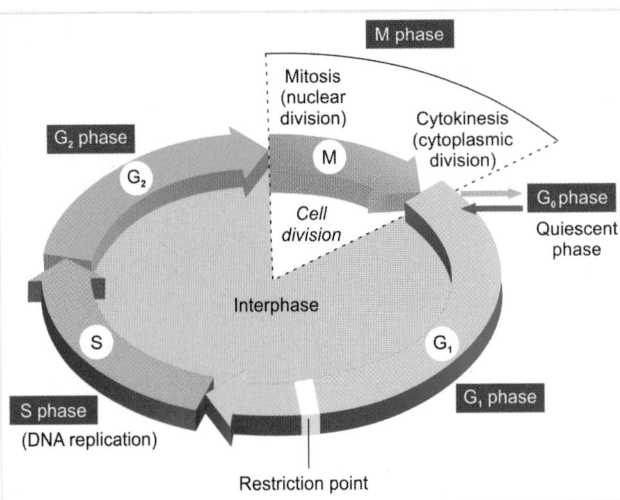

FIG. 1: Diagrammatic representation of different phases of cell cycle. It consists of G_1 (gap 1), S (DNA synthesis), G_2 (gap 2), and M (mitotic) phases. The quiescent cells that are not actively cycling are in the G_0 (gap 0) state.

- **Quiescent cells** (state of inactivity) are those cells that temporarily or reversibly stop dividing and are called to be in **G_0 phase/state**. Cells can enter G_1 phase either from the G_0 quiescent cell pool or after completion of a round of mitosis.
- **Senescent** cells are cells that permanently stop dividing, either **due to aging or due to accumulated DNA damage.**
- **Replicative senescence:** Normal somatic cells (i.e., cells forming the body and not the germ line cells) are capable of only a limited number of cell divisions. After these number of divisions, they enter a **nondividing but viable state** called as replicative senescence.

Q. Explain cell cycle regulation in health and disease.
Q. Discuss the cell cycle and its role in tissue homeostasis.

Cell Cycle Regulators

Cell cycle regulators control progression of cell cycle. Many checks and balances help in highly regulating the cell cycle so that there is a state of balance or **homeostasis between cell proliferation, cell differentiation, and cell death.** The patterns of expression of cell regulator proteins and enzymes depend upon the cell cycle phase. Each phase/stage needs completion of the previous phase/step and activation of necessary factors. Lack of prompt and accurate DNA replication or deficiency of cofactor results in arrest of cell cycle at the various transition points. **Cell cycle is regulated by many activators and inhibitors, as well as checkpoints.** Regulatory molecules involved in cell cycle progression are categorized into two important classes, namely—(i) **cyclins and (ii) cyclin-dependent kinases (CDKs).** These two types form a series of dimeric complexes **(cyclin-CDKs)** that cause progression of cell proliferation (**Fig. 2**). Certain **cyclin-CDKs** have enzymatic (kinase) activity. Whenever needed, **cyclin-dependent kinase inhibitors** (CKI) inhibit cyclin-CDK complexes.

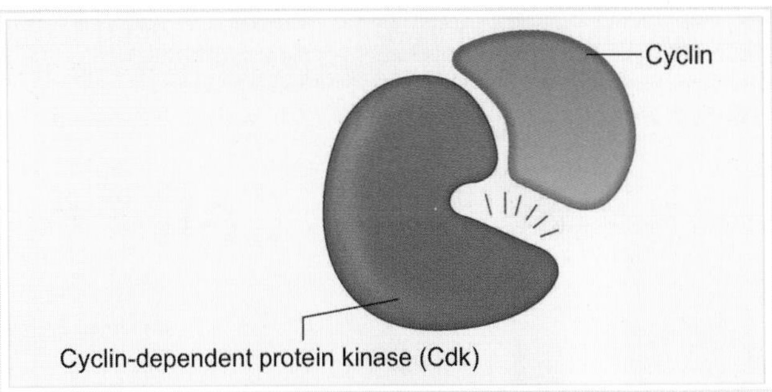

FIG. 2: Formation of cyclin–cyclin dependent kinase (CDK) complex. Progression through the cell cycle depends on CDKs. A CDK must bind to a regulatory protein cyclin before it can become enzymatically active. This activation also needs an activating phosphorylation of the CDK. Once activated, a cyclin–CDK complex phosphorylates key proteins in the cell that are needed to initiate particular steps in the cell cycle.

CYCLINS

Q. Role of cyclins in cell cycle progression.
Q. Write about the role of cyclins in cell cycle transition.

Cell cycle progression is dependent on two important classes of regulatory molecules, cyclins, and CDKs. Cyclins are a family (>15) of cell cycle regulatory proteins. They are named cyclins because of the cyclic nature of their production and degradation. The cyclins are **categorized as cyclins D, E, A, or B**. Different cyclins are produced to regulate specific phases of the cell cycle. The concentrations of cyclin rise and fall throughout the cell cycle due to its synthesis and degradation via the proteosomal pathway (refer **Fig. 4**). There are different categories of cyclins.

- **D-type cyclins** [cyclins D1, (refer **Fig. 8**) D2, and D3] regulate G_1 phase. Once a cell is stimulated to divide (e.g., by growth factors), D-type cyclins are activated first. They are critical for progression through the restriction point, the point beyond which a cell irreversibly progresses through the remainder of the cell cycle.
- **S phase cyclins** include type E cyclins and cyclin A (**Table 1**).
- **Mitotic cyclins** include cyclins B and A.

Major cyclin and CDK complexes regulating the cell cycle, important target proteins and CDK inhibitors are presented in **Table 1**.

Cyclin-dependent Kinases

Apart from cyclins, cell-cycle progression is operated by cyclin-associated enzymes known as cyclin-dependent kinases (CDKs). This is a family of protein kinases (PKs) which are the essential drivers of cell cycle events. They are the central controlling molecules that guide the transitions from one cell cycle stage to the next. As the name indicates, CDKs can function only after associating with proteins called **cyclins** (**Fig. 2**). This phosphorylation can either activate or inactivate target proteins (**Fig. 3**). The cyclin portion of

Table 1: Major cyclin and cyclin-dependent kinase (CDK) complexes regulating the cell cycle, important target proteins and CDK inhibitors.

Phase of the cell cycle	*Active cyclin-CDK Complex*	*Examples of target proteins*	*CDK inhibitors*
Early G_1	Cyclin D (D1, D2, and D3)-CDK4 or 6	Phosphorylates Rb protein, releasing transcription factor E2F	For CDK4: p16, p15, p18, p19 For CDK6: p21, p27, p57
Late G_1/entry of S	Cyclin E-CDK2	Further activation E2F-mediated gene transcription, protein p53, other kinases (initiation of DNA synthesis)	p21, p27, p57
Progression through S	Cyclin A-CDK2	DNA polymerase and other proteins for DNA replication	p21, p27, p57
G_2/entry of M	Cyclin A-CDK1	Specific phosphatases and cyclin B	p21, p27, p57
Progression through M	Cyclin B-CDK1	Nuclear lamins, histone H1, chromatin- and centrosome-associated proteins	p21, p27, p57

(CDK: cyclin dependent kinases; DNA: deoxyribonucleic acid; Rb: retinoblastoma)

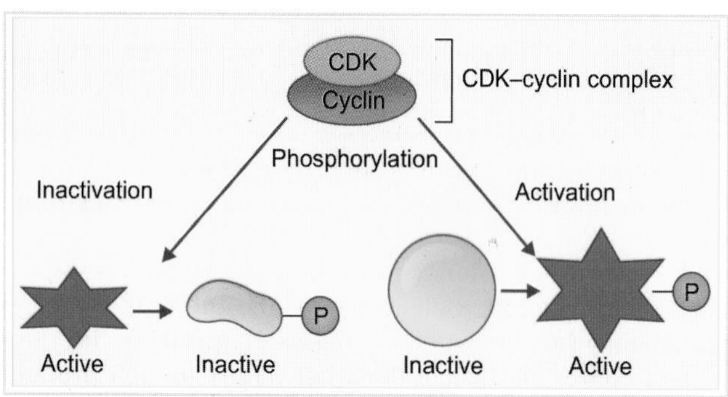

FIG. 3: Actions of cyclin-dependent kinases (CDKs). CDKs control the cell cycle by phosphorylating other proteins. When CDK combines with a cyclin, it can phosphorylate target proteins. Phosphorylation of a protein can either inactivate or activate it.

a CDK–cyclin complex decides which set of proteins to be a phosphorylated and the CDK portion of the complex then causes the actual phosphorylation. CDK–cyclin phosphorylate hundreds of target proteins that perform specific functions at specific times in the cell cycle. Certain cyclins form complexes with certain CDKs and have ability to phosphorylate protein substrates (i.e., kinase activity). Phosphorylation changes the activation status of substrate proteins and permits for initiation of the next phase of the cell cycle. Transiently increased production of a particular cyclin leads to increased kinase activity of the appropriate CDK binding partner. As the CDK completes its round of phosphorylation, the associated cyclin is degraded and the CDK activity subsides. Thus, as cyclin levels rise and fall, the activity of associated CDKs increases and decreases.

- Active CDK2 is responsible for activating target proteins involved in S phase transition (movement from G_1 to S) and for initiation of DNA synthesis.
- CDK1 targets activated proteins needed for the initiation of mitosis.

Different types of cyclins appear in a logical order during the cell cycle and bind to one or more CDKs. The cell cycle thus resembles a relay race in which a distinct set of cyclins appear and leave the track, and the next set takes over.

Different CDK–cyclin Complexes for Different Cell Cycle Transitions (Fig. 4)

In the cell cycle, different CDK–cyclin complexes appear at specific times (**Fig. 4**). The cyclins in these complexes appear at particular stages of the cell cycle and they associate with the appropriate CDKs. They produce their action on target protein. Then they disappear to make way for the succeeding set of cyclins. The precise timed appearances and disappearances of cyclin in the cell cycle is brought out by the two mechanisms—(i) gene regulation that turns on and off the synthesis of particular cyclins, and (ii) regulated protein degradation that removes the cyclins once their action is finished. Cyclin degradation at different phases of cell cycle itself is activated by the CDK–cyclin. Thus, the cell cycle has an intrinsic regulatory mechanism, in which there is activation of one phase followed by irreversible end of that phase.

Cell Cycle Checkpoints (Figs. 1 and 5)

In the cell cycle, there are closely observed (surveillance/vigilance) continuous specific mechanisms aimed to check/sense any DNA or chromosomal damage in the replicating cells. Therefore, there are control mechanisms which give time to cells to repair DNA damage or correct other errors of DNA. These additional controls check for the integrity of the genome before allowing the cell to continue to the next phase of the cell cycle. These are known as **checkpoints**. These checkpoints make sure that only normal cells complete replication (and maintain the genomic stability) and not cells with genetic imperfections. These quality-control *checkpoints* placed at critical points in the cell cycle check the completion of critical events. Damage to DNA of the genome of a cell can cause serious consequences. When cells detect DNA irregularities, checkpoint activation delays the progression to the next stage of the cell cycle and activates DNA repair mechanisms.

If the genetic damage is too severe to be repaired by DNA repair genes, the cells either undergo apoptosis or enter a nonreplicative state called *senescence*—mainly through p53-dependent mechanisms. These cell cycle checkpoints are landmark transitions in the cell cycle and make sure to maintain

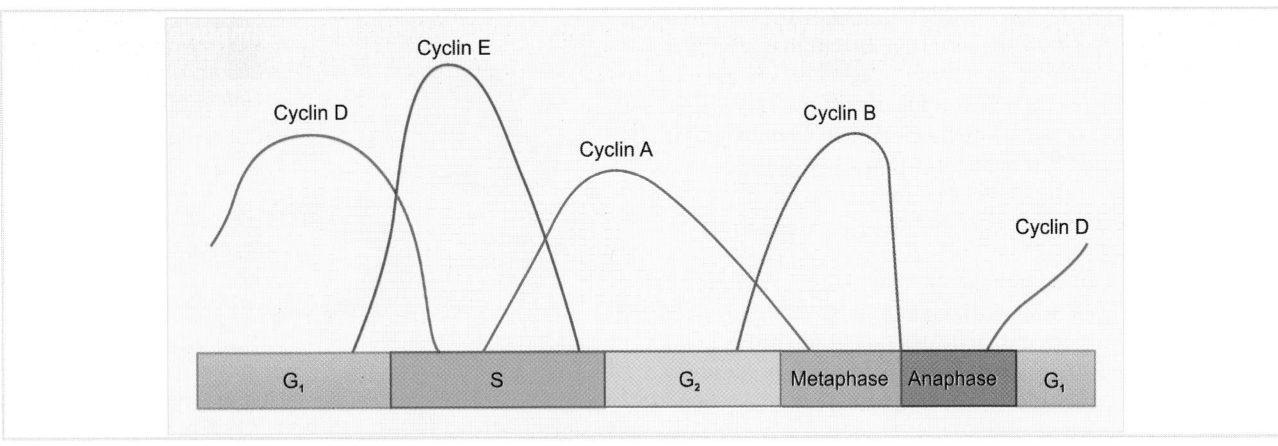

FIG. 4: Different cyclin-dependent kinase (CDK)–cyclin complexes control different cell-cycle transitions. CDKs and cyclins appear during specific stages of cell cycles and prompt the cell to proceed to the next stage.

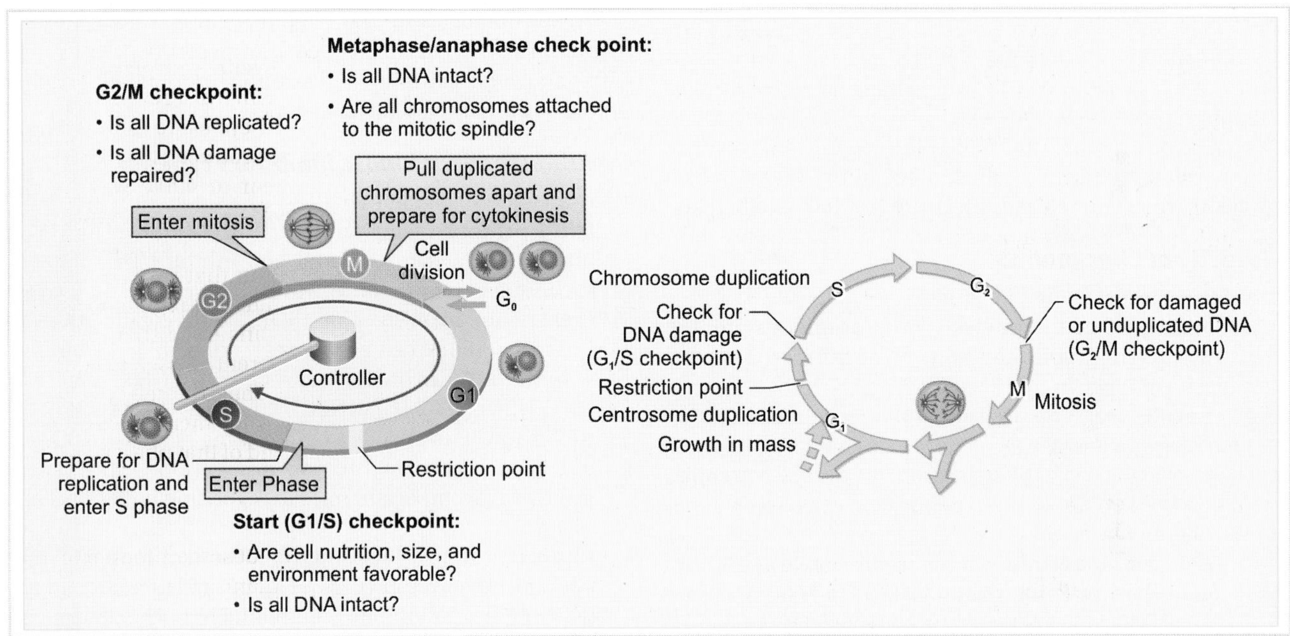

FIG. 5: CDK–cyclin complex's role in mediation of the G_1-to-S phase transition. CDK4 complexed to cyclin D, and CDK2 complexed to cyclin E, phosphorylate the Rb protein. This causes Rb protein to dissociate from E2F. This activates the E2F transcription factor. E2F stimulates the transcription of genes needed for DNA replication, including that for cyclin A. When cells enter S phase, cyclin D is destroyed. Simultaneously CDK2–cyclin A complexes are formed which activate DNA replication.

the genomic stability. Checkpoints are mostly related to DNA damage and mitotic progression. There are two checkpoints:

G_1/S ($G_1 \rightarrow$S) Checkpoint

- **G_1/S checkpoint monitors the integrity of DNA before** DNA replication for next irreversible phase. *G_1-to-S checkpoint* makes sure that cells will not perform the G_1-to-S transition if they have damaged DNA. Radiation or chemical mutagens can produce damage to DNA. When this cell with damaged DNA enters the cell cycle, during G_1 phase, the replication of DNA is postponed. This postponement gives time for DNA repair before the cell proceeds to DNA synthesis; otherwise, replication of the unrepaired damaged DNA can result in dangerous consequences Once the cell passes the R (restriction) point, external forces driving or inhibiting mitosis no longer come into play (i.e., cell proliferation is determined only by intracellular mechanisms). The R point is activated by cyclin D-CDK4/6 phosphorylation of pRb, with consequent release of E2F (refer **Fig. 7**) and proceeds to mitosis. Loss of R-point control is observed in many cancers.
    - **Restriction point** in G_1: The restriction point is related to mitogen deprivation. G_1 restriction point refers to the phase in G_1 at which the cell gets committed to the cell cycle without further need of the growth factor that has initiated cell division. During G_1, the cell decides whether to proceed with mitosis or not. Passage of cell from $G_1 \rightarrow$S occurs when the activity of complexes involving cyclins A and E overpower inhibition by the Cip/Kip family of inhibitors. There are few key

molecular pathways involved in the normal transition from G_1 phase to S phase. First, binding of growth factors to their corresponding receptors on the cell surface initiates a signal transduction cascade. Thus, there is mitogen activation of a growth factor receptor. This activates TFs, which turn on the expression of a suite of downstream genes. Among these downstream genes are those that encode two cyclins namely, cyclin D and cyclin E.

- ○ **If there is DNA damage**, it is sensed by ATM (ataxia telangiectasia mutated) and ATR (ATM and Rad3 related) proteins and activates p53. If the cell is in G_1, p53 increases production of Cip/Kip CKIs family of inhibitors. They block further progress in cell division.

G_2/M ($G_2 \rightarrow$ M) checkpoint

- **G_2/M checkpoint checks DNA after replication** and makes sure that there has been accurate DNA replication before the cell actually divides so that it can safely enter mitosis. Cells pass from $G_2 \rightarrow M$ when cyclin B-CDK1 complexes are activated by removing inhibitory phosphorylation of CDK1. If the cell DNA damage is detected and the cell is in G_2, there are two ways of stopping cell cycle. One way is by p53-mediated down-regulation of cyclin B and CDK1. The other method involves two related enzymes called checkpoint kinases (chk1, chk2), which immediately block progression of cell cycle.

Necessity of Checkpoints

Any defect in checkpoints can produce the following:

- **Instability of cell genomes** (chromosome instability): These include point mutations and chromosome rearrangements such as translocations.
- **Propensity for gene amplification:** Gene amplification (refer Figs. 26 and 27 of Chapter 10) is characterized by an increase in the copies of a gene from the normal two copies to hundreds of copies. This amplification can be seen under the microscope as either:
  - ○ Enlarged area within a chromosome known as a **homogeneously staining region (HSR)**. In HSR, there are increased copies of gene which are inserted/integrated into new chromosomal location which may be distant from the normal location of the involved genes within chromosomes. They contain many tandem repeats of one or more genes. HSR appear as homogeneous in G-banded karyotype, or
  - ○ **Extrachromosomal multiple**, **small**, chromosome-like **structures**/bodies [called **double minutes** (dmin) because of their small size] that lack centromeres and telomeres.

Q. Describe the orchestra of cyclins and cyclin dependent kinases.

Cyclin-dependent Kinase Inhibitors (Fig. 6)

One way of enforcing the cell cycle checkpoints is by *CKIs*. They bring out this by controlling activity of CDK-cyclin complex. There are several different families of CKIs. They strongly inhibit cell proliferation and protect against oncogenesis. CKIs are commonly mutated in human cancers. CKIs exert their effect by either binding to cyclin-CDK complexes

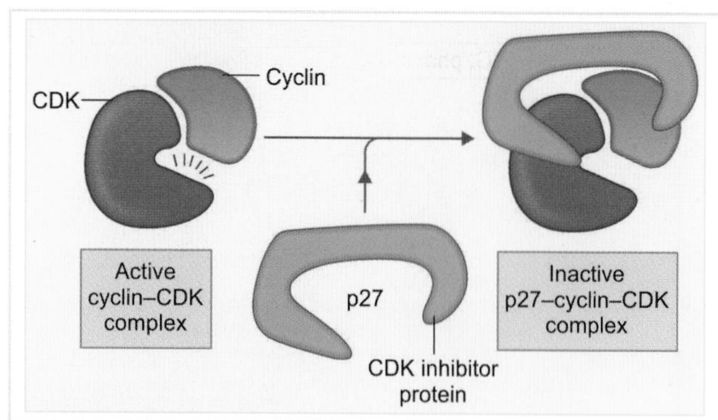

FIG. 6: Cyclin-dependent kinase inhibitors: The activity of cyclin dependent kinases (CDKs) can be blocked by the binding of a CDK inhibitor. For example, in this figure, the CDK inhibitor protein (called p27) binds to an activated cyclin–CDK complex. Its binding prevents the CDK from phosphorylating target proteins needed for the progression of cell cycle through G_1 into S phase.

or directly binding with CDKs and preventing CDK activation by cyclins. Defective CKI checkpoint proteins permits cells with damaged DNA to divide, resulting in mutated daughter cells at risk for developing malignancy.

Cyclin-dependent Kinase Inhibitors Types

There are different families of CKIs.

- **INK4 proteins:** This family of CKIs (known as "INK4 inhibitors") selectively bind and inhibit CDKs namely, cyclin CDK4 and cyclin CDK6 (inhibit cd*k4*) and prevent them from forming complexes with cyclin D. INK4 CKIs thus block cell cycle progression in G_1. There are several INK4 proteins namely, p16 (CDKN2A), p15 (CDKN2B), p18 (CDKN2C), and p19 (CDKN2D). As well, p14ARF is encoded by the same gene as p16INK4a but is an alternate reading frame (i.e., ARF). These proteins play important roles in regulating both CDKs and MDM2.
- **Cip/Kip proteins:** This family of CKIs is composed of three proteins namely, p21 (CDKN1A), p27 (CDKN1B), and p57 (CDKN1C), and inhibits multiple CDKs. **Cip/Kip** proteins bind and block mainly CDK2 and, to a lesser extent, CDK1. Thus, they take up where the INK4 family leaves off and inhibit the rest of the cell cycle (can inhibit all CDKs). The best known Cip/Kip proteins are p21CIP (also called p21WAF1).

Role of Retinoblastoma Gene

One of the most important mechanisms that regulates cell division is by the family of Rb proteins. They mainly act near the $G_1 \rightarrow S$ boundary. One model of these related proteins is p105Rb (pRb=protein Rb and known as Rb) and other members of Rb proteins are related structurally and functionally. pRb prevents progression of the cell cycle by binding members of the E2F family of transcription factors. These E2F factors increase transcription of downstream cyclins (A and E) and also other proteins that promote DNA replication. Binding of E2F by pRb blocks E2F activity. During G_1 phase of the cell cycle, first CDK-cyclin complexes that appear are CDK4-cyclin D and CDK2-cyclin E (**Fig. 7**). These two CDK-cyclin complexes initiate the transition from G_1 to S mainly by phosphorylating the protein product

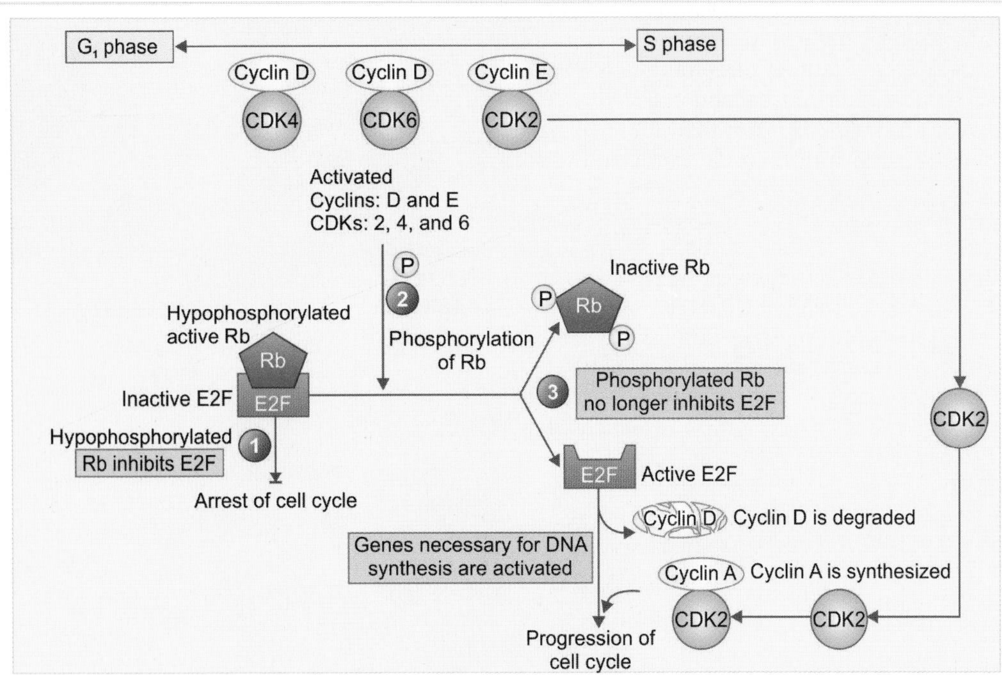

FIG. 7: Role of cyclins, cyclin-dependent kinases (CDKs) and Rb in cell cycle in G_1-to-S phase transition. 1. Normally, active retinoblastoma (Rb) protein bind to E2F transcription factor and this inactivates E2F. Hypophosphorylated Rb is active state of Rb 2. Activated cyclins D and E, along with activated CDKs 2, 4, and 6, phosphorylate Rb. During this process, CDK4 and CDK6 complexed to cyclin D whereas CDK2 complexed to cyclin E. They phosphorylate the Rb protein and make it inactive by phosphorylation. This causes Rb protein to dissociate from transcription factor namely E2F. 3. This releases E2F and activates the E2F transcription factor. E2F is now free to direct transcription of proteins and stimulates the transcription of genes needed for DNA replication, including that for cyclin A. When cells enter S phase, cyclin D is destroyed. Simultaneously CDK2–cyclin A complexes are formed which activate DNA replication. This cause cell cycle to proceed (i.e., progression of cell cycle).

of the *Rb* gene. The unphosphorylated Rb protein inhibits a TF (transcription factor) called E2F. Phosphorylation of Rb by the complex of cyclin D–CDK4/6 cannot inhibit E2F and releases transcription factor E2F . When the brakes on E2F are released, it turns on the expression of various genes required for synthesis/replication of DNA. E2F-mediated upregulation of other cyclins (A and E), which, bind to CDK2, again phosphorylate pRb, allowing the cell cycle to progress. Now the cell progresses from G_1 to S. Thus, the checkpoint ensures that this transition from G_1 to S phase does not occur when cells have damaged DNA.

Role of p53

When the DNA damage in cells is caused by exposure to ionizing radiation or ultraviolet (UV) light, the delay in entry from G_1 to S phase is performed by activation of the *p53 pathway* (**Fig. 8**). p53 is a tumor suppressor gene. Its protein product p53 is a TF which participates in the G_1-to-S checkpoint in mainly three ways:

- p53 turns on transcription of the CDK inhibitor known as p21. The p21 protein binds to CDK-cyclin (CDK4-cyclin D) complexes and inhibits their activity of CDK4-cyclin D complexes. Thus, p21 prevents entry from G_1 to S.
- p53 turns on the expression of genes encoding many DNA repair enzymes. When the cell is arrested in the G_1 phase by p21, the DNA repair enzymes can repair the DNA damage. If DNA is repaired, the p53 pathway is turned off and the cell can proceed into S phase.

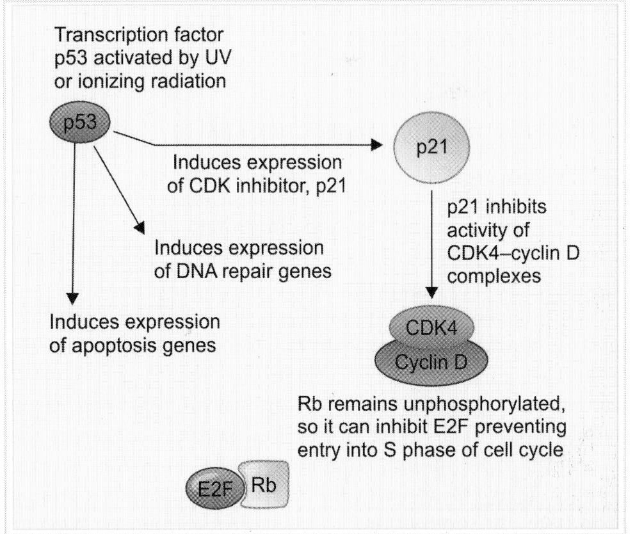

FIG. 8: Role of p53 pathway in G_1-to-S checkpoint. DNA damage activates the p53 transcription factor. This induces expression of the p21 gene. The p21 protein inhibits CDK–cyclin complexes, resulting in a G_1 phase arrest. Activated p53 protein also induces the expression of many DNA repair genes as well as apoptosis genes.

- **The p53 pathway and apoptosis:** If the DNA damage is severe, p53 not only arrests the cell in G_1, but also induces expression of apoptotic gene. This results in cell death by *apoptosis*.

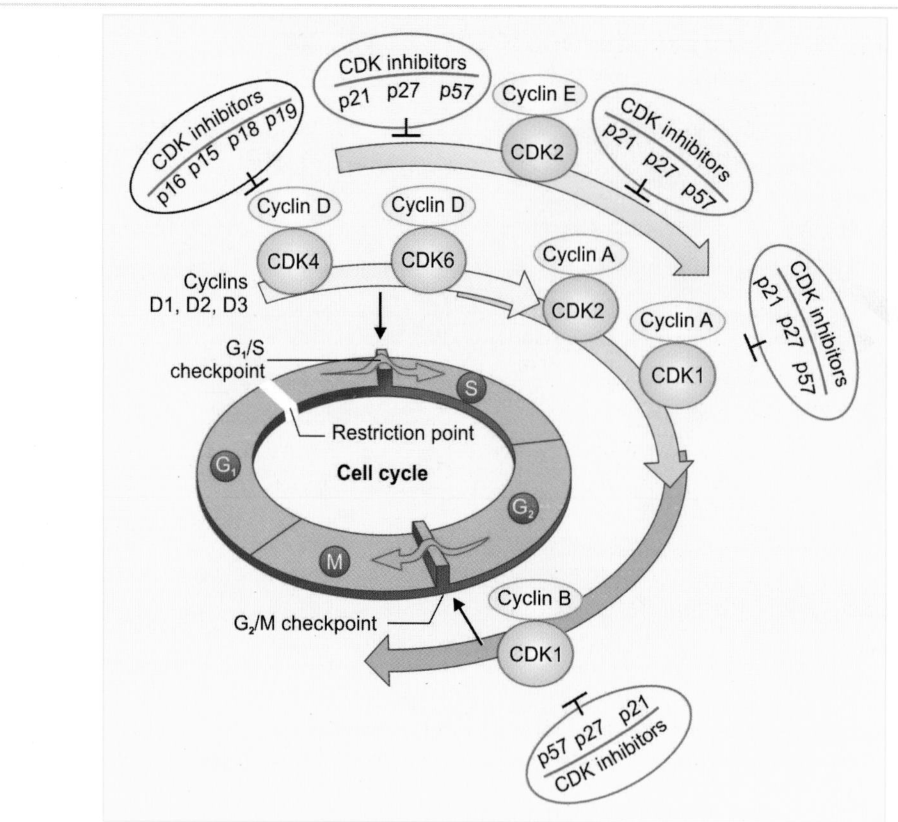

FIG. 9: Role of cyclins, cyclin dependent kinases (CDKs), and cyclin dependent kinase inhibitors (CKIs) in the cell cycle regulation. Different CDK–cyclin complexes control different cell cycle transitions. Cyclin-dependent kinases and cyclins appear during specific stages of cell cycles and prompt the cell to proceed to the next stage. Cyclin D–CDK4, cyclin D–CDK6, and cyclin E–CDK2 regulate the G_1-to-S transition. Cyclin A–CDK2 and cyclin A–CDK1 regulate the S phase. Cyclin B–CDK1 is needed for the G_2-to-M transition. Two families of CDK inhibitors can prevent the activity of CDKs and thereby prevent progression of the cell cycle. One family named "INK4 inhibitors" (composed of p16, p15, p18, and p19) act on cyclin D–CDK4 and cyclin D–CDK6. The other family of Cip/Kip proteins (consists of three inhibitors p21, p27, and p57) and can inhibit all CDKs.

Expression of Cyclin-dependent Kinase Inhibitors

They can be triggered by senescence, contact inhibition, extracellular antimitogenic factors [transforming growth factor-β (TGF-β)], and the tumor suppressor protein p53.

Role of cyclins, CDKs, and CKIs in the cell cycle regulation is summarized in **Figure 9.**

During cell growth and division there is also biosynthesis of the membranes, cytosolic proteins, and organelles necessary to produce two daughter cells. Thus, when the growth factor receptor signaling stimulates progression of cell cycle, it also promotes the metabolic changes that support growth. In the metabolic changes, main being switch to aerobic glycolysis (with the counter-intuitive reduction in oxidative phosphorylation). This is also termed as *Warburg effect* (for details refer pages 487–491).

CELL DIVISION

Genetic information is passed from parent to all the descendant cells through cell division. There are **two types of cell division** namely, **mitosis (somatic cell division** in the cells of the body) and **meiosis (germ cell division)**.

Mitosis

It is the final phase of cell cycle. Mitosis is defined as the **process of somatic cell division to form two identical daughter cells,** each with the same chromosome complement as the parent cell.

Characteristic Features

- It produces **two genetically identical** "daughter cells" having complete set of genetic information.
- These daughter cells have exactly the **same normal number of chromosomes** (i.e., 46) as the original parent cell. The daughter cells are diploid because they contain 46 chromosomes (i.e., $2N = 2 \times 23$).

Sites of Mitosis

It occurs **in all cells except the germ cells** or gametes.

Phases of Mitosis (Fig. 10)

There are **four different phases** of mitosis. They are: (1) Prophase, (2) Metaphase, (3) Anaphase, and (4) Telophase.

1. **Prophase:** The changes occurring in this phase are:
   - Condensation of chromatin.
   - Replication of centrosome.

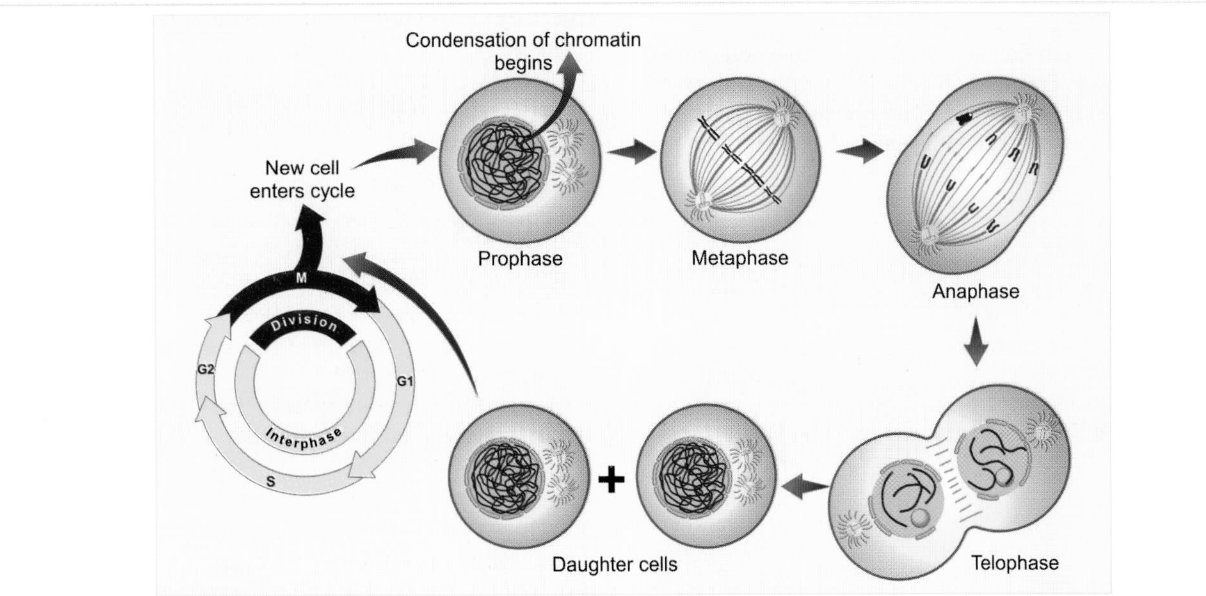

FIG. 10: Various phase of mitosis.

2. **Metaphase:** The changes in this phase are:
   - Gradual breaking of nuclear membrane which later disappears.
   - Movement of the centrosomes and alignment of chromosomes.

A mitotic karyotype can be constructed from cells arrested at metaphase.

3. **Anaphase:** The changes in this phase are:
   - Division and movement of chromosomes.
   - Division of cytoplasm.
4. **Telophase:** During this final phase, two identical, individual daughter cells are formed.

Meiosis

Meiosis the second form of cell division. Like mitosis, interphase of the cell cycle includes G_1, S, and G_2 phases. Interphase is followed by meiosis.

Definition

It is defined as **special form of germ cell division** that **produces reproductive cells** in which **each daughter cell receives half the number of chromosomes** (23) in the genome.

Sites of Meiosis

Meiosis occurs **only in germ cells of the gonads** (sperms in males and ova in females).

Stages of Meiosis

Meiosis consists of two successive stages, namely, meiosis I and meiosis II.

Meiosis I

During this stage, **the number of chromosomes per cell is reduced by half** and is termed the **reduction division**. It is characterized by:

- **Pairing of homologous chromosomes:** In this stage, the replicated homologous chromosomes come together.
- **Recombination:** The **process of exchange of DNA** (swapping of genetic material/crossing over of chromosome segments) **between homologous chromosomes** (chromosomes with identical genetic material) is a unique event known as **recombination (synapsis)**. Recombination results in each chromosome having mixed segments of both maternal and paternal origin. This is responsible for significant **genetic diversity**/variability in humans.

After recombination, the homologous chromosomes separate to opposite poles and the chromatids consist of part of their original DNA and part of DNA from other homologous chromosome. There is no DNA synthesis (no S phase) between the two divisions (meiosis I and II).

Meiosis II

The second division in the meiotic process is termed the **equational division** because the events in this phase are **similar to those of mitosis**. However, meiosis II differs from mitosis in that the number of chromosome has already been halved in meiosis I and the cell does not begin with the same number of chromosomes as it does in mitosis.

Result

The end result of meiosis is different in males and females. **Both sperm and ova are haploid cells (23 chromosomes-N).**

- **Males:** Meiosis in males **produces four spermatozoa** from each original germ cell.
- **Females:** Meiosis I (the first meiotic division) in females gives rise to secondary oocyte and a small cell (polar body) that is discarded. During meiosis II, the secondary oocyte gives rise to one large mature ovum (egg) and a second polar body, which again is discarded. In females, the end result after the second meiotic division is **3 polar bodies and one ovum.**

Main stages of meiosis in males and females are shown in **Figure 11**.

Gametogenesis

It is a process by which diploid cells undergo cell division and differentiate to form mature haploid gametes. The process of gametogenesis **in males is called as spermatogenesis** and **in females as oogenesis.** The differences between them are shown in **Table 2.**

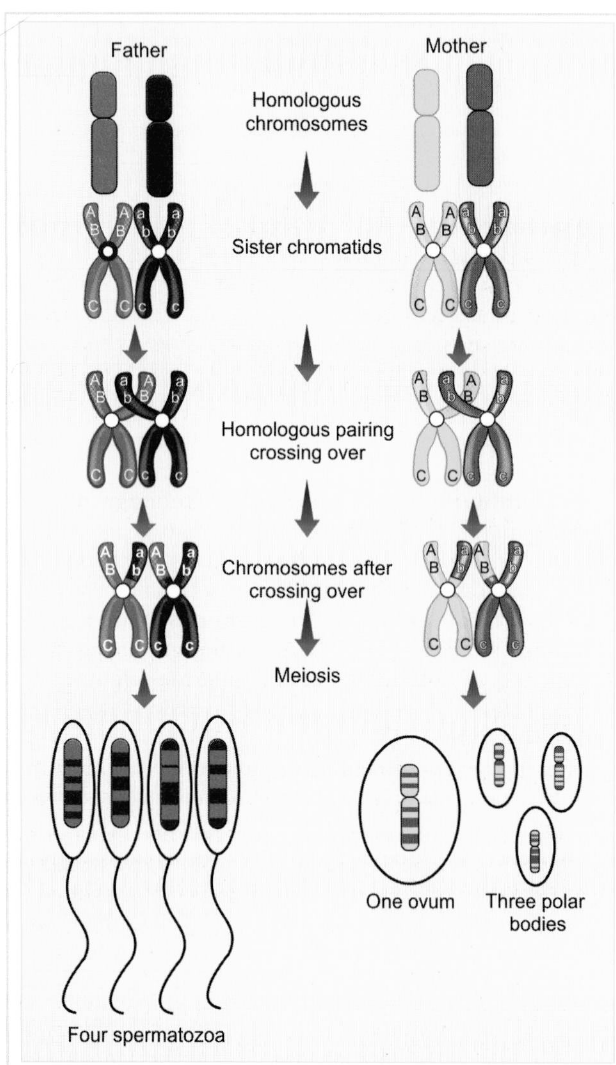

FIG. 11: Main stages of meiosis in males and females. A single homologous pair of chromosomes is shown in different colors. In male, meiosis results in four spermatozoa. In the female, meiosis produces only one ovum (egg) and three polar bodies.

Differences between Mitosis and Meiosis

Meiosis shares certain features with mitosis but involves two distinct steps of cell division that reduce the chromosome number to the haploid state. Meiosis differs from mitosis in several ways (**Table 3**).

STEM CELLS

Q. Explain stem cell therapy in clinical practice.
Q. What are stem cells and their different properties? Write in detail about stem cells in regenerative medicine.
Q. Discuss the role of stem cells in tissue homeostasis.
Q. Elaborate plasticity of stem cell.

One of the puzzles is how is a complex multicellular organism generated from a single fertilized egg? The adult human body is composed of several hundred types of well differentiated cells. During development, totipotent stem cells can give rise to all types of differentiated tissues. Most of the specialized, differentiated (well/fully differentiated) cells are not capable/unable of cell division. These specialized cells need continual replacement. This is true for red blood cells, the epidermal cells in the upper layers of the skin, and the absorptive and goblet cells of the gut epithelium. Such cells are termed as *terminally differentiated*—they lie at the dead end of their developmental pathway. However, they can be replaced by the proliferation of a subpopulation of small number of long-lived, unspecialized (less differentiated), self-renewing cells called **stem cells.** These stem cells are present in **various** adult tissues. Because stem cells retain the capacity to proliferate and replace differentiated cells throughout the life, they play an important role in the maintenance of most tissues and organs. **Stems cells have the capacity to replace damaged cells and maintain cell populations within the tissues where they reside.** In normal tissues (without healing, degeneration, or neoplasia), there is a homeostatic equilibrium between the replication, self-renewal, and differentiation of stem cells, and the death of the mature, fully differentiated cells (**Fig. 12**).

Terminology

- **Totipotent stem cells:** These can give rise to any cell types found in an embryo as well as extraembryonic cells (placenta).

Table 2: Differences between gametogenesis in males and females.		
Features	***Males***	***Females***
Commencement of gametogenesis	Begins at puberty and continues throughout life	Begins in fetal life and does not complete until after ovulation
Time required for completion of single meiotic cell division	Both meiotic divisions are completed in a matter of days	Varies and may take >40 years to complete
Gametes produced per meiosis	4 sperms	1 ovum and 3 polar bodies

Table 3: Differences between mitosis and meiosis.

Characteristics	*Mitosis*	*Meiosis*
Location	Somatic cells	Germ cells
Chromosome number in newly formed daughter cells	Same as that in the original cell (diploid-46)	Reduced by half (haploid-23)
Relationship between daughter cells produced	Genetically identical	Genetically variable due to recombination
Nuclear division	Single	Two
Recombination	Rare and abnormal	Occurs normally
Number of cells produced (end result)	Two	In males: Four sperms In females: Three polar bodies and one ovum

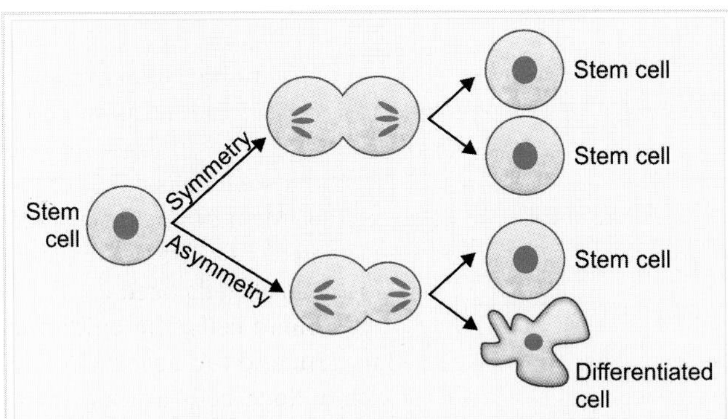

FIG. 12: Asymmetric and symmetric division of stem cells. Asymmetric division gives rise to one stem cell and another differentiated cells, whereas symmetric division give rise to two stem cells.

- **Pluripotent stem cells:** These can differentiate into any of the three germ layers—endoderm, mesoderm, or ectoderm but not into extraembryonic tissues like the placenta.
- **Multipotent stem cells:** They can develop into a limited number of cell types in a particular lineage.

Defining Properties of Stem Cells

Under conditions of homeostasis, stem cells have following important properties:

- **Not terminally differentiated:** Stem cell is not itself terminally differentiated (i.e., it is not at the end of a pathway of differentiation).
- **Capacity for self-renewal:** It can divide without limit (or at least for the lifetime of the individual). Self-renewal permits stem cells to maintain their numbers. Self-renewal may follow either asymmetric or symmetric division. In contrast to stem cells, **progenitor** cells (transit amplifying cells) have little or no capability for self-renewal.
- **Asymmetric division:** It refers to cell replication in which one daughter cell differentiates into a mature specialized cell types, whereas the other daughter cell remains undifferentiated and retains its self-renewal capacity (i.e., remains as a stem cell). Because of this self-renewing population of stem cells, they can serve as a source for the production of differentiated cells throughout life.

Note: In **symmetric division**, both daughter cells retain self-renewal capacity (i.e., as stem cells). Such symmetric divisions are seen early in embryogenesis (i.e., when there is expansion of stem cell populations). It can also occur under conditions of stress, such as in the bone marrow following chemotherapy.

Q. What are the different subtypes of stem cells? Enumerate the role of stem cell in various therapeutic modalities.

Types of Stem Cells

There are mainly two varieties of stem cells namely: (i) embryonic stem cells and (ii) tissue (adult) stem cells.

Embryonic Stem Cells

These are the most undifferentiated. They are present in the inner cell mass of the preimplantation blastocyst. They have almost limitless cell renewal capacity, and can give rise to every cell in the body. Thus, they are said to be **totipotent** (**Fig. 13**). Embryonic stem (ES) cells can be maintained for extended periods without differentiating by culturing in vitro. After culture of these cells, they can form specialized cells of all three germ cell layers (namely ectoderm, mesoderm, and endoderm) including neurons, cardiac muscle, liver cells, and pancreatic islet cells.

Tissue Stem Cells

They are also called **adult stem cells** and are found in many adult tissues, intimately associated with the differentiated cells of a given tissue. They have been identified even in tissues not known to regenerate. Adult stem cells have a more restricted range of cell differentiation than ES cells. Features and common properties of adult stem cells are presented in **Boxes 2** and **3**, respectively. Although adult stem cells are capable of maintaining tissues with high (e.g., skin and gastrointestinal tract) or low (e.g., endothelium) cell turnover, the adult stem cells can usually produce only cells that are normal constituents of that particular tissue (i.e., tissue-specific regeneration).

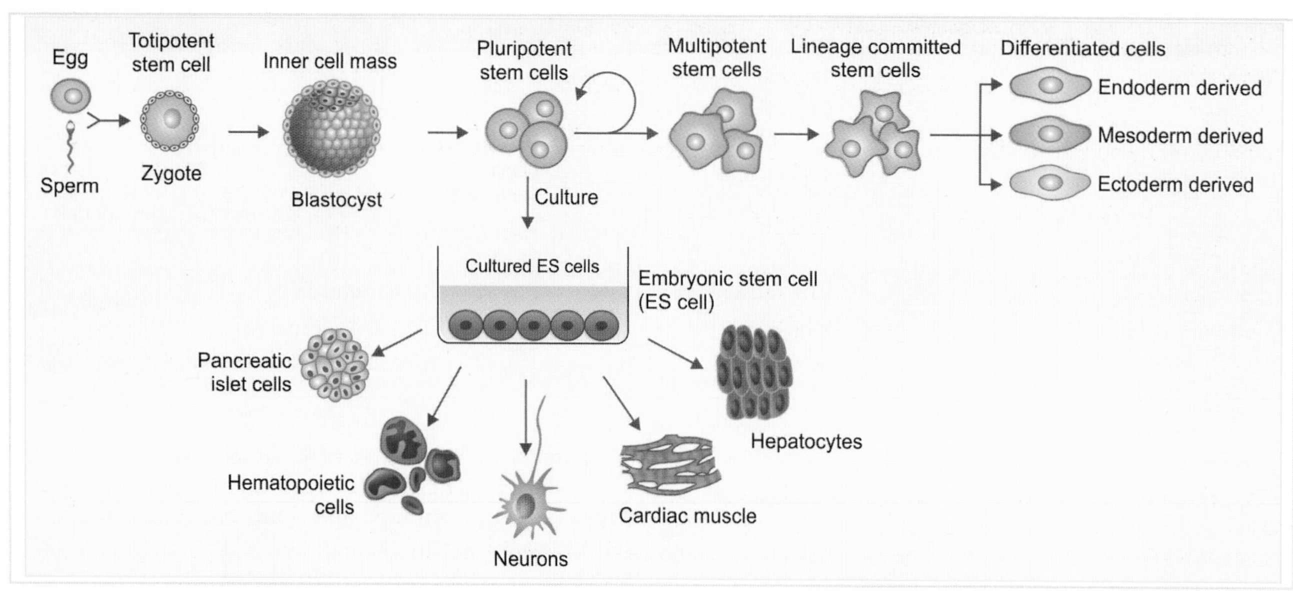

FIG. 13: Embryonal stem (ES) cells. The zygote is formed by the union of sperm and egg. It divides to form blastocysts, and the inner cell mass of the blastocyst produces the embryo. The pluripotent cells of the inner cell mass are known as the ES cells. ES cells can be induced to differentiate into cells of multiple lineages. In the embryo, pluripotent stem cells can asymmetrically divide to give rise to a residual stable pool of ES cells and also generate populations that have progressively more restricted developmental capacity. It can give rise to differentiated cells derived from three lineages (three germ cell layers—ecto, endo, and mesoderm). ES cells can be cultured in vitro and be induced to give rise to cells of all three lineages.

Box 2: Features of tissue or adult stem cells.

- Any organ or tissue may have more than one type of stem cell
- Similar stem cells may be found in different organs
- A stem cell found in tissue may be derived or originated from the bone marrow

Box 3: Common properties of tissue or adult stem cells.

- Capable of division without limit, able to avoid senescence and maintain genomic integrity. However, they have limited capacity of differentiated cells than that of embryonic stem (ES) cells.
- Capable of undergoing intermittent division or to remain quiescent
- Capable to propagate by self-renewal and differentiation of daughter cells
- No lineage markers available
- Specific anatomic localization in some tissues

Stem Cells Niches

The stem cells are normally protected within suitable, specialized tissue microenvironments called *stem cell niches.* They have been detected in many organs such as the bone marrow, where hematopoietic stem cells (HSCs) are gathered in a perivascular niche. These stem cells are kept in inactive state (i.e., quiescent) by the soluble factors and other cells within the niches. When there is a necessity, they expand and differentiate from the precursor pool.

Intestine: Intestinal epithelium, normally undergoes rapid turnovers and it is replaced by intestinal stem cells present in the crypts of Lieberkühn (**Fig. 14A**).

Skin: Cornified skin epithelium and hair follicles regenerate from stem cells in basal epidermis and the bulge region of the hair follicle (**Fig. 14B**).

Cornea: Corneal stem cells are located in the limbus region, between the cornea and the conjunctiva (**Fig. 14C**).

Other sites: Other niches for stem cells include the canals of Hering in the liver; and the subventricular zone in the brain.

Specific Signals Maintain Stem Cell Populations

Every stem cell system needs control mechanisms to make sure that new differentiated cells are produced in the appropriate places and in the right numbers. The controls depend on extracellular signals exchanged between the stem cells, their progeny, and other cell types. These signals, and the intracellular signaling pathways they activate, belong to few basic signaling mechanisms. For example, a class of signal molecules known as the Wnt proteins serves to promote the proliferation of the stem cells and precursor cells at the base of each intestinal crypt (**Fig. 15**).

Hematopoietic Stem Cell

Bone marrow contains hematopoietic, mesenchymal, and endothelial stem cells. HSCs continuously replace all the cellular elements of the blood as they are consumed. HSCs are lineage restricted and can form only all the cells found in blood. They can be obtained directly from bone marrow and also from the peripheral blood after administration of certain colony stimulating factors (CSF). These CSF induce the release of HSCs from bone marrow niches. HSCs can be purified based on cell surface markers. HSCs can be used to repopulate

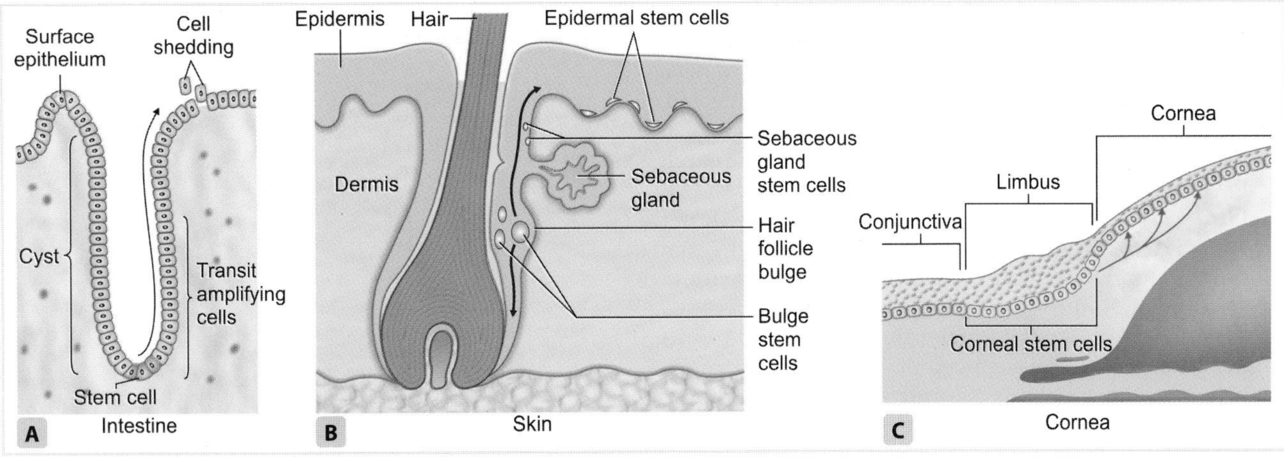

FIGS. 14A TO C: Diagrammatic representation of location of stem cell niches. (A) In small intestine, stem cells are seen at the bottom of the intestinal crypt. (B) In skin, stem cells are located in the bulge area of the hair follicle, in sebaceous glands, and in the lower layer of the epidermis. (C) Corneal stem cells are located in the limbus region, between the cornea and the conjunctiva.

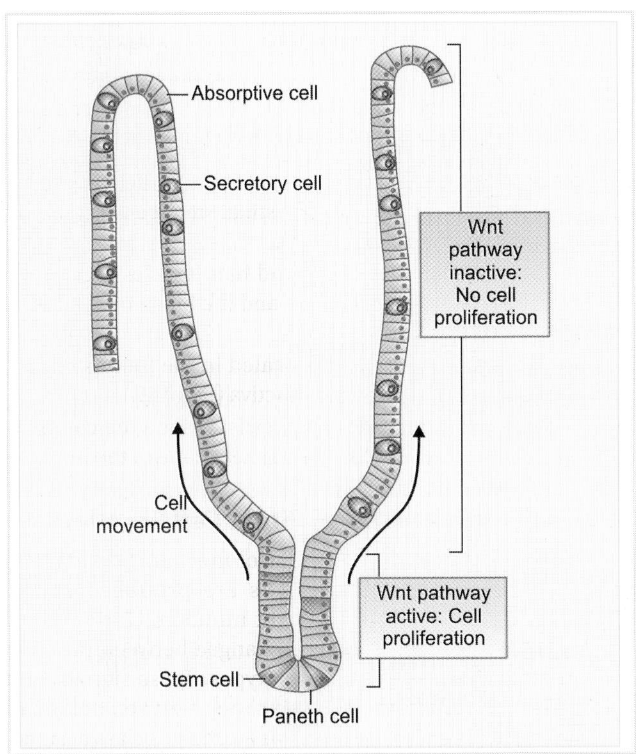

FIG. 15: Control of stem cells in the intestinal crypt. The Wnt signaling pathway maintains the proliferation of the stem cells and precursor cells. The Wnt proteins are secreted by cells in and around the crypt base (e.g., Paneth cells—a subclass of terminally differentiated secretory cells that are generated from the gut stem cells) activate stem cell proliferation.

marrows depleted after chemotherapy (e.g., for leukemia), or to provide normal precursors to correct various blood cell disorders (e.g., sickle cell disease).

Mesenchymal Stem Cells (MSCs)

Apart from HSCs, the bone marrow (and other tissues such as fat) also contains a population of MSCs. These are bone marrow stromal cells and are multipotent stem cells. They can mobilize into the bloodstream and be recruited to (injured) organs. MSCs can be induced to differentiate into multiple or variety of stromal cells types. Thus, they can differentiate into chondrocytes (cartilage), osteocytes (bone), adipocytes (fat), and myocytes (muscle). These cells can be expanded to large numbers. Hence, they can be used as a potential means of manufacturing the stromal scaffolding needed for tissue regeneration. MSCs can also be found in cord blood and many other connective tissues.

Endothelial Progenitor Stem Cells

These cells from bone marrow can produce tissue angiogenesis and may supplement endothelial hyperplasia during regeneration of blood vessels.

A well-established clinical application of adult stem cells is HSC transplantation (or bone marrow transplantation). It plays an important role in the treatment of a many cancers.

Uses of Stem Cells

- Stem cells can proliferate indefinitely and produce progeny that differentiate and hence, help in continual renewal of normal tissue. Stem cells can be **used to repair lost or damaged tissues** through injury. For example, HSC transplantation can be used to treat human leukemia (following bone marrow damage by irradiation or cytotoxic drugs used for treating leukemia).
- Induced pluripotent stem (iPS) cells (refer further) can provide a convenient source of human ES-like cells. They can be used to produce large, homogeneous populations of differentiated human cells of specific types in culture. Such

cells can be **used to test for potential toxic or beneficial effects of candidate drugs**.
- It is possible to produce iPS cells from patients with genetic disease and to use these iPS cells to produce affected, differentiated cell types. These cells can then be studied to learn more about the **disease mechanism** and to **search for potential treatments**.
- Pluripotent stem cells can form organoids: Under appropriate conditions, ES cells, and iPS cells can proliferate, differentiate, and self-assemble in culture to form miniature, three-dimensional organs called organoids. It closely resembles the normal organ in its organization. The development of iPS cells and organoid technology may help us to **study human development and disease**. It also promises as a progress toward use for treatment.

Regenerative Medicine

The achievement in ability to identify, separate/isolate, expand, and transplant stem cells has given birth to a new field of medicine called as regenerative medicine. It is an area of medicine in which there is a potential to fully heal damaged tissues and organs by using stem cells. Theoretically, repopulation of damaged tissues or construction of entire organs can be done by using stem cell replacement by either differentiated progeny of ES or adult stem cells. The therapeutic restoration of damaged tissues having low intrinsic regenerative capacity, such as myocardium after a myocardial infarct or neurons after a stroke, is challenging. Unfortunately, in spite of improving capability to purify and expand stem cell populations, the enthusiasm has not been successful due to the difficulties encountered in introducing and functionally integrating the replacement stem cells into sites of damage.

Induced Pluripotent Stem Cells

There are both technical and ethical difficulties in the obtaining ES cells. More recently pluripotential cells resembling ES cells have been produced. As a major advancement, somatic cell nuclear transfer, in which the adult somatic cells can be directly converted to pluripotent stem cells in culture, provides a direct mechanism for converting somatic cells to stem cells. These stem cells similar to ES cells, have the potential to develop into all tissues of an organism.

Procedure

To obtain such stem cells, few genes have been identified whose products can remarkably reprogram somatic cells to achieve the "stem-ness" of ES cells. These genes are introduced into patient's fully differentiated cells (e.g., fibroblasts). This on culture gives rise to iPS, although at low frequency. These stem cells are called as *iPS cells* (**Fig. 16**). These iPS like ES cells, are capable of differentiating into all cell types. Thus, iPS cells can be induced to differentiate into various lineages (ectoderm, mesoderm, or endoderm).

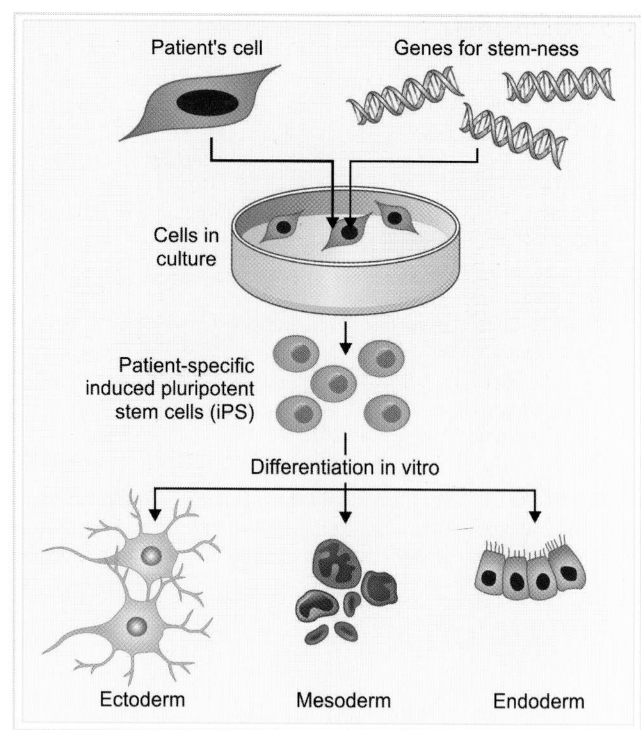

FIG. 16: Steps in the production of induced pluripotent stem cells (iPS cells). They are produced by introducing genes that are responsible for stem cell properties (stem-ness) into a patient's fully differentiated cells. This, on culture, gives rise to iPS. These iPS can be induced to differentiate into various lineages (ectoderm, mesoderm, or endoderm).

Advantage of iPS Cells

One of the advantages of iPS cells is that they and their differentiated progeny can be engrafted without eliciting an immunologically mediated rejection. This is because these cells are derived from the patient itself. For example, in a patient with diabetes, the differentiated progeny of iPS cell is insulin-secreting β cells. In contrast to iPS cells, if the differentiated cells were derived from ES cells obtained from another donor, it can elicit an immunologically mediated rejection reaction.

Applications of Induced Pluripotent Stem Cells

- **Biomedical research:** To study the etiology and pathogenesis of diseases.
- **Personalized medicine:** For drug discovery, potency testing and predictive safety (in pharmacology and toxicology).
- **Cell replacement therapy:** Potential uses of stem cell therapy include
  - Ischemic heart failure
  - Parkinson's disease
  - Alzheimer's disease
  - Diabetes mellitus
  - Age-related macular degeneration

BIBLIOGRAPHY

1. Alberts B, Johnson A, Lewis J, Morgan D, Raff M, Roberts K, Walter P. Molecular Biology of the cell, 6th edition. New York: Taylor & Francis; 2015.
2. Alvarado AS, Yamanaka S. Rethinking differentiation: stem cells, regeneration, and plasticity. *Cell.* 2014;157:110.
3. Blau HM, Daley GQ: Stem cells in the treatment of disease. *N Engl J Med.* 2019;380:1748.
4. De Los Angeles A, Ferrari F, Xi R et al. Hallmarks of pluripotency. *Nature.* 2015;525:469.
5. Fuchs E, Chen T. A matter of life and death: self-renewal in stem cells. *EMBO Rep.* 2013;14:39.
6. Horst A. Molecular pathology, Sound Parkway: CRC Press; 2018.
7. Iwasa J, Marshall W. Karp's cell and molecular biology, 8th edition. Hoboken:John Wiley & Sons: 2016.
8. Jang S, Collin del Hortet A, Soto-Gutierrezy A. Induced pluripotent stem cell-derived endothelial cells: overview, current advances, applications, and future directions. *Am J Pathol.* 2019;189:502.
9. Karp G. Molecular and cell biology: Concepts and experiments. 6th edition. Hoboken: Taylor & Francis; 2010.
10. Kumar V, Abbas AK, Aster JC. Robbins basic pathology, 10th edition. Philadelphia: Saunders Elsevier; 2018
11. Kumar V, Abbas AK, Fausto N, et al. Robbins and Cotran pathologic basis of disease, 10th edition. Philadelphia: WB Saunders; 2021.
12. Martello G, Smith A. The nature of embryonic stem cells. *Annu Rev Cell Dev Biol.* 2014;30:647.
13. Scadden DT. Nice neighborhood: emerging concepts of the stem cell niche. *Cell.* 2014;157:41.
14. Wu J, Izpisua Belmonte JC. Stem cells: a renaissance in human biology research. *Cell.* 2016;165:1572.
15. Strayer DS, Saffitz JE. Rubin's Pathology: Mechanism of Human Disease, 8th edition. Philadelphia: Wolters Kluwer; 2020

CHAPTER 4

Extracellular Matrix

CHAPTER OUTLINE

- Introduction
- Functions
- Forms of extracellular matrix
  - Interstitial matrix
  - Basement membrane
- Components of the extracellular matrix
  - Fibrous structural proteins
  - Water-hydrated gels
  - Adhesive glycoproteins and adhesion receptors

INTRODUCTION

Q. Discuss the role of extracellular matrix in health and disease.

Plasma membrane constitutes the boundary between a living cell and its nonliving environment, the materials present outside the plasma membrane. This extracellular material surrounding immediate vicinity of the plasma membrane of the cells is an **organized network of interstitial proteins and organized extracellular materials**. This is known as **extracellular matrix (ECM)** and forms a significant proportion of any tissue (**Fig. 1**).

FUNCTIONS

The ECM is more than an inert packing material or a nonspecific glue that holds cells together; it often plays an important role in the life of a cell. These include:

- **Mechanical support:** ECM gives mechanical support for cell anchorage and cell migration, and maintenance of cell polarity and shape. It helps in **maintaining normal tissue architecture.**
- **Control of cell proliferation:** ECM controls cell proliferation by binding and displaying growth factors on the surface of cells. It also helps for signaling through cellular receptors of the integrin family. The ECM is a storage place for a variety of latent growth factors that can be activated whenever there is injury or inflammation.
- **Tissue renewal:** ECM provides scaffolding to the cells and tissues, and **maintenance of normal tissue structure needs a basement membrane or stromal scaffold.** Thus, the integrity of the basement membrane or the stroma of parenchymal cells is very important for the regeneration of tissues and healing. Any disruption of ECM results in defective tissue regeneration and repair. For example, collapse of the hepatic stroma (e.g., hepatitis B, C, or alcoholic liver disease) leads to cirrhosis of the liver.
- **Structural and functional role in tissue:** One of the components of ECM is basement membrane. It acts as a boundary between the epithelium and underlying connective tissue. Basement membrane not only provides support to the epithelium but also has its function. For example, in the kidney, glomerular basement membrane (GBM) forms a part of the filtration apparatus.

The ECM is not a static structure. It undergoes constant remodeling characterized by synthesis and degradation. This is observed during morphogenesis, tissue regeneration and repair, chronic fibrosis, and tumor invasion and metastasis.

FORMS OF EXTRACELLULAR MATRIX

There are two main forms of ECM—interstitial matrix and basement membrane.

Interstitial Matrix

It is the ECM present in the spaces between stromal cells in connective tissue, and also between the parenchymal epithelium and the underlying supportive vascular and smooth muscle structures in some organs. The term **matrix implies a structure made up of a network of interacting components**. The ECM consists of a number of proteins (e.g., collagen and proteoglycans), that interact with one another in highly specific ways. Interstitial matrix consists of semi-fluid gel and nonfluid fibrillar and nonfibrillar component. The matrix consists of randomly arranged connective tissues and is synthesized by mesenchymal cells (e.g., fibroblasts) and forms a three-dimensional, relatively amorphous, semi-fluid gel. Man nonfluid constituents of the

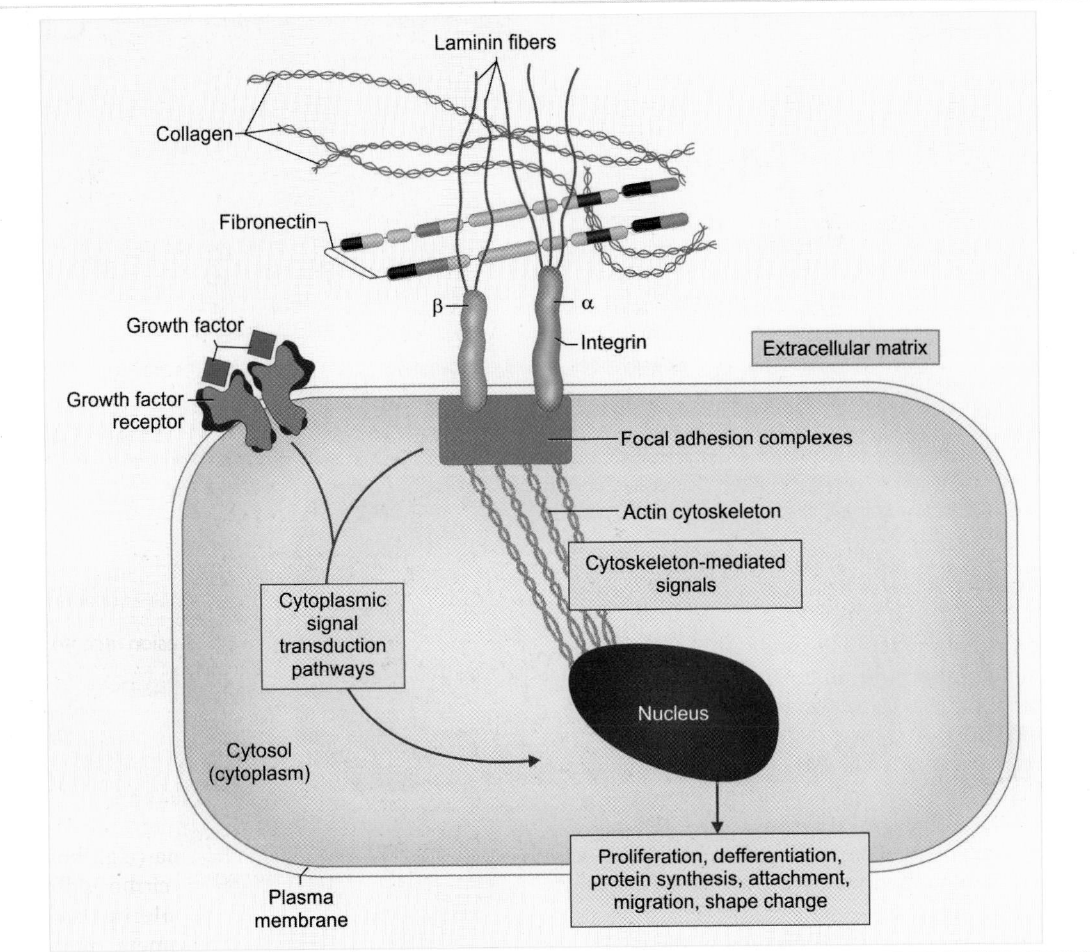

FIG. 1: Extracellular matrix showing its interactions with growth factor-mediated cell signaling. Cell surface integrins interact with the cytoskeleton. Signals from ECM components and growth factors can produce a given response (changes in proliferation, locomotion, and/or differentiation).

interstitial matrix includes fibrillar and nonfibrillar collagens, fibronectin, elastin, proteoglycans, hyaluronate, and others. In some tissues (e.g., gastrointestinal tract, urinary bladder, periarterial soft tissues), fluid within interstitial matrix acts as a cushion for tissue compression that occurs with peristalsis, urination, and pulsatile arterial blood flow.

Basement Membrane

Q. Write a short essay on basement membrane.

One of the best-defined extracellular matrices at the boundary between cells and the connective tissue is the specialized basement membrane (also known as the basal lamina). Basement membranes form under different epithelial layers, around epithelial ducts and tubules of skin, cover smooth and skeletal muscle cells, and peripheral nerve Schwann cells, and surround capillary endothelium and associated pericytes.

Basement membrane is very thin/flat, tough, flexible, lamellar, "chicken wire" mesh of continuous sheet of specialized ECM and most of them measure 50–200 nm in thickness. Though termed as membrane, it is quite porous. It separates cells that synthesize it from adjacent interstitial connective tissue.

Sites: Various sites of basement membrane are as follows:

- It lies beneath the basal surface of epithelial cells/tissues (**Fig. 2A**). Examples include epidermis of the skin, the lining of the digestive and respiratory tracts. It also underlies mesothelium in pleural, peritoneal, and pericardial cavity.
- Glomerular basement membrane between visceral epithelial cells and endothelial cells of the glomerulus (**Fig. 2B**)
- Basal laminae, usually termed *external laminae* but with similar composition as basement membrane, is also seen as thin sleeves surrounding individual muscle cells (**Fig. 2C**), Schwann cells (which wrap around peripheral nerve cell axons) of nerve fibers, and fat (fat-storing) cells. They serve as semipermeable barriers regulating macromolecular exchange between the enclosed cells and connective tissue. Basement membrane is also a key structural and functional feature of the neuromuscular synapse.
- It underlies the inner endothelial lining of blood vessels, lymph vessels, etc.

Periodic acid-schiff stain: Basement membrane appears as a thin lamina that stains by the PAS stain, owing to its high glycoprotein content.

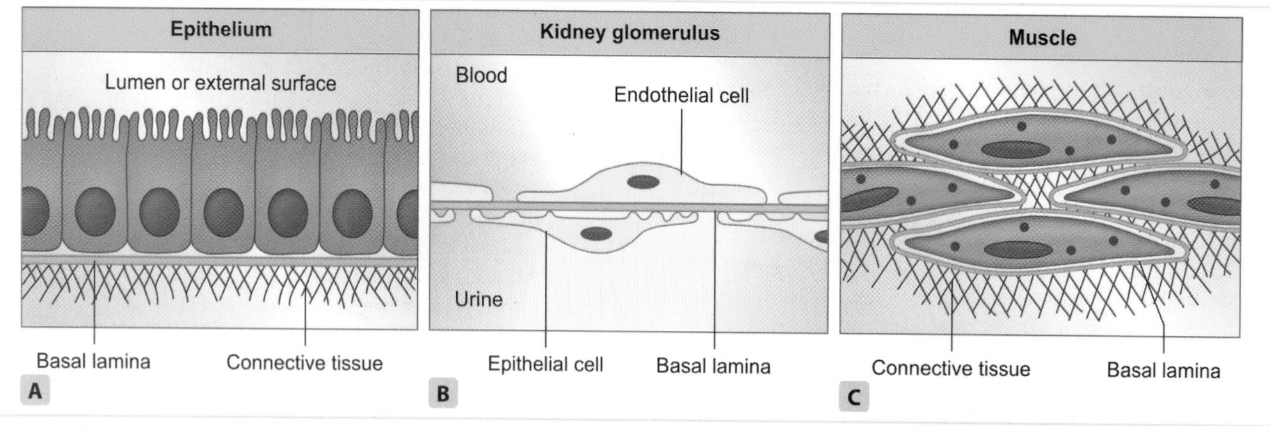

FIGS. 2A TO C: Organization of basement membranes (basal laminae). (A) Basal laminae beneath the epithelia. (B) In glomerulus of the kidney between epithelial cells and endothelial cells as common glomerular basement membrane GBM. (C) Basal lamina surrounds individual cells (e.g., skeletal muscle cells).

Functions: Various functions of basement membrane are as follows:

- **Anchoring (attachment):** The main function of the basement membrane is to anchor/attach the surface epithelial tissue to underlying connective tissue (e.g., the dermis in the skin).
- **Barrier/filter:** Structurally, the basement membrane acts as a boundary between the epithelium and the underlying connective tissue. It acts as a barrier to the passage of macromolecules. For example, it prevents the passage of proteins out of the blood and into the tissues in the capillaries of kidney. Kidney failure developing in long-term diabetics may result from an abnormal thickening of the GBM. It also acts a mechanical barrier (e.g., it prevents invasion of underlying tissues by cancer cells).
- **Mechanical/structural support** for the attached cells, generate signals that maintain cell survival, cell-to-cell interactions (e.g., formation of myoneural junctions), mark routes for certain cell migration along epithelia, separate adjacent tissues within an organ.
- **Maintaining cell polarity:** Basal lamina components help organize integrins and other proteins in the plasma membrane to main cell polarity of epithelial cells.
- **Angiogenesis:** The basement membrane is essential for angiogenesis. The basement membrane proteins accelerate differentiation of endothelial cells.
- **Control of cell proliferation:** It is the store house for growth factors and cell signaling through receptors of the integrin family. Latent growth factors can be activated from injury and inflammation.
- **Scaffold for tissue regeneration:** Maintenance of normal tissue structure needs an intact basement membrane and the integrity of the basement membrane is important for the organized regeneration of tissue.
- **Other activities:** Helps to localize endocytosis, signal transduction, and other activities. Basement membrane also serves as a scaffold that allows rapid epithelial repair and regeneration (e.g., in wound healing, where it forms a surface along which regenerating epithelial cells migrate).

Synthesis: Basement membrane is synthesized conjointly by the overlying epithelium and the underlying mesenchymal cells.

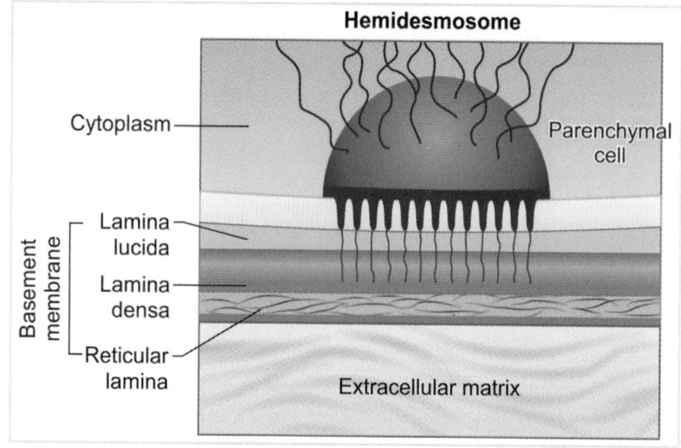

FIG. 3: Diagrammatic representation of basement membrane.

Morphology (Fig. 3): Under the transmission electron microscope (TEM), the basement membrane in most places shows two layers/parts, namely **basal lamina** and the **reticular lamina.** Nearest to the epithelial cells is a thin, electron-dense, sheet-like layer of fine fibrils called as the **basal lamina.** Beneath this layer is a more diffuse and fibrous layer termed as **reticular lamina.**

The terms "basement membrane" and "basal lamina" are sometimes used interchangeably. But "basal lamina" usually should be used for the fine extracellular layer seen ultrastructurally and "basement membrane" is the entire structure beneath the epithelial cells observed with the light microscope.

Composition

The basement membranes contain several proteins. In some organs (e.g., in kidney), it shows three layers, namely: (1) Lamina reticularis/reticularis lamina (the nearest to the epithelial cells), (2) Lamina densa (central region), and (3) Lamina lucida (the nearest to the connective tissue).

Lamina lucida It is the region of the basement membrane near the ECM. It has the transmembrane **laminin receptors**, namely the **integrin** and **dystroglycans** molecules. The lamina lucida also houses the glycoproteins **laminin, entactin**, and **perlecans**.

Lamina densa It is the central region of basement membrane. The lamina densa adheres to the **lamina reticularis** and is the thickest region of the basement membrane. It is composed of:

- **On its epithelial surface: Type IV collagen**, coated by laminin, entactin, and perlecan.
- **On the lamina reticularis surface: Fibronectin** and perlecan.

Additionally, two other **collagen types, XV and XVIII**, are also present in the lamina densa.

Lamina reticularis It is a more diffuse meshwork composed mostly of **type III collagen**, proteoglycans, glycoproteins, as well as of **anchoring fibers (type VII collagen)** and **microfibrils (fibrillin)**. It is bound to the basal lamina by anchoring fibrils of **type VII collagen**. Type I and type III collagen fibers enter the lamina reticularis from its interface with the connective tissue and it attaches the two structures to each other. Thus, it forms a firm bond between the epithelium and the connective tissue.

Some of the proteins are present in all basement membranes and are synthesized and secreted in cells resting on basement membranes. Examples include amorphous **nonfibrillar type IV collagen** (is present only in basement membranes), **laminin, heparan sulfate proteoglycan**, and probably entactin. Other proteins are present only in some of the basement membranes, synthesized and secreted in cells that do not rest on basement membranes. These are usually seen with basement membranes that serve a prominent filtering function. Examples include fibronectin, type V collagen, and chondroitin sulfate. Collagen VII forms **fibrillar anchors** linking hemidesmosome and basement membrane to underlying stroma (structure of various types of collagen are discussed here).

Laminin It is one of the important **noncollagenous components** of basement membranes. Laminin is the large glycoprotein (molecular weight approximately 900,000) composed of three subunits. Laminin attaches to transmembrane **integrin** proteins in the basal cell membrane and projects through the mesh formed by the type IV collagen. Laminin is susceptible to several proteases (trypsin, pepsin) and causes cell adhesion and attachment.

Nidogen and perlecan Respectively, a short, rod-like protein and a proteoglycan, both of these crosslink laminins to the type IV collagen network. They provide the basal lamina's three-dimensional structure. They also help to bind the epithelium to basal lamina and to determine its porosity and the size of molecules able to filter through it.

Clinical Significance of Basement Membrane

- **Genetic defects** in the collagen fibers of the basement membrane cause **Alport syndrome and Knobloch syndrome**.
- Noncollagenous domain basement membrane collagen type I can act as an autoantigen (target antigen) and autoantibodies against this causes an autoimmune disease, namely **Goodpasture's syndrome**.
- A group of diseases due to improper function of basement membrane are grouped under epidermolysis bullosa.
- **Thickening of basement membrane:** It may be found in various diseases.
    - **Membranous nephropathy**
    - **Diabetes mellitus** (both type 1 and type 2): In diabetes mellitus, basement membrane thickening occurs in the capillaries of muscle, retina, skin, and kidney. Besides thickening, in diabetes there may be severe functional changes, resulting in *nephrotic* syndrome (proteinuria, hypoalbuminemia, and edema), retinal exudates, and microhemorrhages. The mechanism of basement membrane thickening in diabetes may be due to formation of advanced glycation end products (AGEs).
- Other changes in basement membrane:
    - **Lipid nephrosis:** It is a glomerular disease characterized by nephrotic syndrome without noticeable changes in the basement membrane under light microscopy. Under electron microscopy it shows effacement (loss of) foot process of visceral epithelial cells lining the GBM.
    - **Alport's syndrome:** It is a hereditary, primary glomerular disease with persistent microscopic hematuria, recurrent gross hematuria, and progressive renal failure. Under electron microscopy, it shows attenuation of the GBM, often with discontinuity of the lamina densa.

COMPONENTS OF THE EXTRACELLULAR MATRIX

Q. Describe the composition of the tissue matrix with emphasis on collagen. What are collagen disorders?

In contrast to most proteins present inside of cells (which are compact, globular molecules), proteins of the extracellular space are typically extended, *fibrous* type. The protein components of the ECM may be divided into three groups (**Table 1** and **Fig. 4**). Each of the proteins of the ECM contains binding sites for one another and for receptors on the cell surface. Because of this, they interact to form an interconnected network that is bound to the cell surface.

The major components of extracellular matrices include collagens, proteoglycans, and a variety of proteins, such as fibronectin, and laminin.

Fibrous Structural Proteins

Collagens

Q. Write a short essay on fibrillar collagen.
Q. Write a short essay on collagen in health and disease.
Q. Write a short essay on types of collagen and their significance.

Collagens comprise a family of insoluble **fibrous glycoproteins** and are **present only in extracellular matrices**. Collagen

Table 1: Main groups of protein in extracellular matrix.

Group	*Examples and nature*
Fibrous structural proteins	Collagens and elastins that provide tensile strength and recoil
Water-hydrated gels	Proteoglycans and hyaluronan that allow compressive resistance and lubrication
Adhesive glycoproteins	Connect extracellular matrix (ECM) elements to one another and to cells

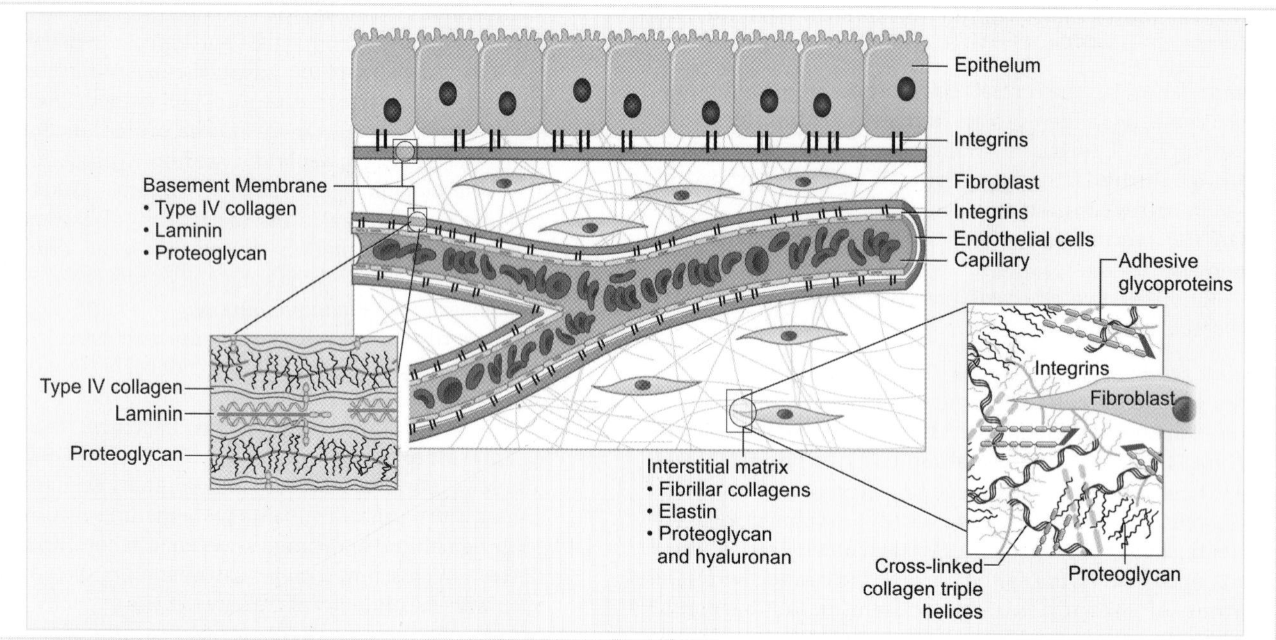

FIG. 4: Diagrammatic representation of main components of the extracellular matrix (ECM). These include collagens, proteoglycans, and adhesive glycoproteins. Epithelial and mesenchymal cells (e.g., fibroblasts) interact with ECM through integrins. Many ECM components (e.g., elastin, fibrillin, hyaluronan) are not shown in this figure.

is the **single most abundant protein** in the human body and constitutes >25% of all proteins. They have **high tensile strength**; they recoil and resist pulling forces. It is essential for the structural integrity of tissues and organs.

Collagen is the major constituent of connective tissue in all organs, most notably in cornea, arteries, dermis, cartilage, tendons, ligaments, and bone.

Production: Collagen is produced **mainly by fibroblasts** found in various types of connective tissues, but they may also be produced by smooth muscle cells and epithelial cells.

Structure: Collagens are composed of three separate polypeptide chains interlaced into a rope like triple helix meaning shape like a corkscrew or spiral staircase **Fig 5**. Collagen can be divided into several types/groups depending on the type of structures they form. There are about 30 collagen types (designated with Roman numerals I–XXX), some of which are unique to specific cells and restricted to particular locations or tissues. Collagen is protein molecules made up of amino acids. Each collagen is formed by type-specific α chains and is composed of three chains. The chains are wound together to form a triple helix of homo- or heterotrimers. All collagen α chains have at least one domain with a repeating α-helical segment. The primary amino acid sequence of collagen is glycine-proline-X or glycine-X-hydroxyproline, in which every third amino acid is glycine (X can be any of the other 17 amino acids, and every third amino acid is glycine). The chains of collagen molecules contain large amounts of proline. Many of the proline (and lysine) residues are hydroxylated (introduction of hydroxyl) following synthesis of the polypeptide chains and form hydrogen bonds between component chains.

Two or more different types of collagen are often present together in the same ECM. Functional complexity is due to the mixing of different collagen types within the same fiber. Though there are many differences among the members of the collagen family, all have at least two important structural features: (1) All collagen molecules are trimers consisting of three polypeptide chains, (2) At least in part of their length, the three polypeptide chains of a collagen molecule are wound around each other to form a rod-like triple helix. The hydroxylated amino acids are needed for maintaining the stability of the triple helix.

Nature of Collagen

Synthesis of collagen: The process of collagen synthesis occurs mainly in the fibroblasts. Collagen synthesis occurs both intracellularly and extracellularly. Salient steps in synthesis of fibrillar collagen are presented in **Figure 5.**

Fibrillar collagens (Fig. 6) Fibrillar collagens (types I, II, III, V, and XI) constitute a sub-group within the collagen family. Their functions are to provide three-dimensional frameworks for tissues and organs. They form linear fibrils stabilized by interchain hydrogen bonding. Fibrillar collagens form a major proportion of the connective tissue in structures such as bone, tendon, cartilage, blood vessels, and skin, as well as in healing wounds and scars. A continuous, uninterrupted, triple helical organization of α-chains is the predominant structure of the rigid, stiff, fibrillar collagens. The tensile strength of the fibrillar collagens is due to lateral crosslinking of the triple helices by covalent bonds. It requires hydroxylation of lysine residues in collagen by the enzyme lysyl oxidase. This lysyl oxidase is a vitamin C-dependent enzyme. The fibrillar collagens turn over slowly in most tissues and are usually resistant to digestion by proteinase, except by specific matrix metalloproteinases (MMPs).

Nonfibrillar collagens Nonfibrillar collagens are a family of structurally-related shortchain collagens that do not form large fibril bundles. They contain interrupting, flexible, noncollagenous domains that may even be the major portion of the protein. They contain a mixture of globular and triple helical domains (**Fig. 7**) and are responsible for their structural diversity and molecular flexibility which is not found in fibrillar collagens. Nonfibrillar collagens are rich in glycine, proline,

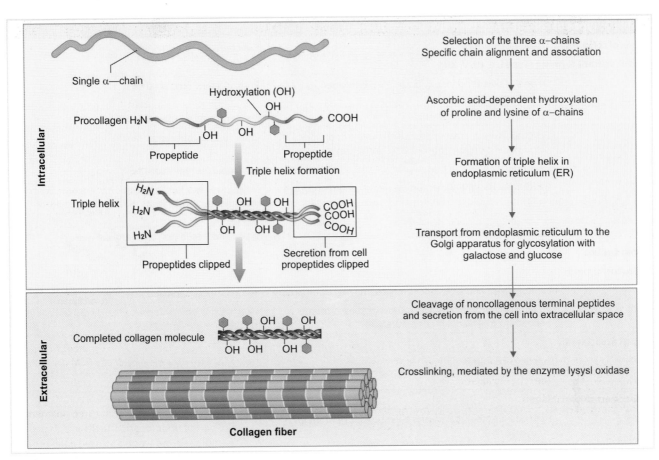

FIG. 5: Steps in the synthesis of fibrillar collagen. NH_2 or H_2N is the free amine group and called as N-terminus. It is the start of a protein or polypeptide. COOH is the carboxy terminals the end of an amino acid chain (protein or polypeptide). OH is hydroxylation.

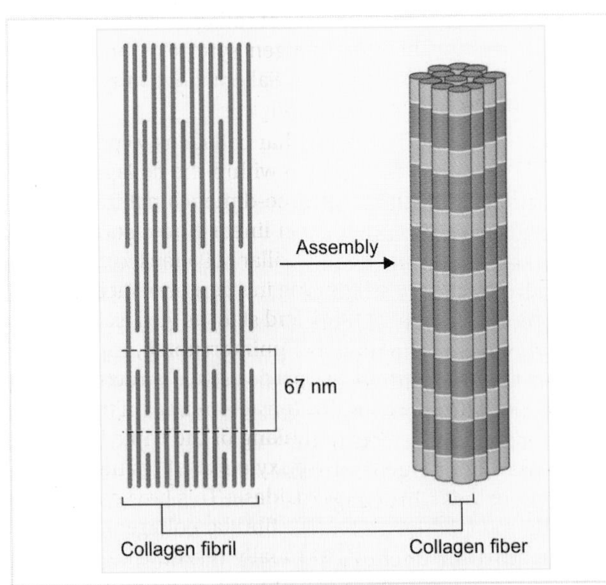

FIG. 6: Diagrammatic appearance of fibrillar collagen.

and hydroxyproline and form triple-helical units. However the helical region is short or interrupted. The nonfibrillar collagens form basal laminas (i.e., basement membranes), anchors, and microfibrils. Significance of nonfibrillar collagen is listed in **Box 1**.

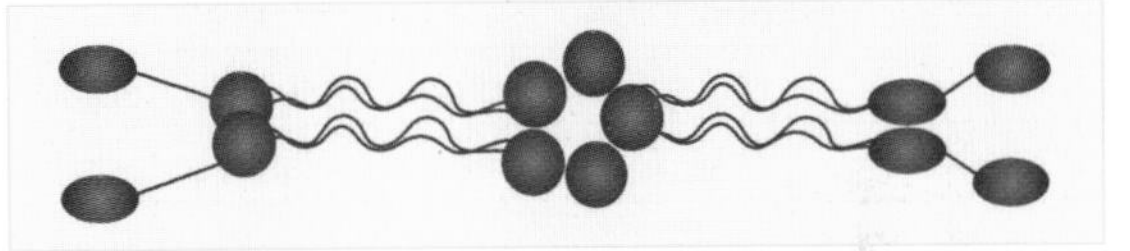

FIG. 7: Diagrammatic appearance of nonfibrillar collagen.

Box 1: Significance of nonfibrillar collagen.

- Contribute to the structures of planar basement membranes (type IV collagen)
- Help regulate collagen fibril diameters or collagen–collagen interactions via so-called "fibril-associated collagen with interrupted triple helices" (FACITs, such as type IX collagen in cartilage)
- Provide anchoring fibrils within basement membrane beneath stratified squamous epithelium (type VII collagen)
- Act as transmembrane proteins (XVII) in hemidesmosomes

Types of collagen and their tissue distribution are presented in **Table 2**.

Abnormalities of collagen

There are numerous steps involved in collagen synthesis and they are carefully executed, tightly regulated, and controlled. However, any genetic mutations can lead to errors in assembly,

Table 2: Types of collagen and their tissue distribution.

Type of collagen	*Tissue distribution*	*Function*
Fibrillar/fibril forming (Type I, II, III, V, XI)		
I	Dermis of skin, tendons and ligaments, bone, dentin, cementum, capsule of organs	Resisting tension placed on it
II	Cartilage (hyaline and elastic)	Resisting tension placed on it
III	Reticular fibers in organs (e.g., spleen, lymph node, liver), blood vessel, skin; commonly found alongside type I	Constructs architectural framework
V	Cell surfaces, hair, and placenta	Accompanies type I collagen
VIII	Endothelial basement membrane, endothelium of cornea	May form a layer for the migration of endothelial and smooth muscle cells, limits the stretching ability of elastin
XI	Same as type I and II collagen	Type I and II collagen forms around it
Nonfibrillar		
Network forming		
IV	Lamina densa of the basement membrane (e.g., glomerulus)	Affords support and acts as a filter
VII	Provide anchoring fibrils within basement membrane beneath stratified squamous epithelium	Attaches the lamina densa to the lamina reticularis of the basement membrane
Fibril associated		
IX	See type II collagen	Combines with type II collagen
XII	See type I collagen	Combines with type I collagen
Transmembrane collagen		
XVII	Hemidesmosome (previously called bullous pemphigoid antigen)	Unknown
XVIII	Lamina reticularis of the basement membrane	Enzymatic cleavage transforms it into angiogenesis inhibitor and endostatin
IX, XII, XIV, XIX, XXI	FACIT (Fibril associated collagens with interrupted triple helices)	
VIII, X	Short chain	
XV, XIII	Multiplexin (Multiple triple helix domains with interruptions)	
Type XIII, XVII	MACIT (Membrane associated collagens with interrupted triple helices)	

post-translational modification, or nutritional deficiencies which can affect enzymatic function.

- **Reduced, delayed, or abnormal synthesis of collagen:** It will result in delay of wound healing (e.g., in scurvy) or **nonhealing of wounds**. The hydroxylated amino acids are needed for maintaining the stability of the triple helix of collagen. Failure to hydroxylate collagen chains produces both structural and functional changes in the connective tissues. Ascorbic acid (vitamin C) is a coenzyme necessary for adding hydroxyl groups to the lysine and proline amino acids of collagen. Scurvy, a disease due to deficiency of vitamin C (ascorbic acid) is associated with poor wound healing and the weakening of the lining of blood vessels (causes easy internal bleeding) due to "weak" collagen. Children with ascorbate deficiency develop skeletal deformities.
- **Excess deposition of collagen** leads to **fibrosis**. Fibrosis is seen in connective tissue diseases such as scleroderma and keloids. Fibrosis can cause chronic damage to many organs such as kidney, lung, heart, and liver, resulting in compromising their function.
- **Mutations of fibrillar collagens:** Genetic defects in collagens can cause diseases of bone (osteogenesis imperfecta), cartilage (achondrogenesis or hypochondrogenesis, chondroplasias or epiphyseal dysplasias), skin, joints, and blood vessels (Ehlers-Danlos syndrome). Mutant interruptions in the triple helix of fibrillar collagens cause minor to lethal pathology in skin, blood vessels, bone, or cartilage. Mutations in the genes of type I collagen can cause assembly defects in the triple helix and can lead to increased bone fractures, hyperextensible ligaments and dermis or easy bruising. Mutations may also produce certain myopathies and muscular dystrophy. Collagen VII forms **fibrillar anchors between** hemidesmosome and basement membrane to underlying stroma. Mutations in these collagens can cause mild-to-severe blistering in junctional and dystrophic epidermolysis bullosa. Examples of disorders associated with abnormal collagen are listed in **Table 3**.

Table 4 shows collagen types, its distribution and associated disease.

Elastin and Elastic Fibers

Elastin is a secreted matrix protein and unlike other stromal proteins, it is not glycosylated (addition of a sugar molecule). This lack of carbohydrate/glucose (glycosylation), its extensive covalent crosslinking, and its hydrophobic amino acid sequence makes it as the most insoluble proteins. The ability of tissues to recoil and recover their shape after physical deformation is due to elastin. Elastin is also crosslinked similar to collagen. However, it has large hydrophobic segments that form a dense globular configuration at rest. When it is stretched, the hydrophobic domains are pulled open, but the crosslinks keep the molecules intact. When the tension is released, the hydrophobic domains of the proteins refold (**Fig. 8**).

Importance: Elasticity is important in cardiac valves and large blood vessels (e.g., aorta), which must stretch to accommodate recurrent pulsatile flow, as well as in the uterus, ligaments, skin, lung, elastic cartilage. Though elastic fiber is important for the function of several vital tissues, it is not efficiently replaced during repair of skin and lung. In emphysema, there is loss of recoil in lung due to degradation of alveolar elastin. Elastin once polymerized into fibers, it is resistant to proteolysis and turns over slowly. However, elastic fibers degenerate and, in skin, decrease owing to a diminished capacity for replacement with aging (responsible for dermal atrophy, wrinkling, and loss of dermal flexibility. Excess exposure to sun increases abnormal elastotic material along with age-related loss of collagen in the dermal connective tissue leads to thickening of skin and forms coarse, furrowed wrinkles.

Stability of elastin: It is due to its: (1) Hydrophobicity, (2) Extensive covalent crosslinking [mediated by lysyl oxidase (enzyme that crosslinks collagen)], and (3) Resistance to most proteolytic enzymes.

Synthesis: Elastic fibers are formed from the condensation of a soluble elastin precursor on a complex of several microfibrillar glycoproteins (mainly **fibrillin**). Morphologically, elastic fibers are composed of a central core of elastin surrounded by mesh-like network composed of fibrillin. Fibrillin also controls the availability of transforming growth factor β (TGF-β).

Diseases produced: Mutated abnormal fibrillin is associated with decreased binding and reduced activation of TGF-β. In

Table 3: Examples of disorders associated with abnormal collagen.

Type of mutated collagen	*Associated disease*
Type I	Osteogenesis imperfecta, Ehlers–Danlos syndrome, infantile cortical hyperostosis (Caffey's disease)
Type II	Collagenopathy, types II and XI, achondrogenesis
Type III	Ehlers–Danlos syndrome, Dupuytren contracture
Type IV	Alport syndrome
Type V	Ehlers–Danlos syndrome (classical)
Type VII	Junctional and dystrophic epidermolysis bullosa
Type XI	Collagenopathy, types II and XI

Table 4: Collagen types, its distribution and associated disease.

Collagen type	*Principle tissue distribution*	*Cells of origin*	*Disease associated*
I	Skin, tendon, vascular ligaments, bone, dentin	Fibroblast, smooth muscle cell, osteoblast, odontoblast	Osteogenesis imperfecta Ehlers–Danlos syndrome (arthrochalasia)
II	Hyaline and elastic cartilage, vitreous of eye	Chondrocyte, retinal cell	Achondrogenesis-II Spondyloepiphyseal syndrome
III	Reticular fibers in organs (e.g., spleen, lymph node, liver), blood vessel, skin; commonly found alongside type 1	Fibroblast and reticular cell	Vascular type Ehlers–Danlos syndrome
IV	Basement membrane, lens capsule of eye	Epithelial and endothelial cell, lens fiber	Alport syndrome
V	Cell surfaces, hair, and placenta	Fibroblast, smooth muscle	Classical Ehlers–Danlos syndrome
VI	Connective tissue	Fibroblast	Bethlem myopathy
VII	Epithelial basement membrane, anchoring fibrils		Epidermolysis bullosa
VIII	Cornea	Corneal fibroblast	
IX	Cartilage		Epiphyseal dysplasia
X	Hypertrophic cartilage		
XI	Cartilage		Stickler syndrome
XII	Hypertrophic cartilage	Fibroblast	
XIII	Reticular dermis	Fibroblast	
XIV	P170 bullous pemphigoid antigen	Keratinocyte	
XV	Endothelial cells		Knobloch syndrome

Marfan syndrome, fibrillin defects lead to skeletal abnormalities and weakened aortic walls (produces aortic dissection/dissecting aortic aneurysm). Mutations in **fibulin** can result in the generalized elastin defect as in cutis laxa.

Water-Hydrated Gels

Proteoglycans

Proteoglycans are distinctive type of protein-polysaccharide complex found in ECM. A proteoglycan consists of a **core protein molecule** (**Figs. 9A** and **B**) to which many chains of polysaccharides called **glycosaminoglycans** (GAGs) are covalently attached. Names of individual proteoglycans are designated by the core protein. Each glycosaminoglycan chain is composed of a repeating disaccharide (i.e., it has the structure –A–B–A–B–, where A and B represent two different sugars). The examples of GAGs include keratan sulfate and chondroitin sulfate and these are sulfated GAGs. In GAGs, the disaccharide/sugar rings are attached by both sulfate and carboxyl groups. These densely packed sulfated sugars are highly acidic nature and bear high negative charge. Proteoglycans of the ECM (basic structures) may assemble to form gigantic complexes by linkage of their core proteins to a long back bone of hyaluronic acid polymer (a nonsulfated GAG). The appearance of this gigantic complex resembles the bristles on a test-tube brush used for cleaning test tubes in laboratory.

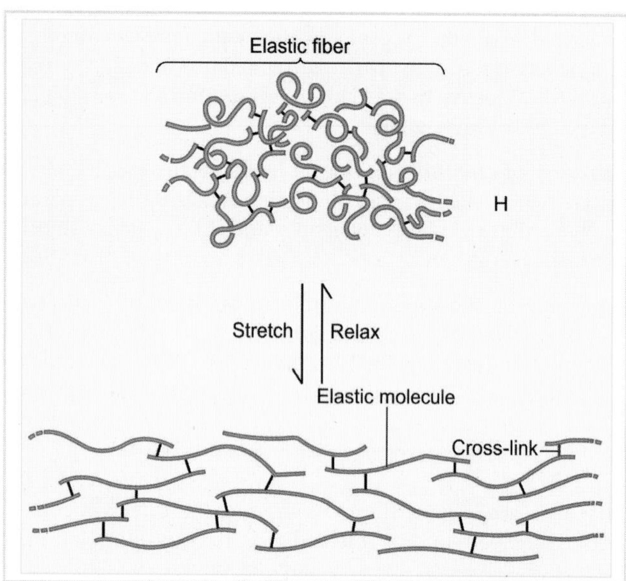

FIG. 8: Structure of elastin. Elastin is also crosslinked similar to collagen. However, it has large hydrophobic segments that form a dense globular configuration at rest. When it is stretched, the hydrophobic domains are pulled open, but the crosslinks keep the molecules intact. When the tension is released, the hydrophobic domains of the proteins refold.

Functions

- **Provides compressibility to tissues:** Because of highly negative charge of sulfated sugars, they attract huge numbers of cations (mostly sodium) which in turn bind to abundant water molecules and produce a viscous, gelatin-like matrix. As a result, proteoglycans form a porous, hydrated gel that fills the extracellular space such as packing material. With this nature of high hydration, these gels give resistance to compressive forces (resists crushing) and in joint cartilage, proteoglycans also provide a layer of lubrication between adjacent bony surfaces.
- **Reservoirs for growth factors:** Proteoglycans serve as reservoirs or as a "sink" for secreted growth factors and other signaling molecules. A number of growth factors bind to proteoglycans [e.g., fibroblast growth factor (FGF), vascular endothelial growth factor (VEGF), hepatocyte growth factor (HGF), and heparin-binding epidermal growth factor (HB-EGF)].
- **Cellular activities:** Some proteoglycans are integral cell membrane proteins. Hence, they are involved in cell proliferation, cell–cell signaling, migration, and adhesion (e.g., by binding and concentrating growth factors and chemokines).

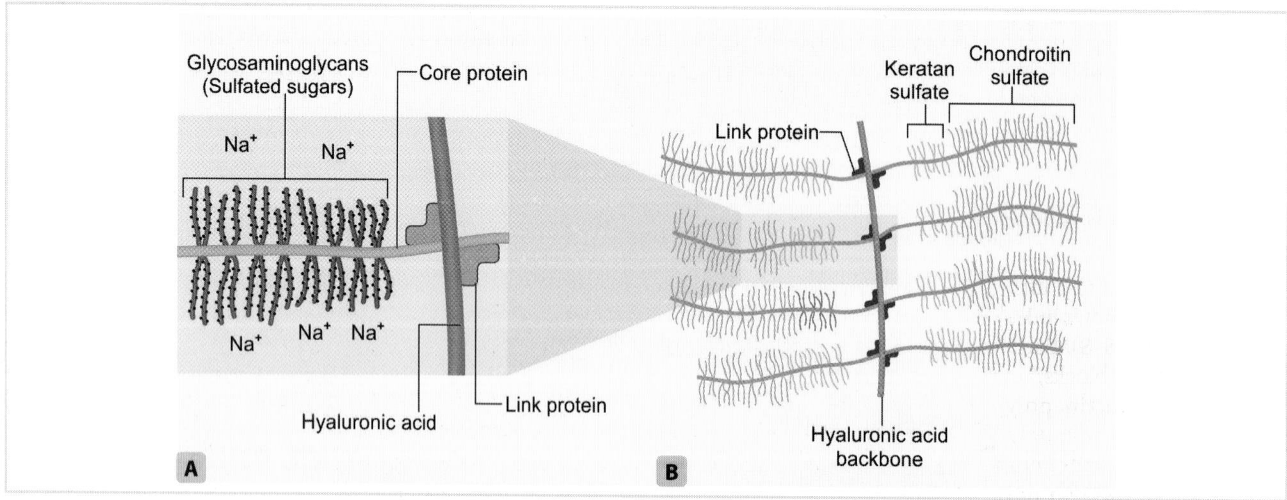

FIGS. 9A AND B: Structure of proteoglycan (diagrammatic). (A) Diagrammatic representation of a single proteoglycan. Basic structure consisting of core protein surrounded by many chains of polysaccharides [called glycosaminoglycans (GAGs)].These GAGs are highly negatively charged sulfated sugars attract sodium and water to generate a viscous compressible matrix. (B) Complex structure shows several basic structures (8 numbers in above figure) attached to a hyaluronic acid backbone Na^+, sodium ions.

Hyaluronan

Hyaluronan is the only GAG not covalently linked to a protein. It is a linear polymer of 2,000–25,000 disaccharides of glucosamine and glucuronic acid. It is very hydrophilic. Hyaluronan can bind protein cores of proteoglycans that contain hyaluronan-binding regions and also with hyaluronan-binding proteins at the cell surface. Some proteoglycans bind along the hyaluronan backbone via a link protein to form large, space-filling, hydrophilic hyaluronan/proteoglycan composites (**Fig. 9B**). These are **aggrecan** and **versican** molecules found in cartilage and stromal tissues, respectively. The viscosity of free hyaluronan in solution gives resilience and lubrication to joints and connective tissue.

Heparan Sulfate Proteoglycan

This proteoglycan is composed of multiple GAG chains covalently bound to a core protein. Heparan sulfate proteoglycan probably plays a major role in filtration and cell attachment. **Syndecans** are heparan sulfate proteoglycans involved in growth factor signaling, coagulation, cell adhesion to the ECM, and tumorigenesis. Regulation of basic FGF (bFGF, FGF-2) activity by ECM and cellular proteoglycans is presented in **Figure 10**.

Composition and connective tissue distribution of GAGs and their interaction with collagen fibers is presented in **Table 5**.

Adhesive Glycoproteins and Adhesion Receptors

They constitute structurally diverse molecules and are involved in cell-cell, cell-ECM, and ECM-ECM interactions. Classical adhesive glycoproteins include fibronectin (a major component of the interstitial ECM) and laminin (a major constituent of basement membrane). Integrins are adhesion receptors [also known as cell adhesion molecules (CAMs)]. CAMs also include immunoglobulin family members, cadherins, and selectins.

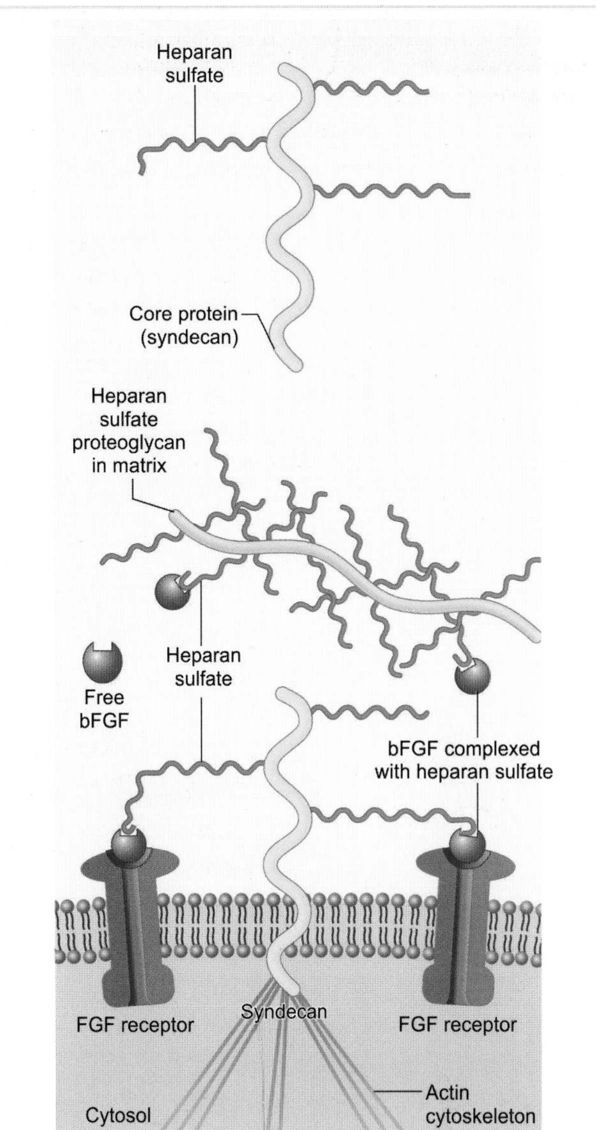

FIG. 10: Diagrammatic representation of regulation of basic fibroblast growth factor (FGF) (bFGF, FGF-2) activity by extracellular matrix (ECM) and cellular proteoglycans. Heparan sulfate binds bFGF secreted in the ECM. Syndecan is a cell surface proteoglycan (heparan sulfate proteoglycans) with a transmembrane core protein and extracellular glycosaminoglycan (GAG) side chains that bind bFGF. The cytoplasmic tail of syndecan interacts with the intracellular actin cytoskeleton. Its side chains bind bFGF released from damaged ECM, thus favors interaction of bFGF with receptors on the surface of cells.

Fibronectin

Q. Write a short essay on fibronectins.

It is a large (450 kD) disulfide-linked heterodimer. This is a versatile, adhesive glycoprotein present in two forms: (1) Hepatocyte-derived, soluble form in plasma, and (2) The insoluble tissue fibronectin (cellular form). It is synthesized by a variety of cells such as fibroblasts, monocytes, and endothelium and is widely distributed in stromal connective tissue.

Structure (Fig. 11) Fibronectin chains form a V-shaped homo- or heterodimer linked at the C terminus (COOH) by two disulfide bonds (S–S). Each chain consists of a linear array of distinct "building blocks," or domains.

Each fibronectin polypeptide is constructed from a sequence of approximately 30 fibronectin (Fn) domains and these domains combine to form five or six larger functional units. Each of the two polypeptide chains that make up a fibronectin molecule contains:

- Specific domains that bind to many distinct ECM components. These include collagens, fibrin, heparin, proteoglycans as well as integrins. The integrins binds through arginine-glycine-aspartic acid (RGD) motifs.
- Binding sites for receptors on the cell surface. These binding sites hold the ECM in a stable attachment to the cell.

Significance In wound healing, tissue and plasma fibronectin provide a scaffold for subsequent ECM deposition, angiogenesis, and re-epithelialization. It can also interact with collagen and promote keratinocyte attachment and migration during re-epithelialization.

Laminin

Laminins are the family of extracellular glycoproteins and are the most abundant glycoprotein in the basement membrane.

Table 5: Composition and connective tissue distribution of glycosaminoglycans and their interaction with collagen fibers.

Glycosaminoglycan	*Repeating disaccharides*		*Distribution*	*Electrostatic interaction with collagen*
	Hexuronic Acid	*Hexosamine*		
Hyaluronic acid	D-glucuronic acid	D-glucosamine	Umbilical cord, synovial fluid, vitreous humor, cartilage	
Chondroitin 4-sulfate	D-glucuronic acid	D-galactosamine	Cartilage, bone, cornea, skin, notochord, aorta	Mainly with collagen type II (***)
Chondroitin 6-sulfate	D-glucuronic acid	D-galactosamine	Cartilage, umbilical cord, skin, aorta (media)	
Dermatan sulfate	l-iduronic acid or D-glucuronic acid	D-galactosamine	Skin, tendon, aorta (adventitia)	Mainly with collagen type I (*)
Heparan sulfate	D-glucuronic acid or l-iduronic acid	D-galactosamine	Aorta, lung, liver, basal laminae	Mainly with collagen types III and IV (**)
Keratan sulfate	D-galactose	D-glucosamine	Cartilage, nucleus pulposus, annulus fibrosus	None

(*** = high, **intermediate and *low level interaction)

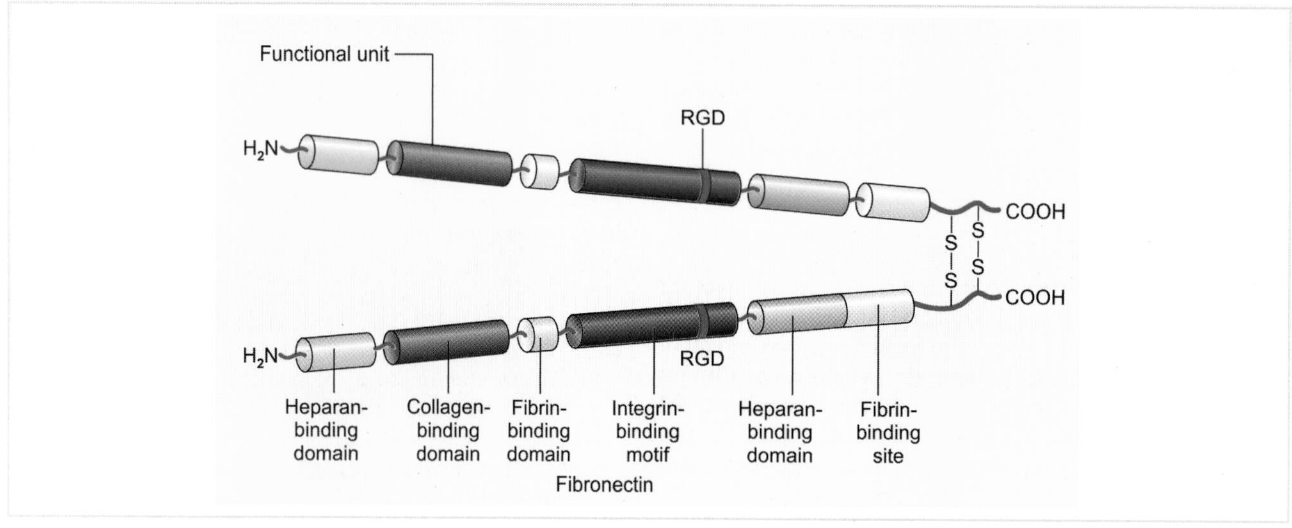

(COOH: carboxy terminal; H_2N, amino terminal; s-s disufide bond)

FIG. 11: Structure of fibronectin. It consists of a disulfide-linked dimer, with several distinct domains. These domains allow binding to various components of extracellular matrix (ECM) and integrins. The integrin binds through arginine–glycine–aspartic acid (RGD) motifs.

Structure (Fig. 12) It consists of three different polypeptide chains (heterotrimer) linked by disulfide bonds and organized into a molecule resembling a cross (cross-like structure) with three short arms and one long arm. It is produced by products of three related gene subfamilies to form α, β, and γ heterotrimers. There are about 18 different laminins, which are formed intracellularly from varying combinations of the five α-, three β- and three γ chains. After secretion, some laminin trimers are further processed by proteinases.

Significance Laminin molecules form sheets and combine with type IV collagen sheets and other basement membrane molecules and form basement membrane. It connects cells to underlying ECM components such as type IV collagen and heparan sulfate. Laminin can bind to both heparan sulfate proteoglycans in basement membranes and to heparan sulfate chains on syndecan receptors (through heparan sulfate proteoglycan binding site). It can also modulate cell proliferation, differentiation, and motility.

Abnormalities and disease Cells can bind to laminin via several integrins, as well as muscle dystroglycan and Lutheran blood grouping receptors. The muscle cell dystroglycan receptor complex binds basement membrane laminin, and mutations in either the receptor or laminin can cause different forms of muscular dystrophy. Mutations in epidermal laminin or the appropriate integrin, or the collagen VII or collagen XVII can produce different forms of a potentially fatal skin blistering disease, termed **epidermolysis bullosa**.

Integrins

Integrins are the large family of transmembrane heterodimeric glycoproteins. It plays a key role in integrating the extracellular and intracellular environments.

Structure (Fig. 13) Integrins are composed of transmembrane α- and β subunits arranged as heterodimers that are noncovalently linked.

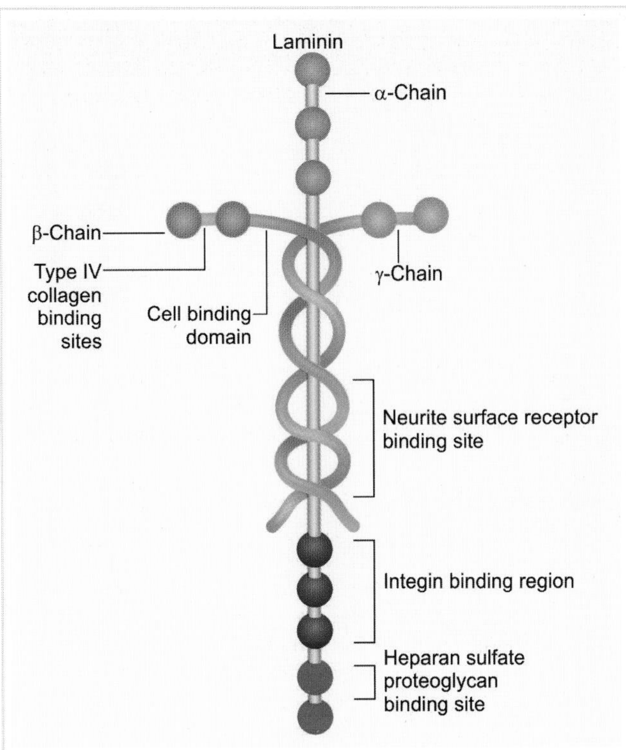

FIG. 12: Structure of laminin molecule. It consists of three chains arranged in cross-like shape. Laminin molecule is one of the major components of basement membranes. It has multiple domains that interact with type IV collagen, other extracellular matrix (ECM) components, and cell-surface receptors.

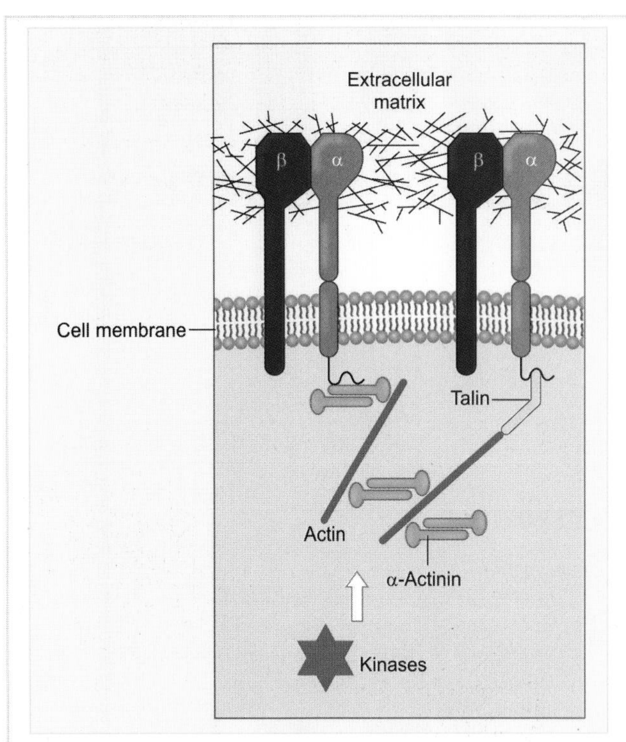

FIG. 13: Structure of integrin. Each α–β heterodimeric integrin receptor is a transmembrane dimer. It links extracellular matrix (ECM) and the intracellular cytoskeleton. It is also associated with linking protein molecules such as talin. These can recruit and activate kinases as well as trigger downstream signaling cascades.

- **Extracellular:** On the outer side of the plasma membrane, integrins bind to diverse molecules (ligands) present in the extracellular environment.
- **Intracellular:** On the intracellular side of the membrane, integrins interact either directly or indirectly with different proteins that influence the course of events within the cell.

Actions Various actions of integrins are as follows:
- **Change in intracellular protein talin:** The cytoplasmic domains of integrins bind to many proteins; one of these proteins is called talin. This protein talin causes separation of the α- and β- subunits of integrin. Outside signals can induce a conformational change in talin on the inside of the membrane. This can lead to the polymerization of actin filaments of the cytoskeleton.
- **Activation of cytoplasmic protein kinases:** Binding of integrins to an extracellular ligand can also trigger the activation of cytoplasmic protein kinases. These kinases can then phosphorylate other proteins and initiate a chain reaction. In few, it may activate specific group of genes in the nucleus.

Functions Various functions of integrins are as follows:
- **Focal attachment to underlying substrates:** Integrins allow cells to attach to ECM components such as laminin and fibronectin via a tripeptide RGD motif. This functionally and structurally links the intracellular cytoskeleton with the outside world (cell-ECM binding).
- **Mediate cell-cell adhesive interactions (cell-cell interactions):** For example, integrins on the surface of leukocytes are required for firm adhesion to and transmigration across the endothelium at sites of inflammation (leukocyte recruitment). Integrins also play a role in platelet aggregation.
- **Others:** Integrin receptors can also trigger signaling cascades that influence cell locomotion, proliferation, shape, and differentiation.

Abnormalities Mutations in talin block its interaction with subunits of integrin and also prevent activation of integrins and adhesion to the ECM.

For more details on integrins refer pages 24–25, 233–234 and 284–286. For the further details on the role of extracellular matrix and collagen in disease refer pages 826–829.

BIBLIOGRAPHY

1. Gartner LP. Color Atlas and Text of Histology, 7th edition. Wolters Kluwer: Wolters Kluwer; 2018.
2. Kierszenbaum AL, Tres LL. Histology and Cell Biology-An Introduction to Pathology, 5th edition. Philadelphia: Saunders Elsevier; 2016.
3. Kumar V, Abbas AK, Aster JC. Robbins basic pathology, 10th edition. Philadelphia: Saunders Elsevier; 2018
4. Kumar V, Abbas AK, Fausto N, et al. Robbins and Cotran Pathologic basis of disease, 10th edition. Philadelphia: WB Saunders; 2021.
5. Mescher AL. Junqueira's Basic Histology-Text And Atlas, 15th edition. New York: McGraw-Hill Education; 2018.
6. Strayer DS, Saffitz JE. Rubin's Pathology: Mechanism of Human Disease, 8th edition. Philadelphia: Wolters Kluwer; 2020.

CHAPTER 5

Basics of Genetics

CHAPTER OUTLINE

- Introduction
  - Genetics
- Chromosomes
  - Morphology of chromosomes
  - Morphological classification of chromosomes
  - Components of chromosome
  - Types of nucleic acids
- Deoxyribonucleic acid
  - Location of deoxyribonucleic acid
  - Structure of deoxyribonucleic acid
  - Structure of nucleotide unit
  - Formation of a strand
  - Histone
  - Nucleosome
- DNA's information content
  - Regions in the deoxyribonucleic acid
  - Nuclear genes
  - Extragenic deoxyribonucleic acid
- Ribonucleic acid
  - Ribonucleic acid structure and types
- Genes
  - Definition
  - Structure of gene
  - Genomic variability
- Gene action: From DNA to protein
  - DNA Transcription and Protein Synthesis
  - Transcription
  - Ribonucleic acid processing
  - Translation
  - Post-translational modification
  - Gene expression
  - Major classes of ribonucleic acid
  - Micro-RNA and long noncoding RNA
- Gene editing technology
  - Engineered targeted nucleases
  - Applications of gene editing

INTRODUCTION

During mid-19th century, the Augustinian monk Gregor Mendel observed that certain features pass from parents to their children/offspring. A child usually looks like their parents and it is due to inheritance of certain characteristics from parents. This **transmission of characteristics from parents to children is known as heredity**. The **basic unit of heredity is gene**, which **consists of portion** of deoxyribonucleic acid **(DNA) molecules**.

Genetics

Genetics is the study which **deals with the science of genes**, heredity, and its variation in living organisms.

The genome is the entirety of the DNA sequence or chromosomes or its "complete genetic complement." Thus, the term ***genome* refers to the total genetic information contained in a cell. Genomics is the sequencing and study of genomes.** The sequencing of the human genome was achieved at the beginning of the 21st century. This has revolutionized the understanding of health and disease. Cytogenetics is the study of chromosomes, traditionally through visualization of the karyotype or set of chromosomes. The human genetic program contains so much information which if converted to words can fill millions of pages of text. This vast amount of information is packaged into a set of chromosomes which occupies the space of a cell nucleus—hundreds of times smaller than the dot on this *i*.

CHROMOSOMES

Chromosomes **appear as colored bodies** and **carry the hereditary material namely genes**. Tjio and Levan in 1956 described that normal human somatic cell contains 46 chromosomes. These chromosomes are arranged in two sets of 23 each per cell. One set is inherited from the father and the other from the mother. Each set of 23 chromosomes have **two types** namely:

1. **Autosomal chromosomes (autosomes):** Each set of chromosomes have 22 autosomes and are **identified by numbers from 1 to 22**. The corresponding individual autosomes in each set are identical to one another in shape and size and are named as homologous pair.
2. **Sex chromosomes:** The **X and Y** chromosomes are known as the sex chromosomes because they determine sex. The human cells contain one pair of sex chromosomes. Females have two X chromosomes (46XX) and males have one X and one Y chromosome (46XY).

Morphology of Chromosomes

- **During rest:** When the cell is not dividing, the individual chromosomes cannot be distinguished.
- **During cell division:** During cell division (mitosis or meiosis), the individual chromosomes **become shorter and thicker** (rod-like) and assume **X shape**. The two identical strands called **chromatids** are held together by narrow region known as **centromere**. The centromere

divides the chromosome into two "arms." The **short arm** labeled the "p arm" (p, from French, *petit*) and the long **arm** of the chromosome is labeled the "q arm". The position of the centromere differs from chromosome to chromosome and gives each chromosome its unique shape.

Morphological Classification of Chromosomes

Depending on the three parameters of length, location of the centromere (constrictions), and the presence or absence of satellites, the chromosomes are classified into various types (**Fig. 1**). Chromosomes appear at the beginning of mitosis and disappear once again when cell division has ended. The nucleus contains two copies of the genome, observed microscopically as 23 chromosome pairs (known as the karyotype). Chromosomes 1 to 22 are called as the autosomes and consist of identical chromosomal pairs. The 23rd "pair" of chromosomes consists of two sex chromosomes (females have two X chromosomes and males an X and Y chromosome). Therefore, a normal karyotype for female is written as 46, XX and for a male as 46, XY.

Components of Chromosome (Box 1 and Fig. 2)

Chromosomes within the nucleus are composed of a **mixture of DNA and** associated **protein** which together forms a tightly packed complex termed as **chromatin**.

Nuclear Chromatin (Box 2)

Chromatin represents the uncoiled chromosome of the interphase nucleus. The individual chromosomes occupy specific positions of the nucleus which are referred to as chromosomal territories. Chromatin consists of DNA, histone, and nonhistone proteins.

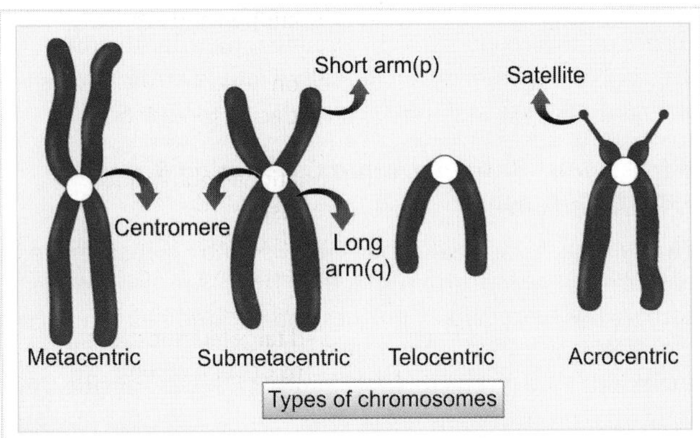

FIG. 1: Morphological types of chromosomes depending on the location of centromere. The centromere is in the center in metacentric, little away from the center in submetacentric, eccentric with satellites in acrocentric, and at one end in telocentric.

Box 1: Salient features of chromatin.

- Represents the uncoiled chromosome of the interphase nucleus
- Composition
  - **Deoxyribonucleic acid** (DNA)
  - Histone
  - Nonhistone proteins
- Types
  - Inactive heterochromatin (dense area under microscope)
  - Active euchromatin (disperse area under microscope)
- Nucleosome
  - The basic unit of chromatin
  - Deoxyribonucleic acid coils in two turns around a central octameric protein core containing two copies each of histone H2A, H2B, H3 and H4
  - Strings of nucleosomes are helically twisted and folded to form chromatin

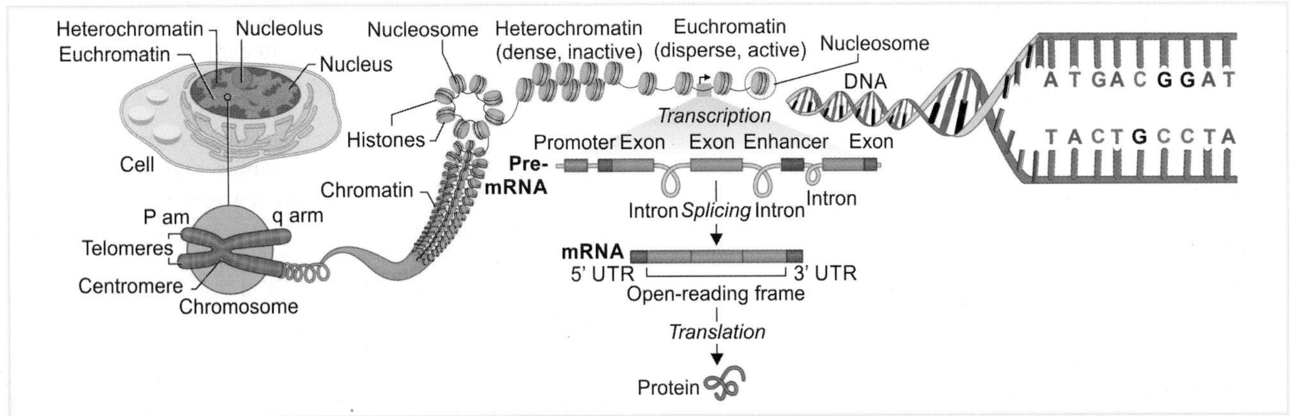

FIG. 2: Diagrammatic representation of deoxyribonucleic acid (DNA), genes, and chromosomes. Under the light microscope, the nuclear genetic material is dispersed into transcriptionally active *euchromatin* or densely packed, transcriptionally inactive *heterochromatin*. Chromosomes can only be seen by light microscopy during cell division. Chromosome during mitosis divides longitudinally into chromatids and consists of a short "p" *("petite")* and long "q" *("next letter in the alphabet")* arms. Individual chromatin fibers are composed of a string of nucleosomes. In each nucleosome, DNA is wound around octameric histone cores. Active gene consists of promoters (noncoding regions of DNA) that initiate gene transcription. Enhancers are regulatory elements that can modulate gene expression. Transcription produces pre-mRNA (precursor messenger ribonucleic acid). Then the intronic sequences in the gene are spliced out of the pre-mRNA to produce the definitive message. The mRNA so formed includes exons and they are translated into protein. The 3′ and 5′ untranslated regions (UTR) may have regulatory functions.

Box 2: Components of chromosome.

- **Deoxyribonucleic acid (DNA):** Nucleotides are the building block of **nucleic acid**. DNA consists of chain of nucleotides.
- **Protein** which consists of approximately equal parts of:
  - Basic core protein namely **histone**
  - Acidic **Nonhistone** protein
- Small amount of ribonucleic acid (RNA)

Table 1: Differences between chromatin and chromosome.

Features	*Chromatin*	*Chromosome*
Packing of deoxyribonucleic acid (DNA)	Loosely packed DNA	Tightly packed DNA
Observed in	Interphase nuclei	Cell division
Composition	Histone and DNA chain	DNA chain only

Classification of Chromatin

Chromatin can be classified as heterochromatin and euchromatin. The heterochromatin consists of condensed portion of chromatin where genes are usually inactive. Euchromatin is less condensed and consists of actively transcribed genes. Heterochromatin and euchromatin (refer **Fig. 2**) are seen in the cells/tissues under light microscope.

Differences between chromatin and chromosome are presented in **Table 1**.

Types of Nucleic Acids

Nucleic acid is a macromolecule composed of a long polymer (chains/**strands**) of individual (monomer) molecules called **nucleotides**. Nucleic acids in combination with proteins form ***nucleoproteins***. Nucleic acids are of two types, namely the DNA and ribonucleic acid (RNA). In cells, information stored in DNA is used to govern activities of cells through the formation of RNA messages.

- **Deoxyribonucleic acid (DNA)** is present in the nucleus of cells. DNA maintains all the information needed for maintenance of the organism and transfers the information to successive generations.
- **Ribonucleic acid (RNA)** carries information from DNA to the cytoplasm of a cell and directs synthesis of the proteins necessary for the function of the organism.

The normality of health depends on the stability of DNA and on accurate duplication of DNA and translation into protein. Gene is the protein-coding unit of DNA.

DEOXYRIBONUCLEIC ACID

Location of Deoxyribonucleic Acid

- **Nuclear/chromosomal DNA:** Most of the DNA is inside the nucleus.
- **Mitochondrial DNA (mtDNA):** Mitochondria contains small amount of DNA.

Structure of Deoxyribonucleic Acid

The structure of DNA was first described by **James D Watson and Francis Crick** in 1953 for which they received the Nobel Prize (1962). The majority of chromosomal **DNA** is a long, **double-stranded** (dsDNA) **helix (**molecule) comparable to a twisted ladder. But it is **single-stranded** (ssDNA) **at the end** of chromosomes composed of a small number of building blocks, where it is called **telomere**. DNA in a double helix is arranged in complementary strands—the sequence of nucleotides in one strand of DNA is a "mirror image" of the nucleotide sequence in the other DNA strand. DNA is a long polymer (consisting of very large molecules, or macromolecules). DNA is composed of subunits or the basic building blocks known as **nucleotides** (**Figs. 3A** to **C**).

Salient features of DNA are presented in **Box 3**.

Structure of Nucleotide Unit (Figs. 3A to C)

Each **nucleotide chain (Box 4)** is made up of **three main components,** namely nitrogenous base, deoxyribose (ribose in case of RNA) sugar, and phosphate molecule. The molecule without phosphate group is called **nucleoside (i.e., only nitrogenous base and deoxyribose)**.

Nitrogenous Base (Nitrogen Containing Bases) of RNA and DNA

Nitrogenous base is so called because nitrogen atoms form part of the rings of the molecule. There are two classes of nitrogenous base namely purines and pyrimidines in a nucleic acid (DNA and RNA). The atoms of the nitrogenous base in nucleosides are given ***cardinal*** numbers; 1–9 for **purines,** and 1–6 for **pyrimidines.** Purine is longer molecule with the *shorter* name and pyrimidine is smaller molecule with the *longer* name. In purine, their atoms are numbered in anti-clockwise direction (**Fig. 4**). In pyrimidine, the atoms are numbered in opposite directions to that of purine (**Fig. 4**). and their atoms are numbered in clockwise direction. The nitrogenous bases are the information-containing parts of DNA because they form sequences. DNA sequences are measured depending on the numbers of base pairs. The terms kilobase (kb) and megabase (mb) are used to abbreviate a thousand and a million DNA bases, respectively. For example, a gene may contain 1,400 bases, or 1.4 kb long.

Purine bases

Two main purine bases found in DNAs and RNAs are: (1) **Adenine** (abbreviated A) and (2) **Guanine** (G). They **contain two rings.**

Pyrimidine bases

There are three major pyrimidine bases, namely: (1) Cytosine (C), (2) Uracil (U), and (3) Thymine (T). They **contain a single ring.**

Both DNA and RNA contain the pyrimidine **cytosine** but they differ in their second pyrimidine base. **DNA contains second** pyrimidine base namely **thymine** (T), apart from **cytosine**(C) whereas RNA contains uracil instead of thymine.

Linked to the 1′ carbon of each sugar is one of four possible bases—2 pyrimidines [thymine (T) and cytosine (C)], and 2 purines [adenine (A) and guanine (G)]. These bases can occur in any sequence order. Thus, they form the variable portion of ssDNA. The building blocks of the single-stranded polymer

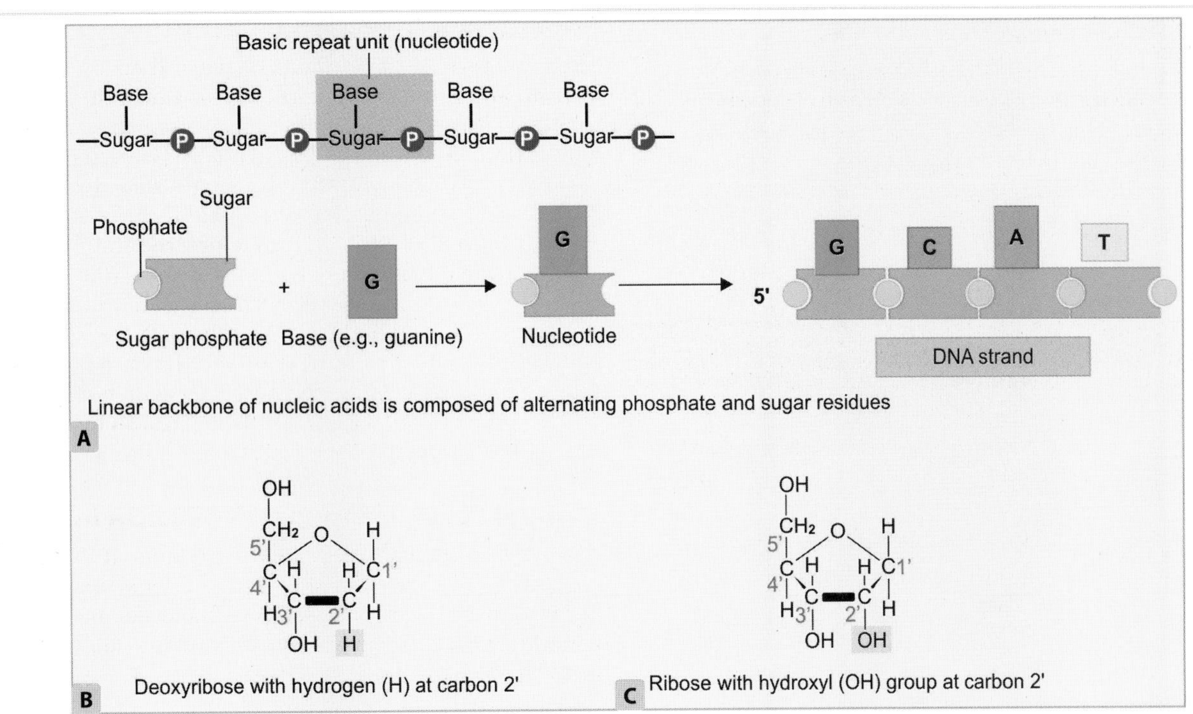

FIGS. 3A TO C: Diagrammatic appearance of repeat units in nucleic acids. (A) The linear backbone of nucleic acids is composed of alternating phosphate and sugar residues. To each sugar a nitrogenous base is attached. The basic repeat unit (shaded) consists of a nitrogenous base + sugar + phosphate = a nucleotide. The sugar has five carbon (C) atoms that are numbered from 1′ to 5′. Sugar in DNA is deoxyribose (B) and sugar in RNA is ribose (C). Sugar ribose differs from sugar deoxyribose in molecule at carbon 2′. In deoxyribose it has hydrogen (H), and ribose has a hydroxyl (OH) group attached.

Box 3: Salient features of deoxyribonucleic acid (DNA).

- Double helical strands consisting of a sugar phosphate backbone and nitrogenous bases attached with the sugar molecule
- Sugar molecule is a pentose attached with the phosphate by third and fifth carbon atom, alternatively
- Four nitrogenous base pairs: Adenine, cytosine, guanine, and thymine
- Adenine binds only with thymine, and guanine binds only with cytosine
- Nucleotides: The unit of pentose sugar, phosphate, and nitrogenous base
- Gene: The specific portion of DNA with particular arrangement of nitrogenous bases and carries the genetic information

Box 4: Components of nucleotide.

- Nitrogenous bases (nitrogen containing bases)
  - Purines Adenine (A) and (2) Guanine (G)
  - Pyramidines (1) Cytosine (C), (2) Uracil (U), and (3) Thymine (T)
- Deoxyribose sugar in DNA and ribose sugar in RNA
- Phosphate molecule

are the four deoxyribonucleotide triphosphates (dTTP, dCTP, dATP, dGTP), each consisting of a sugar molecule (designated as d; 1st letter), one base [designated T (thiamine)/C(cytosine)/ A (adenine)/G(guanine); 2nd letter and a triphosphate group (designated as TP<; 3rd and 4th letter)].

RNA contains uracil (U), usually takes the place of thymine of DNA. Thus, DNA contains thymine whereas RNA contains uracil.

Note: Nucleotides, in addition to their roles as precursors of nucleic acids, ATP, GTP, UTP, CTP, and their derivatives, each serve unique physiologic functions. Synthetic analogs of purines, pyrimidines, nucleosides, and nucleotides modified in the heterocyclic ring or in the sugar moiety have many applications in clinical medicine (e.g., 5-fluoro- or 5-iodouracil, 3-deoxyuridine and 6-mercaptopurine, 5- or 6-azauridine, 5- or 6-azacytidine, and 8-azaguanine in oncology).

Pentose Sugars Present in DNA and RNA

Nucleic acids contain two types of **pentoses,** either ***D-2-deoxyribose*** or ***D-ribose.*** DNA and RNA are distinguished depending on the pentose sugar present (**Fig. 5**).

- **DNA:** It contains **D-2-deoxyribose sugar moiety**.
- RNA contains **D-ribose.**

The pentose sugars have five carbon atoms. The numbers are assigned to the five carbons of the sugars based on their relative positions in the molecule. The carbon atoms are

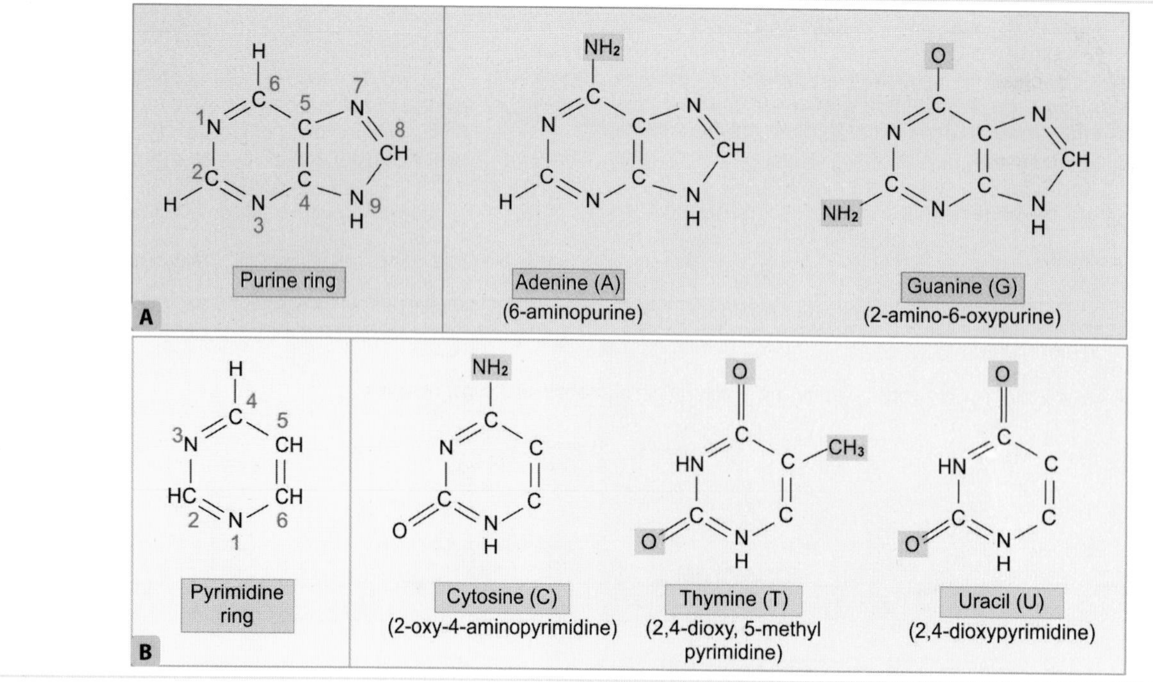

FIGS. 4A AND B: Structure of purine and pyrimidine ring and their bases.

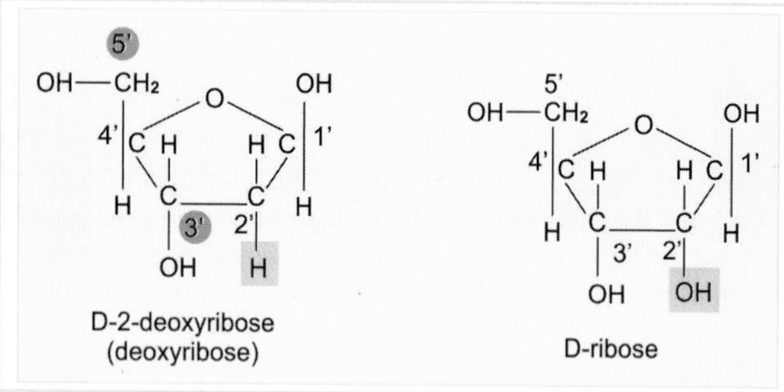

D-2-deoxyribose (deoxyribose)

D-ribose

FIG. 5: Structure of pentose sugars [D-2-deoxyribose in deoxyribonucleic acid (DNA) and D-ribose in ribonucleic acid (RNA)] present in nucleic acid.

numbered from 1 to 5, starting with the first carbon moving clockwise from the oxygen in each sugar (**Fig. 6**).The carbon atoms of the pentose sugars are distinguished from atoms within the nucleotide base by the use of primed numbers from 1′ to 5′ (in contrast to cardinal numbers of nitrogenous bases i.e., -5). It helps in distinguishing sugar atoms from those of the nitrogen base.

Nucleoside

Pentose sugar attachment of a base forms a structure **nucleoside**. A pentose sugar (D-ribose or D-2-deoxyribose) is covalently attached to one nitrogenous base (purine or pyrimidine) to the 1′ site/carbon of ribose sugar via covalent **N-glycosidic bond (Fig. 6)**.

- **N-glycosidic bond:** It joins **nitrogen atom-9** of the purine base or **nitrogen atom-1** of the pyrimidine base with carbon 1′ site of pentose sugar (**Fig. 6**).

Structures two types of nucleosides (of RNA and DNA) are shown in **Figures 7A** to **D**. The term **nucleoside** is used for structures containing only sugar and nitrogen base without a phosphate group.

Attachment of Phosphate to Pentose Sugar

The phosphate group/**molecule** is attached to **5′-carbon** (5′position of the sugar ring) of pentose sugar (**Fig. 7**).

Nucleotide (Figs. 7A to D)

The addition of a phosphate group to the 5′ carbon of pentose (along with the one nitrogenous base) forms a complete *nucleotide*. In other words, nucleoside (i.e., sugar and nitrogen base) and phosphate group form nucleotide.

Formation of a Strand

Phosphate Diester (Phosphodiester) Bonds

Phosphate diester bonds are between sugar molecules. The backbone of the ssDNA polymer is the sugar deoxyribose connected by phosphate groups. In DNA, the 3′ hydroxyl group of the one sugar moiety of one deoxyribonucleotide (i.e., 3′ carbon of one sugar ring) is strongly **linked (joined/attached)** covalently to the 5′ hydroxyl group of the adjacent sugar moiety of deoxyribonucleotide (i.e., 5′ carbon of the next sugar) by a **phosphodiester bonds**/linkage (**Figs. 8A** and **B**). This bond is called as **3′, 5′** (*3′-5′*) -**phosphodiester bonds.** Such covalently joined nucleotides to one another form a long chain (linear polymer), or **strand.** DNA is a polymer of many deoxyribonucleotides. The backbone of the strand (called **sugar-phosphate backbone)** is composed of alternating deoxyribose sugar and phosphate groups (**Figs. 8A** and **B**). The consistent orientation of the nucleotide building blocks gives a chain overall direction, so that the two ends of a single

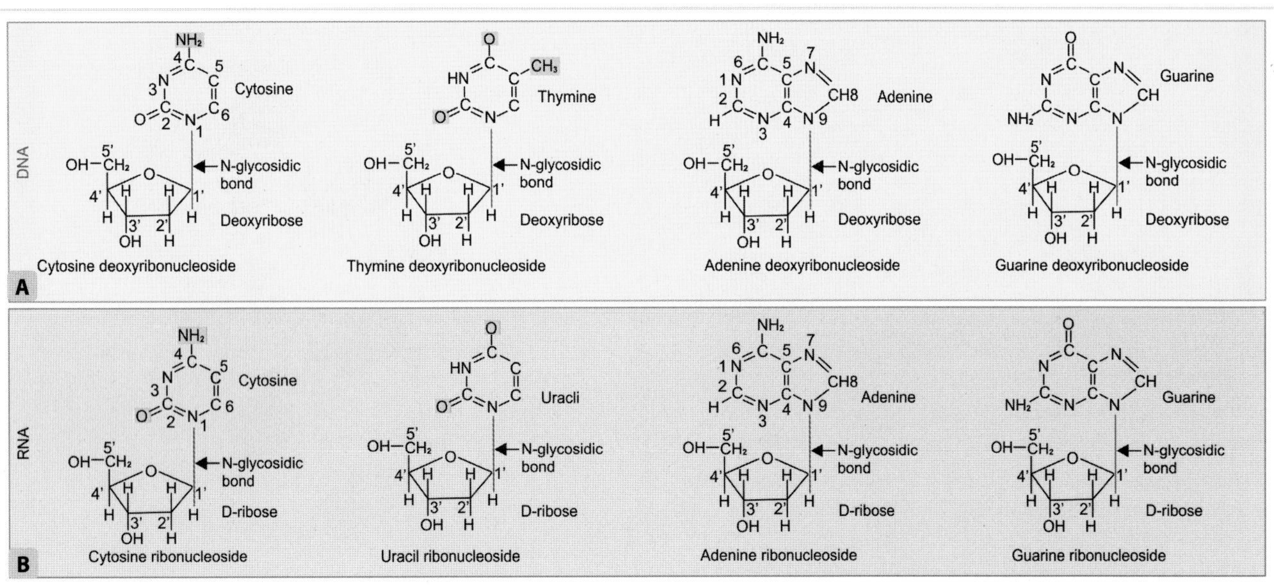

FIGS. 6A AND B: Structures of various nucleosides. The carbon atoms are numbered as 1′ to 5′ (they are labeled as C).

Phosphate

Nuceloside

Purine or pyrimidine base

Phosphate + nuceloside = deoxyribonucleotide (sugar deoxyribose)

A

Phosohate binds with 5' of sugar

Purine or primidine base (e.g., cytosine)

Deoxyribonucleotide

B

Phosphate

Nuceloside

Purine or pyrimidine base

Phosphate + nuceloside = ribonucleotide (sugar ribose)

C

Phosohate binds with 5' of sugar

Purine or primidine base (e.g., uracil)

Ribonucleotide

D

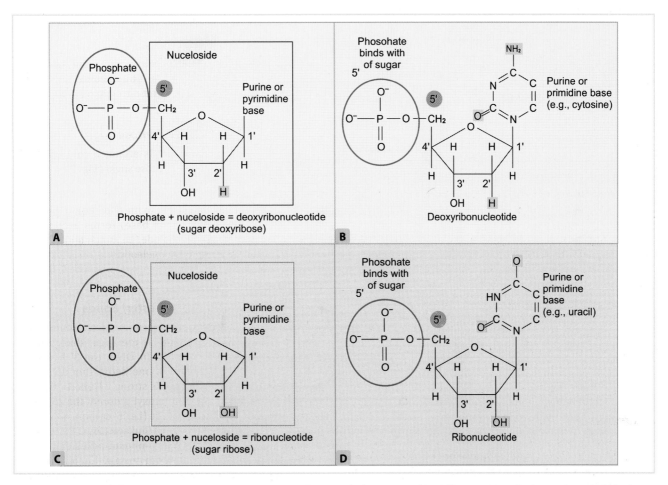

FIGS. 7A TO D: Chemical structure of a nucleotide (deoxyribose and ribose). A nucleotide is composed of a nucleoside linked to a phosphate. The phosphate is shown in the circles. The nucleoside portion of the molecule is depicted in the rectangles in A and C.

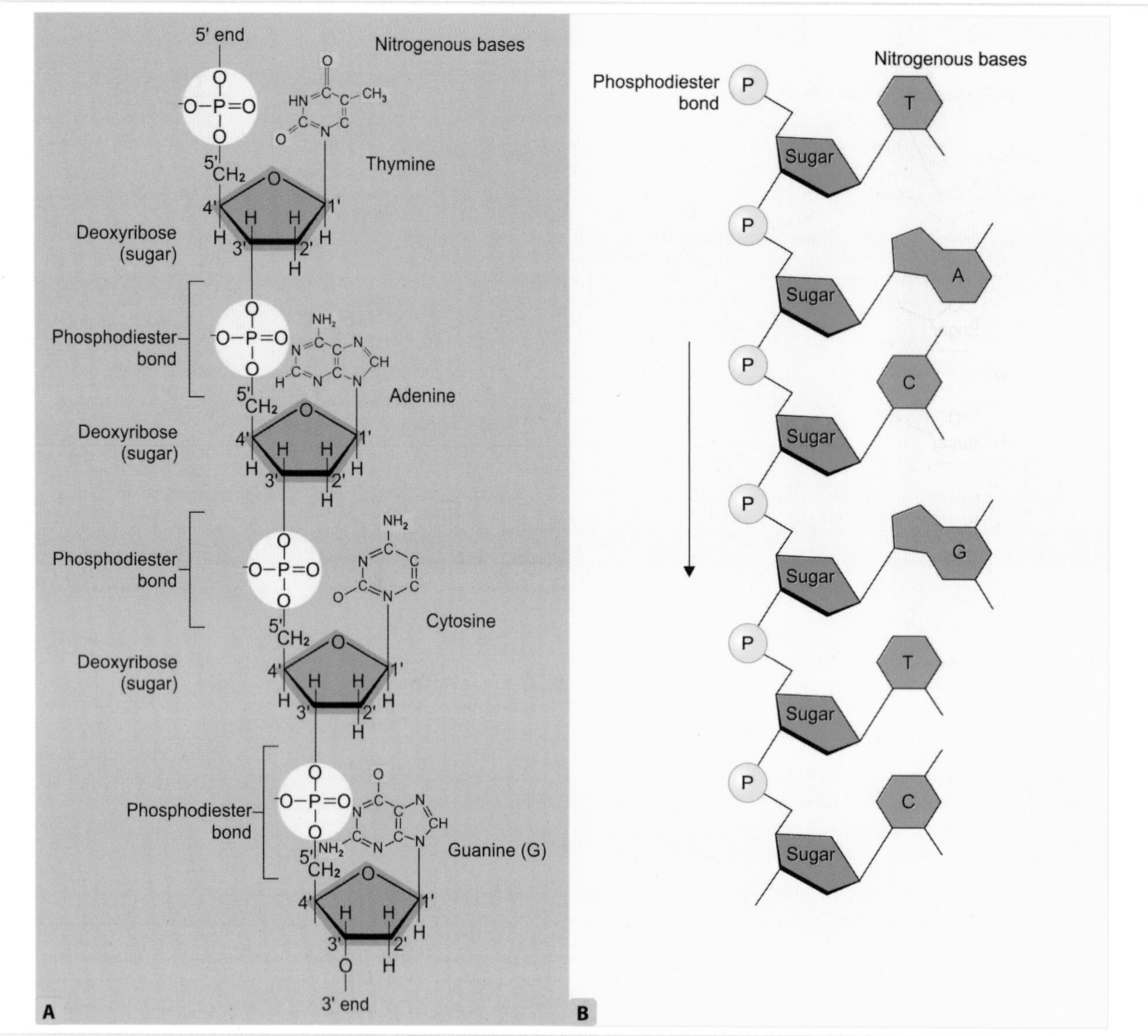

FIGS. 8A AND B: A chain of nucleotides in a single strand of deoxyribonucleic acid (DNA). (A) Shows 4 nucleotides. Molecules are shown in mirror image than depicted in earlier figures. (B) Shows simplified view of one strand with 6 nucleotides. Usually, a DNA chain is described in terms of its bases, written with the 5′-to-3′ direction going from left to right. For example, the chain shown in (A) would be 5′ TACG 3′.

chain are chemically distinct. At one end, the phosphate is located, and this end is called the *5′end* (pronounced "five prime end"). Another end, hydroxyl is located, and this end is called as the *3′end* (pronounced "3 prime end"*)* (**Figs. 8A** and **B**). Because each of the stacked nucleotides in a strand faces the same direction; the entire strand has a direction. Along the DNA chain between the two ends, this 5′-to-3′ polarity is maintained from nucleotide to nucleotide. For this reason, the synthesis of the nucleic acid is said to occur in a 5′-to-3′ direction.

Connecting Nucleotides to Form a DNA Chain

Deoxyribonucleic acid consists of two chains/strands of nucleotides aligned head-to-toe. The head-to-toe configuration derives from the structure of the sugar–phosphate backbone. The opposing orientation of the two nucleotide chains (sugars pointing in opposite directions) in a DNA molecule is known as **antiparallelism (antiparallel configuration)** (**Fig. 9**). For example, if one chain (**Fig. 10**) runs from the 5′ carbon (**Fig. 9**) to the 3′ carbon, the other chain aligned with it runs from the 3′ to the 5′ carbon.

Bonds between nucleotides

The **two nucleotide chains** of DNA are **held together** by two types of molecular forces. These are hydrogen bonds and phosphodiester **bonds** (described previously).

- **Hydrogen bonds:** Chemical attractions called as hydrogen bonds are formed between the nitrogenous bases on the opposite nucleotide strands. They hold the base pairs together. In a hydrogen bond, a hydrogen atom on one molecule is attracted to an oxygen atom or nitrogen atom on another molecule (**Fig. 9**). The locations of the hydrogen bonds are always formed between a purine and pyrimidine nitrogenous base only.

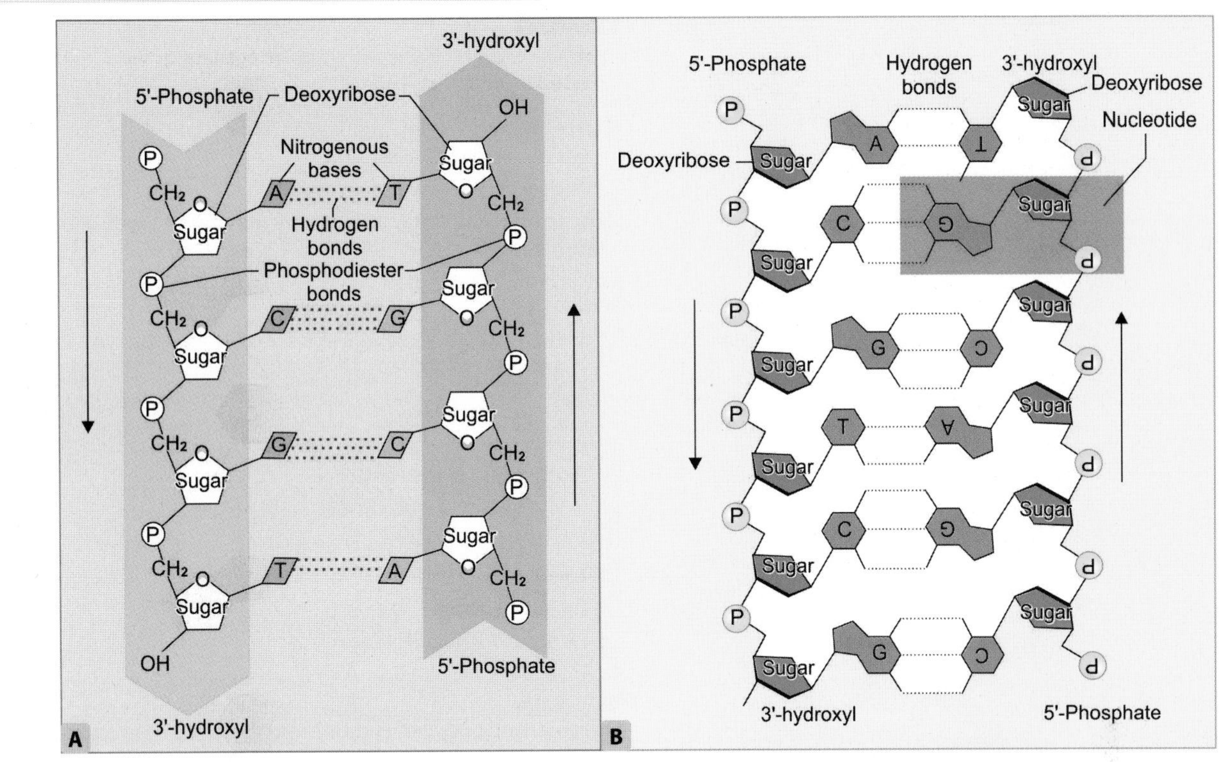

(P: phosphate; A: adenine; T: thymine; G: guanine; C: cytosine)

FIGS. 9A AND B: Deoxyribonucleic acid (DNA) double helix. The chemical structure of a small segment of a double DNA strand showing sugar-phosphate backbone and nucleotide (all four nucleotide) pairing of the DNA double helix.

- Adenine (A) base on one strand always pairs with thymine (T) on the other strand (**A-T or T-A**). Two hydrogen bonds join A and T (**Fig. 9**).
- Guanine (G) base on one strand pairs with cytosine (C) on the other (**G-C or C-G**). Three hydrogen bonds join G and C (**Fig. 9**).

The symmetrical DNA double helix are formed when nucleotides containing A pair with those containing T, and nucleotides containing G pair with those carrying C. The purines have two rings and pyrimidines have one ring. Thus, the consistent pairing of a purine with a pyrimidine results in double helix having the same width throughout. These specific purine–pyrimidine couples are termed as **complementary base pairs.** These complementary pairings produce a highly symmetrical DNA double helix. Though hydrogen bonds are weak individually, over the many bases of a DNA molecule they give great strength. Finally, DNA forms a double helix when the antiparallel, base-paired strands twist about one another in a regular fashion. DNA molecules are very long and the formation of double-stranded, helical structure of DNA gives it 50 times the strength of ssDNA. A single strand of DNA cannot form a helix. The DNA of the smallest chromosome, when stretched out will measure 14 mm (a millimeter is a thousandth of a meter) in length. However, when it is packed into a chromosome that, during cell division, measures only 2 µm (a micrometer is a millionth of a meter) in length.

Histone

Many proteins compress DNA without damaging or tangling it. Scaffold proteins form frameworks which guide DNA strands. The orderly packaging of DNA depends on small proteins called **histones** (refer pages 433–435). These **histones** are the remarkable **group of small proteins** which have an unusually **high content of the basic amino acids arginine and lysine**.

Nucleosome

Nucleosome is the basic unit of chromatin. Each nucleosome consists of approximately 146 base pairs of DNA. The DNA coils around proteins called **histones,** forming structures which resemble beads on a string. A DNA "bead" is termed as a **nucleosome**. The compaction of a molecule of DNA is similar to wrapping of a very long, thin piece of thread around our fingers, to keep it from unraveling and tangling. Each nucleosome consists of eight histone proteins (a pair of each of four types plus the 147 nucleotides of DNA entwined around them). Nucleosomes are repeating units and allow the DNA to fit within the cell nucleus. Sequences of nucleosomes (resembling a string of beads) are wound and packaged to form chromatin. The tightly wound, densely packed chromatin is termed heterochromatin, and open, less tightly wound chromatin is termed euchromatin. A single copy of the human

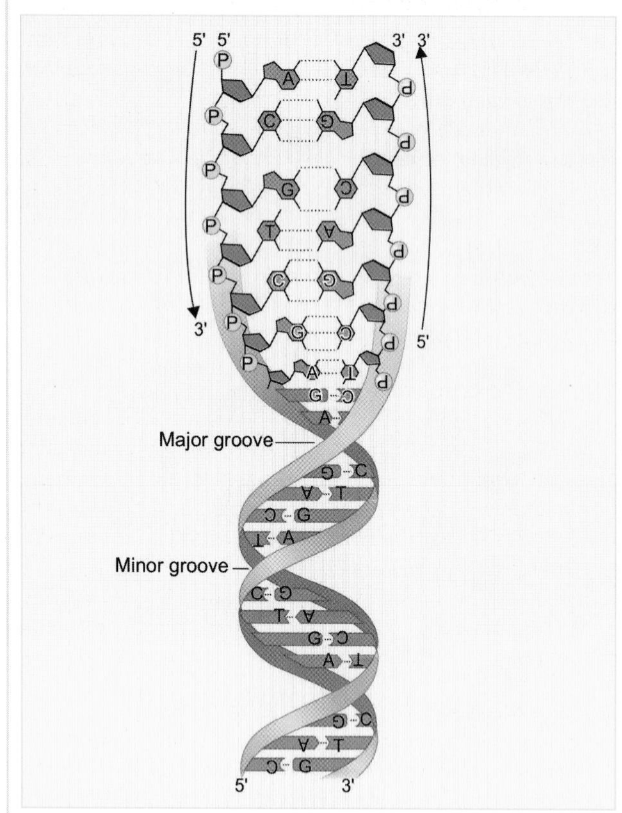

FIG. 10: Deoxyribonucleic acid (DNA) double helix. Antiparallelism in a DNA molecule arises from the orientation of the deoxyribose sugars. One-half of the double helix runs in a 5′ to 3′ direction, and the other half runs in a 3′ to 5′ direction.

genome consists of about 3.1 billion base pairs of DNAs, wrapped/wound around histones. An average human cell contains about 6.4 billion base pairs of DNAs divided among 46 chromosomes. The larger the chromosome, the longer the DNA it contains.

DNA'S INFORMATION CONTENT

Nucleic acids are the basic components of DNA and RNA and are the critical molecules of life. The molecular diagnostic methods are directed toward evaluation/analysis of nucleic acid. DNA is an extraordinarily stable molecule and its double-stranded helix is the most energetically favorable state for DNA. It loses its normal conformational structure only at extremes of heat, pH, or in the presence of destabilizing agents. Both sugar and phosphate groups are hydrophilic, and they form stable hydrogen bonds with surrounding water molecules in solution. In contrast, nitrogenous bases are hydrophobic and are not soluble in water at neutral pH. To form a stable molecule of DNA, it is necessary to make sure that the nitrogenous bases do not come into contact with water. This is achieved by running of two ssDNA polymers in antiparallel direction with twisting around the same axis (i.e., one ssDNA running in the 3′ to 5′ direction, and the other 5′ to 3′). This structural arrangement allows planar hydrogen bonds to form between adenine and thymine, and between guanine and cytosine. As long as the two chains of DNA have base sequences in complementary order, the strands of the helix retain a ladder-like structure with rungs (steps of a ladder) of consistent size. Hence, there is room for water molecules to pass in between.

Box 5: Types of DNA Sequence.

Nuclear (~3 ×10^9 base pairs) Genes (~20,000)
- Unique single copy
- Multigene families
  - Classic gene families
  - Gene superfamilies

Extragenic DNA (unique/low copy number or moderate/highly repetitive)
- Tandem repeat
  - Satellite
  - Minisatellite
    - Telomeric
    - Hypervariable
  - Microsatellite
- Highly repeated Interspersed
  - Short interspersed nuclear elements
  - Long interspersed nuclear elements

Mitochondrial (16.6 kb, 37 genes)
- Two rRNA genes
- 22 transfer RNA (tRNA) genes

Regions in the Deoxyribonucleic Acid

The human genome contains about 3.2 billion DNA base pairs. They consist of coding and noncoding regions. Of the total, only about 20,000 are protein-encoding genes, constituting 1.5% of the genome. Thus, there is 98.5% of the human genome that does not encode proteins. The proteins encoded by coding DNA genes are the fundamental constituents of cells, which will function as enzymes, structural elements, and signaling molecules.

Types of DNA Sequence (Box 5)

When DNA is denatured, it will reassociate as a duplex at a rate which depends on the proportion of unique and repeat sequences present, the latter occurring more rapidly. Analysis of the human DNA has shown that about 60–70% of the human genome consists of single- or low-copy number DNA sequences. The remainder 30–40%, of the genome consists of moderately or highly **repetitive DNA** sequences that are not transcribed. This latter portion consists of mainly satellite DNA and interspersed DNA sequences. The term **DNA sequencing** refers to the **exact order of the nucleotide bases** (adenine, guanine, cytosine, and thymine) **in a molecule of DNA**. Different types of DNA depending on the DNA nucleotide sequences are listed in **Box 5**.

Nuclear Genes

There are about 20,000–25,000 genes in the nuclear genome. The distribution of these genes varies greatly between chromosomal regions with the highest gene density observed in subtelomeric regions. **Chromosomes 19 and 22 are rich in genes, whereas chromosomes 4 and 18 are relatively poor in genes.** The size of genes also varies from small genes with single exons to the *TTN* gene which encodes the largest known protein in the human body and has largest number of exons (363) and also the single largest exon (17,106 bp).

Unique Single-copy Genes

In this type, nucleotide sequences are present only once without any repetition of nucleotide. Most of the human genes are unique single-copy genes and account for 50–60% of human DNA. They code for polypeptides that are involved in or carry out a variety of cellular functions. These include enzymes, hormones, receptors, and structural and regulatory proteins.

Multigene Families

Many genes have similar functions that are produced due to gene duplication events with subsequent evolutionary divergence. These are known as **multigene families.** Some are found physically close together in clusters [e.g., the α- and β-globin gene clusters on chromosomes 16 and 11 (**Fig. 11**)], whereas others are widely dispersed throughout the genome occurring on different chromosomes (e.g., *HOX* homeobox gene family). Multigene families can be divided into two types, **classic gene families** and **gene superfamilies**.

- **Classic gene families:** They show a high degree of sequence homology. Example, the numerous copies of genes coding for the various ribosomal RNAs (rRNAs), which are clustered as tandem arrays at the nucleolar organizing regions on the short arms of the five acrocentric chromosomes, and the different transfer RNA gene families (dispersed in numerous clusters throughout the human genome).
- **Gene superfamilies:** They have limited sequence homology but are functionally related, having similar structural domains. For example, the human leukocyte antigen (HLA) genes on chromosome 6, the T-cell receptor genes, which have structural homology with the immunoglobulin (Ig) genes. Probably, these are derived from duplication of a precursor gene, with subsequent evolutionary divergence, forming the Ig superfamily.

Extragenic Deoxyribonucleic Acid

The 20,000 unique single-copy genes in humans represent <2% of the genome encoding proteins. The remainder of the human genome consists of repetitive DNA sequences that are predominantly transcriptionally inactive. Though it is called as **junk** DNA, some regions show evolutionary conservation and play a critical role in the regulation of temporal and spatial gene expression.

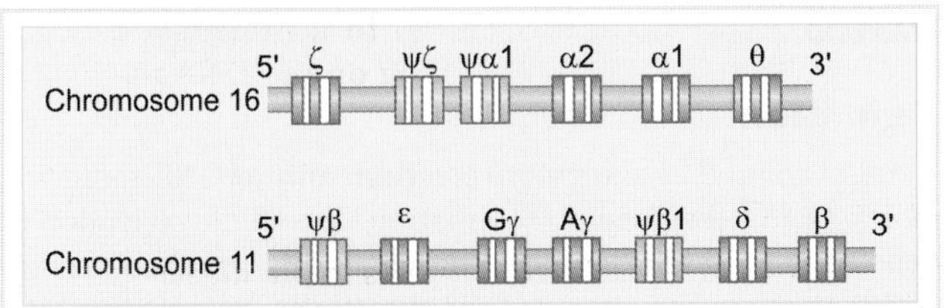

FIG. 11: Diagrammatic representation of the α- and β-globin regions on chromosomes 16 and 11.

Tandemly Repeated DNA Sequences

It is characterized by repetition of nucleotides several times (hundreds to millions). **When repeated sequences are directly adjacent to each other** (sequences are repeated one right after the other), they are known as **tandem repeats.** They consist of blocks of tandem repeats of noncoding DNA sequences that can be either highly dispersed or restricted in their location in the genome. These are noncoding sequences and constitute about 10–15% of human DNA.

Tandemly repeated DNA sequences and repeated DNA sequences can be divided into three subgroups—satellite, minisatellite, and microsatellite DNA.

Satellite deoxyribonucleic acid

It accounts for about 10–15% of the repetitive DNA sequences of the human genome. It consists of very large arrays/series of simple or moderately complex, short, tandemly repeated DNA sequences that are transcriptionally inactive (noncoding ***DNA***). They are clustered around the centromeres of certain chromosomes. This class of DNA sequences can be separated on density-gradient centrifugation as a shoulder, or "satellite", to the main peak of genomic DNA. Hence, they are termed as satellite DNA.

Minisatellite deoxyribonucleic acid

It consists of two families of tandemly repeated short DNA sequences—telomeric and hypervariable minisatellite DNA sequences. These are transcriptionally inactive.

- **Telomeric DNA:** The terminal portion of the telomeres of the chromosomes contains 10–15 kb of tandem repeats of a 6 base pair DNA sequence known as telomeric DNA. The telomeric repeat sequences are needed for the integrity of chromosome in replication and are added to the chromosome by an enzyme known as telomerase.
- **Hypervariable minisatellite DNA:** It is made up of highly polymorphic DNA sequences consisting of short tandem repeats of a common core sequence.

Microsatellite deoxyribonucleic acid

It consists of tandem single, di-, tri-, and tetra-nucleotide repeat base pair sequences located throughout the genome. Microsatellite repeats rarely occur within coding sequences. However, trinucleotide repeats in or near genes are associated with certain inherited disorders. Nowadays DNA microsatellites are used for forensic and paternity tests. They may also be useful for gene tracking in families with a genetic disorder with no identified mutation.

Highly Repeated Interspersed Repetitive DNA Sequences

About one-third of the human genome consists of two main classes of short and long repetitive DNA sequences that are interspersed throughout the genome.

1. **Short interspersed nuclear elements (SINEs):** They constitute about 5% (~750,000 copies) of the human genome.
2. **Long interspersed nuclear elements (LINEs):** They constitute about 5% of the DNA of the human genome. The most commonly occurring LINE, known as LINE-1 (L1 element), consists of >100,000 copies of a DNA sequence of up to 6,000 base pairs that encodes a reverse transcriptase. The function of these is not clear.

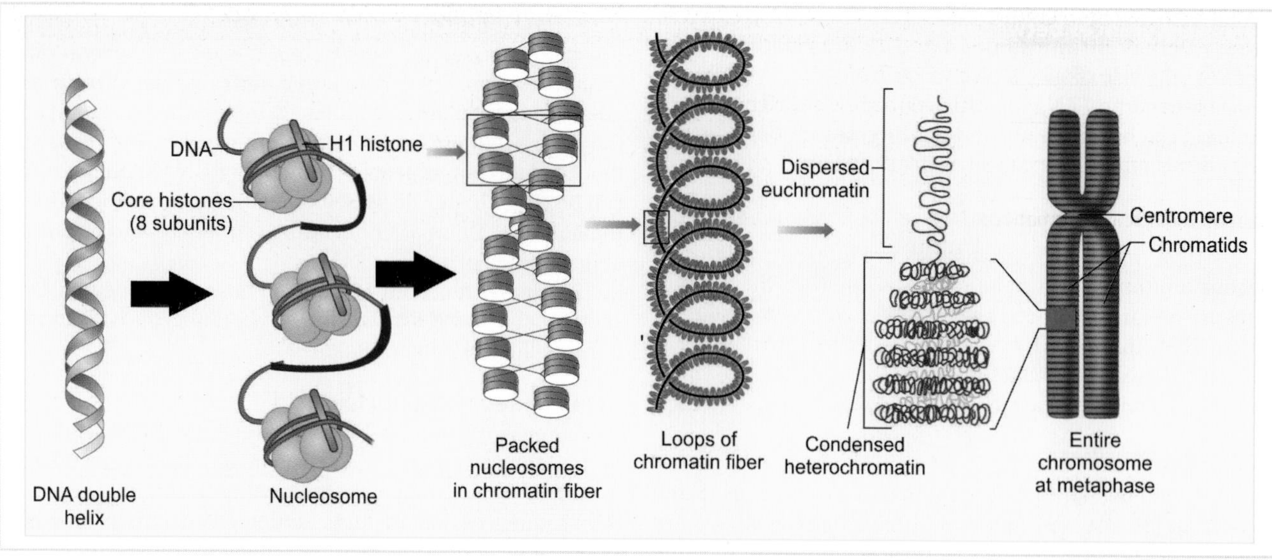

FIG. 12: Diagrammatic representation of levels of organization of chromatin. DNA molecules are wrapped around histones to form nucleosomes and are the lowest level of chromatin organization. Nucleosomes are organized into chromatin fibers, which in turn are organized into looped domains. During mitosis in metaphase, the loops become further compacted into mitotic chromosome.

Mitochondrial Deoxyribonucleic Acid

In addition to nuclear DNA, the mitochondria contain 16.6 kb circular dsDNA, or **mtDNA**. These are very compact and contain little repetitive DNA, and code for 37 genes.

Levels of organization of chromatin are shown in **Figure 12**.

The packaging of DNA into chromosomes involves several orders of DNA coiling and folding. These include primary coiling of the DNA double helix, secondary coiling around spherical *histone* "beads", forming *nucleosomes*, tertiary coiling of the nucleosomes to form the *chromatin fibers* that form long loops on a scaffold of nonhistone acidic proteins, which are further wound in a tight coil to make up the chromosome as visualized under the light microscope.

RIBONUCLEIC ACID

Q. Write a short essay on the types of RNA.

The RNA is chiefly present within the ribosomes and nucleolus. RNA differs from DNA in three main ways:

1. RNA is **single-stranded**.
2. The **sugar** residue within the nucleotide is **ribose**, rather than deoxyribose.
3. Specific pyrimidine base **uracil** (U) is used **in place of thymine** (T).

Ribonucleic Acid Structure and Types

RNA is the bridge between gene and protein. RNA and DNA share an intimate relationship. The bases of an RNA sequence are complementary to those of one strand of the double helix of DNA. This strand of DNA is called the **template strand**. An enzyme, **RNA polymerase,** builds an RNA molecule. The other, nontemplate strand of the DNA double helix is known as the **coding strand**.

Types of Ribonucleic Acid

The **two major types** of RNA (refer **Table 3**) are:

Coding RNA

Messenger RNA (mRNA) contains a coding RNA sequence. It carries the message from the DNA to the ribosomes in the cytoplasm required for the protein synthesis. It contains both exons and introns similar to DNA. During protein synthesis, the introns (noncoding sequences) are cut and removed resulting in a smaller mRNA.

Noncoding RNA (ncRNA)

One of the mechanisms of gene regulation depends on the functions of ncRNAs. These are encoded by genes that are transcribed but not translated. Thus, they do not code for proteins. They are discussed on pages 594-553. They are not translated into protein but can regulate gene expression.

- **Transfer RNA:** It conveys the message carried by the mRNA to the ribosomes.
- **Ribosomal RNA:** They play a significant role in the binding of mRNA to ribosomes and protein synthesis.
- **Micro-RNA (miRNA):** miRNAs are relatively short RNAs (22 nucleotides on average. They are discussed on pages 549-553.

Differences between DNA and RNA are presented in **Table 2** and **Figures 13A to C.**

GENES

Definition

Gene is defined as a **segment/section/unit of DNA** molecule which carries the genetic information. The whole collection of genes constitutes the **genome.** The genetic information present within the base sequence of DNA directs the production of the

Table 2: Differences between deoxyribonucleic acid (DNA) and ribonucleic acid (RNA).

Features	***DNA (deoxyribonucleic acid)***	***RNA (ribonucleic acid)***
Nature of strand	Usually double-stranded	Usually single-stranded
Pyrimidine base	Thymine as a base	Uracil as a base
Sugar	Deoxyribose as the sugar	Ribose as the sugar
Function regarding information	Maintains protein-encoding information (genetic information)	Carries protein-encoding information and controls how information is used
Function as an enzyme	Cannot function as an enzyme	Can function as an enzyme
Stability	Persists and stores genetic information	Transient (less stable than DNA) short-lived carrier of genetic information

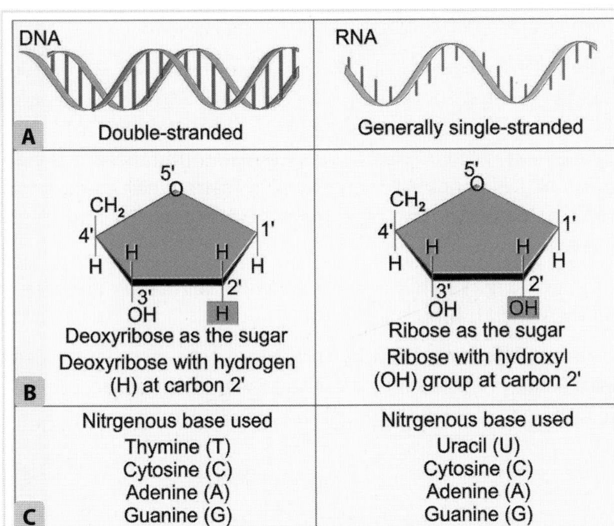

FIGS. 13A TO C: Differences between deoxyribonucleic acid and ribonucleic acid. (A) DNA is double-stranded whereas RNA is usually single-stranded. (B) DNA nucleotides contain deoxyribose and hydrogen (H) at the carbon atom 2′ and RNA nucleotides contain ribose with hydroxyl (OH) group at carbon atom 2′. (C) Nitrogenous bases in DNA include the thymine, cytosine, adenine, and guanine, whereas in RNA instead of thymine there is uracil.

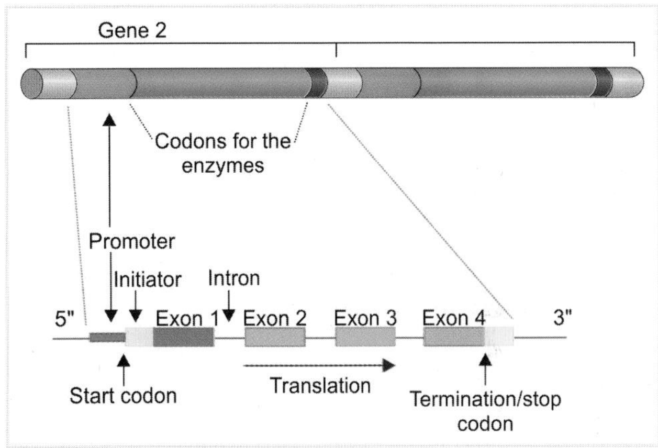

FIG. 14: Diagrammatic structure of gene. Start and termination codons mark the limits of the gene. The coding portion of the gene is exons (four in this example), interspersed with introns.

proteins and enzymes that build the cell. Gene is the basic **physical and functional unit of heredity**. A gene is a sequence of building blocks that specifies the sequence of amino acids in a particular protein. The activity of the protein imparts the phenotype. The human genome contains about **3.2 billion DNA base pairs. But, there are only about 20,000 protein-encoding genes within the genome. Thus, these coding genes constitute only about 1.5% of the genome**. Each gene varies in size (small gene with single exons to gene with up to 79 exons). Chromosomes 19 and 22 are rich in genes, whereas 4 and 18 are relatively poor in genes. The size of genes also shows great variability.

Structure of Gene (Fig. 14)

Genes are located on chromosomes and consist of DNA packaged with histone and nonhistone proteins. DNA also has segments which do not contain genes. Each gene consists of a specific sequence of nucleotides.

Triplet Codons

Genes may be **silent or active**. When genes are active, they **direct the process of protein synthesis**. Genes do not code for proteins directly but **by means of a genetic code**. The **genetic code** consists of a sequence code word called **codons.** The sequence of three (triplet) nucleotide bases in the mRNA that codes for a particular amino acid is called a **triplet codon**. Each triplet codon in sequence codes for a specific amino acid in sequence and so the genetic code is nonoverlapping. The order of the triplet codons in a gene is known as the translational **reading frame**. However, some amino acids are coded for by more than one triplet, so the code is said to be **degenerate**. Each transfer RNA (tRNA) species for a particular amino acid has a specific trinucleotide sequence called the **anticodon.** This anticodon is complementary to the codon of the mRNA. Termination of translation of the RNA is signaled by the presence of one of the three **stop** or **termination codons**.

Regions of Gene

Genes instruct cells to build proteins from 20 types of amino acids. Only about 1.5% of the DNA of the human genome encodes protein. This part is the **exome** which is part of the genome that consists of exons. Rest of the genome controls or regulates how, where, and when to build proteins.

Initiator and stop codons

The boundaries of a gene are known as **start and stop codons**. The start codon tells when to begin protein production and stop (termination) codon tells when to end the protein production. The proteins provide the building blocks and machinery required for assembling cells, tissues, and organisms.

Coding region (Fig. 14)

The nucleotide sequence between the start and stop codons is the core region known as **coding region**.

This region is divided into two main segments, namely exons and introns.

1. **Exons:** This region codes for producing a protein.
2. **Introns:** These are the regions between exons and do not code for a protein (**noncoding region**).

Most of the genes contain both exons and introns, the number of which varies with different genes.

Noncoding DNA

The noncoding regions of the genome provide the critical "architectural planning". The major classes of functional *nonprotein-coding DNA sequences* in the human genome are as follows:

Promoter regions (Figs. 14 and 15): These are regions which bind to transcription factors, either strongly or weakly. Promoters can be broadly classified into two types: (1) TATA box-containing and (2) GC rich.

- **TATA box-containing:** It is about 25 base pairs upstream of the transcription start site and is involved in the initiation of transcription at a basal constitutive level. Mutations in TATA box can alter the transcription start site.
- **GC rich:** It is about 80 base pairs upstream of the transcription start site. It increases the basal level of transcriptional activity of the TATA box.

The regulatory elements in the promoter region are said to be **cis-acting.** The term cis-acting means the transcription factors only affect the expression of the adjacent gene on the same DNA duplex. The term **trans-acting** is used when the transcription factors act on both copies of a gene on each chromosome being synthesized from genes that are located at a distance. Cis-acting elements are DNA sequences in the vicinity of the structural portion of a gene that are required for gene expression. Trans-acting factors are usually proteins, that bind to the cis-acting sequences to control gene expression.

Enhancer regions (Fig. 15A): These are DNA sequences (regions) which increase transcriptional activity of GC and CAAT boxes. CCAAT box (sometimes abbreviated a CAAT box or CAT box) is a sequence of nucleotides found in a conserved region of DNA located "upstream" (5' direction) of the start points of transcription units. Enhancers can enhance the effect of a weak promoter.

Silencers (Fig. 15A): These are negative regulatory elements/ regions which inhibit transcription.

Boundary elements (insulators): These are short sequences of DNA, usually 500 base pairs to 3 kb in size which block or inhibit the influence of regulatory elements of adjacent genes.

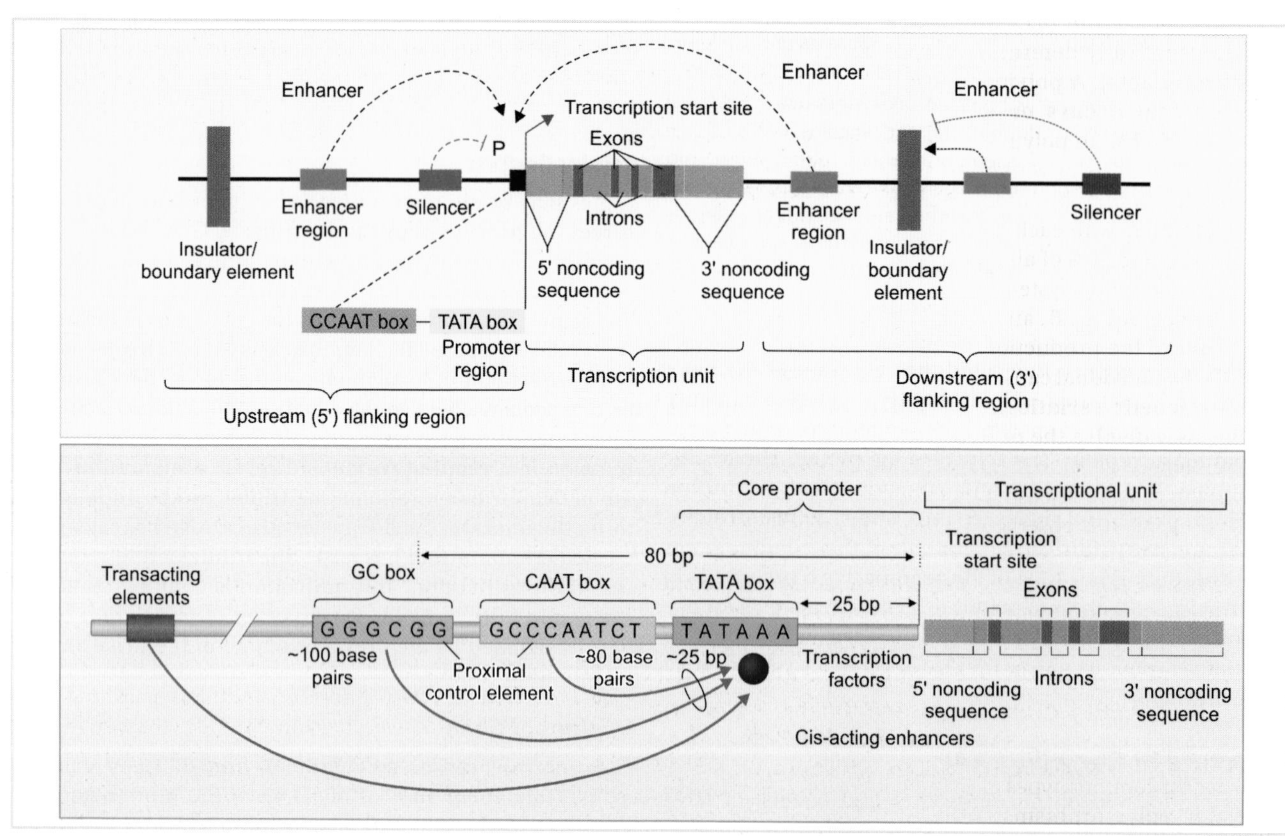

(BP: base pairs)

FIGS. 15A AND B: (A) Various regions of gene. (B) Diagrammatic representation of various factors involved in gene expression.

Binding sites for proteins: They organize and maintain higher order *chromatin structures.*

Noncoding regulatory RNA: Of the 80% of the genome involved in regulatory functions, majority of them is transcribed into RNAs. These include miRNAs and lncRNAs They are discussed on pages 549–553. They are never translated into protein but can regulate gene expression.

Mobile genetic elements (e.g., transposons): More than one-third of the human genome is composed of "jumping genes". These segments can move easily around genome (mobile elements). These are involved in gene regulation and chromatin organization, binding sites for proteins that organize and maintain higher order *chromatin structures.*

Other special structural regions of DNA: These include *telomeres* (chromosome ends) and *centromeres* (chromosome "tethers").

Various factors involved in gene expression are shown in **Figure 15B**.

Genomic Variability

Variation exists between the genomes of any two individuals. The human genome is polymorphic (i.e., there are many DNA sequence variants among different individuals). Only a small fraction of these variations in DNA sequence is responsible for the phenotypic differences that characterize individuals.

Polymorphism

If the **genetic variation/change does not cause obvious effect upon phenotype, it is termed as polymorphism**. Polymorphism is the occurrence in a population of two or more genetically determined (different) forms (alleles, sequence variants). **A polymorphism is defined as genetic variation that occurs or exists in population with a frequency of >1%**. In polymorphic locus, there should be at least two alleles. Alleles with frequencies of <1% are called as rare variants. In humans, at least 30% of structural gene loci are polymorphic, with each individual being heterozygous at between 10% and 20% of all loci. One of the best examples is the ABO blood group system. In ABO, there are at least **four alleles** namely A_1, A_2, B, and O of a single ABO gene. These alleles control the production of antigens on the surface of the RBCs. An individual can have any two of these four alleles.

Many genetic variations *(polymorphisms)* associated with diseases involve the nonprotein coding regions of the genome. Hence, variation in gene regulation seems to be more important in causing disease rather than structural changes in specific proteins. It is observed from genome sequencing that any two individuals are usually >99.5% DNA-identical and are 99% sequence-identical to our ancestor chimpanzees. From this, it appears that individual variation, including variation in susceptibility to diseases and environmental exposures, is encoded in <0.5% of our DNA. This <0.5% of DNA represents about 15 million base pairs.

Types of Polymorphism

The two most common types of DNA variation are—(1) single-nucleotide polymorphisms (SNPs) and (2) copy number variations (CNVs).

Single-nucleotide polymorphisms (SNPs) (Fig. 16) The majority of the DNA variants are single nucleotide substitutions

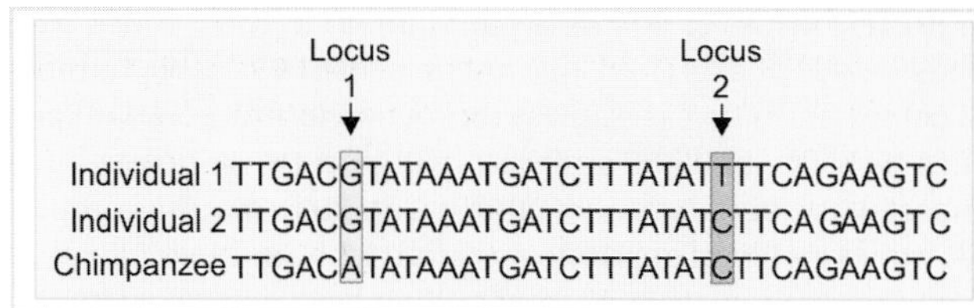

FIG. 16: Single nucleotide polymorphisms at locus 2 between 2 individuals and chimpanzee.

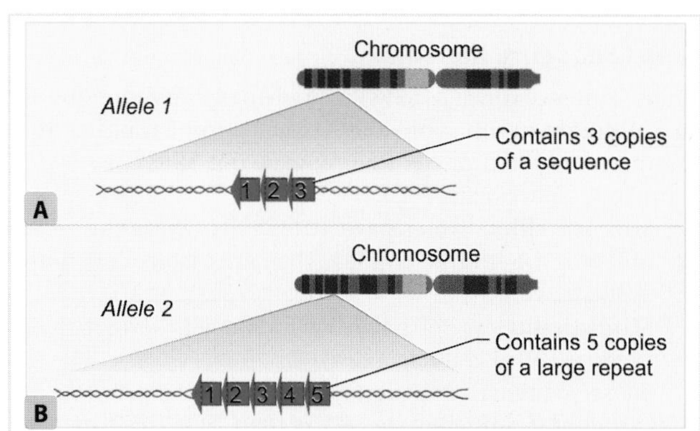

FIGS. 17A AND B: Diagrammatic representation of copy number variation (CNV) in the human genome. (A) Allele 1 in the population contains three copies of a sequence. (B) Allele 2 contains five copies of a large repeat.

and are termed as SNPs. SNPs (pronounced "snips") are inherited, naturally occurring variants at single nucleotide base positions between the DNA sequences in the same gene in two individuals. It has a size of 1 base pair (base pair is one of the pairs A-T or C-G) and always biallelic. Thus, there are only two choices at a given site within the population, such as nitrogenous base adenine (A) or thymine (T) in a nucleotide. There are >6 million human SNPs, with wide variation in frequency in different populations. SNPs account for most of the genetic variation between individuals. The general features include:

- SNPs occur across the genome. They may be in the exons, introns, intergenic regions, and coding regions.
- About 1% of SNPs are found in coding regions. As already mentioned, coding region constitutes about 1.5% of the genome.
- SNPs in noncoding regions can occur in regulatory elements in the genome. This can alter the gene expression and may directly influence disease susceptibility.
- SNPs can also be "neutral" variants. They may not have any effect on gene function or carrier phenotype.
- Even "neutral" SNPs may be useful markers if they are coinheritor with a disease-associated gene and are physically near it. This association of SNP and the causative genetic factor is called *linkage disequilibrium.*
- Most SNPs have a weak effect on disease susceptibility.

Copy number variations (Figs. 17A and B) Copy number variations are a form of genetic variation. They consist of different numbers of large contiguous stretches of DNA (genome). This large-scale structural variation can range from 1,000 base pairs to millions of base pairs. These are large tandem repeats of 50 kb (kb = kilobase pair is a unit of length of nucleic acids = 1,000 base pairs) to 5 mb (mb = mega base pairs = 1,000,000 bp) long that are present in a variable number of copies. In some cases, these loci of polymorphic variant are, such as SNPs, biallelic and simply duplicated or deleted in a subset of the population. In other cases, there may be complex rearrangements of genomic material, with multiple alleles in the human population. Several million base pairs of sequence difference can occur between any two individuals and is usually due to CNVs. About 50% of CNVs involve gene-coding sequences. Thus, CNVs may be responsible for a large portion of diversity of human phenotype.

Short Sequence Repeats

Short sequence repeats (SSRs) are polymorphic variations due to a different number of short sequence repeat units. Most common are the dinucleotide repeats, but SSRs may be tri-, tetra-, or pentarepeats.

- **Microsatellites** (refer page 101): SSRs where the repeat unit is n = 1–15 nucleotides. They are also called simple sequence repeats.
- **Minisatellites** (refer page 101): SSRs with longer repeat units (n = 15–500 nucleotides).

These sequences constitute about 3% of the genome. The most frequent dinucleotide SSR is the $(GT)_n$ (n= n-th term of the sequence; it is pronounced "GT sub n" or just "GT n"). followed by the $(AT)_n$. The most common trinucleotide SSR is the $(TAA)_n$.

GENE ACTION: FROM DNA TO PROTEIN

DNA Transcription and Protein Synthesis (Fig. 18)

Genes are functional elements on the chromosome. The human genome contains >20,000 genes. Many of genes are inactive or silenced in different cell types, reflecting the variable gene expression responsible for cell-specific characteristics. Genes are capable of transmitting information from the DNA template via the production of mRNA to the production of proteins. The central dogma is the pathway describing the basic steps of protein production. There are several steps involved in the synthesis of proteins, namely—(1) **transcription**, (2) splicing, (3) **translation**, and (4) protein modification. Of these, transcription and translation are the main steps. The **genetic information** in cells **flows in one way: DNA → RNA → protein. Transcription** first synthesizes an RNA molecule that is complementary to one strand of the DNA double helix for a particular gene. The RNA copy moves out from the nucleus into the cytoplasm. Then the **translation** process uses the information in the RNA to manufacture a protein by aligning and joining specified amino acids. Finally, the protein folds into a specific three-dimensional form needed for its function. Thus, DNA specifies the synthesis of RNA, and RNA specifies the synthesis of amino acids, which subsequently form proteins. Transcription and translation can occur continuously except during M phase and they supply the proteins essential for life, as well as those that give a cell its specialized characteristics.

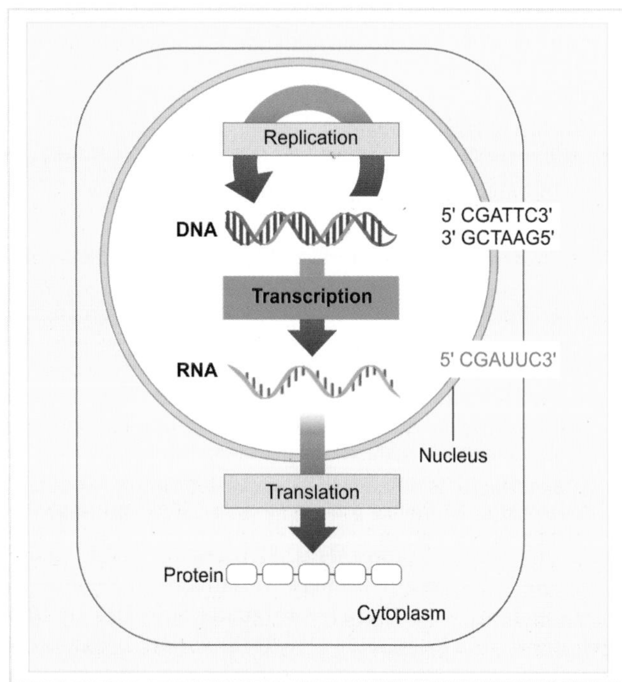

FIG. 18: Main steps involved in protein synthesis.

Transcription

Transcription is a process of conversion of the **genetic information** stored in the genetic code in **DNA** of a gene **to** its equivalent in **mRNA.** In other words, synthesis or production of an RNA copy from a DNA template (one of the DNA strands) is called transcription (**Fig. 19**). The product of transcription is a **transcript—**a molecule of **mRNA.**

When genes are active, proteins called **transcription factors**/proteins **are produced.** *Transcription* produces an RNA transcript of a gene. The template for the RNA transcript is one strand of that portion of the DNA double helix that constitutes the gene. The nucleotide sequence of mRNA is complementary to that of the gene (DNA) from which it is transcribed, the mRNA retains the same information as the gene itself. The enzymes responsible for transcription cells are called **DNA-dependent RNA polymerases**, or simply **RNA polymerases**. These enzymes are capable of incorporating nucleotides, one at a time, into a strand of RNA whose sequence is complementary to one of the DNA strands, which serves as the *template.*

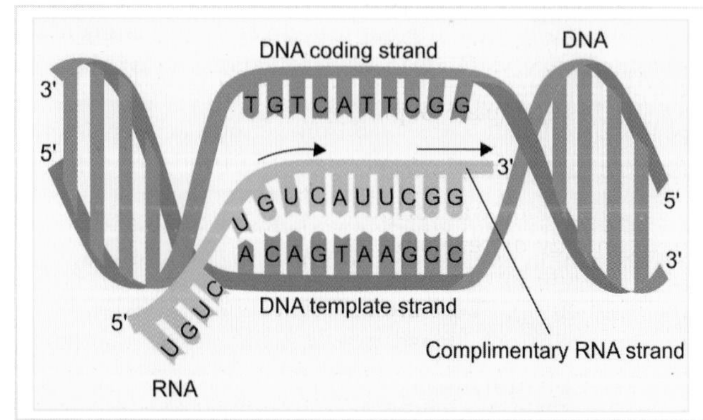

FIG. 19: Formation of messenger RNA from the DNA template strand. First, double stranded DNA is separated into template strand and coding strand. The RNA sequence complementary to the DNA template strand is formed and is the same sequence as the DNA coding strand, with uracil (U) in place of thymine (T).

Before initiating transcription, the first step in the synthesis of an RNA is the association of the RNA polymerase with the DNA template. RNA polymerase molecule binds to a site on the DNA which is called the **promoter or the enhancer region** of a gene (**Fig. 14 and 15A**). The enhancer region may be many thousands of base pairs away from the promoter. A loop in the chromosomal DNA brings the enhancer close to the promoter region and enables the bound proteins to interact. Cellular RNA polymerases themselves cannot recognize promoters and need the help of additional proteins called **transcription factors**. The human genome encodes >1,200 different transcription factors.

- **Separation of double stranded DNA into single stranded DNA:** Before transcription or replication, the double-stranded helix of DNA must be separated into single strands of DNA. This is performed by an enzyme topoisomerase which break or "nick" a DNA strand, releasing the tension of the coiled helix and allowing the DNA to unwind.
- **Assembly of a complementary strand of RNA:** After the separation of DNA into single strands, the DNA strand serves as a template for the mRNA. In any particular gene, only one DNA strand of the double helix acts as the so-called **template strand** (sometimes called the **antisense strand).** RNA polymerase is an enzyme that synthesizes an RNA transcript from a DNA template. Promoters region in the gene provides not only the binding site for the RNA polymerase, but also contains the information that determines which of the two DNA strands is transcribed and the site at which transcription begins.
- **Primary RNA transcript/molecule:** RNA polymerase moves along the template DNA strand toward its 5′ end (i.e., in a 3′ → 5′ direction). As the polymerase progresses, there is temporary unwinding of DNA, and the polymerase assembles a complementary strand of RNA that grows from its 5′ terminus in a 3′ direction. It produces a new complimentary copy of the whole gene and is known as **primary RNA transcript/molecule**. In protein coding genes, this RNA is called as mRNA. The transcribed mRNA molecule is a copy of the complementary strand, or what is called the **sense strand** of the DNA double helix. This mRNA strand is a "mirror image" of the DNA template. Every base in the mRNA molecule is complementary to a corresponding base in the DNA of the gene, except that uracil replacing thymine in mRNA (i.e., AGTC results in a strand of mRNA nucleotide sequence UCAG). Transcription is the first step in protein synthesis and occurs in the nucleus.
- The mRNA migrates from the nucleus to the cytoplasm and is used as a template for protein synthesis.

Control of Transcription

The control of transcription may be influenced either permanently or reversibly by many factors. These factors may be both environmental (e.g., hormones) and genetic (cell signaling). There are different mechanisms of control of transcription. These mechanisms include signaling molecules that bind to regulatory sequences in the DNA known as **response elements,** intracellular receptors known as **hormone nuclear receptors,** and receptors for specific ligands on the cell surface involved in the process of **signal transduction.** All these mechanisms finally affect transcription through the binding of the general transcription factors to short specific DNA **promoter region** that leads to activation of RNA polymerase (**Fig. 20**).

Transcription Factors

A number of genes encode proteins involved in the regulation of gene expression. They have DNA-binding activity to short nucleotide sequences, usually mediated through helical protein motifs, and these are called **transcription factors.** The term **transcription factor** is broadly used to describe proteins

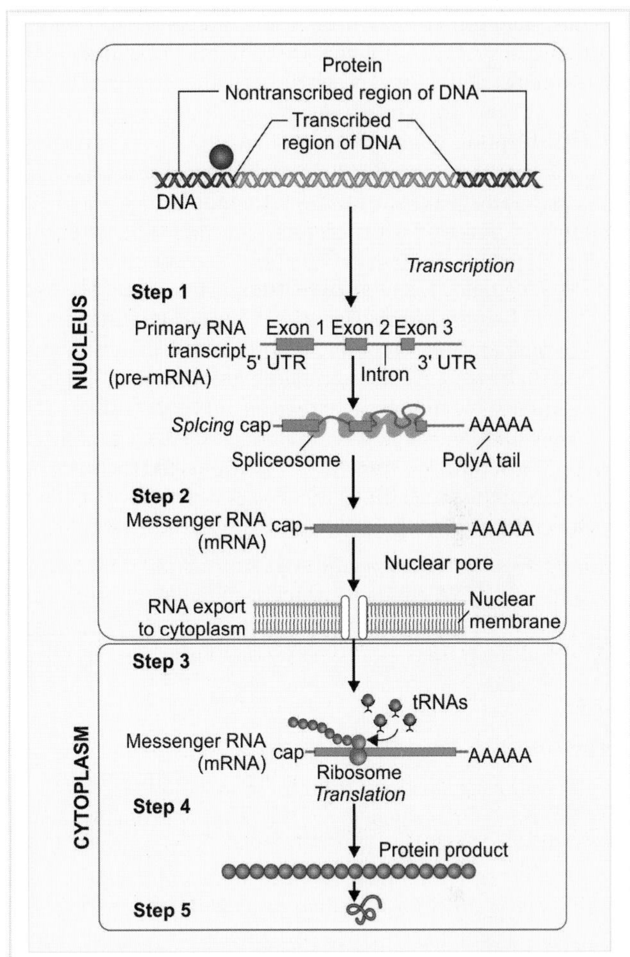

FIG. 20: Various steps involved in protein synthesis. The information encoded in deoxyribonucleic acid (DNA) is converted into the amino acid sequences of proteins by a multistep process. Transcription factors and other proteins bind to the regulatory regions of the specific genes. Ribonucleic acid (RNA) polymerase starts transcription of an activated gene at a specific location, the start site. The polymerase moves along the DNA. Selected sites on the DNA are transcribed into a single-stranded precursor messenger RNA (pre-mRNA) transcript using one of the DNA strands as a template. Formation of this pre-mRNAs (primary RNA transcript) is the step 1. The primary RNA transcript is a copy of the whole gene and includes both introns and exons. The noncoding introns are removed within the nucleus by splicing. After splicing, exons are joined to form the mRNA (step 2). Prior to transport from the nucleus, a methylated guanosine nucleotide is added to the 5′ end of the RNA ("cap") and a string of adenine nucleotides is added to the 3′ ("polyA tail"). This protects the RNA from degradation and facilitates transport into the cytoplasm. The mRNA is then transported from the nucleus to the cytoplasm (step 3). In the cytoplasm, the mRNAs bind to ribosomes and form a template for protein production (step 4). Following translation, the polypeptide folds to form protein of required conformation (step 5). (tRNA: transfer RNA; UTR: untranslated region)

that influence the ability of RNA polymerase to transcribe a given gene. There are two categories of transcription:

1. **General transcription factors:** They are needed for the binding of RNA polymerase to the core promoter and its progression to the elongation stage. General transcription factors are needed for a basal level of transcription.
2. **Regulatory transcription factors:** They serve to regulate the rate of transcription of target genes. The regulatory transcription factors exert their effects by influencing the ability of RNA polymerase to begin transcription of a particular gene. They recognize *cis*-acting elements that are present relatively near the core promoter (the site where transcription begins). These DNA sequences are known as **control elements,** or **regulatory elements.** When a regulatory transcription factor binds to a regulatory element, it affects the transcription of an associated gene.
   - When the binding of regulatory transcription factors to a regulatory element increases the rate of transcription, such a transcription factor is called an **activator,** and the regulatory element that it binds is called an **enhancer.** Such elements can stimulate transcription 10- to 1,000-fold, a phenomenon termed as **upregulation.**
   - When a regulatory transcription factor prevent transcription, they are called as **repressors** and element that it binds is called **silencer**. Their action is called **downregulation.**

Enhancers and tissue-specific gene expression Enhancers or activators are DNA elements which facilitate or ***enhance gene expression***. They provide binding sites for specific proteins that regulate transcription. They facilitate binding of the transcription complex to promoter regions.

Ribonucleic Acid Processing

Transcription produces a primary RNA molecule/transcript that is a copy of the whole gene. The primary RNA (pri-mRNA) molecule produced in the nucleus leaves the nucleus. But before it leaves, it undergoes a number of modifications. These modifications are known as RNA processing and involve—(1) splicing, (2) capping, and (3) polyadenylation.

mRNA Splicing

Messenger RNA (mRNA) splicing is the editing of the nascent precursor messenger RNA (pre-mRNA) transcript into a mature mRNA. During splicing, the noncoding introns (regions not required to make protein) in the precursor (pre) mRNA are excised and the coding exons (segments that are necessary for protein production) are retained. Splicing is a highly regulated process and carried by protein complex called the **spliceosome.** Spicing is followed by joining together of noncontiguous coding exons to form a shorter mature mRNA. Splicing occurs in the nucleus before translation in the cytoplasm. The boundary between the introns and exons consists of a 5′ donor GT dinucleotide and a 3′acceptor AG dinucleotide.

5′ Capping

The 5′ **cap** facilitates transport of the mRNA from the nucleus to the cytoplasm and attachment to the ribosomes. This also protects the RNA transcript from degradation by endogenous cellular exonucleases.

Polyadenylation

Transcription continues till specific nucleotide sequences are transcribed that cause the mRNA to be cleaved and RNA polymerase II to be released from the DNA template. About 200 **adenylate residues**—the so-called **poly(A) tail**—are added to the mRNA. This facilitates nuclear export and translation.

Translation

Translation is the **transmission of the genetic information from mRNA to form protein**. In this step, the information in the RNA is used to make a polypeptide (sequence of a large number of amino acids forming part of or the whole of a protein molecule). Such an informational RNA is termed as **mRNA.** This carries information like a message—from a gene to the cell's protein factories. Translation is a complex process and decodes an RNA molecule to synthesize protein in the cytoplasm. This is the second stage of gene expression. Newly processed mRNA is transported from the nucleus to the cytoplasm.

- During translation process, the cellular machinery decodes the sequence of nucleotides in mRNA into a sequence of amino acids—a **polypeptide.** Translation needs the participation of dozens of different components, including ribosomes. It occurs on **ribosomes** which are nonspecific components of the translation machinery. In the cytoplasm, mRNA attaches to ribosomes. Ribosomes are composed of proteins and **rRNAs (ribosomal RNA).** Translation depends on the **genetic code.** Translation also needs **tRNAs (transfer RNAs),** small RNA adaptwer molecules that place specific amino acids at the correct position in a growing polypeptide chain.
- **Ribosomal RNAs (rRNAs)** such as mRNAs, each is transcribed from one of the DNA strands of a gene. Unlike functioning as an informational capacity of mRNAs, the rRNAs provide structural support and catalyze the chemical reaction in which amino acids are covalently linked to one another.
- **Transfer RNAs (tRNAs)** constitute a third major class of RNA that is required during protein synthesis. During translation, smaller RNA molecules known as tRNAs bind to the ribosome. The tRNAs deliver amino acids to the ribosomes and synthesize a linear **chain of amino acids called a polypeptide (primary protein)** and later form proteins.

Various steps involved in protein synthesis are shown in **Figure 20.**

Post-translational Modification

It is modification of proteins following protein biosynthesis. Many proteins, before they gain their normal structure or functional activity, undergo **post-translational modification.** These modifications include chemical modification of amino acid side chains (e.g., hydroxylation, methylation), the addition of carbohydrate or lipid moieties (e.g., glycosylation), or proteolytic cleavage of polypeptides (e.g., the conversion of proinsulin to insulin). During post-translational modification, the newly synthesized proteins are transported to specific cellular locations (e.g., the nucleus), or secretion from the cell.

Gene Expression

Gene expression is a process that produces a functional protein or RNA from the genetic information in a gene. Gene expression is the means by which genetic information can be interpreted as a phenotype. **Gene regulation is the process that influences or inhibits the expression of a gene.** Gene expression and its regulation are highly complex.

The regulation of gene expression is very essential for the growth, development, and differentiation. Within each cell, genetic information flows from DNA to RNA to protein. Thus, the central dogma of molecular biology is—DNA makes RNA makes protein. Once genetic information has passed into protein, it cannot get out again.

Many cellular processes and corresponding genes are expressed in all cells. For example, ribosomal, chromosomal and cytoskeleton proteins. These genes constitute **housekeeping genes**. Some cells express large amount of a specific protein in certain tissues or at specific times in development (e.g., hemoglobin in RBCs). This differential control of gene expression can occur at a variety of stages.

Regulation of Gene Expression

Gene regulation refers to the phenomenon that can control the level of gene expression so that genes can be expressed at high or low levels. The genome of a cell contains in its DNA sequence called genes which can make many different protein and RNA molecules. Usually a cell expresses only a fraction of its genes. The cells can change the pattern of genes they express in response to changes in their environment, such as signals from other cells.

There are many steps (several mechanisms) in the pathway to regulate the gene expression from DNA to protein. All of these steps in protein synthesis can be regulated (**Box 6**). Acetylation of histones leads to gene expression whereas deacetylation reverses the effect. Usually methylation of DNA leads to inactivation of genes.

Regulation of gene expression occurs at different levels (**Box 6** and **Fig. 21**). Although all of the steps mentioned in **Box 6** can be involved in gene expression, for most genes the initiation of RNA transcription is the most important point of control. Thus, gene regulation at the level of transcription is an important form of control.

- **Transcriptional level control:** Regulation of expression of most genes occurs at the level of transcription.
  - **Control of transcription:** The control of transcription can be affected either permanently or reversibly by a variety of factors. These factors include both environmental (e.g., hormones) and genetic (cell signaling).
  - **Transcription factors:** Many genes encode proteins involved in the regulation of gene expression. They have DNA-binding activity to short nucleotide sequences and are called as **transcription factors.**

Post-transcriptional control of gene expression can also occur at the levels of RNA processing, RNA transport, translation, and mRNA degradation.

- **Ribonucleic acid processing level control** by controlling the splicing and processing of RNA transcripts.
  - **Alternative isoforms:** About 95% of human genes undergo **alternative splicing (also called alternative RNA splicing** is a method cells use to create many proteins from the same strand of DNA) and therefore encode more than one protein. **Alternative polyadenylation** [it is characterized by addition of an alternate poly(A) tail to an RNA molecule and allows a single gene to encode multiple mRNA transcripts] creates further diversity. Some genes have more than one promoter, and these **alternative** promoters may result in tissue-specific isoforms.
- **RNA transport and localization control:** By selecting which completed mRNAs are exported from the nucleus to the cytosol and determining where these mRNAs are localized in the cytosol.
- **Translational control:** By selecting which mRNAs in the cytoplasm are translated by ribosomes.
- **mRNA degradation control:** By selectively destabilizing certain mRNA molecules in the cytoplasm (control). RNA-mediated silencing also plays a key role in controlling post-transcriptional gene expression. (discussed below miRNAs and siRNAs on page 112)
- **Protein activity control:** After translation, a protein must fold a certain way. It may be modified by different folding, shortening of certain polypeptides, by adding sugars, and/or by aggregation Regulation of gene expression can be done by selectively activating, inactivating, degrading, or locating specific protein molecules after they have been made.

Box 6: Mechanism of gene expression regulation.

- Transcriptional level control
- RNA processing level control including alternative isoforms
- RNA transport and localization control
- Translational control
- mRNA degradation control
- Protein activity control

Major Classes of Ribonucleic Acid

Q. What are the types of RNA? Discuss micro-RNA.

There are two major classes of RNA (**Table 3**), namely—(1) the **protein coding RNAs**, or **mRNAs**, and (2) **nonprotein coding RNAs** (they are abundant). The mRNAs, rRNAs, and tRNAs are directly involved in synthesis of protein. The other RNAs are involved in either mRNA splicing (snRNAs) or modulate gene expression by altering mRNA function (mi/siRNAs) and/or expression (lncRNAs).

Micro-RNA and Long Noncoding RNA

Q. Write a short essay on noncoding RNA.
Q. Write a short essay on miRNA in gene signaling.
Q. Write a short essay on miRNA in diagnostic pathology.

Introduction

Noncoding RNAs cal also regulate genes. The two-small **ncRNAs (noncoding RNAs), namely miRNAs (micro RNAs) and** small-interfering RNA [siRNA/silencing (SiRNAs)] inhibit **gene expression.** This is done at the level of specific protein production by targeting mRNAs (messenger RNAs) through one of the several distinct mechanisms.

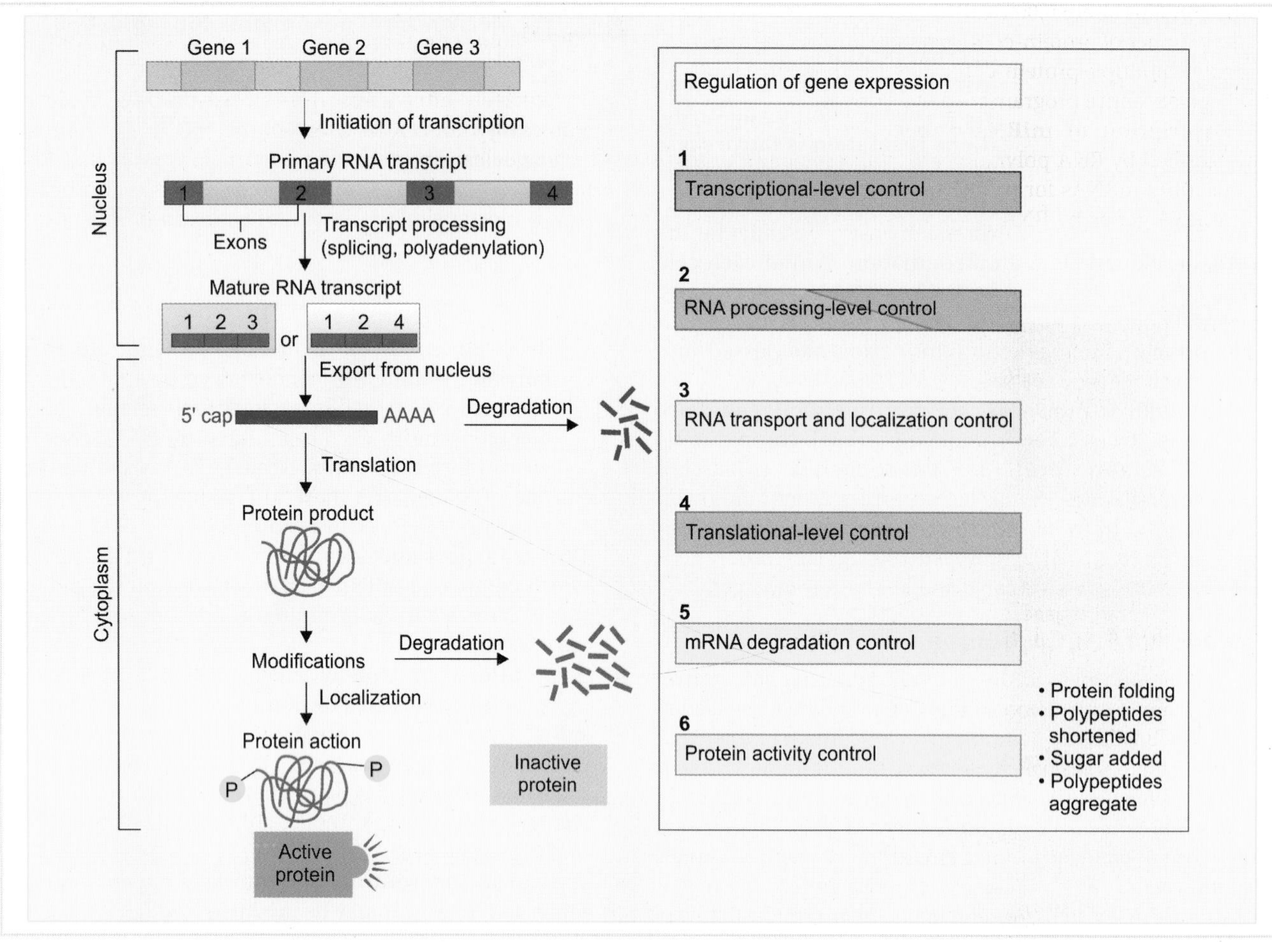

FIG. 21: Different levels of regulation of gene expression. It first involves transcription and mRNA processing in the nucleus. The mRNA is transported to the cytoplasm, where it is translated into a protein.

Table 3: Classes of ribonucleic acid.

Classes of ribonucleic acid (RNA)	*Stability*
Protein Coding RNAs	
• Messenger (mRNA)	Unstable to very stable
Nonprotein Coding RNAs	
• Large ncRNAs	
○ Ribosomal(rRNA)	Very stable
• Long noncoding RNAs (lncRNAs)	Unstable to very stable
• Small ncRNAs	
○ Small ribosomal (sRNA)	Very stable
○ Transfer (tRNAs)	Very stable
○ Small nuclear(snRNA)	Very stable
○ Micro/small-interfering* (mi/siRNAs)	Stable

(nc: noncoding)
*also called as silencing

Both miRNAs and siRNAs represent exciting new **potential agents for therapeutic drug development**. One of the **mechanisms of gene regulation depends on the functions of ncRNAs.** As the term noncoding indicates that these RNAs are encoded by genes which are **transcribed but not translated.** There are many distinct families of ncRNAs. Of these, two important ncRNAs are—(1) small RNA molecules called *miRNAs (microRNAs)* and (2) *lncRNAs (long noncoding RNAs)* >200 nucleotides in length.

Micro Ribonucleic Acids (miRNAs)

These are new type of gene regulators. They are relatively short/small, specialized RNAs, usually an average of 22 nucleotides that prevent the expression of specific genes through complementary base pairing **miRNAs do not encode proteins**. They mainly modulate the translation of target mRNAs into their corresponding proteins. They regulate gene activity at the post-transcriptional level through the modulation of RNA stability and/or translation. **Post-transcriptional silencing of gene expression by miRNA is a mechanism of gene regulation in cells.** Even bacteria have a primitive version of the same general machinery which is used to protect themselves against foreign DNA (e.g., from viruses).

Method of gene silencing by miRNAs (Figs. 22A and B)

miRNAs are generated by specific nucleolytic processing of the products of distinct genes/transcription units. The human genome contains about 6,000 miRNA genes (only 3.5 times less than the number of protein-coding genes). Individual miRNAs can regulate multiple protein-coding genes. Thus, each miRNA can coregulate entire programs of gene expression.

- **Transcription of miRNA genes:** Most miRNAs are transcribed by RNA polymerase II, the same enzyme that transcribes mRNAs for protein production. Transcription of miRNA genes by RNA polymerase II **produces** a long primary transcript called primary miRNA (**pri-miRNA**). This contains one or more miRNA sequences in the form of mostly double-stranded stem loops (**Fig. 22A**).
- Immediately after transcription, pri-miRNAs undergo processing within the nucleus. The pri-miRNA is recognized by the nuclear ribonuclease (RNase) enzyme Drosha. This enzyme crops out pri-miRNA stem-loop structures and form a shorter single RNA strand with secondary hairpin

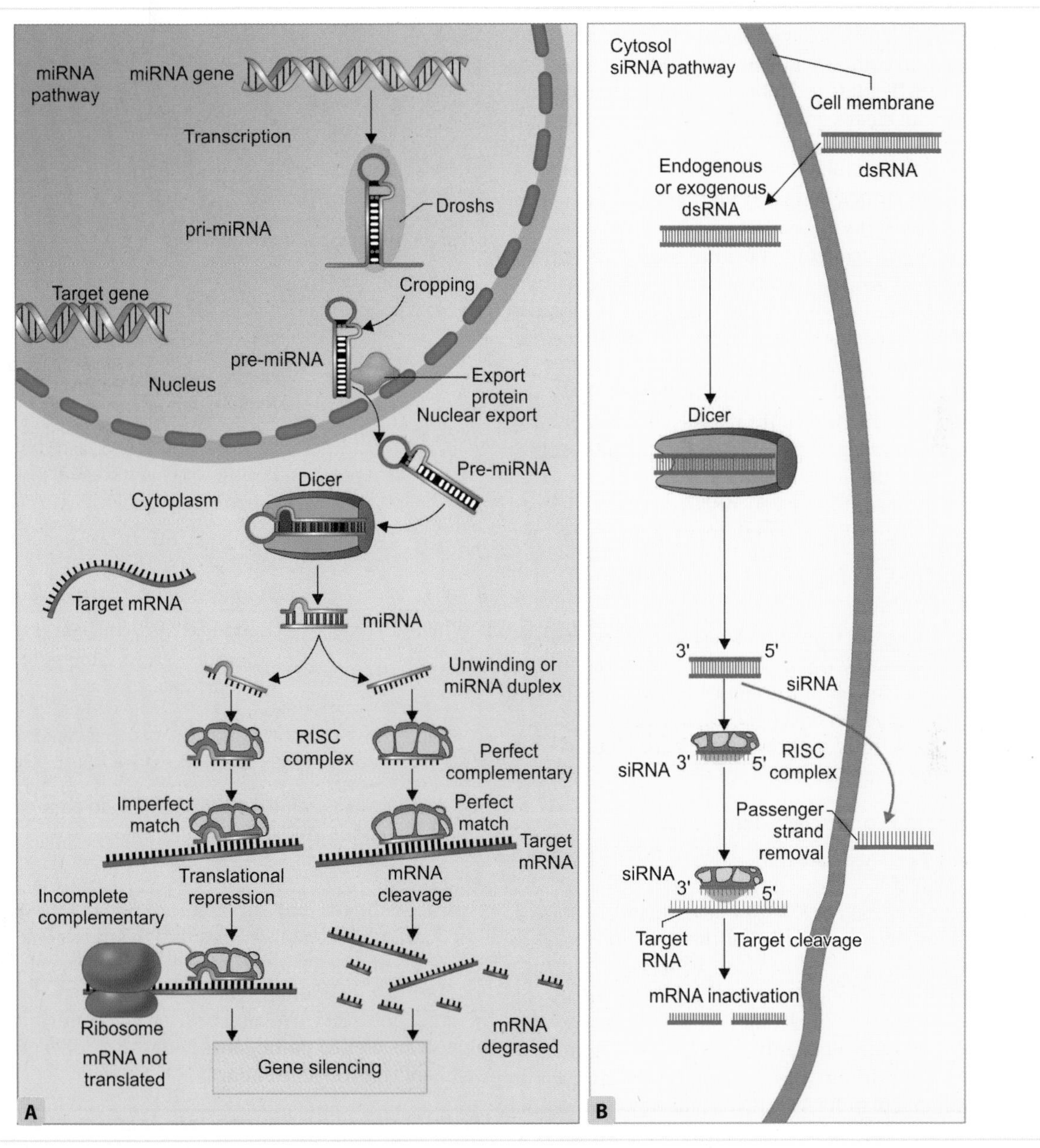

FIGS. 22A AND B: Production of microribonucleic acids (miRNA) and small interfering RNA (siRNA), and their mechanism of action in regulating gene function. (A) miRNA genes are transcribed to produce a primary miRNA (pri-miRNA). It is processed in the nucleus and forms precursor miRNA (pre-miRNA). This pre-miRNA is exported out of the nucleus via specific transporter proteins. In the cytoplasm, enzyme Dicer trims the pre-miRNA to produce mature double stranded miRNAs of 21–30 nucleotides. The miRNA subsequently unwinds, and this results in single strands. These are incorporated into the multiprotein RISC. Base pairing between the single-stranded miRNA and its target mRNA directs RISC to either cleave the mRNA target or to repress its translation. Thus, by both processes, the target mRNA gene is silenced post transcriptionally. (B) siRNAs pathway has many similarities with that of miRNAs. siRNAs result from the nucleolytic processing (also by Dicer) of large double-stranded RNAs (dsRNAs). These dsRNAs are either produced by transcription of both strands either of an endogenous deoxyribonucleic acid (DNA) sequence in the genome or dsRNAs introduced into the cell by an exogenous source such as a virus.

loop structures that form stretches of double-stranded RNA (dsRNA). This is called a precursor miRNA (pre-miRNA).

- This pre-miRNA is actively transported/exported from the nucleus (where they were transcribed) into the cytoplasm (where they will act) via specific transporter proteins. They are processed into progressively smaller segments.
- In the cytosol (cytoplasm), the cytoplasmic RNase enzyme called **Dicer** recognizes pre-miRNAs. Dicer trims the pre-miRNA and generates mature double stranded miRNAs (miRNA duplex) of 21–30 nucleotides. The miRNA duplex subsequently unwinds and forms single-stranded miRNAs. One of the two strands is selected and then incorporated into the multiprotein complex named **RNA-induced silencing complex (RISC)**. RISC includes an enzyme (Argonaute or Ago) that can cleave target mRNAs. Subsequently base pairing between the single-stranded miRNA and its target mRNA occurs and forms a mature, functional 21–22 nt single stranded miRNA. It directs RISC to either cleave the mRNA or to repress its translation.
    - **Direct promotion of mRNA degradation:** If the miRNA and its target mRNA contain perfectly complementary sequences, miRISC cleaves the target mRNA. The two cleavage products are not protected from RNase and are rapidly degraded.
    - **Inhibition of translation of mRNA:** If the miRNA and its target mRNA have only partial complementarity (or complementarity is imperfect), miRNA inhibits translation of the target mRNA.

In either way/case, the target mRNA gene is silenced post transcriptionally. siRNAs (small-interfering RNAs) are produced similarly.

Significance of miRNAs

miRNAs critically control many activities, such as embryogenesis and development, cell cycling, differentiation, apoptosis, and maintaining stem cell pluripotency ("stemness"). They also regulate many steps in oncogenesis. MicroRNAs may act as oncogenes and as tumor suppressors, or both (**Table 4**). For further details refer pages 549–553.

Table 4: Examples of activities of microRNAs (miRNAs) and associated tumors.

Micro ribonucleic acid (miRNA)	*Organ affected by tumor/tumors produced*
Oncogenic miRNAs	
• miR-21	Cancers of solid organs such as breast, colorectal, esophagus, glioblastoma, liver, lung, pancreas, prostate. Chronic lymphocytic leukemia (CLL),
• miR-23	Bladder, breast, CLL
• miR-221	Acute myeloid leukemia (AML), CLL. Bladder, glioblastoma, liver, pancreas, prostate, thyroid
• miR-17–92 cluster	Acute lymphoblastic leukemia (ALL), chronic myeloid leukemia (CML) Colorectal, lung, ovary
Tumor Suppressor miRNAs	
• miR-143	Breast, colorectal, lung, prostate and CLL
• let-7group	ALL, CLL Breast, colorectal, lung, pancreas
• miR-145	Bladder, breast, colorectal, lung, ovary, prostate
miRNAs acting as both suppressors and oncogenes	
• miR-23 group	Oncogenic: Bladder, breast, CLL Suppressor: Prostate
• miR-181 group	Oncogenic: ALL, breast, pancreas, prostate and thyroid Suppressor: AML, CLL, glioblastoma
• miR-125 group	Oncogenic: AML, pancreas Suppressor: Breast, glioblastoma, liver, ovary, prostate, thyroid. Both: ALL

Small Interfering Ribonucleic Acids (siRNAs)

Q. Write a short essay on siRNA.

The siRNAs are short dsRNA (21–23 nucleotides) sequences. siRNAs are the effector molecules of the RNA interference pathway (RNAi). RNAi is a process in which specific RNA molecules inhibit gene expression or translation, by neutralizing targeted mRNA molecules. siRNAs bind to mRNAs in a sequence-specific manner and result in their degradation via an RNase-containing RISC. Its pathway has many similarities with that of miRNAs. siRNAs pathway is presented in **Figure 22B**. Main difference is the source of the small RNA.

- The miRNAs result from the processing of a long, single-stranded transcript, whereas **siRNAs result from the nucleolytic processing** (also by Dicer) **of large** dsRNAs. These dsRNAs are either produced by transcription of both strands either of an endogenous DNA sequence in the genome or dsRNAs introduced into the cell by an exogenous source such as a virus.
- The siRNA pathway may also protect the cell from invading viruses by destroying viral mRNAs. *siRNAs* can be introduced into cells. These serve as substrates for Dicer and interact with the RISC complex in a manner similar to endogenous miRNAs.

Uses

Synthetic siRNAs that can target specific mRNA species can be used as a powerful laboratory tool **to study gene function** (to decrease or "knockdown" specific protein levels by so-called knockdown technology) via siRNA homology-directed mRNA degradation. They can also be used as promising **therapeutic agents to silence pathogenic genes** (e.g., oncogenes involved in neoplastic transformation).

Long Noncoding Ribonucleic Acid (lncRNAs)

About 3% of the human genome encodes proteins. Over 90% of the human genome is actively transcribed and almost all of it as transcripts do not make proteins. It is found that, many DNA sequence changes associated with cancer and other diseases occur within the regions that encode these untranslated RNAs. *These RNAs are called* ***lncRNAs***.

Long noncoding RNAs are defined as RNAs, either primary or spliced transcripts, which do not fit into recognized classes such as structural, protein-coding, or small RNAs. The genome of human also contains a very large number of *lncRNA*.

lncRNAs may be quite large, usually 1,000s or 10,000s of bases. They constitute about 30,000 in number, and their number exceeds by 10–20 times the number of coding mRNAs. *lncRNAs* are present in the nucleus and are physically associated with chromatin. Hence, many of *lncRNA* likely control gene expression. lncRNAs represent exons, introns, and regions between genes.

Modes of action (Figs. 23A to D)

lncRNAs modulate gene expression in different ways.

- **Gene activation:** lncRNAs can promote gene activation by facilitating the binding of transcription factor binding.
- **Gene suppression:** lncRNAs can bind to chromatin and restrict RNA polymerase from accessing coding genes within that region. Example for gene suppression by lncRNA sequence called XIST (refer pages 864 and 865), which normally shuts off one X chromosome. XIST plays an important role in physiological X chromosome inactivation. XIST itself escapes X inactivation but forms a repressive "cloak" on the X chromosome from which it is transcribed, resulting in gene silencing.
    - Long noncoding RNAs can bind transcription factors and prevent gene transcription.
    - lncRNAs can bind to regions of chromatin and restrict RNA polymerase access to coding genes within the region.
- **Promote chromatin modification:** Modification of histone and DNA by acetylases or methylases (or deacetylases and demethylases) may be directed by the binding of lncRNAs.
- **Assembly of protein complexes:** lncRNAs may act as scaffolding to stabilize secondary or tertiary structures and/or multiple subunit complexes that influence general chromatin architecture or gene activity.

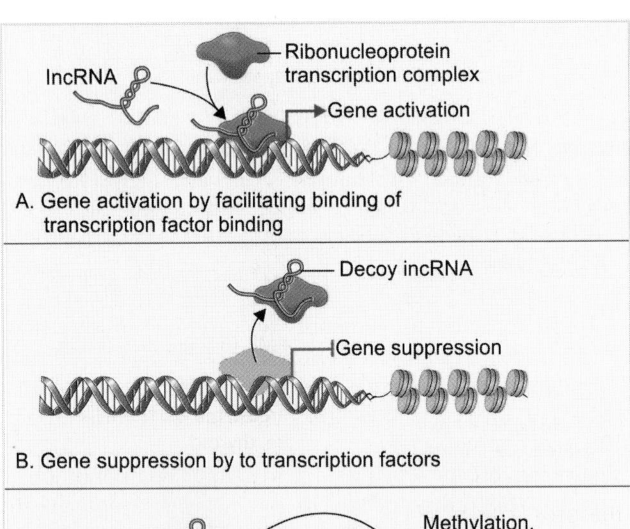

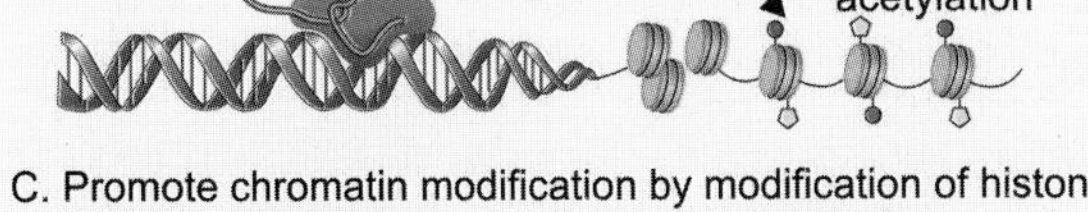

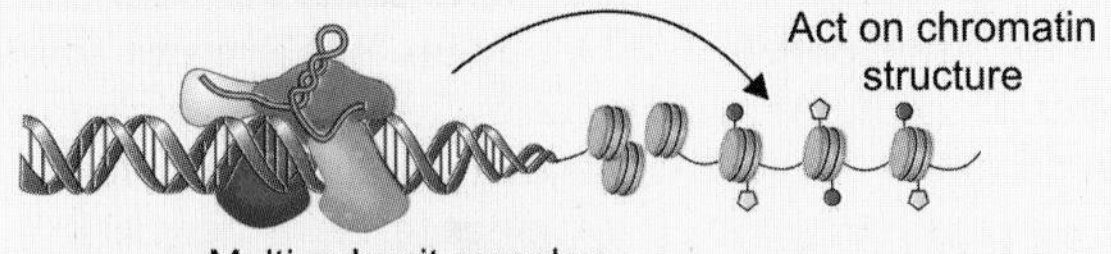

Act on chromatin structure
Multi-subunit complex
D. Assembly of protein complexes by acting as a scaffold to stabilize secondary or tertiary structures and/or multisubunit complexes that influence general chromatin architecture of gene activity

FIGS. 23A TO D: Modes of action of long noncoding ribonucleic acids (lncRNAs). (A) Gene activation by facilitating binding of lncRNAs to transcription factor. (B) Gene suppression by binding to transcription factors. (C) Promoting chromatin modification by modification of histone and deoxyribonucleic acid (DNA) by acetylases or methylases (or deacetylases and demethylases). (D) Assembly of protein complexes.

GENE EDITING TECHNOLOGY

Q. Write a short essay on gene editing technology.

Genome editing (gene editing or genomic engineering) is a group of technologies by which it is able to change a living organism's DNA. It is a type of genetic engineering in which DNA is inserted, deleted, modified or replaced in the genome (DNA sequence). During early genetic engineering, these editing targets was random. In recent years, the emergence of highly versatile genome-editing technologies can rapidly and economically introduce sequence-specific modifications target to specific location in the genome in a broad spectrum of cell types. It is usually aimed at improving, curing, or preventing a genetic disorder.

Mechanism: In this technology, either a protein or an RNA molecule serves as a guide. There are several enzymes capable of degrading nucleic acids (e.g., deoxyribonucleases, RNases, endonucleases). Targeted nucleases (molecular scissors) have the ability to manipulate virtually any genomic sequence. These nucleases create a site-specific double-strand breaks (DSB) at the desired location in the genome. Gene editing technology depends on the nucleases (DNA-cleaving enzyme) that create a site-specific DSB at the desired location in the genome followed by its repair. DNA repair of the break can then result in a point mutation (a base pair change, or insertion or deletion of one or a few pairs) or a knock in of specific DNA sequences. These double-strand breaks (DSB) are repaired by two major pathways namely (i) nonhomologous end joining (NHEJ) or (ii) homologous directed repair/recombination (HDR). NHEJ utilises a variety of enzymes to directly join the broken ends of DNA. However, homologous directed repair/recombination (HDR) uses homologous sequence as a template for regeneration of missing DNA sequences at the broken site.

Engineered Targeted Nucleases

Main requirement for gene editing is to create a DSB at a specific point within the genome.

Restriction endonucleases (restriction enzymes): These are DNA-cleaving enzymes which act by directly binding contiguous DNA base pairs (typically 4, 5, 6, or 8 base pairs). They cleave both strands of DNA, usually DNA within the binding/recognition sequence element.

Specific DSB by using distinct nucleases: Routinely used restriction enzymes can cut DNA but usually recognize and cut at multiple sites. This draw-back can be overcome by creating site-specific DSB by using four distinct classes of nucleases. These include (i) clustered regularly interspaced short palindromic repeats (CRISPR)-CRISPR-associated protein 9 (Cas9), (ii) transcription activator-like effector nucleases (TALENs), (iii) zinc-finger nucleases (ZFNs), and (iv) homing endonucleases or meganucleases.

CRISPR/Cas System

CRISPR-Cas family of enzymes: The newest/novel and most efficient genome editing (DNA editing/gene regulatory) system is called CRISPR/Cas. CRISPR is an acronym for clustered regularly interspaced short palindromic repeats and this system is called CRISPR-associated protein 9 (Cas9) system. CRISPR-Cas are ribonucleoprotein complexes that cleave DNA. Many bacterial genomes contain a CRISPR region and they have a role in adaptive (acquired) immunity in bacteria to protect against viruses. CRISPR immunity also depends on endonucleases called Cas proteins (CRISPR-associated proteins) encoded by the bacterial genome. CRISPRs consist of short sequences that originate from viral genomes and have been incorporated into the bacterial genome. Cas enzymes can cut genome at any desired location and produce double-stranded breaks in DNA. Target site recognition is mediated entirely by the single guide RNA (gRNA) of specific nucleotide sequence targets a nuclease to cleave distinct DNA or RNA sequences. CRISPR-Cas9 is the most flexible and user-friendly genome editing enzyme. These enzymes are important tools in molecular genetics and medical sciences.

Steps in Gene Editing with CRISPRs/Cas9 (Fig. 24)

Gene editing by CRISPs/Cas9 is performed by using artificial guide RNAs (gRNAs). The gRNA sequence is designed to bring the Cas9 endonuclease to a specific target in the genome. The gRNAs have constant region and a variable sequence of about 20 bases. The constant regions of gRNAs bind to Cas9, whereas the variable regions form heteroduplexes (two strands that do not show complementary base pairing) with homologous host cell DNA sequences. Gene editing gives a new purpose to this process by using artificial gRNAs that bind Cas9 and are complementary to a DNA sequence of interest. Once directed to the target sequence by the gRNA, Cas9 nuclease cleaves the bound host DNA and causes a dsDNA break. To perform gene editing, gRNAs are designed with variable regions that are homologous to a target DNA sequence of interest. Both the gRNAs and the Cas9 enzyme can be introduced into the cells with a single easy-to-build plasmid. Simultaneous expression (i.e., coexpression) of the gRNA and Cas9 in cells produces efficient cleavage of the target DNA sequence.

After the highly specific cleavage of particular site in a DNA, repair occurs at that site. Repair may occur by two ways:

1. **Nonhomologous end joining (NHEJ):** In the absence of homologous DNA, the broken DNA is repaired by NHEJ. This is an error-prone method that usually introduces random troublesome/disruptive insertions or deletions (random mutations) in the targeted DNA sequences.
2. **Homologous DNA recombination (HDR):** In contrast, in the presence of a homologous "donor" DNA bridging the region targeted by CRISPR/Cas9, cells may use HDR to repair the DNA break. HDR is less efficient than NHEJ. However, it has the capacity to introduce precise new sequences of interest in DNA sequence.

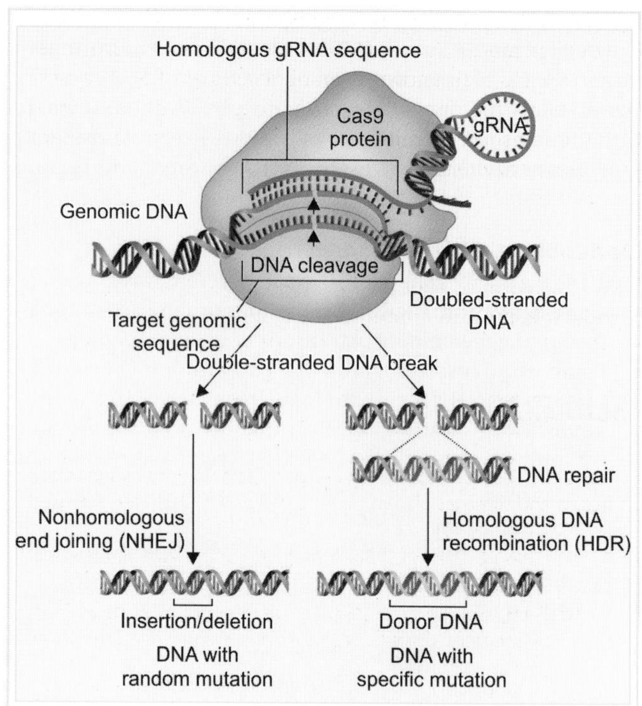

FIG. 24: Mechanism of gene editing with clustered regularly interspersed short palindromic repeats (CRISPRs)/Cas9. Deoxyribonucleic acid (DNA) sequences consisting of CRISPRs are transcribed into guide ribonucleic acids (gRNAs) and processed into an RNA sequence.

Both the guide sequences and the Cas enzyme can be easily introduced into cells. These may be either as a coding DNA (cDNA) or a protein.

Advantage: This new technology in genetic engineering has **impressive flexibility and specificity** and is significantly better than other previous gene editing techniques.

TALE Nucleases

Transcription activator-like effector nucleases (TALENs) are bacterial effectors and are capable of modifying nearly any gene. TALENs are specific DNA-binding enzymes and are artificially produced. It is produced by fusing the DNA cutting domain of a nuclease to TALE domains. TALE arrays consists of about 33–34 amino acid repeats. TALENs have improved specificity and reduced toxicity compared to some ZFNs.

Zinc-finger Nucleases

ZFNs function as dimers. Each monomer recognizes a specific "half site" sequence [typically nine to 18 base pairs (bps) of DNA] via the zinc-finger DNA-binding domain. Zinc-finger motifs occur in several transcription factors. Zinc-finger proteins can target a wide range of possible DNA sequences. Zinc ion is found in 8% of all proteins in humans. In transcription factors, zinc is mostly found at the protein-DNA interaction sites and it stabilizes the motif.

Homing Endonucleases (Meganucleases)

These are naturally occurring enzymes belonging to endonuclease family and are capable to recognize and cut large (long) DNA sequences ranging from 14 to 40 base pairs (hence called meganucleases). They are very specific. The most widespread and well known meganucleases are the members of the LAGLIDADG family of endonucleases. They are named so for the conserved amino acid sequences (motif) present within these enzymes.

Applications of Gene Editing

- **For insertion of specific mutations into the genomes of cells:** It is used to model cancers and other diseases, and rapidly generate transgenic animals from edited embryonic stem cells.
- **Repair mutations causing hereditary/inherited genetic defects:** Less commonly, it is possible to selectively "correct" mutations that cause hereditable disease, or perhaps to just eliminate less "desirable" traits (which is of course worrisome). Hence, application of gene editing technology is a matter of debate.
- Potential applications of CRISPR/Cas9 coupled with HDR may be used for creating pathogenic mutations in inducible pluripotent stem cell.

BIBLIOGRAPHY

1. Almal SH, Padh H. Implications of gene copy-number variation in health and diseases. *J Hum Genet*. 2012;57(1):6-13. [Last accessed on 2021 January 19].
2. Anastasiadou E, Jacob LS, Slack FJ. Non-coding RNA networks in cancer. *Nat Rev Genet*. 2018;18(1):5-18.
3. Hartwell LH, Goldberg ML, Fischer JA, Hood L. Genetics: From Genes to Genomes, 6th edition. New York: McGraw-Hill Education; 2018.
4. Jameson JL, Fausi AS, Kasper DL, et al. Harrison's principles of internal medicine (2 vols), 20th edition. New York: McGraw-Hill Medical Publishing. Division; 2018.
5. Korf BR, Irons MB. Human Genetics and Genomics, 4th edition. West Sussex: Wiley-Blackwell; 2013.
6. Kumar V, Abbas AK, Aster JC. Robbins basic pathology, 10th edition. Philadelphia: Saunders Elsevier; 2018.
7. Kumar V, Abbas AK, Fausto N, et al. Robbins and Cotran pathologic basis of disease, 10th edition. Philadelphia: WB Saunders; 2021.
8. Lewis R. Human Genetics: Concepts and Applications,11th edition. Penn Plaza: McGraw-Hill Education; 2015.
9. Ralston H, Penman ID, Strachan MWJ, Hobson RP. Davidson's Principles and Practice of Medicine, 23rd edition. Edinburgh: Elsevier; 2018.
10. Strayer DS, Saffitz JE. Rubin's Pathology: Mechanism of Human Disease, 8th edition. Philadelphia: Wolters Kluwer; 2020.
11. Turnpenny PD, Ellard S. Emery's Elements of Medical Genetics.15th edition. Philadelphia: Saunders Elsevier; 2017.

SECTION

2

GENERAL PATHOLOGY

CHAPTER 6

Introduction to Pathology

CHAPTER OUTLINE

- Definition
- Learning pathology
- Scientific study of disease
  - Etiology
  - Pathogenesis
  - Pathophysiology
- Morphologic changes
  - Gross
  - Microscopy
- Functional derangements and clinical manifestations
  - Functional derangements
  - Clinical manifestations
  - Laboratory tests and investigations
  - Diagnosis
  - Syndromes
  - Prognosis
  - Complications
  - Sequelae
  - Remission and relapse/exacerbation
- Role of pathologist in diagnosis and management of disease
  - Subdivisions of pathology
  - Role of pathologists
  - Other roles
- History and evolution of pathology
  - Prehistoric times to medieval period
  - Human anatomy and era of gross pathology
  - Era of technology development and cellular pathology
  - Landmarks in modern pathology
  - Modern pathology
  - Telepathology and virtual microscopy

DEFINITION

Pathology is the study of the structural, biochemical, and functional changes in cells, tissues, and organs in disease.

By using morphologic, immunologic, and molecular techniques, pathology attempts to explain the reason for signs and symptoms manifested by patients. It provides a rational basis for clinical management and serves as the bridge between the basic sciences and clinical medicine.

LEARNING PATHOLOGY

Study of pathology can be divided into general pathology and systemic pathology.

General pathology: It deals with the study of mechanism, basic reactions of cells and tissues to injurious stimuli. These basic reactions are generally not specific to tissue. For example, acute inflammation developing against bacterial infections produces a almost similar reaction in most tissues.

Systemic pathology: This deals with the changes in specific diseases/responses of specialized organs and tissues. For example, emphysema is a disease restricted to lungs characterized by abnormal permanent dilatation of air spaces distal to the terminal bronchiole.

SCIENTIFIC STUDY OF DISEASE

Disease process is studied under the following aspects. The common definitions and terms used in pathology are also mentioned here. Main aspects of a disease process that form the core of pathology are (i) causation (*etiology*), (ii) biochemical and molecular mechanisms (*pathogenesis*), (iii) the structural (*morphologic changes*) and functional alterations in cells and organs, and (iv) the clinical consequences (*clinical manifestations*).

Etiology

The etiology of a disease is its initiating cause and modifying factors which are responsible for the initiation and progression of disease process. It describes why a disease arises or what sets the disease process in motion. The causative factors of a disease can be divided into two major categories—genetic (e.g., inherited or acquired mutations in genes, and disease-associated gene variants, or polymorphisms) and environmental (e.g., infectious, hypoxia, nutritional, chemical, physical).

Causative agents: Some diseases are closely linked with etiologic factors and these etiological factors are said to be the causative agents for the disease. For example, microbial pathogens are considered as the causative agents for infectious diseases—*Mycobacterium tuberculosis* causes pulmonary tuberculosis, human immunodeficiency virus (HIV) causes HIV disease, *Entamoeba histolytica* causes amebic dysentery. These diseases cannot develop without pathogens in the body; however, this does not mean that all the individuals exposed to infection will have the same consequences, because many host factors affect the clinical course.

Etiological factors: Even when there is a strong link between disease and etiologic agent, only a proportion of the individuals exposed to the etiological factor may develop the disease. For example, if an individual consumes large quantities of alcohol, he/she may develop liver cirrhosis. In this case, alcohol consumption is considered to be the cause, yet only a proportion of individuals who drink alcohol heavily will develop cirrhosis. The concept of one etiologic agent as the cause of one disease is not applicable to the majority of diseases. The exact causes of most disorders remain incompletely understood.

Multifactorial: Most common diseases are multifactorial due to combination of causes (several different etiologic factors that contribute to their development), i.e., inherited genetic susceptibility and various environmental triggers (e.g., coronary heart disease, hypertension, diabetes, and cancer). For example, coronary heart disease is a result of the interaction of genetic predisposition, elevated blood pressure, exposure to cigarette smoke, diet, and many other lifestyle factors acting together. None of these individual factors can be said to cause the disease.

Idiopathic: When the cause of the disease is unknown, a condition is said to be idiopathic.

Iatrogenic: If the cause of the disease is the result of an unintended or unwanted medical intervention, the resulting condition is said to be iatrogenic.

Risk factor: When the link between a causative/etiologic factor and development of a disease is less than certain but the probability is increased when the factor is present, it is called a risk factor. The identification of risk factors is important for the prevention of the disease.

Pathogenesis

Pathogenesis refers to the sequence of molecular, biochemical, and cellular events that lead to the development of disease. Pathogenesis deals with mechanisms of development, progression of disease, and the sequence of physiologic events that follow the exposure of cells or tissues (i.e., from the beginning of any disease process) to an injurious agent (initial contact with an etiologic agent/causative factor). It is a dynamic interplay of changes in cell, tissue, organ, and systemic function. It produces cellular, biochemical, and molecular abnormalities and ultimate expression of a disease. With the present advances in technology, it is possible to identify the changes occurring at cellular and molecular level that give rise to the specific functional and structural abnormalities of any particular disease. Thus, it describes how a disease process develops or evolves. This knowledge is helpful for designing new therapeutic approaches. New technological advances such as genomics, proteomics, metabolomics are of great value for understanding the pathogenic mechanisms. They may also help in identification of *biomarkers* that may be valuable for predicting the progression and therapeutic response in disease. This is the goal of *precision medicine*. In summary, pathogenesis is a description of how etiologic factors alter physiologic function and lead to the development of clinical manifestations in a particular disorder or disease.

Pathophysiology

In pathology, the study and diagnosis of disease is performed through examination of organs, tissues, cells, and body fluids. Physiology is the study of the mechanical, physical, and biochemical functions of living organisms. Together, as pathophysiology, the term refers to the study of abnormalities in physiologic functioning (i.e., physiological changes) of an individual or an organ due to a disease.

Latent period: Few causative agents produce signs and symptoms of the disease immediately after exposure. Usually, etiological agents take **some time to manifest the disease** (e.g., carcinogenesis) and this time period is called as the latent period. It varies depending on the disease.

Incubation period: In disorders caused by infectious (due to bacteria, viruses, etc.,) agents, the **period between exposure and the development of disease** is called the incubation period. It usually ranges from days to weeks. Most of the infectious agents have characteristic incubation period.

MORPHOLOGIC CHANGES

All diseases start with structural changes (pathologic changes) in cells. Rudolf Virchow (known as the father of modern pathology) proposed that injury to the cell is the basis of all diseases. Morphologic changes refer to the gross and microscopic structural changes in cells or tissues affected by disease. Lesion is the term used for the characteristic changes in tissues and cells produced by disease in an individual. The term "pathology" (pathological feature) is sometimes used as a synonym with morphology.

Gross

Many diseases have characteristic gross pathology and a fairly confident diagnosis can be given before light microscopy. For example, serous cystadenoma of ovary usually consists of one cystic cavity containing serous fluid; cirrhosis of liver is characterized by total replacement of liver by regenerating nodules.

Microscopy

Light Microscopy

Abnormalities in tissue architecture and morphological changes in cells can be studied by light microscopy.

Histopathology: Sections are routinely cut from tissues and processed by paraffin-embedding. The sections are cut from the tissue by a special instrument called microtome and examined under light microscope. In certain situations, (e.g., histochemistry, rapid diagnosis) sections are cut from tissue that has been hardened rapidly by freezing (frozen section). The sections are stained routinely by hematoxylin and eosin (H&E).

Pathognomonic abnormalities: If the structural changes are **characteristic of a single disease or diagnostic of an etiologic process**, it is called as pathognomonic. Pathognomonic features are those features which are restricted to a single disease, or disease category. The diagnosis should not be made without them. For example, Aschoff bodies are pathognomonic of rheumatic heart disease and Reed-Sternberg cells are pathognomonic of Hodgkin lymphoma.

Cytology: The cells from cysts, body cavities, or scraped from body surfaces or aspirated by fine needle from solid lesions can also be studied under light microscope. This study of cells is known as cytology and is used widely especially in diagnosis and screening of cancer.

Histochemistry (special stains): Histochemistry (refer Table 17 of chapter 7) is the study of the chemistry of tissues, where tissues/cells are treated with specific reagent so that the features of individual cells/structure can be visualized, e.g., Prussian blue reaction for hemosiderin (refer Fig. 68 of chapter 7).

Immunohistochemistry and immunofluorescence: Both utilize antibodies (immunoglobulins with antigen specificity) to visualize substances in tissue sections or cell preparations. Former uses monoclonal antibodies linked chemically to enzymes, and latter uses fluorescent dyes.

Morphology is the cornerstone of diagnosis. Now routinely, it is supplemented by analysis of protein expression and genetic alterations. It is especially very useful in the study of neoplasms (e.g., carcinoma of breast). Malignant tumors that are indistinguishable morphologically may result from different genetic abnormalities. Their course may be widely different, as well as they may have different therapeutic responses, and prognoses.

Electron Microscopy

Electron microscopy (EM) is useful to study the changes at ultrastructural level, and for the demonstration of viruses in tissue samples in certain diseases. The most common diagnostic use of EM is for the interpretation of biopsy specimen from kidney.

FUNCTIONAL DERANGEMENTS AND CLINICAL MANIFESTATIONS

Functional Derangements

The effects of genetic, biochemical, and structural changes in cells and tissues are functional abnormalities. For example, excessive secretion of a cell product (e.g., nasal mucus in the common cold); insufficient secretion of a cell product (e.g., insulin lack in diabetes mellitus).

Clinical Manifestations

The functional derangements produce clinical manifestations of disease, namely symptoms and signs.

Symptoms

The subjective feelings of an abnormality in the body are called as symptoms. It is any change in the body or its functions as perceived by the patient. The symptoms are subjective experience of disease and can only be described to an observer by the affected patient. The **prodromal period** of a disease is the time during which an individual develops vague symptoms (e.g., fatigue, loss of appetite) before the onset of specific signs and symptoms. The term **insidious symptoms** is used to describe vague or nonspecific feelings and indicates that there is a change within the body.

Signs

Manifestations of disease that are observed by physician/observer are termed signs of the disease and is an objective evidence of a disease. For example, the feeling of nausea is a symptom, whereas, vomiting is objectively observed and is a sign. Signs are apparent to observers, whereas symptoms may be obvious only to the patient. Some signs are **local** (e.g., redness or swelling in acute inflammation), and other signs are **systemic** (e.g., fever).

Laboratory Tests and Investigations

Some signs and symptoms (e.g., fever, headache) are nonspecific and do not indicate a specific cause. In such situation, further clinical examination and often, laboratory tests (biochemical analysis, hematological, microbiological, cytological examination, etc.,) and investigations (e.g., X-ray, diagnostic imaging) may be required to know the possible causes of the signs and symptoms.

Diagnosis

It is the art or act of identifying (determine the cause) a disease (pathological condition) from its signs and symptoms. Many diseases/disorders are characterized by a particular constellation of signs and symptoms, the knowledge of which is essential for accurate detection and diagnosis.

Syndromes

A **disorder** is an abnormality of function. This term also used to refer an illness or a particular problem (e.g., bleeding disorder, personality disorder, mental disorder). Diseases characterized by **multiple abnormalities** (symptom complex) are called syndromes. A **syndrome** is a group (collection) of medical signs, symptoms, laboratory findings, and physiological disturbances occurring together that are often associated with a particular disease or disorder. For example, carpal tunnel syndrome, irritable bowel syndrome, Klinefelter syndrome, Down syndrome acute respiratory syndrome (SARS). For example, SARS presents with a set of symptoms such as headache, fever, body aches, discomfort, and sometimes dry cough and difficulty breathing.

Epidemiology is the study of patterns or disease occurrence and transmission among populations and by geographic areas. Thus, it is the study of the distribution (frequency, pattern) and determinants (causes, risk factors) of health-related states and events (not just diseases) among specified populations (school, city, state, country, global). **Incidence** of a disease is the term used to indicate the number of new cases occurring in a specific time period. **Prevalence** of a disease is the term used to indicate the number of existing cases within a population during a specific time period.

Prognosis

The prognosis forecasts (predicts) the known or likely **course (outcome) of the disease** and therefore, the fate of the patient.

Complications

It is a **negative pathologic process** or event occurring **during the disease** which is not an essential part of the disease. It usually aggravates the illness. For example, perforation and hemorrhage are complications which may develop in typhoid ulcer of intestine.

Sequelae

It is a pathologic condition **following as a consequence of a disease**. For example, intestinal obstruction following healed tuberculosis of intestine, mitral stenosis following healed rheumatic heart disease.

Remission and Relapse/Exacerbation

Acute disease is characterized by the sudden appearance of signs and symptoms that last only for a short period. **Chronic disease** develops more slowly and the signs and symptoms persists for a prolonged period. Some chronic diseases may persist for a lifetime. Some chronic diseases may pass through several cycles/alteration of remission and relapse/exacerbation. For example, inflammatory bowel disease (Crohn's disease and ulcerative colitis), some autoimmune diseases. An exacerbation is characterized by a relatively sudden increase in the severity of a disease or any of its signs and symptoms. A remission is characterized by a decline in severity of the signs and symptoms of a disease. If a remission is permanent, the patient is said to be cured.

Various steps involved in study of disease are presented in **Figure 1.**

ROLE OF A PATHOLOGIST IN DIAGNOSIS AND MANAGEMENT OF DISEASE

Pathology is a branch of medicine involved in understanding the cause of disease, the processes involved in testing the disease, and the reporting of diagnostic tests.

Subdivisions of Pathology

The study of pathology can be divided into different branches (disciplines) and subspecialties (**Table 1**).

Anatomic Pathology/Histopathology

In anatomic pathology, microscopic examination is an essential tool for the study. It includes histopathology, cytopathology, and autopsy. Histopathology is the classic and most useful method of study. The term histopathology is used synonymously with anatomic pathology or morbid anatomy. Modern anatomic pathology is divided into subspecialties such as renal pathology, dermatopathology, gastrointestinal pathology, cardiac pathology, pulmonary pathology, neuropathology, gynecologic pathology, breast pathology, oral pathology, etc.

Surgical Pathology

It deals primarily with the study of structural changes in tissues/organs removed from the living patients by biopsy or surgical resection. Surgical pathology includes both gross or naked eye examination referred to as gross or macroscopic changes, as well as examination of processed tissue under a compound light microscope. Intraoperative examination is done by use of frozen tissue sections and is employed for rapid diagnosis.

Microscopic examination

It requires tissues to be cut with a microtome into thin sections that can be stained with routine stains such as H&E. Two types

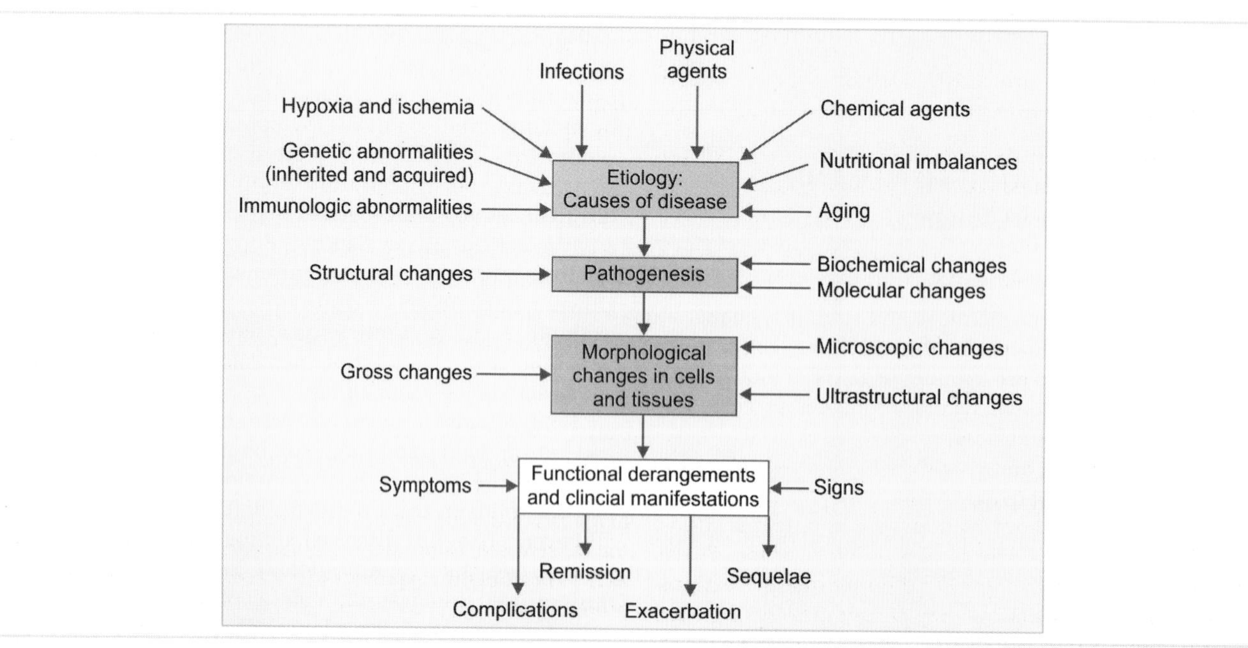

FIG. 1: Steps involved in the study of a disease.

Table 1: Major pathology disciplines and roles.

Discipline/ subspecialty	*Role*
Anatomic pathology	
Histopathology	Study of disease in human tissue samples (e.g., in cancer management through the staging and grading of tumors)
Cytopathology	Study of disease in individual cells
Forensic pathology	Determination of cause and manner of death for legal purposes
Autopsy	Determination of cause and manner of death
Hematology	Study of the blood and bone marrow
Clinical pathology, also called laboratory medicine	It is largely concerned with analysis of blood and other fluids and involves, for instance, clinical biochemistry, microbiology, and hematology
Chemical pathology (clinical biochemistry)	Study of the biochemical tests to diagnose and treat patients. Also, to understand the biochemical basis/mechanisms of the body related to disease. Body fluids such as blood or urine are used for screening, diagnosis, prognosis, and management through chemical and biochemical tests
Medical microbiology	Study of infection
Molecular and genetics pathology	Study of the molecular and genetic basis of diseases and heritable conditions. Variety of tests of molecules within organs, tissues, or bodily fluids are performed
Immunopathology	Study of the immunologic basis of disease
Transfusion medicine	Study of the collection, preparation, storage, and clinical use of blood products

of sectioning methods are most commonly used: *Frozen sections* and *paraffin-embedded* or *permanent sections.*

Frozen sections: Frozen sections are cut by using cryostat (microtome in a refrigerated chamber) or freezing microtome from tissue that has been hardened rapidly by freezing (hence termed frozen section). They can be prepared rapidly (within minutes) during the course of surgery while the patient is still under anesthesia.

Permanent sections: In most instances, pathologists rely on the study of better-preserved tissue by conventional permanent tissue sections with paraffin-embedding technique stained with H&E. These are prepared from tissues that have been fixed, dehydrated, and embedded in paraffin wax as a supporting medium prior to sectioning. Though it needs more time for preparation (about 24 hours), permanent sections have several advantages over frozen tissue sections. These include thinner (typically 5 μm) and better quality sections without any freezing artifacts. They permit greater certainty of interpretation. Some tissues (e.g., those containing fat or bone) cut poorly as frozen sections but may be satisfactorily studied in permanent sections. H&E may be further supported by numerous special stains (histochemistry) for specific tissue components (e.g., mucus, glycogen, collagen, bacteria, and fungi) in certain situations.

Ancillary staining and analytical methods: Histochemistry (special stains), immunohistochemistry, and EM are ancillary techniques in surgical pathology that may be helpful or necessary supplements for diagnosis.

Special stains may aid in the diagnosis of one or another type of tumor (i.e., differential diagnosis) and classification. Examples include special stains for mucins, amyloid, lipids, and glycogen.

Surgical pathology helps to diagnose a disease and determine a treatment plan and has a definitive role in tumor diagnosis. With very few exceptions, definitive therapy for cancer should not be undertaken in the absence of a tissue diagnosis.

Role of Pathologists

Diagnosis

Diagnostic role is a **key aspect of pathology laboratories.** Pathologist examines the changes in the tissue samples/biopsies of the body (removed at surgery or autopsy), in the cells obtained from needle-aspirated specimens, in blood, and other body fluids/secretions [including urine, cerebrospinal fluid (CSF), sputum, pleural/ascitic/pericardial fluid, and synovial fluid]. Some of these changes in test show the causes (e.g., lepromatous leprosy with positive lepra bacilli in the tissue sections, malarial parasites in the peripheral blood smear, *Candida albicans* in vaginal smear).

Tumor Grading, Staging, and Prognosis of Disease

Pathologists help in clinical care by assessing disease severity and prognosis. For example, determining the tumor staging [e.g., the well-known **TNM system** (refer page 544)] and grading of a cancer to estimate tumor prognosis by histopathology; this information determines the precise type and severity (stage) of the cancer. Staging attempts to measure the extent of spread of a malignant tumor within a patient on the basis of tumor size, lymph node involvement, and the presence of other metastases. **Tumor grading is a tumor's degree of differentiation** and growth rate, often graded as I to III, where III represents the least differentiated, fastest dividing tumors; and presumed to have the worst prognosis.

Management of the Disease

Some of the tests are fundamental in deciding and managing treatment plans for patients. Examples include, use of antiestrogenic agents in estrogen receptor-positive breast cancers. A newer approach has been to target the HER2/*neu* antigen which is overexpressed in certain breast and ovarian cancers. The HER2/*neu* antigen is targeted by a therapeutic agent, trastuzumab (Herceptin, Genentech) consisting of a humanized monoclonal antibody that binds to the HER2/*neu.* A complete and accurate pathology report is crucial for precise diagnosis and to decide the best treatment plan for patient. In the present era, importance is given to **identify markers that help to predict the response to new and different therapeutic modalities.**

Monitor the Response to Treatment

Pathology reports may be helpful in monitoring the clinical response to treatment. For example, analyzing blood levels of markers of renal function (renal function tests) in patients with renal failure, minimal residual disease in lymphomas after treatment.

To Comment on Excision Margin in Surgical Specimens

An important concern in surgical pathology is the **adequacy of tumor excision**. Depending on the tissue or type of excision or resected specimen, this decision can be made on either frozen or permanent sections. It is necessary to know the **distances between the edges of the tumor and the excision (resection) margins**. If the tumor forms a discrete mass and the margins of the specimen are well/clearly recognizable/ defined, then determination of excision margins is usually straightforward. Examples of tumors whose excision is likely to have clearly recognizable margins include tumors arising in the gastrointestinal tract, lung, and skin. Excision margins should be identified and painted with ink before any dissection, thus permitting accurate measurement of these distances microscopically. All lymph nodes associated with a cancer specimen need to be dissected out, described along with their location, and processed for histology.

Other Roles

Pathology plays a number of other key roles. One is **quality assurance** within the healthcare system. Pathologists routinely supervise the laboratory to ensure pathology results are appropriate and of the highest standard.

Cytopathology

Cytopathology consists of study of exfoliated cells, [i.e., cells shed off from the lesions (exfoliative cytology)] scraped or brushed cells, or fine-needle aspiration cytology (FNAC) of superficial and deep-seated lesions for diagnosis. This can be a rapid, efficient, and low-risk technique for establishing an accurate diagnosis.

Forensic Pathology and Autopsy

This includes the study of organs and tissues removed at postmortem (autopsy) for medicolegal work and for determining the underlying sequence and cause of death. Forensic pathology is integral to legal system. By this, the course of events that occurred in the patient during life and the probable cause of death can be ascertained. Postmortem anatomical diagnosis helps the clinician to enhance their knowledge about the disease and their judgment. Forensic autopsy is done for medicolegal purposes. In postmortem examination, "the dead teach the living" and has an important role in patient care around the world.

Hematology

Hematology deals with the study of diseases of blood. It includes laboratory hematology and clinical hematology. The hematological diseases include disorders of the red and white blood cells (WBC), platelets, and the coagulation system. It may be non-neoplastic, certain inflammatory diseases, benign, or malignant disorders. Red blood cell (RBC) disorders include disorders of hemoglobin (anemia such as iron deficiency, sickle cell disease) and WBC disorders include quantitative disorders of WBCs and malignant disorders such leukemia, lymphoma or myeloma. The disorders of platelets (e.g., thrombocytopenia) and disorders of blood coagulation (e.g., hemophilia) are also part of hematology. Hematologists receive blood samples for checking any abnormalities. They examine the blood film for any abnormality (e.g., anemia, leukemia) and also perform a bone marrow aspiration and biopsy. Common hematologic test is a complete blood count (CBC), which includes WBC count, RBC count, platelet count, hematocrit/RBC volume (HCT), hemoglobin concentration (HB), differential WBC and RBC indices. Other examples of hematologic tests include prothrombin time (PT), and partial thromboplastin time (PTT).

Clinical Pathology (Laboratory Medicine)

Clinical pathology includes analysis of various fluids including blood and body fluids such as urine, semen, CSF, and other body fluids. Such analysis may be qualitative, semiquantitative, or quantitative. Wide range of laboratory test results assist clinicians in their diagnosis and treatment of disease. These results help hospital departments including intensive care, operating theaters, special care baby units, and oncology.

Clinical Biochemistry

This includes quantitative determination of various biochemical constituents in serum and plasma, and in other body fluids. There is some overlapping between clinical pathology and clinical biochemistry.

Microbiology

This includes the study of disease-causing microbes. Depending upon the type of microorganism studied, it is further developed into bacteriology, parasitology, mycology, virology, etc.

Immunology

In this, abnormalities in the immune system of the body comprising of immunology and immunopathology are studied.

Medical Genetics

It deals with the relationship between heredity and disease. It is useful in blood grouping, inborn errors of metabolism, chromosomal aberrations in congenital malformations, and neoplasms, etc.

Molecular Pathology

Most of the diseases can be diagnosed by the morphological changes in tissues. But, with the present advances in diagnostic pathology, we realize that cellular disturbances develop due to alterations in molecules (genes, proteins, and others) that influence the survival and behavior of cells. Thus, in the present modern pathology it is necessary to understand the cellular and molecular abnormalities that give rise to diseases. The detection and diagnosis of abnormalities at the molecular level [i.e., deoxyribonucleic acid (DNA) of the cell] is performed by molecular pathology. Molecular pathology has revealed the biochemical basis of many diseases, mainly congenital disorders and cancer. These techniques can detect changes in a single nucleotide of DNA and include in situ hybridization (ISH), polymerase chain reaction (PCR), etc. ISH can detect the presence of specific genes or their messenger RNA in tissue sections or cell preparations. Minute quantities of nucleic acids can be amplified by the use of the PCR. DNA microarrays can be used to determine patterns of gene expression [messenger ribonucleic acid (mRNA)]. These methods are used for research purposes as well as a part of diagnostic pathology reports. Molecular pathology, for example, using nucleic acid probes with or without amplification by the PCR, is used to detect expression of specific tumor genes or gene mutations.

Transfusion Medicine

This branch ensures adequate stocks of safe blood when needed for blood transfusions. The blood bank/center confirms that the donated blood is the right match for the patient's blood group. This branch deals with blood and transplant service providing vital support for blood transfusion, organ, and stem cell transplantation.

HISTORY AND EVOLUTION OF PATHOLOGY

Medicine is as old as humankind. In the beginning of mankind, there was a desire and need to know about the causes, mechanisms, and nature of diseases. This knowledge was gained over the centuries from supernatural beliefs to the present knowledge of modern pathology. Pathology has evolved over the years as a distinct discipline or branch apart from others such as anatomy, medicine, surgery, etc. For an undergraduate beginner in pathology, it is necessary to know a brief review of history of pathology and personalities with their outstanding contribution.

Prehistoric Times to Medieval Period

During prehistoric time, religion, magic, and medical treatment were quite linked to each other. It was believed that disease was the outcome of "curse from God" or it had supernatural origin from "evil eye of spirits". The disease was treated by priests through prayers and sacrifices, and magicians by magic power. Some ancient superstitions still exist in some parts of the world.

Religious and Magical Belief

The link between medicine and religion is firmly believed throughout the world. This has resulted in belief in different societies that there are gods and goddesses of healing. For example, *Dhanvantri* is considered as the deity of medicine in India, and orthodox Indians' belief in *Mata Sheetala Devi* as the pox goddess. Same way, Greeks have *Aesculapius and Apollo* as the principal gods of healing.

Philosophical and Rational Approach

This approach was by the methods of observations and this followed the earlier religious and magical beliefs. This philosophical concept to all-natural phenomena was introduced by Greek philosophers namely, *Socrates, Plato,* and *Aristotle.*

Hippocrates

The real practice of medicine began with the great Greek clinical genius *Hippocrates* (460–370 BC). He is regarded as "the father of medicine" and he dissociated medicine from religion and magic. He revolutionized the practice of medicine and established the basic foundations of the role of the physician. He studied patient's symptoms and described methods of diagnosis. He recorded his observations on cases and his writings called *Hippocratic Corpus* remained for nearly 2,000 years as the mainstay of learning of medicine. However, Hippocrates too propagated the prevailing concept on mechanism of disease based on disequilibrium of our basic humors (water, air, fire, and earth). Later, this concept was abandoned. Hippocrates set standards for patient care and the physician's attitudes and philosophies that persist today. Many aspects of the Hippocratic approach to medicine are still with us today. Hippocrates rational and ethical attitudes in practice and teaching of medicine are respected by the medical profession and *"Hippocratic oath"* is taken by all medical students at the time of entry into practice of medicine.

After Hippocrates, Greek medicine reached Rome (now Italy). After 146 BC, Rome controlled Greek world and dominated in ancient Europe. Many terms in medicine have their origin from Latin language which was the official language of countries included in ancient Roman Empire (Spanish, Portuguese, Italian, French and Greek languages have their origin from Latin). Hippocratic teaching was propagated in Rome by Roman physicians. Prominent among them are *Cornelius Celsus* (53 BC to AD 7) and *Claudius Galen* (AD 130–200).

- Celsus first described four cardinal signs of inflammation, namely rubor (redness), tumor (swelling), calor (heat), and dolor (pain).
- Galen postulated humoral theory, later called Galenic theory. According to this theory, the illness was considered as due to imbalance between *four humors* (or body fluids)—blood, lymph, black bile (believed at that time to be from the spleen), and biliary secretion from the liver.

In India, in the centuries before and after Hippocrates, the hypothesis of disequilibrium of four elements of the body (*Dhatus*) similar to Hippocratic doctrine was mentioned in ancient Indian medicine books during AD 200. *Sushruta* (*Sushruta Samhita*) and *Charaka* (*Charaka Samhita*) produced encyclopedic founding works of Ayurvedic medicine. *Charaka* listed 700 plant-derived medicines/remedies and surgical science was documented by *Sushruta*.

Backwardness During Medieval Period

During Middle Ages (or medieval period that lasted from the 5th to the 15th century), there was marked backwardness in medicine. During this period, there were widespread and devastating epidemics. This resulted in reversal of the process of rational thinking back to supernatural concepts and divine punishment for "sins". The dominant belief was that life was due to influence of vital substance under the control of soul *(theory of vitalism)*. During this period, the dissection of human body was strictly forbidden because it was considered to hurt the "soul".

Human Anatomy and Era of Gross Pathology

Renaissance Period

The backwardness during medieval period was followed by the Renaissance period (i.e., revival of learning). This began from Italy in late 15th century and spread to whole of Europe. During this period, there was quest (an attempt to achieve something) for advances in art and science. There was freedom of thought and emphasis on philosophical and rational attitudes again.

Human Anatomy

- The development of human anatomy took place at the beginning of this period with the art works and **drawings of human muscles and embryos** by famous Italian painter **Leonardo da Vinci** (1452–1519).
- **Vesalius (1514–1564) dissected human body** of freshly executed criminals. His pupils, Gabriel Fallopius (1523–1562) described human oviducts (Fallopian tubes) and Fabricius discovered lymphoid tissue around the intestine of birds (bursa of Fabricius).
- The special human anatomic dissection in the form of **postmortem** came into practice in various parts of ancient Europe.

Microscope

- **Antony van Leeuwenhoek** (1632–1723), a cloth merchant by profession in Holland, during his spare time **invented** the first ever **microscope** by grinding the lenses. He also introduced histological staining using saffron to examine muscle fibers.
- **Marcello Malpighi** (1624–1694) observed the **presence of capillaries** by using microscope. He described the Malpighian layer of the skin, and lymphoid tissue in the spleen (Malpighian corpuscles). **Malpighi is known as "the father of histology".**

Morbid Anatomy

Morbid anatomy (pathologic anatomy) is a branch of medical science concerned with the study of the structure of diseased organs and tissues.

- **Giovanni B Morgagni** (1682–1771): The beginning of study of morbid anatomy was by Italian anatomist and pathologist, *Giovanni B Morgagni* (1682–1771). He was an excellent teacher in anatomy, a prolific writer, and a practicing clinician. Morgagni dismissed the ancient humoral theory of disease and published his lifetime experiences based on 700 postmortems and their corresponding clinical findings. Thus, he laid the foundations of clinicopathologic methodology in the study of disease. He introduced the concept of clinicopathologic correlation (CPC), establishing a coherent sequence of cause, lesions, symptoms, and outcome of disease.
- **Sir Percival Pott** (1714–1788) was a famous surgeon in England. He **described tuberculosis of the spine** (Pott's disease). He was also the **first to identify occupational cancer** (cancer of scrotal skin) in the chimney sweeps in 1775 and discovered chimney soot as the first chemical carcinogenic agent.
- During the later part of 18th Century, **John Hunter** (1728–1793) who was a student of Sir Percival Pott became the greatest surgeon-anatomist of all times. His elder brother **William Hunter** (1718–1788) was a reputed anatomist-obstetrician. These brothers **developed the first museum of comparative anatomy and pathology** in the world by collecting surgical specimens and arranged them into separate organ systems. This museum knows as the Hunterian Museum, is now housed in the Royal College of Surgeons of London.
- **Edward Jenner** (1749–1823) who demonstrated **inoculation in smallpox**.
- **Matthew Baillie** (1760–1823) is a prominent English pathologist who published first-ever systematic textbook of morbid anatomy in 1793.
- **Era of gross pathology:**
    - **Richard Bright** (1789–1858) described nonsuppurative nephritis which was later termed as glomerulonephritis or **Bright's disease**.
    - **Thomas Addison** (1793–1860) gave an account of chronic adrenocortical insufficiency and was termed as **Addison's disease**.
    - **Thomas Hodgkin** (1798–1866) observed the complex of chronic enlargement of lymph nodes, often with enlargement of the liver and spleen, which was later, called **Hodgkin's disease** (presently known as Hodgkin lymphoma).
    - **Xavier Bichat** (1771–1802) in France described that organs were composed of tissues and divided the study of morbid anatomy into general pathology and systemic pathology.
    - **RTH Laennec** (1781–1826), a French physician had numerous discoveries. These include **description of several lung diseases** (tubercles, caseous lesions, miliary lesions, pleural effusion, and bronchiectasis), **chronic cirrhotic liver disease** (later called Laennec's cirrhosis), and **invented stethoscope**.
    - **Carl F von Rokitansky** (1804–1878) was a self-taught German pathologist who **performed nearly 30,000 autopsies** himself. He described acute yellow atrophy of the liver, wrote monograph on diseases of arteries and congenital heart defects. Unlike most other surgeons during that time, Rokitansky did not do clinical practice of surgery but instead introduced the concept that pathologists should confine themselves to making diagnosis which became the accepted role of pathologist later.

Era of Technology Development and Cellular Pathology

Correlation of Clinical Features with Autopsy Findings

Up to middle of the 19th century, the major method of study of disease was by correlating clinical manifestations of disease with gross pathological findings at autopsy.

Advances in Pathology

In the 19th century, sophistication in surgical techniques led to advancement in pathology. The anatomist-surgeons of earlier centuries got replaced largely with surgeon-pathologists. **In later half of the 19th century, pathology became a diagnostic discipline** with the evolution of cellular pathology. This was closely linked to technology advancements in machinery for cutting thin tissue sections, improvement in microscope, and development of dyes for staining.

Identification of Microorganisms

- French chemist **Louis Pasteur** (1822–1895) **discovered the disease-causing microorganisms** and this replaced the prevailing theory of spontaneous generation of disease and firmly established **germ theory of disease.**

- In 1873, **GHA Hansen** (1841–1912) in Germany identified **Hansen's (lepra) bacillus** as the first microbe that caused leprosy (Hansen's disease).

Immunity and Phagocytosis

- The **basis of immunization** was initiated by **Edward Jenner** while studying infectious diseases.
- **Metchnikoff** (1845–1916), a Russian zoologist, **discovered the phenomenon of phagocytosis** by human defense cells against invading microbes.

Staining

The **developments in chemical industry** led to switching over from earlier dyes of plant and animal origin to **synthetic dyes**. In 1856, **Perkin** prepared first synthetic dye namely aniline violet. This led to emergence of a viable dye industry for histological and bacteriological purposes. Various pioneers who contributed to the use for dye are as follows:

- **Paul Ehrlich** (1854–1915), German physician, conferred Nobel Prize in 1908 for his work in immunology. He described **Ehrlich's test for urobilinogen** using **Ehrlich's aldehyde reagent** and staining techniques of cells and bacteria. These developments led to the foundations of clinical pathology.
- **Christian Gram** (1853–1938), Danish physician, used **crystal violet for staining bacteria**.
- **DL Romanowsky** (1861–1921), Russian physician, developed **stain for peripheral blood film** using eosin and methylene blue derivatives.
- **Robert Koch** (1843–1910), German bacteriologist **described Koch's postulate and Koch's phenomena**. He also developed techniques of fixation and staining for identification of bacteria. He **discovered *tubercle bacilli*** in 1882 and *Vibrio cholerae* organism in 1883.
- **May-Grünwald** in 1902 **and Giemsa** in 1914 developed **stains for blood and bone marrow**. They applied them for classification of cells in blood and bone marrow.
- **Sir William Leishman** (1865–1926) in 1914 described **Leishman's stain for blood smear/films** and observed Leishman-Donovan bodies (LD bodies) in leishmaniasis.
- **Robert Feulgen** (1884–1955) described **Feulgen reaction for DNA staining**. This laid the foundations of cytochemistry and histochemistry.

Technical Advances

Advances in techniques and machinery led to development and upgrading of microtomes for obtaining thin sections of organs/tissues and staining by dyes for enhancing detailed study of sections. The presence of cells in thin sections of nonliving object cork was first demonstrated by Robert Hooke in 1667. In the 19th century, FT Schwann (1810–1882) was the first neurohistologist, and Claude Bernarde (1813–1878) was pioneer in pathophysiology.

Histopathology

Till the end of the 19th century, the study of morbid anatomy was confined largely to autopsy-based study and thus remained as a retrospective science.

Rudolf Virchow (1821–1905) in Germany **first did the microscopic examination of diseased tissue at cellular level.** This became as the histopathological method of investigation. Virchow hypothesized cellular theory and is aptly known as "**the father of cellular pathology**". According to him:

- All cells come from other cells.
- Disease is an alteration of normal structure and function of these cells.

This led to sound foundation of diagnostic pathology based on microscopy and was followed and promoted by numerous brilliant successive workers. This gave birth to biopsy pathology. Other discoveries by Rudolf Virchow are:

- **Virchow's triad:** Virchow described etiology of thrombosis [(Virchow's triad namely: (1) Slowing of bloodstream, (2) Changes in the vessel wall, and (3) Changes in the blood itself)].
- **Virchow's lymph node:** Metastatic spread of tumor of carcinoma stomach to supraclavicular lymph node.
- **Components and diseases of blood** (fibrinogen, leukocytosis, leukemia).

Frozen section

Julius Cohnheim (1839–1884), student of Rudolf Virchow, **described the concept of frozen section** examination while the patient was still on the operation table. The concept of surgeon and physician as pathologist started in the 19th century and it continued as late as the middle of the 20th century in most clinical departments. During this period, biopsy pathology work was assigned to some faculty member in the clinical department. The notable pathologists of the first half of 20th century had background of clinical training and these include **James Ewing** (1866–1943), **AP Stout** (1885–1967), and **Lauren Ackerman** (1905–1993) in the United States of America; **Pierre Masson** (1880–1958) in France, and **RA Willis** in Australia.

Landmarks in Modern Pathology

- **Karl Landsteiner** (1863–1943) **described major human blood groups** in 1900s and is considered "**the father of blood transfusion**". He was awarded Nobel Prize in 1930.
- **Ruska and Lorries** in 1933 **developed electron microscope**. This helped to identify the ultrastructure of cell and its organelles.
- **George N Papanicolaou** (1883–1962), a Greek-born, American pathologist is known as "**the father of exfoliative cytology**". In 1930s, he developed **exfoliative cytology for early detection of cervical cancer**.
- **William Boyd** (1885–1979), psychiatrist-turned pathologist was an **eminent teacher-author in pathology during the 20th century**. His textbooks, namely "Pathology for Surgeons" (first edition, 1925) and "Textbook of Pathology" (first edition, 1932), dominated and inspired the few generations of students of pathology all over the world due to **his flowery language and lucid style**.
- **MM Wintrobe** (1901–1986) **discovered the HCT technique**.

Modern Pathology

In the later half of 20th century and during the 21st century, advances made it possible to **study diseases at genetic and molecular level**. The evidence-based and objective diagnosis may enable the physician to institute targeted therapy. The major benefits due to these advances in molecular biology are in the field of diagnosis and treatment of genetic disorders, immunology, and in cancer. Some of the discoveries are as follows:

- **Watson and Crick** in 1953 described **the structure of DNA** of the cell.
- **Tijo and Levan in 1956, identified chromosomes and their correct number in humans** (46=23 pairs).
- **Nowell and Hagerford in 1960,** identified **Philadelphia chromosome** t(9;22) in chronic myeloid leukemia. This was the first chromosomal abnormality detected in any cancer.
- **In situ hybridization** was introduced in 1969. In this, a labeled probe is used to detect and localize specific RNA or DNA sequences **"in situ"** (e.g., in the original place). Its **later modification uses fluorescence microscopy** (FISH) to detect specific localization of the defect on chromosomes.
- **Recombinant DNA technique** was developed in 1972 using restriction enzymes to cut and paste part/bits of DNA.
- **Kary Mullis** in 1983, introduced PCR. In this, multiple copies of DNA fragments can be done and this has revolutionized the diagnostic molecular genetics. PCR analysis is more rapid than ISH, can be automated by thermal cyclers and requires less amount of DNA for the test.
- **Barbara McClintock** invented **flexibility and dynamism of DNA** for which she was awarded Nobel Prize in 1983.
- **Ian Wilmut** and his colleagues at Roslin Institute in Edinburgh in 1997, performed **mammalian cloning**. By using this technique, they performed the somatic cell nuclear transfer to create the clone of a sheep named Dolly. However, reproductive cloning for human beings is very risky and absolutely unethical.
- **Stem cell research:** It started in 2000s by harvesting the primitive stem cells isolated from embryos and maintaining their growth in the laboratory. There are two types of stem cells in humans, namely: (1) Embryonic stem cells and (2) Adult stem cells. Stem cells have many applications in the treatment of many human diseases such as Alzheimer's disease, diabetes, cancer, strokes, etc. In future, stem cell therapy may be able to replace whole organ transplant and stem cells "harvested" from the embryo may be used as a replacement of damaged tissue/organ. Hematopoietic stem cells are being used for many diseases of the hematopoietic system.
- **Human Genome Project (HGP):** It consisted of a consortium of countries and was completed in April 2003. By HGP, it is possible to read nature's complete genetic blueprint used in making of each human being (i.e., gene mapping). Clinical trials by gene therapy for the treatment of some single gene defects have resulted in some success, especially in hematological and immunological diseases. Future developments in genetic engineering may be able to design new and highly effective individualized treatment options for genetic diseases and also may suggest preventive action against diseases.
- **Uses of HGP:** They are listed in **Box 1.**

Telepathology and Virtual Microscopy

Q. Write short essay on telepathology.

Telepathology is defined as the **practice of diagnostic pathology at a distance**. In this, a remote pathologist (receiving side) utilizes tissue specimens, histological, and cytological electronic (digital) images which are transferred over a telecommunication network from a different location (sending side).

Box 1: Uses of Human Genome Project.

The understanding of the genome provides clues for:

- **Etiology** of cancers, Alzheimer's disease, etc.
- Defining the **pathogenesis** of a disease and to study the disease processes at **molecular level**
- **Susceptibility** of an individual to a variety of illnesses, e.g., carcinoma breast, disorders of hemostasis, liver diseases, cystic fibrosis, etc.
- Devise new ways to **prevent** a number of diseases that affect human beings
- To **diagnose and treat** disease. Target genes for treatment and management of diseases
- **Human development and anthropology:** Analysis of similarities between deoxyribonucleic acid (DNA) sequences from different organisms helps to **study evolution**
- **For research:** By visiting the human genome database on the World Wide Web, a researcher can examine what other scientists have written about the gene

Components

The various components of telepathology network include:

- A conventional light microscope.
- Devise to capture the image, i.e., a camera mounted on a microscope.
- Telecommunication link between the sending and receiving sites.
- A workstation at the receiving site with a high-quality video monitor.

Advantages/Benefits

Telepathology makes it **faster** and easier to share medical images. Pathologists in different locations can view images simultaneously and discuss diagnoses through teleconferencing. Pathologist can consult other pathologists who are specialized in area of concern, such as liver pathology or lung pathology. It allows pathologists, surgeons, and radiologists to communicate with each other over diagnostic dilemmas and overcoming the barrier of distance.

Main Categories of Telepathology

The types of telepathology include:

Static image-based systems

In static telepathology, images are captured from a digital camera connected to a microscope. An image area is selected and transmitted. A limited number of images (1–40) are captured and stored in the hard drive of the computer or compact disc-read only memory (CD-ROM) for transmission. It is economical, simple, and requires only a standard telephone and internet connection. Disadvantage is that selection of field for images should be done by expert and if done by a nonexpert, may miss the important areas.

Virtual slide systems

Pathology specimen slides are scanned and high-resolution digital images are created for transmission.

Realtime systems

This is also termed robotic interactive telepathology and dynamic pathology. In this, the recipient pathologist remotely guides a robotically controlled motorized microscope by means of a joystick (a device that can be moved forwards, backwards, and sideways to control a machine or computer) and view "realtime" images on a high-resolution monitor. The section can be viewed entirely and this eliminates the inadequate or inappropriate selection of fields. These instruments allow the remote user to move the microscopic field in any direction, to change magnifications, and even to change the focus (particularly useful for cytological preparations). The resolution of the images is practically the same as that obtained with the actual slide under the microscope. This technique is suitable for routine histological preparations, immunostains, cytology preparations, and electron micrographs.

BIBLIOGRAPHY

1. Banasik JL, Copstead LC. Pathophysiology,6th edition. Philadelphia: Saunders Elsevier; 2019.
2. Huether SE, McCance KL. Understanding Pathophysiology,6th edition. Philadelphia: Saunders Elsevier; 2016.
3. Kumar V, Abbas AK, Aster JC. Robbins basic pathology, 10th edition. Philadelphia: Saunders Elsevier; 2018
4. Kumar V, Abbas AK, Fausto N, et al. Robbins and Cotran pathologic basis of disease, 10th edition. Philadelphia: WB Saunders; 2021.
5. Loeffler AG, Hart MN. Human Disease-Pathophysiology for health professional,7th edition. Burlington: Jones & Bartlett Learning Company; 2020.
6. McCance KL, Huether SE. Pathophysiology–The biologic basis for disease in adults and children , 8th edition. Philadelphia: Elsevier; 2019.
7. Mohan H. Text Book of Pathology, 8th edition. New Delhi, JP brothers; 2019.
8. Strayer DS, Saffitz JE. Rubin's Pathology: Mechanism of Human Disease, 8th edition. Philadelphia: Wolters Kluwer; 2020.

CHAPTER 7

Cell Injury, Cell Death, Adaptation and Intracellular Accumulations

7.1 Cell Injury and Cell Death

CHAPTER OUTLINE

- Introduction
  - Types of cellular responses to injury
- Cell injury
  - Definition
  - Causes (etiology) of cell injury
  - The progression of cell injury and death
- Reversible cell injury
  - Cellular (cloudy) swelling
  - Steatosis (fatty change)
- Cell death
  - Necrosis
  - Apoptosis
  - Pathways of cell death other than necrosis and apoptosis
  - Autophagy
  - Major functions of autophagy
  - Categories
  - Autophagy and disease
  - Autolysis
- Mechanisms of cell injury
  - General principles of cell injury
  - General mechanisms and intracellular targets of of cell injury
  - Decreased production of adenosine triphosphate
  - Mitochondrial damage
  - Membrane damage
  - Damage to DNA
  - Oxidative stress: Accumulation of oxygen-derived free radicals
  - Free radicals in health and disease
  - Loss of calcium homeostasis
- Examples of cell injury and death
  - Hypoxia and ischemia
  - Ischemia-reperfusion injury
  - Reperfusion and its effects on myocardial infarction
  - Ischemic preconditioning
  - Neuropathology of hypoxia
  - Cell injury caused by toxins and chemicals
- Protein folding and misfolding
  - Folding of proteins
  - Chaperone proteins
  - Endoplasmic reticulum stress
  - Ubiquitin–proteasome system
  - Abnormal proteins and diseases
  - Basic mechanism of disease by misfolded proteins
  - Diseases due to defective ubiquitination and deubiquitination
  - Gene expression
- Heat shock proteins
  - Types
  - Regulation of heat shock proteins
  - Mechanism of action
  - Functions
  - Clinical significance

INTRODUCTION

All the functions of the body depend on the integrity of cells. The normal cells defend themselves in an unfavorable environment. Normal cells are restricted by a fairly narrow range of functions and structure. This depends on its state of metabolism, differentiation, and specialization; by pressures enforced by neighboring cells; and by the availability of metabolic substrates. Cells must be able to adapt to fluctuating environmental conditions. These includes changes in temperature, solute concentrations, oxygen supply, noxious agents and so on. Normally, cells can handle and adapt to physiologic demands or stress and maintains a steady healthy state called **homeostasis**.

Human is a multicellular "social" organism. Normal cells generate messages, transmit, receive and interpret them. There is a constant cellular communication (cellular crosstalk). These streamlined conversations between, among, and within cells maintains cellular function and specialization. Cells must have a "chemical affection" for other cells to maintain the integrity of the entire organism. When they no longer tolerate this affection, the conversation breaks down, and cells either adapt (sometimes altering function) or become vulnerable to isolation, injury, or disease. Injury to cells and their surrounding environment (i.e., extracellular matrix), leads to tissue and organ injury.

Adaptations: These are reversible functional and structural responses both to normal or changes in physiologic conditions/

states (e.g., pregnancy) and to some adverse or pathologic conditions/stimuli. During adaptations, new but altered steady states are achieved. This allows the cell to survive and continue to function. For example, the uterus adapts to pregnancy (a normal physiologic state) by enlarging the uterus. Enlargement of uterus occurs due to an increase in the size and number of uterine muscle cells (myometrial smooth muscle cells). In pathologic condition, such as high blood pressure, myocardial cells increase in size due to the requirement of increased work of pumping. Cells undergo adaptations to their environment in order to escape and protect themselves from injury. An adapted cell is neither normal nor injured and its condition lies somewhere between these two states. most significant adaptive changes/response in cells consist of (i) an increase in cell size (hypertrophy) and its functional activity, (ii) an increase in cell number (hyperplasia), (iii) a decrease in the cell size and its metabolic activity or function (atrophy), or (iv) a change in the phenotype of cells or reversible replacement of one mature cell type by another less mature cell type (metaplasia). If the stress is completely removed, the cell can return to its original state without having any harmful consequences. Adaptive responses have limits. However, like most of the body's adaptive mechanisms, cellular adaptations to adverse conditions are generally only temporarily successful. Severe or prolonged stressors overcome adaptive processes and can affect essential cell function. This can injure cells resulting in cellular injury (i.e., an injury that exceeds the cell's adaptive capacity) or death. Cellular adaptations can be a common in many diseases.

Cell injury: A cell exposed to persistent sublethal, reversible injury has limited available responses. The stimuli/injury may exceed the limits of adaptive responses or cells may be exposed to damaging insults. Cellular injury can be caused by any factor that disturbs cellular structures, reduces the supply of critical nutrients and oxygen required for survival of the cell or compromised by mutations that affect essential cellular functions. These sequence of events and expression of cell is termed cell injury. Cell injury can be classified as chemical, hypoxic (lack of sufficient oxygen), free radical, intentional, unintentional, immunologic, infection, and inflammatory. Thus, pathology is the study of injury to cells and organs and of their capacity to adapt to such injury. Cell injury is reversible up to a certain point. If the injurious stimulus persists or is severe, the cell suffers irreversible injury and ultimately leads to death of the cell. Adaptation, reversible injury, and cell death (irreversible or lethal injury) may be considered as stages of progressive impairment following different types of insults. For example, whenever there is increased hemodynamic loads, the heart muscle becomes enlarged (hypertrophy is a form of cellular adaptation). The hypertrophied myocardial fibres have increased metabolic demand and are more susceptible to injury. If the blood supply to the myocardium is impaired or inadequate, the myocardial muscle cells first suffers reversible injury and produce certain cytoplasmic changes. If the blood supply is not quickly restored, these myocardial cells suffer irreversible injury and die.

Cell death: The removal of damaged, unnecessary, and aged cells through cell death is a normal and essential process during embryogenesis, the development of organs, and the maintenance of homeostasis into adulthood. But, increased death of cells due to progressive injury is one of the most vital events in the evolution of disease in any tissue or organ. Increased cell death may be due to diverse causes. These include ischemia (reduced blood flow), infection, and toxins. There are two main pathways of cell death namely: (i) necrosis and (ii) apoptosis. Cellular death is confirmed by detecting structural changes in n cells are stained and examined under a microscope. Lack of nutrients to the cell triggers an adaptive cellular response called autophagy that may also terminate in cell death.

Box 1: Types of cellular responses to injury.

- Cellular adaptations: Hypertrophy, hyperplasia, atrophy and metaplasia
- Cell injury
  - Reversible cell injury
  - Irreversible cell injury
- Intracellular accumulations
- Pathologic calcification

Other cellular changes induced by stresses: Stress is an activity, event, or other stimulus that causes stress. Stresses of different types may produce changes in cells and tissues other than typical adaptations, cell injury, and death mentioned above.

- **Intracellular accumulations:** Metabolic derangements and chronic injury may be accompanied by intracellular accumulations of a number of substances. These may be proteins, lipids, and carbohydrates.
- **Pathologic calcification:** Calcium may be deposited at sites of cell death. This results in pathologic calcification (in contrast to physiological calcification which occurs on bone and enamel).
- **Aging:** Normal process of aging is accompanied by characteristic morphologic and functional changes in cells. It ultimately may lead to cellular death or a decreased capacity to recover from injury. Senescence that is growing old, is both inevitable and normal.

Types of Cellular Responses to Injury

Depending on the nature of stimulus/injury, the cellular responses can be mainly divided into four types (**Box 1** and **Fig. 1**).

Different stages of cellular responses to stress and injurious stimuli are shown in **Flowchart 1**.

CELL INJURY

Definition

Cell injury is the effect of stresses due to variety of etiological agents on the cell.

Cellular injury occurs when a stress exceeds the cell's capability to adapt. Injured cells may either recover **(reversible injury)** or die **(irreversible injury)**.

Causes (Etiology) of Cell Injury

Q. Write a short essay on causes of cellular injury.

They range from gross physical trauma (e.g., road traffic accident), to a defect at molecular such as single gene defect (e.g., enzyme deficiency resulting in specific metabolic disease). Following are the main categories of causes of cell injury:

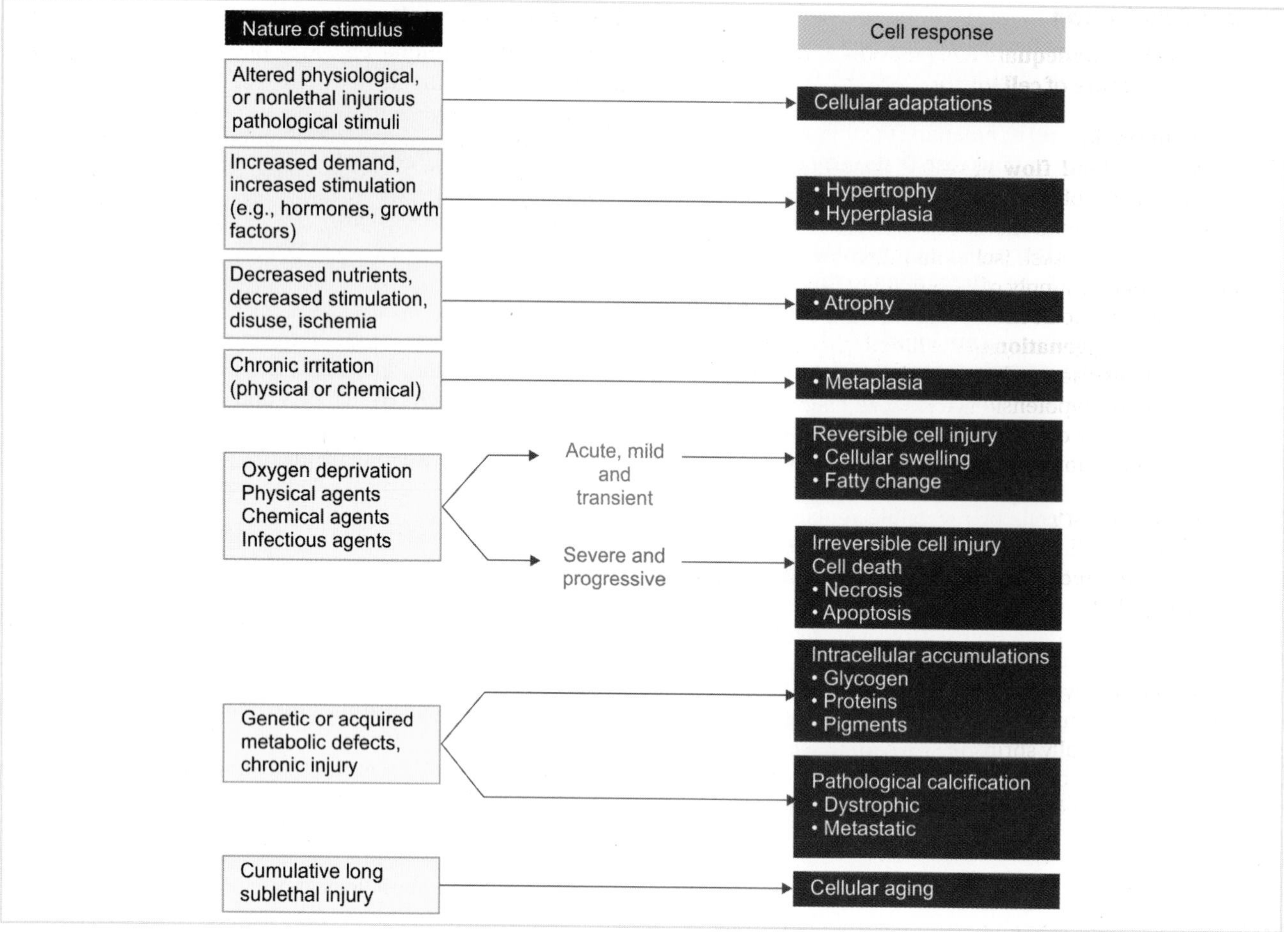

Nature of stimulus
Cell response
Altered physiological, or nonlethal injurious pathological stimuli
Cellular adaptations
Increased demand, increased stimulation (e.g., hormones, growth factors)
• Hypertrophy
• Hyperplasia
Decreased nutrients, decreased stimulation, disuse, ischemia
• Atrophy
Chronic irritation (physical or chemical)
• Metaplasia
Oxygen deprivation
Physical agents
Chemical agents
Infectious agents
Acute, mild and transient
Reversible cell injury
• Cellular swelling
• Fatty change
Severe and progressive
Irreversible cell injury
Cell death
• Necrosis
• Apoptosis
Genetic or acquired metabolic defects, chronic injury
Intracellular accumulations
• Glycogen
• Proteins
• Pigments
Pathological calcification
• Dystrophic
• Metastatic
Cumulative long sublethal injury
Cellular aging

FIG. 1: Types of cellular responses to stimuli/injury.

Normal cell (homeostasis)
Reversible injury
• Cellular swelling
• Fatty change
Stress withdrawal
Stress
Injurious stimulus
Adaptation
• Hypertrophy
• Hyperplasia
• Atrophy
• Metaplasia
Inability to adapt
Cell injury
Mild and transient injury
Severe and progressive injury
Irreversible injury
Necrosis
Cell death
Apoptosis

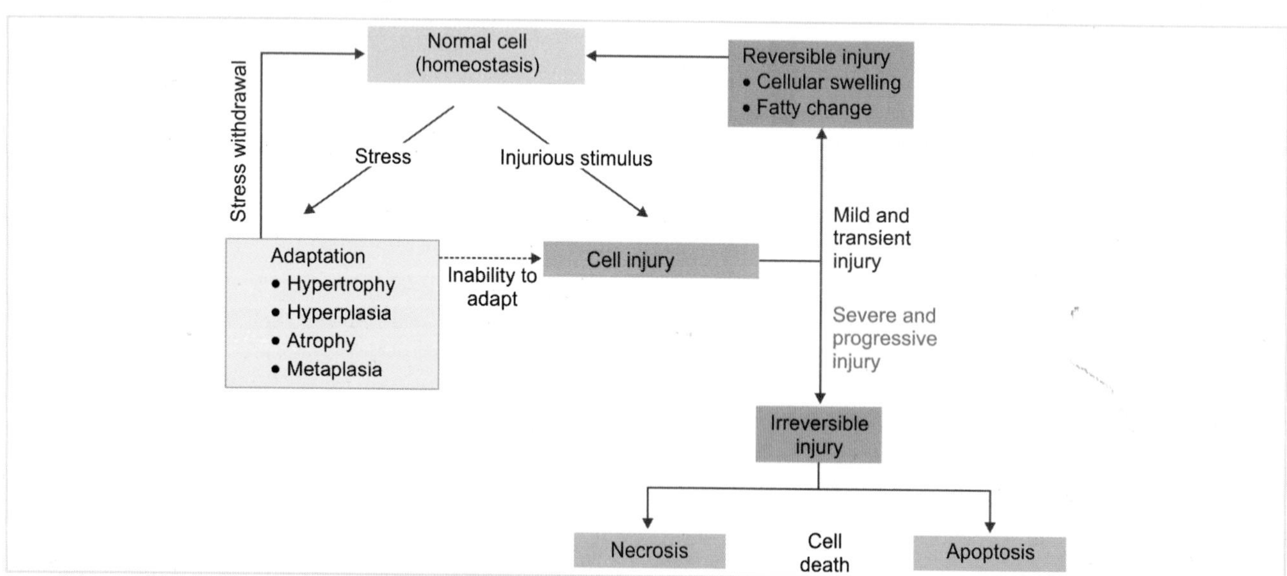

FLOWCHART 1: Different stages of cellular responses to stress/injury.

Oxygen Deprivation

Hypoxia refers to **inadequate oxygenation of tissue**. It is the **most common cause of cell injury.**

Causes of hypoxia

- **Decreased blood flow** is called **ischemia** and results from an arterial obstruction. This obstruction may be due to thrombosis, embolism, atherosclerosis, or external compression of vessel. Ischemia produces reduced blood supply, deficient supply of essential nutrients and leads to accumulation of toxic metabolites in the tissue affected.
- **Inadequate oxygenation of the blood** (hypoxemia): It may be due to lung disease, decreased perfusion of tissues (e.g., cardiac failure, hypotension, and shock), decreased oxygen carrying capacity of the blood (e.g., anemia), severe blood loss, or carbon monoxide poisoning.

Mechanism of Injury

Hypoxia causes cell injury by reducing aerobic oxidative respiration and decreasing the synthesis of adenosine triphosphate (ATP).

Outcome

It depends on the severity of the hypoxic state. Affected cells may adapt, undergo injury, or die. For example, mild narrowing of an artery may initially shrink in size of the tissue (atrophy- a type of adaptation) supplied by that vessel (atrophy). If there is more severe or sudden hypoxia, it causes cell injury and cell death.

Physical Agents

- Mechanical trauma (e.g., blunt/penetrating/crush injuries, gunshot wounds)
- Thermal injury: Extremes of temperature (burns and deep cold).
- Radiation (ionizing radiation and nonionizing radiation)
- Electric shock
- Pressure changes: Sudden changes in atmospheric pressure.

Chemical Agents, Toxins, and Drugs

- Trace amounts of poison: These include arsenic, cyanide, or mercury. They may produce damage to sufficient numbers of cells within minutes or hours and can cause death.
- Simple chemicals (e.g., hypertonic concentrations of glucose or salt). They may cause cell injury directly or by disturbing electrolyte and fluid balance in cells.
- Strong acids and alkalis
- Oxygen at high concentrations is toxic
- Environmental and air pollutants (e.g., insecticides and herbicides)
- Industrial and occupational hazards (carbon monoxide and asbestos)
- Social/lifestyle choices: Addiction to drugs and alcohol and cigarette smoking
- Therapeutic drugs

Infectious Agents

These include viruses, bacteria, fungi, rickettsiae, and parasites. The mechanism by which these infectious agents cause injury varies.

Immunologic Reactions

Normally, the immune system protects us from infectious pathogens. But, immune reactions may also cause cell injury.

- **Autoimmunity:** Immune reactions to endogenous self-antigens are responsible for autoimmune diseases.
- **Hypersensitivity reactions and other immune reactions:** Heightened immune reactions to many external agents (e.g., microbes and environmental agents) may be an important causes of cell and tissue injury.

Genetic Derangements

Genetic defects may cause cell injury because of:

- Chromosomal abnormalities: It may be the presence of as an extra chromosome (e.g., Down syndrome), or as minute as a single base pair substitution leading to an amino acid substitution (e.g., sickle cell anemia). They may produce highly characteristic clinical phenotypes. They may range from congenital malformations to anemias.
- Deficiency of functional proteins (e.g., enzyme defects in inborn errors of metabolism).
- Accumulation of damaged deoxyribonucleic acid (DNA) or misfolded proteins.

They continue to be major causes of cell injury.

Nutritional Imbalances

- **Nutritional deficiencies:** It can be due to inadequate consumption of food or due to food shortages or poor diet. It can be self imposed, as in anorexia nervosa (a psychological disorder).
  - Protein-calorie deficiencies
  - Deficiencies of specific vitamins.
- **Nutritional excesses:**
  - Excess of cholesterol predisposes to atherosclerosis.
  - Obesity is associated with increased incidence of several important diseases, such as diabetes and cancer.
  - Hypervitaminosis

Aging

Cellular aging or senescence in aging decreases the ability of cells to respond to stress and, eventually it results in the death of cells and the individual.

Idiopathic: Cause is not known.

The Progression of Cell Injury and Death

Basic alterations in damaged cells (Fig. 2): All stresses and injurious agents first show their effects at the molecular or biochemical level. Cellular function may be lost long before any cell death. There is a time interval between the exposure to stress/injury and for the morphologic changes of cell injury or death to manifest. The morphologic changes of cell injury (or death) take longer time to appear before any loss of function and viability of tissue (**Fig. 2**). The early changes are slight and can be detected only by highly sensitive methods. By using histochemical, ultrastructural, or biochemical techniques, the changes of cell injury may be seen in minutes to hours after injury. The light microscopy or the gross (naked eye) changes need considerably more time (hours to days) to manifest. Thus, morphologic changes of necrosis take more time to develop than those of reversible damage. For example, in ischemia of the myocardium due to coronary artery disease, the earliest

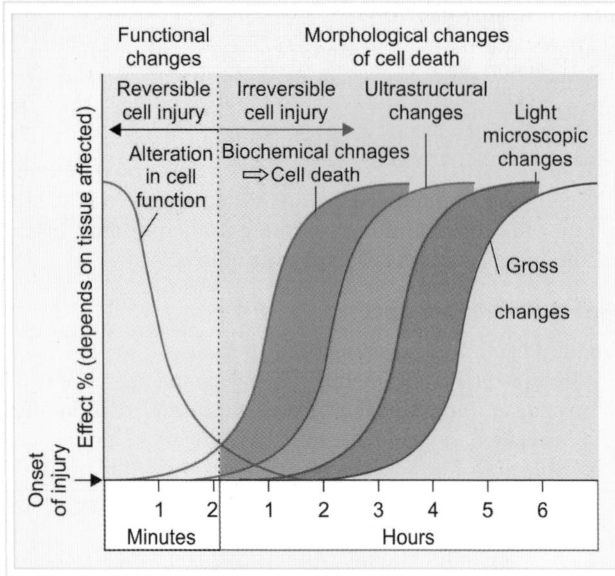

FIG. 2: Sequential changes in cell injury. After the exposure to injurious agent, cells may rapidly lose their function and may become non-functional. These cells may be still viable and show potentially reversible damage of biochemical and morphologic changes. If the duration of injury is prolonged, it may lead to irreversible damage and cell death. During this stage, there will be irreversible biochemical alterations which may cause cell death. Biochemical alterations generally precede all morphologic changes. The morphological features of cell injury or death usually follow the sequential order namely—first ultrastructural, followed by light microscopy, and lastly grossly visible changes.

reversible morphologic change is swelling of myocardial fibres. It may occur within minutes of ischemia to the myocardial cells. They functionally become noncontractile, but may not show morphological features of cell death till 20-30 minutes after ischemia. If the ischemia progresses, the cellular damage may progress to irreversible injury within 1 or 2 hours. First morphological features indicative of the cell death of ischemic myocytes can be appreciated by electron microscopy within 2-3 hours after the death of the cells. However, light microscopic evidence of cell death may not be observed until 4 to 12 hours after onset of ischemia and gross changes can be appreciated still later

REVERSIBLE CELL INJURY

Reversible injury is the early stage or mild form of cell injury during which the deranged function and morphology of the injured cells can return to normal if the causative stimulus is removed. If the stimulus is acute and brief (or short lived) or mild, the cell injury produces changes in the cells which are reversible up to a certain point.

Light microscope features of reversible cell injury: Two patterns of reversible cell injury are (i) cellular **swelling and** (ii) **fatty change**.

Cellular (Cloudy) Swelling

It was originally applied to the gross appearance of the organ involved, but is now applied to the microscopic appearance. It is closely related to **hydropic change** and **vacuolar degeneration**. They represent disturbances in protein and water metabolism. Being a manifestation of a disturbance in protein metabolism, it is also called **albuminous degeneration**.

Causes: It may be caused by many forms of mild injury but usually due to bacterial toxins, chemical poisons and malnutrition. It is due to changes in ion concentrations and fluid homeostasis. There is an increased flow of water into the cells which results in increased water content of injured cells.

Mechanism: Swelling of cells is due an increased inflow (influx) of water into the cytoplasm which results in increased water content of injured cells. Increased water content is consequence of failure of the adenosine triphosphate (ATP)-dependent Na^+-K^+ plasma membrane pump. Pump failure leads to depletion of ATP. ATP depletion result from oxygen deficiency, which interferes with mitochondrial oxidative phosphorylation, or mitochondrial damage by radiation or toxins.

Organs involved: Usually involved organs are kidney, liver, heart, and muscle.

MORPHOLOGY

Gross

Cellular swelling is the earliest feature of almost all forms of cell injury. When it affects many cells, it causes slight enlargement of affected organ and organ appears pallor. Organ appears pale because of compression of blood vessels by the swollen cells. There is increased turgor, and weight of the affected organ. Cut surface has a cloudy appearance and is opaque.

Microscopy

The affected cells may show small clear vacuoles within the cytoplasm. They represent distended and pinched-off segments of the ER. This pattern of nonlethal cell injury is commonly called hydropic change or vacuolar degeneration. When stained with hematoxylin and eosin (H&E), the cytoplasm of injured cells appears red (eosinophilic stained by eosin present in H&E). This is due to loss of RNA, which normally binds to the blue hematoxylin dye in H&E. The eosinophilia becomes more prominent as the injury progresses to irreversible injury causing necrosis.

Best example is cloudy swelling of highly specialized cells of the convoluted tubule of the kidney. The cell is swollen and projects unevenly into the lumen of the tubule. As the process advances the cytoplasm breaks down and its granular material gets discharged into the lumen of the tubule. These granules are proteinaceous in nature.

Electron Microscopy

The ultrastructural (subcellular) changes of reversible cell injury are visible by electron microscopy (**Fig. 3**). The changes in cell organelles are reflected in functional derangements (e.g., reduced protein synthesis, impaired energy production). These changes include the following:

- **Plasma membrane changes:** Plasma membrane may show blebs (focal extrusions of the cytoplasm) and they can detach from the membrane into the external environment without loss of cell viability. Other changes include blunting, and loss of microvilli.

Continued

Continued

- **Mitochondrial changes:** In acute injury such as ischemia (lack of adequate blood flow), mitochondria show swelling. Amorphous densities rich in phospholipid may also appear in the mitochondria, but these effects are fully reversible if injurious agent is removed.
- **Accumulation of "myelin figures"** in the cytosol composed of phospholipids derived from damaged cellular membranes.
- **Changes in endoplasmic reticulum (ER):** The cisternae of the ER become distended by fluid. Membrane-bound polysomes may disaggregate and detach from the surface of the RER.
- **Clumping of nuclear chromatin:** Nuclear alterations, with disaggregation of granular and fibrillary elements.

Steatosis (Fatty Change)

Fatty change is seen in organs that are actively involved in lipid metabolism (e.g., liver). It develops due to disruption of its metabolic pathways by toxic injury (e.g., alcohol). It is characterized by accumulation of triglyceride-filled lipid vacuoles in the cytoplasm. It is discussed in detail on pages 200–202.

CELL DEATH

There are two main types of cell death namely (i) necrosis and apoptosis. They differ in their mechanisms, morphology, and their roles in physiology and disease. Necrosis occurs with severe damage to mitochondria with depletion of ATP and rupture of lysosomal and plasma membranes. Necrosis is observed in many common injuries (e.g., ischemia, toxins, infections, and trauma). Apoptosis has many unique features and is discussed in detail on pages 142–151.

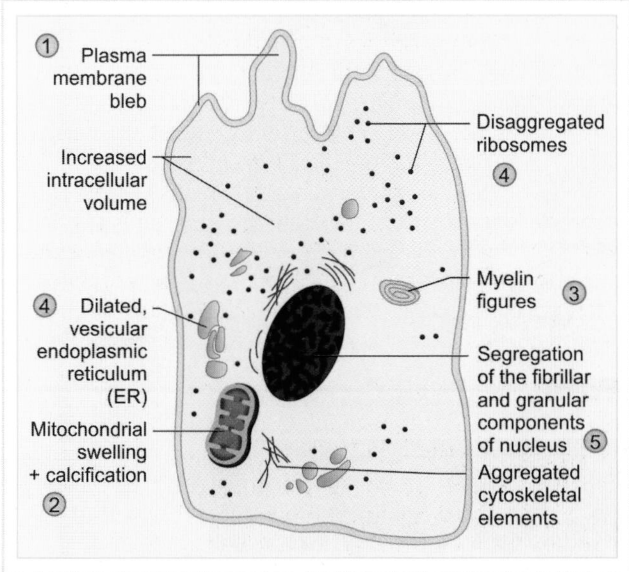

FIG. 3: Ultrastructural changes in reversible cell injury. Main changes include (1) plasma membrane changes, (2) mitochondrial changes, (3) accumulation of "myelin figures, (4) changes in endoplasmic reticulum (ER) and (5) clumping of nuclear chromatin.

Necrosis is considered as "accidental" cell death. The necrosis occurs accidentally because the injury is so severe to be repaired and many cellular constituents fail or fall apart. In necrosis, severe injury produces irreparably damage. If early (reversible) injury persists and progresses it leads to death of involved cells by necrosis. When cells undergo death by necrosis, there is a local inflammatory response at the site and clears the "scene of the accident." Necrosis is not regulated by specific signals or biochemical mechanisms. In contrast, apoptosis is "regulated" cell death. Apoptosis is mediated by defined molecular pathways and it kill cells with surgical precision. There is neither accompanying inflammation nor any collateral damage. The separation of necrosis and apoptosis is neither always very clear nor absolute. In some circumstances, cell death may show morphologic features of both apoptosis and necrosis, or progress from one to the other.

Necrosis

Q. Discuss pathology of necrosis and its various types.

Q. Describe events in a dying cell/discuss irreversible cell injury, nuclear changes in necrosis.

Definition: Necrosis is a pathologic process of accidental cell death that occurs as the consequence of severe injury.

Main causes of necrosis: All the causes of cell injury (refer pages 131–134), if severe can cause necrosis. Main causes include loss of oxygen supply (ischemia), microbial toxins, burns, chemical and physical injury. Leakage of active proteases can cause damage to the surrounding tissues in certain cases such as in acute pancreatitis. All of these initiating causes produce irreparable damage to cellular components.

Characteristics of necrosis: Main characteristics are as follows:

- **Denaturation of cellular proteins:** Denaturation is the process in which the molecular structure of a protein is modified or destroyed.
- **Leakage of cellular contents through damaged membranes:** Severe injury damages the plasma membrane as well as membranes of cytoplasmic organelle.
    - **Damage to lysosomal membrane:** It causes entry or leakage of lysosomal enzymes into the cytoplasm and digest the cell.
    - **Damage to plasma membrane:** The necrotic cells cannot maintain integrity of membrane and their contents, including **cellular enzymes**. It causes leakage of cellular contents into the extracellular space through damaged plasma membrane.
- **Local inflammatory reaction: Leakage of cellular contents into the extracellular space** elicit an inflammatory reaction by host and subsequent repair process in the surrounding tissue (local host reaction). Some specific substances or molecules released from injured cells are termed as damage-associated molecular patterns (DAMPs). Examples of these DAMPs includes ATP (released from damaged mitochondria), uric acid (a breakdown product of DNA) etc. These molecules are normally present within healthy cells. Their release into the extracellular space indicates severe cell injury. These molecules (DAMPs) are recognized by receptors present in macrophages and most other cell types. They bring out

phagocytosis of the debris and also produce cytokines that induce inflammation (refer pages 131–134).

- **Enzymatic digestion of the lethally injured cell:** Inflammatory cells produce more proteolytic enzymes. The cellular enzymes are also released into the extracellular space. The combination of phagocytosis and **enzymes ultimately digest the cell**. This leads to clearance of the lethally injured and necrotic cells. The enzymes which digest the cell are derived from lysosomes of either dying cells themselves or from leukocytes recruited as part of the inflammatory reaction

Laboratory detection of necrosis: Whenever there is necrosis, there is leakage of intracellular proteins through the damaged plasma membrane into the extracellular space. These proteins ultimately reach the circulation. Thus, it is possible to detect tissue-specific cellular injury (necrosis) using blood or serum samples. Examples include: (1) cardiac muscle contains a unique isoform of the enzyme creatine kinase and the cardiac-specific contractile protein troponin, (2) hepatic bile duct epithelium contains a specific isoform of the enzyme alkaline phosphatase, and (3) hepatocytes contain transaminases. Necrosis of these cell types and associated loss of integrity of membrane leads to raised serum levels of these proteins. They are useful as biomarkers. They are used clinically to assess and quantify tissue damage. For example, cardiac-specific troponins can be detected in the blood as early as 2 hours after myocardial cell necrosis. It is elevated even before there is any histologic evidence of myocardial infarction. They are highly sensitive and specific for myocardial injury. Hence, serial measurement of serum cardiac troponins is very useful for the diagnosis and management of patients with myocardial infarction.

MORPHOLOGY

Injured cell in necrosis show changes in the cytoplasm and nuclei (**Fig. 4**). The general changes in H&E stains are as follows:

Cytoplasmic changes: Cytoplasm of the necrotic cells have **increased eosinophilia**. Increased eosinophilia is partly due to the loss of cytoplasmic RNA and partly due to accumulation of denatured cytoplasmic proteins (which bind the red dye eosin). The cytoplasm of necrotic cell may have a **glassy homogeneous appearance** compared to normal cells. This is mainly due to the loss of glycogen. When enzymes have digested cytoplasmic organelles, the cytoplasm becomes vacuolated and gives a "**moth-eaten" appearance** (**Fig. 4**). Necrotic cells may be replaced by large whorled phospholipid precipitates. These are called **myelin figures**. These myelin figures may be either phagocytosed by other cells or further degraded into fatty acids. The fatty acids may undergo dystrophic calcification by the deposition of calcium-rich precipitates.

Electron microscopy (Fig. 4): Ultrastructurally, the cytoplasm of necrotic cells shows (i) discontinuities in plasma as well as organelle membranes, (ii) marked dilation of mitochondria and large amorphous densities, (iii) myelin figures, amorphous debris, and aggregates of fluffy material (due to denatured protein) in the cytoplasm.

Nuclear changes: These may take up one of three patterns. They are produced due to the breakdown of deoxyribonucleic acid (DNA) and chromatin.

Continued

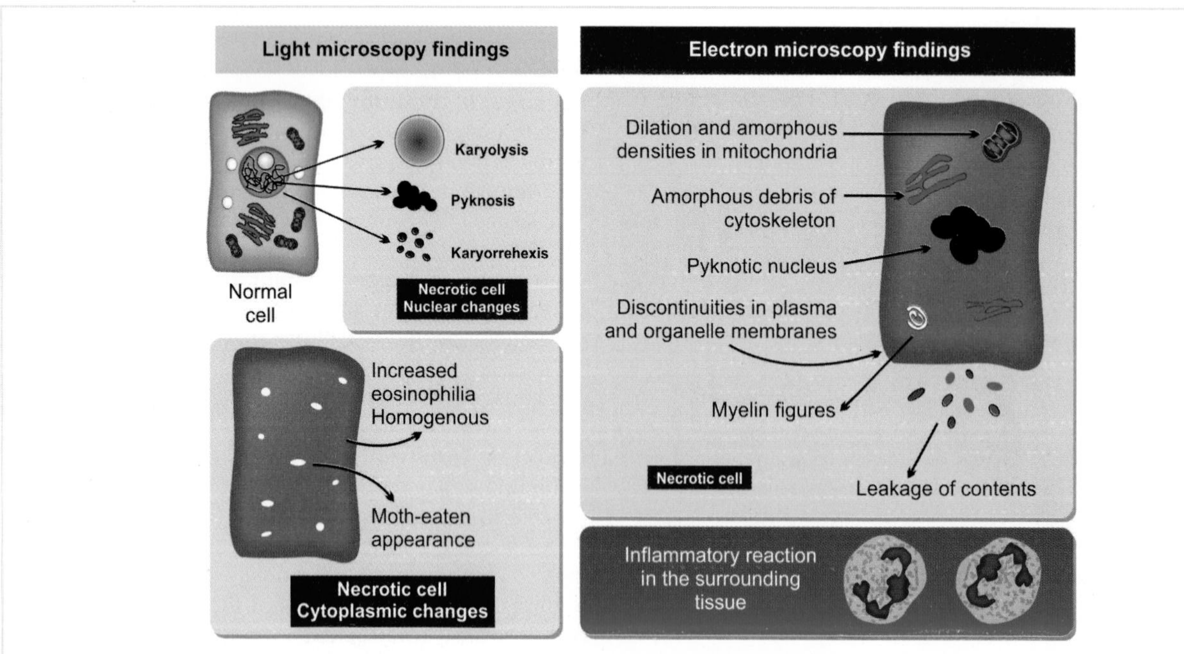

FIG. 4: Diagrammatic representation of light and electron microscopic change in necrosis

Continued

- **Karyolysis:** Normal chromatin appear basophilic due to staining of the chromatin by hematoxylin dye in H&E. **Progressive fading of basophilic staining of the nuclei** may occur in necrotic cells because of enzymatic degradation of DNA by endonuclease. It can lead to ghost nuclei. The nucleus of a necrotic cell may completely disappear within 1 to 2 days.
- **Pyknosis:** A second pattern is called pyknosis and is also seen in apoptotic cell death. Pyknosis is characterized by the **shrinkage of nucleus**. The chromatin of the nucleus condenses into a dense, shrunken deeply basophilic mass (due to increased basophilia) and appears similar to ink drop.
- **Karyorrhexis:** It is the third pattern of nuclear change in necrosis. The pyknotic **nucleus can undergo fragmentation** into many smaller fragments. This change is called karyorrhexis. With the passage of time (1 or 2 days), the nucleus in the necrotic cell totally disappears.

Reversible versus irreversible injury: With reversible injury, injured cells can return to normal if the causative stimulus is removed. When injury progresses and produces irreversible injury, injured **cells cannot return to normal even if the causative stimulus is removed.** Thus, it is important to know the possible events that determine when reversible injury becomes irreversible and progresses to necrosis. If we can identify the point at which the damage becomes irreversible, it will be clinically life saving measure. But the answer is not known. However, probably two phenomena may characterize irreversibility. These are (i) inability to reverse mitochondrial dysfunction (lack of oxidative phosphorylation and ATP generation) and (ii) severe disturbances in membrane function. In necrosis, injury to lysosomal membranes leads to release of lytic enzymes and causes enzymatic degradation of the injured cell.

Patterns (Types) of Tissue Necrosis

So far the changes in individual necrotic cells are discussed. When necrosis involves large numbers of cells, the tissue or organ is said to be necrotic. For example, in myocardial infarct, there is necrosis of a portion of the myocardium with death of many myocardial cells. Different types of necrosis involving tissues or organs produces morphologically distinct patterns. These morphological appearances provide clues regarding the underlying cause. Most of the types of necrosis have distinctive gross appearances (except fibrinoid necrosis) but they can be identified only by microscopic examination.

Coagulative necrosis

Q. Write a short note on coagulative necrosis.

Coagulative necrosis is a **common type of necrosis**. In this type of necrosis, the **outline of dead tissues (underlying tissue architecture) is preserved** (at least for few days). Infarct is a localized area of coagulative necrosis.

Cause: Ischemia caused by obstruction in a vessel may lead to coagulative necrosis of the supplied tissue in all organs. Only **exception being the brain** in which ischemia produces liquefactive necrosis.

Mechanism: In coagulative necrosis, the affected tissue has a firm texture. Probably ischemic injury denatures and coagulates both structural proteins and also enzymes. Thus, it prevents proteolysis of the dead cells by enzymes. Coagulation causes the protein to change from a gelatinous, transparent state to a firm, opaque state, similar to that of a cooked egg white. The cells appear intensely eosinophilic with indistinct or reddish nuclei that may persist for days or weeks. Finally, the necrotic cells are broken down by the action of lysosomal enzymes. These lysosomal enzymes are derived from infiltrating leukocytes and leukocytes also remove the debris of the dead cells by phagocytosis.

MORPHOLOGY

Organs affected: All organs can be affected except the brain. Coagulative necrosis is more frequent in organs supplied by end arteries with limited collateral circulation such as **heart (Fig. 5), kidney (Fig. 6), spleen** (refer **Fig. 38** of Chapter 9) **and limb (dry gangrene)** (refer **Fig. 12A**).

Gross

Appearance: The appearance of necrotic tissue is described as **coagulative necrosis** because it resembles the coagulation of proteins that occurs upon heating. Involved region appears **dry, pale, yellow, and firm. It is wedge shaped in organs like kidney (Fig. 6A) and spleen.**

Microscopy (Fig. 6C)

- **Indistinct outline of dead tissue.** In coagulative necrosis, the normal cells are converted into their "tomb stones", i.e., outlines of the cells are maintained and the cell type can still be recognized but their cytoplasmic and nuclear details are lost.
- After a variable time (depends on the tissue involved and the cause), the lytic activity of intracellular and extracellular enzymes causes the cell to disintegrate. Nucleus may be either absent or show karyolysis.
- Leukocytes are recruited to the site of necrosis and the lysosomal enzymes of the leukocytes digest the necrotic cells. The resulting cellular debris is then removed by phagocytosis by infiltrating neutrophils and macrophages.

Liquefactive necrosis (colliquative necrosis)

In this type of necrosis, **dead tissue is digested and** rapidly **undergoes softening** and transforms into a liquid viscous mass.

Causes: These are as follows:
- **Ischemic injury to central nervous system** [(CNS) i.e., neurons and glial cells in the brain].
- **Suppurative infections:** These include infections by bacteria (e.g., staphylococci, streptococci, and *Escherichia coli*) or, occasionally by fungus. These microbes stimulate the quick accumulation of inflammatory cells (leukocytes), and the enzymes liberated from these leukocytes digest ("liquefy") the tissue.

Mechanism: Liquefaction is due to digestive action of the hydrolytic enzymes released from dead cells (autolysis) and leukocytes (heterolysis).

MORPHOLOGY

Gross

The necrotic cells are completely digested and are converted into a viscous liquid that is eventually removed by phagocytes. The involved area appears soft with liquefied center containing necrotic debris. It may later form a cystic space. Organs affected are:

Brain: Necrotic area is soft and center shows liquefaction (**Fig. 7**). Exact reason for liquefactive necrosis due to hypoxic death of cells within the central nervous system is not known. Probably, the reason for liquefactive necrosis in brain may be the presence of rich digestive hydrolytic (abundant lysosomal) enzymes (or different hydrolases specific to cells of the CNS) and lipids, and also the presence of little connective tissue in the brain.

Continued

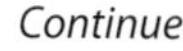

Continued

Abscess anywhere: The bacterial infection causes acute inflammatory reaction and the resulting necrosis of tissue. It produces the liquid viscous material which is frequently thick, creamy yellow because of the presence of leukocytes, and is called **pus** or **purulent exudate. The localized collection of pus is termed abscess.** It is also seen in wet gangrene and pancreatic necrosis.

Microscopy

Pus consists of liquefied necrotic cell debris, dead leukocytes and macrophages (scavenger cells).

Caseous Necrosis

It is a distinctive type of necrosis which shows combined features of both coagulative and liquefactive necrosis. The

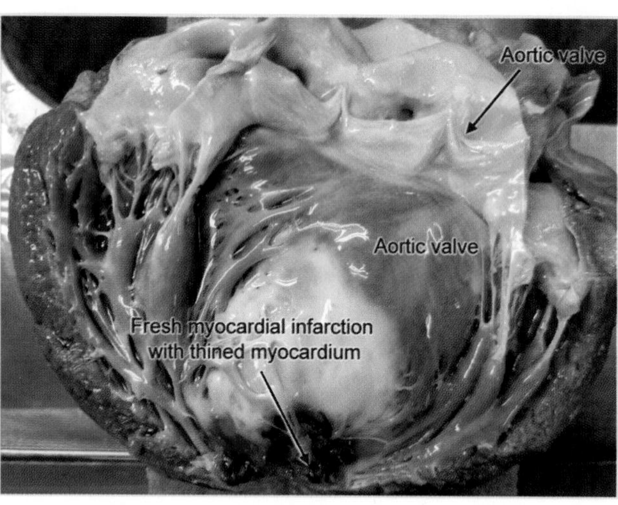

FIG.5: Myocardial infarct at the apex of heart. Acute myocardial infarction with thinning of the wall of the heart at the apex. The lumen of ventricle contains a blood clot.

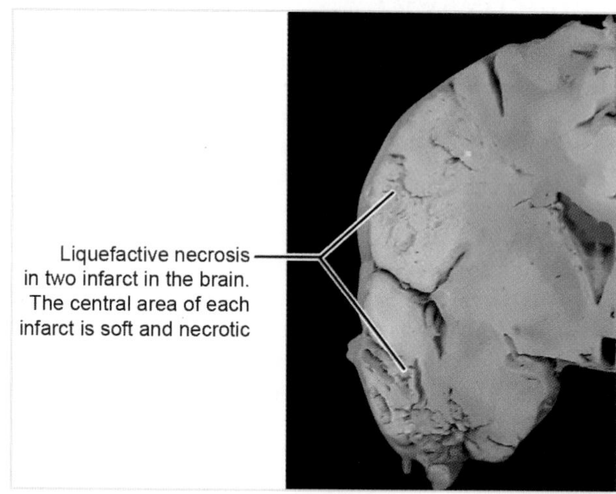

FIG. 7: Liquefactive necrosis. An infarct in the brain shows soft necrotic area with dissolution of the tissue forming a cavity.

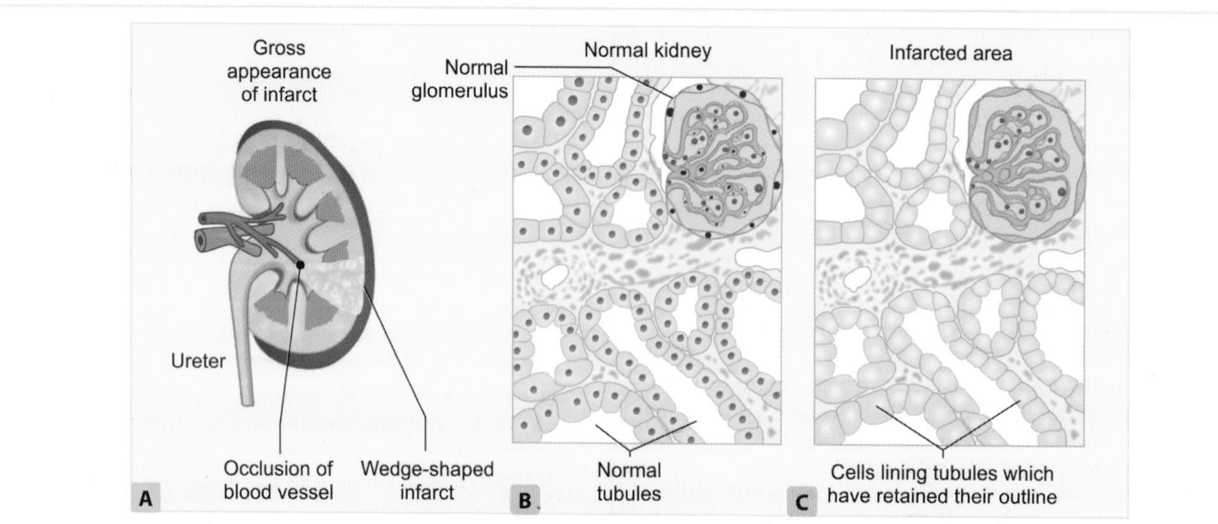

FIGS. 6A TO C: Diagrammatic appearance of gross and microscopy of infract kidney. (A) Gross appearance of infarct of kidney. (B) Microscopy of normal kidney. (C) Diagrammatic microscopic appearance of infarcted area of kidney. Infarcted area shows necrotic cells with preserved cellular outlines with loss of nuclei.

term caseous (cheese like) is derived from the appearance of the area of necrosis which is friable and white.

Causes: Caseous necrosis is characteristic of tuberculosis and is due to the type IV hypersensitivity reaction. It may also occur in certain types of fungal infections.

Mechanism: The dead cells disintegrate, but the debris is not digested completely by hydrolases and persist indefinitely as amorphous, coarsely granular, eosinophilic debris. Unlike, the necrotic cells neither lose their cellular outlines like in coagulative necrosis nor do not disappear by lysis like in liquefactive necrosis. Caseous necrosis is generally attributed to the toxic effects of complex waxes (peptidoglycolipids) in the mycobacterial cell wall. It has been suggested that granuloma formation may actually be orchestrated by mycobacteria and may in fact facilitate their survival against immune response of the host.

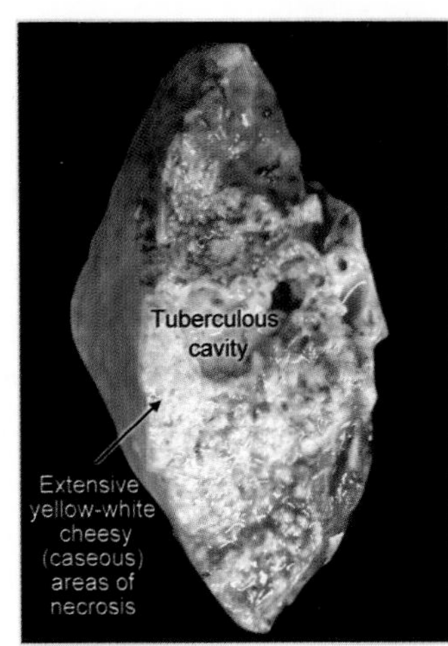

FIG. 8: Tuberculosis of lung. Gross appearance of caseous necrosis. Lung shows cavity with caseous necrosis.

MORPHOLOGY

Organs affected: Tuberculosis may involve any organ, most common in **lung** and **lymph node**.

Gross

Appearance: Necrotic area appears **yellow-white, soft, friable, granular** and resembles **dry, clumpy cheese,** hence the name caseous (**cheese-like**) necrosis (**Fig. 8**).

Microscopy

Caseous necrosis is a collection of fragmented or lysed cells and appears as **eosinophilic**, as amorphous (meaning shapeless/poorly defined), **coarsely granular material** or debris. In contrast to coagulative necrosis, there is complete obliteration of the tissue architecture and it is not possible to identify the cellular outlines. The necrotic area is surrounded by a distinctive inflammatory border. This characteristic focal inflammation lesion is known as a **caseating granuloma**. Caseating granuloma consists of central area of caseous necrosis, surrounded by epithelioid cells; Langhans type giant cells (nuclei arranged in a horse-shoe pattern), lymphocytes and fibroblasts. It is to be noted that granuloma (**Fig. 9**) may be caseating (soft granuloma) or noncaseating (hard granuloma). Noncaseating granuloma dies not show central caseous necrosis. Caseous necrotic material **may undergo dystrophic calcification.**

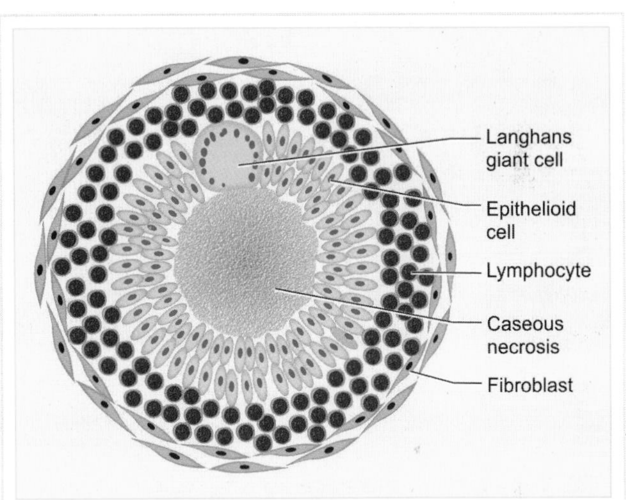

FIG. 9: Microscopic (diagrammatic) appearance of a caseous necrosis.

Fat necrosis

Q. Write short essay on fat necrosis.

Fat necrosis is characterized by focal areas of fat destruction, which affect adipose tissue. It occurs mainly at anatomic locations rich in fat.

Types Fat necrosis may be enzymatic or traumatic type.

Enzymatic fat necrosis: Occurs in adipose tissue around acutely inflamed pancreas (in **acute pancreatitis**).

- **Mechanism (Flowchart 2)**: In acute pancreatitis, the enzymes (one of them is lipase) leak from acinar cells into the substance of the pancreas and the peritoneal cavity and causes tissue damage. Lipase destroys and liquefy the membranes of fat cells and releases triglyceride esters. Lipase splits the triglyceride esters within fat cells and liberates free fatty acids (FFAs). FFAs combine with calcium and produce grossly visible chalky-white areas of calcium soaps (fat saponification).

MORPHOLOGY

Gross

Appears as opaque, irregular, **chalky-white areas** (**Fig. 10A**) embedded in otherwise normal adipose tissue. This helps both the surgeon and the pathologist to grossly identify fat necrosis and usually underlying disorder namely acute pancreatitis.

Microscopy

The necrotic **fat cells appear pale with shadowy outlines surrounded** by basophilic calcium deposits. There is also accompanying acute inflammatory reaction (**Fig. 10B**).

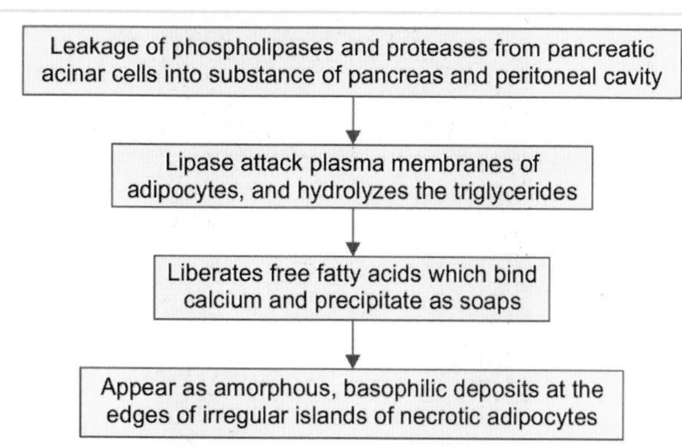

FLOWCHART 2: Pathogenesis of enzymatic fat necrosis.

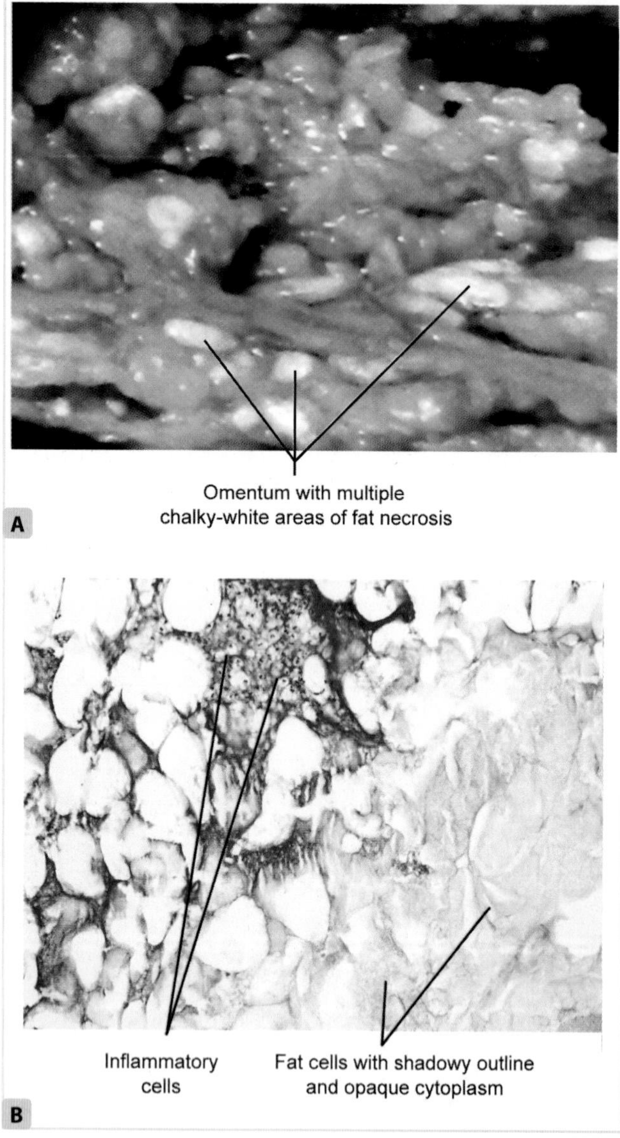

FIGS. 10A AND B: (A) Omentum shows multiple chalky-white areas of fat necrosis seen in acute pancreatitis. (B) Microscopically, fat necrosis shows necrotic fat cells in the right lower part and inflammatory reaction between normal (left upper area) and area of fat necrosis.

Traumatic fat necrosis: Occurs in tissues with high fat content (like in **heavy, pendulous breast, and thigh**) following severe trauma. Fat necrosis may also occur following radiation, surgery or removal of breast implants. In traumatic fat necrosis, triglycerides and lipases are released from the injured adipocytes. Fat necrosis due to trauma is common in breast and may mimic a tumor, particularly if calcification has occurred.

Fibrinoid necrosis

It is a special form of necrosis that develops in walls of arteries. It is characterized by **deposition of pink-staining (fibrin-like) proteinaceous material** in the tissue matrix with a **staining pattern reminiscent of fibrin**. It obscures the underlying cellular detail. In fibrinoid necrosis, there are deposits of immune complexes, together with plasma proteins that has leaked out of vessels. This gives in a bright pink and amorphous appearance in H&E stains. Hence, called "fibrinoid" (fibrin-like) by pathologists.

Causes: Usually seen in **immune-mediated** (deposition of antigen-antibody complexes in the wall of vessels as in systemic lupus erythematosus) **vascular injury/vasculitis** (e.g., polyarteritis nodosa), **malignant hypertension, Aschoff bodies** in rheumatic heart disease, placenta in **pre-eclampsia**, or **hyperacute transplant rejection**.

MORPHOLOGY

Microscopy: The fibrinoid necrosis appears as brightly eosinophilic, hyaline-like deposit in the vessel wall. It is better appreciated under phosphotungstic acid hematoxylin (PTAH) stain (**Fig. 11**).

Gummatous necrosis

In gummatous necrosis, the necrotic tissue is firm and rubbery and is usually found in tertiary syphilis.

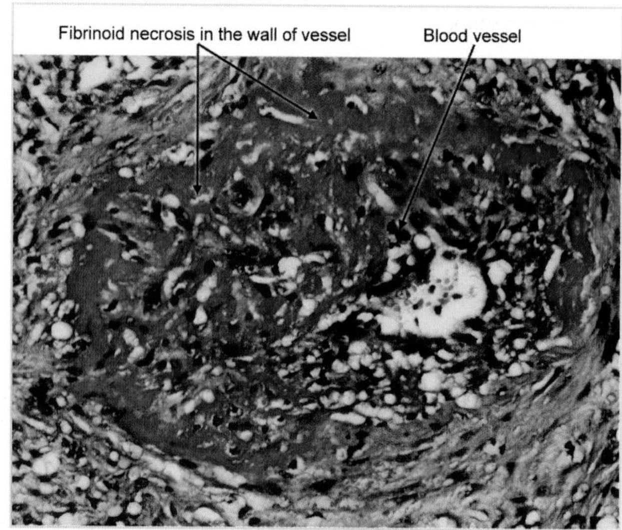

FIG. 11: Fibrinoid necrosis in the wall of blood vessel [phosphotungstic acid hematoxylin (PTAH) stain].

Gangrene (gangrenous necrosis)

Gangrene is not a specific pattern of cell death, but it is commonly used term in clinical practice. It is similar to post-mortem decomposition except that only a portion of the body is dead.

Definition: It is **massive necrosis with superadded putrefaction**. When bacterial infection is superimposed, there is more liquefactive necrosis because of the actions of degradative enzymes in the bacteria and the attracted leukocytes (giving rise to so-called **wet gangrene**).

Types: Two types, namely **dry and wet gangrene**. A variant of wet gangrene known as **gas gangrene** is **caused** by *Clostridia* (Gram-positive anaerobic bacteria).

Dry gangrene

- **Cause: Arterial occlusion** (e.g., atherosclerosis).
- **Sites:** It usually involves a **limb**, generally the distal part of lower limb (leg, foot, and toe).

MORPHOLOGY

Gross

Affected part is **dry, shrunken** (shrivelled) and **dark brown or black** resembling the foot of a **mummy**. The black color is due to the iron sulfide. A **line of demarcation** is seen between gangrenous and adjacent normal area **(Fig. 12A)**.

Microscopy

The necrosis (coagulative type) shows smudging of soft tissue and overlying skin. The line of demarcation consists of granulation tissue with inflammatory cells.

Wet gangrene

Causes: Due to the venous blockage (e.g., strangulated hernia, intussusception, or volvulus). Diabetic patients may develop both dry (due to atherosclerosis of tibial and popliteal arteries) and wet gangrene. It usually follows a minor injury to toe or foot.

Sites: Occurs in **moist tissues or internal organs** (e.g., bowel, lung, mouth, etc.).

MORPHOLOGY

Gross

The affected part is soft, swollen, cold, putrid and black/ dark **(Fig. 12B)**. No clear line of demarcation. It produces a foul odor due to the presence of pus.

Microscopy

Liquefactive type of necrosis and occurs when neutrophils invade the site.

Differences between dry and wet gangrene are presented in **Table 1**.

Gas gangrene: Special type of wet gangrene caused by infection with a gas forming anaerobic Clostridium perfringens. These

Table 1: Differences between dry and wet gangrene.

Characteristics	*Dry*	*Wet*
General features		
Common site	Limbs	Bowels
Examples	Gangrene of lower limb due to atherosclerosis	Volvulus, intussusception
Etiological factors		
Cause of ischemia	Arterial obstruction	Commonly venous obstruction
Rate of obstruction	Slow	Abrupt
Gross features		
Appearance of involved part	Shriveled, dry (mummification) and black	Swollen, soft, and moist/wet
Line of demarcation	Clear cut between gangrenous and healthy part	Not clear cut
Spread	Slow	Rapid
Prognosis	Fair	Poor due to severe septicemia

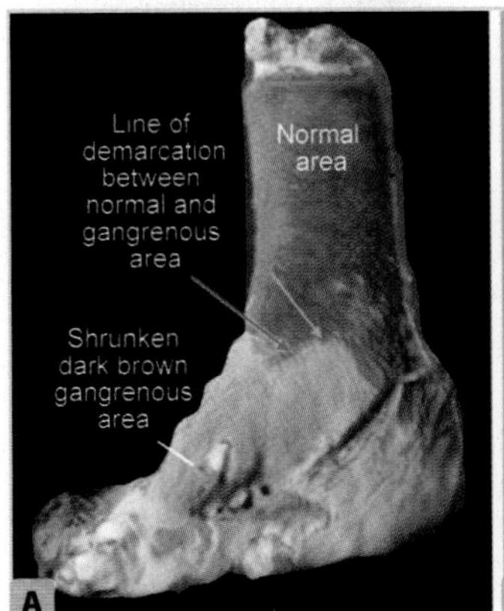

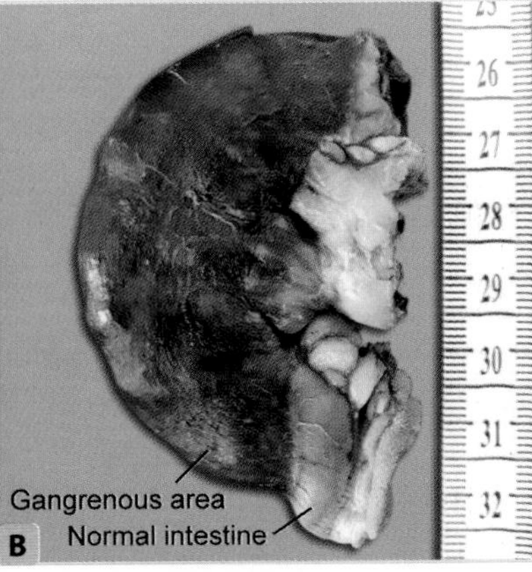

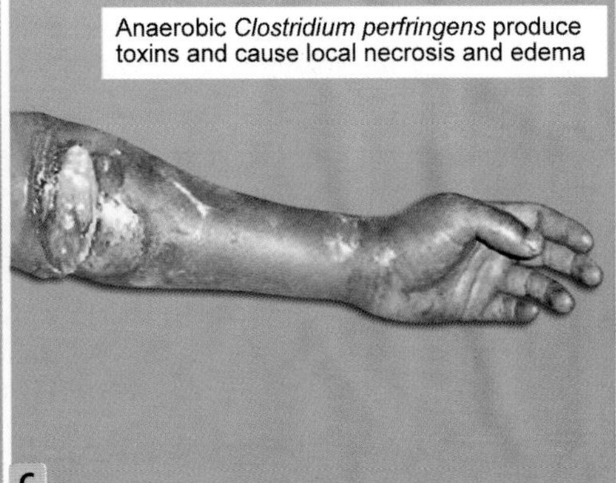

FIGS.12A TO C: (A) Dry gangrene of left leg shows dry shrunken discolored gangrenous foot separated from adjacent normal area by a line of demarcation. (B) Wet gangrene of small intestine. (C) Gas gangrene in upper limb.

organisms enter into the tissues through open contaminated wounds (e.g., muscles, complication of operative procedures on colon). It produces hydrolytic enzymes and a necrotizing toxin. Toxins produced by them cause local necrosis (**Fig. 12C**) and edema, and are also absorbed causing severe systemic manifestations. The hydrolytic enzymes and toxins destroy connective tissue and cellular membranes and cause bubbles of gas to form in muscle cells. It can be fatal if enzymes lyse the membranes of red blood cells, destroying their oxygen-carrying capacity. Fournier's gangrene is a gangrene that involves an infection in the scrotum (including the testicles), penis, or perineum.

Ultrastructural differences between reversible and irreversible injury are presented in **Table 2**.

Fate of necrotic cells: After necrosis, the necrotic cells in the living patient may either persist for some time or their contents may be digested by enzymes and necrotic cells disappear. Dead cells may be replaced by myelin figures. The debris may be either phagocytosed by leukocytes. If necrotic cells and cellular debris are not promptly destroyed and reabsorbed, they may undergo further degradation into fatty acids. These fatty acids can bind calcium salts and other minerals and become calcified. This process of deposition of calcium salts in necrotic cells or tissues is called dystrophic calcification.

Apoptosis

Q. Define apoptosis [programmed cell death (PCD)] and its causes (conditions). Describe different pathways/ pathogenesis/ mechanism of apoptosis. Describe the genetic basis/ factors and genetic pathway of apoptosis.

Q. Describe pathophysiology, apoptosis in tissue homeostasis and significance of apoptosis.

Definition: Apoptosis is a **type of (programmed) cell death induced by a tightly regulated suicide program**.

Apoptosis was first identified in 1972 by its peculiar morphologic appearance of membrane-bound fragments derived from cells. It was named after the Greek designation for "falling off." Later it was discovered in model organisms such as worms that certain cells undergo apoptosis at precise times during development. This phenomenon was called as programmed cell death and is controlled by the action of few genes and this process is required for normal embryogenesis. Thus, apoptosis is a unique mechanism of cell death and is different from necrosis in several respects (refer **Table 4**).

Salient features: In apoptosis, the cells intended to undergo death by apoptosis undergo following changes:

- **Activation intrinsic enzymes of the cell.**
- **Degradation of cells:** Activated enzymes degrade the cells' own nuclear genomic DNA and proteins (both nuclear and cytoplasmic).
- **Formation of apoptotic bodies:** Degraded cells break up into plasma membrane-bound fragments, called apoptotic bodies. These apoptotic bodies contain portions of the cytoplasm and nucleus. These apoptotic bodies fall off from the cells and hence named apoptosis (meaning "falling off").
- **Phagocytosis:** During the process of apoptosis, when the plasma membrane is still intact, its surface components are changes in such a way that produce find or eat me signals for their recognition by phagocytes. The apoptotic cell and its fragments are rapidly ingested by phagocytes before their contents leak out. Therefore, apoptosis does not elicit an inflammatory reaction.

Causes of Apoptosis

Q. Write short essay on causes of apoptosis.

Q. Write the role of apoptosis in health and disease and a note on dysregulated apoptosis.

Apoptosis can occur in two broad situations namely (i) as part of normal physiologic processes (physiologic situations), and (ii) as a pathophysiologic mechanism (pathologic conditions) of cell loss in many diseases. Thus, apoptosis is not necessarily an indication of cell injury.

Apoptosis in physiologic situations

In physiologic situations, cells undergo apoptosis due to (i) the removal or withdrawal of necessary survival signals, such as growth factors and interactions with the extracellular matrix, or (ii) they receive pro-apoptotic signals from other cells or the surrounding environment. Various physiologic situations in apoptosis occurs are as follows:

Removal of excess of the required number of (supernumerary) cells during embryogenesis and developmental processes: Apoptosis is essential for involution of primordial structures as well as remodeling of maturing tissues. For example, structures needed by only one sex disappear in embryos of the other sex. Thus, the Müllerian duct (the progenitor of the uterus), is deleted in males, whereas the

Table 2: Ultrastructural differences between reversible and irreversible injury.

Structure involved	*Reversible injury*	*Irreversible injury*
Plasma membrane changes	Blebbing, blunting, loss of microvilli	Discontinuities in plasma and organelle membrane
Mitochondrial changes	Swelling and appearance of small amorphous densities	Marked dilatation with appearance of large amorphous densities (precipitated calcium), aggregates of fluffy material (denatures protein)
Endoplasmic reticulum	Dilatation with detachment of polysomes	Swelling and fragmentation
Myelin figure (large intracellular whorled phospholipid masses)	May be present	Usually present
Nuclear changes	Disaggregation of granular and fibrillar elements	Pyknosis, karyolysis, and karyorrhexis

Wolffian duct (forms part of the male genital tract), disappears in females. Apoptosis also mediates the disappearance of web tissues (interdigital tissues) between fingers and toes to yield discrete fingers and toes, converts solid primordia to hollow tubes (e.g., GI tract), and produces the four-chamber heart.

Involution of hormone-dependent tissues on withdrawal of hormone: Elimination of cells after withdrawal of hormonal stimuli is by apoptosis. Thus, apoptosis maintains the balance of cellularity in organs that respond to trophic stimuli, such as hormones. Examples include endometrial cell breakdown during the menstrual cycle, ovarian follicular atresia in menopause, the regression of lactational hyperplasia of the breast in women who have stopped nursing their infants is by apoptosis and postmenopausal atrophy of the endometrium after withdrawal/loss of hormonal support.

Maintain a constant number of cell populations: Apoptosis is a normal/ physiologic phenomenon that eliminate cells that are no longer required, or as a mechanism to maintain a constant number of various cell populations in tissues. Physiologic apoptosis mainly affects progeny of stem cells that are constantly dividing. For example, stem cells of the hematopoietic system, GI mucosa, and epidermis. In these organs, apoptosis prevents overpopulation of mature cells by removing excess cells. Thus, it helps in maintain normal organ size and architecture. Probably, there is turnover of about 1 million cells per second in human beings. This process is brought out by death of cells by apoptosis and their removal by phagocytes.

Elimination of potentially harmful cells: In immunology, the clones of **self-reactive lymphocytes** that recognize normal self-antigens are deleted by apoptosis. It helps in avoiding potentially dangerous immune reactions against one's own tissues (autoimmune disease).

Death of host cells after their useful purpose: For example, neutrophils in an acute inflammatory response, and lymphocytes at the end of an immune response.

Eliminates senescent (aged) cells: Cell turnover is needed to maintain the size and function of many organs. For example, as blood cells that are continuously being supplied to the circulating blood, older and less functional white blood cells must be removed to maintain the normal number of the cells in the circulation. The polymorphonuclear leukocytes in chronic myeloid leukemia pathologically accumulate as a result of mutation that inhibits apoptosis and thereby allows these cells to persist. In the small intestine mucosa, cells migrate from the depths of the crypts to the tips of the villi. In the tip of the villi the old mucosal cells undergo apoptosis and are sloughed into the lumen of the intestine.

Role in gametogenesis: Adult male produce about 1,000 new spermatozoa per second. Most of them undergo apoptosis because of intrinsic defects or external damage. Excessive apoptosis of spermatozoa may be responsible for some forms of male infertility. In female, about 99% of neonatal ovarian oocytes are eventually deleted by apoptosis.

Apoptosis in pathologic conditions

Apoptosis eliminates cells that are genetically altered or damaged (injured) beyond repair. This is achieved without producing a host reaction and thus limiting collateral tissue damage. Apoptosis protects from the consequences of a non-functional cell or one that cannot control its own proliferation (e.g., a cancer cell). It is responsible for cell loss in many pathologic conditions:

Elimination of cells with damaged DNA: DNA may be damaged by many injurious agents like radiation, DNA-binding chemicals, cytotoxic anticancer drugs, and hypoxia. They can cause DNA damage either directly or through production of free radicals. If repair mechanisms cannot correct the DNA damage, the cell triggers intrinsic mechanisms that promote apoptosis. DNA damage can lead to malignant transformation of cells. In these situations, apoptosis is a protective phenomenon that prevents the survival of cells with DNA mutations.

- **p53 triggered apoptosis:** Mainly tumor-suppressor gene p53 recognizes cells with damaged DNA and assesses whether it can be repaired. If the damage is too severe to be repaired, p53 triggers apoptosis.
- **Destroying cells with dangerous mutations or with DNA damage** beyond repair by apoptosis prevents the development of cancer.
- Peculiarly cancer cells usually evolve mechanisms to avoid apoptosis that might otherwise eliminate them. In certain cancers, where p53 is mutated or absent, the apoptosis is not induced in cells with damaged DNA.

Elimination of cells with excessively accumulated misfolded proteins: Mutations in the genes encoding proteins or extrinsic factors (damage due to free radicals) may result in accumulation of unfolded or misfolded proteins.

- Excessive intracellular accumulation of these abnormally folded proteins in the ER is known as ER stress, which results in apoptotic cell death.
- Apoptosis caused by the accumulation of misfolded proteins is found in several degenerative diseases of the CNS (Alzheimer, Huntington, and Parkinson diseases) and other organs.

Killing of viral infected cells: Apoptosis acts as a defense against dissemination of infection. When a cell "detects" nonchromosomal DNA replication (as in a viral infection), it initiates apoptosis. By destroying infected cells, the body tries to limit the spread of the virus. In viral infections, the infected cells are lost mainly due to apoptosis induced either by the virus [as in adenovirus and human immunodeficiency virus (HIV) infections] or by host human response by cytotoxic T lymphocytes (CTLs) (as in viral hepatitis). The cytotoxic T lymphocytes (CTLs) specific for viral proteins induce apoptosis of infected cells and thereby attempt to eliminate reservoirs of infection. During this process, apoptosis can produce significant tissue damage.

Many viruses have developed mechanisms that prevent cellular apoptosis and permit their survival. These include carrying genes whose products inhibit apoptosis, viral proteins bind and inactivate cellular proteins (e.g., p53) involved in triggering apoptosis or that interfere with the signaling pathways that activate apoptosis.

Elimination of neoplastic cells/rejection of transplant: The CTL-mediated mechanism is also involved in killing of tumor cells by apoptosis, cellular rejection of transplants, and tissue damage in graft-versus-host disease.

Elimination of parenchymal cells in pathologic atrophy: Obstruction of duct in the parenchymal organs like pancreas, parotid gland and kidney can lead to apoptosis of the parenchymal cells and pathologic their atrophy.

Morphologic and Biochemical Changes in Apoptosis

Q. Describe morphological and biochemical changes in apoptosis

MORPHOLOGY

Electron Microscopy

The ultrastructural features observed in cells undergoing of apoptosis (**Fig. 13**) are:

Cell shrinkage: The size of the cell is reduced and cytoplasm becomes dense. The cellular organelles are more tightly packed than normal. In contrasts, necrosis shows cell swelling and not cell shrinkage.

Condensation and fragmentation of nuclear chromatin: Chromatin condensation is the most characteristic feature of apoptosis. The chromatin aggregates into dense masses of various shapes and sizes. This is observed at the periphery of the nuclei below the nuclear membrane. The nucleus may break into two or more nuclear fragments.

Formation of cytoplasmic blebs and apoptotic bodies: First, the apoptotic cell shows extensive blebbing on the cytoplasmic surface. This is followed by fragmentation of the apoptotic dead cells into membrane-bound apoptotic bodies. The apoptotic bodies are composed of portion of cytoplasm with tightly packed organelles, with or without nuclear fragments of variable size and shapes.

Phagocytosis of apoptotic cells or cell bodies: Phosphatidylserine (PS) is a phospholipid that is normally on the interior aspect of the cell membrane. It is externalized in cells undergoing apoptosis. PS present in apoptotic bodies is recognized usually by macrophages and activates ingestion of apoptotic cells by phagocytosis without release of intracellular constituents. They are degraded by the lysosomal enzymes of phagocytes. This avoids inflammatory reaction and recruitment of neutrophils or lymphocytes.

Continued

Continued

Light Microscopy

In H&E-stained tissue, the apoptotic cells appear as round or oval mass having intensely eosinophilic **cytoplasm**. The **nuclei appear as fragments of dense nuclear chromatin** and shows pyknosis. Apoptotic cells are usually seen against a background of viable cells. Apoptosis occur in single cells or small groups of cells, whereas necrosis characteristically involves larger geographic areas of cell death. Apoptosis **does not elicit an inflammatory reaction** in the host. Shrinkage of cell and formation of apoptotic bodies are rapid process and the apoptotic bodies are quickly cleared by phagocytes. Hence, considerable apoptosis may occur in tissues without its appearance in histologic sections. Absence of an inflammatory response further make it difficult to detect apoptosis under light microscopy.

Mechanisms of Apoptosis

Q. Write short essay on mechanism of apoptosis.

Apoptosis comprises several signaling pathways and are presented in **Table 3**. The different routes to apoptosis intersect and overlap and only extrinsic and intrinsic pathway are described here.

Apoptosis is regulated by biochemical pathway. The survival or apoptosis of many cells depends upon balance between **two opposite sets of signals** namely: **(1) death signal** (proapoptotic) and **(2) prosurvival** (antiapoptotic) signals. Unlike necrosis, apoptosis engages the cell's own signaling cascades and results in its own death (suicide). Apoptosis results from **activation of** a family of cysteine proteases **(enzymes)** called as **caspases** (i.e., they are cysteine proteases that cleave proteins after aspartic residues). Like many proteases, caspases are present as inactive proenzymes. They must be enzymatically cleaved to become active. Therefore, the presence of active caspases is a marker for cells that undergoes apoptosis. Sequential activation of caspases brings out conversion of inactive proenzymes into catalytically effective enzymes, is central to apoptotic pathways. About 14 caspases have been identified, of which about seven are involved in apoptotic signaling. Although the various pathways

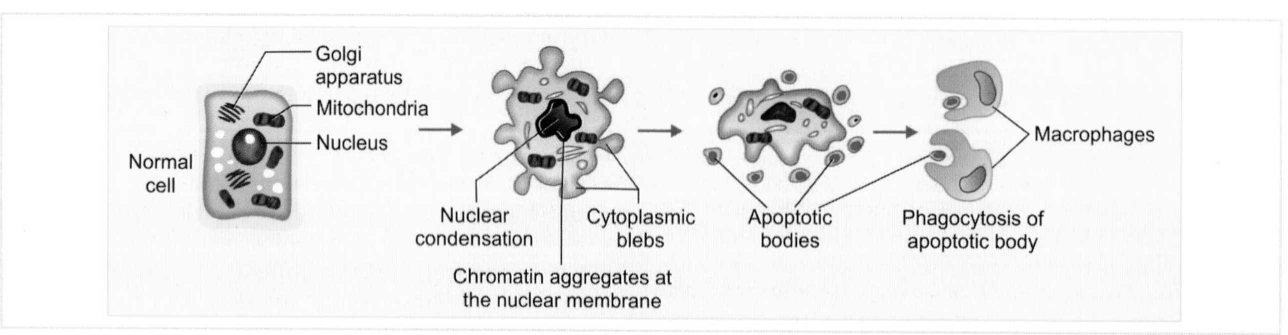

FIG. 13: Electron microscopic changes in apoptosis.

Table 3: Signaling pathways involved in apoptosis.

Pathway of apoptosis	*Mechanism*
Extrinsic pathway	Plasma membrane receptors are activated by their ligands
Intrinsic pathway	Initiated by diverse intracellular stresses and mitochondria play a central role
Inflammatory or infectious processes	Intracellular and extracellular infectious agents can elicit apoptosis,s by diverse routes
Perforin/granzyme pathway	Triggered when cytotoxic T cells attack their cellular targets. They transfer granzyme B from the killer cell to its intended victim
p53-activated apoptosis	Occurs in response to cellular stress or deoxyribonucleic acid (DNA) damage
Endoplasmic reticulum	Calcium signaling plays a central role

		BH domains	Members
Multi-BH Antiapoptotic		4 3 1 2	Bcl-2, Bcl-XL, Mcl-1 and others
Proapoptotic	BH_{1-3}	3 1 2 (No BH4)	Bak, Bax, (Bok)
Proapoptotic	BH_3 only	3 (No BH4)	Bim, Bid, Bad and others

FIG. 14: BCL-2 family of apoptosis-related proteins. These proteins are divided into three groups depending on Bcl-2 homology (BH) domains and function in the protein. Antiapoptotic family members are characterized by the presence of the BH4 domain. By contrast, in proapoptotic Bcl-2 family members, there is no BH4 domain and may have either BH_{1-3} or only BH_3 (termed as BH_3-only proteins).

to apoptosis may start differently, all usually lead to the **killer enzymes: Caspases-3, -6, and -7.**

Role of mitochondria in apoptosis

Mitochondria are organelles that contain proteins such as cytochrome c (in the **inner membrane**) that are essential for life. But **cytochrome c**, when released into the cytoplasm indicates that the cell is not healthy and can initiate the suicidal program of apoptosis. Cytochrome c is a double edged sword. It is required for producing the energy (e.g., ATP) that sustains cell viability. But, if released into the cytoplasm, (indicates that the cell is not healthy), it initiates the suicide program of apoptosis. **Outer membrane** of mitochondria normally contains both **proapoptotic and antiapoptotic proteins** of the Bcl-2 (BCL-2) family (and corresponding genes).

BCL-2 Family The Bcl-2 family is the life/death switch of the cell. The release of mitochondrial proapoptotic proteins is tightly regulated by the Bcl-2 family of proteins. Bcl-2 family consists of >20 proteins (and corresponding genes). This family is named after *BCL2*, which was identified as an oncogene in a B-cell lymphoma. BCL2 is a gene that is frequently overexpressed in certain B cell lymphomas due to chromosomal translocations and other aberrations. The members of the Bcl-2 family can be divided into three subfamilies, depending on their proapoptotic (antisurvival) or antiapoptotic (prosurvival) function and number of Bcl-2 homology (BH) domains in the protein (**Fig. 14**).

- **Antiapoptotic (i.e., prosurvival) members (proteins):** They have four BH domains [labeled BH1, BH2, BH3, and BH4 (called BH_{1-4})]. They are often called to as multi-BH domain proteins. The main members of this group include **BCL-2 *(Bcl-2)*, BCL-XL *(Bcl-xL)*, MCL-1 *(Mcl-1)*** and others. These proteins are present in the outer mitochondrial membranes, cytosol, and ER membranes. They keep the mitochondrial outer membrane impermeable and thereby prevent leakage of cytochrome c and other death-inducing proteins into the cytosol that trigger apoptosis. Growth factors and other survival signals stimulate production of antiapoptotic proteins (**Fig. 15**).

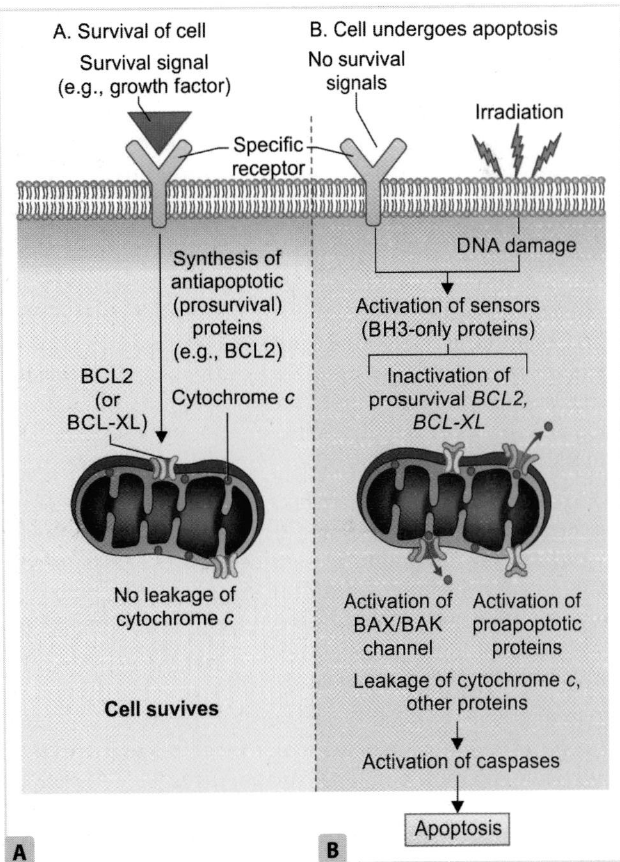

FIGS. 15A AND B: The intrinsic (mitochondrial) pathway of apoptosis. (A) For viability of a cell, survival signals are needed. The signal maintains the cell survival by producing antiapoptotic proteins (e.g., BCL-2). These proteins maintain the integrity of mitochondrial membranes and thereby prevent leakage of mitochondrial proteins. (B) If there are no survival signals, DNA damage, and other insults activate sensors that activate the proapoptotic proteins BAX and BAK. They form channels in the mitochondrial membrane and allow the leakage of cytochrome c and other proteins. This activates caspase and the cell undergoes apoptosis.

- **Proapoptotic (antisurvival) members (proteins):** These are **BH_{1-3} proteins** and contain **three BH domains** (**Fig. 14**). Main members of this group are **BAX *(Bak)* and BAK *(Bax).*** A third member, is Bok (less understood). BAK is mainly a mitochondrial protein, while BAX is largely cytoplasmic. On activation, BAX and BAK oligomerize (Oligomerization is a chemical process that converts monomers to macromolecular complexes through a finite degree of polymerization) within the outer mitochondrial protein and increase the permeability of mitochondrial outer membrane. Probably this is achieved by forming a channel in the outer mitochondrial membrane, allowing leakage of cytochrome c from the intermembranous space.
- **BH_3-only proteins (sensors):** A larger group of proapoptotic proteins belong to BH_3-only proteins. They carry a single (one) BH domain, i.e., third of the four BH domains (BH_3 domain). Hence they are also called as BH_3-only proteins These include Bad *(BAD)*, BIM *(Bim),* Bid *(BID),* Bik *(BIK),* Puma, and Noxa. BH-3 only proteins act as sensors of cellular stress and damage and are called as **BH-3 sensors.** They regulate the balance between the other two groups (antiapoptotic and proapoptotic), thus acting as moderator of apoptosis (regulated apoptosis initiators). Different BH3-only proteins can cause apoptosis by **either inactivating prosurvival** functions of Bcl-2 family members (e.g., **BCL-2, BCL-XL*)* or by directly stimulating death-inducing properties of proapoptotic proteins (e.g., Bax and Bak)**.

Phases of apoptosis

The process of apoptosis are divided into—(1) initiation phase and (2) execution phase. During initiation phase, some caspases become catalytically active and release a cascade of other caspases. In the execution phase, the terminal caspases trigger cellular fragmentation. Regulation of these enzymes depends on a finel balance between the pro-apoptotic and anti-apoptotic proteins.

Initiation phase Apoptosis is initiated by signals derived from two distinct pathways activated by distinct stimuli, namely: (1) intrinsic or mitochondrial pathway and (2) extrinsic or death receptor pathway. Though these two distinct pathways converge, they are usually activated by different conditions, involve different initiating molecules, and play distinct roles in both physiology and disease.

Intrinsic (mitochondrial) pathway of apoptosis (Fig. 16): Mitochondrial damage is the major mechanism in a variety of **physiological and pathological apoptosis**. It is activated by intracellular signals. Survival or apoptosis of cell is determined by permeability of mitochondria. Increased permeability of the mitochondrial outer membrane releases death-inducing (proapoptotic) molecules from the mitochondrial intermembrane space into the cytoplasm. **Mitochondrial membrane permeability is controlled by BCL-2 family** (discussed before) of proteins. Growth factors and other survival signals stimulate the production of antiapoptotic proteins (e.g., BCL-2) and prevent the leakage of death-inducing proteins from the outer membrane of mitochondria. Causes of mitochondrial injury that trigger apoptosis are presented in **Box 2**.

- **Steps in intrinsic (mitochondrial) pathway (Fig. 16):** Mitochondrial injury causes increased mitochondrial permeability and **releases proapoptotic molecules (death inducers) into the cytoplasm**. Thus, the balance shifts to proapoptotic proteins and the apoptotic cascade is activated. The different steps are as follows:
  - **Sensing of mitochondrial damage by BH3-only (sensors) proteins:** The mentioned causes of mitochondrial injury (**Box 2**) or damage is sensed by the BH3-only proteins (BH = BCL-2 homology) and they get activated. BH3-only proteins are activated (upregulated) through increased transcription and/or post-translational modifications (e.g., phosphorylation).
  - **Activation of proapoptotic effectors**: The functions of activated **BH3-only** sensors are:
    1. **Activation of two critical proapoptotic BCL-2 family** effector proteins, namely **BAX** and **BAK**.
    2. BH3-only sensors/proteins may also bind to and **block the function of antiapoptotic proteins** namely BCL-2 and BCL-XL. At the same time, synthesis of BCL2 and BCL-XL may also be reduced because their transcription depends on survival signals. In contrast, growth factors and other survival signals stimulate the production of anti-apoptotic proteins such as BCL2. Thus, they protect cells from apoptosis.

    At the same time, the production of BCL-2 and BCL-XL (**prosurvival proteins)** may decrease because of the relative deficiency of survival signals. The net result is activation of BAX-BAK (proapoptotic) and loss of the protective functions of the anti-apoptotic BCL-2 family members.
    3. *Regulated apoptosis initiators*: These include BAD, BIM, BID, Puma, and Noxa (belongs to BH3-only proteins). The activity of BH3-only proteins is modulated by sensors of cellular stress and damage. If these are upregulated and activated, they can initiate apoptosis.
  - **Creation of channels in mitochondrial membrane:** ***BAX*** and ***BAK*** (proapoptotic proteins) form oligomers that insert into the mitochondrial membrane. This allow proteins from the inner mitochondrial membrane to create channels in the mitochondrial membrane. This allows release of several **mitochondrial** proteins from the inner mitochondrial membrane to leak out into the cytosol (cytoplasm).
  - **Release of cytochrome c:** One of the proteins that leaks from mitochondria into cytosol (cytoplasm) is **cytochrome c.** Once released into the cytosol, cytochrome c binds to a protein called **apoptosis-activating factor-1 (Apaf-1)** and forms an important caspase activator complex called **apoptosome** (multimeric structure). This complex binds to caspase-9, which is the critical initiator caspase of the mitochondrial (intrinsic) pathway.
  - **Activation of caspase cascade**: Binding of apoptosome to caspase-9 promotes autocatalytic cleavage of adjacent caspase-9 molecules. Cleavage activates caspase-9, which triggers a cascade of caspase activation by cleaving and thereby activating other procaspases (such as caspase-3). The active enzymes mediate the execution phase of apoptosis

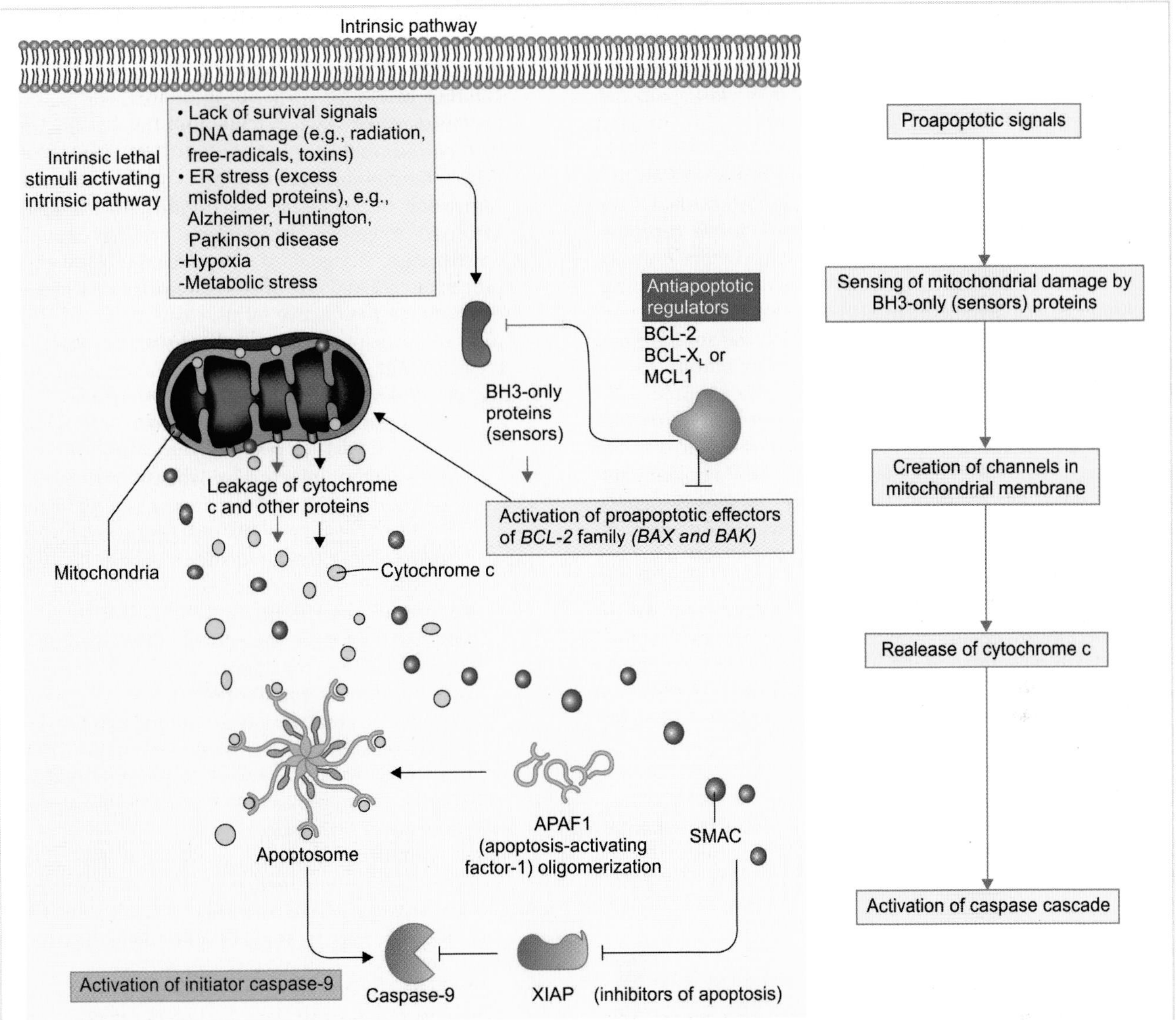

FIG. 16: Steps in the activation of in intrinsic (mitochondrial) pathway of apoptosis. Mitochondrial pathway is the major mechanism involved in the initiation of apoptosis. In this pathway, proteins of the BCL2 family become imbalanced. Normally, BCL2 family regulate mitochondrial permeability. Imbalancing of BCL2 family leads to increased pro-apoptotic proteins compared to anti-apoptotic proteins. This results in the leakage of various substances from mitochondria that lead to activation of caspase [XIAP is a member of the inhibitor of apoptosis family of proteins (IAP)]

Box 2: Causes of mitochondrial injury that trigger apoptosis.

Proapoptotic signals include:

- Deprivation/withdrawal of growth factor or survival signals
- Deoxyribonucleic acid (DNA) damage by radiation, cytotoxic anticancer drugs, hypoxia either directly or through free radical
- Accumulation of excessive amount of misfolded proteins (endoplasmic reticulum stress)
- Increased intracellular free calcium

○ **Blockage of inhibitor of apoptosis**: The cytoplasm of the normal cells contains proteins which block the activation of caspases and function as physiologic **inhibitors of apoptosis (called IAPs)**. The normal function of the IAPs is to prevent the activation of caspases, including executioners like caspase-3 (involved in execution phase), and keep cells alive. Other mitochondrial proteins such as Smac/Diablo also enter the cytoplasm from mitochondria. These proteins bind to and **neutralize** physiologic IAPs present in the cytoplasm. Thus, the neutralization of these IAPs allows the initiation of a caspase cascade.

Extrinsic (death receptor-initiated) pathway of apoptosis (Fig. 17): Extrinsic pathway of apoptosis is **initiated by extracellular signals** and involves receptor-ligand interactions at the cell membrane. Receptors involved in extrinsic pathway of apoptosis are called as death-receptors (i.e., they trigger apoptosis).

Many cells express "death-receptors" molecules on the surface of plasma membrane that trigger apoptosis. Death receptors are **member of the tumor necrosis factor receptor (TNFR) family.** These receptors contain a cytoplasmic domain called the **death domain** because it is essential for delivering apoptotic signals. Death domains consist of specific amino acid sequences in the cytoplasmic tails of these transmembrane receptors. They act as docking (anchoring or binding) sites for the corresponding death domains of other proteins. In the extrinsic (death receptor) pathway, **apoptosis is initiated when** the **death receptors** present get **activated**. It is to be noted that some TNF receptor family members do not contain cytoplasmic death domains. These receptors their function is to activate inflammatory cascades. Their role in triggering apoptosis is less established.

- **Receptors and ligands**
  - **Receptors:** The **well-known** cell membrane **death receptors belong to TNFR family.** The two classic death receptors are the type I TNFR **(TNFR1)** and Fas (CD95). The ligand for receptor **TNFR1** is TNFα. Fas death receptor is expressed on many cell types and the binding ligand for Fas is called Fas ligand (FasL/CD95L).
  - **Ligands:** TNFα is a soluble cytokine, whereas FasL is a membrane protein found at the plasma membrane expressed mainly on activated T lymphocytes (CTLs). CTLs recognize self antigens and functions to eliminate self-reactive lymphocytes and some CTLs kill virus-infected and tumor cells.
- **Steps in extrinsic pathway (Fig. 17)**
  - **Binding of ligand with receptor:** Extrinsic pathway becomes activated when TNFR and Fas/CD95 bind to their corresponding ligands namely, TNFα and CD95L/FasL at the cell surface.
  - **Activation of caspases:** After binding to the ligand-activated receptors, the docking proteins stimulate downstream signaling molecules, especially procaspases-8 and -10. These inactive procaspases are converted to their active forms, caspases-8 and -10. In turn, these caspases activate downstream caspases in the execution pathway of apoptosis. FasL binding to its receptor is described in detail here.
    - **Binding of FasL to Fas receptor:** As described previously, FasL is a membrane protein found at the plasma membrane expressed mainly on activated T lymphocytes (CTLs). When these T cells containing ligand FasL recognize Fas-expressing targets (with Fas receptors), Fas molecules are cross-linked by FasL.
    - **Activation of caspases:** When FasL binds to Fas, three or more molecules of Fas are brought together. The cytoplasmic death domains of Fas receptor bind to an **adapter protein.** This adapter protein also contains a death domain and is called Fas-associated death domain (FADD). FADD in turn binds to procaspase-8 (an inactive form of caspase-8) or caspase-10, via a death domain and generates active caspase-8.
- **Execution pathway:** Activated caspase-8 activates Multiple downstream caspases and mediates the execution phase of apoptosis. Active caspase-8 initiates the same executioner caspase sequence as in the mitochondrial (intrinsic) pathway.
- **Inhibition of extrinsic pathway of apoptosis:** This pathway can be inhibited by a protein called FLIP. Since, this protein does not have protease domain, it cannot cleave and activate the caspase. FLIP [FLICE (FADD-like IL-1β-converting enzyme)-inhibitory protein] act as an inhibitor by binding to procaspase-8 without cleaving or activating it. Some viruses as well as normal cells produce FLIP and use this method of inhibition to protect themselves from Fas-mediated apoptosis.
- **Functions of extrinsic pathway** are listed in **Box 3.**

The extrinsic and intrinsic pathways of apoptosis are initiated by different ways by distinct molecules. However, there may be interconnections between these two. For example, in hepatocytes and pancreatic β cells, caspase-8

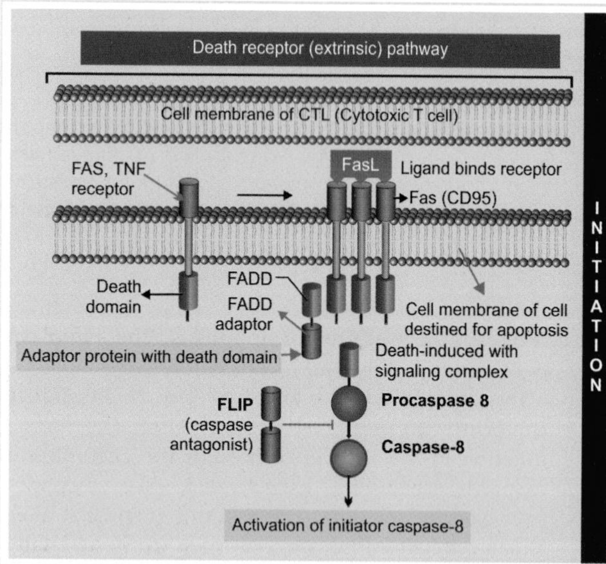

(FADD: Fas-associated death domain; FasL: Fas ligand, FLIP: FLICE[FADD-like IL-1β-converting enzyme]-inhibitory protein)

FIG. 17: Steps in extrinsic pathway of apoptosis. In the extrinsic (death receptor) pathway, signals from plasma membrane receptors lead to the assembly of adaptor proteins into a "death-inducing signaling complex." This activates caspase-8 (initiator caspase of extrinsic pathway).

Box 3: Functions of extrinsic pathway.

Extrinsic pathway of apoptosis is **involved in eliminating:**

- **Self-reactive lymphocytes** thereby avoiding autoimmunity. FasL is expressed on T cells that recognize self-antigens and function to eliminate self-reactive lymphocytes
- **Killing of target cells:** This is by some cytotoxic T lymphocytes (CTLs) that express FasL
  - **Virus infected cells** through CTLs
  - **Tumor cells** through CTLs

produced by Fas signaling (extrinsic pathway) cleaves and activates the BH3-only protein BID (intrinsic pathway). BID activates the mitochondrial pathway. The combined activation of both extrinsic ands intrinsic pathways produces a fatal effect to the cells.

Execution Phase of Apoptosis (Fig. 18)

Q. Write short note on caspase-3.

Q. Explain the action of caspase-3.

The above mentioned **two initiating pathways converge to a cascade of caspase activation, which mediates the final execution phase of apoptosis.** The initiator caspases produced by the **mitochondrial pathway is the initiator caspase-9,** and the **death receptor (extrinsic) pathway is the initiator caspase-8 and -10.**

- The initiator caspases activate another series of caspases called **"effector" or "executioner" caspases (such as caspase-3, -6, and -7)** that mediate the final phase of apoptosis.
- **Caspase-3:** It is the most commonly activated effector caspase. It acts on many cellular components. Once activated, these caspases cleave an inhibitor of a cytoplasmic DNase and thus make the DNase enzymatically active. DNase enzyme degrades structural components of nuclear matrix and causes fragmentation of nucleus [e.g., caspase-activated DNase (CAD), which degrades chromosomal DNA]. Caspase-3 also destabilizes the cytoskeleton as the involved cells begin to fragment into apoptotic bodies.

Removal of apoptotic cells

Phagocytosis: Apoptosis results in formation of apoptotic bodies. These are broken into small fragments that can be easily phagocytosed by phagocytic cells. Apoptotic cells and bodies are engulfed and removed by phagocytic cells (mainly macrophages). The phagocytosis is so efficient that these dead cells and apoptotic bodies disappear within minutes without leaving a trace evidence. Even when the apoptosis is extensive, their rapid removal prevents release of their cellular contents which may elicit inflammation. Macrophages that have ingested apoptotic cells produce reduced amount of pro-inflammatory cytokines. The process of apoptotic cell phagocytosis is called **efferocytosis.**

- **Factors favoring phagocytosis:** The apoptotic cells and apoptotic bodies undergo several changes in their membranes and produce signals that favor phagocytosis of these cells/bodies.
- **Expression of phosphatidylserine (PS):** In healthy cells, phosphatidylserine is present on the inner leaflet of the plasma membrane. In cells undergoing apoptosis, phosphatidylserine turns out and is expressed on the outer layer of the membrane causing easy recognition by receptors present on the macrophage.

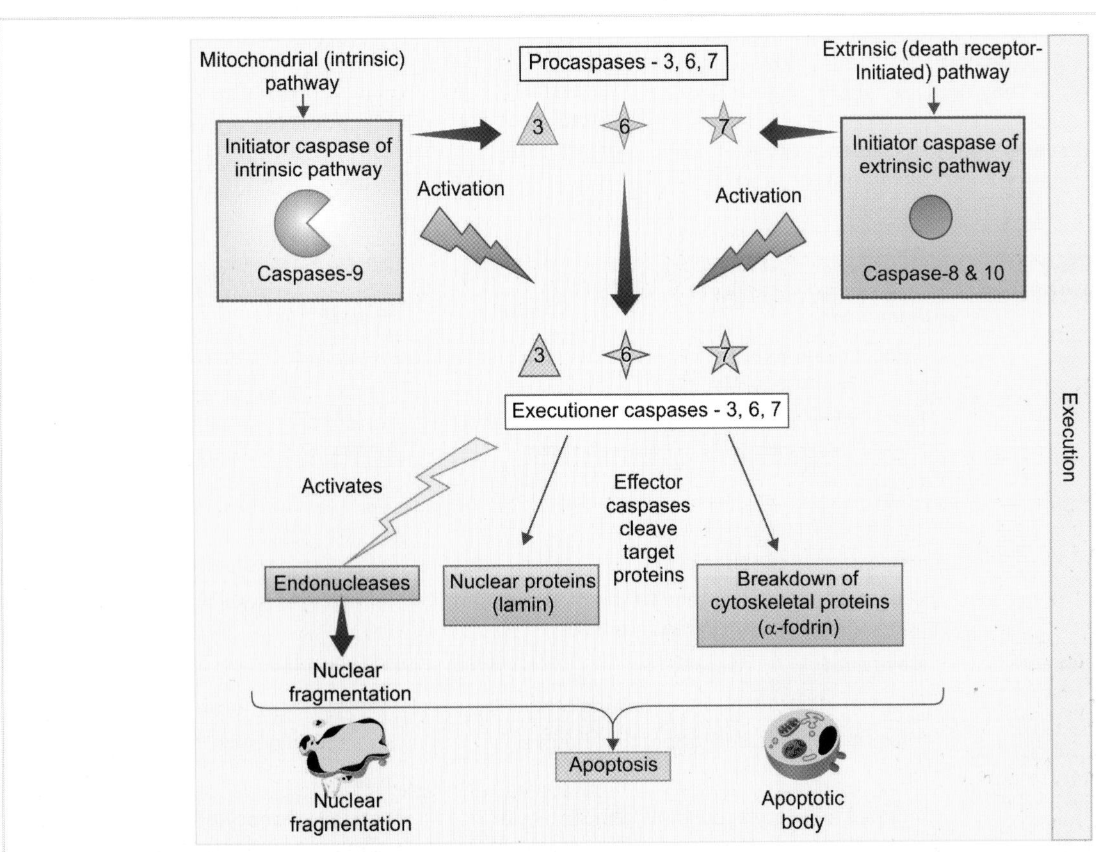

FIG. 18: Execution pathway of apoptosis. Two initiating pathways converge to a cascade of caspase activation. They mediate the final execution phase of apoptosis. The initiator caspases produced by the mitochondrial pathway is the initiator caspase-9, and the death receptor (extrinsic) pathway is the initiator caspase-8 and -10.The initiator caspases activate caspases called "effector" or "executioner" caspases (such as caspase-3, -6, and -7) that mediate the final phase of apoptosis.

- **Secretion of soluble factors: Apoptotic cells secrete soluble factors** (e.g., **thrombospondin**) that recruit phagocytes.
- **Natural antibodies and proteins of the complement system** (notably C1q) may coat apoptotic bodies which aid in phagocytosis.

Diagnosis/detection of apoptosis

- Deoxyribonucleic acid fragmentation assay is carried out by electrophoresis of genomic DNA. Apoptosis produces "step ladder pattern" in contrast to smeared pattern seen in necrosis.
- **T**erminal deoxynucleotidyl transferase biotin d-**UTP N**ick **E**nd **L**abeling (TUNEL) technique for in vivo detection of apoptosis.
- Chromatin condensation seen by H&E, Feulgen, and acridine orange staining.
- Estimation of:
  - Cytosolic cytochrome c
  - Activated caspase
  - Annexin V: Apoptotic cells express phosphatidylserine (PS) on the outer layer of plasma membrane because of which these cells are recognized by the dye Annexin.
  - Propidium iodide assay by flow cytometry/fluorescent microscopy.

Disorders Associated with Dysregulated Apoptosis

Disorders with reduced apoptosis

It may allow the survival of abnormal cells.

- **Cancer:** Apoptosis protects against uncontrolled cell proliferation (e.g., cancer) due to mutations in DNA. Reduced apoptosis may lead to cancer (e.g., follicular lymphoma).
- **Autoimmune disease:** Apoptosis is necessary for correct progression of embryologic development, elimination of self-reactive B and T-lymphocyte clones and many other normal functions. Reduced apoptosis may cause autoimmune diseases.

Disorders with increased apoptosis

This will cause an excessive loss of cells.

- **Neurodegenerative diseases (Alzheimer, Huntington, Parkinson disease)**
- **Ischemic injury:** In myocardial infarction and stroke.
- **Death of virus-infected cells:** Many viral infections, important being acquired immune deficiency syndrome (**AIDS**).

Clinical Significance of Apoptosis in Cancers

- Normally, cells with damaged (mutated) DNA are cleared in the body by undergoing apoptosis.
- Apoptosis may be reduced in some cancers. Best established role of BCL-2 in protecting tumor cells from undergoing apoptosis is observed in **follicular lymphoma**. In this type of nonHodgkin lymphoma of B cell origin, there **is translocation (14; 18) (q32; q21)** which causes **over expression of antiapoptotic protein BCL-2.** This in turn increases the BCL-2/BCL-XL buffer, **protecting abnormal B lymphocytes from undergoing apoptosis** and allows them to survive for long periods.

Differences between apoptosis and necrosis are summarized in **Table 4**.

Pathways of Cell Death Other than Necrosis and Apoptosis

Programmed and regulated forms of cell death serve diverse functions. The balance between cellular differentiation, proliferation, and PCD (programmed cell death) is very important for embryonic development, organ function,

Table 4: Differences between apoptosis and necrosis.

Features	***Apoptosis***	***Necrosis***
Cause	Often physiological, means of eliminating unwanted cells; may also be pathological	Invariably pathological
Biochemical events	Energy-dependent fragmentation of deoxyribonucleic acid (DNA) by endogenous endonucleases	Impairment or cessation of ion homeostasis
Lysosomes	Intact	Leak lytic enzymes
Morphology		
Extent	Single or small cluster of cells	Involves group of cells
Cell size	Cell reduced (shrinkage) and fragmentation to form apoptotic bodies with dense chromatin	Cell enlarged (swelling) and undergo lysis
Integrity of cell membrane	Maintained	Disrupted/lost
Nucleus	Fragmentation into nucleosome-size fragments	Pyknosis, karyorrhexis, karyolysis
Cellular contents	Intact; may be released in apoptotic bodies	Enzymatic digestion; may leak out of cell
Adjacent inflammatory response	None	Usual
Fate of dead cells	Ingested (phagocytosed) by neighboring cells	Ingested (phagocytosed) by neutrophil polymorphs and macrophages
DNA electrophoresis	DNA laddering is seen	Shows smearing effect
Terminal deoxynucleotidyl transferase biotin d-**UTP N**ick **E**nd **L**abeling (TUNEL) staining	Positive	Negative

tumorigenesis, and immune responses during life. When apoptotic cells are not cleared by phagocytic (macrophages) cells, an accidental form of cell death develops. Apoptosis may be physiological or pathological. Necrosis is always pathological and results in the nonspecific release of cellular contents. This can elicit inflammation and organ damage. Therefore, necrosis is considered as a sign of injury, stress, or infection.

Classification of Programmed Cell Death

Necrosis and apoptosis are two usual forms of death. Apart from necrosis and apoptosis, few other pattern alternatives to apoptosis have been described that have certain unusual features. Originally, the term PCD (programmed cell death) was synonymous with apoptosis, but now this includes other forms (**Box 4**). Though their importance in disease is not clear, they are under research, and it is necessary to have a knowledge of these basic concepts.

Necroptosis

Q. Write short essay on necroptosis.

The two best-defined and common forms of cell death are necrosis and apoptosis. In necrosis, the morphological features include cellular swelling, fragmentation of plasma membrane, and nuclear pyknosis, followed by an inflammatory response. In contrast the features in apoptosis are blebbing of plasma membrane and fragmentation of nuclei without inflammation.

Definition: Necroptosis or signaled necrosis is a type of cell death that **shows features of both necrosis and apoptosis**. It **resembles necrosis but is caspase-independent** (apoptosis is caspase dependent). It resembles morphologically necrosis and mechanistically apoptosis. Morphologically, and to some extent biochemically, it resembles necrosis. Both necrosis and necroptosis are characterized by loss of ATP, swelling of the cell and organelles, production of reactive oxygen species (ROS), release of lysosomal enzymes, and rupture of the plasma membrane. Mechanistically, it resembles apoptosis. Both necroptosis and apoptosis are brought out by signal transduction pathways that terminate in death of the cell death. Because of these overlapping features, necroptosis is **sometimes termed as programmed necrosis**. This term is used to distinguish necroptosis from necrosis caused by toxic or ischemic injury to the cell. In contrast to apoptosis, the signals leading to necroptosis are not accompanied by activation of caspase. Hence, it is also sometimes called as "caspase-independent" programmed cell death.

Box 4: List of programmed cell death.

- Apoptosis
- Necroptosis
- Pyroptosis
- Anoikis
- NETosis
- Entosis
- Pyronecrosis
- Autophagy-associated cell death
- Ferroptosis

Mechanism of Necroptosis (Fig. 19): Necroptosis form of cell death can be initiated in several ways. But commonly it starts in a similar manner to that of the extrinsic pathway of apoptosis, that is, by binding of ligand FasL or tumor necrosis factor-α (TNF-α) to respective receptors. The extrinsic pathway of apoptosis also involves downstream of TNFRs. But in necroptosis, binding of a ligand to receptor results in formation of a protein complex. This interacts with two kinases called **receptor-interacting protein (RIP) kinases** namely **RIP1 and RIP3**. This causes phosphorylation of RIP3. Phosphorylated RIP3 can lead to necroptosis by several paths.

- Phosphorylated RIP3 increases the formation of reactive oxygen species (ROS).
- Damage to mitochondria leads to release of apoptosis-inducing factor (AIF) and also reduces the production of adenosine triphosphate (ATP). AIF triggers DNase activity and enters the nucleus. In the nucleus it activates DNA degradation and leads to nuclear pyknosis.
- RIP3 is the important protein in this process. It increases the cytosolic Ca^{2+} that leads to activation of Ca^{2+}-dependent degradative enzymes (e.g., calpains). These enzymes damage the lysosomal membrane and release lysosomal enzymes (e.g., hydrolase) into the cytosol.

Significance: It initiates a series of events that result in death of the cell, much like necrosis.

- **Physiological:** Under physiologic circumstances, necroptosis participates in **development**, especially at the **bone growth plate**. Normally, it is also active in some adult tissues such as the lower portion of the intestinal crypts.
- **Pathological:** If physiologic apoptosis is not available to cells, necroptosis may become the default cell death pathway. It is associated with cell death in steato-hepatitis,vacute pancreatitis,and ischemia-reperfusion injury. It may be an important mechanism of cell death in cancer cells in which apoptotic pathways are blocked. It is important in limiting the spread of certain viral infections that encode caspase inhibitors (e.g., cytomegalovirus). It is believed that some infections kill the cells by this pathway. It may play a role in ischemia/reperfusion injury and other pathologic conditions, especially those associated with inflammatory reactions in which there is production of cytokine TNF. Necroptosis is a double-edged sword and may participate in pathologic processes such as neurodegenerative diseases such as Parkinson disease. However, its exact role in human diseases is not understood.

Pyroptosis

Introduction: The presence of infectious pathogens (microbes) is recognized through receptors present on cells. There are many cellular receptors for microbes which detect pathogens, or the damage induced by them. These receptors recognize simple molecules and regular patterns of molecular structure called **pathogen-associated molecular patterns (PAMPs)** that are part of many microorganisms but not of the host body's own cells. Hence, such cell membrane receptors for microbes are known as "**pattern recognition receptors (PRRs)**".

Pyroptosis is a type of PCD (programmed cell death) and bears some biochemical similarities with apoptosis. Apoptosis and inflammation coexist in pyroptosis. The inflammation is frequently manifested by fever. It is termed pyroptosis because

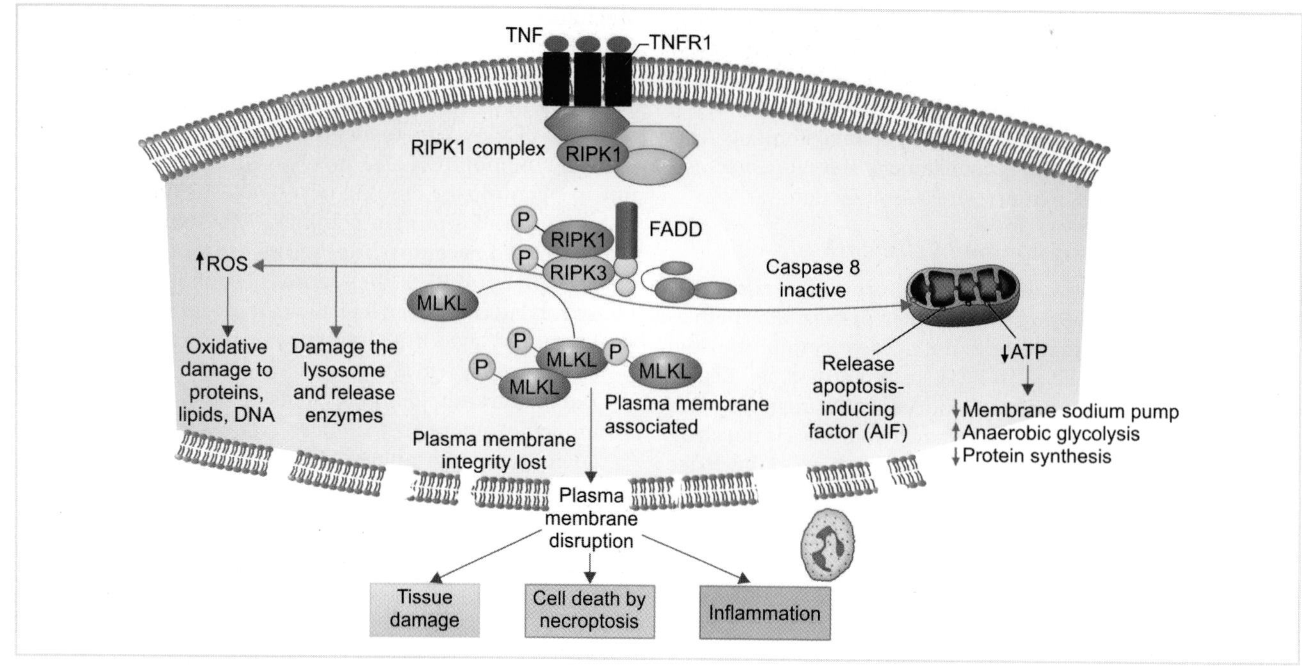

FIG. 19: Mechanism of necroptosis. Binding of a ligand tumor necrosis factor α (TNFα) to a death receptor TNFR1 results in formation of a protein complex that binds receptor-interacting protein kinases [RIPKs (1 and 3). This causes phosphorylation of RIP3. In turn RIPK3 phosphorylates a cytoplasmic protein called MLKL. In response to its phosphorylation, MLKL monomers assemble into oligomers. These oligomers translocate from the cytosol to the plasma membrane. It disrupts the plasma similar to that of necrosis. Phosphorylated RIP3 can lead to necroptosis by several paths namely (i) generating reactive oxygen species (ROS), damaging mitochondria and lysosomes.

of the association of apoptosis with fever (Greek, *pyro* = fire) due to inflammation.

Mechanism of pyroptosis (Fig. 20): Many infectious agents (particularly viruses, but also bacteria and others) interact with diverse **PRRs.**

- **Inflammasomes:** These are a group of multiprotein cytosolic complex of the innate immune system. It consists of an inflammasome sensor molecule, the adaptor protein apoptosis-associated speck-like protein containing a CARD (ASC) (is a procaspase-1 activator which connects inflammasome to procaspase-1), and **inactive procaspase-1**. Inflammasomes recognize/detect pathogenic microorganisms, exogenous agents, and sterile stressors via different kinds of cytosolic PRRs. PRRs respond to either PAMPs that are part of many microorganisms or DAMPs liberated or altered due to cell damage. Inflammasome formation is triggered by a range of substances that emerge during infections, irritative injurious agents (e.g., mineral crystals), tissue damage, or metabolic imbalances. When inflammasome-linked receptors are activated, the inflammasomes activate procaspase-1 and convert it into active form, caspase-1. Caspase-1 is the best-described inflammatory caspase [which was previously called interleukin (IL) 1ß-converting enzyme]. Inflammasome activation causes a rapid, proinflammatory form of cell death called pyroptosis. This caspase-1 proteolytically activates the proinflammatory, fever-inducing cytokines IL-1β and IL-18. This is to be noted that although caspase-1 is a cysteine protease involved in pyroptosis, it is independent of apoptotic signaling, and its activation does not result in apoptosis.
- **Actions of caspase-1**: Once activated, caspase-1 has following actions:
  - Cleaves the enzymes that are needed for glycolysis and this results in depletion of cellular energy. The important intracellular substrates, including cytoskeleton, chaperones, and glycolytic proteins are cleaved.
  - Caspase-1 produces ion-permeable plasma pores. This allows inflow of water and solutes into the cell and leads to cellular swelling and allows leakage of intracellular components out of the dying cell.
  - Produces DNA fragmentation and nuclear pyknosis.
  - Activates many proinflammatory cytokines and along with the dead cell induces inflammation. The inflammation is frequently manifested by fever accompanied by the release of fever producing cytokine IL-1 and may trigger apoptosis. Caspase-1 and the closely related caspases-4 and -5 also produce death of the cells.

Significance: Pyroptosis contributes to **innate immune defense** and has a host-protective role against dangerous pathogens. Probably it is one mechanism by which some infectious microbes cause the death of infected cells. It has been thought that it may be involved in the pathogenesis of metabolic syndrome and the etiology of type 2 diabetes mellitus. Its role in other pathological conditions is not known.

Anoikis

Anoikis (Greek: "homelessness"), is also called "detachment induced apoptosis" or "integrin-mediated death," is a type of apoptosis that develops in epithelial cells. It is necessary for the

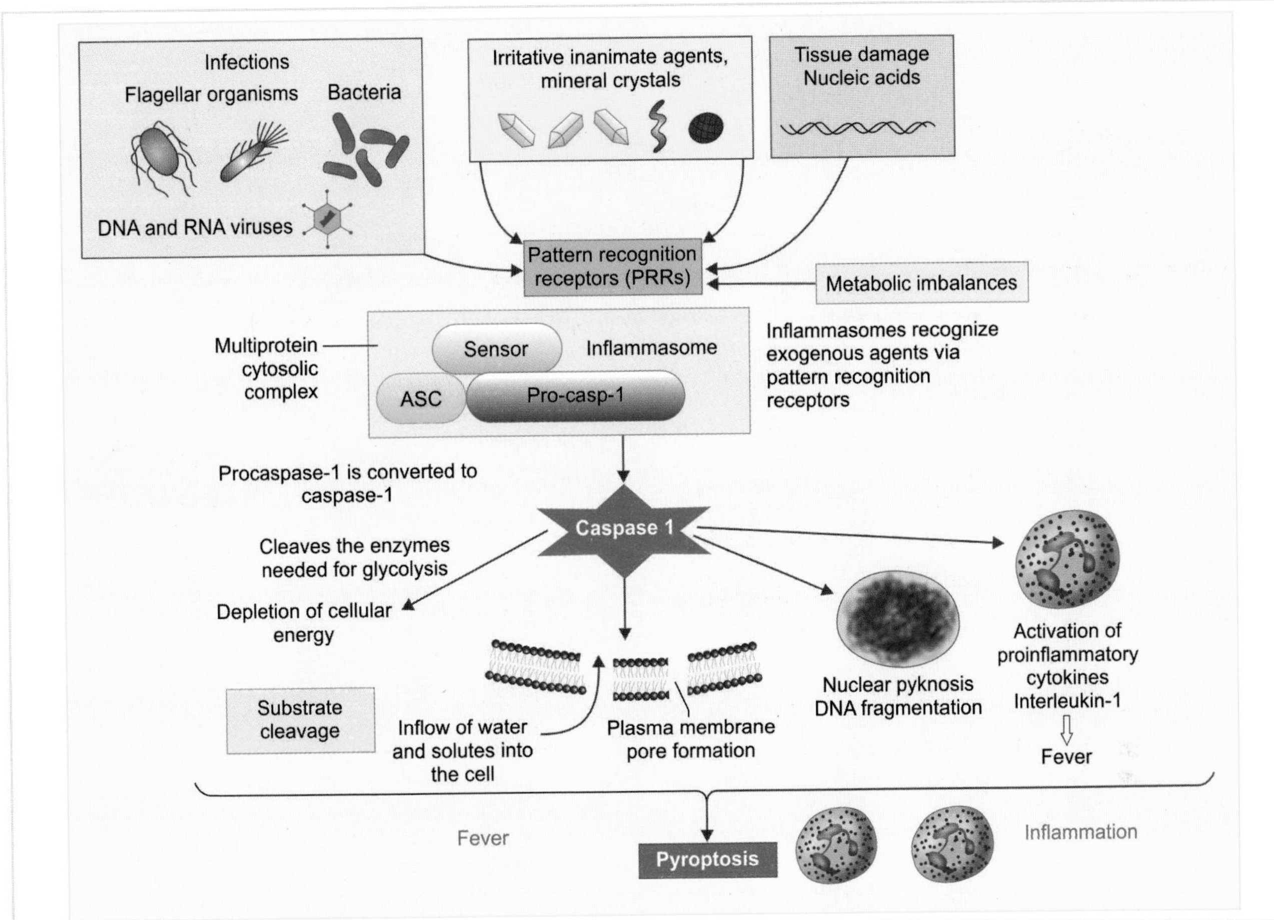

FIG. 20: Mechanism of pyroptosis. When the cell is exposed to injurious agents (both infectious and irritative), inflammasome multiprotein complexes recognize these exogenous agents via diverse pattern recognition receptors (e.g., pattern recognition receptors). Inflammasomes contain, adaptor protein apoptosis-associated speck-like protein containing a CARD (ASC) (is a procaspase-1 activator) which links it to inactive precursor called procaspase-1. When inflammasome-linked receptors are activated, procaspase-1 is converted to active caspase-1. This leads to several consequences. Caspase-1 depletes cellular energy with cleavage of substrate. It creates pores in the plasma membrane and allows leakage of intracellular components out of the dying cell. At the same time, the nucleus is damaged and the important intracellular substrates, including cytoskeleton, chaperones, and glycolytic proteins are cleaved.

cell to correctly bind to the extracellular matrix (ECM) so that the cell is in its correct designated location.

Definition: It is defined as caspase-dependent apoptosis (form of apoptosis) that is induced by inadequate, inappropriate, or nonexistent cell–ECM interactions. It is characterized by detachment of epithelial cells from basement membranes (or ECM) or lack of correct cell adhesion between cells (cell–cell interactions).

Significance of anoikis: Anoikis is activated by loss of cell attachments. It efficiently deletes cells that have been displaced from their proper designated location. It prevents movement of cells or cell clusters from its location to a distant or improper ECM site. Thus, it helps to protect against the development of cancer metastases. Probably tumor associated macrophages may prevent anoikis by expressing adhesion molecules (e.g., integrins) that promote direct physical interactions with tumor cells.

Mechanism of anoikis (Figs. 21A and B): Anoikis is a form of apoptotic cell death triggered by loss of cell's usual binding with familiar ECM constituents.

Normal: Normally, epithelial cells are attached to their native ECM by transmembrane molecules. These include α- and ß-integrins. Integrins mediate prosurvival signals. These transmembrane molecules activate survival signals and block both intrinsic and extrinsic apoptotic signaling pathways.

Loss of attachment: Anoikis involves both intrinsic and extrinsic classical apoptotic pathways. Both the pathways are upregulated or activated when cells becomes detached from each other or from ECM. Anoikis is activated if epithelial cell membrane integrins do not bind to their appropriate ECM partners. When a cell loses contact with neighboring cell or its normal ECM, the cell's integrins are not bound, or not bound by the appropriate ECM moieties. Integrins mediate prosurvival signals and its loss leads to loss of their survival signals. Hence, there is blocking of activation of apoptosis by death receptor signaling and apoptosis may proceed. The detachment of cells from their extracellular ligands makes the cells excessively susceptible to all manners of proapoptotic stimuli. Also, unligated integrins may directly activate caspase-8. For example, cell that is pushed off the tip of an intestinal villus by proliferating cells deeper in the crypts, is stimulated to undergo anoikis. This is due to the loss of integrin-

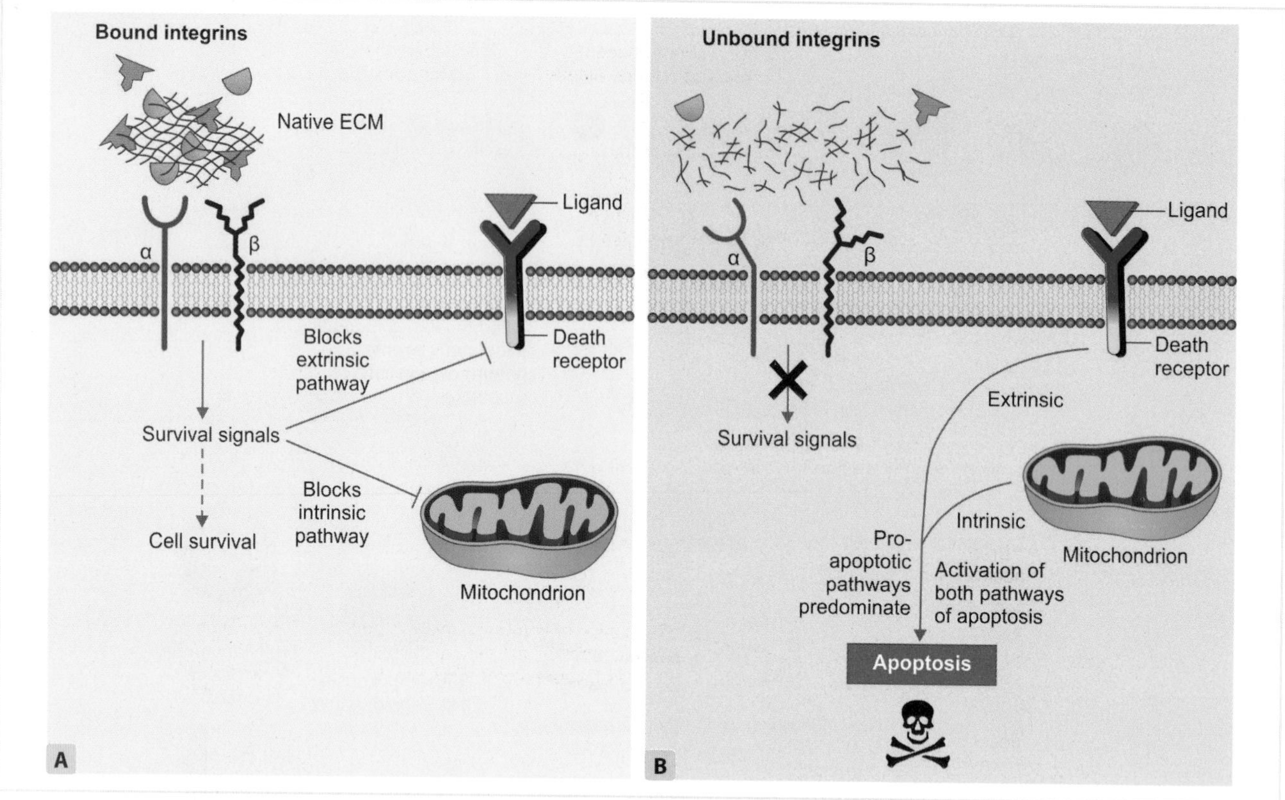

FIGS. 21 A AND B: Diagrammatic representation of mechanisms of anoikis. (A) Normally, epithelial cells are attached to their extracellular matrix (ECM) by transmembrane molecules (including α- and ß-integrins). These transmembrane molecules activate survival signals and block both intrinsic and extrinsic signaling pathways of apoptosis. (B) When the cell's integrins are not bound, or not bound by the appropriate ECM moieties, there is no generation of survival signals. There is also no blockage of apoptosis by death receptor signaling. Therefore, the cell undergoes apoptosis.

mediated survival signaling in the cells at the tip of the villus. Similarly, anoikis may be activated if a detached cancer cell makes contact with inappropriate ECM components. However, in some cancer cells, unbound integrins can maintain survival signaling and so protect from anoikis. This may be achieved by activating TrkB, a suppressor of anoikis.

Neutrophil Extracellular Traps and NETosis

Q. Write a short essay on neutrophil extracellular traps (NETs).

Neutrophils contribute to the defense of the body against infection. Neutrophils engulf ("eat") microbes; produce a range of highly reactive oxygen radicals, which are the most effective means of destroying microbes, and proteolytic enzymes by neutrophils also have an effect on the microbes. NETosis reflects the action of a potent antimicrobial defense mechanism.

Definition: Neutrophil extracellular traps are extracellular fibrillar networks produced by polymorphonuclear granulocytes (mainly neutrophils) in response to infectious pathogens (bacteria and fungi) and inflammatory mediators (e.g., chemokines, cytokines, and complement proteins).

During the formation of NET, the nuclei of the neutrophils are lost, leading to a distinctive form of death of the neutrophils (sometimes termed NETosis). NETs are also formed in the blood during sepsis. Apart from neutrophils, the other polymorphonuclear cells such as eosinophils and basophils also have the ability to undergo a cell death that results in the release of nuclear chromatin and form extracellular traps (ETs). Hence, instead of the more specific terminology of NETs, it was proposed to term as extracellular traps (ETs).

Mechanism (Fig. 22): Neutrophil extracellular traps result from activation of a cell death program, mainly in neutrophils, but also may be in eosinophils and mast cells. This program is termed NETosis. Neutrophils recognize pathogens at the cell surface receptors, and signals acting at the cell surface initiate signaling cascades. These cascades lead to intracellular calcium release, generation of reactive oxygen [by activation of nicotinamide adenine dinucleotide phosphate (NADPH) oxidase], activation of transcription factors that induce the inflammatory response, and activation of autophagy. NETosis needs both autophagy and NADPH oxidase activity and is characterized by destruction of the cell's nuclear envelope and the membranes of most cytoplasmic granules in the neutrophils. This causes **relaxation** (disaggregation/decondensation) **of chromatin** through the action of peptidyl arginine deiminase 4 (PAD4) present in the cytoplasmic granules of neutrophils and eosinophils. Chromatin escapes from the nucleus into cytosol. The intracellular chromatin becomes spread over wide area (dispersed) and the membranes of cytoplasmic

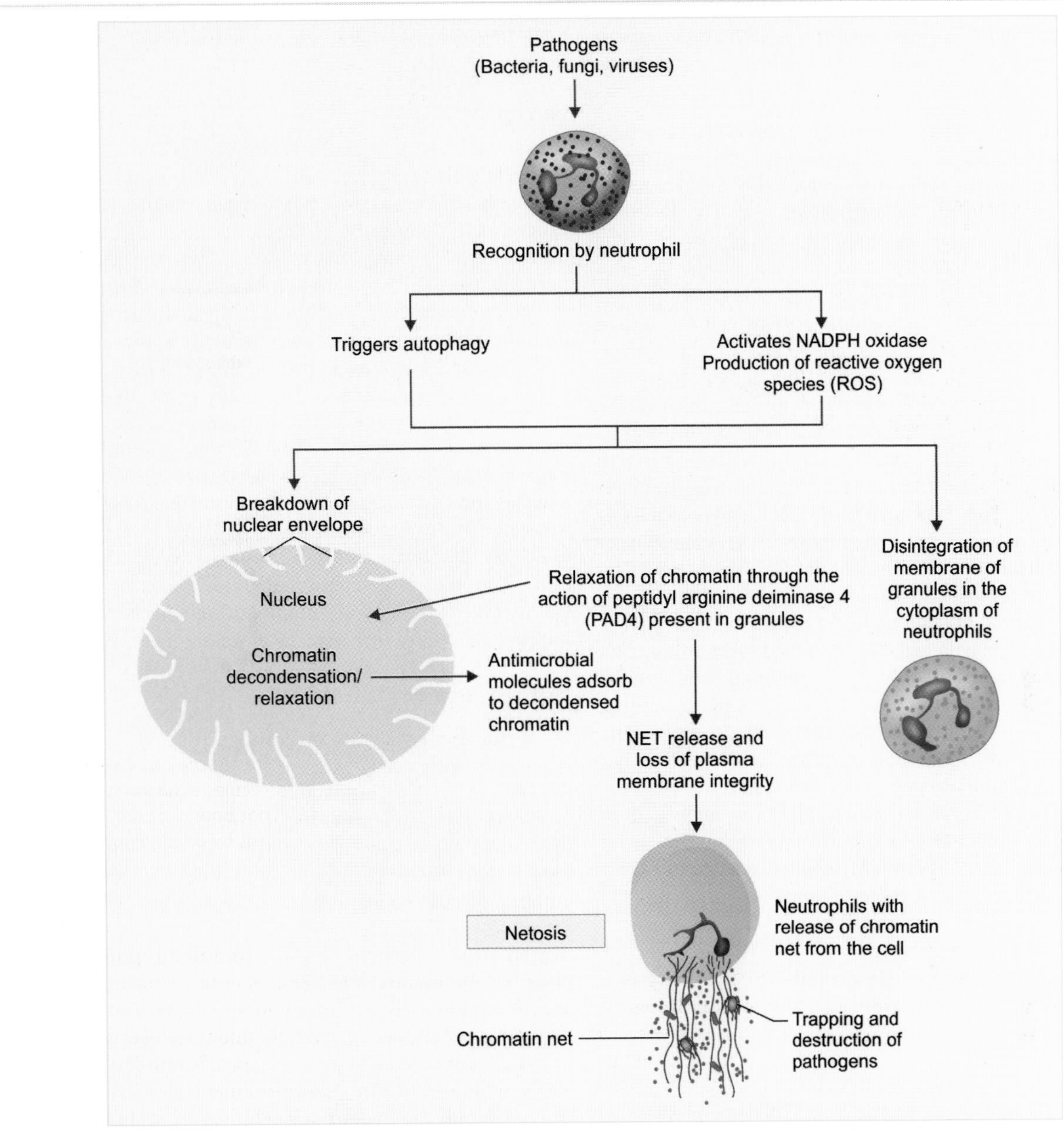

FIG. 22: Steps involved in NETosis. Neutrophils recognize pathogens and activate autophagy and nicotinamide adenine dinucleotide phosphate (NADPH) oxidase. NETosis needs both autophagy and NADPH oxidase activity. The neutrophils NADPH oxidase produces reactive oxygen species (ROS). These changes cause breakdown of membranes of cytoplasmic granules and the nuclear membrane. Peptidyl arginine deiminase 4 (PAD4) present in the cytoplasmic granules of neutrophils and eosinophils causes dispersion and relaxation of nuclear chromatin of neutrophils. NETotic activity releases the neutrophil chromatin traps containing antimicrobial histones and histone cleavage products. These traps can catch and destroy the pathogens.

granules breakup (disintegrate). NETotic activity leads to release of chromatin net from cells as neutrophil chromatin traps (NETs). NET contains both chromatin and strongly microbicidal histones and histone cleavage products. These traps then catch and destroy pathogens.

Neutrophil extracellular traps may be composed of either nuclear or mitochondrial chromatin. Hence, it does not necessarily need self-sacrifice of the neutrophil to contribute the chromatin network of NETs. Unlike apoptotic cells, neutrophils and other cells susceptible to NETosis do not present the signals that are characteristic of apoptosis. Hence, NETotic cells are not removed by macrophages and are capable to stimulate inflammatory responses.

Composition: Neutrophil extracellular traps consist of a viscous meshwork of nuclear chromatin (includes histones and associated DNA) that binds and concentrates granule proteins such as antimicrobial peptides and enzymes.

Function: Neutrophil extracellular traps function as chromatin traps for bacteria and other pathogens. NETs **concentrate antimicrobial substances** (products) **at sites of infection and prevent the spread of the microbes** by trapping them in the fibrils. These formations can kill bacterial, fungal, and protozoal pathogens and it is a nonphagocytic **mechanism of killing microbes**. It constitutes an important host defense from infection.

Significance: The nuclear chromatin in the NETs may be a source of nuclear antigens in systemic autoimmune diseases (e.g., lupus). In these patients, there is immunological reaction against their own DNA and nucleoproteins.

Entosis (Fig. 23)

Entosis is a nonapoptotic cell-death program in which there is a type of cellular cannibalism. In this a cell-eats-cell and causes cell death. In entosis, matrix-detached cells are involved in the invasion of one cell into another. The cells that are not professional phagocytes engulf nearby living cells. This leads to a transient state in which a live cell is contained within a host. The internalized (engulfed) cells may either die or survive. Vacuoles containing the internalized cells (cannibalized cell) may fuse with lysosomes of aggressor cell. These entotic cells are degraded by lysosomal enzymes in which case, target cells usually die. The death is not an inevitable outcome. The cannibalized cell, or parts thereof, may survive the process. The nuclear material of cannibalized cell may become part of the aggressor phagocytic cell. This can lead to multinucleate cells, polyploidy or aneuploidy. Some engulfed cells actually escape the destruction by aggressive cell and re-emerge without suffering any injury, damage, or harm. The phagocytic aggressor cells may engulf cells of either the same or other lineages. For example, hepatocytes may ingest and destroy autoreactive T lymphocytes, thus can inhibit development of autoimmune liver disease. This cell internalization process is more often found "cell-in-cell" cytological feature in tumor cells. Mechanisms of entosis are not known.

Pyronecrosis

Pyronecrosis is a recently described cell death. It is a proinflammatory cell-death pathway and has morphological features characteristic of necrosis. Pyronecrotic cells do not have DNA fragmentation, nor is there a loss of mitochondrial membrane potential.

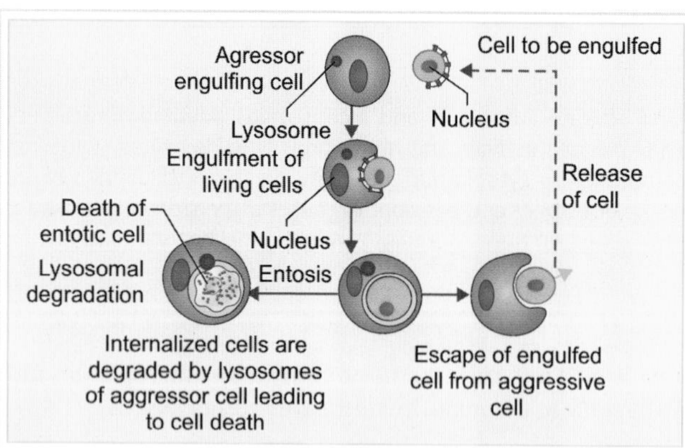

FIG. 23: Steps in entosis. Cells that are not professional phagocytes engulf nearby living cells. The internalized (engulfed) cells may either die or survive. Vacuoles containing the internalized cells (cannibalized cell) may fuse with lysosomes of aggressor cell. These entotic cells are degraded by lysosomal enzymes in which case, target cells usually die. The death is not an inevitable outcome. The cannibalized cell, or parts thereof, may survive the process and escape from aggressive cells.

Ferroptosis

It was discovered in 2012. Ferroptosis is a distinct form of cell death. It is triggered when there are excessive levels of intracellular iron or reactive oxygen species (ROS) which exceeds the defense by glutathione-dependent antioxidant mechanism. This causes unchecked membrane lipid peroxidation. The widespread peroxidation of lipids disrupts the many functions of membrane. These disturbed functions include fluidity, lipid-protein interactions, ion and nutrient transport, and signaling pathways. There is loss of permeability of plasma membrane and this finally result in death of the cell resembling necrosis. As the name indicates (ferro=iron), the process is regulated by specific signals (unlike necrosis) namely iron. Thus, ferroptosis can be prevented by reducing iron levels. Ultrastructurally, ferroptosis shows loss of the mitochondrial cristae and rupture of the outer membrane of the mitochondria. Though its role in normal development and physiology is not clear, ferroptosis may be involved in cell death in a variety of human pathologies such as cancer, neurodegenerative diseases, and stroke.

Autophagy

Q. Write short essay on autophagy.

Autophagy (Greek: "*auto*", self; "*phagy*", eating hence means "self-eating"/"eating oneself") is a highly conserved catabolic process of **digestion** (degradation) **of the cell's own old/ aged organelle or components contents** by lysosomes. In autophagy, cells collect intracellular proteins, cytoplasm and organelles and deliver them to lysosomes, where they are degraded and recycled. Lysosomes play an important **role in organelle turnover** by regulated destruction of the cell's own organelles. Lysosomes degrade many old (senescent organelles) or unnecessary cellular constituents (components) or large protein complexes that have become obsolete for the cell or organism. In 2016, Nobel Prize was awarded to Yoshinori Ohsumi for his discoveries of mechanism of autophagy.

Major Functions of Autophagy

There are two major functions of autophagy.

1. **To remove damaged or unnecessary proteins and organelles:** Autophagy facilitates the **turnover of aged and defunct cellular constituents**. This is commonly referred to as the **protein and organelle quality control function** of autophagy. It maintains functional homeostasis among cellular proteins and organelles in normal conditions as well as during stress. Autophagy is decisive to the balance between cell survival, death, and adaptation. It operates continuously and is required for cell homeostasis and survival. Autophagy acts as on-going physiological quality control mechanism protecting from, e.g., excess production of ROS, by inefficient or damaged mitochondria.
2. **To degrade and recycle intracellular components:** This is performed to sustain metabolism and homeostasis in the absence of external nutrients. This is commonly referred to as the **catabolic function** of autophagy. Autophagy is **a survival mechanism** that is used to protect the cells when

there is **deprivation of nutrients** (e.g., when nutrients are lacking as in starvation or compromised blood supply) and may be associated with atrophy of tissues. This adaptation may be a survival mechanism that preserves the viability/survival of the starved cell during depletion of nutrients. The cells survive by eating its own contents and recycling these contents to provide nutrients and energy. However, if the starved cell can no longer survive by eating its contents, autophagy may lead to cell death by apoptosis.

Both the above functions (quality control and catabolic functions) of autophagy promote cell and tissue homeostasis and survival. In most circumstances this suppresses or delays cell death by both apoptosis and necrosis and promote cellular health. Autophagy occurs at a low basal level in normal cells and tissues. It is greatly upregulated by stress and starvation. This is important for cellular survival and homeostasis. Variations of autophagy can capture and degrade intracellular pathogens and contribute to host defense.

Functional role of autophagy is listed in **Box 5**.

Categories

Autophagic degradation can be divided into three categories, depending on mechanism—how it is carried out and delivered to lysosomes. These include: (1) **macroautophagy, (2) microautophagy, and (3) chaperone-mediated autophagy**. In all the three categories, the final common pathway of destruction of cell components is in lysosomes.

Box 5: Functional role of autophagy.

- Clearance of misfolded or damaged proteins and organelles
- Recycling of cellular organelles and macromolecules during starvation, ischemia
- Host defense (role in infection): Can degrade proinflammatory cytokine production
- Protection from tumorigenesis
- Protect from neurodegeneration

Mechanism of macroautophagy

Cellular stresses (e.g.,nutrient deprivation) activate an autophagy pathway (**Fig. 24**). Autophagy proceeds through several phases (i) initiation, nucleation, and elongation of isolation membrane, (ii) formation and maturation of autophagosome, (iii) usion with lysosome and formation of autophagolysosome and (iv) digestion or degradation.

- First step is **nucleation and formation of an isolation membrane**. It is called as a *phagophore*. During autophagy, an obsolete/used intracellular organelle (e.g., mitochondrion) and portions of cytosol are surrounded by a double membrane derived from the ER (endoplasmic reticulum; other membrane sources such as the plasma membrane and mitochondria may also contribute). Eventually it creates double-membrane-bound vacuoles. In case of autophagy during starvation, it is initiated by cytosolic proteins that sense nutrient deprivation.
- The double membrane progressively expands to encircle a collection of structures (sequestered/segregated intracellular organelles and cytosolic structures) and forms an **autophagosome (or autophagic vesicle)**.
- The outer membrane of this *autophagosome* then fuses with a lysosome to produce an **autophagolysosome**.
- Inside these *autophagolysosomes,* the lysosomal enzymes **digest/degrade the enclosed cellular components/organelle**. The breakdown products are made available to the cell.

After the completion of the digestive process in the autophagolysosome, the organelle is termed a *residual body*. Depending on the type of cell, the contents of the residual body may be completely removed from the cell by exocytosis, or they may remain within the cytoplasm indefinitely as a *lipofuscin granule (wear and tear pigment)*. Lipofuscin granules increase in number as an individual becomes older. These granules are considered a major characteristic of the aging process.

Molecular basis of autophagy The autophagy process is controlled by a group of autophagy-related genes (*ATG/Atgs* genes). More than a dozen *Atgs* genes have been found. The

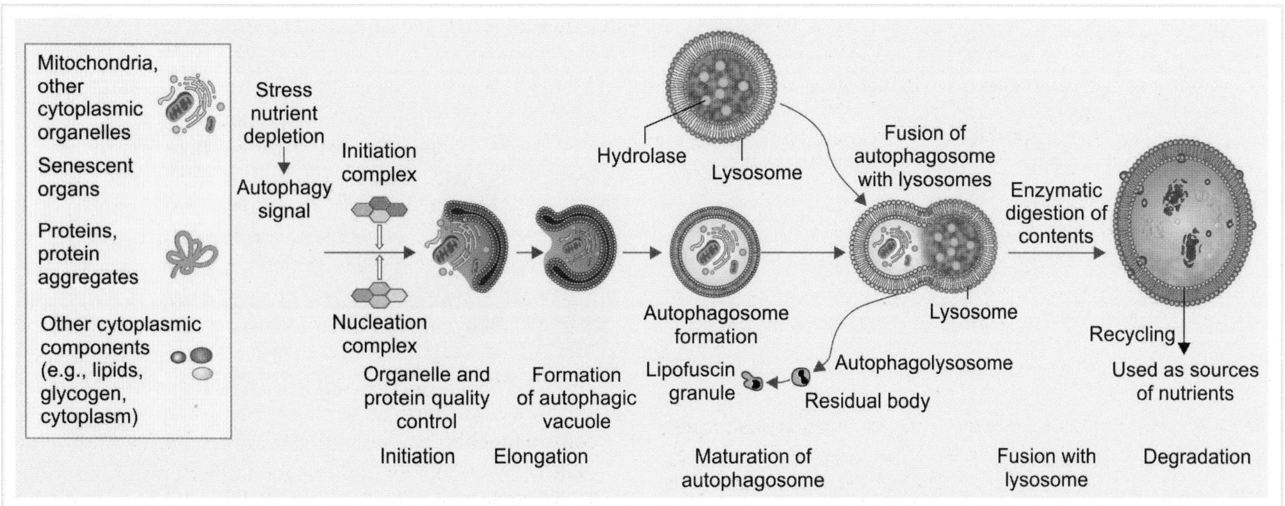

FIG. 24: Steps in autophagy. Obsolete organelles and cellular stresses (such as nutrient deprivation), activate autophagy genes to produce autophagy signal. This initiates the formation of membrane-bound vesicles in which cellular organelles are sequestered. These autophagic vesicles fuse with lysosomes and form autophagolysosome. The organelles are digested in the autophagolysosome by the lysosomal enzymes. The products are recycled and used as nutrients for the cell.

products of these *Atgs* genes are required for the formation of the autophagosome. Environmental factors such as nutrient deprivation or depletion of growth factors activate an initiation complex of four proteins. They along with nucleation complex promote the recruitment of Atgs to nucleate the initiation membrane. The initiation membrane elongates further, surrounds and captures its cytosolic component and close to form the autophagosome. The elongation and closure of the initiation membrane require the co-ordinated action of two ubiquitin-like conjugation systems. These two systems result in the covalent linkage of the lipid phosphatidylethanolamine (PE) to microtubule-associated protein light chain 3 (LC3). PE-lipidated LC3 is increased during autophagy. Hence, it is a useful marker for identifying cells in which there is process of autophagy. The newly formed autophagosome fuses with lysosomes to form an autophagolysosome. Their contents are degraded by lysosomal enzymes. It is observed that autophagy is not a random process but selective, and one of the functions of the lipidated LC3 is to target protein aggregates and effete organelles.

Microautophagy

In this, the cytosolic targets are directly engulfed by invagination of lysosomal membranes (**Fig. 25A**). Then they are transferred into the interior of lysosomes for degradation. This process is important for continuous turnover of membranes and organelles and for maintaining organelle size and composition.

Chaperone-mediated autophagy

Chaperone-mediated autophagy (CMA) is characterized by selective recognition of its targets by chaperone proteins (**Fig 25B**). Target proteins are conjugated to chaperones (e.g., Hsc70). They are recognized by lysosomal receptor proteins (LAMP-2A). Then they are translocated via receptor recognition across lysosomal membranes, without formation of phagosomes. They are received by a second chaperone in the lysosome and degraded. The original, chaperone outside the lysosome (extralysosomal chaperone) survives and work further. This pathway can also be activated when the cell is stressed (e.g., starvation, oxidant stress, toxic exposures, etc.).

Autophagy and Disease

Autophagy is an evolutionarily conserved survival mechanism maintains cellular homeostasis during starvation (state of nutrient deprivation) and removes obsolete or damaged cell organelles. Continuous maintenance of intracellular components is necessary for cell survival and any impairment of any form of autophagy can lead to accumulation of abnormal proteins and defective organelles. Autophagy is involved in many physiologic states (e.g., aging and exercise) as well as pathologic processes. The result may be cell death or disease (cancer, infection, etc.). Thus, autophagy which is a little-appreciated survival pathway in cells may have wide-ranging roles in human disease.

Neurodegenerative diseases: Many inherited neurodegenerative diseases may be associated with mutations in proteins of the autophagic pathways. In diseases such as Alzheimer and Parkinson diseases, autophagy may fail to remove in the same speed as at which protein aggregates accumulate. Alzheimer disease is characterized by impaired autophagosome maturation. Genetic defects in autophagy accelerate neurodegeneration. In Huntington disease, mutant huntingtin impairs autophagy.

Aging: With aging macroautophagy and chaperone-mediated autophagy (CMA) declines. This type of dysfunction in autophagy may be responsible for age-related changes in organ systems (e.g., CNS, heart, etc.).

Pancreatitis: Impaired autophagy may cause inappropriate conversion of trypsinogen to trypsin. This may lead to autodigestion of the pancreas and pancreatitis.

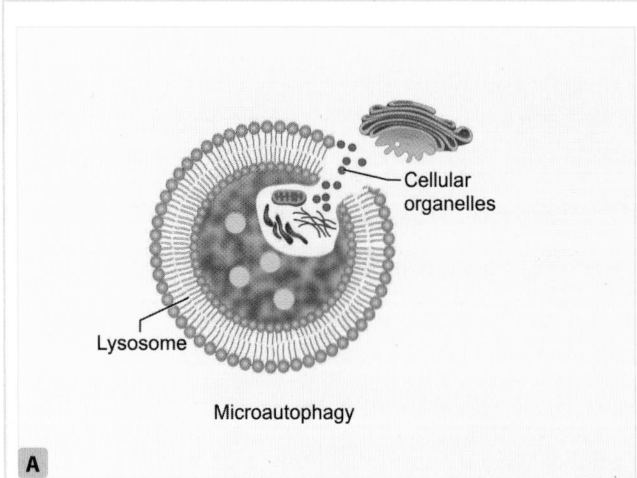

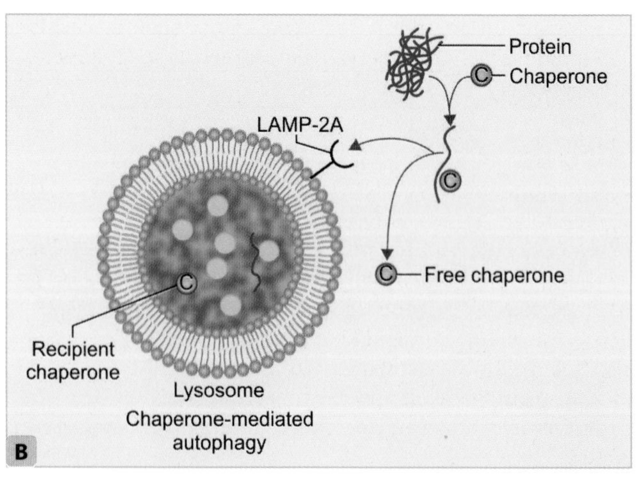

FIGS. 25A AND B: (A) Microautophagy. Cytosolic contents are dircetly engulfed by invagination of the lysosomal membrane. The contents are then degraded by lysosomal enzymes. (B). Chaperone-mediated autophagy. Proteins conjugated to chaperones (e.g., Hsc70) are recognized by lysosomal receptor proteins (LAMP-2A). They are translocated to the lysosomes present inside the cell . They are received by a second chaperone in the lysosome and degraded. The original, chaperone outside the lysosome (extralysosomal chaperone) survives and work further.

Infectious diseases: Autophagy is an important host defense mechanism against pathogens. Many invasive microorganisms may develop mechanism to inhibit the autophagic pathway, thereby avoiding their destruction. Some bacteria may interfere with phagosome-lysosome fusion (e.g., in *Mycobacterium tuberculosis* and *Shigella flexneri*) and thereby survive and replicate. Herpes simplex virus type 1 (HSV-1) encodes a protein that protects the virus from autophagic degradation. Degradation by autophagy is one way by which microbial proteins are digested and delivered to antigen presentation pathways. Macrophage-specific deletion of *Atg5* increases susceptibility to tuberculosis. In contrast, some viruses [e.g., ribonucleic acid (RNA) viruses such as poliovirus and hepatitis C virus] may benefit from increased autophagy. This is because the autophagic vesicles serve as membrane scaffolds for their replication.

Inflammatory bowel diseases: Both Crohn disease and ulcerative colitis are associated with single-nucleotide polymorphisms (SNPs) in the autophagy-related gene *ATG16L1*. There is a strong association between the occurrence of mutations in two genes and the increased risk of Crohn disease. Both these genes normally facilitate autophagic clearance of invasive bacteria. Their mutations impair bacterial clearance and promote increased production of molecules that stimulate inflammation.

Cancer: The role of autophagy in the development and progression of cancer is complex and represents a double-edged sword. Several autophagy genes can behave as tumor suppressors and are deleted or mutated in many tumors. In contrast, if tumor cells are deprived of nutrients or oxygen due to therapy or insufficient blood supply, resulting autophagy can protect cancer cells. Thus, autophagy can both promote cancer growth and act as a defense against cancers. The role of autophagy in cancer is discussed in detail on page 491.

Miscellaneous: Mutations in genes encoding proteins involved in autophagosome–lysosome fusion are observed in some diseases of skeletal muscle (inclusion body myopathy), Paget disease of bone, and frontotemporal dementia. Extensive autophagy may be seen in ischemic injury such as cardiac ischemia and ischemia/reperfusion injury, type II diabetes, stroke, etc.

Autolysis

autolysis (means self-lysis) is destruction of the cell by its own hydrolytic enzymes released from lysosomes. Autolysis is generally reserved for post-mortem change. It develops rapidly in some tissues rich in hydrolytic enzymes such as pancreas and gastric mucosa. It occurs little slowly in tissues such as the heart, liver, and kidney; and slow in fibrous tissue. Microscopically, the cellular details are lost and they appear as cells with homogeneous and eosinophilic cytoplasm.

Differences between necrosis and autolysis are listed in **Table 5**.

MECHANISMS OF CELL INJURY

Q. Write a long essay on the biochemical and molecular mechanism of cell injury.

Table 5: Differences between necrosis and autolysis.

Features	*Necrosis*	*Autolysis*
Definition	Morphologic changes following cell death in living tissue	Self-digestion or disintegration of cells by enzymes liberated from own lysosomes
Occurrence	In living tissue	After death of cells
Inflammatory reaction	Present	Absent
Calcification	May occur	Absent

General Principles of Cell Injury

Cellular response to injury: It depends on: (1) type of injury, (2) duration of injury, and (3) severity of injury. Small doses of a chemical toxin or ischemia for a brief period may produce reversible injury. If dose of same toxin is large or ischemia is for a more prolonged period, it may result either in rapid cell death or slowly progress to irreversible injury and ultimately leading to cell death.

Consequences of injury: It depends on: (1) type of cell involved, (2) adaptability of cell, (3) status of cell, and (4) genetic make-up of the cell. Thus, nutritional and hormonal status, metabolic demands, and functions of the cells decides their response to injury. Vulnerability of the cells to hypoxia is also important. For example, skeletal muscle can tolerate loss of blood supply and hypoxia whereas cardiac muscle cells are more vulnerable. Exposure of two individuals to identical concentrations of a toxin (e.g., carbon tetrachloride), may not produce any effect in on liver cells in one individuals but may lead to cell death in the other. This variation in susceptibility may be due to polymorphisms in genes encoding hepatic enzymes that metabolize carbon tetrachloride (CCl_4) to toxic by-products

Stimulus triggers multiple mechanisms: Any injurious stimulus/injury may simultaneously produce many interconnected mechanisms that damage cells.

Targets and biochemical mechanism of cell injury: These include: (1) mitochondrial damage/dysfunction, (2) disturbance of calcium homeostasis, (3) damage to cellular membranes, and (4) damage to DNA and misfolding of proteins.

General Mechanisms and Intracellular Targets of Cell Injury

Injurious stimuli that cause cell injury lead to complex cellular, biochemical, and molecular changes. Certain mechanisms are common for most forms of cell injury and cell death. **Cell injury results from abnormalities in one or more main cellular components.** The main targets of injurious stimuli are **(i) mitochondria, (ii) cell membranes, (iii) the machinery of protein synthesis and secretion, and (iv) DNA.**

Decreased Production of Adenosine Triphosphate

Adenosine triphosphate (ATP) is required for all processes within the cell. Injury like hypoxia, chemicals (e.g., cyanide), can cause decreased production of ATP. **Effects of decreased ATP** are presented in **Figure 41**.

Mitochondrial Damage (Fig. 26)

Mitochondria are sensitive to almost all types of injurious stimuli (e.g., hypoxia, toxins). **Mitochondria are important players in all pathways that leads to cell injury and death.** This is because mitochondria supplies life-sustaining energy by generating ATP and are also targets of many injurious stimuli. Mitochondria can be damaged by increased cytosolic Ca^{2+}, ROS, and reduced oxygen supply. Thus, they are sensitive to almost all types of injurious stimuli, including hypoxia and toxins. Mutations in mitochondrial genes can cause some inherited diseases.

Consequences of mitochondrial damage

Three major consequences of mitochondrial damage are as follows:

Depletion of ATP Decreased synthesis of adenosine triphosphate (ATP) and depletion of ATP occurs both in hypoxic and chemical (toxic) injury (**Figs. 26** and **27**). ATP is produced in two ways namely (i) oxidative phosphorylation of ADP and (ii) glycolytic pathway.

- **Oxidative phosphorylation of ADP:** It is the major pathway, particularly in nondividing cells (e.g., brain and liver). In this pathway oxidative phosphorylation of adenosine diphosphate (ADP) results in reduction of oxygen and ATP by the mitochondrial electron transport system.
- **Glycolytic pathway:** In this pathway, ATP is generated in the absence of oxygen using glucose derived either from body fluids or from the hydrolysis of glycogen. The ATP generated in much smaller amounts.

Apart from the damage to mitochondrial, other major causes of ATP depletion are reduced supply of oxygen and nutrients (due to ischemia and hypoxia), and the actions of some toxins (e.g., cyanide).

Formation of mitochondrial permeability transition pore: Damage to mitochondria usually leads to the formation of a high-conductance channel in the membrane of mitochondria. They are called as the mitochondrial permeability transition pore (**Fig. 26**). The opening of mitochondrial permeability transition pore causes loss of mitochondrial membrane potential and results in failure of oxidative phosphorylation. This leads to progressive depletion of ATP and ultimately produces cell death by aoptosis.

Changes produced due to depletion of ATP: High-energy phosphate in the form of ATP is needed for almost all synthetic and degradative processes within the cell. These processes include membrane transport, protein synthesis, lipogenesis, and the deacylation-reacylation reactions required for phospholipid turnover. Therefore, depletion of ATP to 5% to 10% of normal levels has numerous effects on many important cellular systems. Various effects of ATP depletion are as follows:

- **Failure of sodium pump**: ATP depletion leads to reduced activity of the plasma membrane energy-dependent sodium pump (Na^+, K^+-ATPase). Failure of sodium pump causes sodium to enter and accumulate inside cells and the reduces the concentration of potassium inside the cell. This in turn produces accumulation of water inside the cell

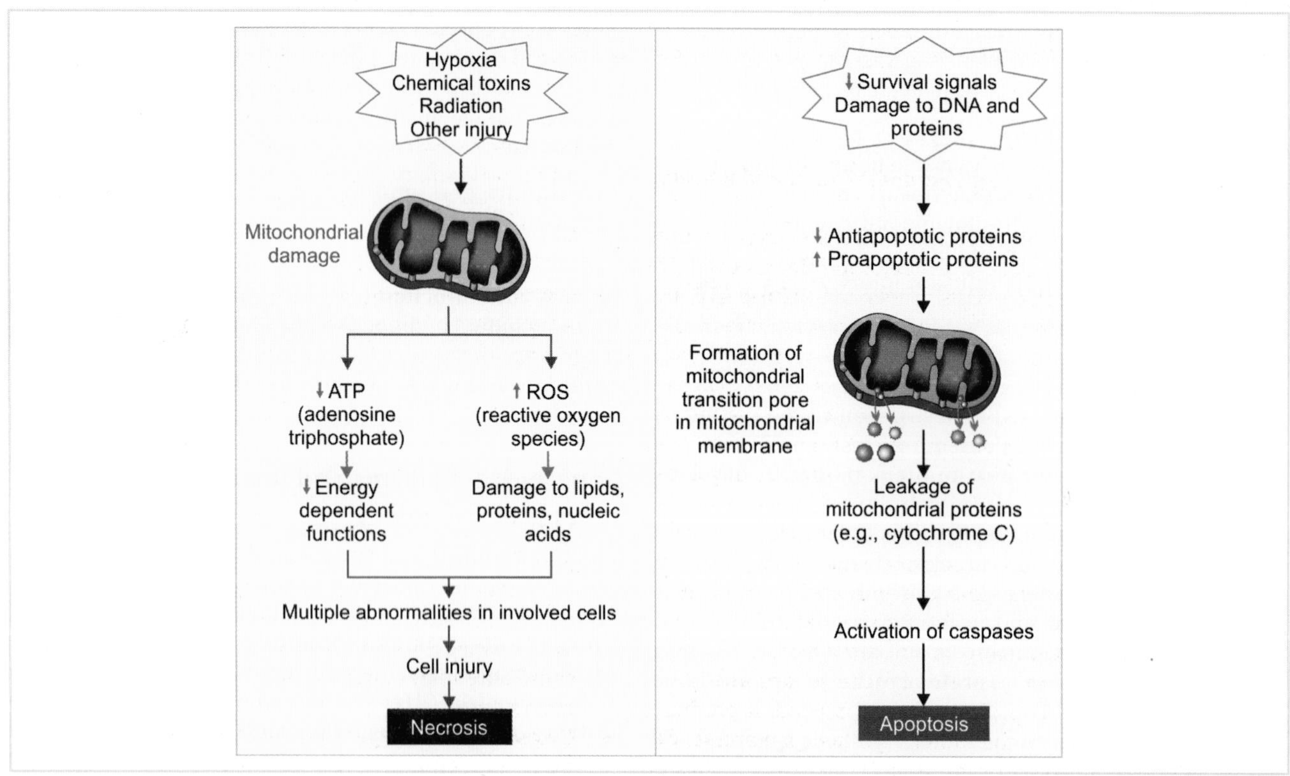

(ATP: adenosine triphosphate; ROS: reactive oxygen species)

FIG. 26: Role of mitochondria and main effects of mitochondrial damage in cell injury and death. Mitochondria are affected by different varieties of injurious stimuli, and their abnormalities lead to necrosis or apoptosis.

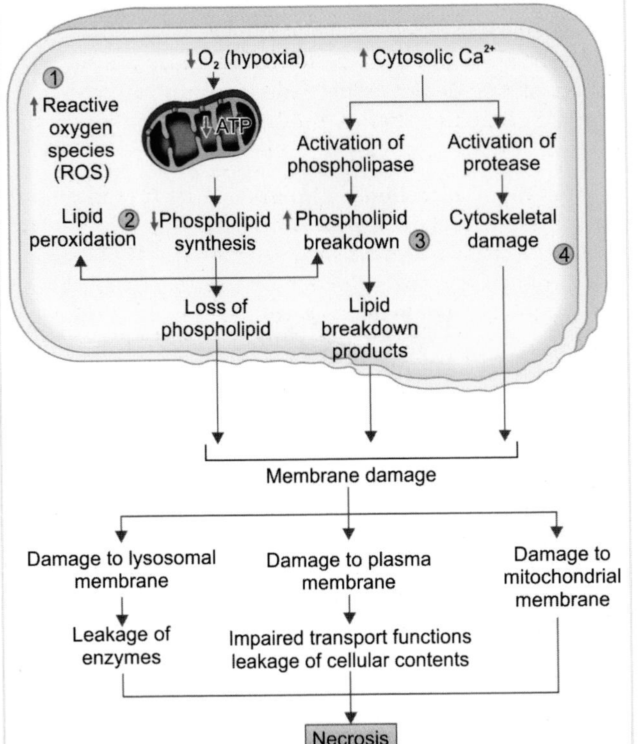

FIG. 27: Various biochemical mechanisms of membrane damage in cell injury. Main mechanisms are (1) reactive oxygen species (ROS), (2) decreased synthesis of phospholipid, (3) increased breakdown of phospholipid and (4) cytoskeletal damage. Decreased O_2 and increased cytosolic Ca^{2+} are generally occur in ischemia, but may be seen in any forms of cell injury. Reactive oxygen species are usually produced on reperfusion of ischemic tissues and cause membrane damage.

and leads to cell swelling and dilatation of endoplasmic reticulum (ER).

- **Altered cellular energy metabolism**: If the oxygen supply to cells is reduced, as in ischemia, it terminates oxidative phosphorylation. This results in reduced cellular ATP and associated increase in adenosine monophosphate (AMP). These changes stimulate the activities of two enzymes namely phosphorylase and phosphofructokinase and leads to increased rates of glycogenolysis and glycolysis, respectively. This is an attempt to maintain the supply of energy by producing ATP through metabolism of glucose derived from glycogen. Utilization of glucose causes rapid depletion of glycogen stores in the cells. Anaerobic glycolysis leads to the accumulation of lactic acid and inorganic phosphates from the hydrolysis of phosphate esters. This in turn reduces the intracellular pH and causes decreased activity of many cytosolic enzymes.
- **Disruption of the protein synthetic apparatus:** If depletion of ATP is prolonged or worsened, it produces structural damage to the protein synthetic apparatus with a reduction in protein synthesis. Damage is manifested as detachment of ribosomes from the rough ER and dissociation of polysomes.
- **Damage to lysosomes:** Finally, if injury produces further ATP depletion, it produces irreversible damage to mitochondrial and lysosomal membranes. The damaged cell undergoes necrosis.

Formation of reactive oxygen species (ROS) Incomplete oxidative phosphorylation also produces reactive oxygen species (ROS). They have many harmful effects and they are discussed on **pages 166–170**.

Leakage of mitochondrial proteins into cytoplasm The mitochondrial membranes contain many proteins **such as cytochrome C and proapoptotic proteins (e.g., BAX and BAK).** Increased permeability of the mitochondrial membrane due to channel formation by proapoptotic BAX and BAK is the initial step in apoptosis by the intrinsic pathway.

Membrane Damage

In most forms of cell injury (except apoptosis), in the early phase there is loss of selective membrane permeability. This finally leads to membrane damage. With the obvious membrane damage, the cell cannot return to normal. Membrane damage may affect the integrity and functions of all cellular membranes. This includes cell membrane and membranes of all cytoplasmic organelles (including mitochondria).

Causes of membrane damage: In ischemic cells, membrane defects may be produced due to depletion of ATP and calcium-mediated activation of phospholipases. The plasma membrane may be also damaged directly. Direct damage may be caused by bacterial toxins, viral proteins, lytic (membrane attack complex/MAC) complement components, and many physical and chemical agents.

Biochemical mechanisms of membrane damage (Fig. 27): These include the following—

- **Reactive oxygen species (ROS).** Oxygen free radicals cause injury to cell membranes by lipid peroxidation (refer **page 166**).
- **Decreased synthesis of phospholipid**: Defective mitochondrial function or hypoxia decreases the production of ATP. This leads to decreased synthesis of phospholipid in all cellular membranes (including the mitochondria) and energy-dependent enzymatic activities.
- **Increased breakdown of phospholipid**: In severe cell injury, there is increased degradation of membrane phospholipids. Severe cell injury increases levels of Ca^{2+} in cytosol (cytoplasm) and mitochondria. This leads to calcium-mediated activation of endogenous phospholipases. The activated phospholipase enzymes degrade membrane phospholipids. This leads to the accumulation of lipid breakdown products. These products include unesterified free fatty acids, acyl carnitine, and lysophospholipids. These products have detergent effect on membranes. They may also cause membrane damage by either inserting into the lipid bilayer of the membrane or exchange with membrane phospholipids. This may cause alteration in permeability and electrophysiology of membranes.
- **Cytoskeletal damage:** Cytoskeletal filaments connect the plasma membrane to the cell interior (refer Figs. 13, 14 and 15 of Chapter 1). **Increased cytosolic calcium (Ca^{2+}) activates proteases which may damage the cytoskeletal elements connecting the cell membrane. When injury produces swelling of cells, especially in myocardial cells,**

damage to cytoskeleton leads to detachment of the cell membrane from the cytoskeleton. These cells stretches the cell and undergo rupture.

Consequences of membrane damage: Cell injury may damage any membrane and damage to different cellular membranes has different effects on cells.

- **Mitochondrial membrane damage (refer page 160):** It results in:
  - Opening of the **mitochondrial permeability transition pore** leading to decreased production of ATP.
  - Release of proteins from damaged mitochondria favor cell death by apoptosis.
- **Plasma membrane damage:** Its consequences are as follows—
  - **Loss of osmotic balance and influx of fluids and ions.**
  - Leakage of cellular contents outside the injured cells.
  - Leakage of metabolites (e.g., glycolytic intermediates) that are required for the reconstitution of ATP. This results in further depletion of stores of energy.
- **Lysosomal membrane damage:** It leads to—
  - **Leakage of lysosomal enzymes into the cytoplasm.**
  - **Activation of lysosomal enzymes:** Acid hydrolases are activated in the acidic intracellular pH of the injured cell. These lysosomal hydrolases include RNases, DNases, proteases, phosphatases, and glucosidases. These lysosomal hydrolases degrade RNA, DNA, proteins, phosphoproteins, and glycogen, and leads to cell death by necrosis.

Damage to DNA (Fig. 28)

Causes of DNA damage: These include exposure to DNA damaging chemotherapeutic (anticancer) drugs, radiation, and ROS. DNA damage may occur spontaneously as a part of aging, mainly due to deamination of cytosine residues to uracil residues.

Cell cycle arrest and activation of repair mechanism: Nuclear DNA damage activates sensors that trigger p53-dependent pathways. Activated p53, arrests the cells with DNA damage in the G1 phase of the cell cycle. This in turn activates DNA repair mechanisms.

Apoptosis: If the DNA damage is too severe to be corrected, DNA repair mechanisms fail to correct the DNA damage. This cell prefers to undergo death rather than survive with abnormal DNA. p53 triggers death of these cells by apoptosis through the mitochondrial (intrinsic) pathway.

Malignant transformation: Cells that survive with damaged DNA has the potential to induce malignant transformation. Mutations in p53 can interfere with its ability to arrest cell cycling or to induce apoptosis. These mutations are associated with many cancers.

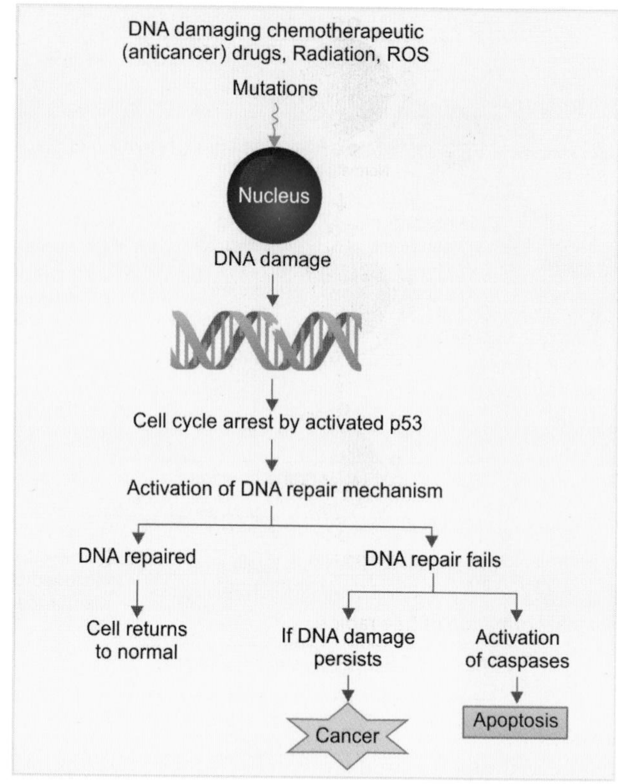

FIG. 28: Causes and consequences of DNA damage due to cell injury.

Oxidative Stress: Accumulation of Oxygen-derived Free Radicals

Q. Write short essay/note on free radical injury and its role in cell tissue injury/disease.
Q. Discuss the role of free radicals in disease causation and antioxidants in their prevention/oxidative stress.
Q. Discuss the role of oxygen radicals in inflammation.
Q. Discuss the role of free radicals in health and disease.
Q. Discuss the role of oxidative stress in cell injury.

General Characteristics

Oxygen is a crucial element for human to survive on Earth and life is impossible without it. It plays a dominant role in the controlled oxidation of molecules containing carbon, and generates energy essential for the survival of all aerobic systems. Thus, oxygen is a blessing. But it can become a curse when some of its derivatives are partially reduced to form reactive oxygen species (ROS is one of the free radicals). Because this can react and cause damage to almost any molecule it reacts with.

Definition of free radical

A free radical is defined as any atom, molecule, or a fragment of an atom or molecule that **contains at least one/single unpaired electron in an outer orbit** (**Fig. 29**). To a certain extent, it can exhibit an independent existence.

Common properties

They are unstable chemical compounds and electrically uncharged. The presence of one unpaired electron makes these molecules unstable and highly reactive.

They can either donate an electron to, or accept an electron from, other molecule. Thus, they behave as oxidants or reductants. Since they have an unpaired electron, they are electrophilic, i.e., have the tendency to attract or acquire electrons. They attack sites of increased electron density, which are usually present in compounds with nitrogen atoms (proteins, nucleic acids) and carbon-carbon double bonds (phospholipids, polyunsaturated fatty acids [PUFAs]). During such an electron interchange, new radicals are formed from previously nonradical molecules and may produce chain reactions.

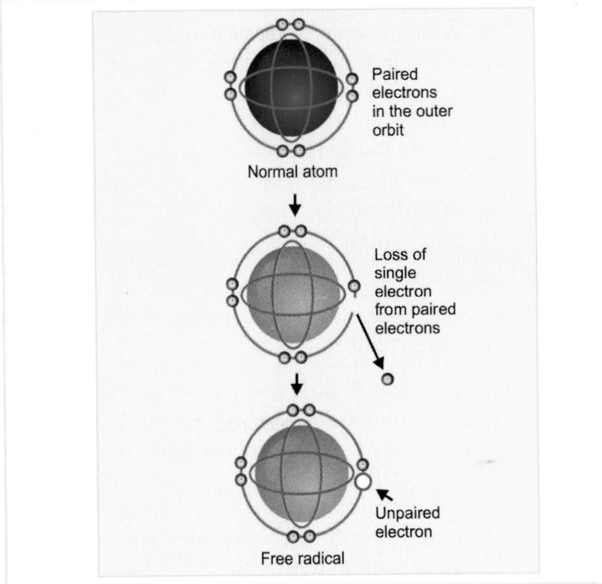

FIG. 29: Formation of free radical.

Generation

Free radical may be produced by one of the two processes namely by: (1) addition of a single electron to a neutral atom or molecule, or by the (2) loss of one electron from a neutral atom or molecule: The free radical molecule can become stabilized either by donating or by accepting an electron from another molecule. If the attacked molecule loses its electron, it becomes a free radical. Free radicals initiate chain reactions and it is difficult to control them. They have low chemical specificity (i.e., they can react with most nearby molecules), hence called as highly reactive. These free radicals are capable of forming injurious chemical bond with DNA, ribonucleic acid (RNA), proteins, lipids, and carbohydrates that are main molecules in membranes and nucleic acids.

Oxidative stress

An important mechanism of membrane damage by free radicals is by disturbing the balance between the production and/or concentration of free radicals [reactive oxygen species (ROS) or reactive nitrogen species (RNS)] and destruction by antioxidant defense systems. This mechanism producing excess of free radicals is termed as **oxidative stress (OS)**. When there is an excessive/higher level of production of free radicals (ROS/RNS), it leads to oxidative stress (OS) and/or nitrosative stress (NS). The term OS is used to cellular abnormalities that are caused by reactive oxygen species (ROS), which belong to a group of molecules called as free radicals. Thus, OS can be caused due to an increase of different reactive species or a depletion of antioxidant defense, or both. OS results in destructive oxidation of different molecules including proteins, lipids, nucleic acids, and others. OS can initiate/activate many intracellular signaling pathways by modulating enzymes and transcription factors. Free radicals injury is an important mechanism of cell damage in many conditions such as chemical and radiation injury, ischemia-reperfusion injury, cellular aging, and killing of microbes by phagocytes, particularly neutrophils and macrophages.

Properties of Free Radicals

- Normally, free radicals produced in the cells are unstable and are rapidly destroyed.
- When free radicals react with any molecules, they convert those molecules into free radicals and thus initiate autocatalytic reactions.
- Excess of free radicals may be either due to increased production or ineffective degradation.

Types of Free Radicals

- **Oxygen-derived free radicals:** These are oxygen-centered radicals and called as **reactive oxygen species (ROS), also called reactive oxygen intermediates**. ROS includes superoxide anion ($O_2^{\bullet}$), hydrogen peroxide (H_2O_2), and hydroxyl ions ($^{\bullet}OH$).
- **Reactive nitrogen species** (nitric oxide derived free radicals): Nitrogen-centered molecules are called reactive nitrogen species (RNS). For example, nitric oxide (NO) is generated by endothelial cells (refer Fig. 17 of Chapter 8), macrophages, neurons, and other types of cells. NO can act as a free radical and can also be converted to highly reactive peroxynitrite anion ($ONOO^-$), NO_2 and NO_3^-.
- **Free radicals from drug and chemical:** Enzymatic metabolism of exogenous chemicals or drugs can generate free radicals which are not ROS but have similar effects (e.g., CCl_4 can generate CCl_3). The accumulation of ROS depends on their rates of production and removal.

Oxidative Chain Reactions

Free radical reactions have three distinct identifiable phases:

1. **Initiation:** It is the initial creation phase, usually cleavage with the assistance of heat, UV, or metal catalysts.
2. **Propagation:** Free radicals are generated and regenerated repeatedly because of the chain reaction.
3. **Termination:** In this phase, two free radicals react with each other to form a stable, nonradical product.

Sources of Free Radical

The sources of free radicals may be intracellular (endogenous). There are many intracellular sources (**Box 6** and **Fig. 30**) of ROS.

Free radicals may also enter biological systems from diverse exogenous sources and most important of them are shown in **Figure 31**.

Production of Free Radicals

Oxygen-derived free radicals

The accumulation of ROS depends on the rates of production and removal. ROS are produced within cells in several ways.

Box 6: Intracellular sources of free radicals.

- **Cellular organelles** with mitochondria (largest source), endoplasmic reticulum (ER) (mainly during ER stress), and peroxisomes. During oxidative phosphorylation, mitochondria utilize oxygen to generate ATP from organic fuel molecules and in the process generate ROS
- **NADPH oxidases** (NOX enzymes)
- **Other enzymes** (xanthine oxidase, lipoxygenase, cyclooxygenase, cytochrome P450, nitric oxidase synthase)

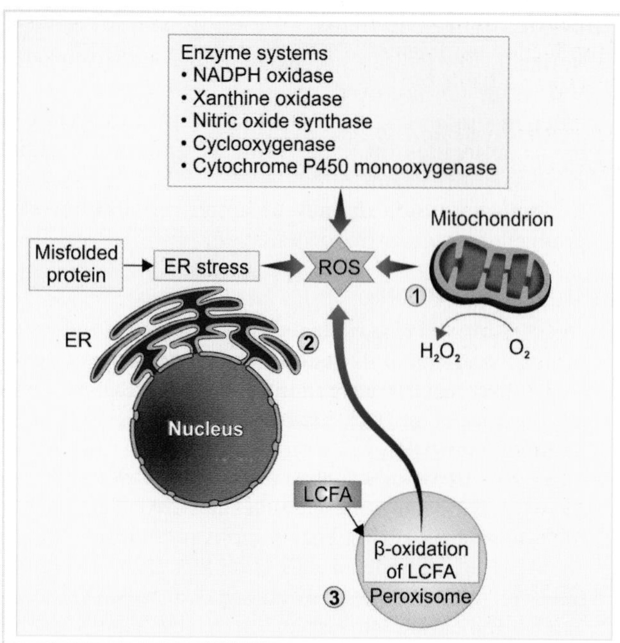

(NADPH: nicotinamide adenine dinucleotide phosphate)

FIG. 30: Intracellular sources and sites of production of ROS. The intracellular sources of reactive oxygen species (ROS) include organelles such as: (1) mitochondria, (2) endoplasmic reticulum (ER) (especially during ER stress), and (3) peroxisomes [metabolizing long-chain fatty acids (LCFAs)]. Various enzymes can also generate ROS during the enzymatic reaction cycles. These enzymes include oxidases and oxygenases.

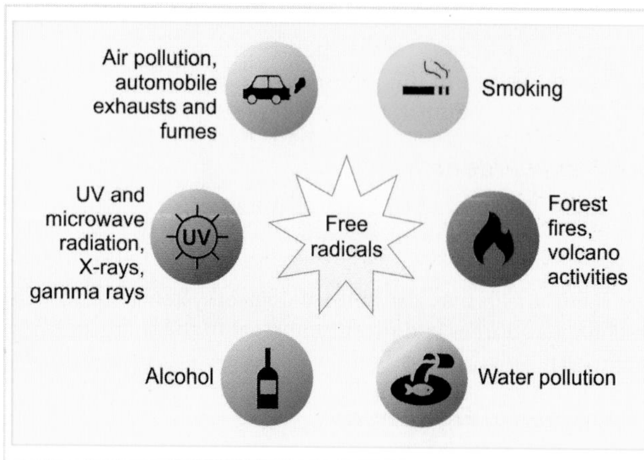

FIG. 31: Exogenous sources of free radicals.

Endogenous (intracellular) sources of ROS

During reduction-oxidation reactions: An reduction-oxidation (redox) reaction is a type of chemical reaction that involves a transfer of electrons between two species. It is commonly used for removing or adding oxygen to a compound. Reduction-oxidation reactions occur during normal metabolic processes. During normal respiration, molecular oxygen (O_2) is reduced by the transfer of four electrons to H_2 to produce two water molecules. This conversion is catalyzed by oxidative enzymes present in the endoplasmic reticulum (ER), cytosol, mitochondria, peroxisomes, and lysosomes. During this process, small amounts of partially reduced, short-lived toxic intermediates are produced in which different numbers of electrons are transferred from O_2. These intermediates include (i) **superoxide anion** ($O_2^{\bullet}$, one electron), (ii) **hydrogen peroxide** (H_2O_2, two electrons), and (iii) **hydroxyl radicals** ($^{\bullet}OH$, three electrons).

Absorption of radiant energy: Examples of radiant energy that can produce free radicals are ultraviolet light and x-rays. For example, ionizing radiation hydrolyze water and produce $^{\bullet}OH$ and hydrogen (H) free radicals.

During inflammation: ROS are rapidly produced in activated leukocytes during inflammation. This is strictly controlled reaction brought out by a plasma membrane multiprotein complex that uses NADPH oxidase for the redox reaction. In addition, some intracellular oxidases (e.g., xanthine oxidase) generate $O_2^{\bullet}$. Defects in production of leukocytic superoxide can lead to chronic granulomatous disease.

Through transition metals: Transition metal or elements are chemical elements that have valence electrons—i.e., electrons that can participate in the formation of chemical bonds. The transition metals were given their name because they had a place between Group 2 and Group 13 in the main group elements. Some transition elements such as iron and copper can donate or accept free electrons during intracellular reactions and they can accelerate or catalyse formation of free radical. For example, in the Fenton reaction (refer Fig 16 of Chapter 8) oxidation of organic substrates by iron and hydrogen peroxide rapidly converts H_2O_2 to $^{\bullet}OH$ (i.e., $H_2O_2 + Fe^{2+} \rightarrow Fe^{3+} + {}^{\bullet}OH + OH^-$). Most of the intracellular free iron is in the ferric (Fe^{3+}) state. Hence, it must be reduced to the ferrous (Fe^{2+}) form to participate in the Fenton reaction. This reduction can be accelerated by $O_2^{\bullet}$. Thus, sources of iron and $O_2^{\bullet}$ may act together to produce oxidative damage to cell.

Other free radicals

Enzymatic metabolism of exogenous chemicals or drugs: Metabolism of some drugs can produce free radicals that are not ROS. But these free radical have effects similar to ROS. For example, CCl_4 can produce a free radical namely $^{\bullet}CCl_3$.

Nitric oxide (NO): It is one of the important chemical mediator produced by endothelial cells, macrophages, neurons, and other cell types. They can act as a free radical. It may also react with **superoxide anion** ($O_2^{\bullet}$) and converted to highly reactive peroxynitrite anion ($ONOO^-$) as well as NO_2 and NO_3^-.

Steps involved in generation of free radicals in all cells include:

- **Superoxide radical:** Superoxide ($O_2^{\bullet}$) free radical is generated as a result of a monovalent reduction (partial reduction) of oxygen (O_2) and the addition of one electron.

$$O_2 + e^- \rightarrow O_2^{\bullet}$$

- **Hydrogen peroxide:** Superoxide ($O_2^{\bullet}$) radicals react with another superoxide radical in a dismutation reaction [by the action of the enzyme superoxide dismutase (SOD)], in which one radical is oxidized to oxygen while the other is reduced to H_2O_2) spontaneously.

$2O_2^{\bullet} + 2H_2O \rightarrow H_2O_2 + O_2$
[catalyzed by Cu (copper), Zn (zinc), Mn (magnesium), SOD (superoxide dismutase)]

Hydrogen peroxide is more stable than superoxide ($O_2^{\bullet}$) and can cross biologic membranes. H_2O_2 is a two-electron product of oxygen reduction. It is able to participate in signal transduction, cell proliferation, differentiation, and response to stress.

- Hydroxyl radical: In the presence of metals (e.g., Fe^{2+}), H_2O_2 is converted by Fenton reaction (refer Fig 16 of Chapter 8) to a highly reactive free radical called hydroxyl radical ($^{\bullet}OH/OH^{\bullet}$). Hydroxyl radicals are defined as the neutral form of the hydroxide ion. They are capable of aggressive reaction with organic and inorganic molecules and cause more severe damage to the cell than any other free radical.
- Superoxide ($O_2^{\bullet}$) is also converted to peroxynitrite ($ONOO^-$) in the presence of NO.

Steps Involved in Generation of Oxygen Derived Free Radicals in Phagocytic Leukocytes (Fig. 32)

In phagocytic leukocytes (Fig. 32): ROS is produced in the leukocytes to destroy the ingested microbes and other substances produced during inflammation.

- During phagocytosis, ROS is produced in the phagosomes and phagolysosomes of the leukocytes (mainly neutrophils and macrophages) by a process similar to mitochondrial respiration. This process is called as respiratory burst (or oxidative burst).
- During this process, superoxide ($O_2^{\bullet}$) is synthesized via reduced nicotinamide adenine dinucleotide phosphate (NADPH) oxidase (NADPH/ respiratory burst oxidase) (phagocyte oxidase) present in the phagosomes and phagolysosomal membrane of the leukocytes.
- Superoxide ($O_2^{\bullet}$) is converted to hydrogen peroxide (H_2O_2).
- Hydrogen peroxide (H_2O_2) in the presence of myeloperoxidase enzyme is converted to highly reactive compound hypochlorous acid also called hypochlorite (HOCl). HOCl is the major component of household bleach.

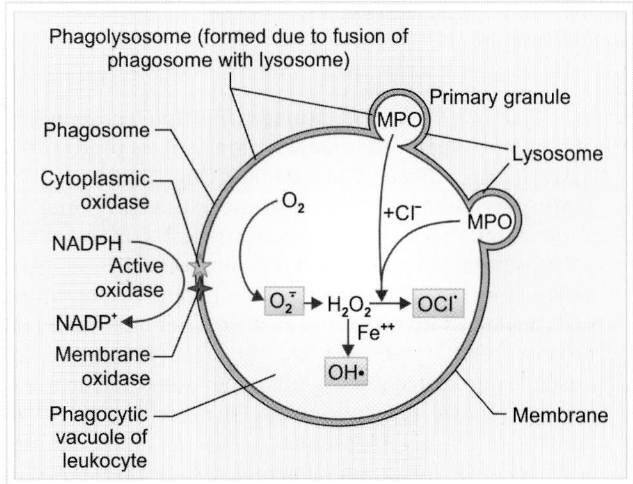

FIG. 32: Production of reactive oxygen species in leukocytes inside the phagocytic vacuole of leukocyte. Hypochlorite ($HOCl^{\bullet}$) and hydroxyl radical ($^{\bullet}OH$) are microbicidal products generated from superoxide.

Main free radicals involved in cell injury, their mechanism of production, and neutralization and pathological effects are presented in **Table 6**.

Mechanisms of Removal/Neutralization of Free Radicals (Fig. 33)

Q. Write short essay on antioxidants (mechanisms of removal/neutralization of free radicals).

Free radicals are generally unstable molecules and usually undergo spontaneous decay. For example, superoxide ($O_2^{\bullet}$) is unstable. It decays (dismutates) spontaneously to O2 and H_2O_2 in the presence of water. Serum, tissue fluids and host cells have many antioxidant mechanisms (**Box 7**), which protect against potentially harmful oxygen-derived free radicals. These mechanism may be divided into enzymatic and nonenzymatic mechanisms. They remove free radicals and minimize the tissue injury.

Enzymatic antioxidants

There are many enzymes that act as free radical-scavenging systems. They break down hydrogen peroxide (H_2O_2) and superoxide ($O_2^{\bullet}$). These enzymes are present near the sites of production of the oxidants and are as follows:

1. **Catalase:** It is present in peroxisomes. Enzyme catalase neutralizes/decomposes hydrogen peroxide (H_2O_2) free radicals by converting it into water and oxygen ($2H_2O_2 \rightarrow O_2 + 2H_2O$). It is one of the most active enzymes having the capacity to degrade millions of molecules of H_2O_2 per second.
2. **Enzyme SODs:** Superoxidase dismutases (SODs) are group of enzymes found in many types of cell. These include both manganese- SOD present in mitochondria, and copper zinc⁻ SOD present in the cytoplasm. They neutralizes superoxide($O_2^{\bullet}$) free radicals by converting it into hydrogen peroxide ($2O_2^{\bullet} + 2H \rightarrow H_2O_2 + O_2$). SOD significantly increases the rate of destruction of superoxide.
3. **Glutathione peroxidases:** These are a family of enzymes and their main function is to protect cells from oxidative damage. Large amount of members of this family found in the cytoplasm of all cells is glutathione (GSH) peroxidase 1. Enzyme GSH peroxidase 1 (enhances GSH) neutralizes and breaks down hydrogen peroxide (H_2O_2), hydroxyl, and acetaminophen free radicals. This enzyme's activity is reflected by the intracellular ratio of oxidized GSH to reduced GSH and this indicates the cell's ability to catabolize free radicals [$2GSH + H_2O_2 \rightarrow GSSG$ (glutathione homodimer) $+ 2H_2O$ or $2GSH + 2^{\bullet}OH \rightarrow GSSG + 2H_2O$].

Nonenzymatic antioxidants

Endogenous or exogenous antioxidants may either block the formation of free radicals or scavenge (inactivate) them after their formation.

Exogenous antioxidants

Examples of exogenous antioxidants include: vitamin E, vitamin A, ascorbic acid, β-carotene and sulfhydryl containing compounds (e.g., cysteine and glutathione in the cytosol).

- **Vitamin E** (α-tocopherol): It is a terminal electron acceptor that aborts free radical chain reactions. Since it is fat soluble, it protects membranes from lipid peroxidation.

Table 6: Main free radicals involved in cell injury, their mechanism of production and neutralization and pathological effects.

Type of free radical	*Mechanisms of production*	*Mechanisms of removal/ neutralization*	*Pathologic effects*
Superoxide ($O_2^{\bar{\cdot}}$)	• In mitochondria: Incomplete reduction of oxygen (O_2) during mitochondrial oxidative phosphorylation • In phagocyte: By phagocyte oxidase in leukocytes	Converted to H_2O_2 and O_2 by superoxide dismutase (SOD)	Direct damage to lipids (peroxidation), proteins (breakdown, misfolding), and DNA (mutations)
Hydrogen peroxide (H_2O_2)	Mainly from superoxide by action of SOD	Converted to H_2O and O_2 by catalase in peroxisomes, glutathione peroxidase in cytosol and mitochondria	Can be converted to $^{\bullet}OH$ and OCl^- and can destroy microbes and cells. It can act away from its site of production
Hydroxyl radical ($^{\bullet}OH$)	Produced from H_2O, by hydrolysis as in radiation; from H_2O_2 by Fenton reaction; H_2O_2, and ($O_2^{\bar{\cdot}}$) by various chemical reactions	Converted to H_2O by glutathione peroxidase	Direct damage to lipids, proteins, and DNA
Peroxynitrite ($ONOO^{\bullet}$)	Interaction of $O_2^{\bar{\cdot}}$ and NO mediated by NO synthase in endothelial cells, leukocytes, neurons etc.	Converted to nitrite HNO_2 by enzymes peroxiredoxins in mitochondria and cytosol	

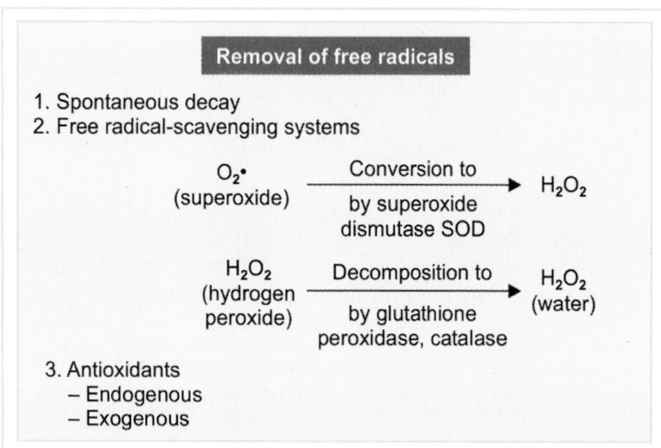

FIG. 33: Mechanism of removal/neutralization of free radicals.

Box 7: Various types of antioxidants.

Enzymatic antioxidants

- Superoxide dismutase* (SOD) converts superoxide ($O_2^{\bar{\cdot}}$) to H_2O_2
- Catalase*(in peroxisomes) decomposes H_2O_2.
- Glutathione peroxidase* decomposes $OH^{\bullet}$ and H_2O_2

Non-enzymatic antioxidants: Either block synthesis or inactivate free radicals

- Exogenous: Vitamin E, vitamin A, vitamin C (ascorbic acid) and sulfhydryl containing compounds (e.g., cysteine and glutathione)
- Endogenous: Storage and transport proteins in the serum, such as transferrin, ferritin, albumin and ceruloplasmin

*Enzymes modulate the cellular destructive effects of free radicals and are also released in inflammation.

- **Vitamin C** (ascorbic acid/ascorbate): It is water soluble and reacts directly with O_2, $OH^{\bullet}$, and some products of lipid peroxidation. It also helps in regenerating the reduced form of vitamin E.
- **Retinoids:** They are the precursors of vitamin A, are lipid soluble. They act as chain-breaking antioxidants.
- **NO•:** It may scavenge ROS, mainly by chelation of iron and combination with other free radicals.

Endogenous antioxidants Iron and copper are reactive metals, which can catalyze the formation of ROS. Their activities are minimized by binding of these ions to storage and transport proteins (e.g., transferrin, ferritin, and ceruloplasmin).

Free Radicals in Health and Disease

Pathologic Effects of Free Radicals (Fig. 34)

Free radicals can produce wide-ranging effects and cause cell injury in many diseases. Free radicals can activate both necrosis and apoptosis. **ROS damages multiple components of cells and produce cell injury.** Various effects of ROS-free radicals important in regard to cell injury (**Fig. 34**) are:

- **Lipid peroxidation of membranes:** Double bonds in membrane (both plasma and organellar membrane) polyunsaturated lipids are susceptible to attack by oxygen-derived free radicals. The interaction of lipid of membrane with oxygen-derived free radical [particularly hydroxyl radical ($^{\bullet}OH$)] yield peroxides. These peroxides are unstable and reactive, and produce an autocatalytic chain reaction (known as propogaation). They produce extensive damage to plasma membranes as well as mitochondrial and lysosomal membranes. Its consequences are similar to injury by ischemia and hypoxia (refer pages 174–175).
- **Crosslinking and other alterations in proteins:** Free radicals promote sulfhydryl-mediated protein crosslinking. This oxidative modification of proteins enhances degradation or loss of enzymatic activity. Free radical reactions may directly cause fragmentation of polypeptide

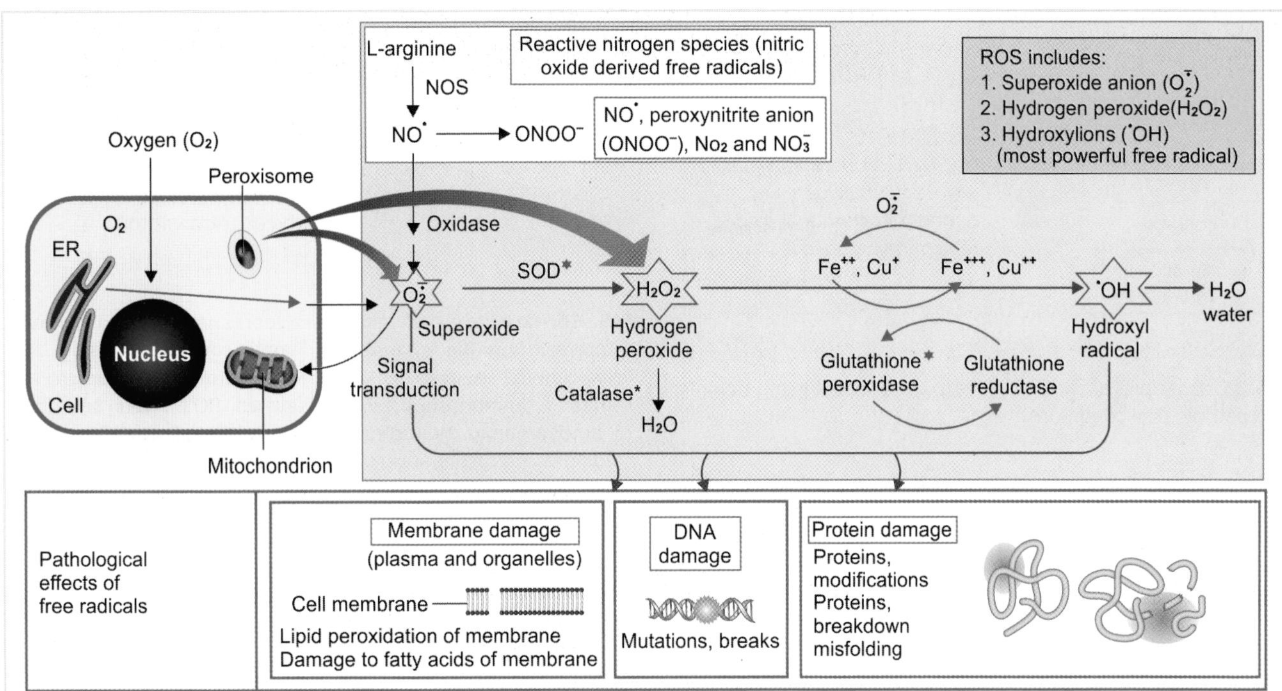

*Antioxidant enzymes.

(NOS: nitric oxide synthase)

FIG. 34: Production of reactive oxygen species (ROS) and antioxidant mechanisms. In the mitochondria, interaction of O_2 and H_2 produces H_2O and during the synthesis of adenosine triphosphate (ATP), superoxide ($O_2^{\bar{\cdot}}$) free radicals are generated from H_2O within the mitochondria. Superoxide ($O_2^{\bar{\cdot}}$) is also converted to peroxynitrite ($ONOO^-$) in the presence of nitric oxide (NO). ROS [hydrogen peroxide (H_2O_2), hydroxyl radical ($^{\cdot}OH$), superoxide ($O_2^{\bar{\cdot}}$) and nitric oxide (NO)] can physiologically modulate some functions of mitochondrial but also may cause cell damage. O_2 is converted to superoxide ($O_2^{\bar{\cdot}}$) by oxidative enzymes in the mitochondria, endoplasmic reticulum (ER), plasma membrane, peroxisomes, and cytosol. Superoxide ($O_2^{\bar{\cdot}}$) is converted to H_2O_2 by superoxide dismutase (SOD) and further to hydroxyl radical (•OH) by the trace metals (e.g., Fe^{++}/Cu^{++})—Fenton reaction. Superoxide catalyzes the reduction of Fe^{++} to Fe^{+++}, thus increasing $OH^{\cdot}$ formation by the Fenton reaction. H_2O_2 is also derived from oxidases in peroxisomes (not shown in Figure). The $NO^{\cdot}$ (radical) is produced by the oxidation of L-arginine. L-arginine is the physiological substrate of nitric oxide (NO) synthesis. NO can be converted to other reactive nitrogen species including the highly reactive peroxynitrite ($ONOO^-$). Both hydroxyl radical ($OH^{\cdot}$) and peroxynitrite ($ONOO^-$) are very reactive; they can modify cellular macromolecules and cause toxicity. The less reactive molecules superoxide ($O_2^{\bar{\cdot}}$) and H_2O_2 can serve as cellular signaling molecules. The major antioxidant enzymes include SOD, catalase, and glutathione peroxidase.

chains. Damaged proteins may not fold properly (abnormal folding of proteins) and stimulate the unfolded protein response.

- **Damage to DNA:** Free radicals can react with thymine residues present in nuclear and mitochondrial DNA and produce single and double strand DNA breaks. They also cause cross-linking DNA strands, and forms adducts. Such DNA damage can lead to cell death by apoptosis, aging, and mutations, leading to malignant transformation of cells.

Note: Though ROS is highlighted above as villain for its role in cell injury and the killing of microbes, ROS in low concentrations are involved in numerous signaling pathways in cells and thus are necessary for many physiologic reactions. Therefore, it is to be kept in mind that these ROS molecules are produced normally. But to avoid their harmful effects, it is necessary to tightly regulate their intracellular concentrations in healthy cells.

Physiological Roles of Free Radicals

- Reactive oxygen species are chemically reactive molecules derived from molecular oxygen. They are produced as natural oxidant species in cells during aerobic metabolism (during mitochondrial respiration) and energy generation. They play an important biologic role and also a role in various diseases.
- Free radicals and reactive intermediates are necessary for a number of cell functions. Normal biological role includes normal cellular communication and cell function. ROS reversibly modulate many intracellular signaling pathways and are involved in signal transduction pathways. ROS can affect protein functions through several mechanisms such as—(1) regulation of protein expression, (2) post-translational modifications, and (3) alteration of protein stability. These mechanisms can—(1) regulate protein stability, (2) increase and decrease protein function, (3) alter protein location, and (4) alter protein-protein interaction. Complete suppression of free radical formation is not desirable, and controlled and moderate free radical production is required for physiological conditions.
- Reduction-oxidation (redox)-dependent regulation and the roles of ROS consist of both normal physiological as well as pathological roles (**Fig. 35**). These include

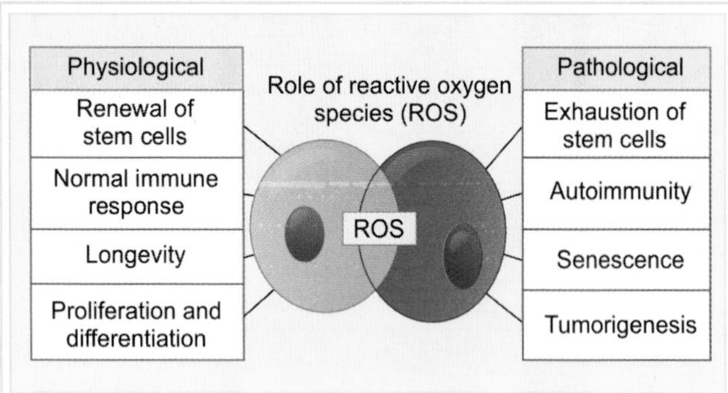

FIG. 35: Examples of role of reactive oxygen species in physiological and pathological conditions.

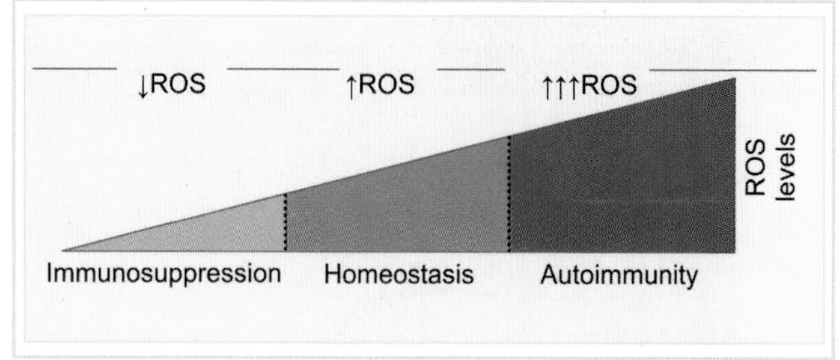

FIG. 36: Low levels of reactive oxygen species (ROS) maintain a normal immune system and homeostasis. Decreasing ROS levels inhibit activation or normal immune responses and results in immunosuppression. Elevated ROS levels contribute to autoimmunity by increasing the release of proinflammatory cytokines and proliferation of some adaptive immune cells.

proliferation and differentiation, immune function, stem cell self-renewal, tumor progression, autoimmunity, stem cell exhaustion, senescence, and longevity.
- Relationship of levels of ROS with normal immune system is depicted in **Figure 36.**

Conditions Associated with Increased Generation of Oxygen-derived Free Radicals

Cell injury produced by free radicals (mainly ROS) is an important mechanism of cell damage in many conditions. **Free radical-mediated cell injury is seen in many types of injury** and includes the following:

Free radicals may be generated within cells in different ways.

- **During inflammation and microbial killing by phagocytes (rapid bursts):** ROS regulation of inflammation is depicted in **Figure 37)** (refer pages 240–242).
- **Enzymatic metabolism of exogenous chemicals or drugs** including chemical carcinogens: For example, a product of carbon tetrachloride (CCl_4) can form free radicals.
- **Absorption of extreme energy sources:** For example, ultraviolet light, radiation, X-rays can also produce free radicals. Ionizing radiation can hydrolyze water (H_2O) into hydroxyl ($^{\bullet}OH$) and hydrogen ($H^{\bullet}$) free radicals.
- **Reduction-oxidation (redox) reaction:** Reduction-oxidation reactions (redox reactions) in normal metabolic processes such as respiration. ROS type of free radicals are produced normally in small amounts in the mitochondria, during the reduction-oxidation (redox) reactions occurring during mitochondrial respiration, and production of energy. Under normal physiological conditions ROS acts as "redox messengers" in the regulation of intracellular signaling. However, when ROS is produced in excess, it may cause irreversible damage to cellular components. All biological membranes contain redox systems and redox systems are important for cell defense (e.g., inflammation, iron uptake, growth and proliferation, and signal transduction).
- **Ischemia-reperfusion injury** induced by restoration of blood flow in ischemic tissue (refer pages 175–176).
- **Transition metals:** Trace metals such as iron and copper can donate or accept free electrons during intracellular reactions and activate the formation of free radicals as in the Fenton reaction ($H_2O_2 + Fe^{2+} \rightarrow Fe^{3+} + OH + OH^-$) (refer Fig. 16 and page 241).

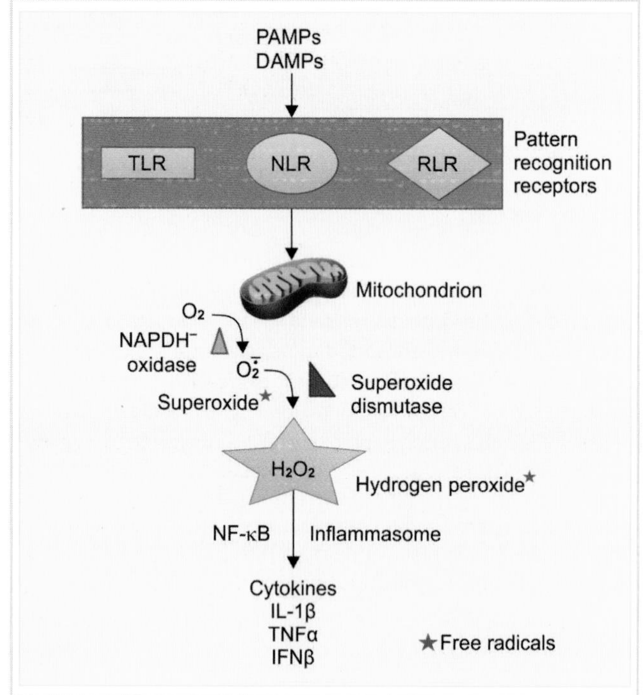

FIG. 37: Reactive oxygen species (ROS) regulation of inflammation needs ROS signaling. Common patterns associated with pathogens (microbes) or cell damage (PAMPS or DAMPS) activate immune surveillance pattern recognition receptors (TLR, NLR, RLR), which increase ROS from NAPDH oxidase enzymes and mitochondria. The release of proinflammatory cytokines [interleukin (IL)-1β, tumor necrosis factor (TNF)-α, interferon (IFN) β] depends on ROS.

- **Cellular aging** (refer pages 210–214).
- **Nitric oxide (NO/**nitrogen monoxide/**NO•):** It is an important colorless gas that is an intermediate in many reactions. It can be produced by endothelial cells, neurons, macrophages, and other cell types. NO is a free radical and can be converted to highly reactive peroxynitrite anion ($ONOO^-$).

$$NO^{\bullet} + O_2^- \rightarrow ONOO^-.$$

Physiological roles of reactive oxygen/nitrogen species in the regulation of cellular function is presented in **Table 7.**

Table 7: Physiological roles of reactive oxygen/nitrogen species.

Physiological function	*Reactive species involved*
Phagocytosis (macrophages)	Superoxide, hydrogen peroxide, nitric oxide
Respiratory burst (neutrophils): Protection against bacterial infection and immune response	Superoxide, hydrogen peroxide, peroxynitrite, hypochlorous acid, hypochlorite
Control of vascular tone and platelet adhesion	Nitric oxide
Spermatogenesis and fertilization	Superoxide, hydrogen peroxide
Apoptosis	Hydrogen peroxide
Cellular growth, differentiation, and proliferation	Nitric oxide, hydrogen peroxide
Biochemical reactions	Hydroxyl radical, hydrogen peroxide
Signal transduction and intercellular communication	Superoxide, nitric oxide

Response of Cells Exposed to Free Radicals

It depends on the type and concentration of free radicals, exposure time, and activation of antioxidant defense mechanisms and repair systems. The cells may respond in three ways:

- **Adaptation:** Cells will upregulate their antioxidant defense systems and undergo adaptive changes.
- **Tissue injury:** Increased oxidative stress (OS) may damage all molecular targets. Cells may respond in different ways such as increased proliferation, halted cell cycle, and senescence.
- **Cell death:** This may be by either necrosis or apoptosis.

Oxidative Stress in the Pathogenesis of Diseases

Overproduction of free radical and the subsequent OS have been associated with a wide variety of pathologies. These include atherosclerosis and cardiovascular diseases; iabetes mellitus and metabolic syndrome; cancer; neurodegenerative diseases, including Alzheimer's and Parkinson's; autoimmune disorders; male and female infertility; as well as psychological impairments such as bipolar disorder, schizophrenia, or attention deficit hyperactivity disorder. The most prominent are shown in **Figure 38**.

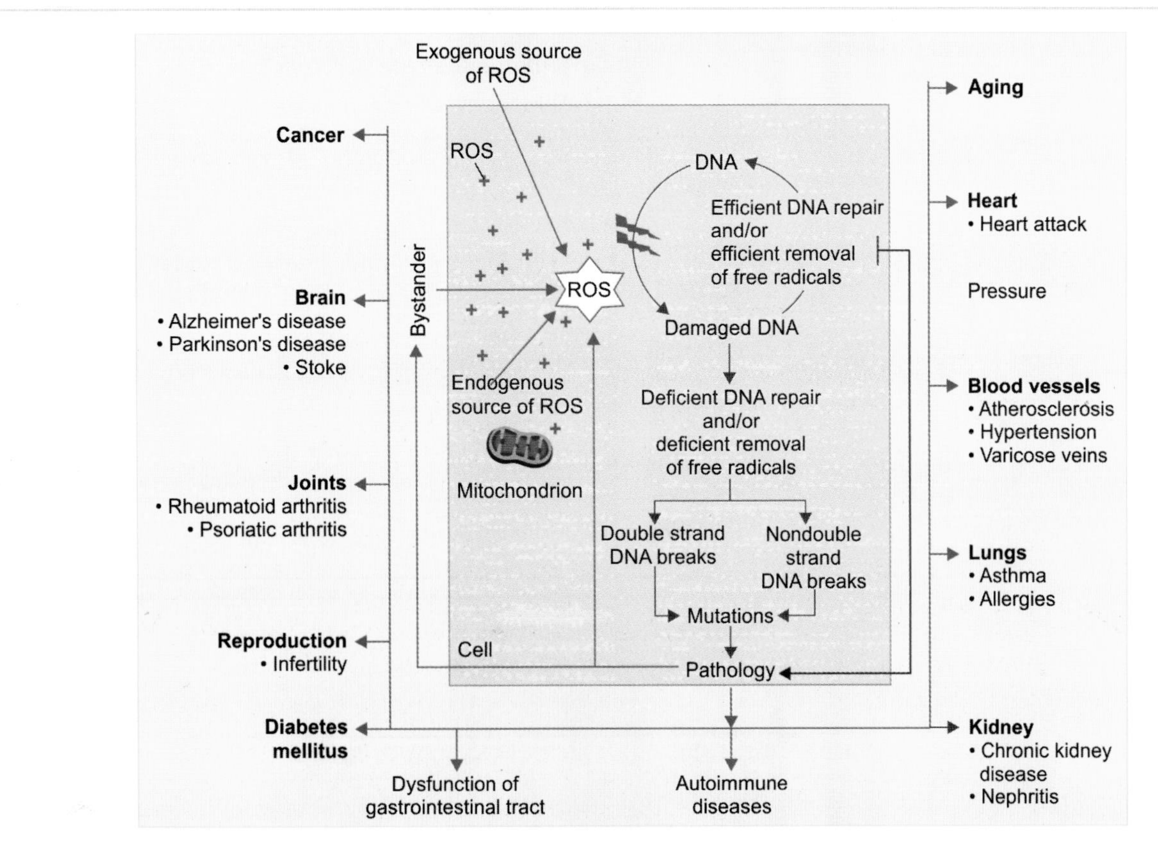

FIG. 38: Oxidative stress in the pathogenesis of diseases. Reactive oxygen species (ROS) play a role in many diseases and age-related conditions (e.g., cancer, neurologic disease, type 2 diabetes mellitus, autoimmune and cardiovascular diseases, infertility, and normal aging). Chronic exposure to ROS and decreased repair of deoxyribonucleic acid (DNA) can lead to permanent DNA mutations. Accumulation of DNA lesions can lead to DNA double strand breaks (DSBs) and disease onset/progression. Diseased cells can in turn produce ROS and decrease the efficiency of the DNA repair mechanism.

Cardiovascular diseases

Reactive oxygen species play roles in the initiation and progression of cardiovascular alterations associated with hypertension, hyperlipidemia, diabetes mellitus, ischemic heart disease, chronic heart failure, and sleep apnea. ROS produce vascular endothelial injury and produces atherosclerosis. ROS can upregulate production of adhesion molecule in the endothelium, which reduces activity of NO synthase and promotes NO breakdown. ROS control endothelial function and vascular tone and reduces endothelial-dependent vasodilation. The endothelial dysfunction may be produced by ROS in inflammation, hypertrophy, proliferation, apoptosis, fibrosis, angiogenesis, and vascular remodeling. Increased OS and increased ROS in diabetes and hypertension can lead to stress-induced arrhythmia and sudden death.

Development of the placenta during pregnancy

It is related to oxygen concentration. ROS can affect trophoblast proliferation, invasion, and angiogenesis. OS influences autophagy and apoptosis. Imbalance in these two processes can be related to pregnancy-related disorders, such as miscarriage, pre-eclampsia, and intrauterine growth restriction.

Oxidative stress is observed in maternal smoking, maternal obesity, and pre-eclampsia and these can be associated with aberrant angiogenesis and placental dysfunction. These in turn can lead to adverse outcomes in pregnancy.

- *Brain disorders*: Ischemic brain injury, Alzheimer's disease, aluminum toxicity, neurotoxins, and stroke
- AIDS-associated dementia
- Cancer
- Deterioration in aging
- Diabetes mellitus

Loss of Calcium Homeostasis (Fig. 39)

Q. Describe the role of calcium in cell injury.

Different Ion Concentrations Inside and Outside of a Cell

Lipid bilayers of plasma membrane are impermeable to inorganic ions. In the living cells, it is capable of maintaining internal ion concentrations different from the concentrations of ions in the surrounding medium. These differences in ion concentration are important for a cell's survival and function. Most important inorganic ions for cells are Na^+, K^+, Ca^{2+}, Cl^-, and H^+ (protons). The movement of these ions across cell membranes plays an important role in many biological processes, but the most important role is in the production of ATP by all cells and in the communication of nerve cells. Na^+ is the most positively charged ion (cation) present in high concentration outside the cell, whereas K^+ is most abundant inside the cell. For a normal cell, the quantity of positive charge inside the cell must be balanced by an almost exactly equal quantity of negative charge. It also applies for the charge in the surrounding interstitial fluid. The high concentration of Na^+ outside the cell is electrically balanced mainly by negatively charged extracellular Cl^-. The high concentration of positively charged K^+ inside is balanced by many negatively charged inorganic and organic ions (anions). These include nucleic acids, proteins, and many cell metabolites.

Ca^{2+} Pumps Keep the Cytosolic Ca^{2+} Concentration Low

Ca^{2+}, like Na+, is also present in low concentration in the cytosol compared to its concentration in the extracellular fluid. But Ca^{2+} is present in much less quantity than Na^+, both inside and

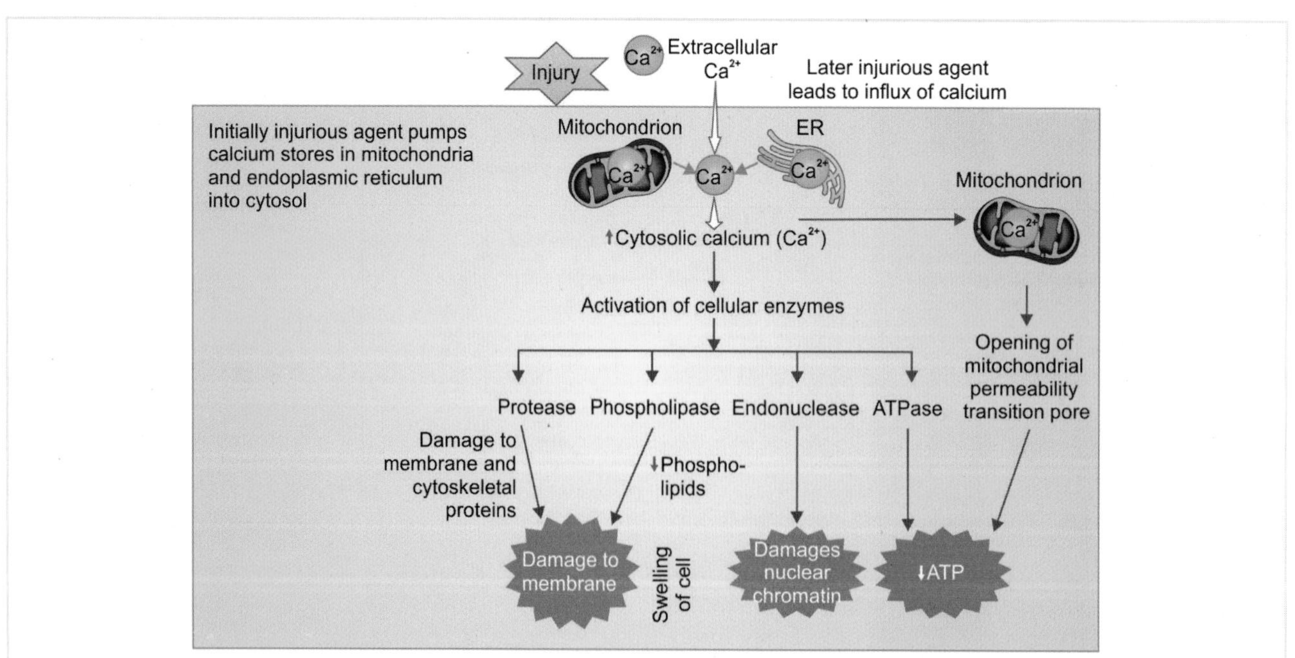

FIG. 39: Effects of increased cytosolic calcium in cell injury. Calcium is normally removed from the cytosol by adenosine triphosphate (ATP)-dependent calcium pumps. In normal cells, calcium is bound to buffering proteins and is present in the endoplasmic reticulum and the mitochondria. Calcium level increases in the cytosol due to—(1) abnormal permeability of calcium ion channels, (2) direct damage to membranes, or (3) depletion of ATP (i.e., hypoxic injury). If the free cytosolic calcium cannot be buffered or pumped out of cells, uncontrolled enzyme activation takes place, causing further damage.

outside cells. Normally, in the cytosol calcium concentration is very low (~0.1 μmol), compared with its concentration in extracellular fluid (1.3 μmol). In normal cells, calcium is bound to buffering proteins (e.g., calbindin or parvalbumin) and is present/sequestered in the endoplasmic reticulum (ER) and the mitochondria. The lower the concentration of free Ca^{2+} in the cytosol, the cell is more sensitive to an increase in cytosolic Ca^{2+}. However, the movement of Ca^{2+} across cell membranes is very crucial. This is because Ca^{2+} can bind tightly to a variety of proteins in the cell and alter their activities.

The big difference in the concentration between in cytosol and outside the cells is mainly achieved by means of ATP-dependent Ca^{2+} pumps present in both the plasma membrane and the ER membrane. Calcium is normally removed from the cytosol by ATP-dependent calcium pumps. This actively removes Ca^{2+} from the cytosol.

Ischemia and Toxins

Calcium ions are important mediators of cell injury. Thus, cells can be protected from injury induced by a variety of harmful stimuli by depleting calcium. Ischemia and certain toxins cause an increase in the concentration of calcium in the cytosol. Initially, it is due to the release of Ca^{2+} from intracellular stores and later due to influx from outside the cell membrane. Increased intracellular calcium stimulates **activation of several damaging enzymes** (e.g., phospholipases, endonucleases, and protease) as well as caspases which causes cell injury. The **net result is apoptosis**. Uncontrolled entry of calcium into the cytosol is an important final pathway observed in many causes of cell death.

Mechanism of Injury by Increased Intracellular Calcium

Intracellular accumulation of calcium salts can occur in both injured and dead tissues. An important mechanism of cellular calcification is the influx of extracellular calcium in injured mitochondria.

Opening of the mitochondrial permeability transition pore: Failure of ATP production opens the mitochondrial permeability transition pore and releases calcium sequestered in mitochondria into cytosol.

Activation of damaging enzymes: If the increased free cytosolic calcium cannot be buffered or pumped out of cells, uncontrolled enzyme activation takes place. Increased cytosolic Ca^{2+} activates many enzymes capable of damaging cells. These enzymes include:

- **Phospholipases: Activation of phospholipase A_2 (PLA_2) produces** membrane damage. Degradation of membrane phospholipids by phospholipase leads to release of free fatty acids and lysophospholipids. The lysophospholipids act as detergents that dissolve the membrane of the cell. Both fatty acids and lysophospholipids are also powerful mediators of inflammation (arachidonic acid metabolites released from these cells). Inflammation may further damage the integrity of the already compromised cell.
- **Proteases: Activation of phospholipase A_2 (PLA_2) together with proteases** breaks down **the plasma membrane and** cytoskeletal proteins. This disrupts cytoskeleton and its attachments to the plasma/cell membrane. This leads to formation of membrane blebs leading to change in the shape of the cell. The combination of electrolyte imbalance and increased permeability of plasma/cell membrane causes accumulation of fluid inside the cell producing swelling of the cell.
    - **Endonucleases:** They cause fragmentation of DNA and chromatin.
    - **ATPases:** These speed up depletion of ATP.

Stimulates apoptosis: Increased intracellular Ca^{2+} levels stimulate apoptosis, by direct activation of caspases as well as by increasing mitochondrial permeability.

EXAMPLES OF CELL INJURY AND DEATH

Hypoxia and Ischemia

Q. Describe in detail the sequence of events in ischemic and hypoxic injury to cells.

Hypoxia is only one component of ischaemia, the two are not equivalent. Hypoxia refers to inadequate oxygenation (oxygen deprivation or lack of sufficient oxygen) of cells/tissue, and decreased blood flow is called ischemia. It includes states of inadequate delivery or utilisation of oxygen such that tissue and cell function are compromised. It is the single most common cause of cell injury and necrosis.

- Ischemia results from a mechanical arterial obstruction. This obstruction may be due to thrombosis, embolism, atherosclerosis or external compression of a vessel. Myocardial infarction and cerebral stroke are the most common cause of mortality and both are due to ischemic cell death. Ischemia can also occur due to reduced venous drainage.
- Pure impairments of oxygen supply (hypoxia), without ischemia is uncommon. Pure hypoxic state differs from ischemia in that ischemia is associated with failure of supply of other substrates and of removal of waste products such as lactate and CO_2 resulting in tissue acidosis Pure hypoxia may occur in young children with respiratory obstruction. Inadequate oxygenation of the blood (hypoxemia) can result from a reduced amount of oxygen in the air, decreased oxygen-carrying capacity of the blood [e.g., reduced hemoglobin (e.g., anemia), or decreased efficacy of hemoglobin (e.g., carbon monoxide poisoning), decreased production of red blood cells (RBCs), severe blood loss, diseases of the respiratory and cardiovascular systems (decreased perfusion of tissues e.g., cardiac failure, hypotension shock)], and poisoning of the oxidative enzymes (cytochromes) within the cells. Hypoxia is also associated with the pathophysiologic conditions such as inflammation, ischemia, and cancer. Hypoxia can induce inflammation and inflamed tissue can become hypoxic. The cellular mechanisms involved in hypoxia and inflammation include activation of immune responses and oxygen-sensing compounds called *prolyl hydroxylases (PHDs)* (refer **Fig. 40**) and *hypoxia inducible transcription factor (HIF) (discussed further).*
- **Ischemic damage is severe and more rapid than due to hypoxia**: In hypoxia blood flow is maintained and during which there is continuation of energy production by anaerobic glycolysis. In contrast, in ischemia there is reduced delivery of substrates for glycolysis. Thus,

in ischemic tissues, the aerobic metabolism stops and anaerobic energy production also fails. This occcurs after exhaustion of glycolytic substrates or inhibition of glycolysis by the accumulation of metabolites. These accumulated metabolites are normally cleared by flowing blood. Thus, ischemia causes more rapid and severe injury to cell and tissue than hypoxia.

Role of hypoxia: Hypoxia plays a role in physiologic processes including cell differentiation, angiogenesis, cell proliferation, erythropoiesis, and overall viability of cells. Mammalian development occurs in a hypoxic environment. There is a link between hypoxia and inflammation in inflammatory bowel disease, certain cancers, and infections. Tumors adapt to low oxygen levels by inducing angiogenesis, increasing glucose consumption, and promoting the metabolic state of glycolysis.

The ability of tissues to maintain oxygen homeostasis is essential for the survival of all cells. The cells need to balance the production of ATP via oxidative phosphorylation against the risk of generating reactive oxygen species (ROS). ROS are capable of damaging cellular DNA, lipids and proteins. Nearly all nucleated cells in human are capable of sensing oxygen concentration and responding to hypoxic conditions. Similar to other physiological systems, adaptation to acute changes in oxygen concentration occurs through alterations (e.g phosphorylation) of existing proteins. Adaptation to chronic changes in oxygenation result from alterations of gene expression. Hypoxia and the cellular response to it are important contributors to a wide range of disorders.

Outcome: Depending on the severity of the hypoxia, cells may adapt, undergo injury, or die.

Mechanism of Injury

Mitochondrial involvement: Hypoxia (inadequate/deficient oxygenation) leads to failure of several energy-dependent metabolic pathways. Oxygen is mainly consumed by mitochondria and the cellular responses to hypoxia are mediated by the production of ROS in the mitochondria. Hypoxia causes cell injury by reducing aerobic oxidative respiration and decreasing the synthesis of ATP. Most of the ATP in the cell is produced from adenosine diphosphate (ADP) by oxidative phosphorylation during reduction of oxygen in the electron transport system of mitochondria. ATP is needed for several cellular functions such as: (1) membrane transport, (2) protein synthesis, (3) lipogenesis, and (4) the diacylation-reacylation reactions necessary for phospholipid turnover. Hence, hypoxia can lead to failure of many essential functions and ultimately can to death of cells by necrosis.

Hypoxia response mechanisms in neoplasia: Hypoxic areas develop in tumors with increasing tumor size and degree of malignancy. Hypoxia increases the levels of cell death by apoptosis and necrosis associated with malignant tumors Hypoxia and the cellular adaptations have a role in a range of tumour-related processes. These include angiogenesis and resistance to adjuvant therapies. Probably hypoxia may exert selective pressure within the tumor micro-environment and contribute to tumor progression. Tumor cells developing a mutation, such as in the *p53* gene, which avoids hypoxia-induced apoptosis may compete with cells without the mutation. This may result in a more aggressive clone.

Hypoxia Inducible Factor-1

Q. Discuss gene expression induced by hypoxia inducible factors.

A range of hypoxia-inducible genes may be activated during hypoxic conditions. Many of these genes have a common method of regulation through activation of transcription factors called the hypoxia-inducible factors (HIFs). Hypoxia-inducible factor is a heterodimeric transcription factor. There are now several molecules in this family. It consists of an alpha (α) subunit and a beta (β) subunit, both of which are members of the basic Helix-Loop-Helix-PAS domain family. There are three isoforms of human HIFα (HIF-1α, HIF-2α, HIF-3α) and three human HIFβ [often called as ARNTs (i.e., aryl hydrocarbon receptor nuclear translocators)] family members. Most attention has focused on HIF-1α. HIF-1α and HIF-2α act to transcription factor that increases the resistance to hypoxic stress and HIF-3α acts as negative regulator of hypoxia inducible gene expression. HIF-1β is constitutively expressed but the mRNA expression of HIF-1α, the half-life of its protein and transactivation domain function are all regulated by cellular oxygen concentrations.

Sites of normal expression: Both HIF-1α and HIF-2α mrna are expressed in many types of cells. HIF-1α RNA is prevalent in all tissues except in peripheral blood leukocytes and HIF-2α RNA is highly expressed in vascular tissue such as lung, heart, placenta and kidney.

Regulation of HIF during normal oxygenation and hypoxic conditions (Fig. 40)

Cells subjected to hypoxia (low O_2 tension/deficiency of oxygen) do not die immediately activate compensatory mechanisms. These compensatory mechanisms are induced by transcription factors of the HIF family. The HIF is a family of transcription regulators that coordinate the expression of many genes in response to oxygen deprivation or hypoxic stress, both in physiological and pathological conditions. The expression of HIF-1 and HIF-1 transcriptional activity are accurately controlled by cellular concentrations of oxygen.

- **Normal function:** HIF-1β is constitutively expressed but HIF-1α is expressed at only low levels when there is normal oxygen (normoxic conditions). In the presence of oxygen, HIFα is hydroxylated on one (or both) of two prolyl sites (proline residues) by oxygen-sensing compounds called *PHDs.* Hydroxylation of either of these sites of HIFα generates a binding site for pVHL [von Hippel-Lindau (tumor suppressor)], which is stably bound to elongin B (*B*), elongin C (*C*), Cul2, and Rbx1 (*R*). This complex is then polyubiquitylates HIFα. Once ubiquitylated, HIFα is then degraded by the proteasome (**Fig. 40A**). Thus, in non-hypoxic cells, the HIF-1 and HIF-2 proteins are ubiquitinated and undergo proteosomal degradation leading to inactivation.
- **During hypoxia (Fig. 40B):** Under low-oxygen (with decreasing cellular oxygen concentrations) conditions (or in cells lacking pVHL), activity of enzyme *PHDs* is impaired because these enzymes require oxygen in order to function. This leads to stabilization and exponential increase in the activity of HIF-1α. Accumulated stabilized subunit HIF-1α then binds to HIFβ often called *ARNT* (a gene that encodes

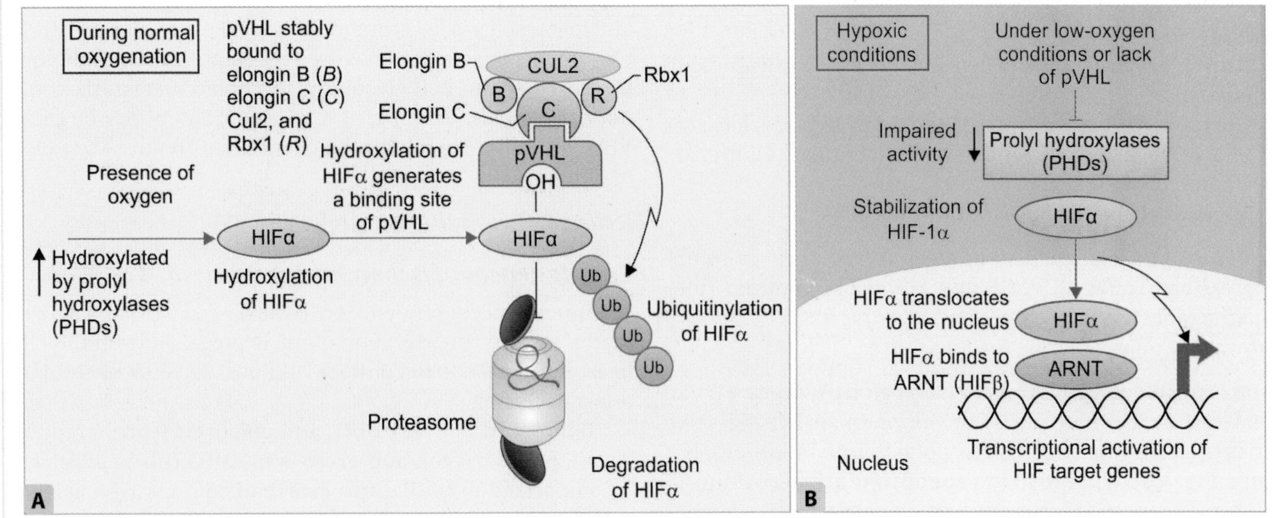

(ARNT: aryl hydrocarbon receptor nuclear translocator)

FIGS. 40A AND B: Regulation of hypoxia-inducible factor (HIF) during normal oxygenation and hypoxic conditions. (A) In the presence of oxygen, proline residues of HIFα are hydroxylated by prolyl hydroxylases (PHDs) enzymes. This creates a binding site for von Hippel–Lindau protein (pVHL), which is stably bound to elongin B (B), elongin C (C), Cul2, and Rbx1 (R). This complex is then undergoes ubiquitinylation and degradation by proteasome. (B) Under low-oxygen conditions, or in cells lacking pVHL, HIFα binds to *ARNT* (a gene that encodes the aryl hydrocarbon receptor nuclear translocator protein), translocates to the nucleus, and activates HIF target genes such as vascular endothelial growth factor (VEGF).

the aryl hydrocarbon receptor nuclear translocator protein). Binding of HIF-1α with HIF-1β, makes them more resistant to proteolytic digestion. Then HIF-1α then translocates to nucleus and bind to core DNA sequences of their target genes. They are rapidly degraded upon subsequent re-oxygenation. HIF-1α activates vascular endothelial growth factor (*VEGF*) and other about 30 genes that contain hypoxia-response elements and promote adaptation to hypoxia. This response promotes a metabolic shift away from oxidative phosphorylation toward oxygen-independent glycolysis, increased vascularization, and decreased *mTORC1* activity by inducing expression of *REDD1* and *REDD2*. *REDD1/2* and *mTORC1* can also potentiate HIF-1α by increasing its transcription and translation. In contrast to HIF-1α and HIF-2α, most of the HIF-3α isoforms lack transactivation capability and may even reduce activity of HIF-1α and HIF-2α.

Actions of hypoxia-inducible factor-1

Hypoxia-inducible factor-1α is the master regulator of transcriptional responses to low O_2 tension and activates genes whose protein products limit production of ROS, Ca^{2+} accumulation and ATP depletion. Thus, HIF-1α tries to protect against mitochondrial injury, DNA damage and OS, and so facilitates survival of the ischemic cell.

- **Vascular endothelial growth factor:** Hypoxia stimulates the synthesis of VEGF. VEGF stimulates the growth of new vessels and attempts to increase blood flow and the supply of oxygen to the tissue. Hypoxia is a major signal for inducing angiogenesis. The HIF family (HIF-1α and HIF-2α) modulate angiogenesis through the gene transcription of vascular endothelial growth factor (VEGF) and vascular endothelial growth factor receptor (VEGFR-1) and the protein expression of VEGFR-2.
- **Other proteins induced by HIF-1:** Hypoxia-inducible factor-1 stimulates the synthesis of several proteins that help the cell to survive in the face of low oxygen.
- **Adenosine triphosphate production:** The adaptive changes in cellular metabolism by HIF include stimulation of the uptake of glucose and glycolysis and diminishing of mitochondrial oxidative phosphorylation. During hypoxia, there is reduced ATP production by aerobic glycolysis. In the absence of oxygen, anaerobic glycolysis can generate ATP using glucose derived either from the circulation or from the hydrolysis of intracellular glycogen. Normal tissues rich in glycogen in the cytoplasm (e.g., the liver and striated muscle) have a greater glycolytic capacity. These tissues are more likely to survive hypoxia and decreased oxidative phosphorylation than tissues with limited glucose stores (e.g., the brain). It is to be noted that anaerobic glycolysis yields less ATP per molecule of glucose burned than oxidative phosphorylation or aerobic glycolysis. On the contrary, rapidly proliferating normal cells and cancer cells depend on aerobic glycolysis to produce much of their energy. This phenomenon is called as the Warburg effect (refer pages 487–491). The metabolites generated by glycolysis and the citric acid cycle [or tricarboxylic acid (TCA) cycle or Krebs cycle] serve as precursors for the synthesis of cellular constituents (e.g., proteins, lipids, and nucleic acids), that are needed for cell growth and division in cancer. If hypoxia persists or become severe, the ischemia can lead to failure of ATP generation and depletion of ATP in cells. Loss of ATP is harmful for many cellular systems.

Application of hypoxia-inducible factor

Normal roles

- **During embryogenesis:** Responsible for angiogenesis in embryo.
- **During repair:** In the wound induced by hypoxia, it causes migration of epithelial cells and angiogenesis during wound repair.
- **Survival of chondrocytes** in the bone plate.

Pathological Consequences of HIFs It has a role in tumor progression (**Table 8**), VEGF and HIF play important roles in pathogenesis of the cancer and also the *PI3K/Akt/mTOR* pathway.

Hypoxia-inducible factor and renal cell carcinoma When renal cell carcinoma (RCC) develops in pVHL-defective patients, there will be impaired polyubiquitylation of HIFα (refer **Fig. 40**). This leads to inappropriate activation of HIF target genes under normal oxygenation. HIF activates a number of genes supposed to play roles in kidney carcinogenesis. These include transforming growth factor alpha (TGF-α), cyclin D1, stromal cell-derived factor 1 (SDF1), CXCR4, matrix metalloproteinases (MMPs) family members, *PDGFB*, and VEGF. The increased expression of factors such as VEGF is likely to be responsible for highly angiogenic nature of clear cell renal carcinomas and they respond to VEGF blocker. HIFα without its partner HIFβ, can also activate Notch signaling and thereby may be involved in renal carcinogenesis.

Hypoxia-inducible factor in other cancers HIF activation may be play via several mechanisms and contribute to tumor pathogenesis. Increased expression of HIF-1α appears to be a marker of more aggressive disease in tumors (e.g., breast and cervical cancer, CNS tumors). By activation of a range of genes, expression of HIF may grant a selective advantage to a tumor. For example, it may promote angiogenesis via VEGF, prolong survival of tumor cells via insulin-like growth factor, and affect metabolism through induced expression of glucose transporters. Inactivation of tumor-suppressor genes (e.g., *p53*) or increased expression of oncogenes (e.g., *HER2*) can lead to increased expression of HIF-1α-regulated angiogenic factors and increased vascularization. Increased expression of HIF-1α may be responsible for increased resistance to chemotherapy, increased tumor cell glycolysis, increased metastasis, and a poor prognosis. The use of angiogenic inhibitors targeting VEGF signaling can inhibit angiogenesis and reduce the growth of tumor.

Table 8: Functions of hypoxia-inducible factor (HIF) and the upregulated genes.

Functions	*Upregulated genes and proteins*
Cell Proliferation	Transforming growth factor (TGF) α, TGF-β3, insulin like growth factor (IGF), IGFBP (insulin like growth factor binding protein), cyclin
Angiogenesis	Vascular endothelial growth factor (VEGF), EG-VEGF (endothelial gland derived VEGF), VEGF receptor 1 (VEGFR1), plasminogen activator inhibitor (PAI)
Hormonal regulation	Erythropoietin (EPO), leptin (LEP)
Metabolism	Glucose transporter 1 (GLUT1), hexokinase (HK) 1 and 2, aldolase A and C (ALD A/C), pyruvate kinase
Breaching of matrix barrier during metastasis	Matrix metalloproteinase 2 (MMP2), fibronectin 1 (FN 1), cathepsin D (CATHD)

Ischemic Preconditioning (refer page 177)

Consequences of Ischemia/Hypoxia (Fig. 41)

The functional consequences of hypoxia and ischemia depend on the severity and duration of the hypoxia. For example, the heart muscle stops to contract within 60 seconds of coronary artery occlusion.

- **Decreased delivery of O_2 and glucose:** Hypoxia reduces supply of oxygen and glucose to cells. This is especially important for cardiac myocytes and neurons, which do not store much energy.
- **Distortion of the activities of pumps in the plasma membrane alter the ionic balance of the cell.**
- **Reduced activity of sodium pump:** The internal cellular milieu of cell is separated from extracellular fluid by the plasma membrane. Plasma membrane has selective ion permeability. This requires—(1) considerable energy (i.e., ATP), (2) structural integrity of the lipid bilayer, (3) intact ion channel proteins, and (4) normal association of the plasma membrane with cytoskeleton. Ischemia reduces activity of plasma membrane ATP-dependent sodium pumps. This results in intracellular accumulation of sodium and efflux of potassium. Na^+ accumulates because lack of ATP impairs the Na^+/K^+ ion exchanger. This effect leads to activation of the Na^+/H^+ ion exchanger. Along with sodium, water also enters into the cytosol and causes cell swelling and dilation of the ER. If ischemia is incomplete or brief, normal ionic equilibrium can be re-established without tissue damage. However, in severe ischemia the cell reaches a "point of no return" and leads to cell death.
- **Influx of calcium:** Ca^{2+} concentration in extracellular fluids is in the millimolar range (10^{-3} M) and cytosolic Ca^{2+} concentration is 1/10,000 of that outside the cell (i.e., about 10^{-7} M). The increase in intracellular sodium activates the Na^+/Ca^{2+} ion exchanger, which increases calcium entry. Normally, excess intracellular Ca^{2+} is extruded by an ATP-dependent calcium pump. Due to acute shortage of ATP, Ca^{2+} accumulates in the cell (refer **Fig. 39**).
- **Overproduction of lactate and decreased intracellular pH:** The reduced aerobic glycolysis causes compensatory increase in anaerobic glycolysis. The end product of anaerobic glycolysis leads to formation of lactic acid and this accumulates in the cytosol. Accumulated lactic acid decreases intracellular pH (acidification), and decreased activity of many cellular enzymes.
- **Disturbance of the protein synthesis:** Prolonged depletion of ATP disrupts the protein synthetic apparatus with a consequent reduction in synthesis of proteins. The cytoplasm shows detachment of ribosomes from the rough ER (RER) and dissociation of polysomes into monosomes.
- **Accumulation of ROS:** Normally, about 1–3% of oxygen entering mitochondria is converted to ROS. Hypoxia increases the generation of ROS, damages the ROS detoxification mechanisms and impaired processing of

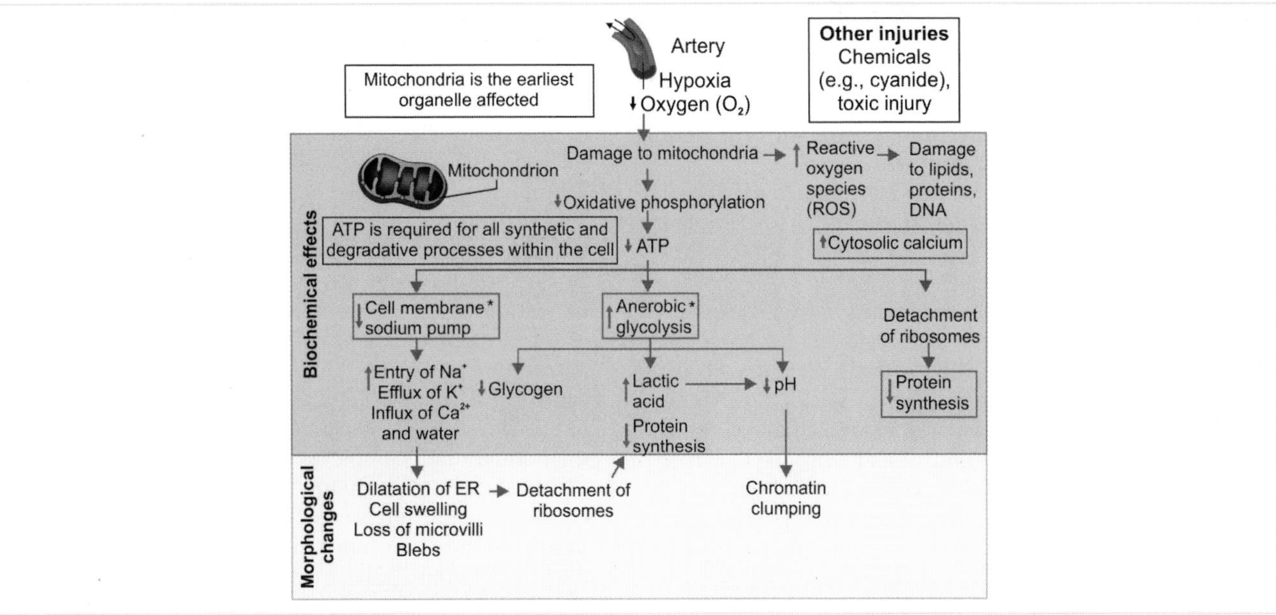

(ATP: adenosine triphosphate; ER: endoplasmic reticulum)
* Indicates the effects of decreased ATP.

FIG. 41: Mechanisms of ischemia-induced cell injury and membrane damage. Loss of oxygen due to occlusion of vessels impairs mitochondrial function. This causes decreased energy [adenosine triphosphate (ATP)] production by aerobic processes. Decreased ATP impairs ATP-dependent ion exchangers. The loss of aerobic processes activates anaerobic glycolysis. This produces intracellular acidosis and increased cytosolic (Ca^{2+}). This in turn activates Ca^{2+}-dependent phospholipases causing destruction of cell membrane.

reactive oxygen intermediates. ROS cause peroxidation of cardiolipin (a membrane phospholipid that is unique to mitochondria) and is sensitive to oxidative damage due to its high content of unsaturated fatty acids. It is known that hypoxia predisposes cells to ROS-mediated damage if blood flow (and oxygen delivery) is re-established. This is called reperfusion injury (see further).

- **Activation of phospholipase A_2 (PLA_2) and proteases: Disrupts the plasma membrane and cytoskeleton.** Raised intracellular Ca^{2+} activates PLA_2. This degrades the membrane phospholipids and release of free fatty acids and lysophospholipids. The lysophospholipids act as detergents and solubilize cell membranes. Both fatty acids and lysophospholipids are also powerful mediators of inflammation, and this may further damage the integrity of the already damaged cell. Calcium also activates proteases that destroy the cytoskeleton and its attachments to the cell membrane. Due to disruption of cohesion between cytoskeletal proteins and the plasma membrane, there will formation of membrane blebs and the shape of cell changes. The cell becomes swollen and may get dissolved.
- **Release of cytochrome c (Cyt c):** Damage to the mitochondria releases Cyt c to the cytosol. In normal cells, there is sporadic opening and closing of the mitochondrial permeability transition pore (MPTP). Ischemic injury to mitochondria causes prolonged opening of the MPTP. This results in release of Cyt c from into the cytosol and may trigger cell death by apoptosis.
- **Irreversible injury:** Ultimately, when a cell can no longer maintain itself as a metabolic unit, hypoxia causes irreversible damage to mitochondrial and lysosomal membranes, and the cell undergoes cell death. Cell death is mainly by necrosis but hypoxia may bring about apoptosis by the mitochondrial pathway. The line between reversible and irreversible cell injury (i.e., the "point of no return") is not well defined.

Ischemia-reperfusion Injury

Q. Write short essay on ischemia-reperfusion injury.

Introduction

- **Decreased blood flow** to a tissue or organ is called **ischemia.**
- Depending on the severity and duration of ischemia, the involved tissue may adapt, undergo injury (reversible), or die (irreversible). Therapies to restore blood flow are the important modality of treating ischemia.
- Reperfusion is the restoration of blood flow after a period of ischemia. If the involved cells of the tissue are reversibly injured, the restoration of blood flow (reperfusion) is often beneficial. However, under certain circumstances the restoration of blood flow to cells that have been ischemic (reversibly injured) but have not died (irreversibly injured), can paradoxically exacerbate and produce injury at an accelerated pace. The process by which reperfusion causes damage is termed as "reperfusion injury".
- The damaging process is set in motion during reperfusion and **reperfused tissues undergo loss of cells** (new damage) **in addition to the cells that are irreversibly damaged (dead) at the end of ischemia.** This damaging process is called as **ischemia-reperfusion injury**.
- **Clinical importance:** It contributes to tissue damage following reperfusion in **myocardial infarction, cerebral**

infarction, and also in other situations (e.g., organ transplantation).

Degrees of Reperfusion Injury

Reperfusion injury can be divided into three different degrees, depending on the duration of the ischemia:

1. **Reversible injury:** If reperfusion (resupply of oxygen) is within a short period of ischemia, there can be complete restoration of the cell's structural and functional integrity. Thus, the cell injury is completely reversible.
2. **Lethal injury during reperfusion:** If reperfusion is established with longer periods of ischemia, it causes cell deterioration and death. Thus, lethal cell injury occurs during the period of reperfusion.
3. **Lethal injury before reperfusion itself:** Lethal cell injury may occur during the period of ischemia itself, which usually was present for longer period. The ischemia itself produced lethal injury and reperfusion is not responsible for this lethal damage.

Mechanism of Reperfusion Injury

Reperfusion injury is due to combination of transient ischemia, consequent tissue damage, and exposure of damaged tissue to the oxygen that arrives when blood flow is re-established (reperfusion). Reperfusion injury can be lethal. In the heart, it may responsible for up to half of the final size of myocardial infarcts. Many factors are involved in reperfusion injury and includes increased production of ROS, RNS [nitric oxide synthase (NOS) and NO•], inflammatory mediators, activation of complement system, platelet-activating factor (PAF), intercellular adhesion molecules, dysregulation of Ca^{2+} homeostasis, etc.

New damage may be initiated during reoxygenation which includes:

- **Increased generation of reactive oxygen and nitrogen species:**
  - **Increased production of free radicals:** Initially, ischemic cellular damage leads to production of free radical species (refer pages 163 and 164). Free radicals may be produced from parenchymal and endothelial cells and from infiltrating leukocytes in reperfused tissue. Free radicals form as a result of mitochondrial damage, causing incomplete reduction of oxygen, or because of the action of oxidases in leukocytes, endothelial cells, or parenchymal cells. Reperfusion provides abundant molecular O_2 which in turn can combine with free radicals already produced to form additional ROS. Thus, new damage may be initiated during reoxygenation by increased generation of reactive oxygen (ROS = recative oxygen species) and nitrogen species (RNS = Reactive nitrogen species).
  - **Decreased antioxidant mechanism:** Ischemia may result in defective cellular antioxidant defense mechanisms, favoring the accumulation of free radicals.
- **Inflammation:** Ischemic injury is associated with inflammation due to release of "danger signals" from dead cells. Ischemic injury produces cytokines (secreted by resident immune cells such as macrophages) and increased expression of adhesion molecules by hypoxic parenchymal and endothelial cells. They recruit circulating neutrophils to reperfused tissue causing inflammation. The inflammation causes further tissue injury. Recruited neutrophils act as an additional source of ROS during reperfusion. Reperfusion prompts endothelial cells to move preformed P-selectin to the cell surface. This increases the binding of neutrophil to intercellular adhesion molecule-1 (ICAM-1) at the surface of the endothelial cell membrane. Recruited neutrophils release large quantities of ROS and hydrolytic enzymes. They cause further injury to the previously ischemic cells.
- **Activation of the complement system:** It is an important mechanism of immune-mediated injury. Some immunoglobulin M (IgM) antibodies may get deposited in the ischemic tissues. When blood flow is restored, complement proteins may bind to the deposited antibodies and complement system may be activated causing inflammation and more injury to cells. Activation of the complement system during reperfusion produces membrane attack complexes which can attract chemotactic agents and proinflammatory cytokines. This also results in recruitment and adhesion of neutrophils.
- **Xanthine oxidase:** Xanthine oxidase activity increases during ischemia, particularly in vascular endothelium. This enzyme converts ATP-derived xanthine into uric acid. This reaction requires oxygen and produces superoxide. During ischemia, abundant purines are formed during catabolism of ATP. On reperfusion, when the oxygen supply returns, these purines produced during ischemia acts as substrates for xanthine oxidase. Since the enzyme xanthine oxidase needs oxygen, restoration of oxygen supply during reperfusion leads to a sudden increase in the production of ROS. The mitochondrial antioxidant systems cannot handle the sudden increase in ROS. Mitochondrial oxidant stress is further aggravated due to—(1) the sudden increase in electron transport, which is due to the renewed availability of oxygen, and (2) the changes in reduced pH and increased intracellular calcium concentrations.
- **Calcium overload:** Intracellular and mitochondrial calcium overload occurs begins during acute ischemia. It it further increased during reperfusion. This is because there is influx of calcium from cell membrane damage and ROS-mediated injury to sarcoplasmic reticulum. Calcium overload leads to opening of the mitochondrial permeability transition pore, ATP depletion and further cell injury (see **Fig. 39**).
- **Ion fluxes during reperfusion:** Ischemia changes ion transporter activities in the cells. This becomes more aggravated with reperfusion. When blood flow is re-established, pH of the cell suddenly becomes normal. The Ca^{2+} overload that began during ischemia becomes exacerbated by reversal of the Na^+/Ca^{2+} exchanger. Increased intracellular Ca^{2+} activates Ca^{2+}-dependent proteases and increases production of ROS. This along with increased mitochondrial ROS opens the mitochondrial permeability transition pore (MPTP) and triggers mitochondria mediated apoptosis.
- **Role of NO and NOS:** NO is produced from arginine by both constitutive and inducible NOSs. NO and NOS are double-edged swords.
  - **Protective role:** NO has a protective effect produced due to (1) dilatation microvasculature by relaxing smooth muscle, (2) inhibition of platelet aggregation, and (3) decreasing leukocyte adhesion to endothelial cells. NO also reduces transferrin-mediated iron uptake. This limits the amount of iron available to

production of OH• from other ROS. These actions are mainly due to the ability of NO to decrease cytosolic Ca^{2+} by moving it from the cell and by sequestering it within intracellular stores.
  - **Damaging role**: During ischemia-triggered ATP depletion, Ca^{2+} overload, and deprivation of nutrient, NO is produced from mitochondrial NOS. NO• also reacts with $O_2^{\bullet-}$ to form $ONOO^-$, which is a highly RNS. Normally, $O_2^{\bullet-}$ is detoxified by SOD and only minute amount of $ONOO^-$ is produced. However, reperfusion both inactivates SOD and supplies abundant $O_2^{\bullet-}$, which together lead to excess production of $ONOO^-$. This free radical causes breaks in DNA strand and produces lipid peroxidation in cell membranes.
- **Inflammatory cytokines:** Reperfusion injury is accompanied by the release of proinflammatory cytokines and promotes inflammation. Proinflammatory cytokines include TNF-α, interleukin (IL)-1 and IL-6. These cytokines: (1) promote vasoconstriction, (2) stimulate adhesion of neutrophils and platelets to endothelium, and (3) have effects at sites distant from the ischemic region itself.
- **Platelets:** Platelets adhere to the microvasculature of injured tissue. These platelets release many factors that have role in both tissue damage and cytoprotection. These include cytokines, TGF-β, serotonin, and NO•.

Reperfusion and its Effects on Myocardial infarction

The ischemic myocardium can be rescued by restoring the myocardial blood flow as quickly as possible by reperfusion.
- **Methods of reperfusion:** It may be achieved by dissolving the thrombus using thrombolytic drugs (plasminogen activator), or angioplasty/stent placement, or coronary artery bypass graft (CABG) surgery.
- **Benefits and outcome of reperfusion:** It depends on rapidity of restoration. Reperfusion within 20 minutes of the onset of ischemia may completely prevent necrosis.

Factors contributing reperfusion injury: These are as follows:
- **Mitochondrial dysfunction**: Permeability of mitochondrial membrane is altered in ischemia. This allows proteins to move into the mitochondria. It results in swelling and rupture of the outer membrane and releases mitochondrial contents. This in turn promotes apoptosis.
- **Hypercontracture of myocyte**: During ischemia, the intracellular levels of calcium are increased. After reperfusion, there is increased and uncontrolled contraction of myofibrils. This produced damage to cytoskeleton and result in death of the myofibrils.
- **Free radicals**: These include superoxide anion, hydrogen peroxide, hypochlorous acid, nitric oxide-derived peroxynitrite, and hydroxyl radicals. They are produced within minutes of reperfusion. They alter membrane proteins and phospholipids and produce damage to the myocytes.
- **Aggregation of leukocyte**: During reperfusion accumulated leukocytes may occlude the microvasculature and may obstruct the reflow of blood. Also, leukocytes release proteases and elastases that cause cell death.
- **Activation of platelet and complement**: They may also contribute to microvascular injury. Complement activation is injures the endothelium and prevents the flow of blood by blocking the microvessels.

MORPHOLOGY OF REPERFUSED MYOCARDIAL INFARCT

Gross
- Reperfused infarcted area appears **hemorrhagic** because the microvasculature is injured during ischemia and it leaks blood with restoration of blood flow.

Microscopy
- **Accelerated acute inflammatory responses:** Neutrophils accumulate more rapidly but also disappear more rapidly.
- **Contraction band necrosis:** It is **one of the characteristic features**. They appear as thick, irregular, transverse, intensely eosinophilic intracellular bands in necrotic myocardial cells. Intense eosinophilic bands of hypercontracted sarcomeres are produced by an influx of calcium across plasma membranes. Increased intracellular calcium increases actinmyosin interactions. Because of absence of ATP , the sarcomeres cannot relax and get stuck in an agonal tetanic state. Thus, though reperfusion can restore reversibly injured cells, but also changes the morphology of irreversibly injured cells.

Stunned myocardium: In reperfused myocytes, the biochemical abnormalities (and their functional consequences) may remain for days to weeks. Such changes are responsible for a phenomenon referred to as stunned myocardium. This is state characterized by prolonged contractile dysfunction produced by short-term ischemia. It usually recovers after several days.

Hibernating myocardium: Myocardium exposed to chronic, sublethal ischemia can enter into a state of lowered metabolism and function. This state is called hibernation. Subsequent revascularization (e.g., by CABG surgery, angioplasty, or stenting) usually restores normal function to such hibernating myocardium.

Complication of reperfusion: Reperfusion injury is mediated by **ROS, calcium overload**, and **severe inflammatory reaction during reperfusion.**

Ischemic Preconditioning

Sudden and complete ischemia may produce cell death before any adaptive mechanisms. However, repeated episodes of ischemia (e.g., in recurrent angina due to coronary artery disease) can stimulate adaptive responses. In the heart, all these **adaptive responses** are termed as **ischemic preconditioning**. The transcription factor HIF-1α is the major regulator of transcriptional responses to hypoxia (low O_2 tension). HIF-1α activates genes which are beneficial. The protein products of these genes limit production of ROS, Ca^{2+} accumulation and ATP depletion. Thus, HIF-1α protects the cell against mitochondrial injury, DNA damage and OS (oxidative stress), and thereby helps in survival of the ischemic cell.

Mechanisms of reperfusion injury are summarized in **Box 8**.

Box 8: Summary of mechanism of reperfusion injury to cells.

Altered ionic composition
- Rapid normalization pH following period of acidic pH
- Increased cytosolic Na^+
- Increased cytosolic Ca^{2+}

Formation of reactive oxygen species produced by
- Mitochondria
- Xanthine oxidase
- Neutrophils

Abnormalities of nitric oxide metabolism
- Decreased endothelial cell nitric oxide synthase (NOS) leading to vasoconstriction
- Increased platelet aggregation and recruitment of neutrophils
- Generation of highly reactive nitrogen species $ONOO^-$ (peroxynitrite)

Altered vascular function and inflammation
- Vasoconstriction and inhibition of vasodilatation
- Increase production of proinflammatory cytokines
- Increased expression of adhesion molecules on the membrane
- Platelet clumping
- Recruitment of neutrophils
- Complement activation

Cell death
- Opening of mitochondrial permeability transition pore (MPTP)
- Activation of apoptosis
- Activation of autophagy

Neuropathology of Hypoxia

Q. Write short essay on neuropathology of hypoxia.

Hypoxia of the brain may contribute to a number of pathological states. In ambient air, partial pressure of oxygen, or oxygen content (PO_2) is 21 kPa [kilopascal (kPa) one thousand times the unit of pressure and stress in the metre-kilogram-second system and is equivalent to 157 mm Hg. Most healthy adults have an arterial PO_2 within the normal range of 12-15 kPa (90-110 mm Hg]. If a PO_2 level is lower than 80 mm Hg, it indicates that an individual is not getting enough oxygen.

Brain depends on aerobic metabolism: Within the brain the tissue PO_2 is low and its values are around 4 kPa (30 mm Hg). It varies from region to region and also depends on the activity of brain. The tissue PO_2 correlates with blood flow. Under normal conditions, there is a link between cerebral blood flow and oxygen consumption. Cerebral tissue requires high energy for maintaining ion gradients and intracellular transport within neurons. Hence, cerebral tissue depends on aerobic metabolism and the brain is extremely vulnerable to the interruption of oxygen supply.

Types of hypoxia in brain: Depending on causation, hypoxia can be divided into (i) hypoxic, (ii) stagnant (hypoxic-ischemic) and (iii) histotoxic types. Pathologist most commonly assess the hypoxic–ischemic type.

Effects of hypoxia and ischemia: The effects of hypoxia and ischemia on the brain differ. Apart from classical types of hypoxic brain disorder, hypoxia and hypoxic cellular response mechanisms have been found to play a role in many disorders of CNS (e.g., neurodegenerative diseases and neoplasms).

Hypoxia damage is less than ischemic damage: The brain is sensitive to reduced oxygen supply and cells with reduce oxygen will die if oxygenation is not restored. Good clinical recovery can occur after hypoxic coma with little residual neurological deficit. This in contrast to the effects of global hypoxic-ischemic coma. Hence, hypoxia as an isolated event without ischemia (i.e., impairment of perfusion) is likely to cause less tissue damage.

Hypoxic-ischemic Encephalopathy Neuropathology

Causes: Global hypoxic-ischemic events develop in associated with general circulatory collapse. This is classically found in encephalopathy after cardiac arrest and as a component of shock states. There may be widespread effects on the brain.

Damage: The extent and severity of damage varies and depends on the following factors:
- Usually, the distribution of damage is depending on the vascular anatomy of the brain and the degree of vulnerability of particular cell types. Neurons are more susceptible to hypoxic-ischemic damage than glia tissue. Neurons within the basal ganglia, particularly the lateral striatum, and the Purkinje cells of the cerebellum are more vulnerable. The boundary zones between vascular territories are susceptible. This is because the cerebral blood flow in these areas is very delicate. For example, boundary zone in the parasagittal cortex supplied by anterior and middle cerebral artery
- The severity of damage depends on factors such as the duration and degree of ischemia, pre-existing vascular disease, blood glucose, age of the patient, and body temperature (hypothermia has a protective role). A more severe or sustained ischemia will lead to necrosis of all components (neurons as well as glial tissue)and produces infarction.

Effects on neurons: Neurons show shrinkage of cells and darkly stained shrunken nucleus. The cytoplasm of neurons shows increased eosinophilia. These cellular events progress to necrosis and loss of neurons. Astrocytes respond with gliosis and this may be demonstrated using immunohistochemistry to glial fibrillary acidic protein (GFAP). In the cerebellum, the loss of Purkinje cells is accompanied by Bergmann gliosis. This is a distinctive pattern of gliosis characterized by increased numbers of reactive astrocytic nuclei along the Purkinje cell layer.

Pathological assessment of ischemic brain: For pathological assessment in a suspected case of ischemic brain damage, it is necessary to follow a systematic assessment of vulnerable areas. Macroscopic abnormalities may be subtle and the brain should be cut only after fixation. Tissue sampling should be done from macroscopically abnormal areas, as well as the areas known to be vulnerable to ischemic brain damage including hippocampus, cerebellum, cerebral cortex (particularly from watershed areas), basal ganglia and central white matter.

Pathways to cell death

Necrosis: In hypoxic-ischemic injury, the main mode of neuronal death is by necrosis. Ischemia leads to reduced PO_2.

- **Glutamate induced excitotoxicity:** Reduced oxygen supply is accompanied by failure of membrane ATPases and membrane depolarisation. Glutamates are found in brain and are its pathways are linked with many other neurotransmitter pathways. In hypoxia, there is efflux of glutamate into the extracellular space and it activates the NMDA (N-methyl-D-aspartate) glutamate receptor, calcium influx into cells and resulting enzyme activation and production of reactive oxygen species (ROS). The glutamate induced excitotoxicity is responsible for many aspects of ischemic neuronal death. Distribution of the NMDA receptors is responsible for some aspects of the selective vulnerability of certain neuronal groups.
- **DNA damage:** DNA damage also develops in hypoxic-ischemic injury. It is produced due to oxidative damage. PARP and poly (ADP-ribose) process occur in hypoxic-ischemic neuronal death. In response to single and double stranded DNA breaks, there is activation of the enzyme poly (ADP-ribose) polymerase (PARP). This enzyme is associated with accumulation of poly (ADP-ribose) groups on a variety of proteins, including histones. Cellular nicotinamide adenine dinucleotide (NAD^+) is utilized during this reaction and produces depletion of NAD. This leads to impaired synthesis of ATP synthesis. This critical depletion of ATP energy may induce cellular necrosis. In apoptosis, this process is prevented because caspases cleave poly ADP ribose polymerase (PARP).

Apoptosis: Some neuronal cells may undergo death by apoptosis, and apoptosis is responsible for delayed neuronal death. Though activation of apoptosis pathways, including caspase 3 can occur in these cells, not all the morphological features of typical of apoptosis and DNA damage appears. Though they appear they appear as a late event.

Other forms of cell death: The outcome of a given cell to stress (reduced oxygen) may depend on the energy level of the cell. The pathway of neuronal death in hypoxic-ischemic injury may vary depending on the severity of the oxygen reduction. Neuronal death shows a continuum between apoptosis and necrosis. Alternatively, there may be other morphological types of necrosis with exotic names, such as aposklesis, abortosis and paraptosis.

Effects of hypoxia-ischemia on development

The effects of hypoxic-ischemic injury are different on the immature brain from that of adult brain. The regions of greatest susceptibility to hypoxia/ ischemia are different from those in the adult. In perinatal global hypoxic-ischemic injury, the areas that are particularly susceptible include pons, subiculum (combined in ponto-subicular necrosis), thalamus and brainstem. Generally, these grey matter damage co-exist with germinal matrix hemorrhages and periventricular leukomalacia. The immature neurons are more likely to die by apoptosis.

Nonperfused brain

The non-perfused brain should not be confused with transient global hypoxic ischemic injury. The non-perfused brain is a state that develops after a global ischemic event when there is no restoration of brain perfusion. The intracerebral pressure reduced to such a level that cerebral perfusion is almost zero. In some cases of raised intracranial pressure, vertebrobasilar blood flow is maintained better than the flow in carotids. This may preserve some functions of brainstem. These patients may be maintained on a ventilator for a variable time after such an ischemic event. Hence, the alternative names for this condition is respirator or ventilator brain.

Pathologic changes: The pathologic alterations are due to non-perfusion rather than specific to the effects of ventilation. Hence, the better term is nonperfused brain. The nonperfused brain is swollen, dusky and grey. It may be softened and subarachnoid space may show fragments of cerebellar cortex. The brain undergoes poor fixation and often centrally remains somewhat pink. Blood vessels appear dilated and red blood cells appear pale. There is no inflammatory response to these changes in the brain.

Cellular response to hypoxia

Two molecules namely neuroglobin and hypoxia-inducible factor (HIF) are important mediators of the cellular response to hypoxia in the brain. They may be important in hypoxic-ischemic injury and other cerebral diseases. HIF is discussed on pages 172–173.

Neuroglobin: Cerebral tissue does not have a mechanism for the storage of oxygen, such as myoglobin. Myoglobin is a small protein found in heart and skeletal muscles that binds oxygen. A noel globin, neuroglobin, has been found in brain. But its role as oxygen-binding protein is uncertain. It may increase oxygen availability to neurons and its distribution correlate anatomically with areas of selective vulnerability of hypoxia. It may be a potential therapeutic target of hypoxic-ischemic brain injury and perhaps also for neurodegenerative diseases.

Cellular responses to hypoxia in disorders of CNS

Ischemic and neurodegenerative diseases Hypoxia is an important component of various forms of ischemic brain damage. HIF has been found to play a role of in cerebral ischemic states. In adult rats, the viable tissue around infarcts caused by permanent middle cerebral artery occlusion shows increased expression of HIF-1α mRNA. Penumbra is a rim of mild to moderately ischemic tissue lying between tissue that is normally perfused and the area in which infarction is evolving. It is observed that HIF-1 and VEGF expression co-localise in the penumbra of an infarct preceding neovascularization. HIF-1 and VGEF play a role in the pathogenesis of acute ischemic brain damage, especially in relation to repair and adaptation. Also, they have a role for hypoxic response mechanisms in chronic vascular insufficiency. In the mouse, it has been found that deletion of the hypoxia response element of the VEGF gene reduces the hypoxia-induced VEGF expression in the spinal cord and causes an adult onset progressive motor neuron degeneration. VEGF may also act as a neurotrophin.

Neurodegenerative disease: Above findings suggest that hypoxia response mechanisms may be involved in neurodegenerative disease and also in dementia states. Alzheimer's disease is the most common cause of dementia and recent evidences suggest that Alzheimer's disease has a vascular component. In Alzheimer's disease, the hippocampus is vulnerable to hypoxic ischemic injury. As mentioned earlier, the levels of neuroglobin vary in different regions of brain. In Alzheimer's, neuroglobin may contribute to ischemic susceptibility in this area, and that a reduced oxygen availability might be a contributing factor.

Brain hypoxia-ischemia is associated with the development of white matter lesions associated with vascular mechanisms. Cellular components of white matter are highly susceptible to ischemia. ICAM-1 and HIF up-regulation is observed in white matter lesions. These lesions are frequent in Alzheimer's disease. This further supports the role of ischemia/hypoxia in the development of this form of dementia.

Hypoxia response mechanisms in neoplasia

Gliomas: The most aggressive of the gliomas is glioblastoma. It is characterised by areas of necrosis (serpentine necrosis) and endothelial proliferation. The tumor cells around such areas of necrosis are hypoxic and demonstrate expression of vascular endothelial growth factor (VEGF). VEGF is important in angiogenesis in glioblastoma. HIF may also play a role in glioma biology. In the diffusely infiltrating astrocytoma, expression of HIF-1 increases with increasing aggressiveness of the tumor and therefore, maximal in glioblastomas. In glioblastoma expression of HIF-1 is most prominent in cells adjacent to areas of necrosis suggesting that it is induced in response to hypoxia.

Hemangioblastoma: In contrast to glioblastoma, hemangioblastoma shows a diffuse expression of HIF-1α. Probably it is related to mutation of the von Hippel Lindau protein resulting in increased stabilisation of the HIF-1α protein (refer **Fig. 40**).

Oligodendrogliomas: HIF-1α expression in oligodendrogliomas correlates with increased micro-vessel density and it has a poorer prognosis.

Demonstration of HIF-1α: Immunohistochemistry to HIF-1α is useful for identifying hypoxic areas in tumours and it may also have some prognostic value.

Cell Injury Caused by Toxins and Chemicals

Toxins include toxic environmental chemicals, poisons and substances produced by infectious pathogens. They cause injury to cells that may produce cell death by necrosis. Chemical injury is one of the frequent problem encountered in clinical medicine. This is a major limitation to drug therapy. Many drugs are metabolized in the liver. Hence, liver is the major target of drug toxicity. TOXIC liver injury is generally the main reason for terminating the therapeutic use or development of a drug.

Mechanism of Cell Injury by Toxins

It can be divided into two types:

Direct toxicity

Some toxins are inherently reactive and can cause cellular injury directly and do not require metabolic activation to exert their effects. These chemicals combine with a critical molecular component or cellular organelle. Common examples include heavy metals (e.g., lead and mercury), toxic gases, corrosives, and antimetabolites. Some toxins have a selective affinity (e.g., carbon monoxide) for a particular cell type or tissue, whereas others produce widespread systemic effects. Severe damage is usually to the cells that use, absorb, excrete, or concentrate the chemicals.

- In **mercuric chloride poisoning**, mercury binds to the sulfhydryl groups of various cell membrane proteins. This inhibits ATP-dependent transport and increases the permeability of cell membrane. The cells of the gastrointestinal tract and kidney are mainly damaged.
- **Lead poisoning**, has widespread effects, including effects on nervous tissue, blood cells, and the kidney.
- **Cyanide** poisons mitochondrial cytochrome oxidase and thus prevents oxidative phosphorylation. Many anticancer chemotherapeutic (cytotoxic) agents used for the management of cancer also produce cell damage by direct cytotoxic effects.
- Some antimetabolites are used as cytotoxic agents. They interfere with normal metabolic processes of the cell.
- Toxins produced by microorganisms also can cause direct cell damage. They usually cause damage by attaching host cell molecules that are needed for essential functions (e.g., protein synthesis, ion transport) of the cell.
- Carbon monoxide tightly and selectively binds to hemoglobin, thereby prevents the RBC from carrying sufficient oxygen. This is an example of selective affinity of toxin.
- Highly acidic or basic chemicals are directly corrosive to cellular structures.

Conversion to toxic metabolites

Many toxic chemicals are not intrinsically active but become injurious only when metabolized into reactive chemicals by the body. These chemicals must be first activated or converted to reactive metabolites and then only they can act on target cells. Hence, such toxins usually affect the cells in which they are activated. The activation of these chemicals is usually performed by cytochrome P450 in the smooth ER of the liver and other organs. These active metabolites may cause membrane damage and cell injury by direct covalent binding to protein and lipids. But the most important mechanism of cell injury by them is by generation of free radicals. Examples include CCl_4 and analgesic acetaminophen.

Carbon tetrachloride was formerly widely used (now banned) as dry cleaning agent in the dry cleaning industry. CCl_4 is converted to a highly toxic free radical CCl_3^-, mainly by liver cells. The free radical is highly reactive and forms abnormal chemical bonds in the cell. It destroys the cellular membranes mainly by membrane phospholipid peroxidation and leads to liver failure.

- In <30 minutes after exposure to CCl_4, it produces sufficient damage to the ER membranes of hepatocytes and reduces the synthesis of enzymes and plasma proteins.
- Within 2 hours, it causes swelling of the smooth ER and dissociation of ribosomes from the RER.
- It is also associated with reduced synthesis of apoproteins and forms complexes with triglycerides and favors secretion of triglyceride. This produces accumulation of lipids in hepatocytes ("fatty liver" or steatosis) and other cells.
- Mitochondrial injury follows, and it reduces the ATP which in turn leads to defective ion transport and progressive swelling of cell.
- There is further damage to plasma membranes by fatty aldehydes produced by lipid peroxidation in the ER. Finally, there is necrosis of hepatocytes.

High doses of acetaminophen (commonly known as paracetamol) that is commonly used analgesic, may produce similar toxic effects on the liver.

PROTEIN FOLDING AND MISFOLDING

Q. Write a short essay on chaperone and protein misfolding diseases.

Q. Describe the mechanisms of defects in protein folding and its role in diseases.

Translation completes the flow of genetic information from DNA to RNA and to amino acids within the cell. When a large number of amino acids are joined together, it forms a chain known as a polypeptide. During the process of formation of protein, the sequence of nucleotides in DNA is converted to the sequence of amino acids. These amino acids form a polypeptide chain. Proteins consist of one or more of these polypeptide chains. Proteins are molecules composed of polypeptide chains made up of amino acid chains. These nascent proteins are synthesized in the ribosomes. The synthesis of a polypeptide is not equivalent to the production of a functional protein.

Folding of Proteins

To be a useful protein, polypeptides in the nascent protein must fold appropriately to form a particular three-dimensional configuration as they exit (or come out of) ribosomes. Protein folding is needed for their biological functions. Protein folding begins within a minute after the amino acid chain winds away from the ribosome. Protein folding occurs usually as a stepwise process. A small protein may fold into its final, functional form in one step within a time frame of milliseconds. However, a vast majority of larger proteins may fold into a series of short-lived intermediates before assuming their final, functional competent forms. If newly produced proteins are left to their own devices, there is great danger of folding abnormally and then aggregating. This can be harmful. To attain correct (or to maintain appropriate) folding, proteins need the assistance of certain proteins referred to as chaperones. Molecular chaperones associate with newly synthesized proteins and help them assume their final, functional, three-dimensional configurations. Some chaperones also help to sustain that conformation over time, thereby prevent accumulation of abnormal proteins. This on-going process of quality control of proteins by chaperones is termed **proteostasis**.

Chaperone Proteins

Proteins that facilitate the protein folding of other proteins within cells are called molecular chaperones. Chaperones are located in every cellular compartment and organelle, bind to the target proteins (also called substrates or client proteins), whose folding they will assist. Chaperones act as catalysts that facilitate assembly without being part of the assembled complex. Chaperonins provide an isolated environment so that correct folding can occur. There are several hundred chaperone proteins. They are organized into distinct families based on structural homologies. Many of these molecules are induced by stress and are called heat shock proteins (Hsps) (discussed on 190–191).

Families of Chaperones

Originally, chaperones were designated by molecular weight (e.g., Hsp70, Hsp90). Many of these molecules are induced by stress and are called heat shock proteins (Hsps) (refer page 190).

There are many chaperone proteins and based on structural homologies, they are organized mainly into two distinct general families.

1. **Molecular chaperones:** They bind to a short segment of a protein substrate and stabilize unfolded or partly folded proteins. Thus, they prevent these proteins from aggregating and being degraded. This group consists of Hsp70 in the cytosol and its homologs [Hsp70 in the mitochondrial matrix and binding immunoglobulin protein (BiP) in the ER].
2. **Chaperonins:** They form folding cylindrical chambers into which all or part of an unfolded protein can be sequestered. Thus, it provides time and an appropriate environment to fold properly. The proper folding of many newly synthesized proteins also needs the help of another class of proteins, the chaperonins, also called Hsp60s.

Functioning of Chaperones

Chaperones in the ER control the proper folding of newly synthesized proteins (**Figs. 42A** and **B**).

- **Correct folding:** As the nascent proteins come out of ribosomes, they are met by one or more chaperones, which direct their folding. If the protein is properly folded and the resulting conformation is sufficient for functionality, the chaperone and the new protein dissociate. The chaperons involved in protein folding proceed to its appropriate location. However, some proteins require additional involvement of cylindrical channels called chaperonins for forming their final tertiary structures.
- **Incorrect folding:** If proteins are misfolded, they are ubiquitinated and targeted for proteolysis in proteasomes. Various proteins help in precise folding. If a protein gets misfolds or "stuck" in an intermediate form, it will affect function of the protein. Then an "unfolded protein response" occurs.

Functions of Chaperones

The chaperone system consists of a proteostasis hub that influences many cellular functions (**Box 9**). They establish and maintain functional protein conformations. The chaperones work closely with the ubiquitin-proteasome system (UPS), and with autophagy machinery to establish an integrated proteostasis network (**Fig. 43**). This network—(1) guides conversion/folding of single polypeptide chains into proteins, (2) maintains active three-dimensional structures by refolding misfolded or unfolded proteins into functional conformations, and (3) at the appropriate juncture, disassemble and destroy potentially toxic protein aggregates that form due to protein misfolding. Chaperone proteins can be used as drugs to treat diseases that result from misfolded proteins.

Chaperonopathies

Chaperonopathies are disorders due to defects in molecular chaperones. These diseases are characterized by defects, excesses, or mistakes in chaperone proteins.

Genetic chaperonopathies

These are due to inherited germline mutations in the molecular chaperones. These include:

- Neuropathies, dilated cardiomyopathy, and polycystic liver and kidney diseases.

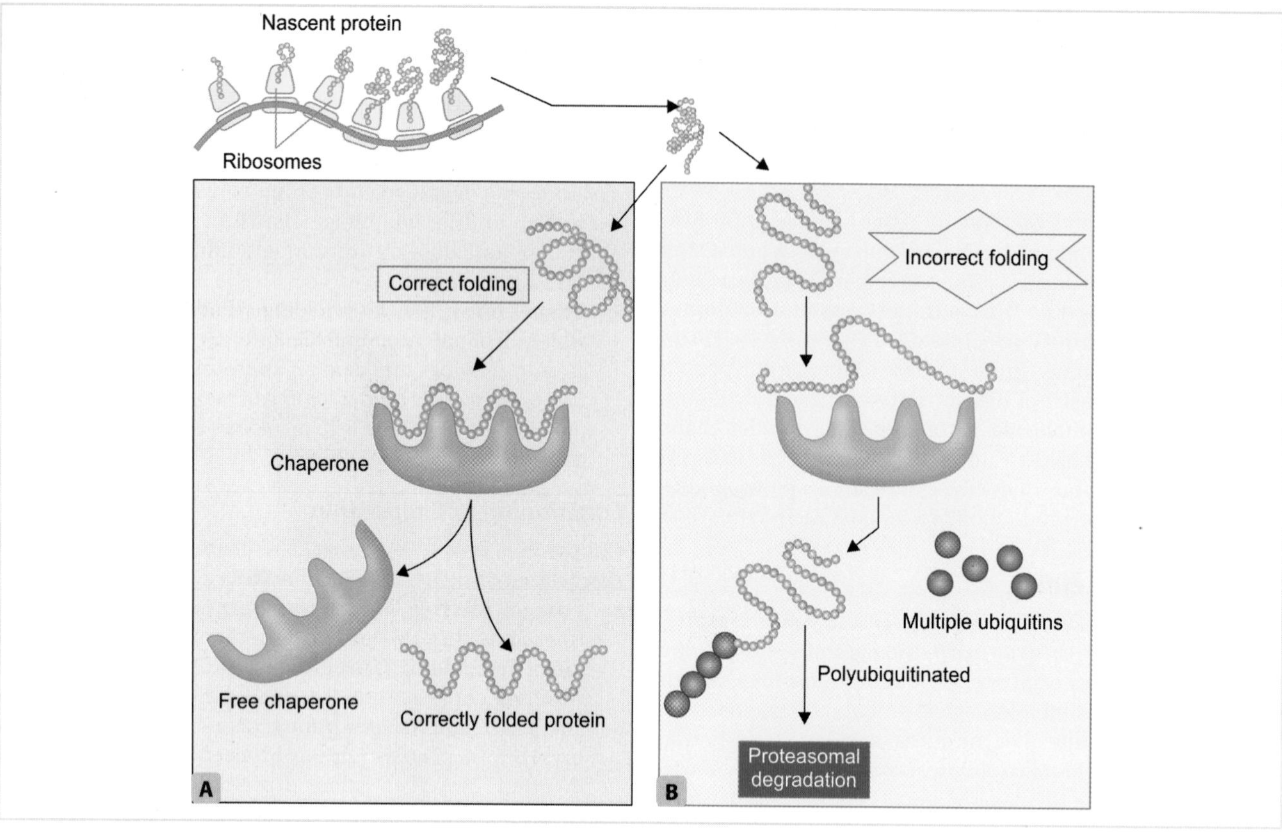

FIGS. 42A AND B: Handling of protein by chaperones. (A) Nascent proteins are correctly folded by chaperones into functional proteins. (B) Incorrectly folded proteins from the ribosomes are polyubiquitinated, which directs them to proteasomes, where they are degraded.

Box 9: Cellular functions that need chaperones.

- Cell cycle progression
- Apoptosis
- Telomere maintenance
- Intracellular transport
- Innate immunity
- Specific degradation of proteins

- X-linked retinitis pigmentosa: There is mutation in a chaperone cofactor.
- Hereditary spastic paraplegia: It is associated with a mutation in mitochondrial chaperone called Hsp60.
- von Hippel-Lindau protein (VHL) is a tumor suppressor. If VHL is mutated, it may bind its chaperone poorly. This leads to its misfolding and inactivation of VHL. These individuals develop tumors of the adrenal, kidney, and brain.
- Cancer: Mutant chaperone genes are responsible for some types of cancer.

Acquired chaperonopathies

There may be several causes.

- **Impairment of stress responses:** It may result in inadequate production of chaperone proteins.
- **High levels of substrate** (misfolded or degraded) proteins may exceed the capacity of the chaperone system.
- **Sequestration or inactivation:** Chaperone molecules may be sequestered in protein deposits. They may be inactivated by exogenous toxins (e.g., an enzyme from a virulent strain of *Escherichia coli* cleaves Hsp70).
- **Tumorigenesis:** Chaperones may also contribute to tumorigenesis. It may be through effects on proteins that regulate the cell cycle and cell death.
- **Others:** Acquired chaperonopathies may be involved in biological aging and in cardiovascular and neurodegenerative diseases.

Endoplasmic Reticulum Stress (Fig. 44)

Q. Write a short essay on ER stress.

Normally, during protein synthesis, chaperones in the ER control the proper folding of newly synthesized proteins. The unfolded or misfolded proteins/polypeptides in a cell are transported into the cytoplasm. In the cytoplsam they are usually ubiquitinated and targeted for proteolysis in proteasomes and thereby prevent their accumulation. However, when misfolded or unfolded proteins get accumulated in the ER, it can stress compensatory pathways in the ER. The misfolded proteins can accumulate in the ER due to inherited mutations or stresses.

Mild Endoplasmic Reticulum Stress

The unfolded or misfolded proteins accumulate in the endoplasmic reticulum (ER). They activate a number of cellular responses, collectively termed the **unfolded protein response**. The misfolded proteins in the ER are detected by sensors present in the membrane of ER [e.g., the kinase inositol-requiring enzyme (IRE)-1]. These sensors form oligomers and

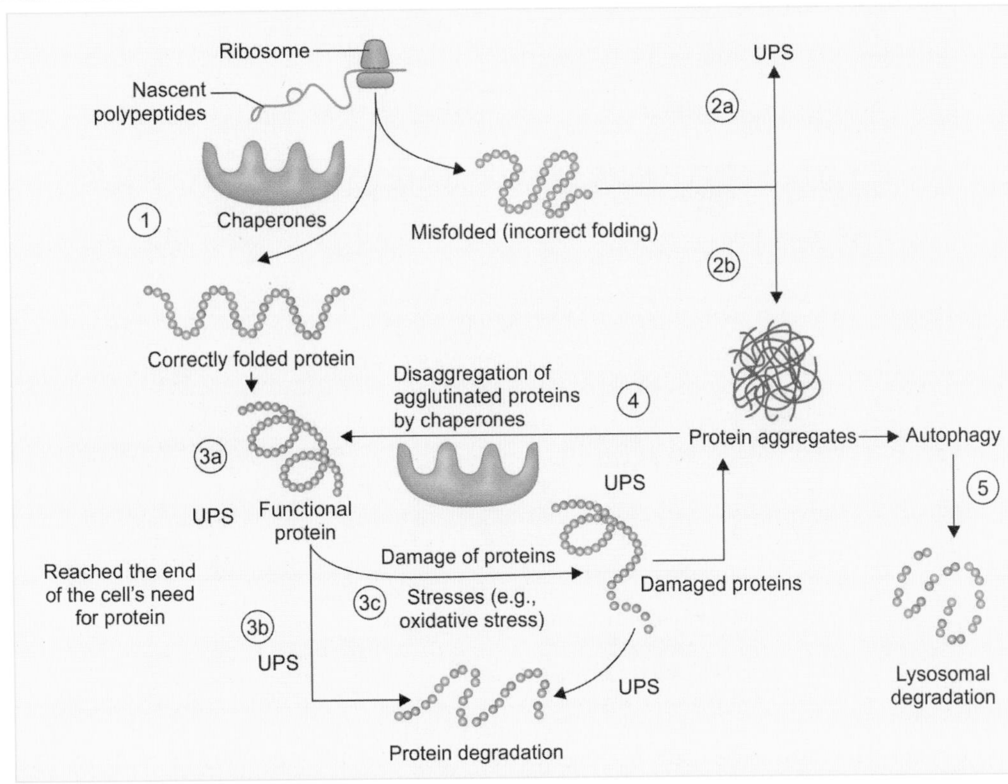

FIG. 43: Shows the roles of chaperones, stress-related modifications, and autophagy in the fate of proteins. (1) Nascent polypeptides are folded into functional proteins with the help of chaperones. (2) A small proportion of proteins may form in a misfolded state. This may be—(2a) degraded by the ubiquitin-proteasome system (UPS) directly, or (2b) may form aggregates. (3) The correctly folded functional protein may have one of three outcomes, namely—it may (3a) continue as a functional protein, (3b) reach the end of the cell's need for it and then be degraded by the UPS, or (3c) be damaged by different stresses (e.g., oxidative stress). In case of damage by stresses, the proteins may be distorted and deformed. These may be degraded by the UPS or may form protein aggregate in the cytosol. (4) Chaperones may cause disaggregation of agglutinated proteins and prevent accumulation of toxic particulates and these proteins may restore their productive function. (5) Protein aggregates may also undergo autophagy and subsequent degradation in lysosomes.

are activated by phosphorylation. This stimulates an adaptive unfolded protein response.

Unfolded protein response

First, accumulated unfolded or misfolded proteins induce a protective cellular response that is called the **unfolded protein response**. This response can protect the cell from the harmful effects of the misfolded proteins. This adaptive response tries to reduce the levels of misfolded proteins in the cell by three mechanisms:

1. **Increased production of chaperones:** Chaperone proteins (or simply called chaperones) in the ER control the proper folding of newly synthesized proteins. The unfolded protein response activates signaling pathways and increases the transcription of genes that encode chaperone proteins and the other folding proteins. This increases the production of chaperones. They stabilize partially folded regions in the protein to their correct form and prevent getting stuck in intermediate form. They in turn quickly restore proper protein folding.
2. **Decrease protein translation:** The unfolded protein response will slow or even stop the corresponding protein synthesis or formation. There is slowing of protein translation and thus reduced the load of misfolded proteins in the cell.
3. **Increased protein degradation:** It is by enhancing proteasomal degradation of abnormal proteins.

Severe Endoplasmic Reticulum Stress

Above cytoprotective responses try to handle the misfolded proteins. However, if the adaptive response is not able to handle the accumulation of misfolded proteins, the cell activates caspases and **induces apoptosis**. This process is termed as **ER stress**.

Terminal unfolded protein response

When the amount of misfolded protein accumulated is too large and cannot be managed by the adaptive response, the excessive activation of ER sensors activates signals. These signals activate proapoptotic sensors of the Bcl-2 Homology 3 (BH3)-only family and also directly activate caspases, leading to apoptosis by the mitochondrial (intrinsic) pathway. The irreparably damaged cell undergoes death by apoptosis. This response is also called as the terminal unfolded protein response.

Ubiquitin–Proteasome System (UPS)

If a protein misfolding occurs in spite of the protection by chaperones, cells have other methods to either refold the protein correctly, or get rid of it.

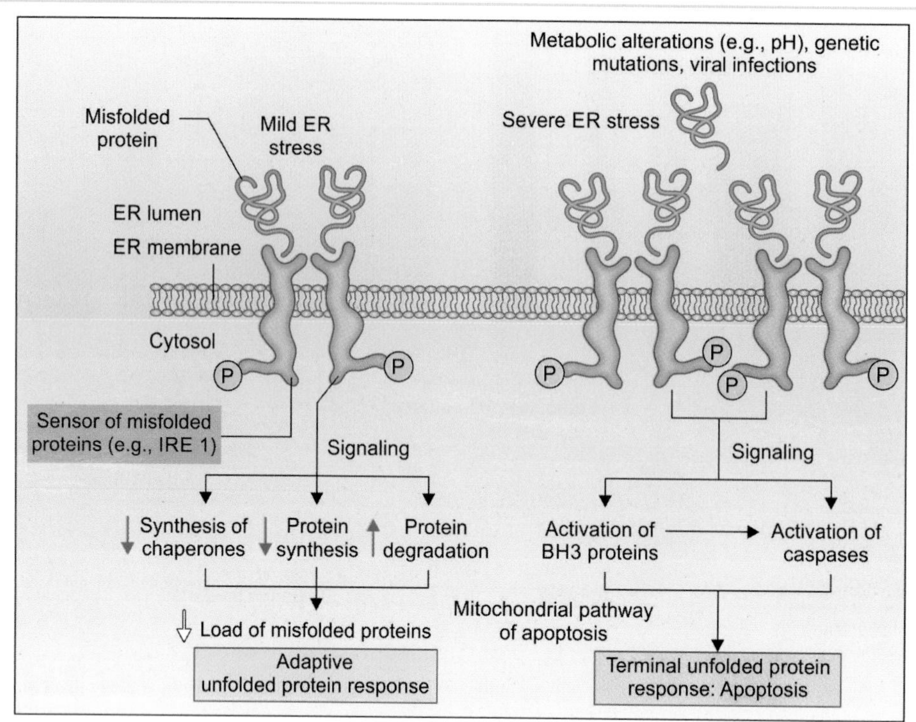

FIG. 44: Response to misfolded proteins and endoplasmic reticulum (ER) stress. The misfolded proteins in the ER are detected by sensors [e.g., kinase inositol-requiring enzyme (IRE)-1] in the membrane of ER and are activated by phosphorylation. In case of mild ER stress, this activates an adaptive unfolded protein response. This can protect the cell from the harmful effects of the misfolded proteins. If the ER stress is severe, and adaptive responses cannot rectify, then activation of ER sensors activates the mitochondrial pathway of apoptosis. This causes cell death by apoptosis and is called the terminal unfolded protein response.

Ubiquitin

Ubiquitin (Ub) is a small 76-amino acid regulatory protein and plays a main role in multiple cellular functions. One of their main roles is in the degradation of many defective intracellular proteins. Their activities are brought out through reversible Ub conjugation with target proteins and can be divided into proteolytic and nonproteolytic (trafficking) pathways. The Ub molecule has seven lysine residues and functional selectivity is due to the diverse patterns of protein linkage to these amino acids. Linkage to some lysines leads to transfer of the tagged protein to degradation by the proteasome. Misfolded proteins are sent out of the ER back into the cytoplasm. Then they are "tagged" or bound to protein Ub. This process is called **ubiquitination**. When there is ligase-catalyzed attachment of four or more additional Ub molecules to the misfolded target protein, it is termed polyubiquitination. A misfolded protein containing one Ub tag maybe straightened and refolded correctly after ubiquitination. "Ubiquitination" is catalyzed by a large family of enzymes called E3 ligases, which attach Ub to the side-chain amino group of lysyl residues on their targets. The polyubiquitinated misfolded proteins are taken to another cellular machine called a proteasome. Functions of Ub-directed protein sorting are listed in **Box 10**.

Fate of Ub-conjugated Proteins

It depends on the number of Ub moieties conjugated and the site of the conjugation linkages on the Ub molecule.

Deubiquitinating Enzymes

Deubiquitinating enzymes (DUBs) are proteases that remove Ub from polyUb chains (**polyubiquitinated proteins**) and their partner proteins. This process is called as deubiquitination. DUBs are important to the function of Ub and they act like regulated cellular switch to counteract the ubiquitination of specific protein targets. Once a protein is degraded in a proteasome or lysosome, the Ub is returned to the cell pool of Ub monomers. About 100 DUBs have been identified that reverse the effects of ubiquitination on many cellular processes. These processes where DUBs are involved include—(1) protein degradation, (2) regulation of cell cycle, (3) gene expression, (4) signaling pathways, and (5) DNA repair.

Proteasome

Cellular homeostasis needs mechanisms to selectively destroy proteins. There is more than one pathway for this process, but the well-known process in which specific proteins are eliminated is the proteasomal apparatus. Proteasome is a highly preserved organelle in the cytoplasm and also probably in the nucleus. Proteasomes are key participants in cell homeostasis and they make up 1–2% of the total mass of the cell.

Structure of proteasome (Figs. 45A and B)

It is a cylinder (barrel-shaped) or tunnel-like multiprotein structure with multiple different protease activities. Their main (but not the only) function is to degrade polyubiquitinated

Box 10: Functions of ubiquitin-directed protein sorting.

- Endocytosis
- Control of cell cycle
- Autophagy
- Regulation of histones and transcription
- Intracellular trafficking
- Repair of deoxyribonucleic acid (DNA) damage
- Cell signaling

proteins. Many (but not all) proteins destined for proteasome destruction are targeted after covalent addition of protein Ub. There are two types of proteasomes, namely 20S and 26S. The degradative unit of both is a 20S destruction chamber. In the 26S proteasome, two 19S "caps" are attached to the proteolytic core or chamber and the caps at the entrance to the proteolytic core regulate entry. The 20S proteasomes lack these caps.

Functions

Proteasomes play an important role in degrading cytosolic proteins and provide quality control of proteins.

- Proteasomes eliminate proteins that have been incorrectly folded (misfolded), denatured (damaged), (similar to those within the ER) or need to be destroyed for some other reason.
- Proteasomes also destroy properly folded proteins that are in excess, reached the end of their usefulness, and no longer needed (proteins whose lifespan needs to be tightly regulated). For example, a cell must destroy excess transcription factors, or the genes that they control may remain activated or repressed for too long.
- They also regulate cell cycle transit by specifically eliminating proapoptotic molecules (e.g., such as p53) and favor of cell survival. They maintain and protect cellular viability. Thus, a proteasome inhibitor (bortezomib) can be utilized to treat patients with certain cancers.
- Proteasomes also destroy proteins from pathogens, such as viruses.
- The 20S proteasomes are necessary for degradation of **oxidized proteins**. In 26S proteasomes, **polyubiquitinated proteins** (polyUb chains) are degraded.
- Immunoproteasome is a type of proteasome that is formed when cells produce interferon-γ (IFN-γ). Immunoproteasome is necessary in processing protein antigens into peptides that attach to major histocompatibility complex (MHC) type I for presentation to the immune system.
- Mutations that interfere with normal proteasomal function can cause death.

Ubiquitin–Proteasome Pathway

Mechanisms of UB conjugation to proteins (Fig. 46)

Ubiquitin and ubiquitination initiate protein degradation. First a Ub-activating enzyme attaches to Ub, which then add Ub to a lysine on the target protein. The process may be repeated multiple times to add a chain of Ub moieties to the original Ub and it forms a polyubiquitin chain (at least four Ubs).

Degradation of proteins by proteasomes

Proteins targeted for destruction or degradation proceed to proteasome. The 26S proteasomes recognize the polyUb-conjugated protein by their one 19S cap (subunit). Proteins are then degraded in the proteolytic core. The polyubiquitinated misfolded protein molecules are progressively straightened (unfolded), dismantled, and funneled into this polymeric proteasome complex. Proteasomes digest proteins into small (peptides of 3–25 amino acids) amino acid (oligopeptides) fragments. These fragments are released through the lower 19S subunit of 26S. These fragments may be further degraded by cytosolic proteases to their constituent amino acids. The amino acids may be recycled to build new proteins or presented to immune cells. During this process, Ub moieties are returned to the cell pool of Ub monomers by DUBs.

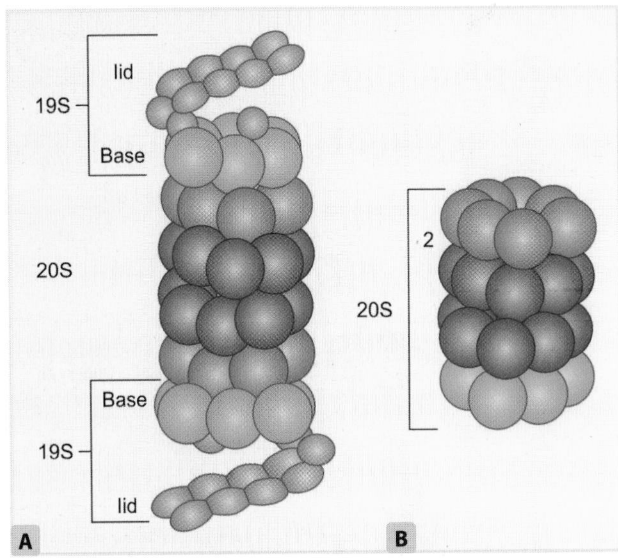

FIGS. 45A AND B: Structure of proteasome. It is barrel-shaped multiprotein structure. There are two types of proteasomes, namely 20S and 26S. (A) In the 26S proteasome, two 19S "caps" are attached to the proteolytic core. The caps at the entrance to the proteolytic core regulate entry. (B) 20S proteasome does not have cap.

Fate of a newly synthesized protein is presented in **Flowchart 3**.

Degradation of misfolded protein by Ub proteasome and effect of endoplasmic stress is presented in **Figure 47**.

Disruption of ubiquitin system

- **By pathogens:** Ub/DUB pathways can be controlled by some pathogens at different points. Some bacterial proteins (called as effectors), may resemble Ub ligases and activate ubiquitination. This may facilitate invasion and pathogenicity of the bacteria into host cells. Some bacteria (e.g., *Salmonella typhimurium, Chlamydia trachomatis*) and viruses (e.g., herpes simplex virus) encode proteins that act as DUBs. They may interfere with cellular ubiquitination and is advantageous for invasion by these pathogens.
- **Protection from ubiquitination:** If some modifications occur in proteins, this modified protein may be protected from undergoing ubiquitination. For example, when the tumor suppressor protein p53 is phosphorylated in response to DNA damage, it gets modified and does not undergo ubiquitination. Thus, phosphorylated p53 is protected from Ub-mediated degradation.

Abnormal Proteins and Diseases

The orders of protein structure include primary structure (the sequence of amino acids in a polypeptide chain); secondary

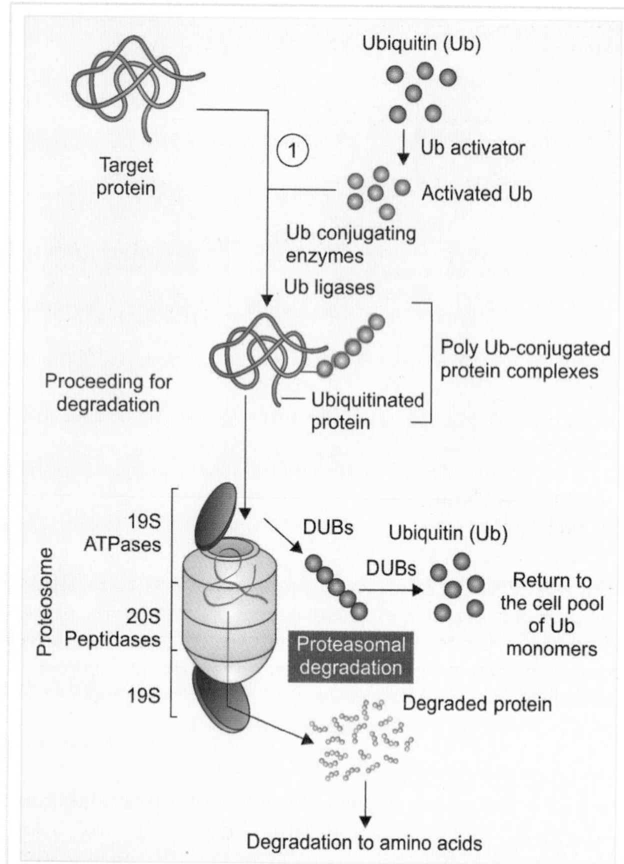

FIG. 46: Steps involved in ubiquitin (Ub)–proteasome pathways. First, a Ub-activating enzyme attaches to Ub, which then adds Ub to the target protein. The process may be repeated multiple times to add a chain of Ub moieties to the original Ub and it forms a polyubiquitin chain. If degradation is to proceed, proteasomes degrade protein into oligopeptides. During this process, Ub moieties are returned to the cell pool of Ub monomers by deubiquitinating enzymes (DUBs). After release from the proteasome, partially degraded proteins may be degraded to amino acids.

structure [the folding of short (3–30), contiguous segments of polypeptide into geometrically ordered units]; and tertiary structure (the assembly of secondary structural units into larger functional units). Many acquired and inherited diseases are characterized by intracellular accumulation of abnormal proteins. A deviation of protein's tertiary structure may occur due to a mutation that alters the amino acid sequence or may be due to an acquired defect in protein folding. Examples of diseases associated with protein aggregation are presented in **Table 9**.

Ways of Accumulation of Misfolded Proteins

Usually, the misfolded proteins are either made to fold properly by chaperones or degraded by proteasomes. The failure of a protein to fold properly usually leads to its rapid degradation. Intracellular accumulation of misfolded proteins may be either due to abnormalities that increase the production of misfolded proteins or abnormalities that reduce the ability to degrade or remove them. Intracellular accumulation of abnormally folded proteins may occur in following ways:

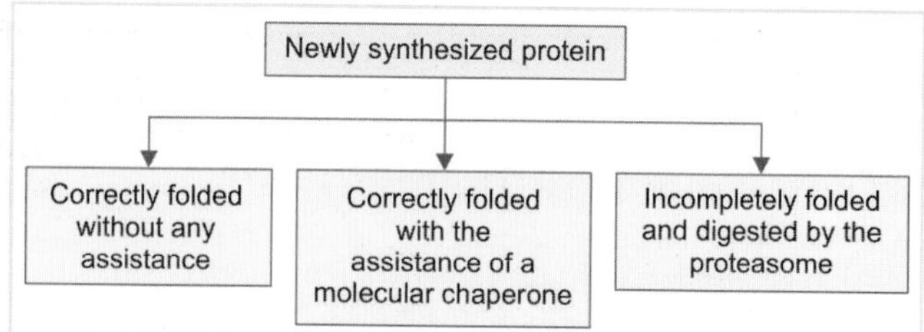

FLOWCHART 3: Fate of a newly synthesized protein.

- **From genetic mutation:** It can lead to the production of proteins that cannot fold properly (e.g., cystic fibrosis).
- **Proteins with more than one conformation:** Some proteins have more than one conformation. The two forms of the same protein have identical amino acid sequences, but fold differently. One of them may become "infectious" and convert the others to more copies of itself. Such an infectious protein is termed as a "prion" (pronounced "pree-on") (refer pages 796–799).
- **Aging or unknown environmental factors:** Aging is associated with a decreased capacity to correct misfolding. In certain disorders of brain, misfolded proteins aggregate, and form masses (e.g., Parkinson's diseases) that clog the proteasomes and block them from processing any malformed proteins. In Huntington disease, extra glutamines in the protein huntingtin cause it to obstruct proteasomes.
- **Production of large amounts of proteins:** Infections (especially viral infections) can produce large amounts of microbial proteins within cells, which are more than the cell can handle.
- **Increased demand for secretory proteins:** For example, increased demand for secretory proteins such as insulin can occur in insulin-resistant states.
- **Changes in intracellular pH and redox state.**
- **Deprivation of glucose and oxygen**: For example, ischemia and hypoxia may increase the burden of misfolded proteins.

Examples for Abnormal Proteins

Defects in protein folding can cause many common diseases, collectively known as **protein misfolding diseases**.

- **Cystic fibrosis:** In some, the misfolding of a protein causes disease due to reduced levels of functional protein in a cell as in cystic fibrosis. It is an autosomal recessive disease. In some cases of cystic fibrosis, there are mutations in a protein called cystic fibrosis transmembrane conductance regulator (CFTR). This produces a **mutated CFTR** protein. Normal CFTR protein is responsible for the transport of chloride ions across the plasma membranes of many types of epithelial cells, including those lining the respiratory tract. Mutated CFTR cannot fold properly and misfolds in the ER. Mutated CFTR attracts too many chaperones and is sent to the cytoplasm. Therefore, CFTR gets degraded. CFTR proteins never reach (transported to) the plasma membrane where normally it will form a chloride channel. Defective chloride transport leads to obstruction of the respiratory tract by thick plugs of mucus. This in turn leads to recurrent infections and the death of most patients from lung disease.

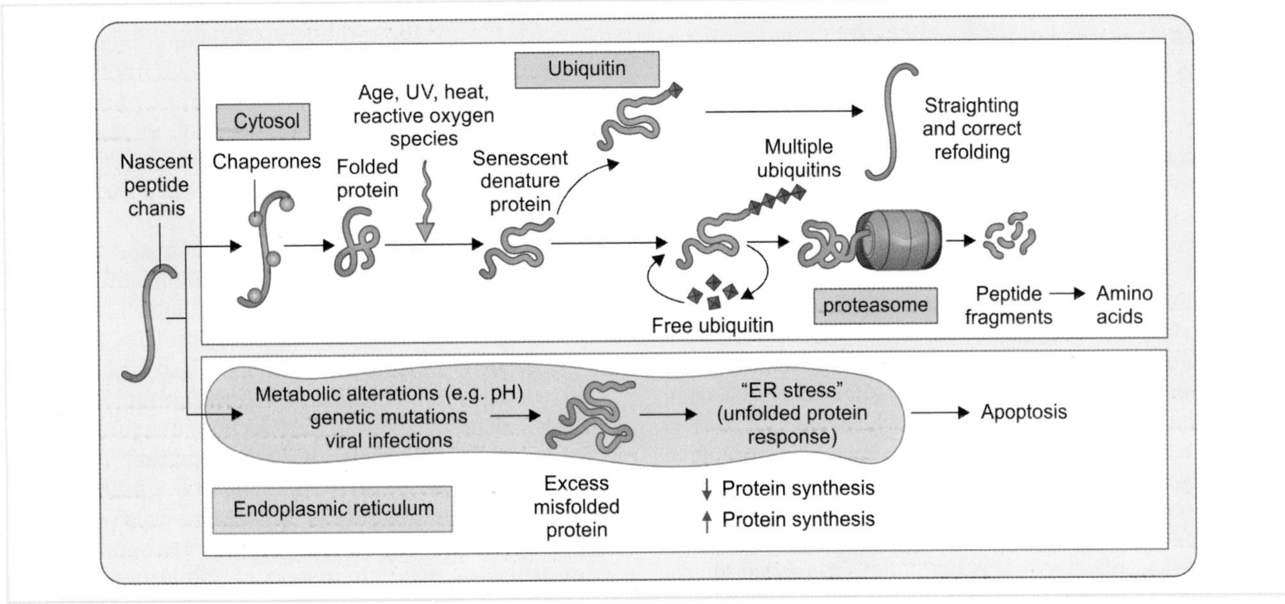

FIG. 47: Degradation of misfolded protein by ubiquitin proteasome and effect of endoplasmic stress. Cytosolic target proteins for turnover (e.g., transcription factors or regulatory proteins), senescent proteins, or proteins denatured due to extrinsic mechanical or chemical stresses are degraded by proteasomes. Increased levels of misfolded proteins within the endoplasmic reticulum (ER) activate a protective *unfolded protein response*. This reduces the protein synthesis, but also increases chaperone proteins which help in refolding of protein. If this mechanism is not adequate, the cell undergoes apoptosis.

Table 9: Examples of diseases associated with protein aggregation.

Disease associated with protein aggregation	*Aggregating protein*
Neurodegenerative diseases	
• Parkinson's disease	α-Synuclein
• Alzheimer's disease	Amyloid-β
• Huntington's disease	Huntingtin
• Spongiform encephalopathies	Prion protein
• Amyotrophic lateral sclerosis	Superoxide dismutase
Non-neurodegenerative	
Localized diseases	
• Type 2 diabetes mellitus	Amylin
• Cataracts	Crystallins
• Injection-localized amyloidosis	Insulin
Systemic diseases (amyloidosis)	
• Amyloid light-chain amyloidosis	Immunoglobulin light chain
• Amyloid A amyloidosis	Serum amyloid A protein
• Senile systemic amyloidosis	Transthyretin

- **Prions:** Certain neurological (neurodegenerative) diseases may develop due to **accumulation of aggregates of misfolded proteins** or their partially degraded products in the cells. They are collectively termed as prions (**pro**teinous **in**fectious agents). These are neurodegenerative disorders (spongiform encephalopathies) caused due to accumulation of abnormally folded prion proteins. The normal α-helical structure is changed to a β-pleated sheet. Abnormal prion proteins may form due to inherited mutations or from exposure to the aberrant form of the protein. The function of the normal prion protein is not known. Probably it plays a role in myelination, antioxidant [superoxide dismutase (SOD)-like] activity, a role in T-lymphocyte-dendritic cell interactions, enhancing neural progenitor proliferation, and in development of long-term memory. Prions have the characteristics of viral or microbial pathogens. They have been implicated in many diseases such as mad cow disease, Creutzfeldt-JaKob disease, Alzheimer's disease, and Huntington's disease.
- **α_1-antitrypsin deficiency:** It is a heritable disorder due to mutations in the gene coding for α_1-antitrypsin. It produces an insoluble protein which cannot be easily exported. The insoluble protein accumulates in liver cells and produces cell injury and leads to cirrhosis.
- **Lewy bodies** (α-synuclein): These are observed in neurons of the substantia nigra in patients with Parkinson's disease.
- **Neurofibrillary tangles** (tau protein): They are seen in cortical neurons of patients with Alzheimer's disease.
- **Mallory bodies** (intermediate filaments): These are hepatocellular inclusions composed of intermediate filaments seen in alcoholic hepatitis, hepatocellular carcinoma, etc., (refer page 205).

Molecular pathogenesis of abnormal protein

during protein synthesis, ribosomes translate messenger RNA (mRNA) and produce a linear chain of amino acids without a defined three-dimensional structure. It is more favorable for cells to produce many folds (even abnormal ones), and then edit the protein than to construct only a single correct conformation. Thus, protein misfolding occurs continuously. However, a substantial proportion of newly formed proteins are inferior, unsuitable for the cells. The possible outcomes of protein synthesis (**Box 11**) are discussed here.

- Correct primary sequence and proper folding into functional conformation.
- Primary sequence may be correct, but the protein does not fold properly.
- A mutant protein (with an incorrect amino acid sequence) folds incorrectly.
- A conformationally correct protein may become unfolded or misfolded. This may occur due to an unfavorable environment such as altered pH, high ionic strength, and oxidation. There may be failure of protein quality control system or quality control system may become overloaded. In both situations, there will be accumulation of misfolded proteins that form amorphous aggregates or fibrils. These may produce cell injury.
- **Production of protein with loss of function:** Some mutations can prevent correct folding of important proteins. These proteins either cannot function properly or cannot be incorporated into the correct site. For example, in cystic fibrosis, abnormal cystic fibrosis proteins are misfolded chloride ion channels, and these are degraded. The protein does not reach its correct site at the cell membrane and causes a defect in chloride ion (Cl^-) transport that produces the disease. Other examples of loss of function include mutations of the low-density lipoprotein (LDL) receptor in few types of hypercholesterolemia and mutations of a copper-transporting adenosine triphosphatase (ATPase) in Wilson disease.
- **Formation of abnormal protein aggregates:** Defects in protein structure may be acquired or genetic. For example, impairment of cellular antioxidant defenses can be associated with protein oxidation. This changes the protein's tertiary structure and during mild-to-moderate oxidative stress, 20S proteasomes recognize and degrade these proteins. However, in case of severe oxidative stress, these proteins may form disordered insoluble aggregates. Such proteins sequester ferrous (Fe^{2+}) ions, which help to produce additional reactive oxygen species (ROS) and in turn further increase the size of the protein aggregate. Disordered protein aggregates may be degraded (e.g., by autophagy) or may become insoluble fibrillar β-pleated sheet structures (e.g., amyloid). Any Ub attached to them is lost and cause a cellular deficit in Ub. This can impair protein degradation. Due to production of toxic ROS and their inhibition of proteasomal degradation, these aggregates may lead to cell death. Examples for this type of mechanism include accumulation of β-amyloid protein in Alzheimer's disease and α-synuclein in Parkinson's disease.
- **Retention of secretory proteins:** Many proteins to be secreted by the cell must be folded correctly for their transport through cellular compartments and release at the cell membrane. Mutations in genes that encode such proteins (e.g., α_1-antitrypsin) can lead to cell injury due to massive accumulation of misfolded proteins within the cell. Failure to secrete this antiprotease into the circulation also results in unregulated proteolysis of connective tissue and loss of parenchyma in the lung (emphysema).
- **Extracellular deposition of aggregated proteins:** Misfolded proteins assume β-pleated conformations instead of random coils or α-helices. These abnormal proteins usually form insoluble aggregates and may be deposited or accumulated extracellularly. Examples include systemic amyloid and neurodegenerative diseases.

Box 11: Possible outcomes of protein synthesis.

Excessive production of misfolded proteins
- Protein with proper folding
- Protein without folding
- Mutant protein
  - With improper folding
  - Misfolded protein with loss of function
  - Retention of secretory protein
- Correct protein becomes misfolded
- Extracellular deposition of aggregated proteins

Diminished degradation of misfolded proteins
- Inhibition of proteasomal degradation

Basic Mechanism of Disease by Misfolded Proteins

Protein misfolding within cells may cause disease by either producing a deficiency of an essential protein or by inducing apoptosis (**Table 10**).

- **Loss of function:** Misfolded proteins usually lose their functional activity and are rapidly degraded. Both can cause loss of function. If this function is essential, it produces cell injury (e.g., cystic fibrosis).
- **Endoplasmic reticulum induced cell death:** Protein misfolding is a fundamental cellular abnormality in a number of diseases. These include several neurodegenerative diseases such as Alzheimer's disease, Huntington disease, and Parkinson's disease, and may also be in type 2 diabetes mellitus (T2DM).

Diseases due to Defective Ubiquitination and Deubiquitination

Ubiquitination and degradation of specific protein is not only important for normal cellular homeostasis but also important for cellular adaptation to stress and injury. Defects in ubiquitination and deubiquitination are responsible for many diseases. Mutations in constituents involved in ubiquitination (Ub) pathway can produce specific diseases, and in many diseases altered UPS activity is important in their pathogenesis (**Table 11**).

Defective ubiquitination is observed in many important neurodegenerative diseases. For example, mutation in parkin, a Ub ligase, is involved in the pathogenesis of some hereditary forms of Parkinson's disease. In these conditions, undegraded parkin accumulates as Lewy bodies.

Cervical Cancer

Regulation of ubiquitination may play a role in the development of tumor. For example, high-oncogenic risk human papillomavirus (HPV 16 and 18) associated with human cervical cancer produces E6 protein. E6 inactivates the p53 tumor suppressor. This is achieved by binding of E6

Table 10: Examples of diseases associated with functional derangement or cell or tissue injury due to misfolded proteins.

Disease	*Cause and protein affected*	*Pathogenesis and effect*
Degradation of mutant proteins with loss of their function		
Cystic fibrosis	Loss of cystic fibrosis transmembrane conductance regulator (CFTR)	Defects in chloride transport and death of affected cells
Familial hypercholesterolemia	Loss of low-density lipoprotein (LDL) receptor	Hypercholesterolemia
Tay–Sachs disease	Lack of the lysosomal enzyme hexosaminidase β subunit	Storage of GM_2 gangliosides in neurons
Misfolded proteins resulting in endoplasmic reticulum (ER) stress-induced cell death		
Retinitis pigmentosa	Abnormal folding of rhodopsin	Loss of photoreceptor and cell death, results in blindness
Creutzfeldt–Jakob disease	Abnormal folding of PrPsc prions	Death of neuronal cells
Alzheimer's disease	Abnormal folding of amyloid β peptide (Aβ peptide)	Aggregation within neurons and apoptosis
Both functional deficiency of the protein and ER stress-induced cell death		
Alpha-1-anti-trypsin deficiency	α_{-1} anti-trypsin with storage of nonfunctional protein	In hepatocytes, it causes apoptosis
	α_{-1} anti-trypsin with absence of enzymatic activity	In lungs, it causes emphysema

Table 11: Involvement of the ubiquitin–proteasome system in disease.

Disease	*Activity of ubiquitin–proteasome system*	*Pathological effect/changes*
Neurologic diseases (associated with loss of neurons)		
Parkinson's disease	Decreased	Lewy bodies
Alzheimer's disease		Amyloid plaques, neurofibrillary tangles
Amyotrophic lateral sclerosis		Superoxide dismutase aggregates in motor neurons
Huntington disease		Polyglutamine inclusions
Autoimmune Diseases		
Sjögren syndrome	Decreased	Chronic inflammation
Metabolic Diseases		
Type 2 diabetes mellitus	Increased	Insulin insensitivity
Cataract formation	Decreased	Aggregated oxidized proteins
Muscle Wasting		
Aging, cancer, and other chronic disease	Increased	Atrophy
Cardiovascular disorders		
Ischemia/reperfusion, pressure overload	Decreased	Apoptosis of myocyte

to Ub ligase and facilitates its association with p53. This in turn causes increased ubiquitination of p53 and increases its degradation. The loss of p53 activity is involved in the genesis of cervical cancer.

Aging and Storage Disorders

Impairment in ubiquitination may also contribute to cellular degenerative changes in aging and to a few storage diseases.

Gene Expression

Ubiquitination also plays a role in gene expression. Nuclear factor-κB (NFκB) is an important transcriptional activator. It can be activated in two different ways by the UPS. The active form of NFκB is a heterodimer (i.e., it consists of two different protein subunits). The below mentioned mechanism releases active NFκB which mediates expression of genes that promote cell survival.

- **Activation of NFκB by proteasome:** Inactive precursor forms of the two NFκB subunits are ubiquitinated and cleaved to their active forms in proteasomes. This is an example in which UPS produces incomplete protein degradation.
- **Degradation of inhibitor of NFκB by ubiquitination:** There is also degradation of IκB, which is the inhibitor of NFκB, by ubiquitination. This step results in release of active NFκB.

Proteasome inhibition allows the persistence of the IκB–NFκB complex and so decreases NFκB-induced transcriptional activation. In cancer cells, tumor cell survival can be impaired by inhibiting proteasome function. Hence, inhibition of proteasome can be used as a target for pharmaceutical manipulation in cancer. Anything that can be done by ubiquitination can be undone or prevented by deubiquitination. DUBs are important for gene expression and can influence many distinct mechanisms. DUBs can activate tumor suppressor proteins and may be important in tumorigenesis. DUBs may be attractive targets for pharmacological intervention in few diseases.

HEAT SHOCK PROTEINS

Q. Write a short essay on heat shock proteins.

Many molecular chaperones are called *heat-shock proteins* (abbreviated as Hsps). Hsps are family of proteins produced in a cell in response to exposure to stress. They were originally discovered in response to heat shock. They are synthesized in dramatically increased amounts after a brief exposure of cells to an elevated temperature (for example, 42°C for cells that normally live at 37°C). Raised temperatures cause protein misfolding/unfolding and boost the synthesis of the chaperones that help these proteins refold. These Hsps protect cells from damage due to protein misfolding under high-temperature conditions. However, Hsps are also known to be expressed in cold, ultraviolet (UV) light, wound healing, toxins, and tissue remodeling. Ub (discussed earlier) is a small 76-amino acid protein which is involved in protein degradation, also has features of a heat shock protein. A conserved protein binding domain of approximately 80 amino acid alpha crystallins are known as small heat shock proteins (sHSP).

Types

They belong to two major groups. Different members of these families function in different organelles.

- **Hsp70 system:** Hsps are named according to their molecular weight. For example, Hsp70 and Hsp40 have 70, 40 kilodaltons size, respectively. This mainly consists of Hsp70 (70-kDa **h**eat **s**hock **p**rotein) and Hsp40 (40-kDa Hsp). These proteins can bind individually to the substrate (protein) and help in the correct formation of protein folding. A special Hsp70 (called *BiP*) helps to fold proteins in the ER.
- **Hsp60 family:** They are sometimes called chaperonins and differ in sequence and structure from Hsp70 and its homologs. This is a large oligomeric assembly which forms a structure into which the folded proteins are inserted. The chaperonin system mainly consists of Hsp60 and Hsp10. These are needed at a later part of the protein folding process, and often work in association with Hsp70 system.

Regulation of Heat Shock Proteins

Activation of Hsp occurs when interaction of transcription factor, namely heat shock factor 1 (HSF1) occurs with heat shock elements (HSEs) in the heat shock protein gene promoter regions.

- In the unstressed state, HSF1 is present in the cytoplasm as a monomeric molecule and cannot bind to gene in the DNA. The activity of HSF1 is regulated by binding to Hsp70. This causes repression of heat shock gene transcription. Another mechanism that regulates heat shock protein synthesis is by the interaction between heat shock protein binding factor 1 (HSBP1). When it binds to even the active trimeric form of HSF1 and Hsp70, it inhibits the capacity of HSF1 to bind to gene in DNA.
- During stress, HSF1 is hyperphosphorylated in a RAS-dependent manner by members of the mitogen-activated protein kinases (MAPK). HSF1 is converted to phosphorylated trimers and can bind gene in the DNA. It translocates from the cytoplasm to the nucleus and initiates the activation process.

Mechanism of Action

Heat Shock Protein70 Family of Molecular Chaperones (Fig. 48)

These proteins act early; when nascent target proteins are formed. They recognize a small stretch of amino acids on a protein's surface. Adenosine triphosphate (ATP)-bound Hsp70 molecules attach to their target protein and then hydrolyze ATP to adenosine diphosphate (ADP). This allows the tighter binding of the Hsp70 molecules to the target. The rapid

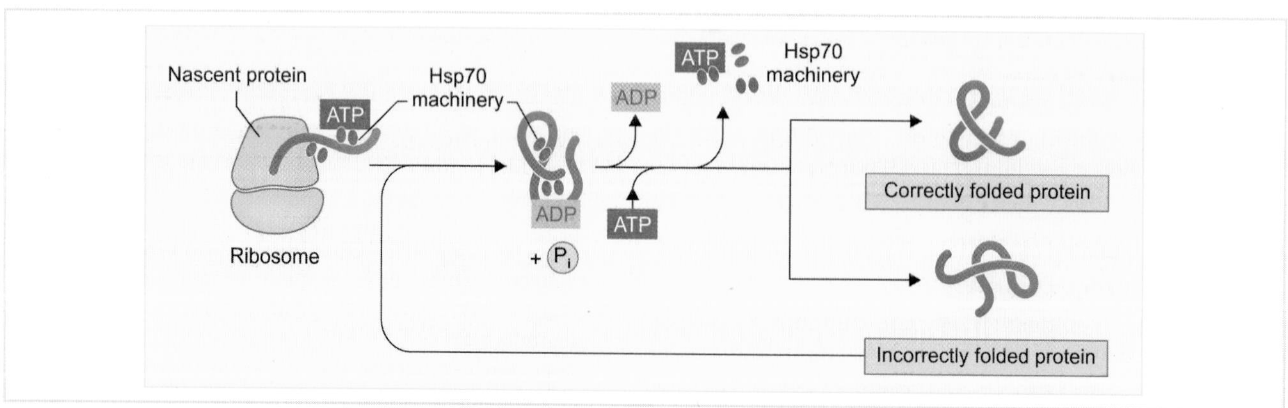

FIG. 48: Mechanism of action of heat shock protein (Hsp)70 family of molecular chaperones. These proteins act early; when nascent target proteins are formed. They recognize a small stretch of amino acids on a protein's surface. Adenosine triphosphate (ATP)-bound Hsp70 molecules attach to their target protein and then hydrolyze ATP to adenosine diphosphate (ADP). This allows the tighter binding of the Hsp70 molecules to the target. The rapid rebinding of ATP to the Hsp70 and release of ADP induces the dissociation of the Hsp70 protein. Repeated cycles of Hsp binding and release help the target protein to refold.

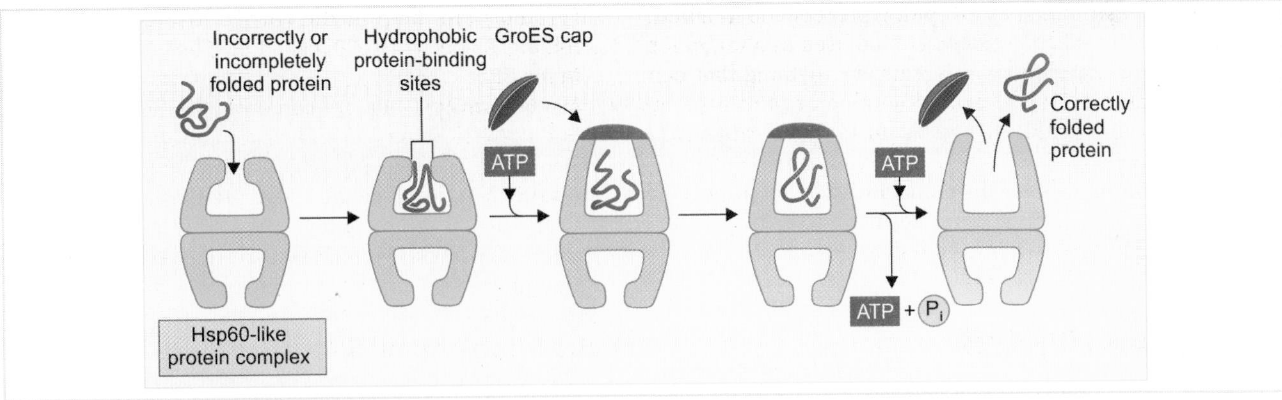

FIG. 49: Structure and function of the Hsp60 family of molecular chaperones. First, a misfolded target protein is captured with the exposed surface of the opening of Hsp60. The initial binding is attached to Hsp60 and itself usually unfold a misfolded protein. The subsequent binding of adenosine triphosphate (ATP) and a cap releases the target protein into an enclosed space. This provides a new opportunity for protein to fold. After about 10 seconds, ATP undergoes hydrolysis and weakens the binding of the cap. Subsequent binding of additional ATP molecules opens the cap and releases the protein. As shown in the figure, only half of the symmetric barrel of Hsp60 operates on a target protein at any one time. This type of molecular chaperone is also known as a chaperonin; it is called as Hsp60 in mitochondria.

rebinding of ATP to the Hsp70 and release of ADP induces the dissociation of the Hsp70 protein. Repeated cycles of Hsp binding and release help the target protein to refold.

Hsp60 Family of Molecular Chaperones (Fig. 49)

First, a misfolded target protein is captured with the exposed surface of the opening of Hsp60. The initial binding is attached to Hsp60 and itself usually unfold a misfolded protein. The subsequent binding of ATP and a cap releases the target protein into an enclosed space. This provides a new opportunity for protein to fold. After about 10 seconds, ATP undergoes hydrolysis and weakens the binding of the cap. Subsequent binding of additional ATP molecules opens the cap and releases the protein. As shown in **Figure 49**, only half of the symmetric barrel of Hsp60 operates on a target protein at any one time. This type of molecular chaperone is also known as a chaperonin; it is called as Hsp60 in mitochondria.

Release of Heat Shock Protein

Heat shock proteins are usually considered as intracellular molecules. Presently it has been found that they can be released into the extracellular compartment. The precise mechanism(s) by which Hsps are actively released by viable cells is not clearly known.

Functions

- **In primordial cells** it is involved in apoptosis, protein synthesis, translocation folding and degradation, and also involved in signaling.
- **Molecular chaperones:** Not all proteins are capable to assume their final tertiary structure by a simple process of self-assembly. This is not due to lack of the required information for proper folding of primary structure of these proteins, but because the proteins undergoing folding should be prevented from interacting nonselectively with other molecules in the compartments of the cell. Several families of proteins function to help unfolded or misfolded proteins to achieve their proper three-dimensional conformation. These "helper proteins" are called **molecular chaperones.** A molecular chaperone binds to and stabilizes an unstable protein, and releases functionally correct protein. It is involved in folding, assembly of oligomers, transport of protein to another subcellular compartment, and controlled switching between active/inactive conformations.
- **Immunity:** Extracellular and membrane bound heat-shock proteins (especially Hsp70) are involved in binding antigens and presenting them to the immune system.

Clinical Significance

- Heat shock factor is a transcription factor and is a modifier of carcinogenesis. HSF1 knockout mice do not develop cancer on exposure to carcinogen.
- Heat shock protein also acts as an antigen presenter. Hence, it can used to boost the efficacy of vaccines.
- Anticancer therapy

7.2 Adaptations of Cellular Growth and Differentiation, and Cellular Aging

CHAPTER OUTLINE

INTRODUCTION

Q. Discuss various cell responses to injury (cellular adaptation)—atrophy, hypertrophy, hyperplasia, and metaplasia.

Adaptation is a process of adjusting physiology, morphology, and behavior in response to new or altered circumstances. These circumstances may be internal and external in origin, in the physical and social environment. Cells adapt to their environment to escape and protect themselves from injury. An adapted cell is neither normal nor injured and its condition lies between these two states. Adaptive responses have limits and when stresses affect the essential cell function, it leads to cell injury.

When the cells are exposed to pathological stimuli (that may harm its normal structure and function), the cells can achieve a new, steady altered state that allows them to survive and continue to function in an abnormal environment. These reversible changes in the size, number, phenotype, metabolic activity, or functions of cells in response to new or altered internal or external conditions or circumstances constitute cellular adaptations. The cellular response to persistent, sublethal stress reflects the cell's efforts to adapt. Cellular stress may be physiological or pathological either due to an increased functional demand or a reversible cellular injury. Physiologic adaptations develop in response to normal stimulation by hormones or endogenous chemical mediators (e.g., enlargement of the breast and uterus during pregnancy), or to the demands of mechanical stress (e.g., muscles). Pathologic adaptations occur to escape injury, but at the expense of normal function (e.g., squamous metaplasia of bronchial epithelium in smokers). Physiologic and pathologic adaptations can take several distinct forms. Types of adaptations are mentioned in **Flowchart 1** and **Fig. 1** of Chapter 7.1.

Hypertrophy

Q. Write a short essay on molecular mechanism of hypertrophy.

Definition

Increase in the size of the tissue or organ due to increase in the size of cells.

Hypertrophied organ has large target cells and there are no new cells. The increase in size of the cells is due to the synthesis and assembly of additional intracellular structural components. Cells capable of division (labile and stable cells) may respond to stress by showing both hyperplasia and hypertrophy. Nondividing cells (e.g., myocardial fibers) can only undergo hypertrophy. In many sites, hypertrophy and hyperplasia may coexist and both lead to increased size of the organ.

Causes (Box 12)

Increased functional demand/workload—**if the cause/stress is not relieved, hypertrophy can progress to functionally significant cell injury.**

Mechanisms of Cellular Hypertrophy

Much of molecular basis of hypertrophy is understood based on studies of the muscles of the heart (cardiac muscle). Hypertrophy results from the action of growth factors and direct effects on cellular proteins. There are two main steps involve in the mechanism of cellular hypertrophy, namely—(1) activation of the signal transduction pathways, and (2) activation of transcription factors. Steps involved in biochemical mechanisms of myocardial (cardiac muscle) hypertrophy are shown in **Figure 51**.

Activation of the signal transduction pathways

Whatever may be the stimulus for hypertrophy (e.g., increased workload, response to endocrine or neuroendocrine

Box 12: Causes of hypertrophy.

Physiological
- **Hypertrophy of skeletal muscle:** For example, the bulging muscles of body builders and athletes in response to increased demand
- **Hypertrophy of smooth muscle:** For example, growth of the uterus during pregnancy from estrogenic stimulation

Pathological
- **Hypertrophy of cardiac muscle:** For example, left ventricular hypertrophy (**Figs. 50A** to **C**) due to hypertension or damaged valves (aortic stenosis, mitral incompetence)
- **Hypertrophy of smooth muscle**
  - For example hypertrophy of urinary bladder muscle in response to urethral obstruction [e.g., prostate hyperplasia (**Fig. 53B**)]
  - Hypertrophy of muscular layer of stomach due to pyloric stenosis

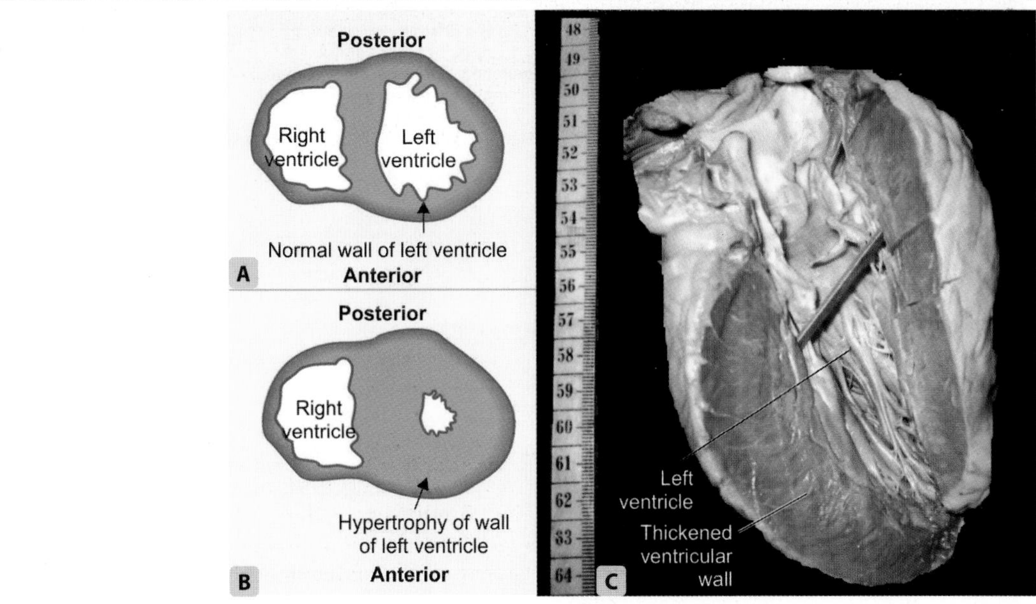

FIGS. 50A TO C: (A) Transverse section of normal heart. (B) Transverse section of heart with thickening of wall of the left ventricle due to hypertrophy. (C) Longitudinal section of heart with left ventricular hypertrophy.

mediators), there are certain processes that usually contribute to generating cellular hypertrophy. Various signaling mechanisms involved in hypertrophy are:

Physiological hypertrophy Increased workload on the myocardium produces **mechanical stretch** and is the major trigger for physiological hypertrophy. Mechanical sensors in the cell detect the increased load. These sensors activate a downstream signaling pathways. These pathways include the phosphoinositide 3-kinase (PI3K)/AKT pathway. These are the most important in physiologic hypertrophy such as exercise-induced, hypertrophy.

Pathological hypertrophy G-protein-coupled receptor-initiated pathways activated by many growth factors and hypertrophy agonists (vasoactive agents) are mainly involved in pathologic hypertrophy.

- **Growth factors:** Some of the signaling pathways stimulate increased production of growth factors and these are key initiators of hypertrophy. These include transforming growth factor-β (TGF-β), insulin-like growth factor-1 (IGF-1), and fibroblast growth factor (FGF) in muscle.
- **Hypertrophy agonists:** Some signaling pathways favor cellular hypertrophy by stimulating increased production of hypertrophy agnoists (vasoactive agents). These favor cellular hypertrophy and include:
  - **Neuroendocrine stimulation:** Adrenergic signaling such as α-adrenergic agonists may be important in initiating or facilitating cardiac hypertrophy.
  - **Other chemical mediators:** Such factors as nitric oxide (NO), endothelin-1, angiotensin II, and bradykinin can support hypertrophic responses.
- **Ion channels:** Ion fluxes may activate adaptation to increased demand. Particularly, calcium channel activity may stimulate a host of downstream enzymes (e.g., calcineurin) to produce cardiac hypertrophy.
- **Hypertrophy antagonists:** Some mechanisms favor cellular hypertrophy, whereas others inhibit it. Those inhibit hypertrophy are termed as hypertrophy antagonists. Atrial natriuretic factors (ANFs) and high concentrations of NO• and other molecules either stop or prevent cell adaptation by hypertrophy.
- **Oxygen supply:** Increased functional demand needs increased energy supply. If there is deficiency of oxygen to tissues, it stimulates angiogenesis and tries to supply oxygen. Thus, angiogenesis is a key component in adaptive hypertrophy.

The mechanisms that produce cardiac hypertrophy involve at least two types of signals—(1) mechanical triggers (e.g., stretch), and (2) soluble mediators (trophic signals) that stimulate cell growth [e.g., growth factors and adrenergic hormones (hypertrophy agonists)]. Mechanical sensors also stimulate production of growth factors and agonists. These signals/stimuli activate signal transduction pathways and induce many genes. These genes stimulate synthesis of many cellular proteins, including growth factors and structural proteins (muscle proteins). This results in the synthesis of more proteins and myofilaments per cell. This will increase the force generated with each contraction of cardiac muscle and makes the cell capable to meet increased work demands. Hypertrophy also may switch contractile proteins from adult to fetal or neonatal forms. For example, the α-myosin heavy chain is replaced by the fetal β form of the myosin heavy chain during muscle hypertrophy. Fetal forms produce slower and more energetically economic contraction.

The signals generated in the cell membrane activate signal transduction pathways. Two of these biochemical pathways involved in muscle hypertrophy are—(1) the phosphoinositide 3-kinase (PI3K)/Akt pathway [most important in physiological hypertrophy (e.g., exercise-induced hypertrophy)] and (2) signaling downstream of G-protein-coupled receptors (activated by many growth

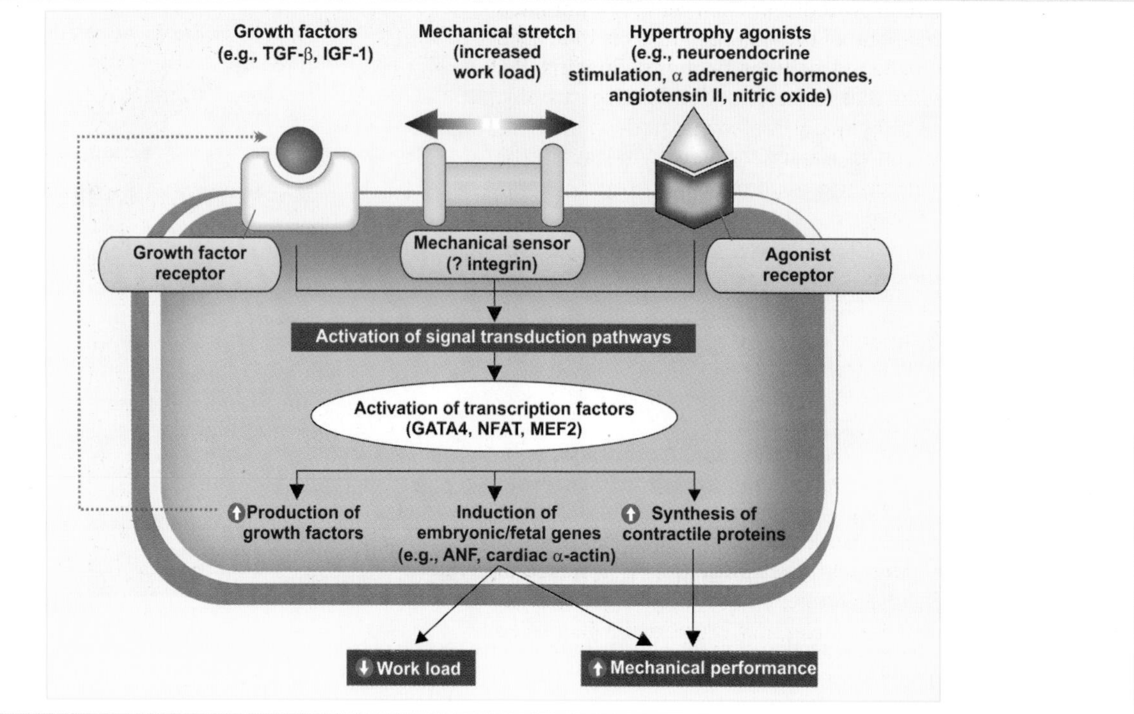

(ANF: atrial natriuretic factor; DNA: deoxyribonucleic acid; GATA4: transcription factor that binds to DNA sequence GATA; IGF-1: insulin-like growth factor; NFAT: nuclear factor activated T cells; MEF2: myocardial enhancing factor 2; TGF-β: transforming growth factor-β)

FIG. 51: Biochemical (molecular) mechanisms of myocardial hypertrophy showing major known signaling pathways and their functional effects. Mechanical sensors are main stimulators for physiologic hypertrophy, whereas other stimuli such as agonists (initiators) and growth factors play important role in pathologic hypertrophy. These factors activate signal transcription pathways and synthesize transcription factors. These transcription factors bind to DNA sequences and activate synthesis of muscle proteins that are responsible for hypertrophy. These pathways include—(1) production of growth factors, (2) induction of embryonic/fetal genes, and (3) increased synthesis of contractile proteins.

factors and vasoactive agents, and are more important in pathological hypertrophy).

Activation of transcription factors

Effector pathways in hypertrophy The different mechanisms (e.g., mechanical stretch, growth factors, and hypertrophy agonists) that initiate signaling pathways activate a set of transcription factors. These transcription factors include GATA4, nuclear factor of activated T cells (NFAT), and myocyte enhancer factor 2 (MEF2). These transcription factors increase the synthesis of muscle proteins that are responsible for hypertrophy. The activated transcription factors activate a limited number of downstream pathways to bring about the effects.

- **Increased synthesis of contractile proteins:** The production of proteins that promote hypertrophy tends to increase. This is necessary to meet the increased functional demand. After a hypertrophic signal, there is increased synthesis of certain proteins. This occurs very quickly through increased translational efficiency, and without changes in ribonucleic acid (RNA) levels. It occurs early in hypertrophy and quickly raises levels of specific proteins required for the increased functional demand.
- **Induction of embryonic/fetal genes:** Few genes are normally expressed only during early development of embryo and fetus. They are re-expressed in hypertrophied cells and the products of these genes take part in the cellular response to stress. For example, the gene for ANF (atrial natriuretic factor) is expressed in the embryonic heart (both the atrium and the ventricle), but not expressed after birth. In cardiac hypertrophy, ANF gene is re-expressed. ANF is a hormone that causes salt secretion by the kidney, decreases blood volume and pressure. Its re-expression decreases hemodynamic workload and increases the mechanical performance.
- **Switch in gene expression:** Cardiac hypertrophy is also associated with a switch in gene expression. This switch in gene expression is from genes that encode adult-type contractile proteins to genes that encode functionally distinct fetal isoforms of the same proteins. For example, the α isoform of myosin heavy chain (adult-type of contractile protein) is replaced by the β isoform (fetal isoform of contractile protein). This β isoform has a slower, more energetically economical contraction.
- **Increased production of growth factors:** Hypertrophy may also involve increased transcription of genes encoding growth promoting transcription factors (e.g., *Fos* and *Myc*).
- **Increased gene expression:** Concentrations of key proteins are also raised by transcriptional upregulation of their genes. Many signaling pathways activated by cytokines, neurotransmitters, etc., activate range of transcription factors. For example, the phosphatase calcineurin dephosphorylates transcription factor NFAT and moves it to the nucleus to stimulate transcription of target genes.

- **Increased protein degradation:** When cells are stimulated to increase in size, one of the first responses is increased degradation of selected cellular proteins. Specifically, to remove proteins that are not needed for hypertrophy. This is brought out by many proteolytic pathways. These include the ubiquitin-proteasome system (UPS), activation of intracellular proteases, and autophagy.
- **Survival:** During hypertrophy, there is inhibition of cell death (by inhibiting programmed cell death). The cell survival is brought out by stimulation of specific receptors that activate several enzymes (e.g., Akt, PI3K) that promote cell survival. In hypertrophy, binding of IGF-1 to its receptor stimulates Akt activity (**Fig. 50**). This leads to activation of the mammalian target of rapamycin (mTOR) complex and consequent increase in synthesis of protein.
- **Extracellular matrix (ECM):** In certain circumstances, hypertrophy may involve changes in a cell's environment (e.g., remodeling ECM).
- **Recruitment of satellite cells:** Hypertrophy of skeletal muscle is associated with recruitment of perimuscular satellite cells. These stellate cells fuse with myocyte syncytia to provide additional nuclei and support the increased synthetic needs of protein in the enlarging muscle.

Changes in heart in hypertrophy Transcription factors increase the synthesis of muscle proteins.
- Initially, enlargement of the heart is due to **dilation of the cardiac chambers** and is short-lived.
- It is followed by **increased synthesis of cardiac muscle proteins** (**Fig. 52**) and this facilitates the muscle fibers to do more work. The nucleus of the cardiac muscle also becomes hypertrophic and increases the synthesis of deoxyribonucleic acid (DNA). Along with the increase in size of the cell, there is also increased accumulation of protein in the cellular components [plasma membrane, endoplasmic reticulum (ER), myofilaments, mitochondria] but without any increase in the amount of cellular fluid.
- Subsequently, cardiac hypertrophy shows **remodeling of ECM** and increased growth of adult myocytes. Remodeling of cardiac tissue occurs after cardiac stress and can progress to heart failure and death. Probably cardiac fibrosis is due to increased activity of cardiac fibroblasts leading to excessive ECM production. Noncoding RNAs (ncRNAs) as gene regulators is the focus of study for cardiac fibrosis and therapeutic targets.
- Whatever, the exact cause and mechanism of cardiac hypertrophy, it reaches a stage beyond which enlargement of muscle mass is not possible to tolerate the increased burden. At this stage, many regressive changes occur in the myocardial fibers. These include lysis and loss of myofibrillar contractile elements and in extreme cases death of the myocytes. If cardiac hypertrophy is prolonged, it progresses to contractile dysfunction, decompensation, and **finally heart failure**. To prevent such tragic consequences, clinical trials are going-on on drugs that inhibit key signaling pathways involving *NFAT, GATA4,* and *MEF2* genes. It is known that microRNAs (miRNAs) can regulate target gene expression post-transcriptionally. It was found in cardiomyocytes of mice, that miRNA 212/132 family regulates cardiac hypertrophy and autophagy.

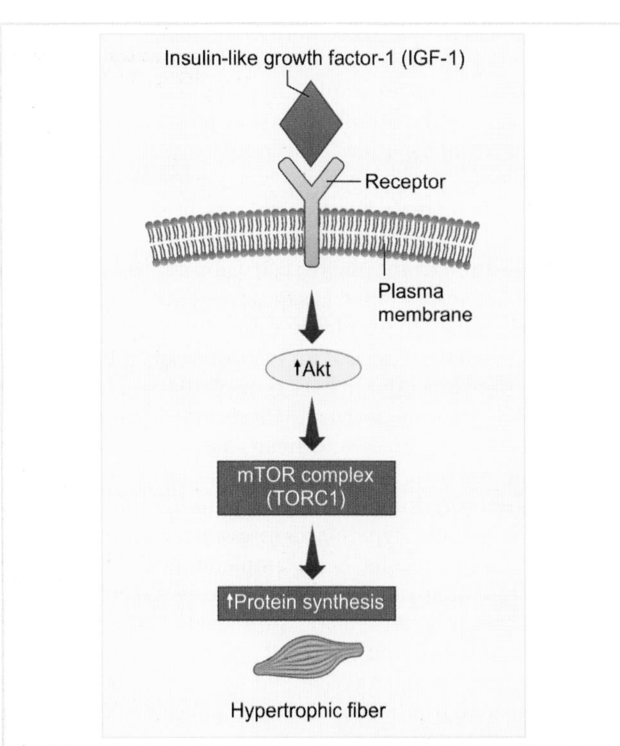

FIG. 52: Mechanism of increased protein synthesis in hypertrophy. Binding of insulin-like growth factor-1 (IGF-1) to its receptor stimulates Akt activity. This leads to activation of the mammalian target of rapamycin (mTOR) complex and consequent increase in synthesis of protein.

MORPHOLOGY

Gross

Involved **organ is enlarged.**

Microscopy

Increase in **size of the cells** as well as the **nuclei**.

Hyperplasia

Definition

Increase in the number of cells in an organ or tissue, resulting in **increased size/mass of the organ or tissue**. Increase in number may be **either of differentiated cells, or in few, due to less differentiated progenitor cells.**

Hyperplasia and hypertrophy are distinct processes. But, they may frequently occur together, and both may be triggered by the same external stimuli. Hyperplasia can occur only in the tissue containing cells capable of dividing (i.e., labile and stable cells and not in permanent cells).

Causes

Physiological hyperplasia

Physiologic hyperplasia may occur due to hormonal/growth factor stimulation or as a compensatory process.

- **Hyperplasia due to hormones:** Hyperplasia due to the action of hormones or growth factors occurs when there is a need to increase functional capacity of hormone sensitive organs. Changes in hormone level can cause proliferation of responsive cells. These hormonal changes may be due to developmental, pharmacological, or pathological influences. For example, hyperplasia of glandular epithelium of the **female breast at puberty, pregnancy, and lactation;** hyperplasia (accompanied by hypertrophy) of the uterus during pregnancy from estrogenic stimulation. The normal increase in estrogens at puberty or early in the menstrual cycle leads to increased number of endometrial and uterine stromal cells. Estrogen administration to postmenopausal women has the same effect.

- **Compensatory hyperplasia**: Compensatory hyperplasia occurs when there is need for compensatory increase after damage or resection. In liver transplantation, individuals donate one lobe of the liver. In these donors, the remaining liver cells proliferate and liver soon grows back to its original size. (e.g., in liver following partial hepatectomy).
- **Increased physiologic requirements:** The bone marrow undergoes rapid hyperplasia in response to a deficiency of mature blood cells. For example, in acute bleeding or premature breakdown of red blood cells (hemolysis), the growth factor erythropoietin are activated. They stimulate the hyperplasia of red blood cell progenitors and produces red blood cell as much as eightfold. Low atmospheric oxygen tension at high altitudes causes compensatory hyperplasia of erythroid precursors in the bone marrow and increased red blood cells (RBCs) (secondary polycythemia). Chronic blood loss (e.g., excessive menstrual bleeding) causes erythroid hyperplasia.
- **Immune responsiveness to many antigens:** It may lead to lymphoid hyperplasia (e.g., the enlarged tonsils and swollen lymph nodes in individuals with streptococcal pharyngitis).

Pathological hyperplasia

Most of the pathologic hyperplasia are caused by excessive or inappropriate actions of hormones or growth factors. They act on target cells leading to hyperplasia. Pathological hyperplasia may also occur due to chronic injury/irritation.

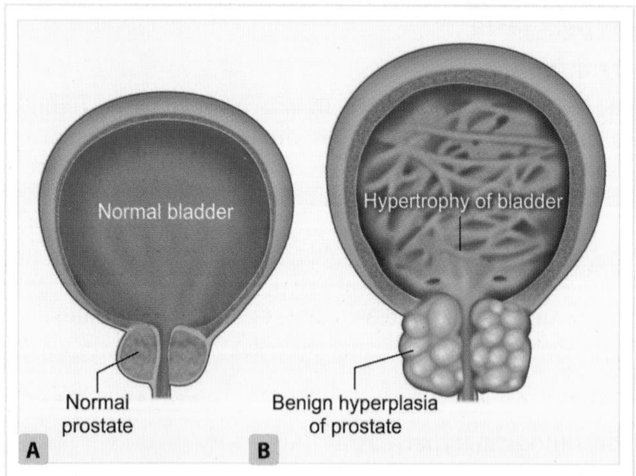

FIGS. 53A AND B: Cut section of prostate along with urinary bladder. (A) Normal prostate. (B) Enlarged prostate due to nodular hyperplasia. The urinary outflow obstruction results in hypertrophy of bladder muscle.

Excessive hormonal stimulation: Endometrial hyperplasia is a classical example for abnormal hormone-induced hyperplasia. Normally, after a menstrual period, the endometrium rapidly proliferates in response to stimulation by pituitary hormones and ovarian estrogen. Usually about 10 to 14 days before the end of the menstrual period, this proliferation is interrupted by the rising levels of progesterone. Sometimes, the balance between estrogen and progesterone may be disturbed. This may lead to absolute or relative increase in the amount of estrogen. This in turn produces hyperplasia of the endometrial glands. This type of pathologic hyperplasia is a common cause of abnormal uterine bleeding. Another common example of pathologic hyperplasia in male is **benign prostatic hyperplasia (Fig. 53A and B).** It develops in response to hormonal stimulation by androgens. Though these types of pathologic hyperplasias are abnormal, the process remains under control. If the hormonal stimulation is eliminated, these hyperplasia can either regress or stabilize. In hyperplasia, there is increase in cell division. This increases the risk of acquiring genetic aberrations. These genetic aberrations can drive unrestrained proliferation of cells and cancer. *Hyperplasia is distinct from cancer. However, pathologic hyperplasia constitutes a fertile soil in which cancerous proliferations may eventually arise.* For example, females with hyperplasia of the endometrium are at increased risk for developing endometrial cancer. Enlargement of the male breast (gynecomastia) may occur in men with excess estrogens [e.g., following estrogen therapy for prostate cancer or in cirrhosis (liver is not capable of metabolizing endogenous estrogens and leads to their accumulation)]. Ectopic production of hormones may be the first presenting symptom of tumor (e.g., erythropoietin secretion by renal tumors leads to erythroid hyperplasia in the bone marrow).

Chronic injury/irritation: Long-standing inflammation or chronic injury may lead to hyperplasia especially in skin or oral mucosa.

Demand-induced hyperplasia: For example, increase in RBC number in response to high altitude.

Viral infections of skin: Hyperplasia may occur in skin in some viral infections.For example, papillomaviruses cause skin warts and mucosal lesions composed of hyperplastic epithelium. The viruses produce factors that interfere with host proteins that regulate cell proliferation. Some hyperplasia due to virus are also precursors to cancer.

Mechanism

- Hyperplasia is characterized by cell proliferation mostly of mature cells, mediated **through stimulation by growth factor or hormones.**
- In some cases, the new cells may be derived from tissue **stem cells/less differentiated progenitor cells.**

For example, after partial hepatectomy, growth factors are produced in the liver. They bind growth factor receptors on the surviving liver cells. This in turn activate signaling pathways and stimulate proliferation of cells. In certain liver diseases (e.g., some hepatitis) the proliferative capacity of the liver cells is compromised and cause cell injury. In such cases, hepatocytes can regenerate from intrahepatic stem cells.

MORPHOLOGY

Gross

Size of the affected organ is **increased**.

Microscopy

Increased number of cells with increased number of mitotic figures.

Atrophy

Definition

Atrophy is the **reduced size of an organ or tissue** resulting from a **decrease in cell size and number**.

Causes

Physiological atrophy

Common during normal fetal development and in adult life.

- **During fetal development:** Some embryonic structures undergo atrophy during fetal development. For example, atrophy of notochord and thyroglossal duct.
- **During adult life** [e.g., involution of thymus, atrophy of brain, gonads, uterus (decrease in the size of the uterus occurs shortly after parturition and also during menopause), and heart due to aging (senile atrophy)].

Pathological atrophy

Pathological atrophy may be produced due to several causes. It can be local or generalized.

Local

Disuse atrophy (decreased workload): Skeletal muscle atrophy can occur when a fractured bone is immobilized in a plaster cast. It can also occur in a patient restricted to complete bed rest. Initially there is decrease in cell size and this is reversible once activity is resumed. More prolonged disuse leads to decrease in the number of skeletal muscle fibers (due to apoptosis) as well as in size. Skeletal muscle atrophy can be accompanied by increased bone resorption. This can lead to osteoporosis of disuse.

Denervation (loss of innervation) atrophy: Normal metabolism and function of skeletal muscle are dependent on its nerve supply. Any damage to the nerves leads to atrophy of the muscle fibers supplied by those nerves (e.g., poliomyelitis)].

Ischemic (diminished blood supply) atrophy: A gradual decrease in blood supply (chronic ischemia) to a tissue can occur due to slowly developing arterial occlusive disease such as atherosclerosis. This leads to atrophy of tissue supplied by that blood vessel. For example, in late adult life, the brain may undergo progressive atrophy. This is mainly due to reduced blood supply as a result of atherosclerosis of carotid arteries. This type of atrophy developing in late adult life is called **senile atrophy**.

Pressure atrophy: Prolonged compression of tissue can cause atrophy. An enlarging benign tumor can cause pressure atrophy in the surrounding uninvolved tissues. Atrophy in these cases may be due to ischemic changes caused by compromise of the blood supply by the pressure exerted by the expanding mass. Atrophy of renal parenchyma can occur in hydronephrosis due to increased pressure.

Loss of endocrine stimulation: Hormone-responsive tissues (e.g., breast and reproductive organs), are dependent on endocrine stimulation for normal metabolism and function. Loss of stimulation by estrogen after menopause leads to atrophy of the endometrium (**Fig. 54**), ovary, and breast. In males, atrophy of the prostrate occurs following chemical or surgical castration (e.g., for treatment of prostate cancer).

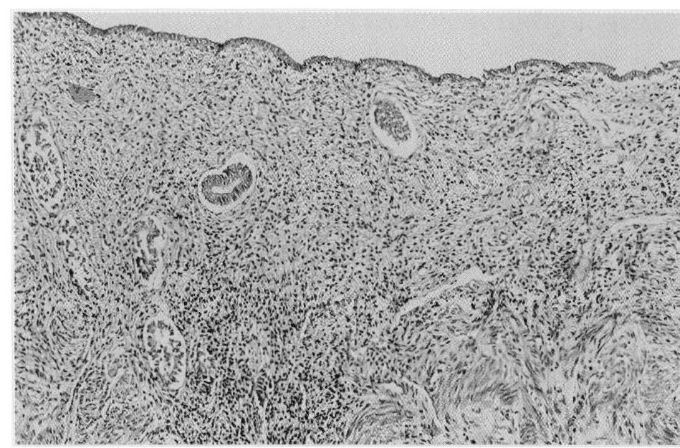

FIG. 54: Atrophic endometrium: The thin atrophic endometrium from an 65-year-old woman composed of only a few atrophic glands.

Absence of growth-stimulating (trophic) signals to maintain size and function: For example, the adrenal cortex, thyroid, and gonads are maintained by trophic hormones from the pituitary gland and undergo atrophy in their absence.

Generalized *Inadequate nutrition*: In severe protein-calorie malnutrition (marasmus), there is utilization of skeletal muscle proteins as a source of energy. This occurs after the depleted other reserves such as adipose stores . The utilization of skeletal muscle proteins produces marked wasting of muscle (cachexia). Cachexia also occurs in patients with chronic inflammatory diseases and cancer. In some cachectic conditions, there is chronic overproduction of the inflammatory cytokine TNF. Probably TNF suppresses the appetite and produces lipid depletion leading to atrophy of muscle.

In all of the above situations causing atrophy, the fundamental changes in the cells are similar. Initially, the cell size is reduced along with the organelles. These adaptations may reduce the metabolic needs of the cell enough to permit its survival. In atrophic muscle, the cells contain less number of mitochondria and myofilaments and a reduced amount of rough ER. A new equilibrium is achieved by balancing the cell's metabolic demands and supply (i.e., the lower levels of blood supply, nutrition, or trophic stimulation). *Early in the process of atrophy, the cells and tissues have diminished function and cell death is minimal*. However, atrophy caused due to gradual reduction in blood supply may progress to the point at which cells are irreversibly injured and die. Cell death is usually by apoptosis. Cell death by apoptosis is seen in atrophy of endocrine organs after withdrawal of hormone.

Mechanisms

In atrophy, there is decreased protein synthesis and increased protein degradation in cells.

- **Decreased protein synthesis**: It is due to reduced trophic signals (e.g., those produced by growth receptors). This increases the uptake of nutrients and increase mRNA translation.

- **Increased protein degradation:** The degradation of cellular proteins occurs predominantly by the ubiquitin-proteasome pathway. Deficiency of nutrient and disuse may activate ubiquitin ligases. These ligases attach the small peptide ubiquitin to cellular proteins. These cellular proteins are then degraded in proteasomes. This pathway is also involved in the accelerated proteolysis seen in a many catabolic conditions such as cancer cachexia.
- **Autophagy:** Atrophy is also accompanied by increased autophagy in many situations. These are characterized by the presence of increased numbers of autophagic vacuoles in atrophic cells. Some of the cell debris within the autophagic vacuoles may resist digestion. These cell debris persist in the cytoplasm of atrophic cells as membrane-bound residual bodies. One of the example of residual bodies is lipofuscin **granules**. When lipofuscin granules are present in sufficient amounts, they produce a brown discoloration to the tissue (**brown atrophy**). Autophagy is associated with various types of cell injury (refer pages 156–159 and Fig. 24 in Chapter 7).

MORPHOLOGY

Gross

The **organ is small and often shrunken.**

Microscopy

The **cells are smaller in size** due to reduction in cell organelles. Later stages, the reduced size of cells is accompanied by reduced number of cells. The reduced number is brought through death of cells mainly by apoptosis.

Differences between atrophy, hypertrophy, and hyperplasia are listed in **Table 12**.

Metaplasia

Definition

Metaplasia is a **reversible change** in which **one adult cell type (epithelial or mesenchymal) is replaced by another adult cell** type.

- Metaplasia is usually a **fully reversible adaptive response** to **chronic persistent injury**. If the noxious stimulus is removed (e.g., cessation of smoking), the metaplastic epithelium may return to normal.
- Metaplasia is mainly **seen in association with tissue damage, repair, and regeneration**.
- Metaplasia is an adaptive response in which one cell type that is sensitive to a particular stress is replaced by another cell type. The **replacing cell type** is usually **more suited to a change in environment** and can withstand the adverse environment better than the original epithelium.

Types and Causes of Metaplasia

Epithelial metaplasia

The most common epithelial metaplasia is columnar to squamous.

Squamous metaplasia In this type, original epithelium is replaced by squamous epithelium.

- **Respiratory tract** [e.g., In the habitual cigarette smoker, chronic irritation due to tobacco smoke, the normal ciliated columnar epithelial cells of the trachea and bronchi undergo squamous metaplasia (**Fig. 55**)].
- **Cornea:** Vitamin A (retinoic acid) deficiency can cause squamous metaplasia in the respiratory epithelium and in the cornea. In the cornea it disturbs the vision.
- **Excretory ducts**: The excretory ducts of the salivary glands, pancreas, or bile ducts are normally lined by secretory columnar epithelium. Stones in these excretory ducts may produce squamous metaplasia.
- **Cervix**: Squamous metaplasia in cervix is associated with chronic infection in the endocervix.

The stratified squamous epithelium in squamous metaplasia is more rough. It can survive better than fragile specialized columnar epithelium. However, squamous metaplasia comes with a price. For example, in the respiratory tract, the epithelial lining becomes more durable. However, mucus secretion and the ciliary action of the columnar epithelium are important protective mechanisms against infection. These are lost with squamous metaplasia. Thus, in most situations, epithelial metaplasia is an undesirable change. Also if the influences or circumstances that predispose to metaplasia, if persistent, can initiate malignant transformation in metaplastic epithelium. For example, development of squamous cell carcinoma in areas of the lungs where the normal columnar epithelium has been replaced by metaplastic squamous epithelium.

Columnar metaplasia Original epithelium is replaced by columnar epithelium.

Table 12: Differences between atrophy, hypertrophy, and hyperplasia.

Features	*Atrophy*	*Hypertrophy*	*Hyperplasia*
Definition	Reduced size of an organ or tissue resulting from a decrease in cell size and number	Increase in the size of the tissue or organ due to increase in the size of cells	Increase in the size/mass of the organ or tissue due to increase in the number of cells
Size of the involved organ	Reduced	Increased/enlarged	Increased
Cells			
Number	Reduced	No change	Increased
Size	Reduced	Increased	No change
Organelles	Reduced	Increased	No change
Rate of cell division	–	–	Increased
Synthesis of deoxyribonucleic acid (DNA), ribonucleic acid (RNA), and protein	–	Increased	Increased

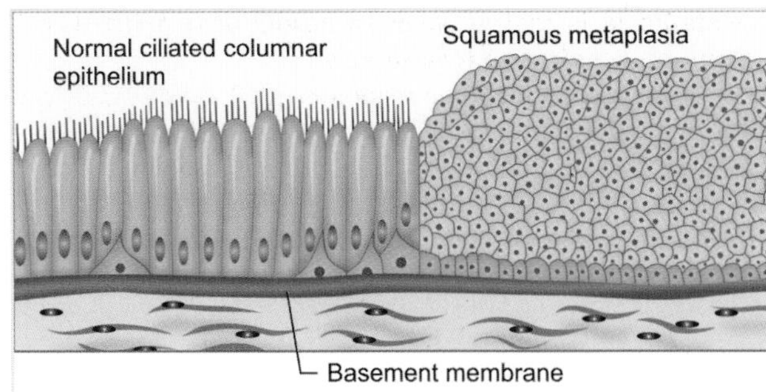

FIG. 55: Squamous metaplasia in which columnar epithelium (left) is replaced by squamous epithelium (right).

- **Squamous to columnar: In Barrett esophagus, the squamous epithelium of the esophagus is replaced by intestinal-like columnar cells** (**Fig. 56**) due to chronic reflux of highly acidic gastric contents into the lower esophagus. Malignant tumors that arise in these areas are typically adenocarcinomas (glandular cancer).
- **Intestinal metaplasia:** The gastric glands are replaced by cells resembling those of the small intestine.

Connective tissue metaplasia

Connective tissue metaplasia is a type of metaplasia. It is characterized by the formation of cartilage, bone, or adipose cells (mesenchymal tissues) in tissues that normally do not contain these elements. This type of metaplasia is not associated with increased risk of cancer.

Osseous metaplasia Formation of new bone at sites of tissue injury is known as osseous metaplasia. Bone formation in muscle, known as **myositis ossificans**, occasionally occurs after intramuscular hemorrhage. This type of metaplasia is less likely to be an adaptive response, and may represent a response of cell or tissue injury. Other examples include cartilage of larynx and bronchi in elderly individuals, scar of chronic inflammation of long duration, fibrous stroma of tumor (e.g., leiomyoma).

Mechanism

In metaplasia, there is no change in the phenotype of an already differentiated cell type. It represents either (i) reprogramming of local tissue stem cells (or undifferentiated mesenchymal cells that are present in normal tissues) or, (ii) alternatively, colonization by differentiated cell populations from adjacent sites. In both situations, the metaplastic change is stimulated by signals produced by cytokines, growth factors, and extracellular matrix components in the cells' environment. In stem cell reprogramming, the external stimuli promote the expression of genes that promote stem cells toward a specific differentiation pathway. Vitamin A (retinoic acid) deficiency or excess, both can cause metaplasia. There is a direct link between transcription factor dysregulation and metaplasia associated with vitamin A. Retinoic acid (refer page 1003) regulates gene transcription directly through nuclear retinoid receptors. They can influence the differentiation of progenitors derived from tissue stem cells.

Myeloid metaplasia: It is occurrence of myeloid tissue (with hematopoietic cells) in extramedullary sites (other than bone marrow) such as spleen and liver.

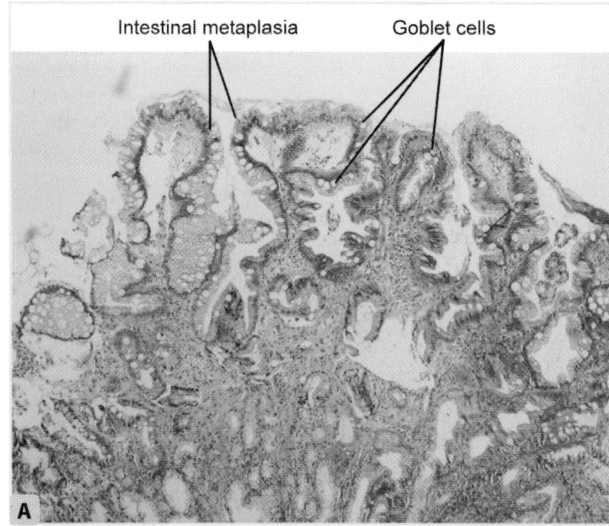

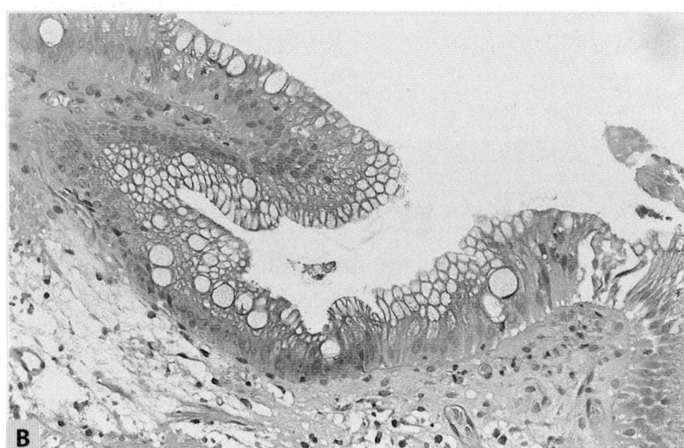

FIGS. 56A AND B: Barrett esophagus with intestinal metaplasia containing goblet cells. (A), low magnification and (B), high magnification

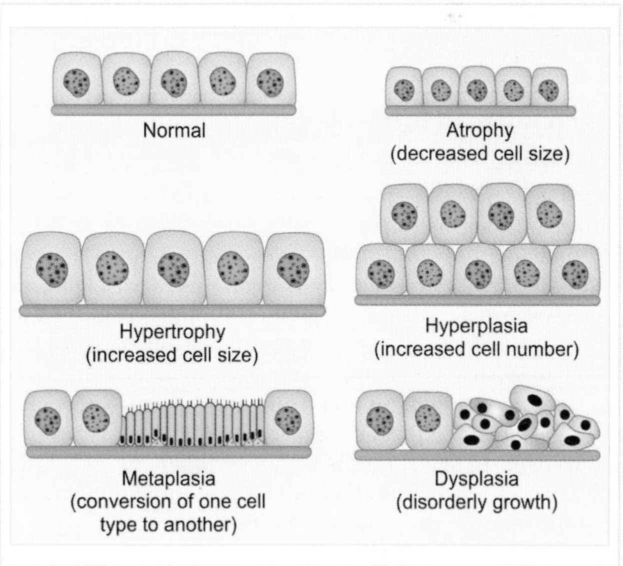

FIG. 57: Various types of cellular adaptations.

Various types of cellular adaptations are diagrammatically shown in **Figure 57**.

7.3 Intracellular Accumulations, Pathologic Calcification and Cellular Aging

CHAPTER OUTLINE

- Intracellular accumulations
  - Mechanism of intracellular accumulation
- Lipids
  - Steatosis (fatty change)
  - Pathogenesis of fatty liver
  - Cholesterol and cholesteryl/cholesterol esters
- Proteins
  - Causes of intracellular accumulation of proteins
- Hyaline change
  - Causes
- Mucoid degeneration
  - Epithelial mucin
  - Connective tissue mucin
- Glycogen
  - Causes
  - Morphology
- Pathologic calcification
  - Definition
  - Dystrophic calcification
  - Metastatic calcification
- Pigments
  - Definition
  - Endogenous pigments
  - Exogenous pigments
- Cellular aging
  - Definition
  - Causes
  - Mechanism of cellular aging
  - Age related pathological changes in various organ systems

INTRACELLULAR ACCUMULATIONS

Q. Write a short essay on intracellular accumulations in cell injury.

Metabolic derangements in cells may manifest as intracellular accumulation of abnormal amounts of various substances. The abnormal amounts of substances may accumulate either within the cytoplasm, within organelles (especially lysosomes) or in the nucleus of the cell. These substances may be normal or abnormal, endogenous (synthesized by the affected cells) or exogenous (produced elsewhere), harmful (causing varying degrees of injury) or harmless (innocuous). Accumulation of the substances can cause reversible cell injury whereas more severe accumulation can lead to irreversible cell injury.

Mechanism of Intracellular Accumulation (Fig. 58)

There are four main pathways which can lead to abnormal intracellular accumulations.

1. **Inadequate removal of a normal substance:** This may be secondary to defects in mechanisms of packaging and transport. For example, abnormal metabolism of lipid can cause excessive amounts of intracellular fat as in fatty change (steatosis) in the liver.
2. **Accumulation of an abnormal endogenous substance:** Genetic or acquired defects in folding, packaging, transport, or secretion of an endogenous substance can cause accumulation of this abnormal endogenous substance. For example, certain **mutated forms of α1-antitrypsin.**
3. **Failure to degrade a metabolite:** An inherited deficiency of critical/key enzymes required for breaking down certain endogenous complex compounds/substrates into soluble products can cause accumulation of complex compounds/substrates (that are not metabolized) in lysosomes. These are termed as lysosomal **storage diseases/disorders**.
4. **Deposition and accumulation of an abnormal exogenous substance:** When a cell has neither the enzymatic machinery to degrade the substance (or phagocytosed particles) nor the ability to transport it to other sites, the abnormal exogenous substance can accumulate within the cells. For example, foreign particulates such as carbon or silica particles or injected tattoo pigments can accumulate in the cells.

Consequences

If the overload can be controlled or stopped, the process of intracellular accumulation is reversible. In inherited storage diseases, there is progressive accumulation and the consequent overload results in injury to cells and can cause death of the tissue involved and the patient.

LIPIDS

Major classes of lipids are triglycerides, cholesterol/cholesterol esters, and phospholipids. All of them can accumulate in the cells. Phospholipids are major components of the myelin figures observed in necrotic cells. Apart from lipids, abnormal complexes of lipids and carbohydrates accumulate in the lysosomal storage diseases (refer pages 834–845).

Steatosis (Fatty Change)

Definition

Steatosis (fatty change) is defined as abnormal accumulations of triglycerides within cytosol of the parenchymal cells.

Organs Involved

Seen in organs involved in fat metabolism namely—**liver**. It may also occur in heart, muscles, and kidney.

Causes

Causes of steatosis of liver are listed in **Box 13**. **Nonalcoholic fatty liver disease (NAFLD)** is a common disease in which fatty liver develops in individuals who do not drink alcohol.

Increased prevalence of NAFLD is seem in **association with insulin resistance** and the **metabolic syndrome**.

Pathogenesis of Fatty Liver

Normal hepatocytes contain some amount of fat derived from the uptake of free fatty acids (FFAs) released from adipose tissue [and gastrointestinal (GI) tract]. A small amount of fatty acids is also synthesized from acetate in the liver cells. Most of FFA is esterified to triglycerides by the action of α-glycerophosphate and only a small part is changed into cholesterol, phospholipids, and ketone bodies. The cholesterol, phospholipids, and ketones are used in the body. Most of newly synthesized triglycerides are secreted by the liver as lipoproteins. Various mechanisms are involved in excess accumulation of triglyceride in the liver and one or more mechanism may be responsible for steatosis of liver.

- **Excessive entry of FFAs into the liver (1 in Fig. 59)**: From peripheral stores FFA enters into liver during starvation and diabetes.
- **Defective metabolism of lipids**: This may be due to:
  - Increased synthesis of fatty acids from acetate by liver (**2 in Fig. 59**).
  - Decreased oxidation of fatty acids into ketone bodies (**3 in Fig. 59**) resulting in increased esterification of fatty acids into triglycerides.
  - Decreased synthesis of apoproteins (e.g., in **CCl_4 and protein malnutrition**) causes decreased formation of lipoproteins from triglycerides (**4 in Fig. 59**).
- **Defective excretion of lipoproteins:** Fatty liver may also develop due to defect in excretion of lipoproteins from liver into the blood (**5 in Fig. 59**).

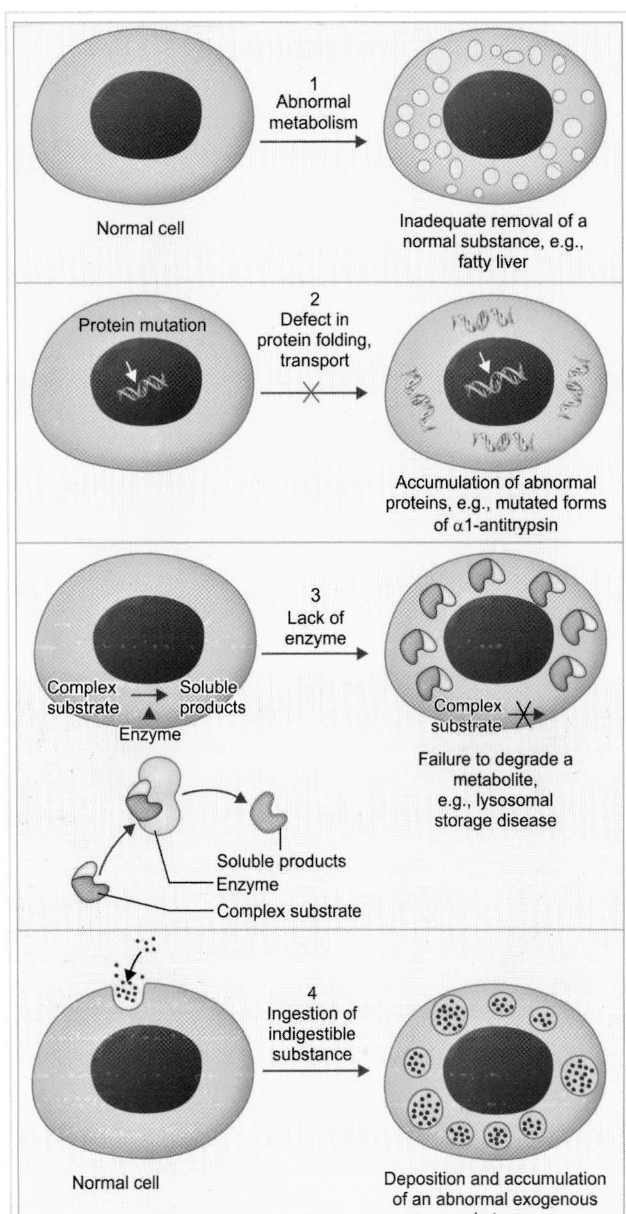

FIG. 58: Mechanisms of intracellular accumulation. (1) Due to abnormal metabolism (e.g., fatty change in the liver). (2) Mutations with alterations in protein folding and transport (e.g., mutated forms of α1-antitrypsin). (3) A deficiency of critical enzymes (e.g., lysosomal storage diseases). (4) An inability to degrade phagocytosed particles (e.g., accumulation of carbon pigment, silica).

MORPHOLOGY

Fatty Liver

- **Gross (Fig. 60):** Liver enlarges and becomes **yellow, soft and greasy to** touch.
- **Microscopy:** First, fat is seen as small **vacuoles in the cytoplasm** around the nucleus (microvesicular steatosis). Later, the vacuoles coalesce, creating clear spaces [macrovesicular steatosis (**Figs. 61A and B**)] that displaces the nucleus to the periphery of the cell (gives a signet ring appearance—not to be mistaken for signet ring cells seen in signet ring carcinoma).

Special stains for fat sections stained with **Sudan IV or Oil Red O** give an orange-red color to the fat. **Osmic acid** (is a fixative as well as a stain) and **Sudan black B** gives a black color.

Heart

Lipid in the cardiac muscle can have **two patterns**:

1. **Alternate involvement:** Prolonged moderate hypoxia (e.g., severe anemia), create grossly apparent bands of involved **yellow myocardium alternating with bands of darker, red-brown, uninvolved myocardium (tigered effect, tabby cat appearance)**.
2. **Uniform involvement:** More severe hypoxia or some types of myocarditis (e.g., diphtheria infection) show more **uniform involvement of myocardial fibers**. It may also be seen secondary to (1) myocarditis, (2) pericarditis, (3) starvation, and (4) fever (scarlet fever, typhoid fever).

Box 13: Causes of hepatic steatosis.

- **Disorders with hepatocyte damage:** Alcoholic abuse, protein malnutrition, starvation, anoxia (anemia, cardiac failure), toxins (carbon tetrachloride, chloroform, etc.), and Reye syndrome. **Alcohol is the most common cause** of fatty change in the liver
- **Disorders with hyperlipidemia:** Obesity, diabetes mellitus, or congenital hyperlipidemia nonalcoholic fatty liver disease

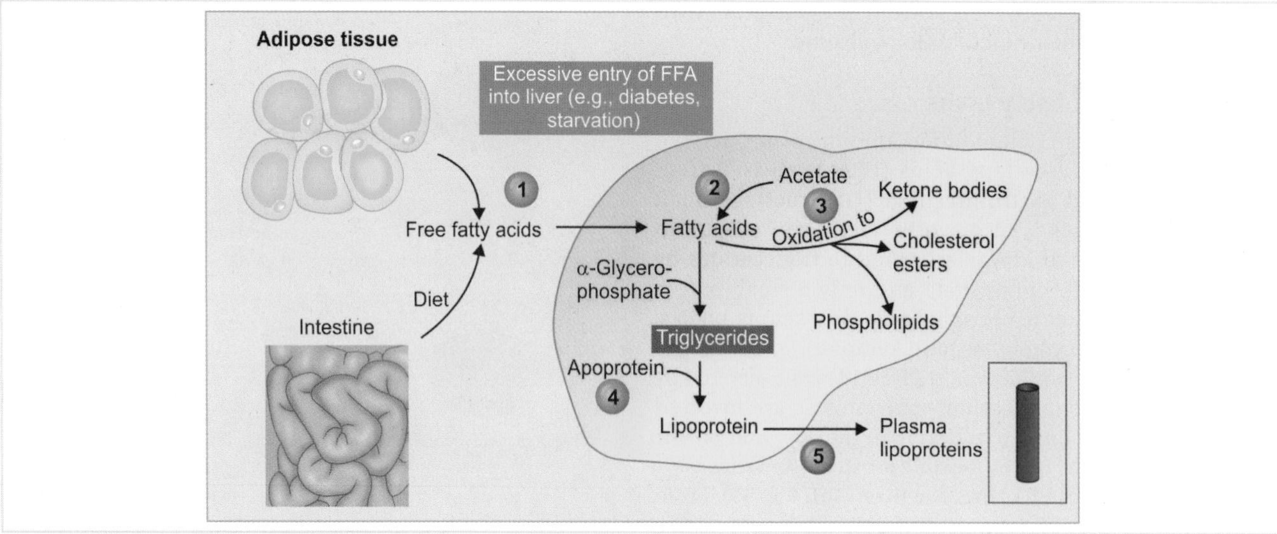

FIG. 59: Various mechanisms that can produce accumulation of triglycerides in fatty liver.

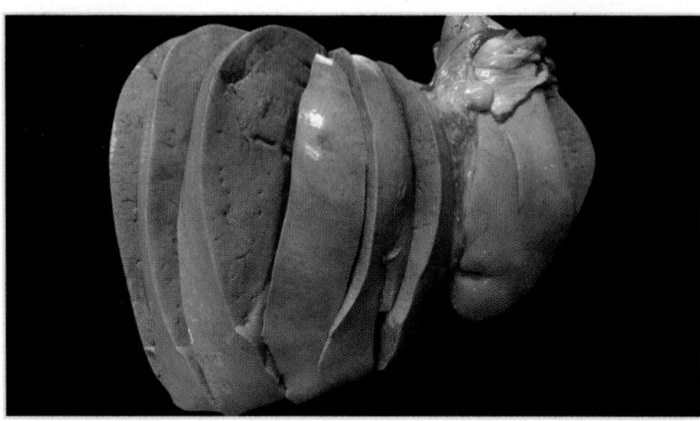

FIG. 60: Fatty liver showing a part of liver with yellow color and sharp border.

Cholesterol and Cholesteryl/Cholesterol Esters

Cholesterol metabolism in cells is tightly regulated in such a way that there is normal generation of cell membranes (in which cholesterol is a main component) without significant intracellular accumulation. However, in pathological conditions, phagocytic cells may intracellularly accumulate lipid (triglycerides, cholesterol, and cholesteryl esters). It may be either due to increased intake or decreased catabolism of lipids. These pathological conditions are briefly discussed here.

Atherosclerosis

It is a disease of **aorta and large arteries** characterized by the presence of **atherosclerotic plaques composed of smooth muscle cells and macrophages within the intima filled with lipid vacuoles. Most of the lipid is cholesterol and cholesterol esters (Fig 62)**. These cells have a foamy appearance and are termed foam cells. Aggregates of these cells in the intima grossly gives a yellow appearance to cholesterol-laden atheromas. Some fat-laden cells may rupture and release cholesterol and cholesterol esters into the extracellular space. These cholesterol or esters may form crystals. They may appear as long needles that produce distinct clefts in tissue sections. Small crystals of cholesterol are phagocytosed by macrophages and activate the inflammasome. This contributes to local inflammation observed in atherosclerosis

Xanthoma

Intracellular accumulation of cholesterol within macrophages is found in acquired and hereditary hyperlipidemic conditions. **The tumor mass produced by the macrophages filled with cholesterol** is termed xanthomas. The xanthomas are found in the subepithelial connective tissue of the skin and the tendons, producing tumorous masses. Microscopically, it consists of clusters of foamy cells in the subepithelial connective tissue of the skin and in tendons.

Cholesterolosis

It is characterized by the **focal accumulations of cholesterol-laden macrophages in the lamina propria of the gall bladder (Fig. 63)**. The mechanism is not known.

Niemann–Pick disease, type C

It is a lysosomal storage disease caused by mutations affecting an enzyme involved in cholesterol trafficking. It is characterized by **accumulation of cholesterol in many organs.** It is discussed in detail on page 841.

PROTEINS

Abnormal pathologic accumulation of proteins can occur within the cells. Under light microscopy, abnormal intracellular accumulations of proteins appear as rounded, eosinophilic droplets, vacuoles, or aggregates in the cytoplasm. When viewed under electron microscopy, they can appear as amorphous, fibrillar, or crystalline structures. In amyloidosis, abnormal proteins are deposited in the extracellular spaces.

Causes of Intracellular Accumulation of Proteins

Excesses, morphologically visible, abnormal/excessive accumulation of proteins within the cells (intracellular) may

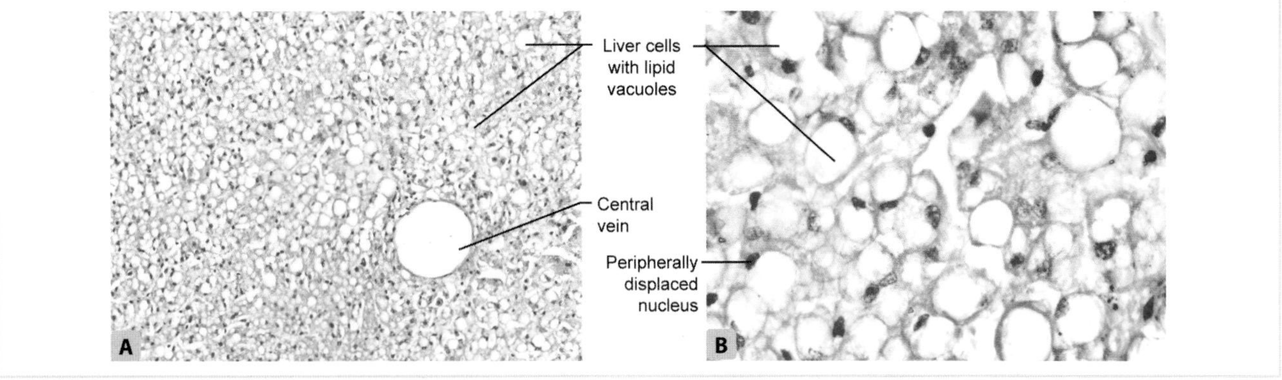

FIGS. 61A AND B: (A) Fatty liver in which the hepatocytes show accumulation of fat which appear as clear vacuole in the cytoplasm. (B) Hepatocytes at higher magnification in which the nucleus is displaced to the periphery by accumulated fat.

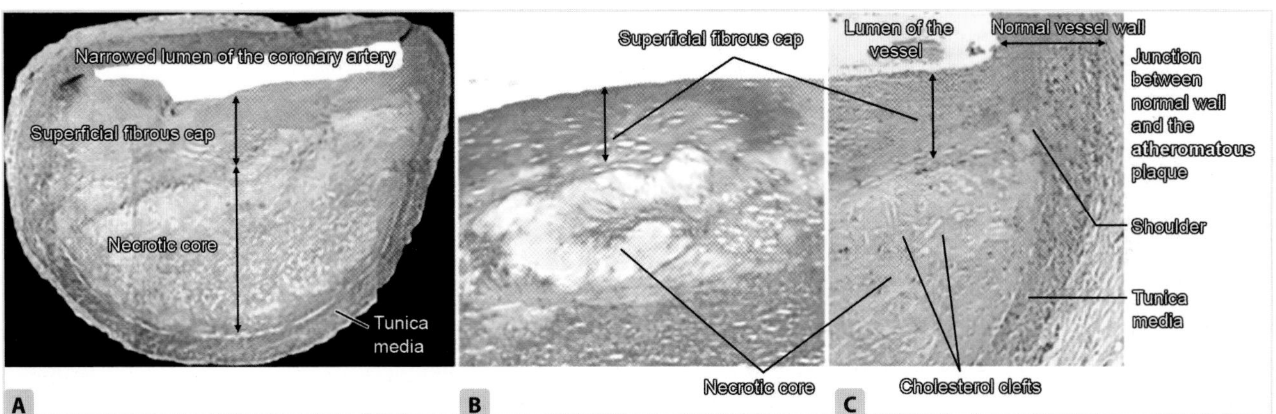

FIGS 62 A TO C: Microscopy of atheromatous plaque: (A) Scanner view of coronary atherosclerosis causing >90% narrowing of the lumen; (B) Shows central necrotic core and superficial fibrous cap; (C) Shows junction between the vessel wall and atheromatous plaque, shoulder region and cholesterol clefts in the necrotic core.

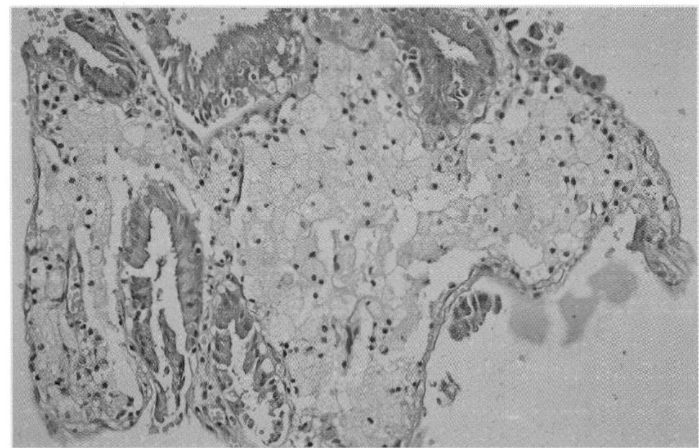

FIG. 63: Cholesterolosis. Focal accumulation of Cholesterol-laden macrophages (foam cells, *arrow*) in gallbladder cholesterolosis.

occur either due to excessive presentation of proteins to the cells or when the cells synthesize excessive amounts of proteins.

Excessive Presentation of Proteins to the Cells

Reabsorption protein in proximal renal tubules: It occurs in renal diseases associated with loss of protein in the urine (proteinuria). In the kidney, trace (small) amounts of protein (albumin) filtered through the glomerulus are normally reabsorbed in the proximal convoluted tubule by a process called pinocytosis (refer page 29 of Chapter 1). However, when there is heavy protein leakage (e.g., nephrotic syndrome) through the glomerulus, there is increased/excessive reabsorption of the protein into vesicles. These vesicles containing this protein appear microscopically as pink hyaline droplets within the cytoplasm of the tubular cell. The process is reversible and with the control of proteinuria, the protein droplets are metabolized and disappear from the cell.

Excessive Synthesis or Accumulation of Proteins

- **Russell bodies:** Plasma cells synthesize immunoglobulins (a type of protein). Whenever the plasma cells newly synthesize excessive amounts of immunoglobulins, they can accumulate within the rough endoplasmic reticulum (RER) present in the cytoplasm of some plasma cells. The RER becomes distended with immunoglobulins and produces large, round, homogeneous eosinophilic (pink hyaline) inclusions called as Russell bodies (**Fig. 64**).
- **Defective intracellular transport and secretion of critical proteins:** α1-antitrypsin deficiency is a heritable disorder in which mutations in the gene coding for α1-antitrypsin yield an insoluble protein. The protein produced is significantly slow in folding process and is

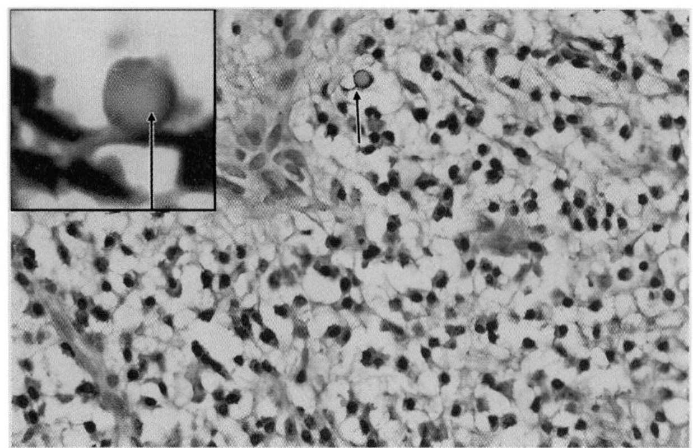

FIG. 64: Russell body (arrow) appear as large, round, homogeneous eosinophilic inclusions in plasma cells. Inset show magnified view of Russell body.

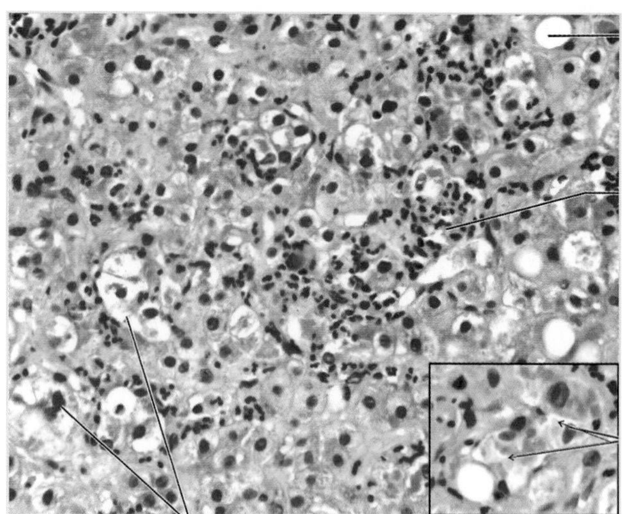

FIG. 65: Mallory's body or alcoholic hyaline appears as an eosinophilic cytoplasmic inclusion seen in liver cells and is characteristic of alcoholic hepatitis .Inset shows higher magnification of Mallory's bodies.

not easily exported/secreted from the cells. This results in the accumulation of partially folded intermediates which aggregate in the endoplasmic reticulum (ER) of the cytoplasm of the liver cells and appear as eosinophilic globular deposits of a mutant protein. This results in the deficiency of the circulating enzyme and there is excessive digestion of elastic tissues which produce emphysema. In many of these diseases, the damage is not only due to the loss of protein function but also due to ER stress caused by the misfolded proteins. This produces unfolded protein response and lead to death of the cells by apoptosis.

- **Accumulation of cytoskeletal proteins:** The internal framework of a cell is composed of protein filaments known as cytoskeletal proteins. They provide structural support to the cells and drive the movement of the cell. There are several types of cytoskeletal proteins and are usually divided into three categories namely—microfilaments [thin actin filaments (6–8 nm), thick myosin filaments (15 nm)], intermediate filaments (10 nm), and microtubules (20–25 nm in diameter), depending on the diameter and the composition of filaments. The intermediate filaments provide a flexible intracellular scaffold that organizes the cytoplasm and resists forces applied to the cell. The intermediate filaments are subdivided into five classes: (1) keratin filaments (characteristic of epithelial cells), (2) neurofilaments (neurons), (3) desmin filaments (muscle cells), (4) vimentin filaments (connective tissue cells), and (5) glial filaments (astrocytes). They are discussed in detail on pages 17–21. Accumulations of keratin filaments and neurofilaments are observed in certain types of cell injury.
  - **Mallory's body or alcoholic hyaline (Fig. 65)**: It is an eosinophilic cytoplasmic inclusion seen in liver cells and is characteristic of alcoholic liver disease. It appears as amorphous pink masses. They represent intracellular accumulation of intermediate filaments of keratin (cytokeratin).
  - **Neurofibrillary tangle (tau protein):** It is found in cortical neurons of the brain of patients with Alzheimer disease and consists of neurofilaments and other proteins.
- **Aggregation of abnormal proteins:** Abnormal or misfolded proteins may aggregate and get deposited in tissues and interfere with their normal functions. These deposits may be intracellular, extracellular, or both. These aggregates of proteins may either directly or indirectly cause the pathologic changes.
  - **Intracellular accumulation of misfolded proteins:** It may be due to either increased production of the misfolded proteins or reduced ability to eliminate them.
    - **Prion diseases**: These are neurodegenerative disorders (spongiform encephalopathies) caused by accumulation of abnormally folded prion proteins. Abnormal prion proteins may be due to either inherited mutations or from exposure to the aberrant form of the protein.
    - **Lewy bodies** (α-synuclein): They are observed in neurons of the substantia nigra of patients with Parkinson disease.
  - **Extracellular accumulation of proteins**: Usually proteins accumulate inside the cells. Apart from abnormal intracellular accumulation, abnormal protein deposits can occur primarily in extracellular spaces in some disorders, such as certain forms of amyloidosis (refer pages 1152–1162). These disorders are sometimes tremed as proteinopathies or protein-aggregation diseases.

HYALINE CHANGE

Q. Write short essay on hyaline change.

Hyaline refers to an alteration within cells or in the extracellular space, which gives a homogeneous, glassy, pink appearance in routine histological sections. It appears reddish and homogeneous with eosin of H&E stain and the term hyaline was used in classic descriptions of diverse and unrelated lesions. The term is ancient but is still used for describing morphological feature.

Causes (Table 13)

Intracellular Hyaline (Table 13)

- **Mallory body (Fig. 62A)** in the liver is alcoholic hyaline **composed of cytoskeletal filaments**. Mallory hyaline/body is observed in: (1) Alcoholic hepatitis, (2) Indian childhood cirrhosis (ICC), (3) Primary biliary cirrhosis, (4) Wilson disease, (5) Hepatocellular carcinoma, (6) Focal nodular hyperplasia of liver.
- **Russell bodies** are **excessive accumulation of immunoglobulins in the RER of plasma cells (Fig. 65)**.
- **Zenker's degeneration:** Hyaline change of rectus abdominalis muscle (becomes glassy and hyaline) in typhoid fever.
- Hyaline droplets in various cells. **Crooke's hyaline body:** Present in basophil cells of pituitary gland in Cushing syndrome.

Extracellular Hyaline (Table 13)

- Collagenous fibrous tissue in **old scars**.
- Hyaline change in **uterine leiomyoma (Fig. 66)**.
- In **chronic glomerulonephritis,** the **glomeruli** show hyalinization.
- Hyaline arteriolosclerosis mainly seen in diabetes and hypertension.
- Hyaline membranes in the lung consist of plasma proteins deposited in alveoli.
- Hyaline casts in urine.
- Amyloid also appears as pink homogenous substance.

Table 13: Examples of hyaline change.

Intracellular hyaline	*Extracellular hyaline*
• Mallory bodies • Russell bodies (e.g., multiple myeloma) • Crooke's hyaline • Zenker's hyaline change	• Collagenous fibrous tissue in scar • Hyaline change in uterine leiomyoma • Hyaline membrane in new-born • Hyaline arteriosclerosis • Hyalinization of glomeruli in chronic glomerulonephritis • Corpora amylacea in prostate, brain, spinal cord in elderly, old infarct of lung

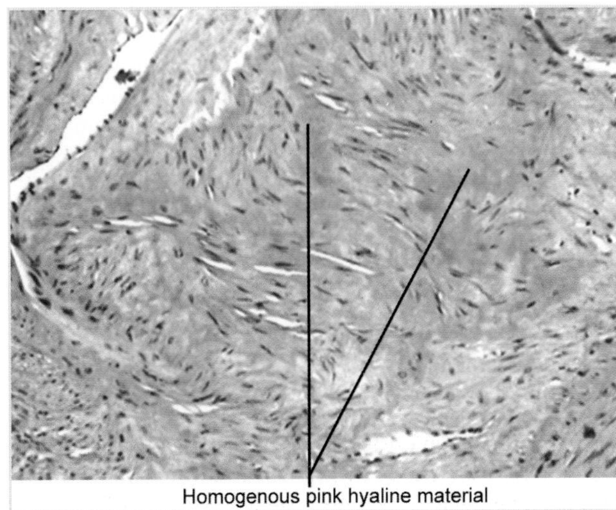

FIG. 66: Hyaline change in leiomyoma of uterus.

MUCOID DEGENERATION

- Mucus is the viscid watery secretion produced by mucous glands. It consists of loose combination of proteins and mucopolysaccharides. Its main constituent is a glycoprotein called mucin.
- Mucus is produced by mitochondria and then they move to Golgi apparatus, where they are converted into mucin. When this process is exaggerated with excessive secretion of mucus it is termed mucoid degeneration.
- Mucin is normally produced by both epithelial cells of mucous membranes and mucous glands, and also by certain connective tissue cells, especially in the fetus (e.g., umbilical cord). Mucoid degeneration may involve both epithelial and connective tissue mucin. Usually, connective tissue mucin is termed as myxoid, i.e., mucus like.
- Both epithelial and connective tissue mucins are stained by alcian blue. Epithelial mucin stains positively with PAS and connective tissue mucin is PAS negative and stains positively with colloidal iron.

Epithelial Mucin

Examples of excessive epithelial mucin secretion are:

- Catarrhal inflammation of the mucous membrane, e.g., inflammation of mucosa of respiratory tract and GI tract
- Obstruction, e.g., mucocele of gallbladder, appendix, and oral cavity.
- Cystic fibrosis of pancreas.
- Mucus secreting tumors, e.g., GI tract and ovary.

Connective Tissue Mucin

Examples:

- Mucoid or myxoid degeneration: Examples of tumors include myxoma, neurofibroma, fibroadenoma and sarcomas.
- Dissecting aneurysm of aorta.
- Myxedema: Myxomatous changes in dermis.
- Myxoid change in ganglion.

GLYCOGEN

Glycogen is a long-chain polymer of glucose. It is formed and mainly stored in the cytoplasm of liver and to a lesser extent in muscles. Glycogen is a readily available energy source and is depolymerized to glucose and liberated as needed.

Causes

Excessive intracellular deposits/accumulation of glycogen can occur due to an abnormality in either glucose or glycogen metabolism.

- **Glycogen storage disease:** Glycogen is degraded in steps by a series of enzymes. Deficient of any enzymes involved in any of these steps may be observed as an inborn (genetic) error of metabolism called as a glycogen storage disease or glycogenoses (refer pages 845–848).
- **Diabetes mellitus:** Storage of glycogen in cells is normally regulated by blood glucose levels, and hyperglycemic states are associated with increased glycogen stores. Thus, in uncontrolled diabetes mellitus (a disorder of glucose metabolism), there is impaired cellular uptake of glucose, which results in high serum and urine glucose levels. It is

accompanied by excessive accumulation of glycogen in hepatocytes, epithelial cells of the renal proximal tubules (renal tubules reabsorb the excess filtered glucose and store it intracellularly as glycogen), β-cells of the islets of Langerhans, and cardiac muscle cells.

Morphology

In routine hematoxylin and eosin (H&E) stained sections, glycogen appear as clear vacuoles within the cytoplasm of the affected cells. Glycogen gets dissolved in aqueous fixatives and appears as vacuoles in the cytoplasm. Hence, for its identification, tissues should be fixed in absolute alcohol. Special stains such as Best's carmine or the periodic acid–Schiff (PAS) imparts a rose to violet color to the glycogen. Diastase digestion of a parallel section before staining serves as a further control by hydrolyzing the glycogen.

PATHOLOGIC CALCIFICATION

Q. Describe the mechanism of dystrophic calcification/ abnormal calcification/pathological calcification.

Definition

Abnormal **deposition of calcium salts in tissues other than osteoid or enamel**. It is also associated with deposition of small amounts of iron, magnesium, and other minerals.

Types of pathologic calcification are: (1) dystrophic and (2) metastatic.

Dystrophic Calcification

It is defined as deposition of calcium salts in **dying/injured or dead tissues**. It occurs in spite of normal levels of serum calcium. There is no derangements in calcium metabolism.

Causes

- **Necrotic tissue:** Calcification in **caseous, coagulative, liquefactive, enzymatic fat necrosis**, in **dead eggs** of *Schistosoma*, cysticercosis and hydatid cysts.
- **Damaged tissue**:
    - **Heart valves:** Occurs in aging or damaged heart valves. Dystrophic calcification of the aortic valves causes aortic stenosis in elderly individuals.
    - Advanced atherosclerosis, **goiter of thyroid, dense old scar, cysts (e.g., epidermal and pilar cysts of skin).**
- **Monckeberg's medial calcific sclerosis:** It is characterized by calcification in the media of the muscular arteries (**Fig. 67A**) in old people (over the of age 50 years). It usually starts along the internal elastic membrane. The calcifications do not narrow the lumen of the involved vessel lumen are usually not clinically significant. They are commonly observed in vessels of the myometrium in females.
- **Psammoma bodies:** The calcium salts appear as gritty, clumped granules that can become hard as stone. When several layers of mineral get deposited progressively (or clump together) on a single necrotic cell to create lamellated shape, they resemble grains of sand and are called **psammoma bodies** (**Fig. 67B**). Examples of conditions in which psammoma body are usually found includes (1) Papillary carcinoma of thyroid, (2) Papillary serous cystadenoma of ovary, (3) Papillary serous cystadenocarcinoma of ovary, (4) Meningioma, (5) Papillary carcinoma of the kidney.

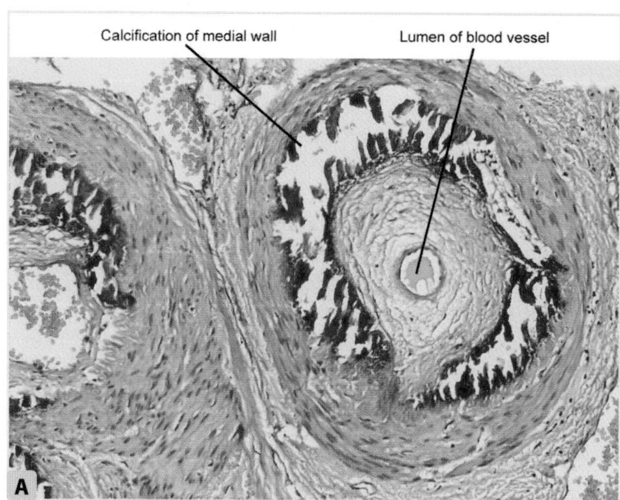

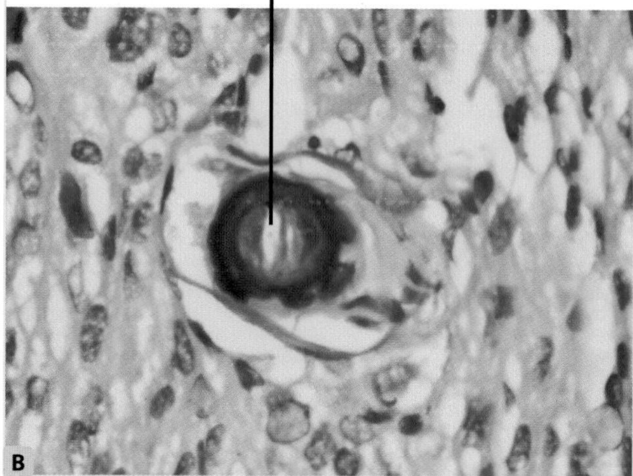

FIGS. 67A AND B: (A) Monckeberg's medial calcific sclerosis in which the tunica media of arteries in the myometrium of uterus show calcification. (B) Photomicrograph of meningioma with psammoma body.

Diagnostic Importance

Dystrophic calcification develops slowly and is a definite marker for the site of dead cells. Dystrophic calcification may be useful in diagnostic radiography. For example, mammography is based mainly on the detection of small calcifications in breast cancers; congenital toxoplasmosis, an infection involving the CNS, is suggested when calcification is seen in an infant's brain.

Mechanism (Flowchart 4)

The exact pathogenic mechanisms responsible for dystrophic calcification are unknown.

Initiation: Probably progressive deterioration of dead cells exposes denatured (changed) proteins and releases enzymes. The membrane bound enzyme phosphatases breakdown organic phosphates. The denatured proteins preferentially bind with phosphate ions.The phosphate ions then react with calcium ions to form deposits of phosphate carbonate

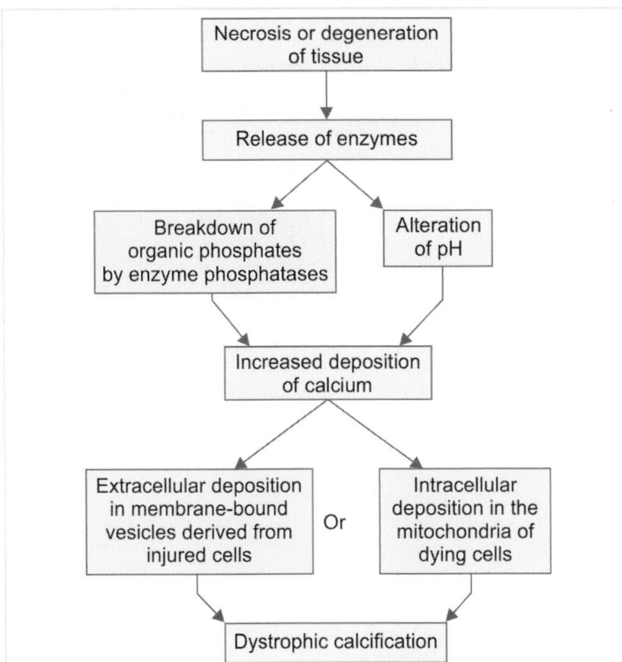

FLOWCHART 4: Mechanism of dystrophic calcification.

precipitates. Dystrophic calcification may begin either with extracellular deposition of the crystalline calcium phosphate in membrane-bound vesicles (derived from injured cells), or the intracellular deposition of calcium in the mitochondria of dying cells. The extracellular deposition of calcium (of calcium phosphate) in vesicles is because of affinity of calcium for membrane phospholipids, and phosphate (of calcium phosphate) deposits are due to the action of membrane bound enzyme phosphatases.

Propagation: Later, the calcium crystals are propagated and form larger deposits.

MORPHOLOGY

- **Gross:** Appear as fine, white granules or clumps, feels gritty and sand-like.
- **Microscopy:** Under routine H&E stain, calcium salts have a basophilic, amorphous granular, sometimes clumped appearance (**Fig. 67A**). These may be intracellular and / or extracellular. In the course of time, **heterotopic** bone may develop at the site of calcification. In **psammoma body** (**Fig. 67B**), single necrotic cell may constitute seed crystals. They become covered by the mineral deposits. The progressive addition of outer layers may create lamellated structure. Some papillary cancers (e.g., thyroid, serous papillary carcinoma of ovary) and benign tumors like psammomatous meningioma are liable to develop psammoma bodies. In asbestosis, calcium and iron salts gets deposited about long slender spicules of asbestos in the lung. This produces a striking, beaded dumbbell shaped structures known as **asbestos bodies.**

Metastatic Calcification

Deposition of calcium salts in apparently **normal tissues.** It is associated with hypercalcemia **secondary to deranged calcium metabolism.**

Causes

- **Increased secretion of parathyroid hormone** (PTH): It may occur in primary parathyroid tumors or secretion of PTH-related protein by some malignant tumors (paraneoplastic syndromes in squamous cell carcinoma of lung, renal cell carcinoma). In these conditions increased secretion of parathyroid hormone (PTH) is associated with bone resorption leading to hypercalcemia.
- **Destruction of bone tissue:** It may be due to increased turnover (e.g., Paget disease of bone), immobilization, or increased bone catabolism associated with primary tumors of bone marrow (e.g. multiple myeloma, leukemia), or diffuse metastatic tumors to bone (e.g., breast cancer).
- **Vitamin D-related disorders:** The causes include vitamin D intoxication, sarcoidosis (in which macrophages activate a vitamin D precursor), and idiopathic hypercalcemia of infancy (Williams syndrome characterized by abnormal sensitivity to vitamin D).
- **Renal failure:** Causes retention of phosphate, leading to secondary hyperparathyroidism.
- **Others:** These include aluminum intoxication (occurs in patients on chronic renal dialysis), and milk-alkali syndrome (due to excessive ingestion of calcium and absorbable antacids such as milk or calcium carbonate).

Sites

It can occur throughout the body but mainly seen in the interstitial tissues of the vasculature of the following regions:

- **Lungs: Alveolar septa of the lung** and usually do not produce dysfunction, However, severe calcifications may be detected on X-ray and may produce respiratory dysfunction. Metastatic calcification can also occur in pulmonary veins.
- **Kidney: Basement membrane of the renal tubules** extensive deposits in the kidney (nephrocalcinosis) can produce renal damage.
- **Blood vessels:** On the internal elastic lamina of **systemic arteries and pulmonary veins.**
- **Stomach: Interstitial tissues of the gastric mucosa.**

Mechanism

In metastatic calcification, calcification occurs at the sites where there is excretion of acid. This leads to the local production of hydroxyl ions produces an internal alkaline compartment. This. Hydroxyl ions result in precipitation of calcium hydroxide and hydroxyapatite and a form a mixed salt.

Morphologically, the calcium salts in metastatic calcification resemble those in dystrophic calcification. Thus, they may occur as noncrystalline amorphous deposits or as hydroxyapatite crystals.

Differences between dystrophic and metastatic calcification are presented in **Table 14.**

Table 14: Differences between dystrophic and metastatic calcification.

Features	Dystrophic calcification	Metastatic calcification
Tissue affected	Dead and degenerated tissue	Living tissue
Calcium metabolism	Normal	Deranged
Serum calcium level	Normal	Raised
Site of calcification	Necrosis (e.g., caseous necrosis), dead parasites, atherosclerotic plaque, etc.	Lung, mucosa of stomach, kidneys, and blood vessels

PIGMENTS

Q. Discuss pigment disorders.
Q. Discuss pigments and a special note on lipofuscin.

Definition

Pigments are **colored substances**, which are either normal constituents of cells (e.g., melanin), or are abnormal (e.g., carbon), and accumulate in cells.

Different types of pigments are listed in **Table 15**.

Table 15: Different types of pigments.

Endogenous pigments	Exogenous pigments
• Bilirubin	• Carbon (anthracotic)
• Melanin	• Tattooing
• Hemosiderin	• Arsenic
• Hemoglobin derived pigments, lipofuscin	• ß-carotene

Endogenous Pigments

Melanin

Melanin is an endogenous, brown-black, nonhemoglobin-derived pigment melanin is the only endogenous brown-black pigment. It is produced by the melanocytes and dendritic cells by the oxidation of tyrosine to dihydroxyphenylalanine by the enzyme tyrosinase. It is stored as cytoplasmic granules in the phagocytic cells namely, melanophores. Normally, it is present in the hair, skin, mucosa at some places, choroid of the eye, meninges, and adrenal medulla. Various disorders of melanin pigmentation produce generalized and localized hyperpigmentation and hypopigmentation (**Table 16**).

Table 16: Causes of hyper- and hypopigmentation.

Generalized hyperpigmentation	Generalized hypopigmentation
• **Addison's disease** • **Chloasma:** Hyperpigmentation on the skin of face, nipples, and genitalia during pregnancy • **Chronic arsenical poisoning** (raindrop pigmentation of the skin)	• **Albinism:** Generalized hypopigmentation due to genetic deficiency of tyrosinase enzyme
Focal hyperpigmentation	***Localized hypopigmentation***
• **Cäfe-au-lait spots** In neurofibromatosis and Albright's syndrome • **Peutz–Jeghers syndrome:** Focal perioral pigmentation • **Melanosis coli:** Pigmentation of the mucosa of the colon • **Tumors of melanocytes:** Benign (nevi) and malignant (melanoma) tumors • **Lentigo:** Premalignant condition	• **Leukoderma:** Autoimmune disorder with localized loss of pigmentation of the skin • **Vitiligo:** Local hypopigmentation of the skin • **Acquired focal hypopigmentation:** Leprosy, healing of wounds, discoid lupus erythematosus (DLE), radiation dermatitis, pityriasis alba, pityriasis versicolor, idiopathic guttate hypomelanosis, etc.

Alkaptonuria

Homogentisic acid is a pathological black pigment formed in rare metabolic autosomal recessive disorder termed alkaptonuria. It is characterized by deficiency of an oxidase enzyme needed for breakdown of homogentisic acid. This leads to accumulation of homogentisic acid pigment in the skin, connective tissue, cartilage, capsules of joints, ligaments, and tendons. The pigment is melanin-like and the pigmentation is known as **ochronosis** (refer page 936 and Fig. 14 of Chapter 13). The homogentisic acid is excreted in the urine (homogentisic aciduria). The urine of patients of alkaptonuria, if allowed to stand for some hours in air, turns black due to oxidation of homogentisic acid.

Hemosiderin

Definition

It is a hemoglobin-derived, golden yellow to brown, granular or crystalline pigment, and is one of the major storage forms of iron.

Iron is normally transported by a specific transport protein called transferrin. It is stored in the cells in association with a protein, apoferritin and forms ferritin micelles. Ferritin is present in most of the cell types. When there is excess of iron, ferritin forms hemosiderin granule.

Causes of excessive iron

Local or systemic excess of iron causes hemosiderin to accumulate within cells.

- Local excesses:
  - **Bruise:** It is the classical example of localized excess of iron. Hemoglobin liberated from extravasated red blood cells at the site of injury are phagocytosed by macrophages. These cells break down the hemoglobin and iron is released. The iron released from heme is incorporated into ferritin and eventually hemosiderin After removal of iron, the heme moiety of hemoglobin is converted first to biliverdin ("green bile") and then to bilirubin ("red bile"). These conversions and the resulting color changes are responsible for colors seen in a healing bruise. It usually changes its color from red-blue to green-blue to golden-yellow before it is resolved.

- **Brown induration of lung** in chronic venous congestion of lung (refer Fig. 6 of Chapter 9).
- **Systemic excesses: Systemic overload of iron** is known as **hemosiderosis.** The main causes:
  - **Increased absorption of dietary iron:** It is due to an inborn error of metabolism called **hemochromatosis**.
  - **Excessive destruction of red cells** (e.g., hemolytic anemias) cause release of abnormal quantities of iron.
  - **Repeated blood transfusions**: Transfused red blood cells represents an exogenous iron load.

MORPHOLOGY

Site of Accumulation

- **Localized:** Found in the macrophages of the involved area.
- **Systemic:** Initially found in **liver, bone marrow, spleen, and lymph nodes**. Later deposited in macrophages of other organs (e.g., skin, pancreas, kidney).

Microscopy: Hemosiderin pigment represents aggregates of ferritin micelles. Normally small amounts of hemosiderin is present in the mononuclear phagocytes of the bone marrow, spleen, and liver. Under light microscocpe, hemosiderin appears as a coarse, golden, granular pigment within the cytoplasm.

Special stain: **Prussian blue** (Perl's stain) histochemical reaction in which hemosiderin converts colorless potassium ferrocyanide to blue-black ferric ferrocyanide (**Fig. 68**).

Other Pigments

- **Hemochromatosis:** Severe accumulation of iron is associated with damage to liver, heart and pancreas. The triad of cirrhosis of liver, diabetes mellitus (due to pancreatic damage), and brown pigmentation of skin constitute **bronze diabetes.**
- **Hemozoin:** It is a brown-black pigment containing heme in ferric form. This pigment is seen in chronic malaria and in mismatched blood transfusions.
- **Bilirubin** is the normal major pigment found in bile. It is noniron containing pigment derived from hemoglobin.
- **Lipofuscin.**
  - Lipofuscin is an **insoluble golden-brown endogenous pigment**. It also called as **lipochrome or wear and tear pigment**.
  - **Composition:** It is composed of mixture of lipids, phospholipids, and proteins. **It is accumulated by accretion (a gradual increase) of peroxidized unsaturated lipids and oxidized cross-linked proteins.** The term lipofuscin is derived from the Latin word (*fuscus*, brown), and refers to brown lipid.
  - **Significance:** It indicates a product of free radical injury and lipid peroxidation. Lipofuscin does not injure cell or its functions. It is observed in cells undergoing slow, regressive changes and is particularly prominent in the **liver and heart (often called brown atrophy of heart)** of aging patients or patients with severe malnutrition and cancer cachexia.
  - **Appearance:** Microscopically, it appears as a yellow-brown, finely granular cytoplasmic pigment, often present in the perinuclear region **(Fig. 69)**.

Exogenous Pigments

Anthracosis

It is the accumulation of exogenous carbon particles in the lung and regional lymph nodes. Almost all urban residents inhale carbon pigment generated by the burning of fossil fuels. These carbon particles are engulfed by the alveolar macrophages in the lung. They are also transported to regional hilar and mediastinal lymph nodes and are stored indefinitely within macrophages. In coal-workers it may produces mild-to-severe disease of the lung depending on the severity of exposure.

Tattoos

Tattoos (derived from the Samoan, "tatou") are artificial introduction of insoluble metallic and vegetable pigments into the skin. In the skin they are mainly phagocytosed by dermal macrophages and persist for a lifetime.

Commonly used histochemistry (special stains) in histopathology are listed in **Table 17**.

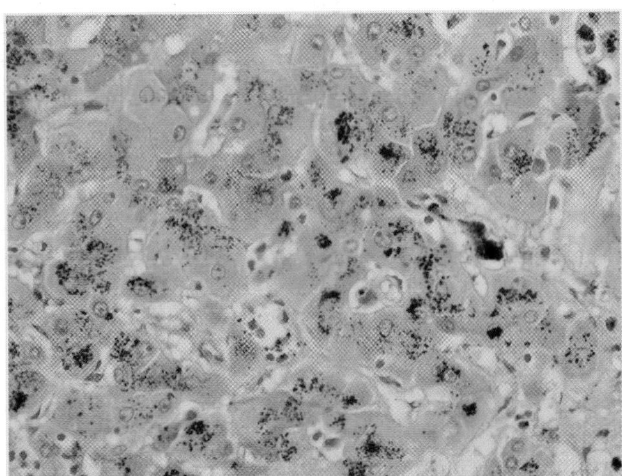

FIG. 68: Perl's stain. Liver with hemosiderin (blue) deposits.

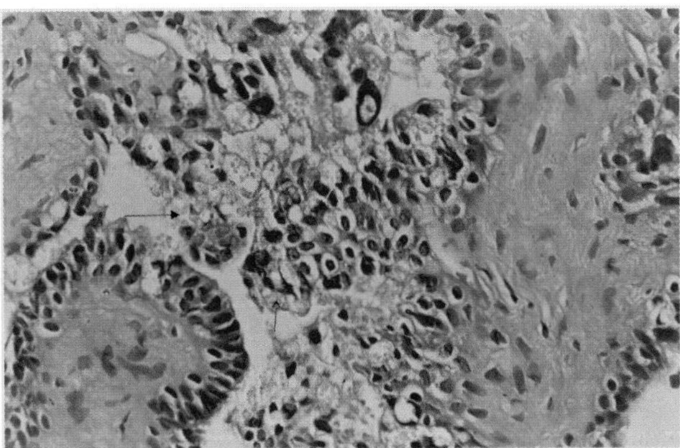

FIG. 69: Lipofuscin in seminal vesicle. Lipofuscin is seen as a yellow-brown, finely granular cytoplasmic pigment in the perinuclear region of the cell.

Table 17: Commonly used special stains in histopathology.

Stain	*Substance*	*Interpretation*
Amyloid		
Congo-red under polarizing microscope	Amyloid	Apple green birefringence
Carbohydrates		
Periodic acid–Schiff (PAS)	Glycogen, mucin, mucoprotein, glycoprotein, fungi, basement membranes of glomeruli and tubules	Magenta color
Mucicarmine/best's carmine	Epithelial mucin	Red color
Alcian blue	Acid mucin	Blue
Lipids		
Sudan III	Lipid	Orange
Oil Red O		Red
Osmium tetroxide		Brown black
Connective tissue		
Van Gieson	Extracellular collagen	Red
Masson's trichrome	Collagen, smooth muscle	Collagen = blue, smooth muscle = red
Phosphotungstic acid hematoxylin (PTAH)	Cross striation of skeletal muscles, glial filaments, fibrin	Dark blue
Verhoeff's elastic	Elastic fibers	Black
Microorganisms		
Gram's stain	Bacteria	Gram +ve = blue Gram –ve = red
Ziehl–Neelsen's (acid-fast) stain	Tubercle bacilli and other acid-fast organisms	Red
Fite-Faraco	Lepra bacilli	Red
Silver methenamine	Fungi	Black
Pigments and minerals		
Prussian blue stain (Perl's stain)	Hemosiderin	Blue
Masson Fontana	Melanin	Black
Von Kossa	Calcium	Black
Alizarin Red S	Calcium	Orange red
Rubeanic acid	Copper	Greenish-black

CELLULAR AGING

Q. Explain the pathophysiology/pathogenesis of aging/ cellular aging.

Q. Describe the mechanisms of cellular aging.

Definition

It is the gradual, insidious, and progressive decline in structure and function (involving molecules, cells, tissues, organs, and organisms) that begins to unfold after the achievement of sexual maturity.

Cellular aging begins from conception and continues till death. With aging, physiological and structural changes develop in almost all systems. Cellular aging is the **result of a progressive decline** in **cellular function and viability.**. Though one of the features of aging is cosmetic changes, it is also one of the major independent risk factors for many chronic diseases (e.g., cancer, Alzheimer's disease, atherosclerosis, and ischemic heart disease).

Causes

Cellular aging is mutifactorial. It is **caused by genetic abnormalities and environmental factors. The accumulation of cellular and molecular damage is due to the effects of exposure to exogenous influences.**

- **Genetic abnormalities:** It causes progressive decline in cellular function and viability.
- **Environmental factors:** These include diet, social conditions, and development of age-related diseases (e.g., atherosclerosis, diabetes, and osteoarthritis). They cause progressive accumulation of sublethal injury over the years at cellular and molecular level.

- Cellular aging may lead to death of the cell or decreased capacity of cells to respond to injury and increasing difficulties in maintaining physiological homeostasis.

Mechanism of Cellular Aging (Flowchart 5)

DNA Damage

DNA may be damaged by a variety of exogenous (e.g., physical, chemical, and biologic) agents and endogenous factors (e.g., ROS). They threaten the integrity of DNA of both in the nucleus and mitochondria.

Reactive oxygen species: One of the toxic products that causes DNA damage is free radical, mainly **ROS**. ROS may be either produced in excess, or there are reduction of antioxidant defense mechanisms. **Excessive production of ROS** may be due to environmental influences (toxins and ionizing radiation) and mitochondrial dysfunction. ROS can produce DNA damage associated with aging. **Reduction of antioxidant defense mechanisms** may occur with age (e.g., vitamin E, glutathione peroxidase). The oxidative damage may be an important cause of senescence in aging. Free radicals may damage DNA, causing breaks and genome instability. Damaged cellular organelles also accumulate as the cells age.

Defective repair mechanism: Most DNA damage is repaired by DNA repair enzymes. However, some DNA damage persists and accumulates as cells age, especially if repair mechanisms become inefficient over time. DNA repair is important in the aging process. By next-generation DNA sequencing, it was found that the average hematopoietic stem cell undergoes 14 new mutations per year. This accumulating DNA damage may be the reason for most cancers (most commonly hematologic malignancies) in the aged individuals. DNA repair mechanisms are defective in certain diseases. Patients with Werner syndrome show premature aging. They have a defective gene product which is an enzyme called DNA helicase, a protein involved in DNA replication and repair and other functions requiring DNA unwinding. A defect in DNA helicase leads to rapid accumulation of chromosomal damage. This DNA damage may mimic some aspects of the injury that normally accumulates during cellular aging. Genetic instability in somatic cells is also characteristic of few disorders in which patients have some of the manifestations of aging at an increased rate. These include Bloom syndrome and ataxia-telangiectasia, in which the mutated genes encode proteins involved in repairing double-strand breaks in DNA

Cellular Senescence

All normal cells (other than stem cells) have a limited capacity for replication. After a fixed number of divisions (about 60–70 cell divisions), all cells become arrested in a terminally nondividing state, known as **replicative senescence**. In aging, there is progressive replicative senescence of cells. Cells from children are capable of more rounds of replication than do cells from older people.

The following two mechanisms may be involved in cellular senescence.

Telomere shortening

One mechanism of replicative senescence is by progressive shortening of telomeres and this finally results in arrest of cell cycle. **Telomeres** are **protective, short repeated sequences**

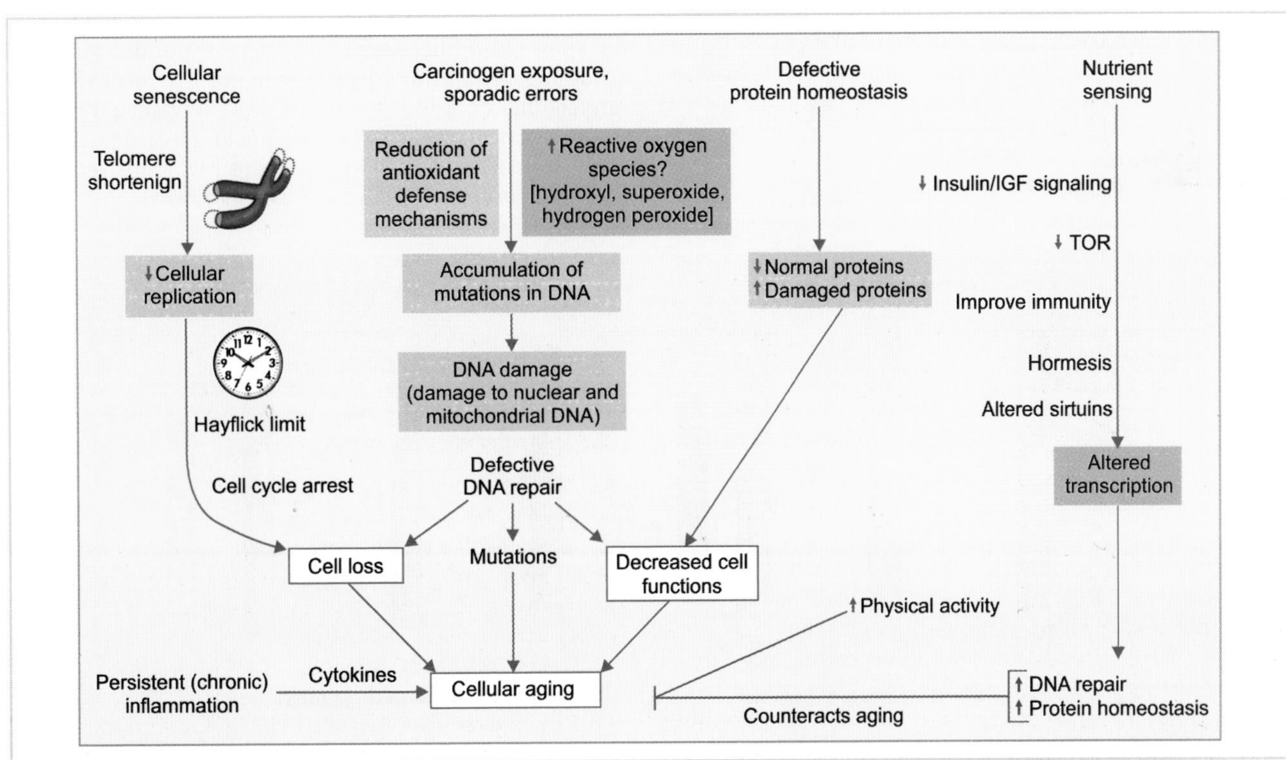

(IGF: insulin-like growth factor; TOR: target of rapamycin)

FLOWCHART 5: Mechanism of aging. DNA damage, cellular senescence, and defective protein homeostasis are the main mechanisms of cellular aging. Nutrient sensing, by caloric restriction, counteracts aging by activating various signaling pathways and transcription factors.

of DNA (TTAGGG) present **at the end regions of linear chromosomes.** Telomeres ensure the complete copying of chromosomal ends during the S-phase of the cell cycle. They protect the ends of chromosomes and prevent fusion and degradation. With each cell division in somatic cells, a small section of the telomere is not duplicated and telomeres become progressively shortened (**Figs. 63A** and **B**). When telomeres are sufficiently shortened, the ends of chromosomes cannot be protected and DNA at the end of chromosomes are broken. Such cells stop dividing (**cell cycle arrest**) leading to a terminally nondividing state. Telomeres represent a "biological clock", which prevent uncontrolled cell division and cancer. **Telomere shortening** may be one of the mechanisms **responsible for decreased cellular replication.** **Hayflick limit** is the number of times a normal human cell population will divide until cell division stops.

Q. Describe telomere/telomerase activity in health and disease.

Telomerase Telomerase is an **enzyme** that **regenerates and maintains telomere length** by addition of nucleotide. Telomerase is a specialized RNA–protein complex which uses its own RNA as a template for adding nucleotides to the ends of chromosomes. Telomerase is absent in most of the somatic cells and expressed in germ cells and is present at low levels in stem cells. Hence, as mature somatic cells age, their telomeres become shorter and they exit the cell cycle. This results in an inability to produce new cells to replace damaged ones. On the other hand, the germ cells (high telomerase activity) have extended replicative capacity (**Figs. 70A** and **B**). In cancers, the telomerase may be reactivated in tumor cells resulting in maintenance of length of telomeres and allows the cells to proliferate indefinitely. It may be an essential step in formation of cancer. Shortening of telomere also may decrease the regenerative capacity of stem cells. Shortening of telomere is also associated with premature development of diseases (e.g., pulmonary fibrosis , aplastic anemia).

Refer pages 470–471 for telomere role in neoplasia.

Activation of tumor suppressor genes

Apart from shortening of telomere, activation of tumor suppressor genes may be involved in controlling replicative senescence. One of the tumor suppressors gene is that encoded by the CDKN2A (cyclin-dependent kinase inhibitor 2A) locus. The CDKN2A locus encodes two tumor suppressor proteins namely p16 (p16INK4a) and p14arf. The expression of p16 or INK4a, is correlated with chronologic age in almost all humans. In the cell cycle, p16 controls progression of G1- to S-phase. Thus, p16 protects cells from uncontrolled mitogenic signals and drive the cells along the senescence pathway.

Defective Protein Homeostasis

Protein homeostasis depends on two mechanisms: (i) maintenance of proteins in their correctly folded structure and (ii) degradation of misfolded, damaged, or unneeded proteins. The maintenance of proteins in correctly folded form is mediated by chaperones by structure whereas degradation is via the autophagy-lysosome system and ubiquitin proteasome system (UPS). This is discussed in detail pages 185–188. As age progresses, both normal folding and degradation of misfolded proteins are impaired. The cells are not able to maintain normal protein homeostasis due to increased turnover and decreased synthesis. In mutant mice deficient in chaperones (which promote normal protein folding) of the heat shock protein family, it was found that they age rapidly, and conversely, those that overexpress such chaperones are long-lived. It is also true with the processes that destroy misfolded proteins namely autophagy and proteasomal degradation of proteins. It was observed that administration of rapamycin, which inhibits the mTOR (molecular target of rapamycin) pathway, increases the life span of middle-aged mice. Rapamycin also promotes autophagy. Abnormal protein homeostasis decreases the intracellular proteins. It can lead to many damaging effects on cell survival, replication, and functions. Also, it can lead to accumulation of misfolded proteins and increased loss of functional proteins. Both can trigger apoptosis.

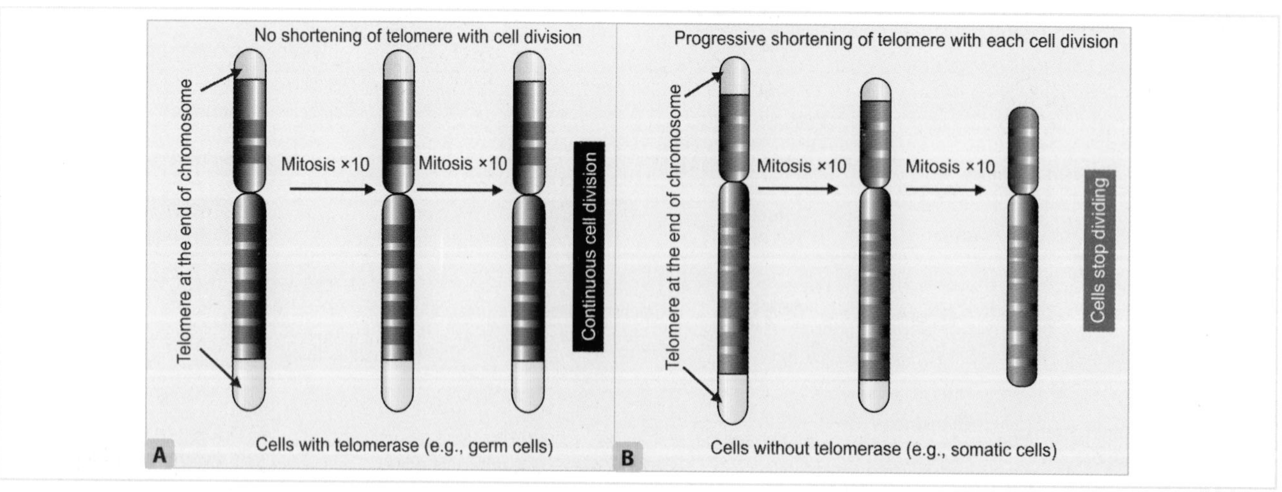

FIGS. 70A AND B: Role of telomerase in maintaining chromosomal length.

Box 14: Systemic physiologic changes of aging.

Heart

- Decreased number of heart muscle fibers with increased size of individual fibers (hypertrophy)
- Reduced filling capacity
- Decreased stroke volume
- Decreased sensitivity of baroreceptors
- Decrease in number of pacemaker cells and increase in fat around sinoatrial (SA) node (decreased heart rate)
- Deposits of aging pigment "lipofuscin"
- Valves thicken and become less compliant
- Left ventricular hypertrophy secondary to hypertension

Blood vessels

- Arteries:
  - Decreased elasticity of vessels caused by calcification of connective tissue (increased pulmonary vascular resistance)
  - Thickening and stiffening of media of large arteries due to collagen cross linking
- Veins: Degeneration of vein valves and minimal changes not impeding function

Respiratory

- Reduced chest wall compliance due to calcification of costal cartilage
- Reduced alveolar ventilation and reduction in forced expiratory volume in one second (FEV_1)
- Reduced strength of respiratory muscles
- Air trapping and reduced ventilation due to degeneration of lung tissue (reduced elasticity)
- Reduction in number and activity of cilia
- Reduction in glandular cells in large airway
- Reduced cough reflex
- Decreased levels of secretory immunoglobulin (Ig) A
- Senile hyperinflation of lungs due to reduced elasticity

Renal/urinary

- Reduced glomerular filtration rate due to nephron degeneration (reduced to almost one-third to one-half by age 70 years)
- Reduced ability to concentrate urine and clearance of drugs
- Reduced ability to regulate hydrogen ion (H^+) concentration
- Decline in number of renal tubular cells
- Decreased bladder capacity from 500 to 250 mL
- Decreased tone and elasticity of bladder resulting in incomplete emptying

Gastrointestinal

- Reduced muscular contraction
- Reduced esophageal emptying
- Reduced bowel motility manifested by constipation
- Thinning of stomach mucosa
- Reduced production of hydrochloric acid (HCl), enzymes, and intrinsic factor
- Reduced production of hepatic enzyme and metabolic capacity
- Decreased pancreatic enzymes leading to reduced absorption of nutrients like iron, calcium, and folic acid

Continued

Continued

Neurologic/sensory

- Nerve cell degeneration and atrophy
- Reduction of 25–45% of neurons throughout life
- Reduced number of neurotransmitters and slowing of neuronal transmission
- Reduced rate of conduction of nerve impulses
- Changes in sleep cycle (takes longer to fall asleep)
- Loss of taste buds
- Decreased sense of smell
- Loss of auditory hair cells and sclerosis of eardrum

Musculoskeletal

- Reduced muscle mass and contractile force
- Increased bone demineralization and gradual loss of bone mass due to bone resorption
- Increased joint degeneration, erosion, and calcification
- Decreased water content in cartilage resulting in decreased mobility
- Osteoporosis

Immune

- Reduced inflammatory response
- Reduction in T cell function due to involution of thymus gland
- Decreased Ig production
- Increased incidence of autoimmune disorders
- Increased susceptibility to and severity of infections

Integumentary (Skin)

- Reduced subcutaneous fat resulting in wrinkles
- Reduced elastin
- Atrophy of sweat glands and dry skin due to decreased sebaceous and sweat glands
- Atrophy of epidermal arterioles causing altered temperature regulation
- Epidermal cells decreased in number (thinner epidermis)
- Skin becomes thin and loses its elasticity
- Rete ridges of dermoepidermal junction flatten out resulting in fragile skin

Hematological changes

- Decreased total body water and blood volume
- Decreased red blood cell (RBC) count
- White blood cell (WBC) same in number but lymphocytes decreased in number and effectiveness

Eyes

- Presbyopia
- Lens opacification

Endocrine

- Impaired glucose tolerance that predisposes to diabetes mellitus
- Decreased vitamin D absorption
- Decreased testosterone
- Decreased thyroid function
- Decreased gonadal function

Increased rate of development of cancer due to a failure of the immune system to reject cancer cells as foreign

Dysregulated Nutrient Sensing

It has been found that caloric restriction (eating less) alters signaling pathways that influence aging and can slow down aging and prolong life. This has created interest in solving the role of nutrient sensing in aging. Tthough not completely understood, two major neurohormonal circuits may be involved in regulating the metabolism.

Insulin and insulin-like growth factor 1 (IGF-1) signaling pathway

IGF-1 as its name indicates mimics intracellular signaling by insulin. IGF-1 is produced in many cell types in response to growth hormone secretion by the pituitary gland. IGF-1 signaling has multiple downstream targets. Most important involved in aging are two kinases: AKT and its downstream target, mTOR, which, as the name implies, is inhibited by rapamycin. Reduced activation of IGF receptor signaling inhibit aging. The actions of reduced IGF-1 signaling includes: (1) lowering the rate of cell growth and metabolism, (2) reduction in errors in DNA replication, (3) better DNA repair, (4) improved protein homeostasis, and (5) probably reduced cellular damage. This effect can be mimicked by rapamycin. TOR is target of rapamycin activity. TOR is a nutrient-sensitive, central controller of cell growth and aging. Decreased TOR activity has been found to slow the aging process and increase life span.

Sirtuins

Sirtuins are a family of nicotinamide adenine dinucleotide (NAD)-dependent protein deacetylases. There are about seven types of sirtuins and are distributed in different cellular compartments. They have necessary functions to adapt bodily functions to various environmental stresses such as deprivation of food and damage to DNA. Sirtuins probably promote the expression of several genes whose products increase longevity. The actions of the protein products of these are: inhibition of metabolic activity, reduction of apoptosis, stimulation of protein folding, and counteracting the harmful effects of oxygen free radicals. Sirtuins may also increase insulin sensitivity and glucose metabolism. Hence, they may be targets for the treatment of diabetes. Caloric restriction increases longevity both by reducing the signaling intensity of the IGF-1 pathway and by increasing sirtuins. An increase in sirtuins, particularly sirtuin-6, has two functions: they (1) contribute to metabolic adaptations of caloric restriction and (2) promote genomic integrity by activating DNA repair enzymes through deacylation. Anti-aging effects of sirtuins not completely understood and if confirmed, sirtuin-activating pills may increase longevity. It has been suggested that a constituent of red wine may activate sirtuins and may increase life span.

Persistent Inflammation

As age advances, there is accumulation of damaged cells, lipids, and other endogenous substances. These may activate the inflammasome pathway, producing persistent low-level inflammation. Persistent inflammation may be responsible for chronic diseases, such as atherosclerosis and T2DM. Cytokines produced during inflammatory reactions may themselves produce alteration in cells that promote aging. Chronic metabolic disorders may speed up the aging process. Stresses may accelerate aging probably by increased production of glucocorticoids. Thus, aging can be delayed either by reducing the metabolic damage or by increasing the repair response to that damage.

Age Related Pathological Changes in Various Organ Systems

Q. Write a short essay on age related pathological changes in various organ systems.

Frequency of some diseases increases with age. They can be broadly divided into two types, namely—(1) age-dependent and (2) age-related. There is considerable variation in the degree to which body systems are affected by aging.

Age-dependent Diseases

These diseases develop to some extent in all individuals with time. Examples include presbyopia, degenerative arthritis, osteoporosis, endocrine changes associated with atrophy of ovaries and testes, and hyperplasia of the prostate.

Age-related Diseases

All systems of the body show age-related changes. It can be generally described as a decrease in functional reserve or impaired ability to adapt to environmental demands. They develop not as part of the aging process because they do not affect all individuals. Examples include atherosclerosis, hypertension, cataracts, Alzheimer's disease, many types of cancer, actinic and seborrheic keratoses of the skin, and diverticulosis of the colon, etc. Frequency of some diseases increases with age, although their onset is not age-related. Examples include chronic lung disease from smoking, and gallstones.

Systemic changes of aging are presented in **Box 14.**

BIBLIOGRAPHY

1. Albasri A, Aleskandarany M, Benhasouna A, et al. CTEN (C-terminal tensin-like), a novel oncogene overexpressed in invasive breast carcinoma of poor prognosis. *Breast Cancer Res Treat.* 2011;26: 47-54.
2. Al-Ghamdi S, Cachat J, Albasri A, et al. C-terminal tensin-like gene functions as an oncogene and promotes cell motility in pancreatic cancer. *Pancreas.* 2013;42:135-40.
3. Akhlaq M, Thorpe H, Ilyas M. (2014). 'Tensins in Health and Disease'in Pignatelli M and Gallaghar P. *Recent Advances in Histopathology*: 23, New Delhi, JP medical pubishers, pp.169-181.
4. Banasik JL, Copstead LC. Pathophysiology,6th edition. Philadelphia: Saunders Elsevier; 2019.
5. Bonaldo P, Sandri M. Cellular and molecular mechanisms of muscle atrophy, *Dis Model Mech.* 2013;6:25-39.
6. Busl KM, Greer DM. Hypoxic-ischemic brain injury: pathophysiology, neuropathology and mechanisms. *NeuroRehabilitation.* 2010;26(1):5-13. doi: 10.3233/NRE-2010-0531. [Last accessed on 2021 January 26].
7. Cao X, Voss C, Zhao B, Kaneko T, Li SS. Differential regulation of the activity of deleted in liver cancer 1 (DLC1) by tensins controls

cell migration and transformation. *Proc Natl Acad Sci*. 2012;109: 1455-60.

8. Choi AMK, Ryter S, Levine B. Autophagy in human health and disease. *N Engl J Med*. 2013;368:651-62.
9. Doherty J, Baehrecke EH. Life, death and autophagy. *Nat Cell Biol*. 2018;20:1110-7.
10. Galluzzi L, Kepp O, Kroemer G. Mitochondrial control of cell death: a phylogenetically conserved control. *Microb Cell*. 2016;3:101-8.
11. Galluzzi L, Kepp O, Chan FK, et al. Necroptosis. Mechanisms and relevance to disease. *Annu Rev Pathol*. 2017;12:103-130.
12. Giroux V, Rustgi AK. Metaplasia: tissue injury adaptation and a precursor to the dysplasia-cancer sequence. *Nat Rev Cancer*. 2017;17:594-604.
13. Green DR: The coming decade of cell death research: five riddles. *Cell*. 2019;177:1094-1107.
14. Hausenloy DJ, Yellon DM. Myocardial ischemia-reperfusion injury: a neglected therapeutic target. *J Clin Invest*. 2013;123:92-100
15. Hotchkiss RS, Strasser A, McDunn JE, et al. Cell death. *N Engl J Med*. 2009;361:1570-1583.
16. Huether SE, McCance KL. Understanding Pathophysiology,6th edition. Philadelphia: Saunders Elsevier; 2016.
17. Kierszenbaum AL, Tres L. Histology and Cell Biology-An Introduction to Pathology, 5th edition. Philadelphia: Elsevier; 2019.
18. Kumar V, Abbas AK, Aster JC. Robbins basic pathology, 10th edition. Philadelphia: Saunders Elsevier; 2018
19. Kumar V, Abbas AK, Fausto N, et al. Robbins and Cotran pathologic basis of disease, 10th edition. Philadelphia: WB Saunders; 2021.
20. Kuroiwa T, Okeda R. Neuropathology of cerebral ischemia and hypoxia: recent advances in experimental studies on its pathogenesis. *Pathol Int*. 1994;44(3):171-81. doi: 10.1111/j. 1440-1827.1994.tb02590.
21. Lambeth JD, Neish AS. Nox enzymes and new thinking on reactive oxygen: a double-edged sword revisited. *Annu Rev Pathol*. 2014;9:119-145.
22. Levine B, Kroemer G. Biological functions of autophagy genes: a disease perspective. *Cell*. 2019:176:11-42.
23. Loeffler AG, Hart MN: Human Disease-Pathophysiology for health professional, 7th edition. Burlington: Jones & Bartlett Learning Company; 2020.
24. Lopez-Otin C, Blasco MA, Partridge L, et al. The hallmarks of aging. *Cell*. 2013;153:1194-217.
25. Marques FC, Volovik Y, Cohen E. The roles of cellular and organismal aging in the development of late-onset maladies. *Annu Rev Pathol*. 2015;10:1-23.
26. McCance KL, Huether SE. Pathophysiology. The biologic basis for disease in adults and children, 8th edition. Philadelphia: Elsevier; 2019.
27. Mohan H. Text Book of Pathology, 8th edition. New Delhi, JP brothers; 2019.
28. Nagata S. Apoptosis and clearance of apoptotic cells. *Annu Rev Immunol*. 2018;36:489-517.
29. Nakamura M, Sadoshima J. Mechanisms of physiological and pathological cardiac hypertrophy. *Nat Rev Cardiol*. 2018;15: 387-407.
30. Oakes SA, Papa FR. The role of endoplasmic reticulum stress in human pathology. *Annu Rev Pathol*. 2015;10:173-94.
31. Radosevich JA. Apoptosis and Beyond. The Many Ways cells Die, Hoboken,Wiley Blackwell; 2018.
32. Schenk RL, Strasser A, Dewson G. BCL-2. Long and winding road from discovery to therapeutic target. *Biochem Biophys Res Commun*. 2017;482:459-69.
33. Shi J, Gao W, Shao F: Pyroptosis: gasdermin-mediated programmed necrotic cell death. *Trends Biochem Sci*. 2017:42:245-254.
34. Simon EJ, Dickey JL, Reece JB, Campell NA. Campell Essential Biology with Physiology, 6th edition. New York: Pearson; 2019.
35. Tang D, Kang R, Berghe TV, et al. The molecular machinery of regulated cell death. *Cell Res*. 2019;29:347-364.
36. Tonnus W, Meyer C, Paliege A, et al. The pathologic features of regulated necrosis. *J Pathol*. 2019;247:697-707.
37. Tyner WJ. Phosphoproteomics microarray screen reveals novel interaction between MPL and Tensin2: implications for biology, disease and therapeutics. *Cell Cycle*. 2011;10:2.
38. Van Opdenbosch N, Lamkanfi M. Caspases in cell death, inflammation, and disease. *Immunity*. 2019;50:1352-1364.
39. Weinlich R, Oberst A, Beere HM, et al. Necroptosis in development, inflammation, and disease. *Nat Rev Mol Cell Biol*. 2017;18:127-136.
40. Strayer DS, Saffitz JE. Rubin's Pathology: Mechanism of Human Disease, 8th edition. Philadelphia: Wolters Kluwer; 2020.

CHAPTER 8

Inflammation and Healing

8.1 Acute Inflammation

CHAPTER OUTLINE

- General features of inflammation
- Historical highlights
  - Cardinal signs of inflammation
  - Causes of inflammation
- Recognition of microbes and damaged cells
  - Molecules produced by microbes and damaged cells
  - Recognition of molecules produced by microbes and damaged cells
  - Circulating proteins
- Acute inflammation
  - Reactions of blood vessels in acute inflammation
  - Leukocyte recruitment to sites of inflammation
  - Definition
  - Type of leukocytes
  - Functions of leukocytes
  - Leukocyte adhesion to endothelium
  - Leukocyte migration through endothelium
  - Chemotaxis of leukocytes
  - Therapeutic significance
  - Phagocytosis and clearance of the offending agent
  - Summary of leukocyte events in acute inflammation
  - Termination of the acute inflammatory response
  - Mechanism of tissue injury in acute inflammation

GENERAL FEATURES OF INFLAMMATION

Definition: Inflammation is a complex **local response of the living vascularized tissues to injury (infections and tissue damage).**

It brings cells (phagocytic leukocytes) **and molecules which are necessary for host defense (antibodies, and complement proteins) from the circulation to the site of injury (where they are required), to eliminate the offending injurious agents.** Inflammation is essentially a protective response and is essential for survival. It helps the host in removing both the initial cause of cell injury (e.g., microbes, toxins) and the consequences of such injury (e.g., necrotic cells and tissues). It mainly consists of responses of blood vessels and leukocytes.

Inflammation is largely confined to the site of infection or damage but can develop some systemic manifestations (e.g., fever in bacterial or viral infections).

Sequential steps in an inflammatory reaction (Fig. 1): Whenever an individual encounters injurious agent (e.g., microbe or dead cells), it tries to contain or eliminate injurious agent/ stimuli and accompanying injured (damaged) tissue components. This is mainly achieved by inflammatory response. Inflammation is characterized by production of inflammatory mediators and movement of fluid (plasma proteins) and leukocytes from the blood into extravascular tissues. The sequential steps in inflammatory reaction are as follows:

1. **Recognition of the noxious (causative) agent:** Recognition of injury is the stimuli for inflammation. Sentinel cells constitute the body's first line of defense. The cells involved in inflammation are: (i) tissue-resident sentinel cells, (ii) phagocytes (neutrophils, macrophage) and others. Tissue resident sentinel cells include macrophage [e.g., Kupffer cells (liver), alveolar macrophages (lungs), microglia (brain), dendritic cells and mast cells]. When pathogenic microbes invade the tissues, or tissue cells die, the phagocytes residing in tissues at the site of injury try to eliminate the injurious agents. At the same time, receptors of the phagocytes and other sentinel cells in the tissues (tissue-resident sentinel cells) recognize the presence of the foreign or abnormal substance. They react by producing and liberating cytokines, lipid messengers, and other mediators of inflammation. These mediators then trigger the subsequent steps in the inflammatory response.

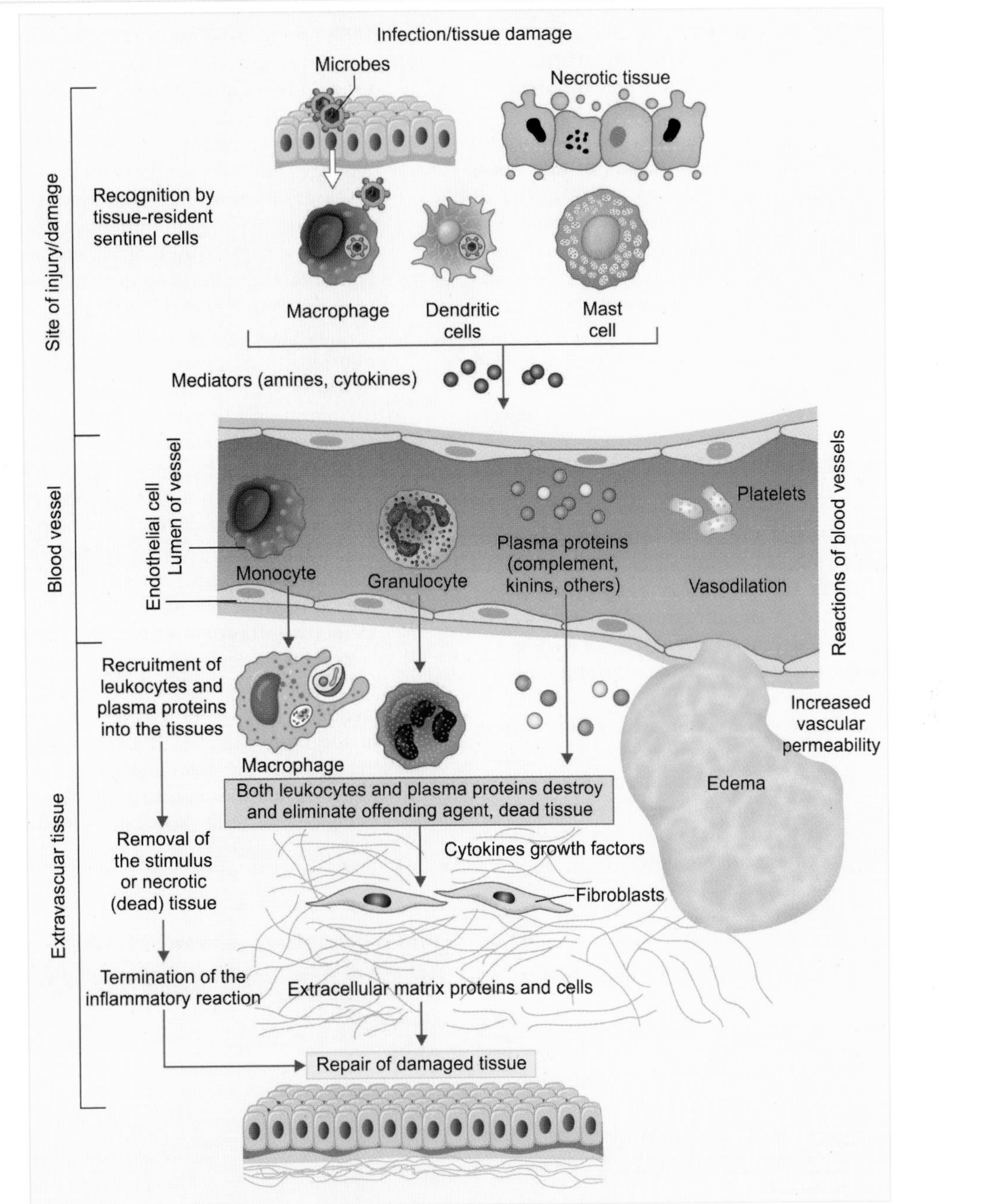

FIG. 1: Sequential steps in an inflammatory reaction. Tissue-resident sentinel cells (neutrophils macrophages, dendritic cells, and other cell types) first recognize microbes and damaged cells. They release mediators and initiate the vascular and cellular reactions of inflammation. The inflammatory reaction is terminated and after the elimination of injurious agent or dead tissue and is followed by repair by regeneration and/or scar tissue.

2. **Recruitment of leukocytes and plasma proteins into the tissues:** Some of these mediators liberated at the site of injury act on small blood vessels in the vicinity and promote the flowing out of plasma and the circulating leukocytes to the site where the offending agent is located. Since blood travels every tissue through blood vessels, leukocytes and proteins components (e.g., complement) present in the circulating blood can be delivered to any site of invasion by microbes or tissue injury. Initial leukocytes that reach the site of injury are mainly circulating neutrophils and followed later by monocytes and lymphocytes. The plasma proteins also quickly escape from the circulation to the extravascular site where the offending agent is located. The migration of cells and escape of plasma proteins from blood needs coordinated changes in blood vessels (vascular response of inflammation) and secretion of mediators. This leads to rapid flooding of injured tissues with inflammatory cells (particularly neutrophils), plasma proteins, cytokines, chemokines, and platelets. These changes are characteristic of acute inflammation.

3. **Removal of the stimulus or necrotic tissue at the site of inflammation:** It is achieved mainly by phagocytic cells (neutrophils and monocytes) that have escaped from blood vessels and reach the site of injury. These phagocytes ingest and destroy microbes and dead cells.
4. **Termination of the inflammatory reaction:** The purpose of inflammation is served by elimination of microbes, altered/damaged cells, foreign particles, and antigens. It is necessary to terminate the reaction and prepare the way for a return to normal structure and function. Termination of the inflammatory response is mediated by intrinsic anti-inflammatory mechanisms. They limit tissue damage and allow healing and repair.
5. **Repair:** This consists of a series of events that heal damaged tissue. During repair, the injured tissue is replaced by regeneration from surviving cells and the residual defects are healed with connective tissue (scarring). This leads to return to normal physiologic function of the involved tissue.

Fundamental properties of the inflammatory response: These include the following:

- **Components of the inflammatory response:** Main components involved in the inflammatory reaction in tissues are (i) blood vessels and (ii) leukocytes (see **Fig. 1**).
  - **Reaction of blood vessels:** In response to inflammatory stimuli, blood vessels undergo dilatation and increases their permeability, and allow the selected circulating proteins to enter the site of infection or tissue damage.
  - **Emigration of leukocytes:** The endothelium lining blood vessels also undergo changes and permit the circulating leukocytes to adhere to them and then migrate into the extravascular tissues.
  - **Phagocytosis:** The migrated leukocytes get activated and begins the process of phagocytosis. These leukocytes ingest and destroy microbes, dead cells, any foreign bodies present and other unwanted substances present in the tissues.
- **Beneficial effect:** Inflammation is a mostly protective, beneficial host response to foreign invaders (infections) and necrotic tissue. Main benefits of inflammation are presented in **Box 1**.
- **Harmful consequences of inflammation: In some circumstances, the inflammatory reaction may cause tissue damage and disease.**
  - **Temporary damage:** Inflammation (e.g., due to infections) may be often accompanied by local tissue damage and its associated signs and symptoms (e.g., pain, swelling, and impairment of function). Usually, these harmful effects are self-limited with little or permanent damage. They often disappear as the inflammation subsides.
  - **Misdirected, excessive or prolonged inflammation:** Inflammatory reaction may be misdirected, inadequately controlled or is more prolonged (e.g., in infections by **microbes that resist eradication** such as tuberculosis). These may contribute to diseases in which the normally protective inflammatory reaction damages the involved tissue becomes the cause of the disease. For example, inflammatory reaction against own tissues as in autoimmune diseases; against normally harmless environmental substances as in allergic conditions. The inflammatory reaction. Few examples of diseases in which the inflammatory response plays a significant role in tissue injury and associated with injurious consequences of inflammation are presented in **Table 1**. Inflammatory reactions are responsible for common chronic diseases such as rheumatoid arthritis, atherosclerosis, and lung fibrosis and also life-threatening hypersensitivity reactions to insect bites, foods, drugs, and toxins. These damaging effects of inflammatory reactions can be overcome by using anti-inflammatory drugs. These drugs ideally would control the harmful sequelae of inflammation without interfering with its beneficial effects.
  - **Defective inflammation:** Too little inflammation, which is usually characterized by increased susceptibility to infections. It is usually seen in leukopenia/neutropenia (reduced number of leukocytes) due to replacement of the bone marrow by cancers and suppression of the marrow by chemotherapies for cancer and graft rejection. It also occurs in immunocompromised hosts.
  - **Exaggerated and sustained acute inflammation:** If acute inflammatory response is exaggerated or

Box 1: Main benefits of inflammation.

- Prevention of infection and further damage to tissue by microorganisms
- Limitation and control of the inflammatory process
- Interaction with components of the adaptive immune system. This will elicit a more specific response to causative pathogen (s).
- Preparation of the area of injury for healing

Table 1: Examples of diseases caused by inflammatory reactions.

Disease	*Cells and molecules that produce injury*
Acute	
Acute respiratory distress syndrome (ARDS)	Neutrophils
Asthma*	Eosinophils and IgE antibodies
Glomerulonephritis	Antibodies and complement; neutrophils, monocytes
Septic shock	Cytokines
Chronic	
Atherosclerosis	Macrophages and lymphocytes
Arthritis	Lymphocytes and macrophages; ? antibodies
Pulmonary fibrosis	Macrophages and fibroblasts
Autoimmune diseases	Cytokines; lymphocytes (mainly T cells), macrophages, NK cells; antibodies, complements
Inflammation may also contribute to many primarily metabolic, degenerative, or genetic disease: e.g., type 2 diabetes, Alzheimer disease, cancer.	

(IgE: Immunoglobulin E; NK: natural killer)

*Asthma can present with acute inflammation or a chronic illness associated with repeated bouts of acute exacerbation of asthmatic attack.

sustained, with or without clearance of the offending injurious agent, it causes tissue damage. Examples include bacterial pneumonia due to acute inflammation or joint destruction in septic arthritis.

- **Local and systemic inflammation:** Most of the situations, the inflammatory response is localized to site of infection or tissue damage. Local inflammatory reactions may have systemic manifestations (e.g., fever in bacterial or viral pharyngitis). Rarely for example in some disseminated bacterial infections, the inflammatory reaction is systemic and produces widespread pathologic abnormalities. This reaction is called sepsis and is one form of the systemic inflammatory response syndrome (refer page 323).
- **Mediators of inflammation:** Irrespective of the cause, inflammatory reaction occurs in a stereotypical pattern, mainly consisting of vascular and cellular reactions. These reactions are brought out by soluble factors called as chemical mediators of inflammation. These mediators are produced by various cells or derived from plasma proteins. These are produced or activated in response to the inflammatory stimulus. Microbes, necrotic cells (whatever may be the cause of necrosis), and hypoxia can bring out production of inflammatory mediators and produce inflammation. Chemical mediators initiate and also amplify the inflammatory response. They determine the pattern, severity, and clinical and pathologic manifestations of inflammation.
- **Types of inflammation:** Inflammation may be divided into **acute or chronic**. Originally, the distinction between acute and chronic inflammation was based on the duration of the reaction. But, there are several differences between acute and chronic inflammation and are listed in **Table 2**.
    - **Acute inflammation:** It is a rapid, self-limited, response to injurious agents. It typically develops within minutes or hours after exposure to injurious agent and is of short duration (several hours to a few days). It is characterized by the exudation of fluid and plasma proteins (edema) and the emigration of leukocytes, predominantly neutrophils. The offending stimulus (e.g., bacteria and fungi, dead cells) are usually eliminated and the reaction subsides. This is followed by repair of the residual injury.
    - **Chronic inflammation:** It may follow acute inflammation or arise de novo. It develops as a response to agents that are difficult to eradicate (e.g., silica), some bacteria (e.g., tubercle bacilli) and other pathogens (such as viruses and fungi), and also against self-antigens and environmental antigens. Predominant cells are lymphocytes and monocytes/macrophages. Inflammatory cells are associated with the proliferation of blood vessels, tissue destruction, and fibroblast proliferation. Its duration is long and is associated with more tissue destruction and scarring (fibrosis). Sometimes, chronic inflammation may coexist with unresolved acute inflammation (e.g., peptic ulcers, chronic osteomyelitis).
    - **Subacute inflammation:** Sometimes, the term subacute inflammation is used to describe the inflammation between acute and chronic.

Table 2: Differences between acute and chronic inflammation.

	Acute inflammation	***Chronic inflammation***
Onset	Rapid in onset (usually in minutes or hours)	May follow acute inflammation or be slow in onset (days)
Duration	Short duration. Lasts for hours or a few days	Longer duration; may be months
Predominant cells	Neutrophils (also called polymorphonuclear leukocytes)	Lymphocytes, monocytes/ macrophages, and sometimes plasma cells
Characteristics	Exudation of fluid and plasma proteins (edema), and the emigration of leukocytes	Inflammatory cells associated with the proliferation of blood vessels, tissue destruction, and fibroblast proliferation
Injury/damage to tissue and fibrosis	Usually mild and self-limited and can progress to a chronic phase	Usually severe and progressive with fibrosis and scar formation
Signs: Local and systemic	Prominent	Less prominent

HISTORICAL HIGHLIGHTS

Cardinal Signs of Inflammation

The word "inflammation" is derived from the Latin verb *inflammare* (literally meaning "to set afire") in reference to heat and redness of the involved tissue in inflammation. Clinical features of inflammation were described in an Egyptian papyrus during 3000 BC. The four cardinal signs of inflammation as mentioned by Roman encyclopedist (writer) of the first century AD **by Celsus (Aulus Cornelius Celsus)** are—*rubor* (redness), *tumor* (swelling), *calor* (heat), and *dolor* (pain). These chief (cardinal/basic) signs are hallmarks (characteristics) of acute inflammation. In the 19th century, a fifth clinical sign, **loss of function** (functio laesa), was later added by Rudolf Virchow. They are listed in **Table 3**.

Scottish surgeon John Hunter (1793) noted that inflammation is not a disease but a stereotypic (chain) response that has a beneficial effect on its host. Russian biologist Elie Metchnikoff (1880s) detected phagocytosis by observing the ingestion of rose thorns by amebocytes of starfish larvae and of bacteria by leukocytes. He put forward the concept that the purpose of inflammation was to bring phagocytic cells from the blood vessel to the injured area to engulf invading bacteria. This concept was criticized by George Bernard Shaw in his play "The Doctor's Dilemma", in which one physician's cure-all is to "stimulate the phagocytes!". Sir Thomas Lewis, while studying the inflammatory response in skin, found the concept that chemical substances, such as histamine (produced locally in response to injury), mediate the vascular changes of inflammation. This fundamental concept is an important discovery of mediators of inflammation.

Table 3: Cardinal signs of inflammation.

Nos.	*Cardinal sign*	*Mechanism*
1	Rubor (redness)*	Increased blood flow and stasis
2	Calor (heat)*	Increased blood flow
3	Tumor (edema/ swelling)*	Increased vascular permeability causing escape of a protein-rich fluid from blood vessels
4	Dolor (pain)*	Mediators: Prostaglandins and kinins
5	Loss of function (functio laesa)†	

*First four are described by Celsus,
†Fifth sign was added by Rudolf Virchow

This concept is used for the therapeutic anti-inflammatory drugs in clinical medicine. Julius Cohnheim first described emigration of leukocytes through microvasculature walls in inflammation.

Causes of Inflammation

Inflammatory reactions may occur in response to a variety of stimuli and includes both exogenous and endogenous causes (**Box 2**). Important causes are discussed below.

Box 2: Exogenous and endogenous causes of inflammation.

Exogenous Causes
- **Infections** (bacterial, viral, fungal, and parasitic) and **microbial toxins.**
- **Trauma** (blunt, penetrating, or crush injuries)
- **Physical agents**
  - Thermal injury (e.g., burns, frostbite, or hyperthermia)
  - Irradiation/radiation
  - Electric shock
  - Sudden changes in atmospheric pressure
- **Chemical injury**
  - Strong acids and alkalies
  - Insecticides and herbicides
  - Environmental toxins
  - Pharmaceutical agents
  - Oxygen, water, glucose, salt
  - Drugs of abuse
- **Foreign bodies** (e.g., sutures, talc)
- **Nutritional derangements**

Endogenous Causes
- **Tissue necrosis**
  - Ischemia (e.g., myocardial infarction)
  - Anoxia
- **Immune reactions**
  - Hypersensitivity reactions
  - Autoimmune diseases
  - Transplant organ rejection
- **Genetic derangements**

Infections: Infections by bacteria, virus, fungus, parasites, and microbial toxins are the most common and important causes of inflammation. Different infectious pathogens produce varied inflammatory responses. These responses vary from mild acute inflammation to severe systemic reactions that may be sometimes fatal. Mild reaction causes little or no permanent damage and successfully eradicates the causative infection. Prolonged chronic reactions produces severe tissue injury. The outcomes of infections depend mainly on the type of pathogen and the host response.

Tissue necrosis: Cells may undergo death by necrosis due to ischemia (reduced blood flow as in myocardial infarction), trauma, physical chemical injury (e.g., thermal injury, as in burns or frostbite; irradiation; exposure to some environmental chemicals) and immunological injury. Irrespective of the cause for necrosis, it brings out inflammatory reaction. It is triggered by many molecules released from necrotic cells.

Foreign bodies: Foreign bodies bring out inflammation by themselves or because the tissue injury or trauma they produce or the microbes carried along with them. Examples for exogenous foreign body are sutures, splinters, dirt. Even endogenous substances are capable of eliciting inflammatory reaction, if they get deposited in tissues. Examples include urate crystals (in gout), cholesterol crystals (in atherosclerosis), and lipids (in obesity associated metabolic syndrome).

Immune reactions: Normally, immune system protectives individual from environmental antigens. However, immune reaction may be against own tissues (self-antigens) and or inappropriately directed and damages the tissue as in hypersensitivity reactions (e.g., against environmental substances such as in allergies, or against microbes). The injurious immune responses, causing inflammation is a major cause of tissue injury in these diseases (refer Chapter 15). The stimuli that produce inflammatory responses in autoimmune diseases (against self-antigens) and hypersensitivity (e.g., against environmental antigens) cannot be eliminated. Hence, both autoimmune and allergic reactions often tend to be produce persistent chronic inflammation and are difficult to cure. These disorders are important causes of morbidity and mortality. The inflammation is mainly produced by cytokines released from T lymphocytes and other cells of the immune system.

RECOGNITION OF MICROBES AND DAMAGED CELLS

Inflammation may be initiated by exogenous microbes and other injurious agents as well as endogenous causes such as damaged or necrotic cells. **The first step** of innate immunity such as in inflammation and taking part in adaptive immune response **is the recognition of microbes, necrotic cells** and **foreign substances.**

Molecules Produced by Microbes and Damaged Cells

The innate immune system recognizes **molecular structures** that are **produced by**—(1) **microbial pathogens, or** (2) endogenous molecules that are produced by or released from **damaged and dying cells.** These molecules are discussed here.

Pathogen-associated Molecular Patterns

The innate immune system recognizes **molecular structures** that are **produced by microbial pathogens.** Microbes have few highly conserved common molecular structures shared by entire classes of pathogens. The microbial structures/ substances that stimulate innate immunity are often **shared by classes of microbes** and are called pathogen-associated molecular patterns (PAMPs). PAMPs are essential for the infectivity of these pathogens. PAMPs are part of many microorganisms but not of the host body's own cells.

Different types of microbes (e.g., viruses, gram-negative bacteria, gram-positive bacteria, fungi) express different PAMPs (**Table 4**). These PAMP structures include nucleic acids that are unique to or more abundant in microbes than in host cells [e.g., double-stranded ribonucleic acid (RNA) found in replicating viruses and unmethylated CpG deoxyribonucleic acid (DNA) sequences commonly found in many bacteria]; proteins that are found in microbes (e.g., initiation by N-formyl methionine, which is typical of bacterial proteins); and complex lipids and carbohydrates that are synthesized by microbes but not by human cells [e.g., lipopolysaccharide (LPS) in gram-negative bacterial cell wall, lipoteichoic acid in gram-positive bacteria, mannose-rich oligosaccharides found in microbial but not in human glycoproteins and peptidoglycans].

In case of infections, the presence of PAMPs on infectious pathogens (microbes) is recognized by membrane-bound or endosomal families of **pattern recognition receptors** (PRRs) present on cells (e.g., phagocytes). The **innate immune system recognizes microbial products that are usually essential for survival of the microbes** (double-stranded viral RNA is an essential intermediate in the life cycle of many viruses; LPS and lipoteichoic acid are structural components of bacterial cell walls that are required for bacterial survival).

Danger (Damage)-associated Molecular Patterns (DAMPs)

The **innate immune system also recognizes endogenous molecules that are produced by or released** (liberated) **from damaged and dying cells** (or cells altered due damage). These substances are called **damage-associated molecular patterns (DAMPs)**. All host cells contain cytosolic receptors which can recognize these molecules. Examples of sources of damage-associated molecules are presented in **Box 3**. Examples of source and type of DAMPs are presented in **Table 5**.

DAMPs may be produced as a result of cell damage caused by infections. But they may also be produced by sterile injury to cells caused by many other causes, such as chemical toxins, burns, trauma, or loss of blood supply. DAMPs are usually not released from cells undergoing death by apoptosis. In some situations, endogenous molecules that are produced by healthy cells are released when the cells are damaged. These molecules then can stimulate innate responses. These molecules are a subset of DAMPs and are called as **alarmins** because their presence outside cells alarms the immune system that something is causing cell death.

In case of damaged or necrotic cells, DAMPs derived from damaged cells are released extracellularly after tissue injury. These DAMPs are also recognized by PRRs located on cell surfaces and intracellularly. The cytosolic receptors activate a multiprotein cytosolic complex called the *inflammasome* (discussed further on pages 224–226).

Box 3: Examples of sources of damage-associated molecules.

- **Cell injury and necrosis:**
  - Adenosine diphosphate (ATP) (released from damaged mitochondria)
  - Deoxyribonucleic acid (DNA) [liberated into the cytoplasm and not sequestered in nuclei (normally it is sequestered)]
  - Uric acid (a breakdown product of DNA)
  - Decreased intracellular K+ concentrations (due to loss of K^+ caused by injury to plasma membrane injury)
  - Proteins
- **Tumor cells:** ATP, DNA, uric acid, and proteins
- **Damage to extracellular matrix (ECM):** Hyaluronan, hyaluronic acid, heparin sulfate

Table 5: Examples of source and type of damage-associated molecular patterns (DAMPs).

Source	*Type of damage-associated molecular patterns (DAMPs)*
Stress-induced proteins	Heat shock protein (Hsps)
Crystals	Monosodium urate
Proteolytically cleaved extracellular matrix	Proteoglycan peptides
Mitochondria and mitochondrial components	Formylated peptides and adenosine triphosphate (ATP)
Nuclear proteins	High-mobility group box 1 (HMGB1), histones

Table 4: Examples of pathogen-associated molecular patterns (PAMPs).

Source	*Type of pathogen-associated molecular pattern (PAMP)*	*Type of microbe*
Nucleic acids	Single-stranded ribonucleic acid (ssRNA) and double-stranded RNA (dsRNA)	Virus
	Cytosine–guanine-rich oligonucleotide (CpG)	Virus, bacteria
Proteins	Pilin and flagellin	Bacteria
Cell wall lipids	Lipopolysaccharide (LPS)	Gram-negative bacteria
	Lipoteichoic acid	Gram-positive bacteria
Carbohydrates	Mannan	Fungi, bacteria
	Glucans (glycogen polysaccharides)	Fungi

Recognition of Molecules Produced by Microbes and Damaged Cells

Q. Write a short essay on pattern recognition receptors.

To recognize PAMPs (produced by exogenous microbes) and DAMPs (produced by host dead cells), the innate immune system uses—**(1) several types of cellular receptors**, present in different locations in host cells (e.g., cellular receptors on the surface of cells such as phagocytes), **and (2) soluble molecules in the blood** (i.e., circulating proteins such as complements) **and mucosal secretions.**

Cellular Receptors: Pattern Recognition Receptors

Several types of cellular receptors present in different locations in cells that recognize PAMPs and DAMPs are called as PRRs.

Definition

Pattern recognition receptors are molecules expressed by cells of the innate immunity. These PRRs are capable of sensing "patterns," triggering the reactions of innate immunity such as inflammation and taking part in adaptive immune responses. Thus, **pattern recognition receptors (PRRs)** are receptors of the innate immune system that recognize molecular patterns present on pathogens but absent in the host. There are many cellular receptors for microbes which detect pathogens or the damage induced by them. Hence, such cellular receptors that recognize the patterns (PAMPs and DAMPs) are known as "**PRRs**".

Cells having PRRs

Pattern recognition receptors are found on:

- **Innate immune cells:** For example, macrophages, dendritic cells, neutrophils, and others
- **Adaptive immune cells:** T and B lymphocytes
- **Other cell types:** They are also found in cells that are not part of the formal immune system (e.g., neuronal cells, epithelial cells, etc.).

Location of receptors

Pattern recognition receptors are located in all the cellular compartments where cells encounter or come across the pathogens. **The plasma membrane receptors detect extracellular pathogens, endosomal receptors detect ingested microbes, and cytosolic receptors detect microbes in the cytoplasm.** Cellular locations of various pattern recognition receptors of the innate immune system are presented in **Figure 2.**

Stimulus for PRRs (Fig. 3)

Infectious agents or damaged/necrotic cells trigger the signaling pathways by recognition of patterns present on them (microbe, necrotic cell) that engage with PRRs in the cells. These **cells with PRRs include phagocytes, dendritic cells (cells in epithelia and all tissues which are involved in capturing microbes), and many other cells.** This leads to an innate or adaptive immune response. The molecular pattern in the infectious agents and necrotic cells are described already on pages 220–221 (refer DAMPs and PAMPs).

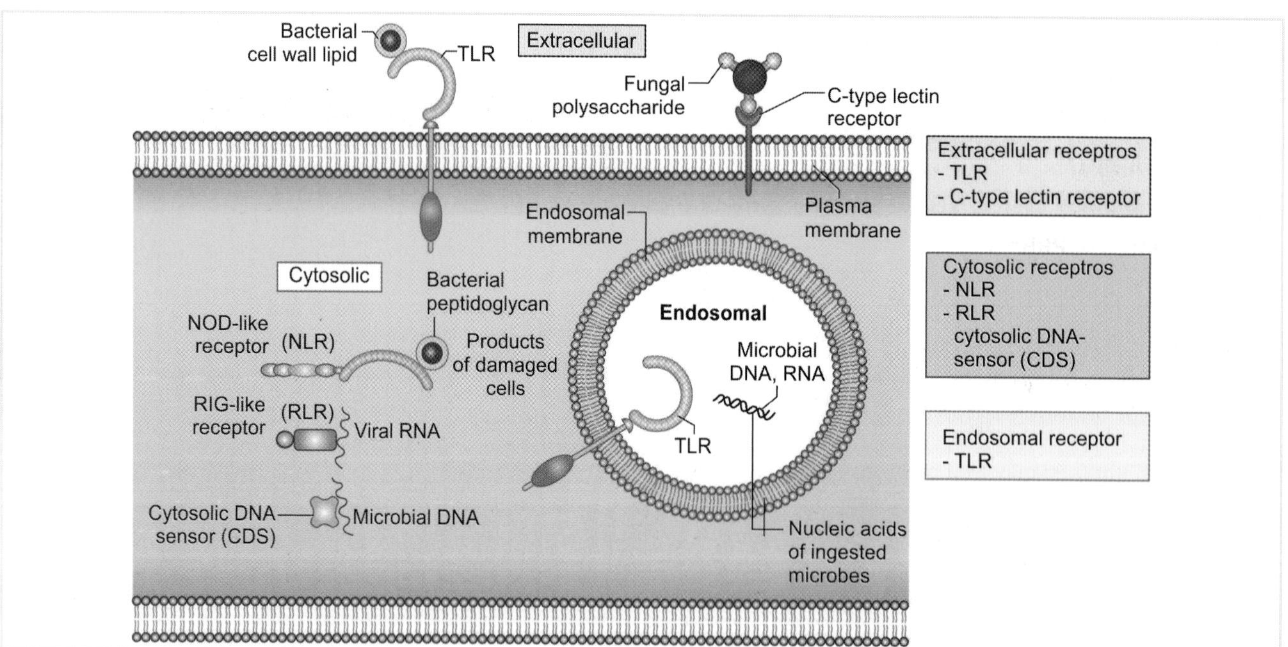

FIG. 2: Cellular locations of pattern recognition receptors of the innate immune system for microbes and products of cell injury. Phagocytes, dendritic cells, and many types of epithelial cells express different classes of receptors that sense the presence of microbes and dead cells. The major classes of innate immune receptors are toll-like receptors (TLRs), nucleotide oligomerization domain (NOD)-like receptors (NLRs) in the cytosol, C-type lectin receptors, RIG-like receptors (RLRs) for viral ribonucleic acid (RNA), named after the founding member RIG-I, and cytosolic deoxyribonucleic acid (DNA) sensors (CDS). TLRs located in different cellular compartments, as well as other cytoplasmic and plasma membrane receptors, recognize products of different classes of microbes. Some pattern recognition molecules (including members of the TLR family and lectin receptors), are located on the cell surface, where they may bind extracellular PAMPs (pathogen-associated molecular patterns). Other TLRs are located on endosomal membranes and recognize nucleic acids of microbes that have been phagocytosed by cells. Cells also contain cytosolic sensors of microbial infection (NLRs, RLRs, and CDS). Cytosolic receptors recognize products of damaged cells (DAMPs: damage -associated molecular patterns) as well as some microbes.

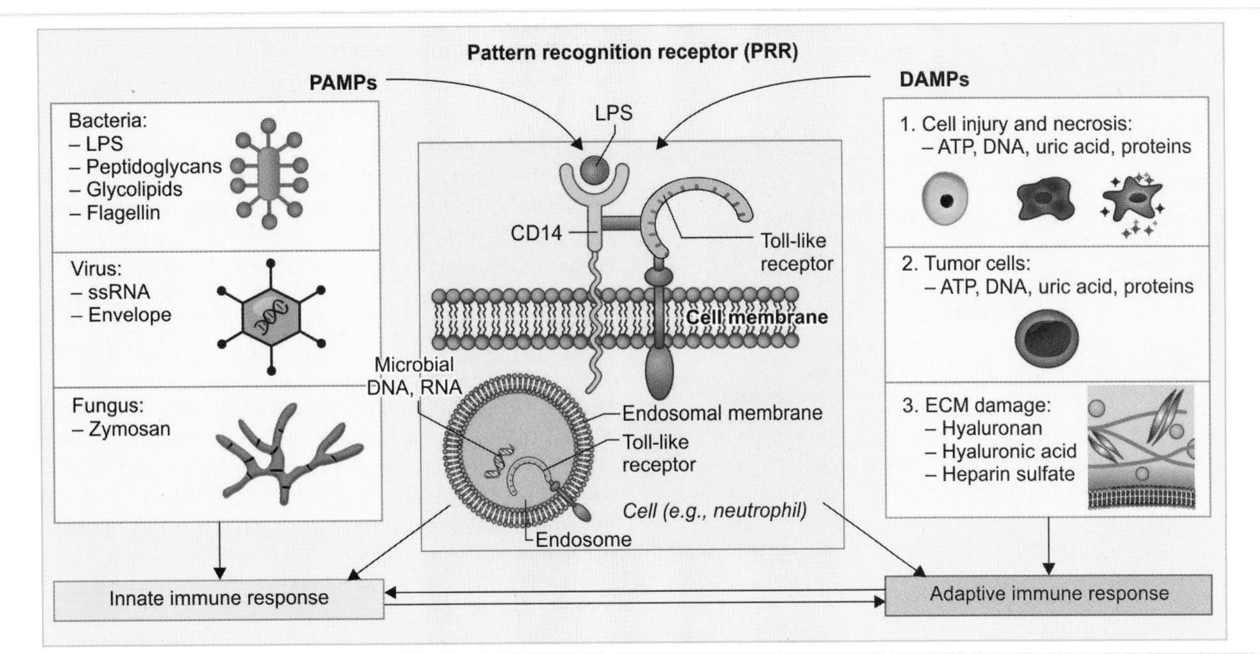

[ATP: adenosine triphosphate; CD14: a member of the family of leucine-rich repeat (LRR) proteins; DNA: deoxyribonucleic acid; ECM: extracellular matrix; LPS: lipopolysaccharide; ssRNA: single stranded ribonucleic acid]

FIG. 3: Pathogen-associated molecular pattern molecules (PAMPs) released by microbes and damage-associated molecular pattern molecules (DAMPs) from damaged cells and tissue bind to receptors belonging to the family of pattern recognition receptors (PRRs) in the cells. This initiates and mediates innate and adaptive immune responses.

Features and types of PRRs

Typically, PRRs consist of one or several C-terminal (carboxy terminal) recognizing or regulatory domains, which sense "patterns". The N-terminal (amino terminal) effector domains of PRRs are associated with signaling molecules. Some PRRs have a central domain. To date, five families of PRRs have been described (**Box 4** and **Fig. 2**).

Consequences of PRRs

Engagement (interaction of molecules) of both PAMPs and DAMPs with PRRs activate intracellular cascades to drive a coordinated immune response (**Fig. 4**). With activation of PRRs, the multifaceted inflammatory response occurs. They activate transcription factors that stimulate the production and expression of many secreted and membrane proteins. The inflammatory response is amplified by—(1) release of mediators of inflammation (proinflammatory responses) such as cytokines and chemokines that induce inflammation, antiviral cytokines [interferons (IFNs)], and membrane proteins that promote lymphocyte activation and immune responses, (2) activation of coagulation and complement cascades, and (3) release of free radicals (**Fig. 4**).

Toll-like receptors (Fig. 3)

Q. Write a short essay on toll-like receptors.

Q. Discuss toll-like receptors in chronic inflammatory disorders.

The well-known pattern recognition receptors (PRRs) are transmembrane proteins that belong to the family of TLRs. They are named after the founding member, Toll, a gene that was discovered in Drosophila.

Box 4: Family of pattern recognition receptors.

- Toll-like receptors (TLRs)
- Nucleotide oligomerization domain leucine-rich repeat proteins [NOD-like receptors (NLRs)]
- C-type lectin receptors (CLRs)
- RIG-1-like receptors (RLRs)
- Absent in melanoma (AIM)-2-like receptors (ALRs)

Location Toll-like receptors are located in plasma membranes and endosomes. They are expressed on the: (1) membranes of macrophages, neutrophils, dendritic cells, lymphocytes, platelets, atherosclerotic plaques, etc., and present in the (2) endosomes of the cells.

Subtypes There are 10 expressed TLR genes in humans. The subtypes and their ligands are presented in **Table 6**.

Properties Toll-like receptors are single-pass transmembrane proteins. Their extracellular region is composed of leucine-rich repeat (LRR) such as CD14.

Recognition of microbial molecules Toll-like receptors recognize a wide range of microbial molecules and can recognize both PAMPs and DAMPs. Each TLR recognizes a distinct set of molecular patterns. The TLRs in the plasma membrane recognize bacterial products [e.g., (LPS) or endotoxin], and endosomal TLRs recognize bacteria and virus taken into phagosome by phagocytosis (e.g., viral and bacterial RNA and DNA). They are capable of detecting PAMPs derived from extracellular necrotic or injured cells. A pathogen bound to TLRs may be engulfed, digested, and presented to

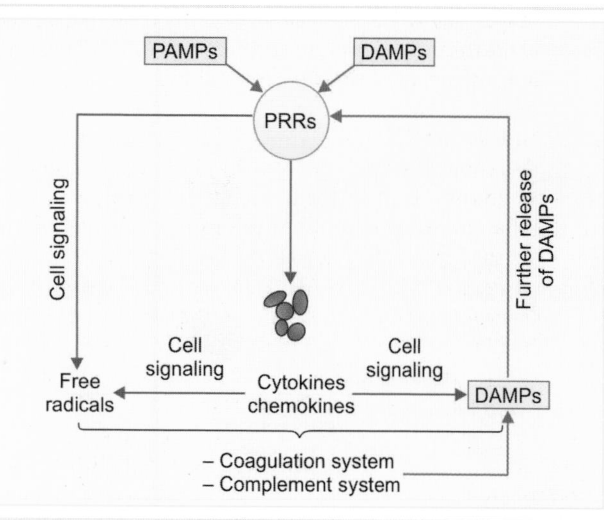

(DAMPs: damage-associated molecular pattern molecules; PAMPs: pathogen-associated molecular pattern molecules)

FIG. 4: Damage-associated molecular pattern molecules from damaged/necrotic tissue and pathogen-associated molecular pattern molecules from microbes interact with pattern recognition receptors (PRRs) present in cell. This initiates cell signaling, leading to enhanced activation of inflammatory mediators and the multifaceted inflammatory response. These inflammatory signals cause further release of DAMPs and maintenance of the inflammatory response.

Table 6: Toll-like receptors (TLRs)—Location and their ligands.

Toll-like receptor (TLR) (location of receptor)	*Ligands (PAMP, DAMP)*
TLR1 (Extracellular)	Triacyl lipopeptides of *Mycobacterium tuberculosis* DAMP
TLR2 (Extracellular)	Diacyl and triacyl lipopeptides of gram-positive bacteria, lipoteichoic acid, peptidoglycan, yeast zymozan DAMP
TLR3 (Intracellular)	Viral double-stranded ribonucleic acid (dsRNA)
TLR4 (Extracellular)	Lipopolysaccharide (endotoxin, LPS) of gram-negative bacteria DAMP
TLR5 (Extracellular)	Flagellin of bacterial flagella
TLR6 (Extracellular)	Diacyl lipopeptides of gram-positive bacteria
TLR7 (Intracellular)	Viral single-stranded ribonucleic acid (ssRNA)
TLR8 (Intracellular)	Viral ssRNA
TLR9 (Intracellular)	Unmethylated CpG nucleotides of bacterial and viral DNA
TLR10	Unknown

(DAMP: danger (damage)-associated molecular pattern; PAMP: pathogen-associated molecular pattern)

lymphocytes in antigenic form. TLRs provide a link between innate and adaptive immunity because they can interact with antigens also.

Consequences of TLRs are same as described for PRRs on pages 223.

Clinical significance: Toll-like receptor engagement activates intracellular pathways to protect against microbial organisms. However, it may lead to excessive activation of cytokine cascades, especially in septic shock. Thus, interleukin (IL)-1 and TLR signaling is involved in many inflammatory and infectious diseases. This has prompted for the development of TLR antagonists.

Nucleotide oligomerization domain-like receptors

Nucleotide oligomerization domain (NOD)-like receptors (NLRs) are intracellular soluble proteins localized in the cytosol (i.e., cytosolic receptors). They are named after the founding members NOD-1 and NOD-2. It is a family of >20 different cytosolic proteins. These are sensors for microbes (PAMPs) and cell injury (DAMPs). These sensors recognize PAMPs and DAMPs and recruit other proteins to form large molecular signaling complexes termed inflammasomes (discussed on pages 224–226) that promote **inflammation.** The inflammasomes cause proteolytic activation of proinflammatory cytokines IL-1. NLRs recognize a variety of substances. These include products of necrotic cells [e.g., uric acid and released adenosine triphosphate (ATP)], ion disturbances (e.g., loss of K+), etc. Several of the NLRs signal via a cytosolic multiprotein complex called the *inflammasome.* Inflammasome activates an enzyme (caspase-1) that converts a precursor form of the cytokine IL-1 and IL-18 to biologically active form. IL-1 is a mediator of inflammation that recruits leukocytes and induces fever. Gain-of-function mutations in one of the cytosolic NLRs produce a periodic fever and rare syndromes, called *autoinflammatory syndromes.* They are characterized by spontaneous inflammation. IL-1 antagonists are effective in the treatment of these disorders.

Inflammasomes

Q. Write a short essay on inflammasome.

Some NLRs contain domains that allow them to assemble with other proteins into large complexes. Inflammasomes are multiprotein complexes and are unit of innate immunity. Inflammasome can recognize products of dead cells (e.g., uric acid, microbial products) and can be formed in the cytosol rapidly in response to infectious invaders and/or tissue injury, i.e., in response to cytosolic PAMPs and DAMPs. Its function is to generate active forms of the inflammatory cytokines IL-1β and IL-18 (**Fig. 5**). The inflammatory cytokines IL-1β and IL-18 are expressed as inactive precursors. These two cytokines must be proteolytically cleaved by the enzyme caspase-1 present in inflammasome to generate active cytokines. Upon activation of the inflammasome, caspase-1 converts pro-IL1β and pro-IL18 into their active forms. Once activated they are released from the cell, IL-1 recruits leukocytes and thus induces inflammation. The recruited leukocytes phagocyte and destroy dead cells. It induces cell pyroptosis (refer pages 151–152), a process of programmed cell death different from apoptosis.

Inflammasomes are composed of—(1) sensor, (2) caspase-1, and (3) an adaptor that links the two (sensor with caspase-1).

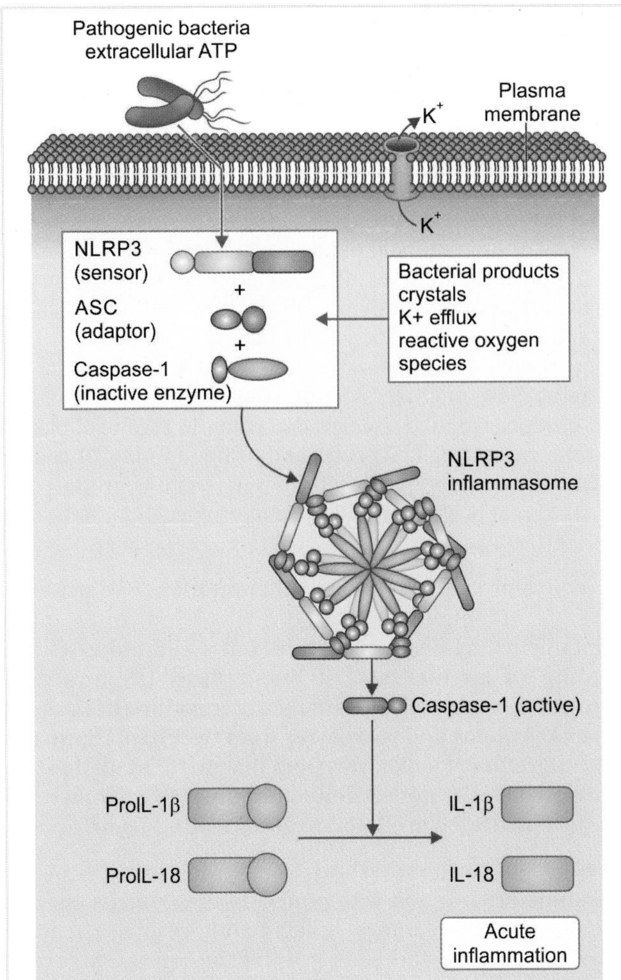

FIG. 5: Components and action of inflammasome. Inflammasome is a multiprotein complex composed of a sensor (e.g., NLRP3), an adaptor (ASC), and an inactive enzyme caspase-1. Various pathogen-associated molecular patterns (PAMPs) or damage-associated molecular patterns (DAMPs) induce proIL-1β and proIL-18 expression through pattern recognition receptor signaling. The activation of the NLRP3 inflammasome converts inactive proIL-1β to active IL-1β and inactive proIL-18 to active IL-18. (ASC: Apoptosis-associated speck-like protein containing a CARD; IL-1: interleukin-1)

- **Activator of inflammasome:** The exact composition of an inflammasome depends on the activator, which initiates assembly of multiple proteins of inflammasome.
  - **Stimuli for inflammasome activation:** Many varieties of cytoplasmic stimuli can stimulate inflammasome formation. These include infections, microbial products, cell stress, environmentally or endogenously derived crystals [may damage lysosomal membranes and release reactive oxygen species (ROS) into the cytosol], extracellular ATP, generation of ROS, and reduction in cytosolic potassium ion (K+) concentrations.
  - **Binding to pattern recognition receptors (PRRs):** The stimuli activate inflammasome formation through **pathogen-associated molecular patterns (PAMPs) and DAMPs.** The molecular patterns bind to a variety of pattern recognition receptors (PRRs). TLRs are one of the important types of PRRs that can detect PAMPs/DAMPs in the extracellular environment and endosome. NLRs (another type PRR present in cytosol) and some other PRRs play an important role in sensing "patterns" in the intracellular compartments. The inflammasome complexes are formed only when the sensors respond to activator (e.g., PAMPs, DAMPs, or changes in the cell indicating the presence of infection or damage). Thus, inflammation mediated by IL-1β and IL-18 occurs when there are PAMPS or DAMPS in the cytosol, indicating infection or cell injury.
- **Sensor proteins:** Inflammasomes can form with several different sensor proteins. The sensor proteins may belong to NLRs family or others that are **not in the NLR family**. NLRs family sensors are found in different inflammasomes and include NLRB, NLRC4, and at least six NLRP proteins. Sensors that are not in the NLR family but are used by inflammasomes include members absent in melanoma (AIM) 2 family. The NLRP3 inflammasome (**Fig. 5**) is the best-studied inflammasome and seems to be activated by many microbes.

Formation of the inflammasome (Fig. 5) Inflammasome is induced by one of the two ways—(1) the sensor proteins in the cytosol directly recognize microbial products, or (2) more commonly, when sensors detect changes in the amount of endogenous molecules or ions in the cytosol (which is indirect indicator of the presence of infection or cell damage).

- **Binding of sensors to adaptor protein:** The sensors such as NLRP3 bind with an adaptor protein called ASC (apoptosis-associated speck-like protein containing a CARD).
- **Recruitment of caspase-1:** The binding of ASC to sensors (e.g., NLRP proteins) recruits an inactive precursor of caspase-1, called procaspase-1. The procaspase-1 proteins are then converted to active caspase-1. Caspases are proteases with cysteine residues in their active site that cleave substrate proteins at aspartate residues. The main function of caspase-1 is to cleave the inactive cytoplasmic precursor forms of IL-1β and IL-18. The active proinflammatory cytokines IL-1β and IL-18 formed in the cytosol are released from cells. The inflammation produced by IL-1 serves a protective function by eliminating the microbes and damaged cells that stimulated the formation of the inflammasome.

Inflammasome and associated disorders

The NLR–inflammasome pathway may play a role in some chronic disorders with inflammation. Recognition of urate crystals by a class of NLRs is responsible for inflammatory reactions to urate crystals (cause of gout). These receptors may detect and respond to cholesterol crystals (in atherosclerosis), lipids (in metabolic syndrome and obesity-associated type 2 diabetes), and amyloid deposits in the brain (in Alzheimer's disease). IL-1 plays a role in atherosclerosis and obesity-associated type 2 diabetes mellitus.

C-type lectin receptors (CLRs)

Glycosylated proteins play a role in cell adhesion. In addition, they also have pathogen recognition functions.

Expression It is mainly expressed on the plasma membrane (refer **Fig. 2, Chapter 8.1**) osf macrophages and dendritic cells (DCs).

Functions These receptors detect fungal glycans and elicit inflammatory reactions to fungi and modulate innate immunity. Similar to TLR, CLRs may recognize both "patterns" and antigens and bridge between innate and adaptive immunity. Soluble type CLRs are related to "acute phase" proteins.

Members These include the mannose receptor, dendritic cell-specific intercellular adhesion molecule (ICAM)-3-grabbing nonintegrin (DC-SIGN), dectin-1, dectin-2, and the collectins.

Mechanism of action Binding of pathogens to these receptors on epithelial and endothelial cells, releases additional DAMPs. This stimulates inflammatory cells and activates coagulation and complement cascades. These, in turn, increase the production of inflammatory mediators (i.e., cytokine, chemokines, and DAMPS).

Retinoic acid inducible gene (RIG)-1-like Receptors (RLRs)

Retinoic acid inducible gene-1-like receptors (RIG-1-like receptors) are expressed in the cytoplasm of macrophages, dendritic cells, and fibroblasts. They consist of a cytoplasmic RNA helicase domain and CARDs (caspase activation and recruitment domains). They survey for microbes and recognize viral RNA in the cytoplasm. A ligand for RLRs includes viral PAMP and dsRNA. Activation of RLRs produces type I IFN.

Absent in melanoma (AIM)-2-like receptors (ALRs)

They are present in the cytoplasm and nucleus. They contain a certain number of HIN200 domains and PYD domain. The term "HIN200" is derived from "hematopoietic expression, IFN-inducible nature, and nuclear localization of *200* amino acids." A ligand for ALRs is dsDNA of bacteria or viruses. Activation of AIM-2 produces AIM-2 inflammasome and proinflammatory cytokines and type I IFNs.

Other cellular receptors involved in inflammation: Apart from direct recognition of microbes, many leukocytes also express other receptors. These include receptors for the Fc tails of antibodies and for complement proteins. These receptors recognize microbes coated with antibodies and complement (the coating process is called opsonization). These receptors gets activated and promote ingestion, destruction of the microbes and inflammation.

Circulating Proteins

Many plasma proteins recognize microbes and function to destroy blood-borne microbes and stimulate inflammation at the site of tissue infection.

- **Complement system:** It reacts against microbes and activates complement products that act as mediators of inflammation.
- **Mannose-binding lectin:** It is a circulating protein which recognizes microbial sugars and promotes ingestion of microbes and activates the complement system.
- **Collectins:** These proteins also bind to microbes and promote phagocytosis of microbes.
- **Others:** Pentraxins and ficolins.

ACUTE INFLAMMATION

Q. Explain the sequential vascular changes/reactions of blood vessels/hemodynamic changes in acute inflammation.

When an injurious agent (e.g., infectious microbe, dead cells) is introduced into a tissue, the local tissue reacts. The phagocytes present in all tissues try to eliminate the injurious agent. At the same time, these foreign or abnormal injurious agents are recognized by the phagocytes and other cells in the tissues. They liberate soluble chemical molecules called as mediators of inflammation that mediate inflammation. Some of these mediators act on nearby small blood vessels and produce vascular changes that result in escape of plasma and the circulating leukocytes at the site of injury. The acute inflammatory response is self-limiting (i.e., it continues only till the threat is eliminated). It usually takes about 8–10 days from onset to healing.

Sequence of Events in Acute Inflammation: The sequence of acute inflammation can be divided into three major components, namely—**(1) dilation of small blood vessels leading to an increase in blood flow; (2) increased permeability of the microvasculature (resulting in escape of plasma proteins and leukocytes from the circulation); and (3) emigration of leukocytes from the microcirculation. The emigrated leukocytes accumulate at the focus of injury, and they are activated to eliminate the offending agent.**

Purpose of Inflammation: The main purpose of the inflammatory reaction is to protect tissues, organs and, the whole body from damage. Inflammation response achieves this by localizing and getting rid of microbes (pathogenic insult), and removal of injured (altered/damaged) cells, foreign particles, and antigens. It also prepares and allows tissue repair to take place and thereby the damaged site return to its normal structure and function. Main function of inflammatory response is to deliver and increase the movement of circulating cells (**leukocytes**), fluids, and plasma proteins from the circulation to sites of infection or tissue injury.

Specific cells are brought to the site of injury to attack and destroy the injurious agents (e.g., infectious microorganisms, toxins, or foreign material), enzymatically digest and remove them, or wall them off. During this process, the cells and tissues are also damaged. The damaged host cells are also digested and removed allowing the process of repair.

Reactions of Blood Vessels in Acute Inflammation

Q. Define inflammation. Describe the vascular changes (reactions of blood vessels) in acute inflammation.

The reactions of blood vessels (vascular changes) in acute inflammation (**Figs. 6** and **7**) have two components, namely—(1) **changes in the vascular flow and caliber** (i.e., dilation of small vessels, leading to an increase in blood flow), and (2) **increased vascular permeability** (i.e., increased permeability of the microvasculature) leading to escape of plasma proteins from the circulation into the site of injury. Alterations in blood flow and diameter of blood vessels, and increased vascular

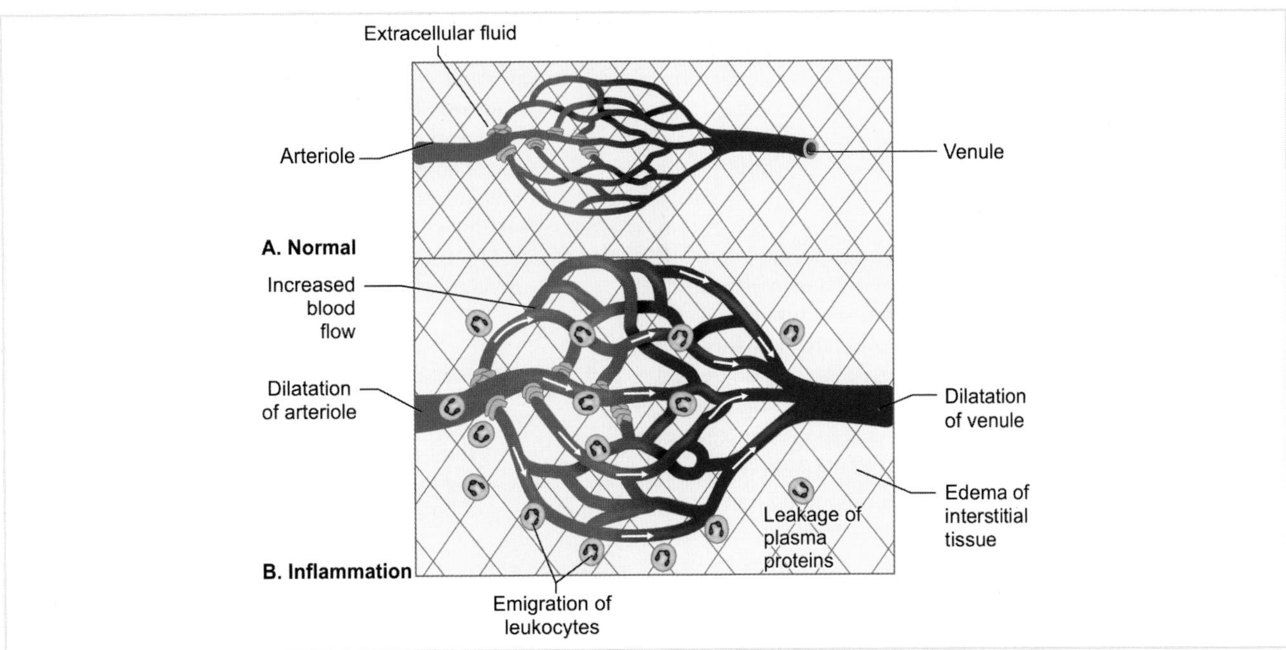

FIG. 6: Local features of acute inflammation compared to normal are—vasodilatation, increased blood flow, leakage of plasma fluid and proteins, and emigration of leukocyte.

permeability **maximize the movement of plasma proteins and leukocytes out of the circulation and into the site of infection or injury**.

Exudation is defined as the process of escape of fluid, proteins, and circulating blood cells from the vessels into the interstitial tissue or body cavities.

Changes in Vascular Flow and Caliber

Immediately after injury, vascular changes develop at variable rates depending on the site of injury and nature and severity of the injury. These vascular changes reflect the classic "**triple response**" first described by Sir Thomas Lewis in 1924. Lewis in his original experiments described a **dull red line** at the site of mild trauma to skin, followed by a **flare** (red halo) and then a **wheal** (swelling). Lewis postulated that a vasoactive mediator produced vasodilation and increased vascular permeability at the site of injury. In inflammation, following changes occur in the vascular flow and caliber.

- **Vasodilation (refer Fig. 6):** It is the earliest feature of acute inflammation; sometimes, it follows a transient constriction of arterioles. The effects of inflammation are observed within seconds.
  - **Effect:** Result is increased blood flow and expansion of the capillary bed. Vasodilation first involves the arterioles and then causes opening of new capillary beds in the area of injury (refer **Fig. 6**). This leads to local heat and redness (erythema) at the site of inflammation.
  - **Mediators involved:** Histamine, prostaglandins, kinins, and nitric oxide (NO) are chemical mediators that act on vascular smooth muscle to produce vasodilation.
- **Increased permeability of the microvasculature:** The increased flow is immediately followed by increased permeability of the microvasculature. This leads to escape of protein-rich fluid from the circulation into the extravascular tissues. This causes edema in the surrounding tissue (discussed below).
  - **Mediators involved:** Histamine, leukotrienes, neuropeptides, and kinins.
- **Slowing of blood flow:** The increased outward movement of plasma into the extravascular space (i.e., exudation with loss of intravascular fluid) and increased diameter of vessel at the injured site leads to three changes. These are (i) slowing of blood flow, (ii) concentration of red cells (RBCs) in small vessels (microvasculature), (iii) and increased viscosity of the blood (viscosity is a measure of a fluid's resistance to flow).
- **Stasis:** The above changes result in engorgement (distention with blood) of small vessels with slowly movement of red blood cells. This condition is termed stasis. Microscopically, they appear as vascular congestion and externally as localized redness (erythema) of the involved tissue.
- **Leukocyte events:** Stasis causes blood leukocytes (mainly neutrophils) to move towards the endothelium and accumulate along the vascular endothelium (pavementing). The endothelial cells get activated by mediators produced at sites of infection/injury and tissue damage. There is increased levels of expression of adhesion molecules and this favors adherence of leukocytes to the endothelium. These leukocyte then migrate through the vascular wall into the interstitial tissue, at the site of injury in a sequence (described later on pages 230–243).

Increased Vascular Permeability (Vascular Leakage)

Q. Write a short essay on mechanism of increased vascular permeability (vascular leakage) in acute inflammation.

Escape of a protein-rich fluid causes edema and is one of the cardinal signs of inflammation. Edema is defined as an excess of fluid in the interstitial tissue or serous cavities; it can be either an exudate or a transudate. An *exudate* is an extravascular fluid that has a high protein concentration and contains cellular debris. In inflammation, edema is due to exudate and it is formed due to increased the permeability of small blood vessels at the site of injury. Pus is as also known as a purulent exudate, is an inflammatory exudate that contains numerous leukocytes (mostly neutrophils), the debris of dead cells, and, causative microbes in many cases. In contrast, a *transudate* is a fluid with low protein content (mostly albumin), few or no cells, and low specific gravity. It is ultrafiltration of blood plasma and occurs due to imbalance between osmotic or hydrostatic imbalance across the vessel wall. It is non-inflammatory in origin and there is no increase in vascular permeability. Differences between transudate and exudate are listed in **Table 7** (**Figs. 7A** to **C**).

Mechanism of Increased Vascular Permeability

Normally, the endothelium acts as a permeability barrier for the movement of fluid between intravascular and extravascular spaces. Endothelial cells are connected to each other by tight junctions and are separated from the surrounding tissue by a limiting basement membrane (**Fig. 8A**). **Disruption of this barrier function is a characteristic of acute inflammation.** Tissue injury is followed by release of specific inflammatory mediators at the site of injury that directly increase permeability of capillaries and postcapillary venules.

Q. Describe the mechanism of increased vascular permeability in acute inflammation.

Several mechanisms (**Fig. 8**) can cause increased vascular permeability:

- **Contraction of endothelial cells:**
  - Contraction of endothelial cells opens the normally closed interendothelial gaps. This gives rise to extravasation (leakage) of intravascular fluids into the extravascular space. It is the most common mechanism of vascular leakage in acute inflammation.
  - **Response:** It occurs immediately after injury and is usually short-lived (15–30 minutes) and hence called as immediate transient response.
  - **Mediators involved:** Histamine, bradykinin, leukotrienes, and other chemical mediators.
  - **Mode of action:** After injury, vasoactive mediators bind to specific receptors on endothelial cells. This produces reversible contraction of endothelial cell and forms gap (see **Fig. 9B**). This leads to extravasation (leakage) of intravascular fluids into the extravascular space.

Delayed prolonged leakage: In some forms of mild injury (e.g., mild burns, irradiation or ultraviolet radiation, and exposure to certain bacterial toxins), vascular leakage starts after a delay of 2 to 12 hours. It lasts for several hours or even days. This is called as delayed prolonged leakage. It may be caused by contraction of endothelial cells or mild endothelial damage. One of the classical example for damage that results in late-appearing vascular leakage is sunburn. Sunburn is a condition characterized by red and inflamed skin that occurs following overexposure to the ultraviolet rays of the sun. Generally the immediate and delayed responses occur along a continuum.

- **Endothelial injury**
  - **Causes:** Endothelial injury may be directly due to the injurious agent or indirectly through neutrophils that adhere to endothelium at the site of injury. Direct injury or damage to the endothelium can be caused by severe injuries. This may be due to direct damage to endothelium as in burns, actions of microbes and microbial toxins. One of the features of acute inflammation is leukocyte (mainly neutrophils) adhesion to endothelium. These neutrophils which adhere to the endothelium during inflammation may also indirectly cause injury to the endothelial cells and thus amplify the damage.
  - **Mode of action:** It produces necrosis and detachment of endothelial cells.

Table 7: Difference between transudate and exudate.

Characteristics	*Transudate*	*Exudate*
Cause	Noninflammatory process	Inflammatory process
Mechanism	Ultrafiltrate of plasma, due to increased hydrostatic pressure with normal vascular permeability	Increased vascular permeability
Appearance	Clear, serous	Cloudy/purulent/hemorrhagic/chylous
Color	Straw yellow	Yellow to red
Specific gravity	<1.018	>1.018
Protein	Low, <2 g/dL, mainly albumin	High, >2 g/dL
Fibrin content and clot formation	Fibrin content is low and does not coagulate	Fibrin content is high and coagulates/clots spontaneously
Cell count	Low	High
Type of cells	Few lymphocytes and mesothelial cells	Neutrophils in acute and lymphocytes in chronic inflammation
Bacteria	Absent	Usually present
Lactate dehydrogenase (LDH)	Low	High
Examples	Seen in congestive cardiac failure	Pus
Character of edema	Pitting type	Nonpitting

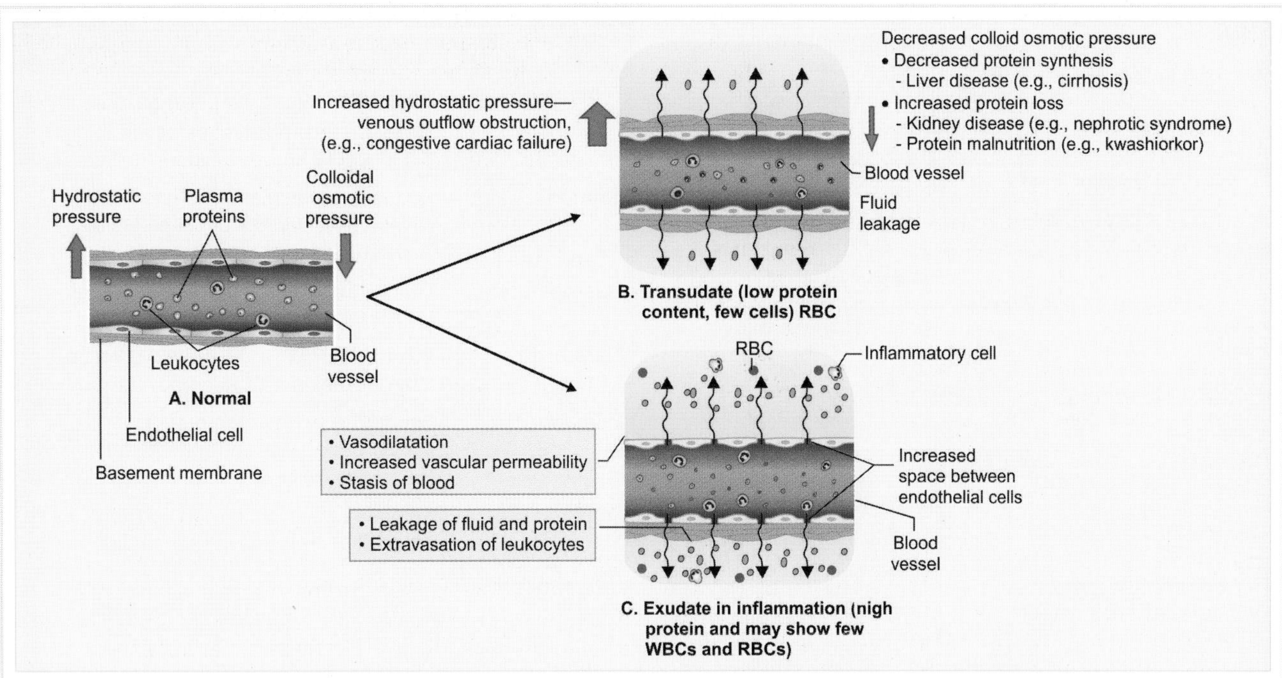

FIGS. 7A TO C: Formation of exudates and transudates. (A) Normal fluid exchange between blood and extracellular fluid: Two sets of forces control the fluid exchange between blood and extracellular fluid. These are hydrostatic pressure and the colloid osmotic pressure. Normal hydrostatic pressure of blood is about 32 mm Hg at the arterial end of a capillary bed and 12 mm Hg at the venous end. The mean colloid osmotic pressure of tissues is approximately 25 mm Hg, which is equal to the mean capillary pressure. Hence, the net flow of fluid across the vascular bed is almost nil. (B) Formation of transudate: A transudate is formed when fluid leaks out of vessels because of increased hydrostatic pressure or decreased osmotic pressure. (C) Formation of exudate in inflammation: An exudate is formed in inflammation. In inflammation vascular permeability is increased due to contraction of endothelial cells that leads to increased interendothelial spaces.

- **Response:** In most of the cases, the increased vascular permeability begins immediately after injury and is sustained for several hours till the damaged vessels are either thrombosed or repaired. Hence, this type of response is called **immediate sustained response**.
  - **Mild direct endothelial injury:** It produces a biphasic response, namely—(1) an early increased vascular permeability within 30 minutes of injury, followed by (2) a second increase in vascular permeability after a delay of 3–5 hours.
  - **Severe direct endothelial injury:** Causes such as burns or caustic chemicals, may produce irreversible damage to the vascular endothelium. The vascular endothelium separates from the basement membrane.
- **Alterations in transcytosis:** Process of transport of fluids and proteins through the intracellular channels (called vesiculo-vacuolar organelle) in the endothelial cell is called transcytosis. These channels may be opened in response to certain factors that promote vascular leakage [e.g., vascular endothelial growth factor (VEGF)]. However, its contribution to the vascular permeability in acute inflammation is not clear.

Though three different mechanisms causing increased vascular permeability are described separately, probably all contribute in varying degrees in responses to majority of injurious stimuli. For example, during different stages of a thermal burn, increased vascular permeability may be caused by contraction of endothelial cells by inflammatory mediators and also by endothelial injury, directly as well as indirectly, through leukocyte-dependent endothelial injury. In case of severe burns, increased vascular permeability by these mechanisms can cause severe loss of fluid which may be fatal.

Mediators causing increased vascular permeability and edema

Histamine, serotonin, C3a and C5a (liberate vasoactive amines from mast cells, other cells), bradykinin, leukotrienes C_4, D_4, E_4, neuropeptides (substance P).

Soluble mediators produced during inflammation stimulate intravascular platelets and inflammatory cells. These mediators include bradykinins, complement and activated components of the coagulation cascade and are also responsible for increased vascular permeability and edema.

Terminologies used in inflammation depending on the appearance of fluid are presented in **Table 8**.

Responses of Lymphatic Vessels and Lymph Nodes

Apart from blood vessels, lymphatics and lymph nodes also participate in acute inflammation. The regional lymphatics and lymph nodes filter the extravascular fluids. Normally, lymphatics drain the small amount of extravascular fluid that escapes out of capillaries. During inflammation, edema (excess fluid in the extravascular space) is produced due to increased vascular permeability. This increases the burden of draining the accumulated edema fluid, emigrated leukocytes, cell debris, and microbes, etc. Lymphatics carry them in the lymph into regional lymph nodes. During inflammatory reactions,

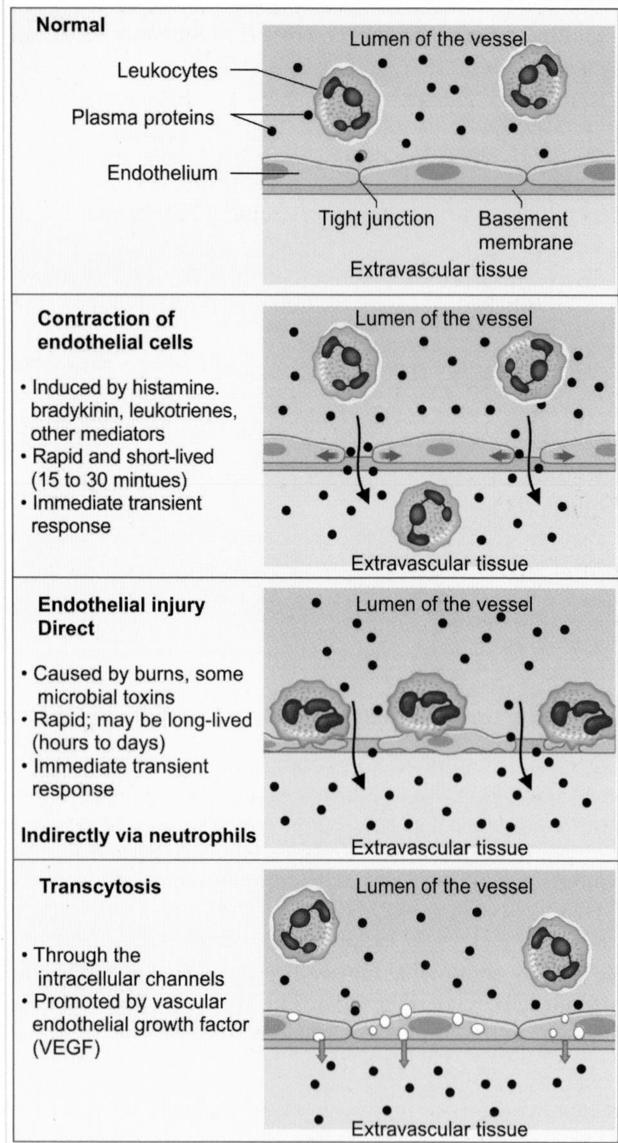

FIG. 8: Various main mechanisms of increased vascular permeability in acute inflammation and their causes and salient features. Some forms of mild injury (e.g., mild burns, irradiation or ultraviolet radiation, and exposure to certain bacterial toxins) produces vascular leakage after a delay of 2 to 12 hours and lasts for several hours or even days. It is termed delayed prolonged leakage. It may be caused by contraction of endothelial cells or mild endothelial damage (read text for details).

like blood vessels, lymphatic vessels also proliferate to handle the increased load. The draining lymphatics may become secondarily inflamed (lymphangitis), as well as draining lymph nodes also become inflamed and enlarged due to increased cellularity (lymphadenitis). This change in lymph nodes is termed reactive or inflammatory lymphadenitis. On clinical examination of a wound in skin, if lymphangitis is present, it appears as red streaks along the course of the lymphatic channels near a skin wound. Its presence indicates infection in the wound. This may be associated with painful enlargement of the draining lymph nodes and indicates lymphadenitis.

Table 8: Terminologies used in inflammation depending on the appearance of fluid.

Terminology	*Features*
Edema	Excessive accumulation of fluid in the extravascular space and interstitial tissues
Effusion	Excessive accumulation of fluid in body cavities (e.g., peritoneum or pleura or pericardial sac)
Serous effusion	Fluid without a prominent cellular response and has a yellow, straw-like color
Transudate	Edema fluid with a low protein content (specific gravity <1.015).
Exudate	Edema fluid with a high protein concentration (specific gravity >1.015) and frequently contains inflammatory cells.
Serosanguineous	Serous exudate, or effusion that contains red blood cells and has a reddish tinge
Fibrinous exudate	Contains large amounts of fibrin, due to activation of the coagulation system.
Purulent exudate or effusion	Contains prominent cellular components. They are observed in pathologic conditions, such as pyogenic bacterial infections, in which polymorphonuclear neutrophils (PMNs) predominate.
Suppurative inflammation	Purulent exudate with significant liquefactive necrosis (pus).

Leukocyte Recruitment to Sites of Inflammation

Q. Describe the leukocyte/cellular changes/events in acute inflammation.

Q. Functions of leukocytes in relation to inflammation and clinical conditions of leukocyte dysfunction.

The changes in blood flow and increased vascular permeability are rapidly followed by arrival of leukocytes into the site of injury in tissue.

Definition

Leukocyte recruitment to sites of inflammation (extravasation) is the **process of migration of leukocytes from the lumen of the vessel to the site of injury in the extravascular tissues.**

Type of Leukocytes

Leukocytic (cellular) event in acute inflammation **delivers leukocytes** capable of phagocytosis **to the site of injury** and is an essential feature of inflammation. The most important phagocytic cells involved are leukocytes, namely **neutrophils and macrophages**.

- **Neutrophils** are produced in the bone marrow. They are rapidly recruited to sites of inflammation and are **short-lived.**
- **Macrophages** (discussed on pages 306–311) are slow to respond and recruit but are **long-lived.**

Both neutrophils and macrophages have many common features and their main functions differ only slightly. Common features include phagocytosis, ability to migrate through blood vessels into tissues, and chemotaxis. However, neutrophils use cytoskeletal rearrangements and enzyme assembly to produce rapid, transient responses, whereas macrophages, being long-lived, make slower but more prolonged responses and that usually depends on new gene transcription. Major distinguishing properties between neutrophils and macrophages are presented in **Table 9**.

Functions of Leukocytes

The extravasated leukocytes perform the main function of eliminating the causative agents. These phagocytic leukocytes ingest and destroy bacteria, other microbes, necrotic tissue, foreign substances, and other injurious agents. Macrophages act as scavenger cells and also secrete growth factors that assist in repair process.

- **Can damage host cells:** Though leukocytes are defensive in inflammation, if they are strongly activated, they can cause damage to host tissue and continue inflammation. This is because the leukocyte products which are used for destruction of microbes and to "clean up" necrotic tissues can also produce "collateral damage" of normal host tissues. For example, invasion of the bloodstream by bacteria can activate systemic inflammation and the resulting systemic inflammatory response (SIRS discussed on pages 319 and 323) may even be fatal.

Migration of leukocytes from the lumen of the blood vessel across the vessel walls and into the surrounding tissue **to the site of tissue injury is a multistep process**. It is a characteristic feature of the inflammatory response and occurs in both acute and chronic inflammatory disease. **It involves mediators and is** mediated/**controlled by** sequential activation of adhesion molecules, their ligands on both neutrophils and the endothelium and cytokines. These **cytokines are called as chemokines.**

This process can be divided into different sequential phases.

- **Leukocyte adhesion to endothelium** in which there is adhesion of leukocytes to endothelium at the site of inflammation.
- **Leukocyte migration across the endothelium and vessel wall:** The leukocytes escape through the vessel wall into the extravascular tissue.
- **Leukocytes migration in the extravascular tissue:** The leukocytes that have escapes through the vessel wall into the extravascular tissue, migration toward the offending agent due to chemotactic stimulus.

Different chemical molecules or mediators are involved in each of these steps.

Leukocyte Adhesion to Endothelium

Q. Describe the role of adhesion molecules in inflammation.

Normal Blood Flow

Normally, blood flows from capillaries into postcapillary venules in an uninterrupted manner with movement of circulating blood cells in parallel layers (called laminar flow). The circulating cells are moved by sweeping movement of laminar flow and prevent the blood cells from attaching to the vascular endothelium. RBCs being the smaller cells tend to move faster than the larger white blood cells (leukocytes). Leukocytes also move rapidly in the flowing blood which

Table 9: Major distinguishing properties between neutrophils and macrophages.

Features	*Neutrophils*	*Macrophages*
Origin of cell	Hematopoietic stem cells (HSCs) in bone marrow	HSCs in bone marrow (in inflammatory reactions) Many tissue-resident macrophages: Stem cells in yolk sac or fetal liver (early in development)
Lifespan in tissues	Several days	Inflammatory macrophages: Days or weeks Tissue-resident macrophages: Years
Responses to stimuli	Rapid, short-lived, mostly by degranulation and enzymatic activity	More prolonged, slower, usually depends on transcription of new gene
Phagocytosis	Rapid ingestion of microbes	Prolonged ability to ingest microbes, apoptotic cells, tissue debris, foreign material
Reactive oxygen species	Rapidly produced by assembly of phagocyte oxidase (respiratory burst)	Less prominent
Nitric oxide	Low levels or none	Induced following transcriptional activation of inducible nitric oxide synthase (iNOS)
Degranulation	Major response caused due to cytoskeletal rearrangement	Not prominent
Cytokine production	Produces none or low levels per cell	Major functional activity, large amounts per cell, requires transcriptional activation of cytokine genes
Formation of neutrophil extracellular traps (NET)	Rapid, by extrusion of nuclear contents	Not formed
Secretion of lysosomal enzymes	Prominent	Less prominent

(HSCs: hematopoietic stem cells)

prevents them from attaching to the vascular endothelium. RBCs occupy the central axial column, and leukocytes are pushed out toward the wall of the vessel. The laminar flow prevents the cells from getting attached to the endothelium.

In inflammation, leukocytes should be stopped and then brought to the offending agent or the site of tissue damage, outside the vessels. Sequence of leukocyte events in inflammation, occurring in the vascular lumen are discussed below.

Margination

During the early phase of inflammation, because of dilation of inflamed postcapillary venules, there is slowing of blood flow (stasis). The vessel shear stress decreases, and more leukocytes (mainly neutrophils) assume a peripheral position (column) and accumulate along the endothelial surface of vessels. This **process of leukocyte redistribution** is termed as margination.

Rolling

Marginated and slowed leukocytes are able to detect and react to changes in the vascular endothelium. If the endothelial cells get activated by cytokines and other locally produced mediators, the endothelial cells express adhesion molecules. Initially, the leukocytes attach loosely/weakly to the endothelium that is expressing adhesive molecules. Then the leukocytes detach and bind again to endothelial surface and move along the endothelial surface with a mild jumping movement. This process of abrupt propelling (instead of smooth gradual) movement of leukocyte along the endothelial surface is termed as rolling. The temporary binding of leukocytes to endothelial cell is also called as **tethering**.

Q. Discuss the role of adhesion molecules involved in inflammatory response.

Q. Describe leukocyte–endothelial adhesion molecules.

Molecules involved in initial weak interaction between leukocytes and endothelial cells

The attachment of leukocytes to endothelial cells is mediated by complementary adhesion molecules. The expression of adhesion molecules is **enhanced by cytokines**. These cytokines are secreted by sentinel cells in tissues in response to microbes and other injurious agents. This makes sure that leukocytes are reach to the tissues where these stimuli are present. The two major families of molecules involved in leukocyte adhesion and migration are the **selectins and integrins**. **Selectins mediate the initial weak interactions between leukocytes and endothelium, and integrins mediate firm adhesion** (described further).

Q. Write short essay on role of selectins and integrins in acute inflammation.

Selectins (Fig. 9)

Selectins are receptors present on leukocytes and endothelium. They have an extracellular domain that binds sugars (hence the lectin part of the name). **Selectins mediate the initial weak interactions between leukocytes and endothelium** during leukocyte events in acute inflammation. The **ligands for selectin receptors are sialic acid-containing oligosaccharides** attached to glycoprotein backbones. The three members of this family of receptors are **E-selectin expressed on endothelial cells, P-selectin present on platelets and endothelium, and L-selectin found on the surface of most leukocytes**. Their corresponding ligands are presented in **Table 10**. Slectins mediate the initial rolling interactions of leukocytes.

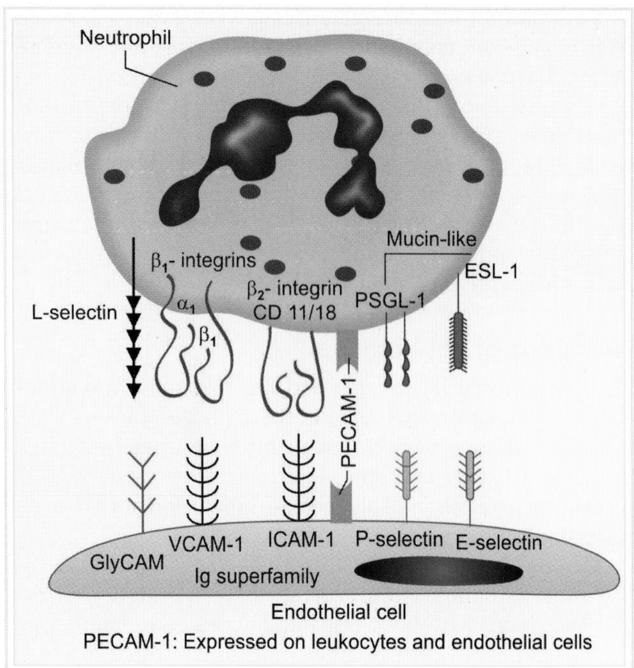

(ESL-1: E-selectin ligand; GlyCAM: glycan-bearing cell adhesion molecule; ICAM-1: intercellular adhesion molecule-1; PSGL-1: P-selectin glycoprotein ligand-1; VCAM: vascular cell adhesion molecule).

FIG. 9: Adhesive molecules on leukocyte and endothelial cell. Inflammatory mediators activate endothelial cells and leukocytes to increase expression of adhesion molecules. Sialyl–Lewis X on neutrophil PSGL-1 and ESL-1 binds to P- and E-selectins on endothelium. It causes initial weak interaction between leukocytes and endothelial cells and causes rolling of neutrophils. Increased integrins LFA-1 (CD11aCD18) on activated neutrophils bind to intercellular adhesion molecule-1 (ICAM-1) on endothelial cells and causes firm adhesion of leukocytes to endothelial cells. Leukocyte function-associated antigen-1 (LFA-1) (synonym CD11aCD18) and macrophage-1 antigen (Mac-1) (CD11bCD18) are β2 leukocyte integrins; very late antigen-4 (VLA-4) is a β1 leukocyte integrin.

Selectins and ligands on endothelial cells Normally, the endothelial selectins [(E-selectins and P-selectins) and ligand for L-selectin (glycan-bearing cell adhesion) molecule (GlyCAM)] are expressed at low levels or not at all on unactivated endothelium. These selectins are upregulated after activation of endothelium by cytokines and other mediators. This is responsible for restricted binding of leukocytes to the endothelium at sites of infection or tissue injury (where the cytokines and other mediators are produced).

- **P-selectin:** In a normal unactivated **endothelial cell**, P-selectin is stored intracellularly mainly in Weibel–Palade bodies of endothelial cells (in platelets they are stored in α-granules). During inflammation, when endothelial cells are exposed to mediators (e.g., histamine or thrombin, oxidants), very quickly within minutes, P-selectin gets mobilized to the endothelial cell surface. Once P selectin is

Table 10: Selectins and complementary selectin ligands involved in rolling.

Type of selectin (protein/synonyms)	*Distribution of selectin*	*Ligand*	*Expression of ligand*
L-selectin (CD62L)	Neutrophils, monocytes, T cells (naïve and central memory) and B cells (naïve)	Sialyl–Lewis X/PNAd on GlyCAM-1, CD34, MAdCAM-1 (MadCAM-1)	On endothelium [high endothelial venule (HEV)]
E-selectin (CD62E)	Endothelium activated by cytokines (TNF, IL-1)	Sialyl–Lewis X (e.g., CLA) on glycoproteins	On neutrophils, monocytes, T cells (effector, memory)
P-selectin (CD62P)	Endothelium activated by cytokines (TNF, IL-1), histamine, or thrombin; platelets	Sialyl–Lewis X on PSGL-1 and other glycoproteins	On neutrophils, monocytes, T cells (effector, memory)

(GlyCAM-1: glycan-bearing cell adhesion molecule-1; MAdCAM-1: mucosal adhesion cell adhesion molecule-1; TNF: tumor necrosis factor; IL-1: interleukin-1; CLA: cutaneous lymphocyte antigen-1; PSGL-1: P-selectin glycoprotein ligand-1)

at the endothelial cell surface, it is available for interaction with **its ligand, namely P-selectin glycoprotein ligand (PSGL)-1 expressed on rolling neutrophils**.

- **E-selectin and the ligand for L-selectin** are expressed on endothelium only after the endothelial cells become activated by mediators such as IL-1 and tumor necrosis factor (TNF) and cytokines. These mediators are produced by tissue macrophages, dendritic cells, mast cells, and endothelial cells themselves following infection by microbes and exposure to dead tissues.
- **L-selectin is expressed solely on leukocytes. Leukocytes express L-selectin** at the tips of their microvilli **and also express ligands for E- and P-selectins.** All of them **bind to the complementary molecules on the endothelial cells.** These interactions are low-affinity form and are easily get detached by the flowing blood. This results in repeated loose binding and detachment of leukocytes and produces rolling movement of leukocytes along the endothelial surface. These weak selectin-mediated rolling interactions slow down the leukocytes along the endothelium.

Selectins ligands on leukocytes Leukocytes have **L-selectin** at the tips of their microvilli and also **ligands for E- and P-selectins.** They bind to the complementary molecules on the endothelial cells. These are low-affinity interactions and can easily disrupt the adhesion by the flowing blood. This is responsible for initial binding and detachment and binding again that results in the process called rolling along the endothelial surface. However, these initial weak selectin-mediated rolling interactions slow down the movement of leukocytes and give them the time to recognize additional adhesion molecules on the endothelium.

Mediators involved The expression of selectins and their ligands is regulated by cytokines produced in response to infection and injury. **Cytokines includes: (1) tumor necrosis factor (TNF), (2) interleukin-1 (IL-1),** and **(3) chemokines (chemoattractant cytokines).** Cytokines are secreted by cells in tissues (tissue macrophages, mast cells, and endothelial cells), in response to microbes and other injurious stimulus and dead tissues. The endothelial selectins (E-selectins) are activated after stimulation by cytokines and other mediators. TNF and IL-1 act on the endothelial cells of postcapillary venules adjacent to the infection. They induce the coordinate expression of many adhesion molecules. Within 1 to 2 hours of injury, the endothelial cells start expressing E-selectin and the ligands for L-selectin. Chemical mediators such as histamine and thrombin, stimulate the redistribution of P-selectin from its normal intracellular stores in endothelial cell granules (namely *Weibel-Palade* bodies) to the cell surface. The low-affinity interactions are easily disrupted by the flowing blood. Thus, during initial interaction between leukocytes and endothelial cell , the leukocytes bind, detach, and bind again and detach. This is responsible for rolling of leukocyte along the endothelial surface.

Firm Adhesion of Leukocyte to Endothelium

Following initial weak interaction between endothelial cells and leukocytes, the endothelium gets activated and leukocytes bind more firmly and finally come to rest at some point (leukocyte arrest). The weak rolling interactions between leukocytes and endothelium slow down the leukocytes. This provide an opportunity for leukocyte to bind more firmly to the endothelium. These leukocytes resting on the surface of endothelial surface resemble as pebbles over the endothelium (**pavementing**) and bloodstream runs without disturbing them.

Molecules involved in firm adhesion of leukocytes to endothelium

Leukocyte surface proteins called integrins (family of leukocyte surface proteins) **and corresponding ligands on endothelium (Table 11) are responsible for firm adhesion of leukocytes to endothelium.**

Integrins

Integrins are transmembrane two-chain glycoproteins. They mediate the adhesion of leukocytes to endothelium and also of various cells to the extracellular matrix (ECM).

Expression of integrins on leukocytes Normally, integrins are expressed on plasma membranes of leukocyte in a low-affinity form. They do not attach to their specific ligands unless the leukocytes are activated by chemokines. Chemokines are chemoattractant cytokines that are produced by many cells at sites of inflammation. Chemokines attach to endothelial cell proteoglycans, and are displayed at high concentrations on the surface of endothelial cells. When the rolling leukocytes come across the chemokines displayed on endothelial cells, the leukocytes get activated. This converts integrins in leukocytes from low-affinity form to a high-affinity form. There are two groups on integrins involved in inflammatory reaction.

- **β2 leukocyte integrins: Leukocyte function-associated antigen-1 (LFA-1)** (synonym CD11aCD18) and **macrophage-1 antigen (Mac-1)** (CD11bCD18)
- **β1 leukocyte integrins: Very late antigen-4 (VLA-4)**

Table 11: Integrins along with complementary ligands involved in endothelial–leukocyte adhesion.

Integrins (proteins/synonyms)	*Distribution of integrin*	*Complementary ligands*	*Expression of ligand*
LFA-1 (CD11a:CD18 /αLβ2)	Neutrophils, monocytes, T cells (naïve, effector, memory)	ICAM-1 (CD54), ICAM-2 (CD102)	On endothelium and upregulated on activated endothelium
Mac-1 (CD11b:CD18 /αMβ2)	Monocytes, macrophages, dendritic cells (DCs)	ICAM-1 (CD54), ICAM-2 (CD102)	On endothelium and upregulated on activated endothelium
VLA-4 (CD49d:CD29/α4β1)	Monocytes, T cells (naïve, effector, memory)	VCAM-1 (CD106)	On endothelium (upregulated on activated endothelium)
α4β7 (CD49dCD29)	Monocytes, T cells (gut homing naïve effector, memory)	VCAM-1 (CD106), MAdCAM-1	On endothelium in gut and gut-associated lymphoid tissues

(ICAM: intercellular adhesion molecule; LFA-1: lymphocyte-associated function antigen; MAC-1: macrophage antigen1; VCAM: vascular cell adhesion molecule; VLA-4: very late antigen-4)

Expression of ligands for integrins on endothelial cells During high-affinity expression of integrins on leukocytes, simultaneously, other cytokines such as TNF and IL-1, activate endothelial cells to increase their expression of corresponding ligands for integrins. The various integrins and corresponding ligands on endothelial cells are presented in **Table 11**. These various ligands in endothelium include:

- **Intercellular adhesion molecule-1:** This is a ligand on endothelium for the β2 leukocyte integrins, namely **LFA-1** (synonym CD11aCD18) and **Mac-1** (CD11bCD18). LFA-1 is expressen on neutrophils and, monocytes and Mac-1 is expressed on monocytes and dendritic cells.
- **Vascular cell adhesion molecule-1 (VCAM-1):** This is a ligand on endothelium that binds to the integrin **VLA-4 on leukocytes** (i.e., β1 integrin VLA-4) (**Table 11**).

Firm binding of leukocytes to endothelium The cytokine-induced **increased expression of integrin ligands on the endothelium, combined with increased affinity** (high-affinity ligands from low-affinity) **of integrins on the leukocytes,** produces a firm integrin-mediated binding of the leukocytes to the endothelium. This occurs in the vessels at the site of inflammation. This in turn stops the rolling of leukocytes, and binding of integrins to their ligands produces signals. These signals produce changes in the cytoskeleton of leukocyte resulting in arrest and firm binding of the leukocytes to the endothelium. The importance of leukocyte adhesion molecules is clearly evident in patients with genetic deficiencies in these molecules. These patients develop recurrent bacterial infections as a consequence of impaired leukocyte adhesion and defective inflammation.

Mediators involved Cytokines are responsible for the recruitment of leukocytes to the tissues where the causative stimuli are present.

- Endothelial cells are activated by cytokines, namely TNF and IL-1, and increase the expression of ligands for integrins on leukocyte. Drugs that block TNF leukocyte recruitment are used for the treatment of chronic inflammatory diseases.
- Chemokines are chemoattractant cytokines that cause leukocyte activation and **convert low-affinity** integrins **on leukocyte to high-affinity state** resulting in firm adhesion of the leukocytes to the endothelium

Adhesive molecules are discussed in detail on pages 284–290. Various steps involved in leukocyte adhesion to endothelium in inflammation are presented in **Flowchart 1**.

Clinical Importance of Leukocyte Adhesion Molecules

- Three main types of leukocyte adhesion deficiency (LAD) have been identified.
- All are transmitted as autosomal recessive disease.
- Characterized by the inability of neutrophils to exit the circulation to sites of infection, leading to **leukocytosis** and **increased susceptibility to infection**.

Leukocyte Migration through Endothelium

Adhesion molecules in endothelial cells keep the endothelial cells to adhere to one another and seal off the vascular space from adjacent tissue. Normally, they act as an endothelial barrier and prevent leukocyte migration through blood vessel. **Across the vessel wall and the endothelium**, leukocytes migration through vascular and extravascular spaces is guided by a **complex interaction of attractants, repellents, and adhesion molecules**. After the firm adhesion and arrest of leukocytes on the endothelial surface, the next step is migration of leukocytes through the vessel wall.

Transmigration or Diapedesis

Leukocytes traverse the endothelium and the vessel wall mainly by squeezing through the intercellular junctions between endothelial cells to gain access to tissues (in the extravascular space). Chemokines act on the leukocytes adherent to the endothelium and stimulate the leukocytes to migrate through endothelium. Responding to chemokine gradients, leukocytes put forth their pseudopods and pass themselves between the adjacent intact endothelial cells (interendothelial gaps/junctions) and then come out of the intravascular space. This **process of extravasation of leukocytes** is called transmigration diapedesis. This mainly occurs in postcapillary venules because this is the site where there is maximal retraction of endothelial cells. Leukocytes migrate through interendothelial gaps toward the chemical concentration gradient. Chemical gradient is created at the site of injury or infection where the chemokines are being produced.

Molecules involved in transmigration

Endothelial cells in the vessels adhere to one another and separate the vascular space from adjacent tissue. This adhesion is brought out by vascular endothelial-cadherin complex forming an adherens junction. These adhesion molecules

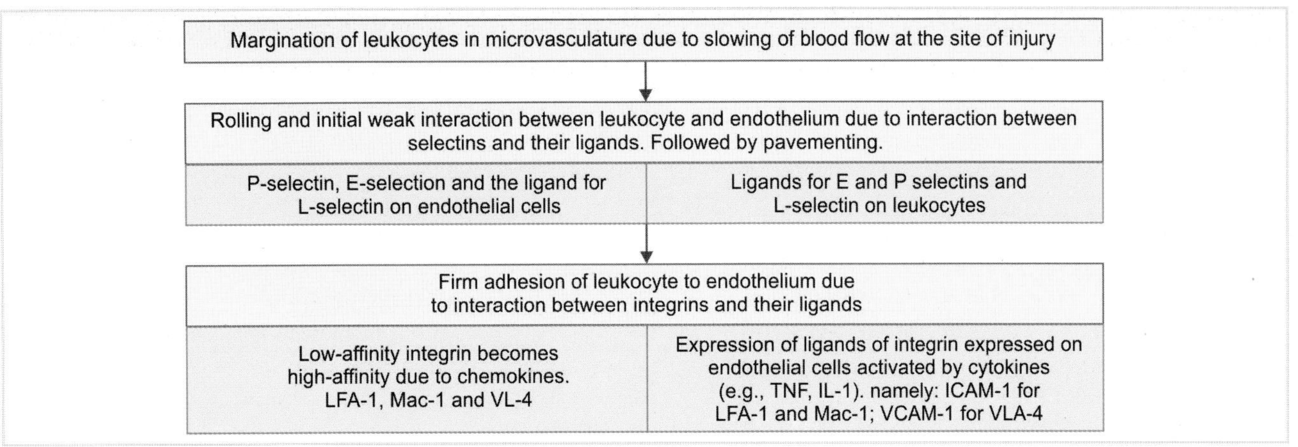

(ICAM: intercellular adhesion molecule; IL: interleukin; LFA-1: lymphocyte-associated function antigen; MAC-1: macrophage antigen-1; TNF: tumor necrosis factor; VCAM: vascular cell adhesion molecule; VLA-4: very late antigen-4)

FLOWCHART 1: Various steps involved in leukocyte adhesion to endothelium in inflammation.

act as an endothelial barrier to transmigration of cells from the vascular space and prevent leukocyte recruitment. There are several adhesion molecules present in the intercellular junctions between endothelial cells (**Fig. 10**). These are involved in the migration of leukocytes. Various molecules involved in adhesion of endothelial cells to each other include occludin, claudins, JAMs, PECAM-1, and CD99. Each of them is adherent to corresponding/homologous molecules on adjacent endothelial cells and forms tight junctions between the endothelial cells.

Immunoglobulin (Ig) superfamily (Table 12). These include mainly **cluster of differentiation 31 (CD31) or PECAM-1 (platelet endothelial cell adhesion molecule)** expressed on leukocytes and endothelial cells; intercellular adhesion molecule (ICAM-1 and ICAM-2) and junctional adhesive molecules (JAMs). **PECAM-1 is expressed on both leukocytes and endothelial cells.** This brings out the binding events needed for leukocytes to traverse the endothelium. Other adhesion molecules of the Ig superfamily are ICAM-1 and ICAM-2. They interact with integrins on leukocytes to mediate recruitment. They are expressed at the surfaces of cytokine-stimulated endothelial cells and some leukocytes.

- **Junctional adhesive molecules** (JAMs) (**Fig. 10**): JAMs are proteins of the Ig superfamily. JAM-A, JAM-B, and JAM-C are present on endothelial cells, leukocytes, and platelets. During inflammation, JAM-A binds the integrin LFA-1 (present on leukocytes), VLA-4 (present on leukocytes) binds to JAM-B, MAC1 (present on leukocytes) connects with JAM-C and allows transmigration of leukocytes.

Migration Across the Basement Membrane

After traversing the endothelium, leukocytes penetrate the basement membrane of the vessel probably by secreting collagenases (enzyme that dissolves collagen) and they enter the extravascular tissue. Usually, leukocyte transmigration does not injure the wall of the vessel. After passage of leukocytes through the basement membranes, the basement membrane of of vessels become continuous again. Various steps of leukocyte events are presented in **Figure 11**.

Various adhesion molecules in leukocyte and endothelial cells are presented in **Figure 12**.

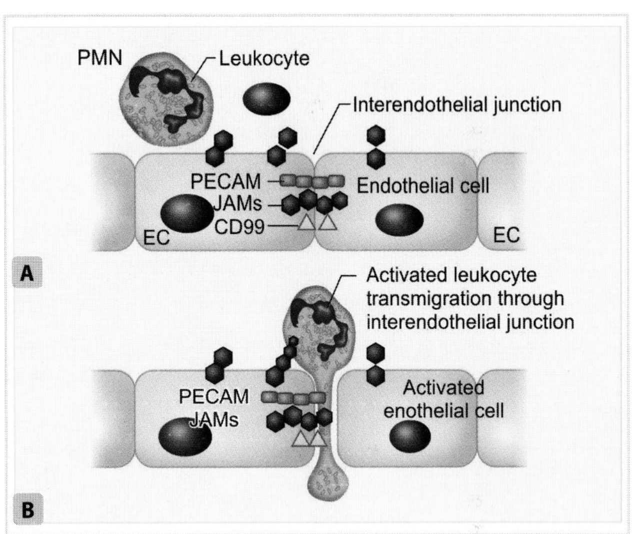

(CD31: cluster of differentiation 31; EC: endothelial cell; PMN: polymorphonuclear neutrophil; PECAM: platelet endothelial cell adhesion molecule, JAMs: junctional adhesion molecules)

FIGS. 10A AND B: Endothelial cell junctional molecules involved in transmigration of leukocyte in inflammation. (A) Junctional molecules produce cell–cell adhesion and function as an endothelial barrier. (B) During inflammation, these molecules allow transmigration of leukocytes.

Chemotaxis of Leukocytes

After leaving the circulation (i.e., intravascular) leukocytes move in the extravascular tissues towards the site of injury by a process called chemotaxis. The process of leukocyte migration toward is brought out by the chemotactic gradient created by chemokines and other chemoattractants.

Definition

Chemotaxis is defined as a dynamic and energy-dependent **process of directed migration** (locomotion) **of leukocytes along a chemical gradient**. The leukocytes move through interendothelial spaces **toward the inflammatory stimulus**

Table 12: Immunoglobulin (Ig) superfamily with complementary ligands.		
Name (synonym)	***Expressed by***	***Complementary ligands***
CD2 (LFA-2)	T cells	LFA-3
ICAM-1 (CD54)	Activated endothelium, lymphocytes, dendritic cells	LFA-1, Mac-1
ICAM-2 (CD102)	Dendritic cells	LFA-1 (CD11a:CD18/αLβ2)
ICAM-3 (CD50)	Lymphocytes	LFA-1
LFA-3 (CD58)	Antigen-presenting cells, lymphocytes	CD2
VCAM-1 (CD106)	Activated endothelium	VLA-4 (CD49aCD29)
PECAM-1 (CD31)	Endothelial cells, leukocytes	CD31 (homotypic interaction*)

*binding of an adhesion to same type of molecule on another cell

(CD: cluster of differentiation; ICAM: intercellular adhesion molecule; LFA: lymphocyte-associated function antigen; Mac-1: macrophage antigen 1; PECAM-1: Platelet/endothelial cell adhesion molecule-1; VCAM-1: vascular cell adhesion molecule-1)

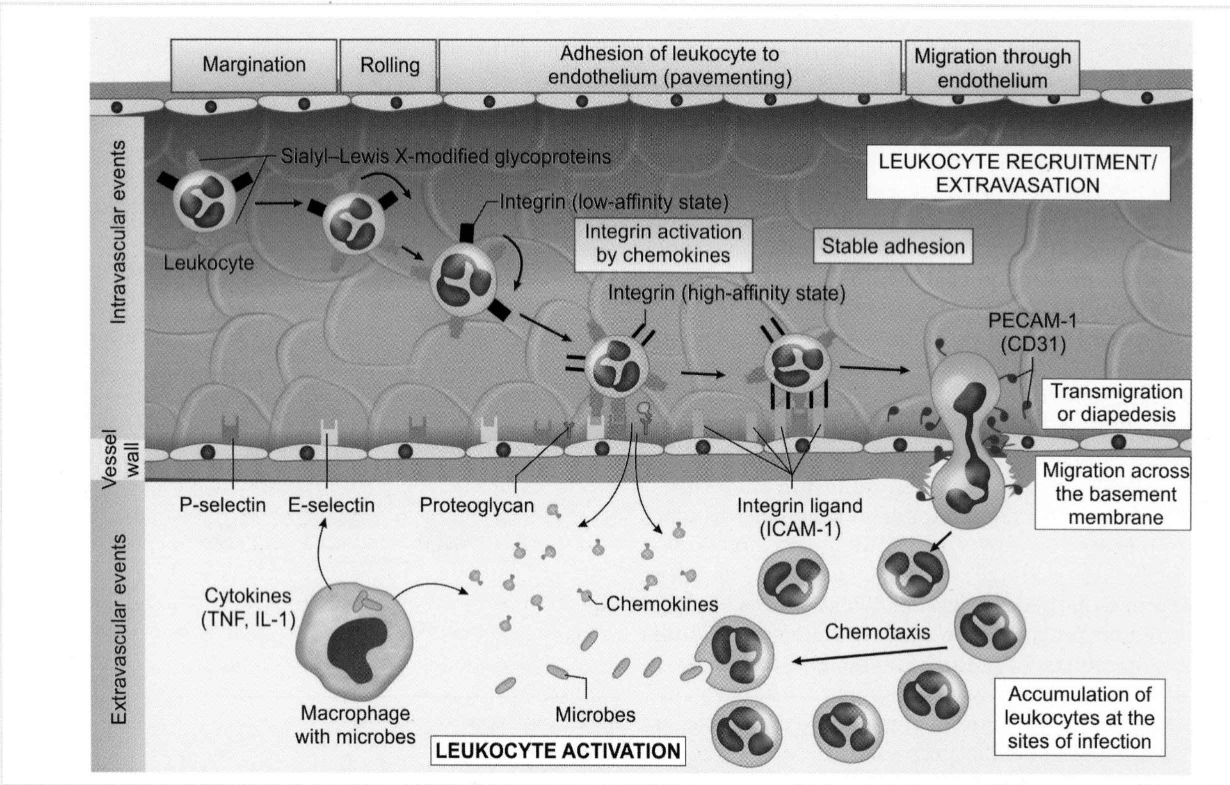

FIG. 11: Various steps of leukocyte migration through blood vessels. The leukocytes first roll, and then firmly adhere to endothelium, followed by transmigration across the endothelium. Leukocytes pierce the basement membrane and migrate toward chemoattractants from the source of injury. Selectins are involved in rolling, integrins in adhesion, and CD31 [cluster of differentiation 31 or platelet endothelial cell adhesion molecule (PECAM-1)] in transmigration.

in the **direction of the** chemical **gradient** of locally produced chemoattractants.

Chemoattractants

These chemoattractants are produced by microbes and host cells in response to infections and tissue damage, and during immunologic reactions. These may be exogenous and endogenous substances.

Exogenous

Bacterial products [e.g., peptides with N-formylmethionine termini such as FMLP (formyl-methionyl-leucyl-phenylalanine)] and some lipids.

Endogenous

These include:

- **Cytokines,** mainly belonging to the **chemokine** family (e.g., **IL-8**). The chemokines are produced at the site of injury or infection. Chemokines act on the adherent leukocytes in the vessel and stimulate them to migrate toward the site of injury. **Chemokines are the key molecules involved in leukocyte recruitment** because they produce a chemotactic gradient by binding to ECM proteoglycans. As a result, high concentrations of chemokines persist at sites of tissue injury and produce a chemical concentration gradient being maximum at the site of injury.
- **Complement components: C5a** and **C3a**

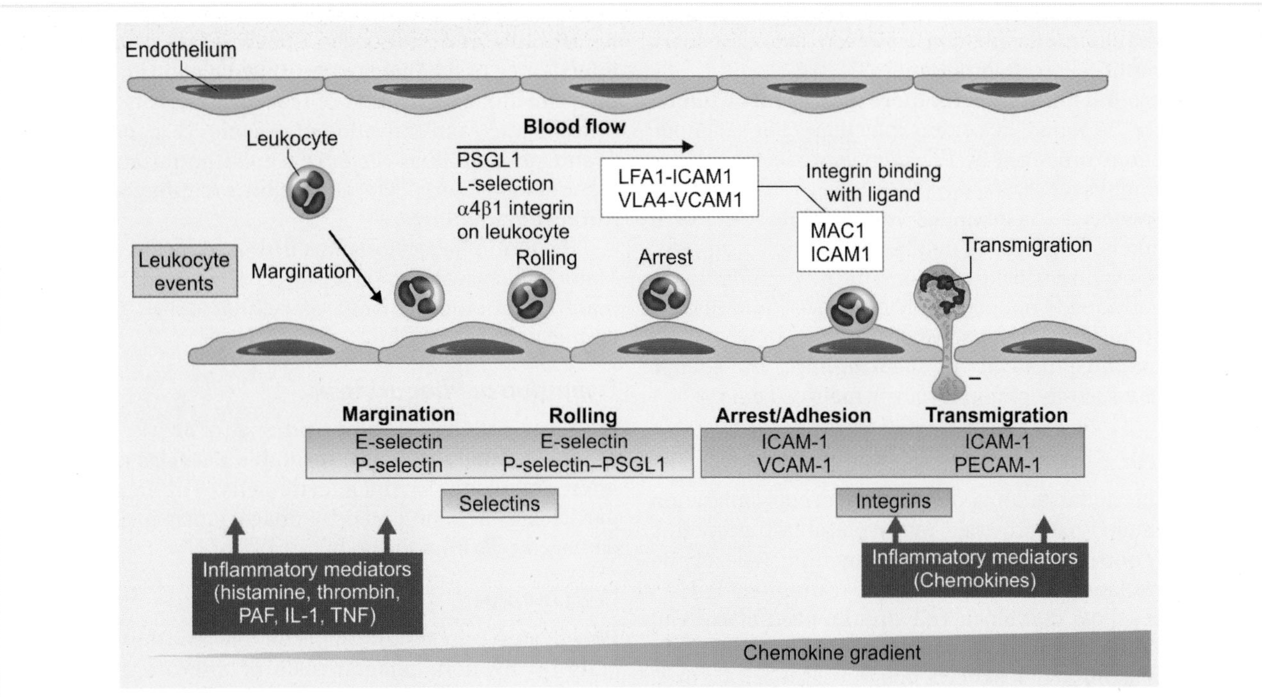

(ICAM, intercellular adhesion molecule; LFA-1, lymphocyte-associated function antigen-1; Mac-1, macrophage antigen-1; PECAM-1, platelet endothelial cell adhesion molecule; PSGL-1, P-selectin glycoprotein ligand-1; VCAM, vascular cell adhesion molecule; VLA4, very late antigen 4)

FIG. 12: Major adhesion molecules and respective ligands involved at various stages of leukocyte events in inflammation.

- **Arachidonic acid metabolites of lipoxygenase pathway: Leukotriene B4 (LTB4).**
- Products of ECM degradation

Mechanism of Chemotaxis

Both endogenous and exogenous chemoattractants act by binding to seven transmembrane G protein-coupled receptors present on the surface of leukocytes. This binding initiates signals that activate second messengers that cause polymerization of actin. This increases the amounts of polymerized actin at the leading (front) edge of the leukocyte and localize the myosin filaments at the back. The leukocyte moves by extending filopodia (thin, dynamic cell extensions consisting of tight bundles of long actin filaments covered with cell membrane) that pull the back of the leukocyte in the direction of extending filopodia. This process resembles the front wheels of a four-wheeler (automobile) pulling the rear wheel during driving. Thus, leukocytes move toward the inflammatory stimulus in the direction of the locally produced chemoattractants.

Endothelial cell junctional molecules involved in transmigration of leukocyte in inflammation are presented in **Figures 10A** and **B**.

Accumulation of leukocytes at the sites of infection and injury

Leukocytes migrate toward the chemotactic gradient produced by chemokines and other chemoattractants and they accumulate in the extravascular site. This is achieved by binding of leukocytes to the ECM proteins through integrins and CD44. CD44 is a ubiquitous multistructural and multifunctional cell surface glycoprotein. It is involved in cell-to-cell adhesion, cell-to-matrix interactions, cell migration, and cell homing. Its principal ligand is hyaluronic acid (HA, hyaluronate, hyaluronan). Apart from neutrophils and macrophages, chemotactic factors are also produced at sites of tissue injury for other cell types, including lymphocytes, basophils, and eosinophils. These chemotactic factors may be secreted by activated endothelial cells, tissue parenchymal cells, or other inflammatory cells. These chemotactic factors include platelet activating factor (PAF), transforming growth factor (TGF)-β, neutrophilic cationic proteins, and lymphokines. **The mixture of chemokines within a tissue mainly determines the types of leukocytes at the site of injury**.

Type of leukocytes infiltrates The type of the leukocyte infiltrate in acute inflammation depends on the age of the inflammatory response and the type of stimulus. Usually, following cells are observed in acute inflammation:

- **Neutrophils:** Predominantly during the first 6–24 hours. Reasons for the early preponderance of neutrophils in acute inflammations are:
  - More in number in the peripheral blood
  - Respond more quickly to chemokines
  - May attach more firmly to the adhesion molecules that are rapidly produced on endothelial cells (e.g., P- and E-selectins).

  Neutrophils are short-lived and after their accumulation at the site of injury, they undergo cell death apoptosis and disappear within 24–48 hours.
- **Monocytes and macrophages:** Neutrophils are replaced by monocytes in 24–48 hours. They are transformed into macrophages. Monocytes live longer and may also proliferate in the tissues. Thus, they are the dominant cells when inflammation is prolonged.

- **Exceptions:** The above mentioned cells are observed in most of the acute inflammation. However, there are certain exceptions of cellular infiltration.
  - **Neutrophil infiltration for more than usual 48 hours:** It may be found in certain infections. For example, infections produced by *Pseudomonas* bacteria, shows neutrophils for several days.
  - **Lymphocytes instead of neutrophils:** In viral infections, lymphocytes may be the first cells to appear. In few hypersensitivity reactions, the predominant cells are activated lymphocytes, macrophages, and plasma cells (indicates immune response).
  - **Eosinophils instead of neutrophils:** In allergic reactions, eosinophils may be the main cell type.

Therapeutic Significance

The molecular understanding of leukocyte events (migration and recruitment) has provided many possible therapeutic targets for controlling harmful inflammation. One of the important cytokines involved in leukocyte recruitment is TNF. Therapeutic agents that block TNF are the most successful therapeutics developed for treating chronic inflammatory diseases. Antagonists of leukocyte integrins also can be used for treating inflammatory diseases. Though, these antagonists can control the inflammation but can prevent the ability of these patients to protect themselves against microbes.

Phagocytosis and Clearance of the Offending Agent

Q. Discuss phagocytosis and defects in leukocyte function.

Q. Discuss the role of phagocytosis in the containment of infection and inflammation.

Recognition of microbes or dead cells by the leukocyte receptors initiates several responses in leukocytes together known as **leukocyte activation**. After leukocytes (particularly neutrophils and monocytes) have reached to the site of infection or tissue injury, they must be activated to perform their functions. Activation of leukocytes results in increased cytosolic Ca^{2+} and activation of enzymes (e.g., protein kinase C and phospholipase A_2). The most important functional responses of leukocyte activation are **phagocytosis and intracellular killing**.

The term phagocytosis was first used by Elie Metchnikoff. Many leukocytes **recognize, internalize, and digest** foreign material, microorganisms, or cellular debris by a process termed as phagocytosis.

Definition of Phagocytosis

Phagocytosis is defined as the process (or activity) of ingestion of large (usually >0.5 μm) insoluble particles and invading microorganisms by phagocytic cells. The large insoluble particles to be eliminated by phagocytosis include aged or damaged cells from the body.

Cells Involved

Phagocytes (cell eating) are effector cells, and the inflammatory cells involved in phagocytosis of micro-organisms and tissue debris include three types of white blood cells, namely neutrophils, monocytes/macrophages, and dendritic cells. These are frequently referred to as "professional phagocytes". Major phagocytes involved in acute inflammation are neutrophils and macrophages.

Steps in Phagocytosis

It consists of three **sequential** steps (**Figs. 13A** to **C**):

1. Recognition (and attachment **of the particle to be ingested by the leukocyte**)
2. Engulfment (and **internalization** with formation of **a phagocytic vacuole**)
3. Killing (of the microbe) or degradation of the ingested material.

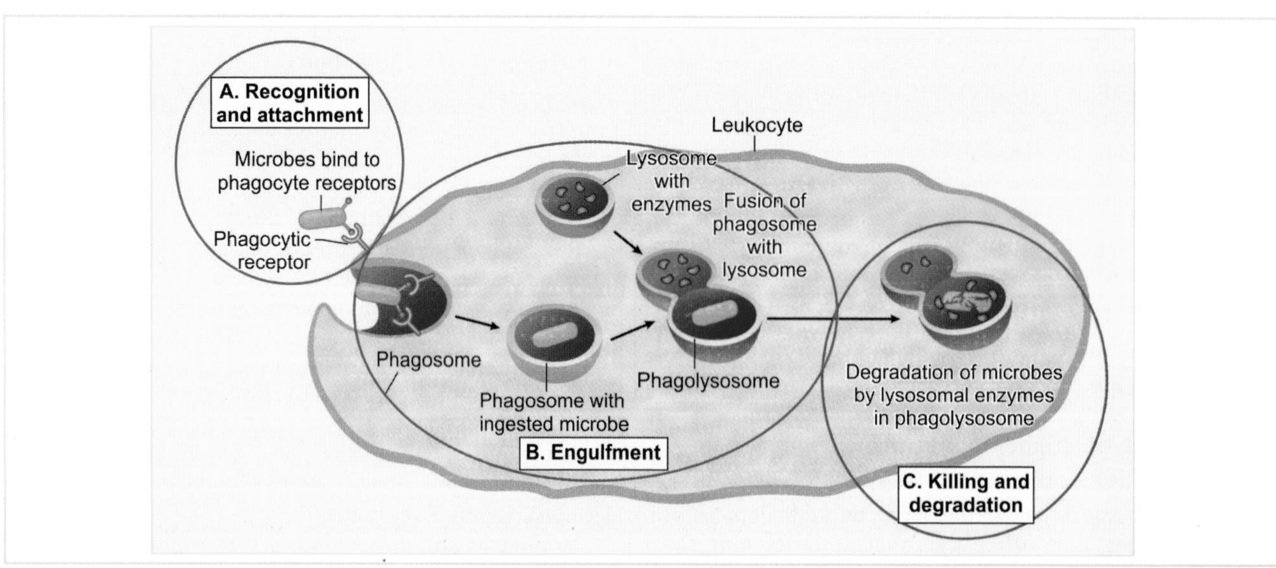

FIGS. 13A TO C: Different steps in phagocytosis. (A) Recognition and attachment which involves binding of receptors on the leukocyte membrane to injurious agent (e.g., bacteria); (B) Engulfment, formation of phagosome, and fusion of lysosomes with phagocytic vacuoles to form phagolysosome; (C) Killing/degradation of ingested particles within the phagolysosomes by lysosomal enzymes and by reactive oxygen and nitrogen species.

Recognition and attachment

Recognition by phagocytic receptors Phagocytosis is initiated when specific receptors on the surface of phagocytic cells (leukocytes) recognize their targets (e.g., components of microbes and necrotic cells).

Receptors on leukocytes Leukocytes express several receptors (**Fig. 14**) that recognize external stimuli. These include:

- **Receptors for microbial products** (e.g., TLRs)
- **G protein-coupled receptors** (recognize N-formyl methionine residues)
- **Receptors for cytokines** (for IFN-γ)
- **Macrophage mannose receptors:** These are lectins that bind to terminal mannose and fucose residues of glycoproteins and glycolipids present on microbial cell walls. In contrast to microbes, glycoproteins and glycolipids in humans contain terminal sialic acid or N-acetylgalactosamine. Therefore, mannose receptor recognizes only microbes and not host cells.
- **Scavenger receptors:** Originally, scavenger receptors were described as molecules that bind and mediate endocytosis of oxidized or acetylated low-density lipoprotein (LDL) particles that do not bind with the conventional LDL receptor. Macrophage scavenger receptors bind modified LDL particle and also interact with a variety of microbes. Macrophage integrins namely MAC-1 (CD11b/CD18), may also bind microbes for phagocytosis.
- **Receptors for various opsonins:** The capacity of phagocytosis is highly increased when leukocyte receptors recognize microbes coated (opsonized) by specific host proteins known as opsonins. Opsonins are plasma components that coat microbes/particles and tag them for phagocytosis. Main opsonins are IgG antibodies, the C3b breakdown product of complement of C3 produced during complement activation, and some plasma lectins (such as mannose-binding lectin) called collectins. Phagocytic cell contains specific high-affinity opsonic receptors. Different opsonins and their corresponding opsonic receptors on leukocyte are presented in **Table 13**.

Clinical significance of opsonins

- After exposure to antigen, B cells get activated and mature into plasma cells, which produce IgG. Defect in maturation of the B cells leads to absence of Ig production. Hence, there is **defective opsonization** in Bruton disease.
- Many pathogens have developed **mechanisms to avoid phagocytosis** by leukocytes. For example, polysaccharide capsules, protein A, protein M, or peptidoglycans around bacteria can prevent complement deposition or antigen recognition and receptor binding.

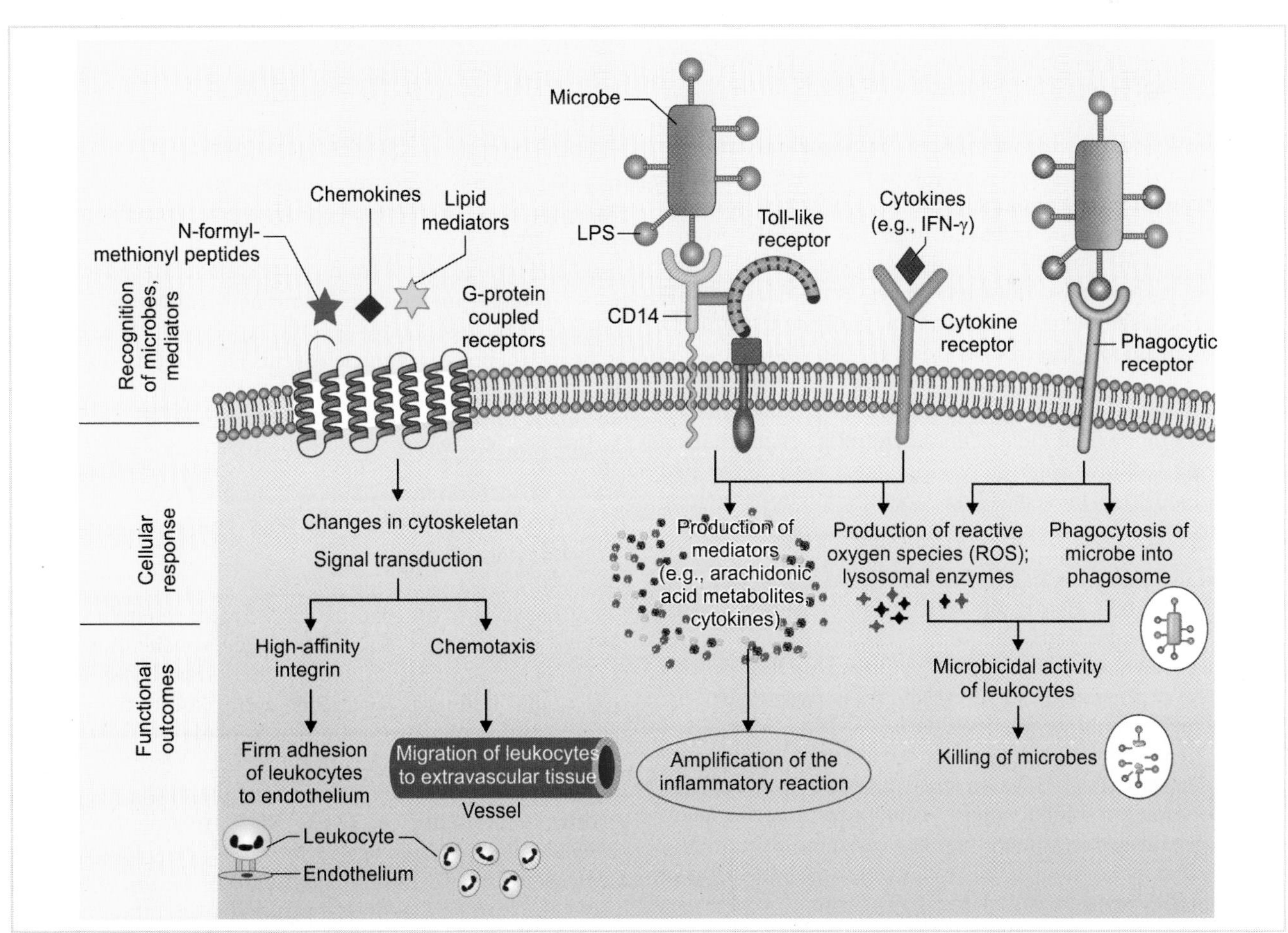

(IFN-γ: interferon-γ; LPS: lipopolysaccharide)

FIG. 14: Various types of leukocyte cell surface receptors are activated in acute inflammation. They recognize different agonists. After the receptors are stimulated, they initiate responses that mediate different leukocyte functions.

Table 13: Different opsonins and their corresponding receptors on leukocyte.

Opsonins	*Receptor on leukocyte*
Immunoglobulin G antibodies	Fc receptor (FcγRI)
Complement components C3	Type 1 and 3 complement receptor (CR1 and CR3)
Collectins	C1q

Box 5: Different methods of killing microbes or degrading ingested material during phagocytosis.

Oxidative bacterial killing:
- Reactive oxygen species
- Reactive nitrogen species

Nonoxidative bacterial killing:
- Lysosomal enzymes and other lysosomal proteins

Engulfment and internalization

Next step in phagocytosis is engulfment and formation of a phagocytic vacuole. The phagocytic process is complex and involves the integration of many receptor-initiated signals. These signal lead to membrane remodeling and cytoskeletal changes. Phagocytosis is dependent on polymerization of actin filaments present in the phagocytic cell. Therefore, many signals that trigger phagocytosis are same as those involved in chemotaxis.

- **Phagosome:** After a microbe/particle is attached to receptors on phagocytes, extensions of the plasma membrane **of leukocyte form pseudopods surrounding the** foreign material/**particle to be ingested**. These pseudopods of plasma membrane form a phagocytic cup and engulf the foreign agent. The plasma membrane then "zippers" around the opsonized particle and pinches off to form a vesicle or vacuole in the cytosol (cytoplasm) called as a phagosome. The phagosome contains the ingested particle/microbe.
- **Phagolysosome:** The membrane of **phagosome** with the foreign material fuses with membrane of cytoplasmic **lysosome to form a phagolysosome**. Lysosomal **granules are discharged or released** into this phagolysosome. The acid pH in the phagolysosome activates these hydrolytic enzymes. These lytic enzymes then degrade the phagocytosed material. Unfortunately, during this process of engulfment, the phagocyte may also liberate some contents of its lysosomal granules into the extracellular space. They may damage the innocent surrounding spectator normal cells. This is called as regurgitation during feeding. Some microorganisms have developed mechanisms to prevent killing by neutrophils by preventing lysosomal degranulation or inhibiting neutrophil enzymes.

Clinical significance of defects in phagolysosome function

***Chédiak-Higashi* syndrome:** It is an autosomal recessive condition characterized by:

- **Increased susceptibility to infections: Due to defective fusion of phagosomes with lysosomes in phagocytes.**
- Leukocyte abnormalities include:
  - Neutropenia (decreased numbers of neutrophils)
  - Defective degranulation and delayed microbial killing
  - Peripheral blood smear: Leukocytes contain giant granules, due to aberrant phagolysosome fusion.
- Gene associated with this syndrome encodes a **large cytosolic protein** called **LYST** (Lysosomal Trafficking Regulator), which **regulates lysosomal trafficking**.
- Albinism: Due to abnormalities in melanocytes
- Nerve defects
- Bleeding disorders due to defect in platelets

Killing and degradation

Intracellular Destruction of Microbes and Debris: Phagocytosis is very effective for clearing foreign debris from the site of tissue injury. Killing (destruction) or degradation is the final step involved in the disposal of ingested infectious (microbial) agents and disposal of dead-cell debris or necrotic cells. Killing and degradation process occurs within phagocytes, namely neutrophils and macrophages. These processes occur most efficiently after these phagocytes undergo activation.

Mechanism of killing microbes or clearing of phagocytosed material There are different mechanisms (**Box 5**) to **kill microbes or destroy or clear the ingested materials** in the phagocyte. Normally, all these potentially harmful substances involved in killing/degradation are preserved in lysosomes. Thus, they are separated (segregated) from the cell's cytoplasm and nucleus to avoid damage to normal cells. They come into play when phagocytosed materials in the phagosome fuse with the lysosome to form phagolysosome. An important mechanism of killing of bacteria (and also causing cellular injury) is by free radicals (oxidative method). Free radicals may be oxygen-derived free radicals [reactive oxygen species (ROS)] or nitric oxide-derived free radicals [reactive nitrogen species (RNS)]. Lysosomes contain powerful enzymes that can digest the foreign debris (or ingested/phagocytosed material) by nonoxidative method. Enzymatic activity is specific. Certain enzymes can digest only specific types of molecules, such as proteins, lipids, or nucleic acids. In contrast to specific digestion of clearing of phagocytosed material by lysosomal enzymatic method, oxygen-derived free radicals can damage/destroy whatever substrate they come in contact with.

Killing of bacteria by reactive oxygen species

Q. Write a short note on free radicals and acute inflammation.

Reactive oxygen species are chemically reactive oxygen-derived free radicals. Reactive oxygen species (also called reactive oxygen intermediates) are signal-transducing, bactericidal, and cytotoxic molecules. Leukocyte-derived ROS, released within phagosomes, are bactericidal.

Phagocytosis is accompanied by metabolic reactions in inflammatory cells. This reaction results in the production of oxygen metabolites. These ROS are reactive oxygen molecules derived from oxygen and chemically more reactive than oxygen itself. They contribute to the killing of ingested bacteria. Normally, they are rapidly inactivated, but they can be toxic to cells if inappropriately generated. The role of oxygen-derived free radicals in inflammatory reaction depends on the balance between their production and inactivation by cells and tissues.

Types of ROS (also called reactive oxygen intermediates): The oxygen-derived free radicals destroy microbes by binding and modifying cellular lipids, proteins, and nucleic acids of microbes (refer Fig. 32 of Chapter 7). Main ROS involved in inflammation are:

- Superoxide anion [$O_2^{\bullet}$ (O_2^-), one electron]: **Weak**
- Hydrogen peroxide (H_2O_2, two electrons): **Weak**
- Hydroxyl ions ($^{\bullet}OH$), three electrons: **Highly reactive**.

Mechanism of production (Fig. 15 and refer Fig. 32 of Chapter 7): The steps in the production of ROS are as follows:

- **Superoxide anion ($O_2^{\bullet}$):** In the phagocytic vacuole of leukocyte, process of phagocytosis rapidly activates reduced nicotinamide adenine dinucleotide phosphate (NADPH) oxidase (also called **phagocyte oxidase**) in the cell membrane of polymorphonuclear leukocyte. NADPH oxidase is a multicomponent electron transport complex that oxidizes NADPH to NADP. Phagocyte (NADPH) oxidase is an enzyme complex consisting of seven proteins. In resting neutrophils, different components of this enzyme are present in the plasma membrane and the cytoplasm. The activating stimuli during phagocytosis, cause the protein component of the enzymes present in the cytoplasm to translocate to the phagosomal membrane. There, they assemble and form the functional enzyme complex. Thus, the ROS are produced within the phagolysosome, where they can act on ingested particles without damaging the host cell. Activation of this enzyme NADPH oxidase is enhanced by prior exposure of cells to a chemotactic stimulus or bacterial lipopolysaccharides (LPS). NADPH oxidase increases oxygen consumption and stimulates the hexose monophosphate shunt. The HMP shunt is an alternative pathway to glycolysis and produces. nicotinamide adenine dinucleotide phosphate (NADPH). During the process, molecular oxygen is reduced to superoxide anion ($O_2^{\bullet}$). In neutrophils, this oxidative reaction occurs during phagocytosis and together, these cell responses are called as **respiratory burst**. The ROS produced within the phagolysosome can act on ingested particles without damaging the host cell.
- **Hydrogen peroxide (H_2O_2):** $O_2^{\bullet}$ is rapidly converted into hydrogen peroxide (H_2O_2) on the cell surface and in phagolysosomes by spontaneous dismutation (a process characterized by simultaneous oxidation and reduction) by **superoxide dismutase** (SOD). H_2O_2 is stable and is a source for generating additional reactive oxidants.

$$O_2^{\bullet} + 2H \rightarrow H_2O_2$$

- **Hypochlorous acid (HOCl) and hypochlorite ($HOCl^{\bullet}$):** Amount of H_2O_2 produced is insufficient and is not able to kill most of the microbes by itself. The enzyme **myeloperoxidase** (MPO) present in the azurophilic granules of neutrophils has a very strong cationic charge and is secreted from granules of neutrophils during exocytosis. Hypochlorous acid is a major oxidant created from hydrogen peroxide and chloride within the activated neutrophils at the site of inflammation. The reaction is catalyzed by the enzyme MPO. MPO can convert H_2O_2 into a powerful ROS in the presence of a halide [**halide** ion is a halogen atom bearing a negative charge/anions and includes fluoride (F^-), chloride (Cl^-), bromide (Br^-), iodide (I^-)] Halide such as chloride (Cl^-), catalyzes conversion of H_2O_2 to hypochlorous acid (HOCl). NaOCl is a potent ROS and is the active ingredient in household bleach (i.e., sodium hypochlorite is a sodium salt of hypochlorite, involved chlorination processes). $HOCl^{\bullet}$ is a powerful (potent) oxidant and a major bactericidal (antimicrobial) agent produced by phagocytic cells. HOCl can pass through membranes, causing damage to membrane proteins and lipids as well as intracellular biomolecules. $HOCl^{\bullet}$ destroys microbes either by **halogenation** [chemical reaction that involves the addition of halide/halogens (e.g., chlorine), to cellular constituents] **or by proteins and lipid peroxidation** (oxidative degradation of proteins and lipids). Hypochlorite also helps to activate neutrophil-derived collagenase and gelatinase, both of which are secreted as latent enzymes. $HOCl^{\bullet}$ also inactivates α_1-antitrypsin. The **H_2O_2–MPO–halide system is the most efficient bactericidal system present in neutrophils**. However, inherited deficiency of MPO only causes a moderate increase in susceptibility to infection.
- **Hydroxyl radical ($OH^{\bullet}$):** Reduction of H_2O_2 via the Haber–Weiss reaction forms $OH^{\bullet}$. Haber–Weiss reaction is a reaction in which toxic oxygen and hydroxyl radicals are formed from hydrogen peroxide and superoxide ($O_2^{\bullet}$) is also converted to hydroxyl radical ($OH^{\bullet}$) $OH^{\bullet}$ is also powerful, destructive (highly reactive) agent (**Fig. 16**). This occurs slowly at physiologic pH. If there is ferrous iron (Fe^{2+}) present, the **Fenton reaction** (oxidation of organic substrates by iron and hydrogen peroxide) rapidly converts H_2O_2 to $OH^{\bullet}$, which is a potent bactericidal agent. Further reduction of $OH^{\bullet}$ produces H_2O (**Fig. 15**).

Cell of Origin: Leukocytes (neutrophils and macrophages).

Mode of action: Oxygen-derived free radicals bind and modify lipids, proteins, and nucleic acids in the cells and destroy cells such as microbes. Functions of ROS include the following:

- **Physiologic function:** ROS in leukocytes **destroys** phagocytosed **microbes and necrotic cells**.
- **Pathological actions:**
    - Endothelial cell damage, which causes increased vascular permeability.
    - Injury to other cells (e.g., tumor cells, parenchymal cells, and red blood cells).
    - Inactivation of antiproteases, such as α1-antitrypsin, e.g., destruction of elastic tissues in emphysema of lung.

Extracellular release and tissue damage: Oxygen-derived radicals destroy microbes. At the same time, they may be released extracellularly from phagocyte leukocytes. This extracellular release may occur after exposure to microbes, chemokines, and antigen-antibody complexes or following a phagocytic challenge. These ROS can produce damage to host tissue during inflammation.

Antioxidant mechanism: Plasma, tissue fluids, and host cells have mechanisms that protect healthy cells from these potentially harmful oxygen-derived radicals. They are known an antioxidant mechanism. These are: (i) the enzyme superoxide dismutase, (ii) the enzyme catalase, (detoxifies H_2O_2), (iii) glutathione peroxidase (detoxifies H_2O_2), (iv) the copper-containing plasma protein ceruloplasmin, and (v) the iron-free fraction of plasma transferrin. Antioxidants are discussed on pages 165–167 (refer Box 7 Chapter 7).

Note: Monocytes, macrophages, and eosinophils also produce oxygen derived free radicals, depending on their state of

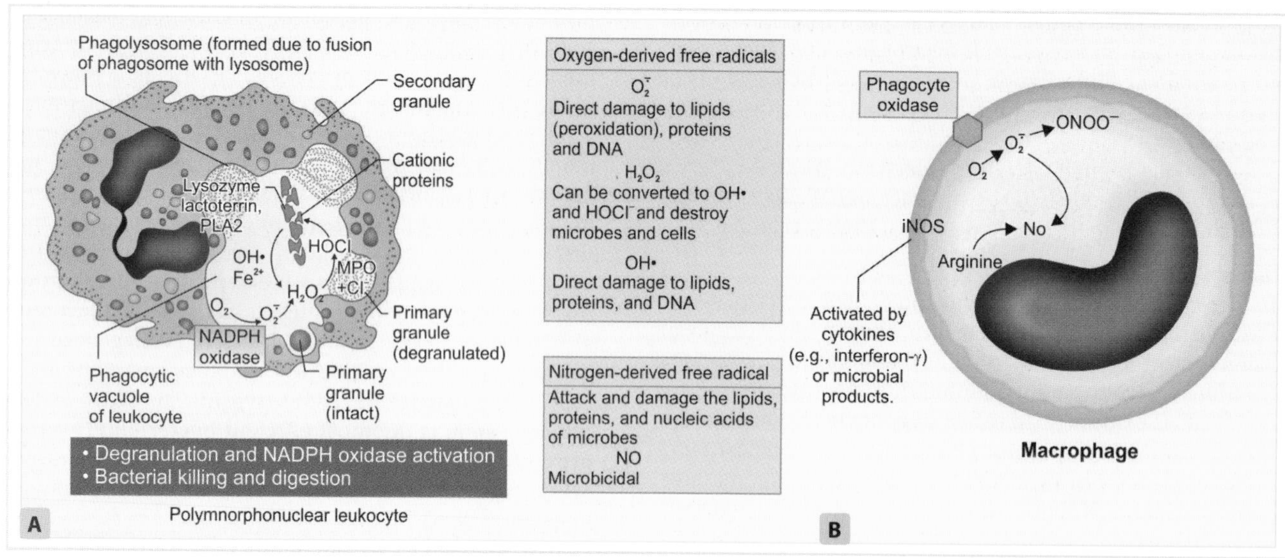

(Fe^{2+}: ferrous iron; HOCl: hypochlorous acid; iNOS: inducible nitric oxide synthase; MPO: myeloperoxidase; O_2^-, superoxide ions; OH: hydroxyl ions; PLA_2; phospholipase A_2; ROS: reactive oxygen species).

FIGS. 15A AND B: Mechanism of destruction of ingested particles within the phagolysosomes by lysosomal enzymes and by reactive oxygen and nitrogen species. (A) Oxygen-derived free radicals in polymorphonuclear leukocytes includes hypochlorite (HOCl•) and hydroxyl radical (•OH) which has microbicidal action. Both are generated from superoxide (O_2^-). (B) Reactive nitrogen species formed in macrophage. nitric oxide (NO) is produced from arginine by the action of iNOS. NO reacts with superoxide (O_2^-) and peroxynitrite (OONO•)

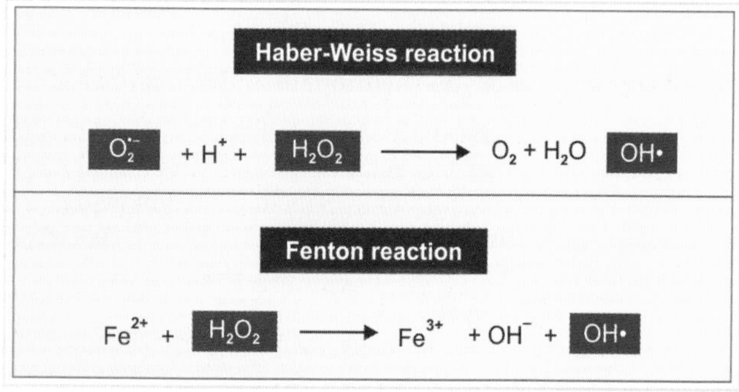

(Fe^{2+}: ferrous iron; Fe^{3+}: ferric iron; H+: hydrogen ion; H_2O_2: hydrogen peroxide; $O_2^{\bullet-}$: superoxide ion; OH–: hydroxide; OH•: hydroxyl radical)

FIG. 16: Haber–Weiss and Fenton reactions produce free radical (in red background).

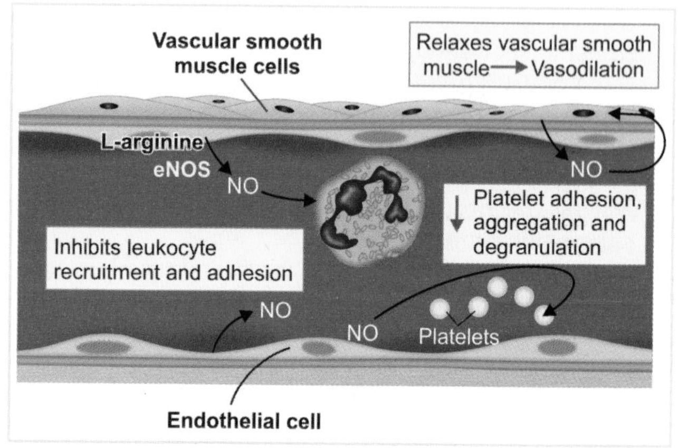

FIG. 17: Role of nitric oxide (NO) in blood vessels and macrophages. NO is produced by NO synthase enzymes. It causes vasodilation, and NO-derived free radicals are microbicidal.

activation and the stimulus. By producing ROS, these cells can have bactericidal and fungicidal activity and are also capable of killing certain parasites.

Reactive nitrogen species (Fig. 17)

Q. Write a short essay on nitric oxide in inflammation.

Q. Write a short essay on role of nitric oxide (NO) in health and disease.

Q. Nitric oxide synthase in human disease.

Q. Pathophysiological role of nitric oxide.

Nitric oxide (NO, or NO•) is a soluble, free radical gas. Nitric oxide (NO) causes vasodilation [hence formally known as endothelium-derived relaxing factor (EDRF)].

Source: Sources of reactive nitrogen species include endothelial cells, macrophages, and neurons in the brain.

Synthesis: Nitric oxide is synthesized from l-arginine (i.e., guanidino nitrogen of l-arginine), by the action of enzyme nitric oxide synthase (NOS).

Types of nitric oxide synthase: There are three different main isoforms/types of NOS—**type I neuronal (nNOS), type II inducible (iNOS), and type III endothelial (eNOS)**.

- **Endothelial NOS** and **nNOS** are constitutively expressed at low levels. The NO produced by them acts to maintain vascular tone and as a neurotransmitter, **respectively**.
- **Inducible (iNOS):** It is involved in **microbial killing**. iNOS is expressed/produced when macrophages are activated by inflammatory cytokines (e.g., IFN-γ) or microbial products. They produce both intracellular and extracellular NO, that have many roles in vascular physiology

and pathophysiology. The iNOS produces NO within macrophages. In macrophages, NO reacts with superoxide ($O_2^{\bullet}$) and produces highly reactive and cytotoxic free radical species, peroxynitrite ($ONOO^{\bullet}$). This is especially prominent when excessive production of NO is parallel with superoxide ($O_2^{\bullet}$) generation. Similar to ROS, nitrogen-derived free radicals attack and damage the lipids, proteins, and nucleic acids of both microbes as well as host cells.

Effects (actions) of Nitric Oxide: Phagocytes and endothelial cells produce $NO^{\bullet}$ and its derivatives. They have many physiologic and nonphysiologic effects. It acts in a paracrine manner on target cells. In physiologic concentrations, NO alone and in balance with superoxide anion ($O_2^{\bar{\bullet}}$), is an intracellular messenger. $NO^{\bullet}$ and other free radicals interact with one another to balance their cytotoxic and cytoprotective effects. $NO^{\bullet}$ can either react with oxygen radicals to form toxic molecules such as peroxynitrite and S-nitrosothiols (which further increase the damage), or it can scavenge/inactivate superoxide anion ($O_2^{\bar{\bullet}}$), thus reducing the amount of toxic radicals.

- **Vasodilatation** by relaxing vascular smooth muscle cells. NO generated by eNOS in endothelial cells. NO relaxes vascular smooth muscles and produces vasodilation. However, the role of NO in the vascular reactions of acute inflammation is not clear.
- **Controls inflammatory responses** by inhibiting/reducing leukocyte recruitment, leukocyte adhesion, and scavenging/removing oxygen radicals.
- NO prevents/**reduces platelet adhesion, aggregation, and degranulation** at sites of vascular injury.
- **Microbicidal killing:** NO also can kill microbes similar to ROS. Inducible (iNOS) type (one of the three types) is involved in microbial killing. Similar to ROS, the nitrogen-derived free radicals attack and damage the lipids, proteins, and nucleic acids of microbes and host cells.

Lysosomal enzymes and other lysosomal proteins Bacterial killing may also occur by nonoxidative mechanism. Phagocytic cells, particularly neutrophils and monocytes/macrophages have granules in cytosol/cytoplasm containing enzymes and antimicrobial proteins. These cytoplasmic granules are actively secretory and are different from classical lysosomes. The content of granules of different cells involved in inflammation are discussed on pages 268–279). Neutrophils contains mainly two types of granules namely: (i) smaller specific (or secondary) granules and (ii) larger azurophilic (or primary) granules. Secondary granules contain lysozyme, collagenase, gelatinase, lactoferrin, plasminogen activator, histaminase, and alkaline phosphatase. The primary granules contain MPO, bactericidal proteins (lysozyme, defensins), acid hydrolases, and many neutral proteases (elastase, cathepsin G, nonspecific collagenases, proteinase 3). Phagocytic vesicles containing engulfed material may fuse with these both types of cytosolic granules (and with lysosomes) of phagocytic cells. The liberated enzymes and antimicrobial proteins degrade/destroy the ingested materials (microbes and dead tissues) by **oxygen-independent antimicrobial activity**. Both types of granules also undergo exocytosis (degranulation) and the enzymes and antimicrobial proteins may be liberated into the extracellular space. This may produce damage to extracellular host tissue. Different enzymes in granules have functions. Acid proteases degrade bacteria and debris within the phagolysosomes. Neutral proteases degrading various extracellular components (e.g., collagen, basement membrane, fibrin, elastin, and cartilage) and causes the tissue destruction observed in inflammatory processes. Neutral proteases can also split C3 and C5 complement proteins and release a kinin-like peptide from kininogen. The released components of complement and kinins act as mediators of acute inflammation. Neutrophil elastase can degrade virulence factors of bacteria and thus fight against bacterial infections. Macrophages also contain acid hydrolases, collagenase, elastase, phospholipase, and plasminogen activator. Various enzymes and antimicrobial (bactericidal) proteins are as follows:

- **Lysosomal acid hydrolases:** Primary and secondary granules present in neutrophils and lysosomes of mononuclear phagocytes contain hydrolases. These hydrolases include sulfatases, phosphatases, and other enzymes which can digest polysaccharides (carbohydrate) and DNA.
- **Bactericidal/permeability-increasing protein (BPI):** This is a cationic protein present in primary granules of neutrophils. It can kill many gram-negative bacteria but is not toxic to gram-positive bacteria or normal host cells. BPI enters into outer membranes of bacterial envelope and increases their permeability. This is followed by activation of certain phospholipases and enzymes that degrades bacterial peptidylglycans.
- **Defensins:** These are cationic proteins present in primary granules of neutrophils and lysosomes of some mononuclear phagocytes. These defensins can kill many gram-positive and gram-negative bacteria, fungi, and some enveloped viruses. Some defensins can also kill host cells. Defensins are also chemotactic for phagocytes, immature dendritic cells, and lymphocytes. Thus, they can also help in mobilizing and amplifying antimicrobial immunity.
- **Lactoferrin:** It is an iron-binding glycoprotein present in secondary (specific) granules of neutrophils and also in most body secretory fluids. Since this chelating agent chelates iron, it competes with bacteria for iron. It may help production of $OH^{\bullet}$ for oxidative killing of bacteria.
- **Lysozyme:** This is a bactericidal enzyme present in many tissues and body fluids, in primary and secondary granules of neutrophils, and in lysosomes of mononuclear phagocytes. Lysozyme hydrolyzes the muramic acid-*N*-acetylglucosamine bond found in the glycopeptide coat of all bacteria. Peptidoglycans present in the cell wall of gram-positive bacteria are sensitive to degradation by lysozyme. However, gram-negative bacteria are usually resistant to it.
- **Eosinophil's bactericidal proteins:** Granules of eosinophils contain several cationic proteins. The most important are major basic protein (MBP) and eosinophilic cationic protein. Both are powerful in killing many parasites, though not bacteria. MBP constitutes about 50% of the total protein of eosinophil granules.

Other microbicidal granule contents include cationic arginine-rich granule peptides (toxic to microbes) and cathelicidins, (antimicrobial proteins found in neutrophils and other cells).

Defects in Leukocyte Function

Inherited defects in microbicidal activity

Inherited (congenital) diseases of defective phagocytic cell function are characterized by recurrent bacterial infections. They are presented in **Table 14**.

Leukocyte adhesion deficiencies (LAD) It is due to inherited defects in adhesion molecules. It impairs leukocyte recruitment to sites of infection and is characterized by recurrent bacterial infections. LAD-1 is caused by defects in the β_2 chain that is shared by the integrins LFA-1 and Mac-1. LAD-2 is caused by a defect in fucosyl transferase that is required to synthesize functional sialyl-Lewis X, the ligand for E- and P-selectins. This leads to a defect in a fucosyl transferase which is an enzyme that attaches fucose moieties to protein backbones. Both LAD-1 and LAD-2 are associated with defect of leukocyte adhesion to endothelium. This prevents the leukocytes from migrating into tissues. These patients are susceptible to bacterial infections, which are generally recurrent and frequently life threatening.

Hyper-IgE syndrome (job syndrome)
- Recurrent abscesses, eczema, eosinophilia, and high serum levels of IgE.
- Autosomal dominant and sporadic cases

Table 14: Inherited (congenital) diseases of defective phagocytic cell function.

Disease	*Defect*
Leukocyte adhesion deficiency (LAD)	
Leukocyte adhesion deficiency 1	Defective leukocyte adhesion because of mutations in the β chain of CD11/CD18 integrins. There is defective β2-integrin expression or function
Leukocyte adhesion deficiency 2	Defective leukocyte adhesion because of mutations in fucosyl transferase required for synthesis of sialylated oligosaccharide (receptor for selectins). There is defective fucosylation and selectin binding
Hyper-IgE-recurrent infection, (Job syndrome)	Poor chemotaxis
Chédiak–Higashi syndrome	Decreased leukocyte functions due to mutations affecting protein involved in lysosomal membrane traffic (defective lysosomal granules) Poor chemotaxis
Neutrophil-specific granule deficiency	Absent neutrophil granules
Chronic granulomatous disease	Decreased oxidative burst. Deficient NADPH oxidase, with no production of H_2O_2
• X-linked	Defect in phagocyte oxidase (membrane component)
• Autosomal recessive	Defect in phagocyte oxidase (cytoplasmic components)
Myeloperoxidase (MPO) deficiency	Decreased microbial killing because of defective MPO–H_2O_2 system. There is deficient production of $HOCl^-/OCl_2^-$

(H_2O_2: hydrogen peroxide; $HOCl^-$: hypochlorous acid; Ig: immunoglobulin; NADPH: nicotinamide adenine dinucleotide phosphate; OCl_2^-: dichlorine oxide)

Chédiak-Higashi syndrome (refer pages 240 and 1119) It is a autosomal recessive condition in which there is defective fusion of phagosomes and lysosomes. This results in defective phagocyte function and susceptibility to infections. The gene associated with this disorder encodes a large cytosolic protein called LYST (lysosomal trafficking regulator). This LYST regulates lysosomal trafficking.

Main leukocyte abnormalities These include neutropenia, defective degranulation, and delayed microbial killing.

Peripheral smear In peripheral blood smears, the **affected leukocytes show giant granules,** which are probably the result from aberrant phagolysosome fusion.

Other abnormalities These include abnormalities in melanocytes (leading to albinism), cells of the nervous system (associated with nerve defects), and platelets (causing bleeding disorders).

Chronic granulomatous disease

Q. Write a short essay on chronic granulomatous disease.

One of the examples of the disease characterized by defect in oxygen-dependent bacterial killing is **chronic granulomatous disease (CGD)** of childhood. It is a group of congenital (inherited) disorders characterized by inherited defects in the genes encoding components of phagocyte oxidase (NADPH oxidase). NADPH oxidase is the phagolysosomal enzyme that is needed for the production of ROS such as superoxide ($O_2^{\bullet}$). This leads to defects in bacterial killing. Patients fail to produce superoxide ($O_2^{\bullet}$) and H_2O_2 during phagocytosis and are susceptible to recurrent infections (especially with gram-positive cocci).

Decreased oxidative burst It is due to **defects in** the genes encoding components of **phagocyte oxidase (NADPH oxidase)** which generates superoxide anion ($O_2^{\bullet}$ S). Variants of phagocyte oxidase defect are:
- X-linked defect: Defect in the gene coding one of the membrane-bound component (gp91phox) of NADPH/ phagocyte oxidase.
- Autosomal recessive: Defect in the gene encoding two of the cytoplasmic components (p47phox and p67phox) NADPH/phagocytic oxidase.

Patients are susceptible to recurrent bacterial infection. Disease is named granulomatous because the initial neutrophil defense is inadequate and there is **chronic inflammatory reaction rich-macrophage** that appears at sites of infection, if the initial neutrophil defense is inadequate. These collections of activated macrophages try to control the infection and form granulomas. These collections of activated macrophages try to wall off the microbes, forming aggregates (called granulomas).

Diagnosis of CGD Following tests can be performed:
- **Nitroblue-tetrazolium (NBT) test:** This test depends on the direct reduction of NBT by superoxide anion ($O_2^{\bullet}$) to form an insoluble formazan. It is positive in normal individuals (with NADPH oxidase), but negative in CGD.
- **Dihydrorhodamine (DHR) test:** In this test, whole blood is stained with DHR, incubated and stimulated to produce superoxide anion ($O_2^{\bullet}$). This free radical reduces DHR to rhodamine in cells with normal NADPH oxidase.
- **Cytochrome C reductase assay:** This is an advanced test that quantifies the amount of superoxide anion ($O_2^{\bullet}$) that can be produced by patient's phagocytes.

MPO deficiency

Decreased microbial killing because of defective MPO-H_2O_2 system. Patients with genetic deficiency in MPO cannot produce HOCl and are extremely susceptible to fungal infections with *Candida*.

Toll-like receptors defects

They are rare. Mutations in TLR3 (a receptor for viral RNA) are characterized by recurrent herpes simplex encephalitis. Mutations in MYD88 (an adaptor protein needed for signaling downstream of multiple TLRs) are associated with destructive bacterial pneumonias.

Acquired Defects of Leukocyte Functions

Quantitative deficiency of leukocyte

Decreased production of leukocytes: The importance of acute inflammatory cells in protection against infection is realized in a patient with depleted or defective neutrophils. They develop frequent and severe infections. Examples include bone marrow suppression due to tumors, radiation, and chemotherapy. The most common is iatrogenic neutropenia due to cancer chemotherapy.

Qualitative/functional Deficiency of Leukocyte

Functional deficiency of phagocytes may occur at any step in the leukocytic events. Thus, it may involve leukocyte adhesion, emigration, chemotaxis, and phagocytosis or killing. These disorders may be acquired or congenital.

- **Defect in leukocyte adhesion and chemotaxis:** It may be observed in conditions such as diabetes mellitus, malignancy, sepsis, malnutrition, chronic dialysis etc.
- **Defects in phagocytosis and microbicidal activity:** It may be observed in conditions such as leukemia, anemia, sepsis, diabetes mellitus, viral infections, malnutrition.

Summary of Leukocyte Events in Acute Inflammation

Main feature of inflammation is leukocyte accumulation [especially polymorphonuclear neutrophils (PMNs)], in affected tissues. Quick recruitment of leukocytes needs a response managed by chemoattractant that causes directed cell migration. A variety of inflammatory stimuli (e.g., proinflammatory cytokines, bacterial endotoxins, and viral proteins) stimulate endothelial cells to allow leukocytes adhere to endothelium. Leukocytes adhere to activated endothelium and get themselves activated in the process. These leukocytes crawl along the interendothelial junctions of the vessel wall and migrate from the vascular space into surrounding tissue. In the extravascular tissue, leukocytes ingest foreign material, microbes, and dead tissue by phagocytosis. Leukocyte events in inflammation are summarized in **Flowchart 2**.

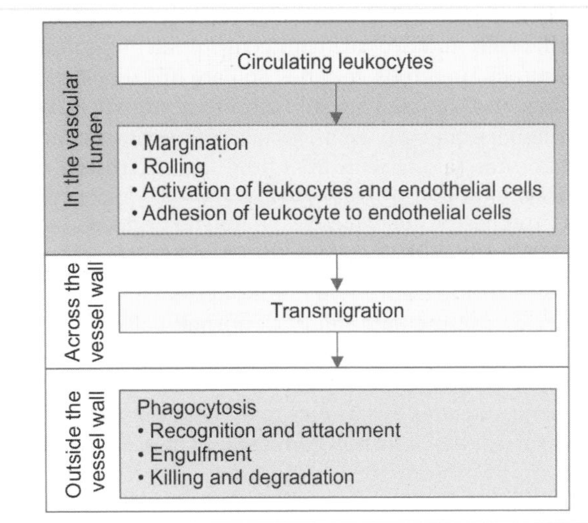

FLOWCHART 2: Leukocyte events in acute inflammation.

Termination of the Acute Inflammatory Response

Inflammation is a powerful mechanism of host defense and is capable of causing tissue injury. Hence, it requires a tight controls to minimize damage to host tissue. **Inflammation is terminated after the elimination of the offending agent.** It is brought out by the following:

- Acute inflammatory process is reduced after the causative agents are removed. This is because of the following properties of the **mediators of inflammation. Mediators—**
  - Are produced only as long as the stimulus persists
  - Have short half-life span
  - Are degraded after their release
- **Neutrophils also have short lifespan** and die by apoptosis within hours to a day or two after leaving the bloodstream.
- There are a variety of **termination mechanisms** which stop the inflammatory process. These include:
  - A switch in the type of metabolite produced from arachidonic acid, namely proinflammatory leukotrienes to anti-inflammatory lipoxins (refer pages 253–254).
  - The liberation of anti-inflammatory cytokines (e.g., TGF-β and IL-10) from macrophages and other cells.

Mechanism of Tissue Injury in Acute Inflammation

Q. Mechanism of tissue injury in inflammation.

Introduction: Main three functions of inflammatory cells in acute inflammation are:

- Phagocytosis of microorganisms and tissue debris
- Enzymes released by inflammatory cells provide antimicrobial defense and debridement
- Inflammatory cells kill bacteria by ROS and nonROS-mediated mechanisms

Inflammatory cell enzymes are needed for antimicrobial defense and debridement. PMNs (polymorphonuclear leukocytes) and macrophages are important for degradation of microbes and cell debris. However, they may also cause tissue injury. PMNs release their contents in the cytoplasmic granule at sites of injury. This is a double edged sword. On one hand, the proteolytic enzymes breakdown and debride the damaged tissue and facilitate tissue repair. On the other hand, these proteolytic degradative enzymes can damage endothelial and epithelial cells and degrade connective tissue. Inflammatory cells contain numerous enzymes and are utilized to degrade microbes and tissue. They are discussed on 268–279. The tissue damage/injury in acute inflammation may be induced by leukocytes (along with ROS produced by them) or the proteases.

Leukocyte-mediated Tissue Injury

Causes of tissue damage by leukocytes

Leukocytes can mediate injury to normal cells and tissues under many situations.

- **During defense against infection:** During normal defense reaction against infectious microbes, the tissues at or near the site of infection can undergo damage. In certain infections where they are difficult to eradicate (e.g., tuberculosis and chronic viral hepatitis), and the duration of inflammation is prolonged, the host response can cause damage to the tissue than to the causative agent.
- **Autoimmune diseases:** In some autoimmune diseases, there is inappropriately directed inflammatory response against own tissue [e.g., rheumatoid arthritis, systemic lupus erythematosus (SLE), Hashimoto thyroiditis].
- **Hypersensitivity reactions:** These disorders are characterized by exaggerated response by the host against usually harmless environmental substances (e.g., bronchial asthma, drug reactions, allergic reactions).

Mechanism of tissue damage

In all leukocyte-mediated tissue injuries, the mechanisms by which leukocytes damage normal tissues are the same as the mechanisms involved in antimicrobial defense.

Releasing injurious molecules When the leukocytes are activated, they cannot distinguish between offender (e.g., microbes) and host. During leukocyte activation and phagocytosis, neutrophils and macrophages produce microbicidal substances (e.g., ROS, NO, and lysosomal enzymes) within the phagolysosome. These injurious molecules/substances are also released into the extracellular space and are capable of damaging normal cells and vascular endothelium. They may exaggerate the effects of the initial injurious agent. Leukocyte granules contain potentially toxic molecules. The contents of granules may be released by leukocytes into the extracellular space by several mechanisms. Normally, activated leukocytes during inflammation secrete their granule contents by degranulation in a controlled manner. If unchecked or inappropriately directed against host tissues, the leukocyte infiltrate itself becomes the offender. **Leukocyte dependent tissue injury is responsible for many acute and chronic human diseases** (refer **Table 1**).

Frustrated phagocytosis If leukocytic phagocyte encounters materials that cannot be easily ingested (e.g., immune complexes deposited on immovable flat surfaces such as glomerular basement membrane), the leukocytes cannot surround and ingest these substances. This is called "frustrated phagocytosis". This further activates leukocytes and release of more amounts of enzyme present in granule and lysosomes into the extracellular environment. Some phagocytosed substances (e.g., urate and silica crystals), may damage the membrane of the phagolysosome and can release damaging contents into the extracellular space. In some instances, phagocytosed substances (e.g., urate crystals) may damage the membrane of the phagolysosome and thereby release contents of lysosomal granule.

Damage by ROS The oxygen derived free radicals (i.e., ROS) destroy microbes, but may be released extracellularly from leukocytes after exposure to microbes, chemokines, and antigen-antibody complexes, or following a phagocytic challenge. These ROS are implicated in tissue damage accompanying inflammation.

Proteinases

The term "protease" is used for a broad group of enzymes that degrade proteins by hydrolysis of peptide bonds and are also called as proteolytic enzymes. There are mainly two types of proteases. Some proteases (proteolytic enzymes) act best on intact proteins, whereas others preferably act on small peptides. The term "proteinase" is used for proteases that show specificity for intact proteins. Proteinases are proteolytic enzymes stored in cytoplasmic granules and **secretory vesicles of neutrophils** (see page 269–270). They split the peptide bonds in polypeptides (proteins). During leukocyte events, PMNs leave/emigrate from the blood circulation into the ECM. They release proteinases from their granules which help them to penetrate the ECM and migrate to sites of injury by chemotaxis. At the site of injury, they degrade matrix, cell debris, and pathogens. Apart from neutrophils, **other sources of proteinases include monocytes, eosinophils, basophils, mast cells, lymphocytes, and tissue cells, including endothelium.**

Categories of proteinases

They are grouped depending on their catalytic activity into different types, namely neutral proteases and acid proteases.

Neutral proteases They are neutral enzymes and include serine proteinases and metalloproteinases. They work in extracellular spaces and are capable of degrading various extracellular components. These components include collagen, basement membrane, fibrin, elastin, and cartilage, and produce tissue destruction observed in inflammatory processes.

- **Serine proteinases:** Serine proteinases are most important for digesting (degrading) molecules/proteins in the ECM. They also degrade cell debris and bacteria in the ECM. Leukocyte elastase mainly degrades fibronectin. Cathepsin G converts angiotensin I to angiotensin II. This brings down its action by causing contraction of smooth muscle and increasing the vascular permeability. Urokinase-type plasminogen activator (uPA) dissolves fibrin clots and generates plasmin at the site of wound, degrades ECM proteins and activates procollagenases and creates route for migration of leukocytes. Serine proteinases also modify cytokine activity. They solubilize membrane bound cytokines and receptors by cleaving active cytokines from inactive precursors. They also detach cytokine receptors from cell surfaces and regulate cytokine activity.
- **Metalloproteinases:** There are about 25 metallo-proteinases. Matrix metalloproteinases (**MMPs**, matrixins) can degrade all components of ECM, including basement membranes. They are subclassified by substrate specificity into interstitial collagenases, gelatinases, stromelysins, metalloelastases, and matrilysin. Proteins with metalloproteinase and disintegrin domains (ADAMs)

regulate neutrophil infiltration. They target disintegrins, polypeptides, and disrupt integrin-mediated binding of cells to each other and to the ECM.

Acid proteases These act in the acidic medium of lysosomes and include cysteine proteinases and aspartic proteinases. These enzymes target many intracellular and extracellular proteins. These targets include—(1) inflammatory products, (2) debris from damaged cells, microbial proteins, and matrix proteins, (3) microorganisms (e.g., bacteria) and debris within phagolysosome, (4) plasma proteins, including complement and clotting proteins, Igs and cytokines, (5) matrix macromolecules (e.g., collagen, elastin, fibronectin, and laminin), and (6) lymphocytes and platelets. Macrophages also contain acid hydrolases, collagenase, elastase, phospholipase, and plasminogen activator.

- **Cysteine proteinases and aspartic proteinases:** These are acid proteinases. They function mainly within lysosomes of leukocytes and degrade intracellular proteins.

Examples of proteins present in the granules of neutrophil, eosinophil, and basophil are presented in **Table 15**. Proteinases involved in inflammation are presented in **Box 6**.

Mechanisms of cell and tissue damage in inflammation are presented in **Flowchart 3**.

Proteinase inhibitors

Control of damage induced by proteases If the initial leukocytic infiltration continues and remains unchecked, the destructive effects of enzymes of leukocyte granules can be released extracellularly and damage tissue during inflammation. This can further continue inflammation. These harmful proteolytic environments of proteinases are normally controlled or regulated by a system of antiproteases in the serum and tissue fluids. These antiproteases constitute few proteinase inhibitors. The proteinase inhibitors and main action are listed in **Table 16**. Most important is α1-antitrypsin, which is the major inhibitor of neutrophil elastase. A deficiency of these inhibitors can lead to sustained action of leukocyte proteases. This is observed in patients with α1-antitrypsin deficiency. Neutrophil elastase destroys infections by degrading virulence factors of bacteria. During wound healing, these antiproteases protect tissue from proteolytic damage by limiting protease activity. ECM remodeling maintains a balance between proteolytic enzymes and their inhibitors. In chronic wounds, continuous recruitment of neutrophils, with their proteases and ROS, may dominate and inactivate these protease inhibitors. This will allow continuation of proteolysis.

Control of damage induced by ROS In case of damage by ROS, the serum, tissue fluids and host cells have antioxidant mechanisms which can protect tissue damage caused by these potentially harmful oxygen-derived radicals.

Proteinase inhibitors and their main action are presented in **Table 16**.

Box 6: Proteinases in inflammation.

Enzyme Class with Examples
- Neutral Proteinases
  - Serine Proteinases
    - Leukocyte elastase
    - Cathepsin G
    - Proteinase 3
    - Urokinase-type plasminogen activator
  - Metalloproteinase
    - Collagenases
    - Gelatinases
    - Stromelysins
    - Matrilysin
    - Metalloelastase
    - ADAMs (A protein with disintegrin and metalloproteinase domains)
- Acidic Proteinases
  - Cysteine Proteinases
  - Cathepsins
  - Aspartic Proteinases

Table 15: Examples of proteins present in the granules of neutrophil, eosinophil, and basophils.

Cell type	*Molecule in granule*	*Examples*	*Function*
Neutrophil	Proteases	Elastase, collagenase	Tissue remodeling
	Antimicrobial proteins	Defensins, lysozyme	Direct killing of pathogens
	Protease inhibitors	α-1-antitrypsin	Regulates proteases
	Histamine		Vasodilation, inflammation
Eosinophil	Cationic proteins	Eosinophil peroxidase	Induces formation of ROS
		Major basic protein (MBP)	Vasodilation, degranulation of basophil
	Ribonucleases	Eosinophil cationic protein (ECP), Eosinophil-derived neurotoxin (EDN)	Antiviral activity
	Cytokines	Interleukin (IL)-4, IL-10, IL-13, tumor necrosis factor (TNF)-α	Modulates adaptive immune responses
	Chemokines	RANTES, macrophage inflammatory protein (MIP)-1α	Attract leukocytes
Basophil/mast cell	Cytokines	IL-4, IL-13	Modulates adaptive immune
	Lipid mediators	Leukotrienes	Regulates of inflammation
	Histamine		Vasodilation, smooth muscle activation

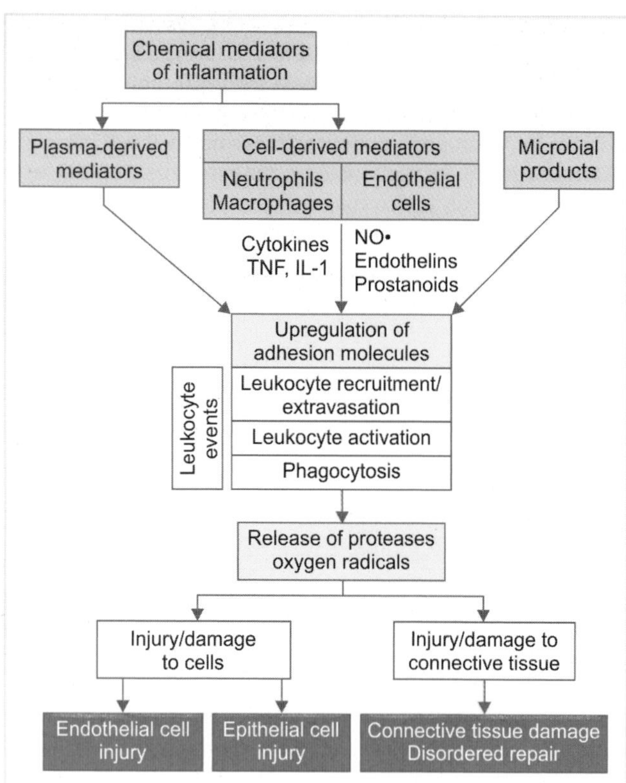

(IL: interleukin; LPS: lipopolysaccharide; NO•: nitric oxide; TNF: tumor necrosis factor)

FLOWCHART 3: Mechanisms of cell and tissue damage in inflammation.

Table 16: Proteinase inhibitors and their main action.

Proteinase inhibitors	*Target and main action*
α_2-Macroglobulin	Nonspecific inhibitor of all classes of proteinases. Mainly found in plasma
Serpins	Major inhibitors of serine proteinases
α_1-Antiproteases (α_1-antitrypsin, α_1-antichymotrypsin)	Inhibit human leukocyte elastase and cathepsin G
Secretory leukocyte proteinase inhibitor (SLPI), Elafin	Inhibit proteinase 3
Plasminogen activator inhibitors (PAIs)	Inhibit urokinase-type plasminogen activator (u-PA)
Tissue inhibitors of metalloproteinases (TIMP-1s)	Specific for tissue matrix metalloproteinases

Box 7: Role of macrophages in inflammation.

- Secretion of cytokines: They can either amplify or limit inflammatory reactions
- Production of growth factors: Stimulate the proliferation of endothelial cells and fibroblasts and the synthesis of collagen
- Enzymes: They remodel connective tissues.
- Important in chronic inflammation and tissue repair

Protection from inflammatory injury by stress proteins

When cells are stressed, many cells undergo irreversible injury and undergo death. Others may undergo severe damage. It is observed that, mild heat treatment before potentially lethal injury provides tolerance to subsequent injury. This is due to increased expression of the heat shock family of stress proteins (Hsps). Stress proteins belong to multigene families and are divided into different types according to molecular size (e.g., Hsp27, Hsp70, Hsp90). They are discussed in detail on pages 190–191. These Hsps are upregulated by diverse threats (e.g., oxidative/ischemic stress, inflammation). They help in protection during sepsis and metabolic stress. In injury and disease, commonly there is damage to proteins and formation of misfolded proteins. Hsps mediate protection from many types of nonlethal stresses. This is achieved by molecular chaperones, increasing protein expression by guiding folding of nascent proteins and preventing misfolding. The stress proteins suppress proinflammatory cytokines and NADPH oxidase, increase nitric oxide-mediated cytoprotection and increases synthesis of collagen.

Other Functional Responses of Activated Leukocytes

Apart from destruction/killing of microbes and dead cells, activated leukocytes play many other roles in host defense. Role of activated leukocytes (especially macrophages) is presented in **Box 7**. Functions of **macrophages** are discussed on pages 310–311. Some T lymphocytes (cells of adaptive immunity) also contribute to acute inflammation. The most important being **T lymphocytes that produce the cytokine IL-17** (called as Th17 cells). IL-17 stimulates secretion of chemokines that recruit other leukocytes in acute inflammation. Individuals without effective Th17 responses are susceptible to fungal and bacterial infections. They also develop skin abscesses which are termed as "cold abscesses", in which there are no cardinal signs of acute inflammation, such as *calor* (heat or warmness) and *rubor* (redness).

[8.2] Mediators of Inflammation

CHAPTER OUTLINE

- Introduction
  - General features of mediators
- Cell-derived mediators
  - Vasoactive amines: Histamine and serotonin
  - Arachidonic acid metabolites (prostaglandins, leukotrienes, and lipoxins)
  - Plasma-derived mediators of inflammation
- Negative regulators of acute inflammation

INTRODUCTION

Q. Discuss the chemical mediators of inflammation.
Q. Discuss the molecular basis of inflammatory events.

Substances that initiate and regulate inflammatory reactions are called **mediators of inflammation**.

Numerous mediators are responsible for inflammatory reactions. These mediators help to trigger, amplify, and terminate various inflammatory processes.

General Features of Mediators

Source of Mediators

Mediators may be either **produced locally** at the site of inflammation by cells **or may be derived from circulating inactive precursors**. The circulating inactive precursors are converted to activated molecules at the site of inflammation (**Table 17**).

- **Cell-derived mediators:** These are most important for inflammatory reactions against injurious agents in tissues.
  - **Mode of production:** Present **either as preformed molecules** that are rapidly released from intracellular granules (e.g., histamine in mast cell granules) **or are synthesized de novo** [e.g., prostaglandins (PGs), leukotrienes (LTs), cytokines] in response to a stimulus.
  - **Major cell types producing mediators of acute inflammation: These are the sentinels that detect invaders and tissue damage. These include tissue macrophages, dendritic cells, and mast cells**. Other cells such as platelets, neutrophils, endothelial cells, and most epithelia also can produce some of the mediators.
- **Plasma-derived mediators:** These include complement proteins and kinins. These are produced mainly in the **liver** and present in the circulation as **inactive precursors**. **They need activation** usually by a series of

Table 17: Main mediators of acute inflammation.

Mediator	*Source*	*Action*
Cell-derived		
Vasoactive amines • Histamine	Mast cells, basophils, platelets	Vasodilation, increased vascular permeability, activation of endothelial cells
Arachidonic acid (AA) metabolites • Prostaglandins	Mast cells, leukocytes	Vasodilation, pain, fever (systemic)
• Leukotrienes	Mast cells, leukocytes	Increased vascular permeability, chemotaxis, leukocyte adhesion, and activation
Cytokines (TNF, IL-1, IL-6)	Macrophages, endothelial cells, mast cells	Local: Endothelial cell activation (increased expression of adhesion molecules). Systemic: Fever, metabolic abnormalities, hypotension (shock)
Chemokines	Leukocytes, activated macrophages	Chemotaxis, activation of leukocyte
Platelet-activating factor (PAF)	Leukocytes, mast cells	Vasodilation, increased vascular permeability, leukocyte adhesion, chemotaxis, degranulation, oxidative burst
Plasma protein-derived		
Complement components [C3a, C5a, C3b, C5b-9 (MAC)]	Produced in the liver and circulate in plasma	Leukocyte chemotaxis and activation, direct target killing by MAC, vasodilation (mast cell stimulation)
Kinins		Increased vascular permeability, contraction of smooth muscle, vasodilation, pain

(IL-1: interleukin-1; TNF: tumor necrosis factor; MAC: membrane attack complex)

proteolytic cleavages to produce their effects. They act against circulating microbes but can also act into tissues.

Stimulus

Active mediators are released or synthesized only in response to various molecules that stimulate inflammation. These stimuli include microbial products and substances released from necrotic cells. Most of these stimuli bind to well-defined receptors and act by **binding to specific receptor** on target cells and generate signaling pathways. Because initiating stimulus such as microbes or dead tissues is required for release of these mediators, inflammatory reaction develops only when and where it is required.

Short-lived

Most of these mediators have a short lifespan and effectively turn off the response and allow the inflammatory process to resolve. They rapidly deteriorate or undergo inactivation by enzymes by intrinsic mechanisms, or discarded or inhibited. Thus, they are **tightly regulated and** there is a **system of checks and balances** ("on" and "off" control mechanisms) that regulates actions of these mediators.

Interrelated

Both cell- and plasma-derived mediators work together and are interrelated. They bring out activation of cells involved in inflammation by binding to specific receptors. They activate as well as recruit cells to sites of injury and also stimulate release of additional soluble mediators in various steps of inflammatory reaction.

One mediator can stimulate the release of another mediator. For example, products released from activation of complement can stimulate the release of histamine, and the cytokine tumor necrosis factor (TNF) acts on endothelial cells to stimulate to produce another cytokine, interleukin (IL)-1, and chemokines. The secondary mediators may have the similar, different, or even opposite actions. Thus, it may either amplify or counteract the initial action of a mediator.

Diverse targets

Target cell type varies depending on the type of mediator. They can act on one or few or many diverse targets, or may have different effects on different types of cells.

Main mediators involved in the inflammatory reaction are listed in **Table 17**.

CELL-DERIVED MEDIATORS

Q. Write a short essay on cell-derived mediators of inflammation.

Vasoactive Amines: Histamine and Serotonin

Q. Write a short essay on vasoactive amines.

They are termed as vasoactive **because of their important actions on blood vessels. The two major vasoactive amines** are **histamine and serotonin**. They are stored as preformed molecules in cells. Hence, they are the first mediators to be released during inflammation.

Histamine

It is a preformed vasoactive mediator. Responsible for immediate transient response.

Source: Mast cells are normally present in the connective tissue adjacent to blood vessels. These tissues are the richest source. Other sources include **blood basophils and platelets.**

Stimuli for release from mast cell granules: Mast cell undergo degranulation in response to a variety of stimuli.

- **Physical injury:** For example, trauma, cold, heat (mechanisms not known)
- **Immune reactions:** When antigens bind to IgE antibodies on mast cells [e.g., immediate (type 1) hypersensitivity (allergic) allergic reactions].
- **Products of complement system:** Anaphylatoxins C3a and C5a
- **Other mediators:** Leukocyte-derived histamine-releasing proteins, neuropeptides (e.g., substance P), cytokines (IL-1, IL-8).

Actions: (i) **Dilation of arterioles** and (ii) **increase of the vascular permeability of venules**. Histamine also causes contraction of some smooth muscles and is less potent for causing spasms of bronchial muscles, for example, in asthma.

Mode of action:

- **Increased vascular permeability:** Histamine is the main mediator involved in the immediate transient phase of increased vascular permeability. It acts by producing interendothelial gaps in postcapillary venules.
- **Dilation of arterioles:** Its vasoactive effects are mediated by binding of histamine to its receptors, called H_1 receptors present on microvascular endothelial cells. Common antihistamine drugs used to treat some inflammatory reactions, such as allergies, are H_1 receptor antagonists. These drugs bind to and block the H_1 receptor.

Serotonin (5-hydroxytryptamine)

It is a preformed vasoactive mediator.

Source: Platelets, some **neurons,** and **enterochromaffin cells** in the gastrointestinal tract.

Stimulus: Platelet aggregation and antigen–antibody complexes.

Actions: Its main function is as a neurotransmitter in the gastrointestinal tract and the central nervous systemt. Its role in inflammation is not clear.

Arachidonic Acid Metabolites (Prostaglandins, Leukotrienes, and Lipoxins)

Q. Write a short essay on role of arachidonic acid metabolites/prostaglandins in inflammation.

Arachidonic Acid

Arachidonic acid (AA) is a 20-**carbon polyunsaturated fatty acid** (5,8,11,14-eicosatetraenoic acid). It is either ingested directly as a dietary constituent (i.e., present in diet) or is synthesized from the essential fatty acid (two essential fatty acids are linoleic and linolenic acid), namely linoleic acid present in the diet. The term essential fatty acid (e.g., linoleic acid) means that there is lack of the ability to or a very limited capacity to produce it thereby making it an essential part of the diet.

Arachidonic acid in cell membrane

In the cells, AA does not occur in free form. Most of AA is normally present as esterified form (in combination with alcohol or acid) in **phospholipids of the cell membrane.** AA in the cell membranes accounts for 5–15% of the fatty acids in phospholipids. Phospholipids in the cell membrane are of different types, namely—(1) phosphatidylcholine (most abundant type of phospholipid found in cell membranes), (2) phosphatidylethanolamine, (3) phosphatidylserine, and (4) phosphatidylinositol (least abundant).

Stimuli

In the body, different stimuli can release **AA from phospholipid molecules of cell membranes of inflammatory cells and injured tissues.** These stimuli include—mechanical, chemical, and physical, or mediators (e.g., C5a).

Mechanism of release of arachidonic acid from cell membrane

Depending upon the specific inflammatory cell and nature of the stimulus, activated cells produce AA by one of two routes (**Flowchart 4**).

- Release AA from the phospholipid (in particular, phosphatidylcholine) of the cell membrane **by stimulus-induced activation of enzyme phospholipase A_2** (PLA_2).
- Release AA from the membrane phospholipid, namely phosphatidylinositol phosphates **by enzyme phospholipase C**. This enzyme cleaves phosphatidylinositol phosphates into diacylglycerol (DAG) and inositol phosphates. DAG is further cleaved into AA by the enzyme DAG lipase.

Arachidonic acid metabolism

Once released from the cell membrane, AA is quickly converted to bioactive mediators. AA is the major precursor of group of mediators/molecules termed as **eicosanoids** because of their derivation from 20-carbon fatty acids [Eicosanoids, from the Greek *eikosi* ("twenty")]. Thus, AA is the precursor of eicosanoids. Eicosanoids bind to G protein-coupled receptors on many cell types and can mediate almost every step of inflammation. AA is further metabolized along two major enzymatic pathways (**Fig. 18**). These are—(1) **cyclooxygenase (COX) pathway**/cyclooxygenation (by enzyme cyclooxygenase) to produce **prostaglandins** (PGs), **prostacyclins** (PGI_2), and **thromboxanes**, or by (2) **lipoxygenase (LOX) pathway**/lipoxygenation (by enzyme lipoxygenases) to produce **leukotrienes** (LTs) and **lipoxins** (LXs) (**Fig. 19**). Thus, eicosanoids are the broad term and include all the derivatives of both the pathways of AA. Eicosanoids includes PGs, PGI_2, thromboxanes, and LTs.

Products of cyclooxygenase pathway-prostanoids

Q. Write a short essay on prostaglandins and their role in inflammation.

Products of cyclooxygenase (COX) pathway are—(1) PGs (PGE2, PGD2), (2) PGI_2, and (3) thromboxane A_2 (TXA_2). These products are collectively termed as prostanoids.

Prostaglandins

Source: Prostaglandins are produced by **mast cells, macrophages, endothelial cells,** and many other types of cells.

Action: Prostaglandins are involved in the **vascular and systemic reactions of inflammation.**

Production: They are produced from AA by the actions of two cyclooxygenase (COX) *(*in the COX pathway) isoforms called COX-1 and COX-2.

- **Cyclooxygenase-1 (COX-1):** It is normally present in most tissues/cells. It is produced in response to inflammatory stimuli. It is the **main enzyme involved in the synthesis of PGs.** In the normal tissues, it may serve a homeostatic (housekeeping) function, namely—(1) cytoprotection of the mucosa in the gastrointestinal tract, (2) regulation of fluid and electrolyte balance in the kidneys, (3) stimulation of platelet aggregation to maintain normal hemostasis, and (4) maintain resistance to thrombosis on vascular endothelial cell surfaces.
- **Cyclooxygenase-2 (COX-2):** It is expressed **usually in low or undetectable level in most normal tissues.** COX-2 is upregulated and increases substantially by cytokines, shear stress, and growth factors. It is the

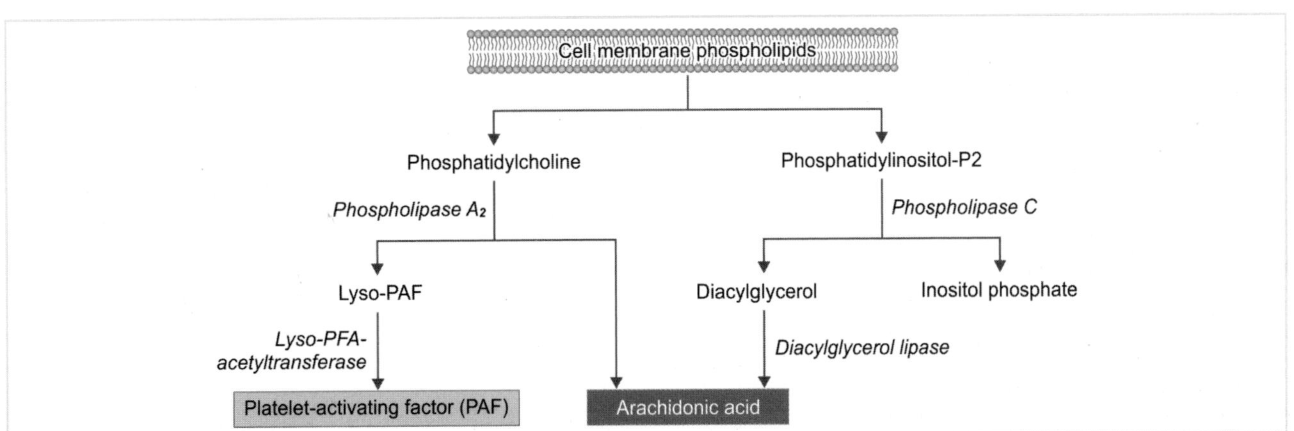

FLOWCHART 4: Mediators derived from cell membrane. Arachidonic acid is derived from phosphatidylinositol phosphates and from phosphatidylcholine. Platelet-activating factor (PAF) is derived from choline-containing glycerophospholipids, namely phosphatidylcholine in the cell membrane.

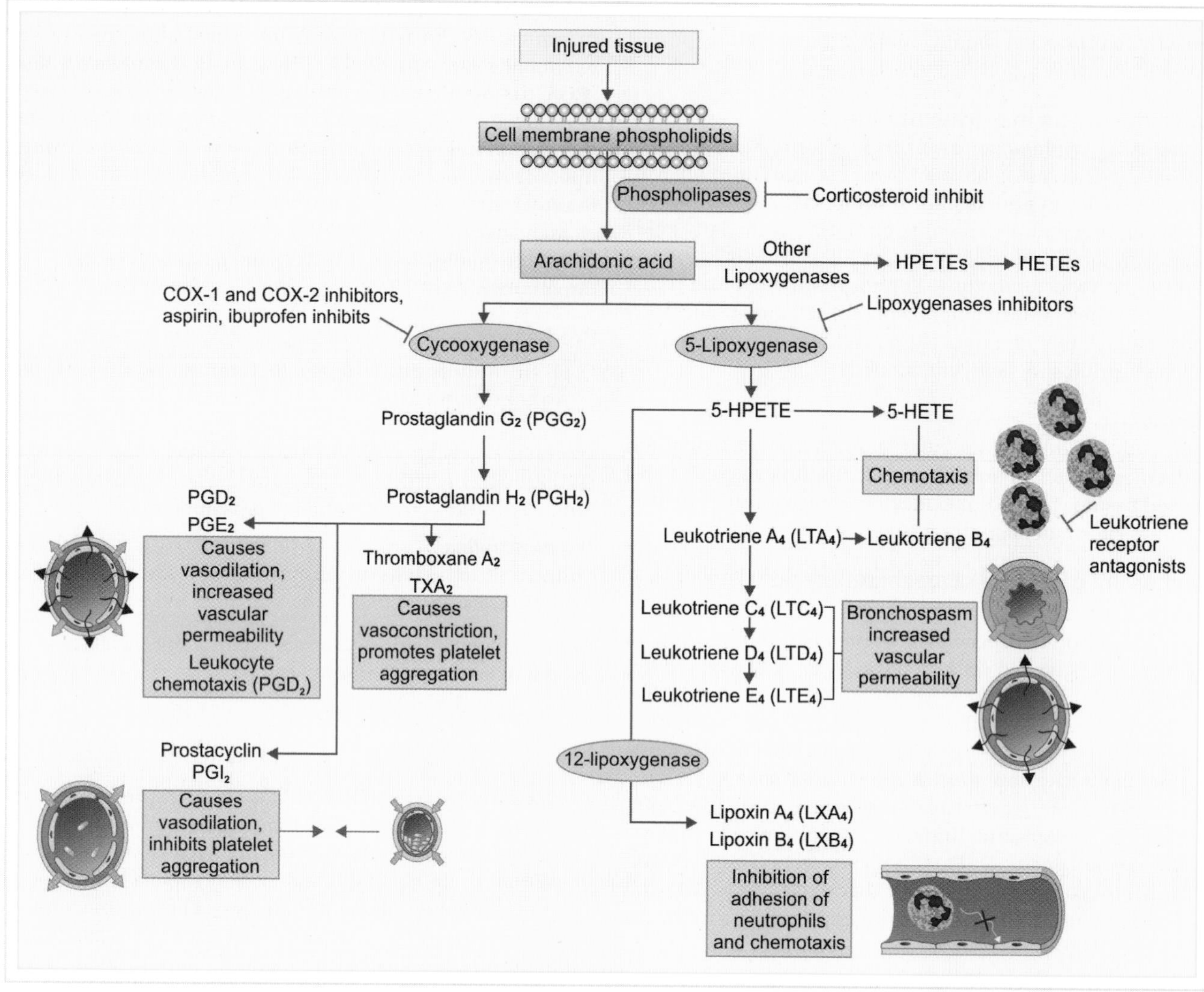

(COX: cyclooxygenase; HETE: hydroxyeicosatetraenoic acid; HPETE: hydroperoxy eicosatetraenoic acid)

FIG. 18: Arachidonic acid metabolites involved in inflammation. The cyclooxygenase pathway generates prostaglandins (PGIs), prostacyclins (PGI_2), and thromboxane (TXA_2). The lipoxygenase pathway forms lipoxins (LXs) and leukotrienes (LTEs). Nonsteroidal anti-inflammatory drugs (NSAIDs) such as aspirin, ibuprofen block COX-1 and COX-2.

main source of prostanoid formation in inflammation and cancer. Thus, it produces the PGs that are involved in inflammatory reactions. Its metabolites are also **important in producing pain**.

- The early inflammatory prostanoid response is dependent on COX-1. As inflammation proceeds, COX-2 takes over as the major source of prostanoids. Both COX isoforms (COX-1 and COX-2) produce prostaglandin G_2 (PGG_2) followed by prostaglandin H_2 (PGH_2), which is the substrate for production of PGI_2, PGD_2, PGE_2, PGF_{2a} and TXA_2.
- **Terminology:** Prostaglandins are named depending on structural features and coded by a letter (e.g., PGD, PGE, PGF, PGG, and PGH). This is followed by a subscript numeral (e.g., 1, 2), which indicates the number of double bonds in the compound.
- **Most important PGs involved in inflammation:** These are PGE_2, PGD_2, PGF_{2a}, PGI_2, and TXA_2. Each of these prostaglandins is produced by the action of a specific enzyme on an intermediate product in the pathway. Some of these enzymes are limited to certain tissues and functions.

Prostaglandin D_2 and PGE_2

Source: Prostaglandin D_2 is the major prostaglandin derived from mast cells; along with PGE_2 (which is more widely distributed).

Actions: Both PGD_2 and PGE_2 cause vasodilation and increase the permeability of postcapillary venules, thereby causing exudation and edema. PGD_2 also is a chemoattractant for neutrophils.

Thromboxane A_2 It is the major platelet eicosanoid.

Source: Platelets have an enzyme called thromboxane synthase, and hence only platelets can produce TXA_2.

Actions: Thromboxane A_2 is a powerful platelet-aggregating agent and vasoconstrictor. Thus, it favors thrombosis. TXA_2 itself is unstable and is rapidly converted to its inactive form TXB_2.

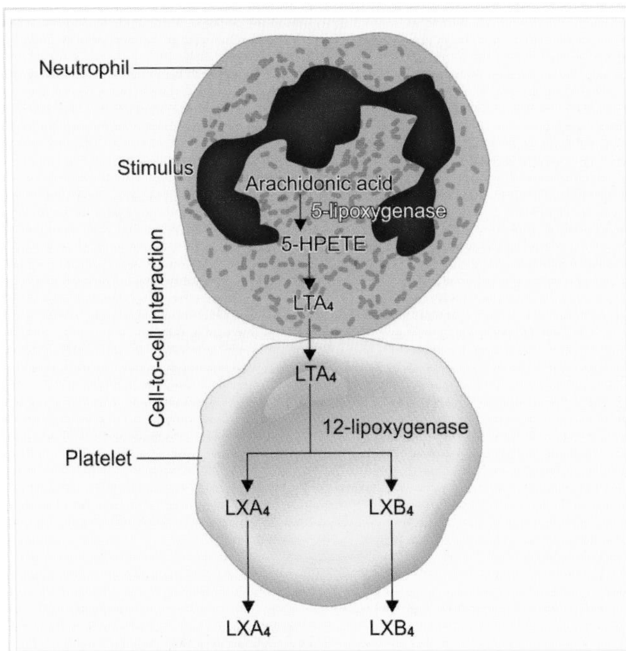

(5-HPETE: 5-hydroxyperoxyeicosatetraenoic acid)

FIG. 19: Synthesis of lipoxins.

Prostacyclin and its stable end product PGF_{1a}

Source: Vascular endothelium contains PGI_2 synthase and forms PGI_2 and its stable end product PGF_{1a} in the endothelium.

Actions: Prostacyclin is a vasodilator and a potent inhibitor of platelet aggregation. Thus, it prevents thrombus formation on normal endothelial cells. PGI_2 also markedly increases the permeability and chemotactic effects of other mediators. An imbalance between thromboxane—PGI_2 may lead to thrombosis in coronary and cerebral artery.

PGF_{2a} stimulates the contraction of uterine and bronchial smooth muscle and small arterioles.

Apart from local effects, PGs are also involved in the pathogenesis of two common systemic manifestations of inflammation, namely **pain and fever.** PGE_2 is hyperalgesic and makes the skin hypersensitive to painful stimuli (e.g., intradermal injection of suboptimal concentrations of histamine and bradykinin) and is also involved in cytokine-induced fever during infections. The quantity and type of PGs produced during inflammation depends partly on the cells present and their state of activation. Thus, mast cells produce mainly PGD_2, macrophages produce PGE_2 and TXA_2, platelets produce TXA_2, and endothelial cells generate PGI_2.

Products of lipoxygenase pathway

Major products of the lipoxygenase (LOX) pathways are hydroxy fatty acid derivatives known as 5-**hydroxyeicosatetraenoic acids (**HETEs), **leukotrienes** (LTs), and **lipoxins** (LXs).

Q. Write a short essay on functions of leukotrienes.

Leukotrienes

Leukotrienes (LTs) are the products of LOX pathway and are the second major family of derivatives of AA**.** LTs play a major role in the development and persistence of the inflammatory response. Synthesis of an LT involves multiple steps. The first LT produced is LTA_4, which in turn gives rise to LTB_4 or LTC_4.

- There are three different lipoxygenases. One of them is enzyme 5-lipoxygenase (5-LOX) that is predominant in neutrophils. The enzyme 5-LOX converts AA to 5-hydroxyperoxyeicosatetraenoic acid (HPETE). 5-HPETEs are converted to their corresponding 5-HETE and LTA_4.
  - The **5-HETE** is chemotactic for neutrophils, and is the precursor of the other LTs.
  - LTA_4 is transformed by distinct enzymes to LTB_4 or LTC_4.

***Source: Leukotrienes* are produced in leukocytes and mast cells.**

- **Leukotriene B_4:** In neutrophils and some macrophage populations, LTA_4 is metabolized to LTB_4.
- **Leukotriene C_4, LTD_4, and LTE_4:** The cysteinyl-containing LT—LTC_4, and its metabolites, LTD_4 and LTE_4, are produced mainly in mast cells. In mast cells, basophils, and macrophages, LTA_4 is converted to LTC_4 and thence to LTD_4 and LTE_4.

***Actions: Leukotrienes* are involved in vascular and smooth muscle reactions and leukocyte recruitment.**

- **Leukotriene B_4:** It is a powerful chemotactic agent for neutrophils, monocytes, and macrophages; and is also activator of neutrophils. It causes aggregation and adhesion of the leukocytes to the endothelium of venules, generates reactive oxygen species (ROS), and releases lysosomal enzymes.
- **Leukotriene C_4, LTD_4, and LTE_4:** These three cysteinyl-LTs cause—
  - Intense vasoconstriction
  - Smooth muscle contraction (bronchospasm in asthma)
  - Increased vascular permeability of venules
  - Many of the clinical symptoms associated with allergic-type reactions.

Thus, they play a central role in the development of asthma.

Vascular permeability and bronchospasm produced by LTs is more than caused by histamine.

The term slow-reacting substance of anaphylaxis (SRS-A) was used previously and is actually a mixture of LTs. It is a smooth muscle stimulant and mediator of hypersensitivity reactions.

Leukotrienes perform their action by acting through high-affinity specific receptors. This is useful for targeted drug therapy.

Lipoxins

Lipoxins are the third type of AA products **generated by the LOX pathway**.

Actions

- **Inhibit inflammation:** In contrast to **PGs and LTs, the LXs suppress inflammation by inhibiting the recruitment of leukocytes.**
- Lipoxins inhibit **neutrophil chemotaxis** and recruitment
- **Inhibit leukocyte adhesion** to endothelium.

Synthesis

They are synthesized in the vascular lumen. They also are unusual in that two cell populations (i.e., cell–cell interactions) are required for the transcellular biosynthesis of these mediators. Several cell types synthesize LXs from LTs. For example, activated leukocytes (particularly neutrophils), produce LTA_4 intermediate in LX synthesis. This LTA_4 intermediate is available for transcellular enzymatic conversion by nearby cells. When platelets interact with the leukocytes/neutrophils, LTA_4 from neutrophils is converted by plastelet and 12-LOX to LXA_4 and LXB_4 (**Fig. 19**).

Pharmacologic Inhibitors of Prostaglandins and Leukotrienes

The eicosanoids play an important role in inflammation. Hence, anti-inflammatory drugs were developed to inhibit the production or actions of eicosanoids and thereby suppress inflammation. The various anti-inflammatory drugs are as follows:

Cyclooxygenase inhibitors: They act by inhibiting both COX-1 and COX-2 involved in COX pathway. They block synthesis of all prostaglandins and are useful in treating pain and fever. The drugs under this category include aspirin and other nonsteroidal anti-inflammatory drugs (NSAIDs), such as ibuprofen naproxen.

- Aspirin: It acts by irreversibly inactivating cyclooxygenases. Low-dose aspirin inhibits COX-1 and blocks TXA2 and prevents aggregartion of platelets. Higher doses of aspirin blok PGI2 synthesis.
- Selective COX-2 inhibitors: These are a newer class of drugs that are 200–300 times more potent in blocking COX-2 than COX-1. COX-1 produces PGs involved in both inflammation and normal homeostasis/physiologic functions (e.g., protection of gastric epithelial cells from acid-induced damage, maintenance of fluid and electrolyte balance in the kidneys). COX-2 produces PGs only in inflammation. Hence, selective COX-2 inhibitors should be anti-inflammatory therapeutic target without having the toxicities of the nonselective inhibitors (e.g., gastric ulceration). However, this is not proved to be totally correct. Probably, COX-2 also plays some role in normal homeostasis and in fact, selective COX-2 inhibitors may increase the risk of cardiovascular and cerebrovascular events. This risk may be due to impaired endothelial cell production of PGI_2, which prevents thrombosis, as well as inhibition of the COX-1-mediated production by platelets of TXA_2, which causes aggregation of platelets. Thus, use of selective COX-2 inhibition may favor vascular thrombosis. These drugs are used in individuals without any risk factors for cardiovascular disease.

Lipoxygenase inhibitors: 5-lipoxygenase is not affected by NSAIDs. Hence, inhibitors of this enzyme pathway have been developed. Drugs that inhibit leukotriene production are used in the treatment of asthma.

Corticosteroid: This is a broad-spectrum anti-inflammatory agent that is used to suppress tissue destruction in many inflammatory diseases. These include allergic conditions, rheumatoid arthritis, and systemic lupus erythematosus (SLE).

- **Action:** Corticosteroids reduce the transcription of genes encoding COX-2, stimulate the synthesis of an inhibitor of PLA_2, proinflammatory cytokines (e.g., IL-1 and TNF), and inducible nitric oxide synthase (iNOS). Thus, this broad-spectrum anti-inflammatory agent blocks the release of AA by inflammatory cells. It is used to suppress tissue destruction associated with many inflammatory diseases (e.g., allergic responses, rheumatoid arthritis, SLE). It is to be borne in mind that prolonged use of corticosteroid is harmful and increases the risk of infection and damage to connective tissue.

Leukotriene receptor antagonists: They block leukotriene receptors and thereby prevent the actions of the LTs. These drugs are useful in the treatment of asthma.

Another therapeutic way of manipulating inflammatory responses is to modify the intake and content of dietary lipids by increased consumption of fish oil. Probably polyunsaturated fatty acids present in fish oil are not converted to active metabolites by both the COX and LOX pathways. In fact, they may favor the production of anti-inflammatory lipid products.

Main actions of AA metabolites (eicosanoids) involved in inflammation are presented in **Table 18.**

Arachidonic acid metabolites involved in inflammation are presented in **Figure 18**.

Platelet-activating Factor

Q. Write short note on platelet-activating factor.

Platelet-activating factor (PAF) is another powerful inflammatory mediator derived from membrane phospholipids.

Source

It is synthesized by **almost all activated inflammatory cell** (basophils, mast cells, neutrophils, macrophages, endothelial cells, platelets themselves, and injured tissue cells). During inflammation and allergic reactions, PAF is synthesized from choline-containing glycerophospholipids present in the cell membrane (refer **Flowchart 4**). Initially, it is formed by the catalytic action of PLA_2, followed by acetylation by an acetyltransferase.

Action

In plasma, PAF activity is regulated by PAF-acetyl hydrolase. PAF stimulates platelets, monocyte/macrophages, neutrophils, endothelial cells, and vascular smooth muscle cells. PAF was discovered as a factor that caused platelet aggregation, but it is now known to have multiple inflammatory functions or effects:

- **Vascular reactions:** At the site of tissue injury, it produces—
  - Powerful **vasodilation** and
  - **Increased vascular permeability**.

Table 18: Main actions of arachidonic acid metabolites (eicosanoids) in inflammation.

Action	*Arachidonic acid metabolites (eicosanoid)*
Vasodilation	PGI_2 (prostacyclin), PGE_2, PGD_2
Vasoconstriction	Thromboxane A_2, leukotrienes C_4, D_4, E_4
Increased vascular permeability	Leukotrienes C_4, D_4, E_4
Chemotaxis, leukocyte adhesion	Leukotriene B_4, HETE (hydroxyeicosatetraenoic acid)
Smooth muscle contraction	Prostaglandins PGC_4, PGD_4, PGE_4

- **Cellular reactions:**
  - **Increases leukocyte adhesion** to endothelium by expressing adhesion molecule **on leukocytes,** specifically integrin. It also causes oxidative burst.
  - It also causes **chemotaxis.**
  - Platelet activating factor produced by the endothelial cell attaches to its receptor on the leukocyte and induces intracellular signaling.
- **Platelet aggregation:** Platelet-activating factor causes aggregation of platelets and degranulation of platelets at sites of tissue injury. Thus, it increases the release of serotonin from platelets and increases the vascular permeability.

Cytokines and Chemokines

Q. Write a short essay on cytokines in inflammation.

These are polypeptides (proteins) which function as mediators in **immune responses** and in **inflammation (acute and chronic)**. Ordinarily, growth factors that act on epithelial and mesenchymal cells are not grouped under the category of cytokines.

Source: Cytokines are secreted by many types of cells (activated lymphocytes and macrophages, dendritic cells endothelial, epithelial, and connective tissue cells). Important cytokines involved in inflammation are tumor necrosis factor, interleukin-1, and chemokines.

Tumor necrosis factor and interleukin-1

Q. Write a short essay on tumor necrosis factors.

These are the two major cytokines involved in inflammation.

Source: Both are produces by activated macrophages and dendritic cells. Apart from these cells, TNF is also produced by T lymphocytes and mast cells, and IL-1 is produced by some epithelial cells.

Stimuli and mode of production: The stimuli for the secretion of TNF and IL-1 includes microbial products, dead cells, immune complexes, foreign bodies, physical injury, and many other inflammatory stimuli.

- **Production of TNF:** It is induced by signals through TLRs and other microbial sensors.
- **Synthesis of IL-1:** It is stimulated by the same signals as that of TNF. However, the production of the biologically active form of IL-1 is dependent on the inflammasome.

Actions in inflammation (Flowchart 5) (refer Fig. 39) Both **TNF and IL-1 play critical roles in recruitment of leukocyte. They promote adhesion of leukocytes to endothelium and their transmigration through blood vessels.**

Local effects:

- **Endothelium:** Both TNF and IL-1 cause *endothelial activation*. These changes include **increased expression of endothelial adhesion molecules** (mainly E- and P-selectins and ligands for leukocyte integrins), increased production of other mediators (e.g., other cytokines and chemokines, and eicosanoids), and increased procoagulant activity of the endothelium.
- **Leukocytes:** Tumor necrosis factor increases the responses of neutrophils to other stimuli (e.g., bacterial endotoxin) and stimulates the microbicidal activity of macrophages.
- **During repair:** Interleukin-1 activates fibroblasts to synthesize collagen during repair.

Systemic effects:

- **Systemic acute-phase reactions:** Interleukin-1 and TNF (and also IL-6) produce the systemic acute-phase responses in association with infection or injury. This also include fever.
- **Systemic inflammatory response syndrome** (SIRS): IL-1 and TNF can produce SIRS resulting from disseminated bacterial infection (sepsis) and other noninfectious serious conditions such as severe burns, trauma, pancreatitis (discussed on page 323).
- Leukocytosis
- **Suppresses appetite:** Tumor necrosis factor can regulate energy balance by promoting lipid and protein catabolism and by suppressing appetite. Hence, continuous production of TNF may lead to *cachexia*. Cachexia is a pathologic state characterized by loss of weight, atrophy of muscle, and loss of appetite (anorexia) and is observed in some chronic infections (e.g., tuberculosis) and cancers.

Clinical importance **TNF antagonists have been found to be effective in the treatment of chronic inflammatory diseases,** particularly rheumatoid arthritis, psoriasis, and few cases of inflammatory bowel disease. However, patients on TNF antagonists are more susceptible to mycobacterial

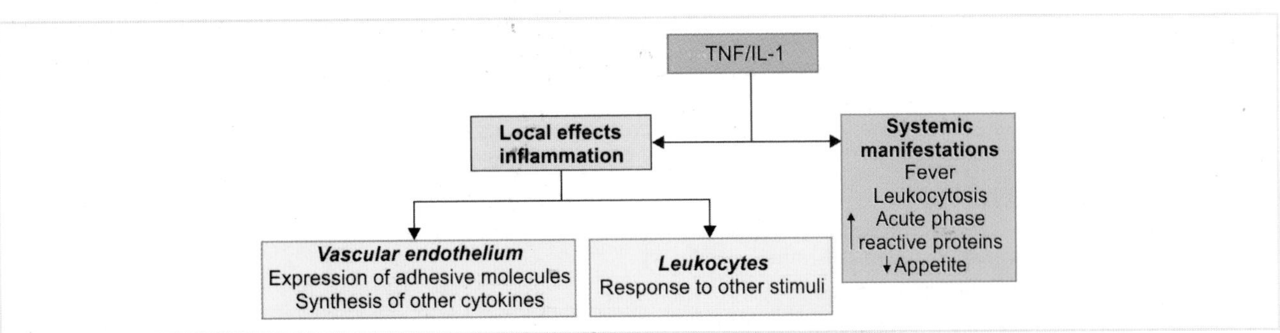

FLOWCHART 5: Important local and systemic effects of tumor necrosis factor (TNF) and interleukin-1 (IL-1).

infection and this is due to decreased ability of macrophages to kill intracellular microbes. Many of the actions of TNF and IL-1 are overlapping. However, IL-1 antagonists are not as effective in inflammatory disorders. It is to be noted that blocking either TNF or IL-1 has no effect on the outcome of sepsis. This is probably because other cytokines may contribute to the systemic inflammatory reaction in sepsis.

Chemokines

Chemotactic cytokines or chemokines are small proteins (8 to 10 kDa), **which selectively attract various (specific types of) leukocytes to the site of inflammation**. They are discussed in detail on pages 297–302.

Classification There are about 40 different chemokines and 20 different receptors for chemokines. Chemokines are classified into four major groups (according to the arrangement of cysteine (C) residues in the proteins), namely—(1) C–X–C chemokines, (2) C–C chemokines, (3) C chemokines, and (4) CX3C chemokines.

Mode of action: The activities of chemokines are mediated by its binding to seven transmembrane G protein–coupled receptors. These G-protein coupled receptors generally show overlapping ligand specificities. Leukocytes usually express more than one type of receptor. Certain chemokine receptors such as CXCR4 (CCR5) act as coreceptors for a viral envelope glycoprotein of human immunodeficiency virus (HIV). Thus, they are involved in binding and entry of the virus into host cells.

Functions in acute inflammation: Chemokines may be attached to proteoglycans on the surface of endothelial cells and in the extracellular matrix (ECM). The production of inflammatory chemokines is induced by microbes and other inflammatory stimuli. Their functions in inflammation are as follows:

- **Leukocyte activation:** The inflammatory chemokines stimulate attachment of leukocyte (leukocyte adhesion) to endothelium. They increase the affinity of integrins by acting on leukocytes.
- **Chemotaxis:** They also stimulate migration (chemotaxis) of leukocytes in tissues to the site of infection or tissue damage.

Though chemokines play a role in inflammation, its antagonists are not effective therapeutic agents to reduce inflammation.

Other cytokines in acute inflammation

- Interleukin-6 produced by macrophages and other cells is involved in local and systemic reactions.
- Interleukin-17 produced by T lymphocytes promotes neutrophil recruitment.

Antagonists against IL-6 and IL-17 are effective for the treatment of inflammatory diseases. For example , anti-IL-6 receptor in juvenile arthritis and anti-IL-17 in psoriasis. Cytokines are also involved in chronic inflammation. Main cytokines involved in acute and chronic inflammation are presented in **Table 19**. Cytokines and chemokines are discussed in detail on pages 297–302.

Lysosomal Constituents of Leukocytes

Neutrophils

Types of granules

- **Smaller specific (or secondary) granules:** They contain lysozyme, collagenase, gelatinase, lactoferrin, plasminogen activator, histaminase, and alkaline phosphatase.
- **Larger azurophilic (or primary) granules:** They **contain myeloperoxidase**, bactericidal factors (lysozyme, defensins), acid hydrolases, and a variety of neutral proteases (elastase, cathepsin G, nonspecific collagenases, proteinase 3).

Monocytes and macrophages

They also contain acid hydrolases, collagenase, elastase, phospholipase, and plasminogen activator. These are active mainly in chronic inflammation.

Plasma-derived Mediators of Inflammation

Mediators derived from plasma proteins belong to three major interrelated systems (enzyme cascades):

- Complement
- Kinin
- Clotting systems **(coagulation cascade)**

Table 19: Main cytokines involved in acute and chronic inflammation.

Cytokine	*Main cellular sources*	*Main actions in inflammation*
Acute inflammation		
TNF	Macrophages, mast cells, T lymphocytes	Expression of endothelial adhesion molecules and secretion of other cytokines; systemic effects
IL-1	Macrophages, endothelial cells, some epithelial cells	Similar to TNF; more involved in generation of fever
IL-6	Macrophages, other cells	Systemic effects: Acute phase response
IL-17	T lymphocytes	Recruitment of neutrophils and monocytes
Chemokines	Macrophages, endothelial cells, T lymphocytes, mast cells, other cells	Recruitment of leukocytes, migration of cells in normal tissues
Chronic inflammation		
IL-12	Dendritic cells, macrophages	Increases production of IFN-γ
IL-17	T lymphocytes	Recruitment of neutrophils and monocytes
IFN-γ	T lymphocytes, NK cells	Activation of macrophages and increases their ability to kill microbes and tumor cells

(IFN-γ: interferon-γ; IL-1: interleukin-1; NK: natural killer; TNF: tumor necrosis factor)

Complement System

Q. Discuss complement system in health and disease.

Q. Discuss structure and functional relationship of complement.

Q. Discuss disorders of the complement system.

The complement system is a **group of soluble plasma proteins and their receptors on cell membrane** (surface). They function mainly in host defense against microbes and are also involved in several pathological inflammatory reactions. During the process of complement activation, it produces several cleavage products of complement proteins. They cause (i) increased vascular permeability, (ii) chemotaxis, and (iii) opsonization. Complement system consists of >20 complement proteins found in the blood and some of them are numbered C1 through C9. These proteins include plasma enzymes, regulatory proteins, and cell lysis proteins. They were first detected as a heat-labile serum factor that kills bacteria and "complements" antibodies. Generally, complement cleavage fragments are designated with letters according to their relative size with "a" fragments smaller than "b" fragments.

Source: Complement components are mainly synthesized in the liver.

Pathways of complement system activation (Fig. 20)

Complement proteins are present in the plasma in inactive forms and enzymes that circulate as proenzymes. Complements are activated in sequence. Many of complements are activated to become proteolytic enzymes that degrade other complement proteins. Thus, they form an enzymatic cascade that is capable of intense amplification. Activation of the first components of complements results in sequential activation of other components of the complement system. This sequential activation is referred to as a cascade. The decisive or **critical step in complement activation is the proteolysis of the third component**, C3 (most abundant complement). Cleavage of C3 can occur by any one of the **three convergent pathways (routes)—(1) classical, (2) alternate, and (3) lectin pathways**. Each of the three pathways produces a C3 convertase, which activates C3, leading to the formation of a C5 convertase. Then all these three pathways continue as **common pathway**.

Classical complement pathway In this pathway, C1 through C9 are utilized and the nomenclature of complements (1 through 9) is followed according to the historical order of discovery.

Activators: It is activated by formation of antigen–antibody (Ag–Ab) complexes and usually triggered by immunoglobulin (Ig) G or IgM antibody–antigen complexes. Antigens can be proteins or carbohydrates from bacterial cell surfaces (products of bacteria) or other infectious agents. Other activators of this pathway include viruses, proteases, urate crystals, apoptotic cells, and polyanions (polynucleotides).

- **Formation of Ag–Ab complexes:** This pathway is primarily activated by antibodies, which are proteins of the acquired immune system. Antibodies must first bind to their targets, called antigens. Antibodies bind to antigens and form **Ag-Ab complexes**.
- **Binding of C1 to Ag–Ab complexes:** Complement C1 is a Ca++ dependent macromolecular complex comprised of C1q , C1r and C1s. Antibodies (IgM or IgG) **of Ag–Ab complexes** (immune complexes) bind C1q and activate C1r and C1s (and form C1 complex consisting of C1q, 2 molecules of C1r and 2 molecules of C1s). Thus, antibodies activate the first component of complement namely C1.
- **Formation of C3 convertase:** C1s cleaves C4, which binds the bacterial surface and then cleaves C2. Resulting split molecules form the **C4b2a enzyme complex** (also termed as **C3 convertase**). In this **classical pathway, C3 convertase** remains covalently bound to the microbial surface. This covalent bond causes attachment of the complement system at specific tissue sites. If there is no formation of covalent bond between C3 convertase and bacterial surface, the C1 complex is inactivated. This will prematurely end the complement cascade in normal host cells or tissues.
- The complement cascade then continues as common pathway.

Note: There is decreased serum C1, C3, and C4; that is all early complement components are reduced.

Alternative Pathway

Q. Write a short essay on alternate pathway of complement activation.

Activators: It is activated by several substances/products found on the microbial surface of infectious organisms [e.g., lipopolysaccharides/LPS (endotoxin) on the bacterial surface], carbohydrate zymosan (on yeast cell walls), complex polysaccharides, cobra venom, aggregates of IgA, viruses, tumor cells, and foreign materials. This pathway uses unique proteins (factor B, factor D, and properdin) to form an alternate pathway C3 convertase that activates C3. Thus, the complement system can be directly activated by certain infectious organisms without the presence of antibody **(no antibody and no Ag–Ab complexes as in classical pathway)**.

- A small amount of C3 in plasma is cleaved to C3a and C3b. This C3b gets covalently bound to carbohydrates and proteins on cell surfaces of microbes.
- C3b binds factor B and factor D to form the **alternative pathway C3 convertase**, C3bBb. C3bBb is labile and degraded by **factors I and H** but stabilized by properdin.
- The complement cascade then converges with the classical pathway.

Note: There is **decreased serum C3 but normal C1 and C4**. The early components of complement (C1 and C4) are used only in the activation of classical complement pathway.

Lectin pathway (mannose-binding pathway) Lectin is a circulating biomolecule in plasma. It binds mannose present on bacterial cell walls and triggers complement activation at C2 and C4. The lectin- or mannose-binding pathway shares some elements similar to the classical pathway but is independent of antibody.

Activators: It is activated by several plasma proteins, particularly mannose-binding lectin (MBL). It is initiated when microbe's bacterial polysaccharides containing the carbohydrate mannose bind MBL in plasma (i.e., bacterial mannose + MBL in plasma). These MBLs are one of the family of calcium-dependent lectins, or collectins. MBL is a multifunctional acute phase protein that resembles IgM (it binds many oligosaccharide structures), IgG (it interacts with

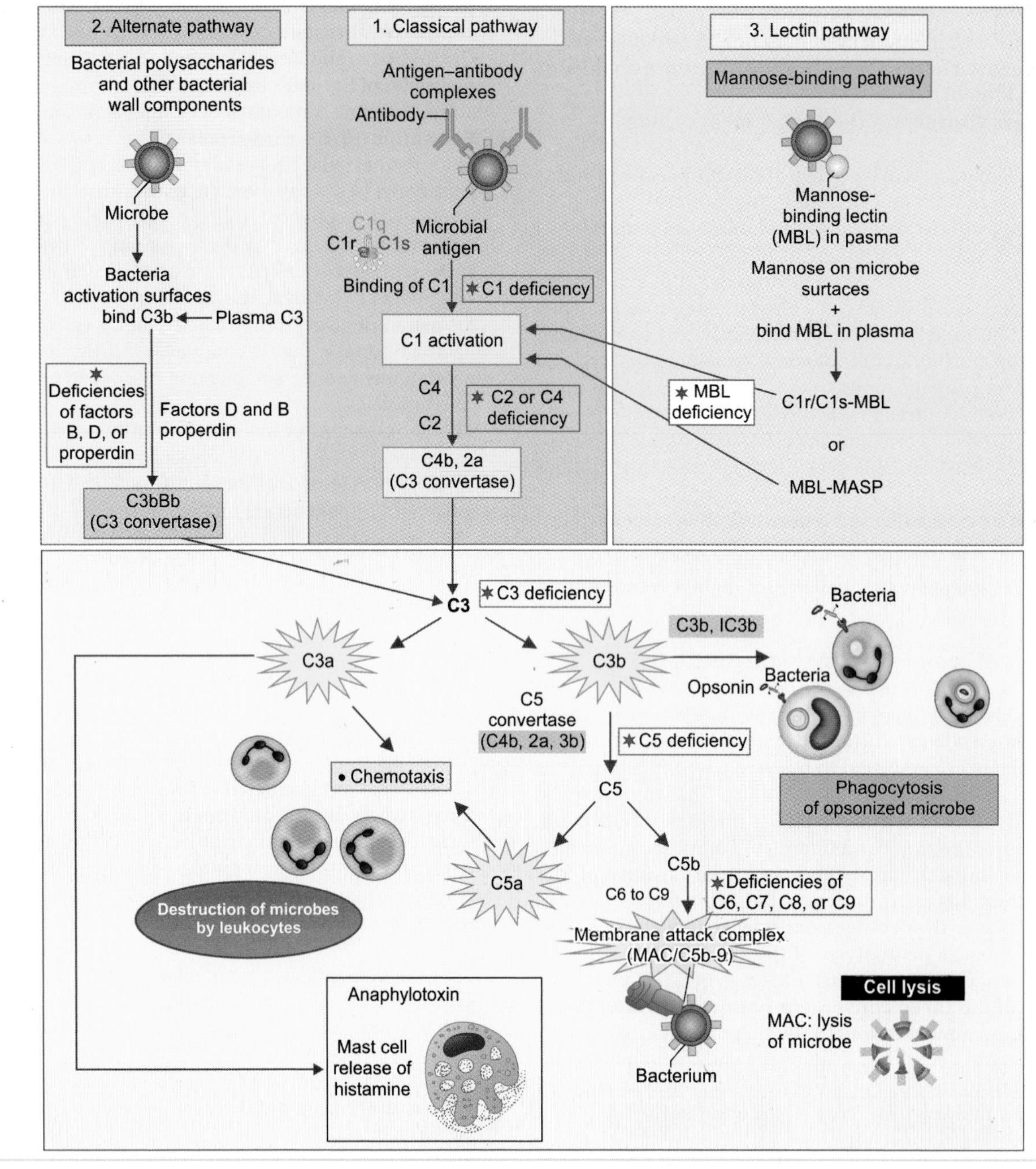

(MASP: MBL-associated serine protease)

FIG. 20: Different pathways of activation and functions of the complement system. All pathways of activation lead to cleavage of C3. Various complement defects that can occur in complement system area depicted in red stars( ). The most severe defect is a C3 deficiency because it blocks all three pathways.

phagocytic receptors) and C1q. This last property of MBL is responsible for its ability to activate complement system. The complement system may be activated by lectin pathway by two methods:

1. **Direct interaction of MBL with complement:** Plasma MBL binds to mannose on glycoproteins or carbohydrates of microbes. MBL interacts directly with C1r and C1s to evoke C1 esterase activity.
2. **MBL forms complex with MBL-associated serine protease and activates complement:** Alternatively, and preferentially, MBL can form a complex with a precursor of the serine protease, MBL-associated serine protease (MASP). There are two MASP—MASP-1 and MASP-2. MBL and MASP bind to mannose groups on glycoproteins or carbohydrates on bacterial cell surfaces. After MBL binds a substrate, the MASP proenzyme is cleaved into two chains and expresses a C1 esterase activity. Thus, infectious agents that do not activate the alternative pathway may be susceptible to complement through the lectin pathway.

C1 esterase activity (either from C1r/C1s-MBL interaction or MBL-MASP), cleaves C4 and C2. This produces classical pathway C3 convertase. The complement cascade then converges with the classical pathway.

Common pathway of convergence C3 is an important and plentiful of the complement proteins. Activation of C3 is central to the complement cascade. **All three pathways of complement activation form an enzyme called the *C3 convertase.*** The following steps are common for all these three pathways.

- **Cleaving C3 and opsonization:** C3 convertase divides C3 into **two functionally distinct fragments,** C3a and C3b. This is an important step. **C3a** is released and is a **proinflammatory protein and anaphylatoxins**. C3a causes release of histamine from mast cells, contraction of smooth muscle, and increased vascular permeability. C3b becomes covalently attached to the cell proteins or molecule and localize, or "fix," on the cell surface where the complement is being activated. C3b and its degradation products [especially inactive C3b (iC3b)] act as opsonins. Opsonins are molecule that favors opsonization. C3b opsonin gets deposited on the surface of microbe and intensifies phagocytosis. This process of coating a pathogen with a molecule that enhances phagocytosis is called opsonization.
- **Cleavage of C5:** More C3b then binds to the previously generated fragments to form *C5 convertase* (complex of C4b, C2a and C3b). **C5 convertase cleaves C5 into C5a and C5b.**
    - C5a is released and is a powerful inflammatory chemical and also an **anaphylatoxin** similar to C3a described earlier. C5a is also a **potent chemotactic agent and stimulates neutrophils and monocytes to migrate to the site of inflammation.** C5a also activates neutrophils by triggering their oxidative activity and increasing their glucose uptake.
    - C5b remains attached to the cell surface.
- **Formation of membrane attack complex:** C5b fragment acts as the nidus for subsequent sequential binding of the late components of complement (i.e. C6, C7, C8 and C9). The C5b combines with C6, C7, C8, and multiple units of C9 to form a large pore like structure (C5b6789) called the membrane attack complex (MAC, composed of multiple C9 molecules).
- **Assembly of MAC (C5b-9) on target cells:** The MAC has a direct cytotoxic effect by attacking cell membranes and disrupting the lipid bilayer. The MAC directly inserts into the plasma membrane by hydrophobic binding of C7 to the lipid bilayer of plasma membrane. This produces a cylindrical transmembrane channel and allows free movement of sodium and water into the target cell. This leads to rupture/lysis of target cell.

Note: The enzymatic activity of complement proteins is so great that it gets to produce millions of molecules of C3b that can get deposited on the surface of a microbe within 2 or 3 minutes after activation of the complement system.

Complement pathway specific activators are summarized in **Table 20**.

Functions (biological activities) of complement components

Complements function in both innate and adaptive immunity and their **main function is defense against microbial pathogens**. During the process of complement activation, several cleavage products of complement proteins are produced at each step. These cleavage products activate the next step in the cascade and also have supporting roles as important inflammatory molecules. Activation of the complement system produces several cleavage products that can either directly destroy pathogens or can activate or increase the activity of many other components of the inflammatory and adaptive immune response. These include increased vascular permeability (by anaphylatoxins e.g., C3a and C5a), chemotaxis (by chemotactic factors e.g. C5a), and opsonization (by opsonins e.g., C3b). The endpoint of complement activation is formation of MAC and this produces direct lysis of cells/microbes (pathogens). Physiologic activities of the complement system include the following.

- ***Anti-infective functions***: Defense against pyogenic bacterial infection can be brought out by:
    - **Leukocyte activation, adhesion, and chemotaxis:** C5a causes **leukocyte activation and adhesion.** C3a and C5a are **powerful chemotactic** agents for neutrophils, monocytes, eosinophils, and basophils.
    - **Opsonization and promote phagocytosis:** In bacterial infections, certain molecules (e.g., IgG or C3b) bind the surface of a bacterium. These molecules are called as opsonins. C3b and its cleavage product iC3b (inactive C3b) act as opsonins. They get attached to the cell wall of microbe and promote phagocytosis by neutrophils and macrophages through surface receptors (i.e., C3b receptor) for these complement fragments. The C3b

Table 20: Complement pathway specific activators.

Classical	*Alternative*	*Lectin*
Immune complexes [immunoglobulin (Ig) M, IgG]	Endotoxin	Repeating simple sugars
C-reactive protein	Aggregates of IgA	G0 carbohydrate glycoforms [carbohydrates linked to proteins through serine or threonine (o-linked) residues]
Apoptotic bodies	Complex polysaccharides	Cytokeratin-1
ß-amyloid fibrils	C3 nephritic factor	
Serum amyloid P	Viruses	
Mitochondrial products	Cobra venom	
Others: Viruses, proteases, urate crystals, and polyanions	Others: Carbohydrate zymosan (on yeast cell walls), tumor cells, and foreign materials	

receptors on phagocytic cell membranes recognize and bind the opsonized (coated by C3b) bacterium. Similarly, viruses, parasites, and transformed cells can activate complement and cause their inactivation or death.

- **Cell and bacterial lysis:** The deposition of the MAC (C5b–C9) on cells and bacterial wall creates pores/holes in the cell membrane. This allows water and ions to enter into the cells and results in osmotic death (lysis) of the cells and bacteria. This property of complement is mainly useful for killing of microbes with thin cell walls (e.g., *Neisseria* bacteria). Patients with deficiency of the terminal components of complement (C6 to C9) are prone to infections by the *Neisseria* species (e.g., *meningococci, gonococci*). In patients with complement deficiencies, *Neisseria* species can cause serious disseminated infections.
- **Increased vascular permeability:** Cleavage products of the corresponding complement components, namely C3a, C5a, and to a lesser extent, C4a are pro-inflammatory molecules. They stimulate histamine release from mast cells. Histamine in turn **increase vascular permeability and cause vasodilation**. C3a and C5a are called **anaphylatoxins, because their actions are similar to mast cell mediators involved in the reaction called anaphylaxis**. Functions of the anaphylatoxins in inflammation are presented in **Flowchart 6**.
- **Activation of AA:** C5a activates the LOX pathway of AA metabolism in neutrophils and monocytes. Thus, it releases more mediators of AA metabolites of LOX pathways.
- **Proinflammatory molecules** (MAC, C5a): These chemotactic factors can activate leukocytes and tissue cells. Thus, they can produce oxidants and cytokines and induce mast cell and basophil degranulation.

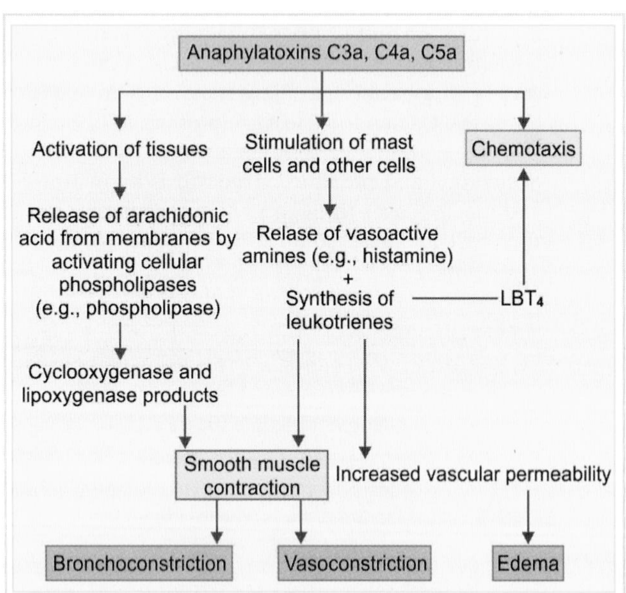

FLOWCHART 6: Functions of the anaphylatoxins in inflammation. Complement activation products, namely anaphylatoxins (C3a, C4a and C5a) are produced during activation of the complement cascade. They regulate vascular permeability, smooth muscle contraction, and chemotaxis.

- ***Interplay between innate and adaptive immune system: Complements play a role in defense against microbes through*** bridging ***innate and adaptive immunity.*** They increase antibody responses and intensify immune memory.
- ***Other functions: These include clearance of—***
  - Immune complexes (Clq, C3) and products of inflammatory injury from tissues
  - Apoptotic cells (Clq, C3).

Regulation of the complement system

The complement system is a potent inflammatory (produces proinflammatory molecules) and cytotoxic system. It is a carefully and tightly regulated process by inhibitory factors. **The activation of complement is controlled by cell membrane-associated proteins on cell surfaces** [e.g., decay accelerating factor (DAF)] and CD59) **and circulating regulatory** (inhibitory) **proteins in serum** (e.g., C1 inhibitor, protein S). These regulating processes are expressed on normal host cells and prevent complement binding to their surface. Thus, they prevent healthy tissues from being injured at sites of complement activation and protect the host from indiscriminate injury. Different regulatory proteins either inhibit the production of active complement component or remove fragments that deposit on cells. Major regulatory mechanisms are as follows:

- **Spontaneous decay:** C4b2a and C3bBb and their cleavage products, C3b and C4b undergo decay thereby decrease their effect.
- **Regulatory proteins in serum:**
  - **Proteolytic inactivation:** Plasma/serum contains inhibitors that inhibit unnecessary activation of complements. These include factor I (an inhibitor of C3b and C4b) and serum carboxypeptidase N (SCPN). SCPN deletes a carboxy-terminal arginine from anaphylatoxins C3a, C4a, and C5a. Removing single amino acid markedly reduces the biological activities of complements.
  - **Binding active components:** C1 esterase inhibitor (C1INH) is a binding protein in the plasma that binds to C1r and C1s and forms an irreversible inactive complex. Other binding proteins in the plasma include factor H- and C4b-binding protein. These form complex with C3b and C4b, respectively and increase their susceptibility to proteolytic breakdown/destruction by factor I.
- **Cell membrane-associated molecules:** These molecules are present on the cell membrane. Examples include two proteins linked to the cell membrane by glycophosphoinositol (GPI) anchors. These are **decay accelerating factor (DAF)** and **protectin (CD59)**. DAF destroys the alternative pathway C3 convertase. CD59 (membrane cofactor protein, protectin) binds membrane-associated C4b and C3b and, inactivates them by factor I and prevents formation of the MAC.

Note: If large amounts of complement are deposited on host cells and in tissues, the regulatory proteins can produce a strong response and produce damage. For example, in autoimmune diseases, patients produce complement-fixing antibodies against their own cell and tissue antigens.

Complement-mediated diseases

Q. Write short essay complement-mediated diseases.

The complement system can produce disease by different mechanisms.

- **Activation of complement** may be due to **antibodies or Ag–Ab complexes** deposited on host cells and tissues. It is an important mechanism of cell and tissue injury.
- **Ineffective complement system**
- **Inherited deficiencies of complement proteins** cause increased susceptibility to infections
- **Amplified inflammatory response by the complement**
- **Deficiencies of regulatory proteins** can cause a variety of disorders. The complement system targets microorganisms and avoids damage to normal cells and tissues. This is achieved by the regulatory system discussed previously. When the mechanisms regulating this balance are disturbed, the resulting imbalances in complement activity can produce tissue injury. This imbalance may be due to malfunction or deficiency caused by mutation. Uncontrolled systemic activation of complement may be observed in sepsis and plays the main role in the development of septic shock.

Immune complex diseases **Activation of complement** may be due to **antibodies or Ag–Ab complexes** deposited on host cells and tissues. It is an important mechanism of cell and tissue injury. In bacterial infections, immune complexes (Ag–Ab complexes) can form on bacterial surfaces. Ag-Ab complexes in association with C1 can activate the classical pathway of complement. Complement then promotes physiological clearance of these circulating immune (Ag–Ab) complexes. However, if these complexes are formed continuously and in excess (e.g., in chronic immune disorders), there will be continuous activation of complement system. This consumes and later depletes the complement. Complement inefficiency may be due to—(i) depletion of complement, (ii) deficient binding of complement, or (iii) defects in complement activation. This results in deposition of immune complexes and inflammation. This in turn may trigger development of autoimmunity.

Ineffective complement system

Infectious disease: Main role of complement system is defense against infection. If the complement system does not function effectively, the individual is susceptible to infection.

- **Defects in antibody production, complement proteins or phagocyte function:** It increases the susceptibility to pyogenic infections with microbes such as *Hemophilus influenzae* and *Streptococcus pneumoniae.*
- **Deficiencies in MAC formation:** It can lead to increased susceptibility to infections, particularly with meningococci.
- **Deficiency of complement MBL:** It results in recurrent infections in young children.

Strategies followed by microbes to overcome their destruction by complement These are as follows:

- Some bacteria have **thick capsules** that protect them from lysis by complement.
- Some **enzymes of bacteria** can also **inhibit the effects of complement components**, especially C5a.
- Few bacteria can increase **catabolism of components**, such as C3b and reduce formation of C3 convertase.
- Viruses may use **cell-bound components and receptors to facilitate their entry** into the cell.
- **Use of complement components to target inflammatory or epithelial cells:** Microbes such as *Mycobacterium tuberculosis*, Epstein Barr virus, measles virus, picornaviruses, human immunodeficiency virus (HIV) and flaviviruses use complement components to target inflammatory or epithelial cells.

Inflammation and necrosis **The inflammatory response is amplified by the complement system.** Anaphylatoxins C5a and C3a activate leukocytes and C5a and MAC stimulate endothelial cells. Thus, they produce excess of oxidants and cytokines that injure tissues.

Complement deficiencies (refer Fig. 20)

Q. Write a short essay on complement deficiencies.

Complement system should be intact and appropriately regulated. Complement activation is required for protection against many infectious agents, particularly bacteria. IgG and complement components, such as C3b, are opsonins and facilitate phagocytosis by neutrophils and macrophages. Thus, complement deficiencies **usually resemble antibody deficiencies**. Encapsulated bacteria (e.g., *Hemophilus influenzae* and *Streptococcus pneumoniae*) are very sensitive to opsonin-assisted phagocytosis. Hence, complement deficiency may cause recurrent life-threatening infections at an early age. Any acquired or congenital deficiencies of specific complement components or regulatory proteins can produce various diseases (**Table 21**). The most common congenital defect is a C2 deficiency, inherited as an autosomal codominant trait.

Congenital deficiencies

C3 complement deficiency: Activation of C3 is central (or critical) step in the complement cascade. All three pathways of complement activation (i.e., classical, alternative, and lectin pathways) activate C3 into C3a and C3b. C3b is a major opsonin and also is the activator of the terminal components of the cascade (C6 through C9). Hence, deficiency of **C3** is the most severe form of complement deficiency.

Mannose-binding lectin (MBL) deficiency: It is the primary defect of the lectin pathway of complement activation. Patients have increased risk of infection with microorganisms with polysaccharide capsules rich in mannose. These include mainly the yeast *Saccharomyces cerevisiae,* and encapsulated bacteria such as *Neisseria meningitides* and *S. pneumonia.*

Properdin deficiency: It is involved in alternate complement pathway and is the most common defect in the alternative pathway. It is an X-linked disorder, whereas all other congenital complement deficiencies are autosomal recessive. It is associated with recurrent infections with *Neisseria meningitides.*

Deficiency of terminal complement components: Deficiencies of any of the terminal components of the complement cascade (C5, C6, C7, or C8 deficiencies) can occur as hereditary disorders. They are associated with increased predisposition to infections with one group of bacteria belonging to the genus *Neisseria,* particularly *Neisseria meningitides. Neisseria* usually produces localized infections (meningitis or gonorrhea), but in patients with deficiency of

Table 21: Examples of defects in complement and complement regulatory system.

Complement deficiency	*Defect/clinical association*
Deficiency of Complement	
Classic pathway	
• C1q, C1r and C1s, C4	Immune-complex syndromes [includes systemic lupus erythematosus (SLE) and SLE-like syndromes, glomerulonephritis, and vasculitis syndromes], pyogenic infections
• C2	Immune-complex syndromes, few with pyogenic infections. Increased risk for recurrent respiratory tract infections with encapsulated bacteria, systemic infections with *Neisseria*
• C2, C4 deficiency	Defective activation of classical pathway. Results in reduced resistance to infection and reduced clearance of immune complexes
C3 and alternative pathway C3	
• C3 deficiency	Defects in all complement functions, immune-complex syndromes, pyogenic infections
• C3b, iC3b, C5, MBL	Pyogenic bacterial infections, membranoproliferative glomerulonephritis
• Factor D (C3 proactivator convertase, properdin factor D esterase)	Pyogenic infections, risk for systemic infections with *Neisseria*
• C3, properdin, MAC proteins	Neisserial infection
Lectin pathway	
• MBL	Other pyogenic, fungal, human immunodeficiency virus and SLE
• MASP-2	Pneumococcal pneumonia
Membrane attack complex	
• C5, C6, C7, C8	Recurrent *Neisseria* infections, immune-complex disease
• C9	Rare *Neisseria* infections
Deficiency of complement regulatory proteins*	
Positive regulation	
• Properdin	Stabilizes alternative pathway C3/C5 convertases Neisserial infection
Negative regulation	
• C1 inhibitor (C1-INH)	Inhibits C1r/C1s, MASPs. Hereditary angioedema, rare immune-complex disease, few with pyogenic infections
• Factor H[#]	Meningococcal bacteremia and meningitis, other pyogenic hemolytic–uremic syndrome, membranoproliferative glomerulonephritis
• Factor I[#]	Pyogenic infections, meningococcal meningitis, pneumococcal bacteremia, and meningitis
• C4-binding protein	Autoimmune disease
Membrane regulatory proteins	
• Decay accelerating factor (DAF) (CD55)	Inhibition by decay acceleration of the classical and alternative pathway C3 convertases. Paroxysmal nocturnal hemoglobinuria (PNH) with hemolysis and thrombosis
• CD59[#]	Blocks C8-C9 and C9 Paroxysmal nocturnal hemoglobinuria (PNH) with hemolysis and thrombosis

(MAC: membrane attack complex; MASP: MBL-associated serine protease; MBL: mannose-binding lectin)

*Causes excessive activation of complement system

#Acquired disorders

terminal complement components, defects have several fold increased risk for systemic infections with atypical strains of these microorganisms.

- **C9 deficiency:** It is the most common terminal pathway defect and is usually asymptomatic.
- Other deficiencies of the terminal pathway: They are extremely rare. They are associated with more aggressive infections.

  Other complement deficiencies are listed in **Table 21**.

Acquired deficiencies Acquired deficiencies have been described in each of the pathways of complement and most of them may be less severe.

- **Acquired deficiencies of early complement components:** Defects in the early components involved in classical pathway (i.e., C1, C2, C4) may occur. It may be observed in patients with some autoimmune diseases associated with circulating immune complexes. Examples include certain forms of membranous glomerulonephritis and SLE.

Deficiencies in early components of complement (e.g., C1q, C1r, C1s, C4) is strongly associated with susceptibility to SLE or SLE-like syndrome. This suggests the role of these early complement components in removal of naturally occurring immune complexes from the circulation. They are prone to increased risk for recurrent infections, sometimes severe, with encapsulated bacteria.

- **Deficiency of middle complement components:** Lack of the middle (C3, C5) components causes increased susceptibility to recurrent pyogenic infections, membranoproliferative glomerulonephritis, and skin rashes.
- **Deficiency of terminal complement components:** Patients who lack terminal complement components (C6, C7 or C8) are vulnerable to infections with *Neisseria* species.

Congenital deficiencies of complement regulatory proteins

C1 inhibitor **It is a complement regulatory protein** that blocks the activation of C1, the first protein of the classical complement pathway. Inherited deficiency of C1 inhibitor is the cause of *hereditary angioedema (HAE)*. **HAE** is a serious autosomal dominant disorder caused by mutation of the C1INH (discussed in detail below on pages 263–265). It leads to chronic complement activation.

Decay accelerating factor and CD59 **Phosphatidylinositol glycan-group A** (PIGA) **is an enzyme essential for the synthesis of certain membrane-associated complement regulatory proteins**. PIGA gene mutation results in **deficient synthesis of glycophosphatidylinositol (GPI)-linked proteins.** These proteins anchor several proteins to the plasma/cell membrane and some are responsible for complement degradation. There are **two complement regulator proteins** that can degrade complements—**DAF or CD55 and membrane inhibitor of reactive lysis or CD59**. These two complement regulator proteins are linked to plasma membranes by a GPI anchor. DAF prevents formation of C3 convertases. CD59 binds to C8 in the C5b–8 complex and blocks the binding and incorporation of C9 into the complex. Further, CD59 also binds directly to C9 and prevents the addition of additional C9 to the complex and stops the complex from forming a transmembrane pore. Thus, CD59 inhibits formation of the MAC.

- An **acquired deficiency of the GPI-linked proteins leads to deficiency of these regulators.** So, there will be **excessive complement activation and lysis of cells** (which are sensitive to complement-mediated cell lysis). This gives rise to a disease called **paroxysmal nocturnal hemoglobinuria (PNH).**

Other complement regulatory proteins There are other regulatory proteins that can proteolytically cleave active complement components. Factor I and factor H are main regulators of the complement cascade. They control the level of spontaneous activation of C3. Both **factor I deficiency** and **factor H deficiency** can be severe, because their deficiency will increase spontaneous destruction of C3 and lead to secondary C3 deficiency.

- **Complement Factor H:** It is a circulating glycoprotein. It inhibits the alternative pathway of complement activation by cleaving and destroying C3b and the turnover of the C3 convertases. Inherited defects in Factor H and many other regulatory proteins that interact with Factor H produces an atypical form of hemolytic uremic syndrome. In this disorder, the complement deposits in glomerular vessels. This damages the endothelial cells and forms platelet-rich thrombi. Polymorphisms in the *Factor H* gene may be associated with age-related macular degeneration. This is an important cause of loss of vision in older adults.

Factor H It is a complement regulator plasma protein that acts as a **cofactor for the proteolysis of the C3 convertase.** Deficiency of factor H results in excessive complement activation. **Mutations in factor H** are associated with a kidney disease called the **hemolytic uremic syndrome** and increased permeability of retinal vessels in *wet* macular degeneration of the eye.

Various complement defects that can occur are depicted in **Figure 20**.

Angioneurotic edema

Q. Write a short essay on angioneurotic edema.

Angioedema or angioneurotic edema is defined as a well-demarcated localized edema (swelling) involving the deeper layers of the skin, including the subcutaneous tissue and submucosal tissues. Urticaria (also known as hives) is produced due to localized edema of dermis secondary to a temporary increase in capillary permeability.

Etiology It can be immunological or nonimmunological-mediated disorder or can be idiopathic. It is usually an IgE-mediated reaction that causes direct release of histamine from the mast cells. It follows a variety of allergens. It may develop because of insect sting, drug reaction, allergy to food, peanuts, cow's milk, chicken eggs, and exposure to other biological products. Rarely, angiotensin-converting enzyme (ACE) inhibitors used for the treatment of hypertension or heart disease which may produce angioedema because of increased levels of bradykinin. Most of the cases are idiopathic. In idiopathic cases, the cause is usually not identified or angioedema is only weakly correlated to allergen exposure.

C1 Esterase inhibitor deficiency C1 esterase inhibitor is a complement protein that inhibits spontaneous activation of classical complement pathway. C1INH also regulates kinin cascade, activation of which increases local bradykinin levels and produces local pain and swelling. Both C1INH and C1 levels are low. C1INH deficiency produces bradykinin. Deficiency of C1INH may be **hereditary** or **acquired disorder**.

Hereditary Angioedema Hereditary angioedema is an autosomal dominant disorder due to inherited deficiency of the plasma protein C1 inhibitor (also called C1 inhibitor or C1INH). It is a rare but serious disorder in children.

It exists in three forms, namely type 1, 2, and 3. Type 1 and 2 are caused by mutations in the *SERPING1* gene (in chromosome 11) and type 3 HAE has been linked with mutation in the factor XII (*F12*) gene.

- **Type 1** deficiency of C1INH: In 85% of patients, no detectable protein (i.e., C1INH).
- **Type 2** deficiency of C1INH: 15% of patients have a dysfunctional protein, namely C1INH.
- **Type 3:** It is less common type of HAE. In this type, C1INH function is normal and patients have a mutant form of factor

XII, which leads to production of excessive bradykinin. It occurs in an X-linked dominant fashion and therefore mainly affects women. It can be exacerbated by pregnancy and use of hormonal contraception. It has been linked with mutation in the factor XII (*F12*) gene. This gene encodes the coagulation protein factor XII.

Pathogenesis (Flowchart 7) C1 inhibitor is an acute phase reactant and functions as a kallikrein-serine protease inhibitor and belongs to serpin family. Serpins inhibit both lectin complement pathway and kinin producing pathways.

- **Continuous activation of complement system:** Deficiency of C1INH causes continuous activation of the complement system. Continuous production of kallikrein-serine protease inhibitor (serpin) normally inhibits the association of C1r and C1s and C1q and prevents the formation of the C1 complex. As already discussed under classical complement pathway, C1 complex activates other proteins of the complement system.
- **Increased production of bradykinin:** Though C1 inhibitor has many functions, its role in the kinin pathway is important for the development of angioedema. C1INH is an inhibitor of many proteases, including kallikrein and coagulation factor XII (both are involved in the production of vasoactive peptide bradykinin). C1INH usually limits bradykinin production by inhibiting both kallikrein and factor XII (Hageman factor) as well as the C1r/C1s components of C1. The common result is degradation of bradykinin. Deficiency of C1INH causes activation of factor XII of the coagulation cascade. Activated factor XII (i.e., XIIa) converts prekallikrein to kallikrein, and kallikrein in turn catalyzes the cleavage of high-molecular weight kininogen (HMWK) into bradykinin. This is associated with increased production and increased bradykinin action. Bradykinin is a potent vasodilator as well as increases vascular permeability. Thus, it produces edema. In individuals with a deficiency of C1 inhibitor, this process proceeds unchecked and leads to gross vasodilation and angioedema.

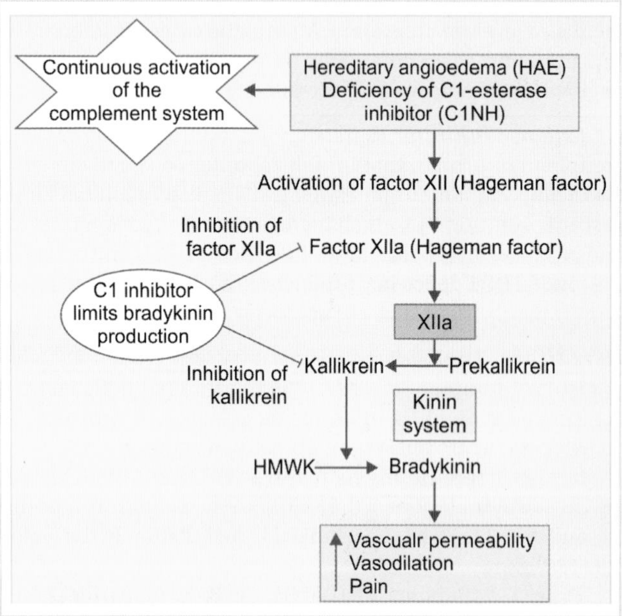

Continuous activation of the complement system
Hereditary angioedema (HAE) Deficiency of C1-esterase inhibitor (C1NH)
Activation of factor XII (Hageman factor)
Inhibition of factor XIIa
Factor XIIa (Hageman factor)
C1 inhibitor limits bradykinin production
XIIa
Inhibition of kallikrein
Kallikrein
Prekallikrein
Kinin system
HMWK
Bradykinin
↑ Vascualr permeability
Vasodilation
Pain

FLOWCHART 7: Pathogenesis of hereditary angioedema (HAE). Deficiency of C1 esterase inhibitor (C1INH) causes continuous activation of the complement system and also increased bradykinin production (responsible for edema).

Clinical presentation All forms of HAE lead to abnormal activation of the complement system.

- Angioedema develops either spontaneously (with no direct identifiable cause) or following infection or mild trauma/injury (e.g., dental work and other stimuli). Onset is usually in early childhood. Affected patients have episodes of edema affecting skin and mucosal surfaces. Most obvious in the face but can also involve the larynx and the gastrointestinal tract.
- There is usually no associated itch or urticaria because it is not an allergic response.
- The attacks become worse at puberty and usually their frequency and severity decrease after the age of 50 and may even disappear totally.
- HAE can also have recurrent episodes (often called "attacks") of abdominal pain, intense vomiting, and weakness.
- The mortality of undiagnosed HAE can be >50%.

Acquired C1 esterase inhibitor deficiency Th2: C1 esterase inhibitor deficiency can also develop in a sporadic acquired form. It results from excessive consumption of C1INH either due to formation of immune complexes or as an autoimmune disorder due to the generation of an autoantibody against C1INH. It may occur with B-cell lymphoma, multiple myeloma, Waldenstrom's macroglobulinemia, and chronic lymphocytic leukemia. It presents in a manner similar to the HAE but the onset occurs in the fifth and sixth decades of life.

Clinical features

- It may occur at any age but most common in young adults.
- It presents with well-defined, nonpitting swelling, usually nonpruritic. It may be associated with urticaria lesions.
- It may involve any area of the body but often affects periorbital, lips (**Fig. 21**), and genital areas.
- Angioedema of the upper respiratory tract may cause laryngeal obstruction which may be life-threatening.
- Involvement of gastrointestinal system may produce abdominal colic, with or without nausea and vomiting.

Diagnosis: Diagnosis depends–

- Clinical features
- Routine blood tests (complete blood count, electrolytes, renal function, liver enzymes) should be routinely performed.
- Mast cell tryptase levels: It may be raised if the angioedema is due to an acute allergic (anaphylactic) reaction.
- **In HAE:** Laboratory evaluation of complement and C1INH levels usually helps in accurate diagnosis. During clinical attacks of angioedema, laboratory findings show low levels of C1INH (in 85% cases) or it is dysfunctional (in 15% cases). The plasma levels of bradykinin are elevated leading to angioedema. The excessive activation of C1 results in a decline in C4 and C2 levels.

Products of Coagulation

inhibition of coagulation was found to reduce the inflammatory reaction to certain microbes and probably indicates that there is a link between coagulation and inflammation. Protease-activated receptors (PARs), expressed on leukocytes are activated by thrombin (the protease which converts fibrinogen to fibrin clot). Platelets have a PAR known as the thrombin receptor and when activated by thrombin, it causes powerful aggregation of platelets during the process of clot formation. There is a close association between clotting and inflammation. Almost all types of tissue injuries that lead to clotting also induce inflammation, and inflammation causes changes in endothelial cells that increase the chances of abnormal clotting (i.e., thrombosis). However, the significant role of products of coagulation in stimulating inflammation is not well established.

Inflammation and clotting system are intertwined with each other. Activated Hageman factor (factor XIIa) activate the four systems involved in the inflammatory response (**Fig. 22**).

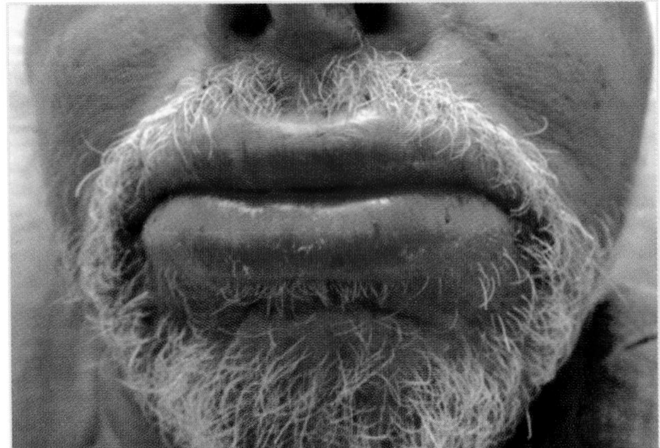

FIG. 21: Angioedema.

1. **Activation of fibrinolytic system:** Factor XIIa stimulates fibrinolytic system by converting plasminogen to plasmin. The role of fibrinolytic system in inflammation are:
   - Activation of complement system.
   - Fibrin split products: Plasmin degrades fibrin to form fibrin split products, which may increase vascular permeability.
2. **Activation of the kinin system** (discussed below)
3. **Activation of the alternative complement pathway:** Factor XIIa can activate alternate complement pathway.
4. **Activation of the coagulation system:** Factor XIIa activates coagulation system and forms thrombin, which has inflammatory properties.

Kinins

Kinins are vasoactive peptides formed in plasma and tissue by the action of specific proteases called kallikreins on specific plasma glycoproteins, called **kininogens**. The enzyme kallikrein cleaves a plasma glycoprotein precursor, high-molecular-weight kininogen to produce *bradykinin*.

Actions of Bradykinin: Their effects are similar to those of histamine (refer page 250).

- **Increases vascular permeability**
- **Pain** when injected into the skin.
- Bradykinin mediates some forms of allergic reaction, such as anaphylaxis.
- Bradykinin and related peptides also regulate multiple physiologic processes. These include blood pressure, contraction and relaxation of smooth muscle, **dilation of blood vessels,** plasma extravasation, and cell migration.
- Most significant function of kinins is their ability to amplify inflammatory responses by stimulating local tissue cells and inflammatory cells to generate additional mediators.

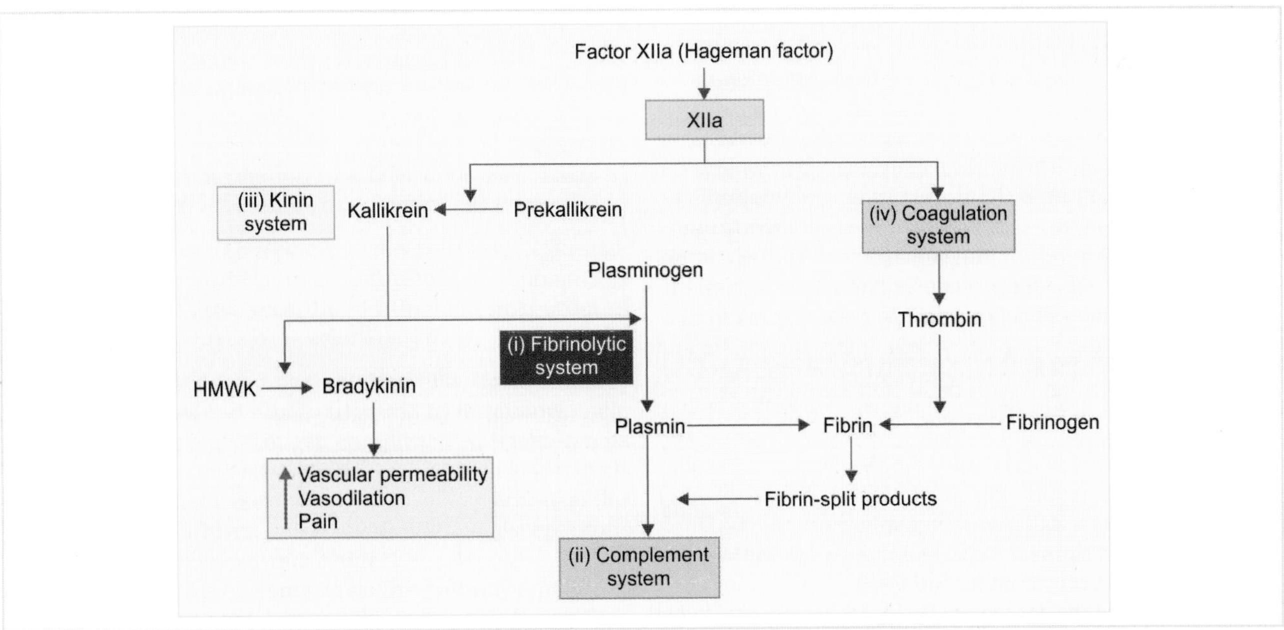

(HMWK: high-molecular-weight kininogen)

FIG. 22: Interrelationships between the four plasma-derived chemical mediator systems. Activation of factor XII (Hageman factor) is a key event leading to (i) conversion of plasminogen to plasmin, resulting in generation of fibrin split products and (ii) active complement products. (iii) Activation of kallikrein produces kinins and (iv) activation of the coagulation system results in fibrin formation.

These include prostanoids, cytokines (e.g., TNF-α and ILs), and NO.

Inactivation: The action of bradykinin is quick and short-lived. They are quickly inactivated by an enzyme called kininase.

Other Mediators

Neuropeptides

Neuropeptides are small peptides belonging to neurokinin family and are secreted by sensory nerves and various leukocytes. They may be involved in the initiation and regulation of inflammatory responses. Neuropeptides such as substance P, neurokinin A (NKA) and B (NKB) are distributed throughout the central and peripheral nervous systems and link the endocrine, nervous, and immune systems. Nerve fibers containing substance P are seen in the lung and gastrointestinal tract. These peptides have several functions such as transmitting pain signals, regulating blood pressure, stimulating secretion of hormone by endocrine cells, extravasation of plasma proteins and edema, increasing vascular permeability, vasodilation, smooth muscle contraction and relaxation, salivary secretion, and airway contraction.

It was noted the association between sensory afferent nerves and inflammation. Injury to nerve terminals during inflammation stimulates increase in neurokinins. This in turn causes release of inflammatory mediators, such as histamine, NO, and kinins.

When Lewis first discovered the role of histamine in inflammation, it was thought that one mediator is enough to carry out the inflammatory reaction. However, we have discovered a large number of them and most important mediators involved in acute inflammation are summarized in **Table 22**.

Table 22: Important mediators involved in acute inflammation.

Action of the mediator	*Name of the mediator*	*Source of the mediator*
Vasodilation	Prostaglandins	Mast cells, all leukocytes
	Histamine	Mast cells, basophils, platelets
	Nitric oxide	Endothelium, macrophages
Increased vascular permeability	Histamine	Mast cells, basophils, platelets
	Serotonin	Platelets
	C3a and C5a (liberate vasoactive amines from mast cells, other cells)	Plasma (produced in liver)
	Bradykinin	
	Leukotrienes C4, D4, E4	Mast cells, all leukocytes
	Platelet-activating factor (PAF)—at low concentration	All leukocytes, platelets endothelial cells
	Neuropeptides (substance P)	Leukocytes, nerve fibers
Chemotaxis and leukocyte activation	Cytokines [tumor necrosis factor (TNF), interleukin (IL)-1, IL-6]	Macrophages, lymphocytes, endothelial cells, mast cells
	Chemokines	Leukocytes, activated macrophages
	C3a, C5a	Plasma (produced in the liver)
	Leukotriene B_4	Mast cells, leukocytes
	Bacterial products (e.g., N-formyl methyl peptides)	Bacteria
Fever	IL-1 TNF	Macrophages, endothelial cells, mast cells
	Prostaglandins	Mast cells, leukocytes
Pain	Prostaglandins	
	Bradykinin	Plasma protein
Tissue damage	Lysosomal enzymes	Leukocytes
	Reactive oxygen species	
	Nitric oxide	Endothelium, macrophage

NEGATIVE REGULATORS OF ACUTE INFLAMMATION

Resolution is expected outcome of all acute inflammation. After the removal of the initial stimulus or agent, resolution of acute inflammation begins with removal of damaged/necrotic tissue followed by proper healing by regeneration. The inflammatory cells undergo apoptosis. However, the response to injury is variable and depends on the genetics, sex, and age of the patient. Negative regulators of acute inflammation include:

- **Gene silencing and reprogramming:** During resolution, there will be decreased proinflammatory mediators and increased anti-inflammatory mediators. This is achieved by—(1) silencing of acute proinflammatory gene expression, (2) increasing anti-inflammatory gene expression, and (3) allowing the inflammatory process to start to resolve. There may be repression of TNF-α, IL-1β, and other proinflammatory genes and increased expression of anti-inflammatory factors, such as IL-1 receptor antagonist (IL-1RA), TNF-α receptors, IL-6, and IL-10.
- **Cytokines:** Many ILs (IL-6, IL-10, IL-11, IL-12, IL-13) reduce production of proinflammatory TNF-α, thereby limit inflammation.
- **Protease inhibitors:** Secretory leukocyte proteinase inhibitor (SLPI) reduce the responses of a variety of cell types such as macrophages and endothelial cells, thereby, reduce the damage to the connective tissue.
- **Lipoxins:** Lipoxins and aspirin-triggered LXs are anti-inflammatory mediators that inhibit synthesis of leukotriene in AA pathway.

- **Glucocorticoids:** Stimulation of the hypothalamic–pituitary–adrenal axis increases the release of immunosuppressive glucocorticoids. These corticoids reduce inflammatory reaction.
- **Kininases:** Kininases are present in plasma. They degrade the potent proinflammatory mediator bradykinin.
- **Phosphatases:** Signal transduction mechanism that commonly regulates inflammatory cell signaling is rapid and reversible protein phosphorylation. Phosphatases and associated proteins reduce their effect by dephosphorylation.
- **Transforming growth factor-β (TGF-β):** Apoptotic cells, mainly neutrophils, induce expression of TGF-β. In turn, TGF-β suppresses proinflammatory cytokines and chemokines and favors the production of anti-inflammatory LX through AA.

8.3 Cells of Inflammation

CHAPTER OUTLINE

CELLS OF INFLAMMATION

Leukocytes are the major cells involved in inflammation. These include neutrophils, lymphocytes (T and B), monocytes, macrophages, eosinophils, mast cells, and basophils. Each type of leukocyte has specific functions, but they overlap and change as inflammation progresses. Inflammatory cells and resident tissue cells interact with each other in an organized continuous response during inflammation. Nomenclature and location of cells of the immune system is presented in **Figure 23**.

LEUKOCYTES

Q. Write a short essay on constituents of granules of leukocytes and their function.

Leukocytes [white blood cells (WBCs)] defend the body against microorganisms causing infection. It also removes debris, including all dead or injured cells. The leukocytes act primarily in the tissues but are circulating in the blood. Leukocytes are the primary effector cells of the immune system.

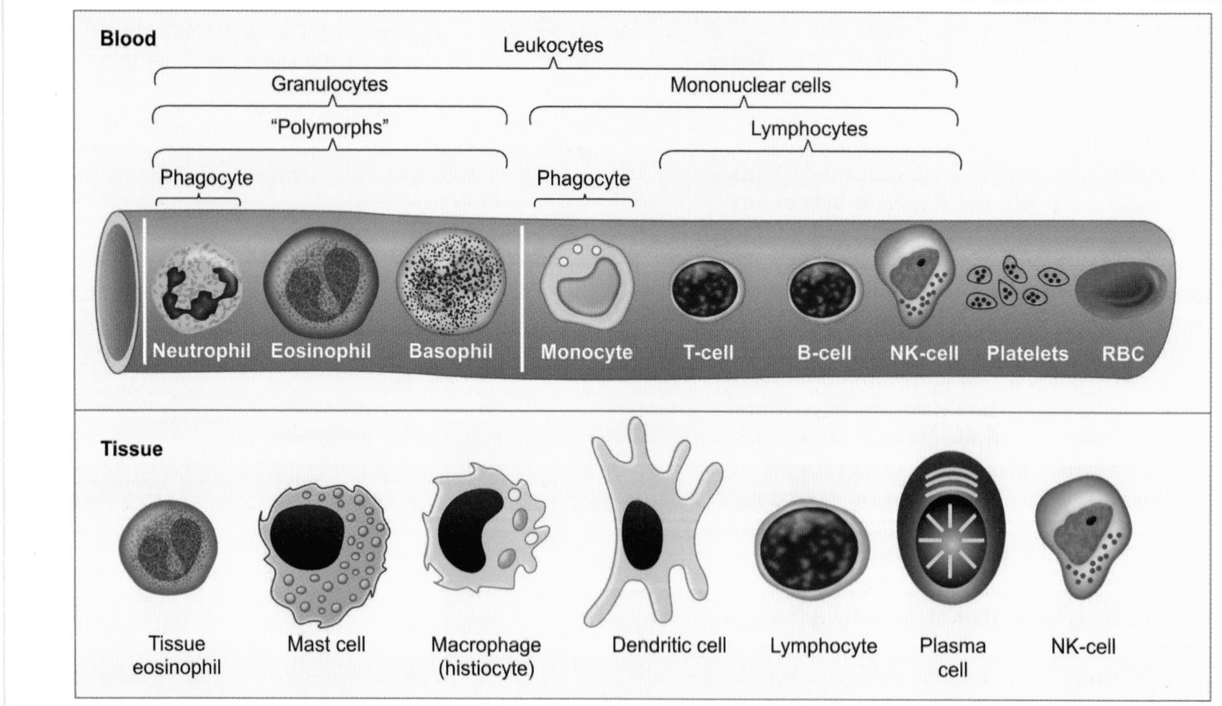

FIG. 23: Nomenclature and location of cells of the immune system (eosinophils are also phagocytes).

Classification

Leukocytes can be classified according to structure as either **granulocytes** or **agranulocytes**; according to function as either **phagocytes** or **immunocytes** (cells that create or are involved in immunity); **and** depending on their developmental path in the bone marrow as **myeloid or lymphoid cells**. Each of the different types of leukocytes in blood has a special function.

Granulocytes

It includes neutrophils, basophils, and eosinophils, and all are phagocytes. Mast cells also are classified as granulocytes. Of the agranulocytes, the monocytes and macrophages are phagocytes, whereas the lymphocytes are immunocytes (involved in immunity).

Properties of Granulocytes

The cytoplasm of granulocytes contains many membrane-bound granules. These granules contain enzymes capable of killing microorganisms and degrading debris ingested during phagocytosis.

- The granules also contain **powerful biochemical mediators** with inflammatory and immune functions. These biochemical mediators and the **digestive enzymes** are released from granulocytes in response to specific stimuli. The biochemical mediators have vascular and intercellular effects, and the enzymes are involved in the breakdown of debris from sites of infection or injury.
- Granulocytes are **capable of ameboid movement**. They migrate through vessel walls (diapedesis) to sites where their action is needed (e.g., inflammation).

Neutrophil

The **neutrophil** is the major cell lineage of WBC in the peripheral blood (i.e., circulating granulocytes) in healthy adult individuals. Neutrophils are also known as **polymorphonuclear neutrophil**/*leukocytes* (polys or **PMN**s). Neutrophils constitute about 45–75% of the total WBC/leukocyte count in adults. PMNs predominate in acute inflammation. They circulate in the blood as spherical cells approximately 12–15 μm in diameter with numerous membranous projections.

Granules of neutrophil (Fig. 24 and Box 8)

Neutrophils have a central segmented nucleus and normally with two to four distinct nuclear lobes (i.e., two- to four-lobed nucleus) and coarse, clumped chromatin. Neutrophils have granulated cytoplasm (contains about 200 granules) with three types of granules, namely primary [large azurophilic (1/3)], secondary [smaller specific (2/3)], and tertiary (very few) granules. These granules contain microbicidal factors. Main types are primary and secondary granules. They are morphologically and biochemically distinct and each has unique activities. These granules (and lysosomes) can fuse with phagocytic vacuoles containing engulfed/ingested material and destroy them. In addition, the granule contents also undergo exocytosis (degranulation), and are released into the extracellular space. These granules do not stain strongly with either basic or acidic dyes (hematoxylin and eosin, respectively). Different granule enzymes perform different functions. Primary inflammatory mediators and granule contents of polymorphonuclear leukocyte are presented in **Box 8**.

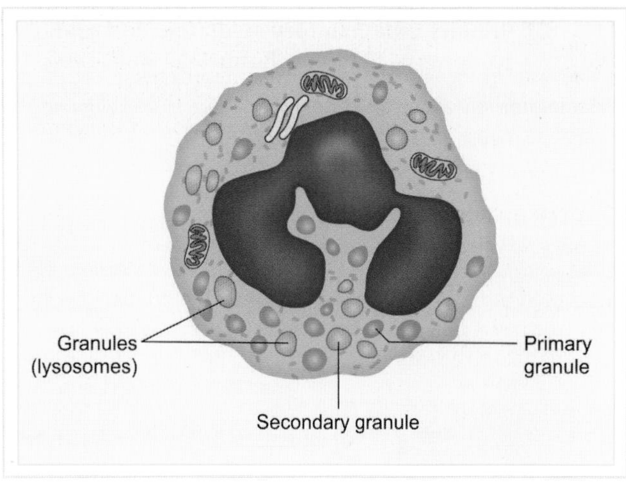

FIG. 24: Diagrammatic representation of neutrophil.

Primary granules (azurophilic granules) They are present in all granulocytes and contain myeloperoxidase which produces antibacterial compounds, acid hydrolases, and bactericidal factors (lysozyme, defensins). The various actions are:

- These granules have **antimicrobial and proteinase activity** and can directly activate other inflammatory cells.
- **Potent acid hydrolases** (these include nucleases, proteases, glycosidases, lipases, phosphatases, sulfatases, phospholipases) **degrade bacteria and debris** within phagolysosomes, by acidification.
- **Neutral proteases** (e.g., neutrophil elastase, cathepsin G, nonspecific collagenase, and proteinase 3) can **degrade various extracellular components** (e.g., collagen, basement membrane, fibrin, elastin, and cartilage). This results in the destruction of tissue in inflammatory processes. Neutrophil elastase fight infections by degrading virulence factors of bacteria. Neutral proteases can also directly cleave C3 and C5 complement proteins producing complement products that are anaphylatoxins (C3a, C5a), and release a kinin-like peptide from kininogen.
- **Lysozyme and** PLA_2 **degrade bacterial cell walls** and **biological membranes**. They are important in killing bacteria.
- **Myeloperoxidase** is a key enzyme in the **metabolism of hydrogen peroxide** and **produces toxic ROS**.

Secondary granules (specific granules) They are the most numerous type and complement activators and enzymes e.g., collagenases. PLA_2, lysozyme, and proteins present in these granules initiate killing of specific cells. Other contents include the cationic lactoferrin, a vitamin B_{12}-binding protein, and matrix metalloproteinase (collagenase) specific for type IV collagen.

Tertiary granules (small storage granules, C granules) They are either phosphatases or metalloproteinases (aid in movement of leukocytes through connective tissue). During chemotaxis, these granules are liberated at the leading front of neutrophils. They contain enzymes such as proteinases, cathepsin, gelatinase, and urokinase-type plasminogen activator (u-PA) that promote migration of leukocytes through basement membranes and tissues.

Box 8: Primary inflammatory mediators and granule contents of polymorphonuclear leukocyte.

Primary Inflammatory Mediators
- Reactive oxygen metabolites
- Lysosomal granule contents

Granules and their Content

Primary (larger azurophilic) granules
- Myeloperoxidase
- Bactericidal factors
  - Lysozyme
  - Defensins
- Acid hydrolases
  - Nucleases
  - Proteases
  - Glycosidases
  - Lipases
  - Phosphatases
  - Sulfatases
  - Phospholipases
- Bactericidal/permeability increasing protein (BPI)
- Neutral proteases
  - Neutrophil elastase
  - Cathepsins G
  - Nonspecific collagenases
  - Proteinase 3
- Glucuronidase
- Mannosidase
- Phospholipase A_2

Secondary (smaller specific) granules
- Lysozyme
- Collagenase
- Gelatinase
- Lactoferrin
- Plasminogen activator
- Histaminase
- Alkaline phosphatase
- Reduced nicotinamide adenine dinucleotide phosphate (NADPH) oxidase
- Elastase
- Complement activator
- Phospholipase A_2
- CD11b/CD18
- CD11c/CD18
- Laminin
- Cathelicidin

Tertiary granules
- Metalloproteinases (collagenase, gelatinase)
- Plasminogen activator
- Cathepsins
- Glucuronidase
- Mannosidase

Pools of neutrophils

There are two pools of neutrophils—*a circulating pool* and a *marginal pool.*

- **Marginal pool:** Neutrophils of the marginal pool are distributed close to the vascular endothelium. Neutrophils stored in the bone marrow outnumber, by about 10 times the quantity of circulating neutrophils.
- **Circulating pool:** Circulating neutrophils are a major cell type among WBCs, making up to 45–75% in an adult healthy individual. However, in healthy children from 4–5 days old to 4–5 years of age, lymphocytes predominate over neutrophils in the blood circulation.

Production

Neutrophils are produced from stem cells in the bone marrow in response to IL-3, granulocyte-macrophage colony-stimulating factor (GM-CSF), and granulocyte colony-stimulating factor (G-CSF). Neutrophils produced in the bone marrow stem cells undergo several stages of maturation. These stages, from least to most mature are—myeloblast, promyelocyte, metamyelocyte, band form, and mature segmented neutrophil. The early form seen in blood is an immature neutrophil called banded neutrophils (*bands* or *stabs*), while mature neutrophils are called *segmented neutrophils* because of the characteristic appearance of their nucleus (with 3–5 segmented nuclei). Normally, an adult individual produces >1×10^{11} neutrophils per day. These stored neutrophils are released into the circulation, where they have a half-life of 4–10 hours. Neutrophils that are not recruited into tissues within about 6 hours undergo cell death by apoptosis.

- **Marrow neutrophil reserve:** Neutrophils undergo full maturation in the bone marrow, and these mature neutrophils are termed the *marrow neutrophil reserve.* Normally, about 14 days are needed for neutrophils to develop from early precursors to mature form. However, this process is accelerated by infection and treatment with colony-stimulating factors. Similar *tumor-associated macrophages (TAMs), tumor-associated neutrophils* (*TANs*) are recently described as a neutrophil population different from conventional neutrophils and granulocyte fraction of myeloid-derived suppressor cells (MDSCs). It is a challenging field of the current research.

Neutrophils in inflammation

Main functions Neutrophils play central role in acute inflammation, phagocytosis of microorganisms and tissue debris and mediate tissue injury. Neutrophils are highly adherent, motile, phagocytic leukocytes. Polymorphonuclear neutrophils (PMNs) are characteristic, typically the first cells recruited to acute inflammatory sites and predominant (most abundant) cells of acute inflammation. Numerous adhesive molecules, cytokines, and chemokines regulate neutrophil activity including IL8, IL17, CXCL1, CXCL2, CXCL3, CXCL5, CXCL6, and CXCL7.

Adhesion to endothelium Circulating neutrophils have receptors on their cell surfaces.These receptors are called *L-selectins,* and are chemokine receptors. First, they allow neutrophils to loosely adhere and roll along the capillary surface in areas of inflammation. Later, they enable them to bind firmly to endothelial cells (refer **Fig. 11**).

Emigration and chemotaxis After adhesion, other interactions between neutrophil integrin receptors and extracellular matrix (ECM) facilitate movement of neutrophils through the capillary wall and into the extravascular tissue. They are early responders to an acute bacterial infection and rapidly (very quickly) accumulate in large numbers at the site of infection or tissue injury. Neutrophils are attracted to areas of inflammation by chemotactic factor (e.g., bacterial products, complement fragments such as C5a, and cytokines).

Phagocytosis Neutrophils recognize microbes or dead cells and this induces several responses in leukocytes that are called as leukocyte activation. Neutrophil receptors recognize the Fc portion of IgG and IgM; complement components C5a, C3b and iC3b; AA metabolites; chemotactic factors; and cytokines. This leads to activation of various types of leukocyte cell surface receptors in acute inflammation (**Fig. 9**). Recognition is the first step in phagocytosis. Neutrophils are the chief phagocytes of early inflammation. In tissues, neutrophils are capable of phagocyting and destroying invading extracellular pathogens (e.g., bacteria, molds) as well as dead tissue/debris. On phagocytosis, the granules of neutrophils undergo degranulation. They degrade the engulfed micro-organisms, other material or dead tissue. Then these neutrophils undergo apoptosis in 1 or 2 days, mainly during the resolution phase of acute inflammation. The dissolution of dead neutrophils releases digestive enzymes present in their cytoplasmic granules. These enzymes dissolve cellular debris and prepare the site for healing.

Neutrophil extracellular traps Neutrophils also defend through the release of deoxyribonucleic acid (DNA)-chromatin structures, known as neutrophil extracellular traps (NETs). Released proteins adhere to the NETs (refer pages 154–156) and act as a scaffold of enzymes to function in extracellular spaces to attack micro-organisms. The process of creating NETs is called NETosis (refer pages 154–156) to attack pathogens in a specific manner.

Damage to tissue Neutrophils produce potent mediators (including granule enzymes) that can destroy microorganisms and numerous toxins are also released by neutrophils during inflammation. These include oxidizing free radicals, defensins, and proteolytic enzymes (e.g., elastase). The main purpose of release of these toxins from neutrophils is to destroy the causative agent. However, generated free radicals and released enzymes from neutrophils can cause extensive damage to normal tissue (e.g., basement membrane and small blood vessels), if the initial leukocytic infiltration is unchecked and continues. This can produce further increase in inflammation. It may occur during inflammatory response such as immunologic cell injury. However, these harmful proteases are normally controlled by a system of antiproteases in the serum and tissue fluids (e.g.,α_1-antitrypsin, α_2-macroglobulin). In chronic bacterial infection bone (osteomyelitis), a neutrophilic exudate may be observed for months and this pattern of inflammation is termed as acute on chronic.

Changes in circulating neutrophils

Initially during an acute infection, there is increase in the number of circulating neutrophils. This is termed **neutrophilia** and is due to the release of stored neutrophils from bone marrow.

- **Immature band forms:** As neutrophils are consumed and demand exceeds production, there is an increase in the number of **immature (band) neutrophils** in the circulating blood. Bands are identified by their absence of nuclear segmentation. This increase in band cells is termed to as a "**shift to the left of normal**" (**Fig. 25**). Usually, the presence of increased band count is used to differentiate bacterial from viral infections (not seen in viral infections), and a greater shift to the left is indicative of a more severe infection.

An adult human produces >1 × 10^{11} neutrophils per day. Each of these neutrophils circulate in the blood for a few hours or days. Neutrophils may migrate to sites of infection immediately after the entry of microbes. After they emigrate to the tissues, neutrophils function only for 1–2 days and then undergo death by apoptosis.

Various effector functions of neutrophils are presented in **Figure 26**.

Eosinophils

Eosinophils (refer **Fig. 23**) contain large, coarse granules and constitute only 1–6% of circulating leukocytes in adults. They express IgA receptors.

Primary inflammatory mediators of eosinophils are presented in **Box 9**.

Functions

Like neutrophils, eosinophils are capable of ameboid movement and phagocytosis. They have a spectrum of pattern-recognition receptors. Eosinophils ingest Ag–Ab complexes and viruses.

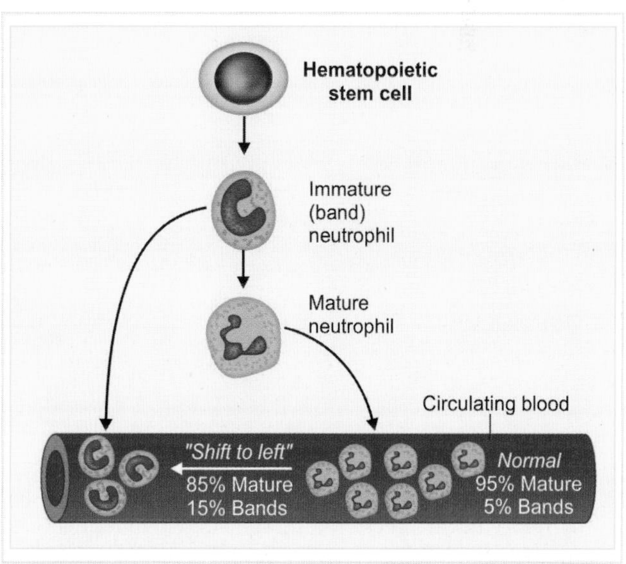

FIG. 25: During acute inflammation, inflammatory cytokines stimulate the release of more immature neutrophils, namely band forms into the circulation from the bone marrow. An increased ratio of bands to mature neutrophils is called as a "shift to the left." A shift to the left is commonly observed in acute bacterial infections.

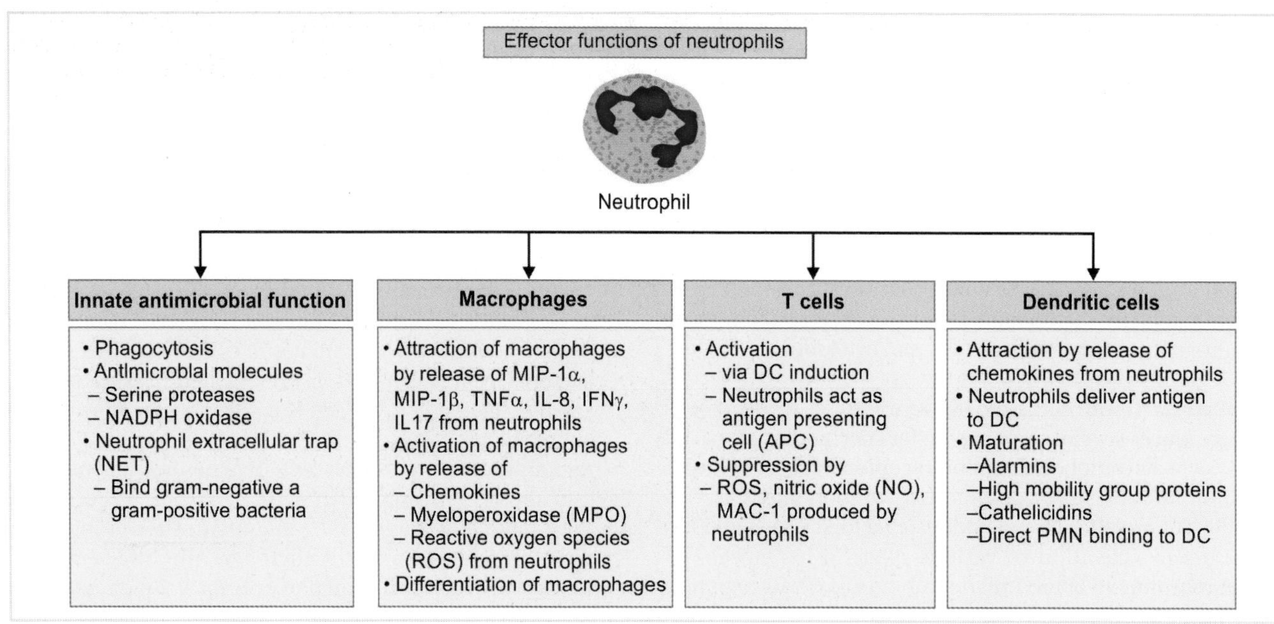

(DC: dendritic cell; IFN: interferon; IL: interleukin; MAC: macrophage antigen; MIP: macrophage inflammatory protein; PMN: polymorphonuclear leukocyte; TNF: tumor necrosis factor)

FIG. 26: Various effector functions of neutrophils.

Box 9: Primary inflammatory mediators of eosinophils.

- Lysosomal granule enzymes (primary crystalloid granules)
  - Major basic protein (MBP, a highly cationic protein)
  - Eosinophil cationic protein (ECP)
  - Eosinophil peroxidase
  - Acid phosphatase
  - Eosinophil-derived neurotoxin (EDN)
  - ß-glucuronidase
  - Arylsulfatase B
  - Histaminase
- Reactive oxygen metabolites
- Phospholipase D
- Prostaglandins of E
- Leukotrienes
- Cytokines [e.g., interleukin-1 (IL-1), IL-6, tumor necrosis factor-alpha (TNF-α), granulocyte–macrophage colony-stimulating factor (GMCSF)]
- Chemokines (e.g., IL-8)
- Platelet-activating factor (PAF)

- **Allergic (IgE-mediated immune) reactions:** They are recruited to tissue mainly in immune reactions mediated by IgE. They are recruited by specific chemokines (e.g., eotaxin) derived from leukocytes and epithelial cells. They produce tissue damage in IgE-mediated immune reactions (e.g., type I hypersensitivity allergic reactions and asthma).
- **Parasite-associated inflammatory reactions:** Eosinophil secondary granules contain toxic chemicals [e.g., major basic protein (highly cationic protein), eosinophil cationic protein, eosinophil peroxidase, eosinophil-derived neurotoxin] which are toxic and highly destructive to parasites and viruses. Its granules also have leukotrienes (LTs), platelet activating factor (PAF), acid phosphatase, and peroxidase.
- **Control/augmentation of inflammatory process:** The eosinophil granules contain a variety of enzymes (e.g., histaminase) that help to control inflammatory processes. Eosinophils contain antigens and also release LTs, prostagalndins (PGs), PAF, and a variety of cytokines (e.g., IL-1, IL-6, TNF-α, GM-CSF), and chemokines (e.g., IL-8) that augment the inflammatory response. Eosinophils may be seen in certain chronic inflammation.
- **Involved in mast cell-mediated reactions**

Basophils

Basophils are the least common leukocyte in the blood (<1%). Basophils are granulocytes characterized by granules that stain blue with basophilic dyes. They have lots of large basophilic cytoplasmic granules containing abundant mixture of biochemical mediators. Basophils have ***many structural and functional similarities to mast cells.*** Mature basophils circulate in the vascular system, whereas mast cells are distributed in connective tissue (especially around blood vessels and under mucosal surfaces). Although they are normally not present in tissues, when stimulated by cytokines, basophils can migrate to connective tissue in some inflammatory sites. But once in the tissue, basophils (then called *mast cells*) do not re-enter the circulation. The average basophil life span is in days, whereas mast cells can live for weeks to months. Mast cells and basophils have IgE receptors that allow them to bind and display IgE antibodies on their cell surfaces. When stimulated (e.g., antigen binding to the IgE antibodies), mast cells and basophils release granules (degranulate) containing proinflammatory chemicals. The cytoplasmic granules contain histamine, chemotactic factors, proteolytic enzymes (e.g., elastase, lysophospholipase), PAF, and an anticoagulant (heparin). Stimulation of basophils induces the synthesis of vasoactive lipid molecules (e.g., LTs) and cytokines.

Functions

They can migrate into tissue to participate in immunologic responses.

- **Type I hypersensitivity reactions:** They are functionally similar to mast cells and present in all supporting tissues. They play an important role in regulation of vascular permeability and bronchial smooth muscle contraction, especially in type I hypersensitivity reactions. Mast cells are found in connective tissues (especially on lung and gastrointestinal mucosal surfaces, in the dermis, and in the microvasculature). They bind to IgE molecules.
- **B-cell differentiation:** Basophils produce IL-6, which induce IL-10 by T helper 1 (Th1) cells and also induce Th2 cells that favors B-cell differentiation. Basophils are rich in cytokine IL-4, which guides B-cell differentiation towards plasma cells that secrete IgE.
- **Basophilia:** The numbers of basophils are increased at sites of allergic inflammatory reactions and parasitic infection (especially ectoparasites such as ticks). IgE receptors on the basophil induce degranulation at sites of IgE-mediated hypersensitivity reactions and is responsible for the local inflammatory response.
- Mast cells and basophils are also involved in wound healing and chronic inflammatory conditions.

Mast Cells

Q. Write short essay on mast cells in health and disease.

Mast cells were first described by Nobel Laureate P Ehrlich in 1908. *Mast* in German refers to fattening of animals. The name of these cells as mast cells came from the erroneous belief that their granules fed the tissue where the cells were located. Mast cells (or tissue basophils) are large cells highly similar to basophils. However, these are generated from a different set of precursor cells in the bone marrow. They migrate in an immature form from bone marrow into connective tissues throughout the body. Basophils migrate to the blood when mature, whereas the mast cells first circulate in the immature form. They bind to IgE molecules.

Granule contents

Similar to basophils, mast cells have many (50–200) large granules. They contain following:

- **Preformed mediators***:* For example, histamine, serotonin, chemotactic peptides for neutrophils and eosinophils, enzymes, and heparin
- **Newly formed mediators:** For example, thromboxane, LTC4, LTB4, PGD_2, and PAF

The granules contain acidic proteoglycans which bind basic dyes such as toluidine blue.

Phenotypes

There are two phenotypes of mast cells—**connective tissue mast cells** and **mucosal (atypical) mast cells**. Differences between two phenotypes of mast cells are presented in **Table 23**.

Table 23: Differences between two phenotypes of mast cells.

Feature	*Connective tissue mast cells*	*Mucosal (atypical) mast cells*
Size	Larger	Smaller
Predominant localization	Skin, submucosa	Mucosa
Tryptase	Present	Present
Chymase	Present	Absent
Histamine	More	Less
Predominant proteoglycan	Heparin	Chondroitin sulfate
Predominant arachidonate	Prostaglandin D_2 (PGD_2)	Leukotriene C_4 (LTC_4)
Dependency on T cells	Absent	Present

Distribution

They are widely distributed in vascularized connective tissues just beneath body epithelial surfaces. Their sites of distribution include the submucosal tissues of the gastrointestinal and respiratory tracts and the dermal layer just below the surface of the skin.

Functions

Upon activation, mast cells release many potent inflammatory mediators that defend against parasite infections, or cause symptoms of allergic diseases (refer pages 1070–1075). They participate in both acute and chronic inflammatory reactions. Mast cells have surface receptor (FceRI) which can bind with the Fc portion of IgE antibody. In immediate hypersensitivity reactions, IgE antibodies bound to mast cells recognize antigen/allergen and they degranulate. Their activation and degranulation affect many cells. These cells include those involved in inflammation (e.g., vascular endothelial cells, smooth muscle cells, circulating platelets and leukocytes, nerves) and healing (e.g., fibroblasts), glandular cells, and cells of the immune system. They release mediators such as histamine and prostaglandins (PGs). This occurs during allergic reactions to food, insect venom, or drugs. Sometimes, it may have catastrophic results (e.g., anaphylactic shock). Their activation causes increased permeability of blood vessels and synthesis of mediators producing smooth muscle contraction. Similar to neutrophils and eosinophils, mast cells are capable for *phagocytosis* and *NETosis.* Mast cells are involved in wound healing, maintenance of the blood–brain barrier, fertility, and angiogenesis.

Primary inflammatory mediators of mast cell (basophil) are presented in **Box 10**.

Lymphocytes

Lymphocytes constitute about 20–45% of circulating leukocytes in adults. They are also present in large numbers in spleen, thymus, lymph nodes, and mucosa-associated lymphoid tissue (MALT). There are two types of lymphocytes, namely B and T lymphocytes. They are discussed in Chapter 15.

Platelets

- Platelets are produced from bone marrow precursors known as megakaryocytes.
- Normal platelet counts ranges from 1, 50,000–4,00,000/cu mm (150–400 × 10^9/L) and it has a normal life span of 8–10 days.

Morphology of Platelets

Light microscopy: On Romanowsky-stained peripheral blood smear, platelets appear as small (diameter of 2–3 µm, approximately 1/5 the diameter of red blood cell), round, anuclear (lack nuclei) cells with prominent reddish-purple granules.

Electron microscopy: Platelets (**Fig. 27**) reveal several glycoprotein receptors, two types of cytoplasmic and a contractile cytoskeleton.

- **Glycoprotein receptors:** The two main platelet membrane receptors are:
  i. ***Glycoprotein (Gp)* IIb-IIIa:** It is the main receptor on cell surface.
  ii. ***Glycoprotein* Ib-IX:** It is a receptor for binding vWF with platelets.
- **Cytoplasmic granules:** Platelets have three types of inclusions.
  i. **Alpha (α) granules** contain fibrinogen, coagulation factors V and VIII, von Willebrand factor (vWF), fibronectin, chemokines, platelet factor 4 (heparin-binding chemokine), platelet-derived growth factor (PDGF) and transforming growth factor-β (TGF-β). They also have adhesion molecule P-selectin on their membranes.
  ii. **Dense granules** contain potent aggregating molecules adenosine diphosphate (ADP), ATP, serotonin, ionized calcium, histamine and epinephrine.
  iii. **Lysosomes** sequester acid hydrolases.
- **Contractile cytoskeleton:** It consists of dense microtubules and circumferential microfilaments, which maintain the disk shape of platelets.

Box 10: Primary inflammatory mediators of mast cell (basophil).

- Histamine
- Leukotrienes (LTC, LTD, LTE)
- Prostaglandins
- Platelet activating factor (PAF)
- Eosinophil chemotactic factors
- Cytokines [e.g., tumor necrosis factor alpha (TNF-α), interleukin (IL)-4]

Functions

Main functions are as follows:

Normal hemostasis: Platelets play main role in normal homeostasis and in initiating and regulating coagulation.

Inflammation: Platelets produce inflammatory mediators (e.g., vasoactive substances such as serotonin) and growth factors that modulate mesenchymal cell proliferation. Following injury to vascular endothelium, the subendothelial fibrillar collagen and interstitial matrix proteins are exposed to platelets. At the site of endothelial injury, platelets adhere, aggregate and degranulate or thrombin is formed after activation of the coagulation system. Degranulation of platelets releases serotonin (5-hydroxytryptamine). Similar to histamine serotonin, directly **increases vascular permeability**. Also the platelet arachidonic acid metabolite TXA_2 causes the second wave of platelet aggregation and mediates **smooth muscle constriction**. On activation, platelets, as well as phagocytic cells (leukocytes), secrete cationic proteins. These cationic proteins neutralize the negative charges on endothelium and promote **increased vascular permeability**.

RESIDENT TISSUE CELLS

Resident tissue cells mainly include dendritic cells, mast cells, tissue eosinophils, macrophages (histiocytes), and plasma cells.

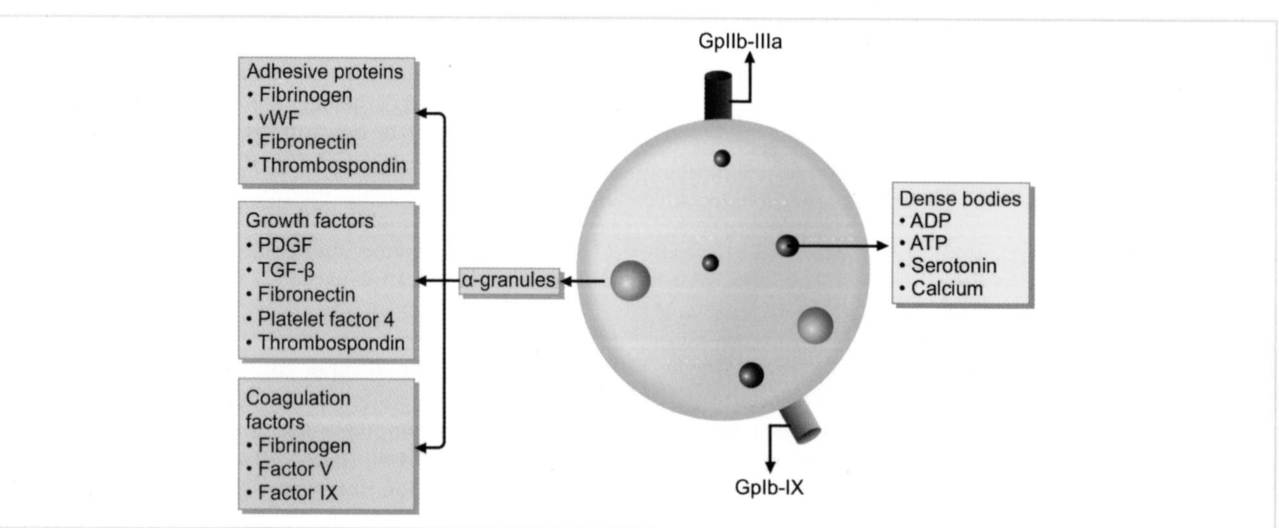

FIG. 27: Cellular constituents of platelets under electron microscope.

Dendritic Cells

Dendritic cells (DCs) are named so because they have numerous fine cytoplasmic processes that resemble dendrites. Dendritic cells are derived from bone marrow progenitors. They circulate in the blood as immature precursors and then settle widely in tissues. In the tissue, they undergo differentiation

Functions: DCs (sometimes called interdigitating DCs) are the most important highly efficient, antigen-presenting cells for initiating T-cell responses against protein antigens. They have a unique position in the immune system and are involved in both innate and adaptive immunity. They sense the presence of microbes and initiate innate immune defense reactions and capture microbial proteins (antigens) for display to naive T cells. Antigens bind to MHC class II on dendritic cells and are presented to lymphocytes, which are subsequently activated to initiate adaptive immune responses. Thus, they serve as sentinels of infection that begin the rapid innate response and also link innate responses with the development of adaptive immune responses. They are discussed in detail on pages 1054–1055.

Plasma Cells

They have an eccentric nucleus with a paranuclear hof/clearing. The nuclear chromatin has a cart-wheel pattern. They synthesize antibodies and are normally not present in peripheral blood. They are increased in chronic inflammations (e.g., syphilis, rheumatoid arthritis, tuberculosis), hypersensitivity states, and multiple myeloma.

Macrophages (discussed separately on page 306–311).

ENDOTHELIAL CELLS

Q. Discuss endothelial cells in health and disease.

Endothelial cells are monolayer of cells that line the innermost layer, namely intima of blood vessels. They separate intravascular and extravascular spaces. It forms the interface between tissues and the blood compartment and regulates the passage of molecules and cells. The endothelial cells are able to serve as a selectively permeable barrier. This barrier fails in vascular diseases, including atherosclerosis, hypertension, renal disease, pulmonary edema, sepsis, and other conditions of "capillary leak".

Vascular endothelial cells are squamous, polygonal, and elongated with their long axis along the direction of blood flow. They produce antiplatelet and antithrombotic agents that maintain the patency of blood vessel. Injury to a vessel wall damages the endothelium and exposes local procoagulant signals for thrombus formation (refer pages 369–370). They secrete vasodilators and vasoconstrictors and regulate vascular tone. Primary inflammatory mediators derived from endothelial cell are listed in **Box 11**.

Endothelial cells act as gatekeepers in recruitment of inflammatory cell during inflammation. Endothelial cells may either promote or inhibit tissue perfusion and inflammatory cell infiltration. Endothelial cells may play important role in inflammation, homeostasis, and thrombus formation. Normal endothelium has limited interaction with circulating leukocytes. When endothelial cells are activated by bacterial products (e.g., endotoxin) or by proinflammatory cytokines released during infection or injury, endothelial cells express several adhesion molecules. These molecules selectively bind to different leukocytes in different pathologic conditions. For example, the adhesion molecules and chemokines produced during acute bacterial infection recruit granulocytes, whereas in chronic inflammatory diseases (e.g., tuberculosis, atherosclerosis), the adhesion molecules recruit monocytes. Endothelial cells are involved in the pathophysiology of many immune-mediated diseases. Complement-mediated lysis of endothelial cells is an example of immunologically mediated tissue injury in type III hypersensitivity reaction. The immune-mediated endothelial injury also plays a role in thrombotic thrombocytopenic purpura or hemolytic-uremic syndrome. The endothelial cells are involved in solid-organ allografts and promote allograft arteriopathy.

Box 11: Primary inflammatory mediators and adhesion molecules/ligands derived from endothelial cell.

Mediators of inflammation
- Nitric oxide
- von Willebrand factor
- Cytokines [e.g., tumor necrosis factor (TNF), interleukin (IL)-1]
- Platelet activating factor
- Endothelins

Adhesion molecules/ligands
- Monocyte chemoattractant protein-1 (MCP-1)
- Vascular cell adhesion molecule-1 (VCAM-1)
- Intercellular adhesion molecule-1 (ICAM-1)
- E-selectin

Transmigration
- Platelet/endothelial cell adhesion molecule-1 (PECAM-1)

Adhesive Molecules in Endothelial Cells

Integrity of endothelial cells depends on many types of adhesion complexes. These adhesive molecules promote cell-substratum and cell-cell adhesions.

- **Cell-substrate adhesion molecules:** These molecules attach endothelial cells to their subendothelial structures (e.g., basal lamina). They form complex with intracellular cytoskeleton and are involved in intracellular signal transduction. For example, integrins are transmembrane molecules which bind endothelial cells to extracellular matrix adhesive molecules, including laminin, fibronectin, fibrinogen, von Willebrand factor and thrombospondin. The cytoplasmic tails of the integrins bind to the intracellular complex of proteins. These proteins regulate adhesion at focal contact sites and associate with actin microfilaments and microtubules of the cytoskeleton.
- **Cell-cell adhesion molecules:** These molecules attach one endothelial cell to its neighboring endothelial cells. Cadherin molecules are present at intercellular adhesion junctions and occluding molecules at intercellular tight junctions. Cadherins bind to the actin cytoskeleton in the cytoplasm through catenins.

Main Functions of Endothelium

Endothelial cells are metabolically active and are involved in several biological functions. Endothelial cells maintains vascular integrity, regulates platelet aggregation, regulate coagulation, regulate fibrinolysis, regulates vascular contraction and relaxation (through paracrine pathways), mediates leukocyte recruitment in inflammation immunoregulation and repair. Endothelial cells form unique mechanotransduction structures and modulate the effects of luminal hemodynamic shear stress on the vessel wall. Because of its mechanical sensing property, endothelial cell membranes may deform. This activates biochemical signaling and causes expression of vasoactive compounds, growth factors, coagulation/fibrinolytic/ complement factors, matrix degradation enzymes, inflammatory mediators and adhesion molecules. The endothelial cells are quiescent but able to proliferate once appropriate genes are activated in response to injury and/or disease. They are highly active metabolically and alter their function as their microenvironment changes. Endothelial cell-derived factors also control some immune responses. Immune responses to endothelial cells are major mechanism of organ rejection following transplantation and play a role in the pathogenesis of graft arteriosclerosis.

Primary inflammatory mediators: These include von Willebrand factor, nitric oxide, endothelins, and prostanoids.

Mediators Involved in Inflammation

These mediators include:

- **Nitric oxide:** Nitric oxide (NO) is a low-molecular weight, soluble, free radical gas which causes vasodilation (was known as endothelium-derived relaxing factor). Nitric oxide (refer page 242–243) inhibits platelet aggregation, regulates vascular tone by relaxation of vascular smooth muscle and reacts with ROS to create highly reactive radical species. Source of nitric oxide is endothelial cells as well as macrophages.
- **Cytokines:** Activated endothelial cells generate cytokines such as IL-1, IL-6, TNF-α, and other inflammatory cytokines. Apart from endothelial cells, other sources of cytokines include macrophages, lymphocytes, and mast cells
- **Arachidonic acid-derived contraction factors:** The COX pathway of AA products (source: mast cells and all leukocytes) such as TXA_2 induces smooth muscle contraction of blood vessel (vasoconstriction). Lipoxygenase pathway metabolite of AA, namely LTC_4, LTD_4, and LTE_4 causes vasoconstriction and increased vascular permeability. For details refer pages 250–254 and Figure 18.
- **Arachidonic acid-derived relaxing factors:** The biological opponent of TXA_2 is arachidonic metabolite PGI_2 (source: mast cells and all leukocytes). It inhibits platelet aggregation and causes vasodilation.

Role in Homeostasis and Thrombus Formation

Endothelial cells play an important role in both homeostasis and thrombus formation (for details refer pages 366–370). They have both antithrombotic and prothrombotic (procoagulant) properties. The balance between these two opposing endothelial properties determines the thrombus formation and is regulated by endothelium through a highly tuned set of regulatory pathways.

Antithrombotic properties

- **Anticoagulant effects:** Heparin-like molecules, thrombomodulin, endothelial protein C receptor (EPCR), and tissue factor pathway inhibitor (TFPI) inactivate the coagulation cascade.
- **Fibrinolytic factors:** Tissue-type plasminogen activator (t-PA) promotes fibrinolytic activity by converting plasminogen into plasmin. Plasmin cleaves fibrin.
- **Antiplatelet effects:** Antiplatelet as a barrier between platelets and subendothelial thrombogenic von Willeband factor (vWF) and collagen. It produces inhibitors of platelet aggregation (e.g., PGI_2, NO, and adenosine diphosphatase).

Prothrombotic properties

- **Platelet effects:** Endothelial damage exposes the subendothelial thrombogenic ECM and favors deposition of platelets. *von Willebrand factor (vWF)* produced by normal endothelial cells is an essential cofactor that helps platelet binding to matrix elements in the subendothelial region. Thus, vWF facilitates adhesion of platelets to the subendothelial region.
- **Procoagulant effects:** Endothelial cells **synthesize tissue factor** in response to cytokines [e.g., TNF or IL-1] or bacterial endotoxin. Tissue factor activates the extrinsic coagulation cascade. Activated endothelial cells increase the catalytic function of activated coagulation factors IXa and Xa.
- **Antifibrinolytic effects:** Endothelial cells secrete inhibitors of plasminogen activator (PAIs). They reduce fibrinolysis and tend to favor thrombosis.

Atherosclerosis

Endothelial cells regulate the growth of underlying smooth muscle cells of tunica media. For example, heparan sulfate glycosaminoglycans secreted by endothelial cells can inhibit smooth muscle proliferation. Endothelial injury or dysfunction can produce growth factors and chemoattractants, such as platelet-derived growth factor (PDGF). These may cause the migration and proliferation of vascular smooth muscle cells into the intima. Dysregulation of these growth-stimulatory molecules may cause accumulation of smooth muscle cells in the intima and produce atherosclerotic plaques.

Endothelial physiological function and endothelial dysfunction properties are presented in **Table 24**.

Endothelins

Q. Write a short essay on endothelin.

Endothelins (ET) are a family of low-molecular weight peptides (proteins) synthesized by endothelial cells. There are 3 types of endothelins, namely endothelins-1 (ET-1), -2 (ET-2), and -3 (ET-3). They are 21 amino acid peptides having powerful vasoconstrictor and pressor agents. They produce prolonged vasoconstriction (potent vasoconstrictor) of vascular smooth muscle.

Table 24: Endothelial physiological function and endothelial dysfunction properties.

Physiological function	*Endothelial dysfunction properties*
Homeostasis and thrombus formation: Maintains vascular integrity, regulates platelet aggregation, regulates vascular contraction, and relaxation	
Platelet resistant	Platelet adhesion
Anticoagulant production: Thrombomodulin, other proteins	Procoagulant production: Tissue factor, plasminogen activator/ inhibitor, factor V, factor VIIIa (von Willebrand factor)
Antithrombotic agent production: Prostacyclin (PGI_2), adenine metabolites	
Fibrinolytic agent production: Tissue plasminogen activator (tPA), urokinase-like factor, tissue factor pathway inhibitor	Antifibrinolysis: Secretion of inhibitors of plasminogen activator (PAIs).
Inflammation: Mediates leukocyte recruitment	
Anti-inflammatory	**Proinflammatory**
Leukocyte resistant	Leukocyte adhesion
Provasodilation	Provasoconstriction
Permeability barrier (selective impermeability)	Increased permeability
Vasoactive factors: Nitric oxide [Endothelium-derived relaxing factor (EDRF)], endothelin	Inflammatory mediator production: Interleukin-1, cell adhesion molecules
Antioxidant	Prooxidant
Atherosclerosis	
Endothelial cells regulate the growth of underlying smooth muscle cells of tunica media.	Produce growth factors and chemoattractants (e.g., platelet-derived growth factor).
For example, heparan sulfate glycosaminoglycans secreted by endothelial cells can inhibit smooth muscle proliferation.	They cause migration and proliferation of vascular smooth muscle cells into the intima and produce atherosclerotic plaques.
Others	
Quiescent	Migration/proliferation
Quiescent smooth muscle cell (SMC)	SMC activation
Matrix stability	Matrix remodeling
Vessel stability	Angiogenesis
Optimize balance between vasodilation and vasoconstriction	Impaired dilation, vasoconstriction
Replication: Antiproliferative	Proproliferative
Other properties of endothelium **Receptors for:** Factor IX, factor X, low-density lipoproteins, modified low-density lipoproteins, thrombin **Growth factor production:** Granulocyte monocyte-colony stimulating factor (GM-CSF), insulin-like growth factors binding protein (IGFBP), insulin-like growth factor, fibroblast growth factor (FGF), epidermal growth factor (EGF), platelet-derived growth factor (PDGF) **Growth inhibitor:** Heparin **Vasoactive compounds:** Angiotensin-converting enzyme (ACE), NO-endothelial nitric oxide synthase (eNOS), NO-induced nitric oxide synthase (iNOS), Prostacyclin, Endothelin-1 **Extracellular matrix (ECM)/ECM degradation enzymes:** Matrix metalloproteinase-9 (MMP-9), collagen XII, thrombospondin **Others:** Extracellular superoxide dismutase (ecSOD), sterol regulatory element binding protein (SREBP)	

Source

Various sources are as follows:

- **Endothelin 1** (ET-1) is found in vascular endothelial and smooth muscle cells, epithelial cells of airways, macrophages, fibroblasts, cardiac myocytes, brain neurons, and islets of pancreas. Endothelin-1 is a potent (powerful) endothelium-derived, peptide vasoconstrictor.
- **Endothelin 2** is observed in ovary and intestinal epithelial cells.
- **Endothelin 3** is identified in endothelial cells, neurons of brain, renal tubular epithelial cells, and intestinal epithelial cells.

Endothelin Receptors

The endothelin exerts their physiological effects in a receptor-mediated fashion. Endothelins bind two distinct seven-transmembrane G protein-coupled endothelin receptors. They are named as endothelin$_A$ (ET_A/ET-A) and endothelin

B receptor (ET_B /ET-B). These receptors are distributed in various tissues and cells, but the levels of expression vary. Both receptors are found on smooth muscle cells, but only one (ETB) on endothelial cells. ET_A receptors are found on vascular smooth muscle cells, and on activation, produce a slow onset sustained vasoconstriction. In contrast, ET_B receptors are seen on both endothelial and vascular smooth muscle cells. Activation of ET_B receptors on endothelial cells causes vasodilation by the release of vasodilators that act on smooth muscle cells. ET_B receptor also inhibits cell growth and vasoconstriction in the vascular system. It functions as a clearance receptor and selective blocking of ET_B receptor inhibits the accumulation of ET-1 in tissue.

Synthesis of Endothelin-1

Endothelin is produced by the vascular endothelium from a precursor (proendothelin-1) by the action of an endothelin converting enzyme (ECE) found on the endothelial cell membrane. Formation and release of ET-1 is stimulated by angiotensin II (AII), antidiuretic hormone (ADH), thrombin, cytokines, reactive oxygen species (ROS), and shearing forces acting on the vascular endothelium. ET-1 release is inhibited by prostaglandin I_2 (PGI_2), nitric oxide, and atrial natriuretic peptide (ANP) (**Fig. 28**). Apart from endothelial cells, it may also be produced by cardiac myocytes. It is also a potent growth factor for cardiac myocytes. It can bind to its receptor and cause cardiac hypertrophy. Its concentration in the plasma is elevated in patients with severe heart failure and is responsible for renal vasoconstriction, sodium retention, and edema.

Mechanism of Action of Endothelin-1 (Fig. 28)

After the release of ET-1 by the endothelial cell, ET-1 binds to its receptors (ET_A and ET_B) on the target tissue (e.g., adjacent vascular smooth muscle). ET-1 binds to its G protein-coupled receptors and the form of inositol trisphosphate (IP_3). Increased IP_3 releases calcium by the sarcoplasmic reticulum in the smooth muscle cells. This leads to contraction of smooth muscle. Normally, ET_A receptor is dominant in blood vessels with respect to action of ET-1 on endothelium. When ET-1 binds to endothelial ET_B receptors, it stimulates the formation of nitric oxide (NO). In the absence of stimulation of endothelin receptors on smooth muscle, the NO causes vasodilation.

Effects of Endothelin on Cardiovascular System

- Systemic administration of ET-1 causes transient vasodilation (initial activation of endothelial receptor ET_B) and hypotension. This is followed by prolonged vasoconstriction and hypertension (due to activation smooth muscle endothelial receptors ET_A and ET_B).
- Endothelin-1 stimulates aldosterone secretion, decreases renal blood flow and glomerular filtration rate, and releases ANP (atrial natriuretic peptide).
- Endothelin-1 stimulates smooth muscle cell proliferation and marked accumulation of subendothelial fibrotic tissue. It can also cause platelet activation and initiate platelet aggregation.

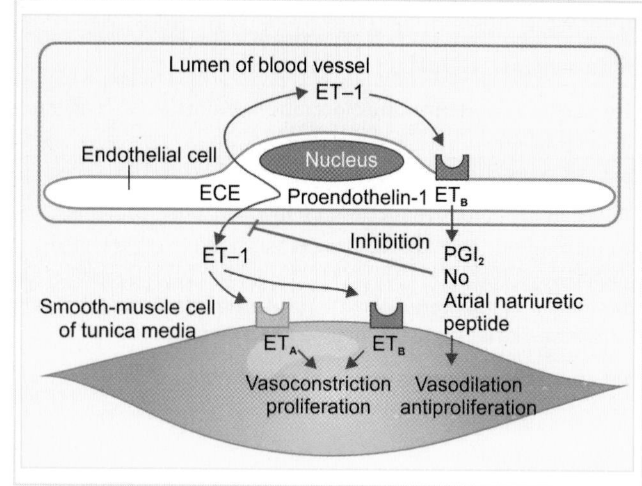

(ET-1: endothelin-1; ECE: endothelin-converting enzyme; NO: nitric oxide; PGI_2: prostacyclin)

FIG. 28: Synthesis of endothelin-1. Details are provided in the text.

Pathological Conditions Associated with Raised Endothelin Levels

- **Systemic hypertension and heart failure:** Endothelin-1 is involved in the pathogenesis of systemic hypertension, coronary vasospasm, and heart failure. Angiotensin-converting enzyme (ACE) is an endothelial product that converts angiotensin I to angiotensin II, a potent vasoconstrictor that is important in the pathogenesis of hypertension. In heart failure, ET-1 is released by the failing myocardium and it can contribute to calcium overload and cardiac hypertrophy. Orally active endothelin antagonists may lower blood pressure in patients with resistant hypertension. Endothelin receptor antagonists may decrease mortality and improve hemodynamics in heart failure.
- **Pulmonary arterial hypertension**: Endothelin-1 is a potent endogenous vasoconstrictor and vascular smooth muscle mitogen. It is elevated in patients with pulmonary arterial hypertension. Nonselective ET-1 receptor antagonist (ERAs such as bosentan, macitentan) target ET-1 is used in the treatment of pulmonary hypertension. Selective ET_A receptor Antagonist Available Is Ambrisentan. Endothelial receptor antagonists (ERAs) block the binding of ET-1 to either endothelin receptor A (ET_A) and/or B (ET_B). ET_A receptors found on pulmonary artery smooth muscle cells (PASMC) produce vasoconstriction. In the normal pulmonary vasculature, ET-B receptors are found on endothelial cells and mediate ET-1 clearance, as well as vasodilation by producing PGI_2 and NO (refer **Fig. 28**).
- **Tumors:** The endothelin peptides (ET-1, ET-2, and ET-3) are potent mitogens for several human tumors. Endothelin-1 has pathophysiological roles malignancies of female genital tract (e.g., ovarian cancer). ET-1 and its

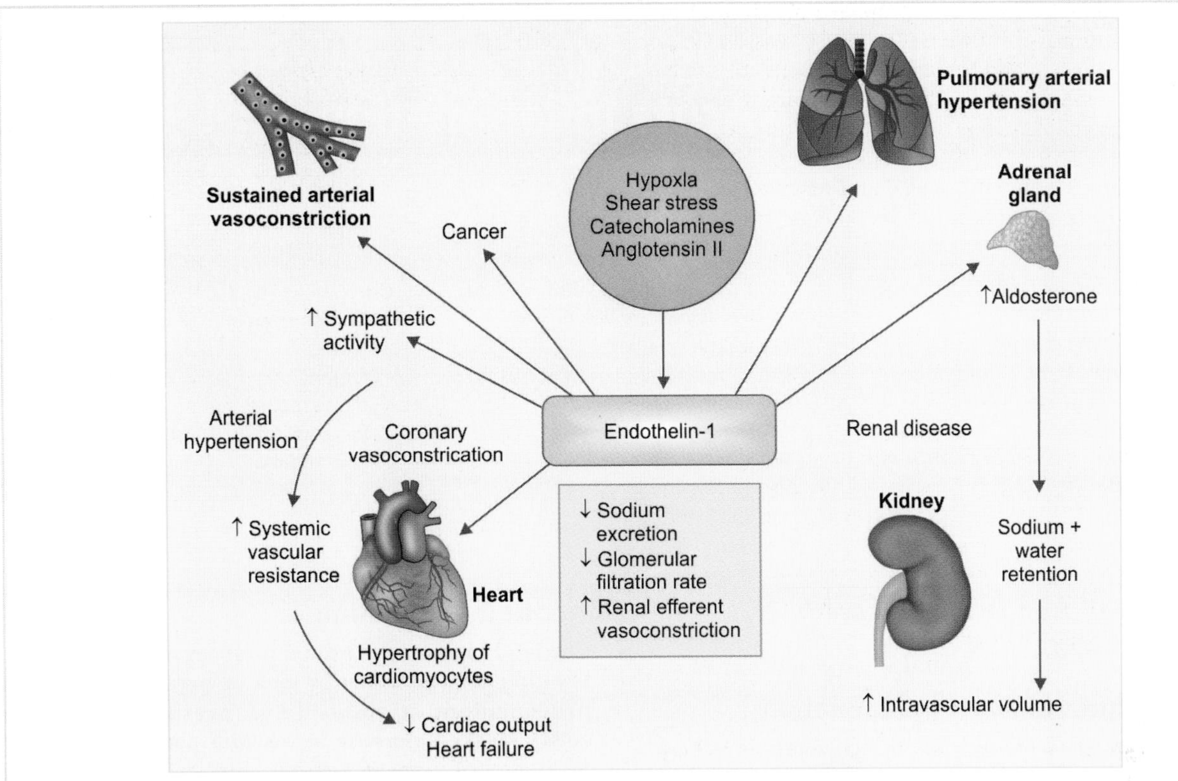

FIG. 29: Systemic and local effects of the major target organs involved in endothelin-1.

ET_A receptor (ETAR) are overexpressed in primary and metastatic ovarian cancers.

- **Others:** ET-1 also activates EGFR, stimulates proliferation, blocks apoptosis, activates integrin-like kinase (ILK), upregulates matrix metalloproteinases (MMPs), and increases vascular endothelial growth factor (VEGF) expression and enhances angiogenesis. Endothelin has neurotoxic effects in HIV infection. Placental ischemia with decreased endothelin may be involved in the pathogenesis of pre-eclampsia. However, endothelin-receptor blockers are teratogenic and are contraindicated during pregnancy.

Systemic and local effects of the major target organs involved with ET-1 are presented in **Figure 29**.

8.4 Morphological Types and Outcomes of Acute Inflammation

CHAPTER OUTLINE

MORPHOLOGICAL TYPES/PATTERNS OF ACUTE INFLAMMATION

General Features of Acute Inflammation

The morphological characteristics of acute inflammatory reactions are—(1) vasodilation and (2) accumulation of leukocytes and fluid in the extravascular tissue. These are responsible for the signs and symptoms of the inflammatory response.

The general features of inflammation are characteristic of most acute inflammatory reactions. However, special morphologic patterns may be superimposed on them This depends on the cause, severity of the reaction, and the tissue and site of involvement. Recognition of these distinct gross and microscopic patterns of inflammation usually gives a valuable clue about the underlying cause.

Serous Inflammation

- Characterized by marked outpouring **(exudation)** of a thin, **cell-poor** serous fluid into spaces produced by injury to surface epithelia or into body cavities such as peritoneum, pleura, or pericardium.
- Serous exudate or effusion is yellow, straw-like in color and usually does not contain microbes. Microscopically, they show either few or no cells. Since they are not infected by destructive organisms, they do not contain large numbers of leukocytes. Accumulation of serous fluid in body cavities is called an *effusion*. The fluid of these effusions in body cavities may be either derived from the plasma (due to increased vascular permeability) or secreted by mesothelial cells (as a result of local irritation) that line the body cavities.
- *Note:* Effusions consisting of transudates can also occur in noninflammatory conditions, such as reduced blood outflow in heart failure, or reduced plasma protein levels in diseases of kidney and liver.
- **Examples:**
  - Skin blister formed in burns or viral infection: The serous fluid accumulates within or immediately beneath the damaged epidermis of the skin.
  - Inflammation of synovium (synovitis).

Fibrinous Inflammation

- **Cause: Fibrinous exudate is observed when there is either a large vascular leak or presence of a local procoagulant stimulus (e.g., presence of cancer cells). Marked increase in vascular permeability** leads to escape of large molecules (high-molecular weight proteins) like fibrinogen from the lumen of the vessel into the extravascular space. It forms fibrin and gets deposited in the extracellular space. The **exudate rich in fibrin** is called fibrinous exudate.
- **Sites:** A fibrinous exudate is mostly observed with inflammation in the lining of body cavities, such as the meninges, pericardium, and pleura. When a fibrinous exudate develops on a serosal surface, such as the pleura or pericardium, it is known as fibrinous pleuritis or fibrinous pericarditis, respectively.
- **Microscopically**, fibrin appears as an eosinophilic or pink meshwork of threads or pink amorphous coagulum.
- **Fate:** Fibrinous exudates may be dissolved by fibrinolysis and removed by macrophages. If the fibrin is not dissolved, it may stimulate the ingrowth of fibroblasts and blood vessels (i.e., granulation tissue) and may lead to scarring. If the fibrinous exudate is not dissolved, it will be converted to scar tissue *(organization)* in the pericardial sac. This produces opaque fibrous thickening of the pericardium and epicardium in the area of exudation. If the fibrosis is extensive, it may obliterate the pericardial cavity. For example, fibrinous pericarditis in rheumatic fever, classically known as "**bread and butter**" pericarditis (**Fig. 30**).

Suppurative or Purulent Inflammation and Abscess

- **Purulent inflammation** is characterized by the production of large amounts of pus or purulent exudate.
- Microscopically, shows neutrophils, liquefactive necrosis **(liquefied debris of necrotic cells)**, and edema fluid.
- **Causes:** Most frequent cause is bacteria (e.g., *Staphylococci*) and these bacteria which produce localized suppuration are called as **pyogenic** (pus-producing) bacteria (e.g., *Staphylococci*). For example, acute suppurative appendicitis.

- **Abscesses:** It is the **localized collections of pus (i.e., purulent inflammatory exudates) in a tissue**, an organ, or a confined space. For example, boil caused by *Staphylococcus aureus*. Abscesses are caused by seeding of pyogenic bacteria into a tissue. Abscesses have a central necrotic focus (consisting of necrotic leukocytes and necrotic parenchymal cells) and are surrounded by a zone of preserved neutrophils around the central necrotic focus. This in turn may be surrounded by tissue showing dilated vessels and parenchymal and fibroblastic proliferation, indicating chronic inflammation and repair. Subsequently, the abscess may become walled off and replaced by connective tissue. If pus accumulates in hollow organs (e.g., gallbladder) or pleural cavity, it is known as empyema. When abscess persists or is at critical locations (e.g., brain), abscesses need to be drained surgically.

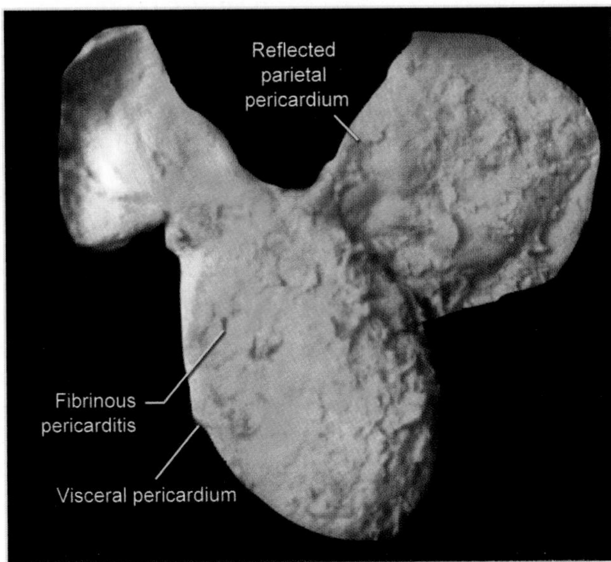

FIG. 30: Fibrinous pericarditis developing in rheumatic fever.

Hemorrhagic Inflammation

When inflammation is associated with severe vascular injury or deficiency of coagulation factors, it causes hemorrhagic inflammation, e.g., acute pancreatitis, (**Fig. 31**) due to proteolytic destruction of vascular walls.

Catarrhal Inflammation

Acute inflammation of a mucous membrane is accompanied by excessive secretion of mucus and the appearance is described as catarrhal, e.g., common cold.

Membranous Inflammation

In this type, epithelium is covered by a membrane consisting of fibrin, desquamated epithelial cells, and inflammatory cells, e.g., pharyngitis or laryngitis due to *Corynebacterium diphtheriae.*

Pseudomembranous Inflammation

- It is characterized by superficial mucosal ulceration covered by sloughed mucosa, fibrin, mucus, and inflammatory cells.
- For example, pseudomembranous colitis due to *Clostridium difficile* colonization of the bowel, usually following broad-spectrum antibiotic treatment.

Necrotizing (Gangrenous) Inflammation

The combination of necrosis and bacterial putrefaction is **gangrene** (refer Fig. 12, Chapter 7), e.g., gangrene foot, gangrenous appendicitis.

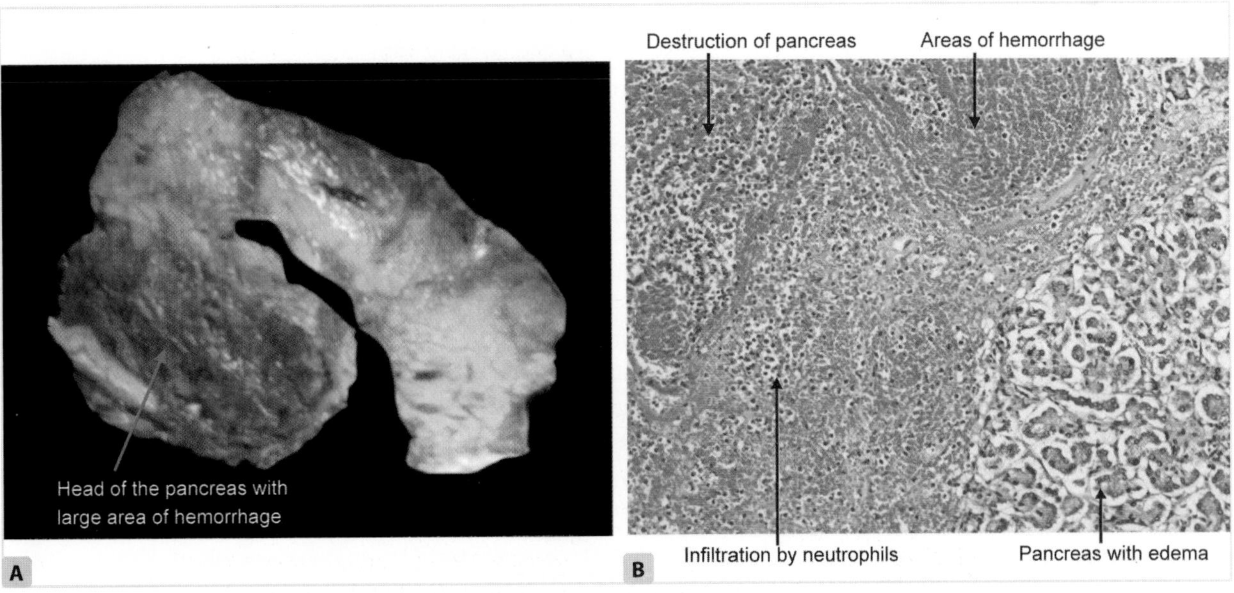

FIGS. 31A AND B: (A) Acute hemorrhagic pancreatitis. Longitudinal section of the pancreas shows dark areas of hemorrhage in the head of the pancreas (left). (B) Microscopic appearance of acute hemorrhagic pancreatitis. Histology shows numerous neutrophils, hemorrhage and destruction of parenchyma (left side) and pancreas with edema (right side).

Ulcer

An ulcer is defined as a local defect, or excavation, of the surface of an organ or tissue. It **is produced by the sloughing (shedding) of inflamed necrotic tissue.** Ulcer develops only when tissue necrosis and resultant inflammation occur on or near a surface.

Common Sites

- Mucosa of the mouth, stomach (e.g., peptic ulcer of the stomach or duodenum), intestines, or genitourinary tract.
- Skin and subcutaneous tissue of the lower extremities. It occurs in individuals with disorders that predispose to vascular insufficiency. These conditions include diabetes, sickle cell anemia, and peripheral vascular disease (e.g., varicose ulcers).

Microscopy

Ulcer usually shows coexistence of acute and chronic inflammation. For example, peptic ulcers of the stomach or duodenum and diabetic ulcers of the legs. During the acute phase, they show dense polymorphonuclear infiltration and vascular dilation in the margins of the defect. With chronicity, the margins and base of the ulcer show proliferation of fibroblast, scarring, and infiltration by lymphocytes, macrophages, and sometimes plasma cells.

Terminology

- **Bacteremia:** It is defined as a condition characterized by the presence of small number of bacteria in the blood. They cannot be detected by direct microscopic examination of blood and are detected by blood culture (e.g., typhoid infection caused by *Salmonella typhi*).
- **Septicemia:** It is defined as the presence of rapidly multiplying, highly pathogenic bacteria in the blood (e.g., pyogenic cocci/bacilli). It is usually associated with systemic effects such as toxemia and neutrophilic leukocytosis.
- **Pyemia:** It is the dissemination of small septic emboli in the blood which produce their effects at the site of their lodgement. Thus, it can lead to pyemic abscesses or septic infarcts.
- **Cellulitis:** It is the term used for diffuse inflammation of the soft tissues due to organisms, produced from spreading effects of substances like hyaluronidase released by some bacteria.

OUTCOMES OF ACUTE INFLAMMATION

The outcome of acute inflammation depends on many variables that can modify the basic process of inflammation. These variables include, (i) the nature and intensity of the injury, (ii) the site and tissue involved, and (iii) the response of the host. Various usual outcomes of acute inflammation (**Fig. 32**) are as follows:

Complete Resolution

Situations in which Resolution Occurs

- It is the process of **complete return of tissue architecture to normal** following acute inflammation. This restoration of the site of acute inflammation to normal is the the most wanted outcome. It occurs under following circumstances:
  - When the injury is limited or short-lived.
  - With no or minimal tissue damage or destruction.
  - When injured tissue is capable of regeneration.

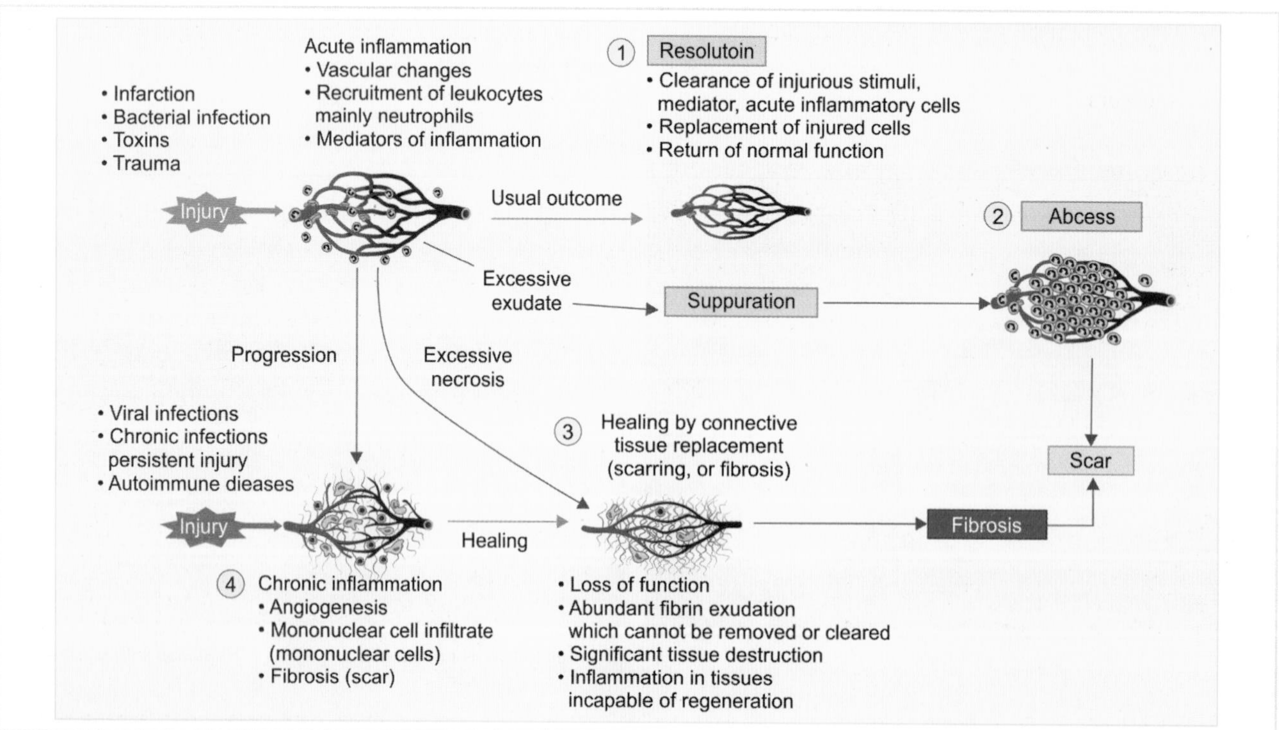

FIG. 32: Outcomes of acute inflammation—(1) resolution, (2) organization (healing by fibrosis and scarring), (3) abscess, or (4) chronic inflammation.

If a tissue is to return to normal, the inflammatory process must be reversed. This includes the following—elimination or removal of stimulus to tissue injury, turning off of the proinflammatory signals, end of acute inflammatory cell influx, restoration of tissue fluid balance, removal of cell and tissue debris, and restoration of normal vascular function. It should be accompanied by regeneration of epithelium, tissue architecture and extracellular matrix (ECM) and restoration of normal and physiological function. The process of resolution involves removal of cellular debris and microbes by macrophages, and resorption of edema fluid by draining through by lymphatics. One of the best example is resolution of lobar pneumonia following prompt treatment.

Abscess

Localized collection of pus is called abscess. If the area of acute inflammation is walled off by inflammatory cells and fibrosis, neutrophil products destroy the tissue and form an abscess.

Lymphadenitis

Localized acute (even chronic) inflammation may cause secondary inflammation a result of either the persistence of the injurious agent or sprocess of healing of lymphatic channels (lymphangitis) and lymph nodes (lymphadenitis). The inflamed lymphatic channels may appear as red streaks, and lymph nodes may be enlarged and painful. Microscopically, affected lymph nodes show hyperplasia of lymphoid follicle and proliferation of mononuclear phagocytes in the sinuses (sinus histiocytosis).

Organization/healing by Connective Tissue Replacement

Situations in which Organization Occurs

- Process of **replacement of dead tissue by living tissue,** which matures to form scar tissue is known as **organization**. Healing by connective tissue replacement (scarring, or fibrosis) occurs
    - When there is plenty of fibrin exudation in tissue or serous cavities (pleura, peritoneum) which cannot be adequately removed or cleared.
    - In the presence of significant destruction of tissue.
    - With inflammation in tissues not capable of regeneration.

Though the body may eliminate or remove the offending agent, if a tissue is irreversibly injured, normal architecture is usually replaced by a scar. This process involves growing of connective tissue into the area of tissue damage or exudate, which is converted into a mass of fibrous tissue (scar).

Progression from Acute to Chronic Inflammation

Chronic inflammation may follow acute inflammation, or it may be chronic from the beginning itself. Acute inflammation may progress to chronic when the acute inflammatory response cannot be resolved.

Situations in which Acute Inflammation Progresses to Chronic

Acute inflammation can transform into chronic when the acute inflammatory response cannot be resolved or organized. This may be due to:

- Persistence of the injurious agent or
- Some interference during the normal process of healing.

Examples:

- Bacterial infection of the lung may begin as acute inflammation (pneumonia). But when it fails to resolve, it can cause extensive tissue destruction and form a cavity with chronic inflammation known as lung abscess.
- Acute osteomyelitis, if not treated properly may progress to chronic osteomyelitis.
- Chronic inflammation with a persisting stimulus results in peptic ulcer of the duodenum or stomach, which may persist for months or years.

8.5 Cell Adhesion Molecules

CHAPTER OUTLINE

- Cell adhesion molecules
  - Characteristics of CAMs
  - Cells of inflammation
  - Importance
  - Types of cell adhesion molecules
  - Integrins
  - Cadherins
  - Selectins
  - Immunoglobulin superfamily (IgSF) cell adhesion molecules
  - Addressins
  - Adhesive molecules and disease
  - Adhesive molecules in stem cell

CELL ADHESION MOLECULES

Q. Write a short essay on cell adhesion molecules.
Q. Explain leukocyte adhesion molecules.
Q. Explain endothelial adhesion molecules.
Q. Discuss the role of adhesion molecules in human diseases.
Q. Explain endothelial-leukocyte adhesion molecules.
Q. Describe the role of adhesion molecules in inflammation.

Cell adhesion molecules (CAMs) are cell surface proteins/compounds that bind the cell to an adjacent cell (termed cell-to-cell adhesion/interaction) and cells to components of the ECM (termed as cell-to-matrix adhesion). Cell adhesion receptors mediate cell communication and cell–cell and cell–matrix interactions. CAMs are the receptors in the enlarged sense.

Characteristics of CAMs

- **Stability:** Cell adhesion may vary from very stable to transient. For example, the cell-to-cell interactions in muscle cells are strong and stable, whereas the adhesion between cells that move through blood vessel walls are weaker and transitory.
- **Binding with ligands:** Cell adhesion results from multiple different adhesion molecule–ligand binding events. This involves crosstalk and cooperation between many different adhesion molecules. Each CAM binds to its specific ligands with different affinities.
- **Domains:** All CAMs are integral membrane proteins. They consist of three types of domains, namely—(1) extracellular, (2) transmembrane, and (3) cytoplasmic domains.
  - **Extracellular domains:** They extend from the cell and bind ligands on other cells or within the ECM.
  - **Transmembrane:** They are present in the cell membrane.
  - **Cytoplasmic domains:** They interact with cytoskeletal proteins and provide an intracellular attachment.
- **Types of binding:** It can be divided into three types
  i. Between adhesion molecules of the same type (homophilic binding)
  ii. Between adhesion molecules of a different type (heterophilic binding), or
  iii. Via an intermediary "linker" that binds other adhesion molecules.

Importance

- **Organization:** The cell-to-cell and cell-to-matrix interactions are vital cell behavior that are largely responsible for the precise, distinctive organization needed for a collection of cells to form a tissue, for tissues to form organs, and for organs to form a system.
- **Communication:** Cell adhesion is the route by which cells communicate with each other and is important in development and morphogenesis, cell migration, and the regulation of gene expression, cell division, and cell death.

Types of Cell Adhesion Molecules

Cell adhesion molecules or cell adhesion receptors consist of four main types of protein (molecular) families—(1) the integrins, (2) the cadherins, (3) the selectins, and (4) immunoglobulin (Ig) superfamily (IgSF).

Integrins

The integrins are important large family of CAMs. They are membrane proteins composed of transmembrane two-chain glycoproteins. They are involved in cell–cell adhesion and cell interactions with the ECM proteins. They play main role in integrating the extracellular and intracellular environments.

Binding

On the outer side of the plasma membrane, the extracellular domains of integrins bind to diverse type of molecules (ligands) that are present in the extracellular environment. These include ECM (extracellular matrix) proteins, namely laminin, collagen, fibronectin, vitronectin, and fibrinogen. On the intracellular side of the membrane, the cytoplasmic domains of integrins interact either directly or indirectly with several different proteins (mainly actin cytoskeleton) inside the cytosol. This influences the course of events within the cell.

Integrins functionally and structurally mediate the link and communication between the extra- (outside world) and intracellular environments. Interactions between integrin and cytoskeleton affect the binding affinity and avidity of integrins for ECM ligands (inside-out signaling), whereas interaction between ECM and integrin leads to changes in the shape and composition of the cell architecture (outside-in signaling). All integrin-ligand binding depends on the presence of divalent cations such as Ca^{2+}, Mg^{2+}, and Mn^{2+}.

Integrin Structure: The α and β Subunits

Integrins are the most important large family of heterodimeric (different monomers) transmembrane two-chain glycoproteins (α and β chains). A homodimer is formed by two identical proteins and heterodimer is formed by two different proteins. Integrins **participate in cell-cell interactions, cell-ECM binding, and leukocyte recruitment**. They are **receptors** composed of noncovalently bound/linked (bond in which electrons are not shared between atoms) two membrane-spanning polypeptide chains namely α and β subunits (chains). There are 18 different α subunits and eight different β subunits. There are different combinations between these two α and β subunits giving rise to 24 different integrins (identified on the surfaces of cells). Each of these combinations has a specific distribution within the body. They have different combinations of **α and β (e.g., $\alpha_1\beta_1$, $\alpha_2\beta_1$, $\alpha_6\beta_4$)** and give integrins with distinct binding properties. The **β_2-type subunit is expressed exclusively by leukocytes** [white blood cells (WBCs)]. Depending on the combination, the integrins act as receptors for a variety of different ECM proteins. The α and β chains share no homology and are distinct polypeptides with specific domain structures. The extracellular domains from both α and β subunits contribute to the ligand binding site of the heterodimer (protein composed of two polypeptide chains of different composition).

Integrins molecules are attached to the actin cytoskeleton inside the cytosol. This attachment is mediated by a network of proteins grouped together on the cytoplasmic side of the focal adhesions. These proteins mediate a physical connection from the cell interior to exterior, as well as serve role in signaling and regulating cell adhesion. This network of proteins includes kinases, phosphatases, and adaptor molecules. In addition to its property of focal attachment to underlying substrates, by binding through the integrin receptors, it can trigger signaling cascades. These may influence cell locomotion, proliferation, shape, and differentiation.

Integrin Activation

Activators for integrins

Chemokines, lipid mediators, and proinflammatory molecules activate cells to express integrin adhesion molecules.

Activation states

Integrins have three major activation states, namely—(1) inactive (low-affinity), (2) active (high-affinity), and (3) ligand occupied. During inactive state, the integrin is bent over causing the burial of ligand-binding site.

- **Low-affinity to high-affinity ligand binding (Figs. 33 and 34):** During active state, integrin receptors become upright and fully expose the ligand-binding pocket. When inactive, integrins bind ligands with low affinity. This low-affinity interaction stimulates intracellular signals and activate the cytoskeletal protein talin (refer Fig. 23, Chapter 1). Protein talin then gets attached to the small cytoplasmic tail (domain) of the β subunit. This interrupts the inhibitory association between the α and β chains and causes the separation of the cytoplasmic and transmembrane regions of the two chains/subunits of integrins (α and β subunits) and convert it into the active conformation. This changes the extracellular domain from a bent to an extended form to allow high-affinity ligand binding.

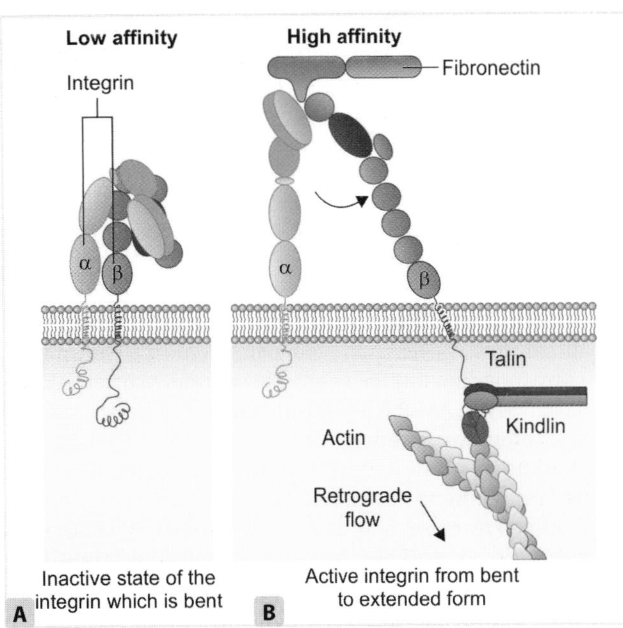

FIGS. 33A AND B: Integrin activation from low-affinity to high-affinity ligand binding. In low-affinity state, the integrin is in bent form whereas in high-affinity, it is upright and attached to ligand (e.g., fibronectin shown in figure).

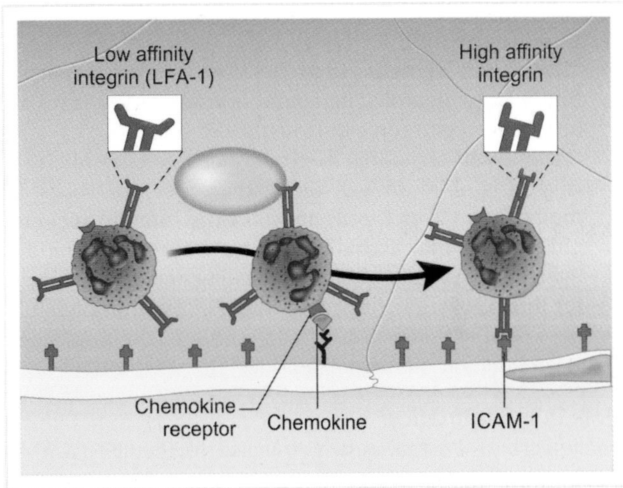

FIG. 34: Integrin activation. Normally, the integrins on leukocytes in blood circulation are in a low-affinity state. If a leukocyte comes in close contact with endothelial cells, initially selectins produce rolling of leukocytes. Then, chemokines will be displayed on the endothelial surface and will bind chemokine receptors on the leukocyte and produce chemokine receptor signaling. This in turn activates the low-affinity integrin on leukocyte integrins into high-affinity state. These leukocytes can then bind with increasing affinity for their ligands on the endothelial cells. It results in firm adhesion of leukocytes to the endothelial cells.

- Integrins bind their ligands with high affinity following inside-out activation described above. However, stable binding needs cytoplasmic domains on integrins to be attached to the cytoskeleton. Integrin–ligand binding leads to the recruitment of enzymes and adaptor molecules that form adhesion complexes linking integrins to the cytoskeleton.

Members

Integrins have different combination of α and β. Synonyms are used which indicate the type of α and β chain. For example, very late antigen 4's (VLA-4) synonym is $\alpha_4\beta_1$, i.e., it contains α4 and β1 chain. CD is the type of protein present in the integrin. The integrin family includes:

- **Lymphocyte function-associated antigen** (LFA-1) ($\alpha_L\beta_2$): The known binding partners of β2 (CD18) integrin chains are α-integrin chains, namely CD11a, CD11b, CD11c, and CD11d. Binding of CD18 and CD11a results in the formation of LFA-1. This LFA-1 is present on neutrophils, monocytes, T-cells (naïve, effector, memory). They bind to corresponding intercellular adhesion molecule-1 (ICAM-1) (CD54), ICAM-2 (CD102) on endothelial cells.
- **Complement receptors** [CR3 ($\alpha_M\beta_2$) and CR4 ($\alpha_X\beta_2$)]: Binding of CD18 and CD11b-d results in the formation of complement receptors. For example, macrophage-1antigen receptor, Mac-1, when bound to CD11b [CD11b/CD18 ($\alpha_M\beta_2$)]. They are proteins found mainly on neutrophils, macrophages, and natural killer (NK) cells. They bind ICAM-1 and ICAM-2.
- **Very late activation (VLA) molecules:** These include VLA-4 ($\alpha_4\beta_1$) on leukocytes and lymphocytes. They bind vascular cell adhesion molecule-1 (VCAM-1) on endothelial cells.

Types of signaling

Characteristic feature of all integrins is that they are able to serve as a bilateral link between the cytoskeleton and the ECM (extracellular matrix).

- **"Outside-in" signaling:** It occurs after the integrin receptor binds to its ligand. The signal is transmitted from the integrin receptor (outside) into the cell (inside).
- **"Inside-out" signaling:** It occurs when a cell stimulus (e.g., triggering of an antigen-recognition receptor/accessory molecule on T or B cell) activates the integrin receptor. This process may activate the integrin receptor to bind its ligand. This results in inside signaling going out. Ligands for integrins are members of the IgSF, (immunoglobulin superfamily discussed on pages 288–289) complement fragments, various serum peptides, etc.

Role in inflammation

The integrins (LFA 1) along with members of the IgSF (ICAM 1, ICAM 2, and ICAM 3) play an important role in the strong adhesion, and leukocyte transmigration through endothelial cells.

Functions of integrins are discussed on pages 24–25 and 233–234.

Cadherins

The name "cadherin" comes from "**calcium-dependent adhesion**". The cadherin superfamily is glycoproteins and each molecule consists of Ca^{2+}-dependent extracellular domain. They mediate Ca^{2+}-dependent cell–cell adhesion and have a unique pattern of tissue distribution. Cell-cell adhesion is primarily mediated by cadherins and is modulated by members of the IgSF (immunoglobulin superfamily). Cadherins play important roles in tissue organization and morphogenesis. The extracellular domains of cadherins repeat and thus they are defined depending on the presence of these cadherin repeats. There are >100 cadherins defined. They are classified into **subgroups—(1) classical type I cadherins, (2) type II cadherins, (3) desmosomal cadherins, (4) protocadherins, and (5) other cadherin-related molecules**.

Basic Structure (Fig. 35)

Cadherins have **three domains.** Most of the cadherins consist of—(1) an N-terminal extracellular domain containing five or six cadherin repeats, (2) a short transmembrane region, and (3) a C-terminal intracellular domain. The cadherin repeat unit in the extracellular domain are linked by Ca^{2+} -binding motifs and is responsible for providing stability to the extracellular domain. The cadherin repeats in the extracellular domain are numbered, with the repeat closest to the N-terminus designated as extracellular cadherin (EC) 1 (**Fig. 35**). The C-terminal intracellular domain is attached to a variety of molecules (e.g., p120, β-catenin) that link cadherins to the cytoskeleton. Intracellular cytoplasmic tail is associated with a large number adapter and signaling proteins.

Cadherin Subgroups

Classical (type I) cadherins

The classical cadherins were the first to be described. They are named after the tissue in which they were detected. The extracellular domain of classical cadherins is composed of an N-terminal predomain followed by five EC domains. These cadherins show hemophilic specificity (e.g., E-cadherin binds E-cadherin more strongly than it binds other classical cadherins).

- The cytoplasmic domains of classical cadherins are connected with proteins involved in endocytosis and intracellular signaling, and also with the actin cytoskeleton. Interactions with actin are important for cadherins to form stable cell–cell adhesions.
- The cytoplasmic tail of classical cadherins is composed of a **juxtamembrane domain** (JMD) and a **C-terminal catenin-binding domain** (CBD). The JMD is attached to

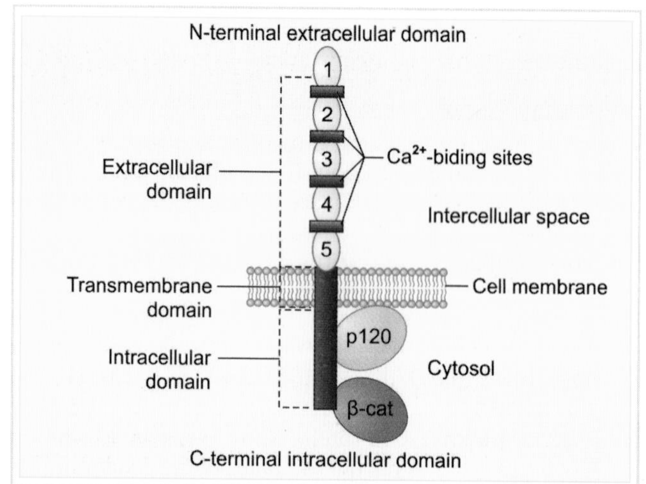

(β-cat: β-catenin; p120: p120 catenin)

FIG. 35: Diagrammatic representation of basic structure of cadherin. In this figure, extracellular domain contains five cadherin repeats that are numbered starting from N-terminal end.

p120-catenin and is required for stabilizing the cadherin molecule at the cell surface whereas the CBD attached to the β-catenin. This β-catenin is responsible for the linking of classical cadherins to the actin cytoskeleton via intermediates such as α-catenin and vinculin.

Type II cadherins

In contrast to type I cadherins, they have an increased tendency toward heterophilic binding with other subfamily members. Their intracellular (cytoplasmic) domain is similar to type I cadherins, except that the **C-terminal** CBD binds to γ-catenin rather than β-catenin.

Desmosomal cadherins

It consists of seven desmosomal cadherins belonging two families, namely three desmocollins (DSC 1–3) and four desmogleins (DSG 1–4). Both subfamilies have five extracellular domains. Desmosomal cadherins form *cis* (interaction between molecules on the same cell) dimers within a desmosome, then interact with dimers on a neighboring cell, with heterophilic interactions between DSC (desmocollins) and DSG (desmogleins) proteins. The DSC and DSG proteins differ from classical cadherins as well from each other in their cytoplasmic domains. Both DSC and DSG groups of desmosomal cadherins contain a membrane proximal intracellular anchor domain, which corresponds to the JMD in type I cadherins, and an intracellular cadherin segment (ICS) similar to the CBD in classical cadherins. The ICS in DSC and DSG proteins, however, binds mainly to γ-catenin and is connected with the intermediate filament cytoskeleton.

Protocadherins

The protocadherins constitute the largest subgroup of the cadherin superfamily and consists of about 70 members. Protocadherins have six or seven extracellular domains, a single transmembrane region and different cytoplasmic domains.

Examples of various cadherins (including other cadherin-related molecules) are presented in **Table 25**.

Table 25: Examples of various cadherins.

Group and member	*Tissue distribution*
Classical	
• CDH1 (E-cadherin)	Epithelium
• CDH2 (N-cadherin)	Neurons
• CDH3 (P-cadherin)	Placenta
Desmosomal	
• Desmogleins (DSG1, DSG2, DSG3, DSG4)	Skin
• Desmocollins (DSC1, DSC2, DSC3)	Skin
Protocadherins	
• PCDH1, PCDH10, etc.	Various tissues
Ungrouped/unconventional	
• CDH4 (R-cadherin)	Retina
• CDH6 (K-cadherin)	Kidney
• CDH13 [T-cadherin (H-cadherin)]	Heart
• CDH17 (LI-cadherin)	Liver, intestine

Selectins

The selectins are C-type lectins that are carbohydrate-binding proteins which require calcium for binding. Selectins are receptors expressed on the surface of leukocytes, platelets, and activated endothelial cells. Selectins promote the attachment and rolling of leukocytes and platelets on the vascular endothelium. They are also important for the recruitment of leukocytes to sites of inflammation and for lymphocyte homing to secondary lymphoid organs.

Types of Selectins

There are three types (members/subfamilies) of selectins (CD62):

1. **L-selectin or leukocyte-selectin** (CD62L), expressed on surface of most leukocytes, except activated T cells.
2. **E-selectin or endothelial-selectin** (also called CD62E), expressed on cytokine-activated endothelial cells.
3. **P-selectin or platelet-selectin** (CD62P), expressed by platelets and activated endothelial cells.

These three types differ from each other in a number of the consensus repeats and in cell expression, respectively. The selectins are involved in heterophilic binding.

Selectin Structure

Selectins are rigid and extended molecules and share a similar molecular structure. They have three domains, namely:

1. **Extracellular lectin-binding (C-type lectin) domain:** The extracellular regions consist of an N-terminal carbohydrate recognition domain (CRD) that binds to carbohydrate moieties. These are carbohydrate-binding proteins. This domain binds sugars (hence the lectin part of the name) and contains a highly conserved Ca^{2+}-dependent CRD (hence the name C-type). This calcium-dependent, or C-type lectin binds sialylated oligosaccharides, specifically the sialyl-Lewis X moiety on cadherins (addressins). This is responsible for rapid attachment of leukocytes to endothelium and rolling.
2. **Epidermal growth factor (EGF)-like domain** and short consensus repeats (SCR) of differing numbers.
3. **Transmembrane domain** consisting of chain of transmembrane glycoproteins.

The size difference of different selectins is due to the number of SCRs (short consensus repeats). L-selectin contains two SCRs, E-selectin has six, and P-selectin contains eight or nine SCRs (**Fig. 36**). The transmembrane and cytoplasmic domains of the selectins are quite different and they bind to different intracellular proteins.

P-Selectin

P-selectin (CD62P, GMP-140, PADGEM) is **constitutively expressed** by **megakaryocytes.** It is **preformed and normally stored in Weibel–Palade bodies of endothelial cells and a-granules of platelets in the cytosol.** Following activation/stimulation of platelets and endothelial cells (by histamine, thrombin, or specific inflammatory cytokines), P-selectin present in the preformed cytosolic granules moves rapidly to the cell surface and fuse with the cell membrane. The **important ligand for P-selectin is sialyl-Lewis X on P-selectin glycoprotein ligand 1 (PSGL-1) on leukocyte surfaces.** PSGL-1 is a sialomucin expressed on microvilli-like projections of leukocytes. Interactions of P-selectin with

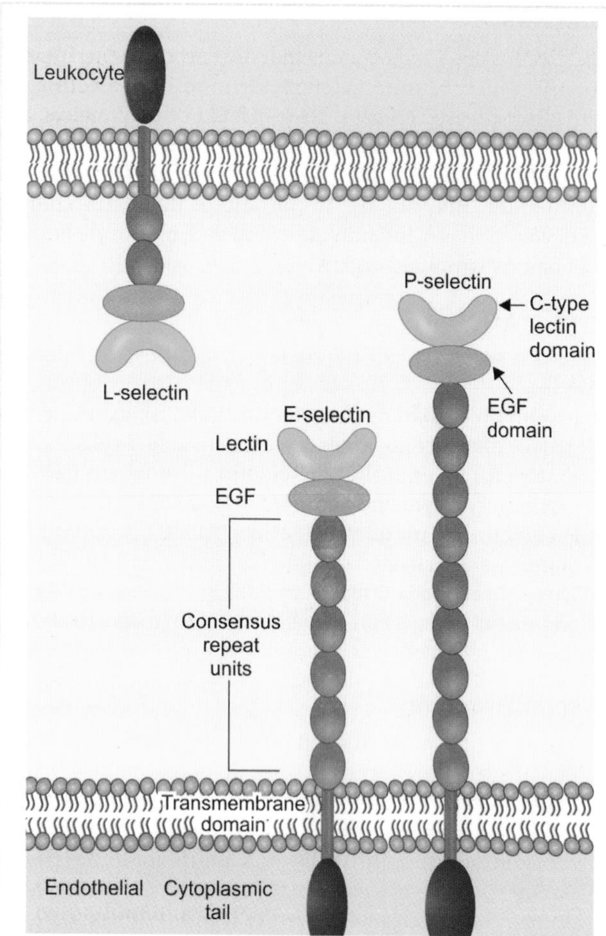

FIG. 36: Diagrammatic representation of selectin family, namely L-selectin, E-selectin, and P-selectin.

PSGL-1 are important for adherence and **rolling of leukocytes on endothelial cells**, or immobilized platelets, expressing P-selectin. P-selectin can also weakly attach to some forms of heparin and heparan sulfate and to some glycoproteins carrying the sialylated Lewis X (SLeX) structure.

E-Selectin

E-selectin (CD62E, ELAM-1) is **not normally expressed on endothelial cell** surfaces. But it is **induced by inflammatory mediators, such as cytokines or bacterial lipopolysachharides** (LPSs). They cause expression of E-selectins on **cytokine-stimulated endothelial cells**. It can **recognize many glycoproteins present on leukocytes including PSGL-1**. E-selectin causes adhesion of neutrophils, monocytes, and certain lymphocytes by binding to Lewis X or Lewis A. The cytoplasmic tail of E-selectin interacts with cytoskeletal elements and signaling molecules.

L-Selectin

L-selectin (CD62L, LAM-1, Leu-8) is a "homing" molecule **constitutively expressed** on the microvilli of many types of **leukocytes**. The intracellular tail of L-selectin attaches to calmodulin and actin cytoskeleton. This attachment is brought through α-actin and the ezrin/radixin/moesin protein family. The extracellular domain of L-selectin **binds to specialized high endothelial venules (HEVs) of peripheral lymphoid tissue and thus regulate lymphocyte trafficking/handling**. It can also bind to glycan-bearing cell adhesion molecule-1 (GlyCAM-1), mucosal addressin cell adhesion molecule-1 (MadCAM-1), and CD34.

Box 12: Members of *immunoglobulin superfamily*.

- Immunoglobulins
- Antigen receptors (TCR and BCR)
- Coreceptors (CD4, CD8, CD21)
- Costimulatory molecules [CD28, CTLA-4 (CD152)]
- B7–1 (CD80), B7–2 (CD86),
- Fc receptors
- Human leukocyte antigen (HLA) molecules
- Cytokine receptors
- Platelet endothelial cell adhesion molecule-1 (PECAM-1) (CD31)
- Intercellular adhesion molecule (ICAM)-1 (CD54), ICAM-2 (CD102), and ICAM-3 (CD50)

Selectin Functions

The selectins act together to **promote adhesion and rolling of leukocytes along the endothelium of vessels**. This occurs under constant changes occurring in the blood flow in the capillaries. Changes in blood flow exert straining forces on the leukocytes and platelets as they interact with each other and endothelial cells. Shear rate is defined as a measure of the extent or rate of relative motion between adjacent layers (two parallel in case of blood flow, i.e., one moving at a constant speed and other one is stationary) of the moving fluid. When the shear rate is low (i.e., the difference between the rate of flow between two adjacent layers is small), leukocytes are unable to roll, but as shear rates increase (i.e., the difference between the rate of flow between two adjacent layers is high) past a threshold, selectin-ligand bonds are strengthened. This phenomenon is termed as "catch bonds". When shear rates increase beyond an optimal level, there will be weakening of selectin-ligand bonds and this shortens the lifetime of selectin-ligand binding. These interactions are termed as "slip bonds". A combination of catch and slip bonds makes the leukocytes to roll along the endothelia between 100 and 1,000 times slower than the mean rate of blood flow. This leukocyte rolling is sustained by the formation of new and the dissociation of old selectin-ligand bonds.

They are also involved in inflammatory processes, and cancer progression and metastasis. Ligands for selectins are mucosal vascular addressins (mucin-type glycoproteins).

Role in Inflammation

The selectins play an essential role in "rolling" of leukocytes and leukocyte transmigration through endothelial cells (refer page 234–235).

Immunoglobulin Superfamily (IgSF) Cell Adhesion Molecules

The IgSF is one of the largest and most diverse protein families in the genome with about 100 members (**Box 12**). Proteins of the IgSF contain one or more Ig-like domains. These domains are homologous to the basic structural unit of Ig (antibody) molecules. Most of IgSF belong to cell surface proteins, and many are CAMs.

Immunoglobulin Domains

Immunoglobulin domains consist of 70–110 amino acids. They are classified into two subtypes—the variable (V) and constant (C) domains. Both V and C subtypes have a characteristic sandwich structure, consisting of two sheets of antiparallel β strands that are bound and stabilized by a disulfide bonds. This produces a compact structure which is relatively insensitive to cleavage by proteolytic enzymes. The V subtype has antigen-binding properties, whereas the C subtype mediates effector functions. Initially, these were called Igs because it was thought that they were specific to the immune system. However, later it was discovered that they mediate a different interaction outside the immune system. These sequences are called IgSF (immunoglobulin superfamily) domains or Ig-like domains, to distinguish them from the domains of Igs.

Structure of IgSF Cell Adhesion Molecules

Most IgSF members consist of three regions (**Fig. 37**), namely—(1) an amino N-terminal extracellular region, (2) a single transmembrane domain, and (3) a carboxyl C-terminal cytoplasmic domain. The extracellular domains of IgSF CAMs have one or more Ig-like domains (in **Fig. 37** shown five in number) and many also have one or more fibronectin type III (FNIII) domains (**Fig. 37**). The transmembrane domains of IgSF CAMs are small. The intracellular domains vary in length and many contain signaling motifs and/or regions that interact with cytoskeletal or adaptor elements. Hence, interactions of IgSF CAMs at the cell surface can produce signaling both within the cell (outside-in signaling) and inside-out signaling.

Interactions of IgSF Cell Adhesion Molecules

The IgSF CAMs (cell adhesion molecules) bind both homophilic and heterophilic ligands. These interactions are usually mediated through the N-terminal Ig-like domains and **bind other Ig-like domains**. However, it may also interact with **integrins and carbohydrates**. In contrast to the high-affinity binding between antibody and antigen, interactions between IgSF CAMs and their ligands are weak. The interaction between molecules on the same cell is termed *cis* and interaction between molecules on another cell surface is termed *trans*. IgSF proteins form *trans* interactions with molecules such as integrins. Immunoglobulin superfamily Ig superfamily adhesive molecules involved in inflammation are discussed on page 235 (refer Table 12 for Ig family of adhesive molecules.)

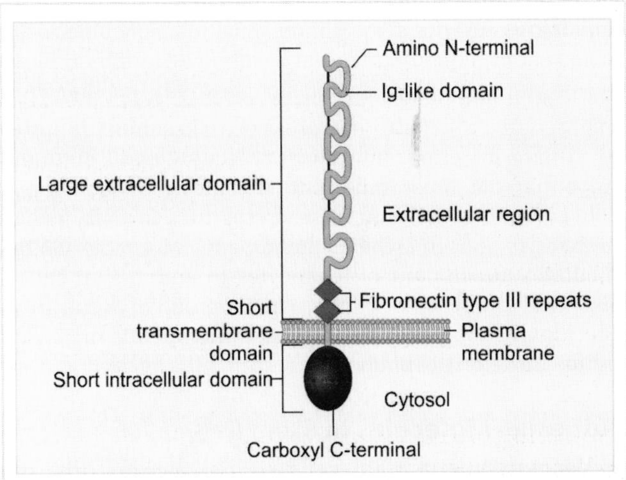

FIG. 37: Diagrammatic appearance of immunoglobulin superfamily (IgSF). It consists of a large extracellular domain containing five Ig-like domains stabilized by disulfide bonds and two fibronectin type III repeats, and short transmembrane and intracellular domains.

Addressins

Vascular addressins are mucin-like glycoproteins. They include GlyCAM-1, P-selectin glycoprotein-1 (PSGL-1), E-selectin ligand (ESL-1), and CD34. They have sialyl-Lewis X, which binds the lectin domain of selectins. Addressins are present on leukocyte and endothelial surfaces. They regulate localization of leukocyte subpopulations and are involved in lymphocyte activation.

Definition of some of the adhesive molecules are presented in **Table 26**.

Role in Inflammation

Platelet endothelial CAM-1 (or CD31) is required for the leukocyte transmigration process through endothelial cells.

Adhesive Molecules and Disease

It is necessary to have normal expression and function of adhesive molecules to maintain health and to defend against disease. Whenever there is interruption or alteration in these normal cell-to-cell and/or cell-to-matrix interactions, it can

Table 26: Definition of terms.

Term	*Description*
Cadherins	Cell surface proteins that mediate calcium dependent cell–cell adhesion. Each cadherin contains an extracellular cadherin (EC) repeat
Ig-like domain	Basic structural unit of IgSF members. It is made up of two sheets of antiparallel β strands which form a sandwich structure and stabilized by a disulfide bond
Immunoglobulin superfamily (IgSF)	Family of proteins that contain at least one Ig-like domain
Integrins	Cell adhesion molecules mediating cell–cell and cell–matrix adhesion. They are made ups of two noncovalently bound subunits (i.e., α and β)
Selectins	Carbohydrate-binding adhesion molecules. There are three types, namely E-, L-, and P-selectin. They mediate early stages of leukocyte migration from the vasculature
Type of binding	
Heterophilic binding	Binding by an adhesion molecule to a different molecule
Homophilic binding	Binding of an adhesion molecule to same type of molecule on another cell

trigger disease process. Movement of leukocytes to the site of inflammation in a tissue depends upon adhesion molecules on both leukocytes and on the endothelium. Impaired expression of adhesion molecule can interrupt this process. However, these adhesion molecules can also be misused by infectious agents and disease processes itself. For example, increased expression of adhesion molecule can produce an inflammatory condition such as asthma and rheumatoid arthritis.

Extravasation

It is the process of leukocyte migration from circulation to the site of inflammation tissue. When a leukocyte responds to an infectious agent in a tissue, its adhesion molecules (L-selectin and integrins) must encounter their corresponding ligands and help leukocyte's movement from blood circulation into tissue.

- **Steps in inflammation:** During extravasation, L-selectin on the leukocyte binds to its ligand on endothelial cell. This causes "**rolling**" of the leukocyte along the endothelium of the blood vessel. This is followed by **activation** of an integrin on the same leukocyte, in an inside-out fashion. The activated integrin can then bind to its ligand on the endothelium, causing a **firm adhesion and arrest** of the leukocyte. This is followed by **emigration**, or movement of leukocyte through the endothelial layer, and **extravasation,** or entry of the leukocyte into the tissue at the site of offending injurious agent. Thus, these traditional three steps of rolling, activation, and firm binding require different adhesive molecules. It is discussed in detail on pages 231–234.
- **Atherosclerotic plaque formation:** The same leukocyte processes of extravasation to tissue site of infection also occur in formation of **atheromatous plaque.** The atherosclerotic process begins with an injury to the intima of the blood vessel, namely the endothelium. Monocytes bind to the injured endothelium in an adhesion-molecule dependent manner and then undergo extravasation into the subendothelium. These monocytes engulf excess lipids (entered from the circulation) and become foam cells. The foam cells accumulate in the intima of the blood vessel and form atheromatous plaque. It can restrict the flow of blood.

Adhesion Molecule Defects

Any impairment of expression of particular adhesion molecules can inhibit leukocyte extravasation to the sites of infection. Also, any abnormal expression of other adhesion molecules can result in the disruption of normal tissue structure.

- **Cancer:** Changes in the expression or function of adhesion molecules can be responsible for progression of cancer. Most cancers arise from epithelial tissue and E-cadherin is very important in organizing the epithelium to each other. The function of E-cadherin is altered in most epithelial tumors. Loss of E-cadherin-mediated cell-to-cell adhesion occurs during tumor progression and is also responsible for subsequent tumor spread or metastasis (refer pages 477–479).
- **Leukocyte adhesion deficiency (LAD):** The importance of functional adhesion molecules is revealed when there is **LAD** I. LAD is a rare inherited defect in the β2 **subunit of integrins**, which is normally exclusively expressed on leukocytes. Therefore, these leukocytes have an impaired ability to emigrate to the sites of infection. These patients develop recurrent bacterial infections and usually do not survive beyond two years of age.
- **Pemphigus:** Pemphigus is an autoimmune condition characterized by formation of blisters due to defect in cell-to-cell adhesion due to defects in adhesion molecule. In pemphigus, there is disruption of cadherin-mediated cell adhesions. Pemphigus is caused by autoantibodies that bind to the proteins in a subfamily of the cadherins, known as the **desmogleins (DSGs)**. Antibody binding to DSGs prevents their function in cell adhesion. Therefore, adjacent epidermal cells are not able to adhere to each other and this leads to blister formation. **Pemphigoid** is a related group of blistering disorders in which autoantibodies to proteins of hemidesmosomes are formed. They impair the attachment of epidermal cells to the underlying basal lamina.

Increased Adhesion Molecule Expression and Inflammation

Normal adhesive molecules are necessary for health. Deficiency and excess produce disease. Increased expression of adhesion molecules (i.e., more than the usual number per cell) can result in enhanced migration of cells to a region and can lead to inappropriate inflammation.

- **Asthma:** ICAM-1 is an adhesion molecule and is a member of the IgSF. Normally, it facilitates adhesion between endothelial cells and leukocytes after injury or stress. Increased ICAM-1 expression is observed in the respiratory tract of patients with asthma and has been implicated in pathogenesis of asthma. Increased ICAM-1 may allow an inappropriately large number of leukocytes to migrate and stimulate chronic inflammation in the respiratory tract.
- **Rheumatoid arthritis:** It is an autoimmune inflammatory condition in which there may be increased expression of adhesion molecules. In rheumatoid arthritis, synovial inflammation is associated with selective involvement of the integrin LFA-1 and of ICAM-2. Inhibition of certain adhesion molecules is used as a therapy for rheumatoid arthritis.

Adhesion Molecules as Receptors for Infectious Agents

Adhesion molecules are widely expressed on human cells. These adhesion molecules may be used as receptor by some infectious agents. Because viruses need a host binding protein to initiate infection, adhesion molecules may sometimes serve this role. Most important etiologic agents of common cold are rhinoviruses and these viruses are also a major cause of exacerbations in asthma. The same ICAM-1 molecule that mediates attachment of leukocytes to endothelial cells is also used as a receptor by these major group of rhinoviruses. Blocking ICAM-1 may be used as a therapeutic method to inhibit infection by rhinovirus.

Adhesive Molecules in Stem Cell

- Hematopoietic stem cells (HSCs) express adhesion molecules of the cadherin family, integrin family, IgSF, CD44 family, and sialomucin family.
- Mesenchymal stem cells (MSCs) express IgSF (ICAM-1, ICAM-3, VCAM-1, ALCAM), CD44, and P-selectin, etc.

8.6 Cytokines and Chemokines

CHAPTER OUTLINE

CYTOKINES AND CHEMOKINES

Q. Discuss cytokines and their role in health and disease/ lymphokines/chemokines.
Q. Discuss the role of cytokines in acute inflammation.
Q. Write a short essay on cytokines and their function.
Q. Describe cytokines and their general properties.

General Features

Cytokines are specialized **low molecular-weight** regulatory molecules **(proteins**/polypeptides or glycoproteins) that function as mediators/regulator in **immune responses,** in **inflammation (acute and chronic),** and **hematopoietic processes**. They are produced at sites of tissue injury and involved in regulation of inflammatory responses. Thus, they are involved from initial changes in vascular permeability to resolution and restoration of integrity of tissue. Cytokines communicate among cells of the immune system. The term "cytokine" is derived from Greek words "*cyto-*" and "*-kinos*", which means "cell" and "movement".

Source

Cytokines are secreted by many types of activated cell (activated lymphocytes and macrophages, endothelial, epithelial, and connective tissue cells). Important cytokines involved in inflammation are discussed further.

Mode of Action

Cytokines are inflammatory hormones that act mainly through three modes—(1) **autocrine (affect** the cells that produce them), (2) **paracrine** (affect the neighboring cells), and (3) **endocrine** (act through the bloodstream on distant cells). Most *cytokines* act in a *paracrine* or *autocrine* manner, whereas only few of them may function at the systemic level, by the *endocrine* way (refer pages 40–41 and Fig. 2 of Chapter 2).

Responses

Cytokine acts on a target cell through a high-affinity cytokine receptor triggering followed by signaling inside the cell. The interaction of a cytokine with its receptor on a target cell can produce a wide variety of responses.

- **Movement of a cell:** Cytokines can cause changes in the expression of adhesion molecules and **chemokine receptors** on the target membrane. This may lead to movement of cells from one location to another.
- **Changes in the activities of a cell:** Cytokines can produce signal in an immune cell to increase or decrease the activity of particular enzymes or to change its transcriptional program. Thus, cytokines may activate the cell to proliferate and differentiate, or to modulate its effector functions.
- **Cell survival or death:** Finally, cytokines can instruct a cell when to survive and when to die.

Characteristic features of cytokines are listed in **Box 13.** Main functions of cytokines are presented in **Box 14.**

Classification

Originally, cytokines were called as lymphokines because they were thought to be derived only from lymphocytes. The term monokine was used for those secreted by monocytes

Box 13: Characteristic features of cytokines.

- Produced by many cell types
- Usually act at short range
- Mediate multiple effects
- Effective at very low concentration
- Transiently produced
- Short half life
- Act through specific receptors
- Can have beneficial or harmful effects

Box 14: Main functions of cytokines.

- **Innate immunity:** Tumor necrosis factor (TNF), interleukin (IL)-1, IL-12, type 1 interferon (IFN), IFN-γ, chemokines. Source includes macrophages, dendritic cells, natural killer (NK) cells, endothelial, and epithelial cells
- **Adaptive immunity:** IL-2, IL-4, IL-5, IL-17, and IFN-γ. They act mainly on CD4+ T lymphocytes
- **Promote lymphocytic proliferation and differentiation**
- **Limit or terminate immune response:** TGF β and IL-10
- **Stimulating hematopoiesis:** Colony stimulating factors (CSF) increase number of leukocytes during immune and inflammatory responses. E.g., granulocyte–macrophage colony stimulating factor (GM CSF), IL-7. These are produced by marrow stromal cells, T lymphocytes, macrophages

and macrophages. The term interleukin (IL) was used because they were produced by some leukocytes and affected other leukocytes. Other cytokines such as interferons (IFNs) were involved in antiviral responses, and colony stimulating factors (CSFs) support the growth of cells in semisolid medias, and chemokines promote chemotaxis.

The term "cytokine" has now replaced all the older terms and covers all of the above. There is no unified cytokine classification system. According to their functional role in inflammation, they may be classified as proinflammatory or anti-inflammatory. Recently, they are classified based on structural similarities observed between related cytokines (**Table 27**). Classification of cytokines according to their mode of action is presented in **Box 15**.

Mechanisms of Action

Cytokines have different mechanisms of action and produce different biological effects. Cytokines have pleiotropy, redundancy, synergism, antagonism, and cascade induction (**Figs. 38A to E**).

Table 27: Principal source, cellular targets, and functions of cytokines.

Group and types of cytokine	*Principal cell source*	*Principal cellular targets and primary biologic effects*
Interleukins		
IL-1	Macrophages, endothelial cells, some epithelial cells	Endothelial cells: Adhesion, activation (inflammation, coagulation) Hypothalamus: Fever Liver: Synthesis of acute-phase proteins T cells: Th17 differentiation
IL-2	Th1 cells, NK cells	T cells, B cell, monocytes: Proliferation/growth and activation
IL-3	T cells, NK cells, and mast cells	Bone marrow hematopoietic precursors: Growth and differentiation
IL-4	Th2 cells, mast cells	Naive T cells: Differentiation to Th2 cell T cells: Differentiation/growth and activation B cells: Isotype switching to IgE
IL-5	Th2 cells, mast cells	Eosinophils: Activation, increased generation
IL-6	Macrophages, endothelial cells, T cells	Liver: Synthesis of acute-phase proteins B cells: Proliferation of antibody-producing cells, adhesion T cells: Th17 differentiation
IL-7	Stromal cells in bone marrow	Stimulates immature lymphocytes to divide to produce B and T cells
IL-8	Macrophages, epithelial cells, platelets	Neutrophils: Chemotaxis and activation
IL-9	Th2 cells	Enhances growth of T helper cells, B cells, and mast cells
IL-10	Macrophages, T cells (mainly regulatory T cells)	Macrophages, DCs: Inhibition of expression of IL-12, costimulators, and class II MHC molecules
IL-11	Stromal cells in bone marrow	Stimulates platelet production
IL-12	Macrophages, NK cells	Naïve T cells: Differentiation into a Th1 cell NK cells and T cells: IFN-γ synthesis, increased cytotoxic activity
IL-13	T cells	B cell: IgE switching, B cell growth Epithelial cells: Increased mucus production Macrophages: Alternative activation
IL-14	T cells	Induces B cell proliferation
IL-15	Macrophages, others	NK cells: Proliferation T cells: Proliferation (memory CD8+ cells)
IL-16	CD8+ T cells	CD4+ cell chemotaxis, suppresses viral replication of human immunodeficiency virus (HIV)
IL-17	T cells	Neutrophils, inflammatory cells: Inflammatory regulation, chronic inflammation GM-CSF and G-CSF production
IL-18	Macrophages	NK cells and T cells: Increase IFN-γ synthesis
IL-19	Macrophages	Stimulates macrophage IL-1 secretion
IL-20	Monocytes	Stimulates hematopoietic stem cells
IL-21	Th2 and Th17 and TFH cells	Activates B cells, stimulates production of NK cells

Continue

Continue

Group and types of cytokine	*Principal cell source*	*Principal cellular targets and primary biologic effects*
IL-22	Th17 cells	Epithelial cells, increased barrier function, defensin production
IL-23	Macrophages and DCs	T cells: Maintenance of IL-17-producing T cells
IL-24	Monocytes, T cells	Monocyte inflammatory cytokine production
IL-25	T cells, mast cells and macrophages	Stimulates production of cytokines by Th2 cells (IL-4, IL-5, IL-13)
IL-26	T cells, monocytes	Uncertain
IL-27	Macrophages and DCs	T cells: TH1 differentiation; inhibition of Th17 cells NK cells: IFN-γ synthesis
IL-31	Th2 cells	Uncertain
IL-33	Endothelial cells, fibroblasts	Th2 cell development
Growth factors		
Stem cell factor (c-Kit ligand)	Bone marrow stromal cells	Pluripotent hematopoietic stem cells: Induced maturation of all hematopoietic lineages
GM-CSF	T cells, macrophages, endothelial cells, and fibroblasts	Immature and committed progenitors, mature macrophages: Induced maturation of granulocytes and monocytes, macrophage activation
M-CSF (CSF1)	Macrophages, endothelial cells, bone marrow cells, fibroblasts	Committed hematopoietic progenitors: Induced maturation of monocytes
G-CSF (CSF3)	Macrophages, fibroblasts, endothelial cells	Committed hematopoietic progenitors: Induced maturation of granulocytes
Chemokines		
CC (CCL 1–28) CXC (CXCL 1–16) XC CX3C	Macrophages, endothelial cells, T cells, fibroblasts, platelets	Leukocytes: Chemotaxis, activation; migration into tissues Recruitment of neutrophils, macrophages, lymphocytes
Interferons		
IFN-α	Plasmacytoid DCs, macrophages,	All cells: Antiviral state, increased class I MHC expression NK cells: Activation
IFN-β	Fibroblasts, plasmacytoid DCs	All cells: Antiviral state, increased class I MHC expression NK cells: Activation
IFN-γ	Th1 cells, NK cells	Monocytes: Classical activation (increased microbicidal functions) B cells: Isotype switching to opsonizing and complement-fixing IgG subclasses T cells: Th1 differentiation Various cells: Increased expression of class I and class II MHC molecules, increased antigen processing and presentation to T cells
IFN-λs (type III interferons)	DCs	Epithelial cells: Antiviral state
Proinflammatory cytokines		
TNF-α	Macrophages, T cells	T cells, B cells, and endothelial cells: Activation (inflammation, coagulation) Hypothalamus: Fever Neutrophils: Activation Muscle, fat: Catabolism (cachexia) Many cell types: Apoptosis Anorexia Shock Cytotoxicity Cytokine induction
TGF-ß	T cells, macrophages	T cells and macrophages: Inhibits activation and growth

(DC: dendritic cells; G-CSF: granulocyte colony stimulating factor; GM-CSF: granulocyte-macrophage colony stimulating factor; Ig: immunoglobulin; IFN: interferon; IL: interleukin; M-CSF: monocyte colony stimulating factor; MHC: major histocompatibility complex; NK: natural killer; Th: T helper cell; TFH cell: T follicular helper cells; TGF: transforming growth factor; TNF: tumor necrosis factor)

Box 15: **Classification of cytokines according to their mode of action.**

- **Type I cytokine family members:** IL-2, IL-3, IL-4, IL-5, IL-6, IL-7, IL-9, IL-11, IL-12, IL-13, IL-15, IL-17, IL-21, IL-23, IL-25, IL-27, stem cell factor (c-Kit ligand), granulocyte-monocyte CSF (GM-CSF), monocyte CSF (M-CSF, CSF1), granulocyte CSF (G-CSF, CSF3)
- **Type II cytokine family members:** IFN-α, IFN-β, IFN-γ, IL-10, IL-22, IL-26
- **TNF superfamily cytokines:** Tumor necrosis factor, lymphotoxin
- **IL-1 family cytokines:** IL-1, IL-1 receptor antagonist, IL-18, IL-33
- **Chemokines**
- **Other cytokines:** Transforming growth factor-β (TGF-β)

(CSF: colony stimulating factor; IL: interleukin; INF: interferon)

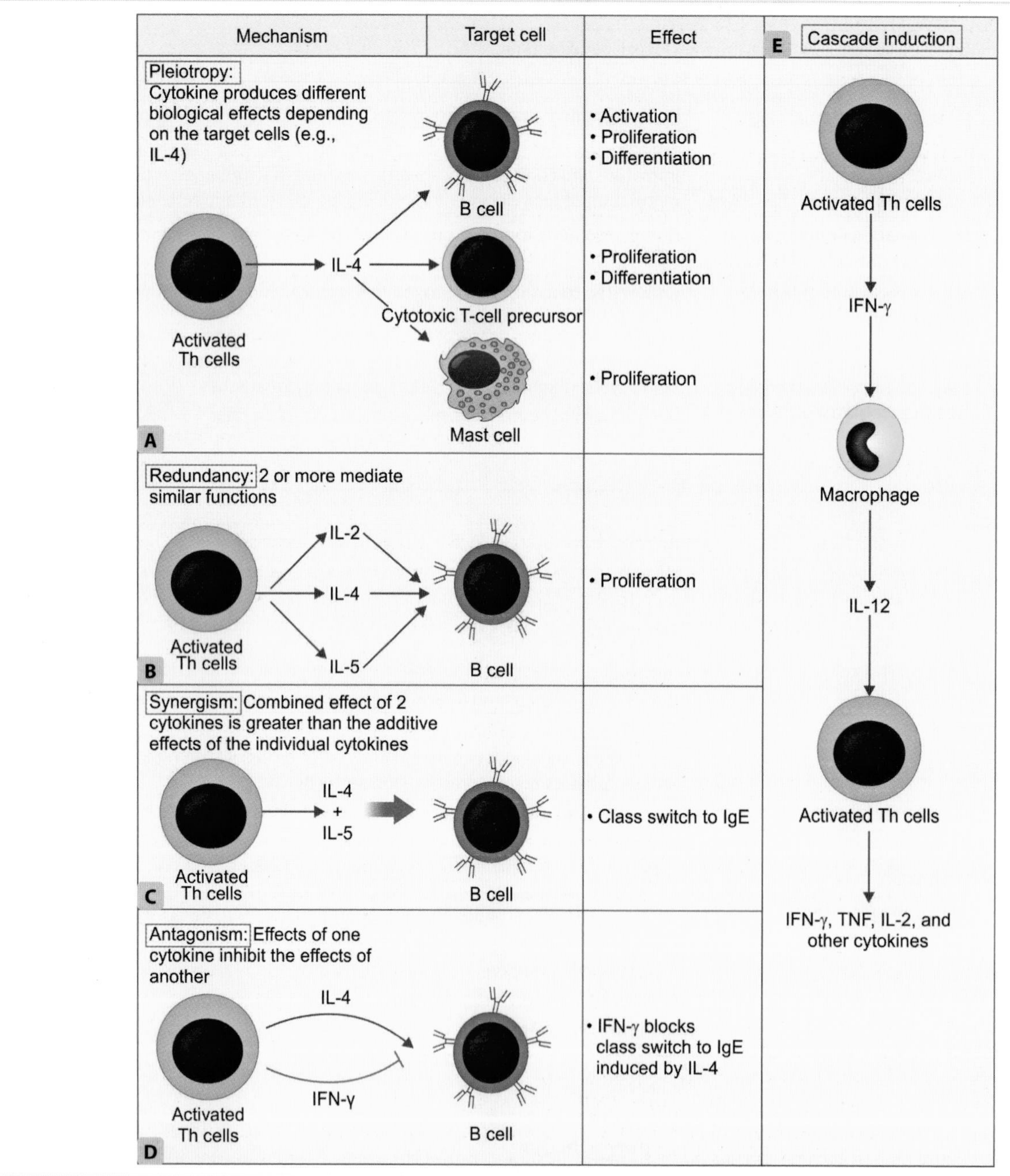

(IFN: interferon; IL: interleukin; Th: T helper; TNF: tumor necrosis factor)

FIGS. 38A TO E: Mechanism of action of cytokine by (A) Pleiotropy, (B) Redundancy, (C) Synergism, (D) Antagonism, and (E) Cascade induction.

- **Pleiotropy:** A cytokine that produces **different biological effects depending on the nature of the target cells** is termed as cytokine with pleiotropic activity.
- **Redundancy:** Two or more cytokines that mediate similar functions are said to be **redundant**.
- **Synergism:** If the **combined effect of two cytokines** on cellular activity **is greater than the additive effects of the individual cytokines,** it is called cytokine **synergy.**
- **Antagonism:** If the effects of **one cytokine** inhibit or **antagonize the effects of another,** it is called antagonism.
- **Cascade induction:** In this, the **action of one cytokine on one target cell induces that cell to produce one or more additional cytokines**.

Macrophages bring out the tissue inflammatory responses through production of cytokines. LPS (lipopolysaccharides) present in the outer membranes of gram-negative bacteria is a potent activator of macrophages, endothelial cells, and leukocytes. LPS binds to specific cellular receptors on the macrophage either directly, or after binding a serum LPS binding protein (LBP). It stimulates the macrophage to produce tumor necrosis factor alpha (TNF-α) and interleukins (IL-1, IL-6, IL-8, IL-12, and others). The cytokines produced by macrophage bring out endothelial cell-leukocyte adhesion (TNF-α), leukocyte recruitment (IL-8), acute phase responses (IL-6, IL-1), and immune functions (IL-1, IL-6, IL-12).

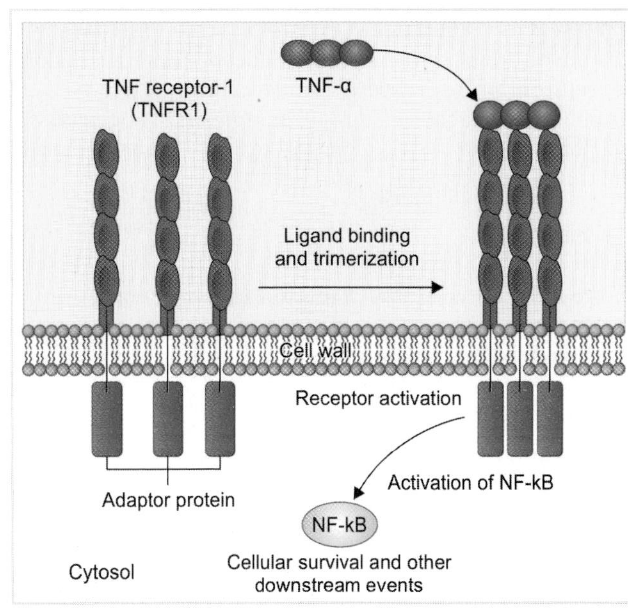

FIG. 39: Binding of tumor necrosis factor (TNF) to tumor necrosis factor receptor-1 (TNFR-1) induces trimerization and activate downstream events. The ligand is TNF-α which as trimer causes three molecules of TNFR receptors to come close together (trimerization). The exact nature of the downstream events that are stimulated depends on the adapter (e.g., death domain in apoptosis) and signal-transducing proteins that are present in the particular cell type.

Tumor Necrosis Factor

Q. Write a short essay on tumor necrosis factors.

Tumor necrosis factor and IL-1 are central to the development and amplification of inflammatory responses. These cytokines activate endothelial cells to express adhesion molecules and also release cytokines, chemokines, and reactive oxygen species (ROS). **TNF is a cytokine that mediates the acute inflammatory response to bacteria and other infectious microbes.** The name was derived from its original identification as a serum substance (factor) that caused necrosis of tumors. Now it is known that this is due to inflammation and thrombosis of tumor blood vessels. TNF is also called as TNF-α to distinguish it from the closely related TNF-β, which is also called lymphotoxin.

Source

Tumor necrosis factor is mainly produced by **activated macrophages, dendritic cells (DCs), mast cells and T cells** (lymphocytes).

Tumor Necrosis Factor Receptors (Fig. 39)

Tumor necrosis factor-α (frequently referred to simply as TNF) is a member of a large family of homologous proteins called the TNF superfamily. The TNF acts through TNF receptors which are the members of a large family of proteins called the TNF receptor superfamily. There are two distinct TNF receptors called type I (TNF-RI) and type II (TNF-RII). Both TNF receptors are present on most cell types. Many of TNF receptors are involved in immune and inflammatory responses. These receptors are present as trimers in the plasma membrane. Different members of the TNF receptor family can induce gene expression or cell death, and some can do both.

- Binding of ligand to some TNF receptor family members, such as TNF-RI, TNF-RII, and CD40 (cluster of differentiation 40 is a member of the TNF-receptor superfamily), leads to the recruitment of proteins called TNF receptor-associated factors (TRAFs) to the cytoplasmic domains of the TNF receptors. In turn TRAFs activate transcription factors such as nuclear factor (NF)-κB and activator protein (AP)-1.
- Cytokine binding, to some family members of TNF-receptor superfamily, such as TNF-RI, may recruit an adaptor protein that activates caspases and triggers apoptosis.

Stimuli for TNF Production

The stimuli for the secretion of TNF and IL-1 includes microbial products, immune complexes, foreign bodies, physical injury, necrotic cells, and many inflammatory stimuli. TNF production by macrophages is stimulated by pathogen associated molecular patterns (PAMPs) and death associated molecular patterns (DAMPs). Pattern recognition receptors (PRRs) such as Toll-like receptors (TLRs), NOD-like receptors (NLRs), and RIG-I-like receptor (RLRs) can induce TNF gene expression, in part by activation of the NF-κB transcription factor. Hence, many different microbial products can stimulate production of TNF. Infections with gram-negative and gram-positive bacteria which express and release the cell wall TLR ligands, LPS and lipoteichoic acid, respectively. This can stimulate production of large amounts of TNF. Septic shock and life-threatening severe infections are mediated mainly by TNF. TNF is also a major contributing factor for inflammation in many inflammatory diseases. Hence, anti-TNF agents have been used for treating many of these diseases. Other stimuli include viruses, protozoa, immune complex, neuropeptide substance P, and reactive oxygen intermediates. It is a powerful proinflammatory cytokine and even endogenous toxin, an endogenous pyrogen, and a regulator of adaptive immune responses.

Biological Effects

It is involved in septic shock, reduced tissue perfusion, depression of myocardial contractility, intravascular thrombosis, metabolic disturbances, apoptosis, angiogenesis and fibrosis. It may have a direct cytotoxic effect on tumor cells and can stimulate antitumor immunity.

Actions of TNF are discussed along with IL-1 on pages 255–256.

Q. Describe interleukins and their role in therapeutics.
Q. Describe the role of interleukins in acute inflammation.

Interleukin-1

Interleukin-1 also mediates acute inflammatory response and it has many similar actions as TNF.

Source

It is mainly produced by activated macrophages (major source). Unlike TNF, IL-1 is also produced by many cell types other than macrophages. These include neutrophils, some epithelial cells (e.g., keratinocytes), and endothelial cells.

Forms

There are two forms of IL-1, namely—(1) IL-1α and (2) IL-1β. Though they have <30% homology to each other, they bind to the same cell surface receptors and have the same biologic activities. IL-1β is the main biologically active secreted form during infections and most other immune responses.

Stimuli for IL-1 Production

Tumor necrosis factor can also stimulate phagocytes and other cell types to synthesize IL-1. IL-1 is stimulated by the same signals as TNF, but the production of the biologically active form of this cytokine is dependent on the inflammasome.

Action

At the systemic level, it exerts the property of endogenous pyrogen. It takes part in the "acute phase" inflammation, costimulation, proliferation, and differentiation of lymphocytes and other cells.

Mechanism of Action

The IL-1 brings out its biologic effects through a membrane receptor called the type I IL-1 receptor (**Fig. 40**). This receptor is expressed on many cell types and includes endothelial cells, epithelial cells, and leukocytes. The signaling events that occur when IL-1 binds to the type I IL-1 receptor result in the activation of NF-κB and AP-1 transcription factors. A second IL-1 receptor, called the type II IL-1 receptor cannot activate downstream signals, and serves as a decoy receptor that limits responses to IL-1.

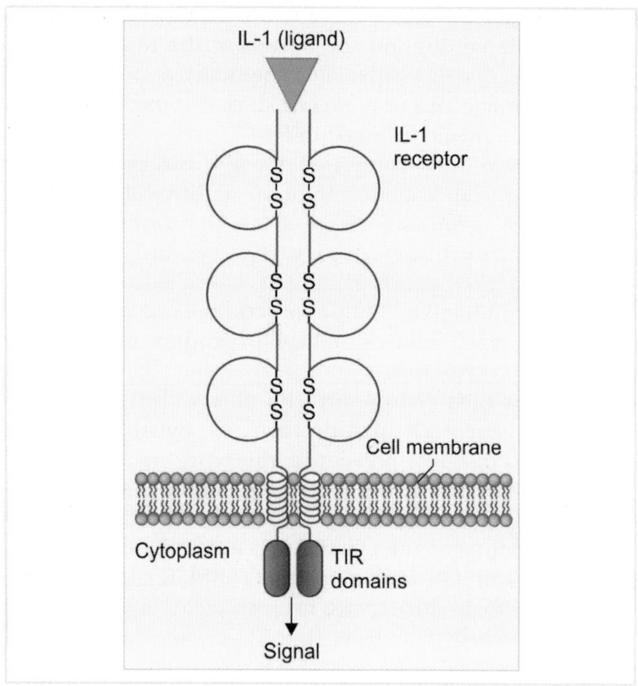

(TIR: toll/interleukin-1 receptor/resistance)

FIG. 40: Interleukin-1 (IL-1) receptor.

Actions of TNF and IL-1

Local Effects

Endothelium: Both TNF and IL-1 act on endothelium to produce changes termed as *endothelial activation*. These changes include **increased expression of endothelial adhesion molecules** (mainly E- and P-selectins and ligands for leukocyte integrins), increased production of other mediators (e.g., other cytokines and chemokines, growth factors, and eicosanoids), and increased procoagulant activity of the endothelium.

Leukocytes: Their actions are as follows:
- **Tumor necrosis factor:** Increases the responses of neutrophils to other stimuli (e.g., bacterial endotoxin) and stimulates the microbicidal activity of macrophages.

During repair: The actions of IL-1 are as follows:
- **Interleukin-1:** It activates fibroblasts to synthesize collagen during repair. It stimulates proliferation of synovial cells and other mesenchymal cells. IL-1 and IL-6 stimulate the formation of a subset of CD4+ helper T cells called Th17 cells.

Systemic Effects

- **Systemic acute-phase reactions:** IL-1 and TNF (and also IL-6) produce the systemic acute-phase responses in association with infection or injury. This also includes fever.
- **Systemic inflammatory response syndrome** (SIRS): IL-1 and TNF can produce SIRS resulting from disseminated bacterial infection (sepsis) and other noninfectious serious conditions such as severe burns, trauma, pancreatitis (SIRS is discussed on page 323).
- Leukocytosis
- **Suppresses appetite:** TNF can regulate energy balance by promoting lipid and protein catabolism and by suppressing appetite. Hence, continuous production of TNF may lead to *cachexia*. Cachexia is a pathologic state characterized by loss of weight, atrophy of muscle, and loss of appetite (anorexia) and is observed in some chronic infections (e.g., tuberculosis) and cancers.

Interleukin-6

Interleukin-6 is another important cytokine in acute inflammatory responses. IL-6 constitutes the IL-6 family of cytokines.

Action

It produces both local and systemic effects.

- It induces the synthesis of acute phase reactants by the liver, stimulates neutrophil production in the bone marrow, and promotes the differentiation of IL-17-producing helper T cells. It takes part in the maintenance of the blood-brain barrier.
- B cells: Proliferation of antibody-producing cells, adhesion.
- T cells: Th17 differentiation.

Source

Interleukin-6 is synthesized by mononuclear phagocytes, DCs, vascular endothelial cells, fibroblasts, T cells, and other cells.

Stimuli

They may be secreted by macrophages in response to PAMPs and in response to IL-1 and TNF.

Significance

Interleukin-6 is a major contributor to inflammation in several inflammatory diseases (e.g., rheumatoid arthritis). Antibodies specific for the IL-6 receptor are used in the treatment of some forms of arthritis. Some lymphoproliferative disorders such as Castleman's disease are caused by human herpesvirus-8 (HHV-8). This virus encodes a homolog of IL-6. Hence, blocking of IL-6 is used to treat these diseases.

Clinical Importance

Tumor necrosis factor antagonists have been found to be effective in the treatment of chronic inflammatory diseases, particularly rheumatoid arthritis, psoriasis, and few cases of inflammatory bowel disease. However, patients on TNF antagonists are more susceptible to mycobacterial infection and this is due to decreased ability of macrophages to kill intracellular microbes.

Interleukin-12

Interleukin-12 is a proinflammatory cytokine.

Source

Interleukin-12 is secreted by activated DCs [antigen-presenting cells (APCs)], NK cells, and macrophages.

Actions

- Naive T cells: Promote differentiation into a Th1 cell during T-cell-mediated responses.
- NK cells and T cells: Stimulate IFN-γ synthesis, increase **NK cell and cytotoxic T lymphocytes (CTL)-mediated** cytotoxic activity.

Main cytokines involved in acute and chronic inflammation are presented in **Table 28**.

Role of cytokines in inflammation is presented in **Table 29**.

Major local and systemic actions of cytokines in inflammation are presented in **Figure 41**.

Chemokines

Q. Describe chemokines and their role in inflammation.
Q. Describe chemokines. Discuss their role in health and disease.
Q. Explain applied aspects of chemokines.

Chemotactic cytokines or chemokines are **a large family of structurally homologous** specialized cytokines of small proteins. They **stimulate leukocyte movement and regulate the migration of leukocytes from the blood to tissues.** They selectively or **primarily act as chemoattractants** (attract **specific types of leukocytes to the site of inflammation)**. There are about 40 different chemokines and 20 different receptors for chemokines. It is named chemokine, meaning cytokine that is chemotactic.

Specificity

Classical leukocyte chemoattractants (i.e., chemotactic factors) have little specificity. In contrast, *chemokines* recruit well-defined (specific) cell types and leukocyte subsets. For example, CXC chemokines can attract neutrophils but not macrophages, while CC chemokines are mainly responsible for the migration of macrophages.

Main Functions

To date, about 40 chemokines have been identified.

- They mainly act on neutrophils, monocytes/macrophages, lymphocytes, and eosinophils, and play an important role in host defense mechanisms.
- Chemokines also regulate the development of lymphoid organ, the functioning of the nervous system, and may stimulate tumor cell metastasis.

Functional Types

Chemokines also can be functionally divided into two classes or groups, homing (homeostatic) and inflammatory chemokines.

1. **Homing (homeostatic) chemokines:** They are normally produced (constitutively expressed) in certain tissues and cells. They are upregulated in disease. They are required for homing leukocytes in particular organs or tissues. They are involved in the organogenesis, migration of progenitor cells, and cell development. They direct trafficking and homing of lymphocytes and DCs to lymphoid tissues during an immune response. However, homeostatic chemokines can also be involved in the carcinogenesis and metastasis of cancer cells.
2. **Inflammatory chemokines:** They are produced under pathological conditions. The proinflammatory stimuli which stimulate their production are generated from sites of infection (elicited by bacterial toxins), injury, or tissue damage. These chemokines take an active part in the inflammatory response. Under the influence of inflammatory chemokines, leukocytes will extravasate from the blood vessel and follow the gradient to proinflammatory stimuli (chemotaxis). They are also recruited in healing of wound healing.

Classification

Chemokines are synthesized as secretory proteins. They consist of 70–130 amino acids, with four conserved cysteines attached by disulfide bonds.

Table 28: Main cytokines involved in acute and chronic inflammation.

Type of cytokine	*Main source*	*Main action in inflammation*
Acute inflammation		
TNF	Macrophages, mast cells, T lymphocytes	T cells, B cells, and endothelial cells: Activation (in inflammation stimulates expression of endothelial adhesion molecules, coagulation) Hypothalamus: Fever Neutrophils: Activation Muscle, fat: Catabolism (cachexia) Many cell types: Apoptosis Anorexia Shock Cytotoxicity Cytokine induction Secretion of other cytokines
IL-1	Macrophages, endothelial cells, some epithelial cells	Similar to TNF; greater role in fever Endothelial cells: Adhesion, activation (inflammation, coagulation) Hypothalamus: Fever Liver: Synthesis of acute-phase proteins T cells: Th17 differentiation
IL-6*	Macrophages, endothelial cells, T cells	Liver: Synthesis of acute-phase proteins (systemic effects) B cells: Proliferation of antibody-producing cells, adhesion
Chemokines	Macrophages, endothelial cells, T lymphocytes, mast cells, other cell types	Recruitment of leukocytes to sites of inflammation; migration of cells in normal tissues
IL-17	T lymphocytes	Recruitment of neutrophils inflammatory cells, inflammatory regulation, chronic inflammation and monocytes
Chronic Inflammation		
IL-12	Dendritic cells, macrophages, NK cells	NK cells and T cells: Increased production of IFN-γ
IFN-γ	T lymphocytes, NK cells	Monocytes: Activation of macrophages (increased ability to kill microbes and tumor cells)
IL-17†	T lymphocytes	Recruitment of neutrophils and monocytes, inflammatory regulation, chronic inflammation

(IFN-γ: interferon-γ; IL: interleukin; NK: natural killer; TNF: tumor necrosis factor)

Note: All the cytokines mentioned under acute inflammation may also contribute to chronic inflammatory reactions. Type I interferons (normal function is to inhibit viral replication) may produce some of the systemic manifestations of inflammation. Some cytokines cause fever (formerly referred to as endogenous pyrogens) and are now called pyrogenic cytokines [e.g., IL-1, IL-6, TNF, and ciliary neurotrophic factor, a member of the IL-6 family]

*IL-6 receptor antagonists are used in the treatment of rheumatoid arthritis.

†IL-17 antagonists are very effective in psoriasis and other inflammatory diseases.

Table 29: Role of cytokines in inflammation.

Proinflammatory cytokines enhance the acute inflammatory process Source: Leukocytes and endothelial cells • Interleukin-1 (IL-1) • IL-6 • Tumor necrosis factor • IL-8 • Interferon-γ	Local effects on endothelium • ↑ Leukocyte adhesion • ↑ Procoagulant activity • ↑ Prostaglandin I_2 synthesis Systemic effects • Fever • Neutrophilia • ↑ Slow-wave sleep • ↓ Appetite
Attenuating (resolution) cytokines have downregulating effect and consequently assist in the resolution of acute inflammation Source: Macrophages and T cells • TGF-β • IL-10	Effect on fibroblast • ↑ Proliferation • ↑ Collagen synthesis

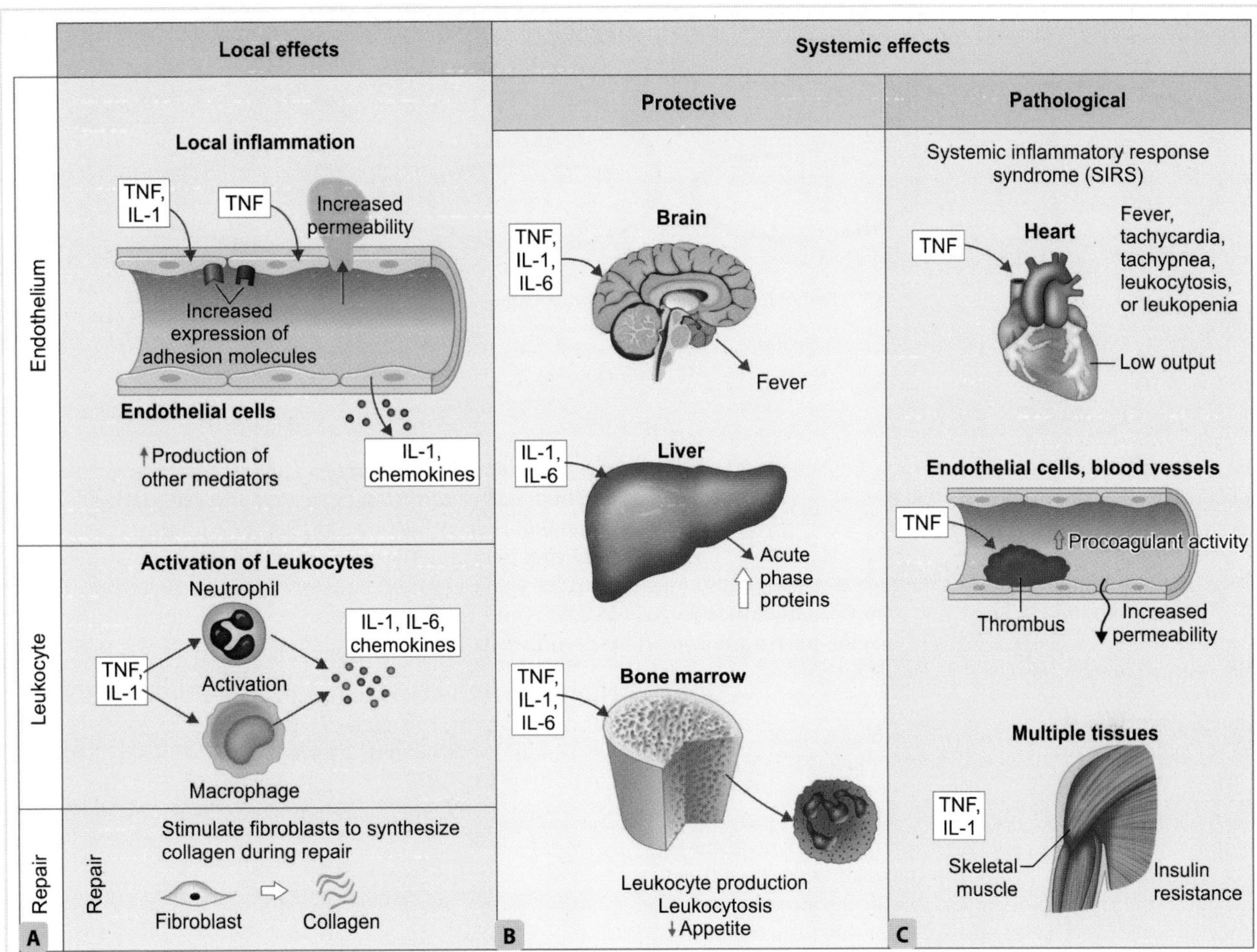

FIGS. 41A TO C: Major local and systemic actions of cytokines in inflammation. Tumor necrosis factor (TNF), interleukin (IL)-1, and IL-6 have multiple local and systemic inflammatory effects. (A) TNF and IL-1 act on leukocytes and endothelium to produce changes of acute inflammation, and both these cytokines induce the expression of IL-6 from leukocytes and other cell types. (B) TNF, IL-1, and IL-6 mediate protective systemic effects of inflammation. These include fever, acute-phase protein synthesis by the liver, and increased production of leukocytes by the bone marrow. (C) TNF can produce the systemic pathologic abnormalities that lead to septic shock. The effects include decreased cardiac function and low cardiac output, thrombosis in the blood vessels, capillary leak producing increased vascular permeability, and metabolic abnormalities due to insulin resistance.

Structural Classification (Fig. 42)

Chemokines are structurally classified into four major groups (main subfamilies) according to the number and arrangement (location) of two of four conserved cysteine (C) residues between other amino acids (X) in the chemokine's protein molecule sequence. These are—(1) C-X-C (*CXC*) chemokines, (2) C-C (*CC*) chemokines, (3) C chemokines, and (iv) CX3C chemokines.

C-X-C Chemokines (or α)

C-X-C chemokines (formerly called as α chemokines) have one amino acid residue separating the first two of the four conserved cysteines. IL-8 (now called CXCL8) is a typical chemokine belonging to this group.

Action These chemokines mainly cause activation and chemotaxis of neutrophils, with limited activity on monocytes and eosinophils. They activate leukocyte and promote their recruitment to the sites of inflammation. It's most important inducers are microbial products and cytokines, mainly IL-1 and TNF.

Source It is secreted by activated macrophages, endothelial cells, and other cell types. Its production is mainly stimulated by microbial products and other cytokines (mainly IL-1 and TNF).

C-C Chemokines

In this chemokine, the first two conserved cysteine residues are adjacent.

Types The C-C (formerly called as β chemokines) chemokines include monocyte chemoattractant protein (MCP-1, CCL2), eotaxin (CCL11), and macrophage inflammatory protein- 1α (MIP-1α, CCL3).

Action Mainly serve as chemoattractants for monocytes, eosinophils, basophils, and lymphocytes. They are less powerful chemoattractants for neutrophils. Most of these

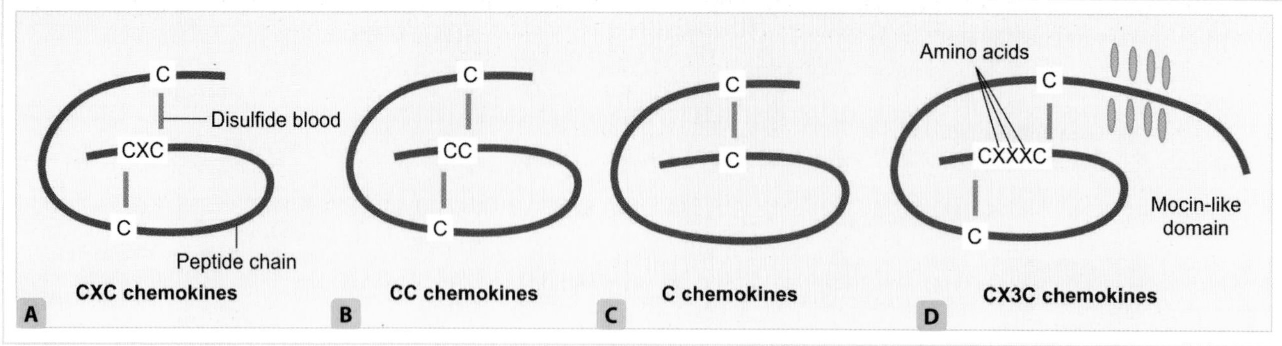

FIGS. 42A TO D: Structure of chemokines.

chemokines in this class have overlapping actions. However, eotaxin selectively recruits eosinophils.

C Chemokines

These lack the first and third of the four conserved cysteines [i.e., single cysteine (XC family)]. The C chemokines (e.g., lymphotactin, XCL1) are relatively specific for lymphocytes. They were originally called as lymphotactin.

CX_3C Chemokines

They contain three amino acids between the first two cysteines [i.e., two cysteines separated by three amino acids (CX3C)]. Fractalkine (CX3CL1) (or neurotactin) is the only known member of this class. This chemokine has two forms—(i) a cell surface-bound protein induced on endothelial cells by inflammatory cytokines that promotes strong adhesion of monocytes and T cells, and (ii) a soluble form, derived by proteolysis of the membrane bound protein, that has powerful chemoattractant activity for the same cells.

Nomenclature of Chemokines

Chemokines were originally named depending on how they were identified and the responses they triggered. Presently, a standard nomenclature is followed and coordinated with names for the receptors the chemokines bind to (**Table 30**). The CC chemokines are named CCL1 through CCL28, and the CXC chemokines are named CXCL1 through CXCL17. Chemokines are named according to their structure, followed by "L" and the number of their gene (CCL1, CXCL1, etc.). Addition of the letter *L* indicates to chemokines themselves and means *Ligand*. However, many of the traditional names for chemokines are still currently used. Chemokine receptors are named according to their structure, "R" (is added) and a number (CCR1, CXCR1, etc.); letter *R* denotes *Receptor.* Most receptors can recognize >1 chemokine and most chemokines can bind >1 chemokine receptor. Binding of chemokine to receptor may produce either agonistic or antagonistic activity. It is to be noted that, the same chemokine. may act as an agonist at one receptor and an antagonist at another.

Chemokine Receptors

Chemokines bring about their actions by binding to ***chemokine receptors.*** These are seven-transmembrane G protein-coupled receptors (**Fig. 43**) present on target cells. These receptors usually show overlapping ligand specificities. Usually leukocytes express multiple receptors **in *different* *combinations on different types of leukocytes, which mediate distinct patterns of migration of the leukocytes.*** Certain chemokine receptors (e.g., CXCR4, CCR5) act as coreceptors for a viral envelope glycoprotein of human immunodeficiency virus (HIV), the cause of acquired immunodeficiency syndrome (AIDS). Thus, they are necessary for binding and entry of the virus into cells.

Numbers of chemokine receptors (refer Table 30)

Various receptors include—

- Ten different receptors for CC chemokines (called CCR1 through CCR10).
- Seven for CXC chemokines (called CXCR1 through CXCR6 and CXCR8).
- One for the C chemokines (called XCR1).
- One for CX3CL1 (called CX3CR1).

Expression of receptors

Chemokine receptors are expressed **on all leukocytes.** On T cells, they are many in number and show diversity. These receptors are produced either constitutively or after induction. They show **overlapping specificity for chemokines** within each family. The pattern of cellular expression and biological action varies widely. This diversity depends on the specific cell types targeted, specific receptor activation, and differences in intracellular signaling.

Biologic Actions of Chemokines

Chemokines may be either immobilized or soluble molecules. Chemokines are produced either—(1) constitutively (normally) by cells in tissues and maintain the distribution of cells in these tissues (e.g., localization of T and B cells in lymphoid organs), or (2) in response to external stimuli and are involved in inflammatory reactions.

Q. Describe role of chemokines in inflammation.

Role of chemokines in inflammation

In inflammatory reactions, chemokines control leukocyte motility and **recruit circulating leukocytes from blood vessels into the site of inflammation in the extravascular sites.** This is achieved by generating a chemotactic gradient. Different groups of chemokines attach to chemokine receptors expressed on different cells. In coordination with the types of adhesion molecules expressed, chemokines control the nature of the inflammatory infiltrate. Chemokines play two roles in inflammation.

Table 30: Examples of chemokines, chemokine receptors, and their main functions.

Chemokine (original name)	*Chemokine receptor*	*Main function*
CC chemokines*		
• CCL2 [monocyte chemoattractant protein (MCP)-1]	CCR2	Mixed leukocyte recruitment
• CCL3 [macrophage inflammatory protein (MIP)-1α]	CCR1, CCR5	
• CCL4 (MIP-1β)	CCR5	T cell, dendritic cell, monocyte, and NK recruitment Coreceptor for human immunodeficiency virus (HIV)
• CCL5 [regulated upon activation, normal T cell expressed and presumably secreted (RANTES)]	CCR1, CCR3, CCR5	Mixed leukocyte recruitment
• CCL11 (eotaxin)	CCR3	Eosinophil, basophil, and T_H2 recruitment
• CCL17 [thymus and activation-regulated chemokine (TARC)]	CCR4	T-cell recruitment
• CCL19 [MIP-3β/EBI1 ligand chemokine (ELC)]	CCR7	T cell and dendritic cell migration into parafollicular zones of lymph nodes
• CCL21 [secondary lymphoid-tissue chemokine (SLC)]	CCR7	
• CCL22 [macrophage-derived chemokine (MDC)]	CCR4	NK cell, T-cell recruitment
• CCL25 [thymus-expressed chemokine (TECK)]	CCR9	Lymphocyte recruitment into intestine
• CCL27 [cutaneous T-cell-attracting chemokine (CTACK)]	CCR10	T-cell recruitment into skin
CXC chemokines*		
• CXCL1 [growth-regulated. oncogene (GROα)]	CXCR2	Neutrophil recruitment
• CXCL8 (IL-8)	CXCR1, CXCR-2	
• CXCL9 [monokine induced by gamma interferon (Mig)]	CXCR3	Effector T-cell recruitment
• CXCL10 [interferon gamma-induced protein (IP-10)]	CXCR3	
• CXCL12 [stromal cell-derived factor 1 (SDF1)]	CXCR4	B cell migration into lymph nodes Plasma cell migration into bone marrow
• CXCL13 [B-cell-attracting chemokine 1 (BCA-1)]	CXCR5	B cell migration into lymph nodes and into follicles T follicular helper cell migration into follicles
C chemokines		
• XCL1 (lymphotactin)	XCR1	T cell and NK cell recruitment
CX_3C chemokines		
• CX3CL1 (fractalkine)	CX3CR1	T cell, NK cell, and monocyte recruitment

(IL: interleukin; NK: natural killer cells)

*CC and CXC subfamilies of chemokines are produced by leukocytes and by many other tissue cells, such as endothelial cells, epithelial cells, resident macrophages, fibroblasts, and other stromal cells. Several CC chemokines are also produced by activated T cells.

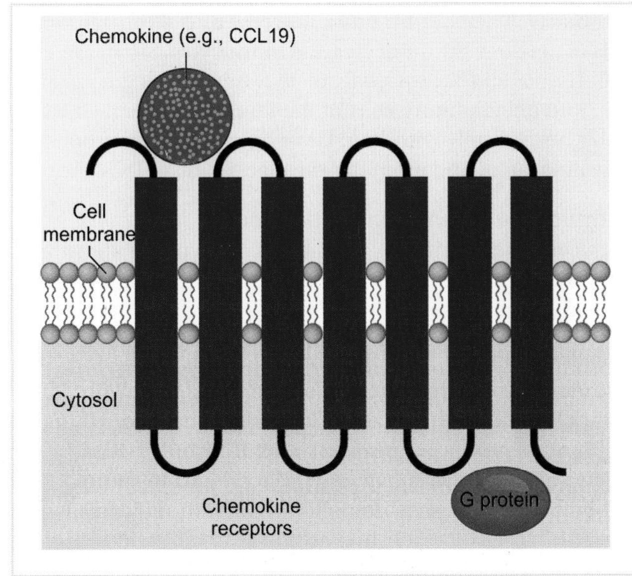

FIG. 43: Diagrammatic representation of chemokine receptor.

- **Increased adhesion of leukocytes to endothelium:** Chemokines are produced at the site of inflammation. They are produced in response to microbes and other injurious stimuli.
  - In the tissues, cytokines create chemotactic gradient by binding ECM proteoglycans on cell surfaces (e.g., endothelial cells). They bind to heparan sulfate proteoglycans on endothelial cells lining the postcapillary venules. High concentrations of chemokines are displayed on the surface of endothelial cells and in the ECM at sites of tissue injury. During inflammation, circulating leukocytes are initially attached (adhered) temporarily to the endothelial surfaces through interactions with adhesion molecule. The endothelial bound chemokines (e.g., TNF and IL-1) are displayed to these leukocytes attached to endothelium.
  - Endothelial display a high local concentration of chemokines, and they bind to chemokine receptors on the leukocytes. Signals from chemokine receptors increases the integrin affinity by conversion of low-affinity integrins to high-affinity integrins on leukocytes.

This leads to firm adhesion of the leukocyte to ligandins (e.g., VCAM-1, ICAM-1, and ICAM-2) on endothelium.
  - Chemokines are also released on cytokine-activated vascular endothelial cells. This can increase VLA-4 integrin-dependent adhesion of leukocytes and result in their firm arrest.
  - Most chemokines produce firm attachment of leukocyte to endothelium by acting on leukocytes to increase the affinity of integrins. But chemokines also serve as chemoattractants, thereby directing the movement of leukocytes to sites of infection or tissue damage. Since they mediate aspects of the inflammatory reaction, they are sometimes termed *inflammatory chemokines.* Leukocyte adhesion to endothelial cells is an important step for migration of leukocytes out of blood vessels into extravascular tissue.
- **Emigration of leukocytes through blood vessels toward the site of infection or tissue damage.** Chemokines produced in the extravascular tissues act on leukocytes that have adhered to the endothelium as well as those emigrated out of the circulation. The chemokines stimulate movement of leukocytes along the concentration gradient of chemokines toward the injurious stimuli. Specific seven transmembrane G protein-coupled receptors (**Fig. 43**) present on the surface of migrating leukocytes recognize matrix-bound chemokines and associated adhesion molecules. This causes cells to move along the chemotactic gradient to a site of injury. This process of responding to matrix-bound chemoattractants is **haptotaxis**. The process of unidirectional movement of leukocytes toward a chemical gradient is called **chemotaxis** (or chemoattraction). Thus, leukocytes move toward infected and damaged cells in tissues, where chemokines are produced.
  - Signals initiated from seven transmembrane G protein-coupled receptors (**Fig. 43**) present on the surface of migrating leukocytes activate second messengers. These second messengers induce polymerization of actin. At the leading front of the pseudopod of leukocyte, there will be marked changes in levels of intracellular calcium. This is associated with assembly and contraction of cytoskeleton proteins in the leukocytes. This results in increased amounts of actin at the leading edge of the leukocyte and localize myosin filaments at the back of leukocyte. The leukocyte moves by extending filopodia (thin projections extending from the edge of migrating leukocyte) that pull the back of the cell in the direction of extension. This is similar to the front wheels of an automobile pulling the back wheel. During leukocyte migration, the cell puts forth a pseudopod toward increasing chemokine concentrations (i.e., along the chemical gradient). The net result is migration of leukocytes toward the inflammatory stimulus in the direction of the locally produced chemoattractants.
  - The variety and combinations of chemokine receptors on cells is responsible for diverse biological functions. Neutrophils, monocytes, eosinophils and basophils share few receptors but express other receptors exclusively. Thus, specific chemokine combinations can recruit selective population of cells.
- **Migration of DCs from sites of infection into draining lymph nodes:** Chemokines are required for this function. DCs are activated by microbes in peripheral tissues. They are carried to the regional lymph nodes to inform T lymphocytes of the presence of infection. This migration of dendritic cells (DCs) depends on expression of a chemokine receptor, CCR7, which is induced when the DCs encounter microbes. The chemokines produced in lymphatics and lymphoid tissues bind to chemokine receptor CCR7.

Maintenance of tissue architecture

Some chemokines are produced constitutively (normally) by stromal cells in tissues. These cytokines are called as *homeostatic chemokines.* These chemokines are responsible for maintenance of normal tissue architecture and organization of various cell types in different anatomic regions of the tissues. Chemokines are involved in the development of lymphoid organs. They regulate the movements of lymphocytes and other leukocytes through different regions of secondary lymphoid organs. For example, T and B lymphocytes in discrete areas of the spleen and lymph nodes.

Chemokines in disease

Chemokines can be involved in many acute and chronic diseases. In disorders with a severe inflammatory reaction, multiple chemokines are expressed in inflamed tissues. Examples include rheumatoid arthritis, inflammatory bowel disease (ulcerative colitis, Crohn disease), pulmonary inflammation (e.g., chronic bronchitis, asthma), autoimmune diseases [e.g., multiple sclerosis (MS), rheumatoid arthritis, systemic lupus erythematosus (SLE)] and vascular diseases, including atherosclerosis.

Colony Stimulating Factors

Colony stimulating factors (CSFs) are cytokines that promote the expansion and differentiation of bone marrow progenitor cells. CSFs are important for the maturation of red blood cells (RBCs), granulocytes, monocytes, and lymphocytes. Examples of CSFs include granulocyte–monocyte colony stimulating factor (GM-CSF), granulocyte colony stimulating factor (G-CSF), and IL-3.

Granulocyte–macrophage Colony Stimulating Factor

GM-CSF is a cytokine secreted by a variety of cell types such as activated T cells, macrophages, endothelial cells, and stromal fibroblasts. They **act on bone marrow and stimulate stem cells to produce granulocytes and monocytes**. Similar to IL-1, IL-6, TNF-α, and TNF-β, GM-CSF may function at the systemic level and affect mature cells of the immune system. GM-CSF acts synergistically with IL-3. GM-CSF is also a macrophage-activating factor and promotes the maturation of DCs.

Granulocyte colony stimulating factor

It is a cytokine secreted by a variety of cell types. It **stimulates stem cells in the bone marrow to produce granulocytes** and release granulocytes and stem cells into the bloodstream. It is also produced by activated T cells, macrophages, and endothelial cells at sites of infection. In inflammation, it acts on the bone marrow to increase the production of and mobilize neutrophils to replace those consumed in inflammatory reactions. G-CSF also upregulates the proliferation, maturation, and survival of granulocytes.

Macrophage colony stimulating factor (M-CSF)

It is a cytokine released by some cell types. It **stimulates the proliferation, differentiation, survival, and functional**

activity of monocytes and macrophages. M-CSF acts synergistically with IL-34. In addition, M-CSF is also involved in processes associated with fertility and pregnancy.

Interferons

Q. Write a short essay on interferon.

Q. Write an essay on interferon and its use in clinical practice.

Interferons (INFs) are the cytokines, which can induce cells to resist viral replication and certain tumor cell proliferation that is called **natural cytostasis.** There are three subfamilies of IFN subfamily, namely type I, type II, and type III.

Type I Interferon

Type I IFN consists of IFN-α and IFN-β. They mediate early antiviral responses.

Source

The sources include—

- *Interferon-α* is an anti-inflammatory cytokine produced by lymphocytes (NK cells, B cells, and T cells), activated macrophages, DCs, and also by virally infected cells following PRR-mediated recognition of viral components.
- *Interferon-β* is secreted by fibroblasts and other cell types.

Actions

These include—

- *Interferon-α* is a potent antiviral agent to promote the cytostasis of target cells. IFN-α is a stimulator of natural killer (NK) cell and macrophage activity. IFN-α can act as a pyrogenic and painful factor by affecting thermosensitive neurons in the hypothalamus that cause fever and pain.
- Interferon-β exerts the same effects as IFN-α, in particular, in defense against viral infections. Also, IFN-β is used in the treatment for some forms of MS.

Type II Interferon

It is more usually **known as IFN-γ.** It belongs to the Th1 profile of cytokines, and shows wide immunoregulatory qualities in the immune processes. IFN-γ is a potent stimulus for macrophage activation and cytokine production.

Source

The *IFN-γ* is produced by activated T and B lymphocytes. It is also produced by NK cells in the primary host response to intracellular pathogens (e.g., *Listeria monocytogenes*) and certain viruses. NK cells migrate to tissues at sites of injury. These NK cells when exposed to IL-12 and TNF-α at the sites of injury, they produce IFN-γ. Thus, there is an amplification pathway by which activated tissue macrophages produce TNF-α and IL-12. This in turn stimulates IFN-γ production by NK cells. Subsequently, IFN-γ activates additional macrophages. IFN-γ is also the key cytokine made by helper T cells of the TH1 subset, which generally support cell-mediated immunity.

Action

In contrast to type I IFN-α and IFN-β, IFN-γ is a proinflammatory cytokine. It may act in a synergic manner with TNF-α, TNF-β, IL-1, IL-6, and other cytokines and chemokines. IFN-γ induces the activation of macrophages, with subsequent destruction of intracellular pathogens, and stimulates the differentiation of cytotoxic T cells. They also stimulate NK cells to produce an antiviral and antitumor response. However, they are usually weaker than those of IFN-α and IFN-β. IFN-γ is a potent immunoregulatory cytokine.

Type III Interferon

Type III IFN is also known as **IFN-λ.**

Action

Like type I IFNs, the type III IFNs upregulate the expression of genes controlling viral replication and host cell proliferation.

Source

This class of IFNs is secreted by a special type called plasmacytoid DCs.

Biological actions of IFN

They inhibit cell proliferation, induce major histocompatibility complex (MHC) Class 1 expression on cell surfaces, increase cytolytic activity of NK cells, macrophages, T lymphocytes, and improve antibody dependent cell mediated cytotoxicity (ADCC), In viral infection, they inhibit replication of viral deoxyribonucleic acid (DNA)/ribonucleic acid (RNA) and have paracrine effects to protect neighbouring cells that are not infected.

Clinical significance

- Mutations in *IFN-α2* and *IFN-β1* genes (9p21.3) is associated with increased susceptibility to viral infections of the respiratory tract and the predisposition to some types of cancer.
- Mutations in *IFN-γ* gene (12q15) increases the susceptibility to viral and bacterial (including mycobacterial) infections and parasitic invasions and are prone to few autoimmune disorders.
- Mutation in *IFN-GR1 (CD119)* gene (6q23.3) leads to severe combined immunodeficiency (SCID)-like symptoms, defects of phagocytosis, and severe inflammatory response to *Mycobacteria* and other pathogens.

Cytokine-based Therapies

Presently, purified cloned cytokines, monoclonal antibodies against cytokines, and soluble cytokine receptors that inhibit cytokine binding to target cells are available for therapy. A number of strategies that interfere with cytokine signaling are employed in the treatment. Some of them address disease-caused, or disease-related, and cytokine deficiencies (by supplementing the host's own cytokines). Few examples are presented as follows.

Use of Cytokines

- **Hepatitis C and B:** Cytokines from the IFN family have been used for treating hepatitis B and C infections. High concentrations of IFN-α have been used to treat hepatitis C and hepatitis B. In hepatitis C therapy, commonly IFN-α is combined with an antiviral drug. It is used in viral infections with a tendency toward chronic state and can be used as an adjuvant in treatment of HIV.
- **Multiple sclerosis:** IFN-β has been used in the treatment of autoimmune neurological demyelinating disease called multiple sclerosis (MS) and has produced significant clinical improvement.

- **Chronic granulomatous disease:** IFN-γ is used in the treatment of the hereditary immunodeficiency disease, namely chronic granulomatous disease (CGD). In this condition, there is a failure to produce microbicidal oxidants (H_2O_2, superoxide, and others) and severe impairment of phagocytic process to kill ingested microbes. These patients suffer from recurring infections with a numerous bacterium (e.g., *Staphylococcus aureus, Klebsiella, Pseudomonas*, and others) and fungi (e.g., *Aspergillus* and *Candida*). Administration of IFN-γ significantly reduces the incidence of infections and the infections that develop are less severe.
- **Others:** These include—
  - Interleukin-2: Can be used for the treatment of malignant tumors such as renal cell carcinoma, malignant melanoma, cutaneous T-cell leukemia.
  - Interleukin-3: Can be used to shorten the duration of cytopenia associated with chemotherapy, irradiation, following hematopoietic stem cell (HSC) transplantation.
  - Interleukin-4: Can be used for humoral immunodeficiency disorder and antitumor effect in solid tumors.
  - Interleukin-5: Can be used for hypogammaglobulinemia and helminth infections.
  - Tumor necrosis factor in the treatment of septic shock and anti-TNF therapy to ameliorate inflammatory arthritis.
  - Interleukin-10: Septic shock and delayed type hypersensitivity reaction by modulating T_H1 response and inhibit IFN production.
- Recombinant ILs, CSFs, and IFNs are widely used in immune disorders, malignancies, chronic recurrent infections, and complications related to chemotherapy in graft transplantation.
- **Side effects of interferons:** Interferons are powerful modifiers of biological responses and their side effects with their use are relatively mild. Typical side effects include flu-like symptoms, such as headache, fever, chills, and fatigue.

Use of Cytokine-related Agents

Apart from use of cytokines to relieve clinical syndromes, cytokine-related reagents are now used to treat pathologies that develop due to excess of cytokines. These reagents fall into two major categories—(1) monoclonal antibodies that block the binding of cytokines to their receptors and (2) soluble receptors that prevent cytokine binding to cell-bound, active receptors.

Anti-TNF-α drugs

Soluble TNF-α receptor and monoclonal antibodies against TNF-α have been used to treat rheumatoid arthritis and ankylosing spondylitis. These anti-TNF-α drugs reduce proinflammatory cytokine cascades and alleviate pain, stiffness, and joint swelling; and promote healing and tissue repair. However, reduced cytokine activity increases the risk of infection and malignancy. It has been observed that the frequency of lymphoma is slightly higher in patients who are long-term users of TNF-α-blocking drugs.

Anti-IL-2 receptor-antibodies

They may be used for the prevention of rejection after allograft transplant.

The use of cytokines and anti-cytokine therapies in clinical medicine holds great promise. The efforts to develop safe and effective cytokine-related strategies continue, particularly for those diseases that have so far been resistant to more conventional approaches. These include inflammation, cancer, organ transplantation, and chronic allergic disease.

Measurement of Cytokines

The detection of secreted cytokine protein is most widely used type of analysis. Concentration of cytokines reflects the severity of diseases especially sepsis, autoimmune disorders, and allergic disorders. Elevated levels of cytokines can be detected in different body fluids such as blood, synovial fluid, cerebrospinal fluid, amniotic fluid, bronchioalveolar lavage (BAL). Commercial kits are available for quantitation of cytokines.

Sample Collection

It depends on the cytokine detection technique.

- Radioimmunoassay: Sample is collected in ethylenediaminetetraacetic acid (EDTA).
- Bioassay: They are available for some cytokines. They have the advantage of being able to distinguish active cytokines from inactive cytokines. The serum for assay should be collected in a pyrogen free tube. It is rapidly centrifuged and freeze at -80°C.
- Flow cytometry: For detection of intracellular cytokine, peripheral mononuclear cells and other body fluids can be used.

Cytokine Detection Technique

They can be detected by radioimmunoassay, bioassay, or by flow cytometry.

Knockout mice can be used for studying cytokine functions in vivo. A knockout mouse model is a mouse in which a target cytokine gene is deleted or deactivated in the genome of a mouse blastocyst. The loss of gene activity usually leads to changes in the phenotype of the adult mice allowing in vivo studies of the functions of the target gene.

8.7 Chronic Inflammation and Systemic Effects of inflammation

CHAPTER OUTLINE

CHRONIC INFLAMMATION

Definition

Chronic inflammation is defined as **inflammation of prolonged duration** (weeks or months) **in which inflammation, tissue damage, and healing occurs at the same time, in varying combinations**.

Chronic inflammation may:
- **Follow an acute inflammation,** which does not resolve (e.g., chronic osteomyelitis), or
- **Begin as insidious, low-grade, chronic** response without any acute inflammatory reaction.

Chronic Inflammation versus Chronic Infection

Chronic inflammation is not synonymous with chronic infection. When an inflammatory response cannot eliminate an injurious agent, infection may persist and become chronic inflammation. Chronic inflammation need not always be due to infection. It may follow an acute inflammatory or immune response to a foreign antigen without any infection.

Causes of Chronic Inflammation

Chronic inflammation may develop under the following situations.

- **Persistent infections:** Microbes that are difficult to eradicate elicit delayed-type of hypersensitivity and produce chronic inflammation, e.g., *Mycobacteria*, and certain viruses, fungi, and parasites. This is a delayed-type of hypersensitivity reaction. Some agents may cause a **distinct pattern of chronic inflammation** known as **granulomatous reaction/inflammation.** In other situations chronic inflammation represents an unresolved acute inflammation. For example, chronic inflammation may occur in acute bacterial infection of the lung that progresses to a chronic lung abscess. Sometimes both acute and chronic inflammation may coexist, as in a peptic ulcer.
- **Immune-mediated inflammatory (hypersensitivity) diseases:** Chronic inflammation may be caused by excessive and inappropriate activation of the immune system. In these diseases, antigens that are normally harmless trigger immune reactions that have no useful purpose but only cause disease. Morphologically, they may have mixed acute and chronic inflammation because of repeated bouts of inflammation. Fibrosis may develop at late stages. These include:
  - **Autoimmune diseases:** In these diseases, self (auto) antigens evoke an immune reaction and produce chronic inflammation and tissue damage (e.g., rheumatoid arthritis, multiple sclerosis).
  - **Allergic reactions:** These are characterized by excessive immune responses against common environmental substances and chronic inflammation (e.g., bronchial asthma).
  - **Unregulated immune response:** In some situations, chronic inflammation is the result of unregulated immune responses against microbes (e.g., inflammatory bowel disease)
- **Prolonged exposure to toxic injurious agents:** These agents may be exogenous or endogenous.
  - **Exogenous:** For example, **silica** is a nondegradable inanimate exogenous material. If persons are exposed to silica particles for long time, it causes an inflammatory lung disease called **silicosis**.
  - **Endogenous: Atherosclerosis** is a disease of arterial intima, probably represents a chronic inflammatory process partly due to endogenous toxic plasma **lipid components**.

Note: There are certain diseases which are not considered as inflammatory disorders, but some forms of chronic inflammation may be important in their pathogenesis. These include neurodegenerative diseases (e.g., Alzheimer's disease), metabolic syndrome (with associated type 2 diabetes mellitus), and certain cancers in which inflammatory reactions promote tumor development.

Morphologic Features

Acute inflammation is characterized by vascular changes, increased vascular permeability producing edema, leukocyte events, and main infiltrating cells are neutrophils. But chronic inflammation is characterized by the following:

- **Mononuclear cells infiltrate:** These include **macrophages, lymphocytes, and plasma cells**.
- **Tissue destruction:** It is caused by the persistence of causative agents or by the presence of persisting inflammatory cells.
- **Healing by fibrosis:** In chronic inflammation, there is an attempt to heal by connective tissue replacement of damaged tissue, associated with angiogenesis (proliferation of small blood vessels). It usually results in fibrosis.

Chronic Inflammatory Cells and Mediators

The morphological characteristic features of chronic inflammation are—**(1) infiltration of leukocytes, (2) tissue damage, and (3) fibrosis**. These features are due to local activation of several cell types and the production of mediators.

Box 16: Role of macrophages in inflammation.

- Secretion of mediators of inflammation: These include cytokines [tumor necrosis factor (TNF), interleukin (IL)-1, chemokines, etc.] and arachidonic acid metabolites and growth factors that act on various cells
- Phagocytosis/ingestion of cell debris (necrotic tissue) and microorganisms (microbes): They are professional phagocytes that act as filters for particulate matter, microbes, and senescent cells
- Destruction of foreign invaders and tissues
- Chemotaxis
- Inflammation and initiation of the tissue repair
- Antigen processing and presentation
- Secretion of immunomodulatory factors
- Activation of other cells (mainly T lymphocytes)
- Function as effector cells that eliminate microbes in cellular and humoral immune responses
- Display signal to T cells and respond to signals from T cells: This is responsible for the feedback loop for defense against many microbes by cell-mediated immune response

Monocytes/Macrophages

Q. Discuss the role of activated macrophage in chronic inflammation.

Q. Write a short essay on macrophages in health and disease.

Granulocytes and agranulocytes

In the circulating blood, WBCs can be divided into granulocytes and agranulocytes depending on the granules in the cytoplasm. The granulocytes have abundant granules and include neutrophils, eosinophils, and basophils. They are discussed on pages 268–279. The agranulocytes consist of monocytes, macrophages, and lymphocytes. They differ from the granulocytes in that they contain relatively fewer granules in their cytoplasm.

Monocytes

Circulating monocytes are the largest normal blood cell. They have a single lobed or kidney-shaped (horse shoe shaped) nucleus. Monocytes are formed and released by the bone marrow into the bloodstream.

Macrophages

Monocytes may come out of the circulation to migrate into tissue. In the tissue, they accumulate at sites of acute inflammation. Macrophages are usually larger and are more active as phagocytes than monocytes. These cells clear pathogens, cell debris, and apoptotic cells at the site of inflammation. Monocytes/macrophages produce potent mediators of inflammation and fever. They influence initiation, progression, and resolution of acute inflammatory responses.

Macrophages also have a main role in regulating progression to, and maintenance of, chronic inflammation. Macrophage is the predominant cell in chronic inflammation. Role of macrophages in inflammation is presented in **Box 16.**

Mononuclear phagocyte system

It was also known by the older (and inaccurate) name of reticuloendothelial system or macrophage system. Monocytes and macrophages form the mononuclear phagocyte system (MPS). Thus, mononuclear phagocyte system includes circulating cells called monocytes, which become macrophages when they migrate into tissues, and tissue resident macrophages which are derived mostly from hematopoietic precursors during fetal life.

- **Monocytes:** Circulating cells called monocytes (in the peripheral blood).
- **Macrophages:** Monocyte that have migrated into tissues and became macrophages. Macrophages are normally diffusely scattered in most connective tissues.
- **Resident tissue macrophages:** These are derived mostly from hematopoietic precursors during fetal life. They are found in specific locations in organs (**Table 31**) They can remain there for months or perhaps years.

Development of monocytes and macrophages (Figs. 44A and B)

Macrophages are widely distributed in many organs and connective tissue of the body (**Table 31**).

- **Monocytes and macrophages:** In adults, cells of the monocyte-macrophage lineage arise from HSCs (hematopoietic stem cells) in the bone marrow.
  - **Monocytes:** HSCs mature into early progenitor with myeloid potential which further differentiate into colony forming unit Mix (CFU-Mix) and then into committed precursor cells [colony forming unit-M (CFU-M)] in the bone marrow. The stimulus is a cytokine called M-CSF (macrophage colony stimulating factor). The CFU-M matures into monocytes and these monocytes enter into blood circulation (see **Fig. 44A**). Thus, the circulating cells of this lineage are known as monocytes.
- **Macrophages:** The blood monocyte migrates into various tissues, especially during inflammatory reactions. In the tissues, monocytes further differentiate/mature into macrophages. Migration of blood monocytes into tissues depends on the same factors as that are involved in emigration of neutrophil. These include adhesion molecules and chemokines. The half-life of blood monocytes is about

Table 31: Tissue-specific resident macrophages and their tissue specific functions.

Tissue	*Name of the resident macrophage*	*Tissue-specific function [in addition to activity as antigen presenting cells (APCs)]*
Liver	Kupffer cell	Scavenge red blood cells (RBCs), clear particles
Spleen	Red pulp macrophage	Scavenge RBCs, recycle iron
Lymph node	Subcapsular sinus histiocyte/macrophage	Trap antigen particles
Lung	Alveolar macrophage	Remove pollutants and microbes, clear surfactants
Brain (central nervous system)	Microglial cells	Neural circuit development (synaptic pruning*)
Bone marrow	Bone marrow macrophage	Maintain niche for blood cell development, clear neutrophils
Kidney	Mesangial cell	Regulate inflammatory responses to antigen filtered from blood
Skin	Langerhans cell	Skin immunity and tolerance
Peritoneal cavity	Peritoneal cavity macrophage	Maintain immunoglobulin (Ig) A production by B-1 B cells†
Intestine	Lamina propria macrophage Intestinal muscularis macrophage	Immunity and tolerance of gastrointestinal tract Regulate peristalsis
Heart	Cardiac macrophage	Clear dying heart cells
Pathological	Tumor-associated macrophages (TAMs)	Can recognize and lyse tumor cells

*Synaptic pruning is the process by which extra neurons and synaptic connections are eliminated in order to increase the efficiency of neuronal transmissions.
†B-1 B cells are a subclass of B lymphocytes involved in the humoral immune response that are not part of the adaptive immune system.

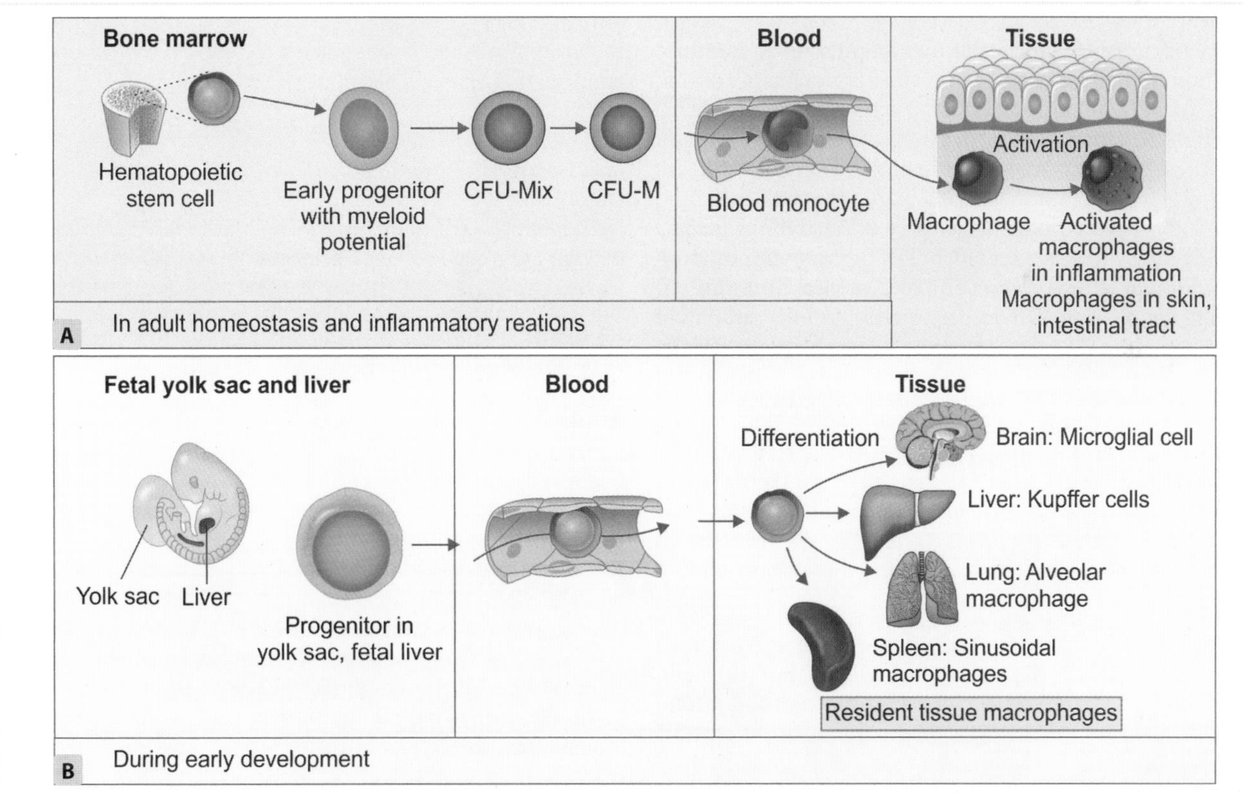

FIGS. 44A AND B: Maturation of mononuclear phagocytes. (A) In the steady state in adults (homeostasis) and during inflammatory reactions, hematopoietic precursors in the bone marrow give rise to circulating monocytes. These monocytes enter peripheral tissues, mature to form macrophages, and are activated locally. (B) In early development, as in fetal life, precursors in the yolk sac and fetal liver give rise to cells that populate the tissues to generate specialized long-lived resident tissue macrophages.

1 day, whereas the life span of tissue macrophages is for several months or perhaps years. Usually, macrophages become the predominant cell population in inflammatory reactions within 48 hours of onset.

- **Resident tissue macrophages:** Many tissues contain resident macrophages derived from progenitors in the embryonic yolk sac or fetal liver precursors during early fetal development (i.e., embryogenesis). These resident tissue macrophages reside and populate tissues in the steady state (in the absence of tissue injury or inflammation). They assume specialized phenotypes depending on the organ where they reside (see **Fig. 44B**). Examples, Kupffer cells lining the sinusoids in the liver, alveolar macrophages in the lung, and microglial cells in the brain. They are long-lived and can remain in the tissue for months or perhaps years. They are replenished (replaced) mainly by the proliferation of resident cells.

Functions of mononuclear phagocyte system

The normal role of cells of the MPS is to ingest, destroy (by phagocytosis), remove old and damaged cells, unwanted materials, and large molecular substances (from the blood). These can be divided into cellular targets or noncellular targets.

- **Cellular targets of macrophage phagocytosis:** These include circulating senescent or damaged/injured RBCs, and platelets (removed mainly in spleen), micro-organisms, dead neutrophils (in the circulation and at sites of inflammation), debris from dead or injured cells, and cells undergoing apoptosis.
- **Noncellular targets:** These include antigen-antibody complexes (circulating immune complexes), foreign protein particles, products of coagulation, and macromolecules (e.g., lipids and carbohydrates synthesized by the body due to faulty metabolism, as in storage diseases).

Macrophage Events in Inflammation

- **Monocytes** also emigrate into extravascular tissues early in acute inflammation, and **within 48 hours**, they are the **predominant cell type**.
- **On reaching extravascular tissue**, the monocyte is **transformed into** a larger phagocytic cell known as tissue **macrophage**. Macrophages are more efficient phagocytes than neutrophils and can ingest several times as many micro-organisms.

Subsets of Macrophages

Depending on Macrophage Activation

Macrophages can be activated by **two major pathways,** namely classical and alternative. These two pathways (**Fig. 45**) produce macrophages with distinct functional capabilities, depending

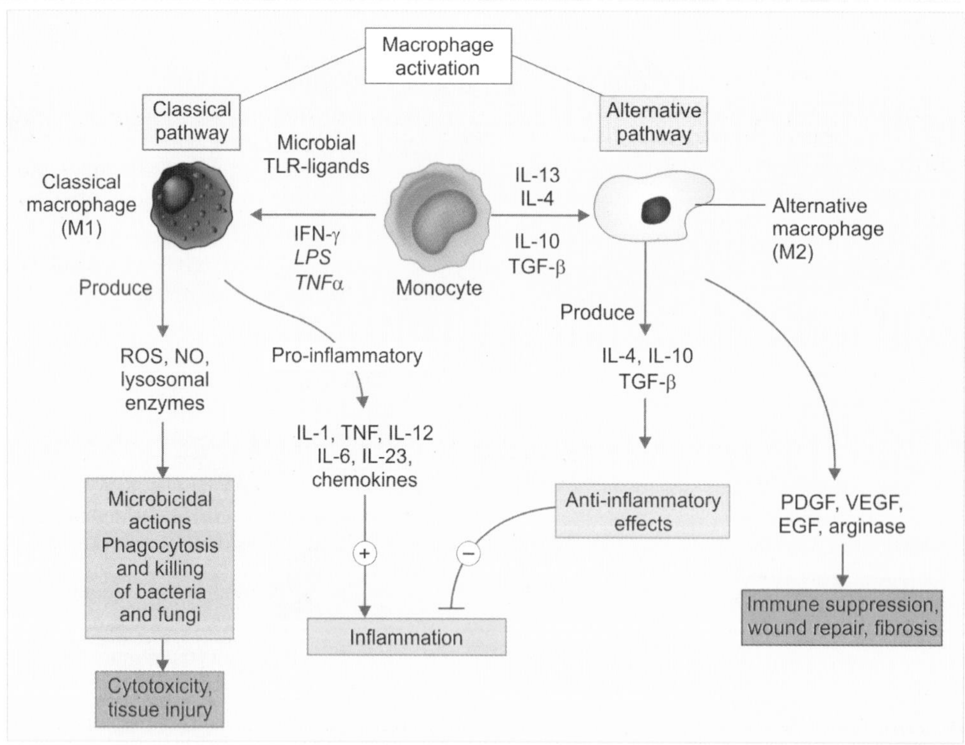

(EGF: epidermal growth factor; LPS: lipopolysaccharide; NO: nitric oxide; PDGF: platelet derived growth factor; ROS: reactive oxygen species; TGF: tumor necrosis factor; TLR: toll-like receptor; VEGF: vascular endothelial growth factor)

FIG. 45: Classical and alternative pathways of macrophage activation. Different stimuli activate monocytes/macrophages to develop into functionally distinct populations. Classically activated macrophages are induced by microbial products and cytokines [e.g., interferon (IFN-γ)] and are microbicidal. They are involved in potentially harmful inflammation. These classical pathway macrophages (M1) phagocytose and destroy microbes and dead tissues and can potentiate inflammatory (proinflammatory) reactions. Alternatively, activated macrophages (M2) are induced by other cytokines [e.g., interleukin (IL)-4, IL-13 produced by T helper (Th) 2 cells and other leukocytes]. They control inflammation and promote tissue repair and fibrosis and also the resolution of inflammation.

on the nature (type) of activating stimuli (signals) they are exposed to.

Classical macrophage activation

In classical activation, activated macrophages become efficient at killing microbes, and these cells are called **M1 macrophages**. Activation is mainly by cytokine **IFN-γ**, TNF-α and lipopolysaccharides (LPS) to promote proinflammatory responses.

- **Mediators of activation:** It is brought out mainly by—
  - Microbial products (e.g., endotoxin): They engage TLRs and other sensors on the macrophages.
  - T cell-derived signals: Mainly cytokines (e.g., **IFN-γ**) in immune responses.
  - Foreign substances (e.g., crystals and particulate matter).
- **Products of activated macrophages:** The products of classically activated (also called M1) macrophages enhance their capability to kill ingested organisms, and secrete cytokines that stimulate inflammation. These include the following—
  - Upregulation of lysosomal enzymes.
  - Nitric oxide (NO)
  - Reactive oxygen species (ROS)
- **Important function:** They are important in host defense against microbes. Their main function is phagocytosis and killing/elimination of ingested microbes. They are involved in many inflammatory reactions.

Alternative macrophage activation

In alternative activation, activated macrophages promote **tissue remodeling and repair** and these cells are called M2 macrophages.

- **Mediators of activation:** Activation is mainly by cytokine other than IFN-γ, such as **cytokines IL-4** and **IL-13** produced by T lymphocytes and other cells.
- **Function:** These macrophages are not actively microbicidal. Their main function is **initiation of the tissue repair**. They secrete growth factors that promote angiogenesis, activate fibroblasts, and stimulate collagen synthesis.

Features of activated macrophage

These are as follows—

- **Morphological features:** Increase in size, adhesion, cytoplasmic granules, and mitochondria.
- **Functional features:** Increase in phagocytic and microbicide activity.
- **Biochemical features:** Increase in metabolic activity, enzymes, cyclic guanosine monophosphate (c-GMP), calcium, prostaglandins (PGs), and interferon (IFN).

Morphological Subsets

Macrophages may also show different morphological appearances after activation by external stimuli (e.g., microbes).

- **Epithelioid cells:** Some macrophages develop abundant cytoplasm. They are called as epithelioid cells because of their resemblance to epithelial cells of the skin.
- **Multinucleated giant cells:** Activated macrophages can fuse to form multinucleated giant cells. This occurs frequently in certain types of microbial infections (e.g., *Mycobacteria*), and in response to indigestible foreign bodies.

Probably, most injurious stimuli first activate the classical pathway of macrophage activation to destroy the offending agents. This is followed by alternative pathway of macrophage activation, which initiates tissue repair.

Products of Activated Macrophages

Usually, the products of activated macrophages **eliminate injurious agents** (e.g., microbes) and **initiate the process of repair**. However, these products are **also responsible for much of the tissue injury** observed **in chronic inflammation**. Several functions of macrophages are important for the development and persistence of chronic inflammation and the accompanying tissue injury.

- **Secretion of proinflammatory mediators:** Macrophages secrete mediators of inflammation. These include cytokines TNF, IL-1, Il-12, IL-6, chemokines, and others, and PGs [arachidonic acid (AA) metabolites]. Thus, macrophages play a central role in the initiation as well as propagation of inflammatory reactions.
- **Defense against microbes:** Macrophages exhibit **antigens to T lymphocytes and respond to signals from T cells.** Thus, it sets up a feedback loop that is needed for defense against many microbes by cell-mediated immune responses.

Macrophages have an impressive collections of mediators which makes them powerful in combination with body's other defense mechanisms against unwanted invaders. On the other hand, inappropriate or excessive activation of these macrophages can induce considerable tissue destruction. It is these inappropriate or excessive activities of macrophages that are responsible for tissue destruction. This tissue destruction is one of the hallmarks of chronic inflammation.

In some situations, if the irritant is eliminated, macrophages disappear from the site of inflammation either dying off or exit via lymphatics into lymph nodes. In others, macrophage accumulation persists and there will be continuous recruitment of macrophages from the circulation. Macrophages are also capable of cell division and may locally proliferate at the site of inflammation.

Macrophage Receptors (Fig. 46)

Macrophages have many signaling receptor proteins located on the surface of or inside the macrophage (**Fig. 46**).

- **Fc receptors (FcR):** These receptors help macrophages locate antigens that have been coated by antibodies (Igs/immunoglobulins). These receptors are termed as *FcRs* because they bind to the part of an antibody called the **constant fragment, or Fc.** FcRs bind at one end of IgG antibody molecules that already have microbes bound at the other end (**Fig. 46**)
- **Receptors for the complement component:** These receptors are for the complement components. For example, complement 3b (C3b) is an opsonin and can coat an antigen and make it more recognizable by macrophages. Coating of antigen by antibodies or by complement is called opsonization. These receptors bind to opsonins that are coated on the surface of microbes. Opsonins are substances that coat particles and tag them for phagocytosis.
- **Pattern recognition receptors (PRRRs):** Macrophages have receptors that can directly recognize bacteria. These innate PRRs bind to particular molecules prevalent in the

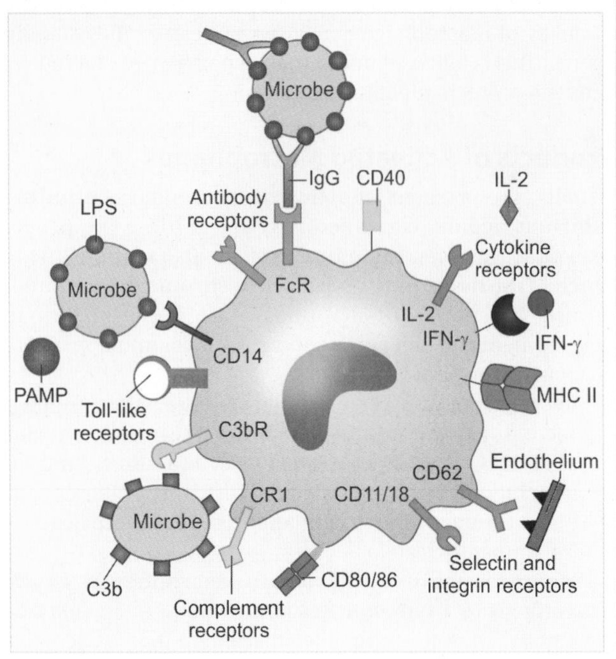

(C3b: complement fraction 3b; IFN-γ: Interferon-γ; IL: interleukin; MHC: major histocompatibility complex; PAMP: pathogen-associated molecular patterns)

FIG. 46: Macrophage surface receptors. Macrophages contains receptors for many extracellular molecules that enhance their function such as, complement (C3b), cytokines (IL-2, INF-γ), selectins (CD62), integrins (CD11/18), and antibody (FcR). Antibody receptors recognize Fc (fragment constant) of antibody. Toll-like receptors (TLRs) recognize patterns of microbial components and trigger intracellular signaling cascades in the macrophage. CD14 acts as a coreceptor [along with the TLRs for the detection of bacterial lipopolysaccharide (LPS)]. Complement receptor binds with C3b. CD 80/86 play a role in the regulation of both the adaptive and the innate immune system. CD11/18 is a component of various integrins and CD62 for selectins. CD40 is a costimulatory protein required for antigen presentation.

bacterial cell wall. Examples include **mannose receptors** and numerous TLRs which are important in innate immunity. They recognize common microbial structures.

- **Other receptors:** These include **selectins, chemokine receptors, and integrins**. They help macrophages to adhere to endothelial cells of capillary walls and enter and move through tissue.

Functions of Macrophages

Macrophages perform several important functions in innate and adaptive immunity.

- **Phagocytosis and microbicidal action:** Most important function of macrophages in host defense is to ingest microbes by the process of phagocytosis and then to kill the ingested microbes. The process of phagocytosis is discussed in detail on pages 238–243.
- **Demolition:** Apart from ingesting microbes, macrophages ingest necrotic host cells. This includes cells that undergo necrosis in tissues due to the effects of toxins, trauma, or ischemia (interrupted blood supply), and neutrophils that undergo apoptosis at the site of infection after clearing the causative stimulus. This is part of the cleaning up process or demolition phase after infection or sterile tissue injury. Macrophages also recognize and engulf apoptotic cells before they can release their contents and induce inflammatory responses. Throughout the life of an individual, unwanted cells undergo death by apoptosis as part of many physiologic processes, such as development, growth, and renewal of healthy tissues. These apoptotic cells are eliminated by macrophages.
- **Secretory function of macrophages:** In addition to phagocytic function, macrophages are activated to secrete substances by microbial products. These include **cytokines** such as IL-1, IL-6, IL-12, and TNF-α. They are of central importance in initiating and **promoting inflammation** and recruitment of other leukocytes (including neutrophils and lymphocytes) from the blood into sites of infections. This amplifies protective response against the microbes. These cytokines also help to coordinate the activities of other immune cells. Some cytokines stimulate the growth and differentiation of other WBC types. Various substances secreted by macrophages and their actions are presented in **Table 32**.
- **Antigen presentation:** Macrophages serve as APCs. For T cells to recognize antigens, these antigens must first be processed and presented on the surface of an APC such as DCs, macrophages, or B cells. Macrophages achieve this task by first engulfing the protein antigen, then processing it into smaller pieces, and finally combining the antigen fragments with special membrane proteins. The macrophages then display these antigen complexes on the cell surface. These are recognized by T lymphocytes (T helper cells) and T lymphocytes become activated. This function is important in the effector phase of T-cell mediated immune responses.
- **Promote repair:** Macrophages promote the repair of damaged tissues. Macrophages secrete many proteins that are important in wound healing. Some of these proteins are enzymes that degrade tissue (e.g., collagenase, elastase, plasminogen activator), whereas others stimulate the growth of new granulation tissue (e.g., fibroblast growth factor helps for synthesis of collagen-rich ECM and fibrosis, angiogenic factors stimulate growth of new blood vessel).

Table 32: Various substances secreted by macrophages and their action.

Secretion by macrophages	*Action*
Interleukin-1 (IL-1)	Promotes inflammation
IL-6	Stimulates B cell growth and inflammation
IL-10	Promotes expression of antigen presenting proteins [major histocompatibility complex (MHC II)]
IL-12	Stimulates helper T cells and NK cells
IL-15 and IL-18	Promote proliferation of NK cells
Colony stimulation factor	Promotes hematopoiesis
Tumor necrosis factor-α (TNF-α)	Promotes inflammation
Fibroblast growth factor	Stimulates wound healing

- **Others:** They destroy senescent RBCs in the spleen. Macrophages act as source of GM-CSF secretion involved in hematopoiesis.

Primary inflammatory mediators of monocyte/macrophages are presented in **Box 17** and effector functions of macrophages are depicted in **Figure 45**. Macrophages are key determinants of the outcome in chronic inflammation (**Fig. 47**).

Role of macrophages in chronic inflammation is presented in **Flowchart 8**.

Various diseases of macrophages are presented in **Table 33**.

Role of Lymphocytes

Microbes and other environmental antigens activate T and B lymphocytes, which amplify and propagate chronic inflammation. Major function of lymphocytes is to mediate adaptive immunity and provide defense against infectious pathogens. Lymphocytes cells are usually seen in chronic inflammation and, when these are activated, the inflammation tends to be persistent and severe. Some of the chronic inflammatory reactions, such as granulomatous inflammation, depend on lymphocyte responses. Lymphocytes are prominent in the chronic inflammation, observed in autoimmune and other hypersensitivity diseases.

CD4+ T lymphocytes can secrete cytokines and promote inflammation and also influence the nature of the inflammatory reaction. These T cells greatly increase the early inflammatory reaction produced by recognition of microbes and dead cells as part of the innate immune response. There are three subsets of CD4+ T cells (Th1, Th2, Th17) that secrete different cytokines (**Fig. 48**) and bring out different types of inflammation. There are three subsets of CD4+ T cells and they secrete different types of cytokines and produces different types of inflammation. Th1 cells produce the cytokine IFN-γ and activate macrophages by the classical pathway. Th2 cells secrete IL-4, IL-5, and IL-13. They recruit and activate eosinophils and are responsible for the activation of the alternative pathway of macrophage activation. Th17 cells secrete IL-17 and other cytokines, which induce the secretion of chemokines. Chemokines recruit neutrophils (and monocytes). Th1 and Th17 cells are involved in defense against many types of bacteria and viruses. They are also involved in autoimmune diseases in which tissue injury is caused by chronic inflammation. Th2 cells are important in defense against helminthic parasites and in allergic inflammation. Type and subtypes of lymphocytes is presented in **Figure 49**.

Interaction of Lymphocytes and Macrophages

Lymphocytes and macrophages interact in a bidirectional way. These interactions play main role in propagating chronic inflammation (**Fig. 50**).

- **Presentation of antigen and activation of T cells:** Macrophages are APCs and display peptide-MHCs for recognition by T cells. The membrane-bound molecules of APCs that function together with antigens to stimulate T cells are called **costimulators**. Macrophages display antigens to T cells and costimulators that activate T cells, and secrete cytokines (IL-12, IL-6, IL-23) that also stimulate T-cell responses.
- **Production of cytokines and activation of macrophages:** Activated T lymphocytes, in turn, produce cytokines (e.g., INF-γ). They recruit and activate macrophages and promote

Box 17: Primary inflammatory mediators of monocyte/macrophages.

- Enzymes (e.g., collagenase, elastase, plasminogen activator)
- Proteins
- Complement proteins
- Chemokines
- Cytokines (e.g., IL-1, IL-6, IL-12, and tumor necrosis factor-α)
- Reactive oxygen species (ROS)
- Antioxidants
- Coagulation factors
- Bioactive lipids

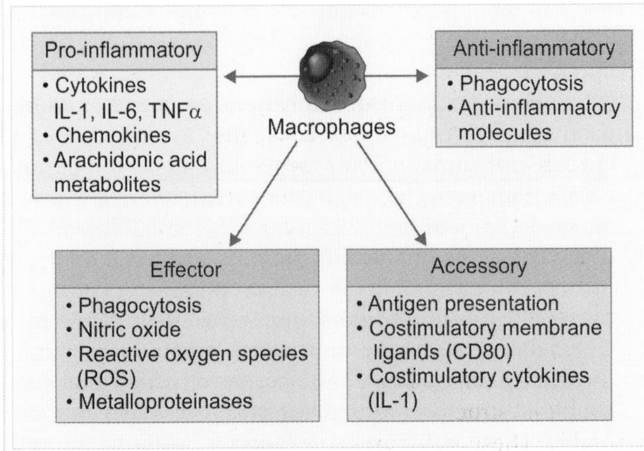

FIG. 47: Effector functions of macrophages.

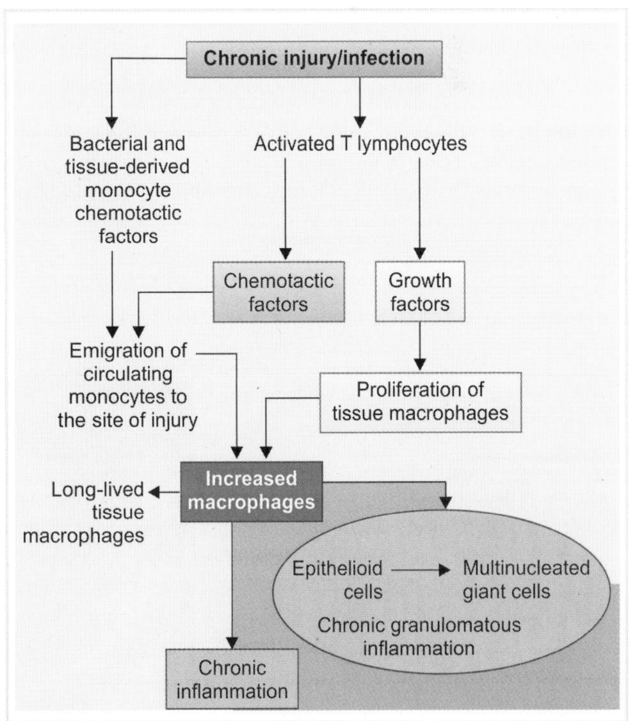

FLOWCHART 8: Role of macrophages in chronic inflammation.

Table 33: Diseases of macrophages.

Reactive proliferation	*Clonal proliferation*	*Monocyte and macrophage dysfunction*
Storage disorders	Langerhans cell histiocytosis	α_1-antitrypsin deficiency
Sinus histiocytosis	Leukemias	Chédiak–Higashi syndrome
Sinus histiocytosis with massive lymphadenopathy	• Acute monocytic leukemia	Chronic granulomatous disease
Hemophagocytic histiocytosis	• Chronic myelomonocytic	Malakoplakia
	• Leukemia	Whipple's disease
	Macrophage deficiency	Corticosteroid therapy

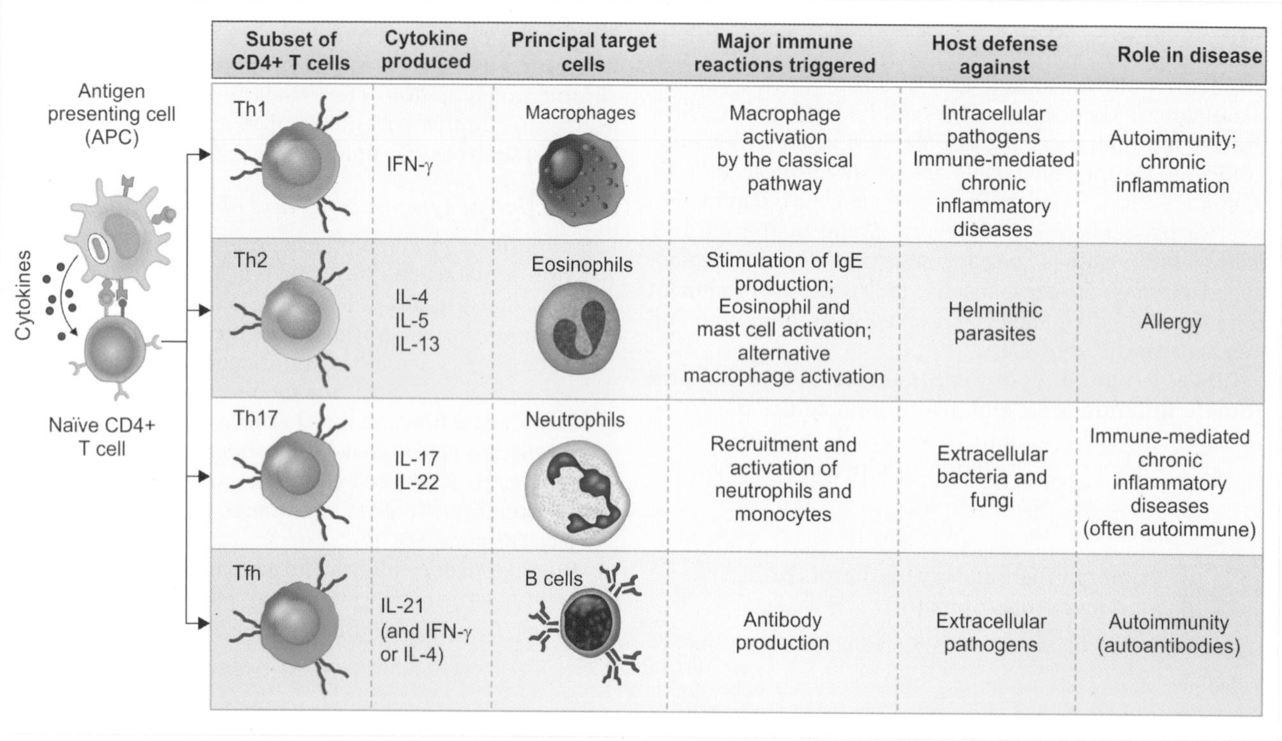

Antigen presenting cell (APC)
Cytokines
Naïve CD4+ T cell

Subset of CD4+ T cells	Cytokine produced	Principal target cells	Major immune reactions triggered	Host defense against	Role in disease
Th1	IFN-γ	Macrophages	Macrophage activation by the classical pathway	Intracellular pathogens Immune-mediated chronic inflammatory diseases	Autoimmunity; chronic inflammation
Th2	IL-4 IL-5 IL-13	Eosinophils	Stimulation of IgE production; Eosinophil and mast cell activation; alternative macrophage activation	Helminthic parasites	Allergy
Th17	IL-17 IL-22	Neutrophils	Recruitment and activation of neutrophils and monocytes	Extracellular bacteria and fungi	Immune-mediated chronic inflammatory diseases (often autoimmune)
Tfh	IL-21 (and IFN-γ or IL-4)	B cells	Antibody production	Extracellular pathogens	Autoimmunity (autoantibodies)

(APC: antigen-presenting cell; IFN: interferon II, interleukin; Th: T helper cell; Tfh cells: T follicular helper cells)

FIG. 48: Major subsets of CD4+ helper T cells and the cytokines produced by them. Naive CD4+ T cells may differentiate into distinct subsets of effector cells in response to antigen, costimulators, and cytokines. The main functions of these subsets and their roles in disease are presented in this figure. T cells may also differentiate into Tfh cells and play critical roles in germinal center formation and function.

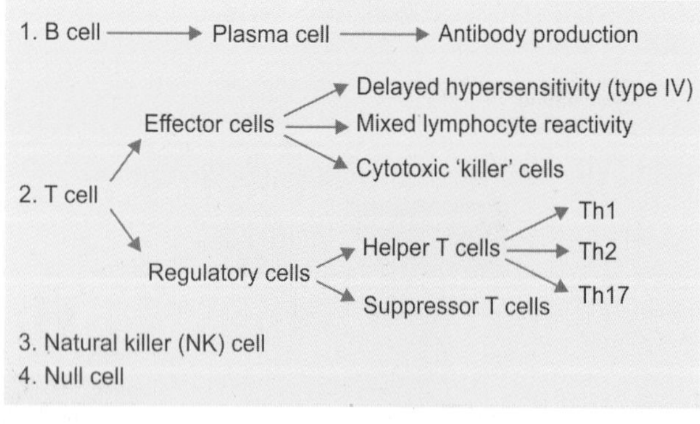

(Th: T helper cell)

FIG. 49: Type and subtypes of lymphocytes.

more antigen presentation and cytokine secretion. This results in a cycle of cellular reactions that incite and sustain chronic inflammation.

- **B lymphocytes:** Activated B lymphocytes and antibody-producing plasma cells are usually present at sites of chronic inflammation. The antibodies present in chronic inflammation may be specific for persistent foreign or self-antigens (autoimmune diseases) in the inflammatory site or against altered tissue components. However, their role in most chronic inflammatory disorders are not known.
- **Tertiary lymphoid organs:** Some chronic inflammatory reactions may show accumulation of lymphocytes, antigen presenting cells (APCs), and plasma cells. They may form lymphoid structures resembling the follicles seen in lymph nodes. These structures are called as tertiary lymphoid

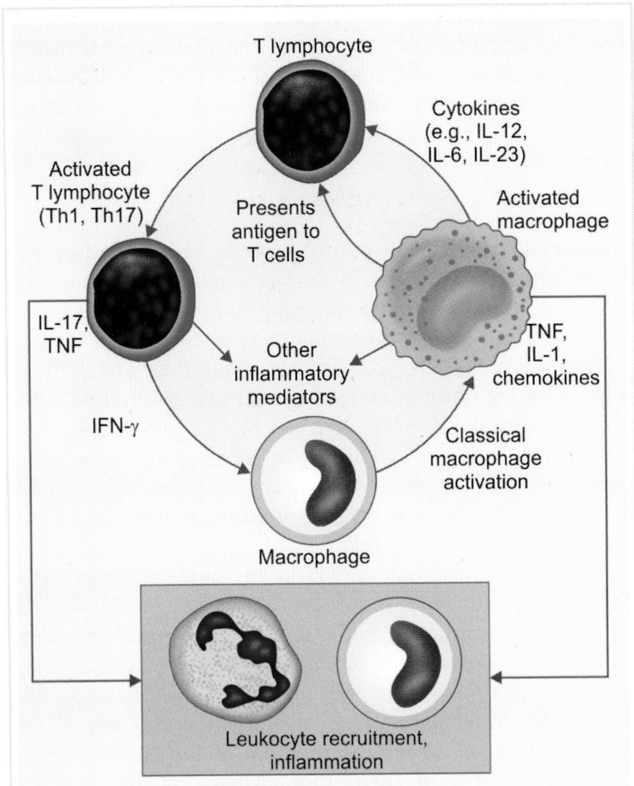

FIG. 50: Macrophage–lymphocyte interactions in chronic inflammation. Activated T lymphocytes [T helper (Th) 1 and Th17] produce cytokines [interferon (IFN)-γ] that activate macrophages. Activated macrophages in turn stimulate T cells by presenting antigens and producing cytokines (e.g., IL-12, IL-6, IL-23). This results in a cycle of cellular reactions that incite and sustain chronic inflammation.

organs. This is usually seen in the synovium of longstanding rheumatoid arthritis, in the thyroid in Hashimoto thyroiditis, and in the gastric mucosa in *Helicobacter pylori* infection.

Other Cells in Chronic Inflammation

Apart from macrophages and lymphocytes, other cell types may be present in chronic inflammation depending on the particular stimuli.

- **Eosinophils:** They are seen in immune reactions mediated by IgE and in parasitic infections. There are recruited by adhesion molecules similar to those for neutrophils, and by specific chemokines (e.g., eotaxin) produced by leukocytes and epithelial cells. The granules of eosinophils contain *major basic protein*, that is a highly cationic protein and toxic to parasites. However, this also damages epithelial cells of the host. Eosinophils are seen in parasitic infections and type I hypersensitivity reactions (e.g., allergies). They are discussed in detail on pages 1070–1075.
- **Mast cells:** They are distributed in connective tissues and are involved in both acute and chronic inflammatory reactions. Because their granules contain many cytokines, they can promote inflammatory reactions. Mast cells originate from precursors in the bone marrow. They have many similarities with basophils circulating in blood. But they do not originate from basophils and are present in tissues, hence, mast cells are more involved in inflammatory reactions in tissues than the circulating basophils. Both mast cells and basophils have receptor FcεRI on their surface. This receptor binds with the Fc portion of IgE antibody. In immediate hypersensitivity reactions (type I), IgE is bound to the mast cell's FcRs. They recognize antigen (allergen) and their interaction causes degranulation of mast cells. They release mediators present in granules such as histamine and PGs. This type of response is observed during allergic reactions to foods, insect venom, or drugs. Sometimes this response produces fatal results (e.g., anaphylactic shock). They are discussed in detail on pages 1074–1075.
- **Plasma cells:** They are rich in rough endoplasmic reticulum (RER) and produce antibodies. They are derived from B lymphocytes. Antibody to specific antigens produced at the sites of chronic inflammation is required for neutralization of antigen, clearance of foreign antigens and particles, and antibody-dependent cell-mediated cytotoxicity.
- **Dendritic cells (DCs):** These are professional APCs that trigger immune responses to antigens. They phagocytose antigens and migrate to lymph nodes. In the lymph node, DCs present these antigens to T lymphocytes. This results in recruitment of specific cell subsets in the inflammatory process.
- **Neutrophils:** They are characteristic cells found in acute inflammation. However, they may be found in large numbers in many forms of chronic inflammation, lasting for months. This may be due to either persistence of microbes (ongoing infection and tissue damage) or cytokines and other mediators produced by activated macrophages and T lymphocytes. For example, in chronic bacterial infection of bone (osteomyelitis), a neutrophilic exudate may be seen for many months. Neutrophils also play an important role in the chronic damage induced in lungs by smoking and other irritant stimuli. This type of inflammation is termed *acute on chronic*. It may be seen in cholecystitis also. Neutrophils are discussed on pages 269–271.
- **Fibroblasts:** These are long-lived, are present everywhere, and their main function is to produce components of the ECM. They are derived from mesoderm or neural crest. Fibroblasts rebuild the scaffolding of the ECM upon which tissue is re-established. Activated fibroblasts produce cytokines, chemokines, and PGs, and regulates the behavior of inflammatory cells in the damaged tissue. This process either results in resolution and wound healing or chronic persistent inflammation.

TYPES OF CHRONIC INFLAMMATION

It can be divided into—(1) chronic nonspecific (nongranulomatous) inflammation and (2) granulomatous inflammation.

Granulomatous Inflammation

Q. Explain the differential diagnosis of granulomatous diseases.

Q. Discuss histopathological assessment of granulomas/ immune granuloma.

Q. Explain cytokines and their role in granulomatous reaction.

Introduction

Polymorphonuclear leukocytes are the predominant cells in acute inflammation. They usually remove or destroy the injurious agents that cause acute inflammatory responses. Sometimes these cells cannot digest the injurious agents. Such a situation may be dangerous, because it can lead to a vicious circle of—(1) phagocytosis, (2) failure of digestion of injurious agent, (3) death of the leukocytes, (4) release of undigested inciting injurious agents, and (5) rephagocytosis by a newly recruited leukocyte (**Fig. 51**).

Definition

Granulomatous inflammation is a distinctive type of chronic inflammation characterized by microscopic collections of activated macrophages (that are transformed into epithelium-like/epithelioid cells)**, often with T lymphocytes. Sometimes it may be associated with central necrosis.**

Older granulomas in addition show rim of fibroblasts and connective tissue as the outermost layer. Granuloma formation is a **cellular attempt to hold an offending agent** that is difficult to eliminate. Thus, it is a **protective response** of the host to chronic infection (e.g., tuberculosis, some fungi) or the presence of indigestible foreign material (e.g., suture or talc). Granulomatous inflammation tries to isolate a persistent offending agent and prevent it from disseminating and restrict inflammation. Some autoimmune diseases may also develop granulomas (e.g., Crohn disease).

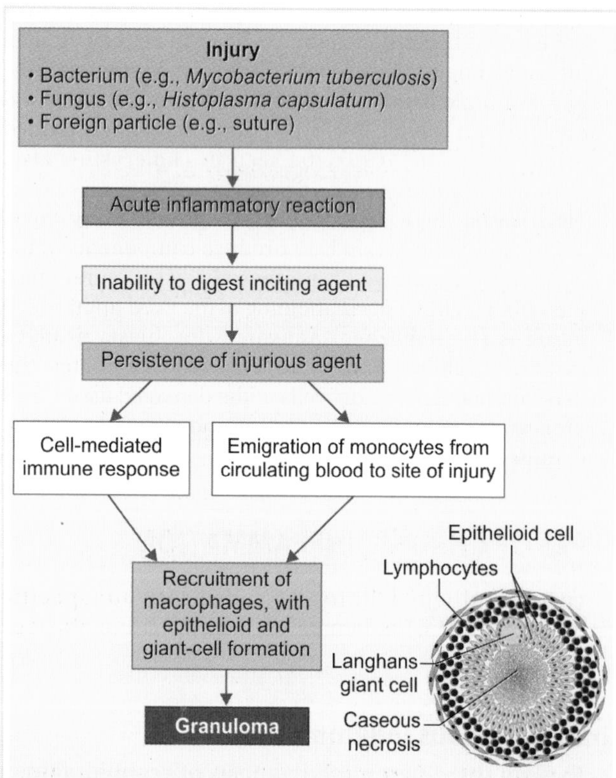

FIG. 51: Mechanism of granuloma formation in granulomatous inflammation.

In some granulomatous disorders such as sarcoidosis, no causative agent has yet been identified. During this process, there is usually strong activation of T lymphocytes leading to macrophage activation. This can cause injury to normal tissues.

MORPHOLOGY OF GRANULOMA

Main cells involved in granulomatous inflammation are macrophages and lymphocytes. Macrophages continuously migrate through extravascular connective tissues. After coming across the substances they cannot digest, macrophages lose their motility and accumulate at the site of injury to form **nodular collections of pale, epithelioid cells forming granulomas (Figs. 52A** and **B)**.

- **Epithelioid cells:** The activated macrophages may develop abundant cytoplasm and begin to resemble epithelial cells. Hence, these **modified macrophages** are called as epithelioid cells.
  - In the routine hematoxylin and eosin (H&E) stained tissue samples, the activated macrophages (i.e., epithelioid cells) have **a pale pink granular cytoplasm** with indistinct cell borders, often appearing to merge into one another.
  - The **nucleus is oval or elongate** and may show folding of the nuclear membrane. The nucleus is less dense than that of a lymphocyte.
- **Giant cells:** Some activated macrophages (i.e., **epithelioid cells) may fuse to form multinucleate giant cells**. They are frequently, but not invariably found in granulomas. These giant cells are formed by cytoplasmic fusion of macrophages. They are found in the periphery or sometimes in the center of granulomas. These giant cells may attain diameters of 40–50 µm and have many small nuclei. Nuclei may be as many as 20 or more. When the nuclei of such giant cells are arranged around the periphery of the cytoplasm in a horseshoe pattern, the cell is called a **Langhans giant cell** [not be confused with Langerhans cell (APCs in skin) and islet of Langerhans in pancreas]. If, a foreign agent (e.g., silica or a *Histoplasma* spore) or other indigestible material persist in the cytoplasm of a multinucleated giant cell, the term **foreign body giant cell** is used. Foreign body giant cells tend to have more central nuclei or haphazardly arranged nuclei.
- **Lymphocytes:** As a cell-mediated immune reaction to antigen, lymphocytes form an integral part of granulomatous inflammation. A collar of lymphocytes surrounds the aggregates of epithelioid macrophages. Some types may be accompanied by plasma cells.
- **Necrosis: Sometimes granulomas are associated with central necrosis** (e.g., tuberculosis). However, the granulomas in Crohn disease, sarcoidosis, and foreign body reactions do not have necrotic centers and are called as *noncaseating (hard) granulomas.*
- **Fibrosis:** Older granulomas may show a rim of fibroblasts and connective tissue. Granulomas may heal by producing extensive fibrosis.

Types of Granulomas

Depending on the pathogenesis they are of two types.

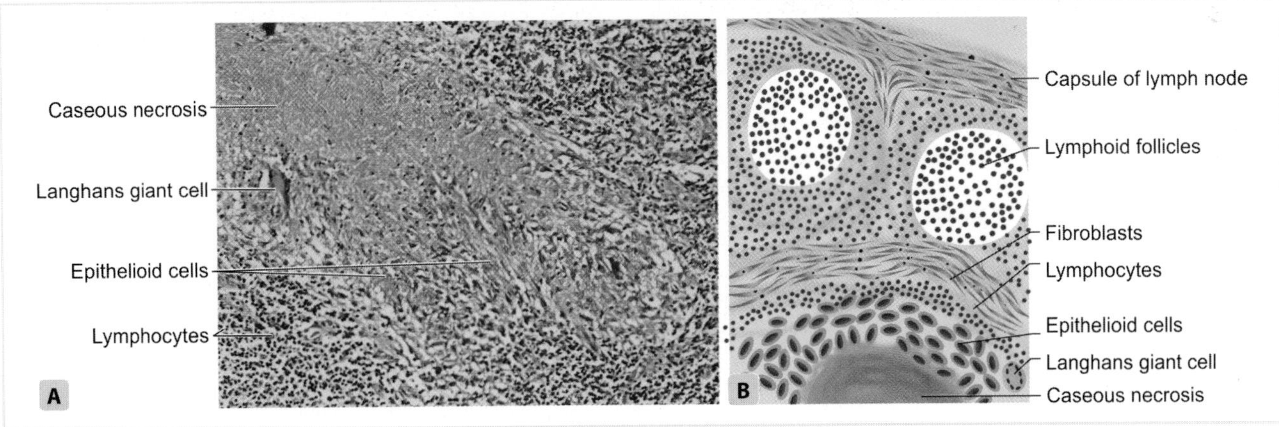

FIGS. 52A AND B: (A) Tuberculous granuloma showing an area of caseous necrosis surrounded by epithelioid cells, Langhans-type giant cell, and lymphocytes. (B) Diagrammatic appearance of granuloma (only a part of it is shown) in tuberculous lymphadenitis.

Immune granulomas

- These are caused by agents/microbes which are capable of generating a persistent T-cell-mediated immune response.
- Immune granulomas usually develop when the provoking/ inciting agent is difficult to eradicate. For example, a persistent microbe (e.g., *Mycobacterium tuberculosis*) or a self-antigen. In these granulomas, macrophages activate T cells (Th1 cells) to produce cytokines, such as IL-2. This in turn activates other T cells and maintains the response, and IFN- γ, which activates the macrophages. T-cell cytokines such as IFN-γ stimulate macrophage function whereas others such as IL-4, IL-10 inhibit macrophage activation. Thus, lymphocytes are crucial for regulating development and resolution of inflammatory responses.

Foreign body granulomas

- It develops against relatively inert or inactive foreign bodies which do not provoke any specific inflammatory or immune response. There is no T-cell-mediated immune response.
- The foreign body which brings out granuloma include suture materials, talc (associated with intravenous drug abuse), or other fibers that are large enough to be phagocytosed by a macrophage but are not immunogenic. Epithelioid cells and giant cells are brought to the surface of these foreign bodies.
- The foreign material can usually be detected in the center of the granuloma, particularly if observed with polarized light (appears refractile).

Granulomas can be further classified depending on the presence or absence of necrosis. Certain infectious agents, such as ***Mycobacterium tuberculosis***, characteristically produce **necrotizing (caseous) granulomas**. Grossly, in tuberculosis this necrotic area has a granular, cheesy appearance and is therefore called caseous necrosis. Microscopically, this necrotic material appears as amorphous, structureless, eosinophilic, mixture of granular debris, with loss of cellular details, and dead micro-organisms. These types of granulomas are called **soft granulomas**. In other diseases, such as sarcoidosis, Crohn disease, and granulomas found in foreign body reactions characteristically do not show necrotic centers. They are said to be **noncaseating** and are termed as **hard granulomas**.

Outcome of Granulomatous Reactions

It depends on the immunogenicity and toxicity of the triggering agent. Cell-mediated immune responses may modify granulomatous reactions by mobilizing and activating more macrophages and lymphocytes. Under the influence of T-cell cytokines (e.g., IL-13 and TGF-β), a granuloma may burn out and become a fibrotic nodule. Granulomas may heal by fibrosis that may be extensive.

Interpretation of Granulomas

Granulomas are detected in certain specific pathologic states. Their recognition is important because it has the limited number of etiological agents that produce granulomas (some life-threatening). Certain microbes (e.g., *M. tuberculosis*, *Treponema pallidum*, or fungi) produce persistent T cell responses to T cell-derived cytokines. These are responsible for chronic macrophage activation and granuloma formation. Granulomas may also occur in some immune-mediated inflammatory diseases such as Crohn disease. This is one type of inflammatory bowel disease. Other unknown cause of granuloma is called sarcoidosis.

Tuberculosis is the model of a granulomatous disease caused by infection. It should always be excluded as the cause when granulomas are identified on microscopic examination. The granuloma in tuberculosis is termed as a tubercle and usually shows central caseous necrosis (due to a combination of hypoxia and free radical-mediated injury) and is rare in other granulomatous diseases.

The morphologic patterns in the various granulomatous diseases may be sufficiently different to make a reasonably accurate diagnosis. However, it is always necessary to perform additional tests/investigations to identify the specific etiologic agent. These include—

- To identify the etiologic agent by special stains for organisms (e.g., acid-fast stains for tubercle bacilli)
- Culture methods (e.g., tuberculosis and fungal diseases)
- Molecular techniques (e.g., polymerase chain reaction in tuberculosis)
- Serologic studies (e.g., syphilis).

Examples of granulomatous inflammation are listed in **Table 34**.

Table 34: Examples of granulomatous inflammation.

Disease	*Cause*	*Tissue reaction*
Tuberculosis	*Mycobacterium tuberculosis*	Caseating granuloma (tubercle): Central necrosis with amorphous granular debris surrounded by epithelioid cells, rimmed by lymphocytes, histiocytes, and fibroblasts. Occasional Langhans giant cells, presence of acid-fast bacilli
Leprosy	*Mycobacterium leprae*	Acid-fast bacilli in macrophages; noncaseating granulomas in tuberculoid leprosy
Syphilis	*Treponema pallidum*	Gumma: Microscopic to grossly visible lesion. Consists of histiocytes; plasma cell infiltrate; central necrotic cells without loss of cellular outline (coagulative necrosis). Spirochetes are difficult to identify in tissue
Cat-scratch disease	Gram-negative *Bacillus*	Rounded or stellate granuloma containing central granular debris and neutrophils; giant cells rare
Sarcoidosis	Unknown etiology	Noncaseating granulomas with plenty of activated macrophages
Crohn disease (inflammatory bowel disease)	Immune reaction against intestinal bacteria, self-antigens	Dense chronic inflammatory infiltrate with occasional noncaseating granulomas in the wall of the intestine

Chronic Inflammation and Tumorigenesis

Several chronic infectious diseases are associated with development of malignancies and indicate that chronic inflammation may facilitate development of tumor (tumorigenesis). For example, schistosomiasis in the urinary bladder predisposes to squamous cell carcinoma of bladder. Inflammation without any specific infection may also be a risk factor for cancer. For example, patients with reflux esophagitis or ulcerative colitis are at higher risk for developing adenocarcinoma in respective organs. The mechanism by which chronic inflammation promotes malignant transformation may be:

- **Increased cell proliferation:** Chronic inflammation stimulates cell division. Probably this increases the possibilities of transforming mutations in proliferating cells.
- **Oxygen and NO• metabolites:** Inflammatory metabolites, such as nitrosamines, may cause genomic damage as in carcinoma stomach.
- **Chronic immune activation:** Chronic antigen exposure changes the cytokine milieu by suppressing cell-mediated immune responses. This probably produces a more permissive environment for the development of malignant tumor.
- **Angiogenesis:** Growth of new vessels (angiogenesis) is associated with inflammation and healing of wound. It is important in sustaining cancers.
- **Inhibition of apoptosis:** Chronic inflammation suppresses apoptosis. Increased cell division and reduced apoptosis may favor survival and increase of mutated cell populations.

GIANT CELLS

Giant cell is defined as any cell having >1 nucleus.

Characteristics of Giant Cells

They have following common features:

- **Size:** Large size varying from 40 to 120 μm in diameter.
- **Nuclei:** They usually contain multiple nuclei (often 15–30 or more). At least they should have >1 nucleus.
- **Phenotype:** It depends on the origin and mechanism of its development.

Types of Giant Cells (Fig. 53)

Various types of giant cells and its associated conditions are mentioned in **Box 18.**

Conditions Associated with Giant Cells

Conditions associated with giant cells are presented in **Table 35**.

Physiological Types of Giant Cells

There are few multinucleate giant cells that are present in normal tissues. These include osteoclasts in the bones, megakaryocytes in the bone marrow, and syncytiotrophoblasts in placenta.

Osteoclasts

- **Osteoclasts** are very large, motile cells with multiple nuclei (about 6–12 nuclei) and contain abundant mitochondria.
- **Origin:** The large size and multinucleated condition of osteoclasts are due to their origin from the fusion of bone marrow-derived monocytes (i.e., hematopoietic progenitor cells of the **mononuclear macrophage–monocyte cell line)**. Osteoclast development needs two polypeptides produced by osteoblasts—(1) M-CSF (macrophage colony-stimulating factor) and (2) the receptor activator of NF-κB ligand (RANKL).
- **Function:** Osteoclasts are **phagocytic cells** that are essential for resorption of bone matrix during bone growth and remodeling (renewal or restructuring). Hence, they are found along bone surfaces where resorption (removal of bone), remodeling, and repair of bone take place. An active osteoclast surrounds an area with many surface projections, called the **ruffled cell border. Lysosomal enzymes** released by osteoclasts erode bony surface.

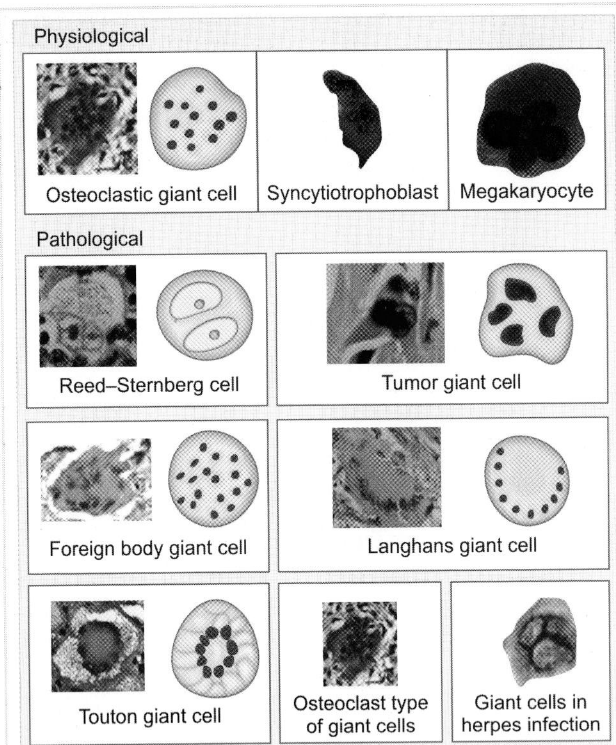

FIG. 53: Various types of giant cells.

- **Control of osteoclastic activity:** Osteoclast activities are controlled by several hormones, such as parathyroid hormone (PTH) from the parathyroid gland and calcitonin from the thyroid gland.

Syncytiotrophoblast

- The chorionic villi from a placenta during pregnancy are surrounded by the trophoblast epithelium. This epithelium consists of an outer layer of the darker-staining multinucleated syncytiotrophoblasts and an inner layer of lighter staining cytotrophoblasts. Syncytiotrophoblast cells arise from the fusion of cytotrophoblast cells. The syncytiotrophoblasts have abundant acidophilic cytoplasm and produce proteolytic enzymes. Proteases released by the syncytiotrophoblasts helps to erode the branches of the spiral uterine arteries during implantation of ovum into uterus. At term, they produce syncytial knots.
- The syncytiotrophoblast secretes human chorionic gonadotropin (hCG) into the maternal lacunae.

Megakaryocyte

- Megakaryocytes are giant cells approximately measuring 50–100 µm in diameter. They have polyploid nuclei that are large and irregularly lobulated (i.e., **irregularly multilobed nucleus**) with coarse chromatin. Their cytoplasm is slightly acidophilic filled with fine azurophilic granules. They contain numerous mitochondria, a well-developed RER, and an extensive golgi apparatus from which arise the conspicuous specific granules of platelets.
- They are produced by an endomitotic nuclear division process in which DNA replication occurs without cell division (polyploid nucleus).

Box 18: Types of giant cells (Fig. 53).

Physiological
- *Osteoclast*
- *Syncytiotrophoblast*
- *Megakaryocyte*

Pathological

Fused macrophages
- Foreign body giant cells: These have multiple uniform nuclei scattered throughout the cytoplasm. They may be seen in reaction to insoluble material
  - Exogenous: E.g., suture material, talc, etc.
  - Endogenous material: E.g., keratin (dermoid cyst of ovary, epidermal cyst), cholesterol, urate crystals (in gout)
- Disorders of lipid metabolism: Touton giant cells have vacuolated cytoplasm due to lipid, e.g., in xanthoma
- Infective or inflammatory conditions: Reaction to certain organisms [e.g., tuberculosis (Langhans giant cells in which nuclei are arranged in a horseshoe pattern), fungal infections, syphilis]
- Fusion of cardiac histiocytes: Aschoff giant cells in immune mediated rheumatic heart disease.

Giant cells resulting from fusion of cells: Viral infection
- Epithelial giant cells: Tzanck giant cells in skin due to viral infection, e.g., herpes virus infection (molding of nuclei to one another)
- Connective tissue, e.g., Warthin–Finkeldey giant cells in measles

Tumor giant cells: They have hyperchromatic nuclei of varying size and shape
- Giant cell tumors: Bone (Osteoclast like giant cell in giant cell tumor)
- Reed Sternberg cells: Hodgkin lymphoma
- Giant cell variants of many malignant tumors, e.g., carcinoma of lung
- Syncytiotrophoblasts-like giant cell

Damaged muscle fibers: Regenerating sarcolemmal cells in damaged skeletal muscles

- **Produces platelets:** Megakaryocytes produce platelets, or thrombocytes, by releasing them from the ends of cytoplasmic processes/fragments called proplatelets. These proplatelets are released directly into the marrow sinusoidal space where they fragment into preplatelets and then into platelets.
- The megakaryocyte can be mistaken for the osteoclast in bone that is multinucleated instead of multilobed.

Pathological Types of Giant Cells (Refer Box 18)

Mechanism of Formation of Giant Cells

It depends on the underlying the etiology. It may be formed due to the following mechanisms:
- **Fused macrophages:** For example, foreign body giant cell, Langhans giant cell, Aschoff giant cell.
- **Giant cells resulting from fusion of cells:** These are formed due to fusion of cell membranes e.g., viral infections.

Table 35: Conditions associated with giant cells.

Non-neoplastic		
Infections	***Inflammatory conditions***	***Neoplasms***
• Measles, herpes, cytomegalovirus (CMV), human immunodeficiency virus (HIV) • Tuberculosis • Leprosy • Fungal infections • Parasitic infestations	• Sarcoidosis • Foreign body reaction • Aneurysmal bone cyst • Giant cell reparative granuloma • Brown tumor of bone in hyperparathyroidism • Simple bone cyst	• Hodgkin lymphoma • Giant cell rich tumors • Malignant melanoma • Giant cell variants of many malignant tumors, e.g., carcinoma of lung • Langerhans cell histiocytosis • Chondroblastoma • Nonossifying fibroma

- **Tumor giant cells:** It is due to chromosomal aberrations in which only nucleus divides without any cytoplasmic division. They may also occur when tumor grows in adverse conditions.
- Damaged muscle fibers.

Fused Macrophages

Giant cells are formed by fusion of macrophages in following conditions:

- **Langhans giant cells:** These are formed by fusion of modified macrophages called epithelioid cells. They measure about 40–50 µm and contain 20 or more nuclei. Their nuclei are arranged around the periphery of the cell in the form of horseshoe or ring. Conditions associated with this giant cells include tuberculosis, tuberculoid leprosy, sarcoidosis, in gumma of syphilis, Crohn disease, deep fungal infections and Leishmaniasis.
- **Foreign body giant cells:** These giant cells are usually larger than Langhans giant cells. They contain numerous uniform nuclei (up to 100) which are distributed throughout the cytoplasm. They may be seen in reaction to insoluble material when the macrophages fail to deal with particles to be removed. As an attempt to remove them, they fuse together and form multinucleated giant cells.
  - Exogenous: For example, suture material, talc, vegetable matter, starch, particles of wood, vegetable matter, microimplant, etc.
  - Endogenous material: For example, keratin (dermoid cyst of ovary, epidermal cyst), hair, cholesterol, fat, deposits of calcium, oxalate, urate crystals (in gout), sequestrum, etc.
  - Microbial infections which are associated with Langhans type of giant cells may also show foreign body giant cells.
- **Touton giant cells:** These multinucleated cells have central area of clear, eosinophilic cytoplasm surrounded by a ring of nuclei. The outer cytoplasm is foamy and vacuolated due to lipid content. The stimuli for their formation are factors that promote lipid uptake. They are found in conditions such as xanthoma, xanthelasma, xanthogranuloma, fat necrosis, and dermatofibroma.
- **Aschoff giant cells:** In rheumatic heart disease, activated macrophages in the heart are called Anitschkow cells. These Anitschkow cells may fuse and form multinucleated (with 2–4 nuclei) giant cells termed as Aschoff giant cells (the cytoplasm fuses and nuclei remain intact within fused cytoplasm). They are seen in Aschoff bodies observed in heart in **rheumatic heart disease**.

Giant Cells Resulting from Fusion of Cells

- **Tzanck giant cells:** These giant cells are formed in the skin due to viral infection. Viral infection stimulates rapid division of nucleus of epidermal cells without any cytoplasmic division. Some nuclei of these giant cells may appear bizarre and atypical. These giant cells may be seen in herpes simplex, herpes zoster and varicella, and cytomegalovirus infections.
- **Warthin–Finkeldey giant cells:** Lymphoid organs **in measles** show marked follicular hyperplasia and enlarged germinal centers. In lymphoid tissues, the virus sometimes causes fusion of infected cells, producing multinucleated giant cells termed as Warthin–Finkeldey giant cells. These are randomly distributed and contain up to 100 nuclei, with both intracytoplasmic and intranuclear eosinophilic inclusion bodies. These cells are pathognomonic for measles. Lymphoid hyperplasia is usually prominent in cervical and mesenteric lymph nodes, spleen and appendix. These are also found in the lung and sputum.

Tumor Giant Cells

They have bizarre shape and size. The nucleus is hyperchromatic, large in relation to cell and nuclei show variation in size and shape. They may be seen in various tumors.

- **Giant cell tumors:** For example, giant cell tumor of the bones (formerly known as osteoclastoma) shows uniform distribution of osteoclastic giant cells in the mononuclear stroma. These osteoclast type of giant cells are not tumor cells, whereas the stromal cells constitute tumor cells.
- **Reed Sternberg cells:** These are large malignant tumor giant cells measuring 20–60 µm in diameter. They have abundant eosinophilic cytoplasm and nuclei are typically two in number (binucleate). These nuclei have a mirror image appearance. They have prominent eosinophilic nucleolus surrounded by a halo. These are seen in various histologic types of **Hodgkin lymphoma**.
- **Giant cell variants of many malignant tumors:** These are large tumor cells with many hyperchromatic nuclei of varying size and shape. They are not derived from macrophages but are formed from dividing nuclei of the neoplastic cells. They are found in many malignant tumors such as carcinoma of lung, uterus, liver, and various soft tissue sarcomas, etc.

SYSTEMIC MANIFESTATIONS (EFFECTS) OF INFLAMMATION

Inflammation is localized response of living vascularized tissue to injury. Features of an effective inflammatory response include—(1) limits the area of damage or injury, (2) destroys the causative pathological agent and removes the damaged tissue, and (3) restores the damaged tissue as well as its function. However, local injury may be associated with prominent systemic manifestations or changes. These manifestations may cause serious impairment of normal functioning. These effects may be due to entry of pathogen into the bloodstream, a separate condition acting synergistically, or indirect effects of both local and systemic features of inflammation. The symptoms associated with inflammation are due to cytokines and include fever, myalgia, arthralgia, anorexia, and sleepy or drowsy feeling. Systemic changes associated with cytokines are collectively known as **acute-phase response.**

Systemic Inflammatory Response Syndrome

The most prominent systemic manifestation of inflammation, is termed the SIRS. It is characterized by activation of the hypothalamic-pituitary-adrenal axis, leukocytosis, and the acute phase response, fever, and shock. It is discussed in detail on page 323.

Hypothalamic–pituitary–adrenal Axis

Several systemic manifestations of inflammation are brought via the hypothalamic–pituitary–adrenal axis. This is mainly observed in response to chronic inflammation and chronic immune disease. Inflammation releases anti-inflammatory glucocorticoids from the adrenal cortex. Thus, any condition in which there is loss of adrenal function can increase the severity of inflammation.

Acute-phase Response

Q. Write a short essay on acute phase response.

Definition

Acute-phase response is a systemic regulated physiological reaction that occurs when pyrogenic and other cytokines are released in response to infection and inflammatory conditions. The clinical and pathologic changes of acute-phase response are listed in **Box 19**.

Box 19: Characteristic feature of acute-phase response.

Clinical features
- Fever
- Myalgia and arthralgia
- Decreased appetite (anorexia)
- Altered sleep patterns (sleepy or drowsy feeling)

Pathological changes
- Leukocytosis
- Changes in plasma levels of acute phase proteins

Causes

Acute-phase response is due to cytokines produced by leukocytes, in response to infections (e.g., bacterial products such as LPS, viral double stranded RNA and by other inflammatory stimuli), or immune reactions. Most important cytokines that mediate the acute-phase reaction are TNF-α, IL-1, and IL-6; other cytokines, such as type I IFNs may also contribute to the reaction.

Fever

Fever is characterized by raised body temperature, usually by 1–4°C above normal temperature of 37°C, i.e., >38°C (1.8–7.2°F above normal temperature of 98.6°F, i.e., >100.4°F). It is one of the most prominent clinical manifestations of the acute-phase response and is a hallmark of inflammation. This is especially observed in inflammation associated with infection. Molecules or substances that cause fever are called pyrogens (Greek *pyro*, "fire").

Pyrogens

These may be **exogenous or endogenous.**

- **Exogenous pyrogens:** They are derived from outside the patient. Most of them are microbial/bacterial products (LPS), microbial toxins, or whole micro-organisms (including viruses). For example, LPS (endotoxin) produced by all gram-negative bacteria. Pyrogenic products derived from gram-positive organisms include the enterotoxins of *Staphylococcus aureus* and the groups A and B Streptococcal toxins. These endotoxin products are called as superantigens. One example is Staphylococcal toxin derived from *S. aureus* of patients with toxic shock syndrome.
- **Endogenous pyrogens (pyrogenic cytokines):** These include cytokines such as IL-1, IL-6 and TNF-α, ciliary neurotropic factor (a member of the IL-6 family) and interferons (IFNs). Endogenous pyrogens are now called **pyrogenic cytokines**. The cytokines increase the enzymes cyclo-oxygenases resulting in conversion of arachidonic acid (AA) into prostaglandins (PGs). Exogenous pyrogens stimulate leukocytes to release of endogenous pyrogens.

Pathogenesis of fever in inflammation (Flowchart 9)

- **Production of pyrogens:** Infection, microbial toxins, mediators of inflammation, immune reactions, etc., stimulate myeloid (monocytes/macrophages) and endothelial cells to produce pyrogenic cytokines. They are released from these cells and enter the systemic circulation. The circulating pyogenic cytokines produce fever by stimulating the synthesis of PGE_2 in the circulation. Some of these systemic PGE_2 escape their destruction by the lung and enter to the hypothalamus via the internal carotid artery. Pyogenic cytokines also produce PGE_2 in peripheral tissues. The increase in PGE_2 in the periphery is responsible for the nonspecific myalgias and arthralgias that usually accompany fever.
- **Interaction of pyrogens with hypothalamic endothelium:** Both exogenous pyrogens and pyrogenic cytokines (endogenous pyrogens, namely IL-1, IL-6, and TNF) interact with the endothelium of capillaries surrounding the hypothalamic regulatory centers and produce PGE_2.
- **Raising the hypothalamic set point by pyogenic cytokines:** The interaction of endothelial cells of hypothalamus with pyrogens (exogenous and endogenous) raises the levels of PGE_2 in the brain. The pyrogens and

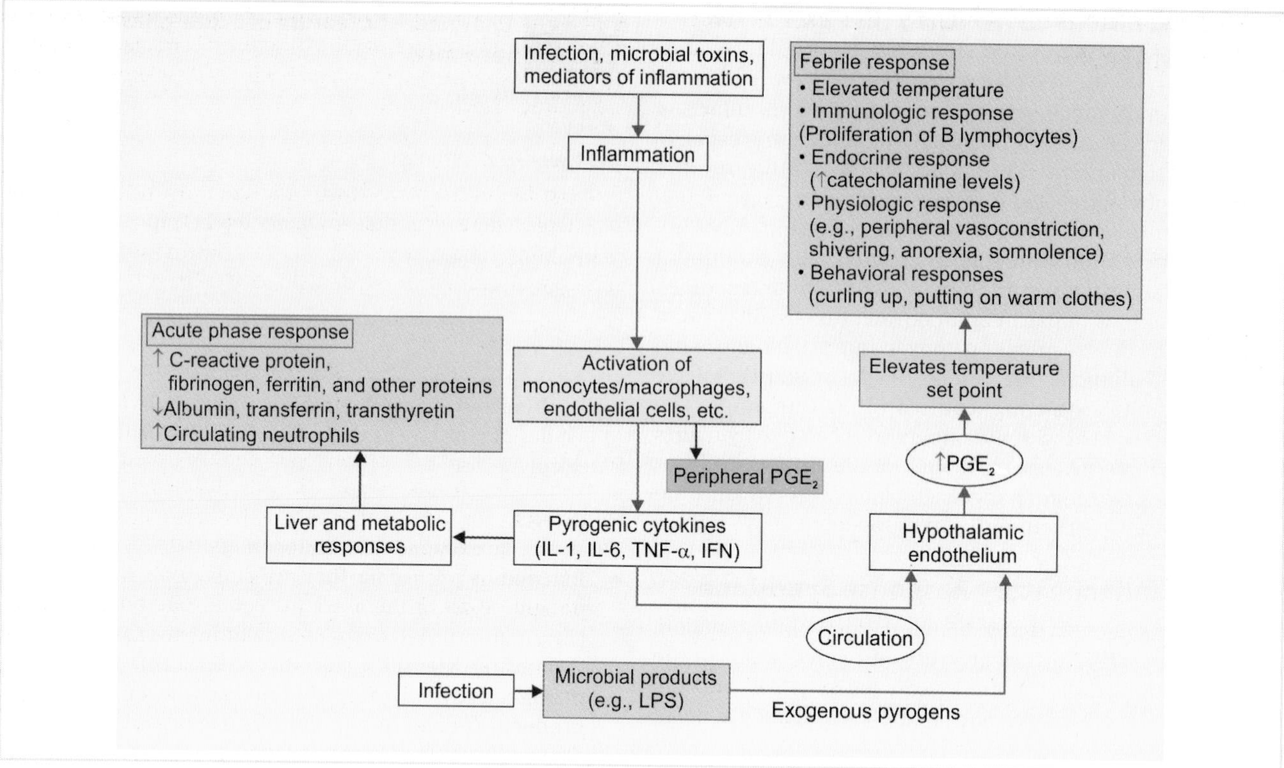

(IFN: interferon; IL: interleukin; LPS: lipopolysaccharide; PG: prostagladin; TNF-α: tumor necrosis factor-alpha)

FLOWCHART 9: Pathogenesis of fever and acute-phase response in inflammation. Inflammation and infection initiate the release of pyrogenic cytokines and exogenous pyrogens. Exogenous pyrogens and pyrogenic cytokines stimulate prostaglandin E_2 (PGE_2) release in the brain. Pyrogenic cytokines also produce PGE_2 in the periphery. PGE_2 acts on the hypothalamus, setting a higher temperature set point and initiates febrile response. Simultaneously, pyrogenic cytokines initiate the acute phase response.

PGE_2 act on hypothalamic thermoregulatory center. The concentrations of PGE_2 are highest near the hypothalamic regulatory centers. Pyrogens and PGE_2 stimulate the production of neurotransmitters that reset the temperature set point. This is the first step in initiating fever [i.e., in raising the hypothalamic set point ("thermostat") for core temperature to febrile levels].

- **Production of fever:** IL-1 can stimulate PG synthesis in hypothalamic thermoregulatory centers. TNF-α and IL-6 also cause fever by a direct action on the hypothalamus. Distinct receptors called as TLRs (similar in many ways to IL-1 receptors) for microbial products are found on the hypothalamic endothelium. Thus, the direct activation of TLRs or IL-1 receptors results in PGE_2 production and fever. Inhibitors of cyclo-oxygenase [nonsteroidal anti-inflammatory drugs (NSAIDs) such as aspirin] reduce the fever by inhibiting IL-1-stimulated PGE_2 synthesis in the hypothalamus. An elevated body temperature is assumed to be a protective host response.

Symptoms associated with fever

These include chills (unpleasant feeling/sensation of coldness in the atmosphere), rigor (intense chills with shivering and piloerection), and sweats (to allow dissipation of heat).

Pain

Pain is an unpleasant sensation localized to a part of the body. Pain in an acute-phase reaction is associated with following:

- **Nociception:** Primary afferent nociceptors (pain receptors) are afferent fibers of peripheral nerve that respond to intense (painful) stimuli and produce the subjective experience of pain. Nociceptors are high-threshold receptors for thermal, chemical, and mechanical stimuli. Individual primary afferent nociceptors can respond to several different types of noxious stimuli. For example, most nociceptors respond to heat; intense cold, intense mechanical distortion (e.g., pinch), changes in pH (acidic), and application of chemical irritants (serotonin, bradykinin, and histamine). Nociception is the detection of noxious stimuli and transmission of this information to the brain. Nociception is mainly a neural response initiated in injured tissues by specific nociceptors. Mediators of inflammation such as kinins (mainly bradykinin), histamine, nitric oxide (NO), prostaglandins (PGs), cytokines (TNF-α and IL-1, -6, and -8), and growth factors activate peripheral nociceptors directly or indirectly. Bradykinin formed during inflammation activates primary sensory neurons via B2 receptors and mediate pain transmission. Another kinin called des-Arg-bradykinin, activates B1 receptors and produces pain. Cytokines produce pain hypersensitivity to mechanical and thermal stimuli. PGs and growth factors may directly activate nociceptors but mostly act by increasing nociceptor sensitivity.
- **Sensitization (pain perception):** The threshold for activating primary afferent nociceptors is lowered when intense, repeated, or prolonged stimuli are

applied to damaged or inflamed tissues. This process is called sensitization. Inflammatory mediators such as bradykinin, nerve-growth factor, few PGs, and leukotrienes contribute to this process. It arises in response to the increased sensitivity to both noxious and normally innocuous stimuli.

- **Suffering and pain behavior.**

Acute-phase Proteins

Q. Write a short essay on acute phase proteins/reactants.

Definition

Acute phase proteins are the proteins in the circulating blood, which are associated to the onset of any infection or tissue injury. They may be either increased (positive) or decreased (negative), and either proinflammatory or anti-inflammatory.

The hepatic acute phase response involves increasing or decreasing protein synthesis. Those that are increased during inflammation are mostly/primarily synthesized in the liver and may be markedly (several hundred-fold) raised/increased during acute inflammatory challenge/response to inflammatory stimuli. Some of the acute-phase proteins are reduced than normal level. Some "acute-phase" proteins enhance inflammation very much and are called proinflammatory and may even contribute to the promotion of sepsis, and other proteins are always anti-inflammatory in nature. All these plasma proteins are called **acute-phase reactants or acute-phase proteins** (**Table 36**) because they are raised in the blood during acute inflammatory reactions, and their increased production is part of the **acute phase response** to infection and other insults. The maximal circulating levels of these acute-phase reactants reach within 10–40 hours after the beginning of inflammation.

Mediators

Stimulation of liver cells to synthesize most of these acute-phase proteins are mediated mainly by IL-1, IL-6, and TNF-α. Circulating levels of various acute-phase reactants during inflammation are presented in **Table 36**.

Significance

Usually, acute-phase proteins have beneficial effects during acute inflammation. However, there are certain disadvantages also.

- Many acute-phase proteins (CRP and SAA) bind to microbial cell walls and **may act as opsonins**. They fix complement and activate complement system. They also bind chromatin, possibly helping to clear necrotic cell nuclei.
- From a clinical point of view, the "acute-phase" proteins are used as markers of any inflammation in the body. Some of them (e.g., α_2 macroglobulin, fibrinogen) are useful for evaluating blood coagulation, intravascular hemolysis, and thrombosis. Deficiency of α1-antitrypsin is used as a diagnostic marker of congenital emphysema.

Three of the well-known of acute-phase proteins are: (1) C-reactive protein (CRP), (2) **fibrinogen, (3) serum amyloid A (SAA) protein**. Their synthesis by hepatocytes is increased by cytokines, especially IL-6 (for CRP and fibrinogen) and IL-1 or TNF (for SAA).

Table 36: Circulating levels of various acute-phase reactants during inflammation.

Acute-phase reactant	*Increased*	*Decreased*
Coagulation components	Fibrinogen*—Coagulation	None
	Prothrombin	
	Factor VIII	
	Plasminogen	
Protease inhibitors	α_1-antitrypsin*—Serine protease inhibitor	Inter-α_1-antitrypsin
	α_1-antichymotrypsin*	
	α_2-macroglobulin*—Antiprotease	
	Cysteine protease inhibitor—Antiprotease	
Transport proteins	Haptoglobin* (binds hemoglobin)	Transferrin (binds iron)
	Hemopexin (binds heme)	Transthyretin (transports thyroid hormone)
	Ceruloplasmin*—Antioxidant, binds copper	Retinol-binding protein (transports vitamin A)
	Ferritin	
Complement components/factors	C1s, C2, C3, C4, C5, C9, factor B, C1 inhibitor	Properdin
Miscellaneous proteins	α_1-acid glycoprotein	Albumin
	Fibronectin	Prealbumin
	Serum amyloid A (SAA) *—Apolipoprotein	α_1-lipoprotein
	C-reactive protein (CRP)—Opsonization	β-lipoprotein
	Mannose-binding protein— Opsonization/ complement activation	
	Thrombopoietin-Raised platelet count	

*anti-inflammatory

Pro-inflammatory "Acute-phase" Proteins

C-reactive protein

C-reactive protein (CRP) is an acute phase reactant (beta globulin) synthesized mainly by the liver. Name is derived from c polysaccharide of capsule of *Pneumococcus.* Its synthesis is stimulated by a number of inflammatory mediators (mainly by cytokines, e.g., IL-6) acting on liver cells These cytokines are produced by phagocytes and dendritic cells (DCs) as part of the innate immune response. CRP plays an important role in host defense. It augments the innate immune response by binding to microbial (bacteria) cell walls or may act as opsonin (opsonizes invading pathogens) and activate the classical complement cascade. They also bind chromatin and help in clearing necrotic cell nuclei. CRP also stimulates repair and regeneration. It activates complements and macrophages.

Significance

- In healthy individuals, plasma concentrations of CRP are very low (<8 mg/dL) but can increase up to 1,000-fold during infections and in response to other inflammatory stimuli. It is helpful for detection of infection and immunocompromised state.
- Raised serum levels of CRP is a **marker for increased risk of myocardial infarction in patients with coronary artery disease**. Probably inflammation involving atherosclerotic plaques in the coronary arteries may predispose to thrombosis and subsequent myocardial infarction.
- Plasma CRP is a **strong, independent marker of risk for myocardial infarction, stroke, peripheral arterial disease, and sudden cardiac death**, even in healthy individuals.
- CRP increases (may be up to 1,000-fold) within 6 hours of acute inflammation. Levels fall within a few days after the inflammation subsides. Sequential measurement of CRP is useful in monitoring disease activity. It is the earliest marker to rise during inflammation amongst all acute phase reactants and returns to normal.
- In some inflammatory diseases, there may be normal or slight elevations of CRP concentration despite unequivocal evidence of active inflammation. These include SLE, systemic sclerosis, ulcerative colitis, and leukemia. However, existing infection in these conditions is associated with significantly raised levels of CRP. It is to be noted that intercurrent infection does not cause a significant CRP response in these conditions.
- CRP is also a useful marker for assessing the effects of risk reduction measures, such as cessation of smoking, weight loss, exercise, and statins; each one of these reduce CRP levels.
- When inflammation decreases, CRP level decreases followed by ESR.

Mannose-binding Lectin

It belongs to the collectin subgroup of the C-type lectin superfamily. It binds carbohydrate mannose "patterns" on the surface of bacteria, fungi, viruses, and protozoans. It activates complement system via the lectin subpathway. It may take part in opsonization.

Hepcidin

It is an iron-regulating peptide synthesized in liver. It is increased as an acute-phase response. In chronic inflammation, plasma concentrations of hepcidin level is chronically elevated. This reduces the availability of iron and is **responsible for the anemia associated with chronic inflammation.**

Anti-inflammatory "Acute Phase" Proteins

- **Fibrinogen:** It is a component of the coagulation system. It is converted into fibrin by thrombin during formation of blood clot. In acute inflammation, the coagulation system protects tissue from bleeding. Fibrinogen may be raised 1.5–2 times during any form of acute inflammation. Fibrinogen binds to red cells to form stacks (rouleaux) and sediment faster at unit gravity than the individual red cells. Increased plasma levels of fibrinogen are responsible for raised **erythrocyte sedimentation rate** (ESR) in infections. Thus, measuring the ESR acts as a simple qualitative index/test used clinically to monitor the activity of many inflammatory diseases. ESR is nonspecific and raised in any inflammatory conditions caused by any stimulus. **Fibrinogen** plays an essential role in wound healing.
- **Serum amyloid A (SAA):** It is an apolipoprotein that plays a role in host defense and stimulates repair and regeneration. During acute inflammation, SAA has beneficial effects by its "urgent bandage" on injured tissue. SAA arises within hours after an inflammatory stimulus, and its level may be markedly increased. But with prolonged production (especially SAA) like in chronic inflammation, it may contribute to the development of causes **secondary amyloidosis** in some cases.
- **α_1-antitrypsin and α_1-antichymotrypsin:** They can inhibit a wide variety of proteases and protect tissues from injury. They control inflammation by neutralizing the enzymes produced by activated neutrophils and prevent tissue destruction. In acute inflammation, they can be markedly elevated. Deficiency of α_1-antitrypsin may be fatal and produces severe emphysema.
- **α_2-Macroglobulin:** It is a large serum protein, acts as an antiprotease, downregulates fibrinolysis, and inhibits thrombin. In acute inflammation, the concentration of α_2-macroglobulin may be increased five times or more than normal. It is synthesized in liver and macrophages. It is increased in nephrotic syndrome.
- **Ceruloplasmin:** It is a ferroxidase enzyme that oxidizes iron. It carries >95% of the total copper in healthy human serum. It is synthesized in liver. It prevents iron uptake by microbes.
  - **Causes of increased ceruloplasmin:** Hemosiderosis, obstructive biliary diseases, pregnancy, estrogen therapy, malignancy
  - **Causes of decreased ceruloplasmin:** Wilsons disease, cirrhosis, malignancy
- **Haptoglobin:** It binds with free hemoglobin released from RBCs. So, if there is liberation of free hemoglobin from RBCs during acute inflammation, haptoglobin prevents loss of iron through the kidneys. It acts as an antioxidant and removes oxygen free radicals.
- **Thrombopoietin:** It is the major growth factor for megakaryocytes (platelet precursors) in the bone marrow. It is also upregulated and as a result systemic inflammation. It may be associated with an raised platelet count (thrombocytosis).

Changes in the Leukocytes

Leukocytosis

Increase in the total leukocyte count in the peripheral blood of >11,000/µL is termed as leukocytosis. It is common in inflammatory reactions, especially those caused by bacterial infections.

- **Leukocyte count: It may be increased up to 15,000 or 20,000 cells/µL**. Sometimes, it may be extremely high reaching 40,000–100,000/µL associated with more immature neutrophils in the blood (referred to as a shift to the left) and are called as leukemoid reactions (i.e., leukemia-like). It is similar to the white cell counts found in leukemia. It is important to distinguish it from leukemia (which is a malignant disease).
- **Cause:** Leukocytosis is most commonly observed in bacterial infections and with tissue injury. It is due to increased release of leukocytes from the bone marrow postmitotic reserve pool. It is caused by release of specific mediators from macrophages and other cells. These mediators include cytokines such as TNF and IL-1. Prolonged infection also causes proliferation of hematopoietic precursor cells in the bone marrow, caused by increased synthesis of CSFs mainly from activated macrophages and marrow stromal cells. The increased output of leukocytes from the bone marrow compensates for the loss of leukocytes in the inflammatory reaction.
- **Bacterial infections** cause an increase in the blood neutrophil count known as **neutrophilia**.

Other features

Presence of **vacuolated neutrophils** may be a sign of bacterial sepsis. The presence of **Döhle bodies** (appear as 1–2 µm blue cytoplasmic inclusions) may be seen in infections, burns, or other inflammatory states. If the neutrophil granules are larger than normal and stain a darker blue, it is termed as "**toxic granulation**". They also suggest a systemic inflammation.

Leukopenia

Leukopenia is characterized by an absolute decrease in number of circulating white cell count. Decreased number of circulating white cells is associated with few infections like **typhoid fever and some viruses, rickettsia, and certain protozoa**. It may be occasionally seen during chronic inflammation, especially in malnourished patients or those who suffer from a chronic debilitating disease such as disseminated cancer.

Lymphocytosis

It is characterized by absolute increase in the number of circulating lymphocytes. In contrast to bacterial infections, viral infections (e.g., infectious mononucleosis, mumps, and German measles) are characterized by lymphocytosis.

Eosinophilia

It is characterized by increase in the number of eosinophils in circulating blood. It is seen in bronchial **asthma, allergy, and parasitic infestations**.

Other Features of the Acute-phase Response

It includes:

- Increased pulse and blood pressure. Decreased sweating mainly due to redirection of blood flow from cutaneous to deep vascular beds. This minimizes the heat loss through the skin. Others symptoms like rigors (shivering) and chills (search for warmth).
- Anorexia and malaise, probably due to cytokines acting on brain cells.
- In severe bacterial infections (sepsis), cytokines (mainly TNF and IL-1) may be produced in large quantities and can result in disseminated intravascular coagulation (DIC), hypotensive shock, and metabolic disturbances, including insulin resistance and hyperglycemia. This clinical triad of is known as *septic shock*. It is one form of a severe, usually fatal disorder termed as systemic inflammatory response syndrome (SIRS).

Systemic Inflammatory Response Syndrome and Shock

Q. Explain systemic inflammatory response syndrome.

Sepsis (disseminated, severe bacterial/microbial infections) shows large number of bacteria and their products in the blood and produces septic shock. A syndrome similar to septic shock may occur as a complication of noninfectious disorders (nonmicrobial conditions) with massive tissue injury such as severe burns, trauma, pancreatitis, and other serious conditions. Both the infectious and noninfectious causes of shock can produce a similar set of clinical findings of systemic inflammation such as fever, tachycardia, tachypnea, leukocytosis, or leukopenia.

Mechanism

In both settings (i.e., severe infection or massive tissue injury), massive ***inflammatory reaction*** stimulates the production of large quantities of several cytokines and other mediators of inflammation into the systemic circulation. These cytokine mainly includes **TNF and IL-1** [others IL-6 and platelet-activating factor (PAF)] into the systemic circulation. Marked blood levels of cytokines produce widespread clinical and pathologic abnormalities. Collectively, these reactions are called *SIRS*. Thus, **SIRS** can develop due to septic shock (by microbes) as well as variety of other noninfectious insults.

SIRS is an exaggerated and generalized manifestation of a local immune or inflammatory reaction.

Features

The persistence of cytokines and other mediators affects the heart and peripheral vascular system by causing generalized vasodilation; increasing vascular permeability, intravascular volume loss, and myocardial depression; and decreasing cardiac output. Cardiac output may then not be enough to supply the body's demand for oxygen and nutrients (cardiac decompensation). SIRS is a hypermetabolic state characterized by two or more signs of systemic inflammation. These include fever, tachycardia, tachypnea, leukocytosis, or leukopenia, in the setting of a known cause of inflammation. SIRS is **often fatal.** Septic shock is triggered by microbial infections and is associated with severe SIRS. In septic shock, clinical SIRS so severe that it is associated with organ dysfunction, disseminated intravascular coagulation (characterized by activation of coagulation pathways causes microthrombi throughout the body, consumption of clotting factors and predisposing to bleeding), hypotensive shock, and metabolic abnormalities such as insulin resistance and hyperglycemia. If severe and persistent, it may lead to multisystem organ dysfunction syndrome (MODS) and death.

8.8 Tissue Repair

CHAPTER OUTLINE

- Introduction
  - Brief history of healing
  - Definitions
- Basic processes of healing
  - Cellular migration
  - Extracellular matrix organization and remodeling
  - Cell proliferation
- Cell and tissue regeneration
  - Requirements for regeneration
  - Cells that proliferate during healing
  - Type of cells or tissues capable of regeneration
  - Mechanisms of tissue regeneration
- Repair by connective tissue deposition
  - Features that favor scarring
  - Steps in scar formation
  - Angiogenesis
  - Activation of fibroblasts and deposition of connective tissue
  - Role of macrophages in repair
- Healing of skin wounds
  - Healing by primary union or by first intention
  - Healing by secondary union or by second intention
- Factors that influence tissue repair
  - Local factors
  - Systemic factors that impair tissue repair
- Complications of tissue repair
  - Defects in healing: Chronic wounds
  - Inadequate granulation tissue formation
  - Excessive scar formation
  - Excessive contraction
  - Others
  - Fibrosis in parenchymal organs

INTRODUCTION

Injury to cells and tissues **results in loss of cells and tissues.** It sets in inflammation (restrict the tissue damage) and the conclusion of inflammation is healing also known as repair. Inflammation initiates replacement of lost tissue by living tissue. The survival of humans depends on the ability to repair the damage caused by toxic insults and inflammation. The inflammatory response to microbes and injured tissues not only tries to remove these injurious agents but also starts the process of repair.

Brief History of Healing

Physicians in ancient Egypt and battle surgeons in classic Greece observed the repair/healing of wounds. The clotting of blood was recognized as the first event in wound healing.

- **Inflammatory cells:** With the advent of the microscope, the inflammatory cells were identified and are considered as necessary in the repair process. The importance of antisepsis to wound healing was also observed.
- **Pus and antiseptics:** From the 2nd century Greco-Roman physician Galen to the works of Pasteur and Lister at the end of the 19th century, the presence of pus at a wound site was considered as beneficial. In 1876, British physician Joseph Lister was invited to take charge as president of the Surgical Section of the International Medical Congress in Philadelphia. Five years later, President Garfield died after being shot by an assassin. He passed away not to damage caused by the bullet but several months later due to formation of pus and sepsis. This was due to tissue probing by physicians who were unaware of the germ theory and antiseptic methods.
- **Extracellular matrix:** The importance of extracellular matrix (ECM), specifically collagen, in wound healing was first recognized while studying scurvy. The disease scurvy is caused by vitamin C deficiency and claimed the lives of millions. In 1747, Dr James Lind, a surgeon in England's Royal Navy, conducted the first controlled clinical trial. He divided sailors suffering from scurvy into six treatment groups and observed that sailors given oranges and lemons had highly benefited. It prevented the reopening of wounds and loss of teeth in these patients. In 1907, the role of vitamin C was discovered by Norwegians—Axel Holst and Theodor Frolich. They observed that guinea pigs, like humans, were not able to synthesize vitamin C (ascorbic acid). Ascorbate was found to be necessary for the stabilization of the collagen triple helix, an important step in wound healing.
- **Regeneration:** Regeneration of the human liver was the basis of the Greek myth of Prometheus, whose liver regenerated daily. In the 1950s, Sir John Gurdon stated that transplantation of somatic cell nuclei into a Xenopus egg could form a normal adult organism. This is the basis of inducible pluripotent stem cells from many tissues.

Definitions

The most favorable outcome expected from inflammation is a return to normal structure and function of the damaged tissue.

Repair/Healing

Repair or healing is a process of restoration of tissue architecture and function after an injury. The term repair is usually used for parenchymal and connective tissues and healing for surface epithelia. However, the terms used interchangeably. Healing can be broadly divided into regeneration and scarring (the deposition of connective tissue) (**Fig. 54**).

1. **Regeneration**: It is a process in which lost tissue is replaced by tissue of similar type. Some tissues are capable of replacing the damaged components and can return to a normal state and this process is termed regeneration. Regeneration can occur by proliferation of differentiated cells. This occurs by the proliferation of cells that survived the injury and retain the capacity to proliferation. For example, hepatocytes in the liver. In other tissues, such as

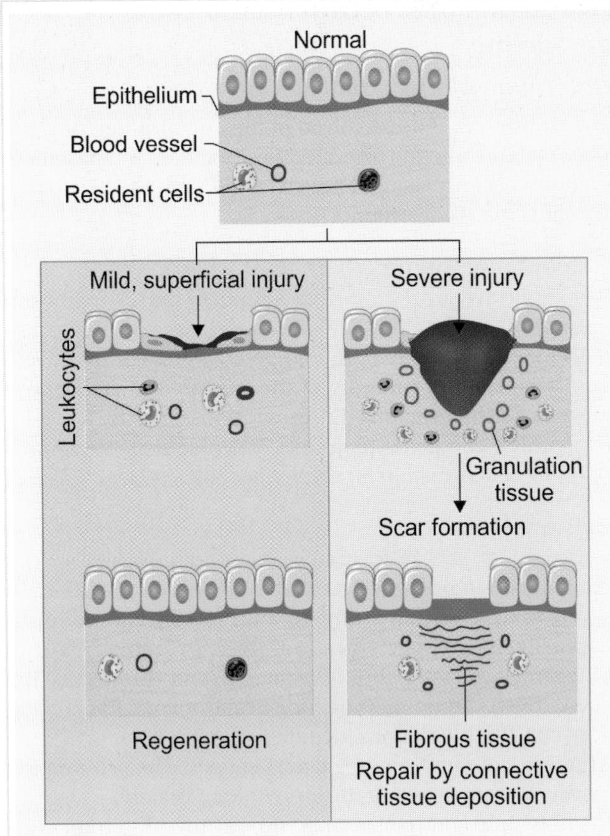

FIG. 54: Repair of damaged tissues by two processes namely regeneration and connective tissue deposition. Resolution occurs by regeneration when the injury is mild and damages to the surface epithelium without the damage to the underlying tissue. If the injury is more severe associated with damage to the connective tissue, repair occurs by connective tissue deposition leading to formation of scar.

the epithelia of the skin and intestines, tissue stem cells and their progenitors can restore damaged tissues. However, the capacity to regenerate most damaged tissues and organs is limited in humans. Only some tissue components are tissues are capable for fully restoration.

2. **Connective tissue deposition (scar formation)**: Regeneration is not possible mainly in two situations: (i) the tissue damaged/injured by inflammation is not capable of regeneration, or (ii) the supporting framework/ structures of the tissue are too severely damaged to support regeneration of the tissue cells. In such situations, repair occurs by the formation of connective (fibrous) tissue. This process may result in scar formation. Though the fibrous scar is not normal, it usually gives sufficient structural stability so that the injured tissue is capable to function.

Extent of Tissue Injury

Depending on the extent of injury and type of tissue involved, the process of healing may vary.

- **Mild and short duration:** In a tissue composed of labile cells, the damaged tissue is healed by regeneration without significant scarring.
- **Severe and chronic:** Healing occurs by fibrous tissue, forming scar.
  - Severe tissue injury damages both parenchymal cells and the ECM framework.
  - Chronic inflammation

BASIC PROCESSES OF HEALING

Many of the basic cellular and molecular mechanisms in wound healing also are involved in other processes such as growth of tumor. After hemostasis in wound, three key cellular mechanisms are involved in wound healing:

1. Cellular migration
2. Extracellular matrix organization and remodeling.
3. Cell proliferation

Cellular Migration

Release of Mediators at the Site of Wound

Cellular migration into a wound and activation of local cells initiates repair process. This is brought out by mediators that are produced either de novo by resident cells or released from preformed molecules present in granules of platelets and basophils. The granules of platelets and basophils contain cytokines, chemoattractants, proteases, and other mediators of inflammation. These mediators control blood supply, degrade damaged tissue and initiate the process of repair.

- **Platelets:** They are activated when collagen is exposed at sites of endothelial damage. They aggregate at the site of injury, form fibrin clot, and limit loss of blood. Activated platelets release platelet-derived growth factor (PDGF) and many other molecules. They facilitate adhesion, coagulation, vasoconstriction, cell proliferation, and clot resorption.
- **Mast cells:** Their granules contain high concentrations of heparin, histamine, and proteinases. These cells are found in connective tissue near small blood vessels. On exposure to foreign antigens, they release the contents of their granules, many of them being angiogenic.
- **Others:** Resident tissue macrophages, mesenchymal cells, and epithelial cells also release mediators that are involved in repair process.

Cell Types Migrating to the Wound

Cell types characteristic of skin wounds are:

Leukocytes: From the circulating blood, leukocytes reach the wound site through different processes such as adhesion to activated endothelium, emigration from the circulation into tissue, and form small focal adhesions with matrix molecules (e.g., fibrin, fibronectin, and collagen). Leukocyte events in inflammation are described in detail on pages 230–245.

- **Polymorphonuclear leukocytes:** Neutrophils are one type of leukocytes that are derived from the bone marrow. They reach the wound site within hours of injury. They degrade and destroy necrotic/nonviable tissue and infectious micro-organisms by releasing their granular contents and producing reactive oxygen species. Then they undergo apoptosis and are removed by macrophages.

- **Monocytes/macrophages:** They maintain a basal resident population in tissues. They are the predominant cell after 48 hours of onset of inflammation and live longer. They phagocytose debris and aid in the formation of granulation tissue and healing by releasing cytokines and chemoattractants.

Dendritic cells: These are resident antigen-presenting cells that regulate innate and adaptive immunity. They can proliferate in some tissues (e.g., skin), and can also be recruited from bone marrow or differentiated from closely related macrophages.

Mesenchymal cells: These cells involved in healing include fibroblasts, myofibroblasts, pericytes, and smooth muscle cells. They are recruited locally and are also derived from mesenchymal progenitors in bone marrow. These cells migrate and proliferate through signals from growth factors and matrix degradation products. They are found by day 3 or 4 in a skin wound. They are involved in the synthesis of connective tissue, tissue remodeling, vascular integrity, wound contraction, and wound strength.

Endothelial cells: They proliferate from existing postcapillary venules and are also derived from the circulating bone marrow progenitors. New capillaries are formed in response to growth factors and are seen in granulation tissue of wound along with fibroblasts after about day 3 of healing process. Formation of capillaries is important for gas exchange, delivery of nutrients, and influx of inflammatory cells.

Epidermal cells: In case of skin wounds, they move across the surface. Re-epithelialization can be delayed if there is damaged basement membrane.

Stem cells: These may be from bone marrow, the skin, stem cells, or progenitor cells in the hair follicle (in the bulge region) and within the basal epidermal layer (interfollicular epidermis). They form the renewable sources of epidermal and dermal cells capable of differentiation, proliferation, and migration.

Mechanisms of Cell Migration

Cell migration in wound healing occurs by receptor-mediated responses to chemical signals (cytokines) and insoluble substrates of the ECM.

- **Leukocytes:** They rapidly move by ameboid locomotion through wave-like membrane extensions called lamellipodia.
- **Fibroblasts:** These are slower-moving cells that extend narrower, finger-like membrane protrusions called filopodia.

Mechanism

- **Binding to the receptors:** Growth factors or chemokines bind to specific receptors on cell surfaces and trigger cell polarization and membrane extensions.
- **Polymerization of actin:** Actin fibrils polymerize and form a network at the membrane's leading edge. This propels lamellipodia and filopodia forward, with traction achieved by engaging ECM substrate.
- **Adhesive molecules:** The leading edge of the cell membrane adheres to the adjacent ECM through adhesive molecules, namely integrins. As cells move forward, older adhesions at the rear are weakened or destabilized. This allows the trailing edge of the cell to retract.

Extracellular Matrix Organization and Remodeling

Extracellular Matrix Organization

Three types of ECM are involved in the organization, physical properties, and function of tissue. These include—(1) basement membrane, (2) provisional matrix, and (3) connective tissue (interstitial matrix or stroma).

Basement membrane

It is a supportive and biological boundary and is important in development, healing, and regeneration. It provides key signals for cell differentiation and polarity and contributes to tissue organization. Integrity of the basement membrane is important for the organized regeneration of tissue. It guides the migration of regenerating cells. It is modified after injury, promoting cell migration for wound healing.

Provisional matrix

Provisional matrix is formed at sites of injury from the accumulated temporary extracellular organization of plasma-derived matrix proteins and tissue-derived components. Plasma-derived provisional matrix proteins include fibrinogen, fibronectin, thrombospondin, and vitronectin. The tissue-derived components include hyaluronan, tenascin, and fibronectin. Their functions include:

- Provisional matrix molecules along with the pre-existing stromal matrix prevent the loss of blood or fluid.
- Provisional matrix assists migration of leukocytes, endothelial cells, and fibroblasts to the wound site.

Stromal (interstitial connective tissue) matrix

Connective tissue stroma is also important for cell migration. It is a medium for storage and exchange of bioactive protein molecules. Connective tissue consists of ECM and the cells that synthesize the matrix.

- **Cells of the matrix:** They are mainly of mesenchymal origin and include fibroblasts, myofibroblasts, adipocytes, chondrocytes, osteocytes, and endothelial cells. Bone marrow-derived cells (e.g., mast cells, macrophages, transient leukocytes) are also present.
- **Stroma:** The ECM of connective tissue is also termed as stroma or interstitium. It consists of fibers formed from collagen molecules. Elastic fibers are responsible for the elasticity to skin, large blood vessels, and lungs. The so-called ground substance consists of a number of molecules, including glycosaminoglycans (GAGs), proteoglycans, matricellular proteins, and fibronectin.

Extracellular Matrix Remodeling

Remodeling is the long-lasting phase of repair process. As the process of repair proceeds, inflammatory cells become less in number and capillaries become reduced. In remodeling, numbers of fibroblast rapidly rise and then fall as an equilibrium between collagen deposition and degradation is restored. Remodeling is discussed in detail on pages 333 and 334.

Cell Proliferation

The regeneration of injured cells and tissues involves cell proliferation. Early in tissue injury, there is a sudden, transient increase in cellularity that raises the immune surveillance and replaces (some) damaged cells. Several types of cells proliferate during tissue repair. These include—(1) the **remnants of the injured tissue** (which try to restore normal structure), (2) **vascular endothelial cells** (to form new vessels that provide the nutrients required for the repair process), and (3) **fibroblasts** (the source of the fibrous tissue that forms the scar to fill defects that cannot be corrected by regeneration).

- **Granulation tissue:** Cell proliferation and migration initiate formation of granulation tissue. Granulation tissue is a specialized, highly vascularized tissue that develops transiently during repair. Cells of granulation tissue are derived from different populations of cells such as circulating leukocytes, and from adjacent, resident capillary endothelial and mesenchymal cells (fibroblasts, myofibroblasts, pericytes, and smooth muscle cells). Local and marrow-derived progenitor cells, which have some features of leukocytes, can also populate wounds, and are capable of differentiating into (transient) endothelial and fibroblasts. However, terminally differentiated cells (e.g., cardiac myocytes, neurons) cannot contribute to repair or regeneration.
- **Stimuli for cell proliferation:** Growth factors and small chemotactic peptides (chemokines) produce soluble autocrine and paracrine signals for cell proliferation, differentiation, and migration. Cell proliferation **is dependent on the integrity of the ECM, and the development of mature cells from stem cells.** There are many different growth factors, some of which act on multiple cell types, while others on specific cell type. Growth factors are usually produced by cells near the site of tissue damage. The main sources of these growth factors are macrophages that are activated by the tissue injury. Others that can produce growth factors include epithelial and stromal cells. Many growth factors bind to ECM proteins and are present at high concentrations at the site of tissue injury. All growth factors activate signaling pathways and cause the cells to undergo cell division. Apart from cell division in response to growth factors, proliferation of residual cells is supplemented by development of mature cells from stem cells, mainly tissue stem cells. These stem cells are present in specialized niches, and injury triggers signals in these niches. This activates quiescent stem cells to proliferate and differentiate into mature cells and repopulate the injured tissue. Major types and properties of stem cells are discussed in detail in pages 342–345.

Cell Proliferation: Signals and Control Mechanisms

The ability of tissues to repair partly depends on their intrinsic proliferative capacity. According to proliferative capacity of the cells, the tissues of the body can be divided into three groups:

1. **Labile (continuously dividing) tissues:** The cells of labile tissues proliferate throughout life, continuously replacing the lost cells by new cells. These new cells are derived from tissue stem cells and rapidly proliferating immature progenitors. The cells of these tissues can regenerate after injury as long as the pool of stem cells is preserved. Examples:
   i. Hematopoietic cells of the bone marrow.
   ii. Surface epithelia: These include the basal layers of the squamous epithelia of the skin, oral cavity, vagina, and cervix.
   iii. Cuboidal epithelia lining the ducts draining exocrine organs (e.g., salivary glands, pancreas, biliary tract).
   iv. Columnar epithelium of the gastrointestinal tract, uterus, and fallopian tubes.
   v. Transitional epithelium of the urinary tract.
2. **Stable (quiescent) tissues:** Cells of stable tissue normally do not proliferate and are in the G_0 stage of the cell cycle. But they are capable of **proliferating in response to injury or loss of tissue** mass. Examples:
   i. **Parenchymal cells** of solid organs: E.g., **liver**, kidneys, and pancreas.
   ii. **Mesenchymal cells:** Fibroblasts, vascular endothelial cells, smooth muscle cells, chondrocytes, and osteocytes. Particularly important in wound healing are endothelial cells, fibroblasts, and smooth muscle cells.
3. **Permanent (nondividing) tissues:** They consist of terminally differentiated nonproliferative cells. These cells **cannot proliferate after birth**. In these tissues, repair is by scar formation. Examples:
   i. **Majority of neurons: Damaged neurons** are **replaced by** the proliferation of the **glial cells**.
   ii. **Cardiac muscle cells**
   iii. **Skeletal muscle cells:** These are usually nondividing, but satellite cells attached to the endomysial sheath have some regenerative capacity for muscle.

Note: Limited stem cell replication and differentiation can occur in some areas of the adult brain, and heart muscle cells can proliferate after myocardial necrosis.

CELL AND TISSUE REGENERATION

Regeneration results in the complete restoration (return) of **an injured** (damaged) **or lost cell and tissue to its original state.** Regeneration is possible if damage is minor, no complications occur, and destroyed tissues are capable of regeneration. It occurs by proliferation of residual uninjured cells and replacement from stem cells. Some tissues are capable to replace the damaged tissue by a process of regeneration and return to a normal state. Regeneration occurs by proliferation of cells that survive the injury and retain the capacity to proliferate. **This proliferation is brought out by growth factors.** For example, skin, intestines, and some parenchymal organs such as liver have capacity to regenerate. In some cases, restoration of damaged tissues is by tissue stem cells. Lower animals like salamanders and fish can regenerate entire limbs or appendages. But in humans, there is limited capacity to regenerate damaged tissues and organs.

Requirements for Regeneration

Regeneration of damaged tissue requires—(1) survival or **integrity of the basement membrane,** (2) **ECM,** (3) **preserved architecture, and** (4) **tissue stem cells** or progenitor cells that can replicate and differentiate.

Cells that Proliferate During Healing

There are many types of cells that proliferate during healing. These include the **remaining cells of the injured tissue** (to restore normal structure), **vascular endothelial cells** (to generate new vessels for supplying the nutrients required for the healing process), and **fibroblasts** (needed for the formation of fibrous tissue to fill defects that cannot be healed by regeneration).

Type of Cells or Tissues Capable of Regeneration

Tissue regeneration can occur in parenchymal organs composed of cells that are capable of proliferation. Regeneration occur in tissues or organs containing **labile cells** (e.g., hematopoietic cells in the bone marrow, surface epithelia) or **stable cells** (e.g., liver, kidney, endothelial cells, fibroblasts). The new cells are derived from tissue stem cells and rapidly proliferating immature progenitors. However, in permanent tissues (e.g., neurons and cardiac muscle cells), the cells cannot regenerate and healing is only by forming scar.

Mechanisms of Tissue Regeneration

Q. Write a short essay on mechanism of regeneration.

Regeneration is the replacement of injured tissues by similarly differentiated tissue. It depends on the type of tissue involved and the severity of injury.

- **Epithelial tissues:** In epithelia of the gastrointestinal tract and skin, injured cells are quickly replaced by proliferation of residual cells and differentiation of cells derived from tissue stem cells. But the underlying basement membrane should be intact for regeneration. The residual epithelial cells produce the growth factors for cell proliferation. The newly produced cells migrate to fill the defect created by the injury, and thereby restore the tissue integrity.
- **Parenchymal organs:** Tissue regeneration can occur in parenchymal organs whose cells are capable of proliferation (i.e., stable cells). However, with the exception of the liver, this is usually not complete but a limited process. Pancreas, adrenal, thyroid, and lung have some amount of regenerative capacity. When kidney is surgically removed, it elicits a compensatory response in the remaining kidney. This consists of both hypertrophy and hyperplasia of proximal duct cells in the kidney. It is absolutely necessary to have structurally intact residual tissue for restoration of normal tissue architecture. By contrast, if the entire tissue is damaged by infection or inflammation, regeneration is incomplete and is associated with scarring.

Liver Regeneration

The human liver has an extraordinary (remarkable or tremendous) capacity to regenerate and hence used as a valuable model for studying the process of regeneration. After partial surgical resection of the liver **(partial hepatectomy)** performed for tumor resection or for living donor hepatic transplantation; the remaining liver grows by compensatory hyperplasia of hepatocytes (regeneration). The mythological image of liver regeneration is the regrowth of the liver of Prometheus. Liver was eaten every day by an eagle sent by Zeus as punishment for stealing the secret of fire, and regrew every night.

For restoration of normal tissue, it is necessary to have structurally intact residual liver tissue. For example, acute chemical injury or fulminant viral hepatitis (e.g., hepatitis A) causes widespread necrosis of hepatocytes. However, if the connective tissue stroma, vasculature and bile ducts survive, liver parenchyma can regenerate to produce restored normal liver. By contrast, chronic injury, liver abscess, chronic viral hepatitis, or alcoholism may be associated with extensive destruction of the liver parenchyma with collapse of the reticulin framework. It leads to scar formation even though the remaining liver cells have the capacity to regenerate.

Two major mechanisms involved in regeneration of the liver are—(1) proliferation of remaining hepatocytes, and (2) repopulation of liver cells from progenitor cells. Which mechanism plays the main role depends on the nature of the injury.

Proliferation of remaining hepatocytes following partial hepatectomy: In humans, resection of up to 90% of the liver can be replaced by proliferation of the residual hepatocytes. The stimulation for proliferation is by cytokines [e.g., interleukin (IL)-6 produced by Kupffer cells], and by growth factors [e.g., hepatocyte growth factor (HGF)] produced by many cell types.

Regeneration following partial hepatectomy occurs in different stages (**Fig. 55**):

- **First or priming phase**: During this phase, cytokines such as IL-6 produced mainly by Kupffer cells act on hepatocytes and make the liver parenchymal cells competent to receive and respond to growth factor signals.

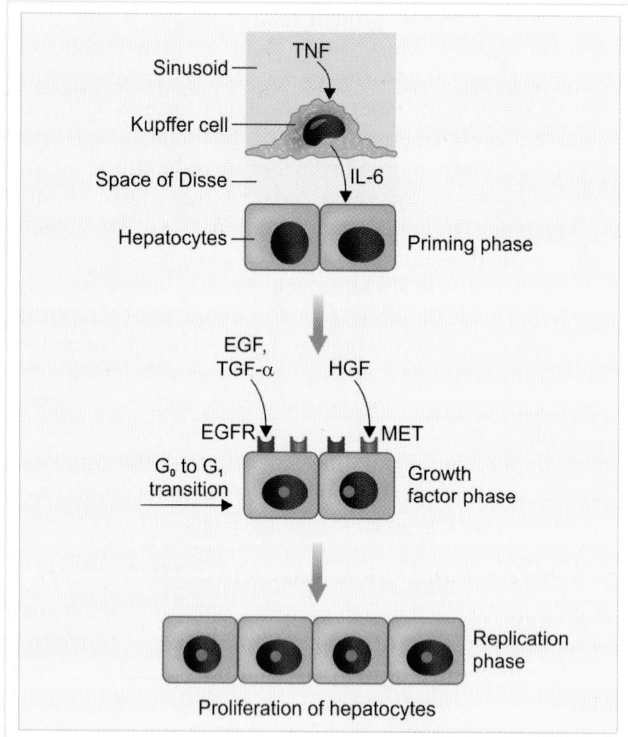

(EGF: epidermal growth factor; EGFR: epidermal growth factor receptor; HGF: hepatocyte growth factor; IL-6: interleukin-6; TGF-α: transforming growth factor-α; TNF: tumor necrosis factor)

FIG. 55: Liver regeneration following partial hepatectomy. The liver regenerates by proliferation of surviving hepatocytes and consists of several phases. Main phase includes (i) priming, (ii) growth factor phase, (iii) replication phase. After the mass of the liver removed by hepatectomy is restored, the proliferation is terminated (not depicted in figure). MET is a receptor tyrosine kinase receptor that binds to its ligand, HGF.

- **Second, or growth factor phase**: During this phase, growth factors such as hepatocyte growth factor (HGF) and TGF-α, produced by many cell types, act on primed hepatocytes. They stimulate hepatocyte metabolism and entry of these hepatocytes into the cell cycle. Since, hepatocytes are quiescent cells, it requires many hours to enter the cell cycle. Thus more time is needed for progression from G_0 to G_1, and reach the S phase of DNA replication.
- **Hepatocyte replication phase**: Almost all hepatocytes replicate during regeneration of liver after partial hepatectomy. During this phase of hepatocyte replication, many genes are activated. Examples include genes encoding transcription factors, cell cycle regulators, regulators of energy metabolism.
- **Replication of nonparenchymal cells**: The hepatocyte proliferation is followed by replication of nonparenchymal cells. These include Kupffer cells, endothelial cells, and stellate cells.
- **Termination phase**: This is the final phase in which hepatocytes return to quiescence phase. Probably antiproliferative cytokines of the TGF-β family are involved in termination signaling.

Liver regeneration from progenitor cells. If there is impairment in the proliferative capacity of hepatocytes (e.g., after chronic liver injury or inflammation of liver), progenitor cells in the liver repopulate the liver cells. In rodents, because of the oval shape of the nuclei of these progenitor cells, they were termed as *oval cells.* Some of these progenitor cells are found in specialized niches called *canals of Hering* (within or peripheral to intralobular bile ducts), where bile canaliculi connect with larger bile ducts and among peribiliary hepatocytes.

REPAIR BY CONNECTIVE TISSUE DEPOSITION

The processes of wound healing involve three basic purposes—(1) fill in, (2) seal, and (3) shrink the wound. Healing may be either by **regeneration or connective tissue deposition or combination of both.** With mild and transient injury, there is regeneration. If the injured tissues are not capable of complete restoration/regeneration, or if the supporting frameworks/structures of the tissue are severely damaged, repair occurs by the connective (fibrous) tissue (forms a *scar*) **or by a combination of regeneration of some residual cells and scar formation.** Repair by connective tissue deposition is the replacement of destroyed tissue with scar tissue. The term *scar* is mostly used in *wound healing* in the skin, but may also be used to describe the replacement of parenchymal cells in any tissue by collagen (e.g., in heart after myocardial infarction). There are two types of reactions in repair—(1) regeneration by proliferation of residual/uninjured/normal cells and maturation of stem cells in tissue, and (2) the deposition of connective tissue which matures to form a scar. Scar tissue is composed of mainly collagen. Though the fibrous scar is not normal, it fills in the lesion and provides or restores sufficient strength (structural stability) to the injured tissue. Though scar is capable of functioning, it may not carry out the original physiologic functions of destroyed tissue.

- **Fibrosis**: The term *fibrosis* is usually applied to describe the extensive deposition of collagen. It is observed in the lungs, liver, kidney, and other organs as a consequence of chronic inflammation, or in the myocardium after extensive myocardial infarction (ischemic necrosis).
- **Organization**: If fibrosis develops in a tissue space occupied by an inflammatory exudate, it is called *organization.* For example, organizing pneumonia of the lung in which inflammatory exudates in the alveoli are replaced by ingrowing capillaries and fibroblasts that mature to form fibrous tissue. Another example is organizing thrombus.

Features that Favor Scarring

Scarring may occur under following conditions:

- Tissue injury or damage is severe, or injury persists (chronic).
- Severe damage to parenchymal cells and epithelia and also the connective tissue framework.
- Nondividing cells are injured.

Steps in Scar Formation

Following injury, wound healing follows many defined sequential steps or events.

Formation of Hemostatic Plug/Clot

Within minutes after injury, a hemostatic plug comprised of platelets is formed at the site of injury. It consists of fibrin clot and is essential to prevent/stop bleeding and also loss of plasma and tissue fluid. Although the clot predominantly consists of plasma fibrin, it also contains the adhesive protein fibronectin. It also provides—(1) a scaffold for infiltrating inflammatory cells, (2) local tensile strength, and (3) maintenance of closure of wound during the evolution of new ECM. A scab or eschar develops after the clot dries on the surface of a wound. It acts as a barrier on wounded skin to invading micro-organisms.

Inflammation

The amount of local tissue destroyed at repair sites vary. For example, a clean surgical incision of a skin lesion has minimal or no devitalized tissue. Medium-sized myocardial infarcts have defined, localized area of necrosis. In contrast, large third-degree burn shows widespread, irregularly defined areas of necrosis. Whenever, there is tissue injury, inflammatory reaction begins which tries to limit the damage and remove the injured tissue. Initially, an acute inflammatory response shows predominance of neutrophils (these are acute inflammatory cells) that are usually present for 6–48 hours (depends on the type of injury) after injury. Activated products of complement, chemokines released from activated platelets, and other mediators produced at the site of injury function as chemotactic agents for inflammatory cells. These chemotactic agents recruit initially neutrophils followed by monocytes during the next 6–48 hours. Neutrophils liquefy the necrotic tissue exudate, and neutrophils may form pus or become trapped in the scab/eschar. These inflammatory cells remove/eliminate/destroy the offending agents (e.g., microbes) that may have entered through the wound, and also clear the debris. Acute inflammation persists as long as necrotic material or bacterial infection persists. Repair can progress only after these elements are removed. **Macrophages play a major role in the repair process** and repair process begins when macrophages predominate at the site of injury. Chemokines facilitate the movement of monocytes from bone marrow to the circulation.

Chemokines and neutrophil granule contents then attract circulating monocytes to the site of injury. Recruited monocytes initially move into tissue and transform into macrophages. Macrophages can assume proinflammatory (M1) or anti-inflammatory (M2) phenotypes. M1 or classically activated macrophages (refer page 309) ingest remnants of neutrophils, clear microbes and necrotic tissue, and also secrete matrix metalloproteinases (MMPs), which facilitate liquefaction. M2 or alternatively activated macrophages secrete growth factors that stimulate the proliferation of fibroblast and many cell types involved in repair. They stimulate collagen secretion, neovascularization, and wound resolution. When the injurious agents and necrotic cells are cleared, the inflammation resolves. Macrophage phagocytosis of apoptotic neutrophils favors their inflammatory to anti-inflammatory transition.

Cell Proliferation

The next stage in repair takes up to 10 days. It involves proliferation of several cell types such as epithelial cells, endothelial and other vascular cells, and fibroblasts. These cells proliferate and migrate to close the wound. Each cell type has particular functions:

- **Epithelial cells:** In response to locally produced growth factors, epithelial cells migrate over the wound to cover it.
- **Endothelial and other vascular cells:** They proliferate and form new blood vessels and this process is termed as angiogenesis (*refer* further).
- **Fibroblasts:** They proliferate and migrate into the site of injury and produce collagen fibers which form scar.

Granulation tissue

The first 24–72 hours of the repair process begins with proliferation of fibroblasts and vascular endothelial cells. A specialized type of tissue, unique and **hallmark (characteristic) of healing wounds,** is formed and is called granulation tissue (**Fig. 56**). This term derives from its pink, soft, glistening, and granular (pebbled) gross appearance of granulation tissue observed below the scab of a skin wound. Granulation tissue is transient, fluid-rich, and specialized tissue of repair. Like a placenta, granulation tissue only develops where and when needed. Granulation tissue grows into the wound from surrounding healthy connective tissue.

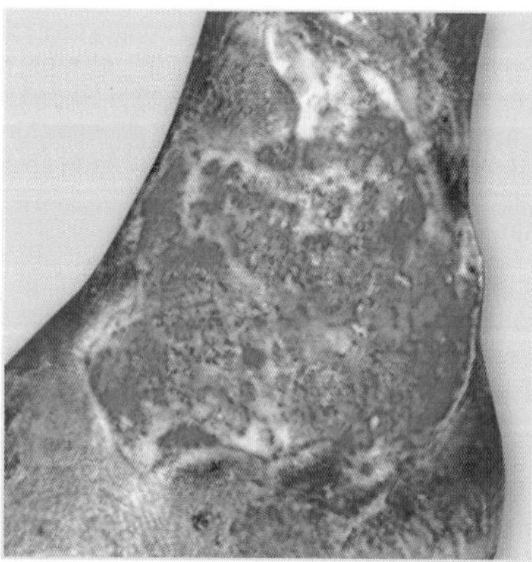

FIG. 56: Pink, soft, granular appearance of granulation tissue on the surface of healing wound.

MORPHOLOGY

Gross: Pink, soft, glistening, and granular (pebbled) on the surface of a healing wound (especially of skin).

Microscopy (Figs. 57A and B) of **granulation tissue consists of combination of proliferating fibroblasts, new blood vessels, loose connective tissue, and interspersed mononuclear leukocytes.**

- **Proliferating fibroblasts**: Fibroblasts also respond early to injury. They secrete collagen and are activated by cytokines such as PDGF, fibroblast growth factor (FGF), transforming growth factor (TGF)-β, etc. Fibroblasts are involved in inflammatory, proliferative and remodeling phases of wound repair. These cells can further differentiate into contractile myofibroblasts.
- **New small blood vessels (angiogenesis)**: These are thin-walled, delicate, leaky capillaries, that allow the passage of plasma proteins and fluid into the extravascular space. This leakage of plasma proteins and fluid is responsible for edema often seen in granulation tissue.
- **Loose connective tissue**: The capillaries of granulation tissue are surrounded by a loose ECM.
- Interspersed mononuclear leukocytes (inflammatory cells), mainly macrophages.

Granulation tissue progressively fills the site of injury. **Amount** of granulation tissue formed depends on the—(1) **size of the tissue deficit** created by the wound and (2) **severity of inflammation**. The cellular constituents of granulation tissue supply immunoglobulins, antibacterial peptides (defensins), and growth factors to the site of injury. It is highly resistant to bacterial infection. This property allows the surgeon to create anastomoses at such nonsterile sites as the colon, in which fully one-third of the fecal contents consist of bacteria.

Deposition of Connective Tissue

Granulation tissue is progressively replaced by deposition of collagen. The amount of connective tissue increases in the granulation tissue as the time progresses. Finally it leads to the formation of a stable fibrous *scar*. This process starts 2–3 weeks after injury and may continue for months or years.

Various steps in wound healing are presented in **Flowchart 10**.

Angiogenesis

Endothelial cell passage during repair through the matrix is an invasive process that requires the co-operation of plasminogen activators, MMPs (metalloproteinases), and integrin receptors. The growth of new capillaries is supported by proliferation and assembly of endothelial cells. There is also a possible contribution of limited numbers of mononuclear, bone marrow-derived endothelial progenitor cells (EPCs), recruited, at least transiently, to support growing vessels.

Definition

Angiogenesis is the process of formation (growth) of new blood vessels from existing vessels.

Angiogenesis is very essential in healing at sites of injury, in the formation of collateral circulations at sites of ischemia, and for increase in the size of tumors beyond the limitation of their original blood supply. Angiogenesis delivers oxygen and nutrients to the site. Much work has been done to

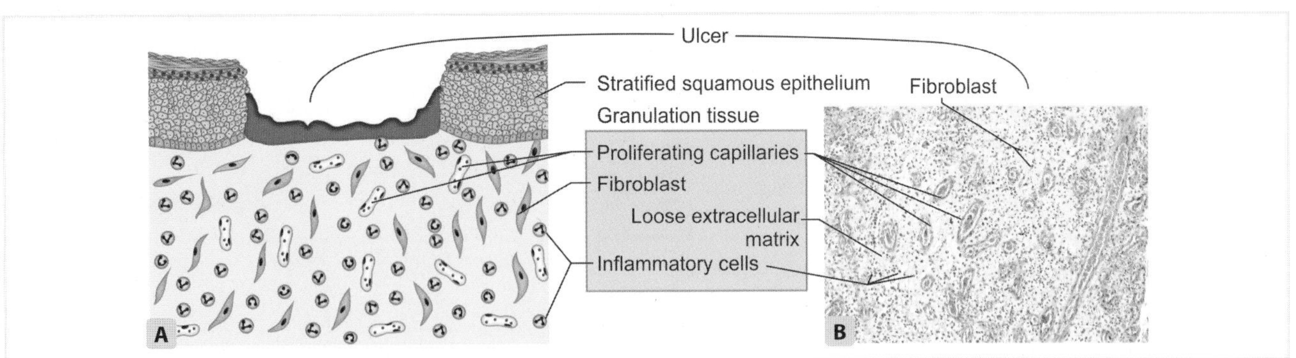

FIGS. 57A AND B: (A) Diagrammatic presentation. (B) Hematoxylin and eosin (H&E). Microscopy of granulation tissue consisting of numerous blood vessels, fibroblasts, and edema.

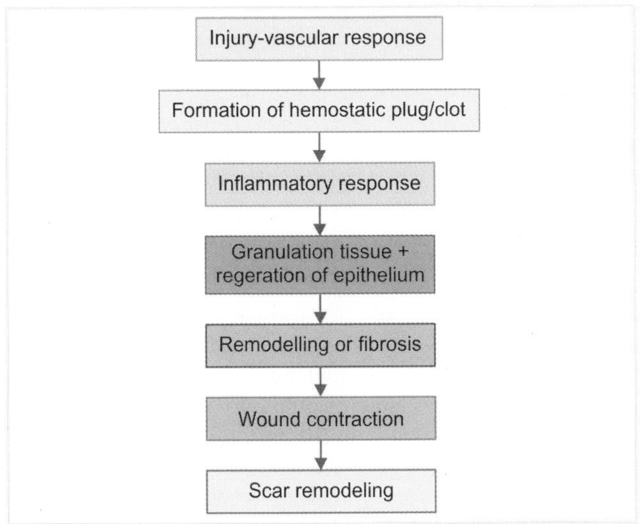

FLOWCHART 10: Various steps in wound healing (e.g., skin wound).

develop therapies to either enhance the angiogenesis process (e.g., to improve blood flow to a heart impaired by coronary atherosclerosis) or to inhibit it (to reduce the growth of tumor or to block pathologic vessel growth, as in wet macular degeneration of the eye).

Steps in Angiogenesis (Figs. 58A to D)

Angiogenesis involves growing of new vessels from existing vessels. Angiogenesis in wound repair is tightly regulated. Various steps in angiogenesis are as follows:

- **Vasodilatation:** It develops in response to nitric oxide (NO) and **increased permeability of the pre-existing vessel caused by vascular endothelial growth factor (VEGF)**.
- **Separation of pericytes** from the abluminal (not adjacent to the lumen) outer surface of blood vessel. Proteolytic enzymes (mediators of angiogenesis) perforate postcapillary venule basement membranes. Breakdown of basement membrane activates quiescent capillary endothelial cells and facilitates formation of a vessel growth. This is characterized by local release of cytokines and growth factors. Disruption or breakdown of basement membranes surrounding endothelial cells and surrounding pericytes determines the sites of endothelial cells growth/sprouting into the surrounding matrix.
- **Migration and proliferation of endothelial cells:** Breakdown of basement membrane leads to reduced adhesion of endothelial cells to their neighboring cells and favors their migration toward the VEGF gradient. This cell is called tip cell (it is the cell that leads to the formation of the new branch) and the endothelial cells that are left behind are called stalk cells. The endothelial cells put out cell extensions, called pseudopodia, that migrate and proliferate from the existing vessel to form capillary sprouts toward the site of injury/wound (angiogenic stimuli). This is brought out by fibroblast growth factors (FGFs), mainly FGF-2. Cytoplasmic flow of endothelial cells enlarges the pseudopodia of endothelial cells, and eventually the cells divide. Vacuoles are formed in the new daughter endothelial cells and they fuse to create new capillary sprouts/tubes with lumen.
- **Maturation of endothelial cells:** Sprout elongation is followed by vessel fusion. Endothelial cells proliferate, loosely following each other, and are presumably guided by pericytes. The entire process continues till the tip cells of blood-vessel sprout encounter another capillary sprout (other vascular branches), with which it will connect. The fusion of migrating tip cells is called anastomosis and is mediated by chaperones.
- **Formation of mature vessel:** Capillary endothelial cells are immobilized when cell–cell contacts form with endothelial cells of another capillary sprout. An organized basement membrane develops on the exterior of the nascent capillary. Maturation of vessel (stabilization) involves the recruitment of pericytes and smooth muscle cells to form the periendothelial layer. Thus, it builds a new circulatory system. At its peak, granulation tissue is the most richly vascularized tissue in the body.
- **Suppression of endothelial proliferation** and migration, and deposition of basement membrane occurs after the formation of new mature capillaries. Once repair is complete, most of the newly formed capillaries undergo apoptosis. It leaves a pale, avascular scar rich in collagen.

During angiogenesis, there is an interplay between endothelial cells and pericytes. To form mature nonleaky capillaries at wound site, it needs endothelial association with pericytes and also signals from angiopoietin I, TGF-β, and PDGF. New capillaries that have not matured are leaky and produce hemorrhage or edema and they may undergo apoptosis.

New capillaries are usually formed by angiogenesis (i.e., sprouting of endothelial cells from pre-existing capillary

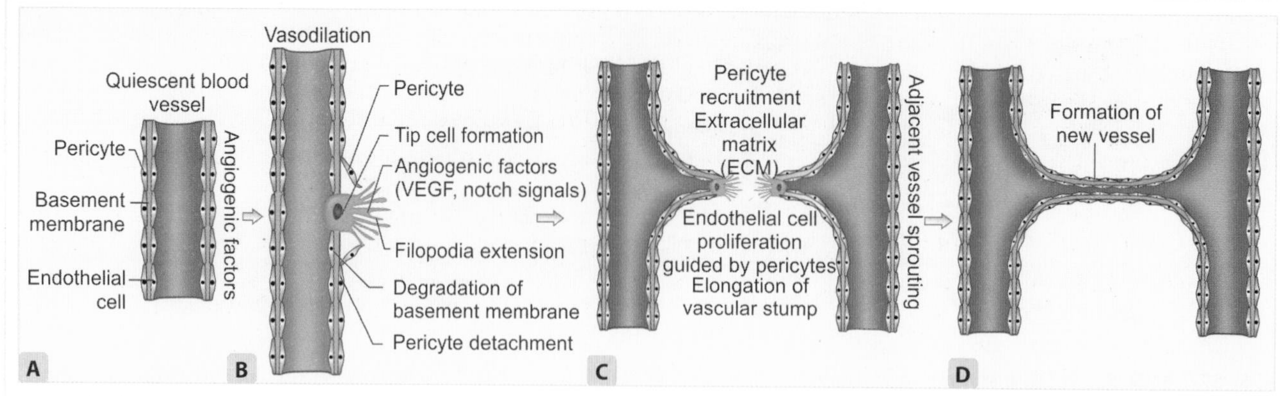

(VEGF: vascular endothelial growth factor)

FIGS. 58A TO D: Mechanism of angiogenesis. (A) Normal blood vessel. (B) Vasodilatation—first, pericytes separate from the outer surface of vessel. Then endothelial cells put out cell extensions, called pseudopodia, that move/grow and proliferate from the existing vessel to form capillary sprouts toward the site of injury/wound (angiogenic stimuli). Cytoplasmic flow enlarges the pseudopodia of endothelial cells, and eventually the cells divide. Vacuoles are formed in the new daughter cells and they fuse to create a new lumen. (C) Endothelial cells proliferate, loosely following each other, and are presumably guided by pericytes. Maturation of vessel (stabilization) involves the recruitment of pericytes and smooth muscle cells to form the periendothelial layer. (D) The entire process continues till the blood-vessel sprouts encounter another capillary sprout, with which it will connect. Thus, it builds a new circulatory system. At its peak, granulation tissue is the most richly vascularized tissue in the body. Once repair is complete, most of the newly formed capillaries undergo apoptosis. It leaves a pale, avascular scar rich in collagen.

venules). Less often, new blood vessels form de novo from angioblasts (EPCs) present in the bone marrow and can be recruited to promote new vessel formation. The latter process is known as vasculogenesis. It is primarily associated with ontogeny (origination and development of an organism) and likely play a minor, if any, role in the angiogenesis associated with the healing of most wounds.

Mechanisms of Angiogenesis

Angiogenesis involves several signaling pathways, cell-cell interactions, ECM proteins, and tissue enzymes.

- **Growth factors: Various growth factors are involved in angiogenesis.**
  - **Vascular endothelial growth factors (VEGFs)**, mainly VEGF-A stimulates both migration and proliferation of endothelial cells. This initiates the process of capillary sprouting in angiogenesis. VEGFs also cause vasodilation by stimulating the production of NO and are also involved in the formation of the vascular lumen in new blood vessels.
  - **Fibroblast growth factors (FGFs),** mainly FGF-2, stimulate the proliferation of endothelial cells. They are also involved in the migration of macrophages and fibroblasts to the damaged site, and stimulate migration of epithelial cells to cover lost epithelium in wound involving epidermis.
  - **Angiopoietins 1 and 2 (Ang 1 and Ang 2)**: These growth factors play a role in angiogenesis and the structural maturation of new vessels.
  - **Growth factors involved in stabilization of blood vessels**: Newly formed blood vessels should be stabilized by the recruitment of pericytes and smooth muscle cells and by the deposition of connective tissue. Multiple growth factors are involved in the stabilization process. These include **PDGF and TGF-β**. PDGF recruits smooth muscle cells whereas TGF-β suppresses endothelial proliferation and migration, and increases the production of ECM proteins.
- **Notch signaling**: Notch signaling pathway "cross talks" with VEGF and regulates the sprouting and branching of new vessels. It ensures that the new formed vessels have the proper spacing so that they can effectively supply blood to the healing tissue. VEGF stimulates the expression of Notch ligands. These ligands bind to the Notch receptor on endothelial cells. Thus, they regulate the pattern of branching of vessels.
- **Extracellular matrix proteins**: ECM proteins **are also involved** in the process of vessel sprouting in angiogenesis. ECM proteins interact with integrin receptors of endothelial cells and **provide the scaffold for vessel growth**.
- **Enzymes in the ECM**: Metalloproteinases (MMPs) are enzymes in ECM that degrade the ECM to permit remodeling and allow extension of the vascular tube.

Edema in healing wounds

Newly formed vessels in angiogenesis are leaky. This is due to incomplete formation of interendothelial junctions and also because VEGF (the growth factor that stimulates angiogenesis) increases vascular permeability. This leakage is partly responsible for the edema that may persist in healing wounds. This edema may persist long after the acute inflammatory response has resolved.

Activation of Fibroblasts and Deposition of Connective Tissue

Formation of connective tissue in healing occurs in two steps—(i) migration and proliferation of fibroblasts into the site of injury and (ii) deposition of ECM proteins synthesized by these cells. These processes are managed by locally produced cytokines and growth factors (e.g., PDGF, FGF-2, and TGF-β).

These factors are mainly derived from inflammatory cells, particularly alternatively activated (M2) macrophages that have migrated to the sites of injury and also present in granulation tissue. The sites of inflammation also contains many mast cells, and may contain lymphocytes. These cells also can secrete cytokines and growth factors. Thus, they may also contribute to proliferation and activation of fibroblast.

Migration and Proliferation of Fibroblasts into the Site of Injury

The cytokines and growth factors stimulate the fibroblasts at the edges of the wound to migrate toward the center. Some fibroblasts may differentiate into cells termed as *myofibroblasts* (discussed in detail below on page 333). These cells contain smooth muscle actin and possess increased contractile activity. This helps to close the wound by pulling its margins toward the center. Both activated fibroblasts and myofibroblasts synthesize increased amount of connective tissue proteins, mainly collagen. Collagen is the major component of the fully developed scar.

Deposition of Extracellular Matrix Proteins

***Transforming growth factor-β* is the most important** cytokine involved in the synthesis and deposition of connective tissue proteins.

- **Synthesis of *TGF*-β:** It is synthesized by most of the cells in granulation tissue, including alternatively activated macrophages. TGF-β levels in tissues are regulated by the post-transcriptional activation, the rate of secretion, and factors in the ECM (mainly integrins), that increase or decrease activity of TGF-β activity. Microfibrils made up of fibrillin also regulate the availability of TGF-β. It is not regulated by the transcription of the TGF-β gene.
- **Actions of TGF-β:** These include—
    - **Stimulates** migration and proliferation **fibroblast.**
    - **Increases the synthesis of collagen and fibronectin.**
    - **Decreases the degradation of ECM** by inhibiting metalloproteinases.
    - **Scar formation and fibrosis**: TGF-β is involved in scar formation after injury. It is also responsible for the development of fibrosis following chronic inflammation in organs such as lung, liver, and kidneys.
    - **Anti-inflammatory effects**: TGF-β also has anti-inflammatory effects. Thus, it limits and terminates inflammatory responses. This is achieved by inhibiting lymphocyte proliferation and the activity of other leukocytes.

Collagen deposition

As healing process progresses, there is decrease in the number of proliferating fibroblasts as well as new vessels. However, the fibroblasts progressively acquire a more synthetic phenotype, and deposit increased amount of ECM. In particular synthesis of collagen is required for the healing wound so that the healed wound is strong and mechanically stable. Synthesis of collagen by fibroblasts starts early in wound healing (days 3–5) and continues for several weeks, depending on the size of the wound. Net amount of collagen accumulated at the wound depends not only on increased synthesis but also on diminished degradation of collagen. When the healing process is complete and scar matures, there is progressive vascular regression. This will convert a highly vascularized granulation tissue into a pale, largely avascular scar.

Connective Tissue Remodeling

Q. Write a short essay on connective tissue remodeling.

The outcome of the repair depends on the balance between synthesis and degradation of ECM proteins. After the formation of scar, there is remodeling (rebuilding) to increase wound strength and to contract the wound.

Increase in wound strength

Wound strength increases due to cross-linking of collagen and increase in size of collagen fibers. There is also a shift of the type of collagen deposited. Though there is a rapid increase in tensile strength at 7–14 days of repair; by the end of 2 weeks, the wound still has a high proportion of type III collagen and has only about 20% of its original strength. Most of the strength of the healed wound is due to synthesis and intermolecular cross-linking of more resilient type I collagen during the remodeling phase. A 2-month-old incision even after healing is still obvious with distinct incision lines and suture marks, vascular and red. In well-sutured wound in the skin and surgical anastomoses in hollow viscera, the wound strength may recover to 70–80% of normal unwounded site by about 3 months. By 1 year, the incision appears white and avascular, but usually still can be identified. As the scar fades further, it usually gets slowly deformed into an irregular line by stresses in the skin.

Wound contraction

One of the characteristics of open wounds is contraction of wound and they may deform as they heal. This depends on the degree of attachment of wound to underlying connective tissue structures. Main role in wound contraction and fibrosis in initial stages is by a specialized cell of granulation tissue called as the myofibroblast. Later, it is due to cross-linking of collagen fibers. As the healing progresses, the connective tissue is degraded and the scar shrinks.

Myofibroblasts Myofibroblasts are modified fibroblast-like cells. They cannot be distinguished from collagen-secreting fibroblasts except by special immunostaining. Myofibroblasts contain abundant actin stress fibers (often α-smooth muscle actin), desmin, vimentin, and a particular fibronectin splice variant (ED-A) that forms polymerized cellular fibronectin. Myofibroblasts possess increased contractile activity and they respond to physical or mechanical forces and agents that cause smooth muscle cells to contract or relax. They appear like fibroblasts but behave like smooth muscle cells. Myofibroblasts along with fibroblasts, contribute to normal wound contraction.

- **Origin:** They are mainly derived by differentiation of fibroblasts. The myofibroblast in wound may also be derived from circulating, marrow-derived fibrocytes and closely related cells in the wound environment, such as perivascular- or perisinusoidal-like pericytes, mesangial cells in the glomerulus, and stellate cells in the liver.

Myofibroblasts usually appear during the 3rd day of wound healing. Then they gradually diminish over the next several weeks. They are associated with an increase in type I collagen and are more prevalent in fibrosis, hypertrophic scars (particularly burn scars), deforming, and pathological wound contracture.

Matrix metalloproteinases (MMPs)

Q. Write a short essay on metalloproteinases (also refer page 477 and 485).

The superfamily of proteinases with the presence of zinc at the catalytic site (metzincins) includes the MMPs and other subfamilies including ADAM (a disintegrin and metalloproteinase) and ADAM with thrombospondin motifs (ADAMTS). MMPs are named so because they are dependent on metal ions (e.g., zinc) for their activity. Members of the metzincin superfamily are the main regulators in tissue during development and remodeling. The degradation of collagens and other ECM components is performed by a family of matrix metalloproteinases (MMPs).

Source of MMPs MMPs are synthesized by different types of cells. These include fibroblasts, macrophages, neutrophils, synovial cells, and few epithelial cells. In contrast to the inflammatory cell proteinases, MMP and ADAM protease activity is only localized. The synthesis and secretion of MMPs are regulated by growth factors, cytokines, and other agents.

Types of MMPs MMPs consist of 25 proteinases with overlapping specificities. Various MMPs include:

- **Interstitial collagenases (MMP-1, MMP-2, and MMP-3)**: They cleave fibrillar collagen.
- **Gelatinases (MMP-2 and 9)**: They degrade amorphous collagen and fibronectin.
- **Stromelysins (MMP-3, -10, and -11)**: They degrade various constituents of ECM such as proteoglycans, laminin, fibronectin, and amorphous collagen.

The activity of the MMPs is tightly controlled. MMPs are produced as inactive precursors (zymogens). Hence, they must be first activated and this is brought out by proteases (e.g., plasmin) presentonly at sites of injury. MMPs aid in migration of cells through the stroma by degrading matrix proteins and thus play main role in wound healing. They are also involved in cell-cell communication and activation or inactivation of bioactive molecules (e.g., immune system components, matrix fragments, growth factors), and influence cell growth and apoptosis.

Inhibitors of metalloproteinases The activity of MMPs is partly controlled or inhibited by a family of specific tissue-based molecules known as tissue inhibitors of metalloproteinases (TIMPs). They are produced by most mesenchymal cells. During formation of scar, MMPs are activated to remodel the deposited ECM, and then they are inactivated by the TIMPs. Thus, a balance between MMPs and TIMPs regulates the size and nature of the scar.

Neutrophil elastase, cathepsin G, plasmin, and other serine proteinases

they can also degrade ECM and are involved in wound debridement during the early phase of healing. They are not important in wound remodeling compared to that of MMPs.

Microscopy of Scar/Fibrosis in Tissues

Components of scar or **fibrosis** in tissues: It is composed of inactive, spindle-shaped fibroblasts, dense collagen, fragments of elastic tissue, and other ECM components.

Connective tissue special stains: To identify different protein constituents of scars and fibrotic tissues, special stains are useful.

- **Trichrome stain**: It contains three stains (hence its name), which stain red cells orange, muscle red, and collagen blue. Thus, it detects collagen fibers in the scar tissue.
- **Elastin stain**: It identifies delicate fibers of elastin, which is the major component of flexible elastic tissue.
- **Reticulin stain**: Reticulin is one of ECM proteins of the connective tissue stroma of normal organs and is also present in early scars. It is composed of type III collagen.

Role of Macrophages in Repair

Macrophages are important cells involved in repair. Their functions in repair include:

- **Clear the offending agents and dead tissue.**
- **Produce growth factors needed for the proliferation of various cells** that promote healing:
  - **Transforming growth factor-β:** It is a cytokine that stimulates fibroblast proliferation into the lesion to synthesize and secrete the collagen precursor procollagen. Thus, it helps in connective tissue synthesis and deposition.
  - **Angiogenesis factors:** These include VEGF and FGF-2. They stimulate vascular endothelial cells to form capillary sprouts/buds that grow into the lesion. Thus, they promote angiogenesis.
  - **Matrix metalloproteinases**: They degrade and remodel ECM proteins (e.g., collagen and fibrin) at the site of damage/injury.
    - **Secrete cytokines required for proliferation of fibroblast and connective tissue synthesis and deposition.**

Macrophages play a main role in repair. They main macrophages involved in repair are the alternatively activated (M2) type. During inflammation, classically activated macrophages (M1 type) dominate and are involved in clearing of microbes and dead tissues. These classically activated M1 type macrophages are gradually replaced by alternatively activated M2 macrophages and terminate inflammation and induce repair.

HEALING OF SKIN WOUNDS

Depending **on the nature and size of the wound** of skin wounds can be classified into two types, namely—(1) healing by first intention (primary union), and (2) healing by second intention (secondary union).

Q. Define the terms "healing", "regeneration", and "repair". Describe the healing of a clean surgical wound/healing by first intention.

Q. Write short essay on healing by first intention.

Healing by Primary Union or by First Intention

Definition

Healing of a **clean, uninfected surgical incision** in the skin joined with surgical sutures is known as healing by **primary union or by first intention.**

In this type of healing, the injury involves only the epithelial layer and the main mechanism of repair is epithelial regeneration. One of the examples is the healing of a clean, uninfected surgical incision approximated by surgical sutures. Surgical incision causes **death of a minimum number** of epithelial and connective tissue **cells**. The **disruption of epithelial basement membrane** continuity is also focal and **minimal**. Re-epithelialization occurs by regeneration and there is a **relatively thin scar** (minimal scarring). This is simplest type of cutaneous wound healing. This type of repair consists of three connected processes—(1) inflammation, (2) proliferation of epithelial and other cells, and (3) maturation of the connective tissue scar.

Stages in the Healing by First Intention (Figs. 59A to D)

First 24 hours

- **Formation of blood clot:** Wounding causes the quick activation of coagulation pathways and produces a blood clot on the surface of a wound. Clot is formed in the space between sutured margins. Blood clot contains not only trapped red cells but also fibrin, fibronectin, and complement components. Clot stops bleeding and acts as a scaffold (temporary platform) for migrating and proliferating cells. The cells are attracted to the site of wound by growth factors, cytokines, and chemokines released into the area. VEGF is also released which causes increased vessel permeability and edema. **Dehydration at the external surface of the clot** leads to formation of a **scab** over the wound.
- **Neutrophil infiltration:** Within 24 hours of wound, **neutrophils** appear at the margins of the incision. Neutrophils use the scaffold produced by the fibrin clot for its migration. They **release proteolytic enzymes which clean out debris.**
- **Epithelial changes:** At the cut edges of the wound, the **basal cells of the epidermis** begin to show increased **mitotic activity**. Epithelial cells from both the edges of wound proliferate and migrate across the wound along the dermis. Within 24–48 hours, epithelial cells from both edges of the wound begin to migrate and proliferate along the dermis. As they progress, the epithelial cells deposit basement membrane components.

Two days

- **Neutrophils are replaced by macrophages. Macrophages play a central cellular role in the repair process.**
- The **epithelial cells** from both sides **fuse in the midline below the surface scab** and epithelial continuity is re-established in the form of a thin continuous surface layer that closes the wound.

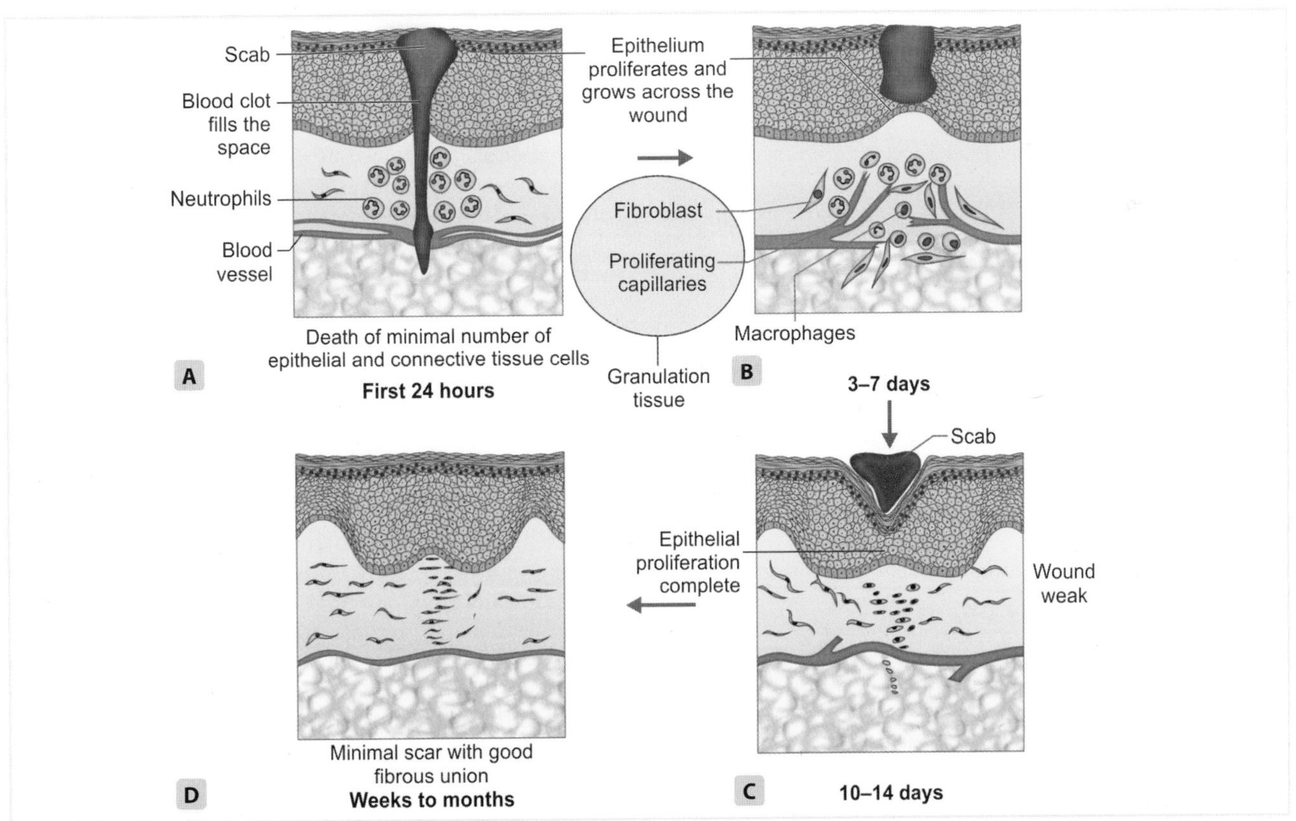

FIGS. 59A TO D: Healing by primary intention. (A) A wound with closely apposed edges and minimal tissue loss. The blood clots and fills the gap between the edges of the wound. (B) Epithelium at the edges proliferates. Minimal amount of granulation tissue is formed. (C) The epithelial proliferation is complete and the wound is weak. (D) Fibrosis with a small scar.

Three to seven days

- Acute **inflammatory response** begins to **subside**. Neutrophils are largely replaced by **macrophages**. These macrophages are key cellular constituents of tissue repair. They clear extracellular debris, fibrin, and other foreign material, and promote angiogenesis and deposition of ECM.
- **Granulation tissue** (neovascularization) begins to invade the incision space. It progressively grows into the **incision space/wound and fills the wound area** by 5–7 days. The newly formed vessels are leaky and allow the passage of plasma proteins and fluid into the extravascular space. Thus, the new granulation tissue is usually edematous.
- **Fibroblasts**: Migration of fibroblasts to the site of injury is stimulated by chemokines, tumor necrosis factor (TNF), PDGF, TGF-β, and FGF. Subsequent proliferation of fibroblast is triggered by multiple growth factors. These include PDGF, epidermal growth factor (EGF), TGF-β, and FGF, and the cytokines IL1 and TNF. The main source of these factors is macrophages, although they may be produced by other inflammatory cells and platelets.
- **Collagen**: The fibroblasts produce ECM proteins, and collagen fibrils are now formed at the incision margins. Collagen is progressively laid down and becomes more abundant and begins to bridge the incision.
- **Surface** epithelial cell proliferation continues and **epidermis** achieves its **normal thickness** and differentiation. It matures with surface keratinization.

Ten to fourteen days

- Leukocytic infiltration, edema, and angiogenesis disappear during the 2nd week.
- **Collagen**: There is continuous **increased accumulation of collagen** and fibroblast proliferation. The **vascular channels** undergo **regression** and increased vascularity, and are markedly reduced. The **granulation tissue scaffolding is converted into a pale, avascular scar.** Wound normally gains about 10% strength of normal skin. Further fibroblast proliferation occurs with collagen deposition.

Weeks to months

- By the end of the 1st month, the **scar** appears as **a cellular** connective tissue covered by intact essentially normal epidermis and without inflammatory infiltrate. However, the skin appendages destroyed in the line of the incision are permanently lost.
- Collagen deposition along the line of stress and **wound gradually achieves maximal 80% of tensile strength** of normal skin.

Healing by Secondary Union or by Second Intention

Q. Write a short essay on healing by second intention.

Definition

When injury produces **large defects** (large wounds) on the skin surface with **extensive loss of cells and tissue**, the healing process is more complicated. Healing in such cutaneous wound is referred to as healing by **secondary union or by second intention.**

Examples include large wounds, abscesses, ulceration, and ischemic necrosis (infarction) in parenchymal organs. They heal by a combination of regeneration and scarring.

Features of Healing by Secondary Intention (Figs. 60A to D)

Secondary healing differs from primary healing in following aspects:

- Larger wounds show **more exudate and necrotic tissue** in the area of wound. The fibrin **clot or scab** formed at the surface of wound is **large**. Full epithelialization of the wound surface is slow because of the larger gap.
- **Severe inflammatory reaction** because of larger defect and greater amount of necrotic tissue, exudate, and fibrin that must be removed. Consequently, they have an increased tendency for secondary, inflammation-mediated injury.
- The **larger defect requires more** amount of (abundant) **granulation tissue to** fill in the gaps and also to provide the underlying framework for the regrowth of tissue epithelium.
- Extensive deposition of collagen and abundant granulation tissue leads to **formation of a large scar**.
- **Wound contraction:** Wound contraction usually occurs in large surface wounds. The contraction reduces the gap between its dermal edges and reduces the surface area of wound. Wound contraction is an important feature in healing by secondary union. It is brought by the action of myofibroblasts. **Myofibroblasts** of granulation tissue **have ultrastructural features of smooth muscle cells**. They contract in the wound tissue and are responsible for wound contraction.
- Initially, the formed provisional matrix contains fibrin, plasma fibronectin, and type III collagen. In about 2 weeks, this is replaced by a matrix mainly composed of type I collagen. Finally, the original granulation tissue is converted into a pale, avascular scar. This scar consists of spindle shaped fibroblasts, dense collagen, fragments of elastic tissue, (devoid of inflammatory infiltrate) and other ECM components. The destroyed dermal appendages in the area of wound are permanently lost.

Wound Strength

Major portion of the connective tissue in repair is fibrillar collagens (mostly type I collagen) and these are responsible for the development of strength in healing wounds.

Time for a skin wound to achieve its maximal strength

- **At the end of the 1st week:** When sutures are removed from an incisional surgical wound, **wound strength** is about **10%** that of normal unwounded skin.
- **Four weeks**: Wound strength quickly increases over the next 4 weeks, and then slows down.
- **Three months:** Wound strength **reaches 70–80% of the tensile strength** of unwounded skin.

Differences between healing by primary and secondary intention are discussed in **Table 37**.

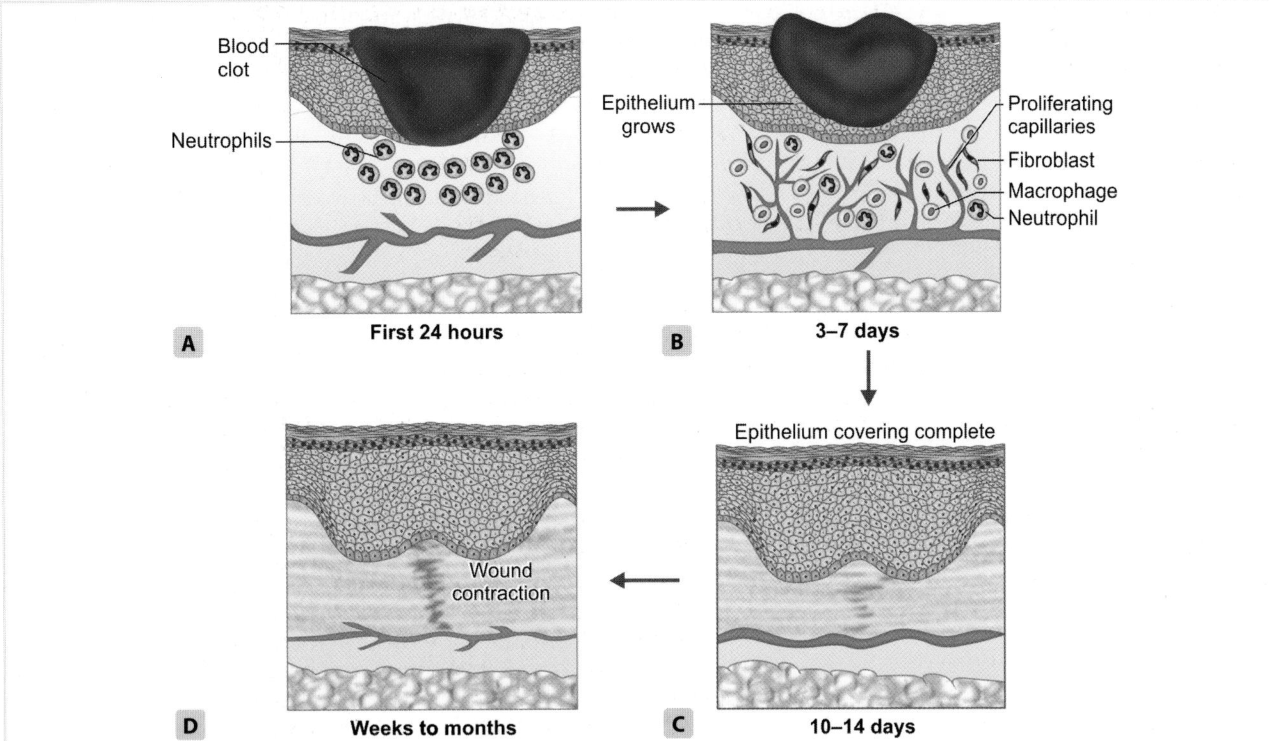

FIGS. 60A TO D: Healing by secondary intention. (A) There is significant loss of tissue and the edges are far apart. Acute inflammation develops both at the edges and base. (B) The cell proliferation starts from the edges and large amount of granulation tissue is formed. (C) The wound is covered on the entire surface by the epithelium. The collagen fibers are deposited. (D) Granulation tissue is replaced by a large scar. There is significant wound contraction.

Table 37: Differences between healing by primary and secondary intention.

Feature	*Primary intention*	*Secondary intention*
Nature of wound	Clean surgical wound	Unclean
Margins	Surgical clean margin	Irregular
Sutures	Used for apposition of margins	Cannot be used
Infection	Absent	May be infected
Amount of granulation tissue	Scanty at the incised gap and along suture track	Abundant and fill the gap
Outcome	Neat linear scar	Irregular contracted scar
Complications	Rare	Infection and suppuration

FACTORS THAT INFLUENCE TISSUE REPAIR

Q. Write a short essay on factors that affect wound healing.

Main three processes in healing are regeneration, repair, and contraction. Any abnormalities in any of the processes can prolong wound healing. Wound healing may be affected by many factors that may reduce the quality or adequacy of the reparative process. Factors affecting healing may be classified as depending on the source of factor extrinsic (e.g., infection) or intrinsic to the injured tissue, and also as systemic or local factors.

Local Factors

Factors that Delay Wound Healing

- **Infection:** It is the single most important cause for delay in healing. Infection causes persistent tissue injury and inflammation.
- **Mechanical factors: Movement of wounded area** may compress the blood vessels and separate the edges of the wound and can result in delayed healing. Increased local pressure or torsion may cause wounds to pull apart (dehisce) and delay healing.
- **Foreign bodies:** Unnecessary sutures or foreign bodies (fragments of steel, glass), or bone can delay healing.
- **Size, type of wound, and extent of tissue injury:** Large excisional wounds or wounds caused by blunt trauma delay healing. Complete restoration can occur only in tissues composed of cells capable of proliferating (labile or stable cells); but in these tissues, extensive injury will lead to incomplete regeneration and partial loss of function. Injury to tissues composed of nondividing (permanent) cells result in scarring (e.g., healing of a myocardial infarct).
- **Location of injury/wound:** It also affects healing. Wound over the skin covering bone with little intervening tissue between skin and bone prevents wound contraction

(e.g., skin over the anterior tibia). The edges of skin lesions (e.g., burns) in such locations cannot be brought together and usually require skin grafts. The character of the tissue in which the injury occurs also is important. For example, small inflammatory exudates in tissue spaces (e.g., pleural, peritoneal, synovial cavities), may be resorbed and digested by the proteolytic enzymes of leukocytes. This will result in resolution of inflammation and restoration of normal tissue architecture. However, when the exudate is large enough to be fully resorbed, it undergoes organization. During organization, granulation tissue grows into the exudate, and ultimately forms a fibrous scar.

- **Poor perfusion/blood supply:** It may be either due to poor arterial supply (e.g., arteriosclerosis) or obstructed venous drainage (e.g., in varicose veins).
  - **Varicose veins** of the legs occur due to failure of the venous valves needed for proper venous return and there is decrease in the venous drainage. Varicose veins can cause edema and produce venous stasis—nonhealing ulcers (venous stasis ulcers) in the leg (usually on the inner aspect of the lower leg).
  - **Bed/pressure sores (decubitus ulcers**) result due to prolonged, localized, dependent pressure. It reduces both arterial and venous blood flow and results in intermittent ischemia.
  - **Peripheral vascular disease**, e.g. arteriosclerosis.
  - **Wounds in lower extremities** (e.g., foot) **of diabetics** usually heal poorly or may even need amputation. This is due to the advanced atherosclerosis of blood vessels in the legs (peripheral vascular disease) and defective angiogenesis which reduce the blood supply and impair repair.
  - Joint (articular) cartilage is avascular and has limited diffusion capacity. Usually it does not produce intense inflammatory response. Thus, repair of articular cartilage occurs poorly in response to progressive, age-related wear and tear.
- Ionizing radiation decreases repair process
- Complications may delay wound healing
- **Excessive bleeding at the wound site:** It prolongs healing. Large clots increase the amount of space that has to be filled by granulation tissue. It also serves as mechanical barrier to oxygen diffusion and blood clot is an excellent culture medium for bacteria. It promotes infection and prolongs inflammation by increasing exudation and formation of pus.

Factors that Favor Wound Healing

- **Size and type of wound:** Small surgical incisional or other injuries heal quickly with less scar formation.
- **Blood supply:** Wounds in areas with **good blood supply,** such as the face, heal **faster than** those with **poor blood supply**, such as the foot.
- **Type of tissue injured:** Complete restoration can occur when there is mild injury to tissues composed of labile (e.g., skin) and stable (e.g. hepatocytes) cells than permanent cells (e.g., myocardial infarct).

Systemic Factors that Impair Tissue Repair

- **Nutritional deficiencies:** Metabolic needs increase during all phases of healing. Hence, optimal nutrition is important and **nutritional status** has serious effects on repair, Nutritional deficiencies delay wound healing. These nutritional deficiencies include:
  - **Protein deficiency**: Hypoproteinemia (e.g., malnutrition) impairs fibroblast proliferation and collagen synthesis. Malnutrition increases risk for wound infection, delays healing, and reduces wound tensile strength.
  - **Vitamin C and A deficiency**: These are cofactors required for collagen synthesis. Prolonged lack of these vitamins inhibits collagen synthesis with poor formation of connective tissue and retard healing.
  - **Trace elements**: Copper, zinc, iron, and manganese are also required as cofactors for collagen synthesis.
- **Age**: Wound healing is rapid in young compared to in aged individuals. Though no specific effect of age alone on repair has been found, aging reduces the stem cell reserves. Scarring is maximum during adolescence and diminishes with age. Healing also declines in postmenopausal women.
- **Metabolic status: Diabetes mellitus** is a metabolic disease associated with delayed healing due to many reasons. Wounds are usually ischemic because of microangiopathy (small-vessel disease) that impairs the microcirculation. Altered (glycosylated) hemoglobin that is increased in diabetics, has an increased affinity for oxygen and thus does not readily release oxygen in tissues. Hyperglycemia also suppresses macrophages and increases the risk for wound infection. Leukocytes require glucose to produce adenosine triphosphate (ATP) that is needed for chemotaxis, phagocytosis, intercellular killing, and initiation of healing. Hence, the wounds heal poorly in diabetics who receive insufficient insulin.
- **Circulatory status: Inadequate blood supply** (due to arteriosclerosis) or venous abnormalities (e.g., varicose veins) that retard venous drainage, delay healing.
- **Glucocorticoids (steroids)**: Exogenous corticosteroids have **anti-inflammatory effects** and also inhibit collagen and protein synthesis, thereby **impair wound healing**. It suppresses both destructive and constructive aspects of inflammation. Administration of steroids may produce weak scars because they inhibit TGF-β synthesis and diminish fibrosis. However, sometimes the anti-inflammatory effects of glucocorticoids are essential. For example, in infections of cornea, use of glucocorticoids (along with antibiotics) will reduce the possibility of opacity due to collagen deposition.
- **Hematological abnormalities**: Quantitative or qualitative defects in neutrophils and bleeding disorders and anemia may slow the healing process.
- **Reduced circulating blood volume**: It inhibits inflammation because of constriction of vessel rather than the required vasodilation to deliver inflammatory cells, nutrients, and oxygen to the site of injury.
- **Obesity**: It can also delay wound healing by impairing leukocyte function and predisposition to infection, decreasing the number of growth factors, and increasing

the levels of proinflammatory cytokines. It is also associated with impaired synthesis of collagen and a decrease in angiogenesis.

COMPLICATIONS OF TISSUE REPAIR

Q. Write a short essay on complications of wound healing/repair.

Complications in wound healing can be due to abnormalities in any of the basic processes involved in healing. These include formation of a deficient scar, excessive formation of the repair components, and formation of contractures. Clinical examples of abnormal wound healing and scarring are discussed here.

Defects in Healing: Chronic Wounds

Defects in healing and chronic wounds are observed in numerous clinical situations and are due to local and systemic factors. Wounds can ulcerate if blood supply is inadequate or if vascularization is insufficient during healing. Common examples are as follows.

- **Venous leg ulcers**: They occur usually in elderly individuals with chronic venous hypertension. This may be due to severe varicose veins or congestive heart failure. These ulcers fail to heal because of poor oxygen supply to the site of the ulcer. Ulcers may show deposits of iron pigment (hemosiderin) resulting from breakdown of red blood cells (RBCs), and may be accompanied by chronic inflammation.
- **Arterial ulcers**: They occur in people with atherosclerosis of peripheral arteries or peripheral arterial disease, especially associated with diabetes. The ischemia causes atrophy followed by necrosis of the skin and underlying tissues. These ulcers develop on the outer part of the lower leg or the foot and are accompanied by pain.
- **Pressure sores**: These are characterized by areas of ulceration and necrosis of skin and underlying tissues due to prolonged compression of tissues against a bone. For example, in bedridden, immobile elderly people with many morbidities. The sores are caused by mechanical pressure and local ischemia.
- **Diabetic ulcers**: They develop in the lower extremities, especially the feet. Diabetes is accompanied by small vessel disease (microangiopathy) that produces ischemia. Other factors such as diabetic peripheral neuropathy (renders the patient insensitive to the progressing ulcer), systemic metabolic abnormalities, and secondary infections are additional factors that contribute to ulcer formation. These produce necrosis of tissue and there is failure to heal. Microscopically, they are characterized by ulceration of epithelium and abundant granulation tissue in the underlying dermis. Diabetes also reduces expression of and cellular responsiveness to growth factors and decreases the healing process. If the ulceration is left unchecked, it proceeds to infection of the underlying bone (osteomyelitis) and progressive loss of the extremity.
- **Neuropathic or trophic ulcers**: Nonhealing wounds also develop in regions devoid of sensation because of trauma or pressure. Such decubitus ulcers (consequence of lying or sitting in one position too long) are common in patients who are immobilized in either beds or wheelchairs. Constant pressure as little as 2–3 hours on the skin over a bony process can produce a local infarct. These ulcers can be both broad and deep, with infection involving into the underlying connective tissue. Neuropathic or trophic ulcers may be seen in diabetic peripheral neuropathy and nerve damage from leprosy.

Inadequate Granulation Tissue Formation

Inadequate formation of granulation tissue or an inability to form a suitable ECM can lead to a **deficient scar formation**. It can produce complications, namely **wound dehiscence** and **incisional hernia**.

Dehiscence (the wound splitting open) or rupture of a wound is most frequent and can be a life-threatening complication after abdominal surgery. In sutured closed wounds, the dehiscence is characterized by pulling apart of wound at the suture line. Dehiscence usually occurs 5–12 days after suturing, when collagen synthesis is at its peak. It is due to local factors such as failure of healing, wound infection, increased abdominal pressure/mechanical stress (strain) on the abdominal wound from vomiting, coughing, pathologic obesity, bowel obstruction or ileus. Obesity can also increase the risk for dehiscence because adipose tissue is difficult to suture. Systemic factors predisposing to wound dehiscence include metabolic deficiency, hypoproteinemia, and the general inactivity that is usually found in metastatic cancer. Wound dehiscence usually is indicated by increased serous drainage from the wound and the patient's feel that "something gave way". It needs prompt surgical attention.

Incisional hernia results from weak scars of the abdominal wall due to a defect caused by prior surgery. They are due to insufficient deposition of ECM or inadequate crosslinking in the collagen matrix. Loops of intestine may be trapped within incisional hernias.

Excessive Scar Formation

Excessive formation of the components of the repair process (i.e., ECM, mostly excessive collagen) at the wound site can result in:

- **Hypertrophic scar**: The accumulation of excessive amounts of ECM, mostly collagen may give rise to a raised scar at the site of wound known as a hypertrophic scar. A hypertrophic scar is raised but remains within the original boundaries of the wound. They usually grow rapidly and contain numerous myofibroblasts, but tend to regress over several months. They usually develop after thermal or traumatic injury, which involves the deep layers of the dermis. They are not associated with race or heredity (in contrast to keloids), but the severity of scarring can decline with age. The scar is restricted within the wound margins, and the development of the scar is usually associated with unrelieved mechanical stress. Hypertrophic scars are usually pruritic (itchy due to activation of mast cells producing histamine) and have a red appearance due to hypervascularity.
- **Keloid**: When the scar tissue grows/progresses beyond the boundaries of the original wound and does not regress, it is termed as a keloid (**Fig. 61**). Thus, keloid is an exuberant/raised, ugly scar that extends beyond the original boundaries of the wound. It recurs with still larger keloid after attempts at surgical excision. Thus, they have properties akin to a benign tumor. Keloids usually develop

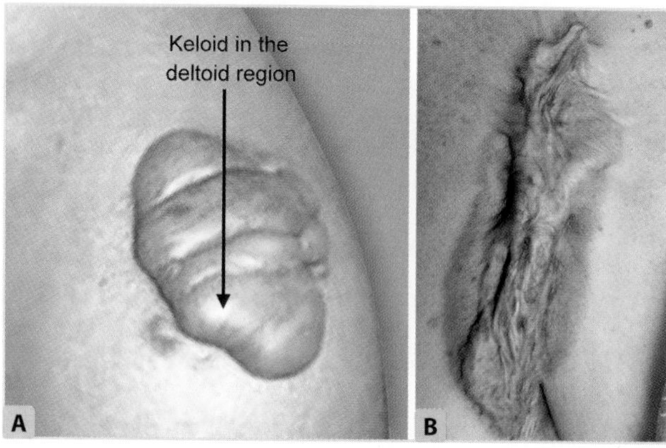

FIG. 61A AND B: (A) Keloid in the upper arm. (B) Large keloid in the sternal region following thoracic surgery.

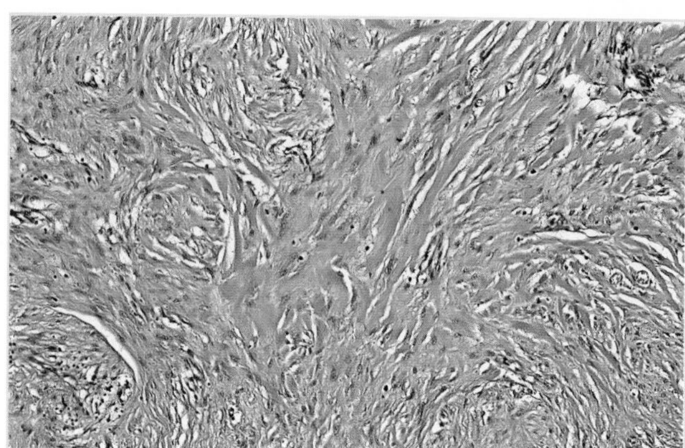

FIG. 62: Microscopic appearance of a keloid. Shows thick haphazardly arranged broad bands of collagen deposits in the dermis.

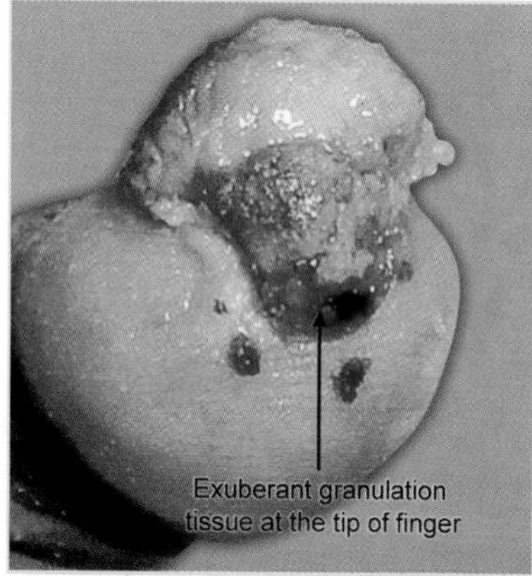

FIG. 63: Exuberant granulation tissue at the tip of the finger.

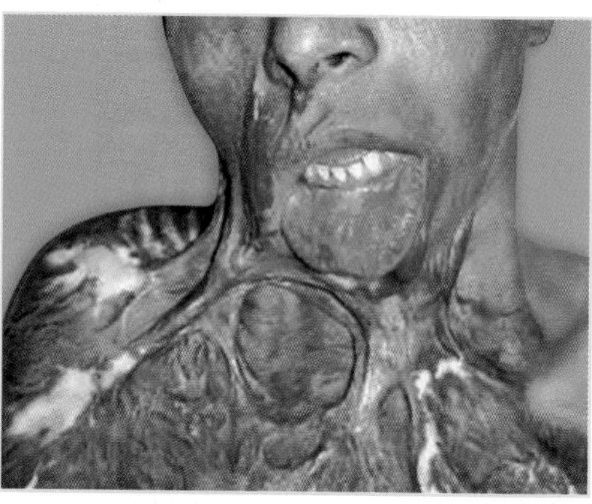

FIG. 64: Wound contracture—severe contracture of a wound on neck and the right side of neck.

during adolescence and early adulthood and involve the upper trunk, neck and head, with the exception of the scalp. Dark-skinned individuals are more prone to developing a keloid, suggesting a genetic basis for this condition. Unlike normal scars, keloids do not reduce collagen synthesis if glucocorticoids are administered. Microscopically, they are composed of haphazardly arranged broad bands of collagen (**Fig. 62**).

- **Exuberant granulation**: It is characterized by the formation of excessive amounts of granulation tissue.

Pyogenic granuloma or granuloma pyogenicum (Fig. 63)

- This consists of the localized formation of excessive amounts of granulation tissue.
- Such exuberant granulation tissue projects above the level of the surrounding skin and prevents re-epithelialization. This mass formed is often named as proud flesh. Excessive granulation must be removed either by cautery or surgical excision for restoration of epithelial continuity (i.e., for re-epithelialization).

Desmoids or aggressive fibromatoses

- Incisional scars or traumatic injuries may be followed by excessive proliferation of fibroblasts and other connective tissue components.
- They are known as desmoids, or aggressive fibromatoses. These are neoplasms that lie at the gray zone of benign and malignant low-grade tumors. They may usually recur after excision.

Excessive Contraction

- A decrease in the size of a wound due to myofibroblasts is known as wound **contraction**. It is an important part of the normal healing process.
- An exaggeration of this contraction is termed **contracture** and produces severe deformities of the wound and the surrounding tissues.
- Site: Contractures are prone to develop on regions that normally show minimal wound contraction. These sites include the palms, the soles, and the anterior aspect of the thorax. Examples of internal contractures include duodenal strictures following healing of a peptic ulcer; esophageal strictures caused by chemical burns, and abdominal adhesions caused by surgery, infection, or radiation. Contracture in cirrhosis of the liver, constricts vascular flow and contributes to the development of portal hypertension and esophageal varices.
- Consequences of contractures:

- ○ **Compromised movements** [e.g., contractures that follow severe burns can compromise the movement of the involved region (**Fig. 64**) and joint movements].
- ○ **Obstruction** [e.g., gastrointestinal tract contracture (stricture) can cause intestinal obstruction].

Many diseases are characterized by contracture and irreversible fibrosis of the superficial fascia. Examples include Dupuytren contracture (palmar contracture), Lederhosen disease (plantar contracture) and Peyronie disease (contracture of the cavernous tissues of the penis). These contractures have no known etiological agent or precipitating injury, even though the basic process of their development is similar to contracture in wound healing.

Others

- **Infection** of wound by microbes.
- **Epidermal cysts** can develop due to persistence of epithelial cells at the site of wound healing.
- **Pigmentation** may develop due to either colored particles left in the wound or due to hemosiderin pigment.
- **Neoplasia** (e.g., squamous cell carcinoma may develop in Marjolin's ulcer, which is the scar that follows burns in skin).

Fibrosis in Parenchymal Organs

Scar and Fibrosis

Fibrosis is the pathologic process characterized by **the excessive**/abnormal **deposition of collagen and other ECM components in a tissue.** Fibrosis is produced due to persistent injurious stimuli such as chronic infections and immunologic reactions. Most often fibrosis is associated with loss of tissue and occurs in internal organs in chronic diseases. The terms *scar* and *fibrosis* may be used interchangeably and the basic mechanisms of fibrosis and formation of scar are the same as those in the skin during tissue repair. **TGF-β is an important fibrogenic agent.**

Fibrotic Disorders

Fibrosis in parenchymal organs may alter their complex structure and is responsible for substantial organ dysfunction. It may even lead to organ failure. For example, persistent inflammation within the pericardium produces fibrous adhesions, which can lead to constrictive pericarditis and heart failure. Examples are:

- Myocardial infarction: In the heart, scar/fibrosis of a myocardial infarction prevents rupture of the heart, but it reduces the amount of contractile tissue. If it is extensive, it may cause congestive heart failure or lead to a ventricular aneurysm.
- Aortic aneurysm: If aorta is weakened and scarred by atherosclerosis, it can produce dilatation (i.e., aneurysm).
- Fibrosis/scarring of heart valves: Mitral and aortic valves injured by rheumatic fever are often stenotic, regurgitant, or both. This can lead to congestive heart failure.
- Other examples: These include cirrhosis of liver, systemic sclerosis (scleroderma), fibrosing diseases of the lung (idiopathic pulmonary fibrosis, pneumoconiosis, and drug- or radiation-induced pulmonary fibrosis), end-stage kidney disease, and constrictive pericarditis.

Factors that affect wound healing are listed in **Table 38.**

Complications of wound healing are shown in **Flowchart 11.**

Table 38: Factors that affect wound healing.

Factors that Delay Wound Healing	
Local factors	***Systemic factors***
• Infection • Mechanical factors • Foreign bodies • Large excisional wounds or wounds caused by blunt trauma • Wounds located in sites where edges cannot be brought together • Poor perfusion • Ionizing radiation • Complications of wound healing	• Poor general health (nutritional deficiencies): Protein deficiency (e.g., malnutrition), vitamin C deficiency, and deficiency of trace elements • Old age • Metabolic status, e.g., diabetes mellitus • Circulatory status, e.g., inadequate blood supply • Drugs, e.g., glucocorticoids • Quantitative or qualitative defects in neutrophils and bleeding disorders
Factors that Favor Wound Healing	
Local factors	***Systemic factors***
• Small surgical incisional or other injuries • Wounds in areas with good blood supply (e.g., face) • Mild injury to tissues composed of labile (e.g., skin) and stable (e.g. hepatocytes) cells • Wounds in which edges are closely brought together	• Good general health (adequate nutrition) • Younger age • Good circulatory status

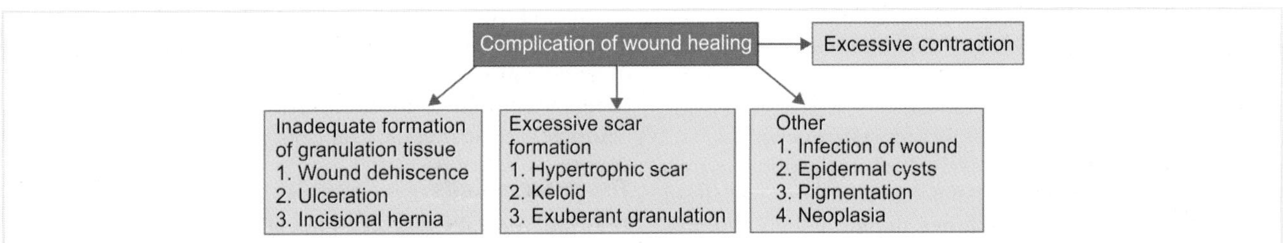

FLOWCHART 11: Complicationsof wound healing.

8.9 Stem Cells

CHAPTER OUTLINE

- Stem cells
  - Defining properties of stem cells
  - Types of stem cells
  - Hematopoietic stem cell (HSC)
  - Mesenchymal stem cells (MSCs)
  - Regenerative medicine
  - Induced pluripotent stem cells

STEM CELLS

Q. Discuss stem cells.

One of the puzzles is—how is a complex multicellular organism generated from a single fertilized egg? The adult human body is composed of several hundred types of well-differentiated cells. During development, totipotent stem cells can give rise to all types of differentiated tissues. Most of the specialized, differentiated (well/fully differentiated) cells are not capable/unable of cell division. These specialized cells need continual replacement. This is true for RBCs, the epidermal cells in the upper layers of the skin, and the absorptive and goblet cells of the gut epithelium. Such cells are termed as *terminally differentiated*—they lie at the dead end of their developmental pathway. However, they can be replaced by the proliferation of a subpopulation of small number of long-lived, unspecialized (less differentiated), self-renewing cells called **stem cells**. These **stem cells are present in various adult tissues**. Because stem cells retain the capacity to proliferate and replace differentiated cells throughout the life, they play an important role in the maintenance of most tissues and organs. **Stems cells have the capacity to replace damaged cells and maintain cell populations within the tissues where they reside.** In normal tissues (without healing, degeneration, or neoplasia), there is a homeostatic equilibrium between the replication, self-renewal, and differentiation of stem cells and the death of the mature, fully differentiated cells (**Fig. 65**).

Defining Properties of Stem Cells

Under conditions of homeostasis, stem cells have following important properties:

- **Not terminally differentiated:** Stem cell is not itself terminally differentiated (i.e., it is not at the end of a pathway of differentiation).
- **Capacity for self-renewal:** It can **divide without limit** (or at least for the lifetime of the individual). Self-renewal permits stem cells to maintain their numbers. Self-renewal may follow either asymmetric or symmetric division. In contrast to stem cells, **progenitor** cells (transit amplifying cells) **have little or no capability for self-renewal**.
- **Asymmetric division:** It refers to cell replication in which one daughter cell differentiates into a mature specialized cell types, whereas the other daughter cell remains undifferentiated and retains its self-renewal capacity (i.e., remains as a stem cell). Because of this self-renewing population of stem cells, they can serve as a source for the production of differentiated cells throughout life.

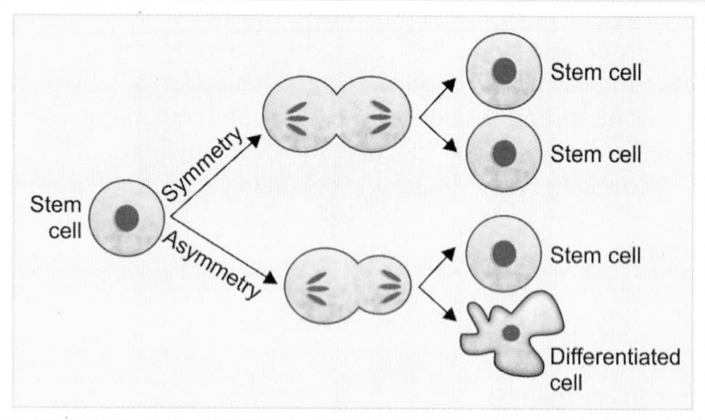

FIG. 65: Asymmetric and symmetric division of stem cells. Asymmetric division gives rise to one stem cell and other differentiated cells, whereas symmetric division gives rise to two stem cells.

Note: In **symmetric division**, both daughter cells retain self-renewal capacity (i.e., as stem cells). Such symmetric divisions are seen early in embryogenesis (i.e., when there is expansion of stem cell populations). It can also occur under conditions of stress, such as in the bone marrow following chemotherapy.

Types of Stem Cells

There are mainly two varieties of stem cells.

Embryonic Stem Cells (ES cells)

These are the most undifferentiated. They are present in the inner cell mass of the preimplantation blastocyst. They have almost limitless cell renewal capacity, and can give rise to every cell in the body. Thus, they are said to be **totipotent** (**Fig. 66**). ES cells can be maintained for extended periods without differentiating by culturing in vitro. After culture of these cells, they can form specialized cells of all three germ cell layers (namely ectoderm, mesoderm and endoderm) including neurons, cardiac muscle, liver cells, and pancreatic islet cells.

Tissue Stem Cells

They are also called **adult stem cells** and are found in many adult tissues, intimately associated with the differentiated cells of a given tissue. They have been identified even in tissues not

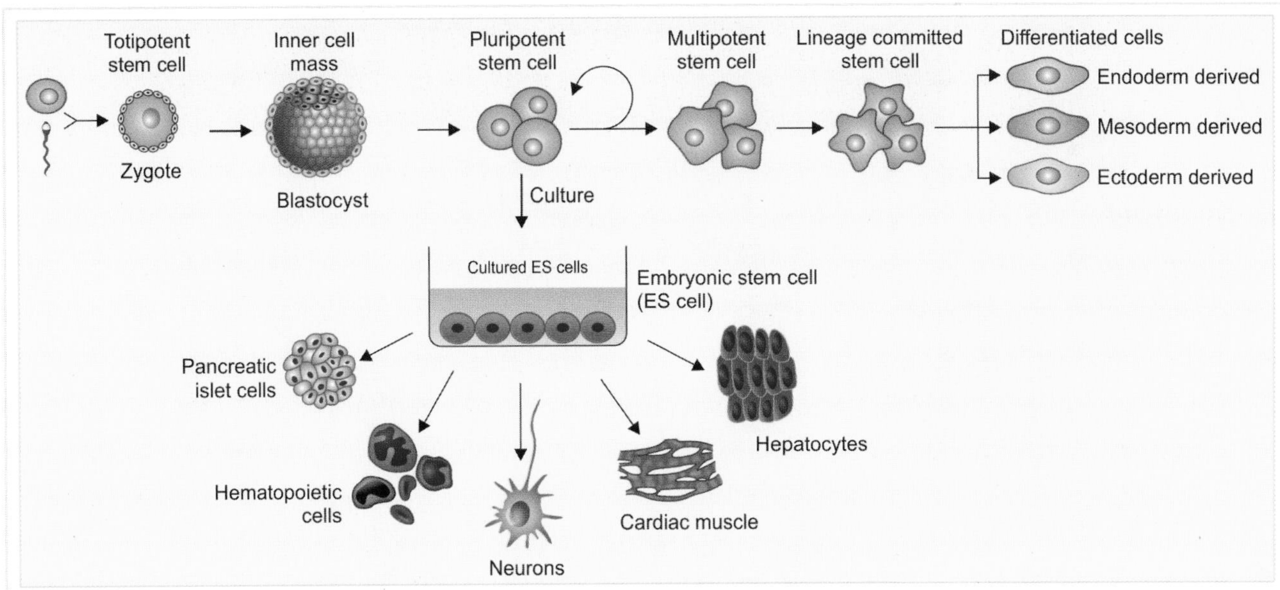

FIG. 66: Embryonic stem (ES) cells. The zygote is formed by the union of sperm and egg. It divides to form blastocysts, and the inner cell mass of the blastocyst produces the embryo. The pluripotent cells of the inner cell mass are known as ES cells. ES cells can be induced to differentiate into cells of multiple lineages. In the embryo, pluripotent stem cells can asymmetrically divide to give rise to a residual stable pool of ES cells and also generate populations that have progressively more restricted developmental capacity. It can give rise to differentiated cells derived from three lineages (three germ cell layers ecto-, endo-, and mesoderm). ES cells can be cultured in vitro and be induced to give rise to cells of all three lineages.

known to regenerate. Adult stem cells have a more restricted range of cell differentiation than ES cells. Features and common properties of adult stem cells are presented in **Boxes 20** and **21**, respectively. Although adult stem cells are capable of maintaining tissues with high (e.g., skin and gastrointestinal tract) or low (e.g., endothelium) cell turnover, the adult stem cells can usually produce only cells that are normal constituents of that particular tissue (i.e., tissue-specific regeneration).

Stem cells niches

The stem cells are normally protected within suitable, specialized tissue microenvironments called *stem cell niches*. They have been detected in many organs such as the bone marrow, where hematopoietic stem cells (HSCs) are gathered in a perivascular niche. These stem cells are kept in inactive state (i.e., quiescent) by the soluble factors and other cells within the niches. When there is a necessity, they expand and differentiate from the precursor pool.

Skin Cornified skin epithelium and hair follicles regenerate from stem cells in basal epidermis and the bulge region of the hair follicle (**Fig. 67A**).

Intestine Intestinal epithelium, normally undergoes rapid turnover and it is replaced by intestinal stem cells present in the crypts of Lieberkühn (**Fig. 67B**).

Other sites Other niches for stem cells include the limbus of the cornea; the canals of Hering in the liver; and the subventricular zone in the brain.

Specific Signals Maintain Stem Cell Populations

Every stem cell system needs control mechanisms to make sure that new differentiated cells are produced in the appropriate places and in the right numbers. The controls depend on extracellular signals exchanged between the stem cells, their progeny, and other cell types. These signals, and the intracellular signaling pathways they activate, belong to a few basic signaling mechanisms. For example, a class of signal molecules known as the Wnt proteins serves to promote the proliferation of the stem cells and precursor cells at the base of each intestinal crypt (**Fig. 68**).

Box 20: Features of tissue or adult stem cells.

- Any organ or tissue may have more than one type of stem cell
- Similar stem cells may be found in different organs
- A stem cell found in tissue may be derived or originated from the bone marrow

Box 21: Common properties of tissue or adult stem cells.

- Capable of division without limit, able to avoid senescence and maintain genomic integrity. However, they have limited capacity of differentiated cells than that of embryonic stem cells
- Capable of undergoing intermittent division or to remain quiescent
- Capable to propagate by self-renewal and differentiation of daughter cells
- No lineage markers available
- Specific anatomic localization in some tissues

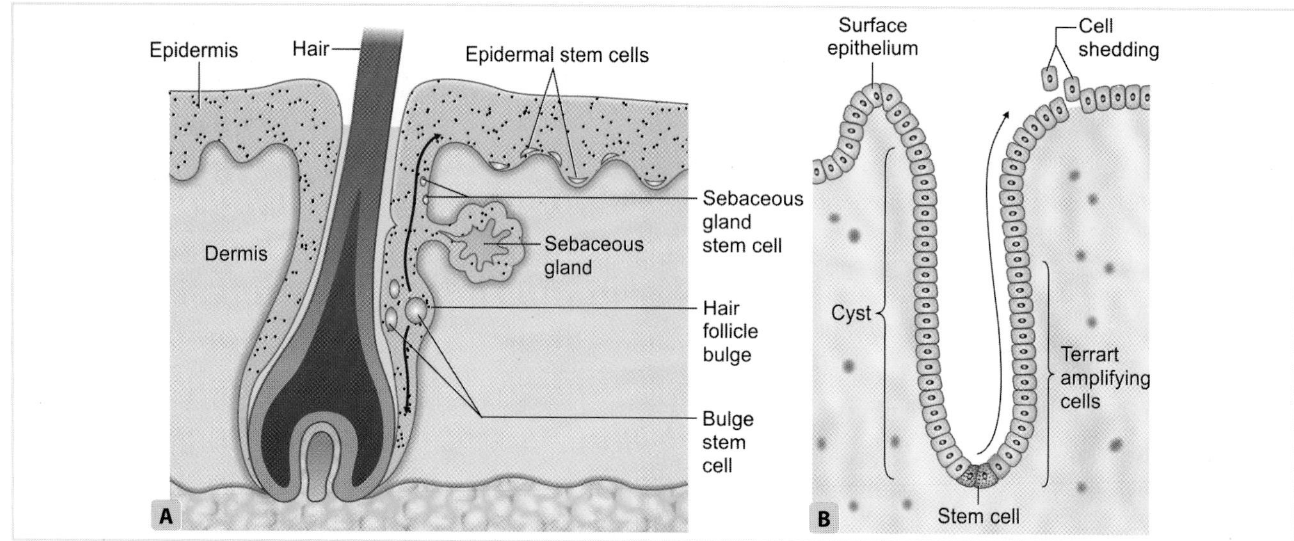

FIGS. 67A AND B: Diagrammatic representation of location of stem cell niches. (A) In small intestine, stem cells are seen at the bottom of the intestinal crypt. (B) In skin, stem cells are located in the bulge area of the hair follicle, in sebaceous glands, and in the lower layer of the epidermis.

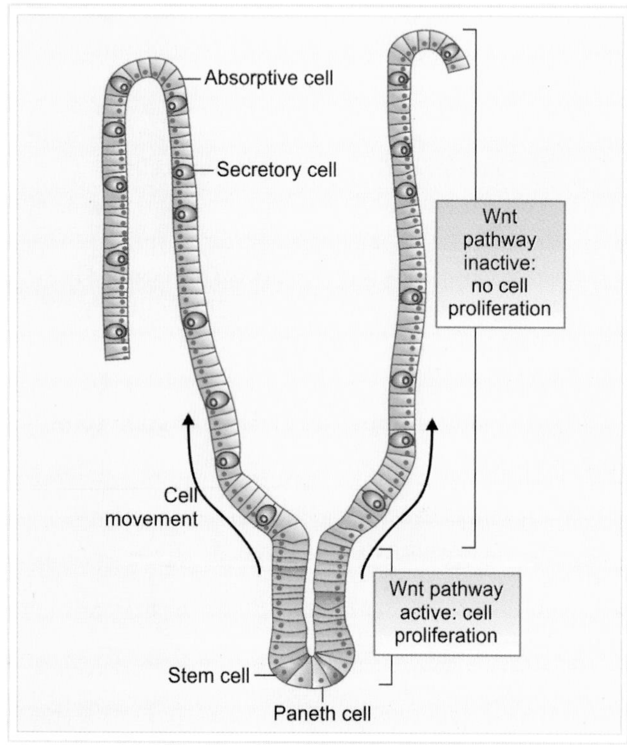

FIG. 68: Control of stem cells in the intestinal crypt. The Wnt signaling pathway maintains the proliferation of the stem cells and precursor cells. The Wnt proteins are secreted by cells in and around the crypt base (e.g., Paneth cells—a subclass of terminally differentiated secretory cells that are generated from the gut stem cells) that activate stem cell proliferation.

Hematopoietic Stem Cell (HSC)

Bone marrow contains hematopoietic, mesenchymal, and endothelial stem cells. HSCs continuously replace all the cellular elements of the blood as they are consumed. HSCs are lineage restricted and can only form all the cells found in blood. They can be obtained directly from bone marrow and also from the peripheral blood after administration of certain colony stimulating factors (CSF). These CSF induce the release of HSCs from bone marrow niches. HSCs can be purified based on cell surface markers. HSCs can be used to repopulate marrows depleted after chemotherapy (e.g., for leukemia), or to provide normal precursors to correct various blood cell disorders (e.g., sickle cell disease).

Mesenchymal Stem Cells (MSCs)

Apart from HSCs, the bone marrow (and other tissues such as fat) also contains a population of MSCs. These are bone marrow stromal cells and are multipotent stem cells. They can mobilize into the bloodstream and be recruited to (injured) organs. MSCs can be induced to differentiate into multiple or variety of stromal cells types. Thus, they can differentiate into chondrocytes (cartilage), osteocytes (bone), adipocytes (fat), and myocytes (muscle). These cells can be expanded to large numbers. Hence, they can be used as a potential means of manufacturing the stromal scaffolding needed for tissue regeneration. MSCs can also be found in cord blood and many other connective tissues.

Endothelial progenitor stem cells from bone marrow can produce tissue angiogenesis and may supplement endothelial hyperplasia during regeneration of blood vessels.

A well-established clinical application of adult stem cells is HSC transplantation (or bone marrow transplantation). It plays an important role in the treatment of many cancers.

Uses of Stem Cells

- Stem cells can proliferate indefinitely and produce progeny that differentiate and hence, help in continual renewal of normal tissue. Stem cells can be **used to repair lost or damaged tissues** through injury. For example, HSC transplantation can be used to treat human leukemia (following bone marrow damage by irradiation or cytotoxic drugs used for treating leukemia).
- Induced pluripotent stem (iPS) cells (refer further) can provide a convenient source of human ES-like cells. They can be used to produce large, homogeneous populations of differentiated human cells of specific types in culture. Such cells can be **used to test for potential toxic or beneficial effects of candidate drugs**.
- It is possible to produce iPS cells from patients with genetic disease and to use these iPS cells to produce affected, differentiated cell types. These cells can then be studied to learn more about the **disease mechanism** and to **search for potential treatments**.
- Pluripotent stem cells can form organoids: Under appropriate conditions, ES cells and iPS cells can proliferate, differentiate, and self-assemble in culture to form miniature, three-dimensional organs called organoids. It closely resembles the normal organ in its organization. The development of iPS cells and organoid technology may help us to **study human development and disease**. It also promises as a progress towards use for treatment.

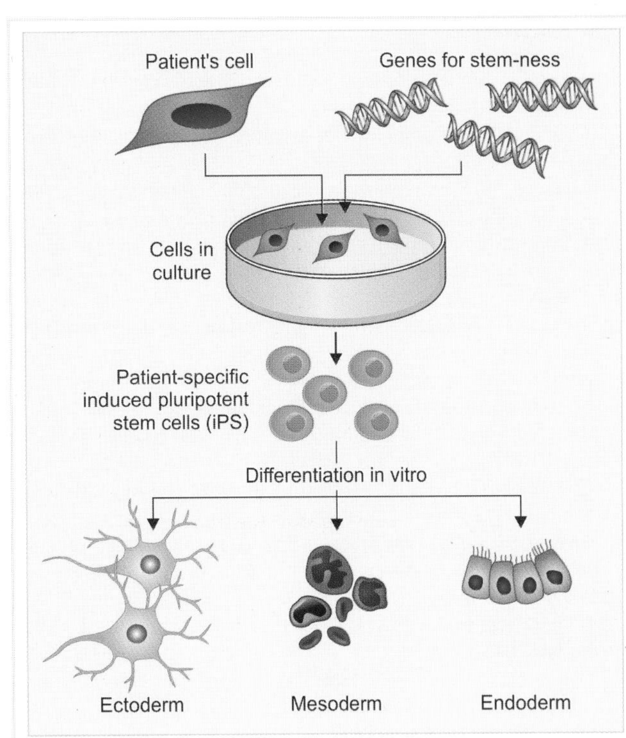

FIG. 69: Steps in the production of induced pluripotent stem cells (iPS cells). They are being produced by introducing genes that are responsible for stem cell properties (stem-ness) into a patient's fully differentiated cells. This, on culture, gives rise to induced pluripotent stem cells (iPS). These iPS can be induced to differentiate into various lineages (ectoderm, mesoderm, or endoderm).

Regenerative Medicine

The achievements in ability to identify, separate/isolate, expand, and transplant stem cells have given birth to a new field of medicine called as regenerative medicine. It is an area of medicine in which there is a potential to fully heal damaged tissues and organs by using stem cells. Theoretically, repopulation of damaged tissues or construction of entire organs can be done by using stem cell replacement by either differentiated progeny of ES or adult stem cells. The therapeutic restoration of damaged tissues having low intrinsic regenerative capacity, such as myocardium after a myocardial infarct or neurons after a stroke is challenging. Unfortunately, in spite of improving capability to purify and expand stem cell populations, the enthusiasm has not been successful due to the difficulties encountered in introducing and functionally integrating the replacement stem cells into sites of damage.

Induced Pluripotent Stem Cells

There are both technical and ethical difficulties in the obtaining ES cells. More recently, pluripotential cells resembling ES cells have been produced. As a major advance, in somatic cell nuclear transfer, the adult somatic cells can be directly converted to pluripotent stem cells in culture. This provides a direct mechanism for converting somatic cells to stem cells. These stem cells, similar to ES cells, have the potential to develop into all tissues of an organism.

Procedure

To obtain such stem cells, few genes have been identified whose products can remarkably reprogram somatic cells to achieve the "stem-ness" of ES cells. These genes are introduced into patient's fully differentiated cells (e.g., fibroblasts). This, on culture, gives rise to iPS cells although at low frequency. These stem cells are called as *iPS cells* (**Fig. 69**). These iPS-like ES cells, are capable of differentiating into all cell types. Thus, iPS cells can be induced to differentiate into various lineages (ectoderm, mesoderm, or endoderm).

Advantages of iPS Cells

One of advantages of iPS cells is that they and their differentiated progeny can be engrafted without eliciting an immunologically mediated rejection. This is because these cells are derived from the patient's own self. For example, in a patient with diabetes, the differentiated progeny of iPS cell is insulin-secreting β-cells. In contrast to iPS cells, if the differentiated cells were derived from ES cells obtained from another donor, it can elicit an immunologically mediated rejection reaction.

BIBLIOGRAPHY

1. Aird W C. Endothelial Cells in Health and Disease. London: Taylor & Francis Group; 2005.
2. Alitalo K. The lymphatic vasculature in disease. *Nat Med.* 2011;17:1371-80.
3. Alvarado AS, Yamanaka S. Rethinking differentiation: stem cells, regeneration, and plasticity. *Cell.* 2014;157:110.
4. Aziz M, Jacob A, Yang WL, et al. Current trends in inflammatory and immunomodulatory mediators in sepsis. *J Leukoc Biol.* 2013;93: 329-42.
5. Blau HM, Daley GQ. Stem cells in the treatment of disease. *N Engl J Med.* 2019;380:1748.
6. Bohlson SS, Garred P, Kemper C, Tenner A. Complement Nomenclature—Deconvoluted, Front. Immunol. 10:1308 ,2019. https://doi.org/10.3389/fimmu.2019.01308 [Last accessed on 2021 February 5].
7. Castanheira FVS, Kubes P. Neutrophils and NETs in modulating acute and chronic inflammation. *Blood.* 2019;133:2178-85.
8. Chavan SS, Pavlov VA, Tracey KJ. Mechanisms and therapeutic relevance of neuro-immune communication. *Immunity.* 2017;46:927-42.
9. De Los Angeles A, Ferrari F, Xi R, et al. Hallmarks of pluripotency. *Nature.* 2015;525:469.
10. Dennis EA, Norris PC. Eicosanoid storm in infection and inflammation. *Nat Rev Immunol.* 2015;15:511.
11. Di Gennaro A, Haeggström JZ. The leukotrienes: immune-modulating lipid mediators of disease. *Adv Immunol.* 2012; 116:51-92.
12. Duffield JS, Lupher M, Thannickal VJ, et al. Host responses in tissue repair and fibrosis. *Annu Rev Pathol.* 2013;8:241-76.
13. Eming SA, Martin P, Tomic-Canic M. Wound repair and regeneration: mechanisms, signaling, and translation. *Sci Transl Med.* 2014;6:265r6.
14. Flannagan RS, Jaumouillé V, Grinstein S. The cell biology of phagocytosis. *Annu Rev Pathol.* 2012;7:61-98.
15. Friedman SL, Sheppard D, Duffield JS, et al. Therapy for fibrotic diseases: nearing the starting line. *Sci Transl Med.* 2013;5:167sr1.
16. Fuchs E, Chen T. A matter of life and death: self-renewal in stem cells. *EMBO Rep.* 2013;14:39.
17. Griffith JW, Sokol CL, Luster AD. Chemokines and chemokine receptors: positioning cells for host defense and immunity. *Annu Rev Immunol.* 2014;32:659-702.
18. Holers VM. Complement and its receptors: new insights into human disease. *Annu Rev Immunol.* 2015;32:433-59.
19. Jang S, Collin del Hortet A, Soto-Gutierrezy A. Induced pluripotent stem cell-derived endothelial cells: overview, current advances, applications, and future directions. *Am J Pathol.* 2019;189:502.
20. Kerrigan MJ, Naik P. C1 esterase inhibitor deficiency. Treasure Island (FL): Stat Pearls Publishing; 2020
21. Klingberg F, Hinz B, White ES. The myofibroblast matrix: implications for tissue repair and fibrosis. *J Pathol.* 2013; 229: 298-309.
22. Kolaczkowska E, Kubes P. Neutrophil recruitment and function in health and inflammation. *Nat Rev Immunol.* 2013;13:159-75.
23. Kotas ME, Medzhitov R. Homeostasis, inflammation, and disease susceptibility. *Cell.* 2015;160:816-827.
24. Kourtzelis I, Mitroulis I, von Renesse J, et al. From leukocyte recruitment to resolution of inflammation: the cardinal role of integrins. *J Leukoc Biol.* 2017;102:677-83.
25. Kumar V, Abbas AK, Aster JC. Robbins basic pathology, 10th edition. Philadelphia: Saunders Elsevier; 2018
26. Kumar V, Abbas AK, Fausto N, et al. Robbins and Cotran pathologic basis of disease, 10th edition. Philadelphia: WB Saunders; 2021.
27. Manthiram K, Zhou Q, Aksentijevich I, et al. The monogenic autoinflammatory diseases define new pathways in human innate immunity and inflammation. *Nat Immunol.* 2017;18: 832-842.
28. Mantovani A, Biswas SK, Galdiero MR, et al. Macrophage plasticity and polarization in tissue repair and remodelling. *J Pathol.* 2013;229:176-185.
29. Martello G, Smith A. The nature of embryonic stem cells, Annu Rev Cell Dev Biol 30:647, 2014Mayadas TN, Cullere X, Lowell CA: The multifaceted functions of neutrophils. *Annu Rev Pathol.* 2014;9:181.
30. McEver RP. Selectins: initiators of leukocyte adhesion and signalling at the vascular wall. *Cardiovasc Res.* 2015; 107:331-9.
31. Muller WA. Mechanisms of leukocyte transendothelial migration. *Annu Rev Pathol.* 2011;6:323.
32. Murawala P, Tanaka EM, Currie JD. Regeneration: the ultimate example of wound healing. *Semin Cell Dev Biol.* 2012;23:954-62.
33. Nagy JA, Dvorak AM, Dvorak HF. VEGF-A and the induction of pathological angiogenesis. *Annu Rev Pathol.* 2007;2:251-75.
34. Nathan C, Cunningham-Bussel A. Beyond oxidative stress: an immunologist's guide to reactive oxygen species. *Nat Rev Immunol.* 2013;13:349-61.
35. Nathan C, Ding A. Nonresolving inflammation. *Cell.* 2010;140: 871-82.
36. Novak ML, Koh TJ. Macrophage phenotypes during tissue repair. *J Leukoc Biol.* 2013;93:875-81.
37. Preedy VR. Adhesive molecule. New Hampshire: CRC Press;2010.
38. Preziosi ME, Monga SP. Update on the mechanisms of liver regeneration. *Semin Liver Dis.* 2017;37:141-51.
39. Rathinam VA, Fitzgerald KA. Inflammasome complexes: emerging mechanisms and effector functions. *Cell.* 2016;165:792-800.
40. Ricklin D, Lambris JD. Complement in immune and inflammatory disorders. *J Immunol.* 2013;190:3831-9.
41. Rock KL, Latz E, Ontiveros F, et al. The sterile inflammatory response. *Annu Rev Immunol.* 2010;28:321-42.
42. Scadden DT. Nice neighborhood: emerging concepts of the stem cell niche. *Cell.* 2014;157:41.
43. Schmidt S, Moser M, Sperandio M. The molecular basis of leukocyte recruitment and its deficiencies. *Mol Immunol.* 2013;55:49-58.
44. Sica A, Mantovani A. Macrophage plasticity and polarization: in vivo veritas. *J Clin Invest.* 2012;122:787-95.
45. Sollberger G, Tilley DO, Zychlinsky A. Neutrophil extracellular traps: the biology of chromatin externalization. *Dev Cell.* 2018;44: 542–553.
46. Stearns-Kurosawa DJ, Osuchowski MF, Valentine C, et al. The pathogenesis of sepsis. *Annu Rev Pathol.* 2011;6:19-48.
47. Strayer DS, Saffitz JE. Rubin's Pathology: Mechanism of Human Disease, 8th edition. Philadelphia: Wolters Kluwer; 2020.
48. Takeuchi O, Akira S. Pattern recognition receptors and inflammation. *Cell.* 2010;140:805.
49. Vestweber D. Relevance of endothelial junctions in leukocyte extravasation and vascular permeability. *Ann N Y Acad Sci.* 2012;1257:184-192.
50. Wick G, Grundtman C, Mayerl C, et al. The immunology of fibrosis. *Annu Rev Immunol.* 2013;31:107-135.
51. Wu J, Izpisua Belmonte JC. Stem cells: a renaissance in human biology research. *Cell.* 2016;165:1572.
52. Wynn TA, Ramalingam TR. Mechanisms of fibrosis: therapeutic translation for fibrotic disease. *Nat Med.* 2012;18:1028-40.
53. Wynn TA, Vannella KM. Macrophages in tissue repair, regeneration, and fibrosis. *Immunity.* 2016;44:450-462.
54. Zlotnik A, Yoshie O. The chemokine superfamily revisited. *Immunity.* 2012;36:705–716.

CHAPTER

9

Hemodynamic Disorders, Thromboembolism, and Shock

CHAPTER OUTLINE

- Introduction
- Edema
  - Definition
  - Types of edema fluid
  - Pathophysiologic categories of edema
  - Mechanism/pathogenesis of edema
  - Increased hydrostatic pressure
  - Decreased plasma osmotic pressure
  - Sodium and water retention
  - Lymphatic obstruction
  - Clinical consequences
  - Special categories of edema
  - Clinical features of pulmonary edema
- Disorders of perfusion
  - Hyperemia
  - Congestion
  - Hemorrhage
- Normal hemostasis
  - Steps in hemostasis
  - Components of normal hemostasis
  - Disorders of hemostasis
- Thrombosis
  - Definition
  - Etiology
  - Terminology of thrombus
  - Fate of thrombus
- Venous thrombosis (phlebothrombosis)
  - Veins involved
  - Pathogenesis of deep vein thrombosis (phlebothrombosis)
  - Thrombophlebitis
  - Consequences of thrombi
- Disseminated intravascular coagulation
  - Etiology
  - Pathogenesis
  - Clinical features
  - Laboratory findings in DIC
- Embolism
  - Definition
  - Types of emboli
  - Pulmonary embolism
  - Systemic thromboembolism
  - Fat and marrow embolism
  - Air embolism
  - Amniotic fluid embolism
  - Miscellaneous pulmonary emboli
- Infarction
  - Definition
  - Causes of infarction
  - Factors that influence the development of an infarct
  - Classification
  - Septic infarctions
  - Infarction in specific locations
- Shock
  - Introduction
  - Definition
  - Classification
  - Etiology and pathogenesis
  - Pathogenesis of septic shock
  - Stages of shock
  - Clinical consequences
  - Prognosis
- Multiorgan system failure

INTRODUCTION

Blood circulation delivers oxygen and nutrients and removes wastes produced by cellular metabolism. Thus, the health of cells and tissues depends on the adequate circulation of blood. Normally, as the blood passes through microvasculature (capillary beds), proteins present in the plasma are retained within the vasculature. There is little net movement of water and electrolytes into the interstitial tissues. This water and electrolyte balance can be affected by various pathologic conditions. These include conditions that alter endothelial function, increases vascular hydrostatic pressure, or decreases plasma protein content. All these lead to edema. Edema is characterized by the excessive accumulation of fluid in interstitial tissues due to net movement of water into extravascular spaces. Depending on severity and location of edema, it may produce minimal or severe effects. For example, edema of the lower limbs may produce only little discomfort where as pulmonary edema (i.e., edema in the lungs) produces accumulation of edema fluid in the alveoli and can result in life-threatening hypoxia.

Table 1: Special forms of edema.

Terminology	*Body cavity involved*
Hydrothorax	Pleural cavity
Hydropericardium	Pericardial cavity
Hydroperitoneum (ascites)	Peritoneal cavity

EDEMA

Q. Write a short essay on mechanisms of edema formation.

Definition

An abnormal accumulation of fluid in the interstitial space within tissues **or body cavities (effusions)** is called edema.

Special forms of edema are listed in **Table 1**.

Water constitutes 50% to 70% of the body weight. It is divided into intracellular and extracellular fluid (ECF). The extracellular is further divided into interstitial and intravascular component. The interstitium contains about 75% of extracellular fluid (ECF).

Types of Edema Fluid

Edema may be **inflammatory or noninflammatory**. The edema fluid may be either transudate or exudate. The differences between transudate and exudate are presented in Table 7 of Chapter 8.

- **Transudate:** It is protein-poor fluid caused by increased hydrostatic pressure or reduced plasma protein.
  - **Causes:** Transudate is observed in heart failure, renal failure, hepatic failure, and certain forms of malnutrition.
- **Exudate:** It is **protein-rich fluid** produced due to increased vascular permeability and is seen in **inflammation**.

Pathophysiologic Categories of Edema (Table 2)

Edema may be localized or generalized in distribution.

Local/Localized Edema

It is limited to an organ or part (e.g., arm, leg, epiglottis, and larynx). Its various causes are as follows:

Table 2: Pathophysiologic categories of edema.

Mechanism	*Causes*
Increased hydrostatic pressure	**Impaired venous return** • Generalized ○ Congestive heart failure ○ Constrictive pericarditis • Regional ○ Ascites in cirrhosis ○ Obstruction (e.g., thrombosis) or compression of veins (e.g., external mass) ○ Arteriolar dilation: Heat, neurohumoral dysregulation
Decreased plasma osmotic pressure (hypoproteinemia)	• Nephrotic syndrome • Ascites in cirrhosis of liver • Malnutrition • Protein-losing gastroenteropathy
Lymphatic obstruction	• Inflammatory • Neoplastic • Postirradiation • Postsurgical
Inflammation	Acute and chronic inflammation, angiogenesis
Sodium retention	• Excessive salt intake with renal insufficiency • Increased tubular reabsorption of sodium: Renal hypoperfusion, increased renin–angiotensin–aldosterone secretion

- **Obstruction of vein or lymphatic** examples include: edema of limb (usually the leg) develops due to venous or lymphatic obstruction caused by **thrombophlebitis, chronic lymphangitis, resection of regional lymph nodes, filariasis**.
- **Inflammation:** It is the **most common cause** of local edema.
- **Immune reaction** examples include: Urticaria (hives), or edema of the epiglottis or larynx (angioneurotic edema).

Generalized Edema

It is systemic in distribution and affects visceral organs and the skin of the trunk and lower extremities. Anasarca is the term used for generalized edema, with conspicuous accumulation of fluid in subcutaneous tissues, visceral organs, and body cavities.

Causes: It is caused due to **disorders that disturb cardio-vascular, renal, or hepatic function and also disorders of** fluid and electrolyte metabolism.

- Heart failure
- Nephrotic syndrome (renal diseases with massive loss of serum proteins into the urine)
- Cirrhosis of the liver.

Mechanism/Pathogenesis of Edema

Normal Fluid Balance

- The smallest vessels of the vascular system and the lymphatic vessels are termed as the *microcirculation*. Normally, the water and salts flows out from the arteriolar end of the microcirculation into the interstitium. This is balanced by flowing in of the water and salts at the venular end.
- As fluid moves through the interstitial space, most of it returns to the capillary bed. Normally, a small amount of fluid (approximately 10% of the fluid) is left in the interstitium and is drained (absorbed) by the adjacent lymphatic vessels, and it reaches the general bloodstream via the thoracic duct. Thus, this mechanism keeps the tissues "dry".
- The movement of water and salts between the intravascular and interstitial spaces is controlled by four distinct forces or pressures. These include: (1) vascular hydrostatic pressure, (2) interstitial fluid colloid osmotic pressure, (3) plasma colloid osmotic pressure, and (4) interstitial fluid pressure. This delicate balance of forces is summarized by **Starling's hypothesis (Fig. 1)**. According to this, the net filtration is equal to the combined forces that favor filtration minus the combined forces that oppose filtration.
- Clinically, **vascular hydrostatic pressure** (the force that drives the fluid out of circulation) and plasma **colloid osmotic pressure** (force which drives the fluid into circulation) are the **most important**.

Mechanism of Edema (Fig. 2)

Any mechanism, which interferes with the normal fluid balance, may produce edema.

- **Increased capillary hydrostatic pressure or decreased** colloid osmotic pressure **produces increased interstitial fluid**.
- If the movement of fluid into tissues (or body cavities) exceeds lymphatic drainage, the fluid accumulates in

the interstitial tissue. If there is involvement of serosal surface (pleural, peritoneal, pericardial) is involved, fluid accumulates with the body cavities as an effusion. Edema may also develop when the permeability of capillaries is increased and they "leak" fluid (e.g., inflammation).

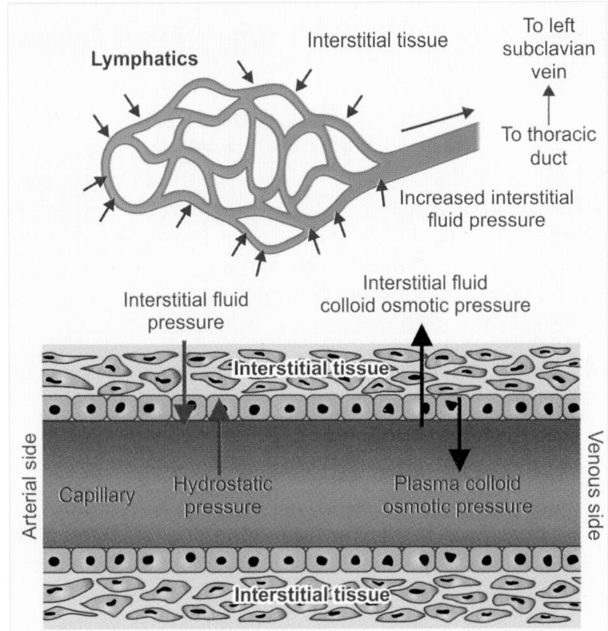

FIG. 1: Factors influencing the movement of fluid across capillary walls. Normally, there is balance between hydrostatic and osmotic pressure so that there is only little net movement of fluid into the interstitium. Mechanisms that can produce edema include increased hydrostatic pressure or diminished plasma osmotic pressure. Normally, lymphatics in the interstitial tissue return much of the excess fluid into the circulation by way of the thoracic duct. If the fluid accumulated exceeds the capacity of lymphatic drainage, it also can produce local edema.

- These pathophysiologic mechanisms may operate singly or in combinations.

Increased Hydrostatic Pressure

Hydrostatic pressure at the capillary end of microcirculation drives the fluid out of the capillary into the interstitial tissue space. Any conditions, which increase the hydrostatic pressure, can produce edema. The increased hydrostatic pressure **may be regional or generalized**.

- **Local increase in hydrostatic pressure:** It can be due to **local impairment in venous return**. Examples:
  - **Deep venous thrombosis (DVT)** in a lower extremity may produce localized edema in the affected leg.
  - **Postural edema** may be seen in the feet and ankle of individuals who stand in erect position for long duration.
- **Generalized increase in hydrostatic pressure:** It produces generalized edema. Most common cause **is congestive heart failure (CHF)**.
  - Congestive heart failure may be failure of the left ventricle, right ventricle, or both.
  - **Right-sided heart failure** results in pooling of blood on the venous side of the circulation—increases the hydrostatic pressure in the venous circulation—increases movement of fluid into the interstitial tissue spaces—shows characteristic **peripheral pitting edema**.
  - **Left-sided heart failure** results in increased hydrostatic pressure (i.e., back pressure) in the pulmonary circulation—produces **pulmonary edema**.

Decreased Plasma Osmotic Pressure

Plasma osmotic pressure normally tends to draw the fluid into the vessels. The plasma osmotic pressure is dependent on plasma proteins, mainly on albumin **(major plasma protein).** Albumin is constitute about 50% of total plasma protein. **Decreased plasma osmotic pressure may be due to:**

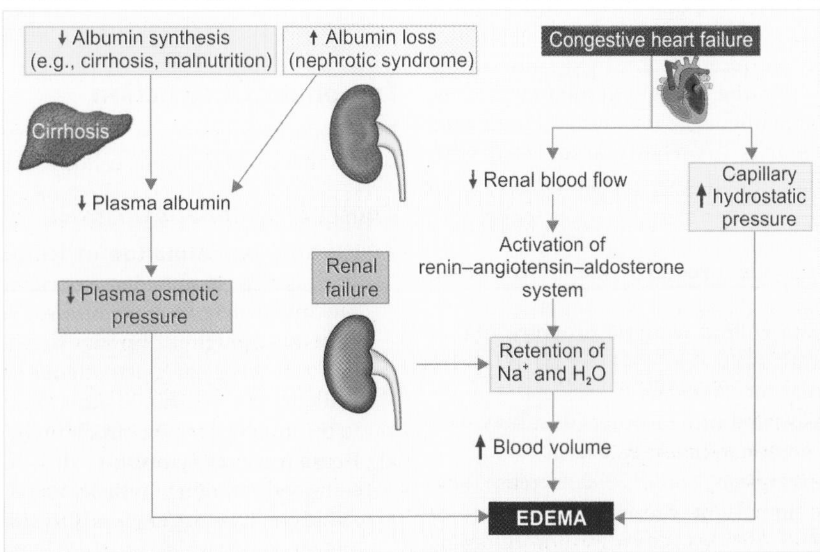

FIG. 2: Pathogenesis of systemic edema from congestive heart failure, renal failure, or reduced plasma osmotic pressure.

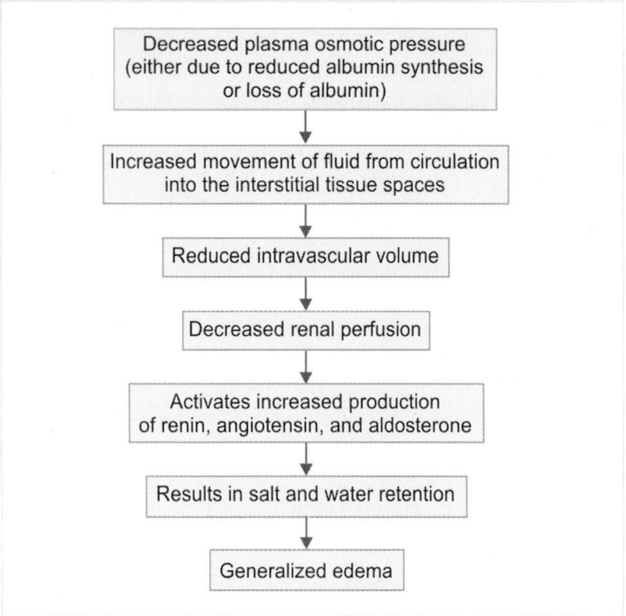

FLOWCHART 1: Mechanism of generalized edema due to reduced plasma osmotic pressure.

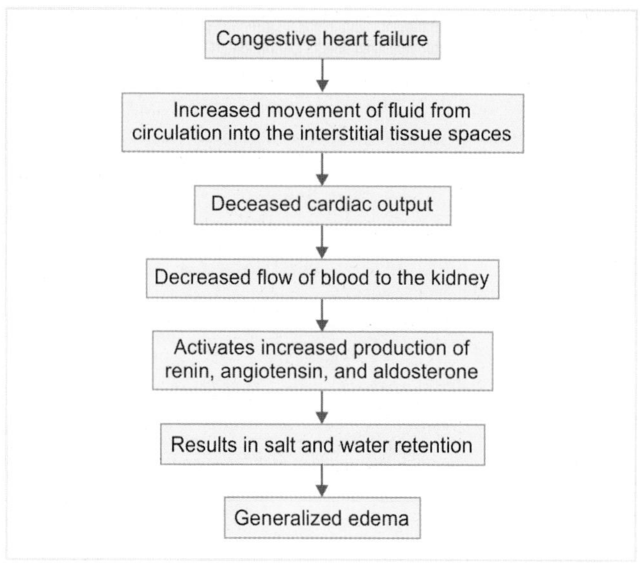

FLOWCHART 2: Mechanism of generalized edema in congestive heart failure.

- **Reduced albumin synthesis:** Occurs in **severe liver diseases** (e.g., cirrhosis) or **protein malnutrition** (due to decreased intake of proteins).
- **Loss of albumin:** May occur in the **urine or stool. Nephrotic syndrome** is an important cause of loss of albumin in urine. **Malabsorption and protein losing enteropathy** are characterized by loss of protein in the stool.

Consequences of decreased plasma osmotic pressure are shown in **Flowchart 1**.

Sodium and Water Retention

Total body sodium is the main cation in the ECF and therefore, the main determinant of volume of extracellular fluid. Hence, increased total body sodium should be balanced by accumulation of more extracellular water to maintain constant osmolality. Control of extracellular fluid volume mainly depends on renal excretion of sodium. This in turn is influenced by (i) atrial natriuretic factor (ANF) and (ii) the renin-angiotensin system of the juxtaglomerular apparatus, and (iii) the activity of sympathetic nervous system. **Increased retention of sodium salt is invariably associated with retention of water**. Sodium and water retention may be a primary cause of edema.

- **Mechanism:**
  - **Increased hydrostatic pressure** due to increased plasma volume
  - **Decreased plasma colloid osmotic pressure** due to dilution effect on albumin.
- **Causes:** May be primary or secondary
  - **Primary:** It is associated with disorders of kidney such as renal failure, glomerulonephritis.
  - **Secondary:** It develops in disorders that decrease renal perfusion, most important cause being congestive heart failure (CHF). This leads to activation of renin-angiotensin-aldosterone axis. In early heart failure, this response is beneficial. This is because the retention of sodium and water and other adaptations [e.g., increased vascular tone and elevated levels of antidiuretic hormone (ADH)] improve cardiac output. This in turn restores normal renal perfusion. However, as heart failure progresses and cardiac output diminishes, the retained fluid only raises the hydrostatic pressure. This leads to development of edema and effusions.

  Mechanism of edema in CHF is given in **Flowchart 2**.
- **Water retention by ADH mechanism**
  - Antidiuretic hormone is released from the posterior pituitary, when there is reduced plasma volume or increased plasma osmolarity.
  - Primary retention of water can occur due to the increased release of ADH.
  - **Increased secretion of ADH** is seen in association with lung cancer and **pituitary disorders**.
  - This can lead to hyponatremia and cerebral edema.

Lymphatic Obstruction

Lymphatic obstruction causes impaired drainage of lymph and produces localized edema, called as **lymphedema**.

Causes of Lymphatic Obstruction

- **Chronic inflammation of lymphatics** associated with fibrosis (e.g., lymphedema occurring at scrotal and vulvar region due to **lymphogranuloma venereum**).
- **Invasive malignant tumors** [e.g., **lymphedema of breast** due to blockage of subcutaneous lymphatics **by malignant cells** gives rise to **orange skin (Peau d'orange) appearance** to the involved region of skin in the breast].
- **Pressure over lymphatic drainage** from outside (e.g., tumors obstructing thoracic ducts).
- **Damage by surgery/radiation:** Patients with breast cancer may develop severe edema of the upper arm as a complication of **surgical removal and/or irradiation of the breast** and **associated axillary lymph nodes**.

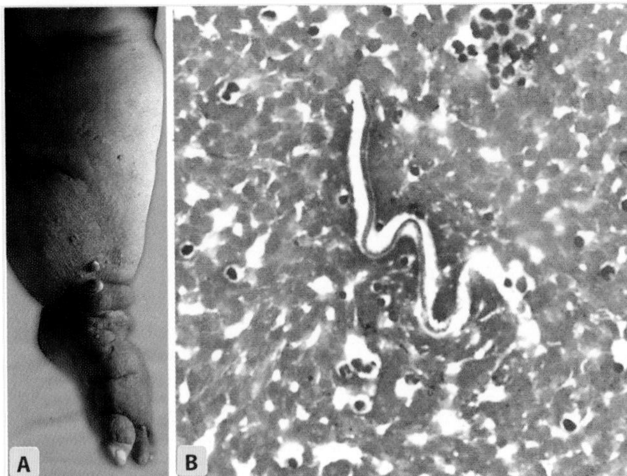

FIGS. 3A AND B: (A) Elephantiasis due to obstruction of lymphatics. (B) *Wuchereria bancrofti* (microfilaria).

- **Parasitic infestations:** In **filariasis** (caused by *Wuchereria bancrofti)*, the parasite (**Fig. 3B**—microfilaria) may cause extensive obstruction of lymphatics and lymph node fibrosis. If the block is in the inguinal region, it can produce edema of the external genitalia and lower limbs (upper arm if axillary region is involved) which may be massive and resemble the leg of an elephant and is known as **elephantiasis (Fig. 3A)**.
- **Hereditary disorder: Milroy's disease** is a hereditary disorder characterized by abnormal development of lymphatics. The edema may be seen in one or both lower limbs.

  Through lymph, proteins in the interstitial space are returned to the circulation. So, **edema fluid** produced due to lymphatic obstruction has a **high protein** concentration. The increased protein content may **stimulate fibrosis** in the dermis of the skin and is responsible for the induration (indurated edema) found in lymphedema.

MORPHOLOGY

Edema can be **easily detected on gross examination**. It may involve any organ or tissue, but is **most common in subcutaneous tissues, the lungs,** and the **brain**. Microscopically, edema appears as a clear space, which separates the extracellular matrix (ECM).

Generalized Edema

It is seen mainly in the subcutaneous tissues.

- **Subcutaneous edema:** It may be diffuse or more easily noticed in regions with high hydrostatic pressures. In most cases, the distribution of **edema is dependent on gravity** and is termed **dependent edema**. Thus, it is prominent in the legs when standing, and in the sacrum when recumbent. **If pressure is applied** by a finger over substantially edematous subcutaneous tissue, it **displaces the interstitial fluid and leaves a depression**. This sign is called as **pitting edema (Fig. 4)**.
- **Edema of renal origin:** It can **affect all parts of the body**. Initially, it is observed **in tissues with loose connective tissue matrix**, such as the **eyelids and scrotal region**. Edema in the eyelids is called **periorbital edema** and is a characteristic of severe renal disease.

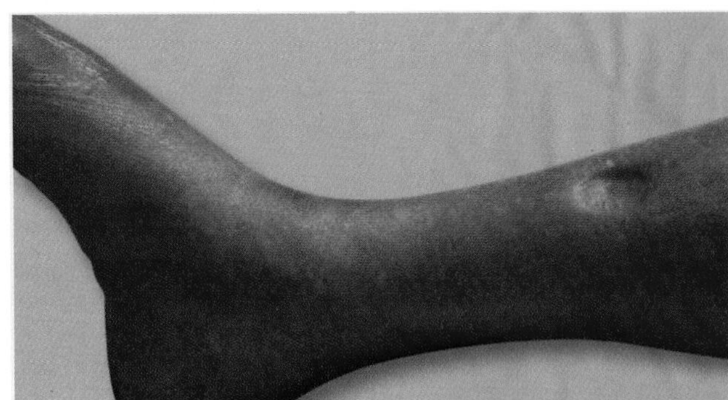

FIG. 4: Pitting edema in which when pressure by finger is applied, it displaces interstitial fluid and leaves a depression at that site.

Clinical Consequences

They range from minimal effects to rapidly fatal effect.

- **Generalized subcutaneous tissue edema:** It indicates the presence of an underlying **cardiac or renal disease**. Severe subcutaneous edema may delay wound healing or the clearance of infection.
- **Myxedema:** It is a form of **non-pitting** edema involving skin of face and visceral organs, **observed in hypothyroidism**. The edema is due to excessive deposition of glycosaminoglycans and hyaluronic acid, in skin, subcutaneous tissue, and visceral organs.
- **Papilledema: Swelling of the optic nerve head** is called as papilledema. The concentric increase in pressure encircling the optic nerve produces stasis of venous outflow which leads to swelling of the optic nerve head. The causes are:
  - Compression of the nerve (e.g., primary neoplasm of the optic nerve)
  - Raised cerebrospinal fluid pressure surrounding the nerve.

Special Categories of Edema

Cerebral (Brain) Edema

Q. Write short essay on cerebral edema.

Definition: Cerebral edema (brain parenchymal edema) results from increased leakage of fluid from blood vessels and injury to various cells in the CNS.

Brain in enclosed rigid cranium and the cranium allows little room for expansion of brain. Hence, edema of the brain is dangerous. **Cerebral edema often increases the intracranial pressure** and compromises cerebral blood supply, distorts the gross structure of the brain, and interferes with the function of central nervous system (CNS). It is often **fatal**.

Cause

Cerebral (brain) edema can be localized or generalized. It depends on the nature and extent of the pathologic process or injury. It **results from increased leakage of fluid from blood vessels and injury to various cells of the CNS**. There are two main pathways of formation of cerebral edema.

- **Vasogenic edema:** It is the most common variety of edema. It is characterized by an increase in extracellular fluid in the brain. It is caused by disruption of blood-brain barrier and increased vascular permeability, mainly in white matter. The tight endothelial junctions of the blood-brain barrier are disrupted. This permits the shift of fluid from the intravascular compartment to the intercellular (interstitial) spaces of the brain. The paucity of lymphatics in CNS impairs the resorption of excess extracellular fluid. Vasogenic edema may be either localized, e.g., adjacent to inflammation (e.g., encephalitis, abscesses), trauma, or neoplasms infarcts; or generalized, as may occur following a global ischemic injury and toxic brain injury (e.g., lead poisoning).

- **Cytotoxic edema:** It is an increase in intracellular fluid (i.e., accumulation of intracellular water) secondary to neuronal, glial, or endothelial cell membrane injury. It may occur with a generalized hypoxic/ischemic damage or with a metabolic derangement in which there is disturbance in the maintenance of the normal membrane ionic gradients. Cytotoxic cerebral edema usually affects the gray matter.

  Usually generalized edema shows elements of both vasogenic and cytotoxic edema. In generalized edema, edematous brain appears soft and heavy. Gyri are compressed and flattened and the intervening sulci are narrowed. The ventricular cavities are compressed. Patients with cerebral edema present with vomiting, disorientation, and convulsions. In severe brain edema, the brain substance may herniate (extrude) through the foramen magnum or occlude the blood supply to the brainstem. Both conditions may damage the medullary centers and lead to death.
- **Interstitial edema:** It develops as a consequence of hydrocephalus, in which fluid accumulates in the cerebral ventricles and periventricular white matter.

Pulmonary Edema

Q. Write short essay on pulmonary edema.

Pulmonary edema is characterized by excessive interstitial fluid in the alveoli (air spaces) and the interstitium of the lung. Pulmonary edema decreases gas exchange in the lung. This leads to hypoxia and retention of carbon dioxide (hypercapnia).

Protective mechanism in lung

Lung is a loose tissue with little connective tissue support. Hence, it needs certain protective mechanisms to keep the normal lung dry and prevent the development of edema. These include:

- Low perfusion pressure in the capillaries of lung. This is due to low right ventricular pressure.
- Effective lymphatic drainage of the interstitial fluid of the lung. These lymphatics are slightly under negative pressure and can drain 10 times the regular lymph flow.
- Presence of tight cellular junctions between endothelial cells. This controls permeability of capillaries.
- Balance among capillary hydrostatic pressure, capillary oncotic pressure, and capillary permeability.
- Surfactant lining the alveoli repels water and keeps the fluid from entering the alveoli.

Classification and causes of pulmonary edema

Pulmonary edema develops when the above-mentioned protective mechanisms are disturbed. Classification of pulmonary edema is presented in **Box 1**. It may be divided into: (1) **due to hemodynamic disturbances (cardiogenic pulmonary edema), or (2) increased capillary permeability due to microvascular injury (noncardiogenic pulmonary edema).**

Hemodynamic pulmonary edema

Causes (Box 1): **Hemodynamic pulmonary edema is caused by *increased hydrostatic pressure*.** Hemodynamic changes in the heart increase perfusion pressure in pulmonary capillaries and block the effective lymphatic drainage. It develops **most commonly in left sided CHF**. Other causes include mitral stenosis and mitral insufficiency.

MORPHOLOGY

Gross

Initially, edema occurs in the basal regions of the lower lobes due to greater hydrostatic pressure in these sites (dependent edema). Lungs appear heavy and wet. They weigh two to three times their normal weight. On cut section, frothy, blood-tinged fluid (mixture of air, edema, and extravasated red cells) oozes out.

Microscopy

The alveolar capillaries are engorged. The alveoli are filled with transudate. This intra-alveolar transudate appears as a homogeneous or finely granular pale pink material, permeated by air bubbles (**Fig. 5**). Alveolar microhemorrhages and hemosiderin-laden macrophages ("heart failure" cells) may be seen.

In long-standing pulmonary congestion (e.g., in mitral stenosis), numerous hemosiderin-laden macrophages may be seen in the alveolar spaces, and the alveolar walls may show fibrosis and thickening. The lungs may become firm and brown *(brown induration)*. These changes impair respiratory function and also predispose to infection.

Pulmonary edema due to microvascular (alveolar) injury

Causes (Box 1): Non-cardiogenic pulmonary edema is produced **due to injury of the alveolar septa**. Primary injury may be due to the vascular endothelium (destruction of endothelial cells or disruption of their tight junctions) or injury to epithelial cells lining alveoli (with secondary microvascular injury). They increase the permeability of capillaries and produce an inflammatory exudate. This inflammatory exudate leaks into the interstitial space and, in more severe cases, into the alveoli. Injury-related alveolar edema is an important feature of a serious and often fatal condition, acute respiratory distress syndrome (ARDS). Various causes include aspiration

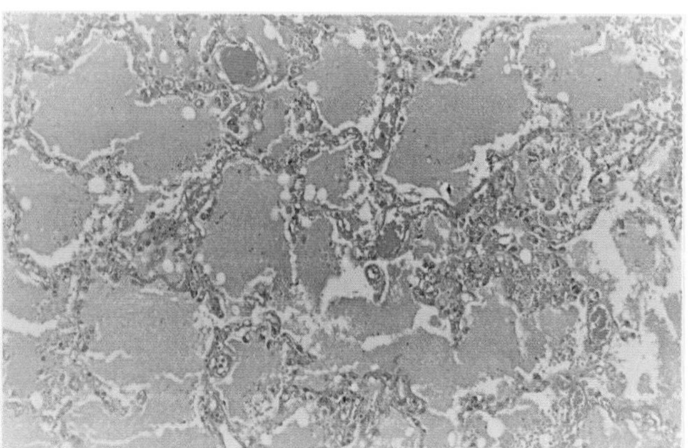

FIG. 5: Pulmonary edema showing pink fluid within the alveoli.

Box 1: Classification of causes of pulmonary edema.

- **Hemodynamic edema (cardiogenic pulmonary edema)**
  - Increased hydrostatic pressure (increased pulmonary venous pressure)
    - Left-sided heart failure (most common cause)
    - Volume overload
    - Obstruction of pulmonary vein
  - Decreased oncotic pressure (less common)
    - Hypoalbuminemia
    - Nephrotic syndrome
    - Liver disease, e.g., cirrhosis
    - Malnutrition
    - Protein-losing gastroenteropathies
  - Lymphatic obstruction (very rare)
- **Edema due to injury to alveolar wall (microvascular or epithelial injury) (noncardiogenic pulmonary edema)**
  - Direct injury
    - Infections: For example, bacterial pneumonia, viral infections
    - Aspiration of liquid: For example, gastric contents, near-drowning
    - Inhaled toxic gases: For example, high concentrations of oxygen, smoke
    - Trauma to the lung
    - Radiation
    - Uremia
  - Indirect injury
    - Systemic inflammatory response syndrome (SIRS): For example, sepsis, burns, pancreatitis, severe trauma
    - Drugs and chemicals: For example, chemotherapeutic drugs (e.g., bleomycin), other drugs (e.g., methadone, amphotericin B), cocaine, heroin, kerosene, paraquat (chemical herbicide)
    - Blood transfusion–related: Transfusion-related acute lung injury (TRALI)
- **Undetermined**
  - High altitude
  - Neurogenic (central nervous system trauma)

of gastric contents, viral infections, inhalation of toxic gases, and uremia.

Types of pulmonary edema

Pulmonary edema may be interstitial or alveolar.

- **Interstitial edema:** It is the earliest phase of pulmonary edema. During this phase, there is exaggeration of normal fluid filtration. Lymphatics become distended. Fluid accumulates in the interstitium of lobular septa and around veins and bronchovascular bundles. Radiologically, it shows a reticulonodular pattern, more severe at the bases of lung. Edema of the lobular septa produces linear shadows ("Kerley B lines") on chest radiographs. Edema results in shunting of blood flow from the bases of the lung to the upper lobes. Edema of the bronchovascular tree produces increased airflow resistance. Generally, this early stage is asymptomatic.
- **Alveolar edema:** When the excessive fluid exceeds the capacity of the interstitial space of the lungs, fluid spills and accumulates into the alveoli. This is termed as alveolar edema. Fluid accumulates initially in the basal regions of the lower lobes. This is because hydrostatic pressure is greatest in these sites (dependent edema). Radiologically, at this stage, alveolar pattern is observed. It is generally more prominent in central portions of the lung and in lower zones. During this phase, patient develops acute shortness of breath (dyspnea) with prominent coughing. Hypoxemia produces cyanosis. On auscultation of chest, bubbly rales are heard. In severe cases, patients cough out pink frothy sputum.

Pathogenesis of pulmonary edema is summarized in **Flowchart 3**.

Clinical Features of Pulmonary Edema

Edema in the interstitium and the alveolar spaces of the lungs impairs gas exchange (leading to hypoxemia) and also creates a favorable environment for bacterial infection. If pulmonary

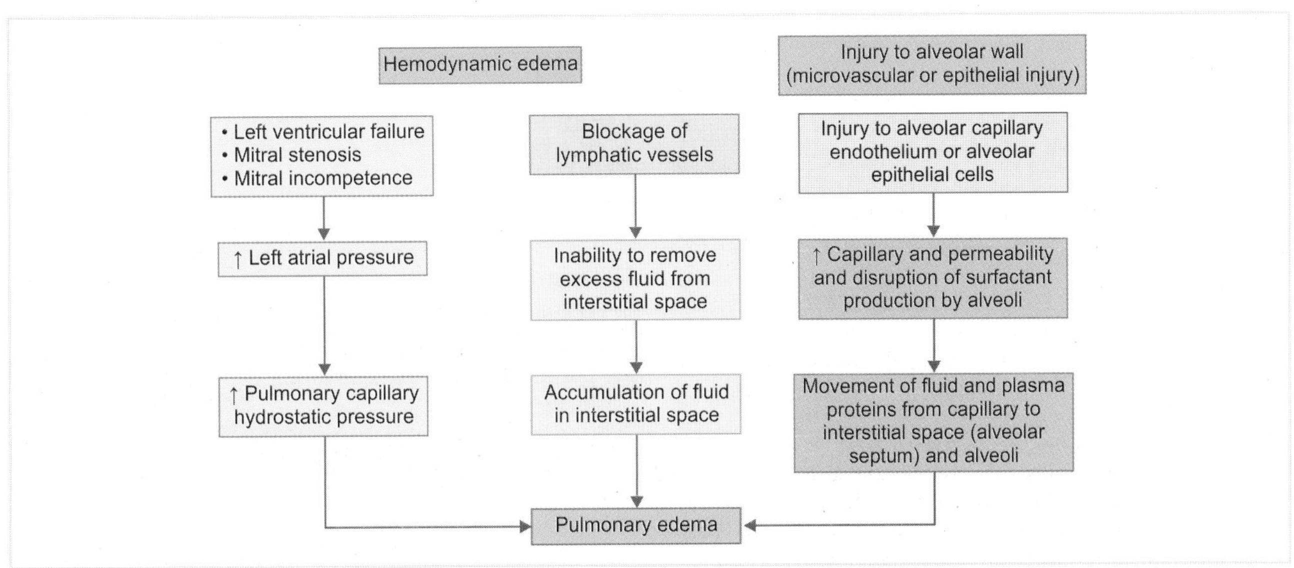

FLOWCHART 3: Pathogenesis of pulmonary edema.

edema is associated with pleural effusions, pleural effusion compresses the underlying pulmonary parenchyma and further compromise gas exchange.

Effusions

Fluid can accumulate in body cavities. Thus, edema may involve the pleural cavity (hydrothorax), the pericardial cavity (hydropericardium), or the peritoneal cavity (hydroperitoneum or ascites). They develop in a wide range of clinical settings. Effusions may be transudative or exudative. Transudative effusions are protein-poor, translucent, and straw colored. One exception is peritoneal effusions that develops due to lymphatic blockage (chylous effusion) may be milky due to the presence of lipids absorbed from the gut and they are protein rich. Exudative effusions are protein-rich and usually cloudy due to the presence of white blood cells.

Pleural space

Pleural effusion (hydrothorax) is accumulation of fluid in the pleural space. The pleural fluid is a straw- colored transudate of low specific gravity and contains few cells (mainly exfoliated mesothelial cells).

Causes: Fluid commonly accumulates in the pleural cavity in generalized edema due to diseases such as the nephrotic syndrome, cirrhosis of the liver and congestive heart failure. Pleural effusion also occurs as response to an inflammatory process (e.g., pneumonia) or tumor in the lung or on the pleural surface.

Pericardium

Pericardial effusion (hydropericardium) is accumulation of fluid in the pericardial cavity. Fluid in the pericardial sac may also accumulate due to either hemorrhage (hemopericardium) or injury to the pericardium (pericardial effusion).

Causes: Various causes of pericardial effusions includes pericardial infections, metastatic neoplasms to the pericardium, uremia and systemic lupus erythematosus. Occasionally, they may occur after cardiac operations (postpericardiotomy syndrome) or radiation therapy for cancer. Rapid accumulation of pericardial fluid may occur with hemorrhage from a ruptured myocardial infarct or dissecting aortic aneurysm or trauma. In such situations, pericardial cavity pressure may exceed the filling pressure of the heart and this is called cardiac tamponade. This can lead to precipitous decline in cardiac output and it is usually fatal. The tolerable limit of pericardial sac is only 90–120 mL. If pericardial fluid accumulates rapidly, it compresses the heart. In contrast, if the process of accumulation of fluid is gradual, pericardial sac can accommodate a liter or more of fluid without immediate serious consequences.

Peritoneum

Peritoneal effusion is accumulation of fluid in the peritoneal cavity and is also called ascites.

Causes: Main causes are cirrhosis of the liver, abdominal neoplasms, pancreatitis, cardiac failure, the nephrotic syndrome and hepatic venous obstruction (Budd-Chiari syndrome). Obstruction of the thoracic duct by cancer may lead to chylous ascites. In this, the fluid has a milky appearance and has a high fat content.

DISORDERS OF PERFUSION

Adequate perfusion of tissues delivers oxygen and nutrients and removes wastes produced by cellular metabolism. Health of cells and tissues depends on the adequate circulation of blood. Hemodynamic disorders are characterized by disturbed perfusion. Hence, it results in organ and cellular injury. Disorders of perfusion includes hyperemia, congestion and hemorrhage. Hyperemia and congestion both are characterized by locally increased volumes of blood within tissues. But, they have different underlying mechanisms and consequences.

Hyperemia

Definition

Hyperemia is an **active process** in which **arteriolar dilation** leads to increased **blood flow to a tissue/organ**. Affected tissues appear red (*erythema*) due to increased delivery of oxygenated blood.

Causes

- **Physiological:** Response to **increased functional demand** (e.g., heart and skeletal muscle during exercise). Neurogenic and hormonal influences play a role in active hyperemia. For example, the blushing bride and the flushing in menopausal lady. Cutaneous hyperemia occurs in febrile states and serves to dissipate heat. The increased blood supply in hyperemia occurs due to dilatation of arterioles and opening of unperfused capillaries.
- **Pathological:** Seen in **inflammation** and is responsible for the two cardinal signs of inflammation namely **heat** (calor) and **redness** (rubor/**erythema**). Vasoactive mediators liberated by inflammatory cells cause dilation of blood vessels and in the skin this gives rise to to cardinal signs "tumor, rubor and calor" of inflammation. For example, in pneumonia, the alveolar capillaries are engorged with RBCs as a hyperemic response to inflammation. Inflammation can also damage endothelial cells and increase capillary permeability. Thus, inflammatory hyperemia is usually associated with edema and local extravasation of RBCs.

Congestion

Definition

Congestion is a **passive process** resulting from **reduced venous outflow of blood** from a tissue/organ.

Types and Causes

- **Systemic** [e.g., CHF (congestive heart failure), congestion involves liver, spleen, and kidneys].
- **Local:** Passive congestion may also be localized. Examples include:
  - Congestion of leg veins due to DVT (deep vein thrombosis)—edema of the lower extremity. Thrombosis of hepatic veins (Budd-Chiari syndrome) produces
  - secondary chronic passive congestion of the liver.
  - Local congestion at various sites due to compression of veins, e.g., tight bandage, plasters, tumors, pregnancy, hernia, etc.

Onset

- **Acute congestion:** It develops during shock, or sudden right-sided heart failure. It may occur in lung and liver. Microscopically, **acute pulmonary congestion** shows engorged alveolar capillaries, edema of alveolar septa, and focal intra-alveolar hemorrhage. In **acute hepatic congestion**, there is distension of central vein and sinusoids. Since, the centrilobular region of the hepatic lobule is at the distal end of the hepatic blood supply, the hepatocytes in the centrilobular region may undergo ischemic necrosis. The hepatocytes at the periportal region are better oxygenated because of their proximity to hepatic arterioles. Hence, they may only develop fatty change.
- **Chronic passive congestion:** It usually produces edema in the organ/tissue in which the venous outflow is reduced.
  - **Appearance:** Congested tissues have a **dusky, reddish-blue color (cyanosis)** due to stasis of red blood cells (RBCs) and the accumulation of deoxygenated hemoglobin.
  - **Consequences:** (i) In long-standing chronic passive congestion, there is **chronic hypoxia**. This may produce ischemic tissue injury and scarring in the involved tissue. (ii) In chronically congested tissues, the **capillaries can rupture and produce small foci of hemorrhage**. Degradation of extravasated RBCs present in the hemorrhage can release hemosiderin. This is phagocytosed by macrophages and these hemosidern-laden macrophages are called heart failure cells. Their presence in tissue is a telltale sign of hemorrhage. (iii) Since congestion is associated with increased hydrostatic pressures, it commonly leads to **edema** in the involved tissue.

Chronic Venous Congestion of Lung

Causes

- **Mitral stenosis** (e.g., rheumatic mitral stenosis).
- **Left-sided heart failure:** It develops secondary to coronary artery disease or hypertension.

Mechanism of chronic venous congestion (CVC) of lung is presented in **Flowchart 4**.

Consequences

Four major consequences are:

- **Microhemorrhages:** The wall of alveolar capillaries may rupture—minute hemorrhages into the alveolar space—release RBCs—hemoglobin breakdown—**liberation of iron containing hemosiderin pigment** (brown color)—alveolar macrophages phagocytose hemosiderin.

Hemosiderin-laden macrophages are known as **heart failure cells**.

- **Pulmonary edema (refer Fig. 5):** It is due to forced movement of fluid from congested vessels into the alveolar spaces.
- **Fibrosis:** It develops due to increased fibrous tissue in the interstitium of lung.
- **Pulmonary hypertension:** It is due to transmission of pressure from the alveolar capillaries to the pulmonary arterial system.

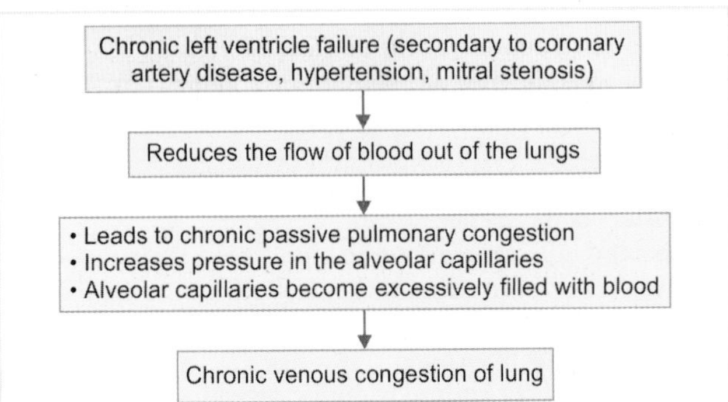

Chronic left ventricle failure (secondary to coronary artery disease, hypertension, mitral stenosis)
Reduces the flow of blood out of the lungs
• Leads to chronic passive pulmonary congestion
• Increases pressure in the alveolar capillaries
• Alveolar capillaries become excessively filled with blood
Chronic venous congestion of lung

FLOWCHART 4: Mechanism of chronic venous congestion of lung.

MORPHOLOGY

Gross

- Lung is **heavy**.
- Cut section (c/s) **rusty brown color** (due to hemosiderin pigment), **firm in consistency** (due to fibrosis)—known as **brown induration of lung (Fig. 6)**.

Microscopy: (Figs. 7A and B)

- **Distension** and **congestion of capillaries** in the alveolar septa of lung.
- **Thickened alveolar septa** due to increase in the fibrous connective tissue—responsible for the firm consistency of the lung.
- **Heart failure cells** are seen in the alveoli.

Chronic Venous Congestion of Liver

Causes

The hepatic veins empty into the inferior vena cava just inferior to the heart, so the liver is vulnerable to acute or chronic passive congestion. Various causes of chronic venous congestion (CVC) of liver are:

- **Right-sided heart failure** is the most common cause.
- **Rare:** Constrictive pericarditis, tricuspid stenosis and obstruction of inferior vena cava and hepatic vein.

Mechanism of CVC of liver is presented in **Flowchart 5**.

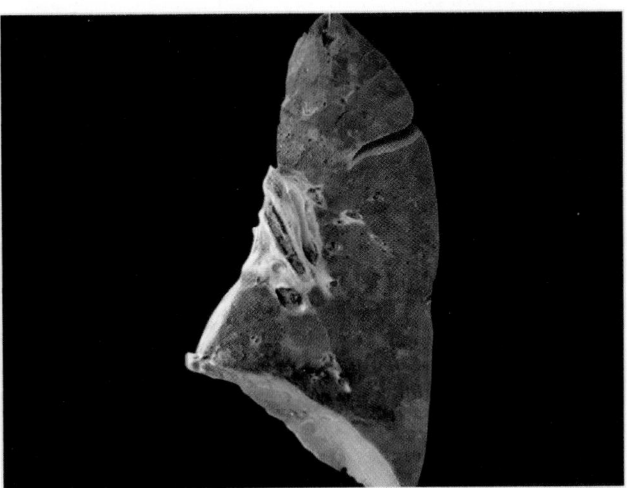

FIG. 6: Chronic venous congestion lung. Gross appearance showing brown induration lung.

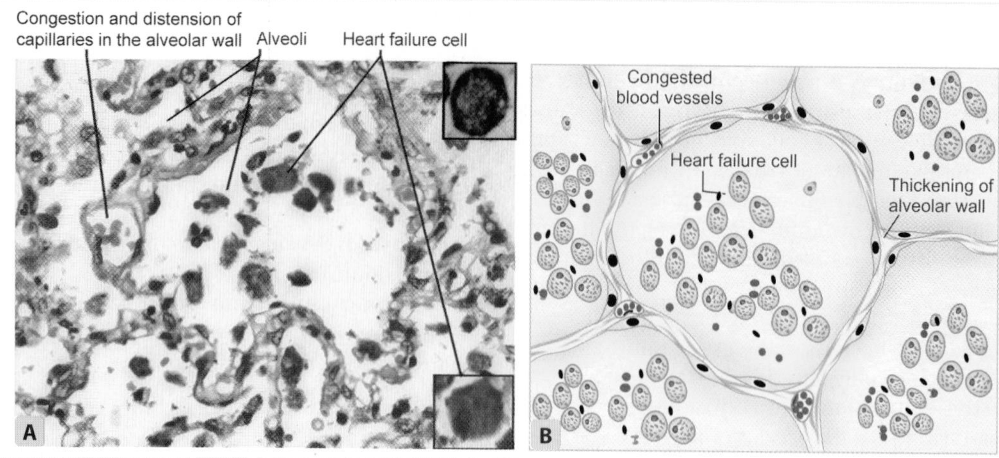

FIGS. 7A AND B: Microscopic appearance of chronic venous congestion lung. (A) Hematoxylin and eosin. (B) Diagrammatic section from lung shows thickened alveolar walls and hemosiderin-laden macrophages (heart failure cells) in the alveolar lumen.

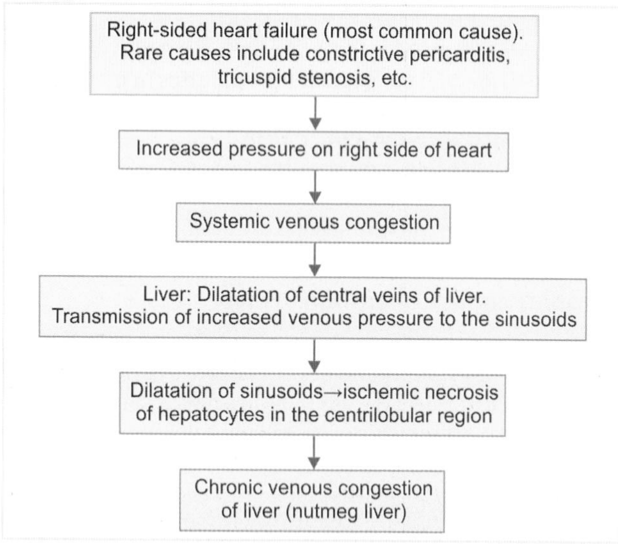

FLOWCHART 5: Mechanism of chronic venous congestion of liver.

MORPHOLOGY

Gross:

- **Liver increases in size** and weight and the **capsule appears tense**.
- **Cut section** shows **alternate** (combination of) **dark and light areas (Fig. 8)** and resembles cross-section of a nutmeg (**nutmeg liver**).
  - **Congested centrilobular regions** (with hemorrhage and necrosis) appear **dark red-brown and slightly depressed (because of cell death)**. Congestion is most prominent around terminal hepatic venule (central veins) within hepatic lobules.
  - **Periportal** (better oxygenated) **region** of the lobules appears **pale** and may show fatty change. The congested red-brown, centrilobular regions are accentuated against the surrounding zones of uncongested tan liver. The result is a reticulated appearance that resembles a cross-section of a nutmeg. Hence, classically known as nutmeg liver.

Continued

Continued

Microscopy (Figs. 9A and B): The central veins of hepatic lobules become dilated. The increased venous pressure in central vein is transmitted to the sinusoids. This in turn dilates sinusoids and produces pressure atrophy of hepatocytes in the centrilobular region.

- **Centrilobular region:**
  - **Congestion and hemorrhage** in the central veins (terminal hepatic venule) and adjacent sinusoids. Hemosiderin-laden macrophages, and variable degrees of hepatocyte dropout and necrosis is also observed.
  - The **severe central hypoxia may produce centrilobular hepatocyte necrosis**.
  - **Thickening of central veins and fibrosis** in prolonged venous congestion.
  - **Cardiac sclerosis/cardiac cirrhosis** may occur with sustained CVC (e.g., due to constrictive pericarditis or tricuspid stenosis). In such cases, the fibrosis is generalized and severe.
- **Periportal region:** It shows **fatty change** in hepatocytes.

Congestive Splenomegaly (CVC Spleen)

Congestion and enlargement of spleen is called as congestive splenomegaly.

Causes

Chronic obstruction to the outflow of venous blood from spleen leads to higher pressure in the splenic vein. This may occur due to increased intravascular pressure in the liver, from cardiac failure or an intrahepatic obstruction to blood flow (e.g., cirrhosis). Higher pressure in the splenic vein produces congestion of the spleen.

- **Intrahepatic obstruction to blood flow: Cirrhosis of the liver** is the main cause (e.g., alcoholic cirrhosis, pigment cirrhosis).
- **Extrahepatic disorders:**
  - **Systemic or central venous congestion** (e.g., tricuspid or pulmonic valvular disease, chronic cor pulmonale, right heart failure or following left-sided heart failure).

Splenomegaly is only moderate and rarely exceeds 500 g in weight.

- **Obstruction of the extrahepatic portal vein or splenic vein:** Due to spontaneous portal vein thrombosis, which is usually caused by intrahepatic obstructive disease, or inflammation of the portal vein (pylephlebitis). Thrombosis of the splenic vein can also develop by infiltrating tumors arising in neighboring viscera, such as carcinomas of the stomach or pancreas.

MORPHOLOGY

Gross (Fig. 10): Spleen is **enlarged, firm and tense**. In long-standing chronic splenic congestion, spleen is markedly enlarged (1,000–5,000 g). Normal weight of spleen is 150 g. **Capsule is thickened**.

- Cut section oozes dark blood.
- Enlarged spleen **may show excessive functional activity** termed as **hypersplenism**—leads to hematologic abnormalities (e.g., thrombocytopenia pancytopenia).

Continued

Continued

Microscopy (Figs. 11A and B):

- **Red pulp**
  - **Dilatation and congestion** in the early stages
  - Hemorrhage and fibrosis in later stages
  - **Capillarization of sinusoids** may occur, in which sinusoids get converted into capillaries.
- **Thickened fibrous capsule and trabeculae**
- Long-standing congestion produces diffuse fibrosis of spleen. It may show **Gamna-Gandy bodies (Fig. 5.3C)**, which consist of **iron-containing, fibrotic, and calcified foci of old hemorrhage**. **Slowing of blood flow** from the cords to the sinusoids—prolongs the exposure of the blood cells to macrophages in the spleen—leads to **excessive destruction of blood cells (hypersplenism)**.

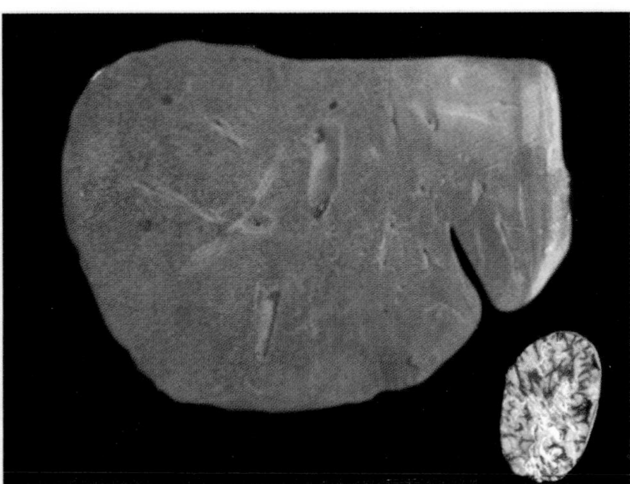

FIG. 8: Chronic venous congestion of liver. Grossly, liver shows alternate dark and light area and resembles the cut surface of a nutmeg (inset).

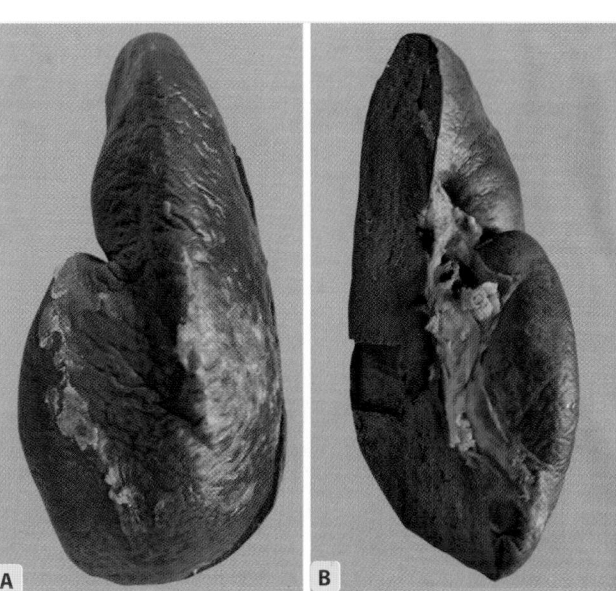

FIGS. 10 A AND B: Gross appearance of chronic venous congestion of spleen. (A) Markedly enlarged firm spleen with thickened capsule. (B) Cut section of spleen with dark color.

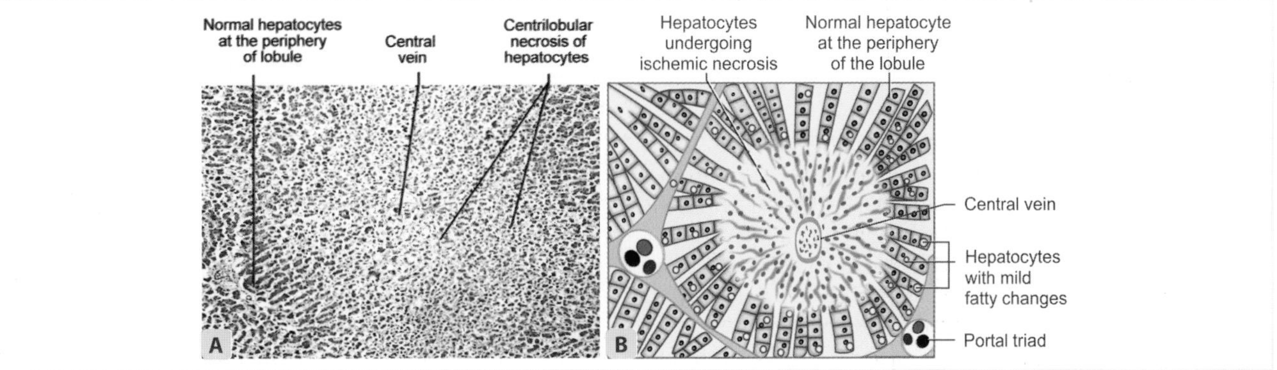

FIGS. 9A AND B: Chronic venous congestion of liver. (A) Microscopy shows centrilobular necrosis with degenerating hepatocytes surrounded by apparently normal hepatic parenchyma in the periportal region (photomicrograph). (B) Diagrammatic presentation of Figure 9A.

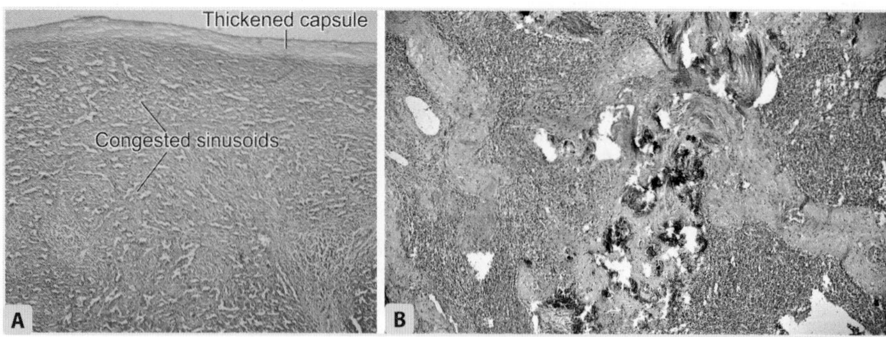

FIGS. 11A AND B: Chronic venous congestion of spleen. (A) Hematoxylin and eosin (H&E). Shows thickened capsule, dilated sinusoids. (B) Gamna–Gandy body.

Hemorrhage

Definition

Hemorrhage (bleeding) is defined as the escape or extravasation of blood from vessels.

Etiology

Blood can be released from the intravascular compartment (circulation) to the exterior of the body or into nonvascular body spaces. The various causes of hemorrhage are:

- **Trauma to the vessel wall:** The most common and obvious cause is trauma that **damages the blood vessels,** e.g., penetrating wound in the heart or great vessels, during labor, etc.
- **Vascular diseases:**
  - **Rupture of aneurysm:** Severe atherosclerosis may weaken the wall of the aorta (mainly abdominal aorta) and produce permanent abnormal dilatation of vessel called as aneurysm. These aneurysms may rupture and bleed into the retroperitoneal space. Aneurysm may be congenital due to weak cerebral artery (berry aneurysm), and may rupture and cause subarachnoid hemorrhage.
  - **Inflammatory lesions of the vessel wall:** Infections (e.g., blood vessels traversing a tuberculous cavity in pulmonary tuberculosis of the lung) bleeding from chronic peptic ulcer, typhoid ulcers, polyarteritis nodosa, septicemia.
- **Neoplastic invasion of vessel:** Invasive neoplasms may erode blood vessels and result in hemorrhage (e.g., hemorrhage following vascular invasion in carcinoma of the tongue).
- **Hemorrhagic (bleeding) diatheses:** The risks of hemorrhage in these clinical disorders/conditions are increased and usually occur spontaneously or follow insignificant injury. There is **defective clot formation**. They have diverse causes, including inherited or acquired defects in vessel walls, platelets, or coagulation factors. Examples include purpura, scurvy, acute leukemias. Scurvy is associated with capillary fragility and bleeding, due to the defective supporting connective tissue structures.
- **Raised pressure within the vessels:** It may occur in systemic hypertension causing bleeding (e.g., cerebral and retinal hemorrhage), or high pressure in the veins (e.g., varicose veins legs, or esophagus, or pulmonary capillaries in CVC of lung).

Box 2: Definition of hemorrhage into various body cavities.

- **Hemothorax:** Hemorrhage into the pleural cavity
- **Hemopericardium:** Hemorrhage into the pericardial space
- **Hemoperitoneum:** Bleeding into the peritoneal cavity
- **Hemarthrosis:** Bleeding into a joint space

Manifestations

The bleeding may occur **externally** (exterior of the body), **or internally**. Internally blood may accumulate within a tissue (e.g., hematoma) or into the serous cavities/body spaces (**Box 2**) or into a hollow viscus. Hemorrhage may be manifested by different appearances and may have various clinical consequences.

Clinical Significance

The blood loss may be acute (large and sudden), or chronic (small repeated blood loss may occur over a period of time).

Effects

The effect of hemorrhage ranges from trivial (e.g., bruise) to fatal (e.g., a massive retroperitoneal hematoma resulting from rupture of a dissecting aortic aneurysm). The effects of hemorrhage depend upon: (1) the amount (volume) of blood loss, (2) the speed/rate of blood loss, and (3) the site of hemorrhage.

- **Amount and speed of hemorrhage**
  - Acute hemorrhage:
    - A sudden/rapid loss of up to 20% of the blood volume or slow loss of even larger amounts usually has little clinical effects in healthy adults because of compensatory mechanisms.
    - A sudden/acute loss of 33% of blood volume may lead to hypovolemic shock resulting in death.
    - Loss of up to 50% of blood volume gradually over a period of 24 hours may not be fatal.
  - **Chronic or recurrent loss of blood:**
    - **External bleeding:** Bleeding into an internal cavity, as in gastrointestinal hemorrhage from a peptic ulcer (arterial hemorrhage), or esophageal varices (venous hemorrhage), or menstrual bleeding, frequently leads to iron deficiency anemia due to loss of iron in hemoglobin.

- Internal bleeding: Iron is efficiently recycled from phagocytosed red cells when the bleeding is internal (e.g., a hematoma). Hence, it does not produce iron deficiency anemia.
  - **Jaundice:** Extensive hemorrhages can occasionally produce jaundice due to massive breakdown of red cells and hemoglobin.
- **Site of hemorrhage:** Bleeding may be trivial in the subcutaneous tissues. However, it can cause death if located in the brain.

NORMAL HEMOSTASIS

Definition: Hemostasis is a well-regulated physiological process by which blood clots form at sites of vascular injury.

Steps in Hemostasis

Hemostasis is initiated to arrest hemorrhage in response to vascular damage (injury) by forming a blood clot. It includes several sequences of events at a site of vascular injury (**Figs. 12A** to **D**).

Normally, blood vessels are lined by a smooth, nonthrombogenic endothelium.

Injury to the endothelium causes transient vasoconstriction and **exposes highly thrombogenic subendothelial** ECM, **initiating the platelet events**. These events form hemostatic plug and prevent or limit any further hemorrhage at the site of vascular injury. Hemostasis is a precisely controlled process and involves platelets, clotting (coagulation) factors, and endothelium of blood vessels at the site pf vascular injury. The general sequence of events of hemostasis at a site of vascular injury is as follows:

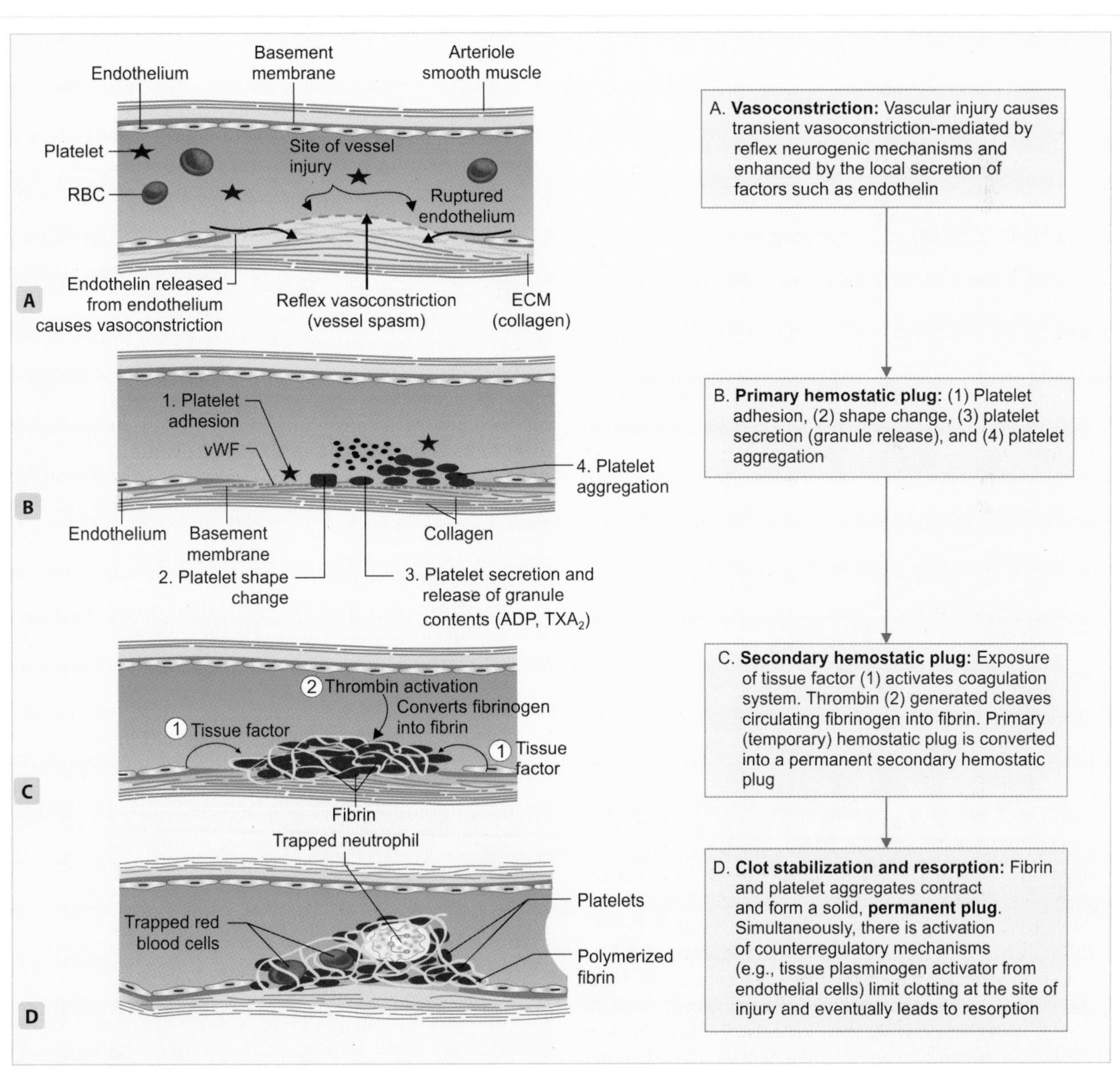

FIGS. 12A TO D: Different steps in hemostasis.

Arteriolar Vasoconstriction

It occurs immediately after vascular injury and markedly reduces flow of blood to the injured site. It is mediated by reflex neurogenic mechanisms and by the local secretion of factors such as **endothelin**. Endothelin is a powerful endothelium-derived vasoconstrictor. This vasoconstriction is transient and bleeding may resume if there is no activation of platelets and coagulation factors.

Primary Hemostatic Plug

Platelets play an important role in hemostasis. Primary hemostasis is the term is used for platelet plug formation at the site of injury. It occurs immediately within seconds of injury and is responsible for cessation of bleeding from microvasculature. It is characterized by the formation of the primary platelet plug that initially seals vascular defects. Platelet plug provides a surface that binds and concentrates activated coagulation factors. Damage or disruption of the endothelium lining the blood vessels after a traumatic vascular injury, exposes subendothelial connective tissue, such as von Willebrand factor (vWF) and collagen. Both vWF and collagen produce sequence of reactions that promote platelet adherence and activation. These lead to the formation of a platelet plug. Primary hemostasis involves three steps: Platelet adhesion and shape change, platelet secretion (granule release) and platelet aggregation.

Platelet adhesion and shape change

- **platelet adhesion at the site of vascular injury:** Initial step is **adhesion of platelets** to subendothelial structures at the site of injury. The link between the receptor sites (GpIb-IX which is an integrin) on the surface of platelet with exposed subendothelial collagen is brought out by an adhesion glycoprotein called **vWF** (**Fig. 13**). vWF is synthesized by both endothelial cells and megakaryocytes. Genetic deficiencies of vWF (von Willebrand disease) or GpIb (Bernard–Soulier syndrome) can produce bleeding disorders.
- **Platelets shape change:** Following adhesion of platelets to the subendothelial region, there is a dramatic change in the shape of platelets. Platelets change their shape from round to spherical smooth discs to spiky "sea urchins" (urchins = young child who is poorly or raggedly dressed) with protrusions, thereby markedly increasing the surface area. This change in shape of platelet is accompanied by:
    - **Conformational changes in platelet surface glycoprotein IIb/IIIa** (GpIIb/IIIa) that **increase its affinity for fibrinogen**.
    - **Translocation of negatively charged phospholipids** (PLs) (especially phosphatidylserine) **to the surface of platelets**. These negatively charged PLs on the surface bind calcium and serve as nucleation sites for the **formation of coagulation factor complexes**.

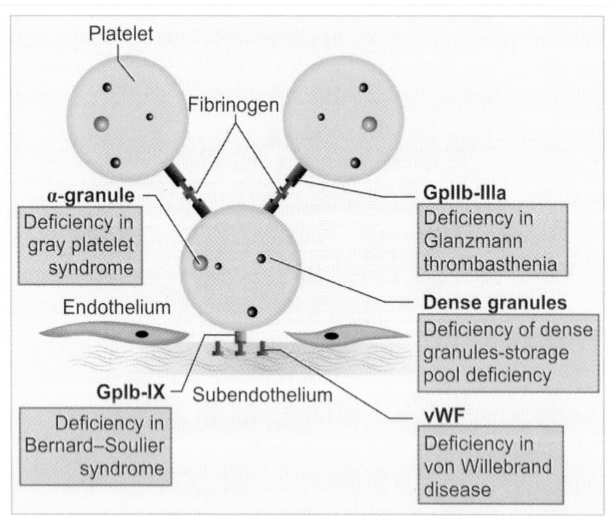

FIG. 13: Platelet adhesion and aggregation. von Willebrand factor serve as link between subendothelial collagen and the glycoprotein Ib-IX (*GpIb-IX*) platelet receptor. Aggregation of platelet is accomplished by fibrinogen bridging GpIIb-IIIa receptors on different platelets. Congenital deficiencies in the various receptors or bridging molecules produce various diseases or disorders.

Platelet secretion (release reaction), activation and recruitment

Soon after platelets change shape, platelets **release granule contents**. These processes of shape change along with release of granule content are together known as **platelet activation**. Platelet activation is brought out by a number of factors, including the coagulation factor thrombin and adenosine diphosphate (ADP).

- **Thrombin** activates platelets by switching on a special type of G-protein-coupled receptor called protease-activated receptor-1 (PAR-1).
- **Adenosine diphosphate** is present in dense body granules of platelets.

Platelet activation and release of ADP leads to additional platelet activation and this phenomenon is called as **recruitment**. ADP causes binding of two G-protein-coupled receptors namely $P2Y_1$ and $P2Y_{12}$. Activated platelets also synthesize prostaglandin thromboxane A_2 (TxA_2). TxA_2 is a causes strong aggregation of platelets. Aspirin inhibits platelet aggregation and produces a mild bleeding defect by inhibiting cyclooxygenase. Cyclooxygenase is a platelet enzyme that is needed for the synthesis of TxA_2. Drugs that inhibit platelet function by antagonizing PAR-1 or $P2Y_{12}$ have been developed. These antiplatelet drugs are used in the treatment of coronary artery disease.

Platelet aggregation

- Platelet aggregation (clumping together) follows platelet activation. The secreted products of platelets recruit additional platelets and cause platelet aggregation (i.e., bridging/adhesion of adjacent platelets) through the receptor sites (Gp IIb-IIIa). This process is mediated by fibrinogen which acts as an intercellular bridge between adjacent platelets. Inherited deficiency of GpIIb-IIIa produces a bleeding disorder called Glanzmann thrombasthenia. Activated platelets also produce the prostaglandin called thromboxane A_2 (TxA_2) which induces strong aggregation of platelets.
- These clumps of platelets so formed quickly (within 3–7 min) stop bleeding from the site of injury and are known as **primary hemostatic plug**. The process of primary hemostatic plug formation is termed as **primary hemostasis**.

Secondary Hemostatic Plug

It is characterized by deposition of fibrin at the site of vascular injury. This process takes an average of 3–10 minutes.

- **Exposure of tissue factor** at the site of injury. Tissue factor is a membrane-bound procoagulant glycoprotein. It is normally expressed by subendothelial cells in the vessel wall namely smooth muscle cells and fibroblasts. Tissue factor binds and activates factor VII. This in turn activates cascade of reactions that generate thrombin. Thrombin is a potent activator of platelets and causes additional platelet aggregation (of primary hemostatic plug) at the site of injury. The initial platelet aggregation is reversible. However, concurrent activation of thrombin stabilizes the platelet plug by causing further activation and aggregation which in turn promotes irreversible contraction of platelets. Platelet contraction is dependent on the cytoskeleton of platelets.
- Thrombin cleaves circulating fibrinogen into insoluble fibrin, thereby forming a fibrin meshwork at the site of vascular injury. The platelets contract, form an irreversibly fused mass. The fibrin formed from fibrinogen cements the platelets and produces a definitive secondary hemostatic plug. The red cells and leukocytes also get trapped in the fibrin meshwork and are found in hemostatic plugs. The process of conversion of the initial temporary primary hemostatic (platelet) plug into a permanent secondary hemostatic plug is known as **secondary hemostasis**. Secondary hemostasis consolidates the initial platelet plug. Entrapped red blood cells and leukocytes are also seen in hemostatic plugs. This is partly due to adherence of leukocytes to P-selectin expressed on activated platelets.
- The solid permanent plug so formed prevents any further hemorrhage. The hemostatic plugs/clots thus formed are confined to the site of injury by the fibrinolytic system. Subsequently, vascular repair is accomplished by thrombolysis and recanalization of the occluded site.

Clot Stabilization and Resorption

Polymerized [large number of units (monomers) bonded together] fibrin and platelet aggregates contract and form a solid, **permanent plug**. This prevents further hemorrhage. Simultaneously, there is activation of counter-regulatory mechanisms [e.g., tissue plasminogen activator (t-PA) released from endothelial cells] which limit clotting at the site of injury and eventually lead to resorption and tissue repair.

Components of Normal Hemostasis

Main components of normal hemostasis as well as pathologic process of thrombosis are: Platelets, coagulation system, and endothelium of the blood vessels. Other components include coagulation regulatory system and fibrinolytic system.

Platelets

Platelets play a main role in hemostasis by forming the initial primary plug that seals vascular defects at the site of injury to vessel. Platelets also provides a surface that binds and concentrates activated coagulation factors. Platelets are disc-shaped anucleate cell fragments and form one of the formed elements of blood. They are shed from megakaryocytes in the bone marrow into the bloodstream. Thy have adhesion molecule P-selectin on their membranes. Their function depends on glycoprotein receptors, a contractile cytoskeleton, and two types of granules in their cytoplasm (refer Fig. 27 of Chapter 8). These are: (i) α-granules and (ii) dense (or δ) granules. They are discussed in detail on page 274.

- **α-Granules:** They contain proteins involved in coagulation, such as fibrinogen, coagulation factor V, and vWF. They also contain protein factors that may be involved in wound healing, and includes fibronectin, platelet factor 4 (PF4, a heparin-binding chemokine), platelet derived growth factor (PDGF), and transforming growth factor-β.
- **Dense (or δ) granules:** They contain adenosine diphosphate (ADP), adenosine triphosphate, ionized calcium, serotonin, and epinephrine

Coagulation Cascade

The coagulation cascade consists of a **series of amplifying enzymatic steps (reactions) and the endpoint is the conversion of soluble plasma fibrinogen to an insoluble fibrin clot**. This cascade is mediated by a number of coagulation factors (**Table 3**).

Recent research has revealed how fibrin formation occurs in vivo rather than how it occurs in the test tube. Clot formation differs in the laboratory test tube and in blood vessels in vivo. However, clotting in vitro and in vivo both follow the same general principles. The cascade consists of several reaction steps. **Each reaction step involves three components namely: (i) a substrate** (an inactive proenzyme form of a coagulation factor), (ii) **an enzyme** (an activated coagulation factor), and (iii) **a cofactor** (a reaction accelerator). The activated platelets provide a negatively charged phospholipid surface needed for the gathering (assembly) of these three components. Assembly of these three components also depends on calcium. Calcium binds to γ-carboxylated glutamic acid residues are present in coagulation factors II, VII, IX, and X. The enzymatic reactions that produce γ-carboxylated glutamic acid requires vitamin K as a cofactor. These are antagonized by drugs such as Coumadin which is used as an anticoagulant.

Table 3: Designations of coagulation factor.

Factor*	Standard name
I	Fibrinogen
II	Prothrombin
III	Tissue factor
IV	Calcium ions
V	Proaccelerin
VII	Proconvertin
VIII	Antihemophilic factor (AHF)
IX	Plasma thromboplastin (PTC)
X	Stuart factor
XI	Plasma thromboplastin antecedent (PTA)
XII	Hageman factor
XIII	Fibrin-stabilizing factor (FSF)
–	Prekallikrein
–	High–molecular-weight kininogen

* When procoagulant clotting factor becomes activated, it is designated by a lower-case letter "a" after the numerical (e.g., activated factor V is Va).

Based on assays performed in clinical laboratories, the coagulation cascade (in vitro) was once traditionally divided into the "intrinsic" and "extrinsic" pathways. Now **intrinsic pathway is called the contact activation pathway and the extrinsic pathway is called tissue factor pathway**. The contact activation pathway actually plays a minor role.

Clotting in vivo

Various steps (Fig. 14A) are as follows:

- **Liberation of tissue factor:** The key step in the initiation of coagulation cascade in vivo is exposure of tissue factor (TF). Tissue factor is a transmembrane surface (i.e., membrane-bound) glycoprotein molecule. TF is present in more or less on all cell surfaces except endothelial cells and circulating blood cells. Thus, under normal conditions when the blood is flowing, blood is never exposed to TF. However, tissue factor is present on the vascular wall and is not normally in contact with blood. Whenever there is **vascular injury/trauma**, blood spills out of the vessel and contacts the tissue factor (also known as thromboplastin or factor III) liberated at the site. Thus, coagulation cascade in vivo is initiated by endothelial injury, which releases tissue factor (TF).
- **Formation of TF–VIIa complex:** Liberated TF binds factor VII. The coagulation cascade reaction would stop immediately without active factor VII (VIIa) to cleave factor IX. However, there is small amount (0.1%) of factor VII that circulates in the active form. This small amount of VIIa from the blood binds TF and forms the TF-VIIa (tissue factor/factor VII) complex. The dynamic association of factor VIIa–TF complexes with TF pathway inhibitor (TFPI) is important in thrombosis. TFPI inhibits initiation of coagulation by binding TF–FXa–FVIIa complex. A major pool of TFPI on the surface of endothelial cells thus probably regulates coagulation.
- **Activation of small amounts of X:** TF–VIIa complex activates small amounts factor X to Xa (activated factor X) in the extrinsic pathway in vitro and converts factor IX into IXa in intrinsic pathway.
- **Conversion of prothrombin to thrombin:** Xa converts small amounts of prothrombin to thrombin that is the central player in clotting.
- **Intensification of conversion of IX to IXa:** Traces of thrombin formed activate factor XI, which in turn intensify conversion of factor IX to IXa (through activation of XI to XIa). When factor IXa is formed, it forms complex with VIIIa.
- **Greater amounts of activation of X:** Greater amounts of activation of X to Xa is by a complex of factors VIIIa and IXa. The presence of VIIIa is important for the function of the Xa complex. While VIIa activation of X is the initial step in coagulation, soon XIa generation becomes the predominant pathway for Xa generation. Two most common forms of hemophilia are due to the absence of the two proteins in this reaction (VIII/hemophilia A and IX/hemophilia B).
- **Formation of prothrombinase complex:** In the presence of calcium, the factor Xa generated (by either VIIa or IXa) binds with cofactor Va to form the prothrombinase complex (Xa and Va complex) on phospholipids from platelet membranes.

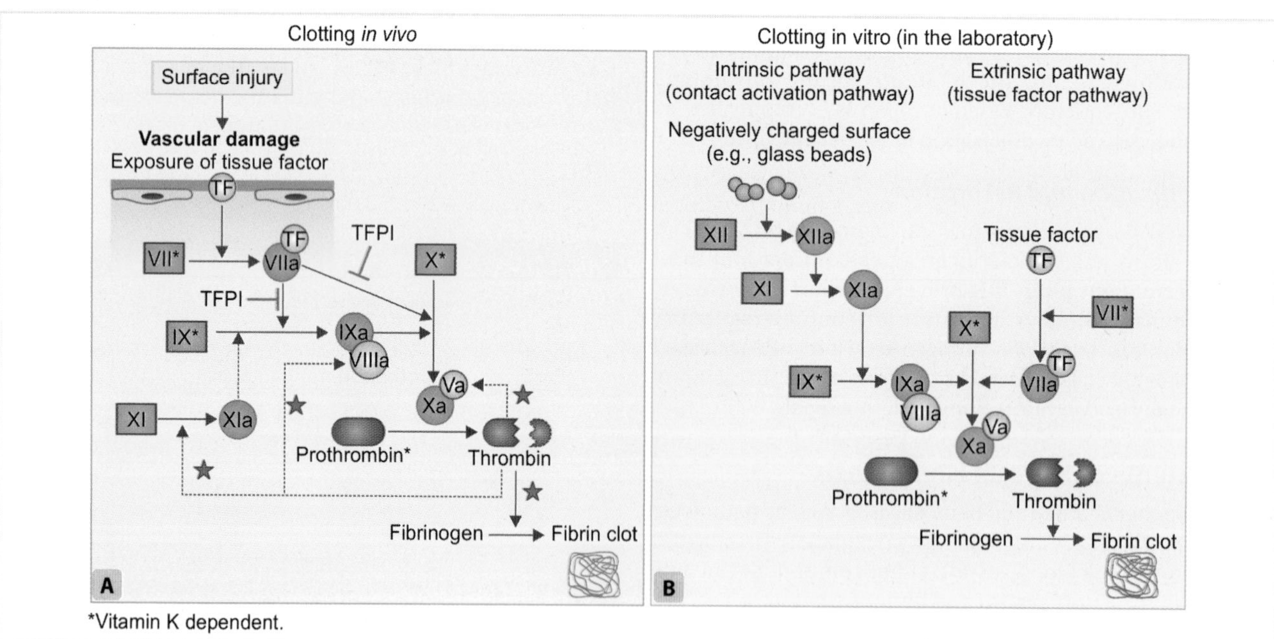

(TFPI: tissue factor pathway inhibitor)

FIGS. 14A AND B: The coagulation cascade in vivo and vitro (in the laboratory). (A) In vivo, the major initiator of coagulation is tissue factor. This is amplified by feedback loops involving thrombin (dotted lines). The coagulation factors in red rectangle are polypeptide coagulation factors in inactive form. The coagulation factors in dark green circle are coagulation polypeptides in active form. The factors in light green circle are polypeptides that acts as cofactors (reaction accelerators). Red star indicates the actions of thrombin in vivo coagulation. (B) Clotting in the laboratory is initiated by adding phospholipids, calcium, and either a negatively charged substance such as glass beads (intrinsic pathway) or a source of tissue factor (extrinsic pathway). Vitamin K is an essential cofactor required for the synthesis of all of the vitamin K–dependent (*) clotting factors. Warfarin acts as an anticoagulant by inhibiting the γ-carboxylation of the vitamin K–dependent coagulation factors.

- **Conversion of prothrombin to thrombin**: Xa and Va complex then catalyzes activation of the inactive zymogen prothrombin (II) to thrombin (IIa). The generation of thrombin is the final step in the initiation of coagulation and is the single most important step in hemostasis.
- **Formation of fibrin**: At sites where the endothelium is disrupted, thrombin converts soluble circulating fibrinogen to insoluble fibrin thrombus. This is achieved in two steps.
    1. First step: Thrombin converts fibrinogen into fibrin monomers which spontaneously polymerize to form fibrin polymers.
    2. Second step: Thrombin also activates factor XIII to factor XIIIa. Factor XIII stabilizes the clot by forming bonds between different fibrin polymers (cross-linked fibrin strands) to stabilize the clot. Thrombin also feeds back to activate factors IX (through XI), VIII, and V; stimulates crosslinking of fibrin; inhibits fibrinolysis; and activates platelets. All these augments the formation of a stable clot.

  Fibrinogen →fibrin monomer →fibrin polymer →fibrin clot

Clotting in vitro

Traditional Coagulation pathway: Coagulation in vitro (in the laboratory) can be activated by two pathways namely extrinsic and intrinsic (**Fig. 14B**). Clotting is vitro is initiated by adding phospholipids, calcium, and either a negatively charged substance such as glass beads (intrinsic pathway) or a source of tissue factor (extrinsic pathway). Both the pathways converge on the activation of factor X.

Extrinsic pathway

- The coagulation factor utilized in extrinsic pathway is factor VII.
- The **prothrombin time (PT) assay** is the laboratory test which assesses the function of the coagulation factors (proteins) involved in the extrinsic pathway (factor VII) and common pathway [factors X, V, II (prothrombin), and fibrinogen]. PT is performed by adding tissue factor ("tissue thromboplastin," usually minced animals' brains), phospholipids, and calcium to plasma, and the time for a fibrin clot to form is recorded.

Intrinsic pathway

- It is activated by exposure of factor XII (Hageman factor) to any thrombogenic surfaces such as glass beads.
- The coagulation factors utilized in intrinsic pathway in order of reaction are: Factors XII, prekallikrein HMWK, XI, IX, and VIII (Table).
- The **partial thromboplastin time (PTT)**/activated partial thromboplastin time (APTT) assesses the function of the coagulation factors (proteins) utilized in the intrinsic pathway (factors XII, pre-K, HMWK, XI, IX, and VIII) and common pathway (factors X, V, II, and fibrinogen). In this PTT assay, clotting of plasma is initiated by adding negatively charged particles like glass beads. These negatively charged particles (e.g., ground glass) activate factor XII (Hageman factor) together with phospholipids and calcium. The time taken to form fibrin clot is recorded.

Common pathway Above two pathways (extrinsic and intrinsic) have in common, factors X, V, prothrombin, and fibrinogen; and this part of coagulation pathway is known as the common pathway. This division is arbitrary because there are many interconnections between these two pathways. Coagulation factors involved in different pathways are listed in **Table 4**.

Table 4: Coagulation factors involved in different pathways.

Extrinsic pathway	*Intrinsic pathway*	*Common pathway*
• VII	• XII • Prekallikrein • HMWK • XI • IX • VIII (cofactor)	• X • V (cofactor) • Prothrombin • Fibrinogen

PT and PTT assays: These two assays are important in the evaluation of coagulation factor functions in patient. However, it is to be noted that they do not recapitulate the events that lead to coagulation in vivo. This should be kept in mind while considering the clinical effects of deficiencies of various coagulation factors.

Most important factors involved in clotting in vivo (Fig. A): These are:

- **Factor VIIa/tissue factor complex**: It is the most important **activator of factor IX.**
- **Factor IXa/factor VIIIa complex**: It is the most important **activator of factor X.**

Significance of coagulation factor deficiencies

Factors deficiencies associated with moderate-to-severe bleeding: Deficiencies of factors V, VII, VIII, IX, and X are associated with moderate-to-severe bleeding disorders. Deficiency of prothrombin is mostly incompatible with life.

Factors deficiencies associated with mild bleeding: These include:

- **Factor XI deficiency** is associated with mild bleeding. The mild bleeding tendency in factor XI deficiency is probably because of the ability of thrombin to activate factor XI (as well as factors V and VIII). This feedback mechanism amplifies the coagulation cascade and causes mild bleeding, if any.
- **Factor XII deficiency** is not associated with bleeding, instead these individuals are prone to thrombosis. By contrast, in some situations factor XII itself may contribute to thrombosis. These paradoxical findings may be because of involvement of factor XII in several pathways. These include the proinflammatory bradykinin pathway and fibrinolytic pathway.

Role of thrombin

Thrombin is the most important multifunctional molecule (**Fig. 15**). This is because, thrombin through its various enzymatic activities control different aspects of hemostasis and bridge clotting to inflammation and repair. Most important activities of thrombin are as follows:

- **Conversion of fibrinogen into fibrin**
    - Thrombin directly converts soluble fibrinogen into fibrin monomers. This monomer fibrin polymerizes into an insoluble fibril namely cross-linked fibrin polymer.
    - Thrombin also augments the coagulation process by activating factor XI, and also two critical cofactors: Factors V and VIII.

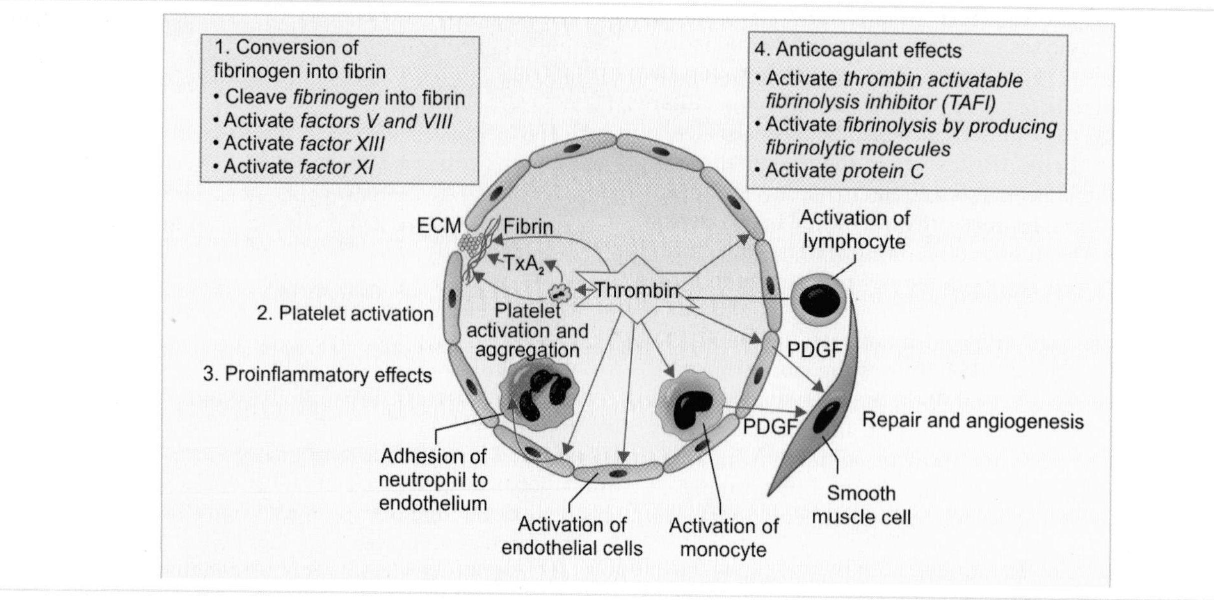

(ECM: extracellular matrix; PDGF: platelet derived growth factor)

FIG. 15: Role of thrombin in hemostasis and cellular activation. (1) Thrombin plays a main role in producing fibrin by cleaving fibrinogen and by activating factor XIII. It activates platelets. Apart from coagulation, it is involved in several other processes. Thrombin receptor is one of the protease-activated receptors (PAR). Through protease activated receptors (PARs), thrombin modulates several cellular activities. (2) It directly induces platelet aggregation and TxA_2 production, and activates endothelial cells, which respond by expressing adhesion molecules and cytokine mediators (e.g., PDGF). (3) Thrombin also directly activates leukocytes. (4) Thrombin participates in production of fibrinolytic molecules. It also mediates the protein C anticoagulant pathway by binding thrombomodulin present on the surface of endothelial cells.

  - It stabilizes the secondary hemostatic plug by activating factor XIII, which covalently cross-links fibrin.
- **Platelet activation:** Thrombin is a potent inducer of platelet activation and aggregation and TxA_2. It is achieved by its ability to activate protease activated receptors-1 (PAR-1). Thus, thrombin links platelet function to coagulation.
- **Proinflammatory effects:** Protease activated receptors (PARs) are also expressed on inflammatory cells, endothelium, and other types of cell types. These proteases activated receptors (PARs) are activated by thrombin modulates several cellular activities. It mediates pro-inflammatory effects. This is involved in tissue repair and angiogenesis. Thrombin activates endothelial cells, which respond by expressing adhesion molecules and cytokine mediators (e.g., growth factors such as PDGF). Thrombin also directly activates leukocytes (neutrophils and monocytes) and lymphocytes. Thrombin also increases vascular permeability by altering shape of endothelial cells and disrupting endothelial cell-cell adhesion junctions.
- **Anticoagulant effects:** Thrombin participates in production of fibrinolytic molecules. As thrombin is swept away in the circulating blood and encounters uninjured vessels, thrombin gets converted to an anticoagulant. This is by binding to thrombomodulin, a protein found on the surface of normal endothelial cells. The thrombin-thrombomodulin complex activates protein C anticoagulant pathway. Protein C is an important inhibitor of factor V and factor VIII. When thrombin encounters normal endothelium, it changes from a procoagulant to an anticoagulant. This property of reversal in function prevents clots from extending beyond the site of the vascular injury. Factor V, an essential coagulation cofactor and has also has anticoagulant activity. This is through its a cofactor function in the activated protein C system, which in turn downregulates factor VIIIa activity.

Uniqueness of thrombin Thrombin is unique in several ways.
- Does not need a cofactor for enzymatic function.
- Provides both *positive and negative feedback*
  - *Positive feedback:* By activating factors V, VIII, XI, and XIII and TAFI. Thrombin activates factor XI and provides a further positive feedback loop. Active factor XI activates IX, finally leading to more thrombin generation.
  - *Negative feedback:* By activating protein C and promoting fibrinolysis.

Factors that limit coagulation

After the initiation of coagulation, the activated coagulation system must be limited to the site of vascular injury so as to prevent dangerous outcome of coagulation in the entire vascular system. Factors that limit coagulation are as follows:
- **Dilution of activated coagulation factors:** Blood flowing past the site of injury washes out activated coagulation factors and is carried in the blood stream to liver. These are rapidly removed by the liver.
- **Absence of negatively charged phospholipids:** The negatively charged phospholipids are required for coagulation. At sites of vascular injury, this is mainly provided by platelets that have been activated by contact with subendothelial matrix. Once the subendothelial matrix is covered by platelets, there is no further availability of negatively charged phospholipids.

- **Factors expressed by intact endothelium adjacent to the site of injury:** The most important counterregulatory mechanisms involve factors that are expressed by intact endothelium adjacent to the site of injury (refer antithrombotic properties of endothelium below on page 366).
- **Coagulation regulatory mechanism** (discussed below)
- **Activation of fibrinolytic system:** Activation of the coagulation cascade also sets into motion a fibrinolytic cascade. This Fibrinolytic system limits the size of the clot and its dissolution later.

Coagulation regulatory mechanism This is achieved by three endogenous anticoagulants.

- **Antithrombin:** It inhibits the activity of thrombin and factors IXa, Xa, XIa, and XIIa. One of the antithrombin is antithrombin III which gets activated by binding to heparin-like molecules on endothelial cells. The heparin used to minimize thrombosis acts by activating antithrombin III (**Fig. 16**).
- **Proteins C and S:** These are vitamin K dependent proteins that act as a complex. Thrombin generated by activation of coagulation cascade, binds with thrombomodulin present on the endothelial cell membrane and activates the coagulation regulatory system called protein C system. Activated protein C (APC) binds with protein S to form APC-protein S complex. This complex inactivates factors Va and VIIIa (**Fig. 16**).
- **Tissue factor pathway inhibitor (TFPI):** TFPI is a protein which inactivates tissue factor—factor VIIa complexes and inactivates factor VIIa (**Fig. 17**).

Fibrinolytic system To prevent uncontrolled clotting, the process of coagulation must be sharply limited to the site of tissue injury. Activated coagulation factors are removed from the circulation by the liver. Activation of the coagulation also initiates fibrinolytic system (**Fig. 18**). Once the clots are formed, this fibrinolytic system is responsible for breaking down blood clots so that the size of the clot is limited. Fibrinolysis is an important process that prevent enlargement of thrombi, it aids wound healing, and prevent thrombosis in an undesirable place. Fibrinolytic system does this by removal of fibrin from the clot. Otherwise the clot may progress and involve the entire circulation with its consequences. Thus, normally several checks and balances ensure that just enough clotting occurs at the right place and time.

Proteins of the fibrinolytic system are involved in diverse processes such as cancer metastasis and memory.

Fibrinolytic proteins: The key proteins in the fibrinolytic system are as follows:

Plasmin: It is a serine protease produced by the liver. Fibrinolysis is largely accomplished through the enzymatic activity of plasmin. Plasmin cleaves bonds in (breaks down) fibrin and fibrinogen and interferes with its polymerization of fibrin. Normally plasmin circulates in blood as an inactive precursor plasminogen. Plasminogen can be converted to plasmin by:

- **Tissue plasminogen activator (tPA):** The most important of the physiologic plasminogen activator (PA) is tissue plasminogen activator (tPA). This is produced by endothelial cells and is most active when bound to fibrin. This characteristic makes tPA as a useful therapeutic agent, because its fibrinolytic activity is mainly confined to sites of recent thrombosis. The effectiveness of tPA to cleave plasminogen to plasmin is more than when plasminogen and tPA are both bound to the fibrin clot. Also, when plasmin is bound to fibrin, it is protected from the action of circulating α_2-antiplasmin.

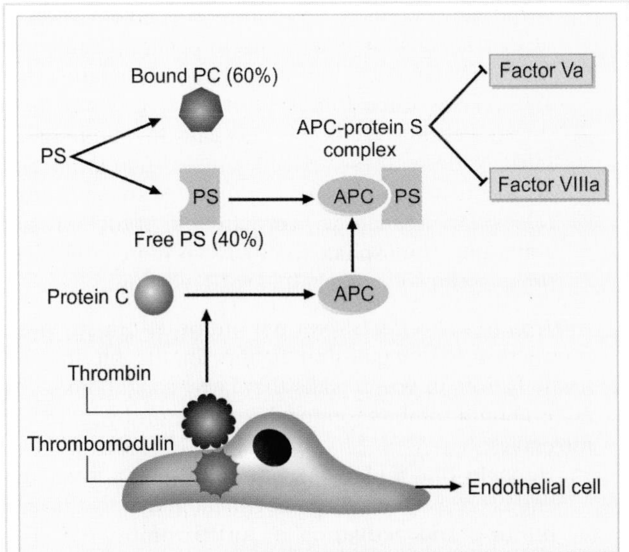

FIG. 16: Protein C and S pathway. Thrombomodulin from endothelial cell membrane binds to thrombin and activates protein C (PC). Activated protein C (APC) combines with free protein S (PS) to form complex which inactivates active factor V and VIII.

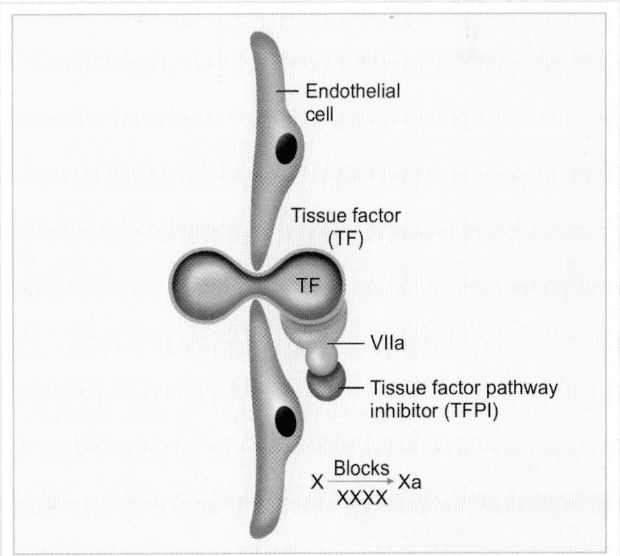

FIG. 17: TFPI inactivates tissue factor: Factor VIIa complexes.

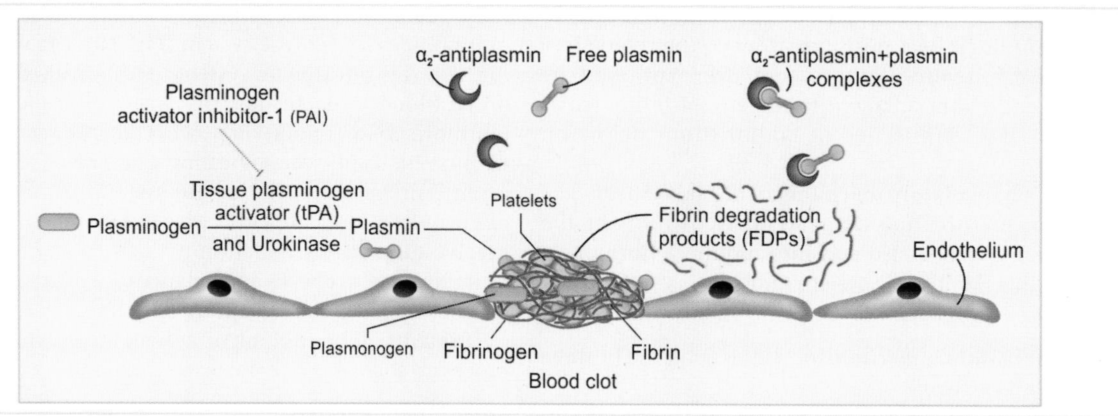

FIG. 18: Fibrinolytic system.

- **Urokinase (UK):** It is secreted in the urine (hence the initial name uro) and in many other cells. It is also a powerful activator of plasminogen.
- **Factor XII-dependent pathway:** It can also activate plasminogen and probably explains the association of factor XII deficiency and thrombosis.

Inhibitors of fibrinolysis: Once activated, plasmin is in tightly controlled by counter regulatory factors. There are several inhibitors of fibrinolysis keep the fibrinolytic system in balance:

- **Plasminogen activator inhibitor (PAI-1):** PAI-1 is synthesized by the liver and endothelial cells. It binds and inactivates tPA.
- **Alpha$_2$ (α_2) antiplasmin:** This is a plasma protein synthesized the liver. It binds and rapidly inactivates free plasmin. thereby limiting the action of plasmin.

When a thrombus is formed, it carries with it the seeds of its own destruction. This is by incorporation of plasminogen into the clot. Tissue plasminogen activator (tPA) released from nearby endothelial cells passes into the clot. The tPA binds to fibrin in the clot and then converts plasminogen to plasmin and this plasmin in turn lyses the clot. Any excess of tPA will escapes into the plasma and is quickly inactivated by plasminogen activator inhibitor (PAI-1). If any plasmin escapes into the plasma, it is quickly inactivated by α_2-antiplasmin. Thus, the process of active fibrinolysis is restricted to the clot or thrombus itself.

Plasmin cleaves fibrinogen and fibrin and produces number of fibrin degradation (FDP) products, also known as fibrin split products (fragments like X, Y, D, E, and D-D). These FDPs clear minor clots in the vessels and restore the blood flow. Elevated levels of FDPs most notably D-D fragment, known as **D-dimers** is used as a marker for thrombosis and is used for the diagnosis of disseminated intravascular coagulation (DIC).

Endothelium

Q. Write a short essay on thrombotic and antithrombotic role of the endothelium.

Endothelial cells play an important role in both hemostasis and thrombus formation. They have both **antithrombotic** (anticoagulant) **and prothrombotic** (procoagulant) activities. The balance between these two opposing endothelial properties determines **whether there is thrombus (clot) formation, propagation, or dissolution**.

Antithrombotic properties

Normally, the endothelial cells have (1) antiplatelet, (2) anticoagulant, and (3) fibrinolytic properties which prevent or inhibit thrombosis (and also coagulation) (**Figs. 19A** and **B**).

1. ***Antiplatelet effects:*** Platelet inhibitory effects of intact endothelium prevent platelet adhesion and aggregation by the following mechanism:
   - **Intact endothelium prevents adhesion of platelets** (and plasma coagulation factors) to the highly thrombogenic subendothelial von Willeband factor (vWF) and collagen.
   - **Production of inhibitors of platelet aggregation** by endothelial cells: These include (i) **prostacyclin (PGI_2)**, (ii) **nitric oxide (NO), and** (iii) **adenosine diphosphatase** [which degrades adenosine diphosphate (ADP)]. ADP is a powerful activator of platelet aggregation. Probably, the major factor that regulates the production of NO and PGI_2 by endothelium is the flow of blood. During normal flow, COX-1 is expressed constitutively by "healthy" endothelium and this produces PGI_2 (inhibits platelet aggregation and also relaxes smooth muscle) from arachidonic acid through cyclooxygenase (COX) pathway. Endothelial nitric oxide synthase (eNOS) converts L-arginine and O_2 to nitric oxide (NO). Compounds that promote release of NO include acetylcholine, bradykini, and adenosine diphosphate (ADP). NO is more labile than prostacyclin and has a half-life of 6 seconds.
2. ***Anticoagulant effects:*** Normal endothelium prevents interaction of coagulation factors in the blood with tissue factors in vessel walls that favor coagulation. The endothelium inhibits (oppose) coagulation by following molecules:
   - **Heparin-like molecules:** Found in the endothelium and exert their anticoagulant effect indirectly through binding and activation of **antithrombin III**. The activated antithrombin III, then inhibits thrombin and coagulation factors IXa, Xa, XIa, and XIIa. Heparin and related drugs used in clinical medicine is based on their ability to stimulate antithrombin III activity.
   - **Thrombomodulin and endothelial protein C receptor:** Thrombomodulin and endothelial protein C receptors are present on the endothelial cells. Endothelial protein

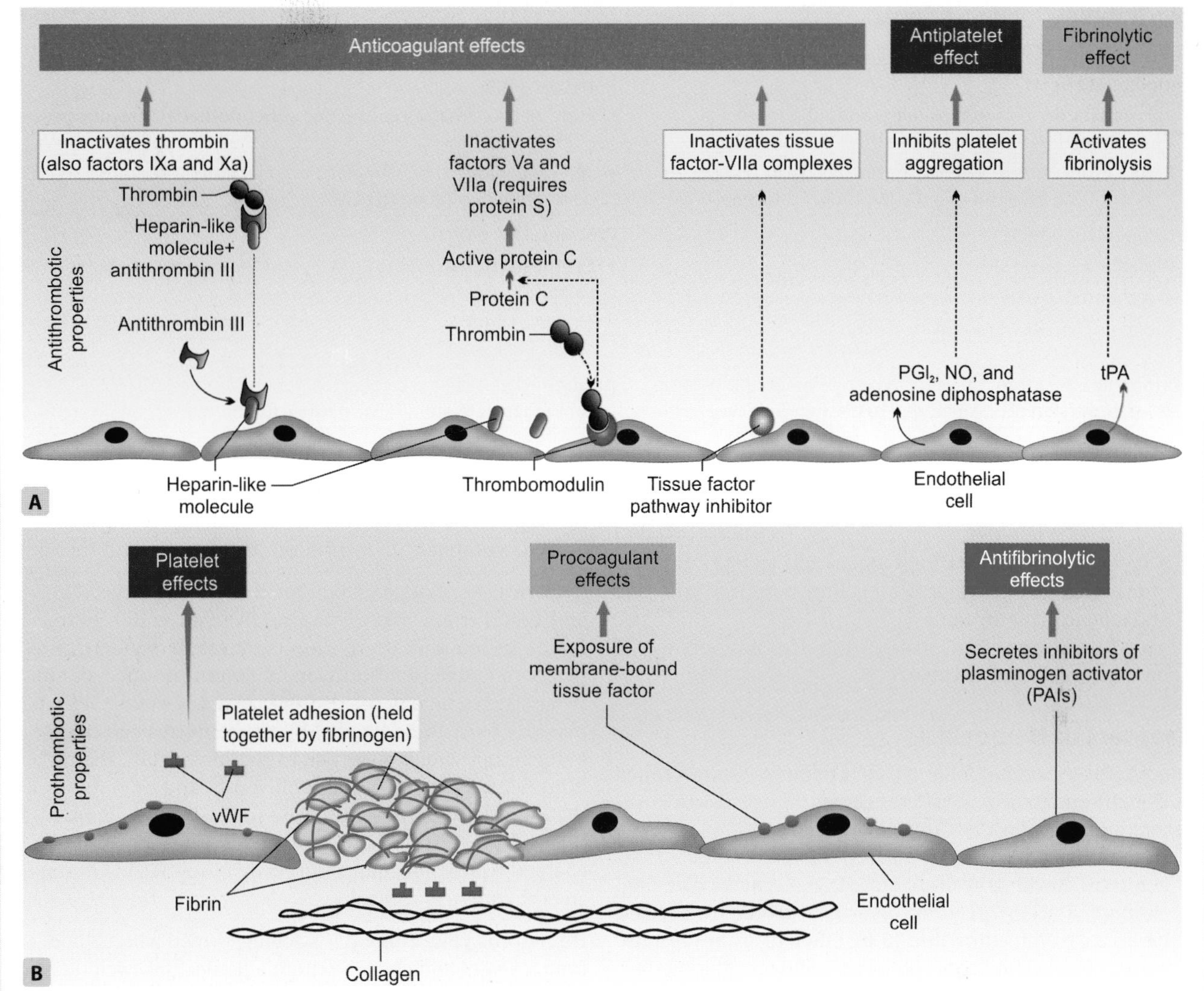

(PGI$_2$: prostacyclin; NO: nitric oxide; t-PA: tissue plasminogen activator; vWF: von Willebrand factor)

FIGS. 19A AND B: Endothelial factors that (A) inhibit and (B) favor thrombosis.

C receptor (EPCR) also known as activated protein C (APC) receptor. Thrombomodulin and endothelial protein C receptor bind thrombin and protein C, respectively. They form a complex on the endothelial cell surface. When thrombin is bound in this complex, it loses its ability to activate coagulation factors and platelets. This thrombin instead cleaves and activates protein C. Protein C is a vitamin K–dependent protease that needs a cofactor, protein S. Activated protein C/ protein S form a complex which is a powerful inhibitor of coagulation cofactors Va and VIIIa.

- **Tissue factor pathway inhibitor (TFPI):** Similar to protein C, tissue factor pathway inhibitor (TFPI) needs protein S as a cofactor. As the name tissue factor pathway inhibitor implies, it binds and inhibits tissue factor/factor VIIa complexes.

3. ***Fibrinolytic Effects*** Endothelial cells synthesize t-PA is main component of the fibrinolytic pathway, which degrades thrombi whenever these are formed.

Prothrombotic properties

Endothelial cells may be damaged or activated by several ways. These include trauma, inflammation, infectious agents, hemodynamic forces, plasma mediators, and cytokines. The damaged or activated endothelial cells promote prothrombotic state by its (1) platelet, (2) procoagulant, and (3) antifibrinolytic effects.

1. ***Platelet Effects***
   - Endothelial damage **exposes the subendothelial thrombogenic ECM** and allows adhesion of platelets from circulation to ECM.
   - *von Willebrand factor* produced by normal endothelial cells is essential cofactor that helps platelet binding to matrix elements.
2. ***Procoagulant Effects***
   - Endothelial cells **synthesize tissue factor** in response to cytokines [e.g., tumor necrosis factor (TNF) or interleukin-1 (IL-1)] or bacterial endotoxin. Tissue factor activates the extrinsic coagulation cascade.

Table 5: Antithrombotic and prothrombotic properties of endothelium.

Antithrombotic properties	*Prothrombotic properties*
Antiplatelet effects • Acts as a barrier between platelets and subendothelial thrombogenic von Willeband factor (vWF) and collagen • Produce inhibitors of platelet aggregation [e.g., prostaglandin I_2 (PGI_2), nitric oxide (NO), and adenosine diphosphatase]	**Platelet effects** • Endothelial damage **exposes the subendothelial thrombogenic** ECM • *von Willebrand factor (vWF)* produced by normal endothelial cells helps platelet binding to ECM
Anticoagulant effects • Heparin-like molecules • Thrombomodulin and endothelial protein C receptor (EPCR) • Tissue factor pathway inhibitor (TFPI)	**Procoagulant effects** • **Synthesis of tissue factor**→ activates the extrinsic coagulation cascade • Activated endothelial cells increase the catalytic function of factors IXa and Xa
Fibrinolytic effect through tissue-type plasminogen activator (t-PA)→conversion of plasminogen to plasmin→cleaves fibrin	**Antifibrinolytic effects** through secretion of inhibitors of plasminogen activator (PAIs)→reduce fibrinolysis

- Activated endothelial cells increase the catalytic function of activated coagulation factors IXa and Xa.

3. ***Antifibrinolytic Effects*** Endothelial cells secrete inhibitors of plasminogen activator (PAIs). They reduce fibrinolysis and tend to favor thrombosis.

Antithrombotic and prothrombotic properties of endothelium are listed in **Table 5**.

Disorders of Hemostasis

Hemostasis is essential for life. It can be deranged in wide range of disorders and its degree of derangement varies. Disorders of hemostasis can be divided into two major groups.

1. **Hemorrhagic disorders:** Failure of the hemostatic system to restore the integrity of an injured vessel causes bleeding. Hemorrhagic or bleeding disorders are characterized by excessive bleeding due to insufficient or hemostatic mechanisms that are not able to prevent loss of blood.
2. **Thrombotic disorders:** Inability to maintain the fluidity of blood results in thrombosis. These disorders are characterized by formation of blood clots (generally called as thrombi) within intact blood vessels or within the chambers of the heart.

Hemorrhagic Disorders

Definition: Hemorrhagic disorder is a general term for a group of conditions (acquired or inherited) in which there is an abnormal tendency to bleeding/hemorrhage due to failure of hemostasis.

They are also known as hemorrhagic disorder/hemorrhagic diathesis (diathesis is a Greek word for a predisposition or tendency) are also known as bleeding disorders. Abnormal bleeding may be due to primary or secondary defects in vessel walls, platelets, or coagulation factors. The bleeding may be heavy and prolonged which may occur after an insignificant injury or it may occur spontaneously.

Terminologies used in bleeding disorders

Petechiae (Fig. 20A): They are small (1–2 mm in diameter), red to purple hemorrhagic spots in the skin, mucous membranes (e.g., conjunctiva) or serosal surfaces. They result from blood leaking through intact endothelial lining of capillaries. They are most commonly found with low platelet counts (thrombocytopenia) or defective platelet function or loss of vascular wall support (e.g., vitamin C deficiency).

Purpura (Fig. 20B): The term purpura means purple. They are slightly larger (>3 mm) than petechiae. The causes are thrombocytopenia, increased vascular fragility and vasculitis.

Ecchymoses/Bruises (Fig. 20C): They are larger (1–2 cm) and result from blood escaping through endothelium into intact subcutaneous tissue. They result from trauma or hemostatic disorder and usually do not produce significant swelling as in hematoma. Extravasated RBCs in the lesions are phagocytosed and degraded by macrophages and release the hemoglobin which gives rise to red-blue color. The pigment from heme is converted into biliverdin and then to bilirubin (blue-green color) and iron from red cells forms hemosiderin (golden-brown color). These changes are responsible for the characteristic color changes in ecchymoses. A good example of an ecchymosis is a "black eye."

Hematoma (Fig. 20D): It is swelling formed when blood leaks from a vessel and collects within a tissue. The swelling results from a large area of hemorrhage in subcutaneous tissue or muscle. It is blue or purple and slightly raised.

Manifestations: Presentation of abnormal bleeding varies widely.

- **Massive bleeding:** At one end of the spectrum of hemorrhagic disorder, it may produce massive bleeding. This may occur with ruptures of large blood vessels such as the aorta or of the heart. In these situations, the tragic or fatal event may overwhelm the normal capacity of hemostatic mechanisms and can lead to death. Examples of diseases associated with sudden, massive hemorrhage include aortic dissection and aortic abdominal aneurysm and myocardial infarction complicated by rupture of the aorta or the heart.
- **Bleeding disorders:** Deficiencies of coagulation factors (e.g., hemophilia) are usually inherited and if untreated, they can lead to severe bleeding disorders
- **Evident during hemostatic stress:** At the other end of the spectrum of hemorrhagic disorder, it may produce minimal defects in clotting. It may become evident only with conditions that cause hemostatic stress. Examples include surgery, childbirth, dental procedures, menstruation, or trauma. Mild bleeding is most commonly found in diseases such as inherited defects in vWF, consumption of aspirin, and uremia (renal failure). In uremia, there is alteration of platelet function by some uncertain mechanisms.

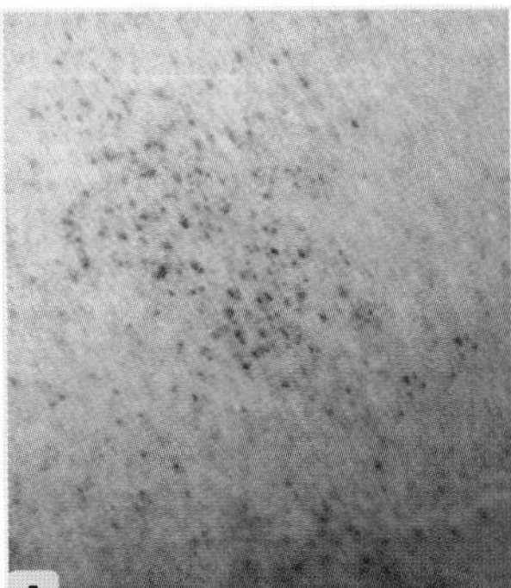

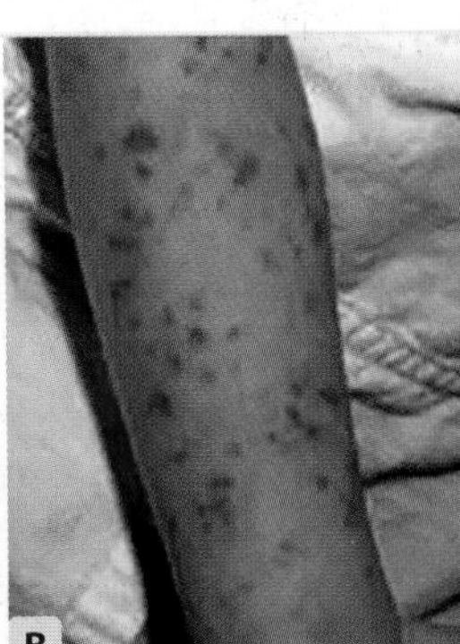

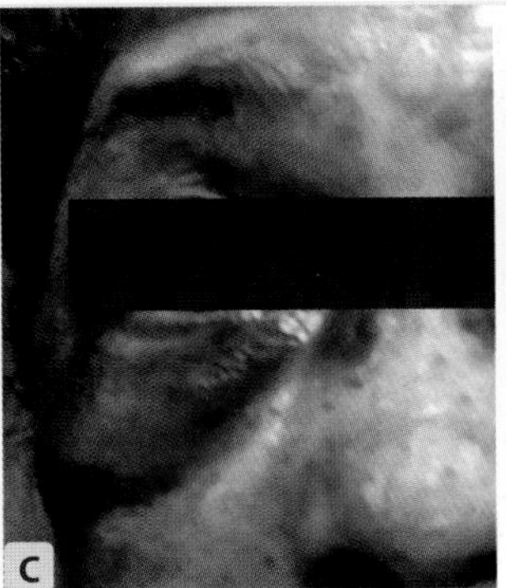

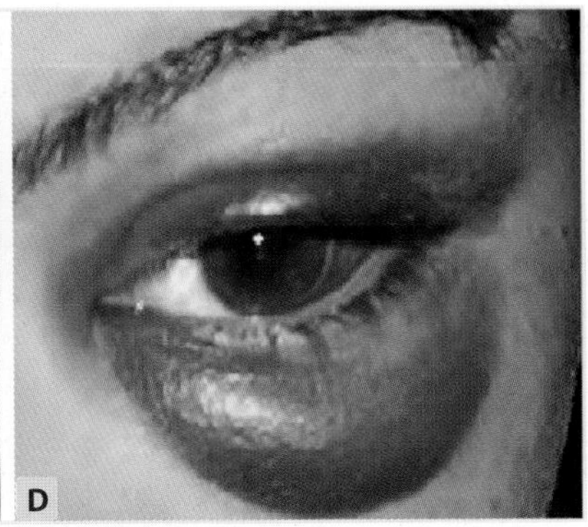

FIGS. 20A TO D: (A) Petechiae which appear as small (1–2 mm in diameter), red to purple hemorrhagic spots in the skin, mucous membranes or serosal surfaces; (B) purpura—slightly larger (>3 mm) than petechiae; (C) ecchymoses are larger (>1–2 cm) and result from blood escaping; (D) hematoma is swelling formed when blood leaks from a vessel and collects within subcutaneous tissue or muscle.

Classification of hemorrhagic disorders: They may be broadly classified as disorders of primary hemostasis and disorders of secondary (coagulation) hemostasis. General principles related to abnormal bleeding and its consequences are as follows:

- **Defects of primary hemostasis**: This include bleeding due to platelet defects, vascular defects or von Willebrand disease. They usually present with small bleeds in skin or mucosal membranes. These bleeds generally produce petechiae (minute 1- to 2-mm hemorrhages), or purpura [slightly larger (≥3 mm) than petechiae]. The capillaries of the mucosa and skin are susceptible to rupture following minor trauma. Normally, the platelets seal these defects almost immediately. Mucosal bleeding associated with hemorrhagic defects in primary hemostasis may present with epistaxis (nosebleeds), gastrointestinal bleeding, or excessive menstruation (menorrhagia). One of the fatal complications of very low platelet counts (thrombocytopenia) is intracerebral hemorrhage.
- **Vascular disorders:** Generalized defects which involves small vessels (e.g., vasculitis) usually present with palpable purpura and ecchymoses. They may also occur with diseases that lead to blood vessel fragility (e.g., amyloidosis, scurvy).
- **Defects of secondary hemostasis**: These are due to defects in coagulation factor. They usually present with bleeding into soft tissues (e.g., muscle) or joints. Bleeding into joints (hemarthrosis) following minor trauma is characteristic of hemophilia.

Clinical significance of hemorrhage: It depends on the amount of the bleed, the rate of bleeding, and location of bleeding.

- Rapid loss of blood volume up to 20% may produce little impact in healthy adults.
- With greater loss of blood, it can lead to hemorrhagic (hypovolemic) shock.
- If minor bleeding in the subcutaneous tissues located in the brain, it can cause death. This is because the skull is unyielding and increased intracranial pressure due to intracranial hemorrhage may compromise the blood supply or causes herniation of the brainstem.
- Chronic or recurrent external blood loss (e.g., peptic ulcer, hemorrhoids or menstrual bleeding) causes iron loss. It can lead to iron deficiency anemia. However, if red cells are retained in the body (e.g., hemorrhage into body cavities or tissues), iron is recycled and used for the synthesis of hemoglobin.

THROMBOSIS

Q. Write short essay on thrombogenesis.

Q. Write short essay on pathogenesis of thrombus formation and its progression.

Q. Describe the current concepts of thrombogenesis.

Definition

Thrombosis is defined as the **process of formation of a solid mass** in the **circulating blood from the constituents of flowing blood**.

The **solid mass formed** is called as **thrombus** and it consists of an aggregate of coagulated blood containing platelets, fibrin, and entrapped cellular elements of blood. Thrombosis is one of the curse for humans, because it is responsible for the most serious and common forms of cardiovascular disease.

Etiology

Three primary abnormalities can lead to formation of a thrombus and constitute Virchow's triad (**Fig. 21**). These include:

1. **Injury to endothelium** (changes in the vessel wall).
2. **Stasis or turbulent blood flow** (changes in the blood flow).
3. **Hypercoagulability of the blood** (changes in the blood itself).

Injury to Endothelium (Changes in the Vessel Wall)

Endothelial injury may be either physical damage or endothelial dysfunction (or activation).

Physical endothelial injury

It is important for formation of thrombus in the **heart or the arterial circulation**. Normally, high flow rates in the heart and arterial circulation prevent adhesion of platelet to endocardium/endothelium and wash out any activated coagulation factors. The endothelial cell injury **promotes adhesion of platelets at the site of injury**.

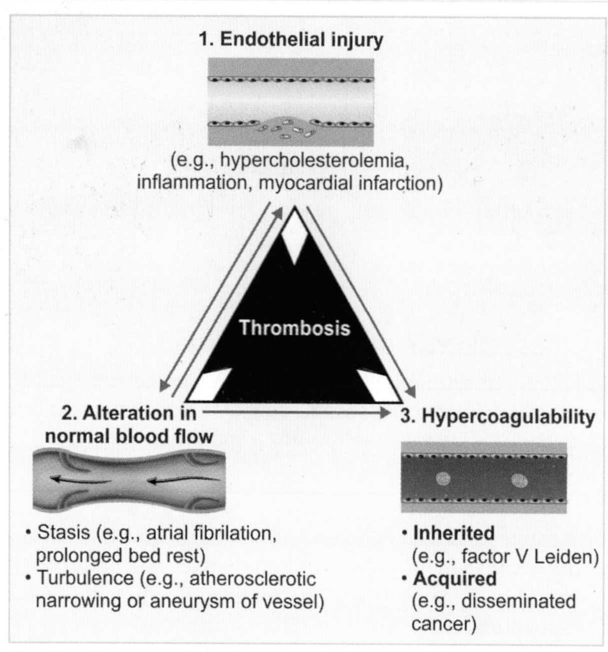

FIG. 21: Virchow's triad in thrombosis. (1) Endothelial injury is the most important factor. (2) Alteration in blood flow (stasis or turbulence). (3) Hypercoagulability.

Usually, cardiac and arterial thrombi are rich in platelets, and platelet adherence and activation. It is considered that platelets are necessary for thrombus formation under high shear stress (e.g., observed in arteries). This is the basis for using aspirin and other platelet inhibitors in coronary artery disease and acute myocardial infarction.

Causes

Heart:

- **Chambers of heart:** It may occur with endocardial injury due to myocardial infarction with damage to the adjacent endocardium or catheter trauma. Mural thrombi can develop in the left ventricular wall, over areas of myocardial infarction. Factors that predispose to thrombus formation over the endocardial region of infarcted area are: (i) damage to endocardium as a part of extension of transmural infarct and (ii) alterations in blood flow associated with an akinetic or dyskinetic segment of the myocardium.
- **Valves:** Small thrombi on the valves are called as vegetations.
  - **Infective endocarditis:** Thrombi on valves (e.g., mitral, aortic valve) damaged by a blood-borne bacteria or fungi
  - **Damaged valves** (e.g., due to rheumatic heart disease, congenital heart disease)
  - **Libman–Sacks endocarditis** in systemic lupus erythematosus
  - **Nonbacterial thrombotic endocarditis:** They are sterile vegetations on noninfected valves with hypercoagulable states.

Arteries [e.g., ulcerated **atherosclerotic plaques**, traumatic or inflammatory vascular injury **(vasculitis)**].

Capillaries: Causes include **acute inflammatory lesions**, vasculitis and disseminated intravascular coagulation **(DIC)**.

Mechanism: Physical loss of endothelium exposes thrombogenic subendothelial von Willeband factor (vWF), tissue factor and collagen. This tigger formation of thrombus. Platelets adhere to the site of endothelial injury and release prothrombotic tissue factor. There is local depletion of antithrombotic factors such as PGI_2.

Endothelial activation or dysfunction

Definition: Endothelial activation or dysfunction is defined as an **altered state,** which promote thrombosis by shifting the pattern of gene expression in endothelium to one that is prothrombotic.

Causes: Endothelial activation or dysfunction can be induced by different causes. These include physical injury, infectious agents, abnormal blood flow, inflammatory mediators, metabolic abnormalities (e.g., hypercholesterolemia, homocystinemia), and toxins (e.g., absorbed from cigarette smoke). Endothelial activation play an important role in triggering arterial thrombotic events.

Mechanism: Endothelial dysfunction can **disturb the balance between prothrombotic** and **antithrombotic activities of endothelium by:**

- **Procoagulant changes:** These are as follows:
  - **Downregulate the expression of thrombomodulin:** Inflammatory cytokines activate endothelial cells that downregulate the expression of thrombomodulin present on the endothelial cells. Thrombomodulin is the main modulator of thrombin activity and enhances the procoagulant and proinflammatory actions of thrombin.
  - **Downregulate the expression of other anticoagulants:** For example, protein C and tissue factor protein inhibitor. These changes promote a procoagulant state.
- **Antifibrinolytic effects:** Activated endothelial cells secrete plasminogen activator inhibitors (PAIs). They prevent fibrinolysis, and downregulate the expression of t-PA. These changes favor the development of thrombi.
- **Producing more procoagulant factors**, e.g., platelet adhesion molecules, tissue factor, PAIs or
- **Synthesizing less anticoagulant effectors**, e.g., thrombomodulin, PGI_2, t-PA.

Alterations in Normal Blood Flow

Normally, blood flows through a blood vessel in layers and the velocity of the layers varies. This normal blood flow is termed as **laminar** (**Fig. 22**). Blood in the center moves faster than blood in the outer layers. This is because, the blood in the center layer is in contact with blood only, whereas the outermost layer is also in contact with the intima of the blood vessel wall, which produces friction against the cellular components (platelets and other cellular elements) of the blood. Many blood cells stick or adhere to the intima from this outer layer because of minimal flow.

Causes of alterations in blood flow

Turbulence (disturbed movement of blood): The streamlined laminar flow may be disrupted by normal anatomy and by pathologic processes creating turbulent flow. Turbulent flow is an interruption in the forward current of blood flow by crosswise flow (**Fig. 23A**). Turbulence results if blood flows around an obstruction in the vessel (**Fig. 23B**) or over a roughened intimal

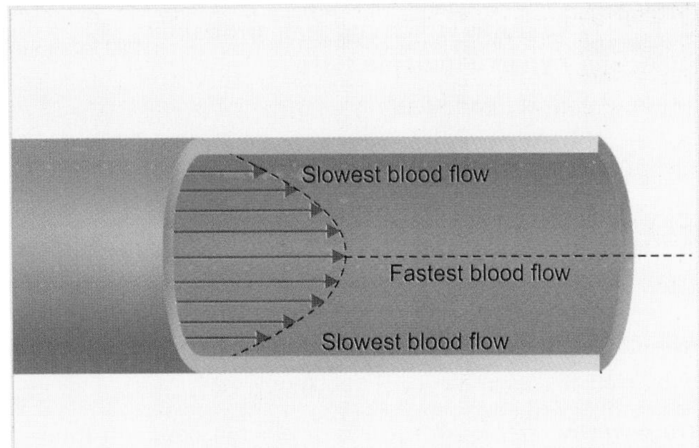

FIG. 22: Laminar blood flow in normal vessel. In laminar flow, all the elements of the blood move in streamlines which are parallel to the axis of blood vessel. The layer of blood in contact with vessel wall is slow-moving or motionless whereas the maximal velocity is observed in the blood that moves along the axis of the blood vessel.

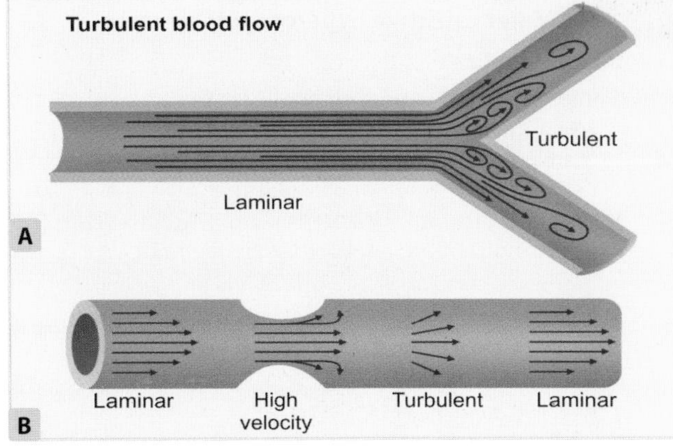

FIGS. 23A AND B: Turbulent flow at the bifurcation of a blood vessel (A) and around the obstruction in the vessel (B).

surface (e.g., atheromatous plaque). It can produce thrombus in the arteries and heart.

Stasis: It is a **major cause for venous thrombosis**.

Mechanism

Stasis and turbulence produce thrombus by the following mechanism:

- **Promote endothelial** injury/**activation** and increases the procoagulant activity and leukocyte adhesion. This is partly brought out by flow induced changes in the expression of adhesion molecules and proinflammatory factors.
- **Bring platelets into contact with the endothelium** due to disruption of normal laminar flow.
- **Prevent cleansing and dilution of activated clotting factors** by fresh flowing blood.
- **Prevent flowing in of clotting factor inhibitors**.

Clinical disorders associated with turbulence and stasis

Heart:

- **Acute myocardial infarction:** In acute myocardial infarction, thrombi can develop in the areas of noncontractile (infarcted) myocardium and sometimes in cardiac aneurysm. Both are associated with stasis and alterations in blood flow. These changes promote the formation of cardiac mural thrombi.
- **Arrhythmias/atrial fibrillation**: For example, rheumatic mitral valve stenosis produced dilatation of the left atrium. This in conjunction with atrial fibrillation (due to disordered atrial activity) produces slower blood flow or stasis in the dilated atrium. It impairs left atrial contractility and predisposes to formation of mural thrombi. Usually it occurs in the left atrial appendage.
- **Dilated cardiomyopathy:** Primary myocardial diseases are associated with mural thrombi in the left ventricle. This may be due to endocardial injury and altered hemodynamics associated with poor contraction of myocardium.

Arteries:

- **Ulcerated atherosclerotic plaques** and vascular injuries: Atherosclerosis of vessels exposes subendothelial vWF and tissue factor and also produces turbulence of blood flow. Vasucular injuries such as vasculitis and trauma may also produce thrombus at the site of damage.
- **Aneurysms:** Abnormal permanent aortic and arterial dilations are called *aneurysms*. They produce local stasis and are therefore prone for thrombosis.

Veins: Thrombi develop in the saphenous veins with varicosities or in deep veins.

Other causes

- **Hyperviscosity**, e.g., with **polycythemia vera** increases resistance to flow and causes stasis in small vessels.
- **Red blood cell disorders**, e.g., **sickle cell anemia** can cause vascular occlusions and stasis in small vessels. This predisposes to thrombosis.

Hypercoagulability

Definition

Hypercoagulability state (also known as thrombophilia) is defined as a **systemic disorder associated with increased tendency to develop blood to clot. It is usually caused by alterations in coagulation factors**.

Causes

Hypercoagulability plays an important role particularly in venous thrombosis. Causes can be divided into primary (genetic) and secondary (acquired) disorders (**Box 3**).

Possibility of hypercoagulable state should be considered if a patient develops unexplained thrombotic episodes in one of the contexts listed in **Box 4**.

Primary (genetic) causes of hypercoagulability

Inherited causes of hypercoagulability must be considered first, whenever a patient younger than 50 years of age present with thrombosis. This applies even if there are acquired risk factors.

Factor V Leiden: A single-nucleotide (point) mutation in the *factor V* gene is one of the main genetic cause of hypercoagulable state. Factor V gene is called factor V Leiden,

Box 3: Major causes of hypercoagulable state.

- **Primary (genetic)**
  - **Common: Increased prothrombotic factors**
    - Factor V mutation: Factor V Leiden (substitution of Arg to Gln in amino acid residue 506; results in resistance to activated protein C)
    - Prothrombin mutation (G20210A noncoding sequence variant; results in increased level of prothrombin)
    - High levels of factors VIII, IX, XI, or fibrinogen (genetics not known)
  - **Rare: Deficiency of antithrombotic (anticoagulant) factors**
    - Antithrombin III deficiency
    - Protein C deficiency
    - Protein S deficiency
  - **Very Rare**
  - Fibrinolysis defects
  - Homozygous homocystinuria (deficiency of cystathione β-synthetase
- **Secondary (acquired)**
  - **High-risk for thrombosis**
    - Prolonged bed rest or immobilization
    - Myocardial infarction, atrial fibrillation
    - Tissue injury (e.g., surgery, fracture, burn)
    - Disseminated intravascular coagulation
    - Cancer
    - Prosthetic cardiac valves
    - Heparin-induced thrombocytopenia
    - Antiphospholipid antibody syndrome
  - **Lower risk for thrombosis**
    - Nephrotic syndrome
    - Hyperestrogenic states (pregnancy and postpartum)
    - Oral contraceptive use
    - Cardiomyopathy
    - Smoking
    - Sickle cell anemia

after the city in the Netherlands where it was discovered. This mutation renders factor V resistant to cleavage and inactivation by protein C (activated protein C [APC]). Hence, this disorder is also termed as **APC resistance**. Factor V Leiden is inherited as autosomal dominant disorder. Frequency of this mutation is higher (about 60–65%) in individuals with recurrent DVT. Due to this defect, an important antithrombotic counter regulatory pathway is lost.

Prothrombin gene mutation A single nucleotide change (G20210A) in the 3′-untranslated region of the prothrombin gene is another common mutation associated with hypercoagulability and thrombosis. This disorder is associated with high levels of prothrombin and threefold increased risk of venous thrombosis.

Antithrombin III (ATIII) deficiency This is an autosomal dominant disorder with incomplete penetrance. It can produce either a quantitative or a qualitative effect on ATIII. These individuals have a risk of a thrombotic event (usually venous) .

Protein C and protein S deficiencies Homozygous protein C deficiency can produce life-threatening neonatal thrombosis with **purpura fulminans**. Patients with heterozygous protein C deficiency may be without any symptoms. Both proteins C and S deficiencies resemble ATIII deficiency

Box 4: Features which suggests probability of hypercoagulable state.

- Recurrence of thrombosis
- Thrombi developing at a young age (younger than 50 years)
- Family history of thrombotic episodes
- Thrombosis in unusual anatomic sites
- Difficulty in controlling thrombus with anticoagulants

Homocysteinemia: An increased plasma concentration of homocysteine is known as homocysteinemia. Raised levels of homocysteine may occur as either inherited or acquired disorder.

- Marked raise of homocysteine levels may be due to an inherited deficiency of cystathionine β-synthetase.
- Acquired causes of homocysteinemia are deficiency of vitamin B_6, B_{12}, and folic acid.

Homocysteine metabolites may form link with a variety of proteins, including fibrinogen and may be responsible for its prothrombotic effects. Homocysteinemia also predisposes to atherosclerosis and thrombosis.

Commonly, thrombophilic genotypes are heterozygous for factor V Leiden and for the prothrombin G20210A variant. They have only a moderate risk of thrombosis and most them are otherwise healthy and are free from thrombotic complications. However, homozygosity and compound heterozygosity factor V and prothrombin mutations genotypes are associated with greater risk. These individuals have a significantly increased frequency of venous thrombosis when there is coexistence of other acquired risk factors (e.g., pregnancy or prolonged bed rest).

Secondary (acquired) causes of hypercoagulability

Pathogenesis of acquired (secondary) causes of hypercoagulability (thrombophilia) is usually multifactorial (see **Box 3**).

- In congestive cardiac failure, prolonged immobilization or trauma, hypercoagulability is usually due to venous stasis or vascular injury.
- In individuals who use oral contraceptives or in hyperestrogenic state of pregnancy, hypercoagulability is probably caused by increased synthesis of coagulation factors and reduced anticoagulant synthesis by the liver.
- Disseminated cancers may release procoagulants and may predispose to thrombosis.
- In advancing age, there may be reduced endothelial PGI_2 production leading to hypercoagulability. The mechanisms that promote hypercoagulability in smoking and obesity is not known.
- In patients with myeloproliferative disorders, heparin-associated thrombocytopenia and thrombotic thrombocytopenic purpura (TTP), hypercoagulability may be due to increased platelet activation which probably accounts for excessive clotting.

Heparin-induced thrombocytopenia (HIT) syndrome

Q. Write short essay on heparin-induced thrombocytopenia syndrome.

Heparin is the widely used anticoagulant for prevention or treatment of thrombosis. HIT is a distinct type of drug-induced thrombocytopenia. Thrombocytopenia occurs in about 10% of patients receiving heparin and it is important to diagnose this entity to prevent its fatal consequences. Heparin can cause two clinically distinct types of HIT syndromes:

Type I: Thrombocytopenia develops immediately (2–5 days) following heparin therapy and is clinically insignificant with mild, transient, self-limited thrombocytopenia. It follows a relatively benign course and resolves after heparin is discontinued. It is probably due to direct platelet aggregation induced by heparin by nonimmune mechanisms.

Type II: HIT syndrome is a serious, potentially life-threatening disorder. It develops following the administration of unfractionated heparin. Risk of HIT is less frequent when low-molecular-weight heparin preparations are used. HIT syndrome is associated with severe consumptive thrombocytopenia, platelet activation and thus a hypercoagulable state. It usually develops 1 to 2 weeks after starting heparin therapy (or earlier if the patient has been previously sensitized to heparin). Surprisingly, thrombocytopenia is associated with life-threatening thrombosis in both veins and arteries, known as **"white clot syndrome"**.

Pathogenesis (Fig. 24): Platelet factor 4 (PF4) protein is normally found in platelet alpha granules and it is released on activation of platelets. Heparin binds to PF4 released from platelets and forms a complex (heparin/PF4 complex) in the circulation. This complex undergoes a conformational change and forms neoantigen. Immunoglobulin (Ig) G antibodies are formed against these complexes of heparin and PF4. PF4-IgG immune complex attaches to and cross-links the Fc receptors on the platelet surface. This leads to activation of platelets and aggregation. This promotes thrombosis even in the presence of marked thrombocytopenia. Platelet activation causes further release of more PF4 and creates more target antigen for HIT antibodies. The HIT antibodies also bind to PF4-like proteins on the surface of endothelium. This activates endothelium and promotes prothrombotic state. Platelets bound by HIT antibodies are removed by macrophages in the spleen (hence the term thrombocytopenia in the name of the syndrome). Though most common manifestation is thrombocytopenia, the most dangerous complication is thrombosis affecting both veins and arteries. It develops in about 50% of patients. The sequelae of thrombosis are necrosis of the skin, gangrene of the limbs, stroke, and myocardial infarction. If heparin is not immediately discontinued, thrombosis of large arteries may lead to vascular insufficiency and emboli from DVT can result in fatal pulmonary thromboembolism.

Diagnosis: By demonstration of antiPF4-heparin antibodies.

Antiphospholipid antibody syndrome

Q. Write short essay on antiphospholipid antibody syndrome (APLA/APS)

Definition: Antiphospholipid antibody syndrome ***(APLA/APS)*** is an autoantibody-mediated acquired thrombophilia characterized by the following:

- Presence of one or more family of antibodies in the patient's plasma known as **antiphospholipid (aPL) autoantibodies**.
- Venous or arterial thromboses, or pregnancy complications such as recurrent abortion (miscarriages), unexplained fetal death, and premature birth.

Types: APS may be of **primary or secondary type**.

- **Primary APS:** In primary APS, patients do not have any predisposing cause or well-defined autoimmune disorders. Their only manifestation is hypercoagulable state. About 50% of the patients with APS are of primary type.

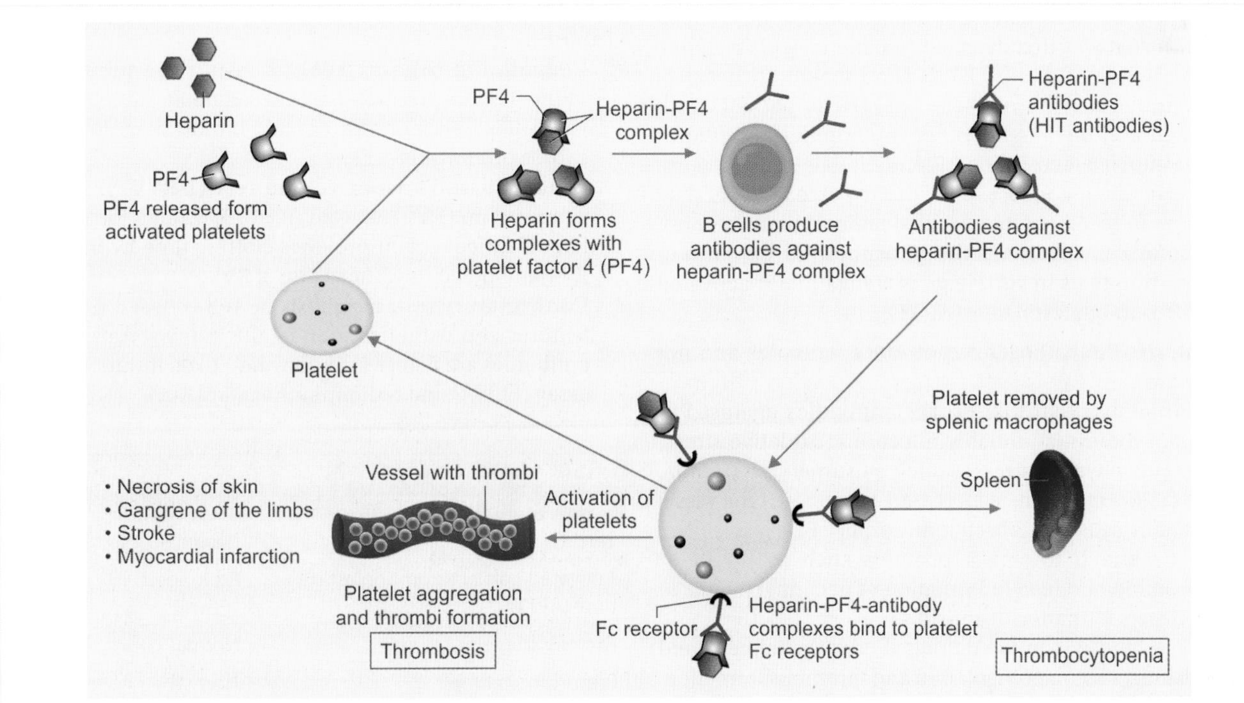

FIG. 24: Pathogenesis of heparin-induced thrombocytopenia.

- **Secondary APS:** These are found in association with a well-defined autoimmune disease [most commonly systemic lupus erythematosus (SLE)]. Because of this association with an underlying condition, they are termed as secondary APS. Because of their association with SLE, they were **formerly known as lupus anticoagulant syndrome**.

Antibodies: APS is characterized by the presence of one or more family of antibodies in the patient's plasma.

- **Antiphospholipid antibodies:** The major **aPL** auto**antibodies** detected in patient's sera are directed **against anionic** (negatively charged) **membrane PLs** and/or **proteins associated with PLs** (PL-binding plasma proteins). Proteins recognized by aPL antibodies include cardiolipin, β_2-glycoprotein I (β_2GPI) and prothrombin. PLs are components of the cytoplasmic membrane of all living cells.
    - **Antibodies against PLs:** The antibodies are directed against negatively charged PLs such as cardiolipin, phosphocholine, and phosphatidylserine.
    - **Antibodies against proteins associated with PLs:** β_2-glycoprotein is found in plasma and has a strong avidity for PLs present on the surfaces of endothelial cells, monocytes, platelets, thrombin, and trophoblasts. Probably **antibodies against β_2-glycoprotein (antiβ_2-glycoprotein antibodies)** play a major role in the pathogenesis of APS. These antibodies bind to β_2-glycoprotein on endothelial cells, monocytes, and platelets and activate these cells. Antiβ_2-glycoprotein antibody can also bind to cardiolipin antigen. Since cardiolipin antigen is used in the serological test for syphilis, patients having this antibody may give a **false-positive serological reaction for syphilis** (caused by *Treponema pallidum*).
- **Lupus anticoagulant (LA) antibodies:** It is another group of antibodies that prolong clotting times in vitro, which are not corrected by adding normal plasma. It was named so because it was first detected in patients with systemic lupus erythematosus (SLE). It is a misnomer; because these antibodies are neither restricted to patients with SLE (and may be found in other autoimmune conditions, or in otherwise asymptomatic individuals) nor they are anticoagulant. It is associated with a hypercoagulable state rather than bleeding. It was called anticoagulant because it paradoxically **prolongs the phospholipid-dependent coagulation tests** in vitro [e.g., prolongation of activated partial thromboplastin time (APTT)].

Pathogenesis: The pathogenesis of APS is complex and not exactly known.

- The initiating event that evokes antibodies against PL-binding proteins is probably infections, oxidative stress, and major physical stresses such as surgery or trauma. These factors may induce increased apoptosis of the vessel endothelial cells and subsequently expose PLs.
- The PLs attach to serum proteins such as β_2GPI or prothrombin and lead to formation of neoantigen. This in turn triggers formation of anti-PLs.
- Anti-PLs bind PLs in the damaged endothelial cells and initiate intravascular coagulation and thrombus formation.
- **Complement activation and inhibition of fibrinolytic processes:** In patients with APS, there may be activation of complement and inhibition of fibrinolytic processes. These events may produce the prothrombotic state. Complement activation is probably responsible for APS-related fetal injury. Fetal loss in APS is not caused by thrombosis, but probably due to antibody-mediated interference with the growth and differentiation of trophoblasts. This can lead to a failure of placentation.
- **Additional factors:** aPLs have also been detected in 5–15% of apparently normal individuals. This indicates that these antibodies alone are not sufficient to cause the full-blown APS. It indicates that a "second hit" is required and it may be by infection, smoking, or pregnancy may trigger the event.

Clinical features: They are varied.

- **Hypercoagulable state:** It is the most common acquired hematologic cause of **recurrent thromboembolic events**. Depending on the site of thrombus it may present as pulmonary embolism (PE) (due to venous thrombosis of lower limb), pulmonary hypertension (due to recurrent subclinical pulmonary emboli), valvular heart disease (cardiac valve vegetation), stroke, bowel infarction, or renovascular hypertension. Renal involvement may cause hypertension, renal microangiopathy, and renal failure due to multiple glomerular capillaries and arterial thromboses. Thromboses may occur due to various mechanisms such as platelet activation, endothelial cell activation, and altered coagulation factor assembly on membranes.
- **Repeated spontaneous abortions (miscarriages):** Recurrent fetal loss in pregnancy of patients with APS is not due to thrombosis in the uteroplacental vasculature, but is due to antibody-mediated interference with the growth and differentiation of trophoblasts. This causes a failure of placentation due to antibody-mediated inhibition of t-PA activity. t-PA is necessary for the invasion of uterine blood vessels by placental trophoblastic tissue.
- **Cardiac valve vegetations**
- **Thrombocytopenia**

Laboratory tests: Various laboratory tests are presented in (**Table 6**).

- **Coagulation tests in APS:** Its results are presented in **Table 4**. aPLs produce a hypercoagulable state in vivo. In vitro, they interfere with PLs and inhibit coagulation. This causes prolonged APTT.
- **Dilute Russell's viper venom test (DRVVT):** Russell's viper venom (RVV) activates factor X leading to fibrin clot. Lupus anticoagulant prolongs clotting time by binding to RVV and preventing the action of RVV.
- **Confirmatory test:** Diagnosis of APS is based on clinical features and demonstration of aPL in the serum. The aPL antibodies are detected by enzyme-linked immunosorbent assay (ELISA) and radioimmunoassay (RIA).

Table 6: Coagulation tests in antiphospholipid antibody syndrome.

Test	*Result*
Activated partial thromboplastin time (APTT)	Prolonged
Factor VIII levels	Normal
Prothrombin time	Normal
Thrombin time	Normal
Fibrinogen level	Normal

Treatment is by various forms of anticoagulation. Laboratory criteria for diagnosis include: (1) LA, (2) anticardiolipin (aCL), and/or (3) anti-β_2GPI antibodies on two occasions, 12 weeks apart.

Terminology of Thrombus

Mural thrombus

It is attached to the wall and projects into the lumen, without complete occlusion of the lumen (refer **Figs. 26B** and **28**). **It occurs in heart chambers or in the aortic lumen**. Thrombi developing on one or both ventricles shortly before death is termed agonal thrombi.

Occlusive Thrombus

It **occludes the lumen of the blood vessel** (refer **Fig. 28**) and prevents the flow of blood. It usually occurs in veins or smaller or medium sized arteries.

Vegetation

It is a **thrombus on heart valve** (**Fig. 25**) and appears as polypoid mass projecting into the lumen (e.g., infective endocarditis).

MORPHOLOGY

Size and shape of thrombi: It depends on the site of origin and its **underlying** cause.

Attachment: Thrombi are focally attached to the underlying surface of vessel/endocardium, mainly at the point of initiation.

Types of Thrombi: Thrombi may be **arterial/cardiac or venous type**.

- **Arterial or cardiac thrombi:** They often begin at sites of turbulence or endothelial injury. From the site of initiation, arterial thrombi tend to grow retrograde direction (i.e., toward the heart).
- **Venous thrombi:** They characteristically develop at sites of stasis of blood. Venous thrombi extend from its site of origin in the direction of blood flow (i.e., toward the heart).

Continued

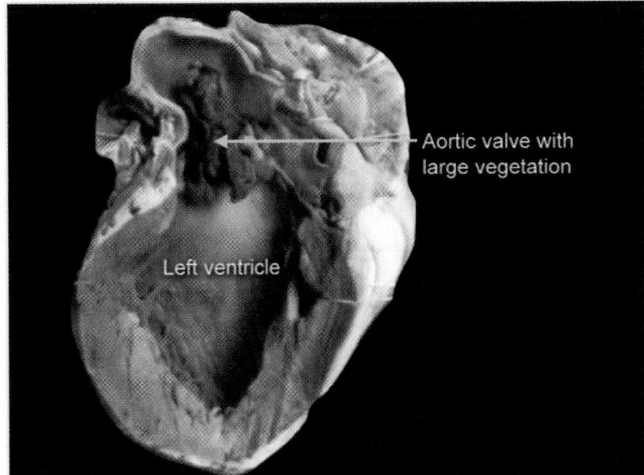

FIG. 25: Acute infective endocarditis showing vegetations on aortic valve and destroyed the valve. Vegetations are thrombi on heart valves.

Continued

Thus, both arterial and venous thrombi propagate toward the heart. The propagating portion of a thrombus is usually attached poorly to the original thrombus. Hence, the propagating portion is prone to fragmentation and embolization. Differences between arterial and venous thrombus are shown in **Table 7**.

Layers in Thrombus

The layers observed in thrombi are:

- **First** layer of the thrombus on the endothelium/ endocardium is a **platelet layer**.
- **On top of the platelet layer, fibrin** is precipitated to **form upstanding laminae** which anastomose to form an intricate structure which **resembles coral** (coralline thrombus).
- In **between the upstanding laminae** and anastomosing fibrin meshwork, the **RBCs get trapped**. **Retraction of fibrin produces a ribbed appearance** on the surface of thrombus.

Lines of Zahn

Both gross and microscopy of thrombus show **alternating light** (pale or white) area of platelets held together by fibrin, **and dark retracted area** of fibrin meshwork with plenty of trapped RBCs. These alternating laminations of light and dark are known as **lines of Zahn** (**Figs. 26A** and **B**). Lines of Zahn indicate that a thrombus has formed in flowing blood. Thus, they help in distinguishing antemortem thrombi from the bland nonlaminated postmortem clots.

Site of Thrombi

Thrombi can develop anywhere in the cardiovascular system.

Heart

Cardiac thrombi: Usually develop at sites of turbulence or endocardial injury.

- More common in the atrial appendages.
- Abnormal myocardial contraction (as in arrhythmias, dilated cardiomyopathy, or myocardial infarction) or endomyocardial injury (due to myocarditis or catheter trauma) favor formation of cardiac mural thrombi.

Valves: Thrombi on heart valves are called **vegetations**. They are more common on **mitral or aortic valves**.

Vegetations may be infected or sterile. Vegetations may be produced by blood-borne bacteria or fungi on the previously damaged valves (e.g., due to rheumatic heart disease). Bacteria and fungi may directly damage valve and predispose to infected vegetations. The predisposing factor is endothelial injury and disturbed blood flow.

- **Infected vegetation:** When vegetation contains organisms, these are called infective vegetations. Sometimes these vegetations may become large as in **infective endocarditis** (especially in acute infective endocarditis).

Continued

Table 7: Differences between arterial and venous thrombus.

Characteristics	*Arterial thrombus*	*Venous thrombus*
Main cause	Injury to endothelium	Stasis
Rate of blood flow	Rapid	Slow
Usual type of thrombus	Mural	Occlusive
Common sites	Aorta, coronary, cerebral, and femoral arteries	Superficial varicose veins and deep veins of leg
Gross		
Color	Gray-white	Red-blue
Lines of Zahn	More prominent	Less prominent
Composition	Friable meshwork of platelets, fibrin, red blood cells (RBCs), and degenerating leukocytes	More trapped RBCs and relatively few platelets
Propagation	Retrograde manner from point of attachment of thrombus (i.e., toward heart)	In antegrade manner from point of attachment toward the direction of blood flow (i.e., toward the heart)
Effects	Ischemia causing infarction of area supplied by the artery containing thrombus	Thromboembolism, edema, and ulceration

Note: Aspirin—prevents arterial thrombosis

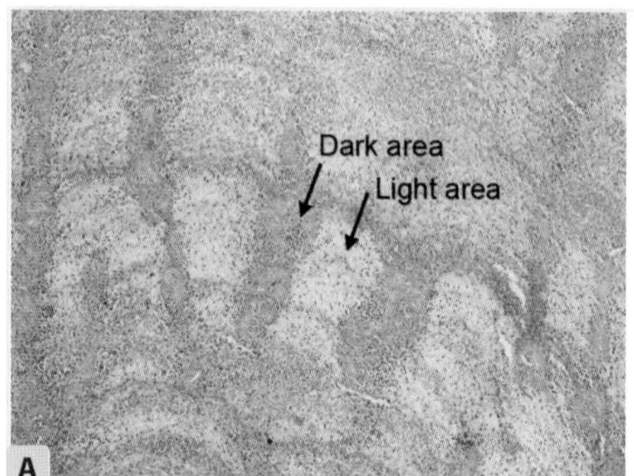

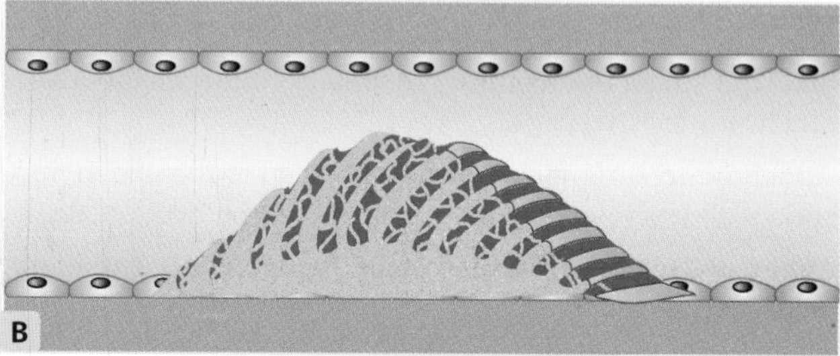

FIGS. 26A AND B: Appearance of thrombus: (A) Microscopic. (B) Diagrammatic, showing alternating dark and light areas (lines of Zahn).

Continued

- **Sterile vegetations:** This type of vegetation develops on noninfected valves and does not contain microorganisms or fungi. In individuals with hypercoagulable states, sterile vegetations are called **nonbacterial thrombotic endocarditis**. Less commonly, sterile verrucous endocarditis **(Libman-Sacks endocarditis)** can occur in patients with SLE.

Blood Vessels

- **Arteries:** Arterial thrombi usually develop at sites of turbulence or endothelial injury. They develop over the ulcerated atherosclerotic plaque and inside aortic aneurysmal dilation. Arterial thrombi tend to be **white.**
  - Aorta or larger arteries usually develop mural thrombi.
  - Thrombi developing in the medium or smaller arteries are frequently occlusive. They develop (in decreasing order of frequency) in the coronary, cerebral, and femoral arteries.

Continued

Continued

  - **Arterial thrombi** usually consist of a friable meshwork of platelets, fibrin, red cells, and degenerating leukocytes. They are usually superimposed on a ruptured atherosclerotic plaque, or sites vascular injuries (e.g., vasculitis, trauma).

Veins

Venous thromboses (phlebothromboses) are usually occlusive, and form a long cast of the lumen. They occur usually at sites of stasis, and contain more trapped RBCs (and relatively few platelets). They are therefore known as red, or stasis thrombi. They should be distinguished from postmortem clots. Venous thrombi are firm, are focally attached to the vessel wall. They show lines of Zahn and this helps in distinguishing them from postmortem clots. They are most common in the veins of the lower extremities (90% of cases). However, they can also develop in veins of upper extremities, periprostatic plexus, or the ovarian and periuterine region. In special circumstances, they can occur in the dural sinuses, portal vein, or hepatic vein.

Continued

Table 8: Differences between antemortem venous thrombi and postmortem clots.

Characteristics	*Antemortem venous thrombi*	*Postmortem clots*
Attachment to vessel wall	Focally and firmly attached	Not attached
Consistency	Dry, granular, firm, and friable	Gelatinous, soft and rubbery
Shape	May or may not fit the vascular contours	Have the shape of the vessel in which it is found
Appearance	Alternate dark and white areas	Currant jelly (supernatant coagulated plasma) and chicken fat (settled RBCs) appearance
Lines of Zahn	Present	Absent
Mechanism	Changes in blood flow (stasis) and hypercoagulability	Occurs in stagnant blood in which gravity fractionates the blood

Continued

Postmortem Clots

Postmortem clots can be sometimes mistaken for antemortem venous thrombi on gross examination. Determination of whether a clot is formed during life (antemortem thrombi) or after death (postmortem clot) is important in a medical autopsy and in forensic pathology. Differences between antemortem venous thrombi and postmortem clots are listed in **Table 8**. After death, the RBCs settle and produce two layers (**Fig. 27**).

- **Lower layer:** It contains **many RBCs**, which have settled by gravity—forms a dark red lower portion. This has a reddish and gelatinous appearance which resembles **currant jelly**.
- **Upper layer:** It is **poor in cells and is yellow-white**. It is firm representing coagulated plasma without RBCs. It is called **chicken fat** because of its color and consistency.

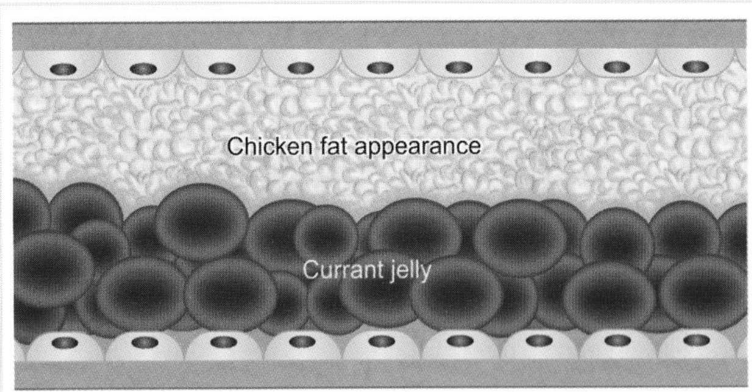

FIG. 27: Two layers of postmortem clot. Upper layer of coagulated plasma without RBCs (chicken fat appearance) and lower layer with settled RBCs (currant jelly appearance).

Fate of Thrombus (Fig. 28)

If a patient survives the initial thrombosis, following complications can occur:

- **Dissolution/lysis of thrombi without any consequences.**
    - **Recent thrombi may undergo rapid shrinkage and may totally disappear** due to activation of fibrinolysis.
    - **Old thrombi** are **more resistant to lysis**. This is because of the extensive fibrin deposition and crosslinking that makes them more resistant to lysis. Hence, it is necessary to administer therapeutic fibrinolytic agents such as t-PA (e.g., in acute coronary thrombosis). It is usually effective only when administered during the initial few hours of a thrombotic event.
- **Propagation of thrombi:** It is the **process in which thrombi grow and increase in size**. The thrombus which was initially **mural, may become occlusive** thrombus. The propagating portion of a thrombus is poorly attached to the wall and therefore, **prone to fragmentation and embolization.**
    - **Arterial thrombi grow retrograde** from the point of attachment
    - **Venous thrombi extend in the direction of blood flow.**

  Both arterial and venous thrombi propagate toward the heart. Usually the propagating portion of a thrombus is poorly attached and is susceptible to fragmentation and embolization.
- **Embolization:** Thrombi may get detached from their sites of origin and form emboli. These emboli can travel to other sites through the circulation and lodge in a blood vessel away from the site of thrombus formation. The **consequences depend on the site of lodgment**. Large venous thrombi may get detached and travel to the pulmonary circulation to the lungs as pulmonary emboli.
- **Organization:** If thrombi are not dissolved (either spontaneously or by therapy), these older thrombi become organized **by the ingrowth of endothelial cells, smooth muscle cells, and fibroblasts**. Small, organized thrombi may be incorporated into the vessel wall.
- **Canalization/recanalization:** New lumen/channels lined by endothelial cells may form in an organized thrombus. These capillary channels may form thoroughfare channels and can re-establish the continuity of the original lumen. A thrombus with continued recanalization may get converted into a smaller mass of connective tissue. This may become incorporated into the vessel wall. Finally, remodeling and contraction of the mesenchymal elements in the thrombus amy lead to formation of fibrous lump within the involved vessel.
- **Mycotic aneurysm:** Rarely, the central region of the thrombi may undergo enzymatic digestion due to lysosomal enzymes released from trapped leukocytes and platelets. If bacteremia develops, these thrombi may become infected and produce an inflammatory mass. This region of the vessel becomes weak and can produce mycotic aneurysm.

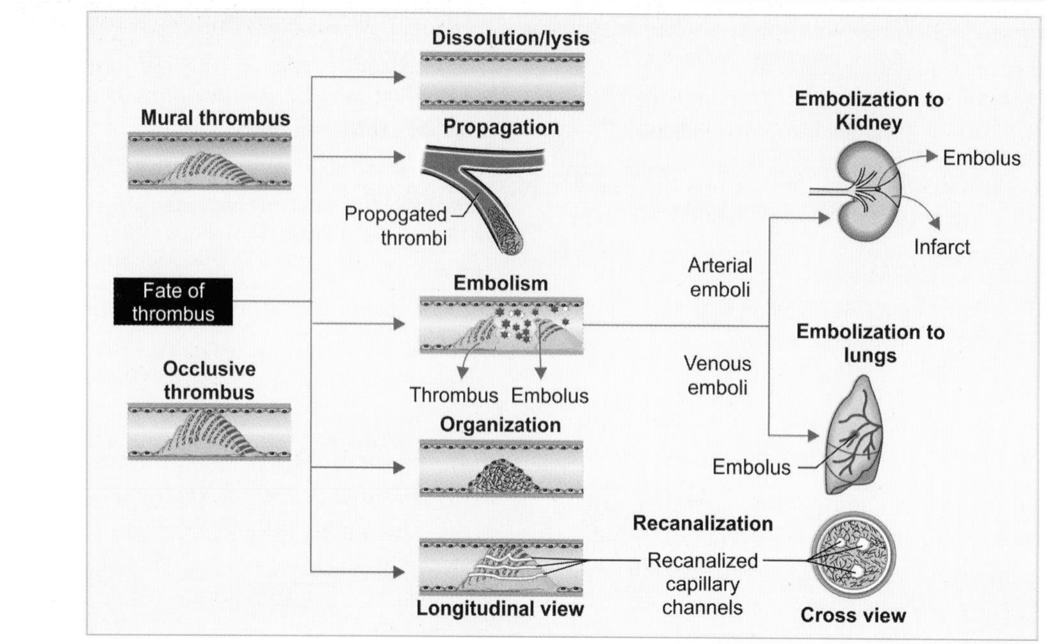

FIG. 28: Fate of thrombus.

VENOUS THROMBOSIS (PHLEBOTHROMBOSIS)

Veins Involved

Most commonly superficial or deep veins of the leg are involved.

Superficial Venous Thrombi

- **Site:** They develop in the varicosities involving **saphenous veins**.
- **Effects:** It can cause **local congestion, swelling (edema), pain, and tenderness**. The **local edema** and impaired venous drainage **predispose** the overlying **skin to infections** from slight trauma and to the development of **varicose ulcers**. Embolization is very rare.

Deep Venous Thrombosis

- Lower extremity DVTs are found in **association with venous stasis and hypercoagulable states**.
- **Sites:** Larger veins in the leg at or above the knee (e.g., popliteal, femoral, and iliac veins).
- **Effects:**
  - Even though DVTs can cause local pain and edema, the venous block produced by them is usually rapidly balanced by the development of collateral channels.
  - **More prone to embolization** into the lungs and produce pulmonary infarction. About 50% of DVTs are asymptomatic and are detected after embolization.

Pathogenesis of Deep Vein Thrombosis (Phlebothrombosis)

Deep venous thrombosis is caused by the same etiological factors that favor arterial and cardiac thrombosis. These include endothelial injury, stasis, and a hypercoagulable state. Common hypercoagulable states predisposing to deep vein thrombosis (DVT) are listed in **Box 5**.

Box 5: Common predisposing factors for deep vein thrombosis

Hypercoagulable states

- **Bed rest and immobilization:** Reduces the milking action of the leg muscles and produces stasis
- **Congestive heart failure:** Causes impaired venous return.
- **Trauma, surgery, and burns:** Associated with immobilization, damage to vessels, release of procoagulant from injured tissues, increased hepatic synthesis of coagulation factors, and decreased t-PA production.
- **Disseminated cancers:** Factors involved are: tumor-associated inflammation and coagulation factors (tissue factor, factor VIII), procoagulants (e.g., mucin) released from tumor cells. For example, migratory thrombophlebitis or Trousseau syndrome.
- **Thrombotic diathesis of pregnancy:** Factors involved includes decreased venous return from leg veins and systemic hypercoagulability associated with the hormonal changes of late pregnancy and the postpartum period.
- **Advanced age**

Different stages in the development of DVTs (**Fig. 29**) are:

- **Primary platelet thrombus:**
  - Damage to the intima of the vein causes adhesion of platelets at damaged site—platelets aggregate to form **pale platelet thrombus.**
  - Venous stasis favors accumulation of coagulation factors, which is activated to form fibrin.
- **Coralline thrombus:** The fibrin and thrombin formed encourages further accumulation of platelets. The **platelets along with fibrin form upright laminae** growing across the stream. Between the laminae, stasis promotes further deposition of fibrin with trapped RBC and white blood cells (WBCs). This **produces alternate layers of fused platelets and fibrin with trapped blood cells**. The contraction

of fibrin produces a **characteristic ribbed (ripple) appearance** on the surface of thrombus. These **raised platelet ridges are known as lines of Zahn**.

- **Occluding thrombus: Further growth of thrombus progressively** occludes the lumen **of the vein and forms occluding thrombus.**
- **Consecutive clot:** Occlusive thrombus **stops the blood flow**. Since, thrombi can develop only in the streaming blood, the **blood column beyond the occluding thrombus clots to form a consecutive clot**. Thereafter, the consecutive clot may be halted and endothelialized or it can spread (**propagate**).
- **Propagated clot:** There are two methods of propagation (**Figs. 30A** and **B**):
  - **Thrombus formation in each tributary:** The consecutive clot when reaches the entrance of venous tributary may form another coralline thrombus over the clot. This causes occlusion of opening of tributary. A consecutive clot will again form up to the opening of next venous tributary. Thus, **several thrombi with associated consecutive clots** may be formed.
  - **Clotting *en masse* beyond the thrombus:** Another method of propagation is **formation of long column of consecutive clots** attached to only one thrombus. These consecutive **clots may break and produce fatal massive PE.**

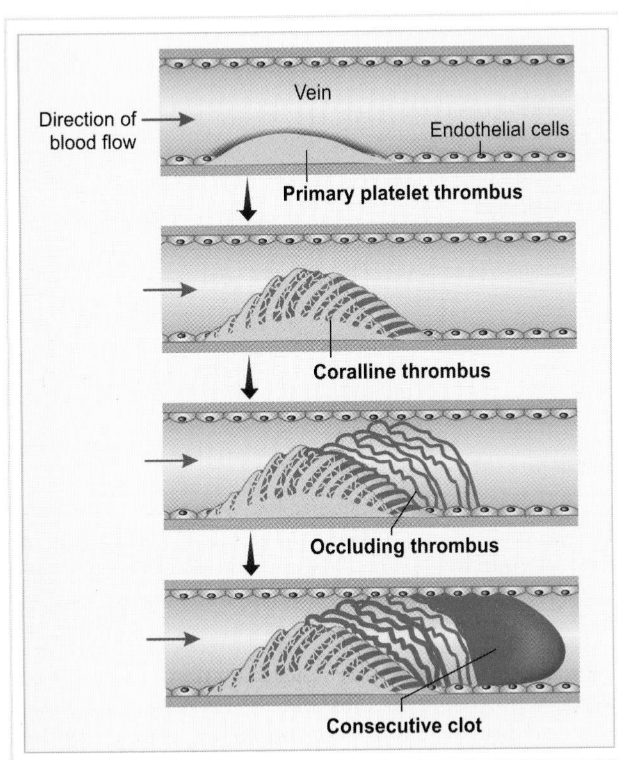

FIG. 29: Various stages in the pathogenesis of phlebothrombosis.

Thrombophlebitis

Inflammation of the wall of vein causes damage to the endothelium and **may lead to thrombus formation.** The thrombus formed is firmly attached to the wall of the vein and does not embolize. Sterile inflammation may be produced by direct trauma, chemicals, or ionizing radiation. Bacterial inflammation of veins may be produced in the veins near the infected areas.

Thrombophlebitis Migrans (Migratory Thrombophlebitis or Trousseau Syndrome)

- **Characterized by recurrent thrombotic episodes** involving the superficial and deep veins, especially of the extremities.
- May develop as a **complication of deep-seated cancers** such as cancer of pancreas (tail and body), lung, stomach, and female genital tract.
- First described by Trousseau who had pancreatic cancer, when he noticed it on himself and suggested that it is a **sign of visceral cancer**. It is known as Trousseau's syndrome.

Consequences of Thrombi

They depend on the site of the thrombosis. **Thrombi clinically manifest when they obstruct arteries or veins, or give rise to emboli.**

- **Obstruction of involved vessel:** Thrombi can cause obstruction of involved arteries and veins.
  - **Arterial thrombi:** They may cause **infarctions** in the region supplied by the involved vessel. Occlusion at certain locations (e.g., a coronary artery) can be life-threatening.
  - **Venous thrombi:** Small venous thrombi may cause no symptoms. Larger thrombi can cause **congestion and edema in region distal to obstruction** by thrombus. Forced dorsiflexion of the foot produces tenderness in the calf associated with DVT and is known as **Homan sign**.
- **Embolization:** Arterial, cardiac, and venous thrombi can undergo fragmentation and detach to form emboli. It is the major complication and these are thromboemboli. The consequences of embolism depend on: (1) site of lodgment of emboli, (2) tissue affected, and (3) source of thromboemboli.

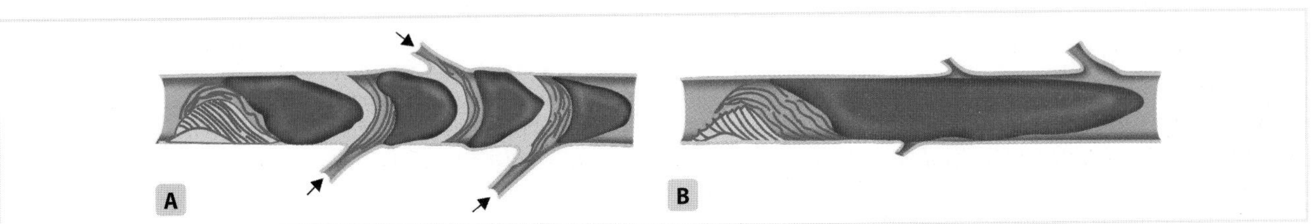

FIGS. 30A AND B: Propagation of venous thrombi. (A) Thrombus formation in each tributary. (B) Clotting en masse beyond the thrombus.

Box 6: Conditions associated with both arterial and venous thrombi.

- Homocystinuria
- Disseminated intravascular coagulation (DIC)
- Cancer
- Antiphospholipid antibody
- Heparin-induced thrombocytopenia
- Paroxysmal nocturnal hemoglobinuria (PNH)
- Hyperhomocysteinemia
- Essential thrombocythemia
- Polycythemia vera
- Dysfibrinogenemia

  - **Arterial and cardiac thromboemboli:** The most common sites of lodgment of emboli are the brain, kidneys, and spleen because of their rich blood supply. The various effects are mentioned in page 384 and 385.
  - **Venous emboli:** They may lodge in the lungs causing various consequences of **PE** (refer page 383 and 384).

Conditions associated with both arterial and venous thrombi are listed in **Box 6**.

DISSEMINATED INTRAVASCULAR COAGULATION

Q. Write short essay on etiology, pathogenesis, clinical features and laboratory investigations of disseminated intravascular coagulation.

Definition: Disseminated intravascular coagulation (DIC) is **thrombohemorrhagic widespread disorder** characterized by the **excessive activation of coagulation and the formation of thrombi in the microvasculature**. It may be acute, subacute, or chronic.

Etiology

DIC is not a specific disease but rather a complication of many conditions associated with systemic activation of thrombin. DIC develops as a secondary complication of wide variety of disorders (**Box 7**). Sometimes the coagulopathy may be localized to a specific organ or tissue. Due to the formation of thrombi in the microcirculation, there is consumption of platelets, fibrin, and coagulation factors. This leads to secondary activation of fibrinolysis. DIC can manifest with signs and symptoms due to tissue hypoxia and infarction caused by microthrombi; hemorrhage, due to reduction of factors needed for hemostasis and activation of fibrinolytic mechanisms; or both.

Pathogenesis (Fig. 31)

Disseminated intravascular coagulation is a disorder that shows combination of (i) thrombosis and (ii) hemorrhage. To understand the pathogenesis, it is necessary to review the normal process of blood coagulation and removal of clot described on page 20. DIC can develop as a result of pathologic activation of coagulation or impairment of coagulation regulatory (clot-inhibiting) mechanisms. Usually the activation of coagulation is the primary mechanisms of DIC.

Box 7: Major disorders associated with disseminated intravascular coagulation.

Obstetric complications
- Retained dead fetus
- Septic abortion
- Abruptio placentae
- Amniotic fluid embolism
- Toxemia and pre-eclampsia

Neoplasms
- Carcinomas of pancreas, prostate, lung and stomach
- Acute promyelocytic leukemia

Infections
- Gram-negative bacterial sepsis
- Meningococcemia and other bacteria
- Fungi, viruses, Rocky Mountain spotted fever, malaria

Massive tissue injury
- Traumatic
- Burns
- Fat embolism
- Surgery

Vascular disorders
- Aortic aneurysm, giant hemangioma

Immunologic reactions
- Transfusion reactions
- Transplant rejection

Respiratory distress syndrome

Miscellaneous
- Snakebite, liver disease, acute intravascular hemolysis, shock, heatstroke, hypersensitivity, vasculitis

Thrombi/Clot Formation

Two main mechanism initiate DIC: (1) release of tissue factor or other procoagulants into the circulation, and (2) widespread injury of endothelial cells. Major disorders associated with disseminated intravascular coagulation (DIC) are listed in **Box 7**.

1. Entry of procoagulant into the circulation

Source of procoagulant substance: In majority of conditions source of procoagulant is tissue factor, which activates coagulation system. Tissue factor can be derived from a variety of sources.

- **In obstetric conditions**: The sources of procoagulants (tissue factors) that produce DIC in obstetric conditions (complications) is from the placenta, dead retained fetus, or amniotic fluid. These procoagulants may enter the circulation.
- **In massive tissue injury by trauma or burns**: They release of procoagulants.
- **In carcinoma**: Acute promyelocytic leukemia and adenocarcinomas of the lung, pancreas, colon, and stomach are most frequently associated with DIC. Mucus released from certain adenocarcinomas may also behave as a procoagulant by directly activating factor X.

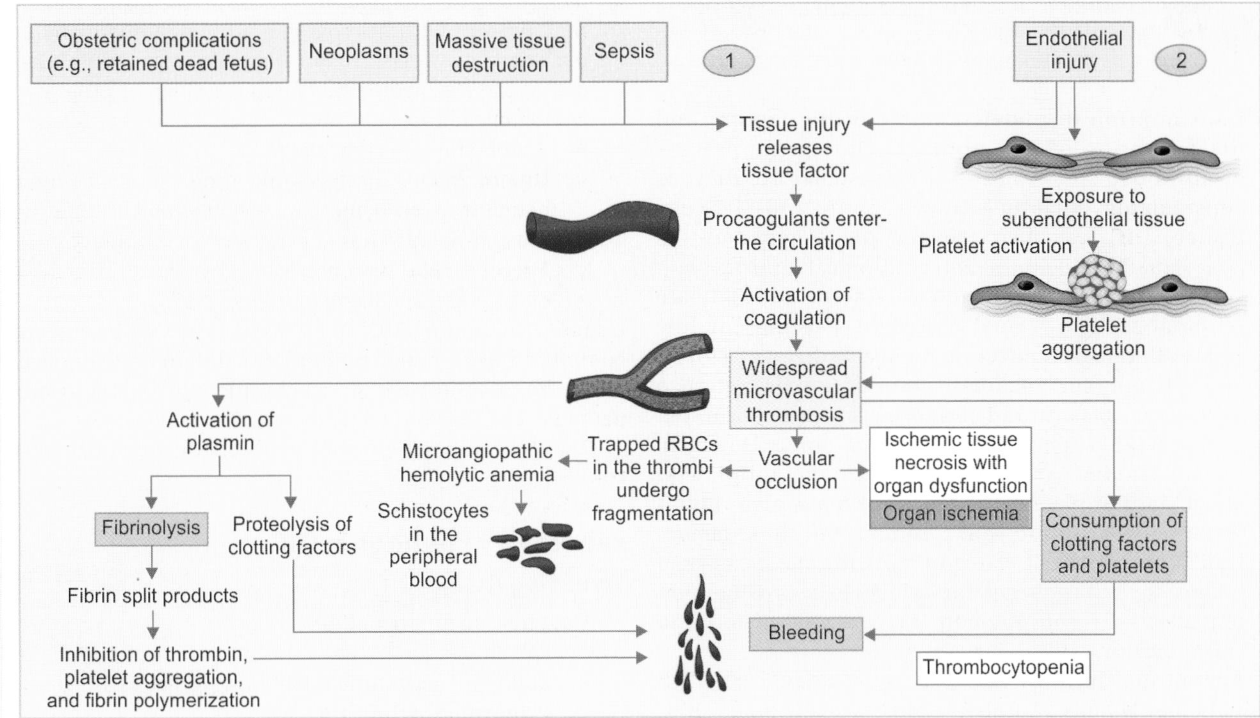

FIG. 31: Pathophysiology of disseminated intravascular coagulation. Two main mechanism initiate DIC: (1) release of tissue factor or other procoagulants into the circulation, and (2) widespread injury of endothelial cells. DIC is characterized by widespread microvascular thrombosis, ischemic tissue necrosis and bleeding.

Triggers: The triggers in conditions that predispose to DIC are usually multiple and interrelated. Examples include the following:

- **Bacterial infections**: In these situations, endotoxins from bacteria can inhibit the endothelial expression of thrombomodulin directly or indirectly by stimulating immune cells to produce TNF. Bacterial infections can also activate factor XII. Antigen-antibody complexes are formed in response to infection. They can activate the classical complement pathway and the resulting complement fragments can secondarily activate platelets and granulocytes.
- **Massive tissue injury:** The major trigger in massive trauma, extensive surgery, and severe burns is the release of procoagulants such as tissue factor.
- **Widespread endothelial injury**: Hypoxia, acidosis, and shock may coexist in severely ill patients. This can cause widespread endothelial injury, and supervening infections can produce further complications.

2. Widespread endothelial injury

Endothelial injury can initiate DIC in many ways.

- **Exposure of thrombogenic subendothelial matrix**: Endothelial injuries can cause necrosis of endothelial cells and expose the thrombogenic subendothelial matrix. This activates the platelets and the coagulation pathway.
- **Activation of procoagulant activity**: Even slight injury to endothelium can free the procoagulant activity of endothelium.
- **Tumor necrosis factor (TNF)**: TNF is one mediator of endothelial injury that is involved in DIC occurring with sepsis.
    - **Expression of tissue factor**: TNF activate endothelial cells to express tissue factor on their cell surfaces and to decrease the expression of thrombomodulin. This shifts the checks and balances that govern hemostasis from anticoagulation toward procoagulation.
    - **Expression of adhesion molecules**: TNF also upregulates the expression of adhesion molecules on endothelial cells. This stimulate the adhesion of leukocytes to endothelial cells. Leukocytes can damage endothelial cells by releasing reactive oxygen species and preformed proteases.
- **Other causes of endothelial injury**: Widespread endothelial damage may also be produced by deposition of antigen-antibody complexes (e.g., systemic lupus erythematosus), extremes of temperature (e.g., heat stroke, burns), or microorganisms (e.g., meningococci, rickettsiae).

Development of thrombi: Both procoagulant substances (tissue factor) and endothelial injury activate coagulation system resulting in widespread fibrin-platelet thrombi formation in the microvasculature.

Consequences of thrombi formation

The possible consequences of DIC are mainly divided into two categories:

1. **Widespread deposition of fibrin within the microcirculation**: This leads to:
    - **Ischemia**: Microvascular deposits of fibrin thrombi produces ischemia of the more severely affected or more vulnerable organs. This may produce microinfarcts or large areas of infarction and multiorgan failure.
    - **Microangiopathic hemolytic anemia**: RBCs trapped in the intravascular fibrin-thrombi deposits undergo

fragmentation as they squeeze through the narrowed microvasculature. These RBCs appear as schistocytes in blood smears; but, frank hemolytic anemia is unusual in DIC.

2. **Consumption of platelets and clotting factors and the activation of plasminogen**: During the process of fibrin deposition in the microvasculature, there is consumption of clotting factors, fibrin, and platelets. Hence, DIC was also referred to as consumptive coagulopathy or defibrination syndrome. Fibrin-thrombi activate secondary fibrinolytic system and activate plasminogen and generates plasmin. Plasmin not only cleaves fibrinogen and fibrin, but it also digests factors V and VIII and reducing their concentration further. Also the cleavage of fibrin and fibrinogen generates fibrin split products (FSPs) [or fibrin degradation products (FDP)]. FSPs are potent anticoagulant and have antiplatelet effect (inhibit platelet aggregation). FSPs also inhibit fibrin polymerization, and thrombin. All these factors lead to a hemorrhagic diathesis. Thus, the major causes of hemorrhagic/bleeding diathesis include (i) consumption of platelets, (ii) consumption of coagulation factors and (iii) activation of fibrinolytic system.

An unusual form of DIC occurs in association with giant hemangiomas (Kasabach-Merritt syndrome). It is characterized by formation of thrombi within the giant cell hemangioma because of stasis and recurrent trauma to fragile blood vessels.

MORPHOLOGY

Thrombi: Microvascular thrombi in DIC can cause diffuse circulatory insufficiency and organ dysfunction. Thrombi are mostly seen in the brain, heart, lungs, kidneys, adrenals, spleen, and liver, in decreasing order of frequency. However, thrombi may be seen in any tissue.

- **Kidney**: Affected kidneys may show **small thrombi in the glomeruli**. This may produce reactive swelling of endothelial cells. In severe cases, thrombi may cause microinfarcts or even **bilateral renal cortical necrosis.**
- **Lung:** Numerous **fibrin thrombi** may be observed **in alveolar capillaries**. Sometimes this may be accompanied by pulmonary edema and fibrin exudation. This may produce "hyaline membranes" similar to that seen in acute respiratory distress syndrome
- **Central nervous system**: Fibrin thrombi may produce **microinfarcts**, occasionally accompanied by hemorrhage. This can produce variable neurologic signs and symptoms.
- **Adrenal**: In meningococcemia, fibrin thrombi may occur within the microcirculation of the adrenal cortex. This may lead to the massive adrenal hemorrhages observed in **Waterhouse-Friderichsen syndrome** (WFS). WFS is a group of symptoms resulting from the failure of the adrenal glands to function normally as a result of massive bleeding into the adrenal gland.

Clinical Features

DIC is serious, often fatal, clinical condition.

- **Onset**: The onset of DIC may be fulminant (e.g., in sepsis, amniotic fluid embolism), or insidious and chronic (e.g., in cases of carcinoma, retention of a dead fetus).
- Symptoms vary depending on the predisposing factor. It may present with microangiopathic hemolytic anemia, dyspnea, cyanosis, respiratory failure, convulsions, coma, oliguria, acute renal failure, sudden or progressive circulatory failure and shock.
- Signs and symptoms are related to:
    - **Hemorrhagic diathesis/bleeding:** Most common, manifest as ecchymoses, petechiae or bleeding from mucous membranes or at the sites of venipuncture.
    - **Microvascular thrombi:** Tissue hypoxia and infarction of the organ leading to multiorgan failure.

Usually, in acute DIC (e.g., associated with obstetric complications or major trauma), the dominant features are a bleeding diathesis, whereas chronic DIC (e.g., in cancer patients), DIC presents with thrombotic complications.

Diagnosis is based on clinical observation and laboratory studies.

Laboratory Findings in DIC

Screening Assays

- **Coagulation abnormalities:**
    - **APTT:** Increased as a result of consumption and inhibition of the function of clotting factors.
    - **Prothrombin time:** Increased.
    - **Thrombin time (TT):** Increased because of decreased fibrinogen.
    - **Fibrinogen level**: Decreased.
- **Bleeding time:** Increased due to decreased platelet count.
- **Platelet count:** Decreased due to utilization of platelets in microthrombi.
- **Peripheral smear:** Microangiopathic hemolytic anemia with schistocytes.

Confirmatory Tests

Fibrinolysis abnormalities: These includes:

- **Fibrin degradation/split products (FDP)**: Secondary fibrinolysis results in generation of FDPs, which can be measured by latex agglutination.
- **D-dimer test:** It is specific for diagnosing DIC.

Prognosis: It is highly variable and mainly depends on the underlying disorder. Definitive treatment is to remove or treat the underlying cause for DIC.

EMBOLISM

Definition

An embolus is a **detached intravascular** solid, liquid, or gaseous **mass** that is **transported in the blood to a site distant from its point of origin**. In the distant site **it usually causes tissue dysfunction or infarction**.

Types of Emboli

Classification—Depending on:

- **Physical nature of the emboli:**
    - **Solid: Thromboemboli**, atheromatous material *(cholesterol emboli)*, **tumor emboli**, tissue fragments, bacterial clumps or parasites, foreign bodies.

- **Liquid: Fat**, bone marrow, and amniotic fluid.
- **Gaseous: Air** or other gases.

- **Whether infected or not**
  - **Bland:** Sterile.
  - **Septic:** Infected.
- **Source (Fig. 32):** The emboli may be **endogenous** (form within the body) or **exogenous** (introduced from outside).
  - **Cardiac emboli:** Usually they arise from left side of the heart. Example, emboli from: (1) atrial appendage, (2) left ventricle in **myocardial infarction**, (3) vegetations on the valves in **infective endocarditis**.
  - **Vascular emboli:**
    - **Arterial** emboli (e.g., atheromatous plaque, aneurysms).
    - **Venous** emboli (e.g., deep vein thrombus, tumor emboli).
    - **Lymphatic** emboli (e.g., tumor emboli).
- **Flow of emboli**.

Q. Write a short essay on paradoxical emboli.

Paradoxical emboli: They are rare and the **emboli originate** in the **venous circulation** and **bypass the lungs** by traveling **through a right-to-left shunt** such as an **atrial septal defect (incompletely closed/patent foramen ovale) or interventricular defect.** Then, they **enter the left side of the heart** and **block the blood flow to the systemic arteries** (refer pages 384–385).

Q. Write a short note on retrograde embolism.

Retrograde emboli: Emboli, which **travel against the flow of ,** are known as retrograde emboli. For example, **prostatic carcinoma metastasis to the spine.** It occurs through retrograde spread via intraspinal veins which carry the emboli from large thoracic ducts and abdominal veins due to increased pressure in the body cavities (e.g., during coughing or straining).

Majority of emboli are dislodged thrombi. Hence it is termed as thromboembolism. Emboli travel through the blood till they come across vessels that is too small to allow their further passage. They lodge in that vessels and cause partial or complete vascular occlusion. Depending on site of origin, emboli can lodge anywhere in the vascular tree. The clinical consequences of emboli vary widely. It depends on the size and the position of the lodged embolus, and the vascular bed involved.

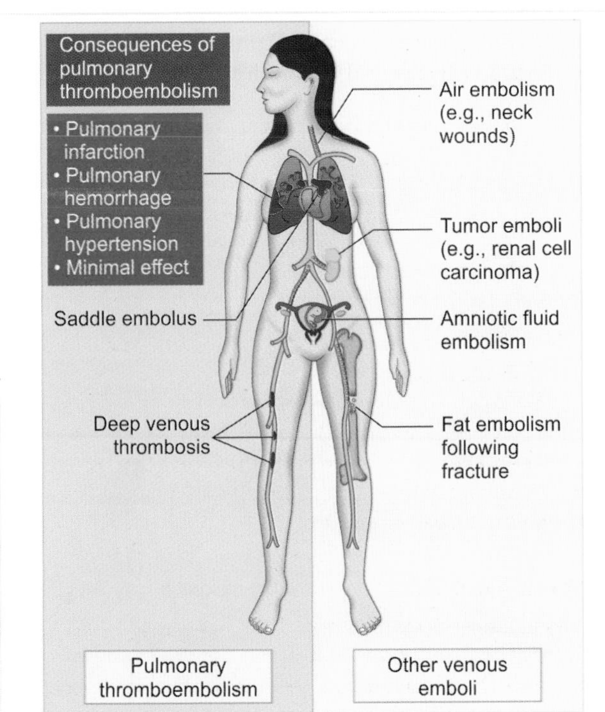

FIG. 32: Sources and effects of venous emboli.

Pulmonary Embolism

Q. Write a short essay on pulmonary embolism.

Definition

PE is defined as an **embolism in which emboli occlude pulmonary arterial tree**.

Site of Origin of Emboli (Fig. 32)

- **Deep leg veins:** DVTs (deep vein thrombosis) are the source in >95% of cases of pulmonary emboli. Deep leg veins include **popliteal, femoral, or iliac veins**.
- **Other sites:** Pelvic veins, vena cava.

Risk of pulmonary embolism: Major risk factor is after surgery. The risk increases with advancing age, obesity, prolonged operative procedure, postoperative infection, cancer, and pre-existing venous disease (refer **Box 3**).

Mechanism of pulmonary thromboembolism is presented in **Flowchart 6**.

Fate of Pulmonary Embolism

Fate depends on the size of the embolus, the embolic load, the adequacy of the pulmonary vascular reserve, the state of the bronchial collateral circulation and the thrombolytic process.

- **Resolution or organization: Small** pulmonary **emboli** may travel into the smaller branches of pulmonary arteries and may **resolve completely**. Most (60–80%) of them are clinically **silent**. With passage of time they become **organized** and are incorporated into the wall of pulmonary vessel.
- **Massive pulmonary embolism:** When emboli **obstruct 60% or more of the pulmonary circulation**, it is known as massive pulmonary embolism.

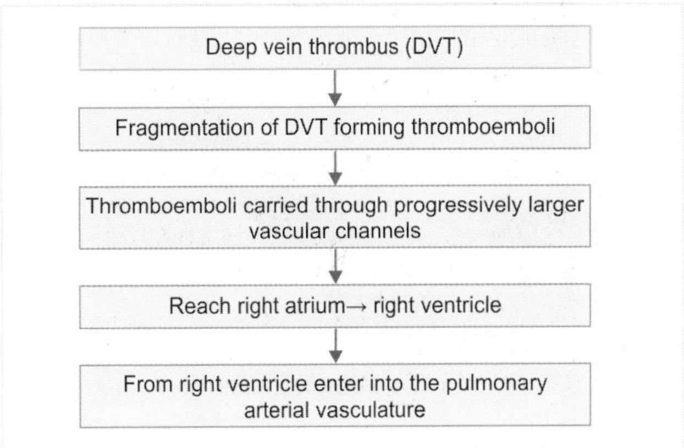

FLOWCHART 6: Mechanism of pulmonary thromboembolism.

- **Saddle embolus:** It is a **large pulmonary embolus** which **lodges at the bifurcation of the main pulmonary artery** (**Fig. 33**). It produces acute massive obstruction of the blood flow to both lungs.
- **Effects:**
  - **Acute right ventricular failure**.
  - **Shock:** Right ventricular failure—reduction in left ventricular cardiac output—sudden severe hypotension (or shock)—may result in sudden death.
- **Multiple recurrent pulmonary emboli:** These **may fuse to form** a **single large mass**. Usually, the patient who has had one PE is likely to have recurrent emboli.
- **Paradoxical embolism** (*refer above*).

Consequences (Fig. 32)

It depends on the size of the embolus, the health status of the patient and whether embolization occurs as an acute or chronic process.

Clinically silent

About 60% to 80% of pulmonary emboli are clinically silent. This is because, these emboli are small and do not produce significant damage. With time, these emboli may undergo organization and may be incorporated into the vascular wall.

Sudden death

When pulmonary emboli obstruct 60% or more of the pulmonary circulation, it can cause sudden death due to **acute right heart failure (cor pulmonale), or cardiovascular collapse**.

Pulmonary hemorrhage

Obstruction of medium sized pulmonary arteries by emboli and subsequent rupture of these obstructed vessels can **result in pulmonary hemorrhage**. Usually, these emboli do not cause pulmonary infarction. This is because the lung is having dual blood supply, i.e., it is supplied by both the pulmonary arteries and the bronchial arteries. Presence of intact bronchial circulation is usually sufficient to perfuse the area affected by embolic event. However, if the bronchial arterial flow is compromised (e.g., by left-sided cardiac failure), infarction may develop.

Pulmonary hemorrhage or infarction

Embolic obstruction of small end-arteriolar pulmonary branches may produce pulmonary hemorrhage or infarction. This is especially in the patients with left-sided cardiac failure or chronic lung disease.

Gross (refer Fig. 39):

- **Type:** Usually **hemorrhagic type, because of blood supply to the infarcted (necrotic) area by the bronchial artery**.
- **Shape: Pyramidal** in shape with the base of the pyramid on the pleural surface. When the blood in the infarcted area is resorbed, the center of the infarct becomes pale.
- **Fate:** Granulation tissue grows from the edges of the infarct and results in organization of infarct and forms a **fibrous scar**.

Clinical Features

- Cough, stabbing pleuritic pain, shortness of breath, and occasional hemoptysis. Pleural effusion is a common complication and pleural fluid is often blood stained.

Pulmonary hypertension

- **Multiple recurrent pulmonary emboli—may cause mechanical blockage of the arterial bed—result in pulmonary hypertension and right ventricular failure.**

Systemic Thromboembolism

Definition

It is defined as an embolism in which **emboli occlude systemic arterial circulation**.

Systemic arterial embolism **usually produces infarcts** in the region supplied by the involved vessel.

Sources of Systemic Emboli (Fig. 34)

- **Heart:** Most common source of thromboemboli.
  - **Intracardiac mural thrombi:** Most common source. Examples:
    - Myocardial infarct of left ventricular wall

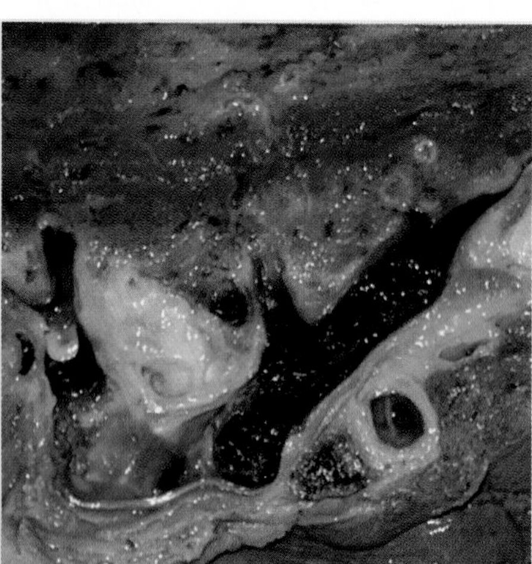

FIG. 33: Saddle embolus at main pulmonary artery and its bifurcation. Most common source of thromboembolus is the deep venous thrombosis in the lower extremities.

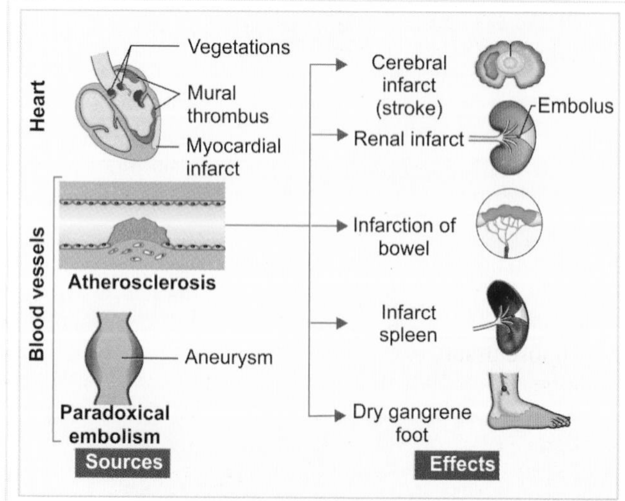

FIG. 34: Common sources and effects of systemic arterial emboli. It usually arises from the left side of the heart or from major arteries. Usual consequence is either infarction or gangrene at the site of lodgment.

- In mitral stenosis, dilatation of left atrium and atrial fibrillation predisposes to thrombus and embolization.
 - **Paradoxical emboli:** Rare source
 - **Valvular source:** Examples, **bacterial endocarditis** (valvular vegetation from aortic or mitral valves) or prosthetic valves.
- **Blood vessels:** Thrombi on **ulcerated atherosclerotic plaques** or from aortic **aneurysms**.
- **Unknown origin**.

Consequences

- The arterial emboli can travel to a wide variety of sites. This is in contrast to venous emboli, which lodge mainly in one vascular bed namely the lung.
- The arterial emboli tend to pass through the progressively narrow arterial lumen and lodge at points where the vessel lumen narrows abruptly (e.g., at bifurcations or in the area of an atherosclerotic plaque).
- **Fate of thromboembolus at the site of arrest:**
 - **Propagation and obstruction:** Thromboemboli may grow (propagate) locally at the site of arrest and produce severe obstruction leading to **infarction of the affected** tissues (**Fig. 34**).
 - **Fragmentation and lysis.**

Major Sites Affected by Arterial Thromboemboli (Fig. 34)

- **Lower extremity (75%):** Embolism to an artery of the leg may produce **gangrene**.
- **Brain:** Arterial emboli to the brain may produce **ischemic necrosis** in the brain (strokes).
- **Intestine:** Emboli in the mesenteric vessels may produce **infarction of the bowel**.
- **Kidney:** Renal artery embolism may cause small peripheral **infarcts** in the kidney.
- **Blood vessels:** Emboli originating from bacterial vegetation may cause inflammation of arteries and produce **mycotic aneurysm**.
- **Other sites:** Spleen and upper extremities are less commonly affected.

Fat and Marrow Embolism

Q. Write short essay on fat embolism.

Fat and marrow embolus **consists of microscopic globules of fat with or without bone marrow** elements. Release of these elements into the circulation produces fat embolism. Bone marrow may embolize to the lungs along with hematopoietic cells and fat.

Causes

- **Trauma to adipose tissue with fracture:** Severe trauma to adipose tissue, particularly accompanied by **fractures of bone** release fat globules or fatty marrow (with or without associated hematopoietic marrow cells) into ruptured blood vessels. Fat embolism occurs in about 90% of individuals with **severe skeletal injuries**, but <10% of them have clinical findings.
- **Soft tissue trauma and burns.**
- **During vigorous cardiopulmonary resuscitation**. This is a procedure in which fractures of the sternum and ribs commonly occur.

Manifestation

In **most of the cases**, it is **asymptomatic**. **Sometimes**, it may manifest as potentially **fatal fat embolism syndrome**.

Fat embolism syndrome: It is the term applied when the patients develops **symptoms due to severe fat embolism**. It develops in only minority of patients.

Pathogenesis

Fat embolism syndrome involves both mechanical obstruction and biochemical injury.

Mechanical obstruction

Pathogenesis of fat embolism by mechanical obstruction shown in **Flowchart 7**.

Biochemical injury (Flowchart 8)

- The chemical composition of the fat present in the lung in fat embolism is different from that in adipose tissue.

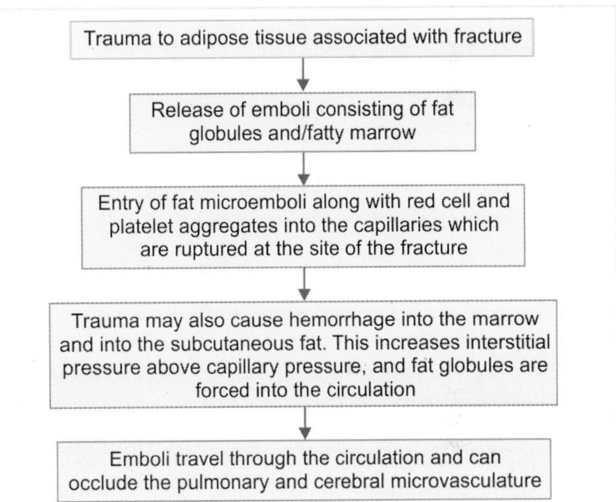

FLOWCHART 7: Pathogenesis of fat embolism by mechanical obstruction.

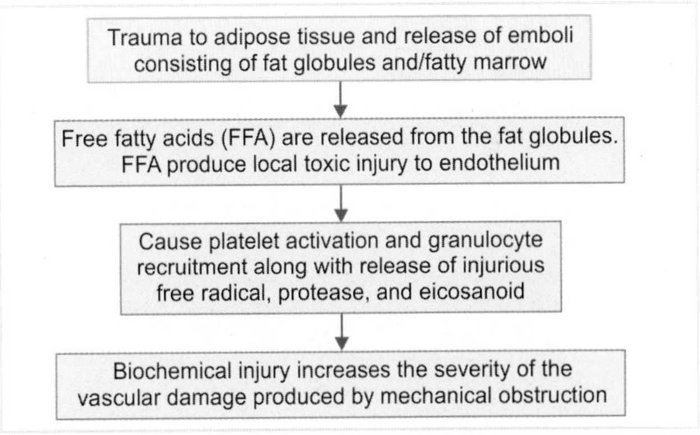

FLOWCHART 8: Pathogenesis of fat embolism by biochemical injury.

- The mechanical obstruction alone cannot explain this difference. So, pathogenesis probably involves mechanical obstruction associated with biochemical injury.

Consequences of Fat Embolism

It depends on the size and quantity of fat globules and whether the emboli are arrested in the pulmonary or systemic circulation. The paradoxical fat emboli may reach systemic circulation (e.g., through patent foramen ovale) and get deposited in brain, kidney, etc.

- **Sites of arrest of fat emboli:**
  - Emboli in the venous side lodge **in the lungs**.
  - **If emboli pass into systemic circulation**, they may be arrested in **brain**, **kidneys**, and other organs.
- **Autopsy findings: Numerous fat globules** can be found impacted **in the microvasculature** of the lungs (in pulmonary emboli) (**Fig. 35**) and brain and sometimes other organs (in systemic emboli).
  - **Lung:** The lungs typically show the changes of **ARDS**.
  - **Brain:** The lesions include **cerebral edema, small hemorrhages**, and occasionally microinfarcts.
- **Demonstration of fat embolism:** Fat is dissolved during routine tissue preparations by the solvents (xylene/xylol) used in paraffin embedding. The microscopic demonstration of fat microglobules requires **frozen sections and special stains for fat** (e.g., Sudan III and IV, Oil Red O, and osmic acid).

Clinical Presentation

The most severe form of fat embolism syndrome may be fatal.

- **Time of development:** It develops 1–3 days after the traumatic injury.
- **Respiratory symptoms:** These include sudden onset of **tachypnea, dyspnea, and tachycardia** which may lead to **respiratory failure**.
- **Neurologic symptoms:** These include **irritability, restlessness,** delirium, and coma.
- **Hematological findings:**
  - **Thrombocytopenia:** Rapid onset of thrombocytopenia produces **diffuse petechial rash** (found in 20–50% of cases) and may be a useful **diagnostic** feature.
  - **Anemia:** It is due to aggregation of red cells and/or due to hemolysis.
- **Chest radiography:** It shows diffuse opacity of the lungs—may progress to an **opacification of lungs** (whiteout)—characteristic of **ARDS**.

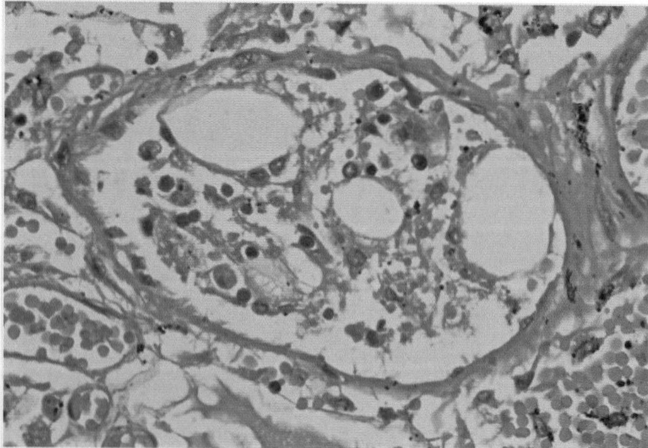

FIG. 35: Fat embolus in the pulmonary circulation. Fat appear as clear spaces (empty vacuoles) and cellular elements of the embolus are hematopoietic cells.

Air Embolism

Q. Write a short essay on air/gas embolism.

Air embolism occurs when **air is introduced into venous or arterial circulation**. Bubbles of gas can coalesce within the circulation and form frothy masses. These may obstruct flow of blood and produce ischemic injury in the distal area.

Causes

Air embolism develops when a communication occurs between the vasculature and outside air. This creates a negative pressure gradient and vessel sucks in the outside air.

- **Trauma/injury:** Air may enter the venous circulation through **neck wounds and chest wall injury**.
- **Surgery/invasive procedures:** These include invasive surgical procedures such as **thoracocentesis**, punctures of the great veins during **obstetric or laparoscopic procedures**, into the **coronary artery during bypass surgery**, endovascular and interventional procedure, during mechanical ventilation, and hemodialysis. Air may be introduced into the cerebral circulation by neurosurgery in the "sitting position." It creates a gravitational gradient and air is likely to enter into the circulation
- **Criminal abortion.**

Amount of Air Required

It is usually **more than 100 mL** to have a clinical effect of air embolism. Entry of 300–500 mL of air at 100 mL/s may be fatal.

Mechanism

In the circulation, air/gas bubbles tend to coalesce to form frothy masses—which physically obstruct vascular blood flow and produce ischemic injury at distal sites. Mere entry of air into the pulmonary vasculature does not obstruct perfusion of downstream region. Microemboli of air trapped in pulmonary capillaries produce a severe inflammatory response and release cytokines. These cytokines damage the alveoli. Air bubbles in the CNS can produce mental impairment and sudden development of coma.

Microscopy

Air bubbles are seen as empty spaces in capillaries and small vessels of the lung/brain.

Decompression Sickness

It is a form of gas embolism and may be acute or chronic.

Acute decompression sickness

Cause It develops when individuals are **exposed to sudden decrease in atmospheric pressure**. Risk factors include:

- Individuals when exposed to high atmospheric pressure, such as **scuba and deep-sea divers and underwater construction workers** (e.g., tunnels, drilling platform construction), during rapid ascent to low pressure.
- Individuals in **unpressurized aircraft** during rapid ascent.
- **Sport diving.**

Mechanism of acute decompression sickness is shown **Flowchart 9**.

Acute decompression sickness is treated by placing the affected individual in a chamber under sufficiently high pressure to force the gas bubbles back into solution. Subsequently slow decompression is achieved that allows gradual resorption and exhalation of the gases. This prevents the reformation of obstructive bubbles

Chronic decompression sickness

Caisson disease

- A chronic form of decompression sickness is known as **Caisson disease** (named for the pressurized vessels/diving bells used in the bridge construction).
- Workers in these pressurized vessels may develop both acute and chronic forms of decompression sickness.
- **Characteristic features:** Avascular necrosis—gas embolus in vessel produces obstruction to blood flow—causes multiple foci of **ischemic (avascular) necrosis of bone**. The more commonly involved bone includes the head of the femur, tibia, and humerus.

Amniotic Fluid Embolism

Q. Write short essay on amniotic fluid embolism.

Amniotic fluid embolism **develops when amniotic fluid along with fetal cells and debris enter the maternal circulation.** The entry occurs through open (ruptured) uterine and cervical veins or a tear in the placental membranes (**Fig. 36A**). Amniotic fluid embolism constitutes the fifth most common cause of maternal mortality.

Time of Occurrence

It is a rare, dangerous maternal threatening complication, which occurs **at the end of labor and the immediate postpartum period**.

Consequences

From the venous circulation, amniotic fluid emboli enter the right-side of the heart and finally rest in pulmonary circulation. Amniotic fluid has a high thromboplastin activity and initiates a potentially **fatal DIC**.

MORPHOLOGY

- **Amniotic fluid contents within pulmonary vasculature:** Amniotic fluid emboli are composed of squamous cells (**Fig. 36B**) shed from fetal skin, lanugo hair, fat from vernix caseosa, and mucin derived from the fetal respiratory or gastrointestinal tract.
- **Other findings:** These include marked pulmonary edema, **diffuse alveolar damage**, and features of DIC.

Clinical Features

- **Abrupt onset:** It develops during immediate postpartum period, and is characterized by sudden onset of severe

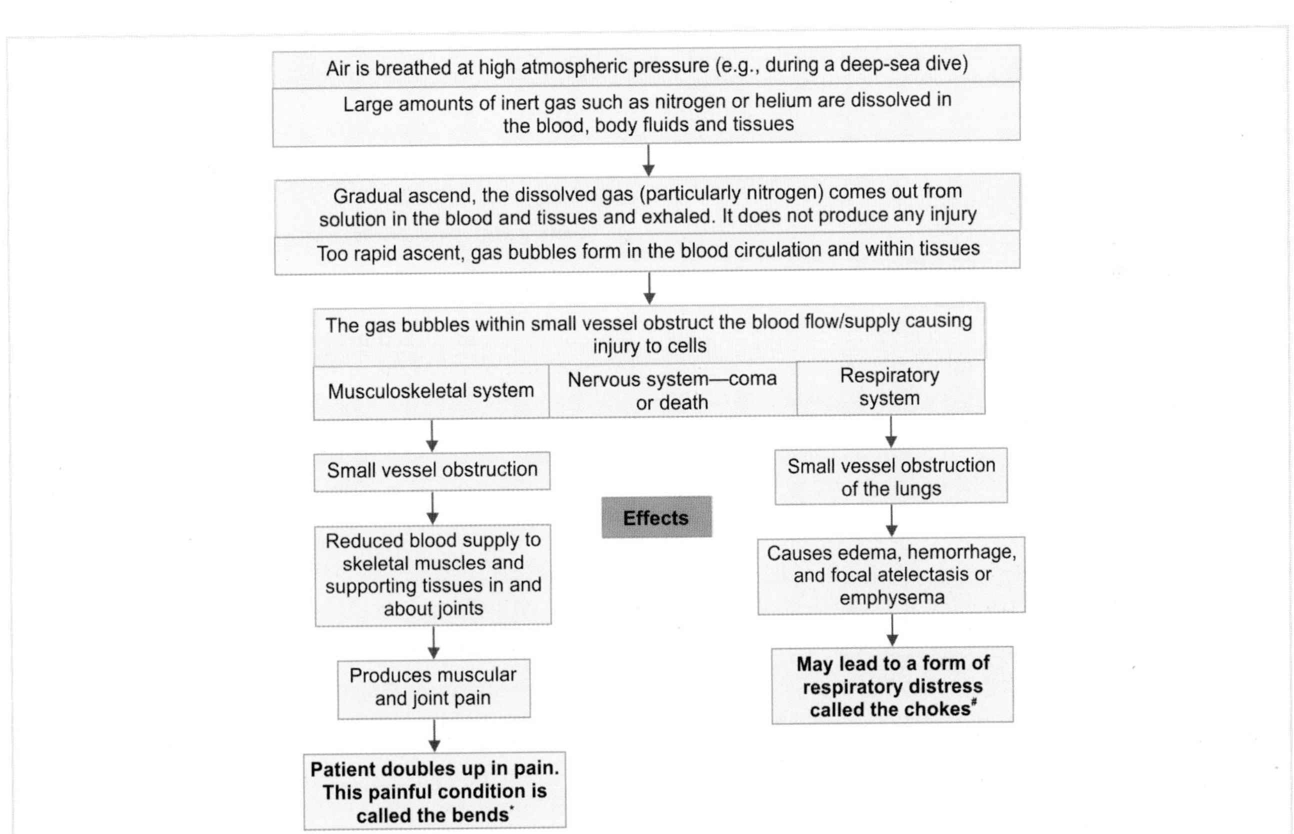

* Bends term was used because in 1880s, characteristically bent of backs was observed in those affected by decompression sickness which was in a manner similar to a then-popular women's fashion pose called the *Grecian bend*.

\# Air bubbles in the vasculature of lung cause edema, hemorrhage, and focal atelectasis or emphysema. This leads to a type of respiratory distress called the *chokes*.

FLOWCHART 9: Mechanism of acute decompression sickness.

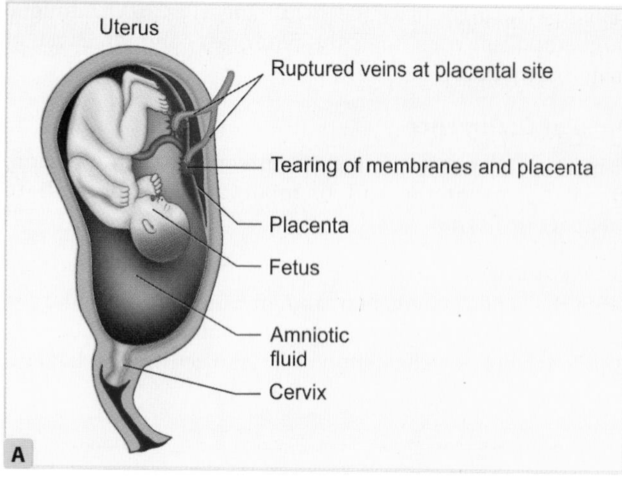

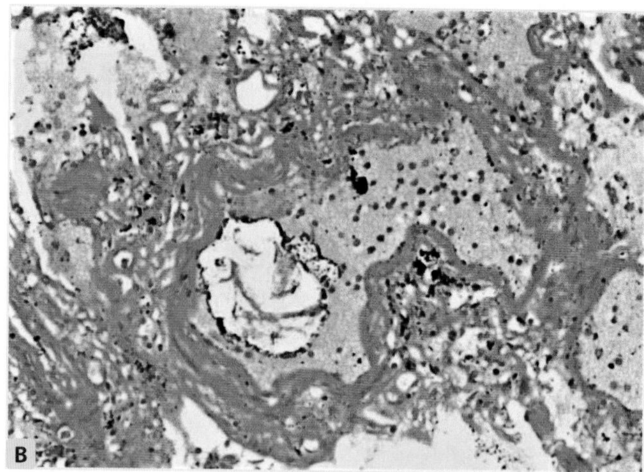

FIGS. 36A AND B: Amniotic fluid embolism. (A) Amniotic fluid enters through open (ruptured) uterine and cervical veins or a tear in the placental membranes. They lodge in the pulmonary vasculature. Section of lung shows a pulmonary artery filled with fetal anucleated squamous cells.

dyspnea, cyanosis, and neurologic impairment ranging from headache to seizures. Patient develops shock, coma, and death.

- **Bleeding:** If the patient survives the initial acute crisis, patient develops bleeding due to DIC.
- **Acute respiratory distress syndrome:** Morbidity and mortality in amniotic fluid embolism is due to biochemical activation of coagulation factors, components of the innate immune system, and release of vasoactive substances, rather than mechanical obstruction of pulmonary vessels by amniotic debris. The vasoactive substances produce acute pulmonary hypertension and right heart failure. This in turn leads to hypoxia, left heart failure, pulmonary edema, and diffuse alveolar damage.

Miscellaneous Pulmonary Emboli

- **Foreign bodies:**
  - **Talc emboli:** It may occur in intravenous drug abusers who use talc as a carrier for illicit drugs.
  - **Cotton emboli:** It may occur due to cleansing of the skin by cotton prior to venipuncture.
- **Schistosomiasis:** The ova of schistosoma may gain entry into the circulation from bladder or gut and lodge in the lungs.
- **Tumor emboli:** It may occur during hematogenous dissemination of cancer.
- **Atheromatous emboli** (cholesterol emboli): Fragments of atheromatous plaque may embolize.
- **Platelet emboli:** During early stages of atherosclerosis, there is platelet deposition in the intimal surface of blood vessels. They may form platelet emboli.
- **Infective emboli:** In infective endocarditis, the vegetations seen on the diseased heart valves may become infected. These infected vegetations may break off and form infective emboli. Their effects are due to both emboli and infective agent that may weaken the wall of the vessel—may lead to the formation of a **"mycotic" aneurysm** (refer page 377). **Mycotic is a misnomer because the infective agent is usually bacterial, not fungal.**

Table 9: Common and important infarcts.

Organ/tissue affected	*Infarction*
Heart	Myocardial infarction
Brain	Cerebral infarction
Lung	Pulmonary infarction
Bowel/intestine	Intestinal infarct
Extremities	Gangrene

INFARCTION

Q. Write a short essay on infarct.

Definition

An infarct is a **localized area of ischemic necrosis** caused by occlusion of either the arterial blood supply or the venous drainage. The **process of producing** infarct is known as **infarction**.

Mostly infarct is coagulative type of necrosis due to sudden occlusion of arterial blood supply. If the patient survives, the infarct heals with a scar.

Common and important infarcts are shown in **Table 9**.

Causes of Infarction

Arterial Causes

Most important cause of infarct.

- **Occlusions of lumen:** It is the most common cause and may be due to: (1) **thrombus** or (2) **embolus** (refer **Fig. 32**).
- **Causes in the wall** (e.g., local vasospasm, **hemorrhage into an atheromatous plaque** or thromboangiitis obliterans).
- **External compression of vessel:** Tumor.

Venous Causes

- **Occlusions of lumen** may be due to: (1) thrombus or (2) embolus.

- **Extrinsic vessel compression:** Tumor, torsion of a vessel (e.g., in testicular torsion or bowel volvulus), **strangulated hernia**.

Factors that Influence the Development of an Infarct

The outcome of vascular occlusion may range from no or minimal effect to the death of a tissue or individual. The **major factors** that determine the outcome of infarct are:

Anatomy of the Vascular Supply

- **Dual/parallel blood supply:** The most important factor that determines whether occlusion of a vessel will cause infarction is the availability of an alternative blood supply. Organs or tissues with double or parallel blood supply are **less likely to develop infarction.** These are relatively resistant to infarction. For example, lungs have a dual blood supply one by pulmonary and other by bronchial artery, The dual blood supply to the lung protects it against thromboembolism-induced infarction. Liver has dual blood supply by hepatic artery and portal vein circulation, and the hand and forearm, have dual radial and ulnar arterial supply.
- **End-arterial blood supply:** Kidney and spleen have blood supply, which are end-arteries with little or no collaterals. Obstruction of vessels in these organs usually causes tissue death and **infarction**.

Rate of Occlusion

Slow occlusion is **less likely to produce infarction than rapid occlusion**. This is because it provides time to develop alternate perfusion pathways. For example, there are three major coronary arteries in the heart namely left circumflex, left anterior descending and right coronary arteries. Normally, they have small interarteriolar anastomoses with minimal functional flow and they interconnect these three major coronary arteries. If one of these coronaries is occluded slowly (i.e., by an enlarging atherosclerotic plaque), flow within this collateral circulation may increase. It may be sufficient enough to prevent development of infarction, even though the larger coronary artery is eventually occluded. If the occlusion is sudden (e.g., by sudden development of thrombus over an ulcerated atheromatous plaque), it may produce infarction.

Vulnerability of Tissue to Hypoxia

- **Neurons are highly sensitive to hypoxia**. They undergo necrosis even if the blood supply is occluded for 3–4 minutes.
- In heart, myocardial cells are also quite sensitive to hypoxia, but less sensitive than neurons. Myocardial cells die after only 20–30 minutes of ischemia. However, the morphological changes in the myocardial fibres of infarcted region are detectable after 4 to 12 hours. On the contrary, fibroblasts within infarcted myocardial region remain viable even after many hours of ischemia.

Oxygen Content of Blood

In a normal individual, partial obstruction of a small vessel may not produce any effect, but in a patient with anemia or cyanosis same may produce infarction. Thus, abnormally low blood oxygen content of blood (irrespective of cause) increases both the likelihood and extent of infarction.

Classification (Table 10)

Infarcts are classified according to color and the presence or absence of infection. Depending on the color, infarcts area classified as white (anemic/pale) and red (hemorrhagic). Depending on the presence or absence of infection , they are classified as septic or bland.

White/Pale Infarcts

They occur:
- With **arterial occlusions**
- In **solid organs**
- Organs with **end-arterial circulation without a dual blood supply** (e.g., heart, spleen, and kidney)
- **Tissue with increased density** which prevents the diffusion of RBCs from adjoining capillary beds into the necrotic area.

Red/Hemorrhagic Infarcts

They occur:
- With **venous occlusions**, e.g., ovary and testicular torsion.
- In **loose textured, spongy tissues**, e.g., lung: They allow red cells to diffuse through and collect in the necrotic zone.
- In **tissues with dual (double) blood supply**, e.g., lung, liver, and small intestine: It allows blood flow from an unobstructed parallel blood supply into a necrotic zone.
- In **tissues previously congested** due to decreased venous drainage.
- Organs with extensive collateral circulation, e.g., **small intestine and brain.**
- **Reperfusion of infarcted area:** When **blood flow is re-established to a site of previous arterial occlusion** and necrosis, e.g., may occur in heart when the infarcted area is reperfused following coronary angioplasty of an obstructed coronary artery.

MORPHOLOGY

White/pale Infarcts

Organs involved include **heart (Fig. 37 and refer Fig. 5 of Chapter 7), kidneys, spleen,** and dry gangrene of the extremities.

Gross

- Usually **wedge-shaped (Fig. 38)**

Continued

Table 10: Classification of infarct.

According to color	*Presence or absence of infection*	*According to the age of infarct*
White/pale (anemic)	Septic, when it is infected	Recent or fresh
Red (hemorrhagic)	Bland, when it is free of infection	Old or healed

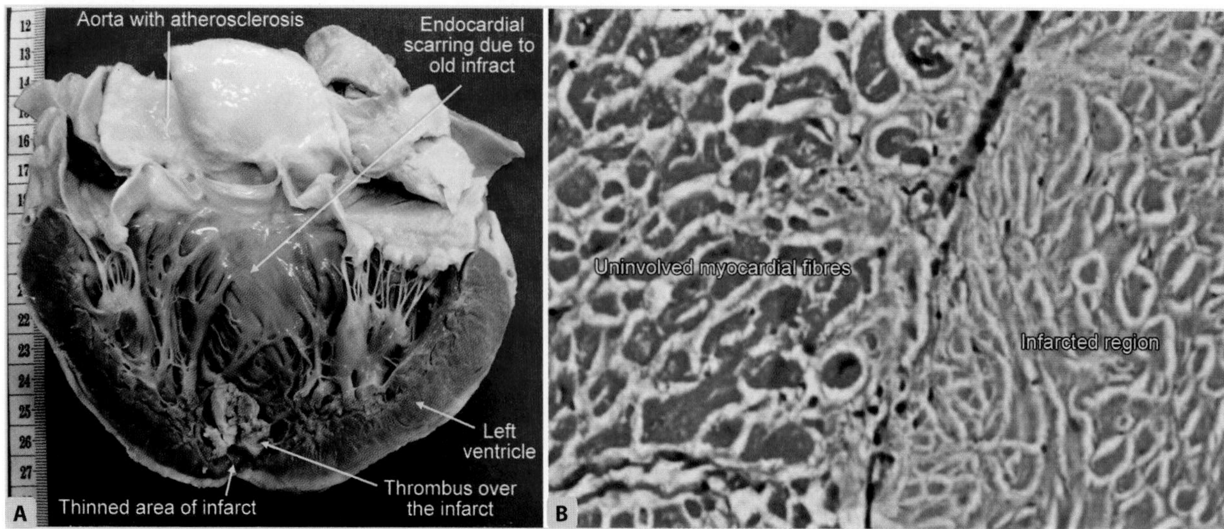

FIGS. 37A AND B: (A) Myocardial infarct with a thrombus over the infarcted area. (B) Microscopic appearance of fresh myocardial infarct of 14 hours' duration. It shows normal darkly stained myocardial fibres on left and ghost outlined of infarcted myocardial fibres without any inflammatory reaction on right half.

Continued

- **Occluded blood vessel** is seen **at the apex of the infarcted region** and the **periphery/surface** of the organ **forms the wide base.** When the base of infarct is a serosal surface, the serosa may be covered by a fibrinous exudate. This is due to acute inflammatory response to mediator release from injured and necrotic cells.
- **Acute (fresh) infarcts** are **poorly defined** and **slightly hemorrhagic**.
- After 1–2 days, the infarct becomes soft, sharply demarcated, and light yellow in color.
- **Margins of infarct appear well-defined** because of narrow rim of congestion caused by inflammation
- **As time passes**, infarcts due to arterial occlusions in organs without a dual blood supply, progressively become **paler** and more **sharply defined**.

Red/Hemorrhagic Infarcts

Gross (Fig. 39)

Appears as **sharply circumscribed** area of necrosis, **firm** in consistency, and **dark red to purple** in color. Extravasated RBCs in hemorrhagic infarcts are phagocytosed by macrophages. They convert heme iron into hemosiderin. If the amount of hemorrhage and hemosiderin formed is small, grossly it may not produce any significant color changes in the infarcted tissue. However, extensive hemorrhage can produce a firm, brown coloration due to more amount of hemosiderin.

Microscopy of Infarct

- **Both pale and red infarcts** characteristically show **ischemic coagulative necrosis (Fig. 40A and B)**.
- If the vascular occlusion has occurred shortly (minutes to hours) before the death of the individual, there may not be any histologic changes. Microscopic changes of **frank necrosis** appear after about **4–12 hours (Fig. 37B)**.

Continued

Continued

- **Acute inflammation cells** infiltrate the necrotic area from the viable margins all-round the infarcts within a few hours. It becomes **prominent within 1–2 days**.
- Followed by a **reparative process,** which begins **at the preserved margins**. The **necrotic cells** in infarcts and extravasated red cells are **phagocytosed by macrophages**.
- In tissues having tissue stem cells, **parenchymal regeneration** can occur at the periphery where stromal architecture is preserved.
- **Granulation tissue** may **replace the infarcted area** which **matures to** form **scar tissue**.
- If the infarct is large (e.g., in heart or kidney), the necrotic center may persist for months.
- In contrast to other organs, infarct in the brain shows **liquefactive necrosis**.

Septic Infarctions

They may occur in two situations:

- **Infection:** Infarct may get infected when it is **seeded by pyogenic bacteria**, e.g., infection of pulmonary infarct.
- **Septic emboli:** They contain organisms and can produce septic infarct, e.g., vegetations of bacterial endocarditis may cause septic infarct of spleen.

The organisms present in a **septic infarct** convert infarct into a frank **abscess**.

Infarction in Specific Locations

These infarcts are often fatal and are described briefly.

Myocardial Infarcts

Myocardial infarcts may be transmural (involving the entire thickness of myocardium) or subendocardial (involving inner one-third of myocardium). A transmural infarct (**Fig. 37**) results from complete occlusion of a major extramural

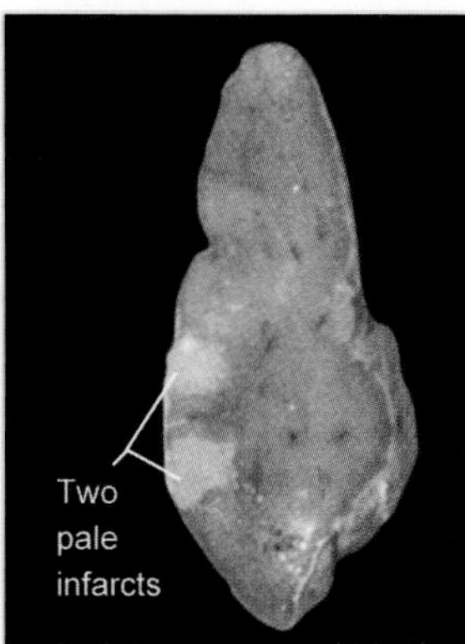

FIG. 38: Infarct spleen showing two wedge-shaped pale/white infarcts.

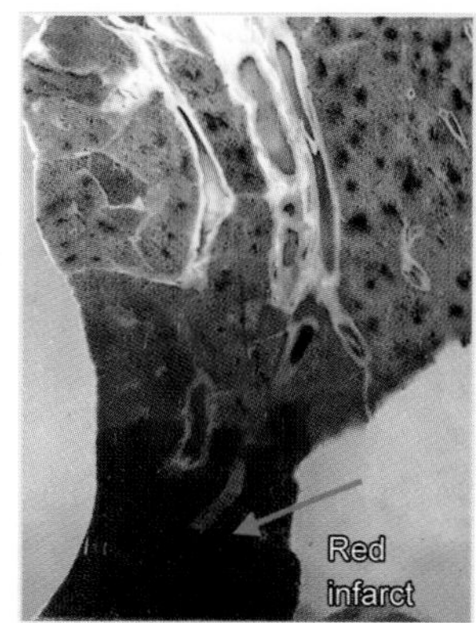

FIG. 39: Lung showing sharply circumscribed, dark red to purple hemorrhagic infarct.

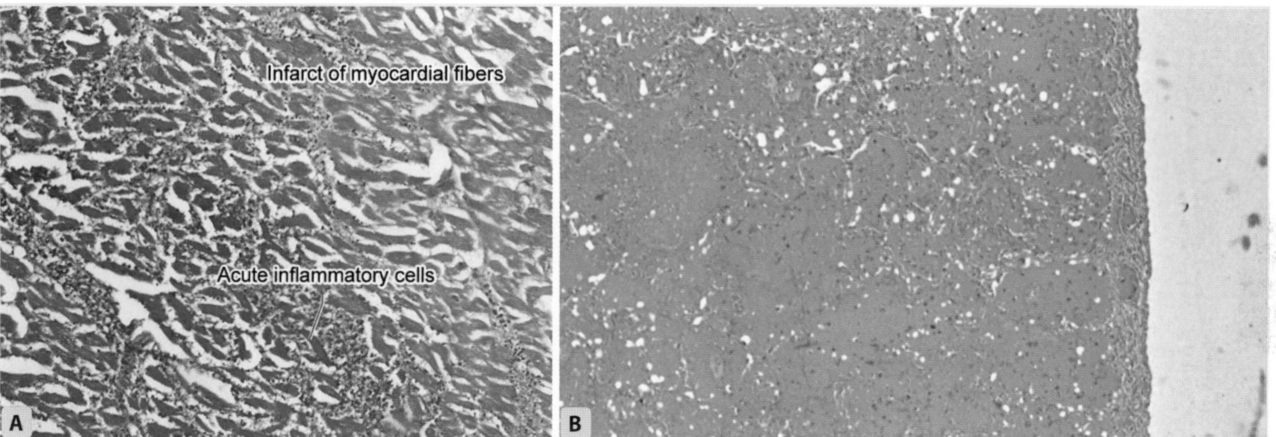

FIGS. 40A AND B: (A) Microscopic appearance of acute myocardial infarction showing coagulative necrosis with acute inflammatory infiltrate. (B) Microscopically, the hemorrhagic area of red infarct in the lung shows ischemic necrosis of the alveolar walls, bronchioles, and vessels.

coronary artery. Subendocardial infarction develops when the requirement for oxygen exceeds that of supply. It occurs due to prolonged ischemia caused by partially occluding, atherosclerotic, narrowing of coronary artery. Subendocardial infarction may be observed in shock, anoxia, or severe tachycardia (rapid pulse). Microscopically it shows coagulative type of necrosis (refer **Fig. 40A**).

Pulmonary Infarcts

About 10% of pulmonary emboli produce clinical symptoms due to pulmonary infarction. The infarction usually follows the occlusion of a middle-sized pulmonary artery and occurs only if circulation from bronchial arteries is inadequate to compensate for supply lost from the pulmonary arteries. Pulmonary infarction is usually observed in patients with CHF (congestive heart failure).

Morphologically, pulmonary infarct is hemorrhagic type. During early stages, it appears as a raised, red-blue area and the corresponding pleural surface is usually covered by a fibrinous exudate. The alveoli are lined by necrotic tissue and hemorrhage occurs into the alveoli associated with lysis of red cells within 48 hours. Gradually, the infarct becomes paler and eventually red-brown (due to hemosiderin). With the passage of time, fibrous replacement begins at the margins producing a gray-white peripheral zone. Ultimately, infarct is converted into a contracted scar. Microscopically, the hemorrhagic area shows ischemic necrosis of the alveolar walls, bronchioles, and vessels (refer **Fig. 40B**). If the infarct is produced due to an infected (septic) embolus, the infarct shows dense collections of neutrophils. These infarcts are termed as **septic infarcts,** some of which be converted into abscess.

Cerebral Infarcts

Infarction of the brain may be due to local ischemia or a generalized reduction in blood flow (e.g., systemic hypotension in shock). Generalized reduction in blood flow causes infarction in the border zones between the distributions of the major cerebral arteries **(watershed/border zone infarct).** Watershed infarcts develop in the regions of the brain that lie at the most distal reaches of the arterial blood supply (i.e., the border zones between arterial territories). If prolonged, severe hypotension can result in widespread necrosis of brain. The occlusion of a single blood vessel in the brain (e.g., embolus) causes ischemia and necrosis in a well-defined area of the brain supplied by the vessel. The occlusion of a large artery in the brain produces a wide area of necrosis.

Morphologically, cerebral infarct may be pale (**nonhemorrhagic**) or red. Microscopically, cerebral infarct shows liquefactive necrosis.

- **Pale infarct:** Grossly, by 48 hours, the infarcted tissue appears pale, soft, and swollen, and the gray-white matter junction becomes indistinct. From 2 to 10 days, the infarcted region becomes gelatinous and friable, and boundary between normal and infarcted tissue becomes more distinct. From 10 days to 3 weeks, the infarcted tissue liquefies and produces a fluid-filled cavity (refer Fig. 7 of Chapter 7). This continues to expand till all of the necrotic tissue is removed. This may resolve and lead to a large fluid-filled cavity in the brain (cystic infarct).
- **Red infarcts** develop with embolic occlusions.

Intestinal Infarcts

Transmural infarction of intestine may be caused by acute arterial obstruction. The demarcation between normal and infarcted bowel is sharp, and initially the infarcted region appears severely congested and dusky to purple-red. Later, blood-tinged mucus or frank blood accumulates in the lumen of the intestine, and the wall becomes edematous, thickened, and rubbery.

The earliest changes observed in intestinal ischemia are necrosis or sloughing of surface epithelium of the tips of the villi in the small intestine and necrosis of the superficial mucosa in the large intestine. When the ischemia is severe, submucosa and muscularis show hemorrhagic necrosis. Small mucosal infarcts heal within a few days, whereas more severe injury leads to ulceration. Small ulcers eventually undergo re-epithelialization. However, large ulcers heal by scarring, and may give rise to strictures. Severe transmural necrosis can produce massive bleeding or bowel perforation. This usually leads to irreversible shock, sepsis, and death.

SHOCK

Q. Define shock. Enumerate the types of shock. Discuss the pathogenesis and its stages and morphological changes in various organs in shock.

Q. Discuss shock with special reference to systemic inflammatory response syndrome.

Q. Discuss the recent concepts about shock.

Q. Write short essay on pathogenesis of multiorgan failure.

Introduction

Shock is the most common, important, and very serious medical condition. It is the final common pathway for several clinical events, which are capable of causing death. These events include severe hemorrhage, extensive trauma or burns, large myocardial infarction, massive pulmonary embolism, and severe microbial sepsis. Characteristic features of shock are presented in **Flowchart 10**.

Definition

Shock is a pathological state of circulatory failure that impairs tissue perfusion leading to cellular hypoxia.

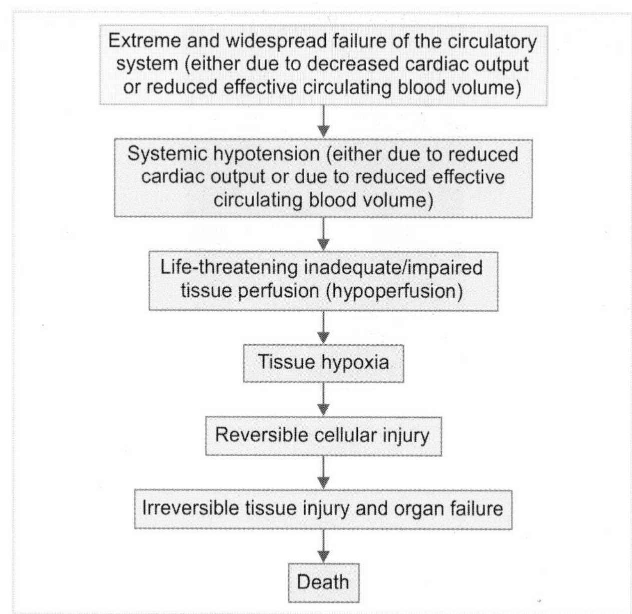

FLOWCHART 10: Characteristic features of shock.

In shock, there is severe hemodynamic and metabolic disturbance. This leads to failure of the circulatory system to maintain an appropriate blood supply or perfusion of vital organs. Tissue perfusion and oxygen supply fall below levels required to meet normal demands. There is failure to adequately remove metabolites. Initially, the cellular injury is reversible; however, prolonged shock leads to irreversible tissue injury and can be fatal.

Classification

According to etiology (cause) shock can be classified into three major general categories (**Table 11**).

Etiology and Pathogenesis

Hypovolemic Shock

Hypovolemic shock results from low cardiac output due to:

- **Loss of blood** (e.g., **massive hemorrhage**).
- **Loss of plasma** (e.g., **severe burns**).
- **Loss of fluid: Vomiting, diarrhea, severe gastroenteritis,** e.g., cholera.

The pathogenesis of hypovolemic shock is presented in **Flowchart 11**.

Cardiogenic Shock

Cardiogenic shock results from low cardiac output due to:

- **Intrinsic myocardial damage** (e.g., **massive myocardial infarction**, ventricular arrhythmias).
- **Extrinsic pressure or compression of heart** (e.g., cardiac tamponade).
- **Obstruction to the outflow blood from ventricles** (e.g., pulmonary embolism).

The pathogenesis of cardiogenic shock is presented in **Flowchart 11**. The left-sided heart failure also reduces the entry of blood from pulmonary vein into the left atrium. This leads to movement of fluid from pulmonary vasculature

Table 11: Major types of shock.

Types of shock	*Principal mechanisms*	*Clinical example*
Hypovolemic shock		
Inadequate blood or plasma volume—decreased circulating blood volume—low cardiac output—hypotension, and shock	Loss of blood volume	Massive hemorrhage, trauma
	Loss of plasma volume	Massive burns
	Loss of fluid	Vomiting, diarrhea, severe gastroenteritis
Cardiogenic shock		
Failure of myocardial pump due to intrinsic myocardial damage, extrinsic compression, or obstruction to outflow—low cardiac output—reduced cardiac output and blood pressure	Myocardial damage	Myocardial infarction, ventricular rupture, arrhythmia, cardiac tamponade, pulmonary embolism
	Mechanical	• Valvular failure (stenosis or incompetence) • Hypertrophic cardiomyopathy • Ventricular septal defect
	Arrhythmic	Ventricular arrhythmias
Septic shock		
Shock associated with systemic inflammation	Activation of cytokines, peripheral vasodilation, and pooling of blood. Endothelial activation/injury; leukocyte-induced endothelial damage, and disseminated intravascular coagulation	Overwhelming microbial infections [bacterial (gram-negative sepsis, gram-positive septicemia), fungal, viral, rickettsial]. Superantigens (e.g., toxic shock syndrome). Trauma, burns, pancreatitis
Others		
Neurogenic shock	Result of loss of vascular tone and peripheral pooling of blood	Anesthetic accident or a spinal cord injury
Anaphylactic shock	Acute widespread systemic vasodilation and increased vascular permeability results in tissue hypoperfusion and hypoxia	IgE-mediated type I hypersensitivity reaction

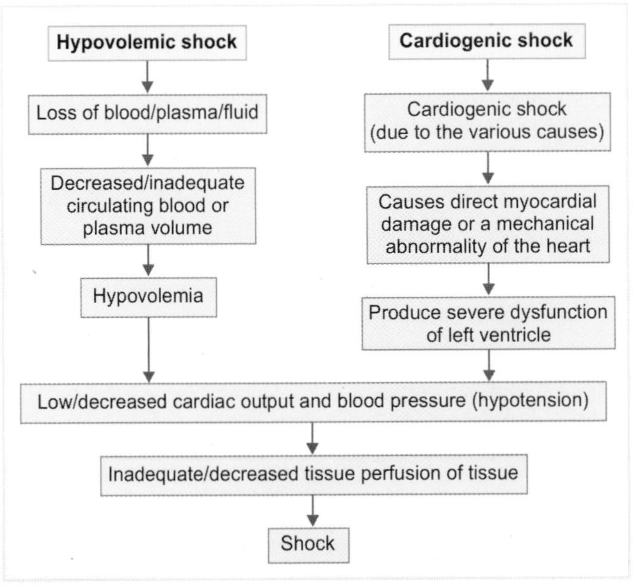

FLOWCHART 11: Pathogenesis of hypovolemic and cardiogenic shock.

into the pulmonary interstitial space and into the alveoli resulting in **pulmonary edema.**

Sepsis, Septic Shock, and the Systemic Inflammatory Response Syndrome

Q. Describe the pathogenesis of septic shock.

These 3 conditions are interrelated and somewhat overlapping. Definition of these according to the Third International Consensus Definitions for Sepsis and Septic Shock (2016) is presented as follows:

Sepsis

It is a dysregulated host response to infection that leads to a life-threatening acute organ dysfunction.

Septic shock

It is defined as a subset of sepsis in which there is intense circulatory, cellular, and metabolic abnormalities and are associated with a greater risk of mortality than with sepsis alone.

Systemic inflammatory response syndrome (SIRS)

It is discussed in detail on page 323. In cancer patients treated with chimeric antigen receptor T-cell (CAR-T) therapy, a similar iatrogenic syndrome called *cytokine release syndrome* can develop.

Pathogenesis of Septic Shock

Q. Discuss in detail pathogenesis and pathology of septic (endotoxic shock).
Q. Discuss multiorgan failure.

Causative organisms: Septic shock may be caused by **gram-positive** (most common) **or gram-negative bacteria, fungi**, and, very rarely, protozoa or rickettsia. Hence, the older term "endotoxic shock," is not appropriate. The common gram-positive bacteria include ***Staphylococcus aureus,* enterococci, *Streptococcus pneumoniae,*** and gram-negative bacilli which are resistant to usual antibiotics.

Pathophysiology of septic shock: The incidence of shock is increasing. It is due to improvements in life support for critically ill patients, increased numbers of immunocompromised hosts (as a result of chemotherapy, immunosuppression, advanced age, or human immunodeficiency virus infection), and the increasing number of patients infected with multidrug-resistant organisms in the hospitals. About 50% of patients with septic shock require treatment in intensive care units. The mortality rate in septic shock is about 50%.

Diverse microorganisms can cause septic shock. This indicates that a variety of microbial constituents can trigger the process of septic shock. Various cells (e.g., macrophages, neutrophils, dendritic cells, endothelial cells), and soluble components of the innate immune system (e.g., complement) recognize and are activated by many substances derived from microorganisms. After activation, these cells and factors initiate many inflammatory and counter-inflammatory responses. They interact in a complex fashion to produce septic shock and organ failure. The host response to septic shock involves multiple mechanisms that lead to decreased oxygen delivery at the tissue level. Several factors play major roles in the pathophysiology of septic shock and are listed in **Box 8**.

Inflammatory and Counter-inflammatory Responses

Initiation of inflammation (triggering of proinflammatory response)

In sepsis, various components of the pathogens interact with pattern recognition receptors (PRRs) on the cells of the innate immune system and trigger proinflammatory responses (**Flowchart 12**).

Box 8: Major factors contributing to the pathogenesis of septic shock.

- Inflammatory and counter-inflammatory (immunosuppressive) responses
- Endothelial cell activation and injury
- Induction of a procoagulant state
- Metabolic abnormalities
- Organ dysfunction

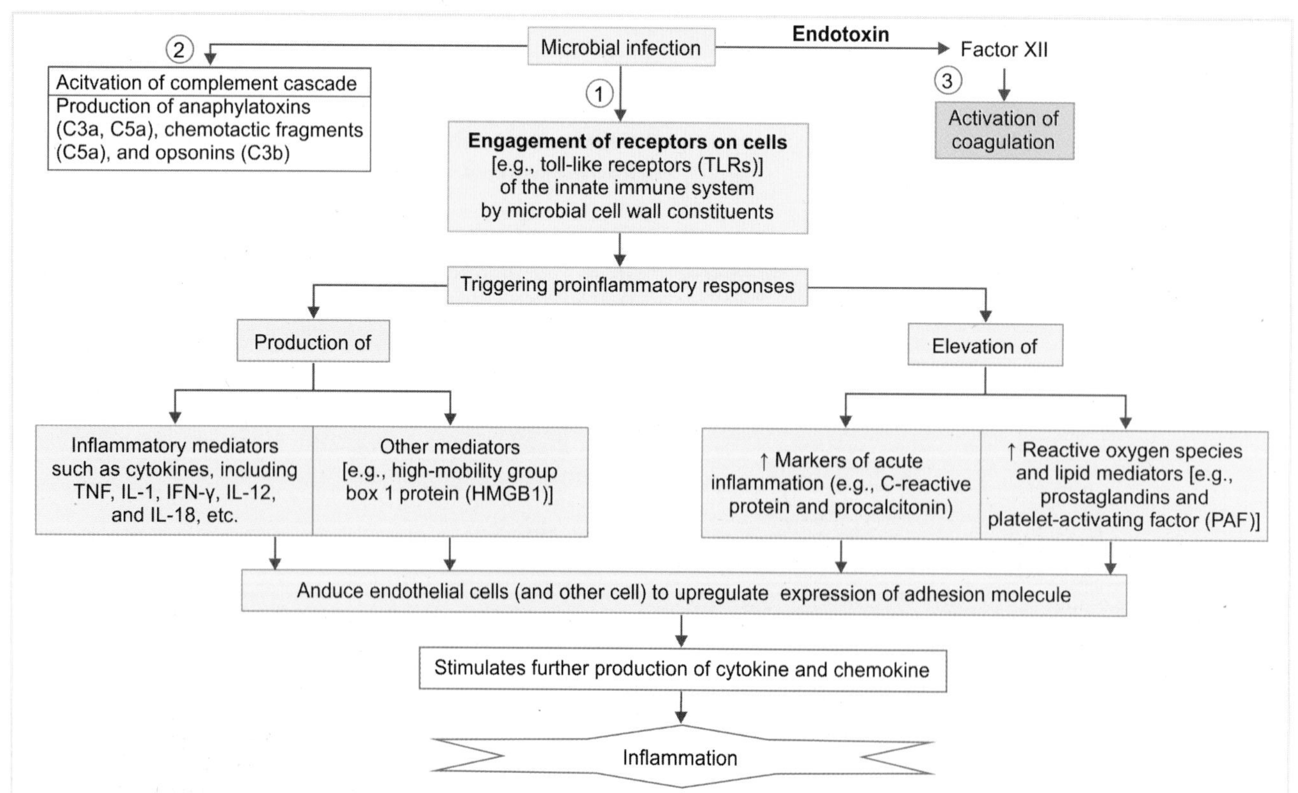

FLOWCHART 12: Proinflammatory responses in septic shock.

Activation of cells of immune system

- **Pattern recognition receptors on immune cells:** There are four main classes of PRRs [Toll-like receptors (TLRs), RIG-I-like receptors, C-type lectin receptors (CLRs), and nucleotide-binding oligomerization domain-like receptors (NLRs/NOD-like receptors are present in the cytoplasm)]. These PRRs are present on cells of the innate immune system (e.g., macrophages, neutrophils, dendritic cells, endothelial cells). G protein-coupled receptor (GPCR) is another receptor that belongs to a large family of signaling proteins. Dectin-1 is a recently discovered pattern-recognition receptor belonging to C-type lectin receptors and is expressed on phagocytes.
- **Microbial components sensed by PRRs (Table 12):** Various components in the microbial cell wall of pathogens such as bacterial peptides, **pathogen-associated molecular patterns (PAMPs)** and **damage-associated molecular patterns (DAMPs)** are recognized by PRRs. A common PAMP is the lipid A moiety of lipopolysaccharide (LPS or endotoxin). It attaches to the LPS-binding protein on the surface of monocytes, macrophages, and neutrophils. G-protein–coupled receptors detect bacterial peptides.
- **Initiation of inflammatory response:** In sepsis, the inflammatory response is typically initiated by interaction between PAMPs expressed by microbial pathogens with PRRs expressed on the cells of the innate immune system. Binding of these receptors leads to increased expression of the genes encoding inflammatory mediators via activation and nuclear translocation of the transcription factor nuclear factor-κB (NF-κB).
- **Release of proinflammatory molecules:** The activated receptors on cells of the immune system trigger/initiate the **production of proinflammatory molecules** to eliminate the causative pathogen. These molecules include:
    - **Inflammatory mediators** such as cytokines including tumor necrosis factor (TNF), interleukin 1 (IL-1), IL-12, IL-18, and **interferon (IFN)-γ**. Also, **cytokine-like** mediators such as **high mobility group box 1 protein (HMGB1)** are also released.
    - **Markers of acute inflammation** (e.g., C-reactive protein, procalcitonin): These are also elevated and are useful indicators of septic shock.
    - **Reactive oxygen species and lipid mediators** such as prostaglandins and platelet-activating factor (PAF) are also released.
- **Effect of inflammatory mediators: Released** proinflammatory effector molecules **activate endothelial cells** (and other cell types) to **upregulate expression of adhesion molecule**. This in turn **stimulates further production of cytokine and chemokine.** The inflammatory response results in tissue damage and necrotic cell death. This in turn releases damage associated molecular patterns (DAMPs) such as HMGB1, etc. These molecules promote the activation of leukocytes. This produces greater endothelial dysfunction, expression of intercellular adhesion molecule (ICAM) and vascular cell adhesion molecule-1 (VCAM-1) on the activated endothelium, coagulation activation, and complement activation.

Table 12: Pattern recognition receptors on the cells of the innate immune system and related components of the microorganism sensed.

Receptors on cells of the immune system	*Component of microorganism detected*
Toll-like receptors (TLRs)*	Pathogen associated molecular patterns (PAMPs)
G-protein-coupled receptors	Bacterial peptides
C-type lectin receptors (e.g., Dectins)	Fungus

* Also recognize endogenous damage-associated molecular patterns (DAMPs) released from injured cells)

Activation of complement cascade The microbial components (directly as well as through the proteolytic activity of plasmin) also activate soluble components of the innate immune system namely complement system. The activated complement system **produces anaphylatoxins (C3a, C5a), chemotactic fragments (C5a), and opsonins (C3b)**. All these complement products contribute to the proinflammatory state.

Activation of coagulation Microbial components can also activate coagulation directly through factor XII and indirectly through altered endothelial function. This causes widespread activation of thrombin and this may further increase inflammation by triggering protease-activated receptors (PARs) on inflammatory cells.

Activation of counter-regulatory inflammatory responses

Simultaneous with inflammatory response there is also triggering of counter-regulatory inflammatory responses. The intensity of each of these reactions depends on multiple factors and includes the host factors (e.g., genetics and underlying diseases) and the pathogen (e.g., virulence and burden of infection). Patients who survive early septic shock but remain dependent on intensive care occasionally demonstrate evidence of a suppressed immune system.

The hyperinflammatory state produced by sepsis **also activates counter-regulatory (anti-inflammatory) and immunosuppressive responses.** This involves both innate and adaptive immune cells. Thus, in a patient with sepsis, there may be **fluctuation between hyperinflammatory and immunosuppressed states**. Various mechanisms of the anti-inflammatory and immune suppressive responses are listed in **Box 9**.

Consequences of inflammatory and counter-inflammatory responses

- **Tissue damage:** Though the purpose of inflammatory responses (proinflammatory reactions) is to eliminate the causative pathogen, they may also be responsible for "collateral" direct organ/tissue damage.
- **Susceptibility to secondary infections:** Counter/anti-inflammatory response develops later in the course and is responsible for the increased susceptibility to secondary infections that occurs later in the course.

The interplay between inflammatory and counter-inflammatory responses causes direct damage to organs by the pathogen and damage to organs due to the host's immune response. The host's ability to resist as well as tolerate both direct and immunopathological damage will determine whether uncomplicated infection becomes sepsis and septic shock. These responses interact in a complex, incompletely

Box 9: Various mechanisms of the anti-inflammatory and immune-suppressive responses.

Anti-inflammatory responses
- Shift from proinflammatory (Th1) to anti-inflammatory (Th2) cytokines
- Production of anti-inflammatory mediators [e.g., soluble TNF (tumor necrosis factor) receptor (STNFR), interleukin (IL)-1 receptor antagonist, and IL-10])
- Switch of phagocytes to an anti-inflammatory phenotype that promotes tissue repair
- Lymphocyte apoptosis
- Immunosuppressive effects of apoptotic cells
- Induction of cellular anergy
- Regulatory T cells and myeloid-derived suppressor cells can reduce inflammation
- Neuroinflammatory reflex releases acetylcholine secretion by a subset of CD4+ T cells. This acts on receptors on macrophages and reduces release of proinflammatory cytokine

Immune suppressive responses
- Widespread apoptosis of lymphocytes (especially of B cells, CD4+ T cells, and follicular dendritic cells)
- Immunosuppression by apoptotic cells
- Induction of cellular anergy

understood fashion to produce septic shock and multiorgan dysfunction.

Endothelial Cell Activation and Injury

Endothelial cell activation/injury is caused **by either microbial constituents and or proinflammatory state** (leukocyte-derived inflammatory mediators).

Consequences of endothelial cell activation (Flowchart 13):

- **Impaired tissue perfusion:** Inflammatory cytokines produced during inflammatory response cause **loosening of endothelial cell tight junctions**. This causes **widespread vascular leakage of protein-rich fluid from vessels into the interstitial tissue** resulting in the accumulation of **edema** fluid in the interstitial tissue throughout the body. **Edema** impairs/reduces both supply of nutrient and removal of waste. This **impairs tissue perfusion** and may be exacerbated by attempts to support the patient with intravenous fluids. Tissue perfusion may be further intensified by intravenous fluids administered in a patient with septic shock.
- **Systemic hypotension:** Endothelial activation also **upregulates production of NO and other vasoactive inflammatory mediators** (e.g., C3a, C5a, and PAF). These may cause **relaxation of vascular smooth muscle and systemic hypotension**.
- **Microvascular dysfunction:** Sepsis is associated with an increase in capillaries with intermittent flow, and heterogeneity of flow in various capillary beds. There is loss of the normal autoregulation of flow based on tissue metabolic environment. These changes further cause an imbalance between oxygen requirement and oxygen delivery.

Induction of a Procoagulant State (Fig. 41)

Sepsis is commonly associated with coagulation disorders that is enough to produce the dangerous complication of DIC (disseminated intravascular coagulation) in up to 50% of patients in septic shock. Sepsis causes expression of many factors that favor coagulation or procoagulant state. Abnormalities in coagulation may possibly isolate invading micro-organisms and/or prevent the spread of infection and

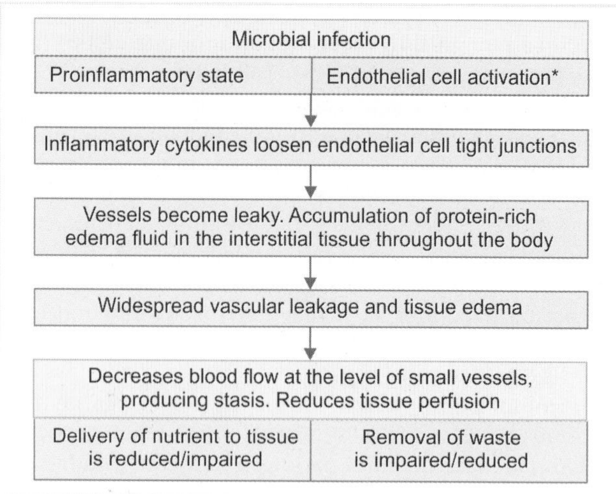

FLOWCHART 13: Endothelial cell activation and injury in septic shock.

*Endothelium cell activation also upregulates production of nitric oxide (NO) and other vasoactive inflammatory mediators (e.g., C3a, C5a, and PAF)—causes relaxation of vascular smooth muscle and systemic hypotension.

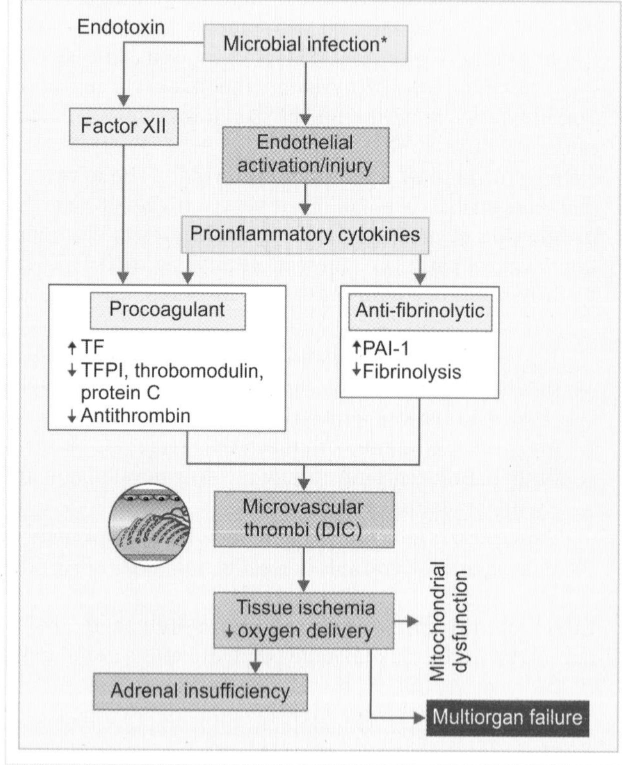

(TF: tissue factor; TFPI: tissue factor pathway inhibitor; PAI-1: plasminogen activator inhibitor-1; DIC: disseminated intravascular coagulation)

FIG. 41: Factors predisposing procoagulant state and its consequences.

inflammation to other tissues and organs. In sepsis, various factors produce a procoagulant state by favoring coagulation as well as reducing antifibrinolytic activity.

- **Factors favoring coagulation:**
  - **Activation of factor XII** by microbial components such as **endotoxin**.
  - **Proinflammatory cytokines (e.g., IL-6) favor** procoagulant state by:
    - **Increasing the production of tissue factor (TF):** This is produced by monocytes and probably by endothelial cells.
    - **Decreasing the production of endothelial anticoagulant factors:** For example, as tissue factor pathway inhibitor (TFPI), thrombomodulin, protein C and antithrombin.
    - **Neutrophil extracellular traps (NETs):** Probably NETs stimulate both intrinsic and extrinsic pathways of coagulation and promote the procoagulant state.
- **Reducing antifibrinolytic activity:** Proinflammatory cytokines (e.g., IL-6) also reduce fibrinolysis (removal of fibrin) by increasing the expression plasminogen activator inhibitor-1(PAI-1).

Consequences of activation of coagulation system

- **Microvascular thrombi:** Activation of coagulation system leads to **systemic activation of thrombin and the deposition of fibrin-rich thrombi in small vessels**, often throughout the body. This **produces dangerous complication DIC** in about 50% of septic patients. This compromises tissue perfusion. The consumption of coagulation factors and platelets leads to deficiencies of these factors and cause **bleeding and hemorrhage**.
- **Diminished the clearing of activated coagulation factors:** The vascular leak and tissue edema reduces the flow of blood flow in the small vessels. This causes stasis and reduces the clearing of activated coagulation factors.

Metabolic Abnormalities

- **Insulin resistance and hyperglycemia:** Hyperglycemia is due to gluconeogenesis stimulated by **the action of proinflammatory cytokines** (e.g., TNF and IL-1), stress-induced hormones (e.g., glucagon, growth hormone, and glucocorticoids), and **catecholamines.** The proinflammatory cytokines reduce the release of insulin, promote insulin resistance in the liver and other tissues, and impair the surface expression of glucose transporter type 4 (GLUT-4).
  - **Consequences: Hyperglycemia decreases neutrophil function**, reduces its bactericidal activity and causes increased expression of adhesion molecule on endothelial cells.
- **Decreased glucocorticoid production:** Initially in sepsis, there is increased glucocorticoid production, and is later followed by decreased production due to adrenal insufficiency. **Adrenal necrosis may also develop due to DIC (Waterhouse–Friderichsen syndrome).**
- **Lactic acidosis:** Cellular hypoxia and reduced oxidative phosphorylation may lead to greater glycolysis. This causes increased production of lactate and leads to lactic acidosis.

Organ Dysfunction

The mechanisms responsible for organ failure/dysfunction in sepsis is due to impaired tissue oxygenation.

- **Decreased supply of oxygen and nutrients to the tissues:** Several factors contribute to decreased oxygen supply to the tissues in septic shock. These include systemic hypotension, interstitial edema, microvascular dysfunction, and thrombi in the small vessels (microvascular thrombosis). Oxidative stress causes damage to the mitochondria and impairs oxygen use.
- **Decreased contractility of myocardium and cardiac output:** It is **due to increased levels of cytokines and secondary mediators**. This along with increased vascular permeability and endothelial injury can lead to the **acute respiratory distress syndrome**.
- **Multiorgan failure (refer page 400): Finally, above factors lead to failure** of multiple organs, mainly the **kidneys, liver, lungs,** and **heart** resulting in death.
- **Outcome:** The severity and outcome of septic shock mainly depends on (i) the severity and virulence of the microbial infection, (ii) the immune status of the patient, (iii) the presence of any other comorbid conditions, (iv) and the pattern and level of mediator production. The septic shock remains a clinical challenge even in the advanced clinical care centers.

Another group of proteins secreted by bacteria is called **superantigens**. They produce a syndrome similar to septic shock (e.g., *toxic shock syndrome*). Superantigens are polyclonal T-lymphocyte activators which stimulate increased release of cytokines. These cytokines can produce diverse clinical features, ranging from a diffuse rash to vasodilation, hypotension, shock, and death.

The summary of various mechanism involved in the pathogenesis of septic shock is presented in **Figure 42**.

Stages of Shock

Shock is a progressive disorder, which if not treated, leads to death. In sepsis-related death, there is increased apoptosis of lymphocyte and enterocytes and cellular necrosis is minimal. Death usually follows the failure of multiple organs. Death in hypovolemic and cardiogenic shock are better understood than due to septic shock. Most of situations shock tends to evolve through three (somewhat artificial) stages except when shock is massive and rapidly lethal (e.g., severe loss of blood in ruptured aortic aneurysm). These stages are clearly observed in hypovolemic shock but are also common in other types of shock.

Nonprogressive (Compensated/Reversible) Phase

During the initial phase, homeostatic compensatory mechanisms **redistribute the blood supply** in such a way that the effective **blood supply to the vital organs is maintained**. This is achieved by neurohumoral mechanisms, which try to maintain cardiac output and blood pressure.

- **Compensatory changes:** The neurohumoral mechanism produces the following compensatory changes:
  - **These mechanisms are:** baroreceptor reflexes, secretion of catecholamines and antidiuretic hormone (ADH), activation of the renin–angiotensin–aldosterone axis, and generalized sympathetic stimulation.

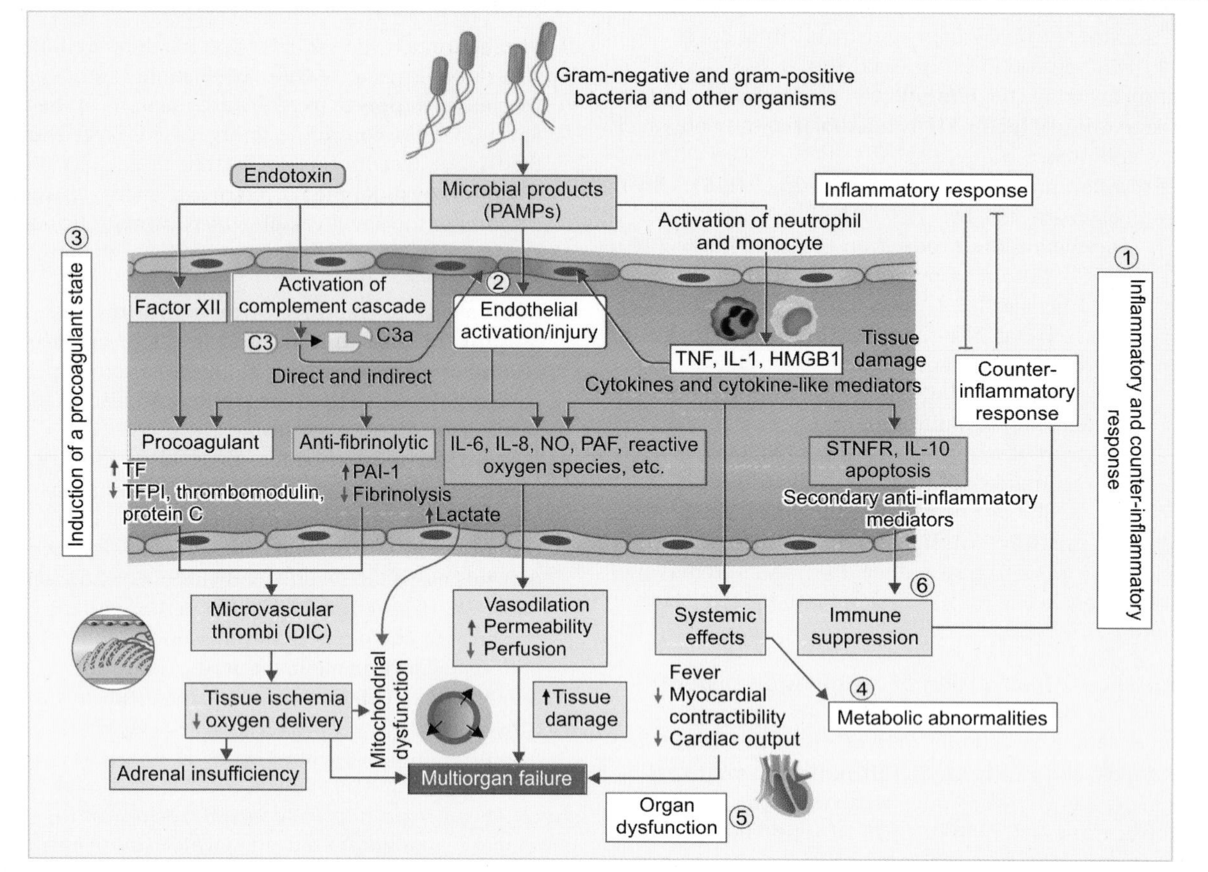

(DIC: disseminated intravascular coagulation; HMGB1: high mobility group box 1 protein; NO: nitric oxide; PAF: platelet activating factor; TF: tissue factor; STNFR: soluble tumor necrosis factor receptor)

FIG. 42: Pathogenesis of septic shock. Microbial products initiate endothelial cell activation/injury, activate endothelial cells, complement activation, activation of neutrophils and macrophages, factor XII. These initiating events lead to end-stage multiorgan failure. Major factors contributing to the pathogenesis of septic shock are: (1) Inflammatory and counter-inflammatory responses, (2) Endothelial cell activation and injury, (3) Induction of a procoagulant state, (4) Metabolic abnormalities, (5) Organ dysfunction and (6) Immune suppression.

- **Widespread vasoconstriction** except vital organs. **Coronary and cerebral vessels** usually **maintain relatively normal blood flow, and oxygen delivery**. Cutaneous vasoconstriction—produces the coolness and pallor of the skin. However, in septic shock, initially there may be cutaneous vasodilation and the patient may have warm and flushed skin.
- **Fluid conservation by kidney.**
- **Tachycardia.**

Progressive Phase

- **If the underlying causes are not corrected**, shock **passes to the progressive phase**.
- Characterized by **widespread tissue hypoperfusion** and **hypoxia.** The intracellular aerobic respiration replaced by **anaerobic glycolysis**. This causes **increased** production of **lactic acid** and leads to metabolic **lactic acidosis.** This in turn **decreases** the tissue **pH**, dilatation of arterioles with peripheral **pooling of blood into the microcirculation**. This **decreases** the **cardiac output** and produces **anoxic injury** to endothelial cell. This favors development of **DIC**, widespread tissue hypoxia and **damage of vital organs**.

Irreversible Phase

- **Without intervention, the shock eventually** enters an **irreversible stage**.
- At this phase, **cellular and tissue injury is so severe** that even if the hemodynamic defects are corrected, **survival is not possible**.
- Widespread cell injury results in leakage of lysosomal enzymes, which aggravate the shock state.
- **Myocardial contractile function worsens** partly due to NO synthesis.
- If ischemic intestine allows microbes from the intestinal flora to enter into the circulation, it may lead to **superimposed bacteremic shock**.
- The patient develops **acute tubular necrosis** and results in death.

MORPHOLOGY (Table 13)

The cellular and tissue changes in shock are mainly due to hypoxic injury and are caused by a combination of **hypoperfusion** and **microvascular thrombosis**. Shock is associated with specific changes in many organs. Though any organ can be affected in shock, most commonly involved organs are the brain, heart, kidneys, adrenals, and gastrointestinal tract.

Changes in Cardiogenic or Hypovolemic Shock

These are mainly due to hypoxic injury. Morphological changes are particularly evident in adrenals, kidneys, lungs, brain, heart, and gastrointestinal tract.

Adrenal

- **Lipid depletion in cortical cell:** It is due to conversion of the relatively inactive vacuolated cells to metabolically active cells. The active cells utilize stored lipids for the synthesis of steroids.
- **Focal hemorrhage:** It occurs in the inner cortex of adrenal in **severe** shock.
- **Massive hemorrhagic necrosis** of the entire adrenal gland is found in the Waterhouse–Friderichsen **syndrome,** which is **associated with severe meningococcal septicemia**.

Kidney

Acute tubular necrosis (acute renal failure) is a major complication of shock.

- **Gross:** Kidney is **enlarged, swollen, congested**, and the **cortex may appear pale**. Cut section shows blood pooling in the outer region of the medulla.
- **Microscopy:** Fibrin thrombi can develop in any tissue but usually seen in glomeruli of the kidney.

Continued

Continued

    - **Tubules:** Dilation of the proximal tubules and **focal necrosis of tubular epithelial cells (Fig. 43)**. Frequently, the tubular lumen may show **pigmented casts** formed due to leakage of hemoglobin or myoglobin.
    - **Interstitium:** It shows **edema** and **mononuclear cells** in the interstitium and within tubules.

Lungs

- Lungs are relatively resistant to hypoxic injury and are usually not affected in pure hypovolemic shock.
- However, when shock is due to bacterial sepsis or trauma, it shows **diffuse alveolar damage** which can lead to ARDS, also known as **shock lung**.
- **Gross:** The lung is **firm and congested. Cut surface** shows **oozing out** of **frothy fluid**.
- **Microscopy:**
    - **Edema:** It first develops around peribronchial **interstitial** connective tissue and later in the **alveoli.**
    - **Necrosis:** Endothelial and alveolar epithelial cells undergo necrosis and lead to formation of **intravascular microthrombi.**
    - **Hyaline membrane:** It is usually seen lining the alveolar surface. It may also line alveolar ducts and terminal bronchioles.

Heart

- **Gross:** It shows **petechial hemorrhages** in the epicardium and endocardium.
- **Microscopy: Necrosis** of the myocardium is seen which may range from minute focus to large areas of necrosis. Prominent **contraction bands** are seen by light microscopy.

Liver

- **Gross:** Liver is enlarged. C/s shows a **mottled** (blotched) appearance due to marked pooling of blood in the centrilobular region.

Continued

Table 13: Summary of main morphological features of shock.

Organ	*Changes*
Adrenal	Lipid depletion in the cortical cells
Kidney	Acute tubular necrosis (ATN)/acute renal failure
Lungs	Relatively resistant to hypoxic injury. However, in septic shock shows diffuse alveolar damage (shock lung) with hyaline membrane
Heart	Coagulative necrosis and contraction band necrosis
Liver	Congestion and necrosis of centrilobular region of the liver
Brain	Encephalopathy (ischemic or septic) and cortical necrosis
Gastrointestinal tract	• Diffuse gastrointestinal hemorrhage • Erosions of the gastric mucosa and superficial ischemic necrosis in the intestine

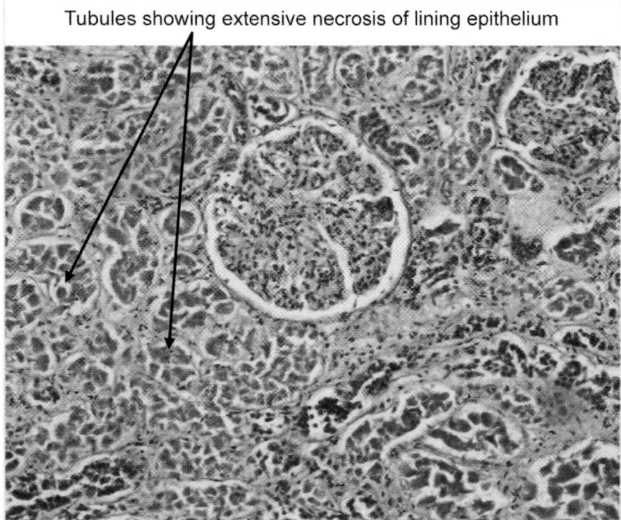

FIG. 43: Acute tubular necrosis showing tubules with necrosis of tubular epithelial cells. The glomerulus appears normal.

Continued

- **Microscopy:** The centrilobular region of the liver shows **congestion and necrosis.**

Brain

Encephalopathy (ischemic or septic) and cortical necrosis.

Gastrointestinal Tract

Shock produces **diffuse gastrointestinal hemorrhage**. **Erosions of the gastric mucosa** and superficial **ischemic necrosis** in the intestine lead to gastrointestinal bleeding.

Changes in Septic Shock

- Septic shock can lead to **DIC** which is characterized by **widespread** formation of fibrin-rich **microthrombi**, particularly in the brain, heart, lungs, kidney, adrenal glands, and gastrointestinal tract.
- The utilization of platelets and coagulation factors in DIC produces **bleeding manifestations**. It may show **petechial hemorrhages** on serosal surface and the skin.

Clinical Consequences

The clinical features of shock depend on the cause.

- **Hypovolemic and cardiogenic shock:** Usually present with features of hypotension and hypoperfusion. The features include **altered sensorium, cyanosis, oliguria, weak rapid pulse, tachypnea**, and **cool, clammy extremities**.
- **Septic shock:** The **skin initially may be warm and flushed** because of peripheral vasodilation.

The initial underlying cause that precipitates the shock may be life-threatening (e.g., myocardial infarct, severe hemorrhage, or sepsis). Later, the organ dysfunction involving **cardiac, cerebral, and pulmonary** function worsens the situation. The **electrolyte disturbances and metabolic acidosis** may further exacerbate the situation.

Patients who survive the initial complications may develop **renal insufficiency** characterized by a progressive decrease in urine output and severe fluid and electrolyte imbalances.

Prognosis

The prognosis depends on the cause and duration of shock.

- Patients with hypovolemic shock may survive with appropriate management.
- Septic shock, or cardiogenic shock associated with massive myocardial infarction, usually have high mortality rate.

MULTIORGAN SYSTEM FAILURE

Q. Write short essay on multiorgan system failure.

Definition: Multiorgan system failure (multiorgan failure syndrome/multiple organ dysfunction syndrome) is defined the simultaneous presence of physiologic dysfunction and/or failure of two or more organs. Organ failure is defined as failure of organ that persists beyond 24 hours.

Causes: It is commonly associated with critical illness. It usually occurs in severe sepsis (regarded as the final stage of severe sepsis), shock of any kind, severe inflammatory conditions such as pancreatitis, and trauma. It occurs commonly in critically ill patients in intensive care unit (ICU). In ICU, a single-organ failure is treated aggressively (e.g., by mechanical ventilation or by renal replacement therapy) and has reduced rates of early mortality in critical illness. In multiple organ dysfunction syndrome usually two or more organs are affected and homeostasis cannot be maintained without intervention. Different alterations of functional activities are responsible for the development of multiple organ dysfunction syndrome.

Mechanism: Pathogenic mechanisms of multiorgan failure syndrome are complex and can differ from patient to patient. These include endothelial activation, immune dysfunction, microcirculatory dysfunction, mitochondrial damage, increase of cell death, hemolysis, hypoperfusion, cellular hypermetabolism, thrombosis, hypoxia, and uncontrolled distribution of pathogens.

Mortality risk increases with the increase of failing organs. The prognosis worsens as the duration of organ failure increases.

BIBLIOGRAPHY

1. Banasik JL, Copstead LC. Pathophysiology, 6th edition. Philadelphia: Saunders Elsevier; 2019.
2. Chen H, Schrier R. Pathophysiology of volume overload in acute heart failure syndromes. *Am J Med.* 2006;119:S11.
3. Chapman JC, Hajjar KA. Fibrinolysis and the control of blood coagulation. *Blood Rev.* 2015;29:17.
4. Coleman DM, Obi A, Henke PK. Update in venous thrombo-embolism: pathophysiology, diagnosis, and treatment for surgical patients. *Curr Probl Surg.* 2015;52:233.
5. DeLoughery TG. Hemostasis and Thrombosis, 4th edition. Switzerland: Springer Nature; 2019.
6. Ellery PE, Adams MJ. Tissue factor pathway inhibitor: then and now. *Semin Thromb Hemost.* 2014;40:881.
7. Hotoleanu C. Genetic risk factors in venous thromboembolism, *Adv Exp Med Biol—Adv In Internal Med.* 2017;906(253).
8. Huether SE, McCance KL. Understanding Pathophysiology, 6th edition. Philadelphia: Saunders Elsevier; 2016.
9. Kumar V, Abbas AK, Aster JC. Robbins basic pathology, 10th edition. Philadelphia: Saunders Elsevier; 2018
10. Kumar V, Abbas AK, Fausto N, et al. Robbins and Cotran pathologic basis of disease, 10th edition. Philadelphia: WB Saunders; 2021.
11. Loeffler AG, Hart MN. Human disease-Pathophysiology for health professional,7th edition. Burlington: Jones & Bartlett Learning Learning Company; 2020.
12. McCance KL, Huether SE. Pathophysiology- The biologic basis for disease in adults and children, 8th edition. Philadelphia: Elsevier; 2019.
13. McCance KL, Huether SE, Brashers VL, et al. Pathophysiology: The biological basis for disease in adults and children. Missouri: Elsevier Mosby; 2014.
14. Montagnana M, Lippi G, Danese. An overview of thrombophilia and associated laboratory testing. In: Favaloro EJ, Lippi G, editors: Hemostasis and thrombosis: methods and protocols, methods in molecular biology, 2017;1646:113.

15. Nisio MD, van Es N, Buller H. Deep Vein thrombosis and pulmonary embolism, *Lancet.* 2016;388.
16. Prince M, Wenham T. Heparin-induced thrombocytopenia, *Postgrad Med J.* 2018;94:453.
17. Rao LVM, Esmon CT, Pendurthi UR. Endothelial cell protein C receptor: a multiliganded and multifunctional receptor. *Blood.* 2014;124(10):1553-62.
18. Rao LVM, Pendurthi UR, Rao LVM. Endothelial cell protein C receptor dependent signaling. *Curr Opin Hematol.* 2018;25:219.
19. Rudinga GR, et al. Protease-activated receptor 4 (PAR4): a promising target for antiplatelet therapy. *Int J Mol Sci.* 2018;19:572.
20. Strayer DS, Saffitz JE. Rubin's Pathology: Mechanism of Human Disease, 8th edition. Philadelphia: Wolters Kluwer; 2020.
21. Versteeg HH, Heemskerk JWM, Levi M, et al. New fundamentals in hemostasis. *Physiol Rev.* 2013;93:327.
22. Vojacek JF. Should we replace the terms intrinsic and extrinsic coagulation pathways with tissue factor pathway? *Clin Appl Thromb Hemost.* 2017;23:922.
23. Walter JB, Talbot IC. General pathology, 7th edition. Edinburgh: Churchill Livingstone; 2009.

CHAPTER

Neoplasia

10

10.1 Nomenclature, General Characteristics of Neoplasms, and Epidemiology of Cancer

CHAPTER OUTLINE

INTRODUCTION

Neoplasia literally means new growth, and a new growth formed is known as a neoplasm (Greek, *neo* = new + *plasma* = thing formed). The term "tumor" was originally used for the swelling caused by inflammation, but it is now used synonymously with neoplasm. Oncology (Greek, *oncos* = tumor) is the study of tumors or neoplasms.

Willis Definition

"A neoplasm is an abnormal mass of tissue, the growth of which exceeds and is uncoordinated with that of the normal tissues and persists in the same excessive manner after cessation of the stimuli which evoked the change."

In the present era, a neoplasm can be defined as a genetic disorder of cell growth which is triggered by a series of acquired or less commonly inherited mutations involving a single cell and its clonal progeny.

Salient Features of Neoplasia

- **Origin:** Neoplasms arise **from cells** that normally maintain a **proliferative capacity**.
- **Genetic disorder:** Cancer is due to **permanent genetic changes** in the cell, known as **mutations**. These mutations may occur in genes which regulate cell growth, apoptosis, or deoxyribonucleic acid (DNA) repair.
- **Heritable:** The genetic alterations are passed down to the daughter tumor cells.
- **Monoclonal:** All the neoplastic cells within an individual **tumor originate from a single cell/or clone of cells that has undergone genetic change**. Thus, tumors are said to be monoclonal.
- **Carcinogenic stimulus:** The stimulus responsible for the uncontrolled cell proliferation **may not be identified or is not known**.
- **Autonomy:** In neoplasia, there is **excessive** and **unregulated proliferation** of cells that do not obey the normal regulatory control. The cell proliferation is **independent of physiologic growth stimuli**. But tumors are dependent on the host for their nutrition and blood supply.
- **Irreversible:** Neoplasm is irreversible and **persists even after the inciting stimulus is withdrawn or gone**.
- **Differentiation** (*refer* page 7–8 of chapter 10.1): It refers to the **extent to which the tumor cells resemble the**

Box 1: Six P's of neoplasm.

- **P**urposeless
- **P**rogressive
- **P**roliferation unregulated
- **P**reys on host
- **P**ersists even after withdrawal of stimulus (autonomous)
- **P**ermanent genetic change in the cell

cell of origin. A tumor may show varying degrees of differentiation ranging from relatively mature structures that mimic normal tissues (well-differentiated) to cells so primitive that the cell of origin cannot be identified (poorly differentiated).

Main characteristics of neoplasm are presented in **Box 1**.

Classification

Neoplasms are derived from cells that are normally capable of multiplying. Thus, mature neurons and cardiac myocytes that are not able to multiply after birth do not give rise to tumors. Commonly the terms "benign" and "malignant" are used for a tumor's overall biological behavior rather than its morphologic characteristics. Tumors are classified as **benign and malignant, depending on** the **biological behavior** of a tumor.

Benign Tumors

- They have relatively innocent microscopic and gross characteristics.
  - **Remain localized without invasion or metastasis.**
  - **Well-differentiated:** Their cells **closely resemble their tissue of origin**.
  - **Prognosis:** It is **very good**, can be cured by surgical removal in most of the patients and the patient generally survives. However, benign tumors in critical locations can be dangerous. For example, a benign intracranial tumor of the meninges (meningioma) can produce pressure effect on the brain. Minute benign tumor of the ependymal cells of the third ventricle (ependymoma) can block the circulation of cerebrospinal fluid. This may lead to lethal hydrocephalus. A benign mesenchymal tumor of the left atrium (myxoma) can cause sudden death by blocking the orifice of the mitral valve. Rarely, a functioning, benign endocrine adenoma can be life-threatening (e.g., sudden hypoglycemia associated with an insulinoma of the pancreas or the hypertensive crisis produced by a pheochromocytoma of the adrenal medulla.

Malignant Tumors

- **Cancer is the general term** used for malignant tumors. The term "cancer" is derived from the Latin word for *crab*, because similar to a crab, malignant tumors adhere to any part that they seize on, in an obstinate (stubborn) manner.
  - **Invasion:** Malignant tumors invade **or infiltrate into the adjacent tissues or structures**.
  - **Metastasis:** Cancers **spread to distant sites** (metastasize), where the malignant cells reside, grow anew and again invade into the surrounding tissue.
    - **Exception: Basal cell carcinoma** of the skin, which is histologically malignant (i.e., it invades aggressively), but rarely metastasizes to distant sites. **Glioma** is malignant tumor of central nervous system (CNS).
  - **Prognosis:** Most malignant tumors cause death. Though the term"malignant"suggests a bad prognosis, not all cancers need not follow a deadly course. Some cancers, if discovered at early stages can be cured by surgical excision, some by systemic administration of drugs or therapeutic antibodies.

Microscopic Components of Neoplasms

Tumors (both benign and malignant) consist of two basic components:

Parenchyma: It is made up of neoplastic cells. The **nomenclature and biological behavior of tumors** are **based primarily** on the **parenchymal component** of tumor.

Stroma: It is the **supporting, non-neoplastic tissue** derived **from the host**.

- **Components: Connective tissue, blood vessels, and cells of the adaptive and innate immune system** (e.g., macrophages and lymphocytes).
- **Inflammatory reaction:** Stroma may show inflammatory reaction in and around the tumors. It may be due to ulceration and secondary infection in the tumors, especially in the surface of the body. This type of inflammatory reaction **may be acute, chronic, or rarely granulomatous reaction**. Some tumors show inflammatory reaction even in the absence of ulceration. It is due to **cell-mediated immunologic response of the host against the tumor** as an attempt to destroy the tumor. For example, **lymphocytes in the stroma are seen in seminoma testis and medullary carcinoma of the breast**.
- **Importance of stroma:** It is required for growth, survival, and replication of tumor (through blood supply) cells.
- **Tumor consistency depends on amount of stroma:**
  - **Soft and fleshy:** These tumors have **scanty stroma**.
  - **Desmoplasia (Fig. 1 and Box 2): Parenchymal tumor cells may stimulate the formation of an abundant collagenous stroma** is referred to as desmoplasia.

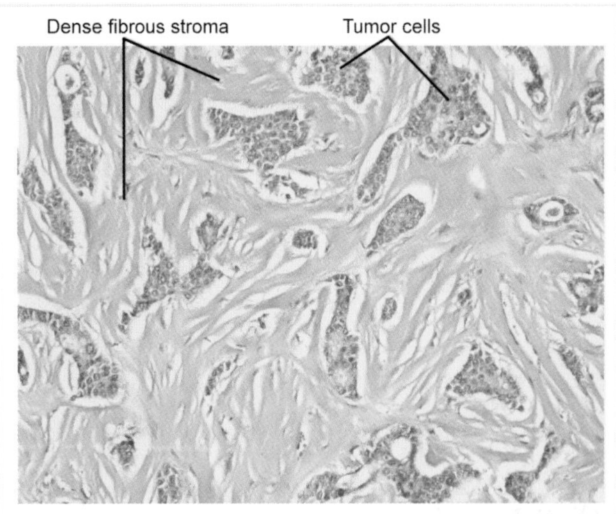

FIG. 1: Carcinoma of breast with abundant stroma separating malignant cells.

Box 2: Examples of tumors with desmoplasia.

- Some carcinomas (e.g., scirrhous) of female breast
- Cholangiocarcinoma
- Pancreatic cancer, some adenocarcinoma of colon
- Linitis plastica (diffuse type of carcinoma of stomach)
- Some colonic carcinomas (especially on left side)

For example, some carcinomas in female breast have **stony hard consistency** (or **scirrhous**).

Table 1: Nomenclature of few benign and malignant mesenchymal tumors.

Cell of origin	*Benign*	*Malignant*
Fibrous tissue	Fibroma	Fibrosarcoma
Fat cell	Lipoma	Liposarcoma
Blood vessel	Hemangioma	Angiosarcoma
Cartilage	Chondroma	Chondrosarcoma
Bone	Osteoma	Osteogenic sarcoma
Smooth muscle	Leiomyoma	Leiomyosarcoma
Skeletal muscle	Rhabdomyoma	Rhabdomyosarcoma

NOMENCLATURE OF NEOPLASMS

Benign Tumors

They are generally **named by attaching the suffix "oma" to the cell of origin**.

Mesenchymal Tumors

They usually follow the nomenclature as shown in **Table 1**. For example, benign tumor of fibroblast-like cells is called a fibroma, a benign tumor of cartilaginous cells is a chondroma.

Epithelial Tumors (Figs. 2A to D)

Their nomenclature is **not uniform but more complex**. They are classified in different ways: **(i) cells of origin, (ii) microscopic pattern and (iii) macroscopic architecture.**
Adenoma: It is a **benign epithelial tumor arising from glandular epithelium**, although they **may or may not form glandular structures**. Few examples are as follows:

- **Adrenocortical adenoma:** It shows heterogeneous mass of adrenal cortical cells growing as a solid sheet without any glands. Termed adenoma because the cell of origin is glandular epithelium.
- **Follicular adenoma of thyroid:** It usually shows microscopically numerous tightly packed small glands.

Papilloma: It is a **benign epithelial neoplasm** that produces microscopically or macroscopically **visible finger-like, exophytic or warty projections** from epithelial surfaces, e.g., squamous papilloma (**Fig. 2B**).

Cystadenoma: It is a tumor forming large cystic masses, e.g., serous cystadenoma of ovary (**Fig. 2C**).

- **Papillary cystadenoma:** It is a tumor which consists of papillary structures that project into cystic spaces, e.g., papillary serous cystadenoma of ovary (**Figs. 2D** and **3**).

Polyp (Fig. 4A): It is a neoplasm that grossly produces **visible projection above a mucosal surface and projects into the lumen**. It may be either **benign or malignant**. It may have a stalk (**pedunculated** polyp) or may be without a stalk (**sessile** polyp), e.g., polyp of stomach or intestine.

- **Adenomatous polyp:** If the polyp consists of glandular tissue, it is called an adenomatous polyp (e.g., adenomatous polyp of colon).

Borderline Tumors

The term borderline tumor is used mainly for surface tumors of ovary (e.g., borderline serous or mucinous or endometrioid tumors). These tumors have **behavior intermediate between benign and malignant tumors**.

Malignant Tumors

They are termed as carcinoma or sarcoma depending on the parenchymal cell of origin.

Sarcomas

They are **malignant tumors arising in mesenchymal tissue**. These tumors have little connective tissue stroma **and** are fleshy (Greek, *sar* = **fleshy**), e.g., fibrosarcoma, liposarcoma, osteosarcoma, chondrosarcoma, leiomyosarcoma, and rhabdomyosarcoma.

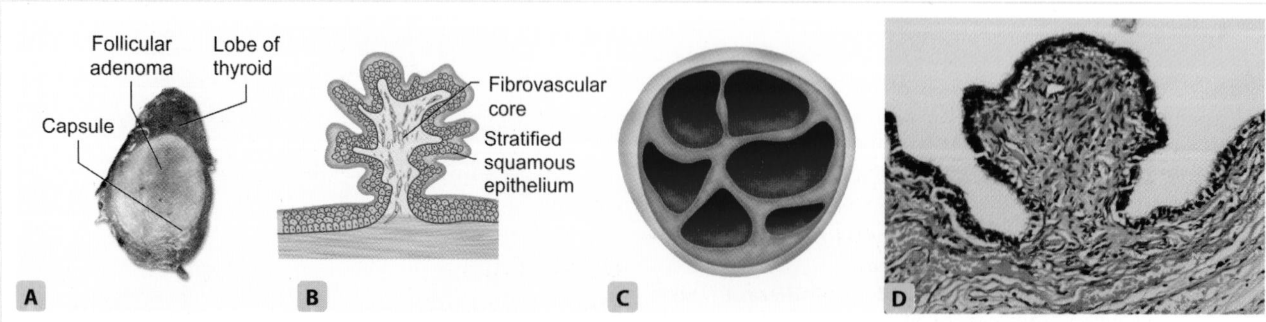

FIGS. 2A TO D: Morphological (gross/microscopic) appearance of some benign epithelial tumors. (A) Gross appearance of follicular adenoma of thyroid. (B) Squamous papilloma composed of finger-like projections. (C) Cut section showing cystadenoma (e.g., mucinous cystadenoma of ovary). (D) Microscopy of papillary cystadenoma of ovary showing a papilla projecting into the cystic cavity.

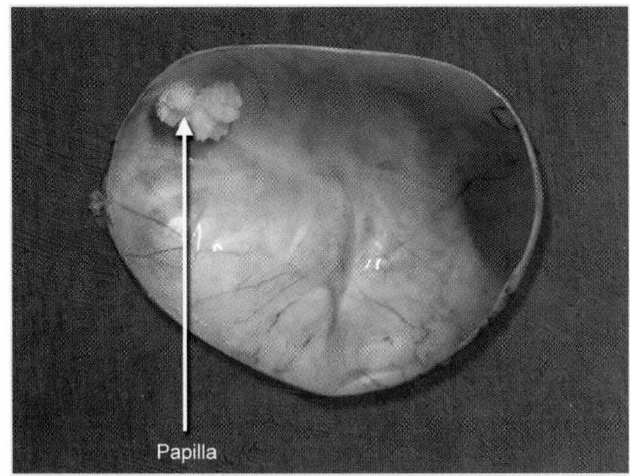

FIG. 3: Serous cystadenoma of ovary. Cut section shows uniloculated cyst with a focus of papilla.

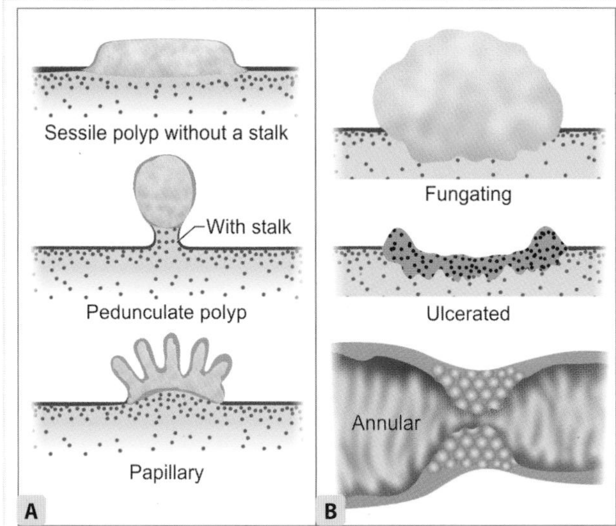

FIGS. 4A AND B: Gross types of tumors. (A) Usually benign growth pattern. (B) Likely to be malignant growth pattern.

Table 2: Nomenclature of carcinomas.

Germ layer	*Tissue/cell*	*Malignant tumor*
Ectoderm	Epidermis	Squamous cell carcinoma
Mesoderm	Renal tubules	Adenocarcinoma
Endoderm	Lining of the gastrointestinal tract	Adenocarcinoma

Table 3: List of malignant tumors with suffix "oma".

Inappropriate terminology for malignant tumor	*Site*
Hepatoma	Liver
Melanoma	Skin
Seminoma/dysgerminoma	Testis/ovary
Lymphoma	Lymph nodes and extranodal lymphoid tissue
Mesothelioma	Pleura, peritoneum

Table 4: Examples of some eponymously named tumors.

Eponymously named tumors	*Cell or tissue of origin*
Burkitt lymphoma	B-cell lymphoma
Ewing sarcoma	Neuroectodermal origin arises in the bone
Grawitz tumor	Renal cell carcinoma arising from renal tubular epithelium
Kaposi's sarcoma	Malignant neoplasm of vascular endothelium
Hodgkin lymphoma	Malignant tumor of post-germinal B cells
Brenner tumor	Benign tumor arising from surface epithelium of ovary

Carcinomas

They are **malignant neoplasms arising from epithelial cell**, which may be derived from any of the three germ layers (**Table 2**). For example, *squamous cell carcinoma* is a malignant tumor, in which the tumor cells resemble stratified squamous epithelium. *Adenocarcinoma* consists of neoplastic epithelial cells arranged in a glandular pattern. Sometimes, when the tissue or organ of origin can be identified, it is added to the nomenclature of the tumor. For example, renal cell adenocarcinoma or bronchogenic squamous cell carcinoma.

1. **Undifferentiated malignant tumor:** It is a malignant tumor composed of undifferentiated cells, where the **cell of origin cannot be made out on light microscopic examination**.
2. **Carcinosarcoma:** It is a rare malignant tumor which shows **mixture of carcinomatous and sarcomatous elements**.
3. **Inappropriate terminology for malignant tumor (Table 3):** Historically the suffix "oma" is applied to benign tumors. However, current terminology is so varied that tumor names do not specify biological behavior with any precision. In certain malignant tumors, the suffix "oma" is inappropriately used and **sounds like a benign tumor**.

Eponymously Named Tumors

Tumors in which historically the histogenesis was poorly understood are often named after the person (eponymous) who first described or recognized the tumor (**Table 4**).

Leukemia and Lymphoma

Malignant tumors arising from blood-forming cells are termed as leukemias (literally meaning white blood). Malignant tumors of lymphocytes or their precursors are termed as lymphomas.

Other Tumors

Mixed Tumors (Fig. 5)

Most neoplasms consists of parenchymal cells all of which closely resemble one another. However, some types of tumors may show more than one line of differentiation and show distinct

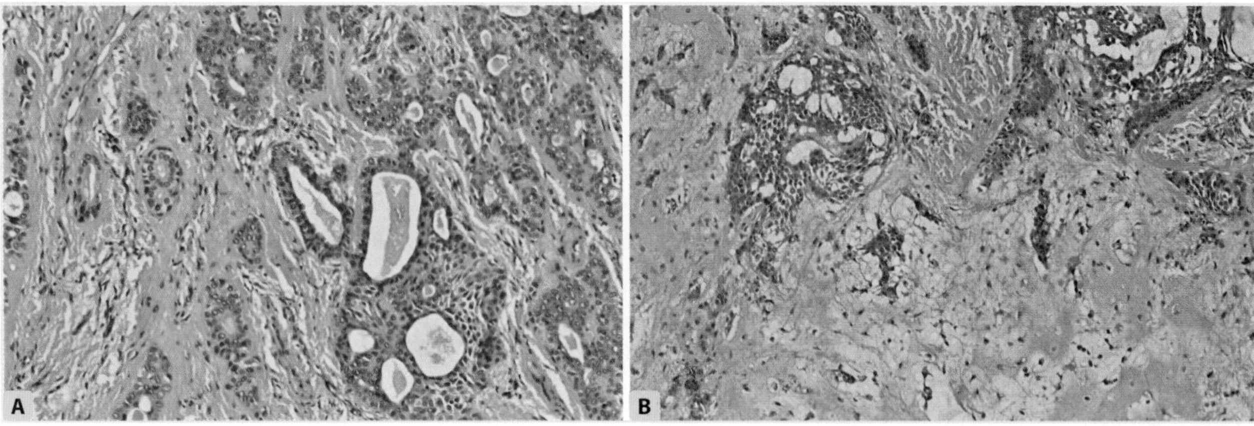

FIGS. 5A AND B: Pleomorphic adenoma. (A) Showing epithelial cells and myoepithelial cells. (B) Shows epithelial cell separated predominantly myxoid stroma with chondroid matrix.

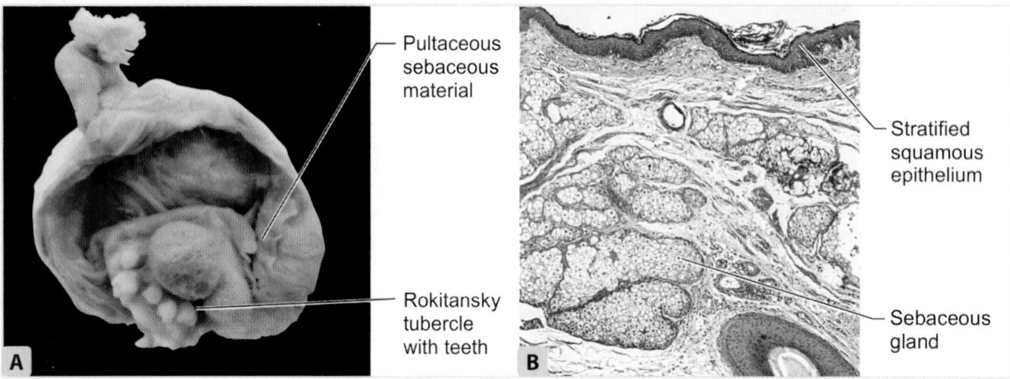

FIGS. 6A AND B: (A) Mature cystic teratoma (dermoid cyst) of the ovary; (B) Microscopic appearance of dermoid cyst of ovary. It shows a cyst lined by skin with adnexal structures (hair, sebaceous glands).

subpopulations of cells. One of the classic example is the mixed tumor of the salivary gland. Mixed tumors are **derived from a single germ layer** but show **divergent differentiation** along two lineages, **Mixed tumor of salivary gland** (pleomorphic adenoma) consists of epithelial components scattered within a myxoid stroma that may contain islands of cartilage or bone. All of these tissue components or elements are derived from a single neoplastic clone capable of producing both epithelial and mesenchymal cells. Majority of neoplasms, including mixed tumors are composed of cells from a single germ layer (mesoderm, endoderm, or ectoderm).

Teratomas

They are special types of mixed tumors **derived from totipotent germ cells** (normally present in **ovary, testis,** and sometimes abnormally present in sequestered embryonic rest in midline). These cells have the capacity to **differentiate into any of the cell types** found in the adult body. Thus, teratoma contains recognizable **mature or immature cells** or tissues representative of more than one germ cell layer and sometimes all three. These cells or tissues are arranged in a helter-skelter fashion. The **tissue derivative from various germ cell layers** may include:

- **Ectoderm** (e.g., skin, neural tissue, glia)
- **Mesoderm** (e.g., smooth muscle, cartilage, bone, fat)
- **Endoderm** (e.g., respiratory tract epithelium, gut, thyroid)

Classification of teratoma

- **Benign/mature teratoma:** It consists of **all mature and well-differentiated tissue**, e.g., ovarian cystic teratoma (dermoid cyst), in which differentiation is mainly along ectodermal lines. It produces a cystic tumor lined by skin with adnexal structures (hair, sebaceous glands) and tooth structures (**Figs. 6A** and **B**).
- **Immature/malignant teratoma:** It consists of **immature or less well-differentiated tissue**.
- **Monodermal teratoma and somatic-type tumors arising from dermoid cyst,** e.g., struma ovarii (**Figs. 7A** and **B**) and carcinoid developing in ovary.
    - **Teratoma with malignant transformation:** It is the **development of malignant nongerm cell tumors** from one or more germ cell layer **in a teratoma,** e.g., squamous cell carcinoma developing in a teratoma of testis.

Sites of teratoma are presented in **Box 3**.

Hamartomas

Definition

It is a **disorganized mass of benign-appearing cells, indigenous to the** particular **site**. Most hamartomas have clonal chromosomal aberrations that are acquired through somatic mutation. Hence, they are considered as benign neoplasms.

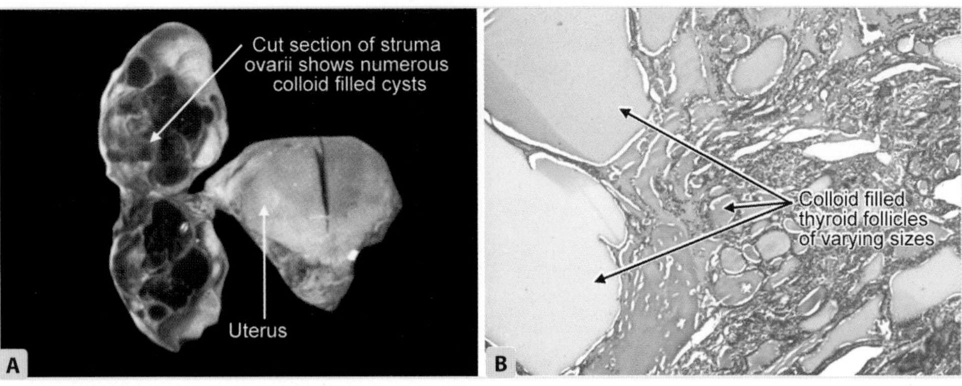

FIGS. 7A AND B: (A) Cut section of struma ovarii involving the ovary; (B) Struma ovarii composed of thyroid follicles containing variable amount of colloid.

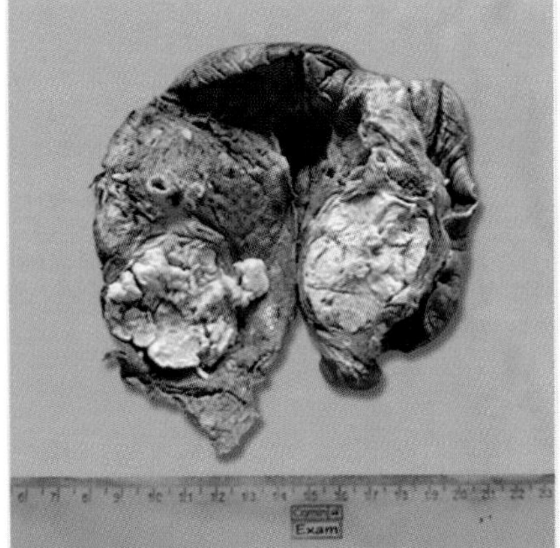

FIG. 8: Pulmonary chondroid hamartoma.`

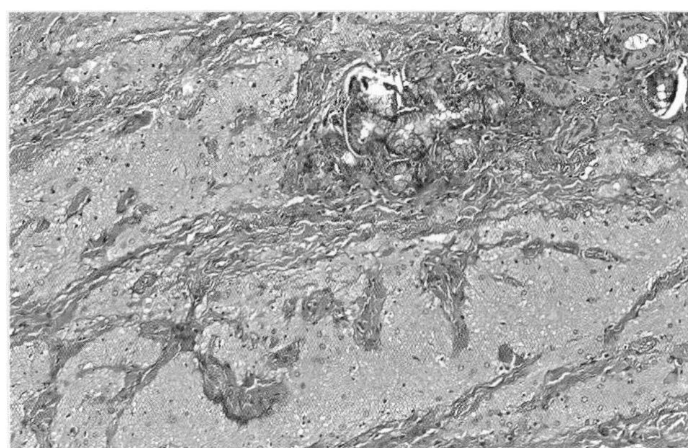

FIG. 9: Nasal neuroglial heterotopia showing mass of mature neuroepithelial tissue in the nose. Portion of nasal seromucous glands also seen.

Box 3: Sites of teratoma.

- Gonads
  - Ovary
  - Testis
- Extragonadal, e.g., mediastinum

Example: Pulmonary chondroid hamartoma (**Fig. 8**) consists of islands of disorganized, but histologically normal cartilage, bronchi, and vessels.

Choristoma

Definition

It is an **ectopic island of normal tissue—heterotopic** rest (normal tissue in an abnormal site) and is a congenital anomaly.

Example: Presence of small nodular mass of normally organized pancreatic tissue in the submucosa of the stomach, duodenum, or small intestine. Nasal neuroglial heterotopia (glial choristomas so-called nasal glioma) characterized by a mass of mature central neuroepithelial tissue in the nose unconnected to the brain proper (**Fig. 9**).

Embryonal Tumors (Blastomas)

They are the **types of tumor that develop only in children** (usually below 5 years of age), and **microscopically resemble embryonic tissue** of the organ in which they arise (**Table 5**).

Table 5: Different types of embryonal tumors and their site.

Type of embryonal tumor	*Site*
Retinoblastoma	Eye
Nephroblastoma or Wilms' tumor	Kidney
Neuroblastoma	Adrenal medulla or nerve ganglia
Hepatoblastoma	Liver
Medulloblastoma	Cerebellum

Nomenclature of the more common forms of neoplasia is listed in **Table 6**.

CHARACTERISTICS OF BENIGN AND MALIGNANT NEOPLASMS

It is **very important to differentiate** benign from malignant tumors mainly because of the different prognostic outcome. In general, benign and malignant tumors can be distinguished on the basis of four fundamental features, namely—**(1) differentiation and anaplasia, (2) rates of growth, (3) local invasion, and (4) metastasis**.

Table 6: Nomenclature of common tumors.

Tissue of origin	Benign	Malignant
Composed of single parenchymal cell type		
Tumors of mesenchymal origin		
Connective tissue and derivatives	Fibroma	Fibrosarcoma
	Lipoma	Liposarcoma
	Chondroma	Chondrosarcoma
	Osteoma	Osteogenic sarcoma
Vessels and surface coverings		
Lymph vessels	Lymphangioma	Lymphangiosarcoma
Mesothelium	Benign fibrous tumor	Mesothelioma
Blood vessels	Hemangioma	Angiosarcoma
Brain coverings	Meningioma	Invasive meningioma
Nerve sheath	Neurofibroma, neurilemmoma	Malignant peripheral nerve sheath tumor
Blood cells and related cells		
Hematopoietic cells		Leukemia
Lymphoid tissue		Lymphoma
Muscle		
Smooth muscle	Leiomyoma	Leiomyosarcoma
Striated muscle	Rhabdomyoma	Rhabdomyosarcoma
Tumors of epithelial origin		
Stratified squamous	Squamous cell papilloma	Squamous cell carcinoma
Basal cells of skin or adnexa		Basal cell carcinoma
Epithelial lining of glands or ducts or organs	Adenoma	Adenocarcinoma
	Papilloma	Papillary carcinoma
	Cystadenoma	Cystadenocarcinoma
	Papillary cystadenoma	Papillary cystadenocarcinoma
Respiratory passages	Bronchial adenoma	Bronchogenic carcinoma
Renal epithelium	Renal tubular adenoma	Renal cell carcinoma
Liver cells	Hepatic adenoma	Hepatocellular carcinoma
Urinary tract epithelium (transitional)	Transitional cell papilloma	Transitional cell carcinoma
Placenta epithelium	Hydatidiform mole	Choriocarcinoma
Testicular epithelium (germ cells)	–	Seminoma, embryonal carcinoma
Tumors of melanocyte	Nevus	Malignant melanoma

Continued

Continued

Tissue of origin	Benign	Malignant
More than one neoplastic cell type—mixed tumors, derived from one germ cell layer		
Salivary glands	Pleomorphic adenoma (mixed tumor) of salivary origin	Malignant mixed tumor of salivary gland origin
Renal anlage		Wilms' tumor (nephroblastoma)
More than one neoplastic cell type derived from more than one germ cell layer		
Totipotential cells in gonads or in embryonic rests	Mature teratoma, dermoid cyst	Immature teratoma

Differentiation and Anaplasia

Differentiation

A tumor may mimic its tissue of origin to a variable degree. Some closely resemble their parent cells (e.g., hepatic adenomas), while others consist of cells that are so primitive that the tumor's origin cannot be identified.

Definition

Differentiation is defined as **the extent to which neoplastic parenchymal cells resemble** the corresponding **normal parenchymal cells**. This includes both morphological and functional differentiation. Differentiation **determines the grade of the tumor**.

Benign tumors

- **Well-differentiated:** The neoplastic cell **closely resembles the normal cell of origin**. It may be not possible to recognize it as a tumor by microscopic examination of individual cells [e.g., lipoma(**Fig. 10A**) and leiomyoma (**Fig. 10B**)]. Only the growth of these cells into discrete lobules discloses the neoplastic nature of the lesion.
- **Mitoses:** They are **rare** and of normal configuration. During normal mitosis, the parent cell splits into 2 perfectly identical daughter cells, each containing one copy of DNA.

Malignant neoplasms

- Show a **wide range of differentiation** of parenchymal cells.
- Varies from **well-differentiated to completely undifferentiated**.

Grading Cancers are usually graded either as well, moderately, or poorly differentiated, or numerically often by strict criteria as grade 1, grade 2, or grade 3.

- **Well-differentiated** tumors:
    - Well-differentiated adenocarcinomas of colon may form normal-appearing glands (**Fig. 11**).
    - Squamous cell carcinomas may show cells which appear similar to normal squamous epithelial cells (**Fig. 12**).
- **Poorly differentiated tumors:** They consist of **cells** that have **little resemblance to the cell of origin.**

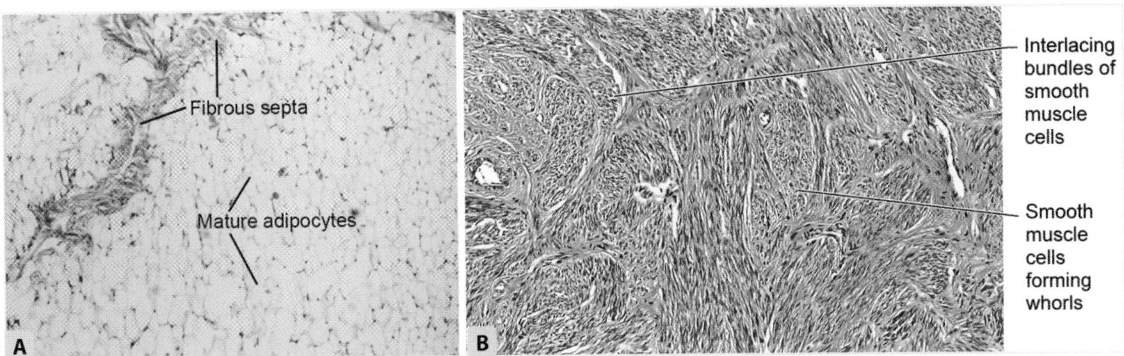

FIGS. 10A AND B: Examples of benign tumors. (A) Lipoma is a well-differentiated tumor composed of lobules of fat cells that are identical in appearance to normal fat cells. **(B)** Microscopic appearance of leiomyoma showing well-differentiated, regular, spindle-shaped smooth muscle cells arranged in interlacing fascicles.

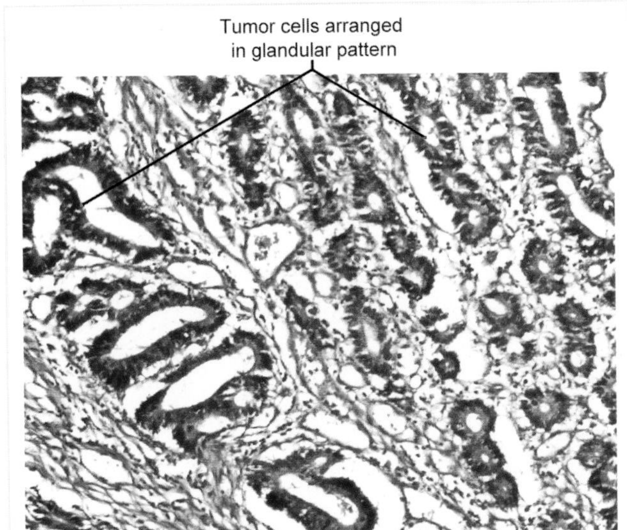

FIG. 11: Well-differentiated adenocarcinoma of the colon. It shows cancerous glands that are irregular in shape and size invading the muscular layer of the colon.

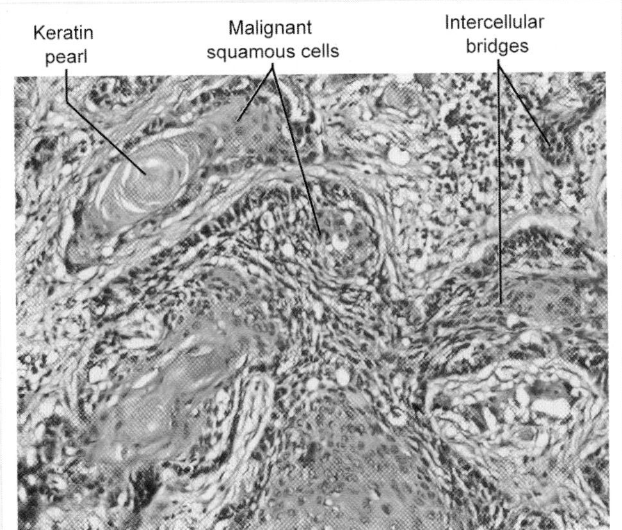

FIG. 12: Well-differentiated squamous cell carcinoma of the skin. The tumor consists of cells which are similar to normal squamous epithelial cells, with intercellular bridges and keratin pearls.

- **Moderately differentiated:** These tumors show differentiation in between the well and poorly differentiated tumors.

Growth pattern: Malignant neoplasms usually show disorganized growth. This may be expressed as sheets of cells, arrangements around blood vessels, papillary structures, whorls, rosettes, etc. Malignant tumors usually show ischemic necrosis due to compromised blood supply.

Anaplasia

- Anaplasia **literally means "to form backward/backward formation"**, i.e., **reversal of differentiation of cell to a more primitive level**.
- Malignant neoplasms composed of undifferentiated cells are called as anaplastic tumors.
- **Lack of differentiation** (both structural and functional) **is called as anaplasia** and is **characteristic of malignancy**.
- The degree of anaplasia in a cancer cell correlates with the aggressiveness of the tumor.
- Thus, more anaplastic the tumor, the more aggressive it becomes.

Microscopic features of cancer (malignant) cells (Figs. 13 and 14)

Pleomorphism It is defined as **variation in the size and shape of cells and cell nuclei**. It is a feature of malignancy. Thus, cells within the same malignant tumor range from large cells (many times larger than the neighbor cells) to extremely small (primitive appearing) cells.

Abnormal nuclear morphology These include the following—

- **Extremely hyperchromatic nuclei** of tumor cells are **due to abundant chromatin** and **increased amount of DNA per cell** compared to that of a normal cell. Microscopically, these **nuclei stain darkly (hyperchromatic nuclei)**.
- **Nuclear shape and size are variable** and may be irregular. **Chromatin is coarsely clumped** and distributed along the nuclear membrane. **Large prominent nucleoli** are usually seen.

Mitoses (mitotic activity) Presence of mitotic figures (rates) **indicates the higher proliferative activity** of the parenchymal cells. However, the presence of mitoses, does not indicate the lesion as malignant. For example, mitosis is usually found in normal tissues exhibiting rapid turnover, such as the epithelial lining of the gastrointestinal tract and nonneoplastic proliferations in hyperplasias (one of the cellular adaption).

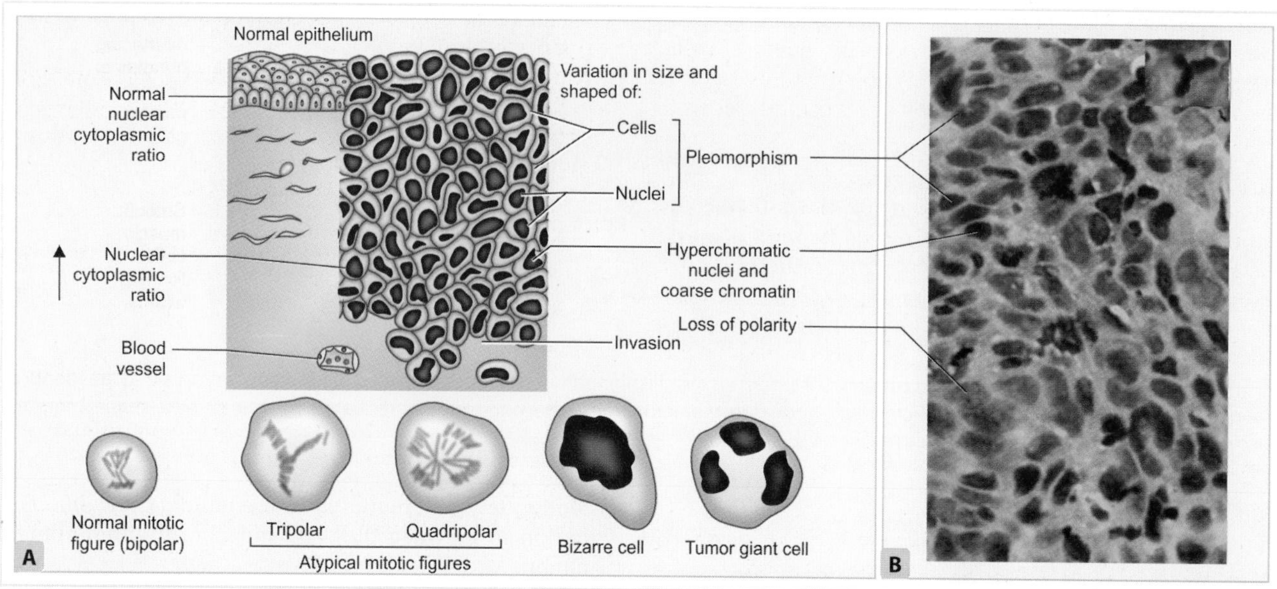

FIGS. 13A AND B: Microscopic features of cancer (malignant) cells. (A) Diagrammatic. (B) Photomicrograph showing nuclear and cytoplasmic pleomorphism, hyperchromatic nuclei, high nuclear cytoplasmic ratio, and loss of polarity. Inset of (B) shows tripolar mitotic figure.

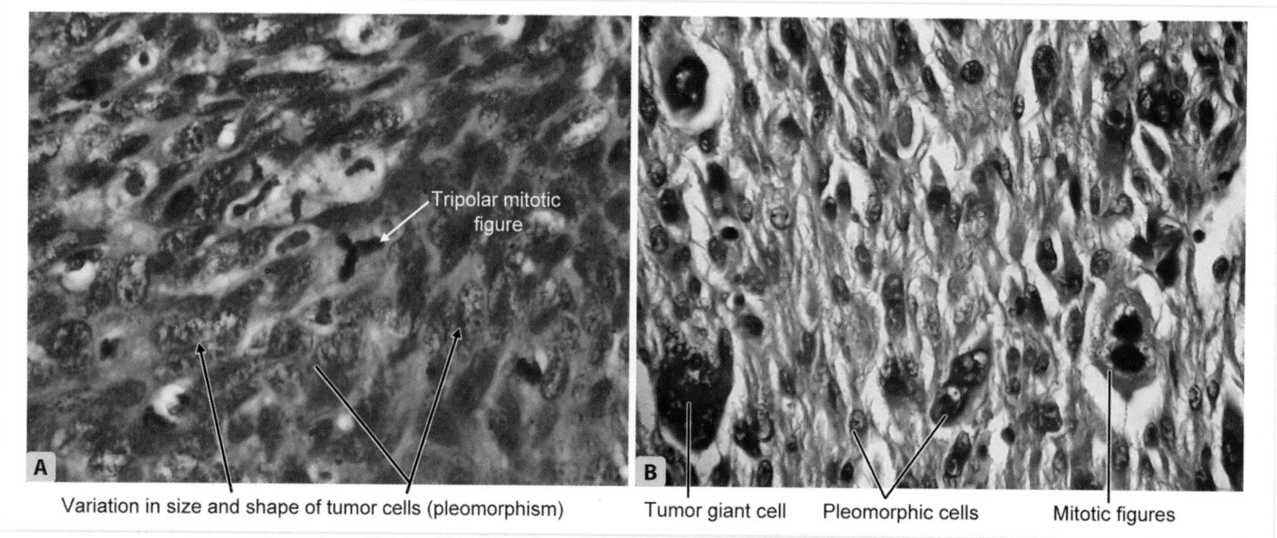

FIGS. 14A AND B: (A) Poorly differentiated carcinoma consisting of tumor cells showing variation in size of cells and nuclei. One tumor cell in the center shows an abnormal tripolar spindle. (B) Sarcoma showing cellular and nuclear pleomorphism, tumor giant cells, and mitotic figure.

- **Number of mitotic figures:** Compared to benign and few well-differentiated malignant tumors, undifferentiated tumors usually show abundant (many/high) mitotic figures. In few tumors (e.g., leiomyosarcomas), a diagnosis of malignancy is based on finding even a few mitoses.
- **Atypical (abnormal) mitotic figures (Figs. 14A and B):** Normal mitosis produces bipolar spindles, and one cell divides into two. When the mitotic spindles are more than two, it is called as atypical. Presence of atypical bizarre mitotic figures is an important morphological feature of malignancy.

Nuclear cytoplasmic (N:C) ratio In a normal cell, N:C ratio is 1:4 or 1:6. In a malignant cell, the nuclei are enlarged, become disproportionately large for the cell, and the nucleus-to-cytoplasm ratio may be **increased** (**Figs. 13A** and **B**) and may reach even up to 1:1.

Loss of polarity **Orientation of cells to one another** is known as polarity. The anaplastic cells lose the normal polarity leading to markedly disturbed orientation (architecture) of tumor cells. Thus, the orientation of anaplastic cells with each other or to supporting structures like basement membrane is markedly disturbed. Sheets or groups of malignant cells grow in a disorganized fashion.

Growth pattern Malignant neoplasms usually show disorganized growth. The tumor cells may form sheets of cells, arranged around blood vessels, papillary structures, whorls, rosettes, etc. Malignant tumors often show central ischemic necrosis due to compromised blood supply.

Bizarre cells, including tumor giant cells Some tumors may show **bizarre cells with a single large polymorphic nucleus** and others may have **two or more large, hyperchromatic nuclei (Figs. 14A and B)**. These tumor giant cells should not be confused with Langhans or foreign body giant cells. In contrast to tumor giant cells, these are derived from macrophages and contain many small, normal-appearing nuclei.

Necrosis and apoptosis Many rapidly growing malignant tumors undergo large central areas of ischemic necrosis and/apoptosis.

Functional Changes

Well-differentiated tumors usually retain the functional characteristics. Function may be in the form of secretion and vary depending on the tumor type.

Secretion of normal substances

These include:

- **Hormones:** Benign tumors and **well-differentiated carcinomas of endocrine glands frequently secrete the hormones** characteristic of their cell of origin (e.g., steroid hormones from an adrenocortical adenoma). These hormones can be detected and quantified. Thus, they are useful for the diagnosis and follow up the response of such tumors to treatment.
- **Normal products**, e.g., **well-differentiated squamous cell carcinomas** produce keratin and form characteristic **epithelial pearls** (refer **Fig. 12**). Well-differentiated hepatocellular carcinomas produce bile.

Fetal proteins

Some tumors may secrete fetal proteins, **which are not produced by comparable normal cells in the adult**, e.g., carcinoembryonic antigen (CEA) by adenocarcinomas of the gastrointestinal tract.

Ectopic hormones

Tumors may produce **substances** which are **not indigenous to the tissue of origin,** e.g., bronchogenic carcinomas may produce adrenocorticotropic hormone (ACTH), parathyroid-like hormone, insulin, glucagon, and other hormones. This may give rise to paraneoplastic syndromes.

Differences between carcinoma and sarcoma are given in **Table 7**.

Rate of Growth

Factors Determining the Rate of Growth

- **Degree of differentiation:**
  - **Benign tumors** are well-differentiated and **usually grow slowly.**

Table 7: Differences between carcinoma and sarcoma.

Features	*Carcinoma*	*Sarcoma*
Definition	Malignant tumor of epithelial origin	Malignant tumor of mesenchymal origin
Meaning of the term	"Carcinoma" came from the Greek word "*karkinos*" which means crab and "*oma*" which means growth	"Sarcoma" came from the Greek word "*sarc*" meaning flesh and "*oma*" which means growth
Site of origin	Mostly from inside lining of colon, breast, and lung or prostrate	Arise from musculoskeletal system, such as bones, muscles, and connective tissues
Incidence	More common cancer (>90% of cancers)	Less common (<1%)
Age	More common in middle and old age	Can occur at any age
Rate of growth	Usually not very rapid	Usually rapid
Route of spread	Initially lymphatics and later hematogenous	• Spread by satellite nodules • Usually hematogenous and lymphatic spread is rare
Site of metastasis through blood	Liver, lung, brain, bone, and adrenals	May spread to lungs
Gross appearance	• Varies, depends on the subtype (e.g., cauliflower-like in squamous cell carcinoma) • Carcinomas infiltrate all nearby structures (nerves, veins, and muscles)	Fleshy, grow in ball-like masses and tend to push nearby structures such as arteries, nerves, and veins away
Hemorrhage and necrosis	Usually not extensive	May be extensive
Microscopy	Pattern varies and parenchymal cells may be arranged in glands, acini, sheets, cords, papillae depending on the subtype	Tumor cells are arranged in different patterns depending on the subtype
Radiosensitivity	High	Radioresistance
Prognosis	Depends on the location and stage	Depends on the location and stage
Examples	Carcinoma breast, squamous cell carcinoma of skin and mucus membranes, carcinoma stomach and colon	Osteosarcoma, chondrosarcoma, liposarcoma

- **Most malignant tumors grow more rapidly.** But there are many exceptions and growth rate is not a reliable for discriminating benign from malignant tumors. Some cancers may show remarkably variable growth rates. Thus at one end of the spectrum, they may be slow-growing tumors associated with survival for many years, even without treatment. Other end of the spectrum, they may grow rapidly and may lead to death of patient within months or weeks.
- **Dependency:** Growth also depends on:
  - **Hormonal stimulation**, e.g., uterine leiomyomas may suddenly grow during pregnancy and may undergo atrophy after menopause.
  - **Adequacy of blood supply.**
- **Balance between cell production and cell loss:** This in turn is determined by three main factors:
  1. **Doubling time of tumor cells:** It is the **time required for the total cell cycle**, i.e., cells to double by mitosis,
  2. **Growth fraction:** It is the **proportion of cells in the proliferative or replicative pool** within the tumor.
  3. **Rate of tumor cell death:** Rate of growth depends on balance between cell production and cell loss. When **both the rate of cell production and the rate of cell loss** (by apoptosis) **are high,** it is termed as **high cell turnover.**

Metaplasia, Dysplasia, and Carcinoma In Situ

These terminologies indicate recognizable changes in differentiation. It may be an adaptation to chronic injury (metaplasia), a premalignant change (dysplasia), or represent a cancer that has not yet invaded (carcinoma in situ).

Metaplasia

It is reversible change in which one type of differentiated cell is replaced by another type of differentiated cells (refer pages 198 and 199). It is a cellular adaptation that develops in association with tissue damage, repair and regeneration, e.g., gastroesophageal reflux damages the squamous epithelium of the esophagus which is replaced by glandular (gastric or intestinal is better able to withstand acidic environment) epithelium, columnar epithelium of endocervix is replaced by stratified squamous epithelium. Usually the replacing cell type is better able to withstand alteration in the local environment than the original cell type. Malignancy may develop in these metaplastic epithelia. For example, squamous metaplasia of the bronchial epithelium in chronic smokers, may progress to squamous cell carcinoma of the lung.

Local Invasion

Benign Tumors

- **Localized:** Most benign tumors **grow as expansile masses** that remain localized to their site of origin.
  - **No infiltration** into adjacent tissue or capsule (if present).
  - **No metastasis.**
- **Capsule (Fig. 15):** It is a rim of compressed connective tissue derived mainly from the extracellular matrix (ECM) of the surrounding normal tissue. ECM is deposited by stromal cells such as fibroblasts. These cells become activated by hypoxic damage produced from the pressure of the expanding tumor.

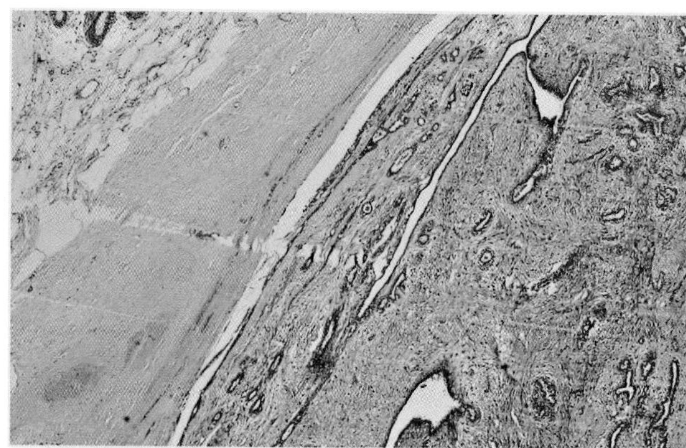

FIG. 15: Microscopic appearance of fibroadenoma of the breast with a well-defined fibrous capsule (left side).

  - **Capsule makes tumor a palpable and movable mass** and can be surgically enucleated.
  - **Benign tumors without capsule (unencapsulated)**, e.g., hemangiomas, uterine leiomyoma. Hemangiomas are benign neoplasms composed of tangled blood vessels. They are usually not capsulated and permeate the site of origin (e.g., the dermis of the skin and the liver). If they are extensive, they can not be resected.

Malignant Tumors

- **Lack of capsule:** Malignant tumors are poorly demarcated from the surrounding normal tissue and lack true capsule. There is no well-defined cleavage planes between tumor and surrounding normal tissue. Slowly expanding malignant tumors may develop an apparent fibrous capsule and they push along a broad front into adjacent normal structures. However, microscopically these "pseudoencapsulated" tumors almost always reveal sheets of tumor cells penetrating the margin and infiltrating adjacent structures.
- **Invasion (Figs. 16 and 17): Two most reliable features** that differentiate malignant from benign tumors are **local invasion and metastases**.

Dysplasia

The **cells that show cytological features of malignancy** and the term dysplasia is used for these changes (**features**). It literally means disordered growth and thus consists of disordered cellular growth and maturation. Dysplasia mostly occurs in epithelial tissues. Normally, the cells of an epithelium show uniform size, shape, and nuclei and these cells are arranged in a regular fashion, e.g., a squamous epithelium consists of plump tall basal cells that progress to flat superficial cells.

Features of Dysplasia Dysplasia represents the morphologic expression of a disturbance in growth regulation. However, unlike cancer cells, dysplastic cells are not entirely autonomous, and with intervention, the cells can revert to normal. In dysplasia, the normal pattern is disturbed and it shows following changes:

- **Cellular** and nuclear **pleomorphism** characterized by loss in the uniformity of the individual cells.
- **Large hyperchromatic nuclei.**
- **High/increased nuclear-to-cytoplasmic ratio.**

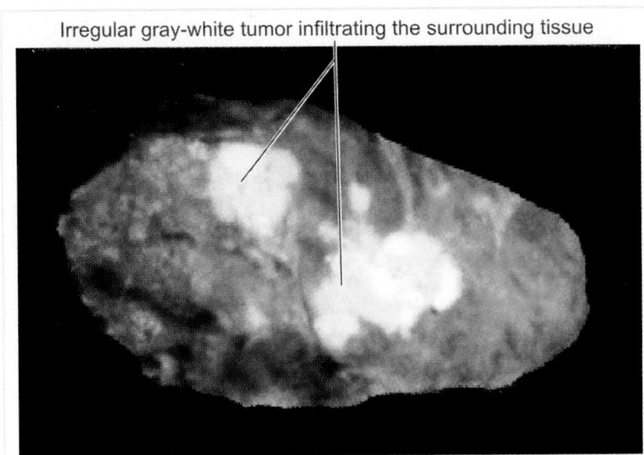

FIG. 16: Mastectomy specimen with irregular, gray-white infiltrating duct carcinoma.

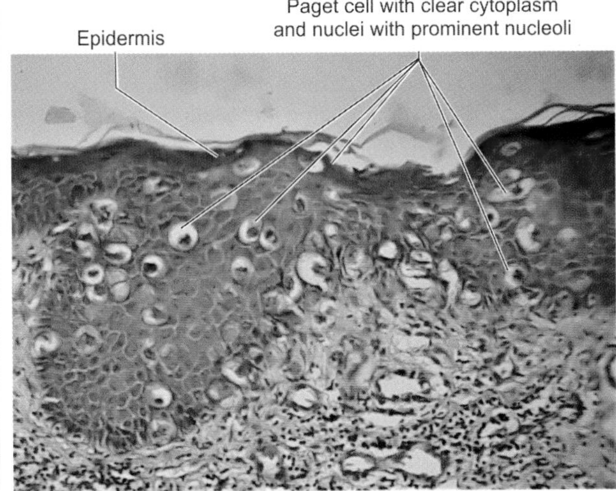

FIG. 17: Paget disease of breast. Skin lesions in the nipple shows clusters of malignant cells known as Paget cells in the epidermis without infiltrating the basement membrane. These cells represent extension from underlying ductal carcinoma via the lactiferous sinuses.

- **Loss of polarity (architectural orientation),** i.e., disorderly arrangement of cells from basal layer to the surface layer, e.g., in dysplastic squamous epithelium, the normal progressive maturation may fail in part or entirely, leading to replacement of the epithelium by basal-appearing cells with hyperchromatic nuclei.
- **Increased mitotic activity:** Mitotic figures are normally confined to the basal layer. In dysplasia, mitotic figures are more than those in the normal tissue and may be seen at all levels (instead of only basal cells), including surface cells.

Sites of Dysplasia

- **Squamous epithelium:** Most common sites of dysplastic changes are seen in the squamous epithelial lining of the **uterine cervix, respiratory tract, and skin**. Dysplasia is most common in hyperplastic squamous epithelium and in areas of squamous metaplasia, such as in the bronchus or the cervix.
- **Other epithelium:** Dysplasia can occur in epithelium other than squamous epithelium.
  - **Columnar mucosa:** Dysplasia can occur in the columnar mucosal cells of the colon in ulcerative colitis.
  - Ductal lining cells in breast.
  - Metaplastic epithelium of Barrett esophagus.
  - Prostate glands: Prostatic intraepithelial neoplasia.
  - Urothelium of the bladder.

Asymptomatic In this stage, they are usually asymptomatic.

Classification, Fate, and Significance **Dysplasia (Fig. 18)** can be classified as **(i) mild, (ii) moderate,** and **(iii) severe dysplasia,** depending on the thickness of epithelium involved by the dysplastic cells.

- **Mild-to-moderate dysplastic changes,** which do not involve the entire thickness of epithelium, **may be reversible,** if the cause is removed. The **dysplasia may be a precursor to malignant transformation, but dysplasia need not progress to cancer.**
- Like metaplasia, dysplasia may develop as a response to chronic irritation or prolonged/persistent inflammation. It may regress or disappear after removal of the inciting stimulus, e.g., dysplasia in bronchial epithelium may regress after cessation of smoking or dysplasia in cervix due to human papilloma virus (HPV) may regress following disappearance of HPV from the cervix.
- Dysplastic changes may be seen adjacent to foci of invasive carcinoma. In some situations, such as in long-term cigarette smokers and individuals with Barrett esophagus, severe epithelial dysplasia may antedate the appearance of cancer.

Carcinoma in situ

When dysplastic changes are marked and involve the entire or full thickness of the epithelium, it is a preinvasive neoplasm and is termed as carcinoma in situ. But the lesion does not penetrate the basement membrane of the lining epithelium.

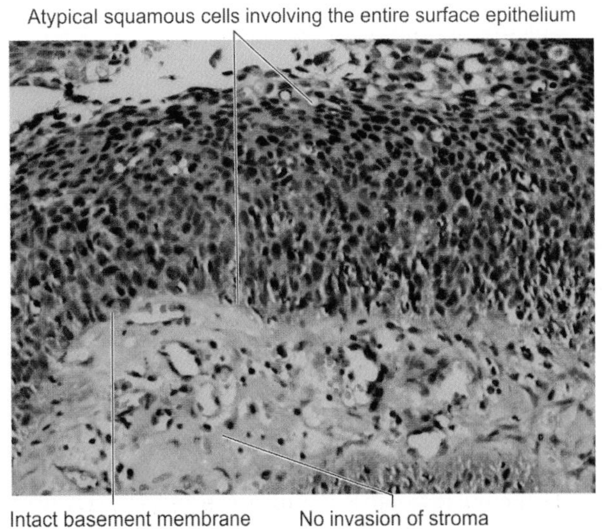

FIG. 18: Moderate dysplasia involving uterine cervix. It shows failure of normal differentiation, marked nuclear and cellular pleomorphism extending toward the surface of epithelium.

Some carcinomas evolve from a **preinvasive stage** called as carcinoma in situ. The tumor cells cannot reach the potential routes of metastasis, such as blood vessels and lymphatics until the basement membrane has been breached or invaded. Carcinoma in situ is usually seen in the (i) skin, (ii) breast, (iii) bladder, and (iv) uterine cervix. When cancer arises from cells that are not confined by a basement membrane, such as connective tissue cells, lymphoid tissue and hepatocytes; there is no defined in situ stage.

Definition Carcinoma in situ is defined as:

- A **preinvasive epithelial neoplasm**.
- Shows **all the cytological features of malignancy**.
- **Involves the entire thickness of the epithelium**.
- Remains **confined within the epithelial basement membrane.**

Once the dysplastic/tumor cells breach the basement membrane, the **tumor is said to be invasive** and carcinoma in situ may take years to become invasive. Most in situ tumors, with time penetrate the basement membrane and invade the subepithelial stroma.

Local invasion

Invasion of adjacent tissue/organ: Malignant tumors within the tissue of origin may also invade beyond the confines of that organ to involve adjacent tissues/organs.

- **Consequences of invasion into the organ of tumor origin (Fig. 19A):** Occasionally, the growth of the cancer may be so extensive that it replaces the normal tissue and produces functional insufficiency of the organ (e.g., hepatocellular carcinoma). Brain tumors (e.g., astrocytomas, glioblastoma) may infiltrate the brain until they compromise vital regions. The direct extension of malignant tumors within an organ can also be life-threatening because of their location (e.g., intestinal obstruction produced by carcinoma colon).
- **Consequences of invasion into the adjacent organ:** The invasion of the tumor into the adjacent organ may impair their function. For example, squamous carcinoma of the cervix may grow beyond the genital tract to obstruct the ureters or produce vesicovaginal fistulas. Neglected cases of breast cancer can produce extensive ulceration of surface skin. Even a small tumor can produce severe consequences when they invade vital structures. For example, a small lung cancer can penetrate the bronchus and cause a bronchopleural fistula or erode a blood vessel causing severe hemorrhage. The pancreatic carcinoma can directly extend into the celiac nerve plexus producing severe pain. Tumor cells that reach serous cavities (e.g., those of the peritoneum or pleura) can spread by direct extension or can be carried by the fluid to new locations on the serous membranes. For example, the seeding of the peritoneal cavity by ovarian cancer.
- **Tissues that resist invasion:** They include mature cartilage (e.g., epiphysis) and elastic tissue of arteries.
- **Pagetoid infiltration (Fig. 17):** It is invasion within epithelium and is seen in Paget's disease of the nipple.
- **Invasion of blood vessels and lymphatics**
- **Perineural invasion** [e.g., cancer of prostate (**Fig. 19B**) and pancreas, adenoid cystic carcinoma of salivary glands].

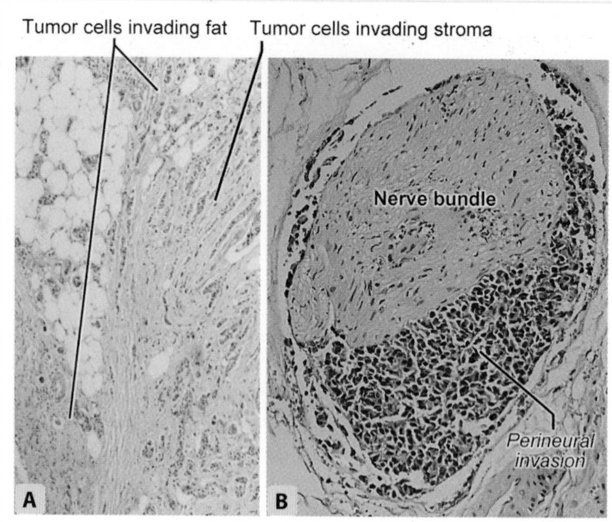

FIGS. 19A AND B: (A) Microscopic appearance of breast carcinoma showing invasion of breast stroma and fat by nests and cords of tumor cells; (B) Perineural invasion in prostatic carcinoma.

Consequences of invasion into the organ/tissue of origin

- Makes **surgical resection difficult**.
- **Functional insufficiency** may occur, if much of the normal tissue is replaced by cancer, e.g., hepatocellular carcinoma may cause liver insufficiency.
- **Compromise vital regions:** Brain tumors (e.g., astrocytomas, glioblastoma) may infiltrate and compromise vital regions. Ocular tumors may lead to impairment of vision.
- **Life-threatening location** (e.g., intestinal obstruction due to carcinoma of colon).
- **Impairment of function of adjacent organ:** The invasive cancers may secondarily impair the function of an adjacent organ. For example, carcinoma of the cervix may grow beyond the genital tract and obstruct the ureters or produce vesicovaginal fistulas.
- **Agonizing pain:** For example pancreatic carcinoma may directly extend to the celiac nerve plexus causing intractable pain.

Metastasis

Q. Discuss mechanism of metastasis (refer also pages 477–483).

Two unique properties of cancer cells are—(1) the ability to invade locally, and (2) the capacity to metastasize to distant sites. These two characteristics are responsible for the majority of deaths from cancer. The properties of invasiveness and metastasis are separable.

Definition

Metastasis is defined by the spread of a tumor to sites that are physically discontinuous (located in a distant tissue) **with the primary tumor.**

This **process of spread of tumor is known as metastasis** *(Greek word meaning "displacement")* and the resulting **secondary deposits are called metastases.** The invasive property permits the cancers to penetrate into blood vessels, lymphatics, and body cavities, and spread to distant sites.

Significance

- Metastases clearly **identify a tumor as malignant** because benign neoplasms never metastasize. **Exceptions** include two malignant tumors, which are locally invasive, but rarely metastasize.
    - **Gliomas** (malignant neoplasms of the glial cells) in the CNS.
    - **Basal cell carcinomas of the skin**.
- Metastases **strongly reduce the possibility of cure of cancer.**
- Metastatic spread is the most **common cause of cancer death.**

Factors Favoring Metastasis

- Poorly differentiated tumor
- More rapidly growing tumor
- Large primary tumor.

Note: Leukemias (called "blood cancers") and lymphomas are malignant tumors derived from blood-forming cells that are normally capable of entering the bloodstream and travel to distant sites. Hence, leukemias and lymphomas (sometimes called as "liquid tumors") usually disseminated at the time of diagnosis and are always considered as malignant. All other tumors (called "solid" tumors) arise from cells that do not normally circulate in the bloodstream.

Morphological Appearance

- Microscopically, **metastases resemble the primary tumor**. But occasionally, they may be so anaplastic that their cell of origin cannot be made out.
- **Unknown primary: Sometimes metastases may appear without any clinically detectable primary tumor** and even the microscopic examination of metastases may not reveal the characteristic features of primary site of origin of tumor, e.g., metastases from adenocarcinoma may be so anaplastic that there is no evidence of any gland formation. In such situations, **electron microscopic examination, immunohistochemistry** by specific tumor markers will be **helpful to establish** the correct origin **primary tumor**.

Pathways of Spread

Invasiveness of cancers allows them to penetrate blood vessels, lymphatics, and body cavities. It provides an opportunity for spread/dissemination of cancers through the various pathways (**Box 4**).

Box 4: Pathways of spread.

- Lymphatic spread
- Hematogenous/blood spread
- Seeding of body cavities and surfaces
- Direct transplantation

Lymphatic spread

- **Most common pathway** of spread for carcinomas. Sarcomas may also sometimes spraed through lymphatics. Tumors as such do not contain functional lymphatic vessels. But, lymphatic vessels located at the margins of invading cancers are enough for the lymphatic spread of tumor cells.
- **Regional node involvement:** Usually, the location of a primary tumor determines the distribution of the initial metastases to the lymph nodes from that tumor. Basement membranes are present only in large lymphatic channels whereas, lymphatic capillaries lack them. The walls of lymphatics in the region of cancer are readily invaded by cancer cells and form a continuous growth within the lymphatic channels (lymphatic permeation). Once the tumor cells gain access into the lymphatic vessels, they may detach to form tumor emboli and are carried to the regional draining lymph nodes. In the lymph node, the **tumor emboli** enter through afferent lymphatics at its convex surface and first **lodge and grow in the subcapsular** (marginal) **sinus**. **Subsequently, the entire lymph node** may be replaced by the metastatic tumor. Lymph nodes with metastatic deposits may be enlarged to many times their normal size.
- **Pattern of lymph node involvement follows the natural routes of lymphatic drainage**. One of the best examples for pattern of regional lymphatic metastasis is breast cancer. The initial metastases are almost always lymphatic. Breast cancers in the upper outer quadrant (lateral aspect) of the breast first spread to axillary lymph nodes; medial breast lesions drain through the chest wall to the internal mammary thoracic lymph nodes (along the internal mammary artery). Thereafter, in both instances, it may spread to the supraclavicular and infraclavicular nodes. Lung carcinomas in the respiratory passages metastasize first to the regional bronchial lymph nodes and then to the tracheobronchial and hilar nodes.
- **Sentinel lymph node:** It is the **first regional lymph node that receives lymph flow from a primary tumor.** During surgery, it can be identified by injecting blue dyes or radiolabelled tracers near the primary tumor. Biopsy of sentinel lymph node is done to know the presence or absence of metastatic lesions by examination of frozen sections. Thus, it helps to determine the extent of spread of tumor and planning the treatment. Sentinel node examination is used to assess the spread of breast carcinoma, melanomas, colon cancers, and other tumors.
- **Skip metastasis:** Occasionally lymphatic metastases are found in lymph nodes far from the primary tumor site. When **local lymph nodes are bypassed** and **lymphatic metastases develop in lymph nodes distant from the site of the primary tumor**; these are called "skip metastasis." It is probably because either microscopic metastases are missed or variation in normal patterns of lymphatic drainage. For example, the first sign of some abdominal **cancers** may be **first detected by an enlarged supraclavicular lymph node**. **Virchow's lymph node** is metastasis to supraclavicular lymph node from cancers of abdominal organs (e.g., cancer stomach). Lymphatic drainage tends to reflect embryologic origin of the organ.

For example, testes develop in the abdominal cavity and descends to the scrotum during development of fetus. Hence, malignant tumors of testis usually spread to abdominal periaortic lymph nodes and not to the inguinal lymph nodes, which drains the scrotal region.

- **Retrograde metastasis: Tumors spreading against the flow of lymphatics** may cause metastases at unusual sites, e.g., **carcinoma prostate metastasizing to supraclavicular lymph node**.
- **Microscopic pattern of deposits:**
  - Initially, **tumor cells** are deposited in the **marginal sinus and later extend throughout the node**.
  - **Micrometastases** (microscopic involvement of lymph nodes) **consist of single tumor cells or very small clusters.**
  - After arrest of malignant within the node, these cells may be destroyed by a tumor-specific immune response.
- **Significance of lymph node metastases: Prognostic value**, e.g., in breast cancer, involvement of axillary lymph nodes is very important for assessing prognosis and for type of therapy. However, all regional nodal enlargements need not be due to metastasis because necrotic products of tumor and antigens may produce sinus histiocytosis in lymph node. Therefore, histopathological identification of tumor within an enlarged lymph node is needed.

Hematogenous spread

Hematogenous spread is usual for sarcomas but is also found in carcinomas. Blood-borne metastasis usually occurs in **osteosarcoma, choriocarcinoma,** and **renal cell carcinoma.**

Vessels invaded Cancer cells easily invade **capillaries and venules**, but thick-walled arterioles and arteries are relatively resistant. However, arterial spread may occur in certain situations. These include: (i) when tumor cells pass through pulmonary capillary beds or pulmonary arteriovenous shunts or (ii) when cancers in the lung (primary or metastatic) give rise to tumor emboli. Before cancers can form viable metastases, circulating tumor cells (CTCs) must lodge in the vascular bed at the site of metastasis.

Tumors with affinity for venous invasion Few carcinomas have tendency to grow within veins. However, they may not be accompanied by widespread dissemination.

- **Renal cell carcinoma:** It can invade the renal vein and grow in a snake-like fashion up the inferior vena cava, sometimes reaching the right side of the heart.
- **Hepatocellular carcinoma:** It may invade branches of portal and hepatic vein and grow within the main venous channels.

Pattern of involvement With venous invasion, the pattern of metastases follows the venous flow.

Target organ for metastasis Usually, the location of a primary tumor determines the distribution of the initial metastases from that tumor.

- **Liver and lungs:** They are the **most frequently involved** organs; liver, because **all portal area drains to the liver**. Tumors which penetrate systemic veins, eventually drain into the vena cava. Since **all caval blood flows to the lungs**, it is the other common site for secondaries by hematogenous spread.
- Through pulmonary veins, cancer cells from the primary lung cancer and metastatic deposit in the lungs may be carried to the left side of the heart. From here the tumor emboli may be carried in systemic circulation to form secondary masses elsewhere in the body.
- **Bone metastasis:** Cancer metastasizing to bone-prostate, lung, breast, liver, intestine, kidney, and thyroid.
  - **Vertebral column is a common site** and the spread is through the paravertebral plexus, e.g., carcinomas of the thyroid and prostate.
  - Radiograph appearance of bone metastasis.
    - **Osteolytic lesion:** It is characterized by radiolucencies (e.g., lung cancer) and may lead to pathological fractures and hypercalcemia.
    - **Osteoblastic lesion:** It is characterized by radiodensities (e.g., prostatic cancer, breast, thyroid) and increased serum alkaline phosphatase due to reactive bone formation.
- **Other common sites: Brain—**most common primary is lung cancer, kidney, and adrenals.
- **Organs relatively resistant** include **skeletal muscle** (though rich in capillaries) **and spleen**.

Note: Anatomic location of a tumor and its venous drainage cannot always explain the systemic distributions of metastases. For example, prostatic carcinoma favorably spreads to bone, bronchogenic carcinoma tends to spread to the adrenal glands and the brain, and neuroblastoma spreads to the liver and bones.

MORPHOLOGY

Gross appearance (Fig. 20)

Appear as multiple round nodules of varying sizes found throughout the organ.

Microscopy

The metastatic deposits generally resemble the structure of primary tumor.

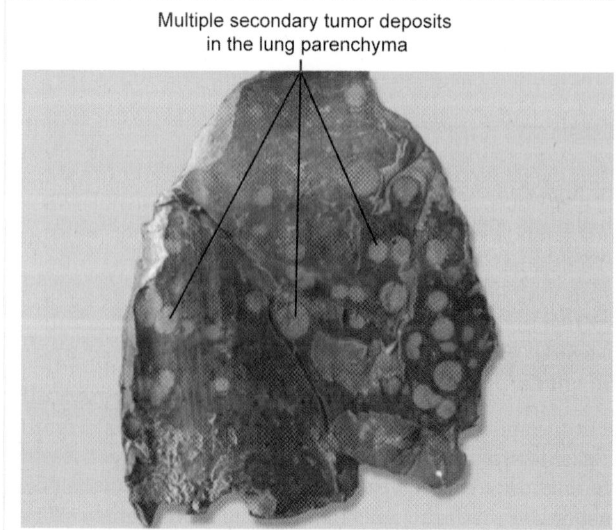

FIG. 20: Lung with multiple metastatic cancer.

Seeding of body cavities and surfaces

Malignant tumors that arise in organs adjacent to body cavities (e.g., ovaries, gastrointestinal tract, and lung) may shed malignant cells into body cavities and surfaces.

Transcoelomic spread:

- **Malignant tumor arising in organs adjacent to body cavities** (e.g., ovaries, gastrointestinal tract, and lung), **may seed body cavities**. The malignant cells may exfoliate or shed from the organ surfaces into the body cavities and cytological examination of this fluid may show malignant cells. Tumor cells in these cavities grow in masses and usually produce fluid (e.g., ascites, pleural fluid), sometimes in very large quantities. Mucinous adenocarcinoma may also secrete copious amounts of mucin in these locations.
- Body cavities include peritoneal (most common), pleural cavities (common), pericardial (occasionally), joint space, and subarachnoid space.
  - **Peritoneal cavity:** Example: (1) **Ovarian tumors,** such as primary carcinomas of surface epithelial origin and (2) **Malignant gastrointestinal tract tumors** may spread to involve peritoneal cavity → ascites.
  - **Pleural cavity:** Peripherally situated **lung tumors** → pleural effusions.
  - **Cerebrospinal fluid (CSF): Glioblastoma** commonly spreads through CSF in the subarachnoid space to the spinal cord.
- After seeding the body cavities, the tumor cells may remain confined to the surface of the abdominal viscera without penetrating into the substance of the involved viscera.
- **Pseudomyxoma peritonei:** Sometimes, mucus-secreting appendiceal carcinomas (**Fig. 21**) or mucinous carcinomas of ovary may fill the peritoneal cavity with a gelatinous neoplastic mass. This condition is called as *pseudomyxoma peritonei*.

Spread along the epithelial lined spaces It is not common, examples.

- **Carcinoma endometrium may spread to ovary** (or vice versa) **through fallopian tube.**
- **Carcinoma of kidney may spread to lower urinary tract via ureters.**

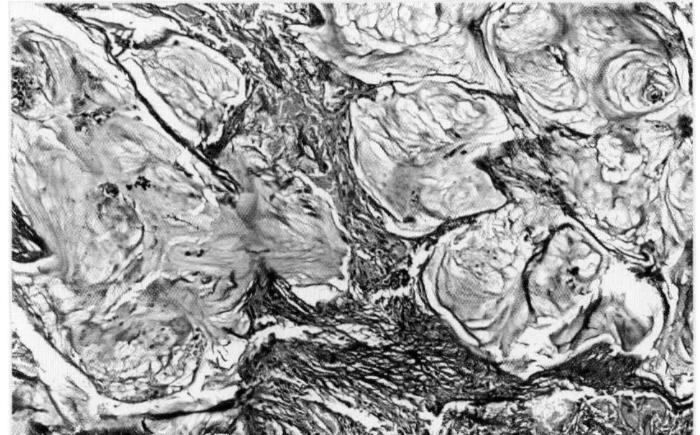

FIG. 21: Pseudomyxoma peritonei. Mucus-secreting appendiceal carcinomas showing peritoneal cavity filled with a gelatinous material.

Direct transplantation

- Tumor cells may be directly transplanted (e.g., by surgical instruments like scalpel, needles, sutures) or implantation by direct contact (e.g., transfer of cancer of lower lip to the corresponding opposite site in the upper lip). Iatrogenic spread of tumor cells on surgical instruments may occur. For example, biopsies of testicular masses are never done because if it is malignant it may spread.
- Even though this method is theoretically possible, they are **rare**.

Drop metastasis

Q. Write a short essay on drop metastasis.

Definition Drop metastases are defined as intradural extramedullary spinal **metastases** that arise from intracranial lesions.

Mechanism of spread It occurs through CSF when the tumor extends into the subarachnoid space and exfoliates tumor cells into the subarachnoid space.

Sites of drop metastasis Due to the gravitational effects, these lesions usually occur in the dorsal lower-thoracic to lumbar spine. Other sites include nerve roots, cauda equina, nerve root sleeves, and the fundus of the thecal sac.

Tumors that produce drop metastasis

- It is frequently observed in **medulloblastoma**.
- It is a rare complication of glioblastoma, the most common form of malignant primary brain tumor. Interventions such as surgical manipulation may increase the likelihood of drop metastases.
- Very rarely, secondaries to the brain from small-cell as well as nonsmall-cell lung cancer, breast cancer, kidney cancer, melanoma, and lymphoma.

Clinical diagnosis Drop metastases should be suspected when the patient presents with rapidly progressive neurologic deficit especially in pediatric patients (e.g., medulloblastoma). Prognosis of drop metastasis is poor.

Investigations These lesions may be missed on X-ray films and sometimes on computed tomography (CT) scans. Hence, the investigation of choice is spinal magnetic resonance imaging (MRI) with contrast. It is usually presented as diffuse enhancing nodules along the spine and cauda equina.

Management of drop metastasis These include neurosurgery, radiation, and steroid therapy.

Differences Between Benign and Malignant Tumors

Differences between benign and malignant tumors are summarized in **Table 8**.

HISTORICAL ASPECTS OF NEOPLASIA

Normal cells, even those that divide the most rapidly (e.g., bone marrow cells, intestinal mucosal cells), are superbly controlled with regards to their rate and location of their proliferation and accumulation.

Deoxyribonucleic acid (DNA) mutations can occur within a single cell due to several causes. When sufficient mutations

Table 8: Differences between benign and malignant tumors.

Characteristics	*Benign*	*Malignant*
Microscopic features		
Differentiation/anaplasia	Well-differentiated	Well-to-poorly differentiated. Anaplasia is characteristic
Pleomorphism	Usually not seen	Commonly present
Nuclear morphology	Usually normal	Usually hyperchromatic, irregular outline, and pleomorphic
Nucleoli	Usually absent	Usual and prominent
Mitotic activity	Rare and if present, they are normal bipolar	High and may be abnormal or atypical (tripolar, quadripolar, multipolar)
Tumor giant cells	Not seen	May be seen and show nuclear atypia
Nuclear cytoplasmic (N:C) ratio	Normal (1:4 to 1:6)	Increased (may be as much as 1:1)
Polarity	Maintained	Usually lost
Chromosomal abnormality	Not found	Usually seen
Gross features		
Border/capsule	Mostly circumscribed or encapsulated	Usually poorly defined
Areas of necrosis and hemorrhage	Rare	Common, often found microscopically
Clinical features		
Rate of growth	Usually slow	Relatively rapid
Local invasion	Usually well-demarcated without invasion/ infiltration of the surrounding normal tissues	Locally invasive, infiltrate surrounding normal tissue
Metastasis	Absent	Frequent
Biological behavior/prognosis	Usually prognosis is good	Prognosis is poor; usually death due to local invasion or metastatic complications

occur, the cell escapes growth control and eventually acquires additional mutations. These mutated cells become cancer cells and permit local invasion and subsequent spread through vascular and lymphatic channels.

In the beginning, cancer was considered to be due to a mysterious act of God.

- Cancer is an ancient disease. Bone tumors was found in prehistoric times and the disease was mentioned in early writings from India, Egypt, Babylonia, and Greece.
- Hippocrates distinguished benign from malignant growths. He also coined the term *karkinos*, from which our term **carcinoma** is derived. Hippocrates described cancer of the breast, and in the 2nd century AD and Paul of Aegina commented on its frequency.
- In the late 18th century, specific causes of cancer were first identified and John Hill of London proposed that exposure to tobacco caused cancer. Sir Percival Pott in 1775 first described that scrotal cancer among chimney sweeps in London is caused due to the soot. This is the first description of occupational cancer. More than a century later, bladder cancer was reported in aniline dye workers in Germany.
- F Peyton Rous (1911): First described an avian cancer caused due to a filterable agent (virus).
- In 1920s, it was found that human exposure to X-rays via fluoroscopy led to cancer.
- Berenblum (1941): First proposed the two-step (initiation/ promotion) theory of chemical carcinogenesis.
- Watson and Crick (1953): They discovered DNA as the genetic material of cells and provided the basic structure of DNA.
- AG Knudson (1971): He proposed the two-hit hypothesis in which involvement of two mutated alleles of the retinoblastoma (*Rb*) gene was demonstrated in the development of retinoblastomas. He termed these genes as tumor suppressors.
- In 1974, the gene responsible for defective DNA repair in the skin disease xeroderma pigmentosum was linked to visceral cancers.
- Bishop and Varmus (1976) demonstrated proto-oncogene. They proposed that **proto-oncogenes** are mammalian genetic homologs of viral transforming genes called **oncogenes**. When mutated, these cellular proto-oncogenes may become growth-promoting oncogenes that can lead to cancer.

Substantial progress has been achieved in understanding neoplasia. However, much of the knowledge in cancer has been derived from experiments in cells in culture, laboratory animals, and genetically modified species.

EPIDEMIOLOGY OF CANCER

Q. Discuss geographic and environmental factors in etiology of cancer.

Differences among individuals are very important in determining the diseases to which they are susceptible and their reactions to the diseases once contracted. Epidemiology is the branch of medicine which deals with study of patterns of disease in human populations (aggregates of people).

The epidemiology provides yet another important dimension. Information may be gained by examining the occurrence, incidence, prevalence, transmission, and distribution of diseases in populations. Epidemiology has several roles in cancer knowledge.

Cancer arises from an interaction of multiple etiological factors. Study of occurrence of cancer in populations has provided knowledge about its origins. It is possible to prevent many types of cancer by avoiding high-risk behavior and exposure to carcinogens, or cancer-causing substances. Examples include:

Smoking: The knowledge about the role of cigarette smoking with development of smoking-related cancer (e.g., cancer of lung, oropharynx) was primarily obtained from epidemiologic studies.

Lifestyle cancers: Lifestyle behavior, dietary and environmental factors [e.g., exposure to ultraviolet (UV) radiation, infections], and occupational exposure can contribute to cancer development. Common lifestyle cancers include colorectal and bladder cancer. Dietary fat and fiber content may be important in the causation of colorectal cancer. Epidemiology helps in prevention of these cancers either by avoiding the exposure or changing the lifestyle behavior.

Knowledge about the causes of cancer can be gained by epidemiologic studies. Environmental, racial (possibly hereditary), and cultural influences on the occurrence of specific neoplasms can also be obtained. Certain diseases are associated with an increased risk for developing cancer. They can provide clues to the pathogenesis of cancer.

Cancer Incidence

The incidence of cancer varies with age, geographic factors, and genetic factors. There is a progressive increase in the numbers of cancer cases and deaths in India. Incidence of the most common forms of cancer varies with region and other associated factors. Oropharyngeal cancers are common in India to use of nonsmoking tobacco products. Decreased use of tobacco products has reduced death due to lung cancer in developed countries. Improved method of detection and treatment has decreased death rates for colorectal, female breast, and prostate cancers. The decrease in cancer of uterine cervix is directly related to widespread use of the Papanicolaou (PAP) smear test for early detection of this tumor and its precursor lesions. The use of the HPV vaccine may nearly eliminate cervical cancer in coming years in western countries.

Environmental Factors

Q. Enumerate various occupation-associated disorders (refer pages 970–973) and enhanced risk of carcinogenesis.

"Environment" is defined as anything people interact with. Environment includes sunlight, workplace exposure, drugs, exposures from lifestyle choices, natural and medical radiation, and substances in the air, water, and soil. **Both genetic and environmental factors contribute to the development of cancer.** However, **environmental influences are the predominant risk factors for most cancers**. The geographic

Table 9: Examples of occupational cancers.

Agents	*Associated malignant tumors*
Arsenic and its compounds	Carcinoma of lung and skin
Asbestos	Carcinoma of lung, esophageal, gastric, and colon; mesothelioma
Nickel compounds	Carcinoma of lung and oropharynx
Beryllium and its compounds	Carcinoma lung
Chromium compounds	
Radon and its decay products	
Benzene	Acute myeloid leukemia
Cadmium and its compounds	Carcinoma of prostate
Vinyl chloride	Angiosarcoma of liver

variation in cancer incidence is mostly due to different environmental exposures. **Environmental factors may be the dominant risk factors for many common cancers. This suggests that many cancers are potentially preventable.** This is supported by the geographic variation of specific forms of cancer due to differences in environmental exposures. Most of the evidence indicates that these geographic differences have environmental rather than genetic origins. There are several environmental factors that contribute to cancer and of course we are surrounded by carcinogenic agents. These environmental factors include infectious agents, smoking, alcohol, diet, obesity, reproductive history, and exposure to carcinogens. They are hidden in the ambient environment, in the workplace, in food, and in personal practices. They can be as universal as sunlight or mainly confined to urban atmosphere (e.g., asbestos) or particular occupations (**Table 9**).

Important Environmental Factors that Predispose to Cancer

Infectious agents

About 15% of cancers may be caused directly or indirectly by infectious agents. For example, *human papillomavirus* (HPV), spreads through sexual contact and is the etiological factor for carcinoma of cervix as well as some head and neck cancers.

Q. Write a short essay on diet and cancer.

Diet

Certain features of diet can be a predisposing factor. Obesity is the modest risk factor for many different cancers. Carcinogens may be present in food (e.g., grilled meat, high-fat diet, alcohol), water (e.g., arsenic), environment (e.g., UV rays, asbestos), drugs medications (e.g., methotrexate), etc. Though not proved, diet may be a risk factor for colorectal carcinoma, prostate carcinoma, and breast carcinoma. **Three factors in the diet are probably involved in the development of cancer:**

i. **Exogenous carcinogen in diet:** *Aflatoxin* causes a specific mutation in codon 249 of the *TP53* gene and is involved in the development of hepatocellular carcinomas. The role of food additives, artificial sweeteners, and contaminating pesticides in the genesis of cancer is not known.

ii. **Endogenous synthesis of carcinogens from dietary components:**
   - **Nitrosamines and nitrosamides: It was implicated mainly in the genesis of gastric cancer.** Nitrosamines and nitrosamides in the diet can induce gastric cancer. These compounds are formed in the stomach from nitrites and amines or amides from the digested proteins in the diet. Sources of nitrites include sodium nitrite (added as food preservative), and nitrates (present in common vegetables), and these are reduced to nitrosamine and nitrosamides in the gut by bacterial flora.
   - **High animal fat intake:** This along with consumption of red meat and low dietary fiber intake has been implicated in the causation of carcinoma colon. Probably high fat intake increases the bile acids level in the gut. This modifies intestinal flora and favors the growth of microaerophilic bacteria. Bile acid metabolites produced by the action of these bacteria may be carcinogenic.

iii. **Lack of protective factors:**
   - **High-fiber diet** may have a protective role in carcinoma colon. This may be due to—(1) increased bulk of stool and reduced transit time, which reduces the exposure of mucosa to probable carcinogens, and (2) certain fibers in the diet may bind to carcinogens and protect the mucosa. However, it is not proved.
   - Correlation between total **dietary fat intake** and breast cancer is also not clear.
   - **Antioxidants:** Fruits and vegetables, consumption of vitamin C and E, β-carotenes and selenium which have antioxidant properties, have been presumed to have anticarcinogenic effect. However, there is no convincing evidence that antioxidants act as chemopreventive agents. Retinoids are effective agents in the therapy of acute promyelocytic leukemia (APML), and there are reports mentioning the associations between low levels of vitamin D and cancer of the colon, prostate, and breast.
   - Epidemiologic studies suggest that a **folate-rich diet** decreases the risk of colorectal cancer.

In conclusion, dietary influences on cancer development are highly controversial. There is no definitive evidence to indicate that a particular diet can cause or prevent cancer. Association has been mentioned that physical activity decreases the risk of developing cancer of breast and colon whereas, obesity increases the risk for endometrial, esophageal, and kidney cancer.

Tobacco products and smoking

Nicotine in tobacco and other tobacco leaf components cause cancer. **Carcinogens in tobacco can act as initiators, as well as promoters.** Risk increases with amount and duration of tobacco use. Tobacco may be used either for **smoking** or as **smokeless tobacco**.

- **Smoking:** It may be in the form of cigarette, *beedi,* cigar, or pipe smoking, or reverse smoking (smoking a cheroot with the burning end inside the mouth is practiced in certain regions of India). Smoking (e.g., cigarettes) is associated with increased risk of cancer in the lung (most important), mouth, pharynx, larynx, esophagus, pancreas, and bladder. During 1930, lung cancer was an uncommon tumor. There is dramatic rise in death rate from cancer of the lung in men from 1930 and at present it is the most common cause of death from cancer in men. This is attributable to smoking.
- **Smokeless tobacco:** It is in the form of **betel quid**/pan that contains several ingredients such as areca nut, slaked lime, and tobacco, which are wrapped in a betel leaf. It is commonly used in India and Southeast Asia, and is associated with marked increase in oral cancer. **Betel quid appears to be the major carcinogen**. However, it may also be related to slaked lime and the areca nut. Other methods of tobacco consumption include snuff dipping and tobacco chewing.

Alcohol

Alcohol abuse is an independent risk factor for cancers of the oropharynx, larynx, esophagus, and liver (following alcoholic cirrhosis). Alcohol acts synergistically with tobacco as either a cocarcinogen (increasing the risk) or a promoter (decreasing the lag time). They increase the risk for cancers of the upper airways and upper digestive tract.

Reproductive history

Lifelong cumulative exposure to estrogen stimulation (especially unopposed by progesterone), increases the risk for cancers of the estrogen-responsive tissues, namely endometrium and breast.

- **Obesity:** Obesity is associated with increased cancer risk.

Examples of occupational cancers are presented in **Table 9**.

Age and Cancer

Age is an important factor that influence the risk of cancer. Cancer can occur at any age, but is most common in older adults. Generally, the frequency of cancer increases as the age increases. This may be due to the accumulation of somatic mutations and decline of immunocompetence that accompanies aging.

However, >10% of all deaths among children younger than 15 years of age is due to cancers. The major fatal cancers in children are leukemias, tumors of the CNS, lymphomas, and sarcomas of soft-tissue and bone.

Acquired Predisposing Conditions

Acquired conditions may predispose to cancer. These include **disorders associated with chronic inflammation, immunodeficiency states, and precursor lesions.**

Chronic Inflammation

Cancer risk rises in certain tissues when there is increased cellular proliferation caused by chronic inflammation or hormonal stimulation. Rudolf Virchow in 1863 first proposed a relationship between chronic inflammation and cancer. Many chronic inflammatory conditions act as a risk factor for the development of malignant tumors (**Table 10**). Tumors arising in chronic inflammatory conditions (both infectious and noninfectious) are mostly carcinomas and others include mesothelioma and lymphoma. Tissue injury caused by chronic inflammatory disorders are accompanied by a compensatory proliferation of cells to repair the damage. Some cases of chronic inflammation may be accompanied by an increase the pool of tissue stem cells. These stem cells may be susceptible to transformation. Chronic inflammation

Table 10: Chronic inflammatory states and associated cancers.

Chronic inflammatory state	*Associated cancer*	*Etiology*
Asbestosis, silicosis	Mesothelioma, carcinoma of lung	Asbestos fibers, silica particles
Reflux esophagitis, Barrett esophagus	Carcinoma of esophagus	Gastric acid
Gastritis/ulcers	Gastric adenocarcinoma, mucosa-associated lymphoid tissue (MALT) lymphoma	*Helicobacter pylori*
Inflammatory bowel disease (mainly ulcerative colitis)	Colorectal carcinoma	Exact etiological agent not known
Hepatitis	Hepatocellular carcinoma	Hepatitis B and/or C virus
Chronic cholecystitis	Cancer of gallbladder	Bile acids, bacteria, gall stones
Opisthorchis, cholangitis	Cholangiocarcinoma, and carcinoma colon	Liver flukes (Opisthorchis viverrini)
Pancreatitis	Carcinoma of pancreatic	Alcohol, germline mutations (e.g., in the trypsinogen gene)
Lichen sclerosis	Squamous cell carcinoma of vulva	Not known
Sjögren syndrome, Hashimoto thyroiditis	MALT lymphoma	Autoimmune disorder
Osteomyelitis	Carcinoma in draining sinuses	Bacterial infection
Chronic cervicitis	Carcinoma of cervix	Human papilloma virus (HPV)
Chronic cystitis	Bladder carcinoma	Schistosomiasis
Chronic thyroiditis	Papillary thyroid carcinoma	Hashimoto thyroiditis
Prostatitis	Prostate carcinoma	Chronic prostatitis
Inflammation provoking agent	Ovarian carcinoma	Endometriosis

(MALT: mucosa-associated lymphoid tissue)

activates immune cells and they may produce reactive oxygen species (ROS). ROS may damage DNA. The inflammatory mediators released in chronic inflammatory disorders may promote cell survival, even those cells with genomic damage. The relationship between chronic inflammation and cancer has practical importance. For example, *Helicobacter pylori* gastritis lead to the development of a gastric cancer. Prompt diagnosis and effective treatment of *Helicobacter pylori* gastritis with antibiotics can silence the chronic inflammatory condition thereby eliminate the development of a gastric cancer.

Cancer incidence of common types of cancer is presented in **Table 11**. It varies depending on geographic location and other factors.

Table 11: Most common types of cancers.

Common location of tumor in descending order according to the incidence	
Males	***Females***
Prostate	Breast
Lung and bronchus	Lung and bronchus
Colon and rectum	Colon and rectum
Urinary bladder	Uterine corpus
Melanoma of the skin	Thyroid
Kidney	Melanoma of skin
Non-Hodgkin lymphoma	Non-Hodgkin lymphoma
Oral cavity	Kidney
Leukemia	Ovary
Pancreas	Pancreas
All other sites	All other sites

Precancerous Conditions/Precursor Lesions

Q. Write a short essay on pre-cancerous state.

Precancerous conditions (precursor lesions) are **non-neoplastic disorders** that are localized disturbances of epithelial differentiation. Lining epithelial cells in certain locations may develop morphologic changes and these are associated with a **well-defined increased risk of developing cancer**; such lesions are termed as precursor lesions. These changes may be in the form of hyperplasia, metaplasia, or dysplasia. These lesions may develop secondary to chronic inflammation or hormonal disturbances (in endocrine-sensitive tissues), or may occur spontaneously. On molecular analyses, these precursor lesions have some of the genetic lesions found in their associated cancers. However, in majority of these lesions, no malignant neoplasm develops except that they have an increased risk. However, recognition of precursor lesions is important because their removal or reversal lowers cancer risk.

- **Chronic atrophic gastritis** of pernicious anemia.
- **Solar or actinic keratosis of the skin, Bowen's disease of the skin.**
- **Chronic inflammation (refer Table 10):** Chronic ulcerative colitis (carcinoma colon), cirrhosis of liver (hepatocellular carcinoma), *H. pylori* gastritis (gastric cancer and lymphoma), chronic irritation from jagged tooth or ill-fitting denture (cancer of the oral cavity), and old burn scar—Marjolin's ulcer (squamous cell carcinoma).

- **Leukoplakia** (erythroplakia) of the oral cavity, vulva, and penis. These may progress to squamous cell carcinoma in the respective sites.
- **Barrett esophagus**.
- **Squamous metaplasia and dysplasia of bronchial mucosa** observed in chronic smokers (risk factor for lung carcinoma), intralobular and intraductal carcinoma of the breast, carcinoma in situ of cervix.
- **Endometrial hyperplasia** and dysplasia in women with unopposed estrogen stimulation (a risk factor for endometrial carcinoma).
- **Precancerous benign tumors:** Benign tumors are not precancerous. However, each type of benign tumor is associated with a certain level of risk, ranging from high to nil.
    - Most benign tumors do not become malignant. However, occasionally a few forms of benign tumor develop into malignant. For example, villous adenoma of the colon as it increases in size, is associated with an increased risk for developing colorectal carcinoma.
    - Malignant change is extremely rare in leiomyomas of the uterus but rarely it can begin in a leiomyoma.
    - Carcinoma developing in long-standing pleomorphic adenomas.
- Malignant peripheral nerve sheath tumor in patients with neurofibromatosis.
- Congenital abnormalities may predispose to cancer, e.g., the undescended testis is more prone to neoplasms than the normally located testis.
- Immunodeficiency states: Patients with deficits in T-cell immunity have increased risk for cancers, mainly those due to oncogenic viruses.

Precancerous lesions of gastrointestinal tract are presented in **Box 5**.

Immunodeficiency and Cancer

Immunodeficient patients, particularly those with deficits in T-cell immunity have a increased risk for cancer. These are mainly due to oncogenic viruses. These patients have increased incidence of chronic infection with viruses. The virus-associated cancer include lymphomas, certain carcinomas, and some sarcomas and sarcoma-like proliferations.

Interactions between Environmental and Genetic Factors

The risk for developing cancer is modified by interactions between genetic factors and environmental exposures.

Box 5: Precancerous lesions of gastrointestinal tract.

Esophagus
- Barrett esophagus, achalasia, postingestion of caustic soda lye (alkaline burn)

Stomach
- *H. pylori*, especially if treated with proton pump inhibitors (PPI) without eradication of *H. pylori*
- Gastric polyps
- Ménétrier's disease (hypertrophic gastropathy)
- Achlorhydria, pernicious anemia
- Postgastrectomy, postvagotomy, postgastrojejunostomy

Small intestine
- Hereditary cancer syndromes, familial adenomatous polyposis (FAP) (especially postcholecystectomy), Peutz–Jeghers syndrome

Colon (large intestine)
- Hereditary cancer syndromes, FAP, Gardner's, hereditary nonpolyposis colorectal cancer (HNPCC, Lynch syndrome)
- Inflammatory bowel disease, especially chronic extensive ulcerative colitis
- Sporadic adenomatous polyps, especially villous and tubulovillous polyps

Hereditary and Genetic Contribution to Cancer

In some families, there is associated family history of cancer. In these individuals, it is transmitted like an inherited trait and is usually associated with mutations in germ cell line. These mutations mostly affect the function of "tumor suppressor gene (TSG)" (discussed later on pages 453–468).

Environmental Factors

About 95% of the cancers are sporadic cancers without any family history. These cancers are mostly related to environmental factors or acquired predisposing conditions.

Usually cancers have both hereditary and genetic contributions and these factors often interact. Such interactions may be complex when development of tumor is affected by small contributions from multiple genes. Also, genetic factors may change the risk for developing cancers induced by environmental factors. For example, inherited variation in enzyme cytochrome P-450 system that metabolizes procarcinogens to active carcinogens and risk of breast cancer in females who inherit mutated copies of the *BRCA1* or *BRCA2* tumor suppressor genes. These individuals have greater risk.

10.2 Molecular Basis of Cancer: Role of Genetic and Epigenetic Alterations

CHAPTER OUTLINE

GENETIC ALTERATIONS IN CANCER

Cancer has a genetic origin and is a genetic disease caused by mutations that alter the function of a limited subset of about 20,000 human genes. Thus, it arises through a series of somatic alterations in DNA that result in uncontrolled proliferation of cells with altered DNA. These genes are called as cancer genes because they contribute directly to the malignant behavior of cancer cells.

Definition of cancer genes: Cancer genes can be defined as genes that are recurrently affected by genetic aberrations in cancers.

The extent of these genetic aberrations can be assessed advanced technology in DNA sequencing and other methods that can assess genome-wide analysis of cancer cells. Certain genomic changes are likely to be observed in almost every cancer.

Nonlethal Genetic Damage

Carcinogenesis develops with nonlethal genetic damage (mostly in DNA) to the cells known as mutation is essential for carcinogenesis. This is because lethal damage cause death of cells.

Type of Genetic Damage

Cancer genes are formed from the mutations of normal genes. The cause of the **mutations** that is responsible for carcinogenesis **may be either inherited** or **acquired**.

1. **Inherited germline mutations:** Causative mutations sometimes are inherited in the germline and occurs in certain families. Therefore, these mutations are present in every cell in the body. The affected individual is at a higher risk for developing cancer. In families with germline mutations, these mutations are passed from generation to generation and cancer behaves like an inherited trait (**Table 12**).

Table 12: Inherited predisposition to malignant tumors.

Mode of inheritance and examples	***Gene***
Autosomal dominant	
Retinoblastoma	*RB*
Li–Fraumeni syndrome (various tumors)	*TP53*
Familial adenomatous polyposis/colon cancer	*APC*
Breast and ovarian tumors	*BRCA1, BRCA2*
Hereditary nonpolyposis colon cancer	Mismatch repair genes *(MSH2, MLH1, MSH6)*
Melanoma	*CDKN2A*
Neurofibromatosis 1 and 2	*NF1, NF2*
Multiple endocrine neoplasia 1 and 2	*MEN1, RET*
Nevoid basal cell carcinoma syndrome	*PTCH1*
Autosomal recessive syndromes of defective deoxyribonucleic acid (DNA) repair	
Xeroderma pigmentosum	Different genes involved in nucleotide excision repair (NER)
Ataxia-telangiectasia	*ATM*
Bloom syndrome	*BLM*
Fanconi anemia	Different genes involved in repair of DNA crosslinks

2. **Acquired mutations:** In most of the cancers, the mutations that give rise to cancer genes are acquired during life and occur spontaneously. Hence, these mutations are confined only to the cancer cells. They may occur spontaneously and may be random. The acquired mutation may be caused by

environmental exposures. Environmental exposure may be exogenous or endogenous agents.

- **Exogenous agents:** These include viruses or environmental chemicals or radiation. It results in sporadic cancers.
- **Endogenous agents:** These may be endogenous products of cellular metabolism that have the capacity to produce damage to DNA (e.g., reactive oxygen species) or alter gene expression through epigenetic mechanisms (e.g., oncometabolites).

Clonal Origin

Tumors is formed by a clonal expansion or proliferation of a single type of precursor (progenitor) cell that has undergone genetic damage or transformation. These genetic change in DNA are heritable and are passed to daughter cells. Thus, all these tumor cells present within an individual tumor have the same set of mutations that were present at the time of initial genetic damage or transformation. These tumor-specific mutations are usually identified by DNA sequencing (e.g., when there is subtle DNA damage such as point mutations) or by chromosomal analyses (e.g., when there are changes that are visible by karyotyping such as chromosomal translocations and copy number changes).

Principal Target Genes

There are hundreds of discovered cancer genes and new ones are still being discovered. Numerous complex cancer genes make it difficult to remember all of them and many of their names have unpronounceable acronyms (abbreviations). This can be simplified by classifying these cancer genes into one of four major functional classes— (1) oncogenes, (2) tumor suppressor genes (TSGs), (3) genes that regulate apoptosis, and (4) genes that regulate interactions between tumor cells and host cells. There four genes are the main targets of genetic damage and they undergo cancer causing mutations.

Oncogenes

Oncogenes are genes that lead to tumor formation in cells by promoting increased cell growth.

Proto-oncogenes are **normal cellular genes**, which encode a number of nuclear proteins that **regulate normal cell proliferation, differentiation, and survival**. Proto-oncogenes have multiple roles, but all act at some level in signaling pathways involved in proliferation of cells.

Oncogenes and Oncoproteins

Oncogenes are mutated or overexpressed versions of normal cellular genes, which are called *proto-oncogenes.* They lead to tumor formation and these **altered/mutated versions of proto-oncogenes are termed as oncogenes.** These oncogenes promote autonomous cell growth in cancer cells. Most oncogenes encode transcription factors which are involved in pro-growth signaling pathways, or factors that increase the survival of cells. These oncogenes usually produce increased encoded **gene product called oncoprotein** and cause tumors. These mutations are called as **"gain-of-function" mutations because they can transform cells even in the presence of a normal copy of the same gene.** Thus, oncogenes behave like dominant genes over their normal counterparts, because mutation of a single allele is sufficient to produce a pro-oncogenic effect.

- **Oncogenes** have the ability to **promote cell growth in the absence** of external normal growth-promoting/**mitogenic signals/stimuli**.
- **Products** of oncogenes are called **oncoproteins**, which resemble the normal products of proto-oncogenes. This may either produces increase in one or more normal gene product that promote tumorigenesis or the gene products may have a completely new function that is oncogenic. These mutations are gain of function mutations and they can transform cells in spite of the presence of a normal copy of the same gene (one normal allele). Thus, usually oncogenes are dominant over their normal counterparts.
- **Oncoprotein production** is **not under normal regulatory control.** The cells proliferate without the usual requirement for external signals and are freed from checkpoints and **growth becomes autonomous. Oncoproteins act like accelerators that speed the replication of cells and their DNA. In contrast, tumor suppressors act as brakes that slow or arrest this process.**

Growth promoting protooncogenes are discussed in detail on pages 441–453.

Tumor Suppressor Genes

Tumor suppressor genes are genes that normally prevent uncontrolled growth or **cell proliferation. The protein product of tumor suppressor is associated with suppression of any of the various hallmarks of cancer.** Tumor suppressor proteins form a network of checkpoints and act as negative growth regulators. As discussed earlier, **oncogenes stimulate proliferation of cells,** whereas, **the protein products of most TSGs** (tumor suppressor genes) **apply brakes and prevent uncontrolled cell proliferation.** When they are mutated or lost from a cell, there will be loss of function of negative growth regulators (i.e., **failure of growth inhibition**). These cells can undergo transformation to develop tumor. So, a second mechanism of carcinogenesis results from failure of negative growth regulator (growth inhibition), due to deficiency of normal TSGs and their products. The functions of TSGs can also be lost by shutting down the expression of these genes through epigenetic mechanisms (involving DNA and histone methylation).

General characteristic features of TSGs are as follows:

Mechanism of action

Most tumor suppressors inhibit cell growth through one or other mechanism. Mutations that affect TSGs usually cause a "loss of function".

- **Apply brakes to cell proliferation:** Many tumor suppressors (e.g., two important TSGs *RB* and *p53*) are part of a regulatory network and they **apply the brakes on cell cycle progression and DNA replication.** They recognize genotoxic stress from any source and prevent proliferation of these cells. Thus, an oncogene in normal cells with intact TSGs may result in quiescence, or permanent arrest of cell cycle (oncogene-induced senescence), rather than uncontrolled proliferation. These cells may ultimately undergo apoptosis. Abnormalities in these genes lead to failure of growth inhibition.

- **Other mechanisms:** Some tumor suppressors prevent cellular transformation through other mechanisms. These include **by altering cell metabolism** [e.g., the serine-threonine kinase 11 (*STK11*)] or **by maintaining genomic stability** (e.g., the DNA repair factors *BRCA1* and *BRCA2*). **Mutations of TSGs may be hereditary and spontaneous.**

Loss of heterozygosity

- Usually, for tumor to develop, **both normal alleles of TSGs must be inactivated (damaged/mutated)**.
- Heterozygous state (one allele normal and other allele inactive) is sufficient to protect against cancer.
- Cancer develops when the cell loses heterozygosity [known as loss of heterozygosity (**LOH**)] for the normal TSG by **deletion or somatic mutation**. Tumor can develop when the cell becomes homozygous (both alleles are inactive) for the mutant allele. Thus, mutated TSGs usually behave in a recessive fashion. However, sometimes, loss of a single allele of a TSG can lead to cell proliferation. When loss of gene function is caused by damage to a single allele, it is called haploinsufficiency. This reduces the quantity of the encoded protein enough to release the brakes on cell proliferation and survival.

Groups of tumor suppressor genes

Tumor suppressor genes can be grouped into two—(1) Governors and (2) Guardians.

1. **"Governors":** They (e.g., *RB* gene) act as important brakes on cellular proliferation. Their mutations remove the brake for cellular proliferation and lead to formation of neoplasia.
2. **"Guardians":** They (e.g., *p53)* sense the genomic damage. Some guardian genes initiate a complex "damage control response" and prevent the proliferation of cells with genetic damage. If the genetic damage is too severe to be repaired, these genes induce apoptosis of those cells. For example, p53 protein ensures that cells advance their cell cycles only if the physiologic state of the cell is appropriate. Thus, p53 sense unrepaired damage to a cell's genome and shuts off the cell division cycle. If there is severe genomic damage or physiological abnormalities, the p53 pathway can induce programmed cell death (refer pages 142–150), thereby putting on the brakes to cell proliferation.

Tumor suppressor genes are discussed in detail on pages 453–468.

Genes that Regulate Apoptosis

Apoptosis is a programmed cell death and **is one of the normal protective mechanism by which a cell with DNA damage (mutation) undergoes cell death.** Many types of signals such as DNA damage, potent oncoproteins such as MYC, and loss of adhesion to the basement membrane (termed anoikis), can initiate apoptosis.

Genes that regulate apoptosis mainly act by increasing the survival of cell, rather than stimulating proliferation of cells. In cancer cells, the genes that protect against apoptosis (i.e., antiapoptotic genes) are often overexpressed (gain-of-function mutations in genes whose products suppress apoptosis), whereas, those that promote apoptosis (i.e., proapoptotic genes) are either under expressed or functionally inactivated by mutations (loss-of-function mutations in genes whose products promote cell death by apoptosis). Mutations or abnormalities in the genes that regulate apoptosis may result in accumulation of neoplastic cells due to less death and increased survival of the cells. There may be gain-of-function mutations in antiapoptotic genes (their products suppress apoptosis) and loss-of-function mutations in proapoptotic genes (their products promote cell death). The *apoptosis-regulating genes* can behave as **proto-oncogenes** (loss of one copy is enough) or **TSGs** (loss of both copies required). They are discussed in detail on pages 453–468.

Genes that Regulate Interactions between Tumor Cells and Host Cells

Apart from the four genes mentioned above, genes that regulate interactions between tumor cells and host cells are also recurrently mutated or functionally altered in certain malignant tumors. Important in this group are genes that enhance or inhibit recognition of tumors cells by the host immune system.

Genes Involved in DNA Repair

Normally DNA repair genes repair any defects in DNA (i.e., any mutations). Loss-of-function mutations of these DNA repair genes may lead to carcinogenesis. This is brought out indirectly by impairing the ability of the cell to recognize and repair nonlethal genetic damage in other genes. Thus, the cells affected acquire mutations at an increased rate. This state is referred to as a mutator phenotype and is characterized by genomic instability. They are discussed in detail on page 504.

Carcinogenesis: A Multistep Process (Fig. 22)

Normal cells do not multiply, accumulate or spread according to their own wish. Even the cells that divide the most rapidly (e.g., myelocytes, intestinal mucosal cells), are also under strict control. Carcinogenesis is the process of development of cancer. Cancer arises with accumulated genomic and changes in gene expression that begin within a single cell. In most of the cases, single mutation is not enough to transform a normal cell into a cancer cell. It occurs in a stepwise fashion over time. When repeated division of cell, mutations accrue. Eventually, the cell's progeny escapes the normal growth control and acquire more mutations. Thus, carcinogenesis is a multistep process that results from the accumulation of multiple genetic alterations (i.e., complementary mutations). Finally, these cells invade locally and subsequently spread through vascular and lymphatic channels.

Malignant neoplasms have several phenotypic peculiarities referred to as cancer hallmarks (discussed in detail on pages 441–513). These includes excessive growth, local invasiveness, and the capability to form distant metastases. These hallmarks are the results of genomic alterations that change the expression and function of key genes which produce a malignant tumor. The number of mutations present in cancer differs according to the type of tumor. The mutations in cancer cells can be divided into two major classes: drivers (pathogenic) and passengers (neutral or hitchhikers) mutations.

Driver Mutations

A relatively small number of genetic changes are fundamental to oncogenesis. Driver mutations are functionally important in driving tumor progression forward. They propel development of tumor

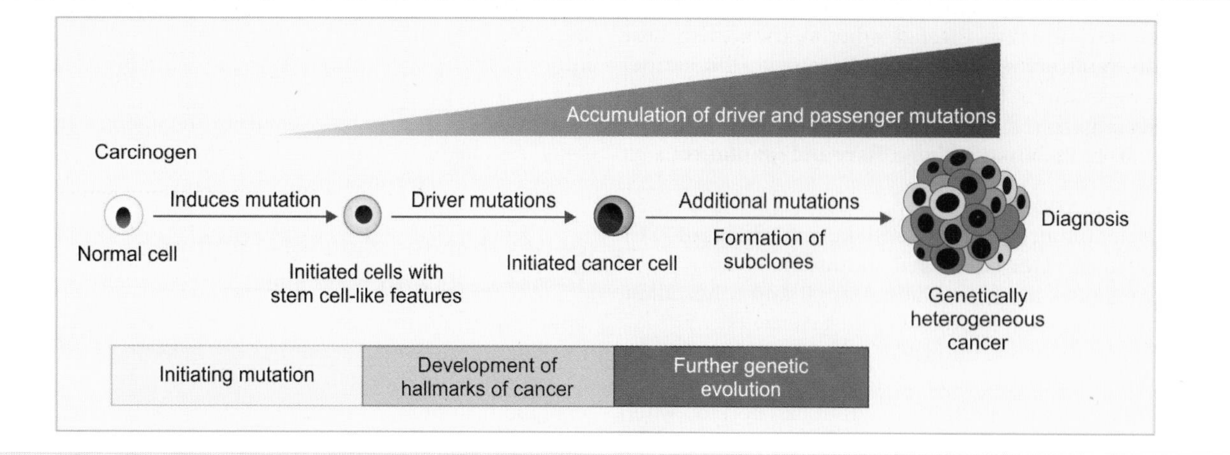

FIG. 22: Multistep process of development of cancer.

- **Driver mutations: These** are those mutations that convert normal cellular genes into oncogenes and thereby **produce malignant phenotype.** Driver mutations contribute to the acquisition of **hallmarks of** cancer. They produce mutational alteration of gene function or amplification in expression. These driver **mutations change the function of cancer genes** and serve to stimulate and sustain progression of cells through their growth and division cycles. They **directly contribute to the development or progression of a cancer.**
- **Initiating mutation: It is the first driver mutation that starts a cell on the path to malignancy.** It is often maintained in all the cells of the subsequent cancer. **Usually,** they are **acquired** and occasionally inherited.
- **Additional driver mutations:** No single mutation can fully transform and cause development of a cancer. The "initiated" cell acquire many additional driver mutations. Each of these additional driver mutations also contributes to the development of the cancer.
- **Time needed for the development of cancer after mutations:** The time required for the occurrence of cancer is unknown in most cancers. Probably it is lengthy and even in aggressive cancers it may appear after a decade. For example, in suddenly manifesting childhood acute lymphoblastic leukemia, cells having initiating mutations may be found in blood samples even a decade before diagnosis. The presence of initiated cells during this long preclinical prodrome points out that cancers arise from cells with stem cell-like properties. These cells are **cancer stem cells**. These cells have a capacity for self-renewal and long-term persistence.
- **Means of driver mutations:** The driver mutations tend to be **tightly clustered within cancer genes**. Tumor cells may acquire driver mutations through several means such as point mutations and nonrandom chromosomal abnormalities (e.g., gene rearrangements, deletions, and amplifications).
- Some driver mutations affect genes coding region whereas others affect noncoding sequences. These

Noncoding sequences include regulatory regions and areas encoding different variety of untranslated RNAs.

Passenger Mutations

Passenger mutations are acquired mutations. They are neutral in terms of fitness and do not affect cellular behavior, in contrast to driver mutations. They may simply occur as consequences of the rampant stochastic mutations that accumulate in patient's tumors. They are termed as "passenger mutations" because of little likelihood of contributing to tumor development. They are nonrecurrent, occur at random, and are sprinkled throughout the genome unlike tight clustering of driver mutations within cancer genes.

Loss-of-function mutations in genes that maintain genomic integrity is a common early step in malignancy, particularly in solid tumors. Mutations which lead to genomic instability increase the chances of acquiring driver mutations (that are needed for malignant behavior) and also greatly increase the frequency of mutations that have no phenotypic consequences (called "passenger" or "hitchhikers" mutations).

Importance of passenger mutations

- **Carcinogen-associated cancers:** It is found that particularly in cancers caused by exposure to carcinogen (e.g., sun exposure in melanoma and lung cancer related to smoking), the number of passenger mutations is more common than driver mutations. In carcinogen-associated tumors, most genomic damage is directly caused by the carcinogen.
- **Creation of genetic variants:** More bad effect of passenger mutations is that they create genetic variants. Though initially passenger mutations are neutral, they may provide selective advantage to tumor cells during therapy. In many instances, in tumors that recur after drug therapy, most of the tumor cells showed mutations that lead directly to drug resistance due to conversion of neutral passenger mutation into a driver mutation. The same resistance mutations also can be generally found before therapy, but only in a very small fraction of cells. The **selective pressure of therapy (e.g., treatment with an effective therapeutic drug) on tumor "converts" a neutral passenger mutation into a driver mutation.** This creation of genetic variant leads to drug resistance which benefits the tumor but is harmful to the patient.

Tumor is initiated in a single cell. Once cancer is established, it evolves genetically during its growth and progression. **Survival of fittest is the theory of biological evolution by the Charles Darwin**. This Darwinian law of selection also applies to tumor cells in that the cancers continue to undergo Darwinian selection and therefore continue to evolve. During early phase of growth, all the cancer cells in a tumor are genetically identical. Thus, they consist of a single type of transformed cell. Usually the tumor comes to clinical attention when cancer expands to form a mass of about 1 g, or about 10^9 cells. During this phase, cancer has gone through a minimum of 30 cell doublings. During this expansion process, individual tumor cells acquire additional mutations at random. Thus, although cancers are clonal in origin, usually by the time cancer become clinically evident their constituent cells are genetically extremely heterogeneous (see **Fig. 22**). These diverse or heterogenous tumor subclones compete for nutrients and those tumor cells that are most fit to survive this Darwinian struggle dominate the tumor mass. This tendency of tumors to become more aggressive over time is termed as tumor progression.

Tumor progression: Cancers during their course usually become more aggressive and acquire greater malignant potential. This phenomenon is referred to as tumor progression. At the molecular level, tumor progression results from accumulation of independent mutations in different cells. Some of these mutations may cause death of the cells and others may affect the function of cancer genes. Mutations that affect function make the affected cells more skilled to grow, survive, invade, metastasize, or evade immune reaction. Due to this selective advantage, subclones with these acquired mutations may come to dominate one area of a tumor. This domination may be at the site of the primary tumor or at the site of metastasis.

Genetic heterogeneity: Malignant tumors begin as having monoclonal (single clone of cells) origin. But due to continuing mutation and Darwinian selection, they become genetically heterogeneous by the time they clinically present. In advanced tumors showing genetic instability, the extent of genetic heterogeneity may be very large. Evidence for heterogenicity was observed in solid cancers such as renal cell carcinoma. DNA sequencing of multiple regions of the primary renal cell carcinoma and its metastatic deposits from the same patient was performed. They revealed two types of mutations: (i) Mutations present in all tumor sites and probably were present in the cell at the moment of transformation, and (ii) Mutations that are unique to a subset of tumor sites. These were probably acquired after the initial transformation during the outgrowth and spread of the tumor.

Two most harmful properties of cancers are their tendency over time to become— (1) more aggressive and (2) less responsive to therapy. Survival of the fittest cancer cells can explain both the natural history of cancer, and also changes in tumor behavior following therapy. Thus, genetic heterogeneity is responsible for progression of cancer as well as its poor response to therapy. When cancer recurs after chemotherapy, this recurred tumor is almost always resistant if the same treatment is given again. This acquired resistance is due to the outgrowth of subclones that have, by chance, mutations (or epigenetic alterations) that allows them to survive and make them resistance to drug.

Dysregulation of Cancer-associated Genes

Genetic lesions in cancer: Mutations causes genetic damage. Cancers can occur with activating mutations of proto-oncogenes or inactivation of tumor suppressor genes (TSGs). These mutations in cancer may be minute/subtle (e.g., point mutations involving single nucleotides) or may involve segments of chromosomes. The mutations involving segments of chromosomes may be large enough to produce gross changes in chromosome structure that can be detected in a routine karyotyping. Genetic abnormalities in some neoplasms are nonrandom and highly characteristic. Specific chromosomal abnormalities occur in most leukemias and lymphomas and in some nonhematopoietic tumors. Some tumors show point mutations.

Point Mutations

Point mutation is a remarkably subtle alteration, characterized by replacement of one **nucleotide base by a different nucleotide base within a gene**. Though humans have evolved highly efficient mechanisms to recognize and repair nucleotide base changes in DNA, single base changes do occur normally.

Effect: Point mutations can **either activate or inactivate the protein products of the affected genes**. This depends on the precise position of point mutation and consequence.

Activation by point mutation: A proto-oncogene can be converted into oncogene by point mutations. Missense mutation is a point mutations that may lead to hyperactive proteins (i.e., activate protein products). It generally produces a gain of-function by altering amino acid residues in a domain that normally control the protein's activity. For example, point mutations convert the RAS gene (proto-oncogene) into a cancer gene and it is one of the most common in human cancers. Activated HRAS was the first oncogene identified in bladder cancer in humans. This gene had a point mutation in codon 12. This point mutation led to the substitution of valine for glycine in the H-Ras protein. Activating, or gain-of function, mutations in proto-oncogenes are usually somatic rather than germline mutations. Mutations in germline in proto-oncogenes (important regulators of growth during development) usually are lethal in utero. However, there are several exceptions to this rule. For example, c-ret is involved in the pathogenesis of certain heritable endocrine cancers, and c-met, which encodes the receptor for hepatocyte growth factor, is associated with a hereditary form of renal cell carcinoma. For example, when the regulatory subunit of RAS proteins is mutated.

Loss of function by point mutation: It is a nonsense mutation and can generate stop codons (nonsense mutations), that lead to truncated versions of a tumor suppressor. This renders its protein product inactive. In case of tumor suppressor genes (TSGs), point mutations reduce or disable the function of the encoded protein of TSG. Most commonly affected TSG by point mutations in cancer is TP53 ("guardian" type TSG). Another example of nonsense mutation in EphB2 tumor suppressor gene (TSG) associated with prostate cancer.

Chromosomal Changes

Some chromosomal abnormalities are associated with particular neoplasms. These chromosomal abnormalities include changes in the number or structure. These will definitely lead to the dysregulation of genes and is plays an integral role in the pathogenesis of that tumor type. Usually changes in chromosome number (aneuploidy) and structure are considered to be late phenomena in cancer progression. However, in some cases (e.g., in cells that have lost their telomeres), it can be an early event that initiates the malignant transformation process.

- **Specific recurrent chromosomal abnormalities:** These are observed in most leukemias and lymphomas, many sarcomas, and few carcinomas.
- **Gain or loss of chromosomes:** Whole chromosomes may be gained or lost in some cancers.

Detection of chromosomal changes: Chromosomal changes in cancer are usually identified through karyotyping. In this process, the metaphase chromosomes prepared from clinical specimens are morphologically identified. Presently, karyotyping of cancer cell karyotypes are being prepared in research laboratories from deep sequencing of cancer cell genomes. Probably, in future these conventional karyotyping will be succeeded by other methods even in clinical laboratories.

Importance of study of chromosomal changes in tumor cells: It has following uses:

1. Genes in the proximity of recurrent chromosomal breakpoints or deletions are most likely to be either oncogenes (e.g., *MYC, BCL2, ABL*) or tumor suppressor genes (e.g., *APC, RB*).
2. Certain karyotypic abnormalities have **diagnostic value or important prognostic or therapeutic implications.** For example, detection and quantification of BCR-ABL fusion genes or their mRNA products are required for the diagnosis of chronic myeloid leukemia (CML) and are used to monitor the response to BCR-ABL kinase inhibitors.

Gene rearrangements: Gene rearrangement is a mutation in which there is change in the structure of the native chromosome. Gene rearrangements may be produced by different classes of events such as chromosomal translocations or inversions. Specific chromosomal translocations and inversions are highly associated with certain malignancies. They are particularly observed in neoplasms derived from hematopoietic cells and other kinds of mesenchymal cells.

Chromosomal translocations

Proto-oncogenes can be activated by any type of chromosomal rearrangement such as translocations, inversions, amplifications, and small deletions. However, the most common mechanism of activation of proto-oncogenes is by chromosomal translocation. Important examples of oncogenes activated by chromosomal translocations are presented in **Table 13.**

Mechanism of activation of proto-oncogenes by chromosomal translocations In chromosomal translocations, piece of one chromosome is joined with a part of another. These gene rearrangements produce tumors in one of the two ways: (1) **translocation leading to over expression**. (2) ***translocation producing a chimeric (fusion) protein.*** It can occur in two ways:

- **Translocation leading to over expression by promoter or enhancer substitution:** Promoter or enhancers are the regulatory elements in a gene. In this method of proto-oncogene activation, the translocation leads to overexpression of a proto-oncogene by exchanging its regulatory elements with those of another gene, usually one that is highly expressed.
- **Translocation producing a chimeric (fusion) gene:** In this, the coding sequences of two genes are fused in part or in whole. This leads to the expression of a novel chimeric protein with oncogenic properties.

Chromosomal translocation leading to over expression of proto-oncogene: A normal gene like a proto-oncogene in their native/normal position is under control of normal regulatory elements (e.g., promoter). During translocation, this normal gene (e.g., proto-oncogene) is transferred or placed (from their position of normal regulatory elements) in a region not under the normal control. This new location is regulated less effectively than the native proto-oncogene promoter and may have an inappropriate and highly active promoter or enhancer. Examples of overexpression of a proto-oncogene caused by translocation include two different kinds of B-cell lymphoma.

- **Burkitt lymphoma:** Burkitt lymphoma have translocation (**Fig. 23**) in cells usually between chromosomes 8 and 14

Table 13: Examples of oncogenes activated by chromosomal translocations.

Malignancy	*Translocation*	*Affected Genes*	
Leukemia			
• Chronic myeloid leukemia (CML)	(9;22)(q34;q11)	*ABL* 9q34	*BCR* 22q11
• Acute myeloid leukemia (AML)	(8;21)(q22;q22)	*AML* 8q22	*ETO* 21q22
	(15;17)(q22;q21)	*PML* 15q22	*RARA* 17q21
Lymphoma			
• Burkitt lymphoma	(8;14)(q24;q32)	*MYC* 8q24	*IGH* 14q32
• Mantle cell lymphoma	(11;14)(q13;q32)	*CCND1* 11q13	*IGH* 14q32
• Follicular lymphoma	(14;18)(q32;q21)	*IGH* 14q32	*BCL2* 18q21
Sarcoma			
• Ewing sarcoma	(11;22)(q24;q12)	*FLI1* 11q24	*EWSR1* 22q12
Carcinoma			
• Prostatic adenocarcinoma	(7;21) (p22; q22) (17;21)(p21;q22)	*TMPRSS2* (21q22.3)	*ETV1* (7p21.2) *ETV4* (17q21)

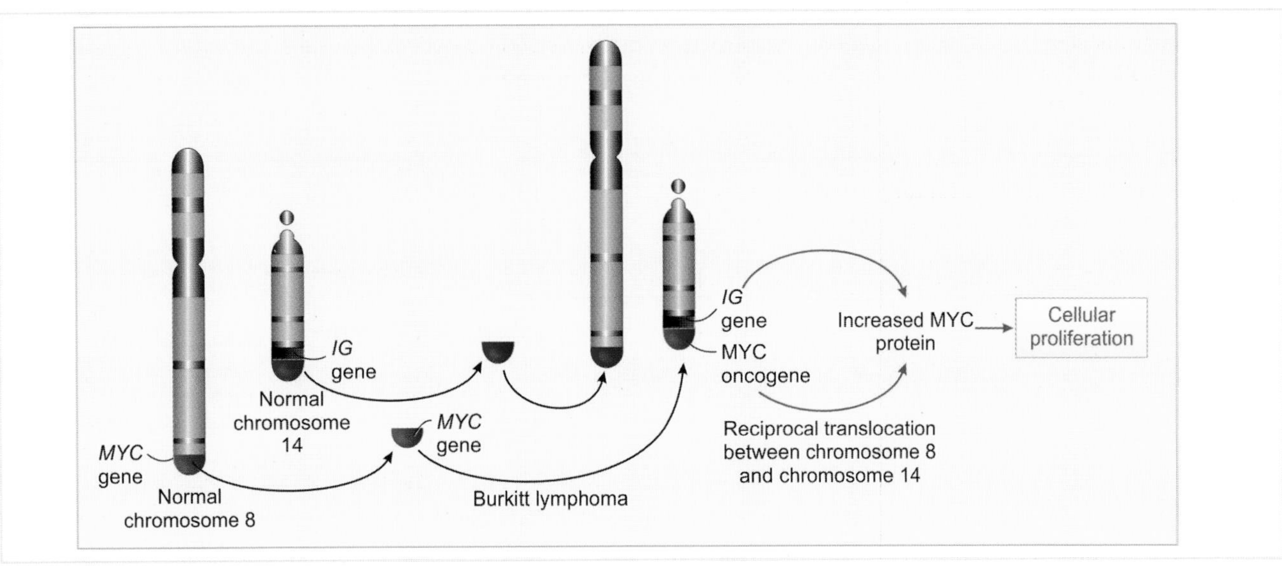

FIG. 23: Chromosomal translocation and activated MYC oncogene in Burkitt lymphoma.

[t(8;14)] in >90% of cases. *MYC* gene is a proto-oncogene involved in cell cycle progression and is present in chromosome 8 (8q24). Normally, MYC is tightly controlled and is most highly expressed in actively dividing cells. Chromosome 14 has regulatory elements (promoter) that control transcription of immunoglobulin heavy chain gene (*IGH* gene). In Burkitt lymphoma, *MYC* -containing segment of chromosome 8 is translocated to chromosome 14 (14q32) and placed adjacent to immunoglobulin heavy chain (*IGH*) gene (i.e., *MYC* juxtapositioned with *IGH*). The genetic notation for the translocation is t(8;14) (q24; q32). This re-location of gene in new regulatory units in the genome can lead to overexpression of the proto-oncogene. The molecular mechanisms of the translocation-mediated overexpression/activation of *MYC* varies. In most cases the translocation removes regulatory sequences of the *MYC* gene (i.e., proto-oncogene) and replaces them with the control regions (i.e., promoter/enhancer sequences) of the *IGH* gene (**Fig. 23**). Consequently, *MYC* coding sequences remain intact, and the MYC protein is constitutively expressed at high levels rather than in a regulated manner. This causes production of excessive amount of MYC protein. is expressed constitutively This probably in association with other genetic alterations, leads to the formation of a dominant clone of B cells which proliferate as a monoclonal neoplasm.

- **Follicular lymphoma:** In follicular lymphoma, there is a reciprocal translocation between chromosomes 14 and 18 (**Fig. 24**). This leads to overexpression of the anti-apoptotic gene, *BCL2*, on chromosome 18. This is also driven by immunoglobulin gene regulatory elements as in Burkitt

Many other chromosomal translocation involving oncogenes and antigen receptor loci in lymphoid tumors have been identified. For these translocations to occur, double stranded DNA breaks must occur simultaneously in at least two places in the genome. This DNA breaks, free DNA ends and they must then be joined to form two new derivative chromosomes. In lymphoid cells, most of these unfortunate molecular changes occur during attempts at normal antigen receptor gene recombination

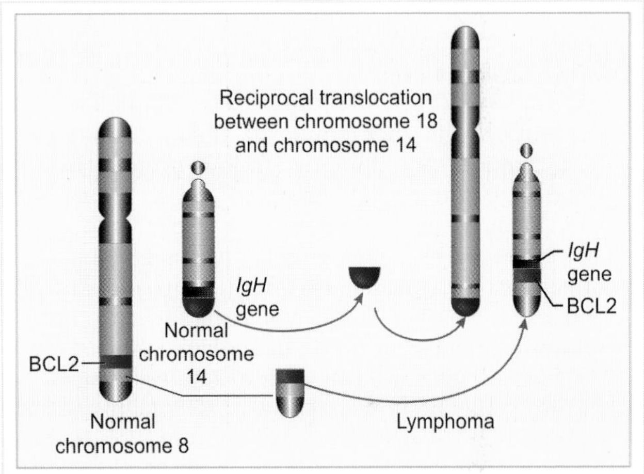

FIG. 24: Chromosomal translocation and activated BCL2 in follicular lymphoma.

(occurs in both B- and T-cell progenitors) or class-switch recombination (which is confined to antigen-stimulated mature B cells). Thus, lymphoid tumors with translocations involving immunoglobulin genes are always are of B-cell origin, and lymphoid tumors with translocations involving T-cell receptor genes are always of T-cell origin. The affected genes are different. But when the translocations involve MYC, there will be overexpression of some protein with oncogenic activity.

Translocation producing a chimeric (fusion) gene: In addition to causing overexpression (discussed before), chromosomal translocation may also create fusion genes. These genes may produce new abnormal chimeric proteins. Thus, a part of one chromosome including part or all of the coding region of a gene (e.g., a proto-oncogene) is transferred to another chromosome, into the coding region of another gene. This result is a fusion (chimeric) gene and produces a new protein. This novel protein shares sequence homology with both the original genes. It drives oncogenesis in a manner that the original genes could not produce. This process is

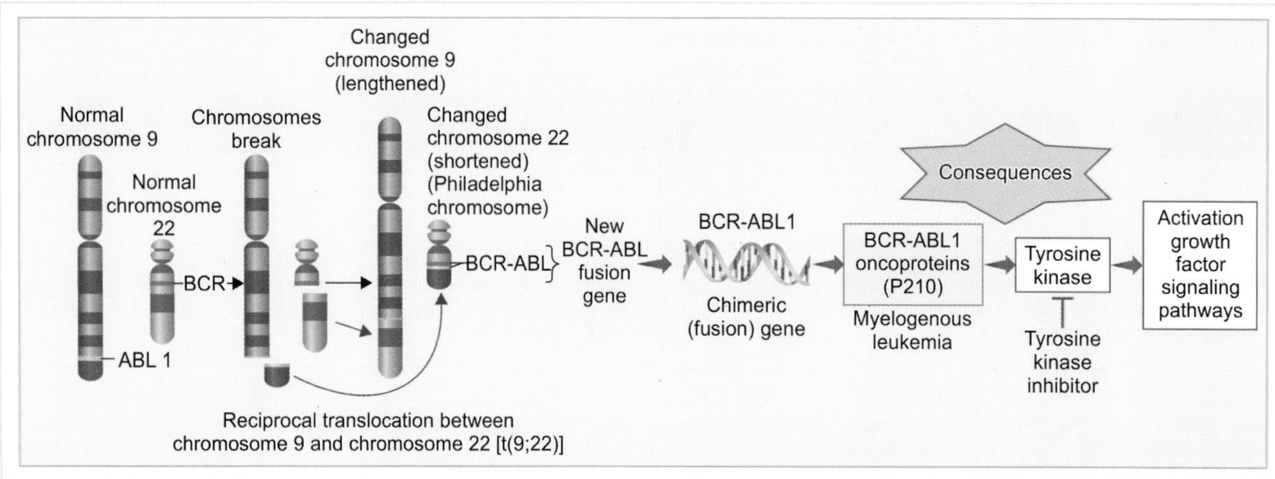

FIG. 25: Balanced reciprocal translocation between long arm of chromosome 9 and chromosome 22 resulting in shortened chromosome 22 known as Philadelphia chromosome.

involved in the pathogenesis of several human leukemias and lymphomas. The first and still the best known example of an acquired chromosomal translocation in a human cancer is the **Philadelphia chromosome**.

- ***Philadelphia (Ph) chromosome (Fig. 25):*** Philadelphia chromosome is an example of oncogene activation by formation of a chimeric (fusion) protein. It is an acquired chromosomal abnormality in all proliferating hematopoietic stem cells (erythroid, myeloid, monocytic, and megakaryocytic precursors). It is found in about 95% of patients with chronic myelogenous leukemia (CML) and a subset of B-cell acute lymphoblastic leukemias. In this, two chromosome breaks occur within the *ABL1* gene on chromosome 9 and within the *BCR* (breakpoint cluster region) gene on chromosome 22. The Ph chromosome consists of a balanced reciprocal translocation between long arm of chromosome 9 and 22, i.e., t(9;22) (q34; q12.2). It increases the length of chromosome 9 and causes shortening of 22. This shortened chromosome 22 is known as Ph chromosome (**Fig. 25**). In this, *ABL1* proto-oncogene from chromosome 9 joins/unites the (juxtaposition to a site) BCR (breakpoint cluster region) gene on chromosome 22. It produces a new hybrid chimeric (fusion) gene (i.e., an oncogene) called *BCR–ABL1*, thus converting ABL1 proto-oncogene into oncogene. BCR-ABL fusion gene encodes a novel tyrosine kinase with potent transforming activity which generates mitogenic and antiapoptotic signals. This product plays a central role in the development of CML. In CML, the tumor cells are dependent on *BCR-ABL1* fusion gene tyrosine kinase activity. This is called oncogene addiction. Cancer cells display functional dependence on activation of specific protumoral signaling pathways in a process referred to as "oncogene addiction".

Other oncogenic fusion genes encode nuclear factors that regulate transcription or chromatin structure. In overactive tyrosine kinases, the mechanism of oncoproteins is well known. But is less known about the mechanism by which nuclear fusion oncoproteins contribute to cancer. One exception with is that observed in acute promyelocytic leukemia (APML). APML is almost always associated with a reciprocal translocation between chromosomes 15 and 17 and produces a PML-RARA fusion gene. It is discussed in detail pages 512–513.

Gene rearrangements in lymphoid tumors: Recurrent gene rearrangements are most common in lymphoid tumors. This may be because of expression of special enzymes in normal lymphocytes that purposefully produce breaks in DNA during the processes of immunoglobulin or T cell receptor gene recombination. Repair of these DNA breaks is prone to errors, and these mistakes sometimes lead to gene rearrangements and activate proto-oncogenes.

Gene rearrangements in mesenchymal tumors: Myeloid neoplasms (acute myeloid leukemias and myeloproliferative disorders) and sarcomas also frequently show gene rearrangements. The cause of the DNA breaks that lead to gene rearrangements in these tumors is not known. Gene rearrangements in myeloid neoplasms and sarcomas produce fusion genes that encode either hyperactive tyrosine kinases (similar to BCR-ABL) or novel oncogenic transcription factors. For example, in Ewing sarcoma there is translocation (11;22) (q24; q12) which produces a fusion gene encoding a chimeric oncoprotein composed of portions of two different transcription factors called EWS and FLI1.

Gene rearrangements in carcinoma: Karyotypically evidence of translocations and inversions are rare in carcinomas. But, recurrent cryptic pathogenic gene rearrangements in carcinomas are revealed by DNA sequencing. The gene rearrangements in solid tumors can produce cancer either by increasing expression of an oncogene or by producing a novel fusion gene.

Deletions

Inactivation by chromosomal deletions are another very common structural abnormality found in tumor cells. Deletion is characterized by a loss of portion of chromatin. It leads to a loss of function phenotype. Deletion may vary from loss of tiny pieces to whole arms of chromosomes. Deletion of specific regions of chromosomes may be led to loss of particular tumor suppressor genes. Amplifications (described further) tend to occur at sites of oncogenes, deletions tend to affect TSGs. In order to produce cancer, tumor suppressors usually require inactivation of both alleles. A common mechanism is inactivating point mutation in one allele, followed by deletion of the other, nonmutated allele. Retinoblastoma may be associated with deletions involving 13q14, the site of the *RB* gene and deletion of the *VHL* tumor suppressor gene on chromosome 3p is a common in renal cell carcinomas. Deletion of 17p is associated with loss of the most important TSG namely *TP53*. There are several other examples of deletions involving tumor suppressor genes and also small insertions of DNA from one site into another. It is to be noted that all deletions need not lead to loss of gene function. Some deletions activate oncogenes through the same mechanisms as chromosomal translocations. For example, in about 25% of T-cell acute lymphoblastic leukemias, there is small deletions of chromosome 1 that juxtapose the *TAL1* proto-oncogene with a nearby active promoter. This leads to overexpression of the TAL1 transcription factor.

Reduction of expression of TSGs or its inactivation: For example, TSGs *p53, PTEN, BRCA1* and *BRCA2* undergo recurrent truncation as a result of chromosome rearrangements in prostate cancer and are usually associated with reduced expression of the TSGs.

Gene amplifications

Overexpression of oncogenes may also result from reduplication and amplification of their DNA sequences. Gene amplification is a chromosomal alteration in which there are an **increased number** (overproduction of **several hundred copies) of gene copies** in the tumor cell. Genetic amplifications are in fact duplications of variable-sized regions of chromosomes. This leads to several fold increase in the expression of a gene (**Fig. 26** and Fig. 45 of Chapter 10.3). These increased numbers of copies can be readily detected by molecular hybridization with appropriate DNA probes. In some cases, the amplified genes produce chromosomal changes that can be detected by microscope. For example, *MYC* gene is amplified in a significant number of epithelial cancers of breast, colorectal, and pancreatic cancer.

Activation by gene amplification causes conversion of proto-oncogenes into oncogenes. Gene amplification produces several hundred copies of the proto-oncogene in tumor cells leading to **overexpression and hyperactivity** of gene product **(normal proteins)**. It has been found mainly in **human solid tumors**.

Patterns of gene amplification (Fig. 27): Two mutually exclusive patterns of gene amplification are as follows:

- **Double minutes: Extrachromosomal multiple, small, structures called "double minutes"**/dmins.
- **Homogeneous staining regions:** Chromosome alteration is referred to a s **homogeneous staining regions (HSR),** if increased copies of gene are inserted or integrated within chromosomes. Increased copies of gene may be inserted into new location in the chromosome, which may be distant from the normal location of the involved oncogenes. HSR regions containing amplified genes does not show normal banding pattern and appear as homogeneous in G-banded karyotype.

Examples of gene amplification: (1) *N-MYC* **gene is amplified in neuroblastomas** (in 25–30% of cases) and associated with poor prognosis; (2) ***HER2/Neu* (also called ERBB2)**

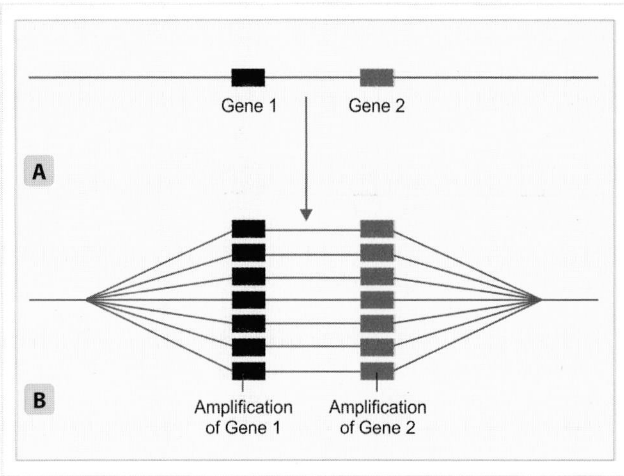

FIGS. 26A AND B: Gene amplification. Two genes are depicted (in blue and red colors). (A) Normal gene. (B) Amplification of these genes.

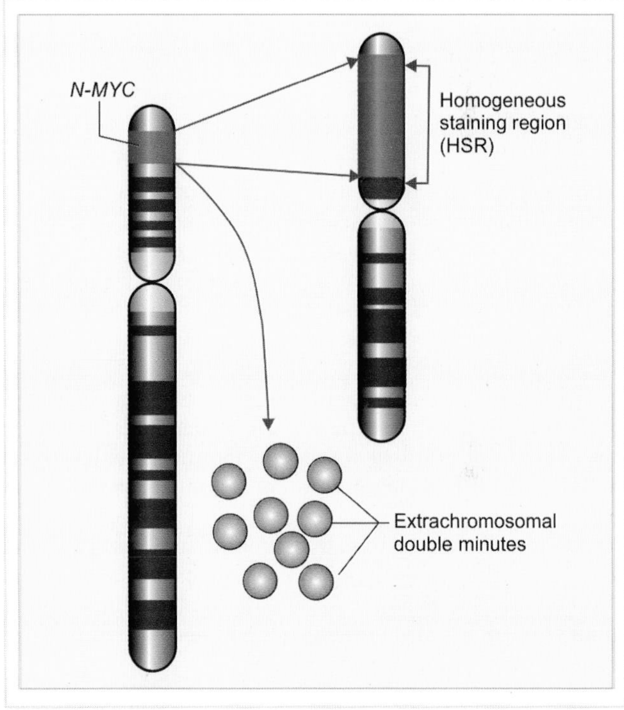

FIG. 27: Amplification of the *N-MYC* gene in human neuroblastomas seen either as extrachromosomal double minutes or as a chromosomally integrated, homogeneous staining region (HSR).

amplification in about 20% of **breast cancer** and also in ovarian cancer. *HER2/Neu gene* encodes a receptor-type tyrosine kinase that structurally resembles the epidermal growth factor (EGF) receptor. Amplification of *HER2/Neu* may be associated with poor overall survival and decreased time to relapse. But antibody targeted against receptor encoded by the *HER2/neu* is now used as adjunctive therapy for these type of breast cancers and are effective. One of the anticancer drugs, namely methotrexate inhibits the enzyme ***dihydrofolate reductase***. After long term treatment with methotrexate, the malignant cells develop drug resistance by amplifying the genes coding for dihydrofolate reductase

Complex chromosomal rearrangements: Sequencing of entire cancer cell genomes allows for comprehensive "reconstruction" of chromosomes from DNA sequences. This has revealed that there is not only a simple chromosomal rearrangement (e.g., small deletions, duplications, or inversions), but also there are more dramatic chromosomal "catastrophes" that arise from chromothrypsis (literally, chromosome shattering). **Dramatic chromosome "catastrophes" are called Chromothripsis** (literally means chromosome shattering). Chromothripsis is seen in about 1% to 2% of cancers and are common in up to 25% of osteosarcomas and in gliomas. It probably develops as a single event in which **dozens to hundreds of chromosome breaks occur within part or across the entirety of a single chromosome or several chromosomes.** Though pathogenesis of these breaks is not clear, probably DNA repair mechanisms are activated when there is chromothripsis. This stitches the pieces of broken chromosomes together in a haphazard way and creates many rearrangements, deletions, and even amplifications. It may be one of the process involved in carcinogenesis. These catastrophic events may simultaneously activate oncogenes and inactivate tumor suppressors leading to carcinogenesis.

Examples of chromosomal alterations in human tumors are listed in **Table 14**.

Table 14: Examples of chromosomal alterations in human tumors.

Type of tumor	*Chromosomal alterations*	*Gene(s)*
Hematopoietic tumors: Translocation		
Chronic myeloid leukaemia	t(9;22)(q34; q11). Alters nuclear tyrosine kinase	*ABL*
Acute myeloid leukaemia	t(8;21)(q22;q22)	*ETO*
Burkitt lymphoma	t(8;14)(q24;q32)	*c-myc-IgH*
	t(2;8)(p12;q24)	*Igk,c-myc*
	t(8;22)(q24;q11)	
Follicular lymphoma	t(14;18)(q32;q21)	*IgH-Bcl-2*
Mantle cell lymphoma	t(11;14)(q13;q32)	*Bcl-1-IgH*
Solid tumors: Translocation		
Ewing's sarcoma/PTEN	t(11;22)(q24;q12)	*EWS-FL1*
	t(21;22)(q22;q12)	*EWS-ERG*
	t(11;22)(q13;q12)	*EWS-WT1*
Synovial sarcoma	t(X;18) (p11.23,q11.2)	*SYT-SSX1*
	t(X;18) (p11.21,q11.2)	*SYT-SSX2*
Malignant melanoma	t(1;19)(q12;p13)	*Not known*
	t(1;6)(q11;q11)	*Not known*
	t(1;14)(q21;q32)	*Not known*
Renal adenocarcinoma	t(X;1)(p11;q21)	*TFE3*
	t(9;15)(p11;q11)	*Not known*
Solid tumors: Deletions (Loss of tumor suppression gene)		
Retinoblastoma	del13q14	*RB*
Wilms' tumor	del11p13	*WT-1*
	del11p15	*Not known*
	del17q12–21	*FWT1*
Bladder, transitional cell carcinoma	del11p13	*Not known*
Lung cancer, small-cell type	del17p13	*TP53*
Colorectal adenocarcinoma	del17p13	*TP53*
	del5q21	*APC*
Breast cancer	del17p13	*TP53*
	del17q21	*BRCA1*
	del13q12–13	*BRCA2*
	del16q22.1	-
Solid tumors: Amplification		
Neuroblastoma	Chromosome 2	*NMYC*
Breast cancer	Chromosome 17 (17q12)	*CERBB2*

(PTEN: phosphatase and tensin homologue)

Aneuploidy

Aneuploidy is the **presence of chromosome numbers that is not multiple of haploid number** (i.e., multiples of 23). It is common in cancers, particularly in carcinomas. In aneuploidy there is either addition or loss of whole chromosomes. It generally results from errors of the mitotic checkpoint. The mitotic checkpoint is the major cell cycle control mechanism that acts to prevent mistakes in chromosome segregation and thereby prevent aneuploidy. The mitotic check point inhibits the irreversible transition to anaphase until all of the replicated chromosomes have made productive attachments to spindle microtubules. Complete absence of the mitotic checkpoint leads to rapid cell death as a consequence of abnormal chromosome segregation. During formation of aneuploidy, chromosomes attach too avidly to mitotic spindles and fail to separate and segregate appropriately. Almost all solid tumors have abnormal karyotypes. Aneuploidy tends to increase the number of copies of key oncogenes and decrease number of copies of potent tumor suppressors.

For example, chromosome 8 is where the *MYC* oncogene is located, is never lost, and usually shows increased/extra copies of *MYC* oncogenes in tumor cells. In contrast, portions of chromosome 17, where the *TP53* gene is located, are often lost. Commonly, tumors lose one copy of a chromosome 10, where the gene for phosphatase and tensin homolog (PTEN, a TSG) is located. Thus, tumor development and progression may be associated with changes in chromosome numbers that increases the dosage of oncogenes and restrict the activity of TSGs.

Uniparental Disomy

It is to be borne in mind that a tumor with a normal karyotype may still have experienced chromosomal loss. This may occur by following mechanisms. One parental chromosome of any particular pair may be lost. This may be replaced by a reduplicated copy of that chromosome derived from the other parent. In other words, one parent's copy of a chromosome may be replaced by a duplicated copy of the other parent's chromosome of the same number. The resulting so-called copy-neutral loss of heterozygosity (CN-LOH) is called uniparental disomy. It is common in many cancers.

Microribonucleic acids (microRNAs) and Cancer is discussed on pages 110–113 and pages 549–553.

EPIGENETIC MODIFICATIONS AND CANCER

Q. Discuss the role of epigenetic changes in carcinogenesis.

Genomics is the study of structural changes in the coding sequences of genes. It is important in the development of cancer. It is known that genesis of tumor may occur due to changes in DNA sequence which lead either to dysfunctional proteins (oncogenes) or loss of proteins (tumor suppressor proteins). However, cancer can develop without changes in DNA sequence.

Definition

Epigenetics is a **reversible, heritable mechanism that controls gene expression independent of DNA base sequences.**

Epigenetics is the broad term used for the mechanisms that control gene expression, independent of DNA base sequences. The term "epigenetics" means "above genetics/genome." In epigenetics gene expression occurs without mutation (i.e., without altering the underlying DNA gene sequence). These regulatory mechanisms simply change the expression patterns, or function of the DNA. In epigenetics, the **changes** are **not due to changes in the nucleotide sequence of the DNA and occur without mutation**. In other words, inheritance that is not encoded in DNA sequence is **epigenetic** as opposed to *genetic*. Epigenetic changes are physiologic processes and maintain normal cellular equilibrium. When these processes go wrong, they produce consequences. In neoplasia, epigenetic mechanisms may suppress and/or facilitate tumor development (**Table 15**).

Epigenetics regulates gene expression by modifying structural configuration of chromatin structure via **histone modification** (e.g., acetylation of specific amino acid residues of histone protein tails) or **modification of DNA via methylation**. **Acetylation of histones leads to activation of gene expression, while DNA methylation is associated with a reduction in gene expression**. Epigenetic modifications do not change or alter the primary sequence of the DNA code but change the chromosomal function. Epigenetics is heritable due to coordination between histone modification and methylation of DNA. However, unlike genetic inheritance, an epigenetic state can usually be reversed. Epigenetic mechanisms play an important role in the establishment, maintenance, and reversibility of transcriptional states. Through epigenetic, the controlled transcriptional on/off states can be maintained through multiple rounds of cell division. The most important epigenetic mechanisms involved in carcinogenesis are to either suppress or to facilitate it, or both. These are listed in **Table 15**.

Table 15: Major mechanisms of epigenetic regulation involved in oncogenesis with example.

Mechanism of epigenetic regulation	*Example of modification*
Covalent (chemical bonds formed by the sharing of electrons between atoms) modifications of deoxyribonucleic acid (DNA)	CpG methylation
Covalent modifications of histones	Acetylation
Remodeling (change or alter the structure)/repositioning (different positioning) of nucleosomes	Incorporation of histone variants
Small noncoding ribonucleic acid (RNAs)	MicroRNAs
Long noncoding RNAs	Pseudogene transcripts

Chromatin Remodeling, Histone Variation, and Histone Modification

Gene activity, or expression, is dependent on a number of complex interacting factors, including the accessibility of the gene promoter to transcription factors.

Structural Configuration of Chromatin

Accessibility of promoter depends on the structural configuration of chromatin. In open chromatin (i.e., euchromatin), gene promoters are accessible to ribonucleic acid (RNA) polymerase and transcription factors. Thus, euchromatin is transcriptionally active. In contrast, heterochromatin (densely packed) is transcriptionally silent.

Chromatin Remodeling (Figs. 28A to C)

One method to change chromatin structure is through **adenosine diphosphate (ATP) dependent chromatin remodeling** (or simply **chromatin remodeling**). **Chromatin remodeling** is the term used for the dynamic changes in the structure of chromatin that occur during the life of a cell. These changes affect nucleosomes position and histone composition and thereby structure of chromatin. The histone composition and the precise positioning of nucleosomes at or near promoters often play a key role in gene regulation. In the process of **chromatin remodeling**, the energy needed to move/reposition the locations and/or compositions of nucleosomes on chromatin (DNA) is derived from ATP hydrolysis. The chromatin remodeling exposes (or obscures) gene regulatory elements such as promoters and makes the DNA more or less amenable to transcription. Therefore, chromatin remodeling is important for both the activation and repression of transcription. There are many families of chromatin remodelers.

Methods of changing chromatin structure by chromatin remodelers

Three effects are possible.

1. **Change in the location of nucleosomes (Fig. 28A):** This may be by shifting the nucleosomes to a new location or a change in the relative spacing of nucleosomes over a long stretch of DNA.
2. **Histone eviction or removal (Fig. 28B):** In this, histone is removed from the DNA. This creates a gap where nucleosomes are not found.
3. **Change in the composition of nucleosomes (Fig. 28C):** By removing standard histones and replacing them with histone variants, it can change the composition of chromosome.

Histone Organization (Packaging the Genome)

Within the nucleus, the DNA is packaged into chromosomes. Nucleosomes are the structural unit of a chromosome. DNA segments are wrapped around the central core of histone proteins to form nucleosome.

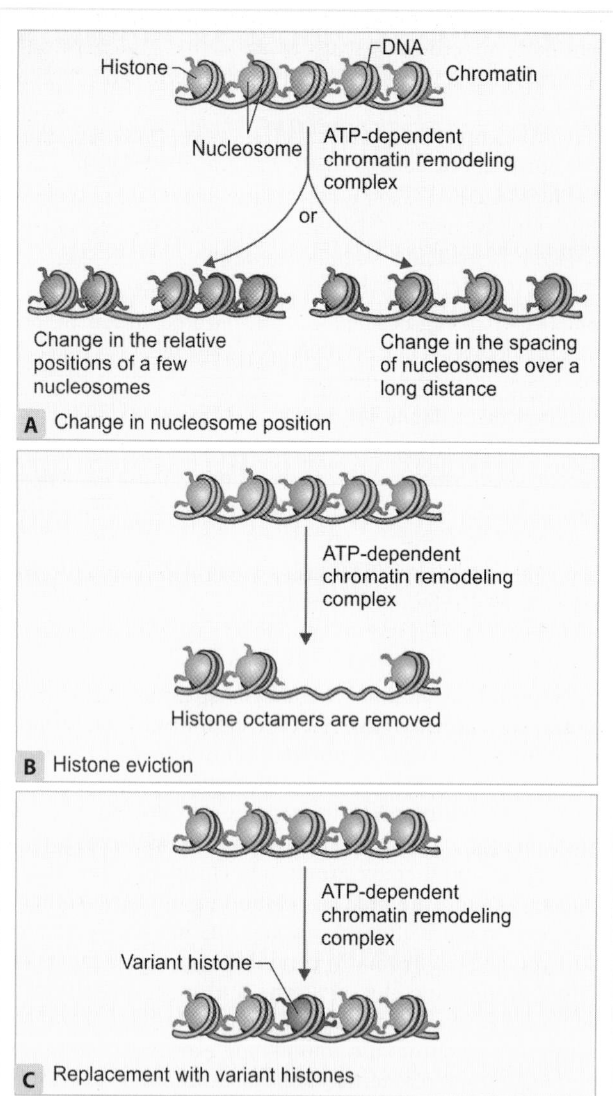

FIGS. 28A TO C: Adenosine triphosphate (ATP)-dependent chromatin remodeling. Chromatin-remodeling complexes may—(A) Change the locations of nucleosomes; (B) Remove histones from the DNA; or (C) Replace core histones with variant histones.

The nucleosome core particle consists of a complex of eight (octamer) histone proteins and 147 base pairs of double-stranded DNA wrapped around the histone octamer. **Histones are a small family of closely related basic proteins** and are the **most abundant chromatin proteins**. Histone proteins form the core of the nucleosome. Each of the core histone proteins consists of a globular domain and a flexible, charged amino terminus called an amino-terminal end/tail (refer **Fig. 30A**) which protrude from the chromatin. The amino acids in the amino-terminal tails of standard histones and histone variants can be modified by acetylation, methylation, and phosphorylation. The C-terminus of histone H2B is involved in chromatin compaction specifically at telomeres. The histone code also controls gene transcription. The histone modifications are an ***important factor in determining the gene expression***.

Classes of Histone (Fig. 29 and Figs. 30A and B)

Histones are divided into five classes (H1, H2A, H2B, H3 and H4) depending on their arginine/lysine ratio. **H1 histones** are the ones least tightly bound to chromatin (**Fig. 29**). Therefore, H1 histone can be easily removed with a salt solution, after which chromatin becomes more soluble. **Nucleosomes contain four major types of histones: H2A, H2B, H3,** and **H4**. The histone octamer consists of two molecules each of histones H2A, H2B, H3, and H4. Almost all cells have the same genetic composition. However, the differentiated cells have distinct structures and functions arising through lineage-specific programs of gene expression. Each nucleosome core particle is separated from the next by about 80 bp of DNA and the linker histone H1.

Chromatin Organization (Fig. 31)

Nucleosomes resemble beads joined by short DNA linkers. The entire structure is generically called *chromatin.*

Heterochromatin and Euchromatin (Fig. 31)

The winding and compaction of chromatin in a cell varies in different genomic regions. When histological section stained by hematoxylin and eosin (H&E) are seen under light microscopy, the nuclear chromatin is seen in two basic forms, namely—(1) histochemically dense and transcriptionally inactive ***heterochromatin*** and (2) histochemically dispersed and transcriptionally active ***euchromatin.*** After the completion of mitosis, most of the chromatin in highly compacted mitotic chromosomes returns to its diffuse interphase condition. However, about 10% of the chromatin generally remains in a condensed, compacted form throughout interphase. This compacted, densely stained chromatin (histochemically

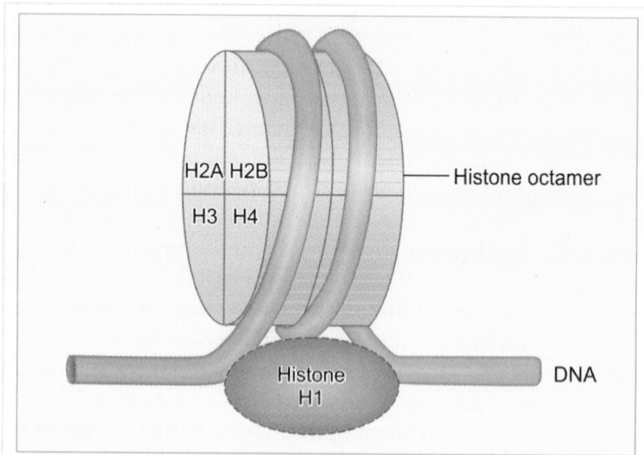

FIG. 29: Schematic diagram of the structure of nucleosome core particle and an associated histone. The core particle consists of about 1.8 turns (~146 base pairs) of negatively supercoiled deoxyribonucleic acid (DNA) wrapped around the surface of a protein cylinder. The protein cylinder consists of two each of histone molecules H2A, H2B, H3, and H4 that form the histone octamer. The H1 linker histone binds (interacts) near the sites where DNA enters and exits the nucleosome. DNA is wrapped around. The position of histone H1, when it is present, is depicted by the dashed outline at the bottom of the figure. The C-terminus (see Fig. 32) of histone H2B (not depicted in figure) is involved in chromatin compaction specifically at telomeres.

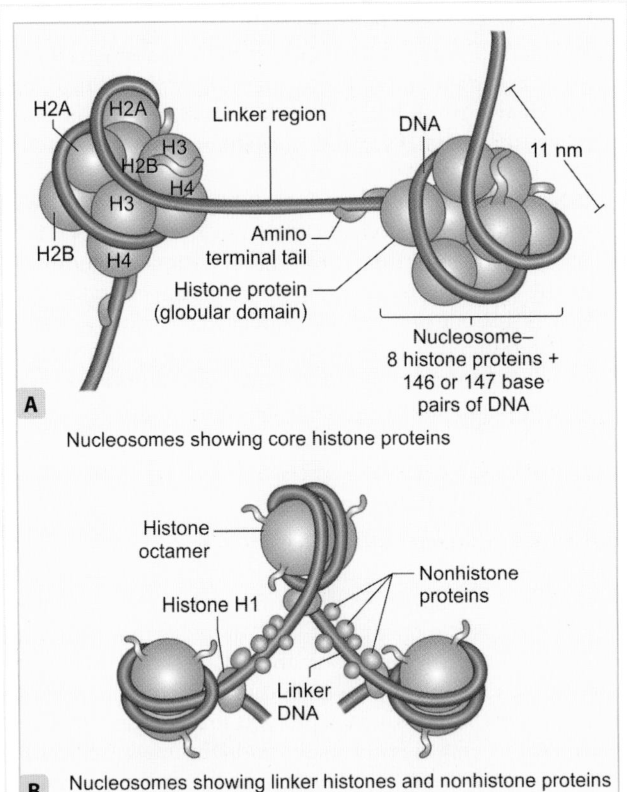

FIGS. 30A AND B: Nucleosome structure. (A) A nucleosome consists of 146 or 147 bp of DNA wrapped around an octamer of core histone proteins. (B) The linker region of DNA connects adjacent nucleosomes. The linker histone H1 and nonhistone proteins also bind to this linker region.

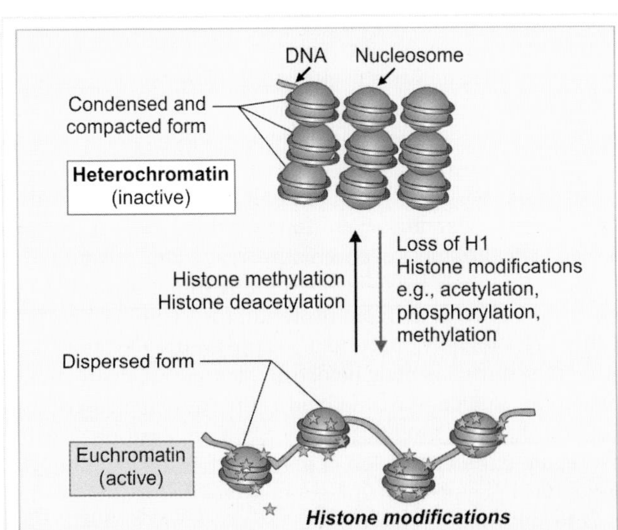

FIG. 31: Heterochromatin and euchromatin. Histone modification can regulate the relative state of deoxyribonucleic acid (DNA) unwinding, thereby allowing the access for transcription factors. Example of histone modifications includes acetylation, methylation, and/or phosphorylation. Histone acetylation "opens up" the chromatin structure, whereas methylation of particular histone residues condenses the DNA and leads to gene silencing. DNA itself can also be also be methylated, a modification that is associated with transcriptional inactivation.

dense) during interphase is called **heterochromatin** (transcriptionally inactive) to distinguish it from **euchromatin** (histochemically dispersed and transcriptionally active), which returns to a dispersed state. Irrespective of euchromatic or heterochromatic region of the genome, both are stably inherited from one cell generation to the next. Because only euchromatin permits gene expression and thereby dictates cellular identity and activity, there are a host of mechanisms that tightly regulate the state of chromatin.

Histone Modification

The carboxyl terminal (C-terminal see **Fig. 32**) two-thirds of the histone molecules are hydrophobic, whereas, their amino terminal thirds are particularly rich in basic amino acids. **These four core histones can undergo at least six types of covalent modification or post-translational modifications (PTMs).** These include—(1) acetylation, (2) methylation, (3) phosphorylation, (4) adenosine diphosphate (ADP)-ribosylation, (5) monoubiquitylation, and (6) sumoylation. These histone modifications play important roles in chromatin structure and function (**Table 16**).

Table 16: Role of modification of histones.

Post-translational modification of histones	***Associated with***
Acetylation (or deacetylation) of histones H3 and H4	Activation (or inactivation by deacetylation) of gene transcription
Acetylation of core histones	Chromosomal assembly during DNA replication
Methylation of histones	Activation gene transcription
Phosphorylation of histone H1	Condensation of chromosomes during the replication cycle
ADP-ribosylation of histones	DNA repair
Monoubiquitylation	Gene activation, repression, and heterochromatic gene silencing
Sumoylation of histones	Transcription repression

(ADP: adenosine diphosphate; DNA: deoxyribonucleic acid; SUMO: small ubiquitin-related modified)

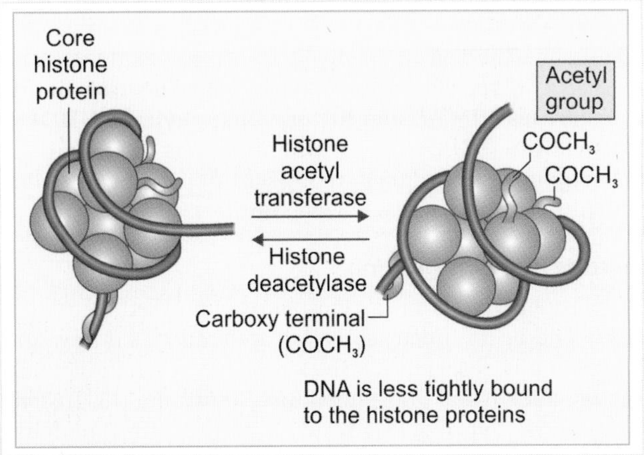

FIG. 32: Effect of histone acetylation. Acetylation of the histone core by histone acetyltransferase causes the deoxyribonucleic acid (DNA) to become less tightly bound to the histones. Histone deacetylase removes the acetyl groups.

Histone Acetylation and Deacetylation

Acetylation of histones leads to gene expression while deacetylation reverses the effect. Usually, methylation of DNA results in the inactivation of genes.

Histone acetylation (Fig. 32)

Acetylation of histones at a gene or chromosomal region leads to open chromatin and is usually associated with increased transcriptional activity and activation of gene expression. Acetylation mainly occurs on the lysine residues in the amino terminal ends (i.e., acetylation of a lysine side chain) of histones. The attachment of the acetyl group (-$COCH_3$) by acetylation of a lysine residue changes the positive charge of the histone molecule. This disrupts the electrostatic attraction between the histone protein and the negatively charged DNA backbone. This leads to an "opening up" transcriptionally permissive chromatin configuration and increase transcription. The acetylation of histones is performed by enzymes called histone acetyltransferases (HATs). Histone deacetylases (HDAC) reverse this process, leading to chromatin condensation. Many transcription factors and coactivators have intrinsic HAT activity. There are three HAT families, namely GNAT, MYST, and CBP/p300 families. There are also more than a dozen other proteins with HAT activity. Several mutations can affect HAT genes. HDACs may be dysregulated in cancers and cause silencing of TSGs as well as derepression (or activation) of oncogenes. The combination of histone modifications and DNA methylation constitutes an intricate regulatory network. Their disruption and plays an important role in oncogenesis.

Histone deacetylation

It causes chromatin condensation, making it inaccessible for transcription. Thus, it inactivates gene expression and silences transcriptional activity. This reaction is catalyzed by enzymes called HDACs. Thus, the degree of histone acetylation depends on the activity of HATs and HDACs. There are about 18 HDACs and they belong to three classes (Class I, II and III).

Histone Methylation

As already discussed, the acetylation of lysine residues of histone changes the charge of histone molecule. But methylation of lysine residues does not change the charge of the histone molecule. However, it changes its basicity and hydrophobicity. **Histone methylation is more stable than histone acetylation** and thus more relevant for epigenetic inheritance. The degree of methylation of histone is depends on the activity of specific **writer enzymes called histone methyl transferases (HMTs) and histone demethylases (HDMs)**. Methylation of histone lysine residues can lead to transcriptional activation or repression, depending on which histone residue is "marked." (refer further)

Histone Phosphorylation

The phosphorylation and dephosphorylation of serine residues of histone of the nucleosome is catalyzed by kinases and phosphatases, respectively. The kinase has several functions, one of which is the phosphorylation of histone H3. *Histone phosphorylation* of serine residues can open or condense chromatin, thereby increase or decrease transcription, respectively.

Other histone modification are presented in **Table 16**.

Other Histone Modifying Factors

Nucleosomes are highly dynamic structures regulated by a range of nuclear proteins and post-translational modifications.

- **Chromatin remodeling complexes:** They can reposition nucleosomes on DNA. This may either expose or obscure gene regulatory elements such as promoters.
- **"Chromatin writer" complexes:** They can carry out more than 70 different covalent histone modifications which are termed as **marks**. These modifications include—(1) methylation, (2) acetylation, and (3) phosphorylation of specific histone amino acid residues as described earlier.
- Histone marks can be reversed by the activity of **"chromatin erasers"**. Other proteins function as **"chromatin readers"**, by binding histones that bear particular marks. They can also regulate gene expression.

Epigenetic Changes in Cancer

Apart from mutations in DNA, epigenetic aberrations (changes) may also be responsible for the malignant transformation of cells. Epigenetic modifications (changes) may alter the expression of cancer genes, or genes that control of differentiation and self-renewal, and also drug sensitivity and drug resistance. Epigenetic mechanisms include (i) histone modifications (histones are the proteins that package DNA into chromatin) by enzymes associated with chromatin regulatory complexes (depending on their nature histone modification may either enhance or decrease gene expression (ii) DNA methylation by DNA methyltransferases which tends to silence gene expression, and (iii) other alterations that regulate the higher order organization of DNA (e.g., looping of enhancer elements onto gene promoters).

General features of epigenetics: The epigenetic state of the cell governs the expression of genes. This in turn determines the lineage commitment and differentiation state of both normal and neoplastic cells. Epigenetic modifications are usually passed on to daughter cells. However, occasionally similar to DNA mutations, epigenetic alterations may occur that result in changes in gene expression. Aberrant DNA methylation in cancer cells may silence some tumor suppressor genes.

Nuclei of cancer cells show abnormal morphologies such as hyperchromasia, chromatin clumping, or chromatin clearing (so-called vesicular nuclear chromatin). These nuclear changes are due to disturbances of chromatin organization. Sequencing of cancer genomes have detected many mutations involving genes that encode epigenetic regulatory genes (proteins) (**Table 17**). Probably, morphologic appearance of cancer cells is due to acquired genetic defects in factors that maintain the epigenome. Epigenome is defined as the complete description of all the chemical modifications to DNA and histone proteins that regulate the expression of genes within the genome. The alterations in cancer cell epigenomes can be broadly divided into the following categories:

1. **Silencing of tumor suppressor genes by local hypermethylation of DNA:** Some cancer cells may show selective hypermethylation of the promoters of tumor suppressor genes (TSGs). This leads to transcriptional silencing of these genes. Usually, hypermethylation involves only one copy/allele of TSG, and the function of the other copy/allele of the affected tumor suppressor gene is lost through another mechanism. These mechanisms include disabling of these

Table 17: Examples of epigenomic regulatory genes that are mutated in cancer

Gene(s)	*Tumor (frequency of mutation)*
DNA methylation	
1. *DNMT3A*	Acute myeloid leukemia (~20%)
Histone methylation	
2. *MLL1*	Acute leukemia in infants (~90%)
3. *MLL2*	Follicular lymphoma (~90%)
4. *CREBBP/EP300*	Diffuse large B-cell lymphoma (~40%)
Nucleosome positioning/chromatin remodeling	
5. *ARID1*	Clear cell carcinoma of ovary (~60%), endometrial carcinoma (~30%–40%)
6. *SNF5*	Malignant rhabdoid tumor (~100%)
7. *PBRM1*	Renal carcinoma (~30%)
Histone H3 variants (nucleosome components)	
8. *H3F3A, HIST1H3B*	Pediatric gliomas (~30%–80%). Varies depending on the site of tumor

TSG by point mutation or deletion. One of the example of tumor suppressor gene that is hypermethylated in many cancers is *CDKN2A*. This is a complex locus and it encodes two tumor suppressors, p14/ARF and p16/INK4a and they enhance activity of p53 and RB respectively.

2. **Global changes in DNA methylation:** Apart from local hypermethylation of tumor suppressor genes, many tumors reveal abnormal patterns of DNA methylation throughout their genomes. For example, acute myeloid leukemia is a tumors commonly showing abnormal DNA methylation. Sometimes, they have mutations in genes encoding DNA methyltransferases or other proteins that influence DNA methylation (see **Table 17**). The most important consequence of methylation is altered expression of multiple genes. Depending on the nature of local changes, these methylated genes may be overexpressed or underexpressed compared to normal genes.
3. **Changes in histones:** Histones causes "packaging" of DNA. Any changes in histone positioning or posttranslational modifications (so-called histone marks) can regulate gene transcription. Cancer cells usually show changes in histones near genes that influence behavior of cells. Similar to DNA methylation, these alterations may have a genetic basis. This may be due to mutations in proteins that "write," "read," and "erase" histone marks or that position nucleosomes on DNA (see **Table 17**). In some malignant tumors, driver mutations occur in the histone genes themselves.

Epigenome and Cancer

Their relationship is discussed below:

- **Lineage restriction:** The lineage-specificity of certain oncogenes and tumor suppressor genes have been found to have an epigenetic basis. Tumor suppressors and oncoproteins can be broadly divided into two classes namely: Those that are (i) mutated or otherwise dysregulated in many cancers (e.g., RAS, MYC, p53); and (ii) mutated in few subset of tumors (e.g., RB in retinoblastoma, VHL in renal cell carcinoma, APC in colon carcinoma). Thus, second category is lineage restricted. Similar to normal cells, the lineage or differentiation state of a cancer cell is dependent on epigenetic modifications. These epigenetic modifications produce a pattern of gene expression that characterizes that particular cell type. Some genes (e.g., encoding Notch receptors) act as a tumor suppressor in one lineage and behave as an oncogene in another. Thus, the *NOTCH1* gene is one of the commonly mutated tumor suppressor genes in squamous cell carcinoma of the skin. This mutation result in loss of function and lead to impaired differentiation. *NOTCH1* gene is also the most commonly mutated oncogene in T-cell acute lymphoblastic leukemia. In this mutations, different parts of the gene result in gain of function and drive the expression of pro-growth genes such as MYC.
- **Therapeutic target:** The knowledge about the role of epigenetic alterations in cancer has showed the new path for the treatment of cancer with drugs that correct epigenetic abnormalities. The knowledge about the role of epigenetic alterations in cancer has showed the new path for the treatment of cancer with drugs that correct epigenetic abnormalities. The epigenetic state of a cell depends on reversible modifications that are carried out by enzymes. Epigenetic changes are probably reversible by drugs that inhibit DNA-modifying or histone-modifying factors. Hence, epigenome is a therapeutic target. These drugs include inhibitors of histone deacetylases, chromatin erasers that remove acetyl groups from histones that can be used in certain lymphoid tumors, and DNA methylation inhibitors can be used to treat myeloid tumors. The principle behind the use of these drugs is partly on the assumption that these drugs may reactivate tumor suppressor genes.
- **Epigenetic heterogeneity:** Probably cancers may show significant epigenetic heterogeneity. Similar to genomic instability which gives rise to genetic heterogeneity in cancers, cancers may also have numerous epigenetic heterogeneity from cell to cell within individual tumors. This may be responsible for drug resistance. For example, epigenetic alterations can produce resistance of lung cancer cells to inhibitors of EGF receptor signaling. When the inhibitors are removed, the lung cancer cells may turn back to their prior inhibitor-sensitive state.

Noncoding RNAs and cancer are discussed in detail on pages 549–553.

Molecular Basis of Multistep Carcinogenesis

Malignant tumors must acquire multiple "hallmarks" of cancer. Hence, cancers result from the stepwise accumulation of multiple mutations. These mutations complement each other to produce a fully malignant tumor. The malignant tumors develop from a sequential accumulation of cancer-promoting and is a multistep process. Genome-wide sequencing of cancers has shown as few as 10 or so mutations in certain leukemias to many thousands of mutations (most of them are passengers rather than driver mutations) in tumors that arise following chronic exposure to carcinogens (e.g., lung cancers following cigarette smoking). Probably, normal epithelial cells can be transformed to malignant cells by the following multiple steps: (1) activation of RAS; (2) inactivation of RB; (3) inactivation of p53; (4) inactivation of PP2A (protein phosphatase 2 A is a tumor suppressive phosphatase and negatively regulates many signaling pathways); and (5) constitutive expression of telomerase. Cells which acquire all these alterations become immortal. They produce invasive, malignant tumor when injected into immunodeficient mice.

In contrast to the events mentioned in the mice in laboratory, in human cancer, probably these never occur simultaneously during the natural development. Instead, they may occur in a stepwise fashion. Supporting evidence for this is adenoma carcinoma sequence in carcinoma of colon. By molecular analyses at each stage has shown that precancerous lesions have few mutations than adenocarcinomas. It is also observed that certain mutations likely to occur early (e.g., mutations in the tumor suppressor gene APC) or late (e.g., mutations in TP53) in the process. Other examples include precursor lesions that progress to epithelial cancers, such as dysplasias of the cervix, epidermis, and oral mucosa, and hyperplasias of the endometrium.

DNA METHYLATION AND INACTIVATION OF GENES

Deoxyribonucleic acid structure can be modified by the covalent attachment of methyl groups, a mechanism called **DNA methylation.** DNA methylation (**Figs. 33A** to **D**) is another regulatory mechanism that silences gene expression.

DNA Methylation at CpGs Regulates Promoter Activity

The amount of a protein in a cell is as important as the structure of that protein. The amount of protein produced depends on the level of transcription of a gene. Transcription, in turn, depends on promoter activity in a gene. The promoters of many genes contain disproportionate concentrations of CpG dinucleotides, called "**CpG islands**". [*Note:* CpG refers to a dinucleotide of C and G in DNA that is connected by an interbase phosphodiester (*p*) linkage/bond]. These CpG islands are commonly 1,000–2,000 base pairs (bp) in length and contain a high number of CpG sites. CpG islands predominate in promoter regions of many genes and in repetitive DNA sequences.

- **DNA methylation: DNA** methylation occurs on the cytosine (C) base. About 20% of CG sequences constituting about 2–7% of the DNA in human DNA exists in methylated form. Cytosine in the sequence CG (CpG) of DNA can be modified by the addition of a methyl group to cytosine. DNA methylation occurs via an enzyme called **DNA methyltransferase** (DNMT). This enzyme attaches a methyl group to the number 5 position of the cytosine base and forms 5′-methyl cytosine. This process is termed methylation. Note that there are two strands in the DNA and this cytosine is present in both strands. Methylation of the cytosine in both DNA strands is called as full methylation (**Fig. 33D**), whereas methylation of only one DNA strand is called hemimethylation (**Fig. 33C**). DNA methylation is tightly regulated by DNMT, demethylating enzymes, and methylated-DNA-binding proteins.
- **DNA methylation usually inhibits (silences or inactivates) the transcription of genes** (thereby loss or inhibition of transcriptional activity), particularly when it occurs in the vicinity of the promoter regions. Inhibition of transcription is because methyl cytosines usually silence the gene immediately downstream. The inhibition of transcription may be due to two reasons, namely—(1) CpG methylation prevents transcription factors from binding the promoter and (2) methylation may recruit transcriptional suppressors to the site. Methylation of DNA correlates with deacetylation of histones and this provides a double means for repression of genes.
- Unmethylated CpG islands are correlated with active genes, whereas suppressed genes contain methylated CpG islands. Thus, DNA methylation may play an important role in the silencing of tissue-specific genes to prevent them from being expressed in the wrong tissue.
- Similar to histone modifications, DNA methylation is tightly regulated.

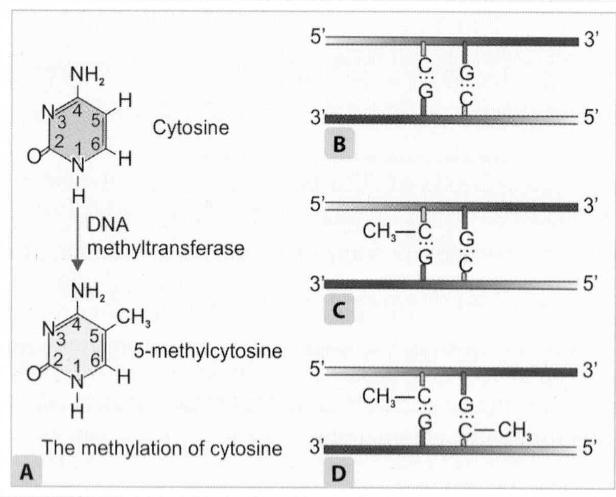

FIGS. 33A TO D: Deoxyribonucleic acid (DNA) methylation on cytosine bases. (A) Methylation occurs via an enzyme known as DNA methyltransferase. It attaches a methyl group to the number 5 carbon on cytosine. The CG sequence can be (B) unmethylated, (C) hemimethylated, or (D) fully methylated.

Methods of Transcriptional Silencing via Methylation

Methylation can affect transcription in two general ways.

- **Methylation of CpG islands may prevent or enhance the binding of regulatory transcription factors to the promoter region.** For example, methylated CG sequences can prevent the binding of an activator protein to an enhancer element, probably by the protrusion of methyl group into the major groove of the DNA (**Fig. 34A**). The inability of an activator protein to bind to the DNA can inhibit the initiation of transcription. However, CG methylation does not reduce the movement of RNA polymerase along a gene. The methylation must occur in the vicinity of the promoter to have an effect on transcription.
- Methylation can inhibit transcription via proteins known as **methyl-CpG-binding proteins**. These proteins contain a domain called the methyl-binding domain. This domain specifically recognizes a methylated CG sequence and binds to it (**Fig. 34B**). After binding to the DNA, the methyl-CpG-binding protein recruits other proteins to the region that inhibit transcription. For example, methyl-CpG binding proteins may recruit HDAC to a methylated

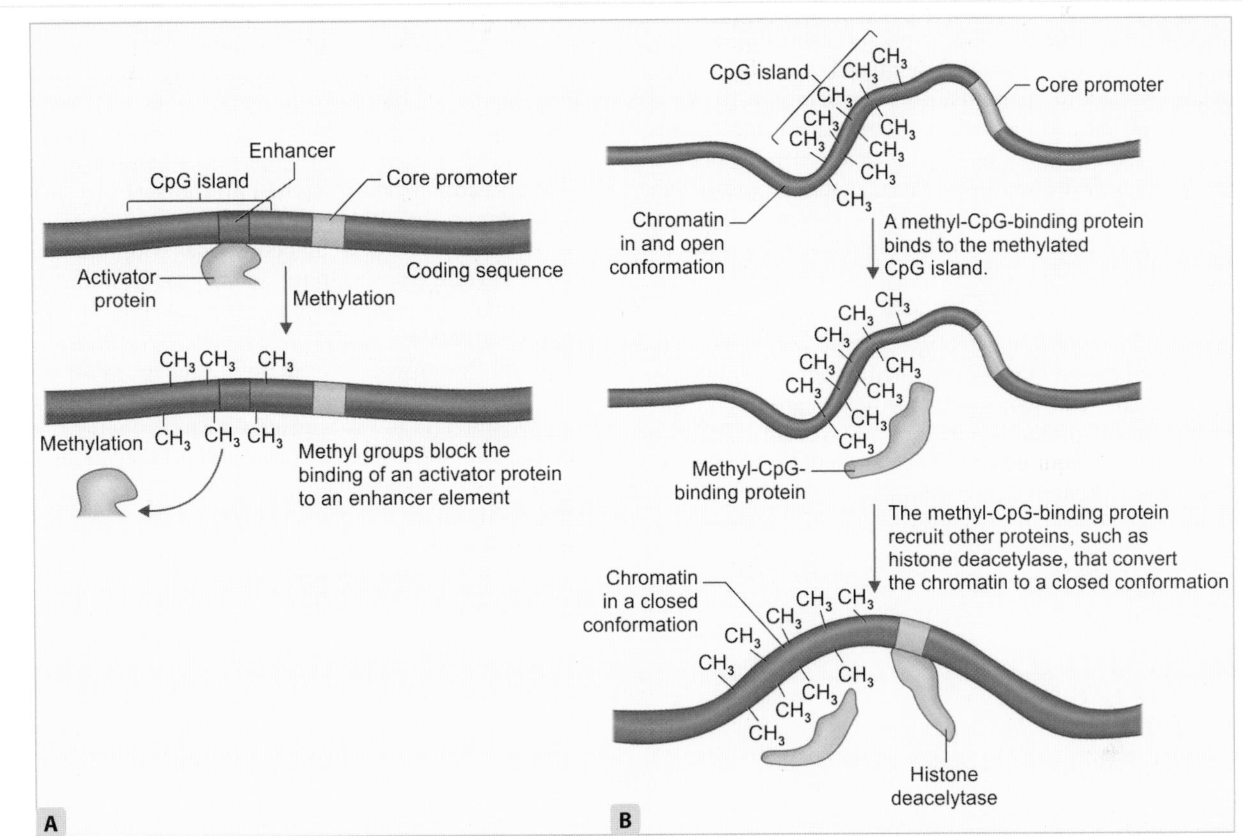

FIGS. 34A AND B: Methods of transcriptional silencing via deoxyribonucleic acid (DNA) methylation. (A) The methylation of a CpG island may inhibit the binding of transcriptional activators to the promoter region. (B) The binding of a methyl-CpG-binding protein to a CpG island may lead to the recruitment of proteins, such as histone deacetylase. This converts chromatin to a closed conformation and thus suppresses transcription.

CpG island near a promoter. Histone deacetylation removes acetyl groups from the histone proteins. This converts chromatin to a closed conformation that makes it more difficult for nucleosomes to be removed from the DNA. In this way, deacetylation tends to inhibit/suppress transcription.

Deoxyribonucleic Acid Methylation is Heritable

The DNA in a particular cell may become methylated by ***de novo*** **methylation** (i.e., the methylation of DNA that was previously unmethylated). When a fully methylated segment of DNA replicates during cell division, one strand will contain the methylated cytosine and the newly made daughter strand will contain unmethylated cytosines. Such DNA, in which only one strand is methylated, is said to be hemimethylated. This hemimethylated DNA is efficiently recognized by DNMT (DNA methyltransferase). This enzyme makes it fully methylated and this process is called **maintenance methylation**. It is named so because it preserves the methylated condition in future cells. However, maintenance methylation does not act on unmethylated DNA. Maintenance methylation is an efficient process. In contrast, *de novo* methylation and demethylation are infrequent and highly regulated events. Once methylation has occurred, methylated DNA sequences are inherited during cell division and they can then be transmitted from mother to daughter cells via maintenance methylation.

Deoxyribonucleic Acid Methylation

Deoxyribonucleic acid methylation in the genome refers to the methylation of cytosine (5-methyl-cytosine, m^5C) within a CpG dinucleotide. CpG is a palindromic sequence. **Palindrome** is a word, number, or other sequence of characters which reads the same backward as forward (e.g., *madam* or *racecar)*. Typically, the cytosines in both strands of CpG dinucleotides are methylated. Because m^5C (methylated cytosine) can undergo spontaneous deamination to thymine, methylated CpG dinucleotides are hot spots for mutation. They are slowly eliminated during evolution. Generally, these CpG islands are unmethylated and overlap the promoter and exon 1 of a gene. High levels of DNA methylation in gene regulatory elements usually result in condensation of chromatin and transcriptional silencing. Binding of transcription factors or the process of transcription protects DNA from methylation.

Deoxyribonucleic Acid Hypomethylation

DNA in most cancer cells is hypomethylated, when compared to their normal tissue counterparts. This is found in repetitive DNA sequences, and also in exons and introns of protein-encoding genes. The degree of DNA hypomethylation may increase as oncogenesis advances from a benign proliferation to a malignant tumor. Undermethylation or hypomethylation destabilizes DNA structure. This favors recombination during mitosis, leading to increased deletions, translocations, chromosomal rearrangements, and aneuploidy. All these chromosomal abnormalities contribute to malignant progression. Hypomethylation of genes involved in cell proliferation may increase transcription of such genes. It is observed in latent human tumor viruses (e.g., HPV, Epstein–Barr virus), in which hypomethylation may lead to tumor development.

Epigenetic Therapy of Cancers

Abnormal epigenetic changes play an important role in the progression of cancer. Epigenetic changes allow expression of normally silenced genes and result in cancer cell dedifferentiation and proliferation. Many diseases are associated with inherited or acquired epigenetic alterations. Epigenetic alterations (e.g., histone acetylation and DNA methylation), unlike genetic changes; are readily reversible. They are therefore amenable to intervention. This epigenetic mechanism can be used for therapeutic purpose.

- **Inhibitors of** HDAC can also be used as epigenetic therapy for cancers. HDAC inhibitors stimulate TSG expression by allowing acetylation of histones in chromatin structure. Epigenetic therapy of cancer by using various inhibitors (individually or in combination) is a great promise. For example, cutaneous T-cell lymphoma is caused due to the re-expression of genes that had previously been silenced in the tumor. The HDAC inhibitor (e.g., vorinostat) is used for the treatment of this cutaneous T-cell lymphoma. These genes encode transcription factors that promote T-cell differentiation as opposed to proliferation, thereby causing tumor regression.
- Hypermethylation of DNA of TSGs is observed in certain cancers. The enzyme DNMT is responsible for DNA methylation and this is targeted for cancer therapy. Many inhibitors of DNMT (e.g., 5-azacytidine) may be used for the treatment of leukemia.
- DNA methylation inhibitors are already being used in the treatment of various forms of cancer.

Role of modification of histones is presented in **Table 16**.

10.3 Cellular and Molecular Hallmarks of Cancer

CHAPTER OUTLINE

INTRODUCTION

Normal cellular proliferation and differentiation are essential to tissue homeostasis. The tissue homeostasis is maintained by the delicate balance between cellular proliferation and differentiation with senescence (senescence is the process by which cells permanently lose their ability to divide) and programmed cell death. The new cells replace dying cells as part of normal tissue function or during tissue repair. Cell proliferation occurs as cells divide, a process that occurs through an orderly set of steps known as the cell cycle. The neoplastic process involves a fundamental disruption of these homeostatic mechanisms and cell proliferation gives rise to cancer development and metastasis.

HALLMARKS OF CANCER

In 2000 and later updated in 2011, Douglas Hanahan and Robert Weinberg rationalized the major biological capabilities that allow cancer cells to grow and produce a tumor and its metastatic dissemination. **All cancers display eight fundamental changes in cell physiology. These are considered as the hallmarks (Box 6 and Fig. 35)** or characteristics **of cancer**. These are typical of a cancer cell. The eight hallmarks may be brought out by genetic and epigenetic alteration. The hallmarks of cancer are necessary biological and functional capabilities acquired by cancer cells during the multistep development of human tumors. These are common to many forms of human cancer (**Fig. 35**). Each one serves a distinct role in supporting the development, progression, and persistence of tumors and their constituent cells.

Enabling Factors

Apart from the eight hallmarks, there are two other distinctive facilitating or accelerating features that contribute to the development of cancer. These are termed as enabling factors because they promote cellular transformation and subsequent tumor progression. These are:

Box 6: Hallmarks of cancer.

- Sustaining proliferative signaling (self-sufficiency in growth signals)
- Evading growth suppressors (insensitivity to growth-inhibitory signals)
- Resisting cell death (evasion of apoptosis)
- Enabling replicative immortality [limitless replicative potential (immortality)]
- Sustained angiogenesis (inducing angiogenesis)
- Activating invasion and metastasis
- Altered cellular metabolism [reprogramming energy metabolism (dysregulating cellular energetics)]
- Evading immune destruction (*evasion of immune surveillance)*

- Genetic instability and mutation (which enables mutational alteration of hallmark-enabling genes)
- Tumor (*cancer*)-promoting inflammation (immune inflammation)

Most cancer cells acquire these properties during their development, usually due to mutations in critical genes. Mutations in genes that regulate some or all of these hallmarks are seen in every cancer.

Note: Gene symbols are italicized but not their protein products (e.g., *RB* gene and RB protein, *TP53* and p53, *MYC* and MYC).

Hallmark 1: Sustaining Proliferative Signaling

Q. Discuss oncogenes in neoplasia.

Q. Discuss the classification, detection, and analysis of oncogenes. Discuss the recent concepts of carcinogenesis and role of oncogenes.

When normal cells receive signals, it guides and checks all their activities and cells enter and progress through cell cycle. However, cancer cells determine their own destinies. They have the capacity to proliferate without external stimuli and multiply independently without any regulatory control. Aberrations

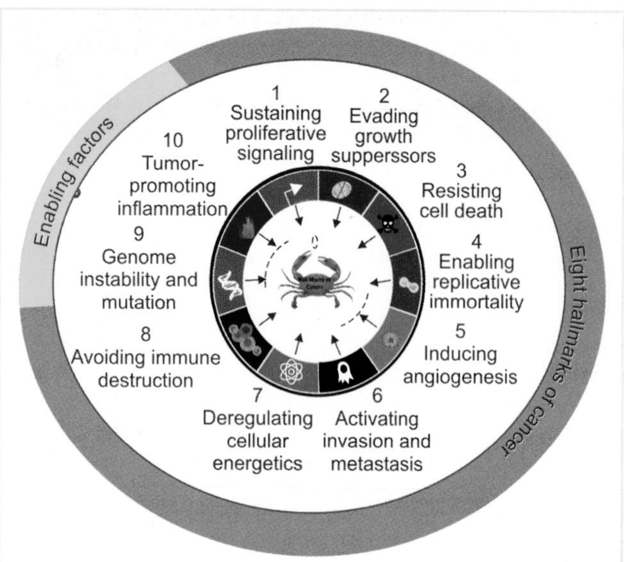

FIG. 35: Eight hallmarks (distinctive functional capabilities) and two enabling factors (genomic instability and tumor-promoting inflammation) of cancer. Most cancer cells acquire these properties during their development by multistep pathogenesis. Usually, they develop due to mutations in critical genes. Certain cancers may be less dependent on one hallmark or another.

in multiple signaling pathways occurs in neoplasms. Many components of these pathways are usually due to activation of oncogenes (mutated proto-oncogenes) and their products namely oncoproteins (**Table 18**). Many tumor suppressors can act by inhibiting one or more components of these same pro-growth signalling pathways. The major signaling pathways that regulate cellular behavior includes the receptor tyrosine kinase pathway, the G protein–coupled receptor pathway, the JAK/STAT pathway, the WNT pathway, the Notch pathway, the Hedgehog pathway, the TGF-β/SMAD pathway, and the NF-κB pathway. Abnormalities in each of these pathways are can lead to the development and progression of various cancers. Proliferation of cells requires not only replication of DNA but also sufficient biosynthesis of membrane, protein, and various macromolecules and organelles so as to produce two complete daughter cells from the original cell. Thus, cell growth pathways involved in oncogenesis also initiate signals that promote and coordinate the biosynthesis of all essential cellular components. The signalling pathways and mechanism of cell signalling are discussed in detail on pages 40 and 41 (refer Fig. 3 of Chapter 2).

Increased Action of Positive Growth Regulators (Oncogenes)

Cells receive and transmit hundreds of different signaling molecules, collectively called the growth factor signals. They are protein products of genes and they participate in many pathways. Signals controlling cell proliferation can activate and inactivate certain genes. Cellular proliferation is brought out through transition of cells from G_0 arrest into the active cell cycle. Normally, the signals acting with cell proliferation or division (proliferative or growth-promoting signals) act in a controllable fashion and is carefully regulated. This maintains normal tissue architecture and function and also prevents unwarranted level of cell division and abnormal growth. To increase proliferation, cells must deregulate the cell cycle. Before entering proliferation, healthy cells must analyze whether they have conditions to proliferate (i.e., enough of nutrients, growth factors, "safe and sound" genome, etc.). If not, the cell cycle breaks (named checkpoints) are switched ON and the cell will not proceed to division. When this control is lost, cells become independent and can divide and grow in an uncontrolled fashion.

Concept of Oncogenes

Early research on transforming retroviruses found that some viral genes could change normal cells to a neoplastic phenotype. It was later found in vitro that transfer of specific genes from human cancer cells (**oncogenes**) could also transform normal recipient cells to neoplastic phenotype. Some of these transforming human tumor genes were found to be mutated version of normal genes (**proto-oncogenes**) that stimulated cellular proliferation. Genes that were isolated from viruses were designated with a *v*- (e.g., *v-myb*), and their cellular counterparts with a *c*- (e.g., *c-myb*). The function of normal proto-oncogene genes is enhanced by the mutations. Hence these mutations are referred to as 'activating' or 'gain-in-function' mutations.

Self-sufficiency in Growth Signals

Cancer may result from an **unregulated cellular proliferation** that chronically instructs cells to grow and divide at inappropriate times and places. These cells acquire the ability to grow independent of normal restraints to multiplication and form cancer. Proliferative signaling is one of the fundamental hallmarks of cancer. Many so-called "driver mutations" (refer pages 425 and 426) can convert normal cellular genes (proto-oncogenes) into oncogenes (by mutational alteration of gene function or amplification in expression). This will stimulate and sustain progression of cells by sustained growth-and-division cycles. Proto-oncogenes and oncogenes are discussed on pages 441–468.

Self-sufficiency in growth usually occurs due to gain-of-function mutations which convert proto-oncogenes to oncogenes. Oncogenes code proteins are called as *oncoproteins.* They promote cell growth, even in the absence of **growth factors and other** growth-promoting external signals. Before we discuss the mechanism of action of oncogenes to produce proliferation of cells, let us briefly review the sequence of events that occur in normal cell proliferation.

Steps in Normal Cell Proliferation

These are as follows:

1. **Binding of a growth factor to its specific receptor** on the plasma/cell membrane (transmembrane receptors).
2. **Transient and limited activation of the growth factor receptor:** After growth factor/ligand binding, the cytoplasmic tails of the transmembrane receptor proteins (**signal transducing proteins**) activate many intracellular signaling cascades on the inner leaflet of the plasma membrane. In order to effectively coordinate signaling cascades, there are variety of molecules present known as adaptor and scaffolding proteins. These proteins play role in intracellular signaling. They recruit various proteins to specific locations and also assemble networks of proteins particular to a cascade.

3. **Transmission of the transduced signal across the cytosol to the nucleus:** This is achieved by second messengers or a cascade of signal transduction molecules.
4. **Induction and activation of nuclear regulatory (transcription) factors:** Signal transducing proteins initiate gene transcription and protein expression. There will be synthesis of other cellular components that are required for cell division. These include organelles, membrane components, and ribosomes.
5. **Entry and progression** of the cell **into the cell cycle**. This ultimately leads to division of cell.
6. **Expression of other genes:** Along with the above changes, there is also expression of other genes that support cell survival and metabolic alterations. These are required for optimal growth.

Classification of Oncogenes

Oncogenes have many roles, but almost all oncogenes encode constitutively active oncoproteins. These oncoproteins are the products of oncogenes and they participate in signaling pathways. They cause proliferation of cells. The normal regulated versions of oncogenes is the proto-oncogenes. Driver mutations may occur in genes involved in any step of this signalling process. The consequence of such mutations is that proteins are produced by them are abnormal and called as oncoproteins, These oncoproteins drive cellular proliferation without the normal restraints.

Mechanisms of cell proliferation: One or more genes that stimulate cell proliferation are usually dysregulated or mutated during onocogenesis. They act in the biochemical pathways that guide entry into and through the cell cycle. The normal proto-oncogenes encode: (i) growth factors, (ii) growth factor receptors, (iii) intracellular signal transduction pathways (transducers), (iv) transcription factors (DNA-binding nuclear proteins), or (v) cell cycle components. In most situations, the corresponding oncogenes encode oncoproteins that serve functions similar to their normal counterparts. Main difference between proto-oncogenes and oncogenes is that, oncogenes are usually constitutively active and the cells are not dependent on growth factors.

Oncogenes act in different stages in the signal transduction circuits. Oncogenes can be classified according to the function of gene product (oncoprotein) (**Box 7**). Categories of oncogenes and examples of associated tumors are presented in **Table 18**.

Box 7: Classification of oncogenes.

- Growth factors
- Growth factor receptors (on cell surface)
- Downstream (intracellular) signal transduction proteins
- Deoxyribonucleic acid (DNA)-binding nuclear regulatory proteins (transcription factors)
- Cell cycle regulators (cyclins and cyclin-dependent kinases)

Table 18: Categories of oncogenes and examples of associated tumors.

Category of oncogene (Proto-oncogene)	*Mode of activation in tumor*	*Examples of associated tumors*
Growth factors (ligands)		
• PDGF-β chain (*PDGFB*) • Fibroblast growth factor (*HST1*) • Fibroblast growth factor (*FGF3*) • TGF-α (*TGFA*) • HGF (*HGF*)	• Overexpression • Overexpression • Amplification • Overexpression • Overexpression	• Astrocytoma • Osteosarcoma • Cancer of stomach, bladder, breast; melanoma • Astrocytoma • Hepatocellular carcinomas, thyroid cancer
Growth factor receptors		
• EGF-receptor family (*ERBB1-EGFR*) • EGF-receptor family (*ERBB2-HER*) • FMS-like tyrosine kinase 3 (*FLT3*) • Receptor for neurotrophic factors (*RET*) • PDGF receptor (*PDGFRB*) • Receptor for KIT ligand (*KIT*)	• Mutation • Amplification • Point mutation/ small duplication • Point mutation • Overexpression, translocation • Point mutation	• Adenocarcinoma of lung • Breast carcinoma • Leukemia • Multiple endocrine neoplasia 2A and B, familial medullary thyroid carcinomas • Gliomas, leukemias • Gastrointestinal stromal tumors, seminomas, leukemias
ALK receptor (*ALK*)	• Translocation, fusion gene formation • Point mutation	• Adenocarcinoma of lung, certain lymphomas • Neuroblastoma
Signal transduction proteins		
GTP-binding (G) proteins • (*KRAS*) • (*HRAS*) • (*NRAS*) • (*GNAQ*) • (*GNAS*)	• Point mutation • Point mutation • Point mutation • Point mutation • Point mutation	• Tumors of colon, lung, and pancreas • Tumors of bladder and kidney • Melanomas, hematologic malignancies • Uveal melanoma • Pituitary adenoma, other endocrine tumors

Continued

Continued

Category of oncogene (Proto-oncogene)	***Mode of activation in tumor***	***Examples of associated tumors***
Nonreceptor tyrosine kinase (*ABL*)	Translocation	• Chronic myelogenous leukemia and acute lymphoblastic leukemia
RAS signal transduction (*BRAF*)	Point mutation	Melanomas, leukemias, colon carcinoma, etc.
Notch signal transduction (*NOTCH1*)	Point mutation, translocation	Leukemias, lymphomas, breast carcinoma
JAK/STAT signal transduction (*JAK2*)	Point mutation, translocation	Myeloproliferative neoplasms, acute lymphoblastic leukemia
Nuclear regulatory proteins/transcription factors		
• Transcriptional activators (*MYC*) • Transcriptional activators (*NMYC*)	• Translocation • Amplification	• Burkitt lymphoma • Neuroblastoma
Regulators of cell cycle		
Cyclins [*CCND1 (Cyclin D1)*]	• Translocation • Amplification	• Mantle cell lymphoma, multiple myeloma • Cancer of breast and esophagus
Cyclin-dependent kinase (*CDK4*)	Amplification or point mutation	Glioblastoma, melanoma, sarcoma

(ALK: anaplastic lymphoma kinase; EGF: epidermal growth factor; GTP: guanosine triphosphate; HGF: hepatocyte growth factor; PDGF: platelet-derived growth factor; TGF: transforming growth factor)

Growth Factors

Normal cell proliferation requires stimulation by growth factors. Cancers may be associated with **excessive production of growth factors** by oncogenes. Normally, cells that produce the growth factor do not express the cognate (corresponding) receptor. This prevents the formation of positive feedback loops within the same cell. This "rule" may be broken by cancer cells in different ways.

Action of growth factor oncoprotein: Cancer cells acquire growth self-sufficiency by secreting growth factors. These growth factors may be **secreted by two mechanisms,** namely—(i) autocrine or (ii) paracrine action.

- **Autocrine action (Fig. 36): Cancer cells** acquire growth self-sufficiency and **themselves may produce growth factors** [growth factor ligands (ligand is a molecule that binds to another molecule)] to which they can respond via the coexpression of cognate (corresponding) receptors. The developing (or developed) tumor cell itself producing growth factors/ligands is called autocrine (or juxtacrine) proliferative signaling (stimulation). This autocrine trigger to cell division is fairly common in many types of cancer and the growth factor oncoproteins may be overexpressed, mostly by gene amplification. For example, in many glioblastomas (malignant glial cell tumors in brain) the tumor cell itself secretes platelet-derived growth factor (PDGF) and expresses the PDGF receptor **tyrosine kinases**. Many sarcomas produce both transforming growth factor (TGF)-α and its receptor, epidermal growth factor receptor (EGFR).
- **Paracrine action (Fig. 37):** Most soluble growth factors are secreted by one cell type and act on a neighboring cell to stimulate proliferation. This is called paracrine action. In **some cancers,** the **cancer cells** send signals to activate normal cells in the supporting tumor-associated stroma (i.e., stromal cells) **to produce growth factors in the tumor microenvironment.** These growth factors produced by the stromal cells reciprocate (move backwards to cancer cells) by supplying the growth factors to the cancer cells and promote their growth.

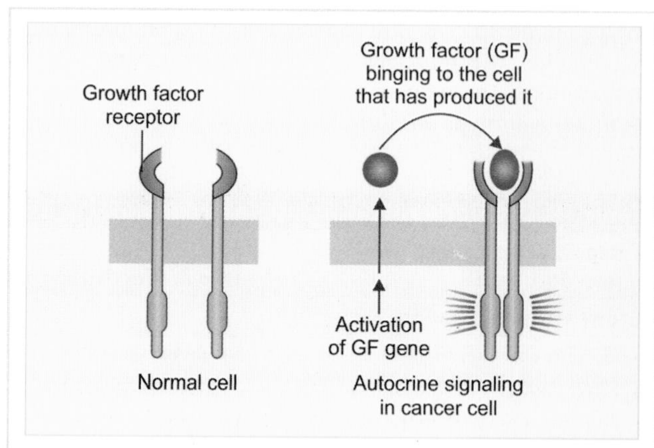

FIG. 36: Autocrine signaling in cancer. Usually, normal cells do not synthesize and release a growth factor ligand with a corresponding receptor. In many types of cancer, an autocrine signaling is observed. In this, tumor cells acquire the ability to produce a ligand (growth factor) for a growth factor receptor that they also display. This produces an autostimulatory or autocrine signaling loop.

Growth Factor Receptors

Growth factor receptors constitute the next group in the sequence of signal transduction. There are several basic classes of receptors that may stimulate or inhibit cell proliferation. Most of the receptors are molecules present on cell/plasma membrane and they respond to growth factors/ligands produced by other cells (paracrine action). Usually, when the growth factors or ligands bind to the corresponding receptor, the interactions cause activation and changes in the receptors. The activated receptors serve as docking (tie-up or anchor) sites for one or more intracellular signaling networks.

Categories of growth factor receptors

The changes that growth factors produce in receptors depend on the specificity of the receptor. Some growth factor receptors have an intrinsic tyrosine kinase activity and get activated by binding of growth factors. Other receptors signal by stimu-

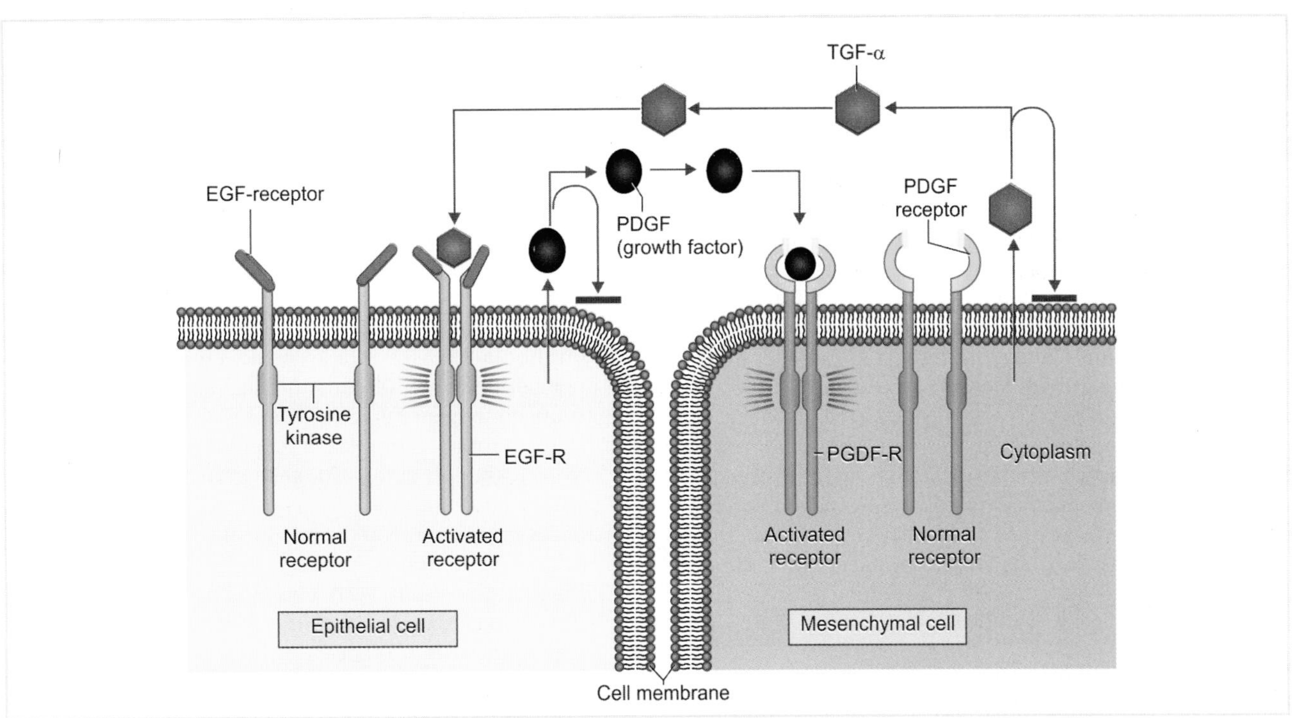

(EGF: epidermal growth factor; EGF-R: epidermal growth factor receptor; PGDF: platelet-derived growth factor; PGDF-R: platelet-derived growth factor receptor; TGF: transforming growth factor)

FIG. 37: Paracrine signaling. In this example, the epithelial cells produce ligand, namely platelet-derived growth factor (PDGF), and the corresponding platelet-derived growth factor receptor (PDGF-R) is displayed by mesenchymal cells. Conversely, mesenchymal cells produce transforming growth factor (TGF)-α [epidermal growth factor (EGF)-related ligand], and it binds to corresponding epidermal growth factor receptor (EGF-R) displayed by epithelial cells. However, the PDGF produced by an epithelial cell does not find its corresponding receptor on the surface of that cell *(horizontal bar)*. This prevents activation by autocrine signaling.

lating the activity of downstream proteins. Depending on the nature of the intracellular signaling cascades initiated by these receptors, they can be classified (refer Fig. 4 of chapter 2) into three major categories—(i) tyrosine kinases, (ii) serine and threonine kinases, and (iii) G-protein-coupled receptors (GPCRs).

- **Receptor with intrinsic tyrosine kinases [receptor tyrosine kinase (RTKs)] activity:** These receptors have intrinsic tyrosine kinase activity within their intracellular tail. These receptor are transmembrane proteins with an extracellular growth factor-binding domain and a cytoplasmic tyrosine kinase domain. Normally, when the growth factor binds to the receptor, the receptor is activated transiently. After ligand/growth factor binding, it induces a rapid change in receptor conformation to an active dimeric state. This stimulates the, tyrosine kinase activity. This leads to phosphorylation (addition of PO_4 molecule) of tyrosine residues in target proteins within the cell (autophosphorylates tyrosine residues in its own intracellular tail). Most of these receptors also autophosphorylate tyrosine residues present in the receptors themselves to magnify signaling. This category includes receptors for many peptide growth factors. Receptor tyrosine kinases (RTKs) are important in a variety of cellular processes including growth, motility, differentiation, and metabolism. For example, receptor for epidermal growth factor (EGF) HER2/ErbB2, and MET.
- **Serine/threonine-specific protein kinases receptors:** These receptors on the cell surface have kinase activity directed toward serine or threonine residues rather than tyrosine. These receptors also phosphorylate many cellular proteins and lead to a cascade of responses. These types of receptors usually associate with nonreceptor tyrosine kinases (**NRTKs**), which mediate further signaling. They include many receptors that undergo structural rearrangements. One of the classical examples for serine-threonine kinase-containing transmembrane receptor is the TGF-α receptor complex.
- **G-protein-coupled receptors (GPCR):** They constitute the most common type of membrane receptors and are members of the so-called 7-membrane-spanning receptor family. These receptors are coupled to guanine nucleotide binding proteins (also called as G-proteins). Hence, these receptors are named as G-protein-coupled receptors. When ligands (growth factors) bind to GPCRs, G-proteins undergo a conformational change that is dependent on the presence of guanosine phosphates. Activation of G-proteins can stimulate a variety of intracellular signals. These include stimulation of phospholipase C and the generation of phosphoinositides (most important being inositol 1,4,5-triphosphate) and diacylglycerol through hydrolysis of membrane phospholipids. GPCRs may be amplified in cancers or they may mediate stimulatory autocrine or paracrine signals.

Oncogenic version of growth factor receptors

Normally, when the growth factor binds to the growth factor receptors, it produces transient dimerization (activity). **Many growth factor receptors function as oncoproteins when they are mutated or if they overexpressed (Figs. 38A and B).**

Receptor proteins are the most important transforming proteins and are implicated in oncogenes of several cancers. In tumors, the genes encoding these receptors are mutated. Mutations can make these receptors constitutively active, independent of their growth factors. **Constitutive** (unrestrained) **dimerization** of growth factor receptors produces continuous mitogenic signals to the cell, **even in the absence of the growth factor**. Elevated levels of receptor proteins at the surface of cancer cells can make such cells hyper-responsive to otherwise limiting amounts of growth factor ligands. This can also result from structural alterations in the receptor molecules that facilitate ligand-independent activation. Most important receptors involved in tumor are the oncogenic versions of **receptor tyrosine kinases**. These mutated receptors lead to constitutive, growth factor-independent tyrosine kinase activity.

Mechanism of activation

In tumors, receptor tyrosine kinases are constitutively activated by multiple mechanisms including **point mutations, gene rearrangements, and gene amplifications**. Examples of few oncogenic mutations involving growth factor receptors are listed in **Table 18**.

Examples—Overexpression of the EGF receptor family:

- **Point mutations: *ERBB1* encodes** one of the EGF receptors (EGFRs). Many different ERBB1 point mutations found in a subset of lung adenocarcinomas. These mutated ERBB1 produce constitutive activation of the EGFR tyrosine kinase.
- **Gene amplification:** *ERBB2* encodes a different member of the receptor tyrosine kinase family, HER2 (HER-2/Neu). It is an EGF-related receptor. Instead of being activated by point mutations, the *ERBB2* (*HER2*) gene is amplified in certain breast carcinomas (~20%). This leads to overexpression of the HER2 receptor and constitutive tyrosine kinase activity. It is also amplified in few adenocarcinomas of the lung, ovary, stomach, and salivary glands. The receptors in these tumors are highly sensitive to the mitogenic effects of small amounts of growth factors.
- **Gene rearrangement (fusion gene):** ALK (anaplastic lymphoma kinase) is a tyrosine kinase receptor. Its oncogenic version of constitutively active form may be produced by gene rearrangement. For example, in 2–9% of lung adenocarcinomas, a deletion on chromosome 2 (2p23) fuses part of the ALK gene on with part of another gene on chromosome 2(2p21) called EML4 (echinoderm microtubule-associated protein-like 4). The resulting ***EML4-ALK* fusion gene** (**Fig. 39**) encodes a chimeric EML4-ALK protein with constitutive tyrosine kinase activity. The EML4-ALK fusion protein is also expressed in breast and colorectal cancers.

Importance of mutated receptor tyrosine kinases

Therapeutically agents that inhibit the enzymatic activities have been found useful.

- **Breast cancers with ERBB2 amplification and overexpression of HER2:** The clinical benefit is obtained by blocking the extracellular domain of HER2 receptor with anti-HER2 antibodies or drugs that inhibit HER2 activity. These inhibitors block tumor growth and also induce apoptosis and tumor regression. This indicates the ability of receptor tyrosine kinase signaling to increase survival and proliferation of cells.

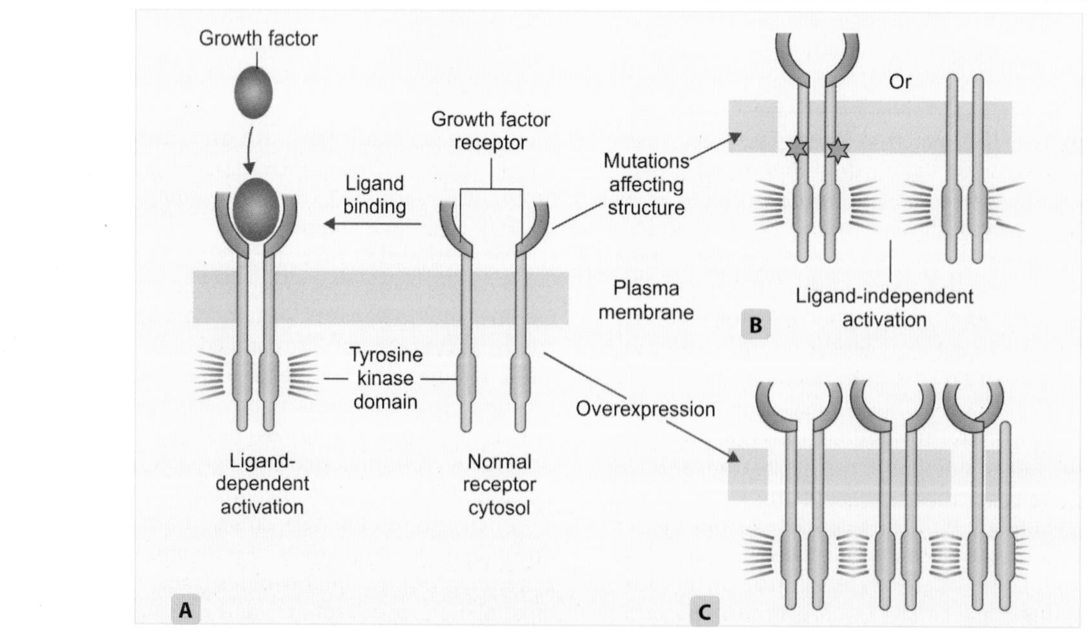

FIGS. 38A TO C: Activation of growth factor receptor. (A) When growth factor ligands (red circle) bind to normally functioning growth factor receptors, they produce cytoplasmic signals (*red spikes*). (B) Mutations in the genes encoding the receptor molecules can cause subtle changes in protein structure, such as amino acid substitutions (blue star). This can produce ligand-independent activation. (C) Tumors may be associated with overexpression of receptor proteins. Excessive numbers of normally structured receptor molecules can also drive ligand-independent receptor activation. They activate by spontaneous dimerization and release signals (*red spikes*).

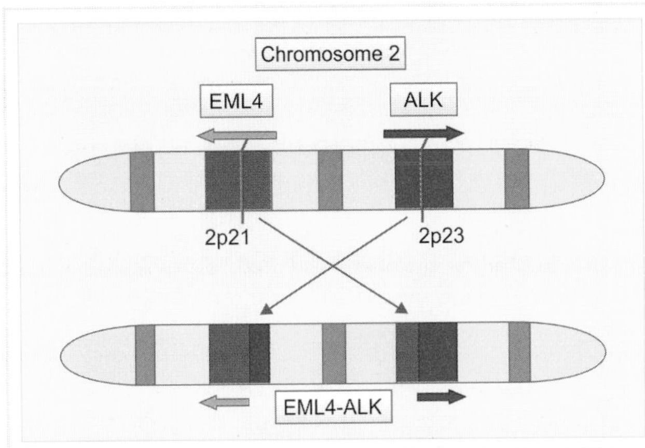

FIG. 39: *EML4-ALK* fusion gene. It is formed by deletion on chromosome 2 (2p23) and fusion of part of the *ALK* gene with part of another gene on chromosome 2(2p21) called EML4 (echinoderm microtubule associated protein like 4).

- **Lung adenocarcinoma:** In patients with lung adenocarcinomas having ERBB1 mutations or EML4-ALK fusion genes, inhibitors of EGFR and ALK also produce similar therapeutic responses respectively. But, these targeted therapies are often not curative in advanced cancers. The tumor cells that withstand therapy usually have other acquired mutations which reduces the effects of the drug. For example, adenocarcinoma of lung cancers that develop resistance to EGFR inhibitors usually have mutations in EGFR that prevent inhibitors from binding, or amplifications in another gene called MET (MET encodes another tyrosine kinase receptor). The presence of subclones within the genetically heterogeneous tumor cell population is responsible for the resistance to targeted therapies. This is one of the most discouraging problems in the treatment of advanced cancers.

Few important receptors involved in cancer are discussed in detail on page 508–513.

Downstream Signal-transducing Proteins

Once a growth factor binds to its receptor, it stimulates downstream signaling pathways. The signals are transmitted from the activated growth factor receptors to the nucleus through various signal transduction molecules. The ability of transforming signals, mainly from the outside of the cell, into a response is called as signal transduction. This response is mediated by biochemical reactions and these are usually referred to as signal transduction pathways or signal transduction cascades. There are different downstream signaling transduction pathways that depend on many factors. Apart from external growth facts, the constitutive activation of components of intracellular signaling cascades operating downstream of these receptors can also occur within cancer cells. These intracellular alterations can stimulate cell proliferation pathways without the ligand-mediated activation of cell-surface receptors. Activation of one or another of these downstream branches (e.g., the pathway responding to the RAS signal transducer) may lead to cancer. **Cancer cells generally acquire growth autonomy due to mutations in genes that encode components of signaling pathways downstream of growth factor receptors.** Two important oncoproteins belonging to this category of signaling molecules are RAS and ABL.

RAS

Q. Write a short essay on *RAS* gene in neoplasia.

Normal RAS Signaling (Fig. 40) Receptor tyrosine kinase signaling pathway is most important pathway. RAS is a signal transducing protein that may be activated by tyrosine kinases via a linker protein, usually Grb2. RAS is a member of a family of small G-proteins. The three members of the RAS family in humans include K-RAS, N-RAS, H-RAS. These were initially found in the genomes of transforming retroviruses. To understand activated RAS and RAS-related oncogenesis, let us briefly study the RAS cycle. Sequential steps in signaling by RAS are as follows:

- RAS proteins (product of *RAS* gene) are attached to the cytoplasmic aspect of the plasma membrane by farnesyl (also the endoplasmic reticulum and golgi membranes).
- RAS are small guanine nucleotide-binding proteins that are present in two structural states depending on the binding of guanosine nucleotides [guanosine triphosphate (GTP) and guanosine diphosphate (GDP)]. Normally, most of the RAS is in the inactive GDP-bound state and in the GTP-bound state, RAS is active. Normally, RAS orderly cycles between an active signal transmitting state (RAS proteins bound to GDP) and in an inactive (quiescent) state and active signal-transmitting state (RAS is bound to GTP).
- When an external growth factor such as EGF and PDGF binds to the growth factor receptors, Grb2 recognizes phosphorylated tyrosine. It triggers conversion of GDP to GTP and subsequent conformational changes occur. This converts/generates RAS to the active state.
- This active signal state of RAS is short-lived, because of its inactivation by intrinsic guanosine triphosphatase (GTPase)-activating protein (GAP). GTPase directs the GTPase activity of RAS and hydrolyzes GTP to GDP. This releases a phosphate group and converts (returns) active GTP bound to quiescent GDP-bound RAS.
- The GTPase activity of activated RAS is greatly enhanced (by about 100-fold the intrinsic GTPase activity) by a family of GAPs from the cytosol. These GAPs act as molecular brakes and prevent uncontrolled RAS activation by favoring hydrolysis of GTP to GDP.

Activated RAS stimulates downstream regulators of cell proliferation by several interconnected pathways. Two important pathways include—(1) RAF/ERK/MAP kinase pathway (MAPK cascade) and (2) phosphatidylinositol 3 (PI3) kinase/AKT (protein kinase B) pathway (PI3K/AKT pathway). These pathways converge on the nucleus and change the expression of genes that regulate growth (e.g., *MYC*). These pathways are important in cell growth. Hence, RAS, PI3K, and other components of these pathways are frequently involved by gain-of-function mutations in different types of cancer. One of the interesting observation is that when mutations in RAS are present in a tumor, there is almost no activating mutations in receptor tyrosine kinases (at least within the dominant tumor clone). This suggests that in such tumors activated RAS can completely substitute for tyrosine kinase activity.

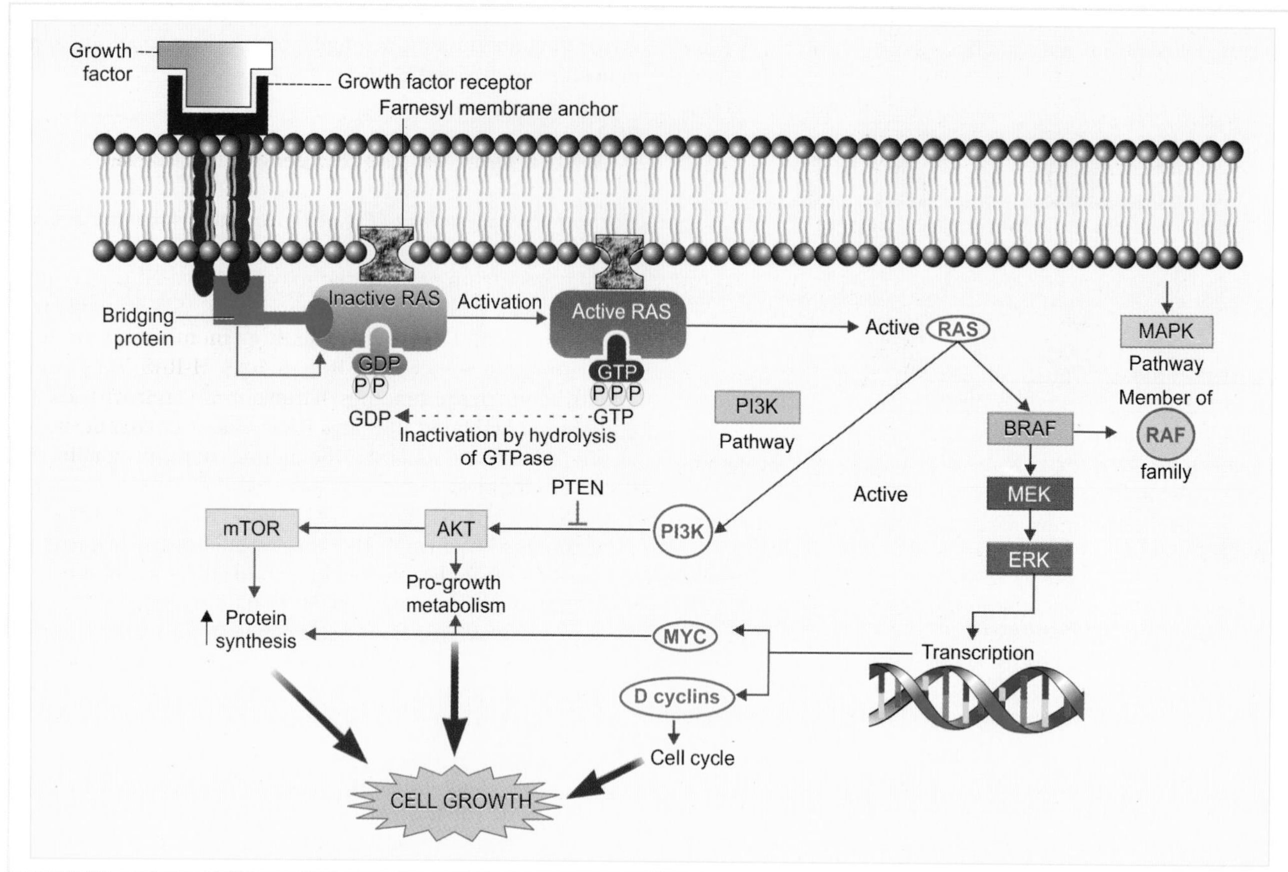

(GDP: guanosine diphosphate; GTP: guanosine triphosphate; GTPase: guanosine triphosphatase; MAPK: mitogen-activated protein kinase; mTOR: mammalian target of rapamycin; PI3K: phosphatidylinositol 3 kinase; AKT: also called protein kinase B)

FIG. 40: Normal RAS cycle and growth factor signaling pathways in cancer. RAS is anchored to the cell membrane by the farnesyl moiety and is essential for its action. When a growth factor binds to growth factor receptor, inactive (GDP-bound) RAS becomes activated to a GTP-bound state. The active GTP state is shortlived because an enzyme GTPase hydrolyzes GTP to GDP. Activated RAS in turn transduces proliferative signals to the nucleus. Growth factor receptors, RAS, PI3K, MYC and D cyclins are oncoproteins. These are activated by mutations in various cancers.

RAS in cancer ***RAS* is the most commonly mutated oncogene in malignant tumors.** About 30% of all cancers have mutated *RAS* genes, and the frequency is more in some specific cancers (e.g., pancreatic adenocarcinoma).

- **Mutated *RAS*: *RAS* family genes are the most commonly activated by point mutations.** Mutated *RAS* does not undergo the inactivation and constitutively turns on (activates) downstream signaling. Normally *RAS* releases downstream signals in response to prior upstream signals by signals arising from activated growth factor receptors. This constitutive activation of *RAS* produces downstream signaling without any stimulation from growth factor receptors. Mutations in *RAS* interferes with breakdown of GTP, which is necessary for inactivation of *RAS*. *RAS* is thus trapped in its activated, GTP-bound form, and the cells continuously proliferate.
- **Tumors with RAS mutations:** About 15% to 20% of all tumors in humans show mutations in RAS. In some types of cancers the frequency of RAS mutations is much higher. Human genome contains three types of RAS genes.
    - ***KRAS:*** Mutation in adenocarcinomas of colon (50%), lung (30%), and pancreas (90%). Other tumors include endometrial, and thyroid cancers.
    - ***HRAS:*** Mutations in bladder and kidney tumors
    - ***NRAS:*** Mutations in melanoma and hematopoietic tumors (30%)

Defect in the negative-feedback mechanisms that reduce the proliferative signaling also may lead to cancer. Loss-of-function mutations in GAPs, also cause a failure to simulate GTP hydrolysis and thereby prevent inactivation of RAS. For example, GAP neurofibromin-1 (*NF1*) is a tumor suppressor that is mutated in the cancer-prone familial disorder neurofibromatosis type 1. *NF1* is a tumor suppressor gene that acts through negative regulation of RAS signaling.

Oncogenic BRAF and PI3K Mutations

Apart from RAS, other downstream factors in the receptor tyrosine kinase (RTK) signaling pathway are also usually involved by gain-of-function mutations in many cancers.

Mitogen-activated protein kinases (MAPKs)

Mitogen-activated protein kinase enzymes bring out many different types of signaling reactions and cause proliferation of cells. MAPKs may be stimulated by upstream proteins such as RAS (after RTK activation), GPCRs, or other mechanisms. Some very important driver mutations of cancer occur among these proteins, leading to constitutive activation.

Mutations in BRAF *BRAF* is a human gene that encodes a protein called B-Raf. *BRAF* is a member of the *RAF* family. *BRAF* is a serine/threonine protein kinase belonging to MAPK family. It is in the top of RAS/mitogen-activated protein kinase (MAPK) cascade ("RAF/ERK/MAP kinase pathway"). *BRAF* mutation is discussed in detail on page 510.

- **Tumors with *BRAF* mutation:** It is associated with unregulated proliferation of cells. BRAF mutation is observed in almost 100% of hairy cell leukemias, 60% of melanomas, 80% of benign nevi, and a lesser percentage in other neoplasms (e.g., colon carcinomas and dendritic cell tumors).
- **Action:** Similar to *RAS* mutations, activating mutations in *BRAF* stimulate downstream kinases and activate transcription factors.

Mutations in other MAPK family members downstream of *BRAF* are not common in cancer.

Mutations of the PI3K family of proteins

Phosphatidylinositol 3 Kinase: Phosphatidylinositol 3 kinase family of enzymes is usually activated by RTKs (receptor tyrosine kinases) and GPCRs (G-protein-coupled receptors). PI3K is a heterodimer composed of a regulatory subunit and a catalytic subunit, of which several tissue-specific isoforms exist. PI3K is recruited by RTK activation to plasma membrane associated signaling protein complexes. These enzymes add a phosphate group to a phosphatidylinositol lipid and produce the small molecule phasphatidylinositol-3-phosphate [PI (3) P] and also heavily phosphorylated derivatives such as phosphatidylinositol 3,4,5-phosphate (PIP3). PIP3 then activates downstream signaling cascade of serine/threonine kinases, including AKT (also called protein kinase B-see **Fig. 40**), which is a key signaling node. AKT has many substrates, one of them is mammalian target of rapamycin (mTOR). mTOR is a sensor of cellular nutrient status and is activated by AKT. mTOR in turn stimulates protein and lipid synthesis. BCL2 associated agonist of cell death (BAD) is a pro-apoptotic protein that is inactivated by AKT and thus enhances cell survival. FOXO transcription factors turn on genes that promote apoptosis and these are also negatively regulated by AKT phosphorylation. Substrates of AKT also include MDM2, and IAP.

Negative-feedback mechanisms operate at multiple sites within the proliferative signaling pathway. For example, phosphatase and tensin homolog (PTEN), is an important/major tumor suppressor second only to p53 in the frequency with which loss of a tumor suppressor function is observed in human cancer. PTEN is a negative inhibitor of PI3 kinase and degrades its product (dephosphorylates PIP3), PIP3. Loss-of-function mutations in PTEN amplify PI3K signaling and promote carcinogenesis.

Mutations of the Phosphatidylinositol 3 (PI3) Kinase: Mutations of phosphatidylinositol 3 kinase (PI3 kinase) in the PI3K/AKT pathway can lead to cancer and are very common in certain cancers. Alterations can involve all components of the PI3K/AKT pathway but similar to the RAS/MAPK pathway, the factors at the top of the pathway—PI3K and its antagonist, PTEN—are most frequently mutated in cancer. PI3K mutations affect the catalytic subunits and usually increase the enzyme activity. For example, about 30% of breast carcinomas are associated with gain-of-function mutations involving the α-isoform of the PI3K catalytic subunit. Loss of function of tumor suppressor gene (TSG) namely *PTEN* may occur through mutation or epigenetic silencing in many cancers (e.g., endometrial carcinomas) and certain leukemias. Function of PTEN in signaling is depicted in **Figure 41**.

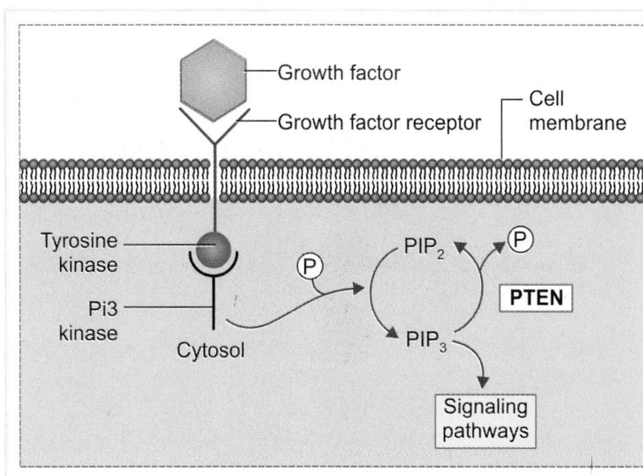

FIG. 41: Function of phosphatase and tensin homolog (PTEN) in signaling. Normal binding of a growth factor to its receptor causes phosphorylation of phosphatidylinositol-4,5-bisphosphate (PIP2) to produce the important signaling molecule phosphatidylinositol-3,4,5-trisphosphate (PIP3). The level of PIP3 is regulated by its dephosphorylation by a tumor suppressor gene called *PTEN*.

Phospholipase C: This family of enzymes is usually activated by many different types of receptors (e.g., GPCRs). They cleave certain phospholipids and produce inositol phosphate signaling intermediates and diacylglycerol. These, in turn, cause multiplication of cells through calcium signaling pathways and protein kinase C, respectively.

Mammalian target of rapamycin kinase: It is a main coordinator of cell growth and metabolism and it lies both upstream and downstream of the PI3K pathway.

- **Stimulation of cell proliferation:** Downstream mTOR signaling can stimulate cell proliferation by reprogramming cancer cell metabolism.
- **Inhibition of cell proliferation:** In some cancer cells, mTOR activation results via negative feedback and inhibits PI3K signaling. When pharmacologically mTOR is inhibited in such cancer cells (e.g., by the drug rapamycin), the associated loss of negative feedback of mTOR results in increased activity of PI3K and its effector, the AKT/PKB kinase. This, in turn, weakens the antiproliferative effects of mTOR inhibition.

Nonreceptor Tyrosine Kinases

Nonreceptor tyrosine kinases (NRTKs) are normally localized to the cytoplasm or the nucleus of a cell (**Fig. 42**). Oncogenic mutations can also occur in several NRTKs. In many occasions, the mutations are the form of chromosomal translocations or rearrangements. These mutations produce fusion genes encoding constitutively active tyrosine kinases. Though localization of these tyrosine kinases is nonmembranous, these oncoproteins activate the same signaling pathways as receptor tyrosine kinase (RTKs). Most important example of this oncogenic mechanism involves the ABL (Abelson) tyrosine kinase.

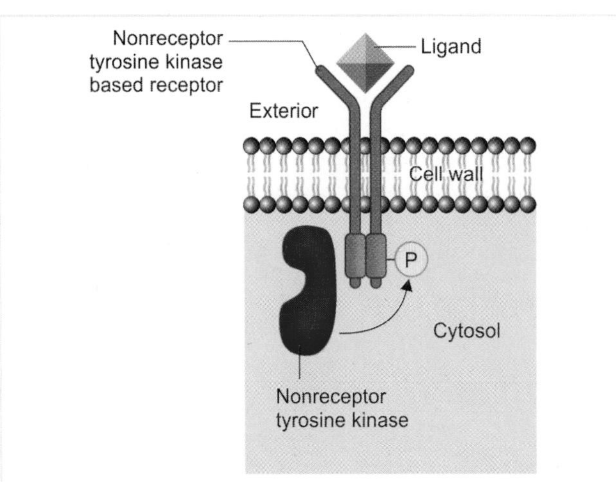

FIG. 42: Nonreceptor tyrosine kinases (NRTKs) receptors. NRTKS are normally localized to the cytoplasm or the nucleus of a cell.

Chromosomal translocation of ABL: Many NRTKs function as signal transduction molecules. One of the classical examples with respect to carcinogenesis is ABL. The ABL proto-oncoprotein has tyrosine kinase activity that is reduced by internal negative regulatory domains. In chronic myeloid leukemia (CML) and certain subsets of acute lymphoblastic leukemia, the *ABL* gene is translocated from its normal position on chromosome 9 to chromosome 22. In chromosome 22, *ABL* fuses with *BCR* (*breakpoint cluster region*) gene. This results in a fusion gene that encodes BCR–ABL hybrid protein (see Fig. 25 of Chapter 10.2). This hybrid protein contains the ABL tyrosine kinase domain and a BCR domain, and produces constitutive activation of tyrosine kinase. BCR moiety promotes self-association of BCR–ABL, and releases the tyrosine kinase activity of ABL.

BCR–ABL protein activates all the downstream signals of RAS and strongly stimulates cell growth. **Patients with chronic myeloid leukemia having this translocation show dramatic clinical response to BCR–ABL kinase inhibitors** (e.g., imatinib mesylate). In an early, perhaps initiating event that drives leukemogenesis, tumor is greatly dependent on a single BCR–ABL signaling molecule. It is an example of the concept of *oncogene addiction* in which tumor cells are highly dependent on the activity of one oncoprotein. Probably, development of leukemia needs other mutations, but the transformed cell continues to depend on BCR–ABL for signals that mediate growth and survival. Though the proliferating component of the tumor is suppressed by BCR–ABL inhibitors, and the patient appears well, rare CML "stem cells" harboring the *BCR–ABL* fusion gene persist. This may be because they do not need BCR–ABL signals for their survival. Hence, treatment with BCR–ABL inhibitors must be continued indefinitely; otherwise, the malignant stem cells generate rapidly proliferating offspring, and the full-blown leukemia may reappear.

TEL-ABL and human leukemia: TEL-ABL (ETV6-ABL1) tyrosine kinase is a rare aberration found in a few hematological malignancies. Similar to ABL-BCR, TEL-ABL is constitutively phosphorylated. It may be due to reciprocal translocation t(9,12) in case of ALL and with a complex karyotype t(9,12,14) in patients with CML. TEL (supposed to be a transcription factor) fuses with ABL proto-oncogene and produces a fusion protein product with elevated tyrosine kinase activity.

Other chromosomal translocations: These include t(5,12) in chronic myelomonocytic leukemia (CMML) producing TEL-PDGF receptor. NPM-ALK fusion products t(2,5) is constitutively activated in anaplastic large cell lymphoma.

JAK 2 mutations

Q. Write a short essay on JAK 2 mutations.

Nonreceptor tyrosine kinases may also be activated by point mutations. This mutation can abolish the function of negative autoregulatory domains that normally prevent the enzyme activity. An example of point mutation is in the JAK2 (Janus kinases 2).

- JAK2 is a member of the Janus kinase family and its cytogenetic location is 9p24.1. It participates in the JAK/Signal transducer and activator of transcription (STAT) signaling pathway, which transduces mitogenic signals from growth factor and cytokine receptors that lack tyrosine kinase activity. Members of cytokine receptors include interferon receptors, granulocyte-macrophage colony-stimulating factor (GM-CSF) receptor family [interleukin-3 receptor (IL-3R), interleukin-5 receptor (IL-5R) and GM-CSF receptor (GM-CSF-R)], the gp130 receptor family [e.g., interleukin-6 receptor (IL-6R)], and the single chain receptors [e.g., erythropoietin receptor (Epo-R), thrombopoietin receptor (Tpo-R), growth hormone receptor (Gh-R), prolactin receptor (PRL-R)].
- JAK/STAT pathway operates by more direct route without the involvement of second messengers. STAT transcription factor binds to the activated receptor, becomes phosphorylated by the JAK kinase. STAT proteins are located in the cytosol and are called as *latent transcription regulators* because they migrate into the nucleus and regulate gene transcription only after they are activated. Once phosphorylated, STAT molecules move/translocate from the cytoplasm to the nucleus. In the nucleus, they bind to specific deoxyribonucleic acid (DNA) sequences [e.g., interferon-stimulated response element (ISRE)] and directly activate transcription. Negative feedback regulates the responses mediated by the JAK/STAT pathway.
- **JAK/STAT activation:** It changes the expression of target genes that bind STAT transcription factors. Many myeloid neoplasms are generally associated with activating point mutations in *JAK2*. This frees the tumor cells of their normal dependence on hematopoietic growth factors such as erythropoietin. Janus kinases play an essential role in regulating hematopoiesis and proliferation of blood cells. Point mutation *JAK2 V617F* leads to activation of the JAK/STAT signaling pathways (**Figs. 43A** and **B**) and leads to development of myeloproliferative neoplasm (MPN) such as polycythemia vera (PV), essential thrombocythemia (ET), and primary myelofibrosis (PMF). This mutation (V617F) is characterized by a change of valine to phenylalanine at the 617 position. This renders hematopoietic cells more sensitive to growth factors such as erythropoietin and thrombopoietin because the receptors for these growth factors require JAK2 for signal transduction. *JAK2 V617F* is a somatic mutation. Thus, it is present only in the hematopoietic cell compartment but not in germline DNA. This mutation is common in most patients with MPN. JAK also activates the MAPK and PI3K signaling pathway, resulting in increased proliferation and survival of cells harboring the *JAK2 V617F* mutation.

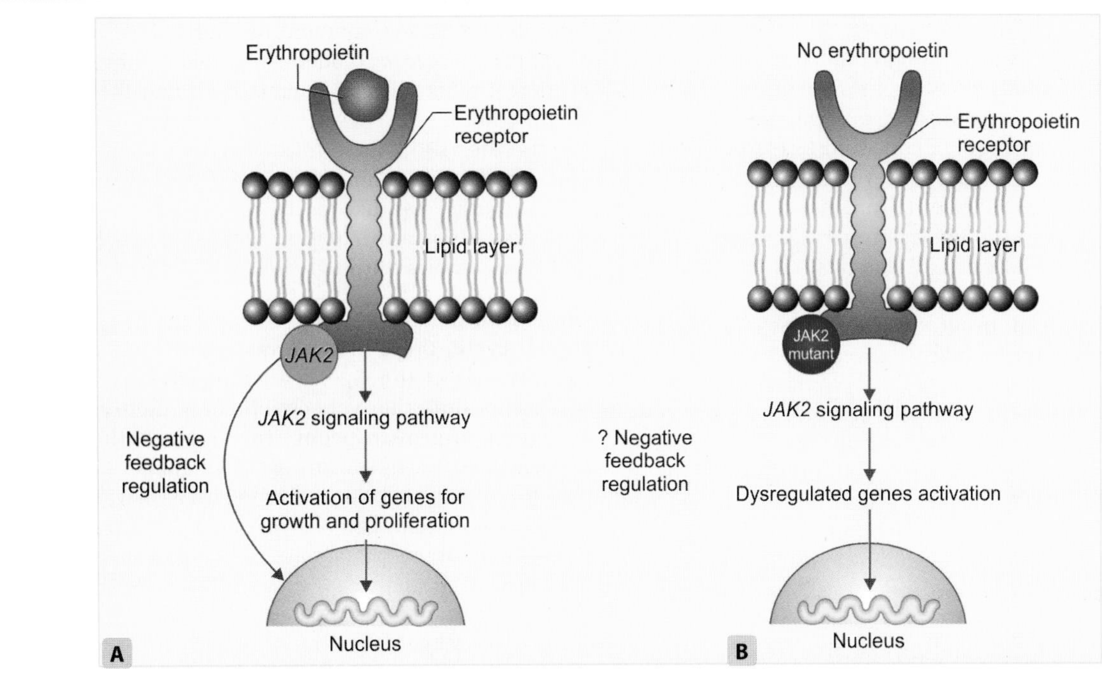

FIGS. 43A AND B: (A) Normal signaling by *JAK2:* Normally, a tyrosine kinase protein called JAK2 (Janus 2 kinase gene), is activated following binding of the growth hormone erythropoietin. *JAK2* then activates a signaling pathway causing cells to replicate. This process is strictly regulated by various feedback pathways. (B) In polycythemia vera (PV), mutation in tyrosine kinase ***JAK2 V617F*** results in dysregulated downstream signaling in the absence of erythropoietin. *JAK2* mutations cause proliferation of not only erythroid lineage but also granulocytic and megakaryocytic lineage.

- This molecular lesion has led to the development of JAK2 inhibitors and also researches on activating mutations in other NRTKs.
- Gain of function mutations of *JAK2* gene may be implicated in the pathogenesis of Crohn's disease.

Nuclear Transcription Factors

The consequence of signaling through oncoproteins (e.g., RAS, ABL) is inappropriate and causes continuous stimulation of nuclear transcription factors. They drive the cells to proliferate without restriction. Thus, whatever may be the upstream driver mutations, transcription factors sit at the end of the of the processes that cause cancer cells to undergo uncontrolled mitosis. Mutations affecting genes that regulate DNA transcription also can produce cancer. The genetic change in transcription factors that drive oncogenesis is usually due to increased production of wild-type (WT) proteins. The term wild type (WT) refers to the phenotype of the typical form of a species as it occurs in nature. Many oncoproteins implicated in oncogenesis such as *MYC, MYB, JUN, FOS,* and *REL* oncogenes, function as transcription factors. Of these, best known is *MYC* that is involved most commonly in human tumors.

MYC

MYC is a proto-oncogene that is expressed in almost all cells and belongs to the immediate early response genes. MYC is a universal transcription factor that may control transcription of as many as 10–15% of all human genes. There are C-MYC, N-MYC, and L-MYC that are key to development of many tumors. Following growth factor stimulation of quiescent cells, MYC is rapidly and transiently induced by RAS/MAPK signaling. Normally, MYC protein (Product of MYC gene) concentrations are tightly controlled at the level of transcription, translation, and protein stability. Almost all pathways that regulate growth have an effect on MYC through one or more of the above mentioned mechanisms. **Dysregulation of MYC promotes tumorigenesis by** cellular proliferation by **promoting the progression of cells through the cell cycle and also alters metabolism that supports cell growth.** MYC has several broad activities, many of which contribute not only to deregulated cell growth but also to several other hallmarks of cancer. MYC activates the transcription of other genes.

Activities of MYC MYC activates the expression of many genes involved in cell growth. These are as follows:

1. **Growth-promoting genes required for cell cycle progression:** Some MYC target genes such as D cyclins are directly involved in progression of cell cycle. For example, cyclin-dependent kinases (CDKs).
2. **Upregulation of ribosomal RNA:** MYC upregulates the expression of ribosomal RNA (rRNA) genes and rRNA processing. Thus, MYC enhances the assembly of ribosomes required for synthesis of proteins.
3. **Upregulates a program of gene expression:** This leads to metabolic reprogramming and the Warburg effect. Warburg effect is one of the hallmarks of cancer (refer page 487–490). MYC upregulates genes involved in metabolism namely multiple glycolytic enzymes and factors involved in glutamine metabolism. Both of them produce metabolic intermediates required for synthesis of macromolecules

such as DNA, proteins, nucleotides and lipids. These are needed for cell growth and division.

4. **MYC is a master transcriptional regulator** of cell growth. Some of the rapidly growing human tumors, such as Burkitt lymphoma almost always have a chromosomal translocation involving MYC consisting (8;14) translocation (see **Fig. 23**). This show highest levels of MYC.
5. **Upregulates of telomerase:** Telomerase is one of enzyme that contribute to the endless replicative capacity (the immortalization) of cancer cells. In some tumors, MYC upregulates expression of telomerase.
6. **Activation of death programme:** MYC may also activate cell death programs in cells with intact p53 and other cell death effectors
7. **Reprogram somatic cells into pluripotent stem cells:** MYC is one of the transcription factors that can reprogram somatic cells into pluripotent stem cells. Probably this nature of MYC may be responsible for cancer cell "stemness." Stemness is another important factor responsible for the immortality of cancers. Given the importance of MYC in regulation of cell growth, it should come as no surprise that it is deregulated in cancer through a large variety of mechanisms. Sometimes deregulation involves genetic alterations of MYC itself.

***Examples of MYC-related cancers*:**

- In **Burkitt lymphoma** (highly aggressive B-cell tumor) and a subset of other B- and T-cell tumors, the *MYC* gene is translocated. This *MYC* is translocated into an antigen receptor gene locus, which contains gene regulatory elements called enhancers. These enhancer regions are highly active in lymphocytes. Instead of driving the expression of B- or T-cell receptors, these misplaced enhancers cause the deregulation and overexpression of MYC protein.
- Amplification and overexpression of *MYC* is also observed in **breast, colon, lung, and many other cancers**.
- MYC-related functionally identical *NMYC* and *LMYC* genes are also amplified **in neuroblastomas (Fig. 27)** and **small cell cancers of lung**, respectively.
- **Oncogenic mutations of the components of upstream signaling pathways:** They cause raised levels of MYC protein by increasing MYC transcription, enhancing MYC messenger RNA (mRNA) translation, and/or stabilizing MYC protein. This in turn produces constitutive activation of RAS/MAPK signaling (many cancers), Notch signaling (several cancers), Wnt signaling (colon carcinoma), and Hedgehog signaling (medulloblastoma). Partly all of these transform cells through upregulation of MYC.
- Many single nucleotide polymorphisms (SNPs) associated with an inherited risk for cancers such as prostate and ovarian carcinoma and certain leukemias may **involve enhancer elements**. These SNPs may stimulate higher levels of MYC RNA expression in response to growth-promoting signals and thereby favor MYC activation.

Cyclins and Cyclin-dependent Kinases

Growth factors bind to their respective receptors and transduce signals, and the transcription factors stimulate the orderly progression of cells through the various phases of the cell cycle. During cell cycle, the cells replicate their DNA in preparation for cell division. The progression of cells through the cell cycle is orchestrated by CDKs. CDKs are activated by binding to *cyclins* (called so because of the cyclic nature of their production and degradation) and they form CDK-cyclin complexes. These complexes phosphorylate critical target proteins that drive cells forward through the cell cycle. There are *CDK inhibitors* (CDKIs) which silence the CDKs and apply negative control over the cell cycle. Expression of these inhibitors is downregulated by mitogenic signaling pathways and this promotes the progression of the cell cycle.

Checkpoints in cell cycle

In cell cycle, there are two main cell cycle checkpoints, namely—(i) at the G_1/S transition and (ii) at the G_2/M transition. Both these checkpoints are tightly regulated by a balance of growth-promoting and growth-suppressing factors, as well as by sensors of DNA damage. If DNA-damage sensors are activated, they transmit signals that arrest cell cycle progression and allow the cell to repair the DNA damage by DNA repair genes. If the cell damage cannot be repaired, it initiates apoptosis. Once cells pass through the G_1/S checkpoint, the cells are committed to undergo cell division. Thus, defects in the G_1/S checkpoint are important in cancer because these defects allow the cells to increased cell division. They may also impair DNA repair. This creates a "mutator" phenotype and lead to development and progression of cancer. All cancers have genetic lesions that disable the G_1/S checkpoint and cause cells to continually re-enter the S phase of the cell cycle. Genetic lesions that disable G_1/S checkpoint may belong to the two following major categories: (i) gain-of-function mutations in D cyclin genes and CDK4 and (ii) loss-of-function mutations in genes that inhibit G_1/S progression.

Gain-of-function mutations in D cyclin genes and CDK4
They promote unregulated G_1/S progression and thus act as oncogenes. Increased expression of cyclin D or CDK4 are common in cancers.

- **Cyclin D genes**: Cyclin D genes have three genes namely D1, D2, and D3 and they are functionally interchangeable. They are usually dysregulated by acquired mutations in cancer. These mutations include chromosomal translocations in lymphoid tumors and gene amplification in a many solid tumors. They are overexpressed in many malignant tumors such as cancers of the breast, esophagus, liver, and a subset of lymphomas and plasma cell tumors.
- ***CDK4* gene:** Amplification of the *CDK4* gene occurs in melanomas, sarcomas, and glioblastomas. In advanced breast cancers associated with excessive CDK4 activity, treatment with CDK4 inhibitors are effective.
- ***Other cyclins and CDKS:*** Mutations can also affect cyclins B and E and other CDKs. But they are less frequent than those involving cyclin D and CDK4. These genes are less important in control of the G_1/S transition.

Loss-of-function mutations in genes that inhibit G_1/S progression CDKIs (CDK inhibitors) are tumor suppressor genes which inhibit formation of cyclin D/CDK complexes. CDKIs are also frequently disabled in many malignant tumors in humans, either by mutation or gene silencing. Example is presented below:

- ○ ***CDKN2A gene (p 16):*** It is a gene that encodes the CDK inhibitor p16.
  - **Germline mutations** of *CDKN2A* occur in 25% of melanoma-prone relatives.
  - **Acquired deletion or inactivation of *CDKN2A*:** It is observed in 75% of pancreatic carcinomas, 40–70% of glioblastomas, 50% of esophageal cancers, and 20% to 70% of acute lymphoblastic leukemias, and 20% of non-small cell lung carcinomas, soft tissue sarcomas, and bladder cancers.
- **Tumor suppressor genes *RB* and *TP53*:** Two very important tumor suppressor genes (TSGs) are *RB* and *TP53*. Both these TSGs also encode proteins that inhibit G_1/S progression. Their mutation is common in cancer.

Note: Increased growth-promoting signals by any of the oncogene discussed above does not by itself lead to sustained proliferation of cancer cells. There are two built-in mechanisms that oppose oncogene-mediated cell growth, namely—(i) senescence and (ii) apoptosis. Genes that regulate these two braking mechanisms must be disabled before the oncogenes cause the cell to proceed to unopposed proliferation.

Different signaling molecules that can be targets for carcinogenic events are presented in **Figure 44**.

Various mechanisms of conversion of proto-oncogene into oncogene and their effects are presented in **Figure 45. Figure 46** shows schematic representation of gene amplification versus overexpression.

Usual cell cycle components and inhibitors mutated in cancer are presented in **Table 19**.

Mechanism of activation of oncogenes: Proto-oncogenes can be altered by many ways. These include: (1) point mutations, (2) amplification, (3) gene rearrangement/translocation, (4) deletion of part or whole of chromosome and (5) altered expression.

Hallmark 2: Evading Growth Suppressors

Q. Discuss tumor suppressor genes in neoplasia.

Q. Role of tumor suppressor genes in carcinogenesis (natural anticarcinogens).

Tumor suppressor genes: According to Isaac Newton, "every action has an equal and opposite reaction". Same holds good for cell growth. As already discussed above, **oncogenes encode proteins that promote cell growth** and cells also possess complex, powerful signaling programs (mechanisms) that suppress cell proliferation. Normally, there are braking mechanisms that serve either to overrule the initiation of, or to subsequently turn off, cell division stimulated by proliferative signals of oncogenes mentioned above. These regulatory mechanisms ensure that cell proliferation is not an entirely cell-autonomous process and guards against tumor development. The molecules that guard and protect against cancer development are called tumor suppressors (the term is used because of their frequent loss-of-function via inactivating genetic mutations that causes cancer). The genes that encode these tumor suppressors are called tumor suppressor genes (*TSGs*). The **products of TSGs apply brakes to cell**

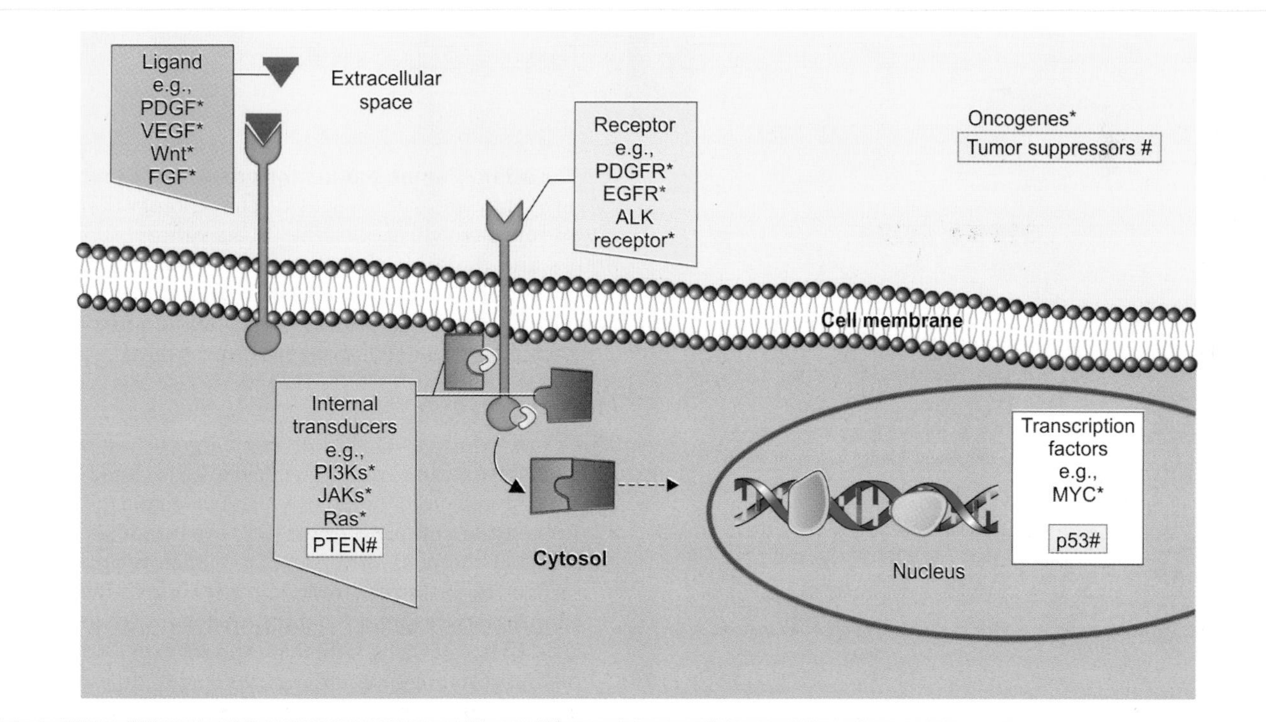

(EGFR: epithelial growth factor receptor; FGF: fibroblast growth factors; PDGF: platelet derived growth factor; VEGF: vascular endothelial growth factor; PDGFR: platelet derived growth factor receptor)

FIG. 44: Different signaling molecules that can be targets for carcinogenic events. The oncogenes or tumor suppressor classes of signaling molecules that can produce cancer include ligands (such cytokines and growth factors); receptors [frequently tyrosine kinase receptors (RTKs)]; intracellular signaling transducers (e.g., RAS, PTEN etc.); and gene regulating factors (e.g., MYC).

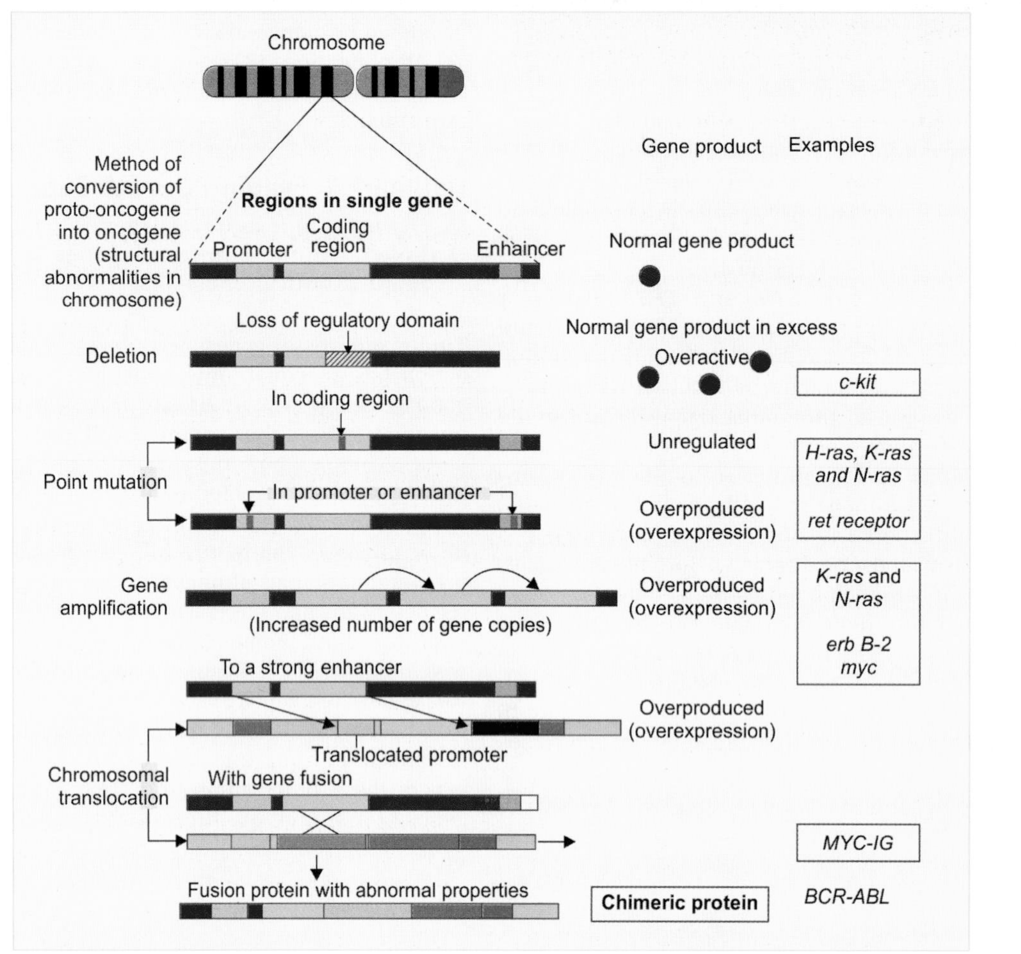

FIG. 45: Various mechanisms of conversion of proto-oncogene into oncogene and their effect.

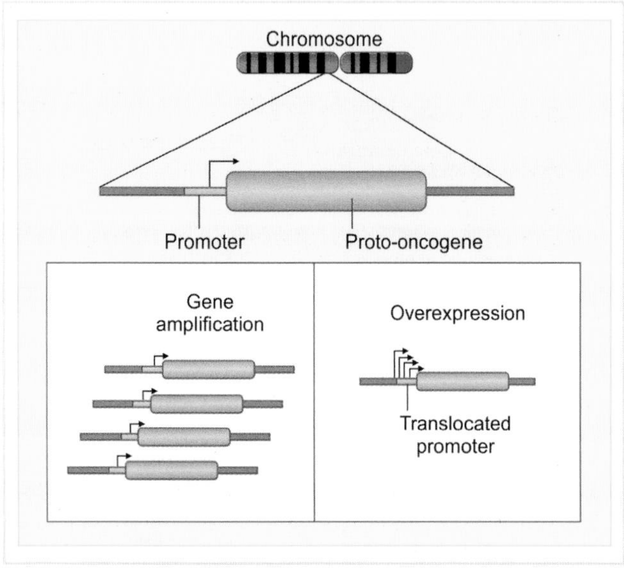

FIG. 46: Schematic representation of gene amplification versus overexpression.

proliferation. Tumor suppressor proteins are the products of TSG. They control a series of checkpoints that prevent uncontrolled growth of cells. The TSGs are the most prominent brakes and the direct regulators of the cell division cycle. The most important in this group are two prototypical TSGs, namely *Rb* and *p53* genes. They encode the retinoblastoma (RB)-associated and TP53 proteins, respectively.

Mechanisms of Actions

There are many TSGs, with diverse targets, functions, and mechanisms of action. Anti-growth signals of tumor suppressors can prevent cell proliferation by several mechanisms.

- **Preventing cell proliferation:** Many tumor suppressors (e.g., RB and p53) form part of a regulatory network that recognizes genotoxic stress from any source. These tumor suppressors respond by shutting down proliferation of cells. In normal cells, if there is expression of an oncogene, the intact tumor suppressor genes lead to quiescence (G_0 phase) or permanent cell cycle arrest (oncogene-induced senescence) rather than uncontrolled proliferation.
- **Entry into a postmitotic differentiated pool:** Another set of tumor suppressors are probably involved in cell

Table 19: Cell cycle components and inhibitors mutated in cancer.

Component	*Normal role*
Cyclins and cyclin-dependent kinases (CDK)	
CDK4 and D cyclins	• Form a complex and phosphorylate retinoblastoma protein (RB) • Allow the cell to progress through the G_1 restriction point of cell cycle
Inhibitors of cell cycle	
CIP/KIP family: p21, p27 (CDKN1A–D)	• Arrest the cell cycle by binding to cyclin–CDK complexes • p21 is induced by tumor suppressor p53 • p27 responds to growth suppressors [e.g., transforming growth factor (TGF)-β]
INK4/ARF family (CDKN2A–C)	• p16/INK4a: Binds to cyclin D-CDK4 and enhances the inhibitory effects of RB • p14/ARF: Enhances levels p53 levels by inhibiting activity of mouse double minute 2 homolog (MDM2)
Cell cycle checkpoint components: Tumor suppressor	
RB	• RB protein binds to E2F transcription factors in its active hypophosphorylated state and prevents G_1/S transition • RB interacts with transcription factors that regulate differentiation of cells
p53 (altered in many cancers and induced by DNA damage)	• Causes cell cycle arrest by upregulating the CDK inhibitor p21 • Promotes apoptosis by upregulating *BAX* and other proapoptotic genes

differentiation. The signal may cause the cells to enter a postmitotic differentiated pool and lose replicative potential. Cells are forced to enter into the nonproliferative but viable state called *senescence* (**nonreplicative senescence**). This is another mechanism of escape from sustained cell growth.

- **Undergo apoptosis:** The signals from TSGs may program the cells to undergo death by apoptosis.

Similar to mitogenic signals involved growth of the cells, signals that causes inhibition of growth inhibition and differentiation by originate outside the cell. These signal use receptors, signal transducers, and nuclear transcription regulators to produce their effects. Tumor suppressors form a portion of these networks. Thus the protein products of tumor suppressor genes may function as transcription factors, cell cycle inhibitors, signal transduction molecules, cell surface receptors, and regulators of cellular responses to DNA damage.

Insensitivity to Growth-inhibitory Signals (Loss of Function of Negative Growth Regulators)

Disruption of TSGs renders cells resistant to growth inhibition and mimic the growth-promoting effects of oncogenes. **Tumor suppressor is a protein or gene which is associated with suppression of any of the various hallmarks of cancer.** As discussed earlier, **oncogenes stimulate proliferation of cells,** whereas **the products of most TSGs apply brakes and prevent uncontrolled cell proliferation.** TSGs are discussed on pages 455–468.

Retinoblastoma Gene (RB Gene)

Q. Write a short essay on retinoblastoma gene.

Retinoblastoma gene (*RB*) is the governor of the cell cycle and is a key negative regulator of the cell cycle. *B* (*RB1*) **gene** was the **first discovered TSG**, which is present **on chromosome locus 13q14**. Retinoblastoma gene *(RB)* is the prototype of TSGs. **RB is inactivated either directly or indirectly in most human cancers. Inactivation of *RB* gene was first detected in retinoblastoma**, which is a rare malignant childhood tumor derived from the retina. Retinoblastoma may occur either as a hereditary (familial) or sporadic (60% of cases) form.

Q. Write a short essay on Knudson hypothesis.

Knudson's (1974) two-hit hypothesis of oncogenesis

It explains the inherited and sporadic occurrence of an identical tumor (e.g., retinoblastoma) (**Fig. 47**). According to Knudson's hypothesis:

- **Two mutations (hits),** involving **both the normal alleles** (hence the two hits) of TSGs **are required to produce the tumor** (e.g., retinoblastoma).
- **In familial cases,** children inherit one defective copy of the *RB* gene in the germline; the other copy is normal. Thus, **one mutation (first hit) takes place in the germline** and **second hit after birth.** Retinoblastoma develops when the normal *RB* gene in retinoblasts is lost due to somatic mutation. In retinoblastoma families, a single germline mutation is enough to transmit disease risk, the trait has an autosomal dominant inheritance pattern.
- In **sporadic cases, both mutations** (two hits) **develop after birth.** Both normal *RB* alleles are lost by somatic mutation in one of the retinoblasts.

The final outcome of both is a retinal cell with loss of both of the normal copies of the *RB* gene and these cells become malignant, causing retinoblastoma. It is to be noted that though the risk for the development of retinoblastoma in retinoblastoma families is inherited as a dominant trait, at the level of the cell, one intact *RB* gene is enough for normal function.

Loss of normal *RB* genes was initially discovered in retinoblastomas. Loss of both alleles (biallelic loss) of *RB* gene is quite common in several tumors such as breast cancer, small cell cancer of the lung, and bladder cancer. Patients with familial retinoblastoma also have a high risk for developing osteosarcomas and some soft tissue sarcomas.

RB gene and retinoblastoma

Familial/hereditary retinoblastoma It constitutes about 40% of retinoblastoma and two hits occur as follows:

- **First hit:** Affected **children inherit** cells with **one defective copy** (mutated allele) of the ***RB* gene in the germline** (one hit) and one normal copy of *RB* gene (the child is heterozygous at the *RB* locus). The product of normal *RB* gene is sufficient to prevent tumor. (Allele is alternative form of the gene found at the same locus in homologous chromosomes).
- **Second hit: Retinoblastoma develops when** the remaining normal *RB* allele is inactivated (mutated) due

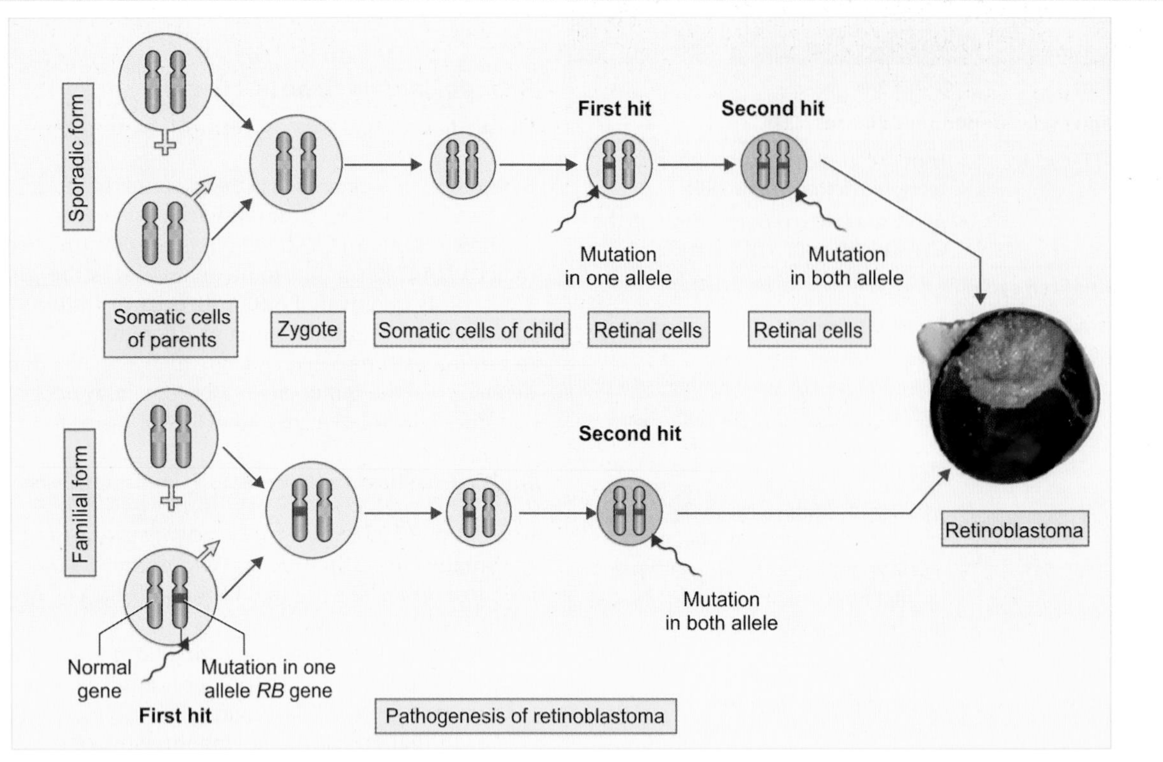

FIG. 47: Pathogenesis of retinoblastoma. Two mutations of the *RB* are required for neoplastic proliferation of the retinal cells. In the sporadic form, both *RB* mutations occur in retinal cell after birth. In the familial form, all somatic cells inherit one mutant *RB* gene from a parent, and only one additional *RB* mutation in a retinal cell is needed for complete loss of *RB* function.

to **spontaneous somatic mutation** (second hit). Because only a single somatic mutation is sufficient for loss of *RB* function in familial retinoblastoma, it is **transmitted as an autosomal dominant trait**.

- Patients with **familial retinoblastoma** have also **increased risk** of developing **osteosarcoma** and other soft tissue sarcomas.

Sporadic retinoblastoma It forms about 60% of cases. The child has two normal *RB* alleles in all somatic cells. To develop retinoblastoma, **both normal *RB* alleles must undergo mutation** and it **needs two hits.**

Normal cell cycle has two gaps (refer pages 66–72 and Fig. 5 of Chapter 3).

Q. Write a short note on the role of RB in the cell cycle.

Gap 1 (G_1) between mitosis (M) and DNA replication (S). Each phase of the cell cycle is carefully monitored. Gap 1 is the transition from G_1 to S and is a **very important checkpoint through which cells must pass before DNA replication commences.** Once the cells cross this checkpoint, they are compelled to complete mitosis. In G_1 phase, **signals determine whether the cell should enter the cell cycle, exit** the cell cycle and differentiate. The cells exit the cell cycle either temporarily (known as quiescence), or permanently (known as senescence). ***RB* plays a key role in this decision process and RB protein** (pRB) **regulates the G_1/S checkpoint.**

- **Gap 2** (G_2) between DNA replication (S) and mitosis (M).

Functions of the *RB* gene (Fig. 48)

Q. Write a short note on the function of retinoblastoma gene.

***RB* gene is the governor of cell cycle** and plays a key role in **regulating the cell cycle** and **also controls cellular differentiation**.

***State of RB gene product: RB* gene product** is a DNA-binding protein expressed in all cells. It is present either in an **active hypophosphorylated** state (in quiescent cells) or **inactive hyperphosphorylated** state (in cells passing through the G_1/S cell cycle phase). Signals that promote progression of cell cycle lead to the phosphorylation and inactivation of RB, while those that block progression of cell cycle maintain RB in an active hypophosphorylated state.

Active RB gene regulates G_1/S checkpoint of cell cycle: Cell cycle is tightly controlled by cyclins and CDKs, which form cyclin-CDK complexes. Before DNA replication, the cell must pass through G_1/S check which is regulated by *RB*.

- **Initiation** of DNA replication (S phase) requires activation of cyclins D/CDK4, cyclin D/CDK6, and cyclin E/CDK2 complexes. Expression of cyclin E is dependent on the E2F family of transcription factors. High levels of these complexes lead to hyperphosphorylation and inhibition of *RB*. This releases E2F transcription factors which causes the expression of genes that are required for progression of cell from G_1 to S phase.

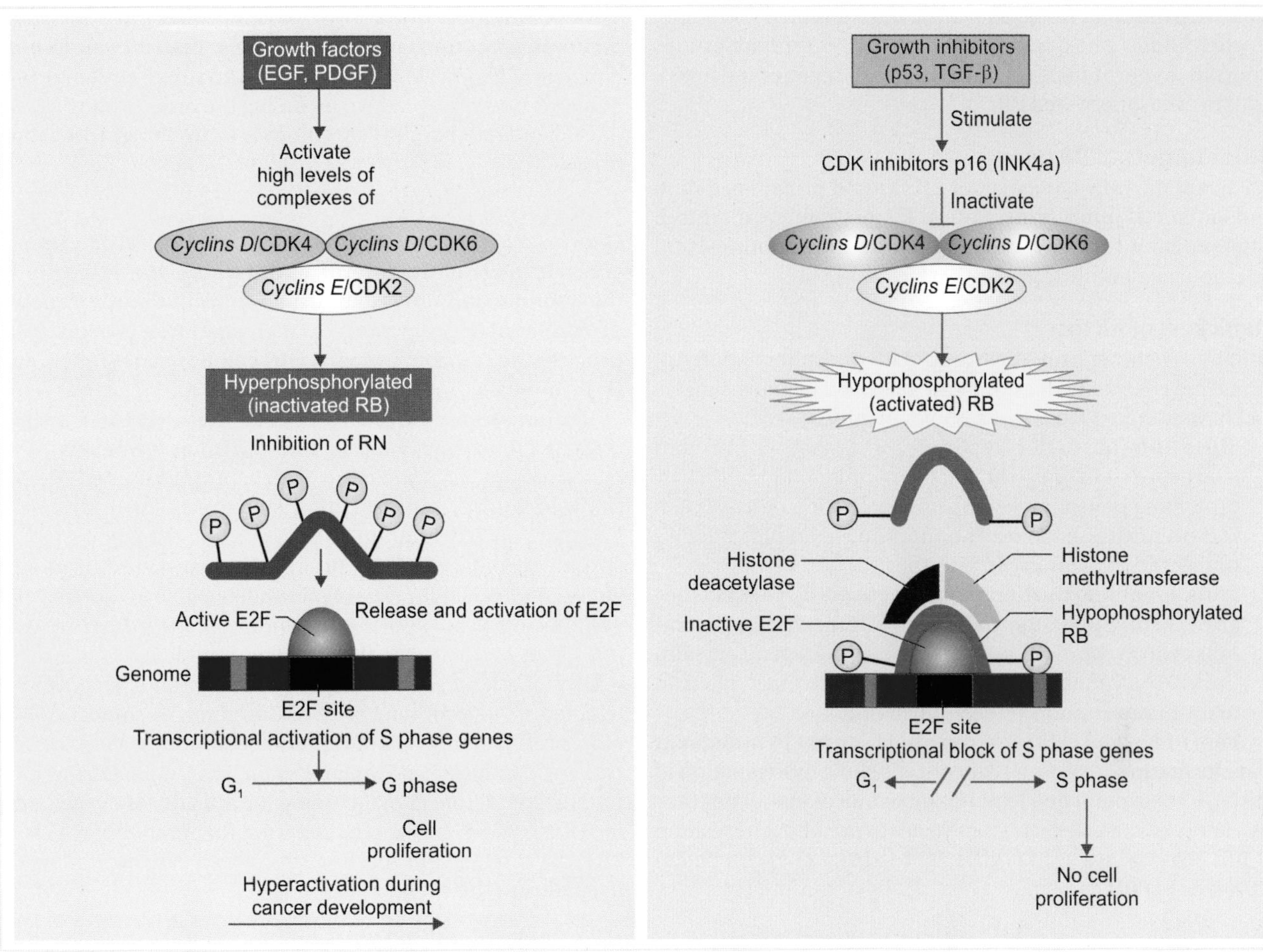

(CDK: cyclin-dependent kinase; EGF: epidermal growth factor; PDGF: platelet-derived growth factor; TGF: transforming growth factor).

FIG. 48: Function of *RB* in regulating the G_1/S checkpoint of the cell cycle. (A) When *RB* is phosphorylated by the cyclin D–cyclin dependent kinase (CDK) 4, cyclin D–CDK6, and cyclin E–CDK2 complexes, it releases E2F. E2F then activates transcription of S-phase genes. The phosphorylation of RB is inhibited by cyclin-dependent kinase inhibitors (CDKIs), because CDKIs inactivate cyclin–CDK complexes. (B) Hypophosphorylated active *RB* combines with the E2F transcription factors and binds to deoxyribonucleic acid (DNA). This recruits two chromatin remodeling factors, namely—histone deacetylases and histone methyl transferases, and inhibits progression from G_1/S phase of cell cycle. Almost all cancer cells show dysregulation of the G_1/S checkpoint due to mutation in one of four genes that regulate the phosphorylation of RB. These genes are *RB, CDK4, cyclin D, and CDKN2A [p16].*

- ***RB* blocks E2F-mediated transcription**: During early G_1 phase, RB is in its hypophosphorylated active form. This **active hypophosphorylated** RB bind and inhibit E2F family of transcription factors, thereby preventing transcription of cyclin E. Two methods of blocking E2F transcription by hypophosphorylated RB are:
  - **Sequesters (segregations of) E2F** prevent it from interacting (combining) with other transcription activators.
  - **RB mobilizes** (recruits) **two chromatin remodeling proteins/enzymes** (histone deacetylases and histone methyl transferases) which bind to the promoters of E2F-responsive genes such as cyclin E. These enzymes modify chromatin at the promoters to make DNA insensitive to transcription factors and thus **block the transcription**.

Inactivation of *RB* gene

Growth factor (mitogenic) signaling upregulates the activity of the CDK/cyclin complexes. It leads to expression of cyclin D and activation of cyclin D-CDK4/6 complexes. The level of cyclin D-CDK4/6 activities are lessened by antagonists (tumor suppressors) such as $p16^{INK4a}$ and $p21.^{WAF1}$ If the mitogenic stimulus is sufficiently strong, cyclin D-CDK4/6 complexes phosphorylate *RB*. This converts active hypophosphorylated *RB* into inactive hyperphosphorylated *RB*.

- **Consequence of inactivation of *RB* gene:** Inactivation of *RB* releases the break and frees the transcription factor E2F from *RB* to activate target genes such as cyclin E. Cyclin E combines with CDK to form cyclin E/CDK complexes that stimulate DNA replication and progression through the cell cycle. When the cells enter S phase of the cell cycle, they divide without additional growth factor stimulation.

- **Reactivation of *RB* gene:** During the subsequent M phase, the cellular phosphatases remove the phosphate groups from hyperphosphorylated RB and regenerate active hypophosphorylated RB.

Other targets of *RB* gene

E2F is not the only one target of RB. The RB protein can bind to a variety of other transcription factors that regulate cell differentiation (e.g., myocyte-, adipocyte-, melanocyte-, and macrophage-specific transcription factors).

Mimickers of *RB* loss

Mutations in other genes that control RB phosphorylation can mimic the effect of RB loss. They are observed in many cancers that have normal *RB* genes. Examples include:

- **Mutation of CDK4** leading to its activation and **overexpression of cyclin D** causes proliferation of cells by promoting phosphorylation and inactivation of RB. Cyclin D is overexpressed in many tumors due to amplification or translocation of the cyclin D1 gene.
- **Mutational inactivation of genes encoding CDKIs:** They also can stimulate the cell cycle by removing important brakes on cyclin/CDK activity. The *CDKN2A* gene encodes the CDK inhibitor p16 and is commonly inactivated in many human tumors by deletion or mutation.

Loss of normal cell cycle control is central to malignant transformation. Almost all cancer cells show dysregulation of the G_1/S checkpoint due to mutation in one of four genes (key regulators of the cell cycle) that regulate the phosphorylation of RB. These genes are **(1) *CDKN2A [p16]*, (2) *cyclin D*, (3) *CDK4*, or (4) *RB*.**

Method of inactivation of RB gene and associated tumors:

- **Loss-of-function mutations involving both *RB* alleles.** It may be:
  - **Germline mutation,** e.g., in **retinoblastomas** and **osteosarcomas**
  - **Acquired mutation,** e.g., in **glioblastomas, small cell carcinomas of lung,** breast cancers, and bladder carcinomas.
- **Change from the active hypophosphorylated state to the inactive hyperphosphorylated state:** The active hypophosphorylated RB state may be shifted to an inactive hyperphosphorylated RB state. This may be due to (1) **gain-of-function mutations that upregulate CDK/cyclin D activity or (2) by loss-of-function mutations that abolish/cancel the activity of CDKIs (p16/INK4a)**.
- **Viral oncoproteins that bind and inhibit RB [E7 protein of human papillomavirus (HPV)]** may occur even without *RB* mutation. In cancers caused due to certain oncogenic viruses, viral proteins directly target RB. For example, E7 protein of the human papillomavirus (HPV) binds to the hypophosphorylated form of RB and thus prevents RB from inhibiting the E2F transcription factors. Free E2F causes progression of cell cycle and produces cervical carcinomas. Thus, functionally RB is deleted and it leads to uncontrolled cell growth (Fig. 102 of pages 537 and 538).

TP53: Guardian of the Genome

Location: TP53 is a **TSG (tumor suppressor gene) located on small arm of chromosome 17 (17p13.1)**. Its protein product p53 is present in almost all normal tissues.

Loss-of-function mutations in *TP53*: These are the most common mutations observed in more than 50% of human cancers. *TP53* mutations occur at variable frequency with almost every type of cancer, including the three leading causes of cancer death namely, **carcinomas of the lung, colon, and breast**.

Functions of p53 (Fig. 49)

***Guardian of the Genome*:** It functions as a **critical gatekeeper gene**. It plays **main role in maintaining the integrity of the genome** and thus is known as **guardian of the genome** or **"molecular policeman"**. ***TP53* regulates (i) cell cycle progression, (ii) DNA repair, (iii) cellular senescence, and (iv) apoptosis**.

In nonstressed healthy/normal cells, p53 has a short half-life (20 minutes) and **is maintained at low levels**). This is because of its association with a protein named MDM2 (murine double minute 2) that targets p53 for destruction. MDM2 is an E3 ubiquitin (Ub) ligase that conjugates p53 to Ub and degrades p53 (**Fig. 50**) by the proteasome. This results almost undetectable levels of p53 undetectable in normal cells. *TP53* has a critical role in the prevention of cancer development. p53 serves as focal point of large network of signals which sense variety of stresses. These stresses include anoxia shortened telomeres, inappropriate progrowth stimuli (e.g., uncontrolled MYC or RAS activity), and DNA damage. They trigger the p53 response pathways. p53 manages the DNA damage and thus plays a central role in maintaining the integrity of the genome. In stressed cells, p53 is released from the inhibitory effects of MDM2 via two major mechanisms, which vary depending on the nature of the stress.

DNA damage and hypoxia: Stress due to DNA damage or hypoxia activates "sensors". They consist of two related protein kinases, namely—(1) ataxia-telangiectasia mutated (ATM) and (2) ataxia-telangiectasia and Rad3 related (ATR). ATM gene was first identified as the germline mutation in patients with ataxia-telangiectasia (inability to repair certain kinds of DNA damage, and have increased incidence of cancer). Though the types of damage sensed by ATM and ATR are different, they have similar downstream effects. Once activated, both ATM and ATR stimulate the phosphorylation of p53 and MDM2 (**Fig. 51**). These posttranslational modifications disrupts the binding and degradation of p53 by MDM2. Thus, the activated sensors (ATM and ATR) release p53 from the inhibitory effects of MDM2 and **p53 becomes activated**. This increases half-life of p53 as well as its ability to drive the transcription of target genes. p53 can trigger transcription of hundreds of genes. These disrupt the binding and degradation of p53 by MDM2, allowing p53 to accumulate.

Oncogenic stress: It may be induced by activation of oncoproteins such as RAS. These stresses produce sustained signaling via progrowth pathways (e.g., MAPK and PI3K/AKT pathways). These signals produce cellular stress and lead to increased expression of p14/ARF (encoded by the *CDKN2A* TSGs). p14/ARF binds MDM2 and releases p53 and resulting in raised p53 levels in the cell.

Prevention of neoplastic transformation Once activated, p53 is a transcription factor that binds DNA in a sequence-specific fashion. Activated p53 in turn activates the transcription of hundreds of target genes with p53-binding regulatory elements. Though the target genes that prevents neoplastic

Normal cell (p53 normal)
Ionization radiation
Carcinogens
Mutagens
Shortened telomere
Cell with DNA damage
Oncogenic stress
hypoxia
p53 normal
p53-activation (↑*p53*)
Loss/mutations of *p53*
p53 accumulates and binds to DNA
p53-dependent genes not activated
• No DNA repair
• No senescence
• No cell cycle arrest
Transcription dependent and independent effects on targets
Cell with mutation
Senescence
p21 (CDK inhibitor)
GADD45 (DNA repair)
BAX, PUMA
(pro-apoptotic)
Uncontrolled cell proliferation
Additional mutations
Cell cycle arrest at G_1
Repair fails
Successful repair
Malignant tumor
Normal cell
Apoptosis

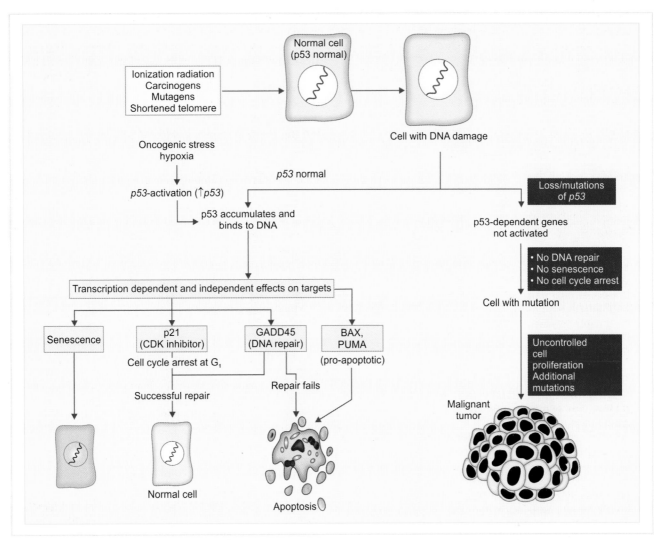

FIG. 49: Role of p53 in maintaining the integrity of the genome. DNA damage DNA-damaging agents or by hypoxia activates normal p53 and arrests the cell cycle in G_1 and induces repair of DNA by transcriptional upregulation of the cyclin-dependent kinase inhibitor *CDKN1A* (encoding the cyclin dependent kinase inhibitor p21) and *GADD45* (growth arrest and DNA damage) genes. Successful repair of DNA allows cells to proceed with the cell cycle. If DNA repair fails, p53 triggers either apoptosis or senescence. In cells with loss or mutations of p53, DNA damage does not induce cell cycle arrest or DNA repair or senescence, and cells with mutation proliferate to form malignant neoplasms.

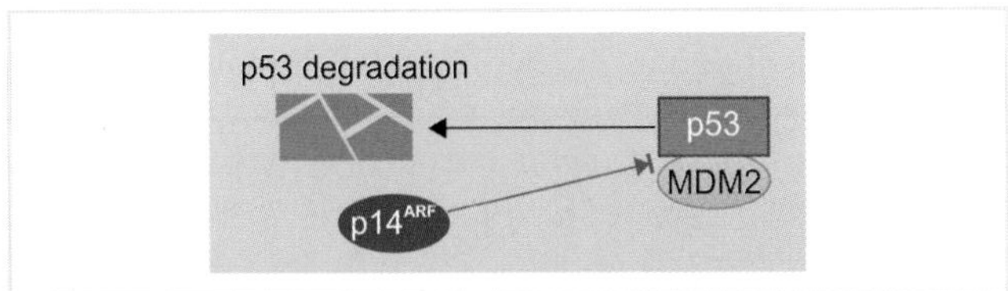

FIG. 50: Interrelation between p53 and MDM2: MDM2 (murine double minute 2) is an E3 ubiquitin ligase. In nonstressed normal cells, MDM2 binds p53 and directs its inactivation. P14 ARF inhibits this interaction between MDM2 and p53.

transformation by p53 are not completely known, they belong to three major categories: (1) genes that cause transient cell cycle arrest, (2) genes that senescence (permanent cell cycle arrest), (3) genes that cause apoptosis (programmed cell death). There is also involvement of genes that enhance catabolic metabolism or inhibit anabolic metabolism.

- **Transient/temporary *p53*-induced cell cycle arrest** (termed *quiescence*): p53-mediated cell cycle arrest is the primordial or primitive response to DNA damage. If there is **damage to DNA**, transient, rapid cell cycle arrest occurs late in the G_1 phase. It is caused mainly by *p53*-dependent transcription of the *CDKN1A* gene (encodes the CDK inhibitor *p21*). The p21 (like p16) protein in turn inhibits CDK4/D cyclin complexes and prevents phosphorylation of RB. Thus, RB is maintained in an active, hypophosphorylated state. This blocks the progression of cells from G_1 phase to S phase, thereby arresting cells. This cell cycle arrest in the G_1 phase gives the cells "breathing time" to repair DNA damage. The p53 protein also activates expression of DNA damage repair genes. **If DNA damage is** successfully **repaired by DNA repair genes,** p53 upregulates transcription of MDM2. This leads to destruction of p53 itself. The resulting **fall in the levels of p53 releases the block in cell cycle** and return of cells to a

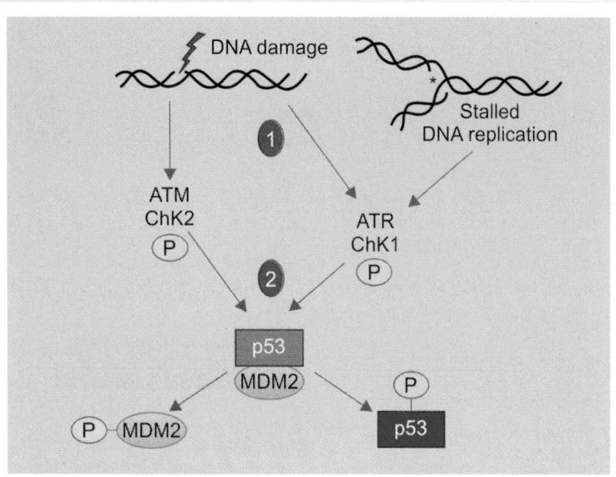

FIG. 51: Connection of p53 with DNA damage and hypoxia. 1. DNA damage and other interference with DNA replication activate ATM (ataxia telangiectasia mutated) and ATR (ATM and Rad3 related) kinases. ATM activates ChK2 and ATR activates ChK1. 2. Both ChK1 and ChK2 phosphorylate p53. This releases p53 from bondage to MDM2 (murine double minute 2).

normal state. If the DNA damage cannot be repaired, the cell may either enter p53-induced senescence or undergo p53-directed apoptosis.

- **p53-induced senescence (permanent cell cycle arrest):** Senescence is defined as a state of permanent cell cycle arrest and is characterized by specific changes in morphology and gene expression that differentiate it from quiescence or reversible cell cycle arrest. Senescence may be stimulated in response to different types of stresses (e.g., unopposed oncogene signaling, hypoxia and shortened telomeres). Senescence needs activation of p53 and/or Rb and expression of their mediators, such as the CDKIs. The senescent cells are not normal and cannot divide. Hence, they are prevented from forming tumors.
- **p53-induced apoptosis (programmed cell death): Cells with irreversible DNA damage undergo p53-induced apoptosis** and it is the ultimate or eventual protective mechanism against development of cancer. It is mediated by upregulation of several proapoptotic genes by p53. These include *BAX* and *PUMA* which cause apoptosis of cells with irreversible DNA damage via the intrinsic (mitochondrial) pathway.

Probably, the duration and the level of p53 activation may be deciding factors that determines whether a cell with DNA damage repairs its DNA, becomes senescent, or undergoes apoptosis. It is assumed that p53 has higher affinity for binding sites in the promoters and enhancers of DNA repair genes than pro-apoptotic genes. Thus, when p53 begins to accumulate, first it stimulates the DNA repair pathway. If the levels of p53 is sustained due to defective DNA repair or other chronic stresses (e.g., oncogenic RAS mutation), it may lead to epigenetic silencing of genes that are required for progression of cell cycle. This leads to senescence. Or if there is enough accumulation of p53, it can stimulate the transcription of the pro-apoptotic genes and the cell undergoes death by apoptosis.

Because of the above activities, p53 is called the "guardian of the genome". RB is a "sensor" of external signals whereas p53 is the central monitor of internal stress. p53 directs the stressed cells towards one of the above pathways.

Method of inactivation of *TP53* gene and Associated tumors

More than 50% of human cancers have defect in *TP53* gene and the remaining cancers usually have defects in genes upstream or downstream of *TP53*.

- **Acquired loss-of-function mutation in both** (biallelic) *TP53* **alleles** in somatic cells is most common and is found in almost every type of cancer. This includes three leading causes of cancer deaths namely carcinomas of the lung, colon, and breast. In most of the cases, mutations affecting both *TP53* alleles in somatic cells are acquired (not inherited in germline).
- **Germline mutations in one *TP53* allele:** It is less common. Individuals may **inherit one mutated/defective *TP53* allele and one additional "hit" in the other normal *TP53* allele** will produce malignant tumors. The resulting disorder called the **Li-Fraumeni syndrome** has germline mutations in one *TP53* and only one additional hit is needed to inactivate the second, normal allele. These individuals usually develop cancer at younger age, have 25-fold greater chance of developing a malignant tumor by age 50 compared with the general population. In contrast to tumors developing in patients who inherit a mutant *RB* allele, patients with the Li-Fraumeni syndrome develop much more varied range of multiple primary tumors. Most common types of malignant tumors include sarcomas, breast cancer, leukemia, brain tumors, and carcinomas of the adrenal cortex.
- **Mutations of proteins that regulate *p53* function:** *TP53* encodes the **protein *p53*, the function** of which is **tightly regulated at several levels by other proteins.** Thus, many **tumors without *TP53* mutations have mutations of proteins that regulate *p53* function.** For example, MDM2 and related proteins of the MDM2 (enzyme that ubiquitinylates *p53*) family degrade *p53* leading to a functional deficiency of *p53*. *MDM2* genes are frequently amplified (in 33% of human sarcomas) or overexpressed in cancers with normal or intact *TP53* alleles.
- **Blocking of *p53* function:** Similar to RB, the **transforming proteins of many** oncogenic **DNA viruses bind and degrade *p53* and** render them nonfunctional even without mutation in *p53*. Proteins encoded by oncogenic HPVs, certain polyomaviruses, and hepatitis B virus bind to p53 and abolish its protective function. For example, viral oncoprotein E6 of high-risk HPVs promote *p53* degradation and cause cervical carcinoma and a subset of squamous cell carcinomas of the head and neck. Thus, transforming DNA viruses suppress two of the well understood tumor suppressors namely RB and p53.

Consequences of Loss of p53 Function:

- **DNA damage goes unrepaired**
- **Driver mutations accumulate in oncogenes and other cancer genes.**
- **Cell blindly follows a dangerous path leading to malignant transformation.**

Therapeutic implications of *TP53*

- **Wild type versus mutated *TP53*:** Irradiation and chemotherapy used for the treatment of cancer, mediate their effects by causing damage to the DNA and producing apoptosis of tumor cells. Tumors with **wild type *TP53*** (**wild type refers to the most common form or phenotype in nature**) alleles are **more susceptible for apoptosis than tumors with mutated *TP53* alleles.** For example, childhood acute lymphoblastic leukemias which have wild type *TP53* alleles respond to radio- and chemotherapy; whereas lung cancers and colorectal cancers with mutated *TP53* allele, are relatively resistant to chemotherapy and irradiation.
- **Consequences of mutated *TP53*:** Tumor cells with mutated *p53* **have a tendency to acquire additional mutations** at a high rate and are **resistant to any mono/single therapy** (radiation/conventional chemotherapy/molecularly targeted therapy).

Other p53 family members: These include *p63* and *p73*. *p53* is universally expressed, whereas *p63* and *p73* show more tissue specificity. For example, *p63* is required for the differentiation of stratified squamous epithelium and p73 has powerful proapoptotic effects after DNA damage produced by chemotherapeutic drugs.

Figure 52 shows gain of function in oncogene and loss of function mutation in tumor suppressor gene.

Transforming Growth Factor-β Pathway (Figs. 53A and B)

***Normal function of TGF-β*:** TSGs (tumor suppressor genes) and their products apply brakes to the cell cycle. One of the molecules that transmit antiproliferative signals to cells is TGF-β. It is an extracellular cytokine and is a member of a family of dimeric growth factor. **In most normal epithelial, endothelial, and hematopoietic cells, TGF-β is a strong inhibitor of cell proliferation**. Normally, it exerts tumor-suppressive activity through effects on the target cells themselves or the extracellular matrix (ECM). It regulates cellular processes by binding to TGF-β receptors I and II. Upon ligand binding, the receptor undergoes dimerization and leads to a cascade of events. This results in the transcriptional activation of CDKIs with growth-suppressing activity and also suppresses growth-promoting genes such as *MYC* and *CDK4*.

Role of TGF-β in cancer: **TGF-β** plays an important role in the pathogenesis of cancer although cell and tissue responses to this cytokine vary. It is present in the microenvironment of cancer cells and inhibits mitogenesis induced by constituents of the ECM. It mainly tends to suppress tumor development by cell communication that modulates cell proliferation, survival, adhesion, and differentiation. Cancer cells may avoid TGF-β-related suppression by the following mechanisms—(i) by mutations in genes for TGF-β receptors or (ii) by interfering with downstream signaling by mutation or by promoter methylation of key proteins

- **Mutations in genes for TGF-β receptors:** In cancers, the growth-inhibiting effects of the TGF-β pathways may be impaired by mutations involving genes for TGF-β receptors. These mutations may alter the type II TGF-β receptor or SMAD ("Small", "Mothers Against Decapentaplegic") molecules. SMAD molecules serve to transduce antiproliferative signals from the receptor to the nucleus. **Mutations of gene for type II receptor** are observed in cancers of the colon, stomach, and endometrium.
    - **Mutational inactivation of SMAD4:** SMADs are tumor suppressors and are intermediary signaling molecules. Mutations in 1 of 10 of SMAD proteins known to be involved in TGF-β signaling, is common in pancreatic cancers.
- **Abnormal downstream signaling of TGF-β pathway:** In other cancers, loss of TGF-β-mediated growth control may occur at a level downstream of the TGF-β signaling pathway. For example, loss of p21 expression and/or overexpression of *MYC*. These tumor cells can then use other elements of the TGF-β-induced program to promote tumor progression. These include suppression of immune system (evasion of host defense mechanisms) or promotion of angiogenesis. Thus, depending on the state of other genes in the cell, TGF-β can prevent or promote proliferation of tumor cells. In late stages of many, TGF-β signaling activates epithelial-to-mesenchymal transition (EMT). EMT promotes migration, invasion, and metastasis.

Various effects of TGF-β are summarized in **Table 20**. Other cytokines [e.g., granulocyte/monocyte colony stimulating factor (GM-CSF) and interleukin-3 (IL-3)] may also be involved in the development of tumor. This may be by overexpression, especially in hematopoietic malignancies.

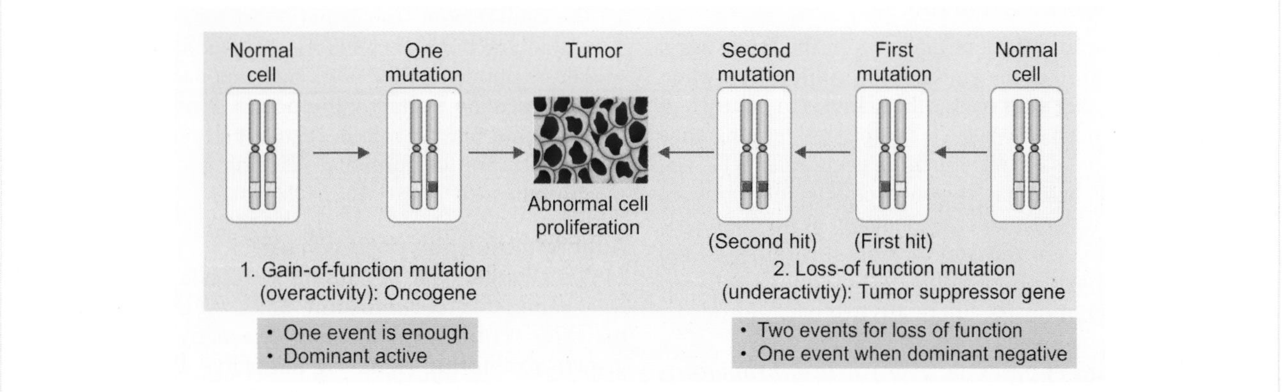

FIG. 52: Diagrammatic representation of gain of function (oncogenes) and loss of function (tumor suppressor gene).

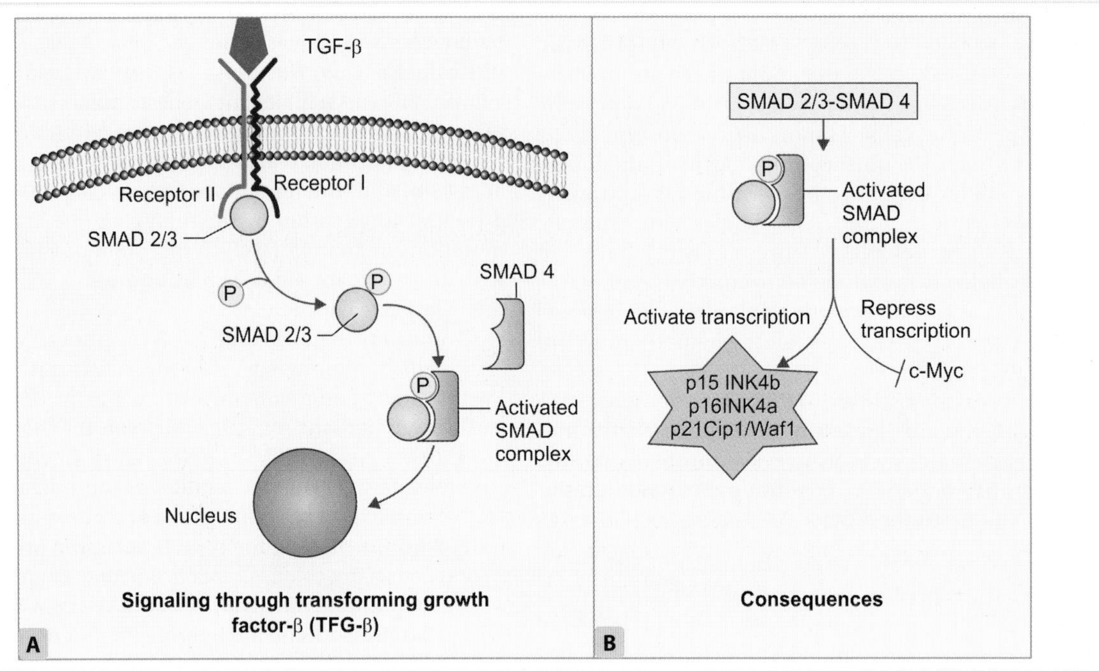

FIGS. 53A AND B: Transforming growth factor-β (TGF-β) pathway and its consequences. (A) TGF-β acts as a tumor suppressor. TGF-β binds its heteromeric receptor to phosphorylate. It activates "Small", "Mothers Against Decapentaplegic" (SMAD) 2 and 3 and in turn binds to SMAD 4 and forms an activated SMAD complex. This translocates to the nucleus and causes transcriptional activation and repression. (B) Consequences. The SMAD 2/3–SMAD 4 complex activates transcription of cell cycle suppressors, and can also repress transcription of the proliferation activator *c-Myc*.

Table 20: Various effects of transforming growth factor-β (TGF-β).

• **Normal tumor-suppressive effects**	
○ **Promotes:** Apoptosis, differentiation, maintenance of cell number	○ **Inhibits:** Inflammation, mitogenesis induced by extracellular matrix
• **Failure of tumor suppression: Promotes:** Autocrine mitogens (production of growth factors), and motility. **Inhibits:** Evasion of immune surveillance	
• **Facilitate tumor cell invasion and metastasis:** Recruitment of myofibroblasts, extravasation of cancer cell, modification of microenvironment, mobilization of osteoclasts	

Contact Inhibition, NF2, and APC

It is observed that in cancer cells grown in the laboratory, there is no inhibition of the cancer cell proliferation when they come in contact with each other. This is in contrast to nontransformed (normal) cells, which stop proliferating once they form monolayers of cells touching each other (cell–cell contacts). This mechanism is known as contact inhibition. In many tissues, cell–cell contacts are mediated by homodimeric interactions between transmembrane proteins called *cadherins*. **E-cadherin** (E for *epithelial*) **mediates cell–cell contact in epithelial layers.** There are two mechanisms by which E-cadherin maintains contact inhibition:

- **By TSG (tumor suppressor gene) *neurofibromatosis type 2 (NF2)*:** One of the TSGs *NF2* and its product, neurofibromin-2 (commonly called *merlin*) acts downstream of E-cadherin in a singling pathway. Neurofibromin-2 is structurally similar to cytoskeletal protein 4.1 of RBC and is related to the ERM (ezrin, radixin, and moesin) family of membrane cytoskeleton-associated proteins. Neurofibromin-2 helps to maintain contact inhibition in cells. Cells without merlin do not form stable cell-to-cell junctions and they are insensitive to normal growth arrest signals produced by cell-to-cell contact.
  - **Somatic mutations** affecting both alleles of *NF2* are associated with sporadic meningiomas and ependymomas and certain neural tumors (e.g., benign bilateral schwannomas of the acoustic nerve).
  - **Germline mutations** in *NF2* predispose to the development of *neurofibromatosis type 2.*
- **By binding to β-catenin:** Catenins (a, β, and γ) are proteins that interact with the intracellular domain of E-cadherin and create a mechanical link between E-cadherin molecule and the cytoskeleton. This is necessary for effective epithelial cell interactions. β-catenin is a signaling protein and is a key component of the WNT signaling pathway. E-cadherin may regulate contact inhibition by binding to β-catenin. β-catenin plays a role in regulating the morphology and organization of epithelial cell lining structures such as the gut.

Adenomatous polyposis coli (APC)

APC is a **gatekeeper of colonic neoplasia** and the locus of *APC* gene is on **chromosome 5q21**. APC is a member of the class of **tumor suppressors**. It acts by **downregulating growth promoting signaling pathways.** Germline loss-of-function mutations involving APC are associated with familial adenomatous polyposis (FAP). APC is a component of the WNT signaling pathway. WNT signalling pathway has an important role in controlling cellular growth and differentiation during embryonic development (see Fig. 9 of Chapter 2).

Role of E-cadherin and β-catenin in adenomatous polyposis coli: Adenomatous polyposis coli (APC) is a rare hereditary disease characterized by the development of numerous adenomatous polyps in the colon. These polyps have a very high incidence of transformation into colonic cancers. These polyps always show loss of a TSG called *APC* (named for the disease). Normal APC exerts antiproliferative effects in an unusual style.

WNT/β-catenin signaling pathway (refer Fig. 9 of Chapter 2): Normally, *APC* gene encodes a cytoplasmic protein namely, APC protein. ***APC protein*** is an important **negative regulator of β-catenin.** The main function of APC is to promote the degradation of β-catenin and it prevents proliferation of cells. **β-catenin** is the key component **of the WNT signaling pathway**. WNT molecules bind to cell surface WNT receptors of the frizzled (FRZ) family. WNTs are soluble factors that bind WNT receptors. Binding of WNT to its receptors stimulates several pathways and the main pathway involve APC and β-catenin. In this pathway, they transmits signals that prevent the APC-mediated degradation of β-catenin. This allows translocation of β-catenin to the nucleus, where it acts as a transcriptional activator. A major function of the APC protein is to regulate the activity of β-catenin.

In quiescent cells: The cells contain a **destruction complex** and APC is an essential part of this complex. In quiescent cells that are not exposed to WNT, cytoplasmic β-catenin is proteasomally degraded by this **destruction complex**.

- **Loss of APC:** *APC* behaves as a TSG. **Both copies of *APC* gene** must be **inactivated** either by mutation or epigenetic (methylation) events. When there is loss (or mutation) of APC (e.g., in colon cancers), degradation of β-catenin by APC **(destruction complex)** is prevented. The **accumulation of β-catenin** forms a complex with T-cell factor (TCF). This leads to inappropriate activation of WNT signaling response even in the absence of WNT factors. In colonic epithelium this leads to changes, namely—(i) increased transcription of growth-promoting genes (e.g., cyclin D1 and *MYC*) and (ii) increased transcriptional regulators (e.g., TWIST and SLUG), which inhibit E-cadherin expression and thus reduce contact inhibition. It **promotes cell proliferation of colonic epithelial cells**.
- **Familial adenomatous polyposis:** One of the syndromes associated with APC inactivation is familial adenomatous polyposis. Individuals born with one mutated allele of APC develop hundreds to thousands of adenomatous polyps in the colon by their teens or twenties. These polyps show loss of the both *APC* allele. Almost always, one or more of these polyps undergo malignant transformation. *APC* mutations are seen in 70–80% of sporadic colon cancers. Sometimes, colonic cancers with normal *APC* genes show activating mutations of β-catenin. This prevents degradation of mutated β-catenin by APC.

The importance of the β-catenin complex in tumorigenesis is evident from the fact that many colon tumors with normal APC genes show mutations in β-catenin. This mutation prevent APC-dependent destruction by β-catenin , and leads to its accumulation and increased expression of β-catenin-dependent target genes. Thus, β-catenin (the target of APC), acts as a proto-oncoprotein. Dysregulation of the APC/β-catenin pathway is found not only in colon cancers but also in other tumors. For example, gain-of-function mutations in β-catenin are observed in about 20% of hepatocellular carcinomas.

Neurofibromatosis type 1: It is a classic tumor suppressor. *Neurofibromin* is the protein product of the *NF1* gene and belongs to a family of GAPs. GTPase-activating domain inactivates (acts as a brake on) RAS signaling. With loss of neurofibromin function, RAS tends to become trapped in an active, signal-emitting state.

***Mutation of NF1*:** *NF1* gene is present on the long arm of chromosome 17 (17q11.2). Germline mutations in the *NF1* gene may be caused by deletions, missense mutations, and nonsense mutations. Individuals who inherit one mutant allele of the *NF1* gene develop many benign **neurofibromas** and **optic nerve gliomas** as a result of inactivation of the second allele of the gene. This condition is called *neurofibromatosis type 1*. Some of the neurofibromas may later develop into **malignant peripheral nerve sheath tumors**. Despite the superficial similarities, neurofibromatosis type 1 and 2, they are not variants of the same disease and have separate genetic origins.

E-cadherin

E-cadherin is a cell surface protein is involved in maintaining intercellular adhesiveness. β-catenin also attaches to the cytoplasmic tail of E-cadherin.

Loss of cell-cell contact may occur following wound or injury to epithelial cells. This disrupts the interaction between E-cadherin and β-catenin (see Fig. 9 of Chapter 2). Similar to WNT signaling, the β-catenin gets translocated to the nucleus and stimulate genes that promote proliferation. In case of injury, this proliferation of cells repairs the wound. Once the wound heals the E-cadherin contacts are re-established and β-catenin binds to the cell membrane and reduces proliferative signaling. Thus, these epithelial cells are said to be "contact-inhibited."

Loss of contact inhibition, by mutation of the E-cadherin/β-catenin axis or by other changes: It is observed in many carcinomas. The loss of E-cadherin can also contribute to the malignant phenotype and allows easy disaggregation of cells. These cells can locally invade or metastasize.

- **Cancers with reduced expression of E-cadherin:** Reduced cell surface expression of E-cadherin is found in many carcinomas. These include **carcinomas of the esophagus, colon, breast, ovary, and prostate**.
- **Germline loss-of-function mutations of the E-cadherin gene**: *CDH1* gene encodes a classical cadherin of the cadherin superfamily. Germline mutations in E-cadherin expression are associated with familial gastric carcinoma, and a proportion of sporadic gastric carcinomas. These can be due to mutation of the *CDH1* gene or other indirect mechanisms.

CDKN2A

CDKN2A is tumor suppressor gene and belong to INK4/ARF family. p14/ARF gene encodes two protein products: The p16/INK4a and p14/ARF.

- **p16/INK4a**: It is a cyclin-dependent kinase inhibitor. It binds and blocks CDK4/cyclin D-mediated phosphorylation of RB. It promotes the inhibitory effects of RB. It reinforces the G_1/S checkpoint and keeps the RB in active stage. Thereby it inhibits cell proliferation.
- **p14/ARF**: This activates the p53 pathway and increases the levels of p53 by inhibiting activities of MDM2 and prevents destruction of p53. p16 is also induces cellular senescence.

Mutations in *CDKN2A*: Germline mutations in CDKN2A are detected in **familial forms of melanoma.** Sporadic mutations are observed in **bladder cancer, head and neck tumors, acute lymphoblastic leukemia, and cholangiocarcinoma.** In some tumors (e.g., carcinoma cervix), p16 is silenced by hypermethylation (epigenetic changes) of the gene rather than mutation.

Other cyclin dependent kinase inhibitors also function as tumor suppressors. They may be frequently mutated or silenced in many human malignancies.

PTEN

PTEN (*p*hosphatase and *ten*sin homolog) is tumor suppressor encoded by a gene on chromosome 10q23. PTEN acts as a tumor suppressor by serving as a brake on the PI3K/AKT part of the RTK pathway. The loss of effective tumor suppression may be due to structural changes in TSG (e.g., due to mutations) or loss of both alleles. However, in some tumor suppressors, the level of protein product of gene is important and one of such a tumor suppressors is PTEN.

PTEN function: PTEN is a membrane-associated phosphatase that dephosphorylates both proteins and lipids. It regulates the many growth factor signals from receptors at the cell surface to nuclear transcription factors. Thus, it mediates many cellular functions (**Fig. 54** and **Fig. 41**).

- **Dephosphorylates PIP3:** PTEN dephosphorylates the active signaling intermediate, PIP3, to its inactive PIP2 form. Thereby, PTEN inhibits the AKT-mTOR pathway (**Fig. 54**).
- **PTEN interaction with p53:** PTEN and p53 interact physically and regulate each other. PTEN may be required for functioning of p53 and also protects degradation of p53 by MDM2.
- **Other functions of PTEN protein:** It is important for the DNA damage repair, response, apoptosis (**Fig. 54**), regulation of cell cycle progression, maintenance of epithelial polarity, and inhibition of EMT. It also controls cell metabolism to limit glycolysis.

Causes of lowered concentration of PTEN: Normally, concentration of PTEN protein is maintained at a steady and high level. PTEN level may be lowered due to inactivation of one or both alleles, altered promoter activity or other epigenetic or posttranslational change.

Consequences of lowered concentration of PTEN (***Fig. 54***): Even slight reduction in PTEN protein concentration can lead to **accumulation of PIP3 and constitutively activate a number of signaling pathways involved in cell proliferation and survival.** Some regulators such as p27, Bad and FOXO are not activated, thus promote cell cycle progression and reduce apoptosis. These may lead to development of cancer. PTEN is the second most frequently mutated gene in cancers, after p53.

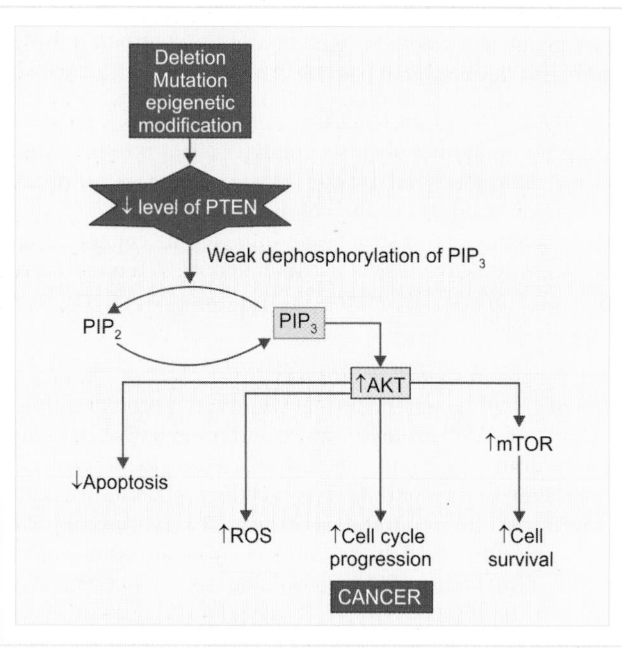

(mTOR: mammalian target of rapamycin; PTEN: phosphatase and tensin homolog; PIP3: phosphatidylinositol-3,4,5-trisphosphate; PIP2: phosphatidylinositol-3,4-bisphosphate; ROS: reactive oxygen species)

FIG. 54: The consequences of decreased concentration of phosphatase and tensin homolog (PTEN). The levels of PTEN activity may be decreased by mutation or by epigenetic mechanism. It leads to accumulation of phosphatidylinositol-3,4,5-trisphosphate (PIP3), due to weak phosphorylation of PIP3 to phosphatidylinositol-3,4-bisphosphate (PIP2). This in turn activates a central signaling intermediate, namely AKT. This promotes cell cycle progression and decreases apoptosis. Activation of mTOR (mammalian target of rapamycin) stimulates cell survival. Thus, loss of PTEN activity favors the development of uncontrolled cell proliferation and cancer.

- **Loss of PTEN causes cancer:** PTEN's tumor suppressor activity depends on the level of PTEN and even small decreases in PTEN activity may allow some tumors to develop. *PTEN* gene function is lost in many cancers through deletion, point mutations, or epigenetic silencing.
- **Cowden syndrome:** PTEN is mutated in an autosomal dominant disorder called Cowden syndrome. It is characterized by frequent benign growths (e.g., tumors of skin appendage), and an increased incidence of epithelial cancers. These include epithelial cancers of the breast, endometrium, and thyroid.

WT1

WT1 is a tumor-suppressor protein and is the product of *WT1* gene located on chromosome 11p13.

Functions of WT1

WT1 protein regulates transcription of several other genes and includes insulin-like growth factor-II (*IGF-II*), *Snail,* E-cadherin (*Cdh1*), and *PDGF.*

- WT1 protein is a transcriptional activator of genes involved in renal and gonadal differentiation.
- Regulates the mesenchymal-to-epithelial transition that occurs in kidney development.

Alterations in WT1

Some genes that regulate development may act as a tumor suppressor in one tissue (e.g., *WT1* in a renal progenitor cell) and an oncogene in a second type of tissue (e.g., *WT1* in a hematopoietic stem cell). *WT1* is an example of "crosstalk" between genes.

- **Loss-of-function mutations in *WT1*:** *WT1* is a tumor suppressor in Wilms tumor. Loss-of-function mutations in the *WT1* gene is associated with the development of a pediatric kidney cancer called **Wilms tumor**. Wilms tumor can occur as both inherited and sporadic forms and both are associated with mutational inactivation of the *WT1* locus. Probably the tumorigenic effect of *WT1* deficiency is related to the role of the gene in the differentiation of genitourinary tissues.
- **Overexpression of *WT1*:** Though *WT1* acts as tumor suppressor in Wilms tumor, overexpression of *WT1* is observed in a variety of **adult cancers (e.g., leukemias, breast carcinomas)**. Normally, these tissues do not express *WT1* at all. Hence, *WT1* may function as an oncogene in these cancers.

PATCHED (PTCH)

PTCH1 is a TSG (tumor suppressor gene) located at chromosome 9q22. It encodes a cell membrane protein called PATCHED1.

Normal function

PTCH is a receptor for hedgehog ligand. PATCHED protein is a negative regulator of the hedgehog signaling pathway (refer page 50). Normally, binding of hedgehog ligands to PATCH receptors relieves this negative regulation of PATCHED protein and activates the Hedgehog signaling pathway (**Fig. 55**). This in turn stimulates downstream transcription factors.

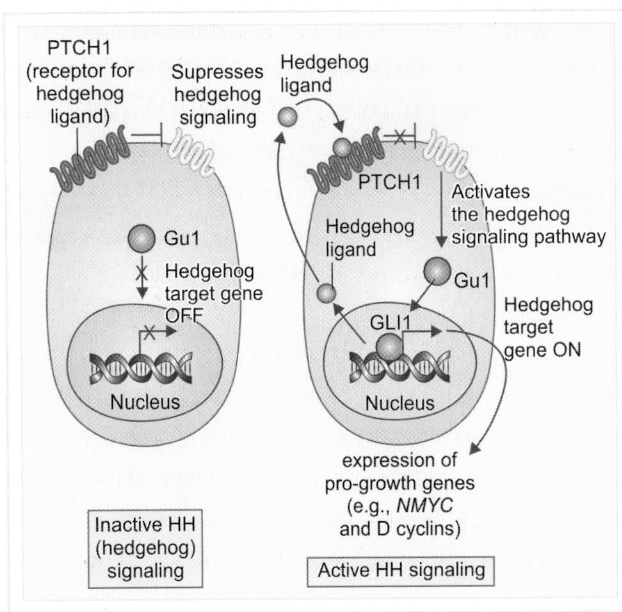

FIG. 55: Role of PTCH in hedgehog signaling. PTCH1 (PATCHED1) protein is a negative regulator of the hedgehog signaling pathway. Normally, binding of hedgehog ligands to PATCH receptors relieves this negative regulation of PATCHED protein and activates the hedgehog signaling pathway. This in turn stimulates downstream transcription factors. GLI1 (cubitus interruptus-like transcription factor involved in glioma formation) proteins mediate activation of hedgehog transcriptional targets Mutations in PTCH result in activation of hedgehog signaling and are causative in basal cell carcinoma and medulloblastoma.

Absence of PATCHED proteins

Absence of PATCHED proteins leads to unopposed hedgehog signaling and increases the expression of many progrowth genes, including *NMYC* and D cyclins.

- **Germline loss-of-function** mutations in *PTCH1* cause Gorlin syndrome. It is an inherited disorder, also known as nevoid basal cell carcinoma syndrome. It is associated with great increase in the risks of developing basal cell carcinoma of the skin and of medulloblastoma (an aggressive tumor of cerebellum that arises in children or adolescents).
- **Somatic mutations**: *PTCH1* mutations are also observed in 20–50% of sporadic cases of basal cell carcinoma and 10–25% of sporadic cases of medulloblastoma. About 50% of such mutations in basal cell carcinomas are caused by ultraviolet (UV) exposure.

Therapeutic target

Hedgehog pathway antagonists are used for treatment of advanced basal cell carcinoma, medulloblastoma, and other tumors associated with hedgehog pathway activation.

von Hippel–Lindau (VHL)

von Hippel–Lindau (*VHL*) TSG **is located at chromosome 3p25 and its product is VHL protein.**

Functions (Fig. 56)

VHL protein is a component of an ubiquitin ligase. Ubiquitin is a type of protein complex that covalently links ubiquitin chains to specific protein substrates. Ubiquitin promotes degradation of the protein substrates by the proteasome. An important protein substrate or target for the VHL ubiquitin ligase is the transcription factor HIF1α (hypoxia-inducible transcription factor 1α). In the presence of oxygen, HIF1α (angiogenic factor) is hydroxylated and binds to VHL. This leads to ubiquitination and degradation of HIF1α.

Consequences of inactivation of VHL (***Fig. 56***): These include:

- **Hypoxic environments**: In hypoxic environments, there will be defect in ubiquitin conjugation and degradation of HIF1α. This leads to increased HIF1α and it accumulates in the nuclei of hypoxic cells. HIF-1α activates many target genes important in cellular responses to **low oxygen environments.** These responses include—(i) increased intake of glucose by cells for anaerobic glycolysis (through activation of the glucose transporter GLUT1, and several glycolytic enzymes), (ii) stimulation of genes encoding the growth/angiogenic factors—vascular endothelial growth factor (VEGF) and (iii) activation of many growth factors (e.g., PDGF).
- **Loss-of-function mutations in VHL:** It also prevents the ubiquitination and degradation of HIF1α, even during normoxic conditions. HIF1 induces many metabolic

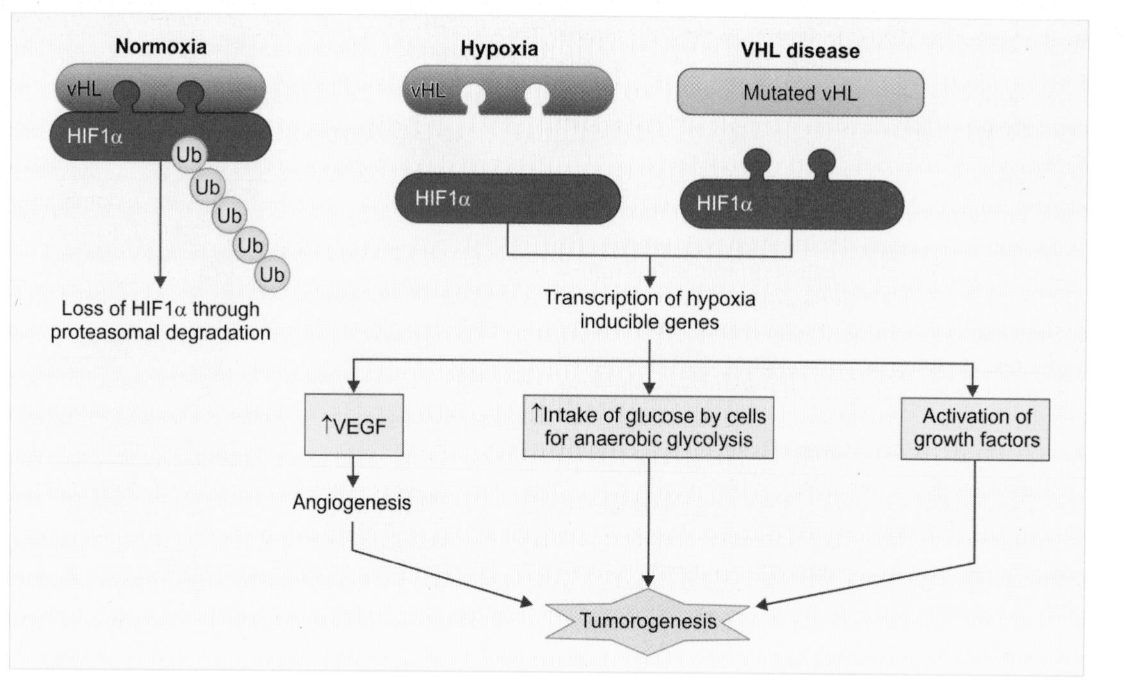

(HIF: hypoxia-inducible transcription factor; Ub: ubiquitin; VEGF: vascular endothelial growth factor; vHL: von Hippel–Lindau)

FIG. 56: Actions of von Hippel–Lindau (VHL) in normoxic, hypoxic, and in disorders associated with mutations of *VHL* gene.

changes that characterize cancer cells. Thus, there is increased levels of angiogenic growth factors and alterations in cellular metabolism that favor growth.

Diseases associated with mutation of VHL

These include:

- **Germline loss-of-function mutations of the *VHL* gene:** These are associated with **von Hippel–Lindau (VHL) syndrome.** This is an autosomal dominant cancer syndrome characterized by **hereditary renal cell cancers (RCC)** (clear cell RCC in about 40% of cases of VHL disease), **pheochromocytomas,** cerebellar **hemangioblastomas, retinal angiomas,** and cysts in various organs (e.g., **renal cysts).** Hereditary RCCs are usually multifocal and bilateral, and appear in younger patients than do sporadic RCCs.
- **Somatic mutations** of the *VHL* gene: It is found in sporadic RCC. Sporadic RCC may have deletions and loss of heterozygosity (LOH) in the short arm of chromosome 3 (3p) in the tumor tissue. In almost all (98%) sporadic clear cell RCCs, one *VHL* allele is lost and *VHL* mutations occur in >50% of tumors.

Serine/Threonine Kinase 11

The serine/threonine kinase 11 (***STK11)* gene** [also known as liver kinase B1 (LKB1)] functions as a TSG (tumor suppressor gene).

Functions of STK11: ***STK11* encodes a serine/threonine kinase that** has several (pleiotropic) effects on multiple facets of cellular metabolism (e.g., glucose uptake, gluconeogenesis, protein synthesis, mitochondrial biogenesis, and lipid metabolism). It **is an important regulator of cell polarity, motility, differentiation, metastasis, and cell metabolism**. PI3Ks are lipid kinases that regulate cellular processes such as proliferation, survival, adhesion, and motility. *STK11* functions as negative regulators of the PI3K/AKT/mTOR pathway and thus their loss of function activates this pathway.

Diseases associated with mutation of STK11

STK11 mutations usually correlate with KRAS activation and promote cell growth. Diseases associated include:

- **Germline loss-of-function** (inactivating) **mutations of *STK11*:** It causes Peutz–Jeghers syndrome. This syndrome is an autosomal dominant disorder characterized by benign polyps of the gastrointestinal tract and an increased risk of multiple epithelial cancers (e.g., carcinomas of gastrointestinal tract and pancreas).
- **Sporadic loss-of-function** (somatic inactivation) **mutations of *STK11*:** They occur through point mutation and deletion on 19p13. They are observed in diverse carcinomas [e.g., nonsmall cell carcinoma of lung (adenocarcinoma) and cervical carcinomas]. *STK11* inactivation is seen in nonsmall cell carcinoma of lung (NSCLC) and are more common in tumors from males and smokers and in poorly differentiated adenocarcinomas.

Examples of TSGs and associated familial syndromes and sporadic cancers are presented in **Table 21**. Main differences between oncogenes and tumor-suppressor genes is presented in **Table 22**.

Mechanism of cancer development by oncogene and mutated TSG is depicted in **Figure 57**.

Table 21: Examples of tumor suppressor genes and associated familial syndromes and sporadic cancers.

Gene (protein)	*Function*	*Familial syndromes*	*Sporadic cancers*
Inhibitors of mitogenic signaling pathways			
APC (Adenomatous polyposis coli)	Inhibits Wnt signaling (degrades β-catenin)	Familial adenomatous polyps (FAP) and carcinomas	Carcinomas of stomach, colon, pancreas; melanoma
NF1 (Neurofibromin-1)	Inhibits RAS/MAPK signaling	Neurofibromatosis type 1 (neurofibromas and malignant peripheral nerve sheath tumors)	Neuroblastoma, juvenile myeloid leukemia
NF2 (Merlin)	Cytoskeletal stability, Hippo pathway signaling	Neurofibromatosis type 2 (acoustic schwannoma and meningioma)	Schwannoma, meningioma
PTCH (Patched)	Inhibitor of Hedgehog signaling (transmembrane receptor)	Gorlin syndrome (nevoid basal cell carcinoma, medulloblastoma, several benign tumors)	Basal cell carcinoma, medulloblastoma
PTEN (Phosphatase and tensin homolog)	Inhibits PI3K/AKT signaling	Cowden syndrome (benign skin tumors, GI, and CNS growths; breast, endometrial, and thyroid carcinoma)	Carcinomas and lymphoid tumors
SMAD2, SMAD4 (SMAD2, SMAD4)	TGF-β signaling pathway; represses MYC and CDK4 expression, inducers of CDK inhibitor expression	Familial juvenile polyposis (hamartomas)	Carcinoma of colon and pancreas
Inhibitors of cell cycle progression			
RB (Retinoblastoma protein)	Inhibits G_1/S transition during cell cycle	Familial retinoblastoma syndrome (retinoblastoma, osteosarcoma, other sarcomas)	Retinoblastoma; osteosarcoma, carcinomas of breast, colon, lung
CDKN2A (p16/INK4a and p14/ARF)	p16: Negative regulator of cyclin-dependent kinases; p14, indirect activator of p53	Familial melanoma	Pancreatic, breast, and esophageal carcinoma, melanoma, some leukemias
Inhibitors of "pro-growth" programs of metabolism and angiogenesis			
VHL (von Hippel–Lindau protein)	Inhibits hypoxia-induced transcription factors (e.g., HIF1α)	von Hippel–Lindau syndrome (cerebellar hemangioblastoma, retinal angioma, renal cell carcinoma)	Renal cell carcinoma
STK11 (Liver kinase B1 (LKB1) or STK11)	Activator of AMPK family of kinases; suppresses cell growth when cell nutrient and energy levels are low	Peutz–Jeghers syndrome (GI polyps, GI cancers, pancreatic carcinoma, and other carcinomas)	Diverse carcinomas
SDHB, SDHD (Succinate dehydrogenase complex subunits B and D)	TCA cycle, oxidative phosphorylation	Familial paraganglioma, familial pheochromocytoma	Paraganglioma
Inhibitors of invasion and metastasis			
CDH1 (E-cadherin)	Cell–cell adhesion, inhibition of cell motility	Familial gastric cancer (diffuse type)	Gastric carcinoma, lobular carcinoma of breast
Enablers of genomic stability			
TP53 (*p53* protein)	Cell cycle arrest and apoptosis in response to DNA damage	Li–Fraumeni syndrome	Majority of cancers
DNA repair factors			
BRCA1 (Breast cancer-1), *BRCA2* (breast cancer-2)	Repair of double-stranded breaks in DNA	Familial carcinoma of breast and ovary; carcinomas of male breast; chronic lymphocytic leukemia (*BRCA2*)	Rare
MSH2, MLH1, MSH6 (MSH2, MLH1, MSH6)	DNA mismatch repair	Hereditary nonpolyposis colorectal cancer (HNPCC, Lynch syndrome)	Carcinoma of colon and endometrium

Continued

Continued

Gene (protein)	*Function*	*Familial syndromes*	*Sporadic cancers*
Unknown mechanisms			
WT1 (Wilms tumor-1)	Transcription factor	Familial Wilms tumor	Wilms tumor, certain leukemias
MEN1 (Menin)	Transcription factor	Multiple endocrine neoplasia-1 (MEN1; pituitary, parathyroid, and pancreatic endocrine tumors)	Pituitary, parathyroid, and pancreatic endocrine tumors

(AMPK: 5′ AMP-activated protein kinase; CNS: central nervous system; DNA: deoxyribonucleic acid; GI: gastrointestinal; HIF: hypoxia-inducible factor; PI3K: phosphatidylinositol 3 kinase; MAPK: mitogen-activated protein kinase; SMAD: "Small", "Mothers Against Decapentaplegic; STK11: serine/threonine kinase 11, TCA: tricarboxylic acid; TGF: transforming growth factor)

Table 22: Main differences between oncogenes and tumor-suppressor genes.

Features	*Oncogenes*	*Tumor-suppressor genes*
Number of alleles* present in normal cells	Two	Two
Mode of action	Dominant	Recessive
Number of alleles mutated to produce oncogenic effect	One	Two
Effect of mutation on the function of the protein product	Enhanced	Reduced
Germline (inherited) mutations identified, i.e., important in genetic predisposition	Rare (e.g., *RET, KIT*)	More common than in oncogene (e.g., *TP53, RB*)
Adjectives used to describe mutations	Activating, gain in function	Inactivating, loss of function

*Allele is an alternative form of the gene found at the same locus in homologous chromosomes.

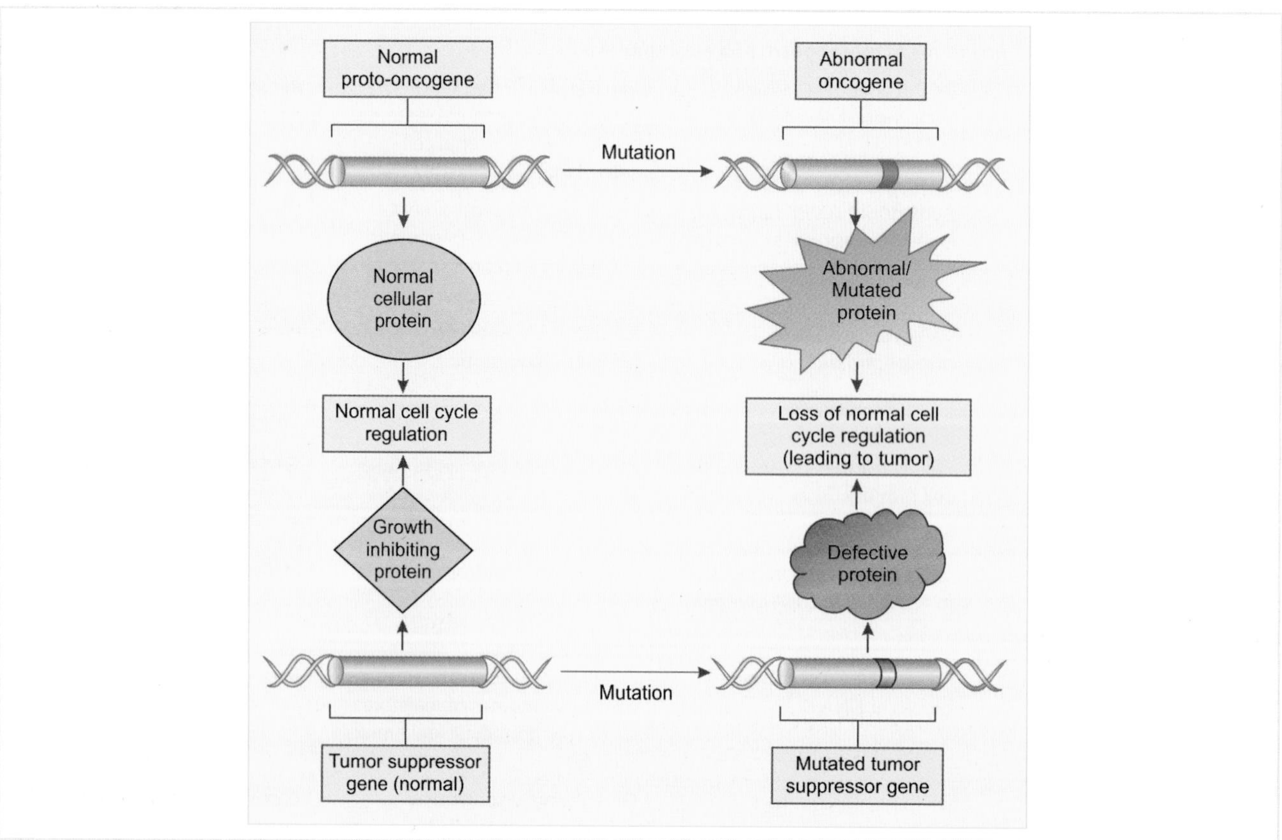

FIG. 57: Mechanism of cancer development by oncogene and mutated tumor suppressor gene.

Hallmark 3: Resisting Cell Death

Review of Apoptosis

The total number of cells (cell population) in any tissue/organ depends on the balance between cell division and cell death. Loss of this intricate equilibrium can produce cancer. One of the mechanisms to prevent aberrant cell proliferation is by inducing cell death, namely apoptosis. Apoptosis (for details refer pages 142–150) is as important as mitosis in maintaining a healthy balance in cell population and functions. Most types of normal cells throughout the body have the ability to activate the normally latent apoptotic cell-death program. **Apoptosis** is a programmed cell death and **is one of the normal protective mechanisms by which it eliminates damaged or abnormal cells** (i.e., **cells with DNA damage/mutation**). This helps to maintain tissue homoeostasis by inducing the apoptosis of aberrant cells, including ones that are inappropriately proliferating and it also occurs in tumors being subjected to cytotoxic chemotherapy. Many types of signals such as DNA damage, potent oncoproteins such as MYC, and loss of adhesion to the basement membrane (termed anoikis), can initiate apoptosis. In apoptosis, or regulated cell death, there is an orderly breaking up of cells into component pieces. These are then accurately consumed by phagocytes without stimulating inflammation. There are two pathways of apoptosis—(i) the extrinsic pathway (triggered by the death receptors FAS and FAS-ligand); and (ii) the intrinsic/*mitochondrial* pathway (initiated by disturbances such as loss of growth factors and DNA damage). Let us briefly review of the intrinsic pathway of apoptosis.

Intrinsic/Mitochondrial Pathway

The integrity of the mitochondrial outer membrane depends on the balance between proapoptotic and antiapoptotic members of the BCL2 protein family. The proapoptotic proteins BAX and BAK are embedded in the mitochondrial outer membrane. The action of proapoptotic proteins is inhibited by the antiapoptotic proteins such as BCL2, BCL-XL, BCL-W, and MCL1. A third set of proteins, belonging to "BH3-only proteins", a key subfamily of the BCL-2 family, inhibit (neutralize) the actions of antiapoptotic proteins like BCL2 and BCL-XL and promote apoptosis by activating the proapoptotic proteins. BH3-only proteins include BAD, BID, BIM, PUMA, and NOXA. One of the key actions of p53 is to trigger apoptosis when there is excessive DNA damage. p53 induces apoptosis by upregulating the expressions of the BH3-only proteins NOXA and PUMA.

When proapoptotic molecules BAX and BAK are activated and are relieved of inhibition by their counterpart antiapoptotic members (BCL2 family), they disrupt the integrity of the outer mitochondrial membrane. It causes formation of pores in the mitochondria and increases the permeability of the mitochondrial outer membrane. This in turn releases molecules that initiate apoptosis, the most important of which is cytochrome C (normally sequestered/segregated in the mitochondria). The cytochrome C leak out from mitochondria into the cytosol and binds to APAF-1 (apoptotic protease activating factor 1). This activates caspase-9, which in turn cleaves and activates executioner caspases such as caspase-3. There is another group of factors that function as negative regulators of the intrinsic pathway and is known as *inhibitor of apoptosis proteins (IAPs)*. IAPs bind to caspase-9 and prevent apoptosis.

Evasion of Apoptosis in Cancer

Q. Write a short essay on the role of apoptosis in neoplasia.

Cancer cells are subject to many intrinsic stresses. These include DNA damage, metabolic disturbances arising from dysregulated growth, and hypoxia caused by insufficient blood supply. These intrinsic stresses can initiate apoptosis. When tumors are treated with chemotherapy or radiation therapy, they kill tumor cells by activating the intrinsic pathway of apoptosis. This further increase stresses several folds. Thus, both before and during therapy, there is strong selective pressure for cancer cells to develop resistance to intrinsic stresses that may induce apoptosis.

Loss of normal apoptosis pathways

The disruption of the apoptotic pathways is one of the essential hallmarks of cancer cells. Major mechanisms by which **evasion of apoptosis by cancer cells occurs is by two ways**—(i) loss of p53 (the key component of early steps in the intrinsic pathway), and (ii) increased expression of antiapoptotic members of the BCL2 family.

Loss of TP53 Function: The TP53 gene and the corresponding protein p53 have a critical role in regulating the Bcl-2 family of proteins. The most common abnormalities involve loss of p53 function. It may be either due to TP53 mutations or overexpression of the p53 inhibitor MDM2.

- **Mutation of *TP53*:** *TP53* is commonly mutated in cancers and their frequency of mutations is higher in tumors that relapse after therapy.
- **Indirect impairment of p53 function:** Apart from mutation of *TP53* in cancers, there may be indirect impairment of p53 function. Most prominent being **amplification of *MDM2***, which encodes an **inhibitor of p53**. Loss of p53 function prevents the upregulation of PUMA (a pro-apoptotic BH3-only member of the BCL2 family) and prevents apoptosis. This leads to survival of cells with DNA damage and cell stress, which under normal state undergo apoptosis.

Overexpression of Anti-apoptotic Members of the BCL2 Family: Overexpression of BCL2 protects tumor cells from apoptosis and this occurs through several mechanisms.

- **Chromosomal translocation:** Typical example of the effectiveness of inhibiting apoptosis in human cancer is follicular lymphoma. The prosurvival (antiapoptotic) protein, Bcl-2, is constitutively activated in B-cell tumor called follicular lymphoma. It shows a characteristic (14;18) (q32;q21) translocation [t(14:8)] that fuses the *BCL2* (located at 18q21) to the transcriptionally active immunoglobulin heavy chain gene (located at 14q32). It produces abundant BCL2. As a result, the normal equilibrium between the survival and death of B lymphocytes is altered and favors the survival of lymphocytes and protects them from undergoing apoptosis. The B lymphocytes survive for abnormally long periods and the accumulated B lymphocytes produce lymphadenopathy. In BCL-2 overexpressing follicular lymphomas, there is reduced cell death rather than uncontrollable cell proliferation. Hence, they tend to be indolent (slow-growing).
- **Loss of expression of micro-ribonucleic acids (micro-RNAs):** In chronic lymphocytic leukemia, BCL2 is

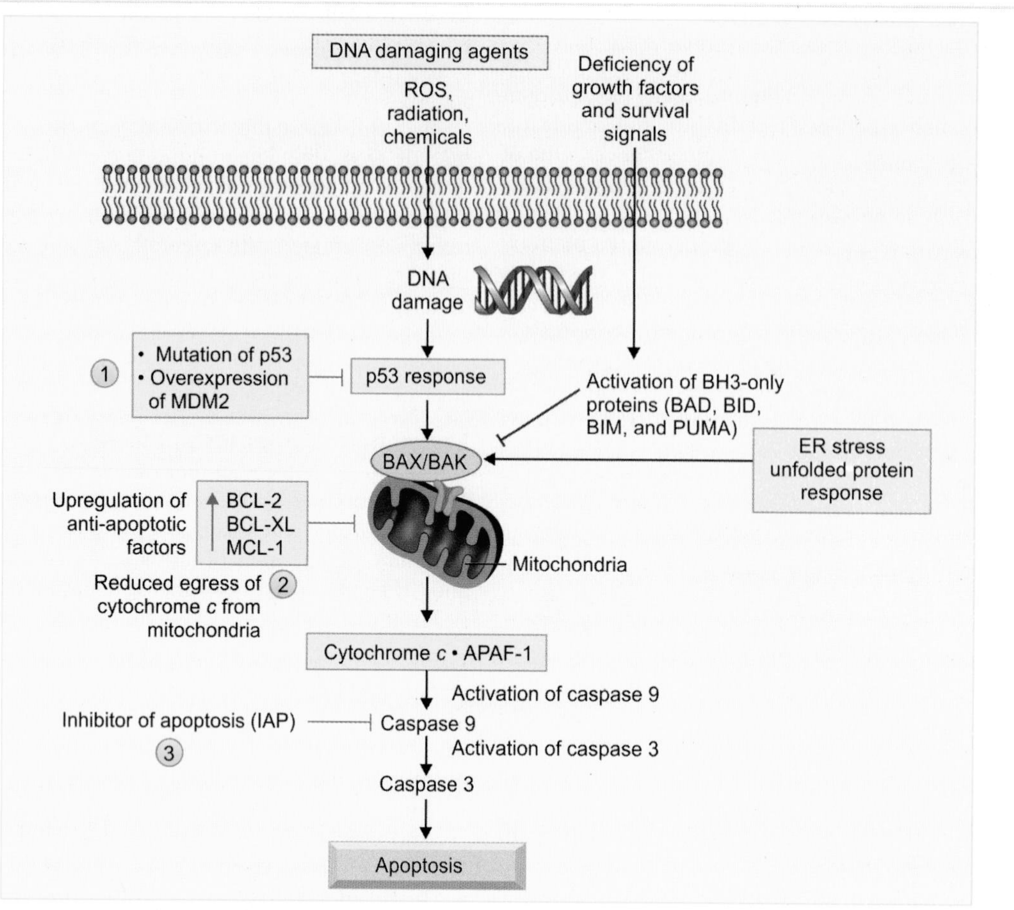

(APAF-1: apoptotic protease activating factor 1; DNA: deoxyribonucleic acid; IAP: inhibitor of apoptosis; ROS: reactive oxygen species)

FIG. 58: Intrinsic pathway of apoptosis and major mechanisms used by tumor cells to resist cell death. DNA damaging agents, deficiency of growth factors and survival signals and endoplasmic reticulum (ER) stress may induce apoptosis. Three major mechanisms may resist apoptosis in tumor cells. (1) Loss of p53 may be caused either through mutation of *TP53* or through antagonism by MDM2. (2) Reduced escape of cytochrome *c* from mitochondria may occur due to upregulation of antiapoptotic factors (they stabilize the membrane of the mitochondria) such as BCL2, BCL-XL, and MCL-1. Other less common mechanism that suppress apoptosis is by (3) unregulating members of the inhibitor of apoptosis (*IAP*) family.

upregulated because of loss of expression of specific micro-RNAs (miRNAs) that normally lessen BCL2 expression.

- **Other mechanisms:** There are other mechanisms that can lead to overexpression of anti-apoptotic members of the BCL2 family, particularly in the setting of cancers that show resistance to chemotherapy. For example, amplification of the MCL1 gene in some cancers of lung and breast.

Clinical significance: The knowledge about mechanisms by which cancers evade cell death can be utilized for the development of targeted therapy. In *TP53*-mutated tumors, it is difficult to restore p53 function because of the difficulty of "fixing" defective genes. However, target therapy can be used in tumors with inactive p53 due to overexpression of its inhibitor, MDM2. In tumors with *MDM2* gene amplification, inhibitor of *MDM2* can reactivate p53 and induce apoptosis. Drugs are available which mimic the activities of BH3-only proteins and inhibit the function of antiapoptotic members of the BCL2 family (particularly to BCL2 itself). They are useful in tumors with BCL2 overexpression such as chronic lymphocytic leukemia.

Intrinsic pathway of apoptosis and major mechanisms by which tumor cells resist cell death are presented in **Figure 58.**

Hallmark 4: Enabling Replicative Immortality

Cellular Senescence

Most of **normal human cells** have a limited capacity to undergo **cell division** (replication) **for about 60–70 times.** The upper limit of the number of mitoses is called the Hay flick (original discoverer of upper limit of mitosis) limit. After this, the cells cannot divide (arrest of growth) and become senescent by permanently leaving the cell cycle and without any cell division (replicative senescence). Senescence is defined as the process by which cells lose their ability to divide but maintain cell viability. Senescent cells are growth arrested cells unable to proliferate but remain viable. This occurs mainly due to progressive shortening of telomeres at the ends of chromosomes.

Telomeres: These are the **special structures present at the ends of chromosomes**. Telomeres are tandem repeats of the sequence TTAGGG, found at the 3' ends of each DNA strand. Telomeres serve as docks (or place) for protein caps that bind the ends of DNA sequences. They prevent the joining of two DNA strands in a chromosome by repair machinery called nonhomologous end joining (NHEJ) reactions. They bind many types of protective protein complexes. **During each cell division**, a small section of the telomere is not duplicated resulting in **progressive shortening**, which is responsible for the limited replicative property of a cell. **Senescence occurs when a cell's telomeres become very short.**

Telomerase: Many cells that replicate frequently (e.g., colon crypt epithelium) express a ribonucleoprotein enzyme called telomerase. This enzyme is responsible for the maintenance of telomeres and this enzyme can prevent shortening of telomeres. Telomerase is active in normal stem cells. But in most somatic cells, telomerase is expressed at very low levels. Telomerase lengthens telomeres and so maintains genomic stability even during continuing cell proliferation.

Limitless Replicative Potential

Immortality of Cancer Cells Unlike normal cells, all cancers contain immortal cells with unlimited (limitless) capacity to replicate (cellular immortalization). It has been found in laboratories that some cell lines from cancers have been proliferating continuously for more than 60 years. Hence, we can expect these cancer cells to continue to grow in laboratory grow indefinitely. **The ability to grow indefinitely by cancer cells** (immortality of cancer cells) **may** be due to three interrelated factors (1) evasion of **cellular** senescence, (2) evasion **of mitotic crisis (catastrophe),** and (3) the capacity for self-renewal.

Evasion of senescence

The mechanisms that produce senescence are not well known. But the senescent state is associated with upregulation of tumor suppressors such as p53 and INK4a/p16. Probably, this occurs in response to the accumulation of DNA damage over time. These tumor suppressors may contribute to senescence in part by maintaining RB in a hypophosphorylated state. This favors cell cycle arrest. In almost all cancers, the RB-dependent G_1/S cell cycle checkpoint is disrupted by a wide variety of acquired genetic and epigenetic aberrations. This may allow the cancer cells to bypass senescence.

Evasion of mitotic crisis (Fig. 59)

Shortening of telomeres Cancer cells that are resistant to senescence have increased replicative capacity. However, these cells are not immortal. These cells eventually enter into a phase referred to as mitotic crisis and undergo death. Mitotic crisis occurs due to progressive shortening of telomeres. Telomeres are special DNA sequences at the ends of chromosome. They bind several types of protective protein complexes. With each cell division, telomeres shorten. Telomerase is an enzyme that is responsible for the maintenance of these telomeres. Most somatic cells do not express telomerase and with each cell division the telomeres of these somatic cell shorten.

Double-stranded DNA breaks and its consequences When the telomeric DNA is markedly reduced beyond a critical size (i.e., completely eroded), the uncapped exposed **ends** of chromosomes are recognized or "sensed" as double-stranded DNA breaks (DSBs) by the DNA repair machinery.

Cells with normal p53: If the affected cells have normal p53 and RB function (competent checkpoints), it arrests the cell cycle. These cells may undergo apoptosis or nonreplicative senescence.

Cells with dysfunctional p53: If the cells have dysfunctional p53 or RB due to mutations (i.e., absence of checkpoints), the NHEJ (nonhomologous end joining pathway-a DNA repair machinery) is inappropriately activated as a last-ditch effort to save the cell.

- **Formation of dicentric chromosome**: NHEJ joins the "naked" shortened ends of two chromosomes. Such an inappropriately activated repair system of NHEJ results in dicentric chromosomes (dicentric chromosome is an abnormal chromosome with two centromeres). NHEJ may fuse the ends of either two sister chromatids or nonhomologous chromosomes.
- **Formation of new double-stranded DNA breaks (DSBs):** As the cell cycle progresses, during anaphase of mitosis, the dicentric chromosomes (fused/bridged chromosomes) are pulled apart. The force of chromosome separation at anaphase, produces new random double-stranded DNA breaks (chromosomal breakage). This activates DNA-repair pathways and leads to the random association of double-stranded ends and again the formation of dicentric chromosomes.
- **Repeated bridge-fusion breakage cycles**: Cells undergo many rounds of this "bridge-fusion-breakage" cycles. This generates genomic damage and genomic instability (i.e., abnormal alteration of genetic material during cell division such as massive chromosomal instability and numerous mutations).
- **Mitotic crisis in cells without telomerase re-expression:** In cells that fail to re-express telomerase, repeated bridge-fusion-breakage cycles, eventually produces mitotic crisis or catastrophe characterized by massive apoptosis (**Fig. 59**). Thus, proliferating cells that escape from senescence are likely to enter mitotic crisis and undergo death.
- **Cells with re-expression of telomerase**: For tumors to grow indefinitely, loss of growth control is not enough. It must also avoid both cellular senescence and mitotic crisis or catastrophe (**Fig. 59**). Most somatic cells, telomerase is expressed at very low levels and thus any cells that escape from senescence are most likely to die in mitotic crisis. If during mitotic crisis, if a cell manages to reactivate or re-express telomerase, the cells escape the bridge fusion-breakage cycle (termination of bridge-fusion-breakage cycles) and the cell is able to survive and avoid death by apoptosis. However, during mitotic crisis genomic instability develops because of damage to oncogenes and tumor suppressor genes. This may lead to accumulation of numerous mutations, helping the cell march toward malignant transformation (i.e., tumorigenesis or cancer formation).
- **Cancer stem cells**: Alternatively, cancers may arise from stem cells, which are normally long-lived partly because of continued expression of telomerase. Whatever the mechanism, telomere maintenance is seen in almost all types of cancers. In 85–95% of cancer, this is due to upregulation of the enzyme telomerase. Few cancers use other mechanisms, termed alternative lengthening of telomeres. This depends on DNA recombination.

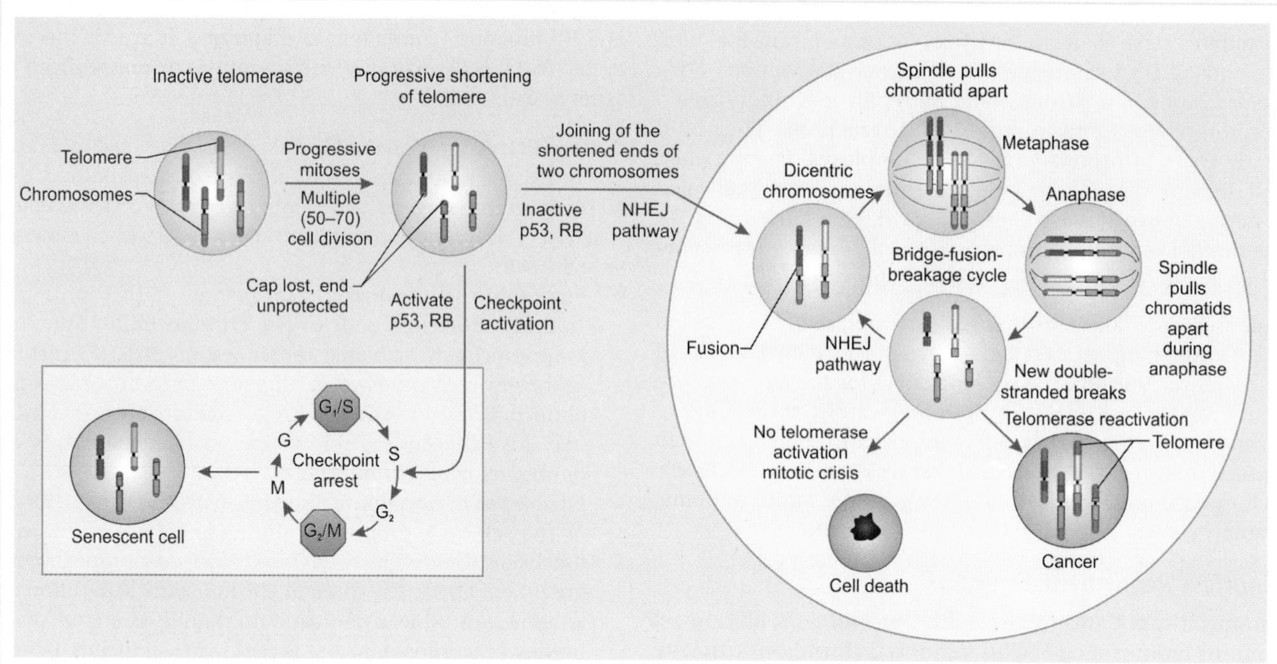

FIG. 59: Evasion of cells from senescence and mitotic crisis caused by telomere shortening. Somatic cells express telomerase at low level or without any expression. Progressive cell proliferation leads to reduction of telomeres at the end of the chromosome. When telomeres are markedly reduced beyond a critical size, they become uncapped. In the presence of normal p53 and competent checkpoints, somatic cells undergo arrest and undergo nonreplicative senescence. In the absence of p53 and checkpoints, uncapped ends of the chromosomes inappropriately activate deoxyribonucleic acid (DNA) repair pathways such as the nonhomologous end joining (NHEJ) pathway. These DNA repair systems join the shortened ends of two chromosomes and leads to the formation of dicentric chromosomes (abnormal chromosome with two centromeres). Nonhomologous end joining (NHEJ) may fuse the ends of either two sister chromatids or nonhomologous chromosomes. When this cell undergoes mitosis, as the fused DNA strands of dicentric chromosomes are pulled apart during anaphase, they produce a chromosome "bridge." The force of chromosome separation may then produce a new double stranded DNA break (DSB)/ chromosomal breakage. DSBs then activate DNA repair pathways and this in turn leads to the random association of double-stranded ends and again forms dicentric chromosomes. These cells undergo many rounds of this bridge-fusion-breakage cycle and produce massive chromosomal instability and numerous mutations. If there is no reactivation of telomerase, these cells will undergo mitotic crisis and death. If there is reactivation of telomerase, the cells escape the bridge-fusion breakage cycle and this promotes their survival and tumorigenesis.

Capacity for self-renewal

Q. Write short essay on cancer stem cells.

Many tissues contain short-lived cells. The continued growth and maintenance of many tissues that contain short-lived cells depends on a resident population of tissue stem cells that are capable of self-renewal. Examples of such tissues include the formed elements of the bone marrow and blood and the epithelial cells of the gastrointestinal tract and skin. The continued growth and maintenance of these short-lived cells depend on a resident population of tissue stem cells. Normal tissues contain stem cells capable of self-renewal and repairing damaged tissue. These stem cells are capable of self-renewal. However, majority of cells in normal tissues do not have this capacity.

Stem cells and their replication: Stem cells have following features.

- **Self-renewal**: Tissue stem cells and germ cells express telomerase, whereas somatic cells express telomerase at low level. This makes these germ cells and stem cells resistant to mitotic crisis, and also somehow avoid the genetic and epigenetic alterations that trigger senescence. Long-lived stem cells also have the capacity for self-renewal. Self-renewal means that each time a stem cell divides at least one of the two daughter cells remains a stem cell.
- **Long-lived:** Stem cells are long-lived.
- **Stem cells with symmetric division:** In a symmetric division, both daughter cells remain stem cells. This symmetric division into two stem cells from single stem cells may be occur during embryogenesis, when stem cell pools are expanding, or during times of stress.
- **Stem cells with asymmetric division:** In asymmetric division, only one daughter cell remains as a stem cell and the other non-stem daughter cells proceeds along some differentiation pathway. These non-stem daughter cell loses its "stemness" but gains one or more functions during this process. Such cells in "transit" to a differentiated state are usually have high proliferative capacity. However, finally they differentiate, stop dividing, and finally may become senescent or undergo apoptosis.

Cancer stem cells (Fig. 60) Stem cell-like properties of cancer cells: All malignant tumors or cancers contain cells that never die (or are immortal and of course they die when the patient dies) and have limitless capacity to replicate or multiply. So,

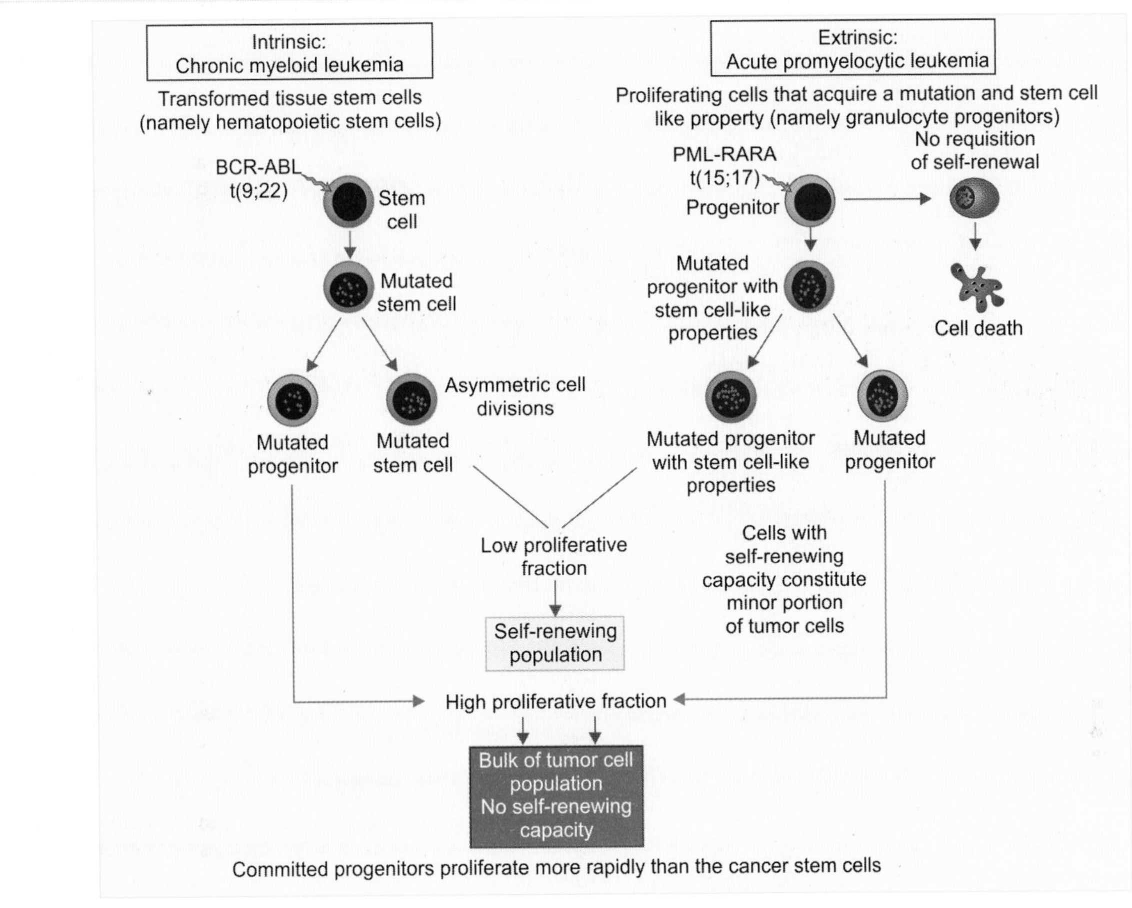

FIG. 60: Cancer cells with self-renewing capacity. Cancer stem cells may arise either from the transformation of tissue stem cells or from the conversion of conventional somatic cells to transformed cells with the acquired stem cell like property. In this example, cancer stem cells may arise from transformed tissue stem cells namely hematopoietic stem cells in chronic myeloid leukemia (CML) with intrinsic "stemness." Cancer stem cells may also arise from proliferating cells that acquire a mutation and stem cell like property namely granulocyte progenitors in acute promyelocytic leukemia. In both examples, the cancer stem cells undergo asymmetric cell divisions and give rise to committed progenitors that proliferate more rapidly than the cancer stem cells. This result in production of most of the malignant cells in both tumors which has no self-renewing capacity.

cancers too may contain cells that self-renew cancer cells. These self-renewing cancer cells are called as **cancer stem cells.** Cancer stem cells (CSCs) are cells (found in solid cancers or hematological malignancies) that have characteristics associated with normal stem cells. They are capable to give rise to all cell types found in a particular malignancy. Cancer stem cells resemble normal stem cells in many ways, but are no longer under homeostatic control. They play a critical role in the initiation, progression, and resistance to therapy of malignant tumors. Only a small proportion of the cells within a malignant tumor are capable of forming tumors. Probably cells resembling stem cells must be present in all cancers. Their presence was demonstrated in hematological malignancies like acute myeloblastic leukemia (AML), but there is also strong evidence for their presence in an increasing number of solid tumors.

Origin of cancer stem cells (Fig. 60): Cancer stem cells may arise either from the transformation of tissue stem cells (e.g., hematopoietic stem cells in chronic myeloid leukemia) or from the conversion of conventional somatic cells to transformed cells with the acquired stem cell like property (e.g., granulocyte progenitors in acute promyelocytic leukemia). Both may occur in different types of tumors. Examples includes chronic myeloid leukemia (CML) and acute promyelocytic leukemia (**Fig. 60**).

- **From transformed tissue/adult stem cells**: CML is characterized by the presence of BCR-ABL fusion gene in a tumor cell subset that has all the properties of a normal hematopoietic stem cell. Thus, CML probably arises a transformed hematopoietic stem cell with a firm capacity for self-renewal. Similarly, certain epithelial tumors may arise from other adult stem cells, such as those that are present in colonic crypts in gastrointestinal tract.
- **From slightly differentiated immediate progeny of the tissue stem cells**: Thus, they may arise form proliferating cells (not directly from stem cells). The oncogenic stimulus or acquired mutation may affect a committed progenitor cell and grants "stemness" (stem cell property). These cells are capable of self-renewal, the resulting transformed progenitor may become a CSC. If it does not activate the self-renewal program, resulting differentiated progeny will be produced and eventually die. For example, granulocyte progenitors in acute promyelocytic leukemia, the cancer stem originate from more differentiated hematopoietic

progenitors that acquire an abnormal capacity for self-renewal. Probably it occurs due to certain mutated transcription factors, such as a PML-RARA fusion protein that is observed with acute promyelocytic leukemia. This may play an important role in acquisition of "stemness." It is well known that expression of few transcription factors can result in the epigenetic reprogramming of a differentiated somatic cell (e.g., fibroblast) into a pluripotent stem cell. Thus, mutations leading to misexpression of certain key transcription factors (e.g., MYC), might convert a somatic cell into a transformed cell with a capacity for self-renewal. Normal stem cells and their more differentiated progeny have a fixed parent-offspring relationship. However, cancer cells present within a tumor can dedifferentiate to a stem cell-like state. Thus, cancers can repopulate their stem cell pools from non-stem cell populations.

- **Dedifferentiation:** Normal stem cells and their more differentiated progeny have a fixed parent-offspring relationship. But cancer cells within a tumor may be able to "de-differentiate" to a stem cell-like state. Thus, cancers can repopulate their stem cell pools from non-stem cell populations. This further complicates the efforts to precisely define and selectively target cancer stem cells.

In both situations, the cancer stem cells undergo asymmetric cell divisions that give rise to committed progenitors. These progenitors proliferate more rapidly than the cancer stem cells. This will result, in most malignant cells (in both tumors) with low or absent self-renewing capacity

Identification of cancer stem cells: The difficulty encountered is in identifying or determining whether any particular cell is a cancer stem cell or not and also their numbers in a particular cancer. Thus, the number of "stem cells" that are calculated to be present in a particular tumor can vary extensively depending on method used to quantify stem cells. This has caused uncertainty about whether CSCs are rare or common in tumors. CSCs can be identified with fluorescence-activated cell sorting (FACS), with antibodies directed at cell-surface markers such as CD133, CD44, ALDH1A1, CD34, CD24 and EpCAM (epithelial cell adhesion molecule).

Cancer stem cells and therapy: Cancer stem cells may be important in therapy for cancer.

- **Targeted cancer therapy (refer pages 572 and 573):** If cancer stem cells are important for the persistence of a tumor, then these cancer stem cells must be destroyed to eradicate the tumor. Similar to normal stem cells, cancer stem cells are resistant to conventional therapies. This is because of a low rate of cell division (i.e., slow cell cycle progression), and high levels of expression of factors that counteract the effects of chemotherapeutic drugs such drug efflux pumps of multiple drug resistance-1 (MDR1) and antiapoptotic Bcl-2 family members. This causes cancer stem cells to be less vulnerable to effects of chemotherapeutic drugs or radiation therapy. Limited success of current therapies for cancer may be partly due to their failure to kill the cancer stem cells that lie at the root of cancer. This may lead to a regrowth of tumors that is manifested as tumor recurrence or disease. Research is in progress to identify unique molecular features of cancer stem cells which will help direct targeting pf cancer stem cells by novel therapeutic agents.
- **Relapse after treatment:** Selectively targeting CSCs may be used for treating aggressive, nonresectable tumors, to prevent metastasis and relapse

Hallmark 5: Inducing Angiogenesis (Increased Angiogenesis)

Q. Write a short essay on the role of angiogenesis in tumor spread.

Q. What are activators and inhibitors of angiogenesis?

Q. Describe the process of angiogenesis and lymphangiogenesis. Discuss in brief, role of angiogenesis in cancer. Enumerate immunohistochemistry (IHC) markers of lymphangiogenesis.

Q. Write a short essay on angiogenesis in neoplasia.

Angiogenesis is the process of formation of new blood vessels from preexisting small blood vessels. Angiogenesis is an essential physiological process for embryologic development, normal growth, and tissue repair. Under homeostatic conditions, there is a balance between factors that favor new blood vessel formation (angiogenic factors/angiogenic promoters) and those that hinder it (antiangiogenic factors/ angiogenesis inhibitors).

Sustained Angiogenesis

Like normal tissues/organs, tumors need a steady supply of oxygen, glucose, and other nutrients, and removal of metabolic waste products to sustain cell viability and proliferation. It is served by vasculature. Probably, the maximal distance across which oxygen, nutrients, and waste can diffuse to and from blood vessels is 1–2 mm zone.

Solid tumors **cannot enlarge beyond 1–2 mm in diameter unless it has the capacity to induce angiogenesis.** In growing cancers, angiogenesis is critical for the growth of these neoplasms.

Importance of angiogenesis in tumor

Solid tumors, even though have all the genetic aberrations that are required for malignant transformation, their **growth requires increased supplies of nutrients and oxygen.** Cancer cells may die by necrosis, apoptosis, or autophagy, if there is no supply of oxygen and glucose. Thus, angiogenesis is an essential feature of malignancy. Hence, most rapidly growing tumors are well-vascularized with evidence of ongoing active angiogenesis. In normal microvasculature, the blood flow is smooth (seamless). Angiogenesis **delivers nutrients and removes wastes**, but newly formed tumor-associated neovasculature/vessels are not entirely normal. They are abnormal (both morphologically and functionally), leaky, torturous, and dilated. These vessels have a haphazard pattern of connection with abnormal (erratic) flow patterns and "dead zones" in which no blood flow is detectable. These features can be appreciated on angiograms. Angiogenesis permits tumor cells approach to these abnormal vessels and thereby also contributes to metastasis. Thus, angiogenesis is an essential feature for a primary tumor to grow and metastasize. The degree of vascularity varies widely in tumors ranging from highly vascularized renal carcinomas to poorly vascularized pancreatic ductal adenocarcinomas.

Effects of Neovascularization on Tumor Growth

- **Perfusion** supplies require nutrients and oxygen and remove waste products.
- Newly formed endothelial cells **secrete growth factors** [e.g., IGFs (insulin-like growth factors), PDGF] which stimulate the growth of adjacent tumor cells.
- Permits access of tumor cells to these abnormal vessels and **contributes to metastasis**.

Mechanism of Angiogenesis

Angiogenesis is controlled by a balance between angiogenesis promoters and inhibitors. In tumors, this balance is shifted in favor of promoters. During early phase of cancer development, most tumors do not induce angiogenesis and tumors remain in a stage of vascular quiescence and starved of nutrients. During this phase, the tumor remains small or in situ, probably for years, till an ***angiogenic switch*** terminates this stage.

Molecular basis of the angiogenic switch

Angiogenesis may be due to increased production of angiogenic factors and/or loss of angiogenic inhibitors. The source of these factors may be the tumor cells or inflammatory cells (e.g., macrophages) or resident stromal cells (e.g., tumor-associated fibroblasts). The local balance of angiogenic and antiangiogenic factors is influenced by many factors. Most tumors experience hypoxia (lack of oxygen) and lack of nutrients and are the main "reasons" for the onset of angiogenesis in tumors.

Factors affecting tumor angiogenesis by increasing the production of pro-angiogenic factors are as follows:

- **Hypoxia:** Relative lack of oxygen due to hypoxia induces expression of **HIFs, mainly** HIF 1α. HIF regulates hundreds of genes, including ones that directly or indirectly induce angiogenesis. HIF 1α is an oxygen-sensitive transcription factor that activates the transcription of proangiogenic growth factor cytokines such as VEGF and basic fibroblast growth factor (bFGF) and stimulate tumor-associated angiogenesis. These angiogenic factors creat angiogenic gradient and stimulate the proliferation of endothelial cells and guide the growth of new vessels towards the tumor.
- **Driver mutations in certain tumor suppressors:** They also can tilt the balance in favor of angiogenesis. For example, normally p53 stimulates expression of antiangiogenic molecules, such as thrombospondin-1 (TSP-1) and inhibit expression of proangiogenic molecules, such as VEGF. When there is loss of p53 in cells, it removes cell cycle checkpoints and alters tumor cell metabolism. It also provides a favorable environment for angiogenesis.
- **Gain-of-function mutations in *RAS*, *MYC* and MAPK signaling:** The transcription of VEGF is influenced by signals from the RAS/MAPK pathway. Hence, gain-of function mutations in *RAS* or *MYC* upregulates the production of VEGF and stimulates angiogenesis. Elevated levels of VEGF can be detected in the serum and urine of a significant fraction of cancer patients.
- **Angiopoietins:** Angiopoietin-2 is a family of vascular growth factor which favors formation of tumor blood vessel, stabilizes growing blood vessels, and stimulates pericytes to surround the developing blood vessels.
- **Proteases:** They are also involved in regulating the balance between angiogenic and antiangiogenic factors. They may be produced either by the tumor cells or by stromal cells in response to the tumor.
  - **Proangiogenic:** Many proteases can release proangiogenic basic fibroblast growth factors (bFGF) present in the ECM.
  - **Anti-angiogenic:** Also, proteases can release the angiogenesis inhibitors (e.g., angiostatin and endostatin) by proteolytic cleavage of plasminogen and collagen, respectively.

Steps in Angiogenesis

Quiescent vessels

Blood capillaries consist of a monolayer of endothelial cells interconnected by adhesion molecules and surrounded by pericytes. Endothelial cells and pericytes at rest produce a common basement membrane and maintain the integrity. The endothelial cells in healthy adult capillaries are quiescent (not dividing), due to the action of pericytes and also the absence of external proliferative factors.

Targeted cancer therapy (**Figs. 61A** to **E**) begins when existing cells (e.g., tumor cells or stromal cells) secrete mediators of angiogenesis (e.g., VEGFs, angiopoietins, and others). The process started by these chemicals resembles vasculogenesis in embryonic development. The main cellular events during angiogenesis (refer Fig. 58 and pages 330–332) are as follows:

- **Sprouting and the definition of tip cells:** Angiogenesis starts from the response of the quiescent endothelial cells to angiogenic factors/signals. The master regulator being VEGF. New vessels sprout from previously existing capillaries. In tumors, the source of VEGF is tumor cells and cells from the tumor microenvironment (e.g., macrophages). VEGF binds to vascular endothelial growth factor receptor (VEGFR) on endothelial cells from a mature vessel. This is characterized by local release of cytokines and growth factors. First step requires the detachment of pericytes and degradation of the basement membranes. Proteolytic enzymes (mediators of angiogenesis) perforate/breakdown postcapillary venule basement membranes. This activates quiescent capillary endothelial cells and facilitates formation of a vessel growth. Disruption or breakdown of basement membranes surrounding endothelial cells and surrounding pericytes determines the sites of endothelial cells growth/sprouting into the surrounding matrix. Endothelial cells in the area of the interrupted (broken down) basement membrane have reduced adhesion to their neighboring cells and favor their proliferation and migration towards the source of the angiogenic cytokines (VEGF gradient). This endothelial cell is called tip cell (it is the cell that leads to the formation of the new branch) and the endothelial cells that are left behind are called stalk cells. The tip cell/stalk cell dichotomy is regulated by the Notch signaling pathway.
- **Migration and proliferation of endothelial cells:** The endothelial cells (tip cells) put out cell extensions, called pseudopodia, that migrate and proliferate from the existing vessel to form capillary sprouts towards the site of angiogenic stimuli. In physiological angiogenesis, endothelial cell sprouting continues in a highly directional and regulated manner. But in cancers it is not so. The sprouting of capillaries is brought out by fibroblast growth factors (FGFs), mainly

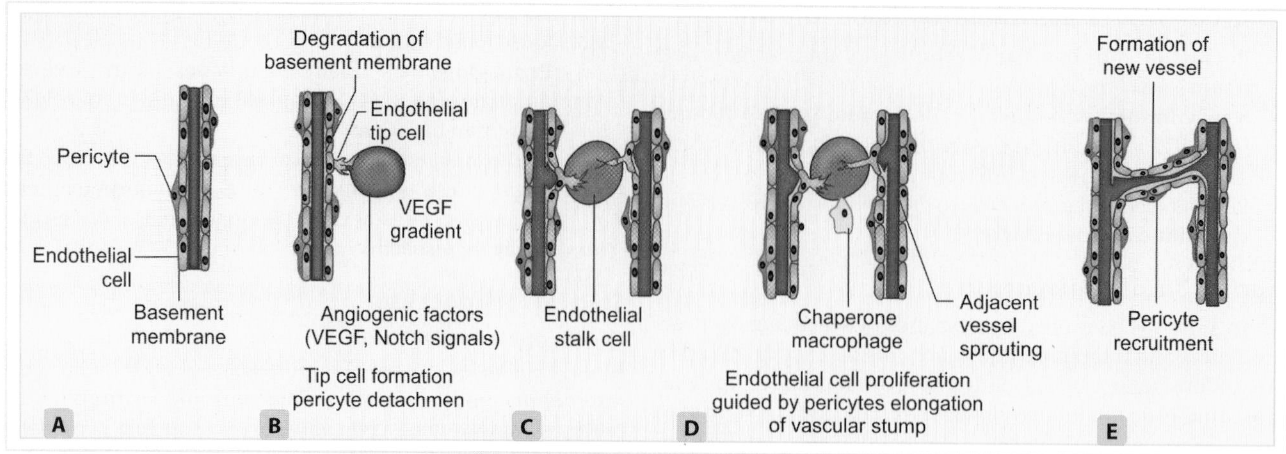

FIGS. 61A TO E: Main events in angiogenesis. (A) Quiescent vessel. (B) Morphological alteration of an endothelial cell from a quiescent vessel in response to a vascular endothelial growth factor (VEGF) gradient. This altered endothelial cell is called the tip cell; and their neighbors, the stalk cells. In this first step, there is also detachment of pericytes and degradation of the basement membranes. (C) The tip cell leads the formation of a new branch. (D) The stalk cells divide and the fusion of endocytic vesicles form lumen. The ligation of the two tip cells is chaperoned by macrophages. (E) Finally, the angiogenic process leads to the formation of a new branch of vessels. This establishes the flow of blood and thereby eliminates the VEGF gradient. For proper blood flow, the new blood vessel requires a maturation process that consists of the reattachment of pericytes and repositioning of a basement membrane.

FGF-2. Cytoplasmic flow of endothelial cells enlarges the pseudopodia of endothelial cells, and eventually the cells divide. At the same time, stalk cells divide and the fusion of endocytic vesicles/vacuoles are formed in the new daughter endothelial cells. These vacuoles fuse to create a new capillary sprouts/tubes with lumen.

- **Lumen formation:** Sprout elongation is followed by vessel fusion. Endothelial cells proliferate, loosely following each other, and are presumably guided by pericytes. The entire process continues till the tip cells of blood-vessel sprouts encounter another similar tip cells of other capillary sprouts (other vascular branches), with which it will connect. The fusion of migrating tip cells is called anastomosis. It produces a capillary network with development of lumen in the advancing cell mass. The ligation of the two tip cells is mediated by chaperones.
- **Maturation and remodeling:** The immature capillaries formed are invested with a basement membrane and blood flow is established. The angiogenic process terminates with the disappearance of the VEGF gradient. To establish proper blood flow, the new blood vessel requires a maturation process that consists in the reattachment of pericytes and repositioning of a basement membrane.

Therapeutic Significance

Angiogenesis is needed for solid tumors that grow to clinically significant sizes. Hence, one of the methods of dealing with cancer is use of therapeutic agents that block angiogenesis. One of the examples is use of monoclonal antibody that neutralizes VEGF activity (e.g., bevacizumab) in the treatment of multiple cancers. However, angiogenesis inhibitors are not as effective as was originally hoped. They can prolong life, but usually for only a few months and are highly expensive.

Inhibitors of Tumor Angiogenesis

There are many powerful endogenous suppressors of tumor-related angiogenesis (blood vessel growth). They limit the growth of tumor.

- **VHL:** The normal VHL protein is a product of *VHL* gene. It is a tumor suppressor and is part of an ubiquitin ligase. It degrades transcription factors, called HIFs. Inactivation of the *VHL* gene causes defect in Ub conjugation and leads to increased HIF 1α. HIF 1α is an angiogenic factor involved in cellular responses to low oxygen. They (i) increase cellular intake of glucose for anaerobic glycolysis, (ii) stimulate angiogenesis (VEGF), and (iii) activate many growth factors. Inactivation of VHL promotes tumor growth mainly by the action of HIF 1α. Activation of HIF 1α also occurs in oxygen-starved regions of many tumors, even without *VHL* mutation. In such situations, degradation of HIF 1α is impaired due to reduced activity of a cofactor for the ubiquitination reaction. VHL has tumor suppressor function independent of HIF 1α. These are brought out by (i) promoting apoptosis, (ii) increasing immobilization of cells by adherence to matrix proteins, and (iii) reducing some cell activation responses.
- **NOTCH:** It is an important stimulator for development of blood vessels in embryo. NOTCH family of endothelial cell receptors, along with their cell surface-bound ligands [especially delta-like ligand 4 (DLL4)] can inhibit tumor angiogenesis.
- **ECM and other angiogenesis inhibitors:** Tumor angiogenesis can be suppressed by constituents of ECM and clotting factors, and their breakdown products.
  - **TSP-1 (Thrombospondin 1):** It is derived from a large ECM glycoprotein. It is a powerful inhibitor of formation of blood vessels.
  - **Angiostatin:** It is a breakdown product of plasminogen, and numerous fragments of ECM constituents (e.g., endostatin, inhibin, etc.) reduce tumor-related blood vessel growth.
- **p53:** It does not directly interfere with tumor angiogenesis but upregulates TSP-1 (thrombospondin 1) expression which has a powerful antitumor angiogenic function. Loss of p53 reduces the activity of TSP-1.

- **Sirtuin (SIRT):** Sirtuin deacetylases are involved in stress responses and longevity. One of the sirtuins, namely SIRT3, increases the activity of mitochondrial antioxidant, manganese superoxide dismutase (MnSOD). This produces less reactive oxygen species (ROS) by mitochondria and decreases HIF-1 activity. This leads to reduced angiogenesis.

Hallmark 6: Activating Invasion and Metastasis

Q. Discuss the cellular basis of invasion and metastasis in neoplasia and also hematogenous spread.

Invasion and metastasis (ability to spread) **are characteristics of malignant tumors** and are the **major causes of cancer-related morbidity and mortality.** Metastatic disease is responsible for >90% of cancer deaths (mortality) and a major barrier to cancer patient survival. Most of the high-grade cancer cells become invasive and migratory. Studies revealed that, each day many locally invasive cancer cells enter the bloodstream. But very few of them produce metastases. It is probably related to the complexity of the process. Cancer cells that emerge from a primary tumor mass must go through a series of steps to enter blood vessels or lymphatics, and produce a secondary growth at a distant site. These steps involve a complex interaction between tumor cells and several different types of host cells and factors. At each step in this sequence, the separated cells are faced with the challenges of avoiding immune defenses and adapt to a microenvironment (e.g., lymph node, bone marrow, or brain) that is entirely different from that of the site of origin of the primary tumor. The "metastatic phenotype" needs the accumulation of complementary genetic and epigenetic changes that together promote the metastatic cascade.

Definition

Invasion-metastatic cascade constitutes the **entire sequence of events from** the beginning of **invasion** to the development of **metastasis**.

Phases

Q. Write a short essay on the role of protease in tumor invasion.

Invasion-metastatic cascade is a **complex, active multistep process. Invasion and metastasis result from complex interactions involving three main components—(i) cancer cells, (ii) stromal cells, and (iii) the ECM (extracellular matrix).**

Invasion-metastatic cascade can be divided into two main phases, namely—(1) **invasion of the ECM** and (2) **metastasis (vascular dissemination and homing of tumor cells)**. Each phase has several sequential steps.

Invasion of extracellular matrix (Figs. 62A to F)

Q. Discuss the role of stroma/matrix in tumor progression (refer page 483–487).

Q. Discuss the metalloproteases.

The structural organization and function of normal tissues depends on interactions between cells and the ECM. Tissue compartments are separated from each other by two types of ECM namely (i) basement membrane and (ii) interstitial connective tissue. Each components consists of different combinations of collagens, glycoproteins, and proteoglycans. Tumor cells especially carcinoma cells must interact with ECM at several steps in the invasion-metastatic cascade. A carcinoma must first breach the underlying basement membrane, invade into adjacent interstitial connective tissue, gain entry into both blood and lymphatic vessels (intravasation) by penetrating the vascular basement membrane, and transit through the vessels. This process is repeated in reverse order when tumor cell emboli extravasate from the vessels at a distant site. It forms micrometastases which later grow into macroscopic tumors. Invasion of the ECM is an active process and consists of four steps:

1. **Loosening of connections between tumor cells**: Normal epithelial cells are attached to each other and maintained as epithelial sheets. This is due to a key epithelial cell-to-cell adhesion molecule (act as intercellular glue), namely **E-cadherins** (epithelial cadherin, also known as cadherin-1, the name cadherin stands for calcium-dependent adhesion). The cytoplasmic portions E-cadherins bind to β-catenin (refer Fig. 9 of Chapter 2). E-cadherins are transmembrane glycoproteins and mediate the homotypic adhesion of epithelial cells. Adjacent E-cadherin molecules keep the cells together and also can transmit antigrowth signals by sequestering β-catenin. Tumor cells usually undergo alterations in their shape as well as their attachment to other cells and to the ECM.
   - **Reduced/loss of E-cadherin function:** It is the first step observed in most epithelial cancers (e.g., adenocarcinomas of the colon and breast), E-cadherin function is lost. This may be due to pathogenic mutations: (i) mutational inactivation of E-cadherin genes (E-cadherin-encoding gene, *CDH1*), (ii) activation of β-catenin genes, or (iii) inappropriate expression of the SNAIL and TWIST transcription factors (suppress E-cadherin expression). E-cadherin expression is silenced, at least transiently, through a process called epithelial-mesenchymal transition (EMT). EMT is essential to the metastasis of carcinomas, particularly breast and prostate cancers. EMT is controlled by the transcription factors SNAIL and TWIST. Apart from the downregulation of epithelial markers (e.g., E-cadherin), the accompanying upregulation of mesenchymal markers (e.g., vimentin and smooth muscle actin) may favor the development of a promigratory phenotype that is essential for metastasis. Loss of E-cadherin causes **loosening of tumor cells**. The separated cells get **detached from the primary cancer**.
2. **Local degradation/proteolysis of basement membrane and interstitial connective tissue:** It is the second step in invasion. ECM is mainly of two types, namely—(1) basement membrane and (2) interstitial connective tissue.
   - **Secretion of degrading enzymes:** Malignant **tumor cells** may either secrete proteolytic enzymes themselves or stimulate **stromal cells** (e.g., fibroblasts and inflammatory cells) **in the cancers to secrete many proteolytic enzymes** that **degrade ECM**. These

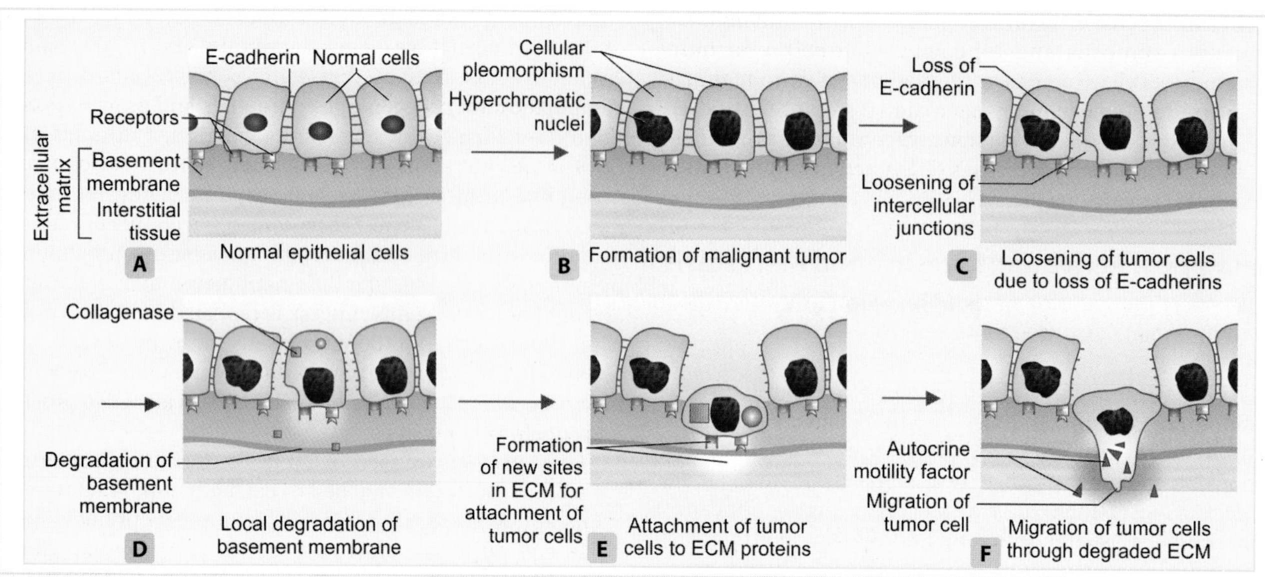

FIGS. 62A TO F: Various steps in the invasion of extracellular matrix (ECM) in invasion–metastasis cascades. (A) Normal cells. (B to F) Tumor cells loosen and detach from each other because of reduced adhesiveness. The tumor cells bind components of the ECM and secrete proteolytic enzymes that degrade the ECM. With binding to proteolytically generated new binding sites in the ECM, tumor cell migration follows. The tumor cells reach the nearby vessels to start the next phase, namely metastasis.

enzymes include **matrix metalloproteinases (MMPs), cathepsin D, and urokinase plasminogen activator (u-PA)** These proteases are involved in tumor invasion. MMPs are a family of zinc-dependent proteases (endopeptidases) **secreted as proenzymes. MMPs** can be proteolytically activated and can degrade ECM. MMPs are normally regulated by tissue inhibitors of MMPs (TIMPs). MMPs regulate tumor invasion by two ways—(i) by remodeling insoluble components of the basement membrane and interstitial matrix and (ii) by releasing ECM-sequestered growth factors (that have chemotactic, angiogenic, and growth-promoting effects). The expression of MMP genes are regulated by inflammatory cytokines, growth factors, hormones, cell-cell and cell–matrix interaction. Tumor invasion, metastasis, and tumor angiogenesis require the participation of MMPs and MMPs expression is increased in association with tumorigenesis. MMPs consist of several subgroups (**Table 23**). MMP-9 is a gelatinase that cleaves type IV collagen of the epithelial and vascular basement membrane. It also stimulates release of VEGF from ECM sequestered pools. In many tumors, invasiveness correlates directly with increased MMP expression. Benign tumors of the breast, colon, and stomach have minimal type IV collagenase activity, whereas their malignant counterparts overexpress this enzyme. Use of metalloproteinase inhibitors as therapeutic agent reduces the tissue degradation. Overexpression of MMPs and other proteases have been found in many malignant tumors. MMPs are a target of therapeutic intervention to inhibit tumor invasion and metastasis.

- **Local degradation of basement membrane and interstitial connective tissue: Tumor cells should** disrupt and penetrate the underlying basement membrane and then pass through the ECM. This is achieved by proteolytic enzymes.

Table 23: Subgroups of active enzymes of matrix metalloproteinases (MMPs) on the cell surface and their actions.

Subgroup of matrix metalloproteinases (MMPs)	*Actions*
Collagenases (MMP-1, MMP-8, and MMP-13)	Degrade types I, II, and III collagens, and other extracellular matrix (ECM) proteins
Gelatinases (MMP-2 and MMP-9)	Degrade molecules such as type IV, V, and XI collagens, laminin, and aggrecan core protein
Stromelysins (MMP-3 and MMP-10)	Degrade basement membrane components (type IV collagen and fibronectin).
Matrilysin (MMP-7 and MMP-26)	MMP-7 cleaves cell surface molecules such as Fas ligand, protumor necrosis factor ligand, and E-cadherin.
Membrane-type MMPs (MT-MMPs)	
• Transmembrane proteins (MMP-14, MMP-15, MMP-16, and MMP-24). • Glycosylphosphatidylinositol (GPI)-anchored proteins (MMP-17 and MMP-25)	Active enzymes on the cell surface

3. **Changes in attachment/adhesion of tumor cells to ECM proteins:** It is the third step in invasion. Normal epithelial cells have receptors such as integrin, for basement membrane components (e.g., laminin and collagen). Integrins are transmembrane proteins that are involved in adhesion of cells to other cells and to ECM. In normal

epithelial cells, integrins that bind basement membrane laminin and collagens are strictly confined to the basal surface of cells. These integrin receptors help to maintain the cells in a resting, differentiated and polarized state. Tumor cells show complex changes in the expression of these integrin receptors. In normal cells, loss of adhesion leads to cell death of these cells by anoikis (anoikis-without a home). But free tumor cells are resistant to anoikis. This is partly due to the expression of other integrins. This integrin reduces the loss of adhesion to ECM, probably by transmitting signals that promote cell survival. Also the matrix itself is modified in such a way that promote invasion and metastasis.

Generation of new sites and stimulation of tumor cell migration: Loss of adhesion in tumor cells does not produce apoptosis and this modifies the matrix in such a way to promote invasion and metastasis. For example, local degradation of the basement membrane proteins, collagen IV, and laminin by MMP-2 or MMP-9 generates **new and strange** sites in the basement membrane that bind to receptors on tumor cells and stimulate migration.

4. **Locomotion/migration of tumor cells through degraded ECM:** It is the fourth and final step in invasion. This pushes the tumor cells through the degraded basement membranes and regions of matrix proteolysis. For solid tumors, invasion requires that the previously stationary cell should become motile. Migration of tumor cells is a complex, multistep process and is the final step of invasion.
   - **Locomotion/migration** drives the tumor cells **forward through the degraded basement membranes** and zones of proteolysis in the **interstitial connective tissue matrix**. Proteolysis is brought out by proteases secreted by cancer cells and nonmalignant tumor-associated cells.
   - **Locomotion involves many receptors and signaling proteins**. Tumor cells attach to the matrix at their leading edge and detach from the matrix at their trailing edge. They contract the actin cytoskeleton and move forward. Cancer cells develop cytoplasmic protrusions that contain an actin core and integrins. These projections are called invadopodia. The motility/locomotion of tumor cell is potentiated and directed by several factors.
     - **Tumor cell-derived cytokines**, These include chemokines and growth factors (e.g., insulin-like growth factors). They act as autocrine motility factors.
     - The **cleavage products of matrix components** (e.g., collagen, laminin) and few growth factors (e.g., IGF I and II) have chemotactic activity for tumor cells.
     - **Stromal cells produce paracrine effectors of cell motility** [e.g., hepatocyte growth factor/scatter factor (HGF/SCF)]. They bind to receptors tyrosine kinase MET on tumor cells and cause motility of tumor cells. For example, the advancing edges of the highly invasive brain tumor, namely glioblastoma, show raised concentrations of HGF/SCF.
     - **Upregulation of C-X-C chemokine receptor type 4 (CXCR4) chemokine receptors**: Tumor cell motility is increased by upregulation of CXCR4 chemokine receptors in cancer cells at the advancing edge. The invading cells stimulate nearby stromal cells to secrete stromal cell-derived factor-1 (SDF-1) (also called CXCL12), the ligand for this receptor.
   - **Migration through interstitial tissue:** The tumor cells invade and traverse through the surrounding interstitial connective tissue and ultimately **reach nearby blood and lymphatic vessels.** Cells gain access to the circulation by penetrating the basement membrane of vessels.

During the initial phase of metastasis, cancer cells penetrate through the endothelial basement membrane and transmigrate into the vascular space. Throughout this phase of the metastatic cascade, cancer cells interact with ECM and several types of stromal cells. These include innate and adaptive immune cells, fibroblasts, and endothelial cells. Successful cancer cells produce signals that modify stromal cells in such a way that they support their malignant behavior. As cancers evolve, they become dominated by cancer cells that serve their malignant purposes.

Vascular dissemination homing, and colonization

Metastasis is a **multistep process** by which tumor produces a secondary growth at a distant site or location. It has several steps (**Fig. 63**).

- **Circulation of tumor cells and tumor-derived DNA in blood:** Following the invasion of surrounding interstitial tissue, malignant cells **frequently escape their sites of origin and enter the circulation.** In solid tumors, even if small, large number (in millions) of tumor cells are shed daily. Both tumor cells and tumor-derived DNA can be detected in circulation by "liquid biopsies," blood samples taken from these patients. The liquid biopsy is the basis currently used to quantitate single tumor cells in the peripheral blood. They are used both as prognostic indicators and to choose chemotherapy. Most of the tumor cells circulate as single cells, whereas others may form emboli by aggregating and adhering to circulating blood component, particularly platelets.
- **Survival in the vascular system:** Once cancer cells are in the circulation, they have two main tasks—(i) to survive and (ii) to find a new site. **Circulating tumor cells (CTCs)** do not spend long time in the vascular system. CTCs can be detected even before the primary tumor becomes pathologically invasive. Their size (20–30 μ) is more than the diameter of pulmonary capillaries (about 8 μ). A single passage of these cells through the pulmonary circulation will filter the majority of them from the blood.
- **Penetration of vascular or lymphatic channels (intravasation into the lumen of vessels):** Malignant cells penetrate (**intravasate**) the basement membrane of blood vessels or lymphatic channels. These vessels provide a route for migration to a faraway site in the body. Cancer cells that travel lonely move more rapidly than do cell clusters. **Factors favoring penetration of vessels are:**
  - Tumor-associated capillaries (stimulated by VEGF produced by tumor and related angiogenic factors) are less well-formed, not completely surrounded by pericytes, and undergo constant remodeling.
  - VEGF increases vascular permeability.
  - Tumor-associated macrophages (TAMs) produce EGF and tumor cells secrete colony-stimulating factor-1 (CSF-1). They increase intravasation.

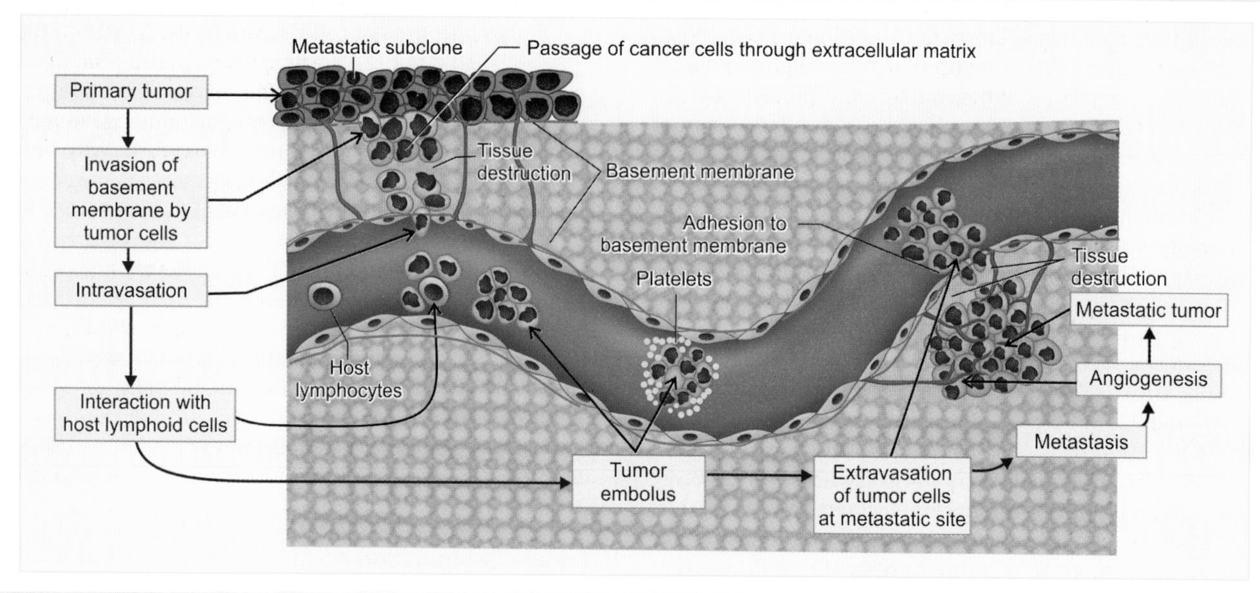

FIG. 63: Various steps involved in vascular dissemination and homing of tumor cells during the metastatic cascade.

  - Matrix metalloproteinases (MMP1 and MMP2) and other tumor and stromal cell products increase the leakiness of tumor-induced blood vessels. They facilitate invasion of vessels by cancer cells.
- **Invasion of the circulation and formation of tumor emboli:** In the circulation, tumor cells are susceptible to destruction by several mechanisms. These include mechanical shear stress, apoptosis stimulated by loss of adhesion (termed *anoikis*), and innate and adaptive immune defenses. In patients with solid tumors such as carcinomas, variable number of viable circulating tumor cells (CTCs) are not rare. Probably, the circulating tumor cells that produce metastases are much more likely to migrate as multicellular aggregates than as single cells. Clumping of tumor cells in the blood is enhanced by homotypic interactions and heterotypic interactions between tumor cells and blood elements, particularly platelets. The clumping may increase the survival of tumor in the circulation. Circulating tumor cells may also express anionic substances (e.g., polyphosphate) that activate factor XII (contact factor). This may lead to deposition of fibrin and further stabilize the tumor emboli. All these factors may favor the arrest of cells en masse within capillary beds. The groups of circulating tumor cells are more likely produce a metastasis rather than any single cell. Presence of cancer cells with stem cell-like properties may be responsible for the continuous growth of metastatic lesions and the "plasticity" that is required for growth of metastatic cells in a new microenvironment.
- **Transit through the circulation**
  - **Arrest within circulating blood or lymph:** It occurs at distant location away from primary tumor. At the site of arrest, tumor cells adhere to endothelial cells.
  - **Exit of cancer cells from the circulation into a new tissue site:** Though tumor cells can easily enter the circulation, cancer cells are not very efficient to leave the circulation, invade, and grow to clinically significant sizes at other distant sites in the body (i.e., metastasis). **Several factors limit the metastatic potential of CTCs.**
- **Destruction of tumor cells by host immune cells:** In the circulation, tumor cells are vulnerable to destruction by host immune cells (discussed further).
- **Difficulty to invade distant sites**: Adhesion of tumor cells to normal vascular beds and invasion of normal tissues in distant sites may be more difficult than the escape of tumor cells from the site of origin of cancer. The blood vessels at the distant site are well-constructed and anatomically complete, rather than new, poorly-formed tumor-induced blood vessels.
- **Difficulty to grow in a metastatic site**: Even if the tumor cells extravasate at distant site, their growth may be difficult in a second site. This may be due to absence of critical stromal support or due to recognition and suppression of cancer cells by resident immune cells. Some primary or metastatic tumors may be present for many years before they are detected clinically. **Metastatic cells** even after their lodging and survival **at distant tissues**, they **may fail to grow**. This phenomenon, is **termed as tumor dormancy**. **Tumor dormancy** is defined as the presence of cancers, whether primary or metastatic, that do not enlarge to the point of being clinically detectable. It is due to prolonged survival of tumor cells without progression (inactivity of tumor). For example, tumor dormancy is observed in melanoma and in carcinoma of breast and prostate. Dormancy of tumor cells at distant sites may be considered as the last defense by host against clinically significant metastatic disease. Growth of both the primary tumor and metastases is usually interrupted by quiescent periods and the time requires for it to grow into a clinically detectable mass is highly variable. This may be due constant variation in the balance between stimulating or permissive signals and the actions of inhibitory factors. Though the exact molecular mechanisms of **escape from tumor dormancy** are not known, probably cancer cells secrete cytokines, growth factors, and ECM molecules. They act on the resident stromal cells and make the metastatic site suitable for the cancer cell. For example, in carcinoma of breast, cancer cells that metastasize to bone usually secrete parathyroid hormone-related protein

(PTHRP). PTHRP stimulates osteoblasts to produce RANK ligand (RANKL). These RANKL in turn activate osteoclasts and degrade the bone matrix and release growth factors embedded within bone matrix (e.g., IGF and TGF-β). These growth factors bind to receptors on the cancer cells. This activates signaling pathways that support the growth and survival of the cancer cells.
- The tumor cells have to penetrate the basement membrane of blood vessels to exit the circulation and these processes involve adhesion molecules (integrins, laminin receptors) and proteolytic enzymes.

Development of metastases

Though the above factors limit metastasis, if neglected, almost all cancers can finally produce macroscopic metastases.

Site of metastases: They **depend on three factors—(i) the anatomical location and vascular drainage of the primary tumor, (ii) the tropism of particular tumors for specific tissues at distant site, and (iii) escape from tumor dormancy (refre page 71 above).**

- **Location and vascular drainage of the primary tumor:** Most metastases develop in the first capillary bed available to the tumor. For example, cancer of colon more likely to give rise to metastases in the liver, the first organ downstream of the tumor, than to metastases elsewhere. So, the frequency of metastases to liver and lung and are common. Natural pathways of vascular or lymphatic drainage cannot entirely explain the distribution of metastases. For example, prostatic carcinoma tends to spread to bone, bronchogenic carcinomas to the adrenal glands and the brain, and neuroblastomas to the liver and bones. Though certain cancers "prefer" certain metastatic sites, the exact localization of metastases cannot be predicted in individual patients with any type of cancer. Tumor cells secrete cytokines, growth factors, and proteases. They may act on the resident stromal cells and make the metastatic site suitable for survival of the cancer cell.
- **Mechanism of organ tropisms:** These include—
  - **Adhesive molecules and ligands:** The ligands for adhesion molecules present in the tumors cells may be expressed preferentially on the endothelial cells of the target organ. One of them is the CD44 adhesion molecule. CD44 is expressed on normal T lymphocytes and this molecule is used by T lymphocytes to migrate to selective sites in lymphoid tissues. This is achieved by the binding of CD44 to hyaluronate on high endothelial venules. Solid tumors can also express CD44 and this enhances their capability of spread to lymph nodes and other metastatic sites. Location at which CTCs leave the capillaries to form secondary deposits depends on the anatomic location and vascular drainage of the primary tumor and the tropism of particular tumors for specific tissues. Exit occurs through the basement membrane of lymphatics or blood vessel. The site at which CTCs leave the vessel or lymphatics must repeat the same events involved in invasion but in a reverse order.
  - **Chemokines:** They may play an important role in deciding the target tissues for metastasis. For example, many cancers (e.g., breast cancer) express the chemokine receptor CXCR4. This is involved in the extravasation of CTCs.
  - **Favorable and unfavorable soil:** Some target tissues may provide a favorable "soil" for the growth of tumor cells. Paget originally proposed "seed-soil" hypothesis. According to this hypothesis, the ability of tumor cells arising from a particular site may develop metastasis in a limited type of foreign metastatic site. The target tissue may have a nonpermissive environment, called as "unfavorable soil". This prevents the growth of tumor deposits. For example, skeletal muscle and spleen though well-vascularized are the rare sites of metastasis.

  Once the cancer cells get arrested at distant sites, extravasation of tumor cells occurs. These cells transmigrate between endothelial cells followed by their exit through the basement membrane. Though exact mechanism of this process is not known, probably it may depend on whether the endothelium is fenestrated (e.g., in tissues such as the liver and bone marrow) or is held together by tight junctions (e.g., as in the brain). Extravasation of cancer cells needs adhesion molecules (integrins, laminin receptors), proteolytic enzymes, and chemokines. These may be derived from tumor cells or from innate immune cells such as monocytes and neutrophils.
- **Formation of micrometastases:** Tumor cells lodge at a distant new site to form micrometastases, e.g., for favored sites of metastasis.
- **Angiogenesis**
- **Local growth of micrometastases into macroscopic tumor**

Molecular genetics of metastasis development (Fig. 64)

Some tumors metastasize whereas others do not and this may be due to inherent differences in the behavior of particular tumors. For example, small cell carcinoma of the lung almost always metastasizes to distant sites, whereas basal cell carcinoma, rarely metastasizes. Generally, large tumors are more likely to metastasize than small tumors. This may be probably because large tumors might have been present for longer periods of time and provide more chances for metastasis to develop. Tumor size and type cannot predict the behavior of individual cancers. It is not known whether metastasis is a matter of chance multiplied by tumor cell number and time or due to inherent differences in metastatic potential in different tumors (a deterministic model).

Many theories have been proposed to explain the mechanism of development of metastatic phenotype.

- **Clonal evolution model:** According to this, metastasis is unavoidable with certain tumors. This is because tumors contain cells with a specific metastatic phenotype. As tumor cells grow, they randomly accumulate mutations. They create subclones with distinct combinations of mutations. Probably only rare tumor cells accumulate all of the mutations needed for metastasis. However, it was difficult to identify metastasis-specific mutations and metastasis-specific patterns of gene expression.
- **Metastatic signature:** It is defined as a set of genes that correlate with and appear to facilitate the establishment of macroscopic metastases (genes "favoring" metastasis) in specific tissues. Some tumors acquire all of the mutations

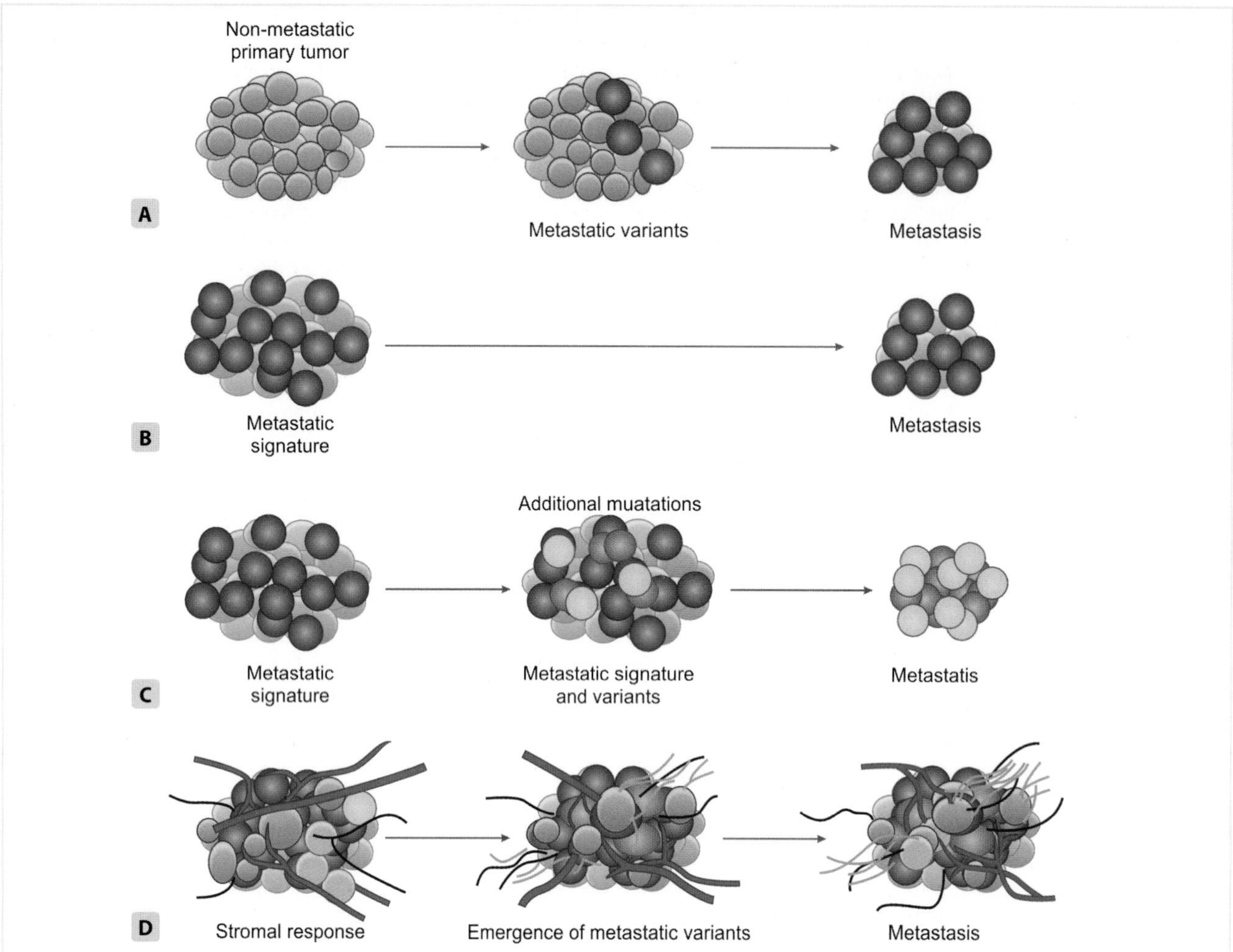

FIGS. 64A TO D: Four theories of molecular mechanisms of metastasis development within a primary tumor. (A) Metastasis is caused due to development of rare variant clones in the primary tumor. (B) Metastasis is caused by the expression of gene in most cells of the primary tumor that favor metastasis (metastatic signature). (C) A combination of (A) and (B). According to this, metastatic variants appear in a tumor with a metastatic gene signature. (D) Metastasis development depends on not only the cancer cells but also on microenvironment such as stroma. The tumor stroma regulates angiogenesis, local invasiveness, and resistance to immune elimination.

required for metastasis early in their development. Probably in these tumors most, if not all, cells develop a predilection for metastatic spread during early stages of carcinogenesis (**Fig. 64B**) and it is an intrinsic property of the tumor. For example, a subset of breast cancers has a metastatic gene expression signature similar to that found in metastases, though there is no clinical evidence of metastasis.

- **Combination of clonal evolution** and metastatic signature: According to this, the metastatic signature is necessary but not sufficient for metastasis. Hence, additional mutations are necessary for development of metastasis (**Fig. 64C**).
- **Involvement of cancer cells along with micro-environment:** The capacity for metastasis does not depend only on intrinsic properties of the cancer cells but also depends on the characteristics of their microenvironment. The microenvironment includes as the components of the stroma, the infiltrating immune cells (IICs), and angiogenesis (**Fig. 64D**).

Q. Write a short note on metastasis genes.

Metastasis genes

Metastasis is a complex process and involves many steps. It is possible that there are genes which control gene expression that promote metastasis. These may include "metastasis oncogenes" or "metastasis suppressor genes." They may promote or suppress the metastatic phenotype and their detection in a primary tumor may have both prognostic and therapeutic importance. Four theories of molecular mechanisms of metastasis development within a primary tumor are, presented in **Figures 64A to D**.

- **Metastasis suppressor gene:** It is defined as a gene, the loss of which promotes the development of metastasis without an effect on the primary tumor. About a dozen genes have been detected that function as "metastasis suppressors" and are lost in metastatic lesions. Most of them probably affect various signaling pathways.

- **Metastasis oncogenes:** Two metastasis oncogenes have been identified, namely *SNAIL* and *TWIST*. They encode transcription factors and their main function is to promote EMT. Activation of epithelial-mesenchymal transition (EMT) is an important cancer cell intrinsic regulatory mechanisms. EMT is associated with cell migrations and tissue invasions during embryogenesis, organogenesis, and also in cancer. In EMT, cancer cells downregulate certain epithelial markers (e.g., E-cadherin) and upregulate certain mesenchymal markers (e.g., vimentin, smooth muscle actin). These molecular changes cause changes that favor the development of a promigratory phenotype that is essential for metastasis. These changes include change in morphology of cancer cells from polygonal epithelioid cell shape to a spindly mesenchymal shape and also increased production of proteolytic enzymes that promote migration and invasion.
    - **Downregulation of epithelial markers:** Loss of E-cadherin expression is the main event in EMT. SNAIL and TWIST are transcriptional inhibitors that downregulate expression of E-cadherin. Probably they are stimulated due to interactions of tumor cells with stromal cells. EMT has been documented mainly in breast cancers. It is not known whether EMT is a general phenomenon in solid tumors.

Role of stromal elements in metastasis

Interaction between tumor cells and stromal elements is important in both invasion and metastasis. For example, macrophages in the stroma secrete matrix-degrading proteases, and cleavage of ECM proteins release angiogenic factors and growth factors (e.g., TGFβ). The tumor cells use these interactions to promote their growth and invasion. These interactions and the stromal cells are potential targets in the treatment of cancer.

Inhibitors of Invasiveness and Metastasis

For each step of invasion and metastasis, there are antagonists that block the spread of tumors.

Inhibitors of tumor cell invasiveness

***Nm23-H1*:** It was the first metastasis suppressor discovered that inhibits tumor cell motility. Nm23-H1 blocks cellular mobility brought out by Ras-related cell activation signaling pathways.

***p63*:** It belongs to the p53 family of tumor suppressors and helps to reduce cellular invasiveness. p63 is usually expressed in some in situ carcinomas (e.g., prostate and breast). It is often suppressed or lost in aggressive, metastatic carcinomas. It acts as a transcriptional regulator and also upregulates expression of some genes that inhibit metastasis (e.g., miR-130B). Movement of tumor cells through connective tissue is important for invasion. This depends on the ability of direct ameboid movement of cells through the ECM. This invasiveness is inhibited by miR-31.

***Suppressors of intravasation*:** Notch is the main inhibitor of tumor angiogenesis and intravasation also depends on Notch. AES (amino-terminal enhancer of split) is a protein that inhibits migration of tumor cells through vascular walls via signaling networks such as Notch activation.

Limiting tumor cell survival in the circulation Many vascular endothelial cells express the Duffy blood group glycoprotein called Duffy antigen/chemokine receptor (**DARC**). During the travel of tumor cells in the circulation, DARC recognizes KAI1 on tumor cell membranes. This triggers senescence programs thus, existence of circulating tumor cell is reduced. Also, cells of the innate immune system can generate cell death programs via TRAIL and CD95. Tumor cells are significantly larger than the caliber of many vascular spaces through which they travel. This imbalance can stimulate the sinusoidal lining cells in the liver to secrete nitric oxide (NO). NO brings out apoptosis in the too large tumor cells that try to pass through vascular channels that are too small.

Blocking extravasation

The miR-31 inhibits tumor cell invasiveness and also can block its extravasation.

Metastatic colonization

Colonization and subsequent growth of tumor are the major rate limiting process in tumor metastasis. Metastasis suppressors such as KISS1 and its receptor, KISS1R may limit this process. The names KISS1 and KISS1R are discovered in Hershey, PA, home of chocolate kisses, hence named so. KISS1, present in tumor cells, binds its cell membrane receptor, KISS1R and causes apoptosis of tumor cells. Other metastatic colonization suppressors include GATA3 in breast cancers (promotes cellular differentiation and retard multiplication), and PSAP in prostate cancers (activates stromal cell to produce antiangiogenic thrombospondin-1). MiR-31 has multiple antimetastatic activities, and effectively inhibits the colonization of cancer cells at distant sites.

Epithelial–mesenchymal Transition

Q. What is epithelial–mesenchymal transition (EMT)? What are its molecular pathways and significance in malignancy?

Q. Discuss epithelial–mesenchymal transition.

Normal epithelial cells are polarized and confined to the mucosa. They are attached to one another by cell to cell interaction as well as cell to basement interaction. The first of the many steps leading to metastasis of epithelial cancer cells is the local invasion. Invasion involves major changes in the phenotype (observable characteristics) of cancer cells within the primary tumor. The organization of the normal epithelial cell layers in tissues does not permit the motility and the invasiveness showed by carcinoma cells. For invasion and metastasis, cancer cells should escape from the confines of the mucosa in which they arise and acquire increased motility. First the cancer cells must shed many of their epithelial phenotypes and detach from epithelial sheets by disrupting the bonds of the cell–cell tight junctions. The carcinoma cells undergo a drastic alteration and assume a new form as single, nonpolarized mobile mesenchymal cells.

Definition

Epithelial–mesenchymal transition is the **process of developmental regulatory program in which epithelial cells acquire a less-differentiated mesenchymal phenotype.**

Classification

Epithelial–mesenchymal transition was first described by Elizabeth Hay in chick development. EMT occur in a range of biological processes and can be classified into three types:

1. *Developmental EMT*: Associated with implantation, embryogenesis, and organ development.
2. *Fibrosis and wound healing EMT*: Takes place during tissue regeneration and organ fibrosis and is largely inflammation-driven.
3. *EMT in cancer*: It is associated with cancer progression and metastasis.

Epithelial–mesenchymal transition is a multifaceted program. It can be activated temporarily (transiently), reversibly or stably, and to differing degrees, by carcinoma cells during the process of invasion and metastasis. **The EMT program regulates invasion and metastasis.** EMT is considered as a prominent means by which neoplastic epithelial cells can acquire the abilities to invade, resist apoptosis, and disseminate. The reverse process is termed as mesenchymal–epithelial transition (MET) and indicates the phenotypic plasticity of cells (i.e., they can move from one state to the other).

Effects of EMT on cells and tissues

Cellular (phenotypic) changes in epithelial cells during EMT (Box 8): The normal and pathological versions of the EMT involve (i) changes in shape, (ii) gain of motility, and (iii) alterations in the gene expression profiles of cells. The transition of epithelial carcinoma cells to mesenchymal phenotype provides migratory, invasive, and stem-like properties.

The EMT process involves many changes in the cell. These include the activation of specific transcription factors, changes in expression and reorganization of cytoskeleton proteins (intermediate filaments), loss of adherens junctions with conversion of a morphology of polygonal/epithelial to a spindly/fibroblastic morphology, increased motility, heightened resistance to apoptosis, production of ECM-degrading proteins, and display of integrins and growth factor receptors on the surface of cells.

Expression of E-cadherin and cytokeratins are characteristics of epithelial cell protein and is lost in EMT, whereas the expression of **vimentin** (an intermediate filament component of the mesenchymal cell cytoskeleton) is induced. Epithelial cells that have undergone an EMT usually secrete fibronectin (an extracellular matrix protein) that is normally secreted only by mesenchymal cells such as fibroblasts. There will be N-cadherin expression (typical fibroblastic marker) and loss of E-cadherin.

Role of E-cadherin E-cadherin is a transmembrane molecule that plays the main role in influencing epithelial versus mesenchymal cell phenotypes. E-cadherin is necessary for adhesion of epithelial cells to one another. In normal epithelia, the extracellular domain of E-cadherin molecules on cell membrane of one epithelial cell form complexes with other E-cadherin molecules on the surface of an adjacent epithelial cell. This homodimeric (and higher-order) bridging between adjacent cells in an epithelial cell layer forms the adherens junctions. These are important for the structural integrity of epithelial cell sheets. The cytoplasmic domains of E-cadherin molecules are attached to the actin fibers of the cytoskeleton via a complex of α- and β-catenins and other ancillary proteins.

Box 8: Cellular changes associated with an epithelial–mesenchymal transition.

Loss of

- Attachment of epithelial adherens junctions involving E-cadherin (loss of cell to cell adhesion/intercellular junctions/tight junctions)
- Cell to basement membrane attachment (loss of epithelial cell polarity)
- Lose epithelial markers: E-cadherin, cytokeratin (intermediate filament) expression
- Epithelial gene expression program

Gain (acquisition) of

- Fibroblast-like shape
- Migratory properties (motility)
- Invasiveness
- Increased resistance to apoptosis
- Mesenchymal gene expression program including EMT-inducing transcription factors
- Mesenchymal markers: Mesenchymal adherens junction protein (N-cadherin), vimentin (intermediate filament) expression, fibronectin secretion
- Protease secretion (MMP-2, MMP-9)
- PDGF receptor expression
- αvβ6 integrin expression
- Stem cell-like traits

The actin cytoskeleton gives tensile strength to the cell. Thus, E-cadherin help an epithelial cell sheet to withstand mechanical forces that try to separate the cells. Once E-cadherin expression is lost, cells acquire a mesenchymal morphology and increased motility.

Role of N-cadherin in EMT N-cadherin binds to other molecules of the same type displayed by nearby cells. N-cadherin molecules are normally expressed by stromal cells and are not expressed by epithelial cells. N-cadherin can be expression on the surface of a carcinoma cell that has undergone an EMT. This increases the affinity of this cancer cell for the stromal cells with N-cadherin, main being the fibroblasts in the stroma found below the epithelial cell layer. This binding assist the invading carcinoma cells to insert themselves between stromal cell populations. The bonds formed between N-cadherin molecules are weaker than those formed by E-cadherin homodimers. This poor binding favors motility of cell.

Induction of EMT: Contribution of the Tumor Micro-environment

Epithelial–mesenchymal transition is most often observed at the invasive front of tumors and enhance tumor invasion. EMT in carcinoma cells can be initiated by a many intra- and extracellular signals. These include growth factors, inflammatory cytokines, oncogenes, and enhanced NF-κB signaling. Execution of an EMT program depends on changes in the expression of many genes.

Triggering factors: Many factors contribute to EMT, but probably diverse stimuli can trigger it.

- **Hypoxia:** Most important factor that triggers EMT is hypoxia. The diffusion of glucose and oxygen are limited to 100–150 μ and in situ tumors (e.g., comedo-type of intraductal carcinomas of breast) may show central area of necrosis. Hypoxia induces HIF-1α which in turn regulates many genes. Examples of these are the proteases, matrix metalloproteinases (MMP1 and MMP2), and lysyl oxidase (LOX). MMP2 degrades basement membrane, and MMP1 and LOX digest ECM and provide the path for the migration of tumor cell. EMT is also associated with expanded stem-like and tumor initiation properties.

- **Autophagy:** It is an important mediator in cancer progression. Autophagy has been shown to induce EMT in some cancers, such as hepatocellular carcinoma.
- **TGF-β:** It is a potent inducer and major regulator of EMT. During EMT induction, TGF-β signaling regulates the expression and activity of several EMT transcription factors (discussed below).

Epithelial to mesenchymal transition regulators

EMT-inducing transcription factors (EMT-TFs): EMTs are programmed (orchestrated) by activation of a series of transcription factors (TFs-these are also involved in embryogenesis). They promote a mesenchymal phenotype during cancer initiation and progression.

There are many genes involved in EMT-inducing transcription factors (EMT-TFs). The transcription factors encoded by these genes include Slug, Snail, Twist and ZEB1/2. These genes are involved in cell mobility during embryogenesis. These transcription factors are reactivated in cancer to modify adult epithelial cells to their mesenchymal embryonic forbearers. These transcriptional factors are induced in various combinations in a number of malignant tumor types. Some of these EMT-TFs are important for programming invasion and others to elicit metastasis.

- **Snail (Snail and Slug) and Twist:** One of the main hallmarks of EMT is down regulation of E-cadherin (that is involved in binding of epithelial cells to each other and suppresses motility). It occurs during the tumor progression process via transcriptional repression. **The** *CDH1* (E-cadherin) gene **is downregulated mainly by two tr**anscriptional repressors namely **Snail** (Snail and Slug) **and Twist**. Snail is a zinc-finger containing transcriptional repressor and Slug (also known as Snail2) were detected at sites of EMT. They release neoplastic epithelial cells from this key suppressor of motility and invasiveness. Loss of E-cadherin causes loosening of epithelial cells so that they can invade and released proteases clear the way for invasion. Apart from down regulation of E-cadherin, they also regulate other epithelial markers and induce mesenchymal genes. Snail is expressed in high grade human breast carcinoma tissues and lymph node positive tumors and overexpression of Snail is associated with decreased relapse-free survival.
- **Twist and ZEB families (ZEB1/ZEB2) transcription factors:** They **downregulate the antiproliferative proteins** p16INK4a and p21CIP1. ZEB1 and ZEB2 are zinc-finger-containing transcription factors that promote EMT. ZEB transcription factors also activate expression of MMP family members (particularly MMP2). This promotes the invasive phenotype.
- **Changes produced by EMT-TFs:** These include the organization of a cell's cytoskeleton. These are involved in the processes of invasion and metastasis.

Role of stromal cells in EMT induction in tumors

Tumor cells and the associated stroma (**Fig. 65**) have dynamic and reciprocal interactions throughout the cancer process (from initiation-progression-metastasis, to resistance and recurrence). Stromal cells include fibroblasts, adipocytes, endothelial cells, and myeloid and lymphoid immune cells. All stromal cells can induce EMT in carcinoma cells via secretion of growth factors, inflammatory cytokines, or proteases.

Macrophages: Macrophages are important cell type in the tumor microenvironment. Tumor-associated macrophages (TAMs) can induce inflammation, angiogenesis, intra- and extravasation, tumor growth, progression and EMT, through production of growth factors and inflammatory cytokines. Macrophages can also regulate the tumor microenvironment through the expression of proteases at the tumor periphery (e.g., matrix-degrading enzymes such as matrix metalloproteinases and cysteine, cathepsins, and urokinase plasminogen activator), LOXs and SPARC (secreted protein acidic and rich in cysteine).

CD8⁺ T cells Other immune cells can also activate EMT. For example, CD8⁺ T cells play a role in immunoediting and the promotion of EMT. Immunoediting (refer page 496) is the process by which the immune system has both host protective and tumor-promoting functions. EMT may be one mechanism involved in immunoediting in cancer.

Carcinoma-associated fibroblasts and endothelial cells

- **Carcinoma-associated fibroblasts (CAFs):** They are frequently present in the stroma. They may promote tumor progression. Resident fibroblasts in the stroma can differentiation into CAFs. During this differentiation,

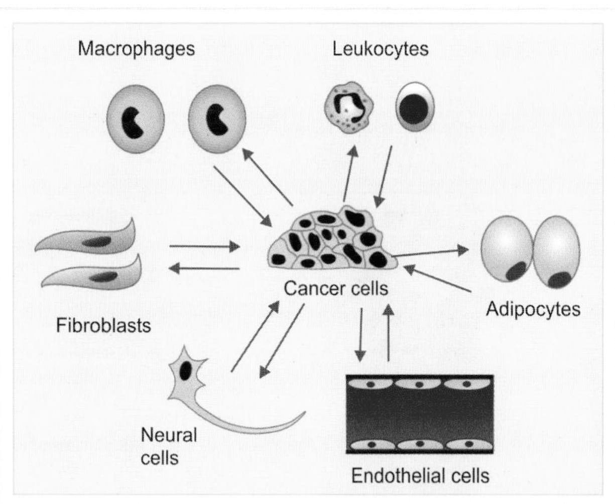

FIG. 65: Stromal cells involved in the cancer cell ecosystem. The developing tumor cells interact with the nonmalignant stromal cells in their environment, via secretion of soluble growth factors, inflammatory cytokines, proteases or other mediators.

stromal fibroblast develop two autocrine signaling loops, mediated by TGF-β and stromal cell-derived factor-1 (SDF-1). Probably CAFs promote tumor activity via inducing EMT by TGF-β produced in the tumor microenvironment.

- **Endothelial cells:** They also induce EMT, by shifting expression from E-cadherin to N-cadherin. This increases migratory properties in carcinoma cells and also responsible for the acquisition of stem cell-like properties.

Reversibility of Epithelial-mesenchymal Transition (Fig. 66) **Plasticity in the invasive growth program:** EMT is induced at the cancer cells of the invasive front of primary tumor EMT is induced by activated stroma and the EMT-inducing signals. The carcinoma cells then proceed with the multiple steps of invasion and disseminate from a primary tumor to distant tissue sites (metastasis). In the metastatic (distant) site, the EMT-inducing signals may no longer present in the cancer cells. In the absence of these signals, carcinoma cells in their new tissue environment (at the distant site) may revert to a more epithelial, noninvasive state. Thus, carcinoma cells after invasion and metastatic dissemination may reverse by passing through the process called MET.

Mesenchymal–epithelial transition (MET)

Epithelial-mesenchymal transition (EMT) is associated with the invasive migratory phenotype in cancer cells. This helps in dissemination of tumor. MET is the reverse process important for colonization of disseminated tumor cells in many cancers. MET transforms motile, nonpolarized mesenchymal cells into nonmotile, polarized epithelial cells. During MET, there is a decrease in mesenchymal markers (e.g., N-cadherin and vimentin) and increase in the epithelial markers (e.g., E-cadherin). EMT is needed for dissemination of tumor cells from the primary tumor, whereas MET is required for the proliferation of the disseminated cancer cell and formation of the secondary tumor.

Thus, both EMT and MET are main events that decide the extent of carcinoma metastasis.

The knowledge about direct role of MET on carcinoma metastasis, may be used for therapeutic targeting the MET process to inhibit formation of a metastatic tumor.

Clinical implications of EMT

Present technologies can analyze epithelial and mesenchymal markers in circulating tumor cells (CTCs). CTCs in the blood are useful disease monitoring or for therapeutic approaches (discussed in detail on pages 564 and 565). Analysis of CTCs can give valuable information regarding the disease state. EMT is associated with the cancer stem cell phenotype and tumor dissemination. EMT status in CTCs can be used as a surrogate biomarker for monitoring therapeutic responses.

Chemoresistance: EMT is associated with resistant phenotype and chemoresistance in many cancer types. These may provide novel therapeutic strategies for treating cancer.

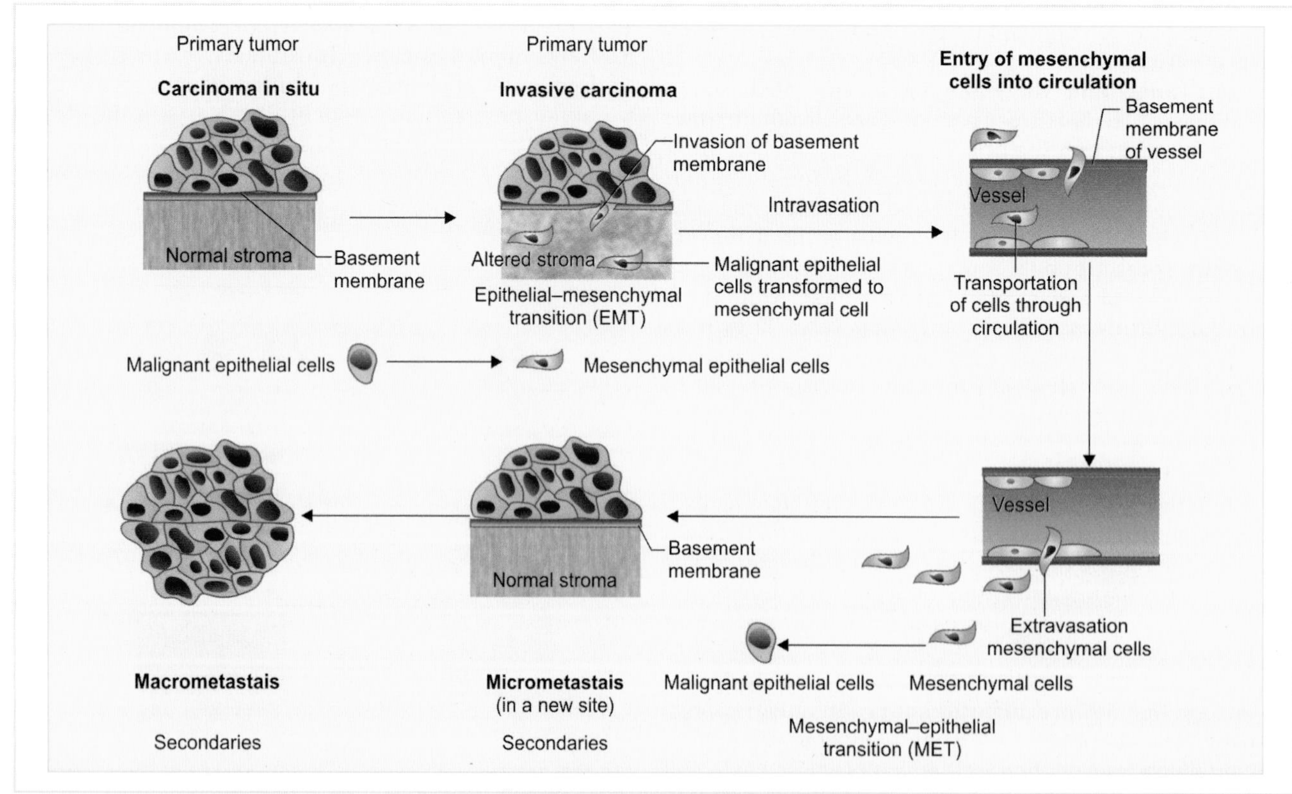

FIG. 66: Reversibility of EMT. Epithelial cancer cells at the invasive edge of a primary carcinoma (pink/brown cells) usually undergo EMT as they invade the stroma and become mesenchymal (red cells). This mesenchymal state of the carcinoma cells allows them to invade locally, intravasate, and subsequently to extravasate into the parenchyma of a distant, seemingly normal tissue. The metastases from these cancer cells revert back to an epithelial phenotype (pink/brown cells) via a mesenchymal–epithelial transition (MET). They may show microscopic features typical of the cells at the center of the primary tumor.

Inhibition of EMT: EMT is involved in tumor progression, metastasis, and chemoresistance. Hence, targeting EMT by EMT inhibitors (EMT-blocking drugs) can be used as an important therapeutic approach for cancer patients.

Hallmark 7: Deregulating Cellular Energetic and Metabolism

All cells should perform several extremely important activities. These include generation of energy; production and repair DNA, RNA, cell membrane, and other lipids, and proteins, etc. These activities depend on the type of cell. Let us review a few basic concepts of cell metabolism.

Normal Cell Metabolism Favors ATP Generation

Metabolism is the sum of all chemical reactions that occur within a cell through which energy is produced. Cells need energy for maintaining metabolic functions, growth and division. Normal cells utilize glucose as their main source to produce adenosine triphosphate (ATP) and to synthesize macromolecules. Glucose enters cells via transporters, main being GLUT1 (glucose transporter). There are two major metabolic pathways of production of energy from glucose.

- **Aerobic respiration** (oxidative phosphorylation): Aerobic respiration is a complex energy-generating process. Under aerobic conditions, normal cells process glucose, first to pyruvate via glycolysis in the cytosol. This is followed by complete oxidation of pyruvate to carbon dioxide (CO_2) and water (H_2O) by oxidative phosphorylation in the mitochondria. Energy yield of aerobic respiration is much higher (36 ATPs) than lactic fermentation (anaerobic glycolysis) but it can only occur in the presence of O_2.
- **Anaerobic glycolysis or lactic fermentation:** Lactic fermentation occurs exclusively in the cytosol in the absence or low oxygen conditions (e.g., intense exercise). Glycolysis is one of the most important pathways for extracting energy from glucose. Glycolysis occurs in the cytosol and does not use oxygen in its reactions, and hence it is called anaerobic. Under anaerobic conditions, glucose is first converted to pyruvate through glycolysis and relatively little pyruvate is dispatched to the oxygen-consuming mitochondria. Then the pyruvate is reduced to lactate, which is released to the bloodstream. This process produces two molecules of intracellular energy-transporting molecules, namely ATP per glucose molecule.

Differences between anaerobic glycolysis, and aerobic glycolysis (Warburg effect) are presented in **Figures 67A and B**. Basic metabolism reactions in cells are depicted in **Figure 68**.

Growth-promoting Metabolic Alterations (Warburg Effect)

Q. Discuss Warburg effect.

Aerobic glycolysis in rapidly dividing (proliferating) cells

In actively dividing normal cells, only a small portion of the cellular glucose passes through the oxidative phosphorylation pathway in mitochondria. This will produce about four molecules of ATP per each molecule of glucose. There is mainly aerobic fermentation of glucose (aerobic glycolysis) and this is needed for growth of cells. Thus, growing cells do not depend on mitochondrial metabolism. Major function of mitochondria in growing cells is not to generate ATP, but rather to generate

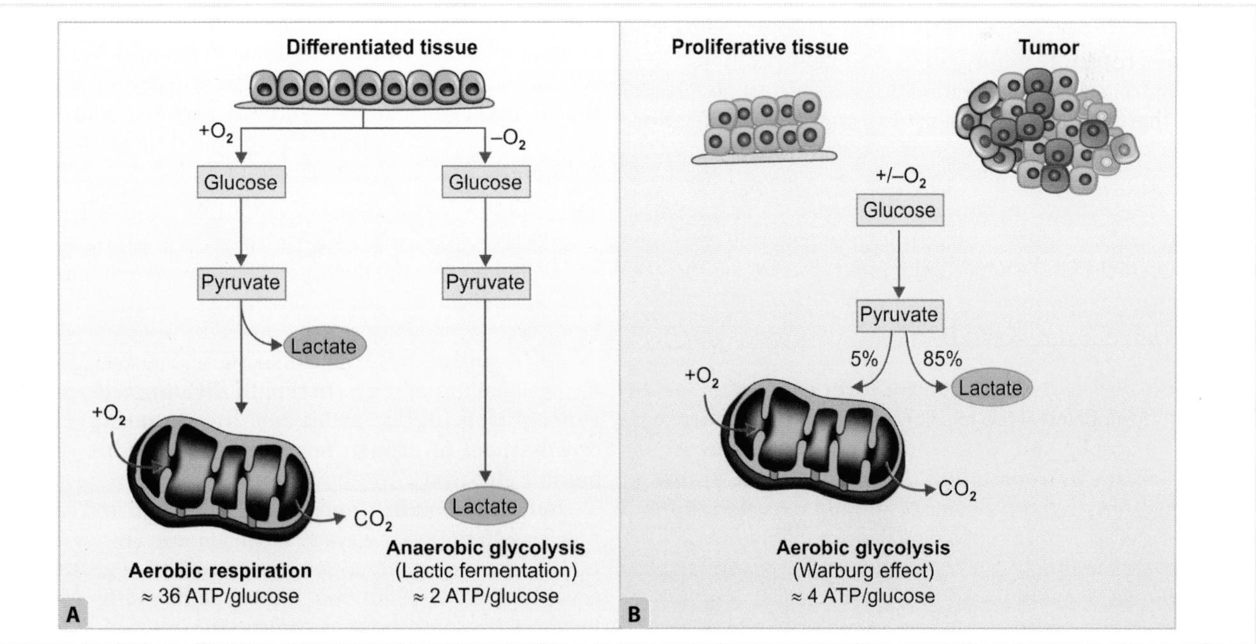

(ATP: adenosine triphosphate)

FIGS. 67A AND B: Differences between anaerobic glycolysis, and aerobic glycolysis (Warburg effect). (A) In the presence of oxygen (oxidative phosphorylation), in nonproliferating tissues, glucose is converted to pyruvate via glycolysis. Pyruvate is then completely oxidized in the mitochondria to CO_2. When oxygen availability is limited, cells can redirect the pyruvate away from mitochondria and generate lactate (anaerobic glycolysis). (B) In cancer, the cells tend to convert most glucose to lactate regardless of the oxygen availability (aerobic glycolysis called as Warburg effect).

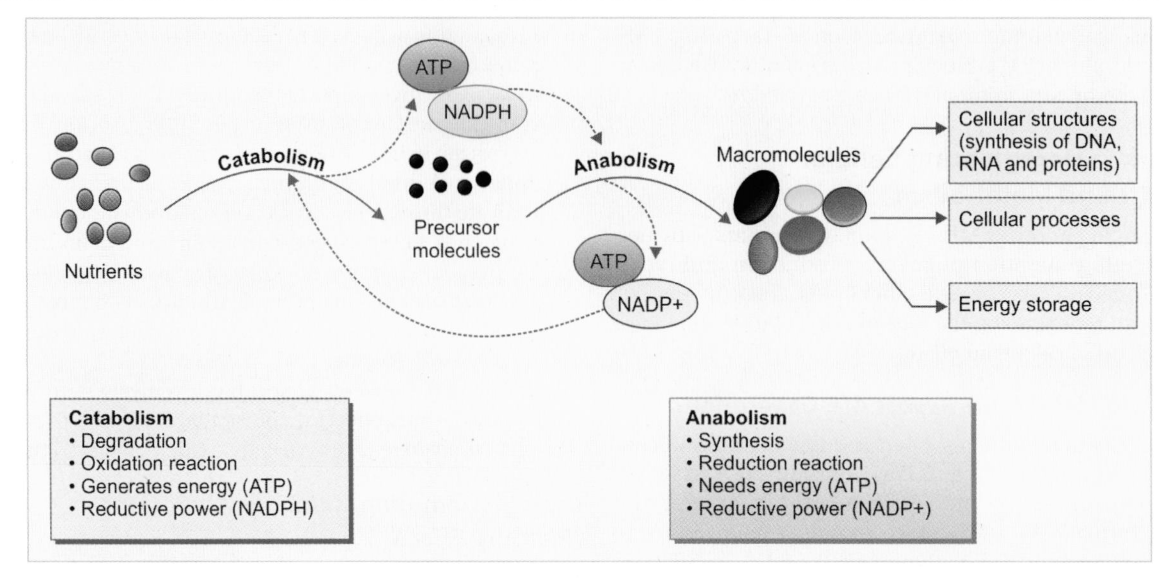

(ATP: adenosine triphosphate; DNA: deoxyribonucleic acid; NADP+: nicotinamide adenine dinucleotide phosphate; NADPH: reduced nicotinamide adenine dinucleotide phosphate; RNA: ribonucleic acid)

FIG. 68: Basic metabolism reactions. Metabolism consists of two major parts—anabolism and catabolism. Catabolism is the metabolic process of breakdown of large complex molecules that generates energy, precursor molecules (building locks). Anabolism is the metabolic process of synthesis of complex molecules and reductive power by which macromolecules are produced.

metabolic intermediates that are used in the synthesis of cellular building blocks. For example, biosynthesis of lipid needs acetyl-Coenzyme A (acetyl-CoA), and acetyl-CoA is mainly produced in growing cells from intermediates such as citrate that are produced in mitochondria. In rapidly dividing normal cells, aerobic glycolysis ceases when the tissue is no longer growing.

Metabolic reprogramming in cancer cells

The uncontrolled cell proliferation is the essence of neoplastic disease. There is not only deregulated control of cell proliferation but also corresponding adjustments of energy metabolism in order to support cell growth and division. Cancer cells have different needs than their normal counterpart and reprogram their metabolism. Their proliferative rate generally exceeds that of normal cells. Cancer cells must quickly synthesize the structural components (e.g., protein, lipid, etc.) that are required for rapid cell growth (that is to sustain their mitotic activity).

Cancer cells show **a distinctive form of cellular metabolism.** It is **characterized by increased amount** (enhanced) **of glucose uptake and increased conversion of glucose to lactose/lactate (fermentation)** via **the glycolytic pathway** (glycolysis) **even in the presence of abundant oxygen supply**. This energy source is for supporting their proliferation. Cancer cells rely on seemingly inefficient glycolysis (generates two molecules of ATP per molecule of glucose) instead of oxidative phosphorylation (generates up to 36 molecules of ATP per molecule of glucose). This process is known as **aerobic glycolysis or Warburg effect.** Growing or rapidly dividing normal cells also show this Warburg effect (refer above). **Warburg effect** was initially **observed by Otto Warburg** (received the Nobel Prize in 1931 for this discovery). He also observed that highly proliferating cells are mainly glycolytic and are heavily dependent on glucose. They usually take up more glucose from outside than do normal cells.

***Biomolecular Biosynthesis*:** The proliferating cells must duplicate its genome, proteins, and lipids, and assemble the components into daughter cells, i.e., they require biosynthesis of biomolecules. The two main extracellular nutrients that support survival and biosynthesis in cells are glucose and glutamine. Proliferating cells must first transform acquired nutrients into different structural intermediates (biosynthetic precursors). Then the biosynthetic precursors produce de novo important biomolecules such as, fatty acids, cholesterol, nucleotides, and nonessential amino acids.

***Metabolic Reprogramming (Fig. 69)*:** Normally, glucose is highly available in the nutrient-rich plasma and the extracellular fluid. But healthy cells cannot import nutrients as they like and glucose intake does not depend on the immediate bioenergetic needs of a cell. Instead importing glucose is strictly regulated by extracellular signals that trigger growth factor signaling pathways. **In rapidly dividing cells, metabolic reprogramming is produced by signaling cascades downstream of growth factor receptors. This results in aerobic glycolysis.**

Cancer cells suffer from glucose addiction and to survive, they should find new ways to make glucose always available. In cancers, the signaling cascade/**pathways of growth factor receptors are deregulated. This is achieved by mutations in oncogenes and tumors suppressor genes** that influence growth signaling steps and get activated. These oncogenic mutations involving growth factor signaling pathways and other key factors such as MYC, facilitate import of glucose to cancer cells from external requirements to a significant degree of independence. In rapidly dividing normal cells, aerobic glycolysis stops when the tissue is no longer growing. In

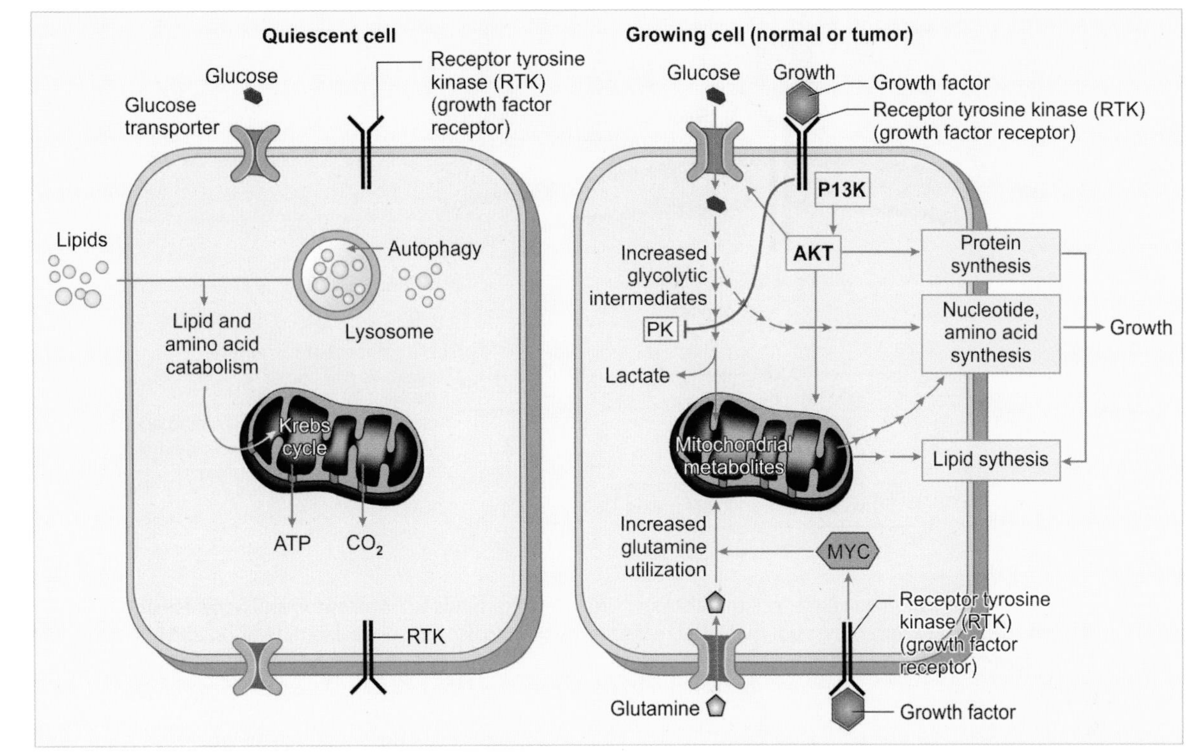

(ATP: adenosine triphosphate; RTK: receptor tyrosine kinase)

FIG. 69: Metabolism and cell growth. (A) Quiescent cells depend mainly on adenosine triphosphate (ATP) produced by Krebs cycle. If starved, it induces autophagy (self-eating) to provide a source of fuel. (B) When stimulated by growth factors, normal cells markedly upregulate uptake of two important nutrients namely, glucose and glutamine. These nutrients provide carbon sources for synthesis of nucleotides, proteins, and lipids. In cancers, oncogenic mutations involving growth factor signaling pathways and other factors such as MYC, deregulate the metabolic pathways. It is termed as the *Warburg effect.*

contrast, in cancer cells this reprogramming continues due to the action of oncogenes and the loss of function of TSG. There is usually crosstalk between progrowth signaling factors and cellular metabolism. These include the following:

- **Growth factor receptor signaling:** Growth factor receptors, after interacting with growth factor, transmit growth signals to the nucleus. Apart from proliferation of cells, signals from growth factor receptors also influence metabolism. One of the growth factors signaling pathways is RTK (receptor tyrosine kinase) and is a master regulator of glucose intake. PI3K/AKT pathway lies downstream the RTK pathway. Mutations that lead to the activation of PI3K/AKT pathway (**Fig. 69B and 68**) bring out many (cell survival, proliferation and mTOR) downstream responses. The most important is mTOR. The **mTOR activation (Figs. 70 and 71)** in conjugation with K-Ras and Myc activation leads to the increased synthesis of glycolytic intermediates. The **mTOR** increases the GLUT1 glucose transporter (increase the uptake of glucose), increases synthesis of lipids. It also increases the activity of cell membrane amino acid (AA) transporters so that increased amino acids are available to synthesize protein needs of cancer cells. Receptor tyrosine kinases also phosphorylate and inhibit pyruvate kinase. This catalyzes the the conversion of phosphoenolpyruvate to pyruvate (last step in the glycolytic pathway). This leads to the buildup of upstream glycolytic intermediates. These macromolecules are used for synthesis of DNA, RNA, and protein.
- **RAS signaling (Fig. 69):** AKT signaling is necessary for glucose uptake when there is proliferation of cells but is not alone that facilitate the access to glucose. *Ras* genes are the most common oncogenes in human cancer. Downstream signals of RAS upregulate the activity of glucose transporters (GLUT1) and multiple glycolytic enzymes. This causes increased cellular glucose consumption (glycolysis) and promotes production of mitochondrial intermediates. These, in turn, lead to biosynthesis of lipid and protein. The hypoxia response system within many tumors also upregulates glucose transporters and multiple enzymes of the glycolytic pathway. Thus, both the Ras oncoprotein and hypoxia can independently increase the levels of the HIF 1α which in turn upregulate glycolysis.
- **MYC (Fig. 69):** Progrowth pathways upregulate expression of the transcription factor MYC. This causes changes in gene expression that support anabolic metabolism and cell growth. Examples of the MYC-regulated genes include many glycolytic enzymes and glutaminase. The enzyme glutaminase is needed for mitochondrial utilization of glutamine. Glutamine is the main source of carbon moieties required for biosynthesis of cellular building blocks.

Cancer cells become highly adaptive and utilize both aerobic glycolysis and mitochondrial oxidative phosphory-

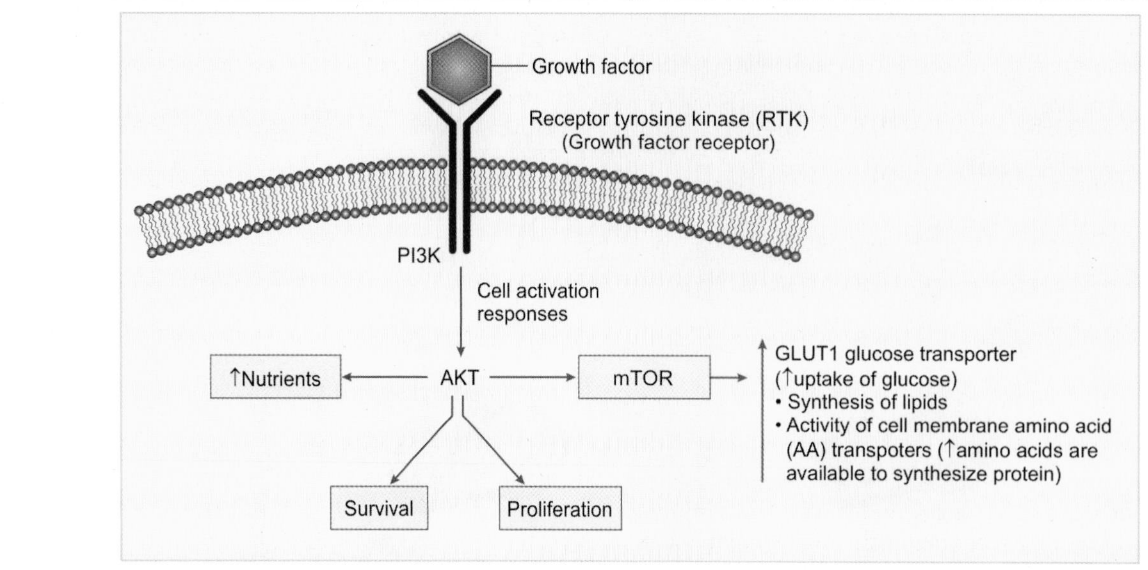

FIG. 70: Effects of metabolic activation on cancer cell metabolism. Growth factor binds to its receptor, and activates phosphatidylinositol 3 kinase (PI3K)/AKT pathway. AKT in turn brings out many [increased entry of glucose, cell survival, proliferation and mammalian target of rapamycin (mTOR)] downstream responses and most important is mTOR.

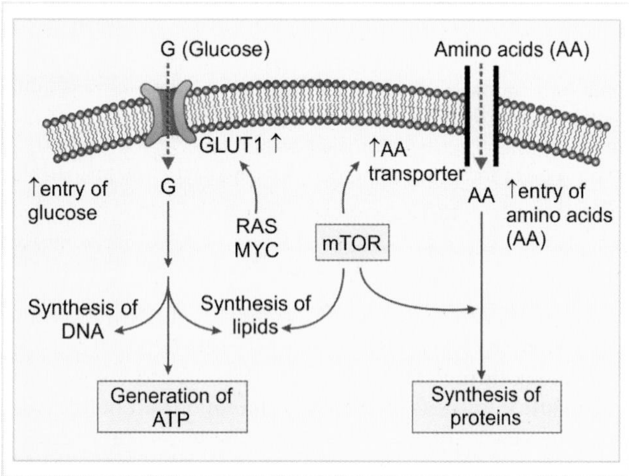

(ATP: adenosine triphosphate; GLUT1: glucose transporter 1)

FIG. 71: Consequences of mammalian target of rapamycin (mTOR) activation in cancer cell metabolism. The mTOR in conjugation with K-Ras and Myc activation leads to the increased synthesis of glycolytic intermediates. The mTOR increases the GLUT1 glucose transporter (increase the uptake of glucose), increases synthesis of lipids/glycolytic intermediates, also synthesizes deoxyribonucleic acid (DNA). mTOR also increases the activity of cell membrane amino acid (AA) transporters so that increased amino acids are available to synthesize protein needs of cancer cells.

lation in varying proportions to generate fuel (ATP) and the biosynthetic precursors needed for proliferation of cells.

Glutamine is the most abundant free amino acid found in serum. It serves as the main way of transport of reduced nitrogen between cells. It is needed for the biosynthesis of nucleotides of nucleic acids. Tumor progression and proliferation is extremely dependent on glutamine.

Advantages of aerobic glycolysis to cancer cells

Aerobic glycolysis allows the **diversion of glycolytic metabolic intermediates** into various biosynthetic pathways **that are needed for the synthesis of cellular components** (e.g., nucleosides and amino acids) **in rapidly dividing tumor cells.** This cannot be met with normal mitochondrial oxidative phosphorylation. Growing cell must duplicate all of its cellular components such as DNA, RNA, proteins, lipid, and organelles, before it can divide and produce two daughter cells. Though oxidative phosphorylation can produce abundant ATP, it cannot produce any carbon moieties that can be used to build the cellular components needed for growth (e.g., proteins, lipids, and nucleic acids). Increased glycolysis diverts glycolytic intermediates into various biosynthetic pathways. These include generation of nucleosides and amino acids. In turn, these are used in the biosynthesis of the macromolecules and organelles needed for assembling new cells.

- Glycolysis-dependent energy production is also associated with **activation of oncogenes** like *MYC* and *RAS* and **mutation of tumor suppressors** (e.g., *TP53).*

Clinical utility

The "glucose-hunger" of tumors is made of use for visualization of tumors in **positron emission tomography (PET) scanning.** Deoxyglucose is an analog of glucose that is transported into the cell by glucose transporters (GLUT1). GLUT1 are highly produced in cancer cells. Deoxyglucose is not metabolized in the glycolytic pathway, so it accumulates. In PET scanning, patients are most commonly injected with positron-emitting radionuclide namely, ^{18}F-fluorodeoxyglucose (18-FDG/ fluorine-18). This is a glucose derivative that is preferentially taken up into tumor cells (also by normal, actively dividing tissues such as the bone marrow) and allows it to be visualized. The increased uptake of 18-FDG indirectly measures the glucose uptake by cancer as well as healthy proliferating cells. Hence, it is used as an imaging biomarker for glucose metabolism. Most tumors are PET-positive, and it is more marked in rapidly growing tumors. So, if a patient has cancer cells spread over the body, the different metastatic foci can be detected and it correlates with a poor prognosis. The 18-FDG-PET signal intensity in tumors correlates closely with the level of PI3K/AKT pathway activity; and PI3K and RTK inhibitors will reduce it.

Rapidly proliferating normal cells (e.g., embryonic tissues and lymphocytes during immune responses) also rely on aerobic fermentation. Thus, "Warburg metabolism" is not specific to cancer, but it is a general property of growing cells that becomes "fixed" in cancer cells.

Inhibition of metabolic pathways that promote growth

We have seen factors that reprogram the metabolism in tumor cells that promote growth. Tumor suppressors usually inhibit metabolic pathways that support growth. Tumor suppressors such as NF1 and PTEN oppose the Warburg effect. Probably, many (and perhaps all) tumor suppressors induce growth arrest by suppressing the Warburg effect. For example, the most important tumor suppressor namely p53, upregulates target genes that inhibit glucose uptake, glycolysis, lipogenesis, and the production of reduced nicotinamide adenine dinucleotide phosphate (NADPH) (main cofactor required for the biosynthesis of macromolecules). Thus, the functions of many oncoproteins and tumor suppressors are definitely closely linked with cellular metabolism.

Apart from the Warburg effect, there are two other links between metabolism and cancer. These are—(i) autophagy and (ii) oncometabolites.

Autophagy

Another program, termed autophagy, is a survival system which may be operative in carcinogenesis. **Autophagy ("self-eating") is the process in which lysosomal enzymes digest the own components of the cell** during stress (e.g., starvation). It serves as a recycling system for cellular organelles that normally helps cells respond to conditions of nutrient deprivation by degrading cellular organelles. Thus, it is a survival mechanism which occurs during a **state of severe nutrient deficiency.** Autophagy generates the metabolites and nutrients that cells are unable to acquire from their surroundings. **During this process, cells arrest their growth. By this mechanism**, the starved cell can live by eating its own contents (e.g., **organelles, proteins, and membranes)** and by recycling these contents to provide nutrients and energy. However, when there is extreme nutrient deprivation, this adaptive mechanism fails. This can lead to hyperactivation of autophagy in the cancer cells and results in autophagic cell death.

Autophagy in cancer

Role of autophagy in the development and progression of cancer is complex and represents a double-edged sword. Autophagy may be useful to tumors that experience episodic depletion of energy and metabolic substrates. Several autophagy genes (e.g., *Beclin-1* and some *Atg* genes) that promote autophagy, act as tumor suppressors and are deleted or mutated in many cancers. Tumor cells may accumulate mutations which derange the pathways that induce autophagy and allow the cancer cells to grow without triggering autophagy. Tumor cells may corrupt the autophagy process to provide nutrients for continued growth and survival. On the other hand, when tumor is under severe nutrient deprivation or oxygen because of therapy or insufficient blood supply, tumor cells may use autophagy to become "dormant" and survive hard times for long periods. Such cells can be resistant to therapies that kill actively dividing cells, and may be responsible for therapeutic failures. Discussed in detail on pages 505–508.

Oncometabolism

Another new mechanism of oncogenesis is mutations in enzymes that participate in the Krebs cycle and is called as *oncometabolism*. One of them being mutations in enzyme isocitrate dehydrogenase (IDH).

Isocitrate dehydrogenase

Role of Isocitrate Dehydrogenase: It is a critical metabolic enzyme **involved in Krebs cycle** [citric acid cycle (CAC) or tricarboxylic acid cycle (TCA)]. The IDH is a potent tumor suppressor and WT IDHs are critical regulators of organ physiology. IDH exists in three isoforms, namely IDH1, IDH2, and IDH 3. IDH1 localizes to both cytosol and the peroxisomes, whereas IDH2 and IDH3, as part of the TCA cycle, are found within the mitochondrial matrix. There is broad involvement of IDHs in the homeostasis of healthy tissue and, when deregulated, in the development of disease.

Citric Acid Cycle: It is the final common pathway for the oxidation of carbohydrate, lipid, and protein. The citric acid cycle provides the main pathway for ATP formation. In citric acid cycle, IDH catalyzes the conversion of isocitrate (ICT) to α-ketoglutarate (αKG). Through production of αKG, IDH promotes the activity of αKG-dependent dioxygenases that epigenetically control gene expression. The αKG-dependent dioxygenases enzymes catalyze many biochemical processes and reactions, resulting in the chemical modification of DNA, RNA, protein, and lipids.

Mutations in IDH and Its Consequences: The steps in the oncogenic pathway involving IDH (**Fig. 72**) are as follows:

- **Mutation in IDH:** Acquired oncogenic mutation in IDH leads to a specific amino acid substitution involving residues in the active site of the enzyme. It results in production of large amounts of a new mutated protein (oncoprotein).
  - Mutated IDH has reduced binding affinity to ICT and loses its ability to function as an IDH. This prevents the normal conversion of ICT to α-ketoglutarate (αKG) by intact (WT) IDH.
  - Instead, it acquires a new enzymatic activity in which αKG is reduced to (*R*)-2-hydroxyglutarate [(*R*)-2HG **or 2-hydroxyglutarate** (2-HG)]. The **(R)-2-hydroxglutarate is an oncometabolite** which is produced at high levels when there is IDH mutation. This results in universal hypermethylation phenotype and malignancy.
- **Inhibition of enzymes of TET family:** (R)-2-hydroxglutarate in turn inhibits α-ketoglutarate-dependent dioxygenase function. (R)-2-HG also acts as an inhibitor of several other enzymes that are members of the ten-eleven translocation methylcytosine dioxygenase (*TET*) family (one of them is TET2).
- **Loss of TET2 activity:** DNA methylation is an epigenetic modification that controls normal gene expression. TET2

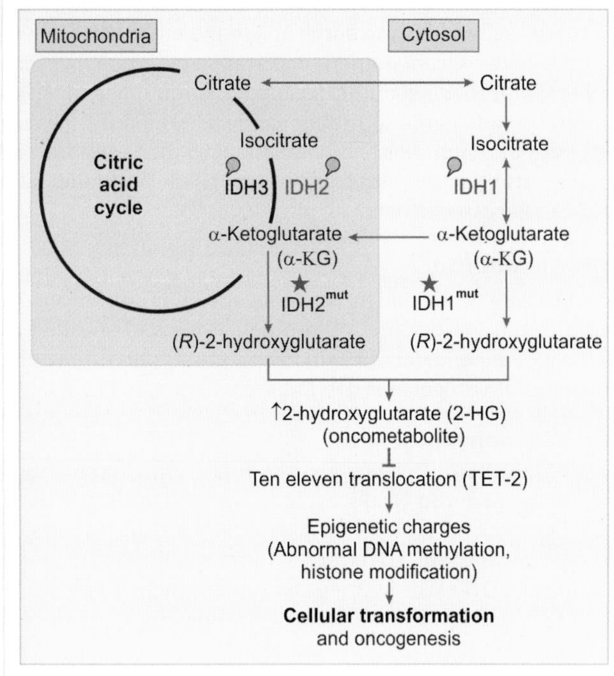

(IDH: isocitrate dehydrogenase)

FIG. 72: Mutated isocitrate dehydrogenase (IDHmut) produces oncometabolite 2-hydroxyglutarate (2-HG). Through epigenetic changes this produces cancer.

is one of the factors that regulate DNA methylation. Loss of TET2 activity leads to abnormal DNA methylation and TET2-related histone demethylation. Inactivating mutations in TET2 usually occur in acute myeloid leukemia (AML), myelodysplastic syndrome (MDS), MPNs, and chronic myelomonocytic leukemia (CMML).

- **Altered gene expression:** Abnormal DNA methylation in turn leads to abnormal expression of some unknown cancer genes, which drive cellular transformation and oncogenesis.
- Transcriptionally induced or downregulated IDH contribute to cancer and neurodegeneration, respectively.
- Cancer-associated mutations in IDH1 and IDH2 are one of the most studied mechanisms of pathological effects of IDH. Oncogenic IDH mutations have been found in many cancers. Examples include gliomas, cholangiocarcinomas, AML, MDS, chondrosarcoma sarcomas, angioimmunoblastic T-cell lymphoma, thyroid carcinomas, and unique subtype of breast cancer known as solid papillary carcinoma with reverse polarity. IDH mutations also contribute to the pathogenesis of skeletal disorders (e.g., Ollier disease and Maffucci syndrome).

***Clinical significance*:** Mutated IDH proteins have an altered structure. Hence, it has ignited drug development efforts to pharmacologically target mutant enzymes that inhibit mutated IDH. These drugs are used to treat leukemias with IDH mutations.

Hallmark 8: Avoiding Immune Destruction

Q. Discuss host defense against tumors.
Q. Discuss tumor immunology.

Normal immune system distinguishes self from nonself molecules and is very effective against infectious agents. Paul Ehrlich (1909) first put forward a hypothesis that tumor cells can be recognized as "foreign" and destroy them by the immune system. Subsequently, Lewis Thomas and Macfarlane Burnet (1957) further developed this concept by coining the term *immune surveillance.* This theory proposed that cells and tissues are constantly monitored ("scanned") by a vigilant immune system for emerging malignant cells. Immunosurveillance is responsible for recognizing and destroying the majority of incipient cancer cells. Probably protective immunologic responses may be elicited against unique "tumor-specific antigens".

William Coley (1891) was a surgeon known as **father of immunotherapy** who supported the immunosurveillance hypothesis. Coley noticed that in some cancer patients who got infections after surgery, their tumors regressed more efficiently than patients who did not get infections. He proposed that infection had stimulated the body's "resisting powers". This concept of immune surveillance was supported by many observations (**Box 9**).

Principles Involved in Immune Reactions in Cancer

Several factors may control the outcome of interactions between tumor cells and the host immune system. The basic principles involved are as follows:

- **Expression of antigens by cancer cells:** Cancer cells express a range of antigens that stimulate the host immune system. These antigens may play an important role in preventing the development of cancers.
- **Immune response is ineffective:** Though the antigens expressed by cancer cells can elicit an immune response, it may be ineffective against established tumors. In fact, in some tumors, immune response may actually promote growth of cancer. This may be due to acquired changes in cancer cells which make them escape from antitumor responses and may encourage protumor responses.
- **Effective of new immunotherapies:** By understanding the mechanisms of immune evasion and "immuno-manipulation" by cancer cells, it was possible to invent effective new immunotherapies that act by reactivating latent host immune responses.

Box 9: Observations that support the concept of immune surveillance.

- Direct demonstration of tumor-specific T cells and antibodies in cancer patients
- Correlation of outcome of the cancer patients with extent and quality of immune infiltrates in cancers. Increasing survival rates in patients with high number of CTL (cytotoxic T lymphocytes/intratumoral lymphocytes) and natural killer (NK) cells in different types of cancers
- Increased incidence of some cancers in immunodeficient individuals [e.g., patients with human immunodeficiency virus/acquired immunodeficiency syndrome (HIV/AIDS), immunosuppressed organ transplant recipients] and mice than in immunocompetent individuals
- Success of immunotherapy in many cancers. Effectiveness of the bacterium *Bacillus Calmette–Guérin* (BCG) vaccine in the treatment of superficial bladder cancer

Tumor Antigens (Fig. 73)

Q. Write a short essay on tumor antigen.

Tumor antigen is an antigenic substance produced in tumor cells. Antigens found in tumors that elicit an immune response have been found in some cancers. Tumor antigens can be classified according to their molecular structure and source. The three main classes of tumor antigens are—(i) neoantigens produced from genes bearing passenger and driver mutations, (ii) overexpressed or aberrantly expressed normal cellular proteins, and (iii) tumor antigens produced by oncogenic viruses.

Neoantigens produced from genes bearing passenger and driver mutations

- Cancer is caused by driver mutations in oncogenes and TSGs (tumor suppressor genes). Most of these mutations are acquired rather than inherited. Apart from pathogenic driver mutations, cancers, due to their inherent genetic instability, also accumulate passenger mutations. These mutations may be mainly numerous in cancers caused by mutagenic exposures (e.g., sunlight, smoking). All of these mutations may produce new protein sequences (*neoantigens*) in the cancer cells. The immune system has not come across these neoantigens. Hence, the immune system can recognize them as foreign and can react against it. Genetic instability in cancers generally likely to develop many passenger mutations throughout their genomes. These mutations are neutral in terms of cancer cell fitness and thus not related to the transformed phenotype. However, some of them may fall in the coding sequences of genes and give rise to protein variants. Then these may serve as tumor antigens when the mutation is in an epitope that binds to the MHC molecules of the individual. The size of the mutational load in a particular tumor is estimated by DNA sequencing of tumor genomes. This mutational load correlates with the strength of the host CD8+ cytotoxic T-cell response and also the effectiveness of immunomodulatory therapies.

Overexpressed or aberrantly expressed normal cellular proteins

- **Self-antigen:** Sometimes, unmutated proteins expressed by tumor cells themselves can stimulate the host immune response. For example, **tyrosinase** is an enzyme involved in biosynthesis of melanin. It is expressed only in normal melanocytes and melanomas. The immune system generally does not respond to this normal self-antigen. This may be probably because normally tyrosinase is produced in very small amounts and by few normal cells. Hence, it is not recognized by the immune system and there is no immune tolerance against this normal self-antigen. However, when it is aberrantly or overexpressed, immune system respond to this antigen.
- **Cancer-testis antigens:** Another group of tumor antigens are proteins that are aberrantly expressed in cancer cells. These proteins are expressed at much greater levels than in normal tissues. This overexpression may be caused by

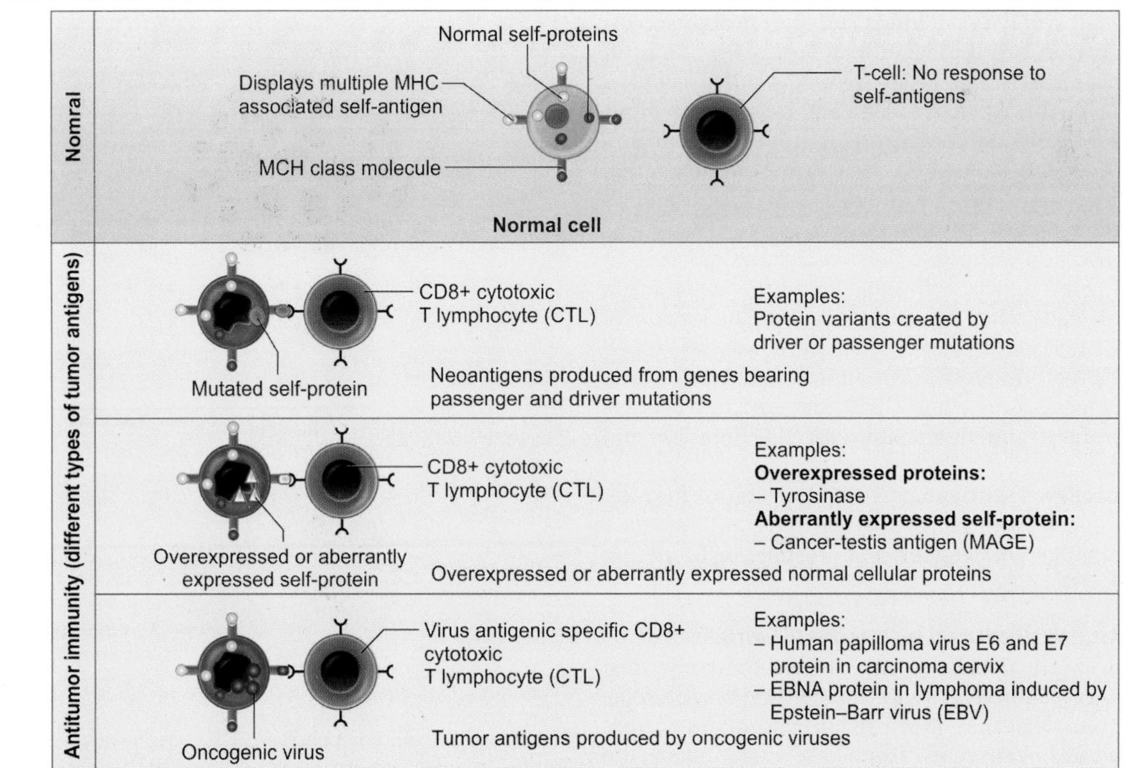

FIG. 73: Tumor antigens recognized by CD8+ T cells. Normal cells with self-antigens are not recognized by T cells. Antitumor immunity develops when CD8+ T cells recognize tumor antigens and get activated. Different types of tumor antigens include—(i) neoantigens produced from genes bearing passenger and driver mutations, (ii) overexpressed or aberrantly expressed normal cellular proteins, (iii) Tumor antigens produced by oncogenic viruses.

gene amplification or acquired epigenetic alterations. They reactivate genes that are normally silenced in adult tissues. One of them is *cancer-testis antigens*. These antigens are encoded by genes that are silent in all adult tissues except germ cells in the testis, hence termed testis antigens. This antigen is present in the testis but is not expressed on the cell surface in a form that can be recognized by CD8+ T cells. This is because sperms do not express major histocompatibility (MHC) class I molecules. Thus, these antigens are tumor-specific and are capable of stimulating antitumor immune responses. These antigens are tumor-specific. Classical example of this group is the melanoma antigen gene (MAGE) family. Originally. MAGE antigen was identified in melanomas, but these antigens are found to be expressed in various types of tumors.

Majority of tumor neoantigens consist of mutated gene products or viral proteins that are endogenously synthesized. They are presented along with MHC class I molecules. These tumor antigens are recognition by CTLs. Hence, main immune mechanism that eradicates tumor is killing of tumor cells by cytotoxic T cells (CTLs) specific for tumor antigens. T Various steps involved in antitumor effector mechanism is discussed below.

- **Oncofetal antigens:** They are proteins that are expressed at high levels on cancer cells and in normal developing (fetal) tissues. However, they are not limited to tumors and may be increased in tissues and blood in various inflammatory conditions, and found in small amount in normal tissues. They are not important targets of antitumor immunity. However, they can be used as markers that aid in the diagnosis of tumor and clinical management. For example, carcinoembryonic antigen (CEA) and α-fetoprotein (AFP).
- **Tumor cell surface glycolipids and glycoproteins:** Most human tumors express higher than normal levels and/or abnormal forms of surface glycoproteins and glycolipids. They may be of diagnostic value and target for therapy. These include gangliosides, blood group antigens and mucins (e.g. CA-125 and CA-19-9, expressed on ovarian carcinomas, and MUC-1 expressed on both ovarian and breast carcinomas).
- **Differentiation antigens:** These molecules are seen in normal cells (normal self-antigens) of the same origin as cancer cells. They do not induce immune responses in tumor-bearing hosts. For example, CD20, which is a normal B-cell differentiation antigen, is expressed by some lymphomas, and anti-CD20 antibody (rituximab) is used for the treatment of mature B-cell lymphomas and leukemias.
- **Overexpressed antigens:** Normal proteins may be overproduced in certain malignant cells (e.g., prostate specific antigen in carcinoma of prostate, HER2/neu in carcinoma of breast).

Tumor antigens produced by oncogenic viruses

Several viruses are associated with cancers and are termed oncogenic viruses. These viruses produce or express proteins (i.e., viral proteins), can be expressed in cancer cells that are transformed by oncogenic viruses. These viral antigens are recognized as foreign by the immune system. The most potent of these antigens are proteins produced by cells latently infected with DNA viruses. Important examples include human papilloma virus (HPV) and Epstein–Barr virus (EBV). The cytotoxic T lymphocytes (CTLs) can recognize viral antigens and play important roles in surveillance against virus-induced tumors. A competent immune system is able to recognize and result in humoral and cellular immune responses. CTLs can recognize and kill virus-infected cells, thus eradicate incipient neoplasia. It is observed that multiple cancers associated with oncogenic viruses, such as HPV-associated cervical carcinoma and EBV-related B-cell lymphomas, develop at significantly higher rates in individuals with defective T-cell immunity (e.g., patients infected with HIV).

Effective Immune Responses to Tumor Antigens (Fig. 74)

- **Death of tumor cells and initiation of immune response:** Immune reactions to cancers are initiated by the death of individual cancer cells. Many cancers, especially the rapidly growing tumors have a high fraction of cells that undergo cell death, either by apoptosis or necrosis. The death of cancer cells may be due to dysregulated growth, metabolic stresses, and hypoxia due to insufficient blood supply. Tumor cell death release "danger signals" (damage associated molecular patterns). This stimulates innate immune cells, including resident phagocytes and antigen presenting cells (APCs).
- **Capture of dead tumor cells by dendritic cells:** Probably some of the dead tumor cells or released tumor antigens are captured and ingested (phagocytosed) by **host antigen presenting cells (APCs)/dendritic** cells and macrophages in the tumor microenvironment.

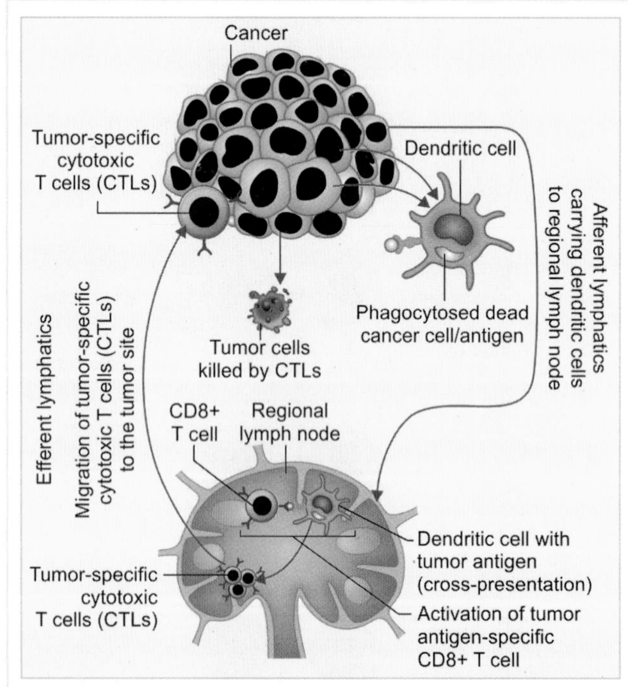

FIG. 74: Cytotoxic T lymphocyte (CTL) response against tumors. Tumor antigens are phagocytosed up by dendritic cells, and carried to regional lymph node and responses are initiated. Cross-presentation of tumor antigens to CD8+ cells produces tumor-specific CD8+ cytotoxic T cell. Tumor-specific CTLs migrate back to the tumor and kill tumor cells.

- **Presentation of antigen by dendritic cells to naïve CD8+ T cells in lymph node:** The dendritic cells and macrophages migrate to draining lymph nodes. The dendritic cells and macrophages present the tumor neoantigens/antigens to naïve CD8+ T lymphocytes (CD8+T cells also called as CTLs) in association with MHC class I molecules. The tumor antigens displayed by dendritic (antigen presenting) cell are recognized by antigen-specific CD8+ T cells. In this pathway, the ingested (phagocytosed) tumor cells (and antigens expressed by these cells) are transported from endosomal vesicles to the cytosol, and present them to naïve CD8+ T cells. This process is termed as **cross-presentation** or cross-priming to indicate that one cell type (the dendritic cell) presents antigens from another cell (e.g., tumor cell) and prime, or activates T cells specific for these antigens. These CD8+ T cells become activated, proliferate, differentiate into active CTLs. Activation of antigen specific CTLs also needs costimulatory molecules. These molecules are upregulated on APCs probably by "danger signals" released from damaged or necrotic tumor cells (DAMPs), can move out of the lymph nodes. They migrate to the tumor site and kill tumor cells.
- **Killing of tumor cells by CD8+ CTLs:** After the activation by interaction with APCs, tumor-specific CTLs migrate from lymph nodes to the site of the tumor. The main mechanism of immune protection against tumor is killing of tumor cells by CD8+ CTLs. These CTLs recognize and kill tumor cells containing neoantigens directly and serially, without any help from other types of cells (**Fig. 74**).
- **Antitumor immune responses CD4+ helper T cells:** CD4+ T cell responses to tumor antigens are common in cancer patients. The presence of T cells, like CTLs, in human tumors **correlates with good prognosis**. The mechanism of antitumor effects of Th1 cells is by enhancing CD8+ T cell/CTLs responses and activating macrophages, through the secretion of tumor necrosis factor (TNF) and interferon-γ (IFN-γ). There is increased incidence of tumors in knockout mice lacking IFN-γ, its receptor, or IFN-γ induced signaling molecules. This indicates the importance of IFN-γ in tumor immunity.
    - **CD4+ regulatory T cells (Tregs):** They are a highly immune-suppressive subset of CD4+ T cells. Tregs play main roles in the maintenance of self-tolerance in healthy individuals. They are involved in maintaining immune homeostasis, i.e., they protect hosts from developing autoimmune diseases and allergy. In **cancers, they promote tumor progression** by suppressing antitumor immunity. High infiltration of Tregs in tumors is associated with a poor prognosis in various types of cancers (e.g., melanoma, nonsmall cell lung, gastric, hepatocellular, pancreatic, renal cell, breast, and cervical cancers).

Antitumor mechanisms

Cell-mediated immunity is the major antitumor mechanism. Although cancer patient's sera may contain antibodies that recognize tumors, under physiologic conditions they do not have protective role.

- **Cytotoxic T lymphocytes** (CD8+ CTLs): CTLs are the **most important cells involved in defense of the host against tumors** (antitumor activity). They play an important role in immunosurveillance in human cancers. Any acquired mutations that prevent CTLs from recognizing tumor cells as "foreign" may be associated with cancer. They react against tumor antigens. They have protective role against virus-associated neoplasms (e.g., EBV- and HPV-induced tumors), and associated with better prognosis in several cancers. In many human tumors, better clinical outcomes are observed in tumors having high levels of infiltrating CTLs and Th1 cells. For example, in patients with surgically resected colorectal carcinomas, the prognosis was better in patients whose tumors contained dense infiltrates of CTLs when compared to those patients with tumors of similar grade and size but had comparatively few infiltrating CTLs. Thus, the immune system acts as a significant obstacle to the progressive growth and dissemination of cancer. Tumor cells undergo a variety of changes to avoid CTL responses. These alterations include—(i) acquired mutations in β2-microglobulin that prevent the assembly of functional MHC class I molecules, and (ii) increased expression of different proteins that inhibit CTL function. These proteins activate immune checkpoints which are regulators of the immune system.
- **Antitumor CD4+ T-cell responses:** It has been identified in some patients. Increased numbers of CD4+ effector T cells (especially Th1 cells), in tumor infiltrates may be associated with a better prognosis in certain cancers (e.g., colorectal carcinoma).
- **Natural killer (NK) cells:** They can kill many types of tumor cells without prior sensitization and thus may be the first-line of defense against tumor cells. They may be involved in immune surveillance against cancers. Tumor cells are susceptible to killing by NK cells in two ways—(i) when they downregulate the expression of class I MHC or (ii) when they upregulate expression of ligands that bind activating NK cell receptors. However, the quality and strength of CTL responses are main importance than NK cells.
- **Macrophages:** Activated macrophages may kill tumors by mechanisms similar to those used to kill microbes (e.g., production of ROS).

Immune Evasion by Cancers

Tumors stimulate specific adaptive immune responses. Immune system is capable of recognizing and destroying cancer cells. Thus, it can prevent or limit the growth and spread of the cancers. When a tumor becomes clinically significant in size, it must be composed of cells that are either not recognized by the host immune system or that the tumor cells express factors that actively suppress the host immunity.

Immunosurveillance

Immune system can identify and control nascent tumor cells. This is performed by a process called cancer immunosurveillance. This concept of **immune surveillance** of cancer was proposed by Macfarlane Burnet in the 1950s. Immunosurveillance is a physiological process by which immune system recognizes transformed cells and destroys clones of tumor cells in order to inhibit the growth of tumor tissue. Thus, immunosurveillance process is observed before the transformed cells grow into tumors and also kills tumor cells after they are formed. Increased frequency of cancers is observed in patients with immunodeficiency (e.g., congenital immunodeficiencies, immunosuppressed transplant recipients, and persons with AIDS). However, most cancers develop in patients without any overt immunodeficiency.

Cancer immunoediting concept

In immunocompetent hosts, highly immunogenic cancer cell clones are normally eradicated. This process is referred to as immunoediting. This leaves behind only weakly immunogenic variants that grow and produce solid tumors. Schreiber and colleagues conducted experiments in genetically engineered mice using a chemical carcinogen (which more closely model the majority of human cancers). It was observed that tumors arose more frequently and/or grew more rapidly in the immunodeficient mice compared to immune-competent mice.

***Induction of tumor using chemical carcinogen*:** The results were as follows:
The above findings showed that tumors that developed in the WT (wild type) **immunocompetent host were subjected to a selective immune-related pressure (editing process)** whereas the others (**lacking adaptive immunity)** are not subjected to immune-related pressure. Tumors occur more frequently and/or grew more rapidly in the immunodeficient mice relative to immune-competent controls. These results show that the immune system not only protects the host against tumor formation, but also edits/selects tumor immunogenicity. For details refer to **Figure 75**.

Concept of cancer immunoediting (Fig. 76)

Schreiber and colleagues developed the concept as a dynamic process composed by three phases. **3 Es of cancer immunoediting** are **elimination, equilibrium, and evasion/escape**.

- **Elimination:** Both innate and adaptive immune cells play a role in immune surveillance. In this phase, the growing cancer cells are completely eliminated (killed) by the action of innate and adaptive immunity.
- **Equilibrium:** During elimination phase, some cancer cells may not be controlled by the innate and adaptive immune cells. The cells that survive elimination grow as with new variants. These tumor cells may be more resistant to the immune response. During this phase, cancer is not clinically detectable and is dormant. There is a state of equilibrium that develops between immune and tumor cells. Patients whose tumors are in equilibrium may either revert to elimination or progress onto the next escape phase.
- **Evasion/escape:** In this phase, cancer cells have escaped the immune system. These cancer cells replicate with promotion of tumor growth, leading to clinically detectable tumors.

Processes in cancer immunoediting Cancer immunoediting consists of **two types of processes namely,** paradoxical anti- and protumoral processes of the immune system. Together, the dual host-protective and tumor-promoting actions of immunity are referred to as cancer immunoediting. It is the result of the cross-interactions between the antitumor response of the immune system and the tumor cells. This leads to the selection of immune-resistant clones/variants.

- **Host-protective action:** A process by which immune system **protects the host against primary tumor development,** and/or
- **Tumor-promoting action:** It **enhances tumor escape either by manipulating tumor immunogenicity or weakening antitumor immune responses**. By cancer immunoediting, the immune system can promote the selection of the tumor subclones that are poorly immunogenic variants (i.e., capable of avoiding host immunity) and suppressing antitumor immunity. Even it can manipulate the immune system for their own malignant purposes. Immune system can also promote tumor progression through chronic inflammation.

Evasion (Escape) of Immune Surveillance

Immune responses frequently fail to prevent the growth of tumors. **Cancer cells can evade the host response** and one factor that may be responsible for this may be a phenomenon called immune tolerance. Normally functioning immune system develops a tolerance toward self-antigens. A tumor may pass under the radar and evade recognition and attack, as it expresses only these normal tissue antigens. Tumors produce many factors that promote immune tolerance and immune suppression. Evasion of host immunity is a hallmark of many cancers. However, if cancer cells express embryonic antigens toward which immune self-tolerance was never established, or express fully novel nonself-antigens created by gene mutation or by an infectious agent; there may be development of immune response.

Mechanism of immune evasion by cancers

The immune system can recognize tumor cells as nonself and destroy them. In an immunocompetent host, tumor cells must develop mechanisms to escape or evade the immune system and immune surveillance. Cancer immune evasion is a strategy used by cancer cells to escape the host immune response. This process increases the probability of cancer cells to survive and grow in the immune competent host. In immunocompetent patients, several mechanisms may avoid the response by immune system to tumors. Various mechanisms of cancer immune evasion are discussed as follows.

Selective outgrowth of antigen-negative variants During progression of tumor, subclones of tumor cells may lose the expression of antigens. These cells may not be recognized by the host immune system. Tumors that elicit effective immune responses, d**uring tumor development, these strongly immunogenic subclones may** become less immunogenic over time or may **be eliminated** by immunoediting (discussed above on page 496). This may lead to **selective outgrowth of antigen-negative (i.e.,** do not express immunogenic antigens) **variants,** because these subclones have a selective survival advantage.

***Loss or reduced expression of MHC molecules by tumor cells*:** Tumor cells may fail to express normal levels of class I MHC molecules. These tumors cells cannot be recognized by CTLs and thereby, escaping attack by these CTLs. Many tumors show reduced synthesis of class I MHC molecules, or proteins needed for expression of class I MHC on the surface of the tumor cell. However, these tumor cells, may trigger NK cells if the tumor cells express ligands for NK-cell activating receptors. Such tumor cells can be destroyed by NK cells.

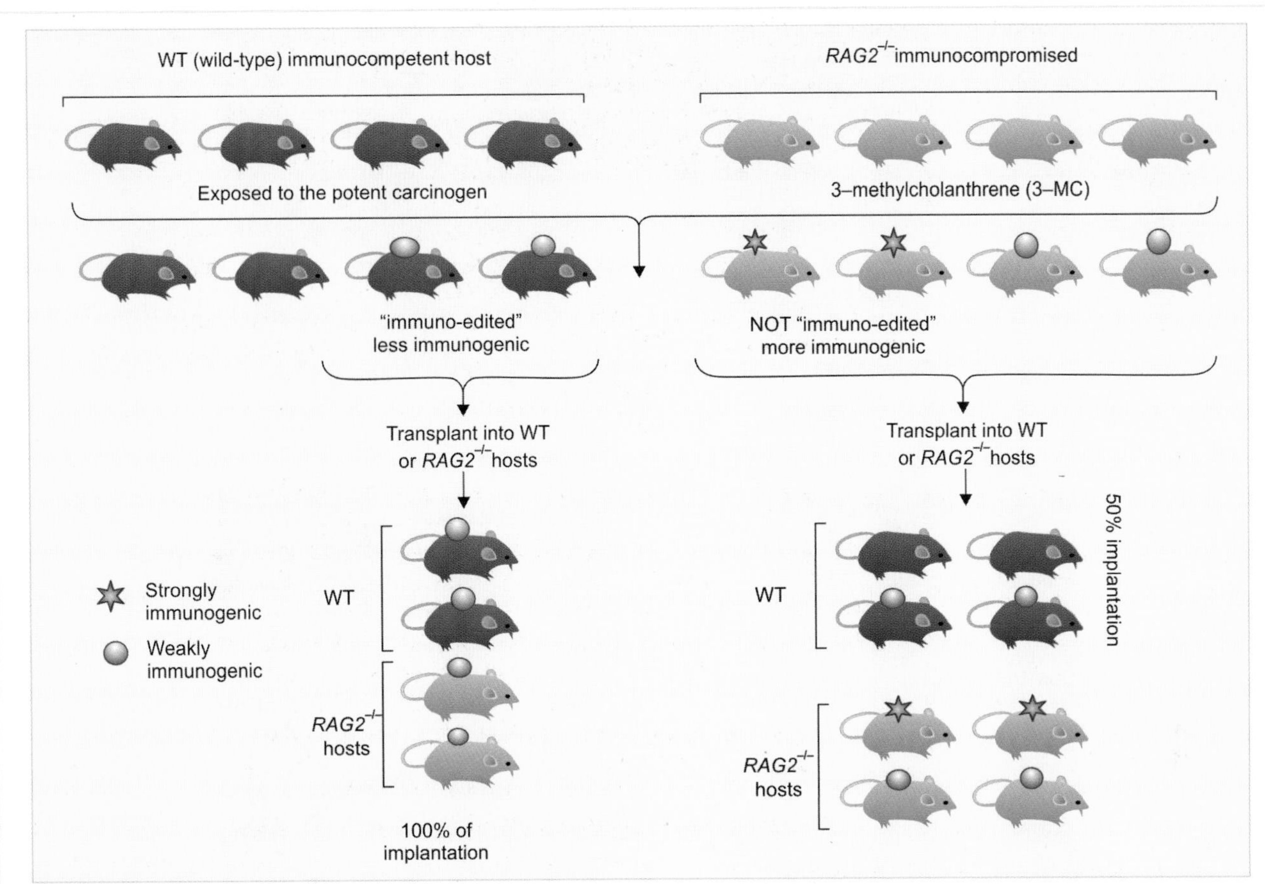

FIG. 75: Effects of immune function on the development of antitumor immune responses by inducing tumor using chemical carcinogen. Both wild-type (WT, i.e., *Rag*$^{+/+}$) immunocompetent and *Rag2*$^{-/-}$ immunocompromised mice were exposed to the potent carcinogen 3-methylcholanthrene (3-MC). (A) Following exposure to 3-MC, the WT immunocompetent (with adequate adaptive immunity) mice developed fewer tumors (*blue*) than did the *Rag2*$^{-/-}$ mutant mice. This is because highly immunogenic cancer cell clones are eliminated on WT immunocompetent and it leaves behind only weakly immunogenic variants (poorly recognized by the immune system). These weakly immunogenic variants grow and generate "immunoedited" tumors. Cancer immunoediting is the ability of the immune system to promote the Darwinian selection of the tumor subclones that are able to avoid host immunity or even manipulate the immune system for their own malignant purposes. (B) In contrast, in immunodeficient *Rag2*$^{-/-}$ mice (they lack adaptive immunity, i.e., T and B cells) developed tumors. The immunogenic cancer cells are not selectively depleted (i.e., no immune-editing). When tumor arises in immunodeficient hosts, the immunogenic cancer cells are not selectively depleted and can, instead, prosper along with their weakly immunogenic counterparts. These are nonedited tumors. (C) Tumor cells were then transplanted into either WT mice or *Rag2*$^{-/-}$ mutant mice. Tumor cells from all of the tumors that appeared initially in the WT mice (*blue*) were able to form new tumors in both WT and *Rag2*$^{-/-}$ recipients (*left*). (D) When the tumors that arose and grew in the *Rag2*$^{-/-}$ mice were transplanted into *Rag2*$^{-/-}$ hosts (recipients), they all formed tumors (*red, blue*). On contrast, when the tumors induced in the *Rag2*$^{-/-}$ mice were transplanted into WT (WT recipient) hosts, only some of these (*blue*) were able to form new tumors and 8 of 20 tumors failed to form. These experiments suggested that chemical carcinogen 3-MC initially produced two types of tumor cells in all of the mice—strongly immunogenic (*red*) and weakly immunogenic (*blue*). Both *red* and *blue* cells formed tumors in the *Rag2*$^{-/-}$ mice (B), but only *blue* cells formed tumors in the WT mice (A). Any initially formed *red* tumor cells were destroyed by the functional immune systems of WT mice. This suggests that the tumors that arise in WT mice were already selected for being weakly immunogenic (immunoedited) and thus, can form new tumors in other WT mice. Weakly immunogenic cells can successfully colonize both immunodeficient and immunocompetent hosts.

Engagement of pathways that inhibit T-cell activation

Q. Write a short essay on immune checkpoint in cancer and immune checkpoint therapy.

Q. Write a short essay on immune checkpoint inhibitors.

Tumor cells can inhibit tumor immunity by upregulating negative regulatory checkpoints.

Immune checkpoints: Immune checkpoints are normal **inhibitory pathways** of immune regulation that suppresses the immune response. Immune checkpoints are very essential **for maintaining self-tolerance** (i.e., to maintain the balance between stimulatory and inhibitory inputs). They regulate an efficient response but at the same time prevent an excess immune response which may lead to autoimmunity. These checkpoints are the inhibitory signals for T-cell activation and prevent the immune system from attacking cells indiscriminately. They also control the size and duration of immune responses so as to minimize collateral tissue damage. Tumor cells can actively inhibit tumor immunity by engaging these "checkpoints" involved in immune responses.

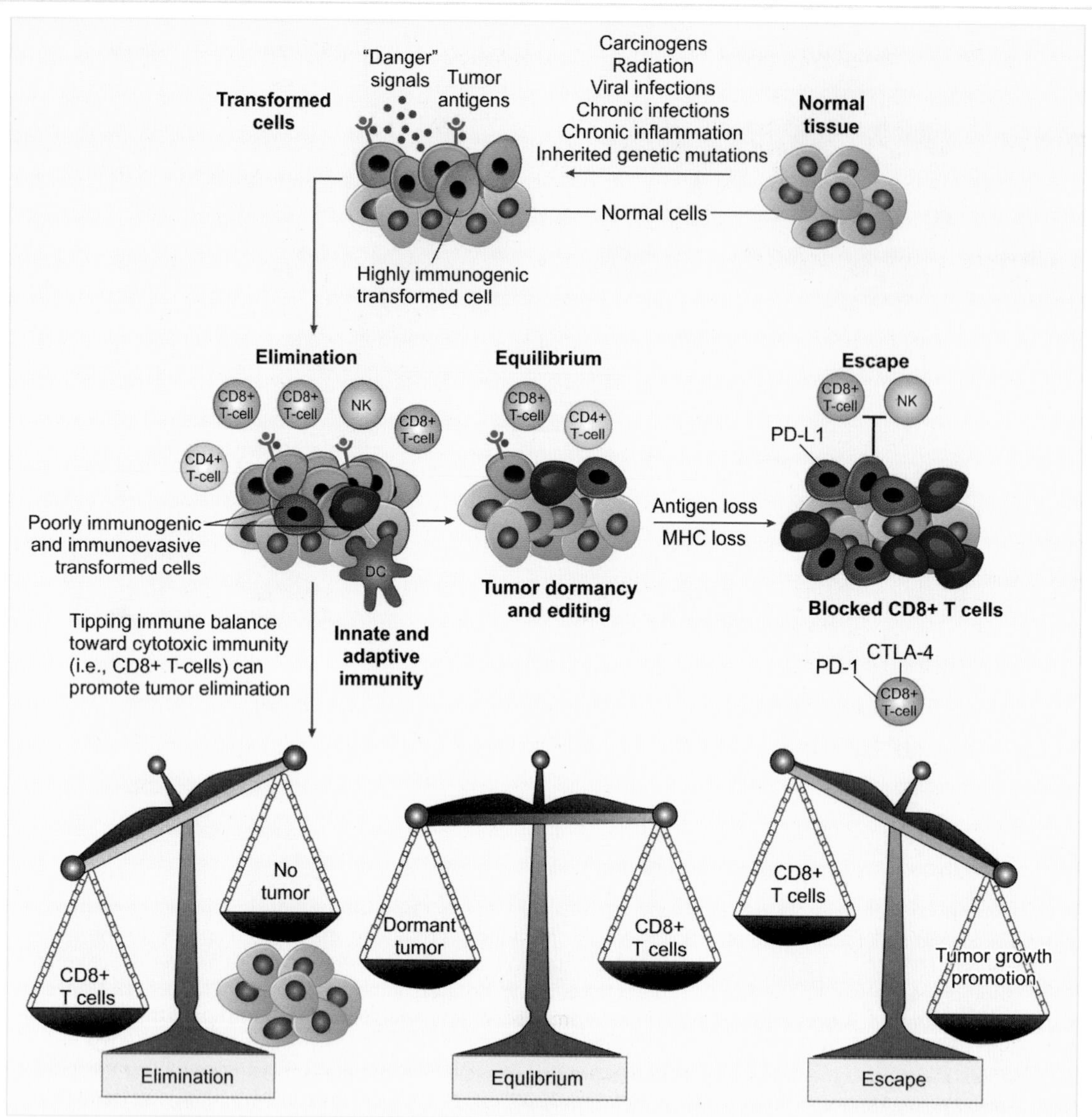

FIG. 76: Three "Es" of cancer immunoediting (refer text for details).

Immune checkpoints in cancer: Immune checkpoint molecules are main modulators of the antitumor T-cell immune response. These immune checkpoint molecules are present on—(i) T cells, (ii) APCs, and (iii) tumor cells. Their interaction activates either inhibitory or activating immune signaling pathways. Some cancers can protect themselves from attack by stimulating immune checkpoint targets. There are several immune checkpoint pathways, involving different ligands and receptors involved in immunoevasion by tumors. Tumors evade antitumor T-cell responses by engaging inhibitory molecules that normally function to prevent autoimmunity or regulate immune responses to microbes.

Inhibitory immune checkpoints (Figs. 77A and B): They play an essential role in maintaining immune self-tolerance. They help to prevent T cells from showing autoimmune reactions. They induce a negative signal to T cells and prevent killing of tumor cells. Two important immune checkpoint receptors are—cytotoxic T-lymphocyte-associated antigen 4 (CTLA4) and programmed cell death protein 1 (PD-1). Apart from CTLA4 and PD-1, there are other molecules that negatively regulate T-cell activation. They suppress effector T-cell activation. Cancers can use these checkpoints to escape attack on them by the immune system. Immune checkpoint inhibitors target regulators of the immune system that inhibit immune responses. Presently, there are two approved immune checkpoint inhibitors, namely—(i) that target the molecules CTLA4 by anti-CTLA-4 antibody and (ii) anti-PD-1 and anti-PD-L1. Anti-CTLA-4 antibody binds to CTLA4 on CTLs and prevents attachment to B7-1 and B7-2. Anti-PD-1 and anti-PD-L1 bind to PD-1 and PDL-1, respectively.

Q. Write short essay on importance of co-stimulation in immune response

- **Cytotoxic T-lymphocyte-associated antigen 4** (also known as CD152): It is member of the CD 28:B7 immunoglobulin family. CTLA-4 is a receptor normally expressed in low levels on naïve effector T cells and regulatory T cells.

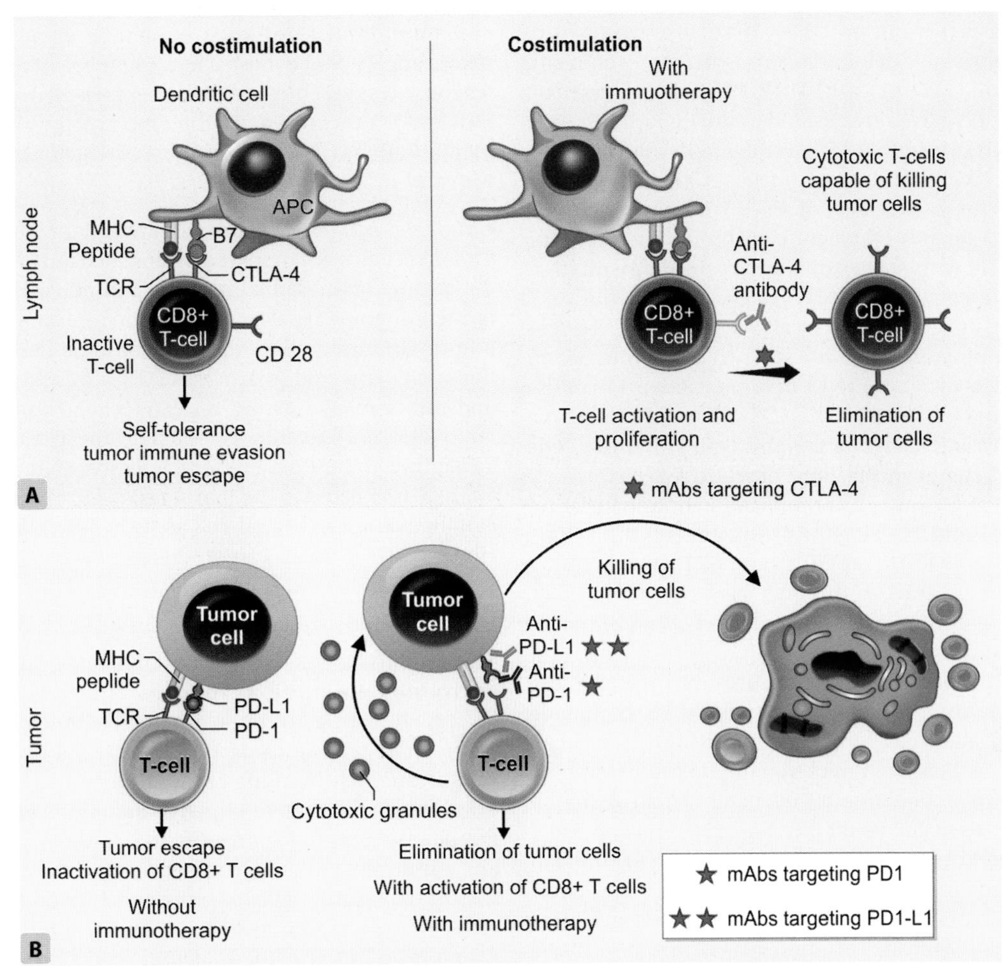

FIGS. 77A AND B: Activation of host antitumor immunity by checkpoint blockade. Patients with tumor usually mount ineffective T cell responses to their tumors by upregulating inhibitory receptors such as cytotoxic T-lymphocyte-associated antigen 4 (CTLA-4) and programmed cell death protein 1 (PD-1) on the tumor-specific T cells, and expression of the ligand PD-L1 on the tumor cells. (A) Blockade of the CTLA4 surface molecule with an inhibitor antibody (anti-CTLA4 antibodies) allows cytolytic CD8+ T cells (CTLs) to engage B7 family coreceptors, leading to T cell activation. (B) Blockade of PD-1 receptor or PD-1 ligand by inhibitory antibodies (anti-PD-1 or anti-PD-L1 antibodies, respectively) abolish inhibitory signals transmitted by PD-1. This leads to activation of cytolytic CD8+ T cells (CTLs) leading to killing of tumor cells.

- **Role of costimulation in T-cell activation (Fig. 77A):** The proliferation and differentiation of naïve T cells need two types of signals, namely antigen-induced signals (first signal) and signals by molecules on APCs. These two molecules together are called costimulators, and the second signal for T-cell activation by APC was called **costimulation**, the first signal being antigen. Well-known costimulatory pathway in T-cell activation involves the T-cell surface receptor CD28, which binds the costimulatory molecules B7 [two homologous proteins, namely B7-1 (CD80) and B7-2 (CD86)] expressed on the surface of activated APCs. After stimulation, CTLA-4 competes with CD 28 to bind with B7.
  - **Antigens without costimulation:** If T cells encounter antigens without costimulation, CTLA-4 binds with costimulatory molecules B7. It turns off the TCR signaling. These T cells either fail to respond or enter a state of prolonged unresponsiveness. Thus, CTLA-4 binding with B7 plays an important role in preventing autoimmunity by downregulating T-cell activation.
  - **Antigens with costimulation:** In this, CD 28 (and not CTLA-4) binds with B7 and results in T-cell activation and proliferation.
- **Action of CTLA4 in cancers:** Tumor cells may downregulate the expression of costimulatory factors on APCs (e.g., dendritic cells). These APCs fail to engage the stimulatory receptor CD28 on T cells and inhibit CD28-mediated costimulatory signals. It also activates the inhibitory receptor CTLA-4 on effector T cells. Thus, it inhibits function of T cell and prevents the killing of tumor cells (refer **Fig. 77A**). Anti-CTLA-4 antibody (e.g., Ipilimumab) can block CTLA-4 and cause prolonged T-cell activation, proliferation, and antitumor response.

- **Programmed cell death protein 1** (**PD-1** also known as CD279): Programmed cell death protein 1 is a member of the costimulatory receptor family of B7-CD28. **PD-1** is **present on CTLs.** There are two types of immunosuppressive cell-surface programmed cell death protein ligand 1 (PD-L1) and PD-L2. PD-L1 is expressed on tumor cells, as well as on activated tumor-IICs (infiltrating immune cells), including APCs (antigen presenting cells), T cells and B cells, and macrophages. **Cancer cells** may upregulate the expression of PD-L1 on their surface. When PD-L1 ligands of cancer cells bind to its **receptor PD-1, on CTLs**, they recruit the tyrosine phosphatase and inhibit T-cell receptor (TCR) signaling in cytotoxic T cells (CTLs), downregulates T-cell activation and reduces cytokine production and T-cell survival. Thus, interaction of PD-1 and its receptor PD-L1 **prevents activation of the cytotoxic mechanisms of the CTLs**. The CTLs become unresponsive and **lose their capability to kill tumor cells** (**Fig. 77B**). In some cancers, there may be overexpression of PD-L1 and PD-L2 due to by amplification or translocation of the PD-L1 and PD-L2 genes respectively. Both PD-1 and PD-L1 serve as therapeutic targets. Drugs targeting (anti-PD-1 or anti-PDL-1) this pathway reactivates T cells. This produces antitumoral responses and kills (eliminate) the tumor cells.

The above discussed antibodies are approved for the treatment of a number of malignant tumors. These include melanoma, nonsmall cell lung cancer (NSCLC), renal cell carcinoma (RCC), head and neck squamous cell carcinoma (HNSCC), urothelial carcinoma, mismatch-repair deficient (dMMR) or microsatellite instability-high (MSI-H) colorectal and other cancers, Merkel cell carcinoma, classical Hodgkin lymphoma, gastric cancer, hepatocellular carcinoma, cervical squamous cell carcinoma, and primary mediastinal large B-cell lymphoma (PMBCL).

Other inhibitory receptors expressed by tumor-specific T cells, include **lymphocyte-activation gene 3 (LAG-3), T-cell immunoglobulin, and mucin domain 3 (TIM-3), V-domain immunoglobulin suppressor of T-cell activation (VISTA)** and T-cell immunoreceptor with immunoglobulin (Ig) and ITIM domains (TIGIT). These also may inhibit antitumor immune responses.

***Costimulatory immune checkpoints*:** They enhance T-cell expansion and survival. Examples are: CD40, OX40 (also known as CD134), 4-1BB (also known as CD137), glucocorticoid-induced TNF receptor (GITR), and inducible T-cell costimulator (ICOS, also known as CD278).

***Blocking of checkpoints (checkpoint blockade) (Fig. 77A and B)*: The checkpoints can be blocked by using appropriate antibodies.** Immune checkpoint inhibitors will **shut off antitumor immunity and release** (relieve) the immunological **brakes on the immune response.** These brakes are evolved to avoid overactivation of the immune system on healthy cells. Currently, checkpoint blockade therapies (e.g., against CTLA-4 and PD-1 that normally limit the killing activity of CTLs) are being used in a variety of solid tumors (melanoma, lung cancer, bladder cancer, and others), and in some hematologic malignancies (e.g., Hodgkin lymphoma). Antibody drugs blocking PD-1 or its ligand PD-L1 (sometimes in combination an anti-CTLA-4 antibody) or conventional or targeted chemotherapy are producing good responses "even potential cures" in a considerable number of patients with metastatic melanoma and significant benefit in some patients with other cancers. Since these checkpoints are blocked to prevent responses to self-antigens, the patients treated with checkpoint blockade therapy may develop various autoimmune manifestations (e.g., colitis), most of which can be controlled with anti-inflammatory agents.

***Chimeric antigen receptors (CARs)*:** Recently personalized tumor vaccines are prepared against neoantigens identified in the tumors of individual patients and new kinds of adoptive immunotherapy are also used. One of the examples of adoptive immunotherapy is the development of patient-derived CTLs that are engineered to express CARs. CARs have extracellular and intracellular domains. The extracellular domains consist of antibodies that bind tumor antigens on the surface of tumor cells and intracellular domains which deliver signals that activate CTLs. CAR T cells kill the tumor cells and are used for treating certain leukemias (e.g., B-cell acute lymphoblastic leukemia). However, CAR T cells can produce serious complications due to cytokines released from the activated CTLs.

Secretion of immunosuppressive factors by cancer cells Tumor cells may secrete many molecules that inhibit the **antitumor immune responses** (immunosuppression). Examples of these immunosuppressive molecules expressed by the tumor cells include TGF-β and PD-1 ligands. They can inhibit the host immune response against tumor cells. For example, TGF-β secreted in large quantities by many tumors is a potent immunosuppressant that inhibits the proliferation and effector functions of lymphocytes and macrophages. Some tumors may secrete galectins, sugar-rich lectin-like factors that reduce T-cell responses, thereby favor immunosuppression. Examples of other soluble factors produced by tumors that may inhibit the host immune response are interleukin-10, prostaglandin E2, metabolites derived from tryptophan, and VEGF. They can inhibit the recruitment of T cells from the vasculature into the tumor bed. Various mechanisms by which tumors escape immune defenses are presented in **Figure 78.**

Induction of immunosuppressive regulatory T-cells (Tregs) Study on mouse and cancer patients suggests that tumors produce factors that favor the development of immunosuppressive regulatory T cells (Tregs). Thus, number of regulatory T cells are increased in tumor-bearing individuals and can be found in the cellular infiltrates in certain tumors. This indicates that they contribute to "immunoevasion". Depletion of Tregs in mice with tumor found to enhance antitumor immunity and reduces tumor growth. However, their role in human tumors is not known.

Tumor growth overpowers the capacity of immune system: Rapid growth and spread of a tumor may overpower the capacity of the immune system. The immune system may not be able to effectively control the tumor and eliminate all the malignant cells.

Therapeutic significance: Knowledge about ineffective adaptive immune responses to cancers can be utilized for therapeutic purposes. Therapeutic strategies be used to treat cancer by stimulating immune responses (e.g., activation of antitumor T cells to effectively kill tumor cells).

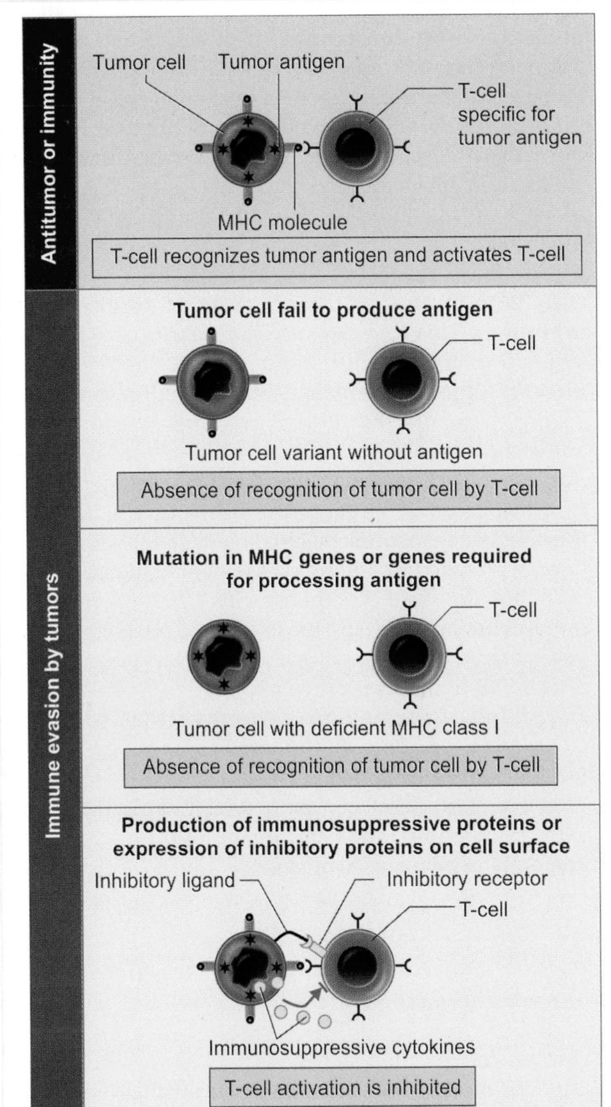

FIG. 78: Various mechanisms by which tumors escape immune defenses. Antitumor immunity develops when T cells recognize tumor antigens and they get activated. Tumor cells may evade immune responses by—(i) loss of expression of antigens, (ii) loss of expression of major histocompatibility complex (MHC) molecules, or (iii) by producing immunosuppressive cytokines or by producing ligands [e.g., programmed death ligand-1 (PD-L1)] for inhibitory receptors on T cells.

Cancer Immunotherapy

Q. Write a short essay on cancer immunotherapy.

Immunotherapy is defined as the treatment of diseases by stimulating or suppressing an immune response.

Cancer immunotherapy or immuno-oncology is a mode of treatment that stimulates the immune system of the patient, facilitating (enabling) a strong immunological response against the tumor. Immune system is classified into innate and adaptive immune system and consists of cells, tissues, and molecules. They protect us from microbial pathogens. However, they are not developed to respond against cancer, because cancer cells arise from our own cells. Usually cancer treatment consists of three modalities either alone or in combination, namely chemotherapy, radiation, and surgery. Cancer immunotherapy is the fourth modality of cancer treatment.

*Various types of cancer immunotherapy (**Fig. 79**)*: Immune-based treatments for cancer can be divided into passive and active immunotherapy. In **passive immunotherapy,** already active immune factors such as tumor-specific monoclonal antibodies (mAbs), cytokines, or antigen-specific adaptive immune cells are delivered to the patient. The aim of **active immunotherapy** is to activate intrinsic factors of the patient's own immune system against the tumor through cancer vaccine, immune checkpoint inhibitors, or oncolytic viruses.

Tumor specific monoclonal antibodies: Monoclonal antibodies (mAbs) have advanced cancer treatment. These antibodies have a high specificity and there are different applications of mAbs in cancer therapy (**Box 10**).

Presently available mAbs used in cancer treatment are listed in **Box 11**.

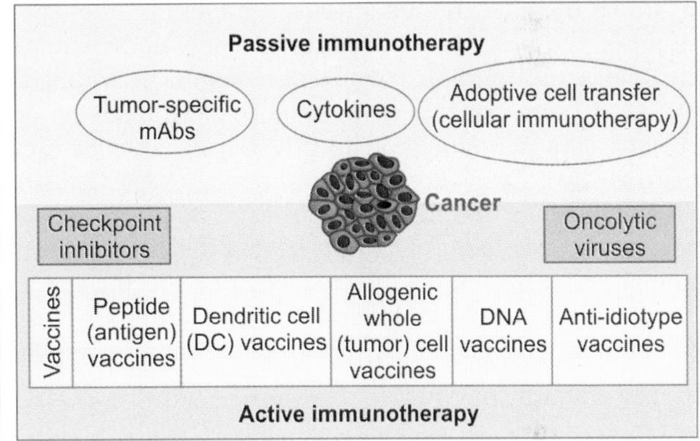

(DNA: deoxyribonucleic acid; mAbs: monoclonal antibodies)

FIG. 79: Various types of cancer immunotherapy.

Box 10: Applications of monoclonal antibodies (mAbs).

- **Variety of effector mechanisms** of antibodies (complement fixation, activation of various effector cells, direct inhibitory effects) by which they act on the target to which they bind
- **Antibodies can target to a specific site.** For example, killing of cells, against inhibitory molecules or effector cells
- **Antibodies can be directed at varieties of targets.** These may be against soluble protein or proteoglycan hormones or cytokines or their cellular receptors. This in turn will antagonize a particular function (e.g., cell growth, invasion, or migration or reverse immunosuppression)
- **Antibodies can be used as antigens** to elicit antitumor responses against immunoglobulin expressing tumors
- **Antibodies can be used to alter the pharmacologic behavior of other substances.** This may either increase or decrease their half-life or alter their distribution. For example, antibodies to digoxin used to treat digoxin toxicity

Box 11: Monoclonal antibodies used in cancer treatment.

- CD20 antibodies
- CD52 antibody
- CD38 antibody
- Vascular endothelial growth factor (VEGF) antibodies
- Human epidermal growth factor receptor 2 antibodies
- Epidermal growth factor receptor (EGFR) antibodies
- Glycolipid antigen disialoganglioside (GD2) antibody
- Interleukin-6 (IL-6) antibody
- Bispecific monoclonal antibodies
- Antibody conjugates
- Signaling lymphocytic activation molecule F7 antibody
- Platelet-derived growth factor receptor κ (PDGFRκ) antibody
- Cytotoxic T-lymphocyte-associated protein 4 (CTLA-4)
- Programmed death-1 (PD-1) antibodies
- Programmed death ligand-1 (PD-L1) antibodies

Cytokine therapy: Cytokines are a group of small extracellular cell-signaling molecules (proteins). They function as paracrine mediators of cell–cell interactions, secreted by one cell to influence the behaviors of another closely approximated cell. They act by binding to cytokine receptors activating the JAK–STAT [Janus kinases (JAKs) and signal transducer and activator of transcription proteins (STATs)] signaling pathway. They regulate inflammatory and immune responses. Cytokines can be used as immune-activating, antitumor passive drug for the treatment of cancer. They evoke a nonspecific immune response and not directed against a specific antigen. Immunostimulatory cytokines such as interleukin-2 and interferon-α (IFNα) stimulate a broad-based immune response and have been approved for treatment of cancer.

Adoptive cell therapy: Adoptive cell therapy (cellular immunotherapy) is a type of passive immunotherapy. In this method, tumor cells from the patient are activated or manipulated in vitro and are subsequently injected back into the patient to attack the tumor. There are different strategies for adoptive cell therapy. These include removal of immune cells from the patient's blood or directly from the tumor, using different types of immune cells such as cytotoxic T cells (CTCs), dendritic cells or NK cells or using genetically engineered immune cells. Presently, dendritic cell therapy (discussed further) and chimeric antigen receptor (CAR) T-cell therapy are approved for the treatment of cancer.

***CAR T-cell therapy*:** It is a cellular immunotherapy. In this, T cells from a patient are genetically engineered ex vivo to express a CAR specific for an arbitrary antigen. The genetically engineered T cells will attack cancer cells (It is discussed on page 500).

Cancer immunomodulatory therapy and its implications

Immunomodulatory therapy can achieve long-term remission and probably even cures (which is unlikely with any other treatment). This may be due to activation of long-life span of tumor-specific memory T cells in patients treated with immunomodulatory therapy. Knowledge gained from clinical trials conducted with immunotherapy are as follows:

- **Tumor neoantigen burden is a good predictor of response to immunotherapy:** Mismatch repair enzymes normally correct errors in DNA replication. It is observed that tumors that are deficient in mismatch repair enzymes that lead to point mutations show the highest mutation burdens of all cancers. These cancers respond well to checkpoint blockade therapy. Thus, anti-PD-1 therapy is used for all metastatic tumors that have mismatch repair deficiency. This leads to a high mutational burden irrespective of the histologic type of cancer.
- **Only 25% to 40% of tumors respond to checkpoint inhibitors**: This may because the tumors which do not respond to checkpoint inhibitors depend on evasion by methods other than engaging checkpoint pathways. For example, tumors that do not respond to anti-PD-1 or anti-PD-L1 therapy, do not express PD-L1, or do not have exhausted PD-1-positive CD8+ T-cell infiltrates.
- **Combination of checkpoint inhibitors with other therapeutic agents:** The higher rates of therapeutic success may be obtained by combined use of different checkpoint inhibitors, or of checkpoint inhibitors with other types of therapeutic agents (e.g., drugs that target oncoproteins like tyrosine kinases). For example, it was observed that melanoma treated with the combination of anti-CTLA-4 and anti-PD-1 respond more effectively than when anti-CTLA-4 is used alone. Both these agents act by different mechanisms (see **Fig. 77**).
- **Toxicity**: Two most common toxicities that develops with checkpoint blockade are autoimmunity and/or inflammatory damage to organs.

Dendritic cells in cancer therapy

Q. Write a short essay on dendritic cell in cancer immunotherapy.

A dendritic cell is called so because it extends and retracts long membranous extensions that resemble the dendrites of a nerve cell.

Importance of dendritic cells*:** Dendritic cells are ***primary phagocytic APC. They are ***capable of initiating immune response and lymphocytic activation, achieved by secretion of cytokine.*** Dendritic cells have the ability to control both immune tolerance and immunity.

***Steps in anticancer immune response*:** Dendritic cells perform the distinct functions of capturing antigen in one location and antigen presentation in another. Dendritic cells act as messengers between the innate and the adaptive immune systems. A series of events occur in the immune response against cancer:

- Dendritic cells recognize tumor antigens and phagocytose these antigens.
- After phagocytosis of antigens, the dendritic cells get activated and tumor antigen bind to newly synthesized MHC proteins.
- MHC molecules then carry the tumor antigens to the dendritic cell surface.
- Dendritic cells effectively present tumor antigens to effector/regulatory T cells capable of destroying cancer cells. Since, dendritic cells present antigens to the adaptive immune systems, these cells are called APCs (antigen presenting cells).

- The effector cytotoxic (killer) T cells reach the tumors and bind to the specific tumor antigen-expressing cancer cells and destroy them.

***Cancer therapy using dendritic cells*:** The antigen processing and presenting property of dendritic cells can be utilized to generate therapeutic immunity against cancer.

Principle: ***Vaccination of cancer patients with tumor antigens may result in enhanced immune responses against the tumor***. Dendritic cell therapy is a cellular immunotherapy in cancer, that induces (activates) dendritic cells to present tumor antigens to lymphocytes. This activates these lymphocytes (tumor-specific CTLs) and they destroy cancer cells having the same tumor antigen on their surface.

Different strategies to activate dendritic cells: Tumor vaccination strategies employ a variety of adjuvants and delivery methods. Dendritic cell can be used for **therapeutic vaccination** (in contrast to prophylactic vaccination) in vivo or ex vivo activation.

- **In vivo activation of dendritic cells:** In this strategy, the dendritic cells are activated by vaccination in vivo.
  - **Injection of tumor antigens plus adjuvant:** Lysates from the patient's own tumor or small peptides of the tumor antigen are given together with highly immunogenic substances, so called adjuvants. These adjuvants usually consist of killed microbial material. These adjuvants mislead (trick) the immune system to think that the tumor antigens are bacterial or viral antigens.
  - **Activation of dendritic cells:** Tumor antigens plus adjuvant are injected into the patient. The dendritic cells of the patient process the injected tumor antigen and express antigenic fragments on their surface.
  - **Immune response against tumor antigen:** The activated dendritic cells in turn promote a T-cell based immune response against cancer cells that carry the tumor antigen.
- **Ex vivo activation of dendritic cells:** This is the second strategy to activate dendritic cells.
  - **Removal of dendritic cells from patient with cancer**: Dendritic cells are removed from the blood of a patient with cancer.
  - **Ex vivo activation of dendritic cells:** The dendritic cells are then activated outside the body. Proinflammatory molecules are used to enhance the numbers of activated dendritic cells. These adjuvants include Toll-like receptor (TLR) ligands [e.g., CpG (5′-C-phosphate-G-3′) DNA and mimics of dsRNA (double stranded RNA)], and cytokines [e.g., granulocyte-macrophage colony stimulating factor (GM-CSF) and IL-12]. Ex vivo activation of dendritic cells is performed in cell cultures in the presence of a specific tumor antigen or a tumor lysate.
  - **Reinfusion of dendritic cells into the patient:** These activated dendritic cells are reinfused (injected) back into the patient usually together with strong adjuvants. Technical challenges with dendritic cell vaccines are—(i) the dendritic cells have to be harvested from each patient and (ii) they require dendritic cell culture, which is difficult to standardize.

Sipuleucel-T (Provenge) is a cell-based therapeutic vaccination that involves the ex vivo activation of dendritic cells previously isolated from the blood of a patient. It is the only dendritic cell therapy that received regulatory approval for clinical practice for the treatment of advanced cancer of prostate. In this, the cultured dendritic cells are exposed to a recombinant fusion protein consisting of tumor-associated antigen prostatic acid phosphatase (PAP, a protein present in almost all prostate cancer cells) and GM-CSF. GM-CSF is an immune-stimulatory cytokine known to activate and promote the maturation of dendritic cells. The activated dendritic cells are then reinfused back into the patient. These dendritic cells stimulate antitumor T-cell responses and attack and kill prostate cancer cells that express PAP. This procedure is repeated three times and has been approved for the treatment of metastatic, hormone-refractory cancer of prostate.

- DNA vaccines and viral vectors encoding tumor antigens: These are under clinical trials.

Preventive vaccine: The development of tumors induced by virus can be reduced by preventive vaccination with viral antigens or attenuated live viruses. For example, newly developed HPV vaccines have been found effective in reducing the incidence of HPV-induced premalignant lesions in the cervix.

Cancer vaccines

Q. Write a short essay on cancer vaccines.

The purpose of therapeutic vaccines is to induce strong antigen specific T-cell responses. In preventive vaccines for infections, vaccines are given to prevent infection in a normal individual. In contrast, most tumor vaccines are therapeutic vaccines; they are given to the individual after the development of the tumor (i.e., having a growing, established tumor). Cancer vaccines are most effective when combined with other immunotherapies (e.g., inhibitors of immune checkpoints).

***Main components of cancer vaccines*:** It consists of (i) a tumor antigen, (ii) an immunological adjuvant, and (iii) a vehicle or carrier.

***Tumor cell vaccines*:** In this method, whole tumor cells rendered safe by irradiation are utilized for preparing vaccine. The source of tumor cells may be autologous (tumor cells from patient itself) or allogenic (tumor cells obtained from other individual). When these tumor cells are injected into the body, it elicits a specific immune response. The immune response acts against tumor cells. These vaccines are studied in tumors such as melanoma, carcinomas of colorectal, kidney, ovary, breast, and lung and leukemia.

***Dendritic cell vaccines*:** Discussed previously on page 503 (above) under dendritic cells in cancer therapy. These vaccines are studied in tumors of prostate, breast, lung, colorectal, kidney, melanoma, leukemia, and non-Hodgkin lymphoma.

***Antigen vaccines*:** This includes peptide vaccines in which only one specific epitope is injected into individual with cancer. It is possible to create vast amounts of antigen in laboratories. Some antigens are specific for a certain type of cancer, whereas other antigens may induce an immune response in several cancers. These vaccines are studied in cancers of kidney, pancreas, ovary, breast, prostate, and colorectal, and melanoma.

Anti-idiotype vaccines: These vaccines are based on the phenomenon that antibodies can also act as antigens and trigger an immune response. This principle is used to produce a vaccine in which the antibodies (that resemble the cancer cells) would be injected into the patient with cancer to elicit an immune response and thereby destroy tumor cells. It is mainly studied in lymphoma.

DNA vaccines: In this method of vaccination, tumor genes are introduced instead of tumor antigen. Cells in the body take up the injected DNA and specific antigens would be produced continuously. The advantage of this constant supply of antigens allows the immune response to continue against the cancer. These vaccines are studied in cancer of prostate and head and neck region, in leukemia, and melanoma.

Immune checkpoint and immune checkpoint therapy/ inhibitors is discussed on pages 498–500.

Oncolytic viruses: Oncolytic viruses are viruses that preferentially infect and destroy cancer cells. The preferences of oncolytic viruses for cancer cells compared to normal cells is due to faster proliferation of cells and are preferable targets for viral replication. Also, cancer cells frequently lose critical antiviral defense mechanisms (e.g., interferon response system disrupted in many transformed cells).

The eight hallmarks of cancer discussed above are acquired functional capabilities of cancer cells that allow them to survive, to proliferate, and to disseminate. The acquisition of these capabilities is made possible by two most prominent *enabling characteristics* or means:

1. Development of **genomic instability** in cancer cells and the resulting mutation of hallmark-enabling genes, and
2. **Inflammatory state** of premalignant and frankly malignant lesions by variety of cells of the innate and adaptive immune system.

Genome Instability and Mutation

Genomic Stability

The maintenance of genomic stability is necessary for integrity of cells. The cell genome is subject to routine DNA damage caused by errors from DNA replication during cell division, endogenous genotoxic stress (e.g., ROS) from byproducts of normal cellular metabolism, and exogenous environmental agents that are mutagenic or carcinogenic (e.g., ultraviolet light, ionizing radiation, or chemical carcinogens). These are usually repaired by the genetic surveillance mechanisms.

Genomic Instability

Q. Discuss genomic instability and cancers.

Oncogenesis involves many genetic changes and main among these is genomic instability or chromosomal instability (CI). Genome [genetic (or genomic)] instability refers to a high frequency of mutations within the genome of a cellular lineage. It is an increased tendency of genome alteration during cell division. Genomic instability disrupts the normal functioning of a cell. Genomic instability is a characteristic of most cancer cells and almost all the eight hallmarks in cancer are related to genetic mutation or genetic instability. Genetic mutation occurs due to copying errors during mitosis and also due to environmental agents such as radiation and chemicals. Cancer frequently results from succession of alterations in the genomes of neoplastic cells. These alterations involve genes that control cell division and tumor suppressors. Genetic instability may occur due to additions or deletions of entire chromosomes, or portions thereof and it gives rise to variable cellular karyotypes. Genetic instability may lead to **aneuploidy** (abnormal chromosome number), **gene amplification** (increased copy number of a gene) and **loss of heterozygosity** (loss of one allele out of a pair). LOH may be due to loss of a whole chromosome, deletion of a fraction of DNA bearing the particular gene or inactivation of that gene. When LOH occurs, the remaining allele is the only one for that locus and controls the phenotype. If this remaining normal allele is undergoes mutation (thereby renders it abnormal), the lack of this second allele the abnormal phenotype (of cancer cells) is unopposed.

Repair of DNA damage

The difference in DNA repair in normal cells and cancer cells.

Normal cells: Normal cells can sense and are extraordinarily able to repair many of the DNA damage (DNA mutations) through cellular DNA (genetic) maintenance machineries. In normal cells. genetic surveillance mechanisms can sense/ detect increased rates of mutation and resolve defects in the DNA. If the resulting DNA defects are not repaired, they can become cell-heritable mutations. However, irreparable genome damage forces genetically damaged cells into either quiescence, senescence (cell aging), or apoptosis (cell death). This ensures that the rates of such spontaneous mutations are usually kept very low in each cell generation and maintains the integrity of the genome.

Cancer cells: Cancer cells can compromise the cellular surveillance mechanisms in several different ways and can increase the rates of mutation.

- **Mutations:** Such higher rates of mutation are achieved through breaking down of genetic maintenance machinery and/or increased sensitivity to mutagenic agent. There are three types of DNA repair systems—(i) mismatch repair, (ii) nucleotide excision repair, and (iii) recombination repair. **Individuals born with inherited defects in any of these DNA repair genes are at greatly increased risk for the development of cancer.** They are discussed in detail on pages 514–527.
- **Epigenetic mechanisms:** Apart from DNA mutations, some epigenetic factors like DNA methylation and histone modifications without modifying the underlying DNA sequence of genes can alter the concentrations of proteins in cancer.

Cancer-enabling Inflammation

One of the basic features of cancer is Infiltration or invasion into the surrounding tissue. This elicits a chronic inflammatory reaction similar to that observed in wound healing.

Tumor-promoting Immune Infiltration (Inflammation)

It is the second important means by which developing cancers can acquire hallmark capabilities. The developing tumors avoid immunological destruction by cells of the adaptive immune system, often by blocking infiltrating cytotoxic T cells.

Mechanisms Promoting Tumor

It is observed that most infiltrating cancers provoke a chronic inflammatory reaction. These cancers are also infiltrated by other cells of the immune system (so-called infiltrating immune cells/IICs) which function as mediators of inflammation. Such inflammation by IICs may represent failed attempts by the immune system to eradicate tumors. However, the IICs may promote cancer. Tumor-associated inflammatory responses can promote multiple steps of tumor progression. Thus, they may help cancers to acquire hallmark capabilities. Various cancer-promoting effects of inflammatory cells (e.g., cancer-associated fibroblasts and endothelial cells) and resident stromal cells are as follows:

- **Supplying bioactive molecules that promote proliferation:** Infiltrating leukocytes and activated stromal cells secrete a variety of growth factors (e.g., EGF), and proteases that can release growth factors from the ECM. They promote proliferation of tumor cells.
- **Removal of growth suppressors:** The growth of epithelial cells is suppressed by cell–cell and cell–ECM interactions. Inflammatory cells secrete proteases and degrade the adhesion molecules that mediate cell–cell and cell–ECM interactions. Thus, they remove growth barrier.
- **Increased resistance to cell death:** Detachment of epithelial cells from cell–cell interactions and basement membranes can cause a type of cell death called *anoikis* (refer pages 152–154). Tumor associated macrophages may prevent *anoikis* by expressing adhesion molecules such as integrins. They can promote direct physical interactions between the tumor cells. Interaction between the stromal cell and cancer cell can increase the resistance of cancer cells to chemotherapy. This may be through activation of signaling pathways that promote cell survival during the stresses such as DNA damage.
- **Stimulate angiogenesis:** Inflammatory cells release proangiogenic factors such as VEGF and stimulate angiogenesis.
- **Favor invasion and metastasis:** Proteases released from macrophages favor tissue invasion by remodeling the ECM. Factors such as TNF and EGF may directly stimulate movement of tumor cell. Factors such as TGF-β released from stromal cells may promote EMT. This may favor invasion and metastasis.
- **Evasion of immune destruction of tumor cells:** Soluble factors such as TGF-β released from macrophages and stromal cells may act as an immunosuppressive tumor microenvironment. They may either favor the recruitment of immunosuppressive T-regulatory cells or suppress the function of CD8+ cytotoxic T cells. Advanced cancers mainly contain alternatively activated (M2) macrophages. Cytokines secreted by M2 macrophages promote angiogenesis, proliferation of fibroblasts, and deposition of collagen. These are commonly observed in invasive cancers. Macrophages may also suppress effective host immune responses to cancer cells by expressing the immune checkpoint factor PD-L1 and by other mechanisms.
- **Release mutagenic chemicals:** Inflammatory cells can release chemicals (e.g., ROS) that can be mutagenic for nearby cancer cells. This may accelerate the malignancy.

Consequences of Inflammatory Reaction

The inflammatory cells can also modify the tumor cells and the local microenvironment and enable many of the hallmarks of cancer. These effects may be either due to direct interactions between inflammatory cells and tumor cells, or through indirect effects of inflammatory cells on other resident stromal cells (particularly cancer-associated fibroblasts and endothelial cells). These include:

- **Systemic signs and symptoms:** In advanced cancers, this inflammatory reaction can be extensive and may produce systemic signs and symptoms. These include anemia (the so-called "anemia of chronic disease"), fatigue, and cachexia.
- **Enable hallmarks of cancer:** Inflammatory cells can also modify the tumor microenvironment to enable many of the hallmarks of cancer mentioned earlier.

Tumor Microenvironment (TME)

Three classes of stromal cell, namely—(i) angiogenic vascular cells (AVC), consisting of endothelial cells and pericytes, (ii) cancer-associated fibroblasts (CAF), and (iii) infiltrating immune (inflammatory) cells are the most important factors within the TME and facilitate tumor progression.

It is observed that most cancers contain distinct subpopulations of cancer cells with a greatly increased ability to seed new tumors. Such tumor-initiating cells (TICs) are termed cancer stem cells (CSCs). In contrast, the bulk of cells in most tumors, lack this tumor-initiating ability. CSCs usually proliferate relatively slowly and often express the distinctive cell-surface markers of tissue stem cells. Therapeutic targeting of these CSCs may be crucial to achieving enduring cancer therapies.

Therapies directed at tumor-induced inflammation and its downstream consequences: Example, one of therapy used is antiinflammatory cyclooxygenase-2 (COX-2) inhibitors. They decrease the incidence of colonic adenomas and useful in patients with familial adenomatous polyposis.

AUTOPHAGY IN CANCER

Q. Write a short essay on autophagy in cancer.

Autophagy is a cellular catabolic degradation process of recycling and removing, mostly of cellular constituents. The cellular proteins, organelles, and cytoplasm are engulfed, digested, and recycled to sustain cellular metabolism. Autophagy was also found to be an important cellular response for generation of energy and amino acids needed during cellular stress (e.g., starvation, infection). In severe nutrient deficiency, autophagy can arrest the cell growth and also digest their own organelles, proteins, and membranes and can be used as carbon sources for energy production (refer pages 156–159). If this adaptation fails, the cells can die. Autophagy is also utilized for the elimination of pathogens and for the degradation of apoptotic cells.

Autophagy is closely regulated in cancer cells. The role of autophagy in the development and progression of cancer is complex and represents a double-edged sword. The connection between autophagy and cancer is not fully understood. Tumor cells usually are able to grow under marginal environmental conditions without stimulating autophagy. This points out that the pathways that induce autophagy may be deranged in cancer. Considerable autophagy may occur in tumors that experience episodic depletion of energy and metabolic substrates.

Oxidative Stress and Autophagy

Autophagy recognizes and removes oxidant damaged cell proteins and organelles. If autophagy is impaired, oxidant injury accumulates and may lead to two important consequences.

- Cellular molecules damaged by oxidant injury can accumulate, aggregate, and produce further oxidant injury. This increases the possibility of **increased rate of DNA mutation and can lead to genomic instability**. Accumulation of damaged cell constituents depends on the autophagy-related protein, p62. Without p62, the oxidized aggregates do not form and do not produce genetic damage. p62 is mainly involved in tumorigenesis and is overexpressed in many human tumors.
- If autophagy is impaired, accumulation of damaged and damaging cell components will lead to cell death. Cell death may be by apoptosis or necrosis. A common cellular response to metabolic stress is cell death by apoptosis. In cancer cells, apoptosis is crucial for suppressing tumorigenesis. p53-dependent apoptosis needs intact process of autophagy. With **impaired autophagy**, **the cell dies**, not by apoptosis, but **by necrosis**. Unlike apoptosis, necrotic cells evoke inflammatory responses, including TAMs that help further tumorigenesis.

Autophagy can influence cancer development, progression, and response to therapy.

Dual and Context-specific Role for Autophagy in Cancer

It is not clear whether autophagy is always bad or good from the point of the tumor. Autophagy may be a tumor's friend or enemy and it depends on how the signaling pathways that regulate it in a given tumor. Autophagy has a dual and context-specific role in cancer.

- **Tumor suppressive:** By preserving cell and tissue health, it can act as tumor suppressive in some circumstances.
- **Tumor promoting:** Autophagy can enable survival of cancer cells (and normal cells) in stress and in response to activation of some oncogenic pathways. Thus, in such situations, autophagy can promote tumor. Autophagy is required for tumor cells to survive metabolic stress.

Autophagy-mediated Tumor Suppression

The protein and organelle quality control function of autophagy plays an important role not only in maintaining tissue health but also suppresses cancer. If there is failure of this function, the accumulated "cellular garbage" is ultimately likely to be prone to develop tumor.

Mechanism of tumor suppression by autophagy: It may be due to—(i) degradation of oncogenic proteins, (ii) suppression of cell death, (iii) inflammation, and chronic tissue damage, and (iv) prevention of mutations and genetic instability.

Genes involved

- Several **autophagy genes** [e.g., essentially beclin-1 and some autophagy-related (*Atg/atg*) genes] that promote autophagy can behave as **tumor suppressors**. They may be deleted or mutated in many tumors. Key activator of autophagy, i.e., *Beclin-1* (*Atg6*), is the gene most commonly mutated or lost in human cancers (e.g., breast, ovarian, and prostate cancers). Overexpression of Beclin-1 reduces the tumorigenicity of human cancer cell lines.
- **Many tumor suppressors**, such as PTEN and the tuberous sclerosis proteins (TSC1, TSC2), **facilitate autophagy**. Main tumor suppressor, **p53**, can **either stimulate** autophagy in some ways **or inhibit** by other ways. Impaired function of the tumor suppressor of autophagy may result in accumulation of materials within the cell that produce chromosomal instability. This can lead to development of cancer.

Pathogenesis of liver cancer due to autophagy defects (Figs. 80A and B)

Deficient autophagy*: Cancer initiation** in the liver probably starts with deficiency in autophagy-related (*Atg5* or *7*) genes or mutation in *beclin1* (thereby producing deficient autophagy). It produces fatty liver disease (steatosis) and causes accumulation of abnormal mitochondria, the autophagy substrate p62, and p62- and ubiquitin-modified protein aggregates. These **p62 aggregates are also called as *Mallory-Denk bodies, which are characteristic of liver disease (e.g., alcoholic hepatitis) and hepatocellular carcinoma. p62 is a signaling adaptor protein that can activate cancer-promoting pathways.

***Activation of pro-oncogenic pathways*:** If the autophagy substrate p62 is degraded, there is tumor suppression in the liver and it does not produce genetic damage.

- The **deregulated levels of p62** due to deficient autophagy can activate the transcriptional factors Nrf2 (nuclear factor erythroid 2-related factor 2) and NFκB (nuclear factor-κB). This can promote the **activation of pro-oncogenic pathways**.
- **Activation of pro-oncogenic pathways by p62:** It can activate transcriptional factors Nrf2 and NFκB.
  - **Activation of Nrf2:** p62 binds Keap1 (Kelch Like ECH Associated Protein 1) which is the negative regulator of Nrf2. This results in activation of transcription factor Nrf2 as well as upregulation of transcription of antioxidant defense genes (promotes survival of cells to oxidative stress).
  - **Activation of NFκB:** p62 also interacts with TRAF6 (TNF Receptor Associated Factor 6) and promotes NFκB activation.

***Genetic damage due to deficient autophagy*:** It has been observed that autophagy-deficient tumor cells have an increased mutation rate, chromosome copy number variations, and genome instability when compared to autophagy-functional tumor cells. Thus, mechanism of tumor suppression is most likely by autophagy preventing genetic instability. Thus, stimulation of autophagy may be beneficial for prevention of cancer and is also the mechanism behind the health benefits

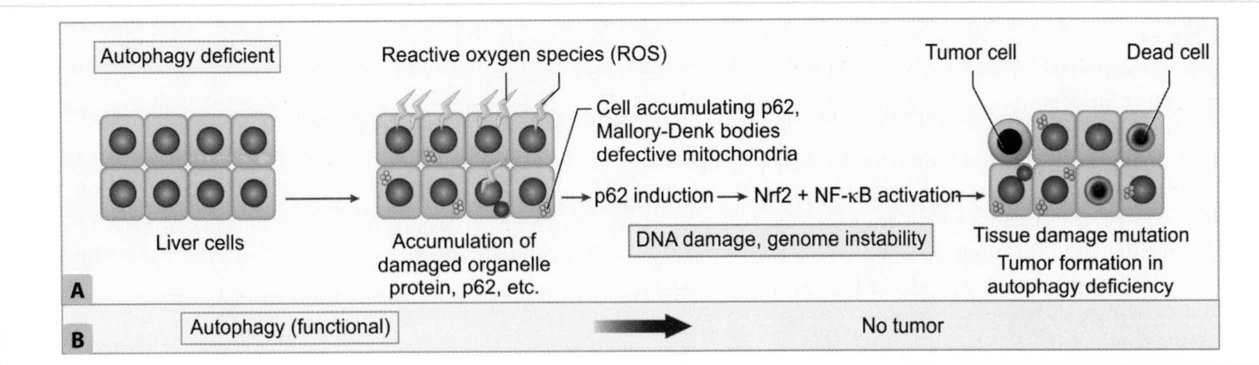

FIGS. 80A AND B: Tumor suppression by autophagy. (A) Tumor develops in cells with deficient autophagy. (B) Tumor suppression may be seen in cells with autophagy-proficient tumor cells (refer text for description).

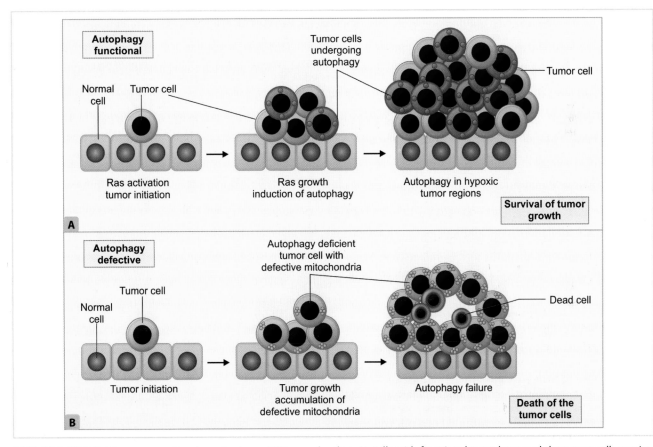

FIGS. 81A AND B: Tumor promotion by autophagy. (A)Tumor develops in cells with functional autophagy and the tumor cells survive, thereby promoting tumor growth. (B) In autophagy defective tumors, there is accumulation of defective mitochondria and these tumor cells undergo death.

of caloric restriction, fasting, and exercise that promote autophagy.

Autophagy and chemoprevention: Several oncogenic proteins (e.g., AKT, Bcl-2, mTOR) can **impair autophagy**. Thus, autophagy may be an antioncogenic process. Cancer prevention by promoting autophagy may be clinically beneficial. As autophagy is needed for the effective management of metabolic stress, promoting autophagy through mTOR inhibition may limit tumor progression.

Tumor Promotion by Autophagy (Figs. 81A and B)

Normal cells and tissues need autophagy to sustain metabolism in starvation. Tumor cells also require autophagy for survival. However, tumor cells usually reside in a metabolically stressed environment, their requirement for autophagy is increased more than in normal cells. For example, autophagy requirement is more for survival of tumor cells that are found in hypoxic region of tumor regions (usually in the center of the tumor). In response to metabolic stress, the tumor cells deficient for autophagy have decreased survival than autophagy-proficient tumor cells. Stressed, autophagy-deficient tumor cells die by necrosis or apoptosis.

Activation of oncogenic pathways promotes cell growth to form tumor and also raise metabolic demand of cells. Tumor cells meet this increased metabolic demand probably by increasing autophagy. High basal autophagy is a common characteristic of human cancer cell lines having activated oncogenic *H-ras* or *K-ras* oncogenes. Examples include human pancreatic cancer cells and tumors that have a high prevalence of activating *K-ras* mutations. Activated Ras causes tumorigenicity and high basal autophagy (**Fig. 81A**). High levels of autophagosomes were found in some aggressive human tumors. High basal autophagy in Ras-driven cancers is needed for survival in stress as well as for tumorigenesis.

Autophagy addiction: Cancer cells can be addicted to autophagy to survive stress and sustain tumor growth. This property can be made of use to improve cancer therapy by inhibiting autophagy.

Analysis of cancer cells and tumors with and without autophagy revealed the possible mechanism of autophagy addiction.

- **Tumor cell with functional autophagy** has functional mitochondria. This functional pool of mitochondria is required for efficient tumor growth. Hence, the **tumor progresses**. Though tumors upregulate glycolytic metabolism, they still need functional mitochondria for anabolic purposes (e.g., citrate production for lipid and new membrane synthesis) and to produce signaling levels of ROS needed for tumor growth.
- **Tumor cells with deficient autophagy (Fig. 81B)** accumulate defective mitochondria. The mitochondria from autophagy-deficient tumor cells are morphologically abnormal and show aberrant ROS production, reduced respiration, and depletion of citric acid cycle [tricarboxylic acid (TCA)] cycle metabolites in starvation.

Role of Autophagy in Cancer Therapy

The survival-promoting function of autophagy in stressed tumor cells and the autophagy addiction of Ras-driven cancers suggests that inhibition of autophagy may be a useful approach to enhance cancer therapy. Most anticancer therapies induce autophagy, either indirectly because they are cytotoxic, or directly because they block pathways that inhibit autophagy (e.g., those upstream of mTOR), and even mTOR itself. This has suggested that therapeutic autophagy induction in combination with autophagy inhibition may enhance efficacy of cancer therapy. Combining autophagy inhibition with nutritional stress or targeted metabolic inhibitors may also be a promising approach for therapy.

Autophagy and Tumor Dormancy

Tumor cells during severe nutrient deprivation or lack of oxygen due to therapy or insufficient blood supply, may use autophagy to become "dormant." This allows the cancer cells to survive nutrient deprivation for long periods and autophagy protects cancer cells and also cause relapse. Such cancer cells may be resistant to therapies that kill actively dividing cells (e.g., chemotherapy, radiotherapy) and can be the cause for therapeutic failures. Thus, autophagy may allow residual or metastasizing tumor cells to tolerate metabolic deprivation. These cells may recover once growth conditions are favorable.

RECEPTORS IN CANCER

Tyrosine Kinase and Tyrosine Kinases Receptor

Q. Write short essay on tyrosine kinase and tyrosine kinases receptor.

Tyrosine kinases are a family of enzymes and are important mediators of the signaling cascade. Tyrosine kinases catalyze phosphorylation of select tyrosine residues in target proteins, using ATP (adenosine triphosphate). They have central roles in different biological processes such as growth, differentiation, metabolism and apoptosis in response to external and internal stimuli.

Biochemical Mechanism of Tyrosine Kinase Activation

Tyrosine kinases are enzymes which phosphorylates tyrosine residue in different substrates.

Types of tyrosine kinase: Tyrosine kinases are mainly classified as (i) receptor protein-tyrosine kinases (RTKs) and (ii) nonreceptor or cytoplasmic protein-tyrosine kinases.

Receptor protein-tyrosine kinases (RTKs) (refer Fig. 4 of Chapter 2): Receptor tyrosine kinases are transmembrane receptors. These RTKs are activated when ligand bind to their extracellular domain. Ligands are extracellular signal molecules and examples of ligands for receptor tyrosine kinase (RTK) include epidermal growth factor (EGF), insulin-like growth factor (IGF1), platelet-derived growth factor (PDGF), fibroblast growth factor (FGF), vascular endothelial growth factor (VEGF), and macrophage-colony-stimulating factor (MCSF). The receptor tyrosine kinase are not only cell surface transmembrane receptors, but are also enzymes having kinase activity. The binding of ligands with RTKs induce receptor dimerization (except Insulin receptor). One ligand may bind with two receptor molecules to form 1:2 ligands: receptor complex (e.g., growth hormone and growth hormone receptor) or two ligands may bind simultaneously to two receptors 2:2 ligand receptor complex (simplest mechanism of receptor dimerization e.g., VEGF and VEGFR). It brings transmembrane segments of receptor and their cytosolic domains (regions) close together. This activates the tyrosine kinase domain and leads to phosphorylation of tyrosine side chains on the cytosolic part of the receptor. The phosphorylation leads to a conformational change in the activation loop that unblocks kinase activity. The resulting enhanced activity of kinase can then phosphorylate additional tyrosine residues in the cytosolic domain of the receptor. The protein kinases phosphorylate specific tyrosine residues of cytoplasmic substrate proteins which binds to sites for various intracellular signaling proteins that relay the signal. The phosphorylation alters the activity, localization, or ability of these substrate proteins to interact with other proteins within the cell.

Nonreceptor or cytoplasmic protein-tyrosine kinases: Nonreceptor tyrosine kinase (NRTK) are cytoplasmic proteins and they show considerable structural variability. The NRTK have a kinase domain and usually have many additional signaling or protein-protein interacting domains (e.g., SH2, SH3 and the PH domain). Examples of non-receptor tyrosine kinase are SRC, ABL, FAK and Janus kinase.

Oncogenic Activation of Tyrosine Kinase

Receptor protein-tyrosine kinases

Normally, cellular tyrosine kinase phosphorylation is tightly controlled by the antagonizing effect of tyrosine kinase and tyrosine phosphatases. This prevents deregulated proliferation. Tyrosine kinases are also involved in the pathophysiology of cancer. Dysregulation of RTK signaling can lead to cancers. It has been observed that various alterations in the genes encoding RTKs such as EGFR, HER2/ErbB2, and MET, is found in cancers. Tyrosine kinase are implicated in several steps of neoplastic development and progression. These signaling pathways may be genetically (e.g., mutation/s, overexpression) or epigenetically altered leading to cancer cells. These alterations provide an oncoprotein status to tyrosine kinase enzymes. This results in the constitutive activation of normally controlled pathways. This in turn leads to the activation of other signaling proteins and secondary messengers and hamper the regulatory functions in cellular responses like cell division, growth and cell death. The tyrosine kinases oncoprotein play a transforming role in many cancers.

Activation by gain-of-function mutations: An important mechanism leading to tyrosine kinase deregulation is gain-of-function mutation in RTK. This leads to abnormal downstream signal transduction that is not subjected to the normal 'checks and balances' that occur with physiological signaling. Overexpression of RTKs has been found in a variety of human cancers.

Mutations within the extracellular domain can produce constitutive activation of receptor tyrosine kinase (hyperactivate the kinase) and subsequently, its downstream signaling. This leads to cell proliferation in the absence of ligand. Examples include:

a. Mutation in epidermal growth factor receptor (EGFR- one of the RTK) is found in glioblastomas, ovarian tumors, non-small cell lung carcinoma and cancers of esophagus and thyroid. Somatic mutations in the EGFR 2 and 3 are associated with human bladder and cervical carcinomas. It was observed that tumors that have activating somatic EGFR mutations are uniquely sensitive to treatment with EGFR tyrosine kinase inhibitors (TKIs).
b. HER2/ErbB2 mutations in lung, bladder, breast and gastric cancer.
c. MET mutations in lung and gastric cancer.
d. Point mutations in the extracellular domain of the FGFR 3 were identified in multiple myeloma.

Overexpression leads to increased local concentration of receptor. This results in elevated RTK signaling and overwhelms the antagonizing regulatory effects. Major mechanism which leads to overexpression of RTKs is by gene amplification. Additional mechanisms of RTK overexpression include transcriptional/translational enhancement, oncogenic viruses, loss of normal regulatory mechanisms such as loss of phosphatases or other negative regulators. Irrespective of the mechanism, overexpression of RTKs, it is associated with poor outcomes in some cancer patients (e.g., EGFR and HER2 in breast cancer).

Nonreceptor or cytoplasmic protein-tyrosine kinases

Chromosomal translocations: BCR-ABL and human leukemia: Many non-receptor tyrosine kinases function as signal transduction molecules. One of the classical example with respect to carcinogenesis is ABL. Tyrosine-protein kinase ABL is encoded by the *ABL* gene. The ABL proto-oncoprotein has tyrosine kinase activity that is reduced by internal negative regulatory domains. In chronic myeloid leukemia (CML) and certain acute lymphoblastic leukemias, a part of the *ABL* gene is translocated from its normal position on chromosome 9 to chromosome 22 t(9,22). In chromosome 22 (Philadelphia Chromosome), ABL fuses with part of the *BCR* gene. This results in a fusion gene that encodes BCR-ABL hybrid protein. This hybrid protein contains the ABL tyrosine kinase domain and a BCR domain and produces constitutive activation of tyrosine kinase. The *BCR-ABL* chimeric gene product has a tyrosine kinase activity several times higher than its normal counterpart. BCR-ABL protein activates all the downstream signals of RAS and strongly stimulates cell growth.

TEL-ABL and human leukemia: TEL-ABL (ETV6-ABL1) tyrosine kinase is a rare aberration found in a few hematological malignancies. Similar to ABL-BCR, TEL-ABL is constitutively phosphorylated. It may be due to reciprocal translocation t(9,12) in case of ALL and with a complex karyotype t(9,12,14) in patients with CML. TEL (supposed to be a transcription factor) fuses with ABL proto-oncogene and produces a fusion protein product with elevated tyrosine kinase activity.

Other chromosomal translocations: These include t(5,12) in chronic myelomonocytic leukemia (CMML) producing TEL-PDGF receptor. NPM-ALK fusion products t(2,5) is constitutively activated in anaplastic large cell lymphoma.

Tyrosine Kinases as Targets for Anticancer Agents

RTKs play a central role in the molecular pathogenesis of cancer. Hence, targeting oncogenic driver mutations of RTKs by anticancer drugs has revolutionized the treatment of cancer. Constitutive oncogenic activation in cancer cells can be blocked by selective tyrosine kinase inhibitors. Thus, it may be a promising approach for innovative genome based therapeutics.

The first tyrosine kinase inhibitor developed and approved was imatinib. It targets the ABL kinase and has revolutionized the treatment of patients with CML. Tyrosine kinase inhibitors are well documented in therapy such as Gleevec, Iressa and Herceptin. There are many monoclonal antibodies that interfere with RTK activation. These include cetuximab in lung cancer, panitumumab in colon cancer, cetuximab in head and neck cancer, trastuzumab and pertuzumab in breast cancer. In spite of present day advances, acquired resistance to targeted therapies inevitably develops. Acquired resistance may be due to either acquired genomic alterations or activation of critical signaling pathways. Efforts are made to personalised cancer therapeutics.

BRAF Mutations

Q. Write short essay on BRAF mutations.

BRAF Gene

BRAF gene is located on the long arm of chromosome 7 (7q34). It codes for the serine/threonine protein kinase, B-Raf. B-Raf is a member of the Raf kinase family and is a downstream target of RAS (**Fig. 82**). B-Raf plays a main role in the MAPK/ERK signaling pathway.

Mutations in BRAF

It a member of the RAF family. BRAF is a serine/threonine protein kinase and is in the top of RAS/MAPK cascade.

- *Tumors with BRAF mutation (**Fig. 83**)*: It is observed in almost 100% of hairy cell leukemias, 60% of melanomas, 80% of benign nevi, and a lesser percentage in other neoplasms (e.g., colon carcinomas, papillary thyroid carcinoma and dendritic cell tumors [Langerhans cell histiocytosis]). Activating mutations in BRAF was found in melanoma with the specific V600E mutation being the most common. BRAF mutations was identified in about 14% of non-small-cell lung carcinoma (NSCLC) with V600E and non-V600E mutations showing relatively equal frequency.

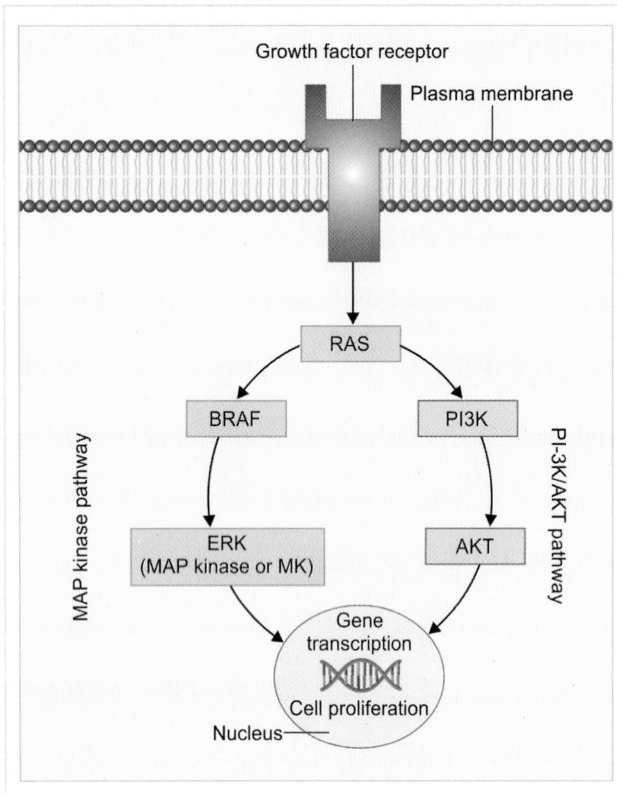

FIG. 82: Pathway of BRAF.

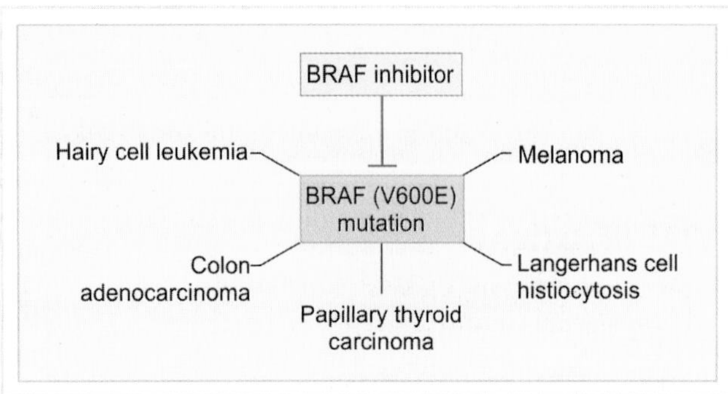

FIG. 83: Different tumors with BRAF mutations.

Point mutations of the *BRAF* gene can be seen in up to 70% of papillary thyroid cancers (PTC). **The most prevalent mutation, the point mutation T1799A in BRAF. It results in an amino acid substitution of a valine to glutamine (BRAF V600E) in the BRAF protein. This increases its basal kinase activity.** There are distinct differences between *BRAF* positive and *BRAF*-negative PTC. This suggests that *BRAF* mutations can be used as a molecular prognostic factor. BRAF proteins with a V600E or other substitutions at the V600 site are characterized by more than 200-fold induction of kinase activity in vitro compared to the wild-type BRAF. The BRAFV600E mutation can be found in some types of microcarcinoma.

- *Action*: Similar to RAS mutations, activating mutations in BRAF stimulate downstream kinases and activate transcription factors.

Mutations in other MAPK family members downstream of BRAF are not common in cancer.

Category of BRAF mutations: More recently, BRAF mutations are further categorized depending on their mechanisms for activation of the MAPK pathway.

1. Class-1: Constitutive active RAS-independent monomer with high BRAF kinase activity involving codon 600.
2. Class-2: Constitutive active RAS-independent dimers with high or intermediate BRAF kinase activity involving codons outside 600, including BRAF fusion mutants.
3. Class-3: Low or no BRAF kinase activity mutations.

New techniques for the molecular analysis of tumors have indicated that the most important part of the work-up of a cancer sample is the identification of molecular targets, rather than histopathologic diagnosis. For example, many histopathologically distinct cancers may harbor the same gain-of-function mutation in the serine/threonine kinase BRAF, a component of the RAS signaling pathway. From these observation, we may think that these diverse "BRAFomas" may be treated with BRAF inhibitors. However, clinical studies found that the effectiveness of BRAF inhibitors widely depending on histologic subtype. The reasons are not clear. For example, hairy cell leukemias with BRAF mutations usually produce show sustained responses, melanomas respond transiently, and colon carcinomas respond little, if at all. These variations, stress the need for the morphologic diagnosis. An example of a treatment based only on molecular features is the use of checkpoint inhibitors in patients with recurrent and metastatic tumors due to defects in mismatch repair genes and not on histopathological findings. However, histopathological examination provides information about other important cancer characteristics (e.g., anaplasia, invasiveness, and tumor heterogeneity). Histopathological examination along with in situ biomarker tests on tissue sections is the best way to assess tumor–stromal cell interactions (e.g., angiogenesis and host immune responses). The host immune responses are assuming increasingly important role in guiding therapeutic interventions that are used to counteract immune evasion by tumors. Thus, it is not the replacement of one set of techniques by another. In future, the most accurate diagnosis and assessment of prognosis in cancer patients will be decided depending on a combination of morphologic and molecular techniques.

Currently, multiple BRAF inhibitors are available with specific targeted affinity for the V600E mutation of BRAF.

Bruton Tyrosine Kinase Gene

Q. Write short essay on Bruton Tyrosine Kinase Gene.

The *BTK* gene encodes for a protein tyrosine kinase called Bruton tyrosine kinase (BTK). *BTK* gene is located on the long arm of the X chromosome at Xq21.22. BTK protein is associated with the pre-BCR and with the B-cell receptor (BCR) complexes that are observed on mature B cells. BTK transduces signals from the pre-B and BCR. When BTK is mutated, the pre-B cell receptor (pre-BCR) cannot deliver the signals that are needed for light chain rearrangement. This leads to arrest of B cell maturation. **Bruton tyrosine kinase regulates B-cell maturation and proliferation. It is** involved in pre-B cell maturation. **BTK is a member of the Tec family of nonreceptor tyrosine kinases (i.e.,** cytoplasmic protein tyrosine kinase). **BTK mediates signaling from a number of receptors, including B- and T-cell receptors.** BTK is also an important transducer of BCR signals that stimulate growth and increase cell survival in benign and malignant mature B cells. The inhibitors of BTK are effective therapies for several B cell malignancies.

- *Congenital X-linked agammaglobulinemia*: It is characterized by a failure of B-cell maturation and development (no mature B cells, <1% of normal) and absence of antibodies (agammaglobulinemia). It is caused due to loss-of-function mutations in the *BTK* gene. **They suffer from recurrent bacterial infections. Without functional BTK, development of B-cell in the bone marrow is arrested and they express the pre-BCR. In these patients, the B cells remain in the pre-B stage.**
- Chronic lymphocytic leukemia: In many CLL patients, CLL cells depend on B-cell receptor signaling and BTK activity for their growth and survival. In CLL, BTK inhibitors inhibit B- cell receptor signaling and produce sustained therapeutic responses.
- *Lymphoplasmacytic lymphoma*: It is an indolent disorder. Like other indolent B-cell tumors, it responds very well to BTK inhibitors. This indicates dependence of the tumor cells on the B-cell receptor signaling pathway.

A recent advance in the treatment of CLL has been the discovery and targeting of the BTK pathway. BTK is an essential component of B-cell-receptor signalling, mediates interactions with the tumour microenvironment, and promotes the survival and proliferation of CLL cells. **Ibrutinib, a** first-in-class **selective BTK inhibitor, has shown very good results in the treatment of a variety of B-cell–associated cancers including CLL, Waldenstrom macroglobulinemia, mantle cell lymphoma, and marginal zone lymphoma.**

KIT Gene

Q. Write short essay on *KIT (CD117)* gene.

CD117

CD117 is also known as KIT, receptor for KIT ligand and stem cell growth factor receptor (SCFR). CD117 (KIT) is a transmembrane protein receptor of tyrosine kinase family with tyrosine kinase activity (cytokine receptor). It is encoded by the *KIT* gene. Stem cell factor (SCF) is a cytokine growth factor expressed by a range of stromal cells and CD117 (KIT) is the cognate (universal) receptor for stem cell factor (SCF).

Distribution of CD117 (KIT) receptor: It is widely distributed (expressed) on germ cells, hematopoietic stem cells, early hematopoietic progenitors and other tissue cells. KIT-dependent cell types include hematopoietic cells, germ cells, mast cells, melanoma cells and the gastrointestinal tract Cajal cells. About 66% of the germ cells and the sperm express KIT receptor. Hence, each type of germ cells can be isolated from human semen by using anti-CD117 monoclonal antibody. About 85% of the B cell progenitors also express KIT receptor, but it is gradually disappearing with cell differentiation and maturation. Thus, during cellular differentiation, expression of CD117 is lost in most cells but is retained on mature mast cells and melanocytes. The KIT receptor can also be found in skin appendages, the breast epithelial cells and the small neurons in the brain.

Functions of CD117: Cellular interaction (engagement) of CD117 by SCF increases a number of cytokine-dependent signaling pathways.

- *Physiological role*: It promotes a several functions in germ and stem cells. These include survival, proliferation, regulation of cell differentiation, resistance of cell apoptosis and migration.
- *Pathological role*: It plays a key role in tumor occurrence, development, migration and recurrence by the downstream signaling molecules. The abnormality of SCF/KIT signaling pathway is found in certain tumors.

Stem Cell Growth Factor

The ligand for KIT is stem cell factor (SCF). SCF is a growth factors and is also called KIT ligand. SCF is a hematopoietic cytokine produced in both soluble and membrane-bound forms. Following binding of SCF to CD117, these forms produce different quantitative and qualitative responses in target cell signaling. Membrane-bound SCF induces a much stronger stimulatory effect than soluble SCF. SCF plays an important role in maintaining the survival of hematopoietic cells, promoting hematopoietic cell proliferation and differentiation, and regulating growth and development of hematopoietic cells.

Signalling Pathway of KIT Receptor

KIT signaling plays a main role in several activities. These include regulation of the RBC production, lymphocyte proliferation, mast cell development and function, melanin formation, and gamete formation. Schematic structure of KIT is shown in **Figure 84**. The extracellular domain of KIT consists of five Ig-like domains (D1 to D5). Binding of SCF to KIT receptor induce homologous dimerization, and activates downstream signal transduction pathway. Subsequently, it regulates gene expression and cell growth, proliferation and differentiation. SCF/KIT downstream signal transduction pathways are very complex and may vary with the cell lines. Currently known signal transduction pathways are as follows:

1. *Ras/Erk signal transduction pathway*: It plays a very important role in cell differentiation and survival.
2. *PI3K signal transduction pathway*: This pathway regulates cell survival and angiogenesis.
3. PLC-γ signaling transduction pathway.

KIT Receptor Mutation in Tumors

Gain of function mutations in KIT is observed in some tumors (**Box 12**). These include point mutation, deletion, duplication

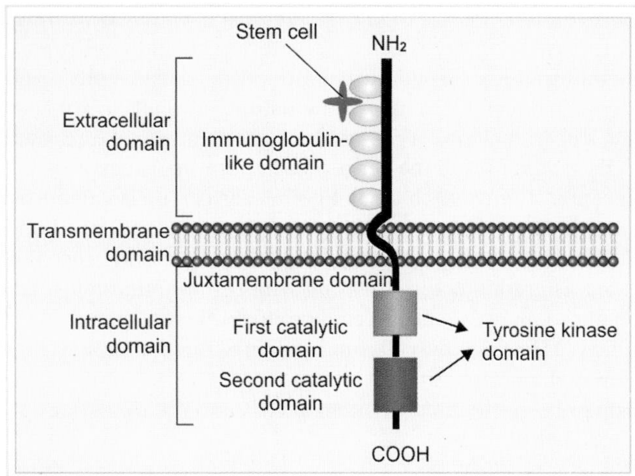

FIG. 84: Structure of KIT (diagrammatic). The extracellular domain consists of five Ig-like domains (D1–D5). The intracellular domain consists of tyrosine kinase domain that is split into two parts by amino acid sequence.

and insertion and can lead to KIT receptor activation. Systemic mastocytosis (increased numbers of mast cells in the skin and, in some instances, in other organs) is a distinctive neoplasm that is associated with mutations in the KIT tyrosine kinase. In addition, the paracrine or autocrine activation of KIT receptor may be found in many other malignancies, such as ovarian cancer, small cell lung cancer and other tumors. Immunohistochemically **CD117 (KIT) is a diagnostic marker used in tumors listed in Box 12.**

Loss of function mutations are associated with the genetic defect called piebaldism. The *KIT* gene mutations in piebaldism lead to a non-functional KIT protein. The loss of KIT signaling disrupt the growth and division (proliferation) and movement (migration) of melanocytes during development, resulting in patches of skin that lack pigmentation.

The KIT is used as a target for tumor treatment. Many cases of GIST respond to tyrosine kinase inhibitor imatinib. Seminomas and leukemias are not inhibited by imatinib and other inhibitors such as dasatinib and nilotinb can be utilized.

Box 12: Tumors associated with gain of function mutations in KIT (%).

- Gastrointestinal stromal tumors (GIST) (>90%)
- Systemic mastocytosis (>90%)
- Nasal T-cell lymphomas (>17%)
- Seminoma/dysgerminoma (> 9%)
- Acute myeloid leukemia (>68%)
- Melanoma
- Other tumors: Lung, breast, endometrium, urinary bladder

Retinoic Acid Receptor

Q. Write a short essay on retinoic acid receptor in cancer.

The retinoic acid receptors include two distinct families, namely retinoic acid receptors (RAR) and retinoid X receptors (RXR). Each family of receptor contains three subtypes—α, β, and γ; all of them can have multiple isoforms, leading to large numbers of possible receptor combinations. They are important regulators of embryonic development and also influence the growth and differentiation of adult cell types.

Ligand

Nuclear retinoic acid receptors mediate most of the effects of **retinoids.** Retinoic acid is synthesized from vitamin A (retinol) and found in embryos and adult vertebrates. Because humans are not able to produce vitamin A, they obtain vitamin A in the form of carotenoids from plants or retinyl esters derived from animal products. The retinoids are the natural derivatives and synthetic analogs of vitamin A. Thus, it includes parent compound retinol, naturally occurring retinoids [e.g., all-trans retinoic acid (ATRA) and 13-cis-retinoic acid] and synthetic retinoids [e.g., etretinate and fenretinide (4-hydroxyphenyl) retinamide or 4HPR]. Retinoids induce the differentiation of various types of stem cells.

Signaling

Retinoic acid functions to regulate gene expression. In cells, retinoic acid enters the nucleus and binds to **two different classes of nuclear receptors—RARs and RXRs**. The receptors are bound to a specific DNA sequence known as the retinoic acid-response element (RARE). Binding of retinoic acid to retinoic acid receptors recruits coactivators (including HAT), leading to transcription activation of specific retinoic acid-regulated genes.

Retinoic Acid Receptor in Cancer

- **Retinoid signaling is often compromised early in carcinogenesis**. This suggests the possibility that a reduction in retinoid signaling may be needed for the development of tumor.
- **Actions of retinoids:** Retinoids can **modulate cellular growth and differentiation as well as apoptosis**. Retinoids inhibit the promotion and progression phases of carcinogenesis and also in the premalignant lesions. Retinoids induce differentiation as well as arrest proliferation of various cancers.
- Epidemiological studies revealed that **lower intake of vitamin A can lead to a higher risk of developing cancer**. Retinoids suppress carcinogenesis in tumorigenic animal models for skin, oral, lung breast, bladder, ovarian, and prostate.
- **Retinoids have been used as potential chemotherapeutic or chemopreventive agents** because of their effect on differentiation and its antiproliferative, proapoptotic and antioxidant activities.
- Retinoids in cancer therapy
  - ATRA (all-*trans* retinoic acid) (tretinoin)
  - 9-cis-retinoic acid (alitretinoin): It differentiates itself from ATRA in its ability to activate both RAR and RXR. It can be effective in the prevention of mammary and prostate cancer.

Retinoids in acute promyelocytic leukemia (Figs. 85A to C)

Normally, when the retinoid binds RARα in the DNA of nucleus, it activates transcription. This leads to differentiation of myeloid progenitors into neutrophils.

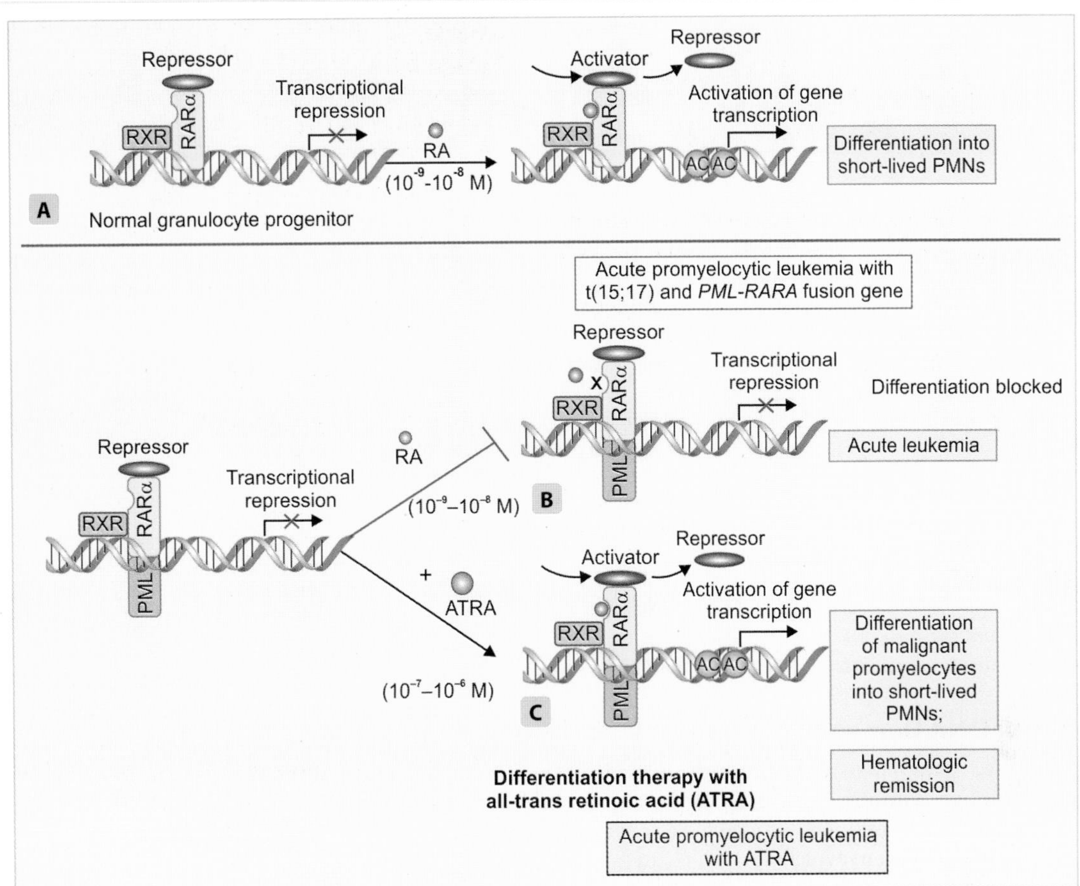

[PMN: polymorphonuclear neutrophil; RA: retinoic acid; RXR: binding partner for normal RARα and PML-RARα fusion protein encoded by a chimeric gene created by the (15;17) translocation in acute promyelocytic leukemia]

FIGS. 85A TO C: Retinoic acid receptor and molecular pathogenesis of acute promyelocytic leukemia *(PML)*. (A) Normal function of retinoic acid is to aid in the differentiation of mainly myeloid precursors in bone marrow. (B) In acute promyelocytic leukemia, translocation t(15;17) results in a *PML*-RARα fusion gene. Its product blocks differentiation of myeloid precursors. (C) When all-*trans* retinoic acid (ATRA) is given, it promotes the differentiation of neoplastic myeloid progenitors into neutrophils and die. This is termed as differentiation therapy.

- **Reciprocal translocation:** APML (acute promyelocytic leukemia) is almost always associated with a reciprocal translocation in which the promyelocytic leukemia gene (*PML*) on chromosome 15 fuses with the *RARα* gene on chromosome 17, i.e., t(15;17).
- **Consequences of reciprocal translocation:** The *PML*-RARα fusion gene encodes a chimeric protein (oncoprotein) consisting of part of a protein called PML and part of the RARα. The *PML*-RARα oncoprotein has reduced affinity for retinoids. Thus, at physiologic levels, these retinoids cannot significantly bind to *PML*-RARα. In this "unliganded" state, RARα can bind DNA, but instead of activating transcription, it inhibits transcription by recruiting transcriptional repressors. These repressor complexes epigenetically silence gene expression. This prevents the expression of genes that are required for differentiation of myeloid progenitors. This in turn leads to accumulation of proliferating myeloid progenitors and they replace normal bone marrow elements.
- **Differentiation therapy with retinoic acid:** When ATRA (all-*trans* retinoic acid) is administered in pharmacologic doses, it binds to *PML*-RARα and produces a conformational change in *PML*-RARα. This displaces the repressor complexes and recruits different complexes that activate transcription. It is also observed that ATRA-bound *PML*-RARα complexes are degraded more rapidly. These changes overpower the block in gene expression and promote the differentiation of neoplastic myeloid progenitors into neutrophils and die (similar to as normal mature neutrophils do). This allows recovery of normal hematopoiesis. Differentiation therapy with retinoic acid in combination with chemotherapy is used for the treatment of APML and can result in a 70–80% cure rate. This is the first example of effective **differentiation therapy**, in which immortal (living for ever) tumor cells are induced to differentiate into their mature progeny of limited lifespans.

10.4 Damage and Repair of DNA and Genomic instability

CHAPTER OUTLINE

- Damage of DNA
  - Mechanism of DNA damage
- DNA repair mechanisms
  - DNA repair pathways
  - Causes of DNA damage
  - Types of DNA damage
  - Methods of DNA repair
  - Double-strand Break Repair
- Genomic instability
  - Threat to DNA integrity
  - DNA mismatch repair factors
  - Nucleotide excision repair factors
  - Homologous recombination repair factors
  - Genetic instability due to defect in DNA repair genes

DAMAGE OF DNA

Q. Discuss DNA repair defects.
Q. Discuss mismatch repair and DNA repair defects.

Mechanism of DNA Damage

Natural processes can cause spontaneous mutations through DNA damage. Various types of DNA damage are presented in **Box 13**. DNA is frequently subjected to chemical and physical assaults. Different types of assaults that cause DNA damage include:

- **Depurination (Fig. 86):** This is characterized by hydrolysis of a purine base, A (adenine) or G (guanine), from the deoxyribose-phosphate backbone. This results in a **apurinic site** which cannot specify a complementary base. Hence, the DNA replication process introduces a random base opposite the apurinic site. This usually causes a mutation in the newly synthesized complementary strand.
- **Deamination (Fig. 87):** It is another naturally occurring process where there is removal of an amino ($-NH_2$) group from nitrogenous bases. This may modify DNA's information content. Deamination can change cytosine (C) to uracil (U), the nitrogenous base found in RNA but not in DNA. Since U pairs with A rather than G, deamination followed by replication may change a C–G base pair to a T–A pair in future generations of DNA molecules (e.g., C–G to T–A change is a transition mutation).

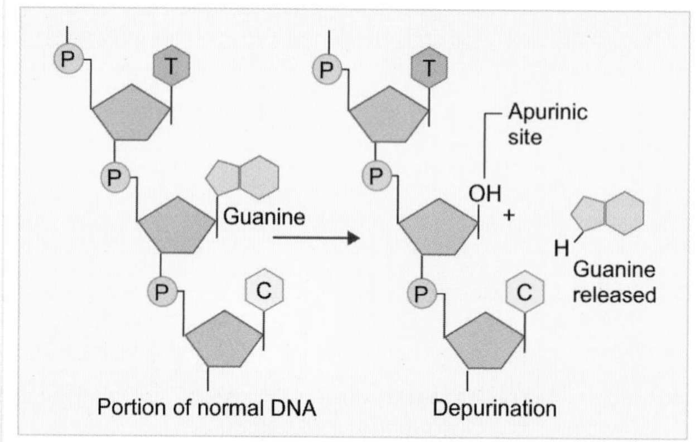

(C: cytosine base; P: phosphate backbone of DNA; T: Thymine base)

FIG. 86: Depurination. DNA contains purine bases namely adenine and guanine. In this type of DNA damage hydrolysis of A (adenine) or G (guanine) bases leaves a DNA strand with an unspecified base (apurinic site).

Box 13: Types of damage to DNA.

- Single-base alteration
- Two-base alteration: UV light-induced thymine-thymine (pyrimidine) dimer
- Chain breaks: Ionizing radiation, radioactive disintegration of backbone molecules, formation of oxygen free-radicals
- Cross-linkage
  - Between bases in same strands or opposite strands
  - Between DNA and protein molecules (e.g., histones)

- **Break of the sugar-phosphate backbone:** It occurs with radiation such as cosmic rays and X-rays (**Fig. 88**). X-rays break the sugar-phosphate backbone and split a DNA molecule into smaller pieces. These smaller pieces may be improperly ligated back together.
- **Thymine dimers:** These dimers can disrupt the readout of genetic information. When DNA is exposed to ultraviolet (UV) radiation, adjacent thymine residues (pyrimidines) on a DNA strand have a tendency to become chemically linked to another to form a covalent complex, that is, a **thymine dimer** (**Fig. 89**).
- **Oxidative damage to any of the four bases (Fig. 90):** Irradiation can produce free radicals (oxygen free radicals with an unpaired electron). They can alter individual bases.

If the above damages are not repaired before DNA replication, all these changes can permanently alter the information content of the DNA molecule.

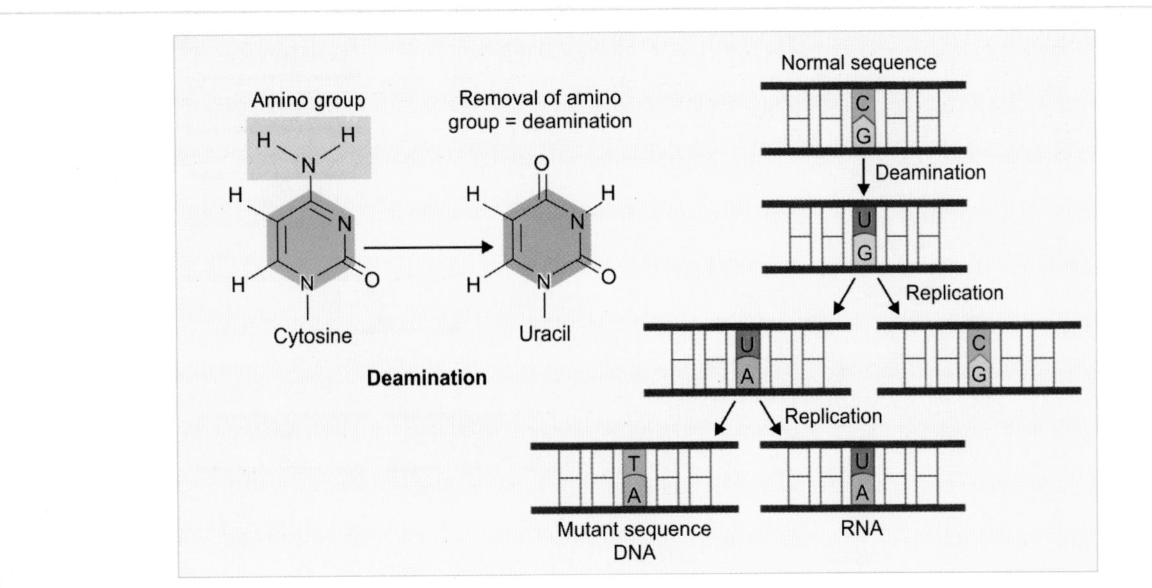

FIG. 87: Deamination. In this removal of an amino group from cytosine (C) initiates a process that causes a transition after DNA replication. Deamination can change cytosine (C) to uracil (U), the nitrogenous base found in RNA but not in DNA. Since U pairs with A rather than G (guanine), deamination followed by replication may change a C–G base pair to a T–A pair in future generations of DNA molecules.

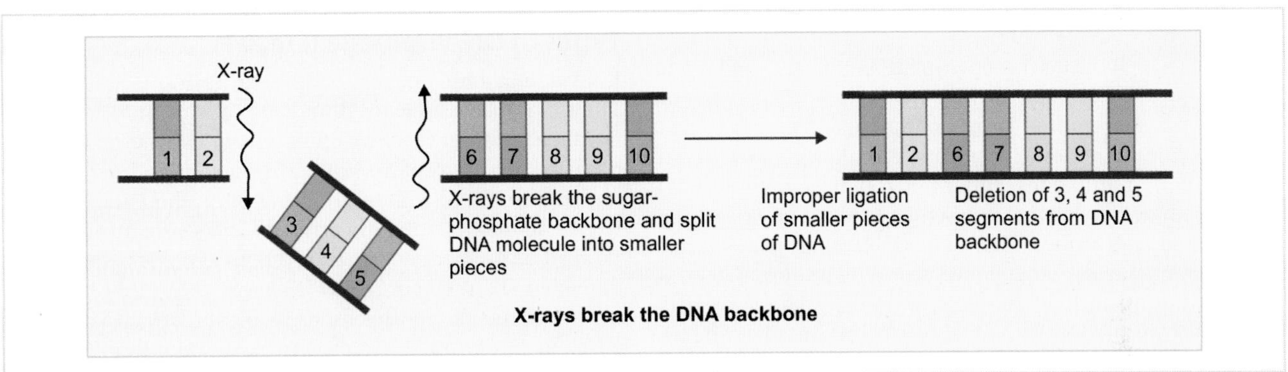

FIG. 88: Break of sugar-phosphate backbone. X-rays break the sugar-phosphate backbone and split a DNA molecule into smaller pieces. These smaller pieces may be improperly ligated back together.

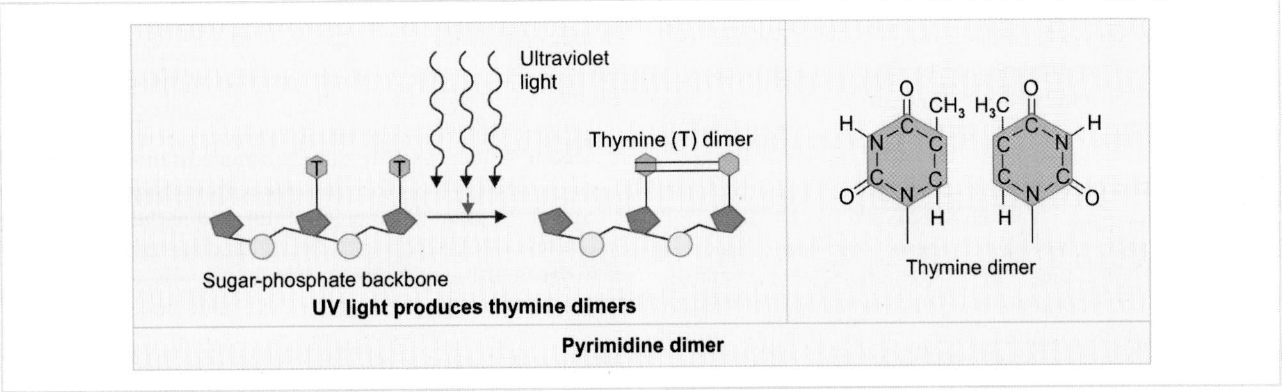

FIG. 89: Ultraviolet (UV) radiation causes adjacent thymines (Ts) to form dimers. Pyrimidine dimers are molecular lesions formed from thymine or cytosine bases in DNA.

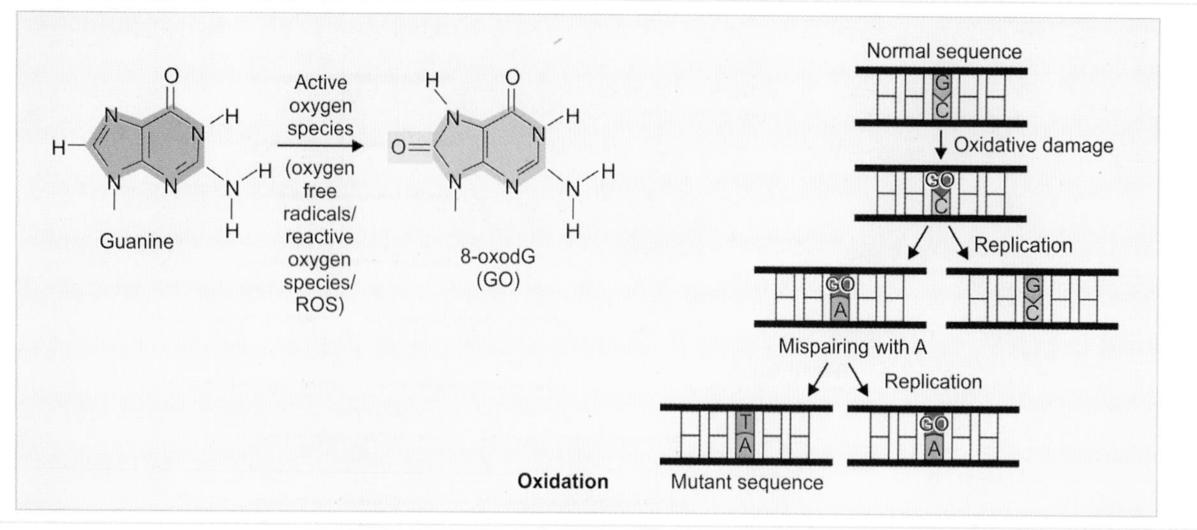

FIG. 90: Irradiation can produce free radicals (oxygen free radicals with an unpaired electron). They can alter individual bases. In this figure, the pairing of the altered base GO with A creates a transversion that changes a G–C base pair to T–A.

DNA REPAIR MECHANISMS

DNA Repair Pathways

Cells have mechanisms for repairing DNA damage, and repair systems can correct almost any type of damage to which a DNA molecule is susceptible. Repair of damaged DNA is critical for maintaining genomic integrity. Repair will prevent the propagation of mutations, either horizontally (somatic cells), or vertically (germ cells). It is essential to efficiently recognize and repair DNA lesions. Normally, DNA repair genes repair nonlethal damage in other genes including proto-oncogenes, tumor suppressor genes, and genes that regulate apoptosis. The majority of DNA repair mechanisms involve several enzymes. These include (i) cleavage of the DNA strand by an endonuclease, (ii) removal of the damaged region of DNA by an exonuclease, (iii) insertion of new base by the enzyme DNA polymerase, and (iv) sealing of the break by DNA ligase.

Causes of DNA Damage

Each human beings have about one hundred trillion (10^{14}) cells. We swim in environmental agents that are damage DNA of our cells which may be mutagenic (causes a mutation). These agents include environmental chemicals, UV and ionizing radiation, and sunlight. Thus, DNA is under persistent attack from many environmental agents (exogenous stresses) as well as internal stresses such as reactive oxygen species (ROS), etc., that can damage cellular DNA. These agents may breakdown the chemical bonds that hold DNA together. However, cancers are relatively rare outcomes of these encounters. Reasons for this is that the cells maintain genomic stability through different mechanisms that detect and repair DNA damage, cause the death of cells with irreparable damage, oncogene-induced senescence and immune surveillance. *TP53* tumor suppressor gene protects the genome from oncogenic damage, (i) by arresting cell division to provide time for repair of DNA damage caused by environmental mutagens, and (ii) by initiating apoptosis in irreparably damaged cells. Genes which repair DNA are called as **DNA repair genes which protect the integrity of the genome**.

Types of DNA Damage (Fig. 91)

DNA damage may occur at different times in the cell cycle. They may be caused by different types of insults and can produce different types of alterations in DNA structure. DNA damage can be repaired and if it is repaired before DNA replication, there will be no mutation in the chromosomes. Hence, to maintain the integrity of a cell's genome, cells have evolved a variety of enzymatic systems that locate and repair damaged DNA. Of course, DNA damage can be of different types and hence requires multiple combination of extremely efficient DNA repair systems to minimize the occurrence of mutations (**Fig. 91**). Various types of DNA damage are (i) single-strand breaks (SSBs), (ii) DNA adducts, (iii) base insertions or deletions, or base mismatches (iv) doublestrand breaks (DSBs). Various methods of DNA repair are listed in **Box 14**.

Most DNA damage is only temporary, because it is immediately corrected by processes collectively called DNA repair. Many repair systems use a general strategy of homology dependent repair. In this mechanism, first they remove a small region from the DNA strand that contains the altered nucleotide. Then use the other normal strand as a template to resynthesize the region removed. This strategy makes use of one of the great advantages of the double-helical structure, i.e., if one DNA strand gets damaged, cells use complementary base pairing with the undamaged strand to recreate the original sequence.

Methods of DNA Repair

Excision Repair

Excision repair is a method of repairing a wide variety of chemical alterations to DNA. In excision repair method of DNA repair, the damaged DNA is recognized and removed, either as free bases or as nucleotides [nucleotide consists of a base (one

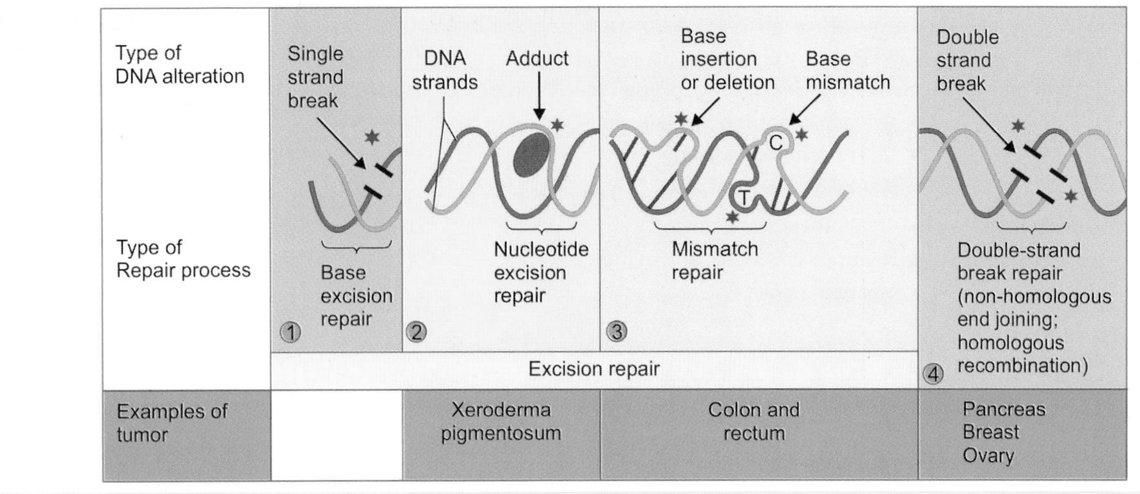

FIG. 91: DNA damage and the mechanisms of DNA repair. Various types of DNA damage are (1) single-strand breaks, (2) double-strand breaks, (3) DNA adducts, (4) base insertions or deletions or (5) base mismatches. The mechanisms that repair these damages are, respectively, (1) base excision repair, (2) nucleotide excision repair, (3) mismatch repair, and (4) double strand break repair.

Box 14: Various methods of DNA repair.

Repair of DNA lesions or base pair mismatches (excision repair) include:
- Base excision repair (BER)
- Nucleotide excision repair (NER)
- Mismatch repair (MMR)

Repair of double-strand DNA breaks: This is via repair pathways involving:
- Nonhomologous end joining (NHEJ)
- Homologous recombination (HR)
- Interstrand crosslink (ICL) repair

of the four bases: Adenine, thymine, guanine, and cytosine) plus sugar and phosphoric acid]. The resulting gap in the DNA is then filled in by synthesis of a new DNA strand, using the undamaged complementary DNA strand as a template. Three types of excision repair are: (i) base excision, (ii) nucleotide-excision, and (iii) mismatch repair (MMR). These repair mechanisms help cells to deal effectively with different kinds of DNA damage.

Base excision repair

One of the component nucleotide is nitrogenous base. The nitrogenous bases are of two types, **purines** and **pyrimidines**. The purines include adenine and guanine; the pyrimidines include cytosine, thymine, and uracil. The BER mechanism repairs DNA damage due to altered base in a nucleotide. Base excision repair (BER) is a homology-dependent repair mechanism and is closely related to nucleotide excision repair (NER). However, BER recognizes only specific forms of damaged bases, whereas other excision repair systems recognize a wide variety of damaged bases that distort the DNA molecule. BER repairs and replaces base of nucleotides with small chemical alterations. Depending upon the number of bases in nucleotides to be replaced during repair, BER pathways may be classified as 'short patch' and 'long patch'

Causes (Table 24): It is mostly caused by chemical injury to DNA bases, such as hydrolysis of base-sugar bonds, reactive oxygen species (ROS) during metabolic processes such as methylation, deamination (removal of an amino group from an amino acid or other compound), SSBs (single strand breaks) and small chemical changes in base structure. Damage to DNA bases are caused by environmental chemicals, ionizing radiation and UV, and metabolic processes such as ROS. Inherited defects in BER have not been detected.

Mechanism (Fig. 92): Base-excision repair removes damaged bases. Both short and long patch pathways are initiated by a specific *DNA* glycosylase. Base excision repair is particularly important in the removal of uracil (U) from DNA. In BER, first altered nitrogenous base is removed from the sugar of its nucleotide. This requires DNA glycosylase. Specific glycosylase recognizes the damaged/altered nucleotide and removes the abnormal base by cleavage of the glycosidic bond between the base and deoxyribose sugar in the DNA backbone. Depending on whether a purine or pyrimidine base is removed and releases the base from the DNA creating an apurinic or apyrimidinic (AP) site respectively. This is followed by making a nick in the DNA backbone (AP endonuclease or an AP lyase) where the altered nitrogenous base is removed. Then a gap is created in their vicinity of the previously damaged strand. DNA polymerase then fills in the gap by copying the undamaged complimentary strand and restores the original nucleotide. Finally, DNA ligase completes the repair process by joining the newly synthesized 'patch' to the pre-existing DNA strand.

About 11 glycosylases have been identified. Germline mutations in one of these, the *MutY* homolog *MUTYH*, lead to a cancer-predisposing syndrome called *MUTYH*-associated polyposis (MAP). Impaired function of MUTYH leads to the inability to repair G:A mismatches in DNA. This leads to an increase of G:C to T:A transversions. MAP is an autosomal recessive disorder characterized by colorectal adenomatous polyps and a very high risk of the development of colorectal cancer.

Table 24: Various types of DNA damage, their common causes and respective DNA repair pathways.

Type of DNA damage	*Causes*	*Pathway of DNA repair*
Oxidation of nucleotide base	• Mitochondrial reactive oxygen species (ROS) • Oxidants produced by phagocytes • UV and ionizing radiation • Smoking	Nucleotide excision repair (NER), base excision repair (BER)
Other damages in nucleotide base	• Chemotherapeutic drugs • Neutrophil bactericidal enzymes • Cigarette smoke • Other environmental chemicals	BER
Distortion of DNA architecture		
Additions	• Errors in transcription • ROS • Ultraviolet (UV) light	NER
Interstrand DNA cross-links	• Ionizing radiation • Arrested DNA replication • Environmental chemicals	Other such as Fanconi-related repair pathways
Single-strand nicks	• ROS • Ionizing radiation • Spontaneous loss of sugar–phosphate bond	BER, NER
Double-strand breaks	• Arrested DNA replication • Ionizing radiation • Chemical damage	Homologous recombination (HR), nonhomologous end joining (NHEJ)

Nucleotide excision repair (Fig. 93)

Each nucleotide is composed of a nitrogenous base, a sugar molecule, and a phosphate molecule. The nitrogenous bases are of two types, **purines** and **pyrimidines**. The purines include adenine (A) and guanine (G); the pyrimidines include cytosine (C), thymine (T), and uracil (U). The helical structure of DNA may be distorted by several ways such as bulky DNA adducts. It causes widespread form of DNA repair. The bulky groups may be added to DNA bases as a result of the reaction of many carcinogens with DNA (chemically-induced cross-links), base oxidation by ROS derived from mitochondria or other sources or by UV and ionizing radiation (**Table 1**). As with all DNA repair pathways, Nucleotide excision repair (NER) involves recognition of the damage, excision of the damaged nucleotides, and repair of the DNA strand. The NER pathway is a complex process involving 20–30 proteins that repair DNA damage. The NER pathway repairs complex lesions through the removal of approximately 30 bases. NER detects for DNA damage in two ways. One method is by constant scanning the genome and the other method is by identifying the alterations that interfere with RNA transcription. Once either NER system recognizes a defect in DNA, both pathways repair the DNA similarly, through an enzyme called ERCC1 (excision repair cross-complementation group 1). NER pathway removes alterations that base excision cannot repair because the cell lacks a DNA glycosylase that recognizes the problem base(s). They repair DNA damage caused by UV light as well as chemically-induced cross-links and bulky adducts. Similar to all DNA repair pathways, NER recognize the damage and operates by a cut-and patch mechanism. NER excises (removes)a variety of bulky lesions (damaged nucleotides), including pyrimidine(thymine)dimers and nucleotides to which various chemical groups have become attached (large chemical adducts) and repair of the DNA strand. The NER pathway repairs (remove) complex lesions through the removal of about 30 nucleotidesbases (e.g., dimers).

Inherited defects in NER: These are associated with two cancer syndromes. In first cancer syndrome, **xeroderma pigmentosum (XP)** the scanning pathway of NER is deficient and in the second **Cockayne syndrome**, NER defect is transcription based.

Mismatch repair

The structure of the DNA double helix follows the AT/GC rule of base pairing. During the normal course of DNA replication, however, by mistake an incorrect nucleotide may be added to the growing DNA strand. This produces a mismatch between a nucleotide in the parental and the newly produced DNA strand. After DNA replication is complete; **MMR genes act as spellcheckers or proofreaders.** These genes **encode proteins involved in the detection, excision and repair of errors that occur during replication of DNA. They excise and replace the mismatched nucleotides.** They play a critical role in maintaining the integrity of the genome by repairing DNA replication errors such as base–base mismatches and insertion/deletion loops that can occur during DNA synthesis.

Mismatch repair pathway is mainly involved in repairing errors that occur during DNA replication. During somatic cell division, the error rate in duplicating the genome is 1 miscopied base per 10^9 bases whereas in germ cells, it is lower and about 1 miscopied base per 10^{11}. *MMR* genes produce MMR enzymes and consists of two overlapping systems. One mainly corrects single base mismatches and another that fixes insertions and deletions that occurs during DNA replication.

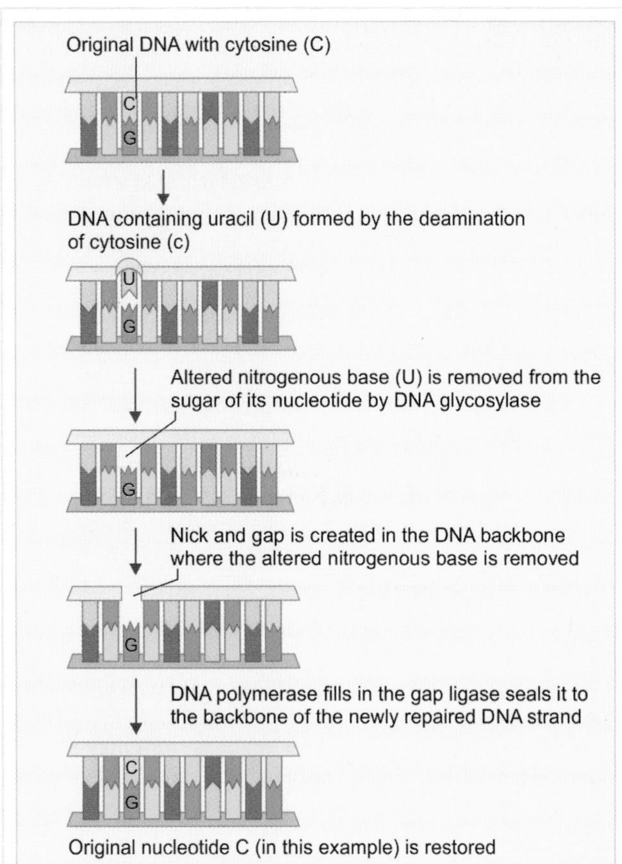

FIG. 92: Base-excision repair removes damaged bases. In this example, aberrant base uracil (U) is formed by deamination (removal of an amino group) of cytosine (C) and is therefore opposite to guanine (G) in the complementary strand of DNA. The bond between uracil and the deoxyribose is cleaved leaving a sugar with no base attached in the DNA. The sugar phosphate backbone is cut to create a nick, and this is extended as a gap. The resulted gap is then filled by DNA polymerase and the corrected DNA strand is sealed by ligase. Thus, correct base (C) is incorporated to the opposite of the other DNA strand containg the G.

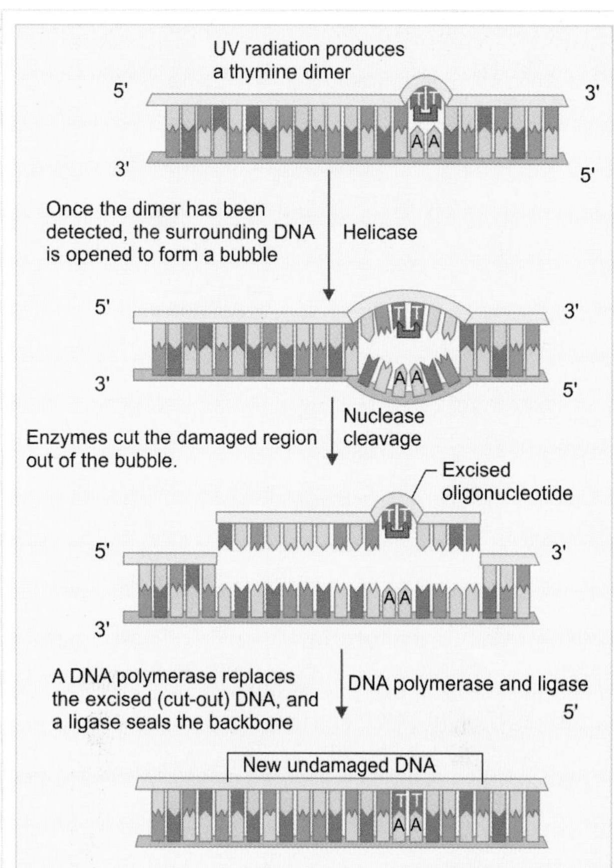

FIG. 93: Nucleotide-excision repair of thymine dimers. Damaged DNA (e.g., thymidine dimer) is detected and then undergoes unwinding around the site of damage by a helicase. The DNA is then cleaved on both sides of a thymine dimer by 3' and 5'nucleases, resulting in excision of an oligonucleotide containing the damaged bases. The gap (excised cut-out area) is then filled by DNA polymerase and the backbone is sealed by ligase. It produces a new undamaged DNA.

In the case of a base mismatch, DNA repair system should determine which base to removed. If the mismatch is due to an error occur during DNA replication, the newly made daughter strand contains the incorrect base, whereas the parental strand is normal. Therefore, mismatch specifically repairs the newly made strand rather than the parental template strand. Prior to DNA replication, the parental DNA has already been methylated. Immediately after DNA replication, some time is needed for the methylation of newly made strand. Therefore, newly replicated DNA is hemimethylated and only the parental DNA strand is methylated. Hemimethylation helps DNA repair system to distinguish between the parental DNA strand and the daughter strand.

Mechanism of repair (Figs. 94 and 95): MMR family consist of enzymes such as MSH6, MSH2, MLH1. After DNA replication is complete; ***MMR* genes act as spell checkers or proofreaders.** They stop DNA replication at the G2/M checkpoint. They recognize the errors and correct the mistake. They can **excise and replace the mismatched nucleotides.** Once corrected, they allow replication to continue. If the DNA damage is irreparable, MMR enzymes activate apoptosis. About six **mismatch repair (MMR) genes** have been identified which are designated as *hMSH2*(mutS homolog 2) located on chromosome 2p16, *hMSH6*(mutS homolog 6) on chromosome 2p16, *hMLH1*(mutLhomolog 1) on chromosome 3p21, *hMLH3*, *hPMS1* (chromosome 2) and *hPMS2*(postmeiotic segregation 2) on chromosome 7p22.

Defective MMR It may be inherited or acquired. Acquired defects in *MMR* genes may develop either due to mutations that develop over time in genome of somatic cells or epigenetic silencing. Inactivation or defect in MMR pathway leads to gradual accumulation of mismatched nucleotide errors in the genome of somatic cells. These **errors may involve proto-oncogenes and tumor suppressor genes**. It is the only form of genetic instability seen in a range of both germline and sporadic cancers. The *MMR* genes act as tumor suppressors and loss f both copies of the genes result in unrestrained growth and ultimately neoplastic transformation. The MMR process also reduces the replication error rate.

Microsatellite instability (MSI): One of the characteristic and important finding in the genome of patients with mismatch repair defects (**defective DNA MMR** gene) is phenomenon

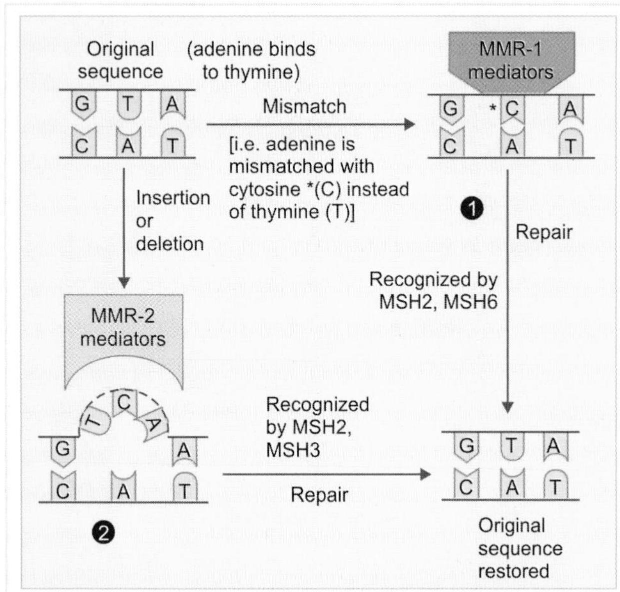

FIG. 94: Mediators of mismatch repair (MMR). (1) Single nucleotide base mismatch in DNA (in this figure "C" (cytosine) is present where a "T" (thymine) should be). This mismatch is recognized by two proteins, MSH2 and MSH6. They recruit a group of MMR repair enzymes, which corrects the defect. (2) If the DNA mispairing is due to a small insertion or deletion, a second group of MMR enzymes, MSH2 and MSH3, recognize the mistake and recruit another group of MMR mediators. They correct the defect and restore the correct nucleotide sequence.

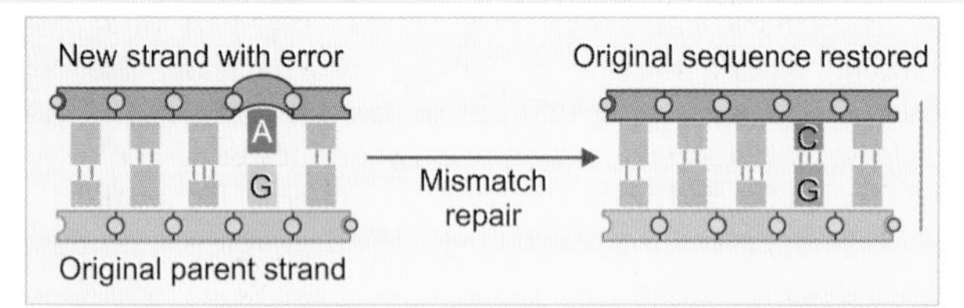

FIG. 95: Mismatch repair replace the incorrect nucleotide and restores the original DNA sequence.

referred to as **microsatellite instability (MSI)**. **Microsatellites** are short sequences of up to 6 base pairs (i.e., **one to six nucleotide bases**) that may be repeated (called as **tandem repeats** i.e., **arranged one after the other**) as many as 100 times and **found in chromosomes throughout the genome**. They are common in the human genome and normally the length of these microsatellites remains constant. They are unusually prone to mutation, including changes in numbers of repeats. Microsatellite mutations are usually detected and repaired by MMR enzymes. However, if they escape repair in germline or somatic cells, individuals likely to develop cancer. In patients with DNA mismatch repair deficiency (due to loss of mismatch repair genes). mutations accumulate in microsatellite repeats. Appearance of abnormally long (expansion due to increase in the number of nucleotide repeats) or short (contraction due to decrease in the number of nucleotide repeats) microsatellites in a DNA (in normal tissue versus tumor) is referred to as **microsatellite instability**. MSI is divided into three groups depending on the alterations in microsatellite length: MSI-High (MSI-H), MSI-Low (MSI-L), and MS-Stable (MS-S).

Minisatellites are longer tandem repeat units (n = 15–500 nucleotides) also termed variable number of tandem repeats (VNTR) because number of repeats in a given minisatellite varies widely among individuals. They are generally found in non-coding regions of DNA.

Mechanism of loss of function of MMR: Loss of MMR function usually occurs through a combination of epigenetic silencing (promoter methylation) or mutation. This is associated with LOH, of MLH1 and less frequently MSH2 or MSH6.

Consequences of loss of function of MMR: Tumors produced show replication error positive (RER$^+$), and this leads to the accumulation of insertion/deletion mutations in mono-, di-, tri-, and tetranucleotide repeats throughout the genome. The altered length of these microsatellite repeats is the "phenotypic" manifestation of an inactive MMR and is referred to as MSI$^+$. This type of genetic instability is found in up to 15% of sporadic colorectal tumors.

Double-strand Break Repair

Breakage of chromosomes is called a DNA double-strand break (DSB). Probably, double-strand breaks in a human cell occur naturally at a rate of between 10 and 100 breaks per cell per day! In DSBs, both strands of the double helix are broken at nearby sites. DSBs are dangerous DNA lesion because if they are not properly repaired, they can lead not only to point mutations, but also to large deletions (and the subsequent loss of genes) and chromosomal rearrangements. Every chromosome contains unique information. If DSB occurs in a chromosome and the broken pieces become separated, the cell has no spare copy it can use to reconstruct the information that is now missing. This type of damage is difficult to repair, and double-strand DNA breaks require a different strategy for repair. In DSBs, both strands of DNA are broken, and they cannot be repaired by excision repair mechanisms described above.

Causes of DSBs (Table 25):

- **Ionizing radiation:** X-rays, gamma rays, and particles released by radioactive atoms are grouped as *ionizing radiation* because they produce ions as they pass through matter. Millions of gamma rays pass through our bodies every minute. When these ionizing radiations collide with a fragile DNA molecule, they can break both strands of the double helix.
- **Chemical mutagens and certain drugs:** DSBs can also be caused by certain chemicals, including several chemotherapeutic drugs used in cancer therapy, and free radicals produced by normal cellular metabolism.
- During replication of damaged DNA.
- Reactive oxygen species that are the by-products of aerobic metabolism.

A single DSB can result in serious chromosome abnormalities with grave consequences for the cell.

Consequences: Double-strand breaks can be harmful in a variety of ways.

- They can result in chromosomal rearrangements such as inversions and translocations.
- DSBs can lead to terminal or interstitial deficiencies. Such genetic changes have detrimental phenotypic effects.

Detection of DSBs: Ataxia telangiectasiamutated (ATM) and ataxia telangiectasia and Rad-3-related (ATR) are the sensors

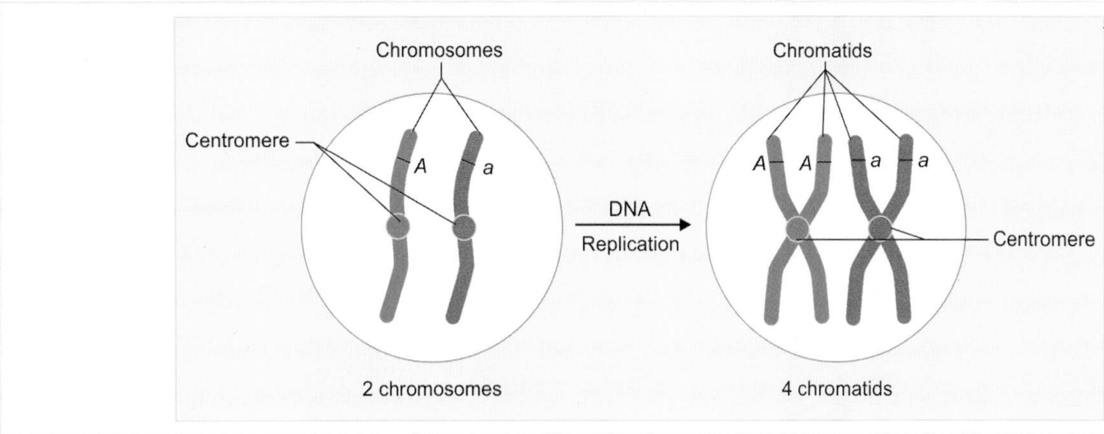

FIG. 96: Chromosomes and chromatids. During S phase of cell cycle all the chromosomes of a cell are replicated (duplicated). Following replication, each chromosome consists of two sister chromatids attached at centromere. These chromatids are genetically identical.

for DSBs, and each recognizes different types of DSBs. ATM detects DSBs that result from DNA damage (e.g., ionizing radiation) and after activation, ATM recruits Checkpoint kinase 2 (Chk2). ATR identifies single-stranded DNA at stopped/stalled replication forks and activates Chk1. Both resulting complexes, ATM/Chk2 and ATR/Chk1, phosphorylates p53. This in turn activate cell cycle checkpoints and halts cell division till the DNA break is fixed. Mutations in ATM and other enzymes involved in DSB repair are associated with a high incidence of cancers.

Before we deal with types of repair of DSBs, let us briefly refresh about chromosomes and chromatids. Chromosomes can exist in duplicated or unduplicated states. In a cell cycle, during S phase, which follows G_1 phase, all of the chromosomes (genetic material) of a cell are replicated (duplicated). Following replication, each chromosome consists of two sister chromatids. Chromatids are the term used to describe the chromosome in its duplicated state. After replication, there are still only 46 chromosomes, however, they look like an X shape. Each chromosome has two sister chromatids (**Fig. 96**). These chromatids are genetically identical and consists of genetic material of each chromosome. However, they are still attached at the centromere and are not yet considered separate chromosomes.

Methods of DSBs repair: Two important mechanisms/methods can repair **double-strand breaks (DSBs)** namely (1) by homologous recombination (HR) repair and (2) by nonhomologous end joining (NHEJ).

Homologous Recombination (Fig. 97)

It is also called homology-directed repair is less common pathway. It occurs when homologous DNA strands, usually from a sister chromatid, are used to repair a DSB in the other sister chromatid. The challenge in repairing a DSB, is finding an intact DNA template to guide the repair. However, if a DSB occurs in a double helix shortly after DNA has been replicated (during S phase of the cycle), the undamaged strands of the intact double helix can serve as a template to guide the repair of both broken strands of DNA. Hence, this mechanism of repair is only operative following DNA replication, when the newly replicated sister chromatids remain associated with each other. Because the two DNA molecules are homologous (i.e., they have identical or nearly identical nucleotide sequences outside the broken region), this mechanism is known as homologous recombination (HR) (the term recombination is described below). It is mostly active in S and G_2 phase of the cell cycle. HR method results in a perfect/accurate repair of the DSB, with no loss or gain of nucleotides (and genetic information). This process involves a complex of proteins including BRCA1, BRCA2, and RAD51.

Recombination repair: Recombination is a process in which random crossing over of double-stranded DNA occurs between two parental homologous chromosomes. Recombination is a distinct mechanism repair to rejoin the broken double-strands of DNA. This occurs by breakage of homologous DNA molecules and rejoining of the parts in new combinations. It is a necessary process in meiosis and involves exchange of genetic information. Recombination also occur during mitosis at a predictable rate. Exposure to ionizing radiation significantly increases the rate of breakage in chromosomes. Usually, these breakages are accurately repaired by recombination repair genes. Disorders associated with recombination repair genes include Bloom syndrome, ataxia-telangiectasia, and Fanconi anemia. *BRCA1* and *BRCA2* are mutated in familial breast cancer and both are associated with many proteins involved in the homologous recombination repair (HRR) pathway.

Disadvantages: The sister chromatids are available only during the S and G_2 phases of the cell cycle. Homologous recombination can result in two major types of genome alterations.

1. **Loss of heterozygosity (LOH):** If HR uses the homologous chromosome as a template for DNA repair, allelic differences between the two chromosomes may be lost (LOH).
2. **Generation of translocation:** Repetitive sequences are abundant throughout the human genome. Hence, if breaks occur in repetitive sequences, HR repair of a

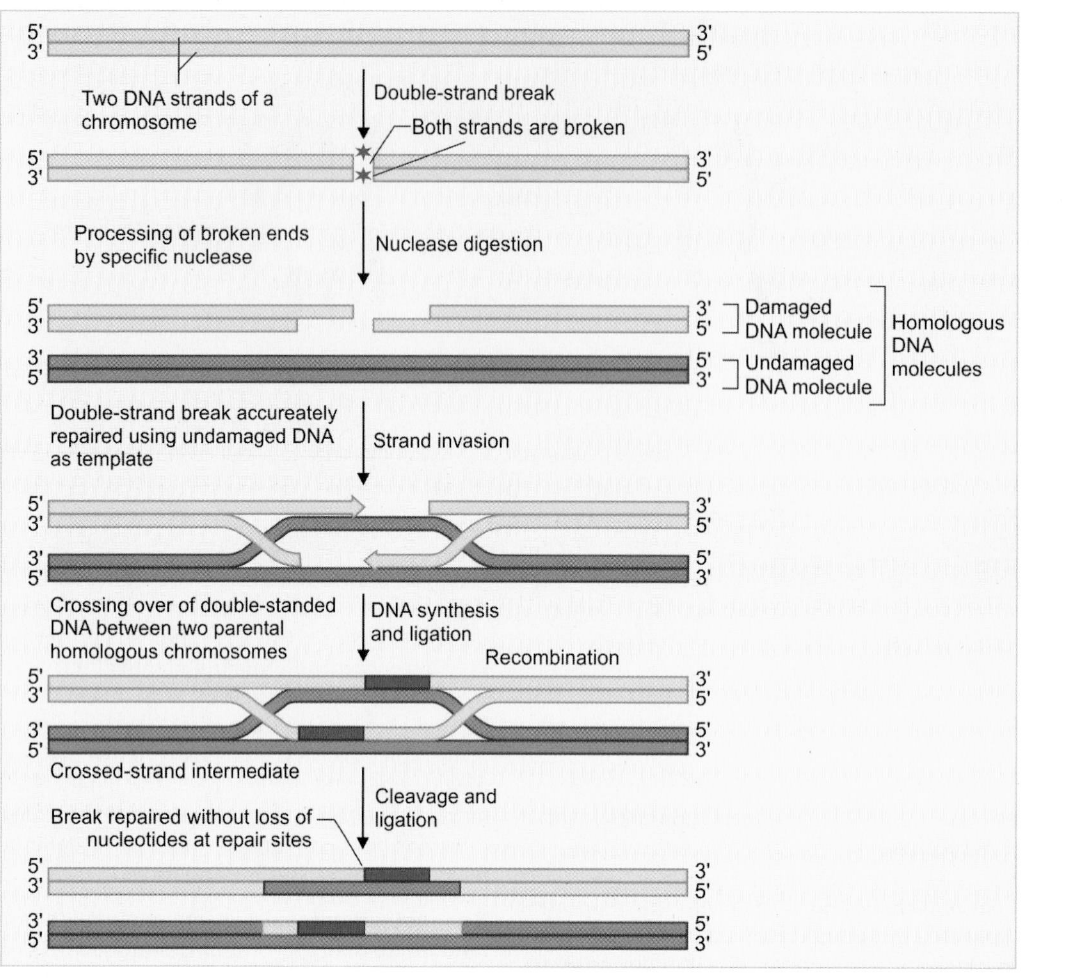

FIG. 97: Repair of double-strand DNA breaks by homologous recombination. In this process, an undamaged chromosome acts a template and restores the normal DNA sequence. Both strands of DNA at a double-strand breaks are digested by nucleases in the 5′ to 3′ direction and a gap is produced between the broken ends. The gaps are then filled by repair synthesis and sealed by ligation and gives rise to a crossed strand intermediate. Cleavage and ligation of the crossed strands then produces recombinant molecules. Homologous recombination repairs DNA double-strand breaks perfectly without any defect. This is the preferred method for repairing double-strand breaks that occurs shortly after the DNA has been replicated (during S phase of cell cycle) but before the cell has divided.

break in one chromosome may lead to use of an identical repetitive sequence on a nonhomologous chromosome as a template for recombination. This generates a translocation. Many genes (e.g., *BRCA1, BRCA2, PALB2*) whose protein products are important for HR are usually mutated or inactivated in many human tumors. This may occur either as part of inherited cancer susceptibility syndromes or epigenetically during oncogenesis.

Steps involved (Fig. 97): Various steps are as follows:

1. Short digestion of DNA strands at the break site.
2. Exchange of DNA strands between the broken and unbroken sister chromatids.
3. The unbroken strands are used as templates to synthesize DNA in the region where the DSB occurred.
4. The crisscrossed strands are resolved, which means they are broken and then rejoined in a way that produces separate chromatids.

Advantage: Because sister chromatids are genetically identical, HRR is an error-free mechanism for repairing a DSB.

Nonhomologous End Joining (Fig. 98)

DNA double strand breaks (DSBs) are repaired mainly by nonhomologous end joining (NHEJ) In NHEJ, the broken ends of both strands of DNA are hurriedly rejoined, before the DNA fragments driven apart and get lost. This pathway needs the participation of several complex proteins that play key roles in the process. This occurs in many cell types and is carried out by a specialized group of enzymes that "clean" the broken ends and rejoin them by DNA ligation. This "quick and dirty" mechanism quickly seals the break in DNA and restores DNA integrity. But it comes with a price, i.e., during "cleaning" the break and make them ready for ligation, nucleotides (deletion of bases) are usually lost at the site of repair (around the site of damage) (**Fig. 98**). It may not reproduce the original sequence (depending on the nature of the break). If this repair disrupts the activity of a gene, the cell can suffer serious consequences. Also, there is no guarantee that the ends that are so joined are in fact the broken ends of the same chromosome and if it joins other chromosome it may result in translocations. Thus, NHEJ

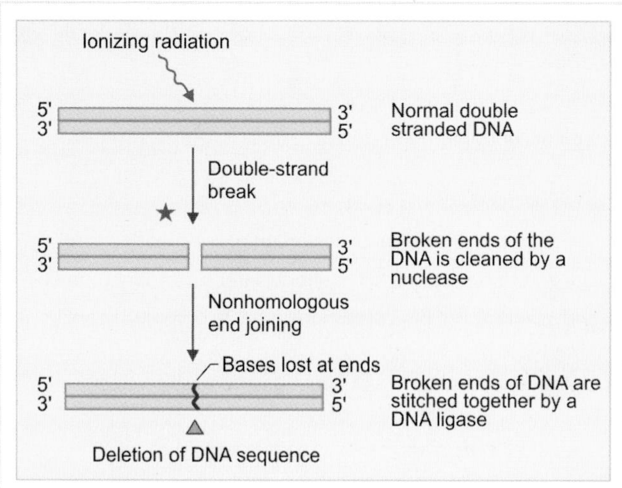

FIG. 98: Nonhomologous end joining method of repairing double stand DNA breaks. The broken ends end of the DNA is first "cleaned" by a nuclease and then stitched together by a DNA ligase. During this repair process, some nucleotides (DNA sequence) are usually lost in the repaired DNA.

can be a risky strategy for fixing broken chromosomes. Unlike HR, NHEJ operates throughout the cell cycle and is more efficient than HR.

Steps (Fig. 98): They catalyze a series of reactions and rejoin the broken strands of DNA. The major steps are as follows:

1. Immediately following the DSB, they are recognized by end-binding proteins (NHEJ repair protein). These proteins (e.g., Ku) recognize additional proteins that form a cross-bridge that prevents the drifting apart of two broken ends.
2. Additional proteins (DNA-PKcs–which is the catalytic subunit of a DNA-dependent protein kinase) are recruited to the region. They process the ends of the broken chromosome by digesting particular DNA strands. This process may result in the deletion of a small amount of genetic material from the region.
3. Any gaps between the broken ends are filled in via DNA polymerase, and the broken ends of DNA are ligated together by DNA ligase IV.

During G_0 phase of the cell cycle, most DSBs are repaired by one of two NHEJ pathways: (i) The Ku (XRCC5/XRCC6 heterodimer)-mediated, and the (ii) ATM-mediated.

Advantage: There is no participation of a sister chromatid. Hence, it can occur at any stage of the cell cycle.

Disadvantage: It can result in small deletions in the region that has been repaired.

Hereditary Cancer Syndromes

Q. Write short essay on inherited cancer syndromes (Hereditary neoplasms).

Certain cancers in a family are strongly linked to an inherited gene mutation. This is part of a hereditary (familial) cancer syndrome in which there is genetic predisposition to certain types of cancer. Individuals carrying mutations (in one or more genes) for hereditary cancer syndromes have a high risk for the development of neoplasms at an early age, as well as the synchronous or metachronous development of multiple tumors of the corresponding tumor spectrum. Approximately 5% of all cancers are part of a hereditary cancer syndrome. These cancers may be inherited as autosomal dominant or recessive pattern (**Table 25**).

GENOMIC INSTABILITY

Threat to DNA Integrity

We swim in environmental agents that are mutagenic (e.g., chemicals, radiation, sunlight). DNA integrity is constantly under threat and is subjected to a huge array of assaults which can damage cellular DNA. These include:

- **DNA-damaging agents:** These may be chemical, physical, and biologic assaults on a daily basis. These include environmental agents (exogenous stresses such as UV light, ionizing radiation (IR), chemical exposure) as well as internal stresses (endogenous such as ROS).
- **Errors occurring during DNA replication.**
- **Distribution of chromosomes between daughter cells during cell division.**

However, cancers are relatively rare outcomes of these encounters. There are different mechanisms to identify/detect and repair damaged or incorrectly copied DNA and thereby maintain genomic stability. There is a mechanism which cause the death of cells with irreparable damage, oncogene-induced senescence and immune surveillance. As discussed earlier, *TP53* tumor suppressor gene protects the genome from oncogenic damage, (i) by arresting cell division to provide time for repair of DNA damage caused by environmental mutagens, and (ii) by initiating apoptosis in irreparably damaged cells. Genes which repair DNA are called as **DNA repair genes which protect the integrity of the genome**. Any failure to repair DNA damage (disruption of these mechanisms) produces permanent alterations, or mutations, in the DNA. If the mutation occurs in a germ cell (destined to become a gamete), the genetic alteration may be passed on to the next generation. Mutations in somatic cells (i.e., cells that are not in the germ line) can interfere with transcription and replication, lead to genetic instability and, ultimately, cancer (malignant transformation of a cell).

DNA repair maintains the integrity of the genome. Normally, DNA repair genes repair nonlethal damage in other genes including proto-oncogenes, tumor suppressor genes and genes that regulate apoptosis. Mutations of these DNA repair genes do not directly transform cells.

- **Loss-of-function mutations** (disability) **involving DNA repair genes** contribute to carcinogenesis (neoplastic transformation) indirectly by **impairing the ability of the cell to recognize and repair nonlethal genetic damage in other genes**. These affected cells acquire mutations at an accelerated rate, a state referred to as a ***mutator phenotype* and it is marked by genomic instability.**
- **Genomic instability:** It refers to an increased tendency (liability) of alterations (mutability/change) in the genome during the life cycle of cells. Most cancer cells have increased susceptibility to random mutation. This allows tumor cells to achieve genotypes that favor cancer maintenance and progression. Genomic instability may

Table 26: Examples of hereditary cancer syndromes with involved genes and associated risk of neoplasms.

Hereditary cancer syndrome	*Gene involved*	*Risk of tumors*
Autosomal-dominant inheritance		
Hereditary nonpolyposis colorectal cancer (HNPCC)/ Lynch syndrome	*MSH2, MLH1, MSH6, PMS2*	Cancer of colon, endometrium, stomach, small intestine, urothelium
Familial breast and ovarian cancer	*BRCA1, BRCA2*	Cancer of breast, ovary, and prostate
Neurofibromatosis type 1	*NF1*	Neurofibroma, optic nerve glioma, malignant nerve sheath tumor
Familial retinoblastoma	*RB1*	Often bilateral retinoblastoma in childhood, later secondary tumors
Multiple endocrine neoplasia type 2 (MEN2a)	*RET*	Medullary thyroid cancer, pheochromocytoma, hyperparathyroidism
Familial adenomatous polyposis (FAP)	*APC*	>100 colonic adenomas, tumors in upper gastrointestinal tract, desmoids
Von Hippel-Lindau disease	*VHL*	Clear cell renal cell cancer and other, usually benign tumors
Li-Fraumeni syndrome	*TP53*	Broad tumor spectrum and includes sarcomas, breast cancer, brain tumors, leukemia
Nevoid basal cell carcinoma syndrome (Gorlin syndrome)	*PTCH*	Basal cell carcinoma
Hereditary paraganglioma-pheochromocytoma syndrome	*SDH (succinate dehydrogenase)*	Paraganglioma
Autosomal-recessive inheritance		
MUTYH-associated polyposis (MAP)	*MUTYH*	Colon cancer, colonic adenoma
Ataxia telangiectasia	*ATM*	Non-Hodgkin lymphoma, leukemia
Fanconi anemia	*FANC, A-H*	Hematological neoplasms
Xeroderma pigmentosum	Genes involved in nucleotide excision repair (NER) enzymes	Skin cancers (squamous cell carcinoma, basal cell carcinoma and melanoma)

be due to either microsatellite instability/**MSI** (single or oligo-nucleotide mutations) or more commonly due to **chromosomal instability** leading to aneuploidy (abnormal number of chromosomes in a cell).

Observations made in familial cancer syndromes, provided understanding regarding the importance of DNA repair genes in oncogenesis. Family cancer syndromes are genetic disorders in which there are inherited genetic mutations in one or more genes. This predisposes the affected individuals to the development of cancers as well as early onset of these cancers. Cancer syndromes usually have a high lifetime risk of developing cancer, but also the development of multiple independent primary tumors.

Inherited disorders of DNA repair gene are characterized by defect in proteins involved in DNA repair. **Individuals with inherited defects in DNA repair genes have a highest risk for the development of cancer.** Mutations in DNA repair genes can also be sporadic and can lead to accumulation of mutations in cancer genes and contribute directly to development of cancer. Few of the inherited disorders of DNA repair gene are discussed below. Human diseases due to DNA repair defect are listed in **Table 25**.

Table 25: Human diseases of DNA damage repair.

Repair of DNA lesions or base pair mismatches
- Defective DNA nucleotide excision repair (NER)
  - Xeroderma pigmentosum (XP)
- Defective DNA base excision repair (BER)
  - MUTYH-associated polyposis (MAP)
- Defective DNA mismatch repair (MMR)
  - Hereditary nonpolyposis colorectal cancer (colon carcinoma) (HNPCC)

Repair of double-strand DNA breaks
- Defective nonhomologous end joining repair (NHEJ)
  - Severe combined immunodeficiency disease (SCID)
- Defective homologous repair (HR)
  - Bloom syndrome (BS)
  - Werner syndrome (WS)
  - Breast cancer susceptibility 1 and 2 (BRCA1, BRCA2)

DNA Mismatch Repair Factors

Hereditary Nonpolyposis Colon Cancer Syndrome

Hereditary nonpolyposis colon carcinoma (HNPCC) syndrome (Lynch syndrome) is autosomal dominant inherited disease and accounts for 2–4% of colorectal cancers.

It is characterized by **familial predisposition to the development of carcinomas of the colon** affecting predominantly the cecum and proximal colon. **It highlights the role of DNA repair genes in predisposition to cancer. It is due to defects in *DNA MMR* gene.**

Molecular pathogenesis

- Normally, during a repair of DNA strand, the products of *MMR* genes act as "spellcheckers." For example, if there is an error in pairing of nitrogenous base G with T, rather than the normal A with T, the *MMR* genes correct the defect. If these "proofreaders," genes are defective, errors accumulate at an increased rate.

- **Mutations in *MMR* genes:** HNPCC (Lynch) syndrome is caused by germline mutations in a *DNA MMR* gene. Mutations in at least four *MMR* genes is associated with HNPCC, but majority of HNPCC involve mutations of either *hMSH2* (human MutS homolog 2) on chromosome 2p and *hMLH1* (human MutL homolog 1) on chromosome 3p. Less common mutations involve *hMSH6* (human MutS homolog 6) or *hPMS2* (human postmeiotic segregation 2) on chromosomes 2p and 7p, respectively. Mutations in MSH6 are usually associated with an increased risk of endometrial cancer. These patients have an 80% lifetime risk of developing colorectal cancer and an increased risk of developing a wide range of other malignancies including ovarian, gastric, brain, pancreatic, endometrial, biliary, small bowel, and urinary tract cancers.
- **Two hits:** In HNPCC, each affected individual inherits one defective copy of one of several DNA *MMR* genes. This is due to germline mutation in one allele of one *MMR* gene. There is no impairment of DNA repair in this heterozygous state (where second copy of DNA MMR gene is normal). Then the second "hit" of DNA *MMR* gene in colonic epithelial cells occurs as an acquired mutation. Once both alleles are mutated, repair of spontaneous replication errors is ineffective. This results in the increased rate of accumulation of mutations in mono-, di-, and trinucleotide repeats throughout the genome. This will result in microsatellite instability (MSI) in about 90% cancers. Thus, **mode of inheritance of DNA-repair genes is like tumor suppressor genes**. DNA repair genes affect cell growth only indirectly. They indirectly allow mutations in other genes during normal cell division.
- **Consequences:** A characteristic finding in the genome of patients with MMR defects is microsatellite instability (MSI). Microsatellites are simple repetitive sequences (tandem repeats) of one to six nucleotides found throughout the genome. In normal individuals, the length of these microsatellites remains constant. But, in patients with HNPCC, these satellites become **unstable during normal cellular replication** leading to insertion or deletion of bases within these regions. Thus, microsatellite increase or decrease in length, creating alleles not found in normal cells of the same patient. ***DNA MMR* genes rapidly correct these errors** to **maintain microsatellite length**. Microsatellites are particularly prone to replication errors. Thus, genes that regulate growth and differentiation, and other *MMR* genes, are disabled by unrepaired mutations in DNA repair genes. Microsatellites are typically formed in noncoding regions. However, some microsatellite sequences are located in the coding or promoter region of genes involved in regulation of cell growth. For example, **MSI** involving:
  - **Type II transforming growth factor (TGF)-β receptor:** Normally, **TGF-β** inhibits colonic epithelial cell proliferation and mutation in type II TGF-β receptor can lead to uncontrolled cell growth.
  - **Proapoptotic gene *BAX*:** Its mutation can lead to loss of *BAX*, which may increase the survival of genetically abnormal clones of cells.
- **Detection:** Deficiency or defect in MMR can be detected by sequencing *MMR* genes, testing for MSI and immunostaining to assess levels of MMR proteins in a tumor. Though HNPCC is responsible for only 2–4% of all colonic cancers, MSI can be detected in about 15% of sporadic colonic cancers. These are due to acquired mutations that in *MMR* genes.

Nucleotide Excision Repair Factors

Xeroderma Pigmentosum

- The first DNA repair disorder recognized was **xeroderma pigmentosum (XP)**. Xeroderma pigmentosum (XP) is an **inherited** (hereditary) **autosomal recessive disorder due to** defective ***NER* (nucleotide excision repair) gene (one of the DNA repair gene)**.
- These patients have a greatly **increased risk** for the development of **cancers** (squamous cell carcinoma, basal cell carcinoma and malignant melanoma) **in sun exposed skin following exposure to the UV light rays** present in sunlight.
- Individuals with XP are extremely sensitive to UV-induced cancers. **UV radiation causes cross-linking of pyrimidine (one of** nitrogenous base in nucleotide of DNA) **residues, preventing normal DNA replication**. Normally, such DNA damage is **repaired by the NER (nucleotide excision repair) system**. Several proteins are involved in NER. Inherited loss of any one of these proteins can give rise to XP. The cells of XP patients are defective in their capacity to excise the DNA cross-links and bulky adducts. The persistence of these UV-induced lesions renders the genome vulnerable to their mutagenic effects.

Homologous Recombination Repair Factors

- Several disorders caused by defects in homologous recombination (HR) factors are associated with an increased risk of cancer. This includes a group of autosomal recessive disorders such as *Bloom syndrome, ataxia-telangiectasia*, and Fanconi anemia. They are characterized by hypersensitivity to DNA-damaging agents. These damaging agents may be ionizing radiation (in Bloom syndrome and ataxia-telangiectasia), or DNA cross-linking agents, such as nitrogen mustard (in Fanconi anemia). Apart from predisposition to cancer, they may present with features such as neural symptoms (in ataxia-telangiectasia), anemia (in Fanconi anemia), and developmental defects (in Bloom syndrome).

Bloom Syndrome

It is an autosomal recessive disorder caused by loss-of-function mutations in a helicase. Helicase is needed for HRR. These individuals have developmental anomalies and an increased risk of developing many different types of cancer.

Ataxia-telangiectasia

It is an autosomal recessive disorder caused due to defects (mutation) in *ATM* gene. *ATM* gene encodes a protein kinase that acts upstream of p53. It is involved in "sensing" DNA damage caused by ionizing radiation and then directing p53 to initiate the DNA damage response. This syndrome is characterized by neurodegeneration (mainly of the cerebellum, hence the ataxia), immunodeficiency, hypersensitivity to radiation (due to an inability to repair double-stranded DNA breaks), and predisposition to cancer (e.g., leukemia and lymphoma). Somatic driver mutations in *ATM* also are also observed in some types of lymphoid neoplasms.

Fanconi Anemia

It is an autosomal recessive disorder that may be caused by mutations in several different genes. Each gene encodes a protein that participates in a pathway that repairs DNA cross-links through HR. It presents with wide clinical spectrum. It is characterized by developmental/congenital abnormalities (short stature, skeletal abnormalities), hypersensitivity to chemotherapeutic agents that cross-link DNA, and increased risk of bone marrow failure (aplasia) and leukemia (e.g., acute myeloid leukemia). They also have increased risk of early onset of cancer such as tumors of liver, squamous cell carcinomas of the esophagus, oropharynx, and uvula.

Familial Breast Cancer

DNA repair genes are also involved in hereditary breast cancer. **Germ line mutations in two genes namely *BRCA1* and *BRCA2*** is responsible **for 25% of cases of familial breast cancer**.

- ***BRCA1* mutations:** It is associated with **breast cancer** and also associated with **higher risk for developing epithelial ovarian cancers. In men,** it is associated with a **slightly higher risk for developing prostate cancer**.
- ***BRCA2* mutations:** It also increases the risk for developing breast cancer (both in men and women), and cancers of the ovary, prostate, pancreas, bile ducts, stomach, melanocytes, and B lymphocytes.

BRCA and recombination

Though exact functions of *BRCA1* and *BRCA2* is not known, cells with a defective *BRCA1* and *BRCA2* genes develop chromosomal breaks and severe aneuploidy. Both genes partly take part in the HR DNA repair pathway. For example, BRCA1 forms a complex with other proteins involved in the HR pathway and also in the ATM kinase pathway. Some germline *BRCA2* mutations was identified as one of several genes mutated in Fanconi anemia, and the BRCA2 protein binds to RAD51, a protein needed for HR. Probably BRCA proteins and Fanconi proteins function cooperatively in a DNA damage response network linked to homologous recombination repair. Defects in this pathway causes activation of the nonhomologous end joining pathway. This leads to formation of dicentric chromosomes, bridge-fusion-breakage cycles, and aneuploidy. This is similar to that occurs in p53-deficient cells and the cells undergo shortening of telomere (refer Fig. 70 of Chapter 7)

Similar to other tumor suppressor genes, cancer can develop when both copies of *BRCA1* and *BRCA2* are inactivated. Though *BRCA1* and *BRCA2* are involved in familial breast cancers, they are rarely inactivated in sporadic cases of breast cancer. Commonly, tumor suppressor genes, such as *APC* and *TP53,* which are frequently inactivated in sporadic cancers.

Genetic Instability Due to Defect in DNA Repair Genes

Loss-of-function mutations (disability) involving DNA repair genes do not directly transform neoplastic cells (carcinogenesis). They indirectly impair the ability of the cell to recognize and repair nonlethal genetic damage in other genes. These affected cells acquire mutations at an accelerated rate, a state referred to as a ***mutator phenotype*** and it is marked by *genomic instability.* Most cancers show some form of genetic instability. This may be at either the nucleotide or chromosome level.

- **At the nucleotide level:** This includes genomic instability due to either **MSI** (single or oligo-nucleotide mutations) ($MIN/MSI^+/RER^+$) or due to poorly understood phenomenon of point mutation instability (PIN).
  - **Point mutation instability:** This form of genetic instability is generally not widely accepted, because of difficulty to confirm the presence of PIN. The diagnostic feature of PIN is the presence of an increased rate in the accumulation of point mutations outside microsatellite repeats.
- **At the level of the chromosomes:** It is termed as **chromosome instability (CIN)** and is more common. It is characterized by the accumulation of structural changes in the chromosome. Aneuploidy is the term used for changes in chromosome number (abnormal number of chromosomes in a cell), but the term CIN is often used to include wider range of changes in chromosome number and/or structure.

DNA damage response (DDR) pathway: This is a signal transduction pathway which recognizes DNA damage and replication stress (accumulation and collapse of stalled DNA replication forks). It repairs the recombinational repair of DSBs, SSBs, and interstrand cross-links (ICLs). Almost all types of replication-independent DNA damage need unwinding of double-stranded DNA by helicases, cleavage of the DNA strand, and repair of the DNA by polymerases.

Genetic Instability at the Chromosome Level

Chromosome instability and aneuploidy

The genetic and/or epigenetic factors which **lead to chromosome instability (CIN)** and aneuploidy in the majority of sporadic malignant tumors is not known.

Mechanisms Implicated in the Development of Genetic Instability in Sporadic Cancers

Epigenetic alterations

Epigenetic alterations in cancer involve DNA hypermethylation of CpG dinucleotides (clustered into regions called CpG islands in the promoters of genes). This will result in the transcriptional inactivation of the associated genes. Almost 50% of all genes contain a CpG rich region that fulfils the criteria of being a CpG island. Methylation of promoter region is a "metastable" change affecting gene expression and it may produce similar effect as mutations.

Telomeres

Telomere shortening

Telomeres are **protective, short repeated sequences of DNA** (TTAGGG) present **at the end regions of chromosomes.** Telomeres ensure the complete copying of chromosomal ends during the S-phase of the cell cycle. With each cell division in somatic cells, a small section of the telomere is not duplicated, and telomeres become progressively shortened (**Fig. 67 of chapter 7**). When telomeres are sufficiently shortened, ultimately the cells stop dividing (**cell cycle arrest**) leading to a terminally nondividing state. Telomeres represent a "biological clock", which prevents uncontrolled cell division and cancer. Telomeres protect the ends of chromosomes and stop them from being recognized by the DNA damage response machinery as DSBs. **Telomere shortening** may be one of the mechanisms **responsible for decreased cellular replication. Hayflick limit** is the number of times a normal human cell population will divide until cell division stops.

Telomerase

Telomerase is an **enzyme** that **regenerates and maintains telomere length** by addition of nucleotide. Telomerase is a specialized RNA-protein complex which uses its own RNA as a template for adding nucleotides to the ends of chromosomes. Telomerase is absent in most of the somatic cells and expressed in germ cells and is present at low levels in stem cells. Hence, as mature somatic cells age, their telomeres become shorter and they exit the cell cycle. This results in an inability to generate new cells to replace damaged ones. On the other hand, the germ cells (high telomerase activity) have extended replicative capacity. In cancers, the telomerase may be reactivated in tumor cells resulting in maintenance of length of telomeres and allows the cells to proliferate indefinitely. It may be an essential step information of cancer. Shortening of telomere also may decrease the regenerative capacity of stem cells. Cells with shortened telomeres which have become resistant to senescence have been shown to undergo chromosome fusion and develop CIN.

Activation of telomerase

Telomerase is expressed at very low levels in most somatic cells and with each cell division their telomeres shorten. Thus, any cells that escape from senescence die in mitotic crisis. However, if cells in crisis reactivate telomerase, these cells can restore their telomeres and survive. The cells damaged by oncogenes and tumor suppressor genes during crisis are at high risk for malignant transformation. Cancers may arise from stem cells which express telomerase. Whatever the mechanism, telomere is maintained in almost all types of cancers, and in 85–95% of cases it is due to upregulation of telomerase

DNA Polymerase

Rate of error in DNA replication is defined as addition of nucleotide that does not match its partner on the template strand of DNA. Normally cellular DNA polymerases are involved in DNA replication and have a very low rate of error. This is partly due to an inherent exonuclease activity. Before proceeding down the template strand, this exonuclease activity allows DNA polymerase to pause, excise mismatched bases, and insert the proper nucleotide. Some cancers, such as carcinoma of endometrium and colon, show mutations in DNA polymerase. This result in a loss of this "proofreading" function and leads to the accumulation of many point substitutions. Cancers with DNA polymerase mutations represent the most heavily mutated of all human cancers. These cancers have a high burden of neoantigens and show excellent responses to immune checkpoint inhibitors.

Regulated Genomic Instability in Lymphoid Cells

Adaptive immunity depends on the ability of B and T cells to diversify their antigen receptor genes. A special type of DNA damage is involved in the pathogenesis of tumors of B and T lymphocytes. Developing B and T cells both express a pair of gene products namely RAG1 and RAG2. These gene products carry out V(D)J segment recombination and allow the assembly of functional antigen receptor genes. Apart from this, mature B cells after encountering antigen, express a specialized enzyme called activation-induced cytosine deaminase (AID). AID is needed for both immunoglobulin gene class switch recombination and somatic hypermutation. These processes are associated with AID-induced DNA breaks or nucleotide substitutions. Both of these are liable to undergo errors such as translocations and mutations. These in turn may produce neoplasm of lymphoid cells.

10.5 Carcinogenic Agents

CHAPTER OUTLINE

- Etiology of cancer (carcinogenic agents)
  - Chemical carcinogens and carcinogenesis
  - Microbial carcinogenesis
  - Radiation carcinogenesis

ETIOLOGY OF CANCER (CARCINOGENIC AGENTS)

Q. Discuss carcinogens.

Definition: A **carcinogen** is an **agent known or suspected to cause tumors** and such agents are said to be **carcinogenic** (cancer causing).

Carcinogenic agents produce genetic damage. Three classes of carcinogenic agents (Flowchart 1) are: (1) Chemicals, (2) Microbial agents, and (3) Radiation.

Chemicals and radiation are involved in causing cancer in humans whereas oncogenic viruses are involved in the pathogenesis of tumors in several animal models and some human tumors.

Chemical Carcinogens and Carcinogenesis

Q. Discuss chemical carcinogens and carcinogenesis.

Sir Percival Pott [English physician and surgeon (in London) in 1775] **first related** cancer of the scrotal **skin in individual who work as chimney sweeps** as children. **It was due to a specific chronic chemical exposure to soot.** Based on this, a rule was made that chimney sweep members must bathe daily and this public health measure controlled scrotal skin cancer. Presently chemical products derived from combustion of organic materials are responsible for a man-made epidemic of cancer, namely, lung cancer in cigarette smokers. Japanese investigators (Yamagiva and Ichikawa, 1915) experimentally produced skin cancers in rabbits by using coal tar. Subsequently, hundreds of chemical carcinogens were discovered.

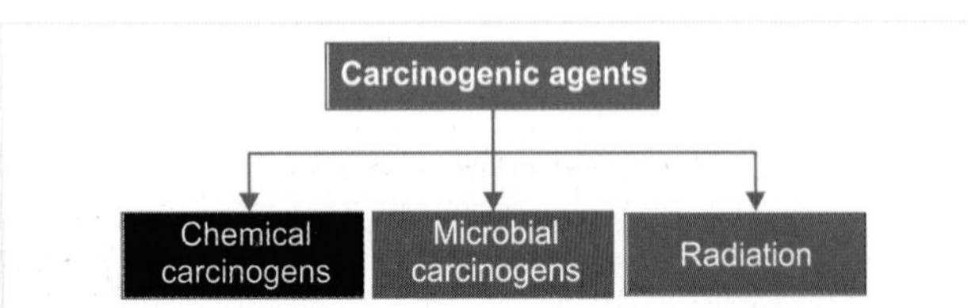

FLOWCHART 1: Major types of carcinogenic agents.

Most of the chemical carcinogens are mutagens. A mutagen is defined as agent that can permanently alter the genetic constitution of a cell. It was observed that many chemical compounds known to be potent carcinogens are relatively inert in terms of chemical reactivity. In the early 1960s, it was shown that most (not all), chemical carcinogens need metabolic activation before they can react with cell constituents.

Ames Assay/Test (Fig. 99)

Mutagenicity testing of chemical is done by **Ames test**. It is an in vitro assay to detect mutagenicity of test compounds and was developed for screening potential chemical carcinogens. Ames test semiquantitatively analyses a chemical's capacity to induce mutations in *Salmonella typhimurium* in a culture medium. It is useful to detect whether a chemical can cause mutations in the DNA of *Salmonella typhimurium*.

- The test uses histidine-synthesis-deficient *Salmonella typhimurium* (i.e., they have mutations in genes involved in histidine synthesis and cannot produce histidine) that need histidine for growth but cannot produce it. The *Salmonella* strains are specially constructed to detect mutations in the genes required to synthesize histidine.
- In this assay, first histidine-synthesis-deficient *Salmonella* strains are grown in the presence of exogenous histidine and then exposed to test compounds.
- If the tested compound is capable of producing mutations in *Salmonella typhimurium*, it allows *Salmonella* to grow on a histidine-free medium (i.e., no need histidine for growth). The mutagenic compound produces mutations in histidine-synthesis genes and revert the bacterial strain to a histidine-independent status. This can be detected by growth of *Salmonella typhimurium* in a media with no or minimal histidine. Only those *Salmonella* that have acquired specific mutations in histidine-synthesis genes are able to form colonies.

Classification of Chemical Carcinogens

Chemical carcinogens constitute a large group of structurally diverse organic and inorganic compounds. **Chemical carcinogens** may be classified into two categories: Direct acting and indirect acting. Major chemical carcinogens are listed in **Box 15**.

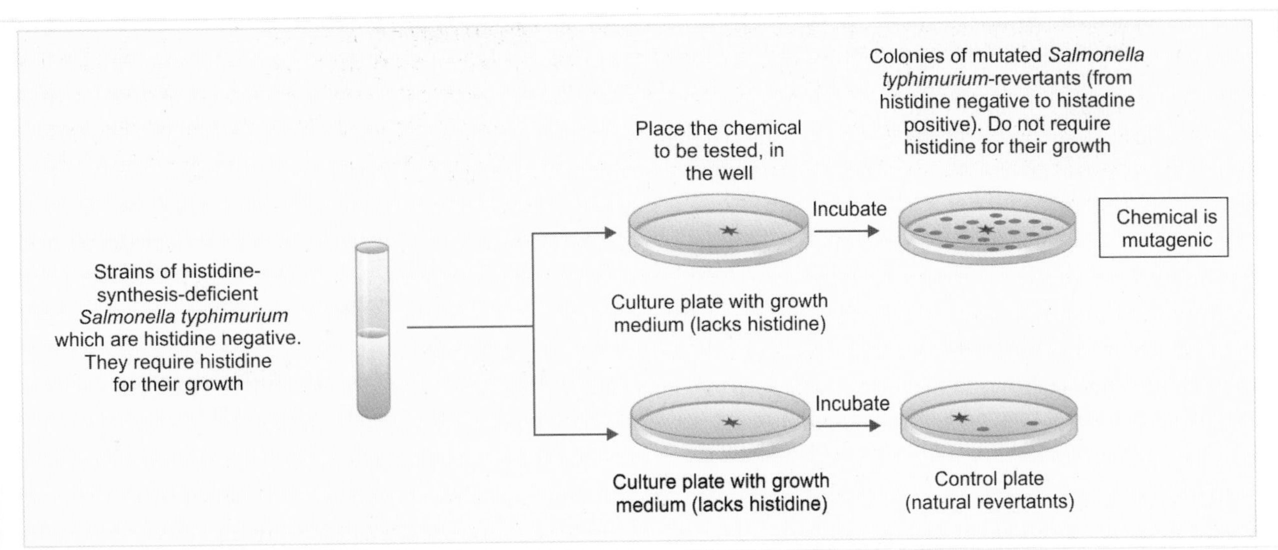

FIG. 99: Ames test. It is an in vitro assay to detect mutagenicity of chemical compounds. If the chemical is mutagenic it induces mutations in strains of histidine-deficienct *Salmonella typhimurium* in a culture medium.

Box 15: Major chemical carcinogens.

Direct-acting carcinogens

Alkylating agents
- β-Propiolactone
- Anticancer drugs (cyclophosphamide, chlorambucil, nitrosoureas, etc.)
- Dimethyl sulfate
- Diepoxybutane

Acylating agents
- 1-Acetylimidazole
- Dimethyl carbamoyl chloride

Indirect-acting carcinogens (procarcinogens)

Polycyclic and heterocyclic aromatic hydrocarbons
- Benz[*a*]anthracene
- Benzo[*a*]pyrene
- Dibenz[*a,h*]anthracene
- 7,12-Dimethylbenz[*a*]anthracene
- 3-Methylcholanthrene

Aromatic amines, amides and azo dyes
- 2-Naphthylamine (β-Naphthylamine)
- Benzidine
- 2-Acetylaminofluorene
- Dimethylaminoazobenzene (butter yellow)

Natural plant and microbial products
- Aflatoxin B_1
- Griseofulvin
- Betel nuts
- Cycasin
- Safrole

Metals
- Beryllium, cadmium, arsenic, chromium, nickel, lead and cobalt

Others
- Nitrosamine and amides
- Vinyl chloride
- Insecticides, fungicides
- Asbestos
- Polychlorinated biphenyls

Other classifications: Chemical carcinogens can also be classified in other ways—
- Natural chemicals, synthetic compounds (manmade), or mixtures of both that are synthesized or used for industrial, agricultural, or commercial purposes.
- Chemical of endogenous origin, (i.e., chemicals that result from natural metabolic intermediates), or exogenous chemicals.
- Chemical carcinogenesis consists of the three sequential and successive steps namely; (i) initiation, (ii) promotion, and (iii) progression. Hence, according to the involvement of carcinogenic chemicals in each of the steps, chemical carcinogens may be classified as initiators, promoters and progressors.
- According to their chemical structure, chemical carcinogens can be classified as polycyclic aromatic hydrocarbons (PAHs), alkylating agents, aromatic amines/amides, amino azo dyes, carbamates, halo-genated compounds, natural carcinogens, metalloids and hormones.
- According to their involvement with DNA as genotoxic (mitogenic) and nongenotoxic (cytogenic).
  - *Genotoxic carcinogens*: These are chemicals, or their metabolites, that are capable of acting directly, or interact with DNA or genetic material. They form DNA adducts and bind to DNA. They generate oxidative damage or induce DNA single- or DSBs. If not repaired, these are fixed as mutations during cell division. Subsequently they lead to mutations, chromosomal aberrations, and/or changes in chromosome number. DNA adducts are covalent (interatomic between two atoms) bonds and if not removed before the replication of DNA, these adducts can lead to mutations. If such mutations occur in oncogenes or the tumor suppressor genes that control cell proliferation, cancer will develop. Examples include polycyclic aromatic hydrocarbons (PAH), alkylating agents, aromatic amines, and amides.
  - *Nongenotoxic carcinogens*: They act as promoters and do not require metabolic activation. They do not react directly with DNA, do not produce DNA adducts. They are negative on mutagenicity tests. Non-genotoxic

carcinogens act by diverse mechanisms. These mechanisms include impact gene expression, disrupt normal cellular homeo-stasis, interact with cellular receptors, and increase cellular proliferation or decrease apoptosis. They are tissue and species-specific. Nongenotoxic carcinogens are further classified as mitogenic and cytotoxic depending on whether their activity is mediated by a receptor (receptor-interacting) or not. Mitogenic compounds produce cell proliferation in target tissues through interaction with a cellular receptor. Cytotoxic carcinogens cause cell death in susceptible tissues followed by compensatory hyperplasia.

Absorption of chemical carcinogens: Following exposure to chemical carcinogens, they may be absorbed in many ways such as ingestion, inhalation, skin absorption, injection, or other possible contamination routes. Then they get distributed across several tissues. Chemical absorbed orally pass through gastrointestinal tract and the liver. Then they are distributed in the body. Chemical inhaled are absorbed in the lungs; are distributed by the blood before reaching the liver; then they pass into the liver at a later stage.

Metabolism of chemical carcinogens: Chemical carcinogens are metabolized as follows—

- **Direct-acting carcinogens:** They directly act on DNA and cause mutations. They form DNA adducts (DNA adduct is a segment of DNA bound to a cancer-causing chemical) without being metabolized. These chemicals are called activation-independent carcinogens and ultimate carcinogens. About 25% of all carcinogens are direct carcinogens. The relative carcinogenic activity depends on its reactions and detoxification reactions. Direct carcinogens usually cause cancer at the site of exposure and at multiple sites.
- **Indirect, procarcinogens or indirect-acting genotoxic carcinogens:** Most chemical carcinogens (~75%) require metabolic activation to be carcinogenic and are called as indirect-acting carcinogens. The terms **procarcinogen is used for the parent compound**, **proximate carcinogen for its metabolite form as well as the intermediate** and **ultimate carcinogen for final form**. The final form of the carcinogen (ultimate carcinogen) causes mutation and neoplastic transformation. Indirect-acting genotoxic carcinogens produce their neoplastic effects, not at the site of exposure (as in direct-acting genotoxic carcinogens) but at the target tissue where they are metabolically activated. Metabolic activation mainly occurs in the liver at the smooth endoplasmic reticulum, where the cytochrome P450 is abundant, and/or in other enzymes located in urothelium, skin, gastrointestinal system, esophagus, kidneys, and lungs. The final product is an electrophilic (a molecule having a tendency to attract or acquire electrons) compound that directly interacts with proteins, RNA, and DNA to form adducts. The P450 system is involved not only for activation of chemical carcinogens but also involved in metabolism of drugs. Though some of these metabolic processes activate reactive electrophiles, many inactivate the chemicals by detoxification pathways. The inactivated chemicals have increased aqueous solubility and are excreted either in urine or in feces. Thus, any exposure to chemical carcinogens, its effect depends on metabolic pathways for activation versus inactivation (detoxification pathways).

Direct-acting Agents

Direct-acting chemical agents **do not require metabolic conversion** to become carcinogenic, but most of them are **weak carcinogens**. Some of the drugs (e.g., alkylating agents) used to cure, (e.g., Hodgkin lymphoma), control, or delay recurrence of some cancer (e.g., leukemia, lymphoma), may produce a second form of cancer (e.g., acute myeloid leukemia) later. Initially, such agents have been used for the treatment of non-neoplastic disorders (e.g., rheumatoid arthritis or granulomatosis with polyangiitis).

Alkylating agents

- **Source: Many cancer chemotherapeutic drugs** (e.g., cyclophosphamide, cisplatin, busulfan) are alkylating agents.
- **Mechanism of action:** Alkylating agents **contain electron-deficient atoms** that **react with electron-rich atoms in DNA**. They transfer alkyl groups (methyl, ethyl, etc.) to macromolecules, including guanines within DNA. These drugs not only destroy cancer cells by damaging DNA, but also injure normal cells.
- **Cancers produced:** Treatment with alkylating chemotherapy carries a significant risk of solid and hematological malignancies at a later time.

Indirect-acting Agents (Procarcinogens)

These chemicals **require metabolic activation** for conversion **to an active ultimate carcinogen**. Most chemical carcinogens act indirectly and they need metabolic activation for conversion into ultimate carcinogens. Most of the potent chemical cacrcinogens are indirect-acting carcinogens.

1. Polycyclic Aromatic Hydrocarbons

Polycyclic aromatic hydrocarbons (PAH) consist of multiple fused benzene rings. They are the most potent and extensively studied indirect-acting chemical carcinogens. Potent to moderately carcinogenic PAHs include benzo[*a*]pyrene, 3-methylcholanthrene, dibenzanthracene, benzo[*a*]pyrene, dibenzo[*a,h*]anthracene, 5-methylchrysene, and dibenz[*a,j*] anthracene. Benzo[*e*]pyrene (the active component of soot and Potts shown it be carcinogenic), dibenz[*a,c*]anthracene, chrysene, benzo[*c*]phenanthrene, and fluoranthene are relatively weak or inactive carcinogens.

- **Source:**
  - Originally derived from coal tar and fossil fuels and are formed during incomplete combustion of organic matter such as coal, mineral oil, and oil shale. Thus, exposure to PAH occurs in the form of automobile exhaust, soot, coal tar, cigarette smoke, and charred food products.
  - *Cigarette smoke*: PAHS are formed during high-temperature combustion of tobacco in cigarette smoking and responsible for lung cancer in cigarette smokers.
  - *Animal fats*: It may be produced during the process of broiling and grilling meats. Broiling is cooking by exposing food to direct heat. This may either on a grill over live coals or below a gas burner or electric coil. Broiling differs from roasting and baking in that the food is turned during the process of broiling so as to cook one side of the food at a time.
  - *Smoked food*: Smoked meats and fish. Smoking is the process of flavoring, browning, cooking, or preserving food by exposing the food to smoke from burning.

- **Mechanism of action:**
  - Polycyclic hydrocarbons are metabolized by cytochrome P450-dependent mixed function oxidases to electrophilic (have electron-deficient atoms) epoxides (electrophilic mutagens).
  - Epoxides react with proteins and nucleic acids (DNA, RNA) (with DNA it forms a DNA adduct). For example, polyvinyl chloride (used in plastic industry) is metabolized to an epoxide and causes hepatic angiosarcomas.
  - Polymorphic cytochrome P450-dependent monooxygenase: The genes encoding these enzymes are polymorphic. The activity and inducibility of these enzymes vary significantly among individuals (refer page 962). These enzymes are required for the activation of procarcinogens into ultimate carcinogen. The susceptibility of an individual to carcinogenesis partly depends on the particular polymorphic variants that an individual inherits. Thus it may be possible to assess risk of cancer in any individual by genetic analysis of these enzymes polymorphisms. For example, the metabolism of benzo[*a*]pyrene (one of polycyclic aromatic hydrocarbons) is by the product of the P-450 gene, *CYP1A1*. For example, particular population may carry a highly inducible form of this gene. Light smokers with the susceptible *CYP1A1* genotype have a higher risk of developing lung cancer compared with smokers without the permissive genotype. The risk of cancer also depends on the variations in metabolic pathways involved in the inactivation (detoxification) of some procarcinogens or their derivatives.
- **Cancers produced:** The specific type of cancer produced depends on the route of administration, e.g., cancers in the **skin**, **soft tissues**, **lung, breast,** skin, and urinary system.

2. Aromatic amines and azo dyes

They are indirect-acting carcinogens.

- **Source:**
  - In the past, the aromatic amines (β-naphthylamine) and azo dyes were used in the aniline dye and rubber industries.
  - Azo-dyes were used for coloring food (e.g., butter and margarine which give yellow color, scarlet red for coloring cherries). **Benzidine** is a member of *aromatic amines* and in the past, benzidine-based azo dyes were synthesized in vast quantities.
- **Mechanism of action:**
  - They are not carcinogenic at the point of application.
  - Both aromatic amines and azo dyes are mainly metabolized in the liver.
  - The aromatic amines are converted to active carcinogens in the liver. However, can be detoxified immediately by conjugation with glucuronic acid in the liver.
  - The conjugated metabolite is excreted in the urine and deconjugated in the urinary tract by the enzyme glucuronidase. The urothelium is thus exposed to the active carcinogen (reactive hydroxylamine) which may cause bladder cancer.
- **Cancers produced: Bladder cancer** (β-naphthylamine and benzidine) and **liver tumors** (azo dyes).

3. Natural microbial product

Aflatoxin B_1 (AFB_1): It is a fungal metabolite and is one of the most potent liver carcinogen.

- **Source:** Aflatoxin B_1 is a natural product of *Aspergillus* mold species, such as ***Aspergillus flavus*** and *Aspergillus parasiticus*. These are molds which grow on **improperly stored grains and peanuts**. The growth of these molds is favored by humid conditions and poor storage. Exposure to aflatoxins occurs via consumption of these contaminated nuts and grain, such as peanuts and corn. There is a strong correlation between the dietary level of food contaminated with aflatoxin and the incidence of hepatocellular carcinoma.
- **Mechanism of action:** AFB_1 is highly mutagenic. AFB_1 is converted to an epoxide metabolite responsible for its mutagenic and carcinogenic action. The epoxides bind to DNA and also produce **mutations of *p53* gene**. Aflatoxin B1-associated hepatocellular carcinoma tend to have a particular mutation in *TP53* that is G:C→T:A transversion in codon 249. This produces an arginine-to-serine substitution in the p53 protein and this interferes with function of p53. It is to be noted that *TP53* mutations are infrequent in liver tumors in regions where aflatoxin contamination of food does not occur, and few of these mutations involve codon 249. The risk of HCC is higher in individuals exposed to both HBV and aflatoxin over individuals exposed to either agent alone.
- **Cancers produced:** Powerful liver carcinogen causes **hepatocellular carcinoma**.

4. Metals

Many metals or metal compounds can induce cancer. Most metal-induced cancers occur in an occupational setting. Compounds like arsenic, nickel, lead, cadmium, cobalt, chromium and beryllium can produce cancer. Most metal-induced cancers occur due to occupational exposure.

- **Beryllium:** It is a carcinogen capable of inducing lung cancer. Occupational exposure to beryllium occurs in workers due to inhalation of beryllium-containing dusts during processing of ores, machining of beryllium metal and alloys, and manufacturing of aerospace materials, ceramics, sports equipment, and electronics.
- **Cadmium:** Cadmium is a heavy metal present in soil, air, and water. Occupational exposures to cadmium occur during the manufacture of nickel-cadmium batteries, pigments, and plastic stabilizers and electroplating processes, metal smelting, and electronic waste recycling. Cigarette smoke also contains cadmium. On absorption, cadmium accumulate in the body because of its poor excretion. Cadmium is stored in liver and kidney. There is no effective pathway of detoxification for cadmium. The half-life of cadmium is about 15–20 years. Cadmium exposure can produce cancers of lung, prostate and kidney. Cadmium may act through non-genotoxic mechanisms to activate proto-oncogenes and disrupt normal cellular processes.
- **Arsenic:** It is distributed widely in the environment. It is found in the earth's crust. It is associated with cancers of skin, lung, urinary bladder, kidney, and liver. Arsenic exposure occurs through drinking contaminated water,

diet, or contact with wood preserved with arsenicals. It may also occur during mining of tin, gold, and uranium; and during application of arsenical pesticides. Chronic exposure to arsenic in drinking water produces altered skin pigmentation and hyperkeratosis of the palms of the hand and soles of the feet. This may progress to skin cancer.

- **Chromium:** Chromium is a carcinogen. Exposure to chromium can occur in workers of industries such as chrome plating, welding, leather tanning, and stainless steel production. Exposure to chromium usually occurs through inhalation and may lead to increased risk of lung cancer.

5. Others

Nitrosamines They are potent carcinogens.

- **Source: Before the advent of refrigerator**, nitrites were added as **a preservative for meats and other foods.** *N*-nitrosamines are present in smoked meats and in meats containing the antimicrobial and color-enhancing agent nitrite.
- **Mechanism of action:** The source of *N*-nitroso compounds may be exogenous and endogenous and in both cases, nitrogen oxides/nitrites are formed. **Nitrites react with amines** (present in meat) **and amides** in the diet and are metabolized by commensal bacteria within the gut and converted to **carcinogenic nitrosamines**. *N*-nitrosamines can react with DNA to initiate carcinogenesis.
- **Cancers produced**: Mainly **gastrointestinal and lung neoplasms.**

Asbestos The term *asbestos* refers to a group of naturally occurring mineral fibers. Asbestos fibers that are classified according to their morphologic characteristics as curly (serpentine) or straight (amphibole) fibers. The carcinogenicity of fiber depends on the shape and length-to-width ratio. Long (>4 μm) and thin (<0.5 μm diameter) fibers are the most carcinogenic. Because of the flame-resistant and durable characteristics of asbestos, they have been used as an insulating agent in schools, factories, homes, and ships, as construction material, and as a raw material for automobile brake and clutch parts. Hence, extensive exposure to asbestos can occur. Inhalation of asbestos fibers results in asbestosis, pleural plaques, **mesothelioma** and **carcinoma of the lung and larynx**. Mesothelioma may involve pleura as well as peritoneum. Mesothelioma is a rare malignant tumor of the membranous lining of the pleura and peritoneum. Cigarette smoking acts synergistically with asbestos exposure to induce lung tumors.

Benzene It is a widely used solvent and is present in petrol (gasoline), automobile emissions, and cigarette smoke. Exposure to benzene occurs in industries involved in rubber production, chemical plants, oil refineries, and shoe manufacturing. Benzene is a volatile aromatic solvent and main exposure is through inhalation. Its exposure is associated with an increased risk of leukemia (e.g., acute myeloid leukemia), myelodysplastic syndromes and non-Hodgkin lymphoma. Apart from being mutagenic, benzene alters cell-signaling pathways that control hematopoiesis in hematopoietic stem cells.

Table 27 shows major group, compound, major source, mechanism of action, and organs affected/cancer, and type of important chemical carcinogens.

Mechanism of Action of Chemical Carcinogens

Molecular targets of chemical carcinogens: Most chemical carcinogens target DNA and are mutagenic. A **mutagen** is an agent, which can **permanently alter the genetic constitution** of a cell.

- All direct and ultimate carcinogens (of indirect carcinogens) **contain highly reactive electrophilic groups and form adducts with DNA, RNA and proteins**. Initiation causes nonlethal damage to the DNA and this damage is repaired by some error-prone fashion. These mutated cell then passes the DNA damage to its daughter cells.
- **Genes affected:** Mutations can occur throughout the genome and any gene may be affected. Most commonly involved genes are proto-**oncogenes** (*RAS*) **and tumor suppressor genes** (*TP53*).

Multistep hypothesis (Fig. 100)

Q. Discuss multi-step hypothesis of chemical carcinogenesis.

Chemical carcinogenesis is a **multistep** process. Once the tumor process is started, it does not require the continued presence of the carcinogen. Complete carcinogens are capable of triggering all three stages of carcinogenesis.

Four major steps involved in chemical carcinogenesis are:

1. Initiation

It is the **first important step** that develops from **exposure of cells** to a sufficient dose of a **carcinogenic agent** (initiator).

- **Reaction with DNA:** Tumor initiators are those carcinogenic compounds that are capable of inducing an initial driving DNA mutation. Sites of reaction of initiation are DNA, RNA and proteins. All initiators are highly reactive electrophiles (electron-deficient atoms) and can react with nucleophilic (electron-rich) sites in the cell. Initiators act in a dividing cell, either directly or following metabolic activation and cause mutagenesis. Examples of carcinogenic initiators include alkylating agents, PAHS, aromatic amines, metals (cadmium, chromium and nickel), aflatoxins, and nitrosamines.
- **Effect of initiation:** Initiators **produces nonlethal permanent (irreversible) alterations or damage to DNA (mutations)** in a cell. If the damage is lethal or severe, it causes cell death.

2. Promotion

- **Promoters:** Chemical carcinogens classified as promoters accelerate or promote the transformation process in a cell when applied repeatedly after initiators.
- **Cell proliferation:** Promoters stimulate the initiated (with permanent DNA damage-mutated) **cells to enter into the cell cycle leading to** cell proliferation. Unlike initiators, the **cellular changes produced by promoters are reversible**.
- **Produce changes only on initiated cell: Tumors develop only if the promoter is applied after the initiator** and not the reverse way. Promoters cannot behave as initiators when used in isolation at the same dosage at which they promote. However, in studies of chemical carcinogenesis it was observed that prolonged exposure and using high doses, almost all promoter agents can induce neoplasia without the prior application of initiators. Examples of this are exposure to phenobarbital, benzene, and asbestos,

which, even without the previous use of initiator agents, lead to neoplastic development

- **Mode of action:** Promoters **cannot directly interact/damage DNA** (mutation) without being metabolically activated. Some promoter is specific to a particular tissue, but others can act on different tissues at the same time.
- **Examples** of chemical carcinogens classified as promoters **include**: Phorbol esters, hormones (such as diethylstilbestrol), phenols, cyclamates, saccharin and drugs.
- **Continuous proliferation** of initiated cells **leads to secondary genetic abnormalities** and tumor growth

Table 27: Examples of chemical carcinogens, their source, mechanism of action and organs affected.

Major group of chemical carcinogen	*Compounds*	*Major source*	*Mechanism of action*	*Organs affected/ Type of cancer*
Direct-acting carcinogens				
Alkylating agents	Anticancer drugs/nitrogen mustards (chlorambucil, cyclophosphamide)	Cancer chemotherapy	DNA adducts, DNA strand breaks, DNA alkylation	Leukemia, nasal tumors
Indirect-acting carcinogens (procarcinogens)				
Polycyclic aromatic hydrocarbons	Benzo[*a*]pyrene	Charcoal broiled foods, cigarette smoke	DNA adducts	Skin, lungs, stomach
	Dimethylbenz[*a*] anthracene	Diesel exhaust	DNA adducts	Liver, skin
Aromatic amines/ amides	• Aniline dyes • 2-naphthylamine (ß-naphthylamine) • Benzidine • 2-acetylaminofluorene	Oil refining, synthetic polymers, dyes, adhesives and rubbers, pharmaceuticals, pesticides, explosives, cigarette smoke, hair dyes, diesel exhaust, burning/pyrolysis of amino acids and protein-rich vegetable matter or cooked food	DNA adducts (DNA adduct is a segment of DNA covalently bond to a chemical)	Liver, urinary bladder
Amino azo dyes	o-Aminoazotoluene; *N*-dimethyl-4-aminoazobenzene	Dyes and pigments	Adducts with DNA and hemoglobin	Liver, lungs, urinary bladder
Natural carcinogens	Aflatoxin B_1	Food contamination (grains, nuts, peanut, butter) by *Aspergillus flavus*	Forms adducts with guanine, react with RNA and proteins	Liver cancer
	Asbestos	Environmental media (air, water and soil); human activities (product manufacture, construction activities and transport)	Mutagenic	Mesothelioma, lung cancer
Metals	Arsenic	Natural and anthropogenic sources (drinking water, gold mining activities, etc.)	Cell cycle checkpoint dysregulation, DNA damage response, defects in cell cycle checkpoints, disabled apoptosis, telomere dysfunction	Skin, lungs, liver, lungs, prostate, kidneys, urinary bladder
	Cadmium	Burning of coal and tobacco	Interferes with antioxidant defense mechanisms, inhibit apoptosis	Lungs, nasal cavity, breast
	Nickel	Industrial processes	Oxidative stress, recombination and repair of DNA	Cancer of respiratory tract
	Chromium	Industrial processes	DNA adducts, oxidative DNA damage	Lungs and nasal cavity
Hormones	Ethinyl estradiol	Medicinal exposure	Cell cycle	Uterus and prostate
	Estradiol	Medicinal exposure	Cell cycle	Breast
	Estrogen	Medicinal exposure	Cell cycle	Cancer of breast, endometrium and ovary
	Tamoxifen	Medicinal exposure	Cell cycle arrest	Breast

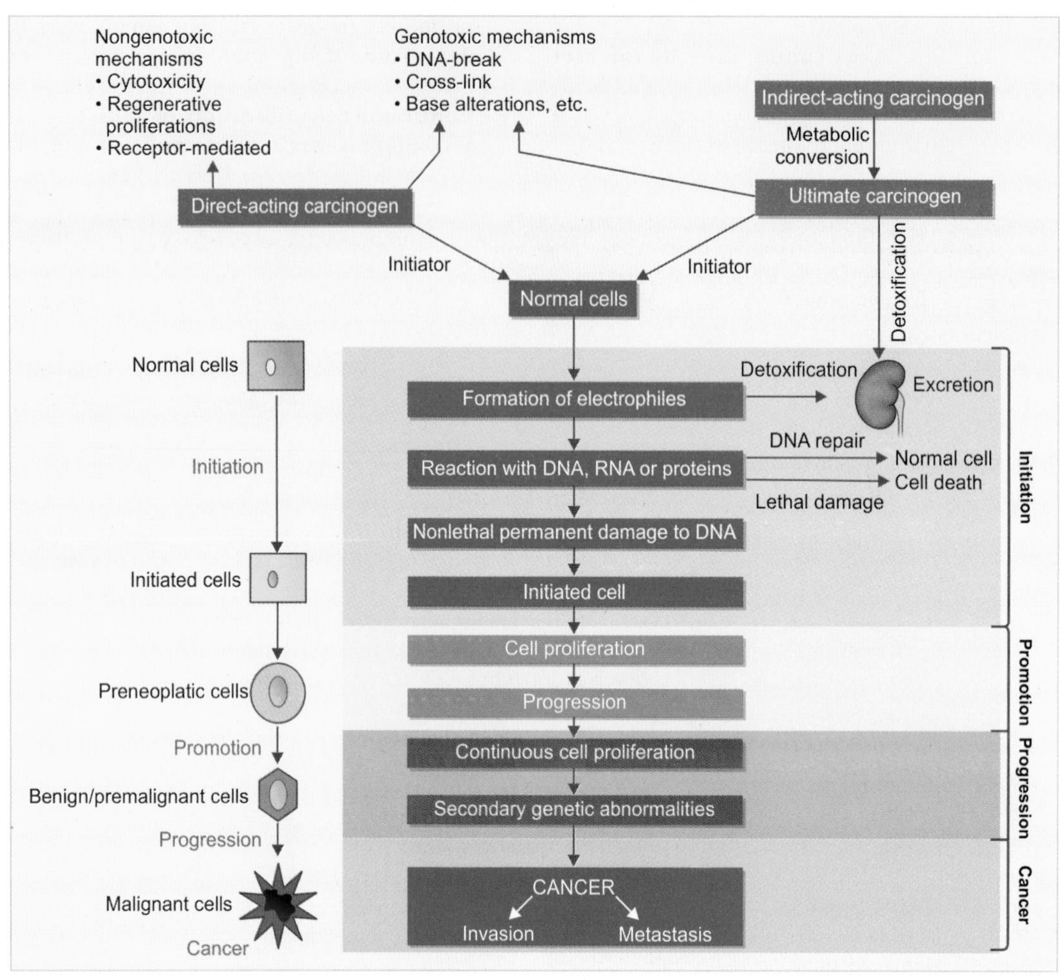

FIG. 100: Multistep theory of chemical carcinogenesis.

becomes independent of the initiator or the promoter (i.e., autonomous). **Many accumulated mutations finally immortalize the cells.**

- Final result of the different steps is the development of neoplasm are invasion and metastases.

3. Progression

- **Continuous proliferation** of initiated cells **leads to secondary genetic abnormalities** and tumor growth becomes independent of the initiator or the promoter (i.e., autonomous). During this stage, sufficient **accumulation of mutations** has accumulated and **finally immortalize the cells**.
- Chemical carcinogens classified as progressors are compounds that move mutated cells from the promotion to progression phase. They convert premalignant mutated cells irreversibly to fully malignant cells.
- Example of progressor agents include alkylating agents, arsenic salts, asbestos, and benzene.

4. Cancer

- Final result of the different steps is the development of neoplasm followed by invasion and metastases.

Examples: The morphologic sequence of hyperplasia, dysplasia and carcinoma in situ found in epithelium (e.g., skin, cervix and colon) indicates multistep carcinogenesis.

Microbial Carcinogenesis

Q. Define and classify oncogenic viruses. Discuss the mechanism of tumor production by viruses.

Q. Classify/list oncogenic viruses. Discuss viral oncogenesis.

Q. Discuss biological/infectious carcinogens.

Q. Discuss viruses and human cancer.

Viruses that cause tumors are called as oncogenic viruses. Many viruses have been proved to be oncogenic in animals, but only about 15% of all human cancers have been associated with viral infection. Few viruses are known to be implicated in human malignancy (**Box 16**). The status of the immune system of the individual is important in controlling oncogenic virus-infected cells. Virus-induced cancers incidence is more in immunosuppressed individuals. In microbial carcinogenesis, initially the infection triggers polyclonal cell proliferation. Later, driver mutations occur in rapidly dividing cells and polyclonal proliferation becomes monoclonal.

Box 16: Classification and types of oncogenic viruses.

RNA viruses
- Human T-cell leukemia virus type 1 (HTLV-1)
- Hepatitis C virus (HCV)

DNA viruses
- Human papillomavirus (HPV)
- Epstein–Barr virus (EBV)
- Hepatitis B virus (HBV)
- Kaposi's sarcoma-associated herpesvirus (KSHV) also called human herpesvirus 8 (HHV-8)
- Merkel cell polyomavirus (MCV)

Classification (Box 16)

They are mainly classified depending on the genetic material into: (i) Oncogenic **RNA viruses,** and (ii) oncogenic **DNA viruses**.

Q. Define carcinogenesis. Discuss the role of RNA viruses in tumorigenesis.

Q. Explain the mechanism involved in tumor production by viruses.

Oncogenic RNA Viruses

Human T-cell leukemia virus type 1

Human T-cell leukemia virus type 1 (HTLV-1) is an enveloped, single-stranded RNA retrovirus. **HTLV-1** infection has been firmly linked with human cancer, namely a rare type of adult T-cell leukemia/***lymphoma* (ATLL). ATLL is a tumor endemic in certain parts of Japan, the Caribbean basin, South America, and Africa. It may be found sporadically elsewhere in the world.**

- **Major target for neoplastic transformation:** Similar to the human immunodeficiency virus (causing AIDS), HTLV-1 has tropism for **CD4⁺ T lymphocytes.** Hence, **CD4⁺ T** cell is the major target for neoplastic transformation.
- **Tumor caused:** Adult **T-cell leukemia/lymphoma** that develops after a long latent period (40–60 years). Only 2–5% of HTLV-1-infected individuals develop disease.
- **Mode of infection:** (i) Sexual intercourse, (ii) blood products, and (iii) breastfeeding.

***Mechanism of Oncogenesis* (Fig. 101):** It is a **multistep process**. HTLV-1 infects CD4⁺ T-cells. **HTLV-1** genome contains the *gag, pol, env,* and long terminal-repeat regions characteristic of all retroviruses. But **does not contain oncogene and its genes cannot integrate** into the host genome. In contrast to other leukemia viruses, **HTLV-1** contains two other genes called as *Tax* and *HBZ* (HTLV-1 basic zipper factor). Many transforming activity of HTLV-1 is due to the protein products of these two genes. **Tax is the protein product of the *Tax* gene**. Tax protein is necessary for viral replication and cellular transformation, because it stimulates transcription of viral RNA from the 5′ long terminal repeat. HBZ is a transcription factor. Both Tax and HBZ alter the transcription of host cell genes and interact with some signaling proteins of host cell. They are probably contribute to the acquisition of cancer and also involved in growth and survival of leukemic cells.

- Increased survival and growth of infected cells:
  - Tax interacts with PI3 kinase and activate the downstream signaling cascade. This promotes both cell survival and metabolic alterations that increases the cell growth.
  - Tax upregulates the expression of cyclin D and represses the expression of many CDK inhibitors. These in turn promote cell cycle progression.
  - Tax can activate the transcription factor Nuclear factor kappa B (NF-κB). This can promote the survival of many cell types, including lymphocytes.
- **Increased genomic instability:** Tax can cause increased **risk of developing mutations and genomic instability** in proliferating CD4⁺ T-cells. This is achieved by interfering with DNA-repair functions and inhibiting cell cycle checkpoints activated by DNA damage. This is responsible for highly aneuploid nature of HTLV-1-associated leukemias.

Steps in the development of adult T-cell leukemia/lymphoma (Fig. 101): The HTLV-1 genome encodes a viral protein called *Tax*. It stimulates cell proliferation, increases cell survival, and interferes with cell cycle controls. Initially, the T cell proliferation is polyclonal, but later they are prone to increased risk for secondary mutations and may progress to the outgrowth of a monoclonal leukemia.

The exact steps involved in the development of adult T-cell leukemia/lymphoma is not clearly known.

1. Infection by HTLV-1 causes the expansion of a nonmalignant polyclonal cell population through stimulatory effects of Tax protein (product of *Tax* gene) on cell proliferation. *Tax* gene turns on cytokines and its receptors such as (i) interleukin (IL)-2 and its receptor [IL-2 receptor (IL-2R)] and IL-15 and its receptor IL-15R. Secretion of cytokines and autocrine stimulation of CD4⁺ T-cells leads to proliferation of **CD4⁺** T cells. Tax also stimulates secretion of granulocyte macrophage colony-stimulating factor (GM-CSF) by CD4⁺ T-cells which in turn stimulates nearby macrophages to produce T-cell mitogens and leads to polyclonal proliferation of CD4⁺ T-cells.
2. *Tax* inactivates ***p53*** and other genes controlling cell cycle (e.g., *CDKN2A/p16* gene, $p16^{INK4a}$). They predispose proliferating T cells to an increased risk for mutations and genomic instability. This genomic instability permits the accumulation of oncogenic mutations and eventually lead to monoclonal neoplastic T-cell population. This proliferation is Tax-independent. The most common driver mutations enhance T cell receptor signaling and stimulate NF-κB activation. NF-κB promotes cell proliferation and resistance to apoptosis.
3. **Role of HBZ:** HBZ plays an essential role in oncogenesis. This is by regulating viral transcription and modulating multiple host factors, as well as cellular signaling pathways. They contribute to the development and continued growth of cancer. HBZ promotes growth and proliferation of leukemic cells. HBZ hinders activation-induced cell death in T cells.

Oncogenic DNA Viruses

Five DNA viruses are strongly associated with cancer in humans. These include human papillomaviruses (HPV), Epstein-Barr virus (EBV), Kaposi sarcoma herpesvirus [(KSHV), also called

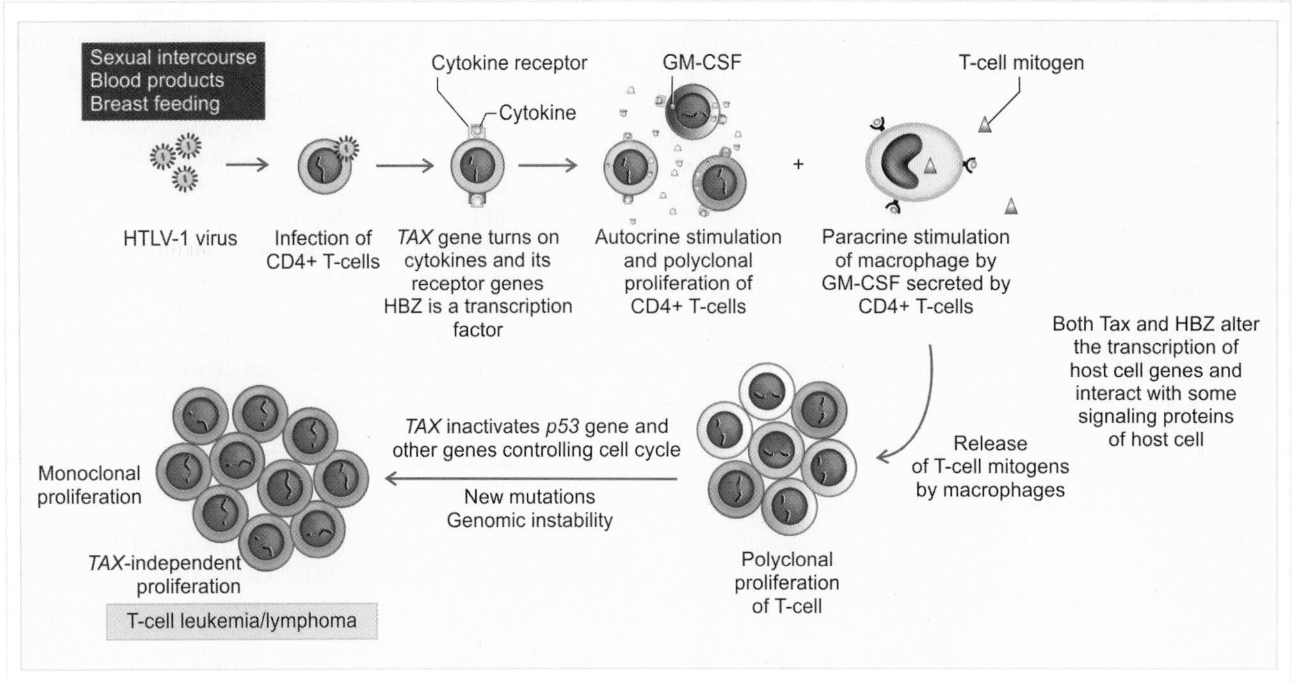

(GM-CSF: granulocyte macrophage colony-stimulating factor; HTLV-1: human T-cell leukemia virus type 1)

FIG. 101: Pathogenesis of human T-cell leukemia. HBZ is a transcription factor. Both Tax and HBZ alter the transcription of host cell genes and interact with certain host cell signaling proteins. In doing so, they appear to contribute to the acquisition of cancer hallmarks, though the mechanisms remain unclear.

human herpesvirus-8 (HHV-8)], a polyomavirus called Merkel cell polyomavirus (MCV), and hepatitis B virus (HBV). Hepatitis C virus (HCV) is a RNA virus and discussion here along with HBV because both viruses share an association chronic liver injury and liver cancer.

Human papillomavirus

Q. Write short essay on oncogenesis by human papillomavirus. Add a note on HPV and genital cancer.

More than 140 known HPV types have been identified and each papillomavirus type is a functionally distinct serotype (means that serum antibodies that neutralize one HPV type do not fully neutralize other HPV types). The papillomaviruses are small (~8 kbp) DNA viruses containing circular, double-stranded genomes.

Cell infected: Human papillomaviruses marked tropism for epithelial tissues. They infect **only the immature squamous cells,** but **its replication occurs in the maturing, nonproliferating squamous cells.** Thus, their full productive life cycle occurs only in squamous cells. The physical state of the virus differs in different lesions.

Classification of HPV There are genetically different types of HPV and are divided into **low-risk and high-risk HPVs**. Low risk type only rarely give rise to tumors, whereas high risk types are found in lesions that progress to malignancy. Types of HPV and associated lesions are presented in **Table 28**.

A. **Low oncogenic risk:**
   - Causes **condyloma acuminatum** in vulva, perineal and perianal region.
   - **HPV genome** is maintained in a **nonintegrated free episomal** (extrachromosomal) **form**.
   - **Virus freely replicates** and **causes the death of the host** cell and it is **known as productive infection**.

B. **High oncogenic risk:**
   - There are about 20 types of high oncogenic risk HPVs. Among these types, **HPV 16 and HPV 18 are the most important** in **cervical carcinogenesis**. At present a new vaccine is available that protects against infection with most oncogenic HPV types. It is likely to reduce the incidence of cervical cancer. Other high risk types include HPV 31 and 33.
   - Can also cause **squamous cell carcinoma** of the **vagina, vulva, penis, anus, tonsil, and oropharynx**.
   - **Integration into the host DNA:** In cancers, the HPV genome (viral DNA) is integrated into the genome of the host cell, which is important for malignant transformation. Similar to HTLV-1, the site of viral integration of HPV in host chromosomes is random. But the pattern of integration is clonal. **Integration causes:**
     - **Overexpression of the oncoproteins E6 and E7**.
     - **Genomic instability** in the host cell.

Various viruses implicated in human tumors are listed in **Table 28**.

Features of infection by HPV Even though **HPV is a causative factor** for squamous intraepithelial lesion (SIL also known as CIN/cerical intraepithelial neoplasia and cancer of the cervix, **only few infected will develop cancer**. Most women infected with HPV clear the infection by immunological mechanisms.

- **Longer the duration of infection, higher the risk of CIN** and subsequent **carcinoma**. Infections with high

Table 28: Various viruses implicated in human tumors and associated lesions.

Type of virus	*Lesions (cofactors)*
ONCOGENIC RNA VIRUSES	
Retroviruses family	
• Human T-cell lymphotropic virus type-1 (HTLV-1)	Adult T-cell leukemia/lymphoma
Flavivirus family	
• Hepatitis C virus (HCV)	Hepatocellular carcinoma (cofactor aflatoxin), splenic marginal zone lymphoma
ONCOGENIC DNA VIRUSES	
Papillomaviruses family	
Human papillomavirus (HPV)	
A. Low-oncogenic risk HPV—benign lesions of squamous epithelium	
• HPV types 1, 2, 4 and 7 • HPV-6 and HPV-11	• Benign squamous papilloma (wart) • Condylomata acuminata (genital warts) of the vulva, penis and perianal region • Laryngeal papillomas
B. High-oncogenic risk HPV—malignant tumors	
• HPV types 16 and 18	• Squamous cell carcinoma of the cervix and anogenital region (cofactors—smoking, oral contraceptives) • Head and neck squamous cell carcinomas, especially of the tonsils and oropharynx
Herpesvirus family	
• Epstein–Barr virus (EBV)	• Burkitt lymphoma (requires cofactor—malaria) • Nasopharyngeal cancer (cofactors— nitrosamines, genetic)
• Human herpesvirus-8 (HHV-8) (KSHV)	• Kaposi's sarcoma (cofactors—AIDS) • Pleural effusion lymphoma, multicentric Castleman disease
Hepadnavirus family	
• Hepatitis B virus	Hepatocellular carcinoma (cofactors—aflatoxin, alcohol, smoking)
Polyomavirus family	
• Merkel cell polyomavirus	Merkel cell carcinoma (cofactors—UV, immunosuppression)

(AIDS: acquired immunodeficiency syndrome)

oncogenic risk HPVs last longer than infections with low oncogenic risk HPVs.

- **HPVs infect immature basal cells of the squamous epithelium, or immature metaplastic squamous cells** present at the squamocolumnar junction.
- **Infects only damaged surface epithelium** and **not the mature intact superficial squamous cells**. In areas of epithelial breaks or damage, the HPV can reach the immature cells in the basal layer of the epithelium.
- **Replication occurs in the maturing nonproliferating squamous cells which normally are arrested in the G_1 phase of the cell cycle** (though the virus infects only the immature squamous cells). However, these mature cells actively progress through the cell cycle when infected with HPV by using the host cell DNA synthesis machinery to replicate its own genome.
- **HPV has to induce DNA synthesis** and must **reactivate the mitotic cycle** in such nonproliferating cells. Viral replication results in a cytopathic effect, **"koilocytic atypia,"** consisting of **nuclear atypia** and a **cytoplasmic perinuclear halo**.

Mode of Action of HPV (Fig. 102) **Episomal form:** In **benign lesions** such as benign warts, condylomata and most **precancerous lesions**; the HPV genome is present as nonintegrated, free (episomal) viral DNA. Extrachromosomal (episomal) form of viral DNA is observed in precursor lesions associated with high-risk HPVs and in condylomata associated with low-risk HPVs.

Integration of viral DNA into the host cell genome: In **cancers**, the HPV genome is integrated into the host genome and is essential for malignant transformation. The effects of integration include (i) increased expression of E6 and E7 genes, (ii) dysregulation of oncogenes near the sites of viral insertion (e.g., MYC). Papillomaviruses normally persist in the basal layer of squamous epithelium. Main step in cervical cancer progression is the accidental integration of viral DNA sequences into the genome of cells in the basal layer. As a result, replication to new virions cannot occur as the cells move upwards from the basal layer to the surface. This interrupts the progress of the virus infectious cycle. Major oncoproteins encoded by high-risk HPV are E5, E6 and E7. **E6 and E7 are most important oncoproteins** responsible for the oncogenesis.

Integration results in overexpression of the two viral genes *E6* and *E7*. They directly drive cellular proliferation. Protein products of E6 and E7 (oncoproteins) are important for the oncogenic effects of HPV.

- **Oncogenic activities of E6 (Fig. 102):** The E6 protein complements the effects of E7.
  - **Inactivation of tumor suppressor *p53* gene:** E6 protein binds and degrades *p53*. It degrades *BAX* (a proapoptotic factor) and **prevents apoptosis**. E6 from high-risk HPV types has a higher affinity for *p53* than E6 from low-risk HPV types.
  - **Activation of telomerase:** E6 stimulates the expression of telomerase reverse transcriptase (TERT). TERT is the catalytic subunit of telomerase. TERT prevents replicative senescence and **cell proliferation** continues (immortalization of cells).
- **Oncogenic activities of E7 (Fig. 102):** The effects of E7 protein are as follows:
  - **Inactivation of tumor suppressor *RB* gene:** The E7 protein complements the effects of E6. **E7 protein binds** to the hypophosphorylated (active) form of **RB protein** and inactivates RB. E2F transcription

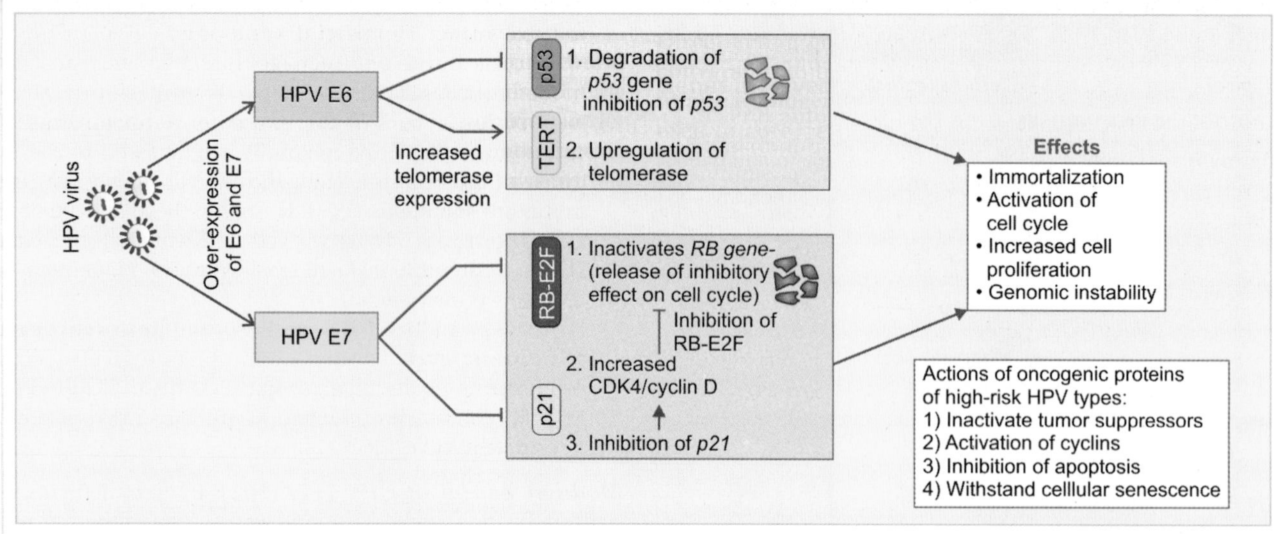

(TERT: telomerase reverse transcriptase)

FIG. 102: Mode of action of HPV proteins E6 and E7 on the cell cycle.

factors are normally sequestered by RB. Inactivation of RB **releases inhibitory effect** E2F transcription factors and permits **cell cycle progression.** E7 proteins from high risk HPV types have a higher affinity for RB than E7 proteins from low-risk HPV types.

- ○ **Inactivation of inhibitors of cell cycle:** E7 also inactivates the cyclin-dependent kinase (CDK) inhibitor. Thus, inactivation of CDK inhibitors (CDKIs) such as **CDKN1A/*p21*** and CDNK1B/*p27* **activates cell cycle.**
- ○ **Activation of cyclins (activators of cell cycle):** Also E7 proteins from high-risk HPVs (types 16, 18, and 31) bind and probably activate cyclins. These include cyclins E and A and facilitates G2/M transition and **activation of cell cycle.**

- **Combined action of E6 and E7:** They induce centrosome duplication and **genomic instability.**

E6 and E7 proteins of noncancer-causing HPV types do not have the above mentioned activities. Some papillomavirus types express an E5 oncogene. Its protein product E5 protein activates cell surface growth factor receptors such as platelet-derived growth factor β (PDGF-β) and epidermal growth factor (EGF) receptor. E5 expression is uncommon in cervical tumors, and its role in human cancer is not known.

Secondary somatic genetic changes occur in these latently infected cells and give rise to malignancy. Infection with HPV itself is not sufficient for carcinogenesis, and it requires the acquisition of mutations in host cancer genes, such as *RAS*. In cells in which the viral genome has integrated show significantly more genomic instability and may contribute to acquisition of prooncogenic mutations in host cancer genes. HPV also acts in harmony with environmental factors. These include cigarette smoking, coexisting microbial infections, dietary deficiencies, and hormonal changes. These may be involved in the pathogenesis of cervical cancers. Many women infected with HPV clear the infection by immunologic mechanisms. Those women who cannot clear the infection may have acquired immune abnormalities (e.g., HIV infection). Hence, women who are coinfected with high-risk HPV types and HIV have a high risk for developing cervical cancer.

HeLa cells: A cell line removed from aggressive cervical cancer in 1951 called as *HeLa cells* (named HeLa cells after the patient **He**nrietta **La**cks). This has become a common source of human cancer cells and is used in the study of cancer. After decades of HeLa cells growing in laboratories, these cells remain dependent on HPV-18 E6 and E7 expression (i.e., oncogene addiction). Inactivation of these oncoproteins results in growth arrest.

Effects of oncogenic proteins of high-risk HPV are listed in **Box 17**.

Epstein–Barr Virus

Q. Write short essay on Epstein–Barr virus, diseases caused and cancers.

Q. Discuss the role of EBV in malignancy.

Denis Burkitt (1958) first described a unique entity with characteristic clinical, pathologic, and epidemiologic features that most frequently arises in the jawbones of children in Africa. This was an unusual B-cell–derived tumor and was named as Burkitt lymphoma and Burkitt suggested that it may be due to virus. In 1964, Epstein, together with then PhD candidate Yvonne Barr, described virus particles of the herpesvirus family in lymphoblastoid cells from patients with Burkitt lymphoma (BL). Hence, the virus is named as EBV.

Epstein–Barr virus is double-stranded DNA virus that belongs to **human herpesvirus** family **and was the first virus identified to cause a malignant** aggressive **tumor in humans namely Burkitt lymphoma.** Other members that belong

Box 17: Effects of oncogenic proteins of high-risk Human papillomaviruses.

- Inactivation of RB and p53: Increased cell proliferation
- Activation of cyclin/CDK complexes: Activation of cell cycle
- Reduction or prevention of cellular senescence
- Genomic instability
- Inhibition of apoptosis

to human herpesvirus family are; herpes simplex viruses types 1 and 2, varicella zoster virus, cytomegalovirus, human herpesvirus types 6 and 7, and Kaposi's sarcoma herpesvirus (KSHV, also known as HSV8). EBV is a member of the gamma herpesviruses because of its tropism for lymphoid cells.

Epstein–Barr virus infects epithelial cells of the oropharynx and B-lymphocytes. The infection of B cells EBV in majority of individual produces a latent infection in which virus does not replicate and the B-cells are not killed. EBV **infects B lymphocytes** and transforms them into lymphoblasts. Primary infections with EBV in some individuals, the lymphoblastoid transformation manifests as short-lived infectious mononucleosis and others may develop few human cancers. EBV has been detected within the cells of a surprisingly diverse other tumors mainly in the immunosuppressed. The **cancers produced by EBV are listed in Box 18.**

Burkitt lymphoma is endemic in certain parts of Africa and occurs sporadically elsewhere. In endemic areas, almost all the tumor cells carry the EBV genome. The infection is usually transmitted through the saliva of EBV-seropositive individuals who replicate the virus in the oropharyngeal epithelium.

Pathogenesis

B lymphocytes are abundant in the tonsillar crypts. EB virus infects these B lymphocytes by binding of EBV envelope glycoprotein gp350 to the B-cell-specific membrane complement receptor CD21 (CR2). This binding mediates virus attachment to B lymphocytes followed by virus entry into the B lymphocyte and systemic dissemination of EBV infection.

The **infection of B-cells may be either productive** (lytic) **or latent.**

- **Productive/lytic infection**: It **develops only in very few patients** and results in death of infected cells and release of virions. These released virions infect other B-cells.
- **Latent infection**: It **occurs in majority of the cases.** The virus becomes latent inside the B-cells and the B-cells are transformed or "immortalized" so that they are capable of proliferation indefinitely. Viral latency is defined as a condition in which the virus expresses one or few gene products but can "reawaken" to express a broader range of viral gene products. Latent infections do not produce progeny virions and the genome circularizes an episome in the nucleus of latently infected B lymphocytes. Latently infected B-cells are highly resistant to immune clearance thereby establishes long-term nonproductive infection. **Immortalization of B lymphocyte is the hallmark of EBV infection. Molecular basis of B-cell immortalization** is related to **two EBV-coded genes** and **viral cytokines.**
  - **LMP-1** (latent-infection-associated membrane protein 1): LMP-1 behaves like a constitutively active CD40 receptor. These receptors after receiving signals from helper T-cell, stimulate the growth of B-cells. LMP-1 **acts as an oncogene** and activates the NF-κB and JAK/STAT signaling pathways This signalling promotes B-cell survival and proliferation. This occur autonomously without T cells or other outside signals in EBV-infected B cells. Also LMP-1 **promotes survival of B-cell** (prevents apoptosis by activating **Bcl-2**) and **proliferation.**
  - **EBNA-2** (Epstein–Barr-induced nuclear antigens 2): *EBNA-2* encodes a nuclear protein that mimics a constitutively active Notch receptor. EBNA-2 is the main viral transcriptional transactivator of both viral and cellular host genes. **It stimulates transcription of many host genes**, including genes that drive the cell cycle (e.g., cyclin D) and the *SRC* family of protooncogenes.
  - **Viral cytokine (vIL-10):** EBV genome contains a gene encoding a homologue of IL-10 (vIL-10). This was "borrowed" or pirated from host genome. It **prevent macrophages and monocytes from activating T-cells and killing viral infected cells.**

Box 18: Cancers produced by Epstein–Barr virus.

- **African form of Burkitt lymphoma**
- **B-cell lymphomas** in immunosuppressed (e.g., HIV infection or immunosuppressive therapy after organ transplantation)
- A subset of **Hodgkin lymphoma**
- **Nasopharyngeal** carcinoma (T-cell tumor)
- Some gastric carcinomas
- **Rare forms** (subset) **of T-cell lymphomas and natural killer (NK) cell lymphomas**
- Very rare sarcomas

Infection of immunologically normal individuals: The EBV proteins involved in immortalization and proliferation of of B-cell are highly immunogenic. EBV-driven polyclonal B cell proliferation is controlled by cytotoxic T cells. These individuals either remains asymptomatic or develop a self-limited episode of infectious mononucleosis. Infectious mononucleosis is characterized by fever, lymphadenopathy, pharyngitis, and fatigue. In infectious mononucleosis, EBV infects B cells and have T-cell lymphocytosis (lymphocytosis in peripheral smear is due to T cells) and usually declines in weeks. However, very few individuals downregulate expression of immunogenic viral proteins such as LMP-1 and EBNA-2. This leads to persistence of memory B cells throughout life.

Infection of individuals with defective T-cell immunity: In these patients, EBV transformed B cells can produce a rapidly progressive and fatal lymphoma.

African form of Burkitt lymphoma

Epstein–Barr virus was the first virus to be firmly linked to the development of a human cancer. Burkitt lymphoma (BL) is a **B-cell neoplasm** and is the **most common childhood tumor in central Africa** and New Guinea. The localization of BL to equatorial Africa is probably due to prolonged stimulation of the immune system by endemic malaria. Normally, EBV induced proliferation of B-cell is controlled by suppressor T cells. Chronic malarial infections may cause lack of an adequate T-cell response resulting in uncontrolled B-cell proliferation. This in turn may undergo further genetic changes resulting in the development of lymphoma. One of the genetic change is a translocation in which c-*myc* is being brought into proximity to an immunoglobulin promoter. Also, EBV proteins inhibit apoptosis and activates signaling pathways of cell proliferation. Features that suggest the strong association between endemic Burkitt lymphoma are (i) presence of EBV genome in more than 90% of endemic tumors, (ii) all affected patients show raised antibody titers against viral capsid antigens, and (iii) correlation of risk of developing the tumor between serum antibody titers against viral capsid antigens. A morphologically similar lymphoma occurs sporadically throughout the world.

Though EBV is involved in the causation of Burkitt lymphoma, there is involvement of additional factors. (1) EBV is a universal virus and infection is not limited to the regions where Burkitt lymphoma is found. (2) The EBV genome is observed in only 15% to 20% of non-endemic Burkitt lymphomas. (3) The patterns of viral gene expression in EBV-transformed (but not tumorigenic) B-cell lines and Burkitt lymphoma cells are significantly different. Burkitt lymphoma cells do not express LMP-1, EBNA-2, and other EBV proteins that causes growth and immortalization of B-cell.

Mechanism of Endemic Burkitt Lymphoma (Fig. 103): **Epstein–Barr virus infects B-cells and stimulate B lymphocyte proliferation which is usually controlled by suppressor T-cells.** Sequence of events in the pathogenesis of endemic African Burkitt lymphoma are:

- Infection of B cells by EBV
- Polyclonal lymphoblastoid transformation of B cells.
    - **Accompanying infections** (such as **malaria** or other infections) **impairs immune competence. This** inhibits suppressor T cells. **Lack of an adequate suppressor T-cell response** allows **uncontrolled proliferation of B-cell. EBV-infected B-cells expressing LMP-1 are eliminated** by T-cell immunity. T-cell mediated immunity is directed against EBV antigens such as EBNA-2 and LMP-1. This destroys most of the EBV-infected B cells. However, a small number of cells downregulate expression of these immunogenic antigens. These cells remain indefinitely, even in the presence of normal immunity. Lymphoma cells may develop from these small population only with the acquisition of specific mutations. Most characteristic being translocations involving the MYC oncogene.
    - Deregulation of *MYC* by translocation i.e., t(8:14) (q24; q32). **Translocations of *MYC* gene,** converts protooncogene into ***MYC*** oncogene, which leads to **overexpression of MYC protein** (oncoprotein). This causes **uncontrolled cell proliferation** of malignant clone of B lymphocytes. The proliferation of the B lymphocytes and the reduction in virus-specific cytotoxic T cells is associated with malaria. This probably increases EBV viral load and increases the risk of the MYC translocations characteristic of BL. **Lymphoma develops** only **when there are chromosomal translocations.** Overexpression of the *MYC* oncogene alone is not enough for malignant transformation of a B cell. Additional mutations occur in these B cells and eventually forms a monoclonal B-cell neoplasm.

Mechanism of nonendemic Burkitt lymphoma: All tumors possess the t(8;14) or other translocations that dysregulate c-*MYC*.

Burkitt lymphoma in immunosuppressed patients Few patients with AIDS or who receive immunosuppressive therapy for preventing allograft rejection develop EBV positive B-cell tumors. These tumors usually develop at multiple sites and in the extranodal region (e.g., gastrointestinal tract , central nervous system). In the beginning these proliferations are polyclonal and later can evolve into monoclonal neoplasms. Burkitt lymphoma in immunosuppressed patients usually express LMP-1 and EBNA-2, which are antigenic. These antigens are normally recognized by cytotoxic T cells. Also, they usually does not show *MYC* translocations. LMP-1 and EBNA-2 are antigenic and can be recognized by cytotoxic T cells. When immunosuppressive drugs in transplant recipients is withdrawn, the T cell function will be restored, and this reduces the potentially lethal proliferations of B cells.

Nasopharyngeal carcinoma

Nasopharyngeal carcinoma (NPC) is a variant of squamous cell carcinoma and is also associated with EBV infection. This tumor is endemic in certain parts of Asia. EBV enters/infects epithelial cells of nasopharynx via infected lymphocytes traveling through lymphoid-rich epithelium. In contrast to Burkitt lymphoma, all the tumor cells in nasopharyngeal carcinomas contain EBV DNA and antibody titers to viral capsid antigens (EBNA) in all affected patients both in endemic and nonendemic regions. The integration site of the viral genome in all of the tumor cells within individual tumors is identical (clonal). This indicates that EBV infection plays an active role in the neoplastic and not that occurs after tumor development. Apart from infection with EBV, genetic or environmental cofactors [e.g., consumption of large quantities of salted fish (that contain nitrosamines) in South East China] or both may also contribute to the development of nasopharyngeal carcinoma. Unlike Burkitt lymphoma, LMP-1 is expressed in nasopharyngeal carcinoma cells and activates the NF-κB pathway. This upregulates the expression of factors such as VEGF, FGF-2, MMP-9 (matrix metalloprotease) and COX-2 leading to cell proliferation and tumor development. Nasopharyngeal carcinomas often show prominent infiltrates of T cells. This may an response against viral antigens such as LMP-1. But this response is ineffective and , suggest that probably immune evasion mechanisms is important in nasopharyngeal carcinoma. Supporting this is expression of the immune checkpoint molecule PD-L1 in cells of nasopharyngeal carcinoma and these tumors responds to PD-L1 inhibitors. Occasionally, EBV-positive carcinomas resembling nasopharyngeal carcinoma may develop at other sites, such as the stomach and the thymus. About 70% of patients are cured by radiation therapy alone.

Hodgkin disease (HD)

The clonal EBV genomes are found in Reed–Sternberg cells and the restricted pattern of latent viral gene expression is observed in about 30–50% of all HD cases. A positive association is also found between a history of infectious mononucleosis and HD. These findings suggest that EBV is plays a role in the development of HD.

Gastric carcinoma

EBV DNA is also present in the epithelial cells, not infiltrating lymphocytes in about 5–15% of gastric adenocarcinomas and over 90% of gastric lymphoepithelioma-like carcinomas.

Non-hodgkin's lymphomas and other malignancies

EBV is present in about 6% of non-Hodgkin's lymphoma (NHL), including some B-cell lymphoma, peripheral T-cell lymphoma, angioblastic T-cell lymphoma, lymphomatoid

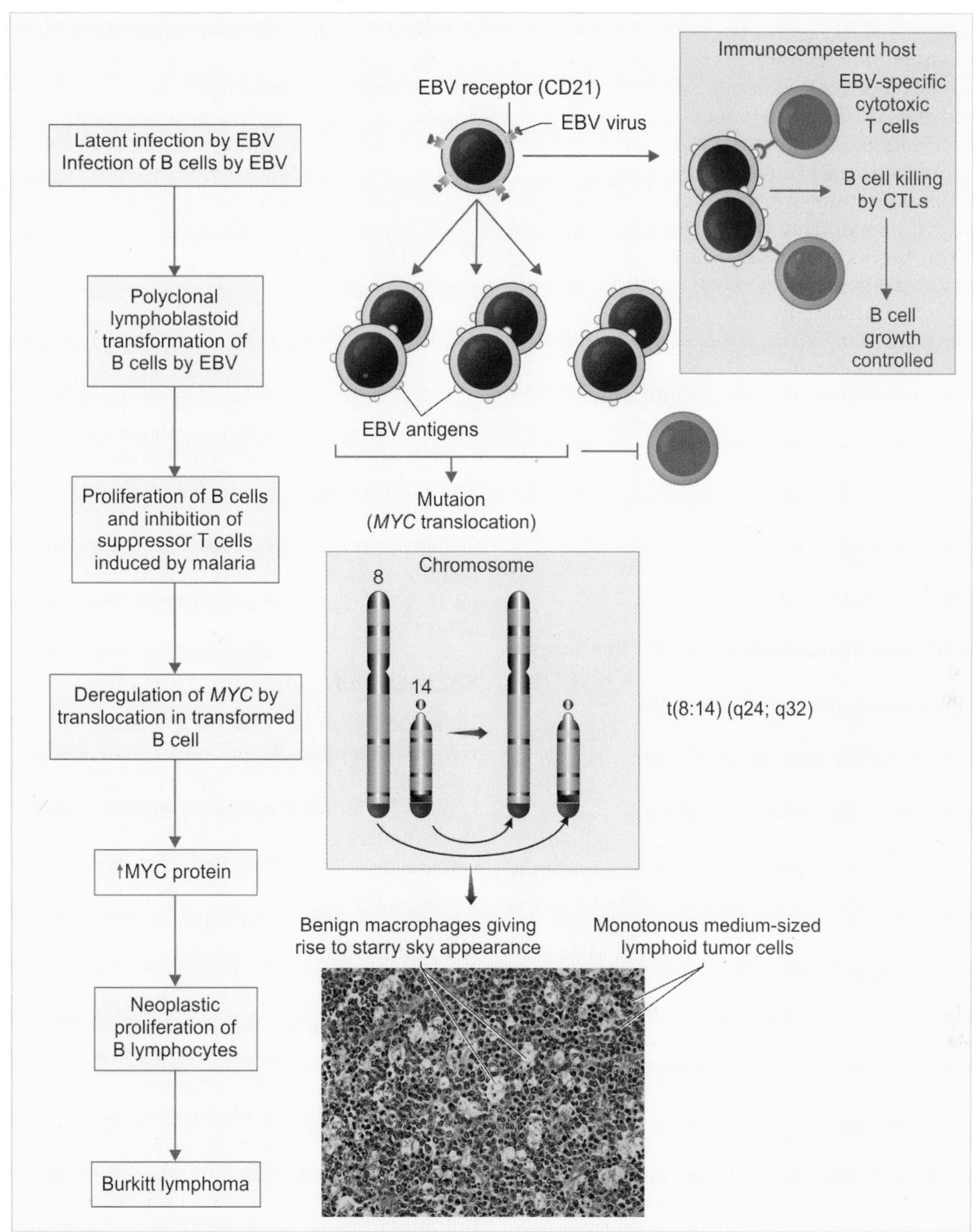

(CTLs: cytotoxic T lymphocytes)

FIG. 103: Mechanism of Epstein–Barr virus (EBV)-induced Burkitt lymphoma.

granulomatosis, pyothorax-associated lymphoma, extranodal NK/T-cell lymphoma (nasal type), aggressive NK cell leukemia/ lymphoma, and inflammatory pseudotumor-like follicular dendritic cell sarcoma.

Hepatitis B and C Viruses

Hepatitis B virus is a DNA virus whereas **HCV is RNA virus.** There is a strong association between chronic infection with HBV and HCV (chronic hepatitis and cirrhosis) with primary **hepatocellular carcinoma**. About **70–85% of hepatocellular carcinomas are caused by HBV or HCV.**

Mechanism

The genomes of HBV and HCV do not encode any viral oncoproteins. The oncogenic effects of both HBV and HCV are **multifactorial**.

- **Immunologically mediated chronic inflammation:** It causes **death of the hepatocytes.**
- **Compensatory liver cell regeneration:** Hepatocellular injury and chronic viral infection leads to the compensatory proliferation of hepatocytes. It is aided by a several growth factors, cytokines, chemokines, and other substances produced by **activated immune cells of inflammation**.

These in turn promote cell survival, tissue remodeling, and angiogenesis.

- **Genomic damage and mutation:** Death of hepatocyte leads to regeneration and genomic damage. Genomic damage and mutation is due to unresolved chronic inflammation and genotoxic and mutagenic mediators (e.g., ROS) produced by activated immune cells.
- Mediators derived from the activated immune cells activate the NF-κB pathway in hepatocytes. Activated NF-κB pathway blocks apoptosis and allows the dividing hepatocytes to undergo genotoxic stress and to accumulate mutations. This appears to be the main mechanism involved in the pathogenesis of virus-induced hepatocellular carcinoma.
- Both HBV and HCV also contain proteins within their genomes that may directly promote the development of liver cancer.
- **HBV:** HBV genome contains a viral regulatory gene known as ***HBx***. Various actions of *HBx* are:
  - Direct or indirect **activation of many transcription factors and signal transduction pathways** (e.g., the ras-raf MAP kinase pathway).
  - **Inactivation of *p53***
  - **HBV DNA can be integrated within the human genome** and can **cause multiple deletions,** which may harbor unknown tumor suppressor genes
  - Consumption of food contaminated with the fungus AFB_1 may act synergistically with HBV infection to induce HCC.
- **HCV:** Apart from chronic injury to liver cells and compensatory regeneration, HCV genome contains **HCV core protein**. This may **activate many growth-promoting signal transduction pathways** and cause tumor. HCV is associated with **lymphoplasmacytic lymphoma**.

Human Herpesvirus 8

Human herpesvirus 8 is also known as KS-associated herpesvirus (KSHV). It is a DNA virus, which **infects the spindle cells of Kaposi sarcoma** and also **lymphocytes**.

Neoplasm produced

- **Kaposi sarcoma (KS):** It is a multicentric **vascular neoplasm** usually presenting with multiple lesions. It is the **most common neoplasm, associated with AIDS**. KS tumor, HHV-8 has also been found in Kaposi sarcoma from HIV-negative patients. All the neoplastic cells of Kaposi sarcoma contain sequences of HHV-8 in both HIV-positive and HIV-negative patients.
- **B-cell lymphoid malignancies:** In addition to infecting the spindle cells of Kaposi sarcoma, HHV-8 is also found to be lymphotropic. Two uncommon B-cell lymphoid malignancies, namely **primary effusion lymphoma** and **multicentric Castleman disease** are also associated with HHV-8.

Mechanism

- **HHV-8 viral genome encodes proteins, which interfere with the *p53* and *RB* tumor suppressor pathways.**
- Some viral proteins may inhibit apoptosis and accelerate cell cycle.
- HHV-8 encodes an inhibitor of the normal regulator of NF-κB (i.e., IκB). This leads to unrestrained activation of NF-κB.
- HHV-8 also **encodes gene products, which downregulate class I major histocompatibility complex (MHC) expression** and infected cells **escape recognition by cytotoxic T lymphocytes**.
- Development and progression of KS depends on lytic HHV-8 infection and latently infected cells. Antiviral drugs that inhibit HHV-8 lytic infection protects against the development of KS.

Merkel Cell Polyomavirus

Polyomaviruses are small, nonenveloped, double-stranded DNA viruses. In 1972, Cyril Toker first described a relatively rare cancer called as Merkel cell carcinoma (MCC). In 2008, Yuan Chang and Patrick Moore discovered a human polyomavirus species, which they called MCV (later designated HPyV5) because of its presence in a very uncommon skin tumor, Merkel cell carcinoma (MCC). MCV DNA integrated into cellular DNA was found in about 50% of MCC. MCC is an aggressive, rapidly lethal skin cancer. It usually presents as a fast-growing, painless, violaceous nodule on sun-exposed skin surfaces (often in the head or neck region) and metastasizes early. Patients with HIV/AIDS and organ transplant patients have a higher risk of MCC.

Bacteria and Cancer

Helicobacter pylori and gastric adenocarcinomas

Helicobacter pylori (*H. pylori*) was first called as *Campylobacter pyloridis*. It is a gram-negative, flagellated spiral or curved bacillus. It attaches to gastric epithelial cells and colonizes the stomach. *H. pylori* is the first bacterium classified as a carcinogen.

Diseases caused by (*H. pylori*): (i) Peptic ulcer, **(ii) gastric adenocarcinoma, and (iii)** MALT (*m*ucosa-*a*ssociated *l*ymphoid *t*issue) lymphoma of the stomach **(gastric lymphoma)**.

Mechanism: Development of *H. pylori*-induced gastric adenocarcinoma is multifactorial. The mechanism includes immunologically mediated chronic inflammation, stimulation of gastric cell proliferation, and generation of ROS that damage DNA. *H. pylori*-induced gastric adenocarcinoma develops similar to that of HBV and HCV-induced hepatocellular carcinoma. *H. pylori* causes chronic inflammation and the inflammatory cells contains numerous genotoxic agents (e.g., excess ROS/free radicals) that produce damage to the host cell DNA and accumulates cellular mutations. Sequence of histopathological changes in the development of gastric carcinoma by *Helicobacter pylori* is presented in **Flowchart 2**. This sequence is observed in only 3% of infected individuals and requires decades to develop carcinoma.

Genes: Similar to HBV and HCV, the *H. pylori* genome contains genes that is involved in oncogenesis. It is observed that strains of *H. pylori* causing gastric adenocarcinoma contains a "pathogenicity island" that contains **cytotoxin-associated A** gene (***CagA***). The product ***CagA*** gene is potentially oncogenic factor called the CagA protein. Though *H. pylori* as such is noninvasive, *CagA* is injected into gastric epithelial cells. In these epithelial cells, it alters a number of signaling transduction pathways that leads to unregulated growth factor stimulation.

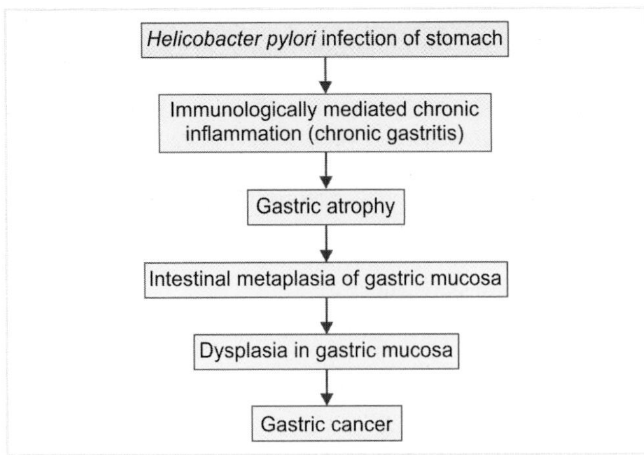

FLOWCHART 2: Sequence of histopathological changes in the development of gastric carcinoma by *Helicobacter pylori.*

Helicobacter pylori and gastric lymphoma

H. pylori produces gastric lymphoma of **B-cell origin.** *H. pylori* transform the B cells and these cells grow in a pattern resembling that of normal MALT. Hence, they are also termed as lymphomas of MALT lymphomas or **MALTomas.**

Molecular pathogenesis: Exact pathogenesis not known. Probably strain-specific *H. pylori* factors and host genetic factors, such as polymorphisms in the promoters of inflammatory cytokines [e.g., IL-1β and tumor necrosis factor (TNF)]. *H. pylori* infection activates *H. pylori*–reactive T cells, which in turn causes proliferation of polyclonal B-cell populations. Later from these proliferating polyclonal B cells, a monoclonal B-cell tumor develops probably due to accumulation of mutations in growth regulatory genes. However, these B-cells remain dependent on T-cell stimulation of B-cell pathways that activate the transcription factor NF-κB. Eradication of *H. pylori* with antibiotics during early course of disease, causes regression of the lymphoma by removing the antigenic stimulus for T cells. *H. pylori* is associated with t(11;18) translocation in MALT lymphomas.

Parasites and Cancer

Askanazy in 1900, observed a link between *Opisthorchis felineus* infection and liver cancer, and Goebel found *Bilharzia* infections (schistosomiasis) with human bladder cancer. Two well-established associations of parasites with human cancer are: **Schistosomiasis with bladder cancer and liver flukes with cholangiocarcinoma**.

Schistosomiasis and Bladder Cancer

Schistosomiasis (also known as bilharzia) is a parasitic disease caused by trematodes from the genus *Schistosoma.* ***Schistosoma*** *haematobium* (see pages 781–784 and Fig. 128 of Chapter 11) produces urinary schisto-somiasis and can cause chronic infections that can lead to kidney damage and to bladder cancer. The ova of the parasite can be found in the affected tissue. *S. haematobium* infections are common in Africa and the Middle East, second only to malaria among parasitic diseases. *S. haematobium* is strongly implicated in **carcinoma of urinary bladder and** histologically **these are usually of squamous cell carcinomas.** Bladder cancers associated with are squamous cell carcinomas. Though the mechanism is not known, most probably it develops as a consequence of a persistent, chronic infection of urinary bladder.

Two parasites which can causes tumor are:

1. **Liver flukes and cholangiocarcinoma:** *Opisthorchis viverrini (O. viverrini)* and *Clonorchis sinensis* are liver flukes (a type of flatworm). These are associated with an increased risk of cholangiocarcinomas. They are found almost exclusively in East Asia and are rare in other parts of the world. Cholangiocarcinoma is more common in regions of endemic liver fluke infection (Hong Kong, Thailand). *O. viverrini* is endemic in northeast Thailand. Infections with these liver flukes occurs by eating raw or undercooked fish. Liver flukes enter the human gastrointestinal tract and they travel via the duodenum into the host's intrahepatic or extrahepatic biliary ducts. Liver flukes lodges in the bile ducts cause bile stasis, inflammation, periductal fibrosis, and epithelial hyperplasia, and sometimes **adenocarcinoma of the bile ducts (cholangiocarcinoma)**.
2. ***Fungi*:** Fungi may cause cancer by producing toxic substances (mycotoxins). **AFB_1** (refer page 531) produced by *Aspergillus flavus* is a potent carcinogen responsible for **hepatocellular carcinoma.**

Hormones

The etiology of many cancers may be influenced by hormonal or dietary factors. Under certain conditions hormones can be associated with carcinogens and hormones may act as cofactors in carcinogenesis. Overweight and obesity are associated with increased risk of cancer and these may be mediated by endocrine dysregulation (e.g., altered adiponectin, leptin, insulin, and IGF-1 levels). Cancers of prostate, ovary, breast, testis, and endometrium are hormonally driven.

Both endogenously synthesized and administered (exogenous) hormones can influence cancer formation. It was found that hormone-dependent cancers could be prevented by removing the primary hormone-synthesis organs. Castration and ovariectomy can helps in tumors with hormone-responsive receptors. Stimulation of hormone receptors (e.g., estrogen receptors) can increase the cellular proliferation rate and promote tumorigenesis.

Estrogen

- **Endometrial carcinoma:** It may develop in females with estrogen-secreting **granulosa cell tumor of ovary** or those receiving exogenous estrogen.
- **Adenocarcinoma of vagina:** Increased frequency of adenocarcinoma of vagina is observed in **daughters of mothers who received estrogen during pregnancy**. Diethylstilbestrol (DES) was given to pregnant women to prevent abortion; however, many of their female offspring developed clear-cell carcinomas of the vagina and cervix after the onset of puberty (due to their exposure to estrogen in utero).
- Hormone replacement therapy and estrogen-only birth control therapy were found to be associated with increased risk of hormone-dependent cancers.

- **Abnormal vascularity of tumor: Estrogens can make existing tumors abnormally vascular** (e.g., adenomas and focal nodular hyperplasia).

Androgens and anabolic steroids: They may cause hepatocellular tumors.

Hormone-dependent tumors

- **Prostatic carcinoma** usually responds to administration of estrogens or castration.
- **Breast carcinomas** regress following oophorectomy.

Radiation Carcinogenesis

Q. Discuss physical carcinogens.
Q. Discuss the mechanisms of radiation carcinogenesis and various radiation induced cancers.
Q. Write short essay on radiation induced cancers.

Definition: Radiation is defined as emission of energy by one body, its transmission through an intervening medium and its absorption by another body. Radiation is energy and is a **well-known carcinogen**. Radiation travels in the form of waves or high speed particles.

Evidence for radiation as carcinogen: These are as follows:

- Incidence of lung cancers in unprotected miners of radioactive elements is 10-fold more than others.
- Survivors of the atomic bombs attack on Hiroshima and Nagasaki had a markedly increased incidence of leukemia after an average latent period of about 7 years. There were also increased mortality rates due to carcinomas of thyroid, breast, colon, and lung carcinomas.
- The nuclear power accident at Chernobyl in the former Soviet Union was associated with high incidence of cancer in the surrounding areas.
- Recently, there was radiation release from a nuclear power plant in Japan damaged by a massive earthquake and tsunami. It will result in significantly increased incidence of cancer in the surrounding geographic areas.
- Therapeutic irradiation of the head and neck can give rise to papillary thyroid cancers.

Oncogenic effects: Radiation has mutagenic effects. It causes chromosome breakage, chromosomal rearrangements (e.g., translocations and inversions), and, less commonly, point mutations. **Double-stranded DNA breaks are the most important form of DNA damage caused by radiation.** It points out the importance of DNA repair genes in carcinogenesis.

Latency: Extremely long latent period is common, and **it has a cumulative effect**. Radiation has also **additive or synergistic effects with other** potential **carcinogenic agents**.

Types of radiation: They are divided into two types, namely (1) UV rays of sunlight, and (2) ionizing radiation.

Ultraviolet Rays

They are derived from the sunlight. UV radiation of sunlight is the short-wavelength portion of the electromagnetic spectrum adjacent to the violet region of visible light.

Categories: Depending on the wavelength, UV light is divided into UVA (320 to 400 nm), UVB (290 to 320 nm), and UVC (240 to 290 nm) radiation. Though UVC is a potent mutagen, most of the UVC light emitted from the sun is absorbed by the ozone layer in the atmosphere. Thus, humans are mostly exposed to UVA and UVB irradiation. **Various effects of UV radiation on cells are; enzyme inactivation, inhibition of cell division, mutagenesis, cell death and cancer.**

Tumors caused: Skin cancer, namely (i) **squamous cell carcinoma**, (ii) **basal cell carcinoma,** and (iii) **malignant melanoma**. They are more common on parts of the body regularly exposed to sunlight and ultraviolet light (UVL). UVB is responsible for skin cancers.

Risk factors: The amount of damage incurred by UV rays depends on:

- **Type of UV rays**
- **Intensity of exposure**
- **Protective mantle of melanin**
    - **Melanin** absorbs UV radiation and has a **protective effect**.
    - Skin cancers (basal cell carcinoma, squamous carcinoma and melanoma) attributed to sun exposure are more common in fair-skinned people (*people of the white race)* and those living in geographic location receiving a greater amount of sunlight (e.g., Australia, New Zealand close to the equator). The skin of people of the darker races contain increased concentration of melanin pigment. This protects by absorbing UV radiation.
- **Type of exposure:** In fair-skinned people, skin cancer occurs on the areas exposed to the sun. These is a direct correlation between total exposure to sunlight and the incidence of skin cancer.
    - Nonmelanoma skin cancers (squamous cell and basal cell carcinomas) are associated with total cumulative exposure to UV radiation.
    - Melanomas are associated with intense intermittent exposure (e.g., sunbathing).

Pathogenesis: UVB light is capable of causing pyrimidine dimers in DNA. Hence, it is carcinogenic. Absorption of the energy in a photon of UV light by DNA produces a chemical reaction. This reaction leads to covalent cross-linking of pyrimidine bases. This particularly occurs in the adjacent thymidine residues in the same strand of DNA. This linking of pyrimidine bases distorts the DNA helix and prevents proper pairing of the dimer with bases in the opposite DNA strand. Usually, pyrimidine dimers are repaired by the nucleotide excision repair (NER) pathway. NER pathway may involve 30 or more proteins. When there is excessive exposure to UVB of the sunlight, the capacity of the nucleotide excision repair pathway is overpowered. This activates error-prone non templated DNA repair mechanisms. Though this allow the cell to survive, it may also introduce mutations. In some cases, this may lead to cancer. Various steps are presented in **Flowchart 3**.

Xeroderma pigmentosum: It is a rare **hereditary autosomal recessive disorder** characterized by **congenital deficiency of nucleotide excision DNA repair** pathway. These individuals are highly sensitive to sunlight damage. They **develop skin cancers** (basal cell carcinoma, squamous cell carcinoma and melanoma) due to impairment in the excision of UV-damaged DNA.

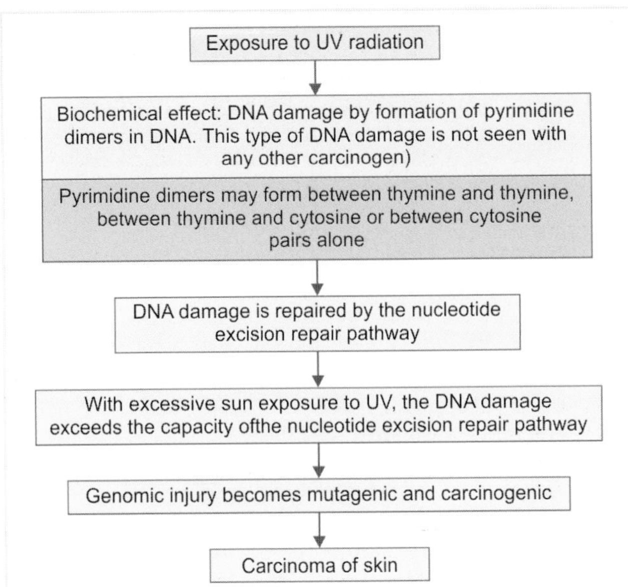

FLOWCHART 3: Steps in the pathogenesis of skin cancer by ultraviolet (UV) rays.

Ionizing Radiation

Definition: Ionizing radiation is defined as radiation that has sufficient energy to ionize molecules by displacing electrons from atoms.

Types: Ionizing radiation can be (i) electromagnetic (e.g., X-rays and gamma rays [γ-rays]), or (ii) particulate consisting of particles (e.g., electrons, protons, neutrons, alpha [α] particles, beta [β] particles, or carbon ions). These are all carcinogenic.

Source of ionizing radiation: Natural sources constitute about 80% of human exposure, whereas medical sources make up about 20%.

- **Natural sources:** Radon exposure is the natural source of exposure risk to humans. With better and more comprehensive screening techniques, the human exposure to radon can be significantly reduced.
- **Medical sources:** The increased medical use of diagnostic X-rays and computed tomography (CT) scanning procedures as well as airport screenings likely to increase the risk of cancer.

Cancers produced

- **Medical or occupational exposure**, e.g., **leukemia and skin cancers**.
- **Nuclear plant accidents:** Risk of **lung cancers**.
- **Atomic bomb explosion:** Survivors of atomic bomb explosion (dropped on Hiroshima and Nagasaki) led to increased incidence of **leukemias**. These leukemias are mainly acute and chronic myelogenous leukemia after about 7 years. Subsequently, increased mortality due to **solid tumors** (e.g., breast, colon, thyroid and lung).
- **Therapeutic radiation:** (i) **Papillary carcinoma of the thyroid** follows irradiation of head and neck and (ii) **angiosarcoma of liver** due to radioactive thorium dioxide used to visualize the arterial tree.
  Mechanism: Hydroxyl free radical injury to DNA.
  Tissues which are relatively resistant to radiation-induced neoplasia: Skin, bone and the gastrointestinal tract.

Radiofrequency and Microwave Radiation

Presently due to manmade activities, humans are exposed to many new physical agents, such as radiofrequency radiation (RFR) and microwave radiation (MR), electromagnetic fields (EMFs), asbestos, and nanoparticles. Evolution has not yet had time to deliver genome-preserving response mechanisms to these new agents.

Frequency range: For RFR, frequency range is 3 kHz to 300 MHz and for MR it is between 300 MHz and 300 GHz.

Actions: Both RFR and MR have not sufficient energies to produce ionizations in target tissues. Hence, the radiation energy is converted into heat as the radiation energy is absorbed.

Sources of RFR and MR: These include mobile phones, radio transmitters of wireless communication, radars, medical devices, and kitchen appliances.

Damage and cancer risk: In recent years, human exposure to RFR has increased dramatically. The exact role of their genotoxic damage is not yet clear. Some studies indicate that long-term usage of mobile phone may be associated with increased risks of developing brain tumors.

Electromagnetic Fields

Definition: An electromagnetic field (EMF) is a physical field produced by electrically charged objects that can affect other charged objects in the field.

Sources: These include electric power lines, electrical devices, and magnetic resonance imaging machines.

Damage and cancer: A low-frequency EMF does not transmit energy high enough to break chemical bonds. Hence, it may not directly damage DNA or proteins in cells. Studies have not detected any association between exposure to EMFs and cancer.

Biological effects of radiation are discussed in detail on pages 999-999.

10.6 Clinical Aspects and Laboratory Diagnosis of Cancer

CHAPTER OUTLINE

CLINICAL ASPECTS OF NEOPLASIA

Both benign and malignant tumors may produce clinical features by its various effects on host.

Local Effects

These are due to encroachment on adjacent structures.

- Compression (e.g., adenoma in the ampulla of Vater causing obstruction of biliary tract).
- Mechanical obstruction: It may be caused by both benign and malignant tumors. For example, tumors may cause obstruction or intussusception in the GI tract.
  - Endocrine insufficiency: It is caused due to destruction of an endocrine gland either due to primary or metastatic cancer. Location of tumor is important in both benign and malignant tumors. A small pituitary adenoma can compress and destroy the surrounding normal pituitary gland. This may produce hypopituitarism.
- Ulceration, bleeding and secondary infections: It may develop in benign or malignant tumors in the skin or mucosa of the GI tract, e.g.:
  - Melena (blood in the stool) in neoplasms of the gut
  - Hematuria in neoplasms of the urinary tract.
- Rupture or infarction of tumor.

Functional Effects

These include:

- Hormonal effects: Patient may present with signs and symptoms related to hormone production. They may be seen in patients with benign as well as malignant neoplasms of endocrine glands. For example, β-cell adenoma or carcinoma developing in islets of Langerhans of the pancreas may produce hyperinsulinism (increased insulin secretion) and cause hypoglycemia which may be sometimes fatal; few adenomas and carcinomas of the adrenal cortex may secrete steroid hormones (e.g., aldosterone, which induces sodium retention, hypertension, and hypokalemia). Hormones are more likely produced by a well-differentiated benign tumor rather than a corresponding carcinoma.
- Paraneoplastic syndromes: Nonendocrine tumors may secrete hormones or hormone-like substances and produce paraneoplastic syndromes (explained below).
- Fever: It is most commonly associated with Hodgkin disease, renal cell carcinoma and osteogenic sarcoma. Fever may be due to release of pyrogens by tumor cells or IL-1 produced by inflammatory cells in the stroma of the tumor.

Tumor Lysis Syndrome

Q. Write short essay on tumor lysis syndrome.

Tumor lysis syndrome (TLS) is a group of metabolic complications that can occur after treatment for leukemias such as acute lymphoblastic leukemia (ALL), acute myeloid leukemia (AML), chronic lymphocytic leukemia (CLL); chronic myelogenous leukemia (CML), poorly differentiated lymphomas such as Burkitt's lymphoma and other non-Hodgkin's lymphoma (NHL), and uncommonly in solid tumors.

Mechanism: It is caused by breakdown products of large amounts of tumor cells following chemotherapy or glucocorticoids or hormonal agent (tamoxifen). The killed tumor cells release intracellular ions and large amounts of metabolic by-products into systemic circulation.

Metabolic Abnormalities

- **Hyperkalemia:** Due to release of the most abundant intracellular cation potassium. Symptoms usually do not manifest until level are high. They include cardiac conduction abnormalities (can be fatal) and severe muscle weakness or paralysis.

- **Hyperphosphatemia:** Due to release of intracellular phosphate.
- **Hypocalcemia:** Due to complexing of calcium with elevated phosphate (hyperphosphatemia) and forms calcium phosphate. Symptom include: tetany, sudden mental incapacity, including emotional lability, parkinsonian (extrapyramidal) symptoms, movement disorders, papilledema and myopathy.
- **Hyperuricemia and hyperuricouria:** Massive death of cells and nuclear breakdown generate large quantities of nucleic acids. The purines (adenine and guanine) of nucleic acids are converted to uric acid via the purine degradation pathway and excreted in the urine. High concentrations of uric acid precipitate as monosodium urate crystals. Acute uric acid nephropathy (AUAN) due to hyperuricosuria can lead to renal failure.
- **Lactic acidosis.**

Risk Factors

1. Tumors with a high cell turnover rate, rapid growth rate, and high tumor bulk are more prone to develop tumor lysis syndrome.
2. Patient-related factors such as elevated baseline serum creatinine, renal insufficiency, dehydration, and other factors affecting urinary flow or the acidity of urine.
3. Chemosensitive tumors (e.g., such as lymphomas).

Diagnosis

Tumor lysis syndrome should be suspected in patients with large tumor burden who develop acute kidney failure along with hyperuricemia (>15 mg/dL) or hyperphosphatemia (>8 mg/dL).

Cairo–Bishop Definition

Laboratory tumor lysis syndrome: Abnormality in two or more of the following, occurring within three days before or seven days after chemotherapy.

1. Uric acid >8 mg/dL or 25% increase
2. Potassium >6 mEq/L or 25%increase
3. Phosphate >4.5 mg/dL or 25% increase
4. Calcium <7 mg/dL or 25% decrease

Clinical tumor lysis syndrome: Laboratory tumor lysis syndrome plus one or more of the following:

1. Increased serum creatinine (1.5 times upper limit of normal)
2. Cardiac arrhythmia or sudden death
3. Seizure

Prevention

- Prophylactic administration of allopurinol before initiating chemotherapy in tumors with high turnover rate
- Proper intravenous hydration to maintain good urine output.

Cancer Cachexia (Wasting)

It is defined as a hypercatabolic state characterized by a loss of muscle mass (with or without loss of fat) that cannot be explained by diminished food intake. It is accompanied by severe weakness, extreme weight loss, fatigue, atrophy of muscles, edema, anorexia and anemia. It develops in about 50% of patients suffering from cancer. It is most common in patients with advanced cancers of gastrointestinal tract, pancreas, and lung. It is responsible for about 30% of death in cancer patients. Mortality is often due to the atrophy of the diaphragm and other respiratory muscles.

Mechanism: It is poorly understood. Though some correlation is found between the size and extent of spread of the cancer and the severity of the cachexia, It is not due to the nutritional demands of the tumor or reduced food intake. It may be due to **inflammatory mediators** such as TNF and other cytokines, like IL-1, IL-6, interferon-γ, and leukemia inhibitory factor. They may be produced by macrophages in the tumor or by the tumor cells themselves. Probably, the muscle loss occurs through a direct effect of inflammatory cytokines on skeletal muscle cells. These cytokines may increase the degradation of major skeletal muscle structural proteins, such as myosin heavy chain, through signaling pathways. This may lead to ubiquitination of target proteins and their proteolysis through the proteasome. Cachectic states may also occur in patients without cancer. Examples include chronic disseminated infections and AIDS. This suggests that inflammatory cytokines may be partly responsible for cachexia. But therapies directed against individual cytokines (e.g., TNF) in cancer patients are not found to reverse cachexia. This findings suggest that apart from cytokines other factors may also be involved in its pathogenesis. Many cancer patients may also lose fat stores. One factor that may be responsible for fat loss may be a protein called lipid mobilizing factor This has been identified in the sera and urine of patients with advanced cancer. This protein sensitize adipocytes to lipolytic stimuli.

PARANEOPLASTIC SYNDROMES

Q. Write short essay on paraneoplastic syndrome.

Malignant tumors invade local tissue, produce metastasis and can produce a variety of products that can stimulate hormonal, hematologic, dermatologic and neurologic responses.

Definition: Paraneoplastic syndromes are **signs and symptom** (produces remote effects) **in cancer patients** that **cannot be explained by the anatomic distribution of the tumor (mass effect/ invasion/ metastasis) or by the secretion of hormones indigenous to the tissue of origin.**

Frequency: Though they occur in 10–15% of cancer patients, it is important because:

1. May be the first clinical (earliest) manifestation of an occult cancer.
2. May be mistaken for advanced metastatic disease leading to inappropriate treatment.
3. May present clinical problems which may be fatal.
4. Certain tumor products causing paraneoplastic syndromes may be useful in monitoring recurrence in patients who had surgical resections or are undergoing chemotherapy or radiation therapy.
5. Paraneoplastic syndrome itself may be disabling. Hence, treatment for these symptoms may have important palliative effects.

The paraneoplastic syndromes develop in many different tumors. A classification of paraneoplastic syndromes and their probable origin is presented in **Table 29**. Most common paraneoplastic syndromes include hypercalcemia, Cushing's syndrome, and nonbacterial thrombotic endocarditis. Tumors most often associated with paraneoplastic syndromes are cancers of lung and breast cancers and hematologic malignancies.

Endocrinopathies

Q. Write short notes on endocrine effects of cancer.

These are frequently observed paraneoplastic syndromes and occurs in cancers that are not of endocrine origin. The hormone secreted by these tumors are called as ectopic hormones.

Table 29: Paraneoplastic syndromes.

Clinical syndromes	*Cause/mechanism*	*Example of associated cancer*
1. Endocrinopathies		
• Cushing's syndrome	ACTH or ACTH-like substance	Small-cell carcinoma of lung, carcinoma of pancreas neural tumors
• Syndrome due to inappropriate antidiuretic hormone secretion (SIADH)	Antidiuretic hormone or atrial natriuretic hormones	Small-cell carcinoma of lung, intracranial neoplasms
• Hypercalcemia	Parathyroid hormone-related protein (PTHRP), TGF-α, TNF, IL-1	Squamous cell carcinoma of lung, carcinoma of breast, renal cell carcinoma, adult T cell leukemia/ lymphoma
• Carcinoid syndrome	Serotonin, bradykinin	Bronchial carcinoid
• Hypoglycemia	Insulin or insulin-like substance	Fibrosarcoma , other mesenchymal sarcomas, carcinoma of ovary
• Polycythemia	Erythropoietin	Renal carcinoma, hepatocellular carcinoma, cerebellar hemangioma
2. Neurologic (neuromyopathic) syndromes		
• Myasthenia	Immunological	Bronchogenic carcinoma, thymoma
• Disorders of the central and peripheral nervous systems	Immunological	Breast carcinoma, teratoma
3. Cutaneous syndromes (dermatologic disorders)		
• Acanthosis nigricans	Immunological; secretion of epidermal growth factor	Carcinoma of stomach, lung and uterus
• Dermatomyositis	Immunological	Bronchogenic and breast carcinoma
• Exfoliative dermatitis	Immunological	Lymphoma
4. Changes in osseous, articular and soft-tissue		
• Hypertrophic osteoarthropathy and clubbing of the fingers	Not known	Bronchogenic carcinoma
5. Vascular and hematologic changes		
• Venous thrombosis (Trousseau syndrome)	Tumor products like mucins which activate clotting	Pancreatic carcinoma, bronchogenic carcinoma and others
• Disseminated intravascular coagulation	Procoagulant substance: Cytoplasmic granules (e.g., acute promyelocytic leukemia cells) or mucus (adenocarcinomas)	Acute promyelocytic leukemia, prostatic adenocarcinomas
• Nonbacterial thrombotic endocarditis	Hypercoagulability	Advanced mucus secreting adenocarcinomas
• Red cell aplasia	Immunologic	Thymoma
6. Renal syndromes		
• Nephrotic syndrome	Tumor antigens, immune complexes	Various cancers
7. Amyloidosis		
• Primary amyloidosis	Immunological (AL protein)	Multiple myeloma
• Secondary amyloidosis	AA protein	Renal cell carcinoma and other solid tumors

(ACTH: adrenocorticotropic hormone; IL: interleukin; TGF: transforming growth factor; TNF: tumor necrosis factor)

Cushing's Syndrome

It is the most common endocrinopathy (paraneoplastic syndrome) and is caused due to excessive ectopic production of corticotropin (adrenocorticotropic hormone [ACTH]) or corticotropin-like peptides. The precursor of corticotropin is a large molecule called pro-opiomelanocortin. About 50% of these patients have carcinoma of the lung, mainly the small-cell type. Lung cancer patients with Cushing's syndrome show elevated serum levels of both pro-opiomelanocortin and corticotropin. The pro-opiomelanocortin is not found in serum of patients with excess corticotropin produced by the pituitary.

Hypercalcemia

It is the most common paraneoplastic syndrome. Symptomatic hypercalcemia is usually related to cancer than to hyperparathyroidism.

Mechanism of cancer-associated hypercalcemia: It may occur by two general processes:

- **Osteolysis:** It is caused by cancer, either due to a primary in bone (e.g., multiple myeloma), or widespread osteolytic metastatic to bone from any primary lesion. However, this hypercalcemia is not a paraneoplastic syndrome.
- **Production of calcemic humoral substances:** This may occur in extraosseous neoplasms. Only this mechanism is considered to be paraneoplastic. Most important mechanism of paraneoplastic hypercalcemia is by the production of a humoral factor namely parathyroid hormone-related protein (PTHRP) by tumor cells. Apart from PTHRP, several other factors, such as IL-1, TGF-α, TNF, and dihydroxyvitamin D may also cause hypercalcemia of malignancy.

Parathyroid hormone-related protein (PTHRP): PTHRP has partial structural homology to parathyroid hormone (PTH) and hence the name. Both PTHRP and PTH bind to the same G-protein-coupled receptor, termed as the PTH/PTHRP receptor (also referred to as PTH-R or PTHRP-R). PTHRP and PTH share some, but not all the biologic activities.

- Similar to PTH, PTHRP increases resorption of bone and renal calcium uptake. It inhibits renal phosphate transport and thereby raise serum calcium levels.
- In contrast to PTH, PTHRP is produced in small quantities by many normal tissues (e.g., epithelial cell types such as keratinocytes). Therefore, there is relatively frequent association of squamous cell carcinomas with PTHRP induced hypercalcemia.

Tumors associated with paraneoplastic hypercalcemia: These include carcinomas of the breast, lung, kidney, and ovary. In breast cancers, paraneoplastic hypercalcemia may be often worsened by osteolytic bone metastases. The most common lung tumor associated with hypercalcemia is squamous cell carcinoma due to production of PTHRP.

Neuromyopathic Paraneoplastic Syndromes

These may present in different forms namely peripheral neuropathies, encephalitis, cortical cerebellar degeneration, a polymyopathy resembling polymyositis, and a myasthenic syndrome similar to myasthenia gravis.

Mechanism: Exact cause is not known, but may be due to cancer-induced immunologic attack on normal tissues. Initially, tumor cells may show ectopic expression of antigens that are normally restricted to the neuromuscular system. The immune system recognizes these antigens as foreign and produces a response. This immune response is usually a T-cell response and in some cases, it may evoke antibodies. They cross-react with neuronal cell antigens and produces tissue damage.

Cutaneous Syndromes

Acanthosis Nigricans

It is characterized by development of velvety, gray-black patches of thickened, hyperkeratotic skin lesions. It can occur rarely as a genetic disease in juveniles or adults. In about 50% of the patients, particularly in adults over 40 years of age, their occurrence is associated with cancer, most commonly carcinoma of the stomach. Sometimes, acanthosis nigricans is accompanied by the abrupt development of multiple seborrheic keratosis and is termed as Leser-Trélat sign. These skin changes may appear even before the discovery of cancer.

Changes in Osseous, Articular and Soft-tissue

Hypertrophic Osteoarthropathy

It may occur in 1–10% of patients with carcinoma of lung. Rarely, it may develop in other cancers. The characteristic features are (i) formation of periosteal new bone, mainly at the distal ends of long bones, metatarsals, metacarpals, and proximal phalanges; (ii) arthritis of the adjacent joints; and (iii) clubbing of the digits.

Causes of clubbing: The cause of osteoarthropathy is not known. Though osteoarthropathy is rarely seen in patients without cancer, clubbing of the fingertips may be observed in patients with liver diseases, diffuse lung disease, congenital cyanotic heart disease, ulcerative colitis, and other disorders.

Vascular and Hematologic Syndromes

Several vascular and hematologic manifestations may develop in association with cancers.

- **Hypercoagulability:** Paraneoplastic syndromes also may manifest as hypercoagulability. This can lead to venous thrombosis and nonbacterial thrombotic endocarditis.
- **Migratory thrombophlebitis (Trousseau syndrome):** It may develop in association with deep-seated cancers (e.g., carcinomas of the pancreas or lung).
- **Disseminated intravascular coagulation:** It may complicate a many clinical disorders. It is most commonly associated with acute promyelocytic leukemia and prostatic adenocarcinoma.
- **Nonbacterial thrombotic endocarditis:** They appear as bland, small, nonbacterial fibrinous vegetations on the cardiac valve leaflets (usually on left-sided valves). They may develop in patients with advanced mucin-secreting adenocarcinomas.

MICRORNA AND NONCODING RNA TYPES

Q. Write short essay on role in mi-RNA in neoplasia.
Q. RNA analysis in tumor biology.

It is observed that many genes do not encode proteins. Instead, their products play important regulatory functions. One class of genes, which do not encode proteins but their products play important role in gene regulation, is small RNA molecules. These are called as non-coding RNAs. Noncoding RNAs participate in carcinogenesis. They regulate the expression of protein-coding cancer-associated genes. Well known among these noncoding RNAs are microRNAs. MicroRNAs (miRs) are small noncoding, single-stranded RNAs called as microRNAs (miRNAs/miR). They are approximately 22 nucleotides in length and function as negative regulators of genes and bring out sequence-specific inhibition of miRNAs. These miRs control normal cell survival, growth, and differentiation. Hence, they may be involved in carcinogenesis.

Ribonucleic acids (RNAs) consists of (i) messenger RNAs (mRNAs), which encode protein sequences, and (ii) small noncoding RNAs (ncRNAs) which are gene transcripts but do not code for proteins. The **noncoding RNAs has three subtypes namely micro-RNAs (miRNAs), small-interfering RNA (siRNA/silencing [SiRNAs]) and piwi-interacting RNAs (piRNAs)** and they inhibit gene expression.

Historically, ncRNAs were not extensively studied compared to protein-coding RNAs. Hence, the functions of ncRNAs were not understood. In 1993, Victor Ambros and his colleagues discovered the activity for miRNAs. Later studies showed that miRNAs regulate gene expression, mRNA degradation, translation, cell proliferation, cancer initiation, and progression.

Piwi-interacting RNAs (piRNAs): They are small ncRNAs with a 26–31 nucleotides. piRNAs regulate gene expression, translation and posttranslational modification. This is achieved by forming a complex with P-element-induced wimpy testis (piwi) proteins. Most piRNAs are processed in the nucleus and cytoplasm. However, piRNAs have been found in mitochondria of cancer cells in humans.

Endogenous small interfering RNAs (endosiRNAs): These are small ncRNAs with a length of 20–24 nucleotides. They regulate target gene expression by forming a complex with genomic sequences to silence gene expression. Retrotransposons are genetic elements capable of reverse transcribing their own mRNAs and inserting DNA copies of themselves into new places within the genome. In healthy somatic cells, retrotransposition by long interspersed nuclear element-1 (also known as LINE-1 or L1) is thought to be held in check by a variety of mechanisms (e.g., DNA methylation). Epigenetic changes in LINE-1s occur early during the process of carcinogenesis. A lower methylation level (hypomethylation) of LINE-1 is common in most cancers, and the methylation level is further decreased in more advanced cancers. In breast cancer, decreased quantity of endosiRNAs epigenetically suppress the expression of long interspersed nuclear element 1 (LINE-1) retrotransposons.

Transfer RNA-derived RNA fragments (tRFs): These are small RNAs derived from processing precursor or mature transfer-RNAs (tRNAs). They contain 5′ leader and 3′ trailer sequences. Three groups of tRFs have been mapped by genome-wide analysis. The tRFs regulate cell proliferation through interacting with cancer susceptibility genes in cancer such human bladder carcinoma and B cell lymphoma.

Long noncoding RNAs (lncRNAs): These are RNA sequences with lengths more than 200 nucleotides. The transcription of lncRNAs is similar to that of mRNAs. Thus, they are transcribed as single stranded RNAs, capped and polyadenylated. The lncRNAs are divide into several subtypes of depending on the locations of the lncRNA with regard to protein-coding genes.

- **Long intergenic ncRNAs (lincRNAs):** They are located between two protein coding genes.
- **Sense lincRNAs:** They are present within introns of a coding gene on the sense strand and antisense lincRNAs are transcripts that overlap with exons of protein-coding genes on the opposite strand. The lncRNAs can regulate cancer initiation and development. They can be used as cancer **biomarkers**.

Mode of action: microRNAs inhibit gene expression posttranscriptionally either by repressing translation or, in some cases, by cleavage of messenger RNA (mRNA). They perform important functions in control of cell growth, differentiation, and survival.

MicroRNAs are discussed pages 109–112.

Synthesis of MicroRNA and Mechanism of Action

miRNAs are generated by specific nucleolytic processing of the products of distinct genes/transcription units. The human genome contains about 6000 *miRNA* genes (only 3.5 times less than the number of protein-coding genes). Individual miRNAs can regulate multiple protein-coding genes. Thus, each miRNA can coregulate entire programs of gene expression. The process of producing mature miRNAs occurs in both the nucleus and cytoplasm.

- **Transcription of miRNA genes:** Most miRNAs are transcribed by RNA polymerase II, the same enzyme that transcribes messenger RNAs (mRNAs) for protein production. In the nucleus, genes encoding miRNAs are transcribed, capped and polyadenylated by RNA polymerase II. Transcription of miRNA genes by RNA polymerase II produces a long primary transcript called primary miRNA (pri-miRNA). This contains one or more miRNA sequences in the form of mostly double-stranded stem loops (Fig. 22 of Chapter 5). Primary miRNAs (pri-miRNAs) consists of 500–3000 nucleotides.
- **Formation of pre-miRNA:** Immediately after transcription, pri-miRNAs undergoes processing within the nucleus itself. The pri-miRNAs are cleaved by the RNAse III enzyme Drosha (nuclear ribonuclease enzyme and its cofactor, double-stranded RNA [dsRNA)-binding protein DGCR (DiGeorge syndrome critical region gene 8). This crops out pre-miRNA and form a shorter single RNA strand of 60–120 nucleotides and is termed as precursor miRNAs (pre-miRNAs).
- **Transport of pre-miRNA from nucleus into cytoplasm:** This pre-miRNA is then actively transported/exported from the nucleus (where they were transcribed) into the cytoplasm (where they will act) via specific transporter proteins called Exportin 5 (XPO5). They are processed into progressively smaller segments.
- **Generation of mature double stranded miRNAs:** In the cytosol (cytoplasm), the cytoplasmic ribonuclease enzyme called Dicer (a double-stranded RNA-specific endoribonuclease) recognizes pre-miRNAs. Dicer trims the pre-miRNA and generates mature double stranded miRNAs (miRNA duplex) of 21–30 nucleotides.

- **Formation of single-stranded miRNAs:** The miRNA duplex subsequently unwinds and forms single-stranded miRNAs. One of the two strands is selected and then incorporated into the multiprotein complex named RNA-induced silencing complex (RISC). RISC includes an enzyme (Argonaute, or Ago) that can cleave target mRNAs. Subsequently base pairing between the single-stranded miRNA and its target mRNA occurs and forms a mature, functional 21–22 nucleotide single stranded miRNA. It directs RISC to either cleave (degrade) the target mRNA or to repress/suppress mRNA translation.
  - Direct promotion of mRNA degradation: If the miRNA and its target mRNA contain perfectly complementary sequences, miRISC cleaves the target mRNA. The two cleavage products are not protected from RNase and are rapidly degraded.
  - Inhibition of translation of mRNA: If the miRNA and its target mRNA have only partial complementarity (or complementarity is imperfect), miRNA inhibits translation of the target mRNA.

In either way/case, the target mRNA gene is silenced post transcriptionally. siRNAs are produced similarly.

Role miRNAs in Carcinogenesis

Q. Write short essay on role miRNAs in carcinogenesis.

miRNAs can also can contribute to carcinogenesis. They may cause cancer by either increased expression of oncogenes or reduced expression of tumor suppressor genes.

MicroRNAs act as oncogenes and tumor suppressor genes.

miRNAs can regulate more than 60% of all human genes. These include oncogenes and tumor suppressor genes. Impaired interactions of miRNAs with oncogenes and tumor suppressor genes usually occurs in early tumorigenesis. This suggests that variations in these miRNAs can be used as an indicators of stages of cancer.

- **Function as tumor suppressor:** The miRNAs can function as tumor suppressor genes by suppressing translation of oncogenes. Examples are as follows:
  - **Lethal-7 (let-7) is a miRNAs having tumor suppressor activity.** The let-7 family interacts with the human KRAS oncogene and suppress the expression of the gene. Impaired expression of let-7 miRNA is observed in some human lung tumors and causes increased expression of the KRAS oncogene, whereas overexpression of let-7 can inhibit cell proliferation by inhibiting KRAS expression.
  - **miR-34a and miR-608:** They target several oncogenes including EGFR, Bcl-xL, B-Myb, and E2F1, to inhibit cell proliferation and growth of glioblastoma.
  - **miR-15a and miR-16-1:** They repress (suppress) expression of proto-oncogene Bcl-2 (B-cell lymphoma 2). Both miR-15a and miR-16-1 are either lost or downregulated in the majority of cases of chronic lymphocytic leukemia (CLL).
  - **miR-1 and miR-206:** They suppress expression of the proto-oncogene of mesenchymal-epithelial transition factor (c-MET) in different types of cancer (e.g., rhabdomyosarcoma).
- **Act as oncogene:** If the target of a miRNA is a tumor suppressor gene, then over activity of the miRNA can reduce the activity of tumor suppressor protein. Thus, some miRNAs may act as oncogenes by suppressing/repressing the expression of tumor suppressor genes and promote cell proliferation. Such miRNAs that promote tumor development are sometimes called as oncomiRs. If a miRNA inhibits the translation of an oncogene, a reduction in the quantity or function of that miRNA can lead to overproduction of the oncogene product.
  - **miR-17-92 cluster:** These are miRNA that encodes six miRNAs. They are highly expressed in several cancers (e.g., lung cancers and anaplastic thyroid cancer [ATC]) cells. The miR-17-92 cluster acts as an oncomiR that suppresses the tumor suppressor PTEN (phosphatase and tensin homolog).
  - **miRNA-155:** When its expression was upregulated in glioma cells, expression of the tumor suppressor forkhead box O3 (FoxO3) was found significantly downregulated.
  - **miR-494 and miR-22 downregulate PTEN expression** in malignant transformed cells
  - **miR-17-92:** Thrombospondins (TSPs) are a multi-gene family consisting of five secreted glycoproteins. They are involved in the regulation of cell proliferation, adhesion, and migration. Expression of TSP-1 acts as a tumor suppressor gene in colorectal cancer. TSP-1 is negatively regulated by miR-17-92 and acts as oncomiRs. Inhibition of the expression of this oncomiRs (i.e., miR-17-92) can upregulate the suppressed/repressed tumor suppressor genes. Hence, these oncomiRs can be used as targets for diagnosis, chemoprevention, and treatment. Also oncomiRs be used as potential molecular markers for cancer early diagnosis and risk prediction.
  - **Amplifications and deletions of miRNA loci** have been observed in many cancers. Downregulation or deletion of certain miRNAs in certain leukemias and lymphomas leads to increased expression of BCL2, an antiapoptotic gene. Thus, by negatively regulating BCL2, such miRNAs function as tumor suppressor genes. miR-200 is important in invasiveness and metastasis; and miR-155, is overexpressed in many human B-cell lymphomas. Deletions affecting certain tumor suppressive miRs, such as miR-15 and miR-16, are frequent genetic lesions in chronic lymphocytic leukemia. Mir34 family of miRNAs are activated by *p53* gene. Dysregulation of other miRNAs that control the expression of the RAS (in lung tumors) and MYC (certain B-cell leukemias) oncogenes also has been identified.
- **Function both as tumor suppressor genes and oncogenes:** Many miRNAs can function as both tumor suppressor genes and oncogenes. For example, in normal tissue miR-125b acts as a tumor suppressor gene and inhibits cell proliferation and cell-cycle progression. miR-125b is downregulated in ovarian, thyroid, breast and oral squamous cell carcinomas. Conversely, miR-125b can also act as an oncomiR. It inhibits apoptosis in tumor cells of neuroblastoma and promotes proliferation of cells and invasion in cancer of prostate.

Altered miR expression, due to amplifications and deletions of miR loci may be found in many cancers. Decreased expression of few miRs increases the translation of oncogenic mRNAs and these miRs have tumor suppressive activity. For example, deletions affecting miR-15 and miR-16 may be found in chronic lymphocytic leukemia (CLL). In CLL, loss of these miRs causes upregulation of the anti-apoptotic protein BCL-2. This increases the survival of tumor cells. Overexpression of few miRs suppress the expression of tumor suppressor genes. These miRs promote development of tumor and are termed as onco-miRs. For example, miR-155 is an onco-miR that is overexpressed in many B-cell lymphomas. They indirectly upregulate many genes that promote proliferation, including MYC.

MicroRNAs in Cancer Detection and Prediction

MicroRNAs as risk indicators

MicroRNA markers can be used as molecular risk indicators for all types of cancer. This is especially useful for rare tumors or tumors without any standard screening and detection tools for the early events of cancer development.

Triple negative breast cancer (TNBC): It is the most dangerous subtype and constitute about 15–20% of all breast cancers. It is usually seen in young women. It is negative for estrogen receptor (ER), progesterone receptor (PR) and Her2/neu. Screening mammograms are either not performed or not useful in young women. Since, presently no method available for accurate early detection of TNBC, it is necessary to develop effective tools for its early detection.

- **miRNAs along oncogene:** The combination of miRNA markers and the oncogene variant may be used as a new detection tool for TNBC. In premenopausal women, the KRAS oncogene is associated with risk of TNBC. Let-7 (Lethal-7) miRNA binds to the 3′-untranslated region of KRAS and suppresses expression of KRAS. Impairment (dysregulation) of binding of let-7 to the KRAS results in increased expression of KRAS and this initiates TNBC.

Glioma: miR-125b was found in the serum of patients with all grades of glioma, with a sensitivity and specificity of 78% and 75% respectively. Hence, miRNA markers may be useful for the detection of glioma.

MicroRNAs for detecting cancer and improving standard diagnostic tools

Multiple miRNAs have been detected in association with various types of cancer such as lung, colon, pancreatic, breast, prostate, brain, and liver cancer. Hence, these miRNAs may be used as biomarkers along with the current standard tests used for the diagnosis of cancer.

- ***Colorectal cancer*:** Presently, colonoscopy is the gold standard for early detection of colorectal cancer (CRC). However, there are certain disadvantages to use colonoscopy for regular screening. These includes, it is expensive, invasive and needs unpleasant bowel preparation. miRNA biomarkers can be used as a non-invasive initial screening method. Many miRNAs are associated with CRC and includes miR-409, miR-7, and miR-93 in plasma samples.
- ***Breast cancer*:** The gold standard screening technique for breast cancer is still mammography. The sensitivity and specificity is about 80–90% and 88–90% respectively. Hence, some cancers of breast can be missed by mammography. In addition, in is not useful for predicting progress to invasive breast cancer in benign breast diseases (BBDs) having increased risk of developing breast cancer (e.g., in ductal epithelial hyperplasia, atypical ductal hyperplasia [ADH] and ductal carcinoma in situ [DCIS]). It was observed that miR-21 and miR-191 were upregulated in breast cancer tissues, while miR-125b was downregulated. Hence, it was suggested that a combined expression profile of the ratio of 2 miRNAs could be used as a biomarker to discriminate between breast cancer and non-tumor tissue.
- ***Lung cancer*:** The most common method for detecting cancer of lung imaging-based screening techniques, particularly, by using low dose helical computed tomography (LDCT; also called spiral CT). However, it gives high false-positive rate and cannot definitely differentiate whether the detected nodules is benign or malignant tumors. MicroRNAs along with spiral CT may provide useful information. miRNAs such as miR-21, miR-31, and miR-210 may be useful to distinguish between malignancy and indeterminate solitary pulmonary nodules (ISPN) with higher sensitivity and specificity.

MicroRNAs in Body Fluids

Detection of miRNAs in serum was first reported in patients with diffuse B-cell lymphoma. The circulating tumor-associated miRNAs in blood are remarkably stable and protected from degradation by endogenous RNase. Detection of tumor derived miRNAs in bodily fluids also can be useful for noninvasive blood-based detection of cancer.

The body fluids useful for detection of miRNA include urine, pancreatic juices, cyst fluids, saliva and sputum, tears, breast milk, bronchial lavage, colostrum, seminal, amniotic, pleural, peritoneal, and cerebrospinal fluids.

Extracellular microRNAs as biomarkers of early detection

There are several reports indicating that the extracellular miRNAs can be used as a potential biomarker for early detection. miRNAs in body fluids can be useful both for diagnostic and prognostic purposes. Examples are as follows:

- ***Plasma*:** miRNA expression patterns in plasma can discriminate patients with non-small cell lung cancer (NSCLC) from healthy individuals. Circulating miRNAs in plasma or serum can be observed in carcinoma of lung, breast, prostate, colorectal region and stomach, and hepatocellular carcinoma. Panels of circulating miRNA in these cancers may be useful for diagnostic and prognostic purposes. However, the circulating miRNAs can be derived from sources other than tumor cells. Thus their levels of can be affected by other, non-neoplastic conditions (e.g., infection, hypoxia, diet and exercise).
- ***Sputum*:** By using a panel of miRNAs (miR-205, miR-210 and miR-708) in sputum, it was found that it can help to distinguish lung squamous cell carcinoma (SCC) patients from normal healthy patients.
- ***Urine*:** Expression of miR-126 and miR-152 in urine can be helpful in detecting the presence of bladder cancer.

MicroRNA Reproducibility and Validation for Cancer Detection

It is expected that miRNAs may emerge as novel biomarkers to increase the ability to manage the patient optimally. In spite of considerable efforts to demonstrate the use of miRNAs as biomarker for the early detection of cancer and improving standard diagnosis tools, there are many challenges faced. Similar to all types of molecular markers, reproducibility is a major issue in using microRNAs for early detection of cancer. To use miRNAs-based biomarkers for clinical diagnosis, there should be increased reproducibility, performance and clinical validation. Currently, there is significant inconsistency in the isolation and detection of extracellular miRNAs, so it requires further research in miRNA before using it in clinical practice.

PROGNOSIS

Q. Write short note on prognostic factors of malignant tumors.

The quantification of the probable clinical aggressiveness and extent of spread of any malignant tumor are necessary for accurate prognostication and for comparing results of various modes of therapy. For example, the treatment of well-differentiated follicular carcinoma localized to the thyroid gland will be different from a highly anaplastic thyroid cancers that has invaded surrounding tissues. The clinical gravity of the disease is judged by using the level of differentiation, or grade, and the extent of cancer spread, or stage. The prognosis of malignant tumors varies and is determined partly by the characteristics of the tumor cells (e.g., growth rate, invasiveness) and partly by the effectiveness of therapy.

Prognostic Indices

Prognosis and the treatment of a malignant tumor depend on:

Tumor Type

It is usually identified from the growth pattern of the tumor and its origin by only histopathological examination.

- Prognosis depends on the histological type (e.g., squamous cell carcinoma, melanoma, adenocarcinoma, leiomyosarcoma).
- Some tumors like lymphomas require further sub-classification into Hodgkin's and non-Hodgkin's lymphoma, each of which is then further sub classified by the cell type.

Grading of Malignant Tumors

Q. Grading and staging of cancer.

It is done by histological examination and is mainly based on the degree of differentiation of the tumor cells. Thus, cancer grading reflects the architecture and cytology of tumors.

- In general, there is a correlation between histologic grade and biologic behavior.
- **Grading system:** Most grading systems classify tumors into two (low grade and high grade) to four grades of increasing malignancy. Low-grade tumors are well-differentiated; high-grade ones tend to be poorly differentiated (anaplastic) neoplasms.
- **Basis of grading:** Gradings depends on the degree of anaplasia and on the number of proliferating cells in a tumor.
    - **Degree of anaplasia:** It is determined from the shape and regularity of the tumor cells and from the presence of distinct differentiated features (e.g., functioning gland-like structures in adenocarcinomas or epithelial pearls in squamous carcinomas). The presence of such characteristics features qualify these tumors as well differentiated. The cells of poorly differentiated malignant tumors bear little resemblance to their normal counterparts.
    - **Number of proliferating cell:** Features of rapid growth includes presence of (i) large numbers of mitotic figures, (2) atypical mitoses, (3) nuclear pleomorphism and (4) tumor giant cells.

Shortcomings of Grading

1. ***Less correlation with behavior*:** There is no perfect correlation between histologic appearance and biologic behavior. Hence, descriptive terms are used. For example, well-differentiated, mucin-secreting adenocarcinoma of the stomach, or poorly differentiated adenocarcinoma of pancreas in general, in soft-tissue sarcomas, grading is of less clinical value than staging.
2. ***Subjective*:** Cytological and histologic grading is subjective and the degree of differentiation can vary in different areas of the same tumor.

Staging is a more important criterion in predicting course of a tumors, to determine therapeutic approach and is proved to be of greater clinical value than is grading.

Staging of Tumors

It refers to the extent of spread of a malignant tumor and is independent of grading. Determining the stage of a cancer helps to predict the clinical behavior of a malignant tumor and to establish mode of treatment (criteria for therapy such as choice of surgical approach, or the selection of treatment modalities). Many cancers are staged using specific protocols that help determine the detectable extent of their spread. Most statistical data related to cancer survival are based on staging of cancer.

- ***Criteria*:** Staging requires both histopathological examination of the resected tumor and clinical assessment of the patient [including additional non-invasive techniques like computed tomography (CT), magnetic resonance imaging (MRI) and positron emission tomography (PET)].
- The criteria used for staging vary with different organs. Commonly the staging of cancers is based on:
    - **Size and extent of local growth of the primary tumor:** In this criteria, the size of primary cancer and extent of local growth (whether within or out of the organ) is assessed. For example, in colorectal cancer, the tumor which has penetrated into the muscularis and serosa of the bowel is associated with a poorer prognosis than with a tumor restricted to superficial mucosa/submucosa.
    - **Extent of spread to regional lymph nodes:** Presence of lymph node metastases indicate poor prognosis than without lymph node involvement.
    - **Presence of or absence of blood-borne (distant) metastases:** The presence of blood-borne distant metastases is bad prognostic sign and is a contraindication to surgical intervention other than for palliative measures.

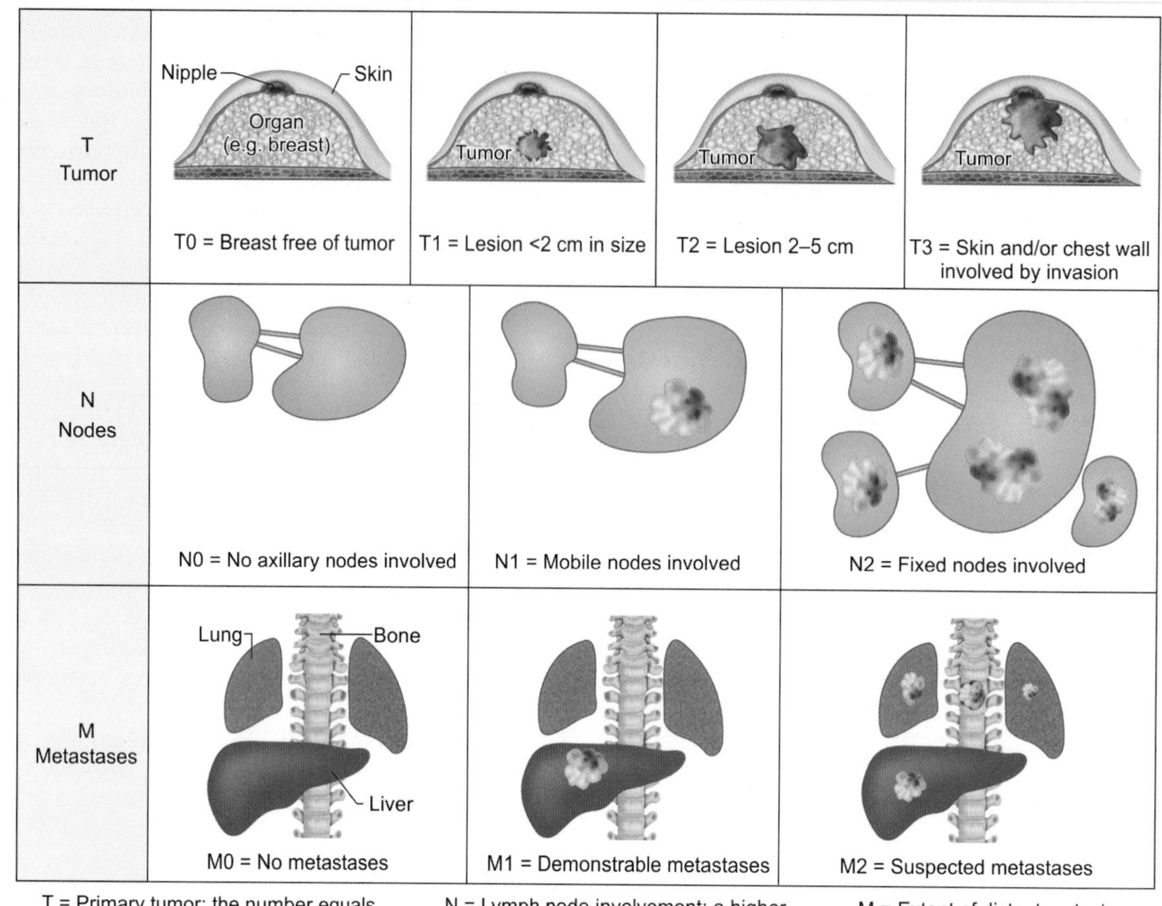

FIG. 104: Tumor staging by TNM system (e.g., breast carcinoma). TNM system is just one of many in current use.

TNM cancer staging systems (Fig. 104)

It is the cancer staging system widely used and it varies for each specific form of cancer. Currently, the major staging system in use is the American Joint Committee on Cancer Staging. This system uses a classification called the TNM system. General principles of TNM system are:

- T refers to the size of the primary tumor and local extent of the primary tumor.
  - It is suffixed by a number which indicates the size of the tumor or local anatomical extent. The number varies according to the organ involved by the tumor. With increasing size, the primary lesion is characterized as T1 to T4. T0 is used to denote an in situ lesion.
- N refers to level of lymph node metastases (status).
  - It is suffixed by a number to indicate the number of regional lymph nodes or groups of lymph nodes showing metastases.
  - N0 would mean no nodal involvement, whereas N1 to N3 would denote involvement of an increasing number and range of nodes.
- M refers to the presence and anatomical extent of distant metastases.
  - M0 signifies no distant metastases, whereas M1 indicates the presence of metastases.

Some tumor types (e.g., central nervous system [CNS] tumors and hematologic malignancies) are staged according to different systems. In modern practice, grading and staging of tumors are supplemented by molecular characterization of the tumor.

LABORATORY DIAGNOSIS OF CANCER

Q. Discuss laboratory diagnosis of cancer

Confirmation of lesion as neoplastic usually requires cytological and/or histopathological examination of the suspected organ or tissue. The approach to laboratory diagnosis of cancer becomes more complex, sophisticated, and specialized as the year passes by. Different laboratory methods available for the diagnosis of malignant tumors are:

Morphological Methods

Mostly the laboratory diagnosis of cancer can be done with ease by morphological examination. Sections taken from a healing fracture can mimic an osteosarcoma. The laboratory evaluation of a lesion can be only as good as the specimen submitted for examination. The specimen must be adequate, representative, and properly preserved.

Histopathological Examination

Histopathological diagnosis is based on the microscopic features of neoplasm and by this method of examination, accurate diagnosis can be made in majority of cases. Both benign and malignant tumors can be diagnosed without much difficulty. However, there are certain tumors which are not easy to diagnose on morphological methods.

- *Clinical data*: It should be provided for accurate pathologic diagnosis e.g.:
  - Clinical and radiological findings
  - Radiation causes changes in the skin or mucosa that mimic changes seen in cancer.
  - Sections taken from the site of a healing fracture can mimic an osteosarcoma.
  - Adequate and representative area of the specimen should be sent.
- Proper fixation.

Frozen section

Q. Write short essay/note on frozen section and its uses.

In this method, tissue is hardened rapidly by freezing (hence termed frozen section) and sections are cut by special instrument called freezing microtome or cryostat (microtome in a refrigerated chamber). By this method, morphological evaluation can be done within minutes. Frozen section when interpreted by an experienced and competent pathologist provide accurate diagnosis. There are certain situations where histological details provided by more time-consuming routine paraffin embedding methods is necessary. In such scenario, it is better to wait a few days. Though this routine embedding method needs few days, it may avoid inadequate or unnecessary surgery.

Uses of frozen section:

- Rapid diagnosis: Frozen section is used for quick histologic diagnosis (within minutes) and useful for determining the nature of a tumor (benign or malignant) lesion, especially when the patient is still on the operation table. It will help to determine whether a lesion is a neoplasm and, if so, whether it is benign or malignant.
- Evaluation of the margins of an excised cancer to know whether excision of the neoplasm is complete. If resection margins are inadequate, additional tissue can be removed immediately, without the need for a subsequent operation.
- Demonstration of fat mainly in nonneoplastic lesions.
- To know the lymph node (sentinel) status for metastasis in carcinoma. Knowing the extent of regional tumor metastases may be useful in deciding the further surgery.
- To determine whether additional workup is necessary for a particular tissue specimen while it is still fresh. For example, if the metastatic tumor found in a lymph node is recognized as a poorly differentiated carcinoma, special fixation and electron microscopy may be needed for proper diagnosis.

Various techniques for tissue sampling

- *Needle biopsy*: It is called as cutting-needle or core-needle or drill biopsy. Using cutting needle, a core of tissue 1–2 mm wide and 2 cm long is obtained for histologic examinations or special studies that permit evaluation of architectural structure. Tissue obtained is small and interpretation may be difficult.
- *Endoscopy biopsy*: It is performed through endoscopy. Usually performed for lesions in gastrointestinal, respiratory, urinary and genital tracts.
- *Incision biopsy*: In this representative tissue sample is obtained by incising the lesions. Incisional biopsy (along with fine-needle aspiration) is often the method of choice for inoperable lesions, or too large for excision, or when excision causes functional or cosmetic impairment.
- *Excision biopsy*: In this entire abnormal lesion is surgically removed. It provides generous amounts of tissue for diagnosis and may be surgical therapy for some tumors (e.g., small- to medium-sized breast cancers).

Pitfalls in biopsy interpretation: These include inadequate tissue sampling and artefacts due to procedure itself (e.g., thermal damage caused by an electrocautery or laser).

Cytological Examination

It is performed on many tissues and usually done for identifying neoplastic cells.

Methods of obtaining cells

Exfoliative cytology: It is the study of spontaneously exfoliated (shed) cells from the lining of an organ into a body cavity. Cytologic (Papanicolaou) smears examination is a method used for the detection of cancer. Historically, Pap smear was used mainly for discovery of carcinoma of the cervix, often at an in situ stage. Now it is widely used for many other cases of suspected malignancy. These include endometrial carcinoma, bronchogenic carcinoma, bladder and prostate tumors, and gastric carcinomas. It is also used for the identification of tumor cells in body fluids (e.g., pleural, peritoneal, joint, and cerebrospinal fluids) and for evaluation of other forms of neoplasia. Tumors cells are less cohesive than others; hence they shed into fluids or secretions. The shed cells are examined for features of anaplasia that indicate origin from a tumor.

Fine-needle aspiration cytology: It involves aspiration of cells and attendant fluid with a small-bore needle. The aspirated cells are spread out on a slide, smears are prepared and stained, followed by microscopic examination of cells. It is widely used, simple and quick procedure. Fine-needle aspiration of tumors is widely used for diagnosis of tumor. This procedure is most commonly performed on readily palpable lesions affecting the breast, thyroid gland, lymph nodes, and salivary glands. With the availability of modern imaging techniques (guided technology such as CT guided), this method is also used for deeper structures (e.g., liver, pancreas, pelvic lymph nodes, retroperitoneal structures). Guided fine needle techniques obviates the surgery and its attendant risks. Though it has some disadvantages such as small size of sample and sampling errors, it can be reliable, rapid, and useful in experienced hands.

Liquid-based cytology (thin prep): This is a special technique for preparation of samples that provides uniform monolayered dispersion of cells on smears. Discussed in detail on pages 564 and 565.

Cytological characteristics of cancer cells

Cancer cells have decreased cohesiveness and show cellular features of anaplasia. Cytologically, differentiation can be made between normal, dysplastic, carcinoma in situ and malignant cells.

Disadvantages of cytological examination

- Diagnosis is based on the features of individual cells or a clump of cells, without the supporting evidence of loss of orientation.
- The invasion which is diagnostic of malignant tumor under histology cannot be assessed by cytology.

Histochemistry and Cytochemistry

These are stains, which identify the chemical nature of cell contents or their products. H&E staining cannot demonstrate certain specific substances/constituents of cells. This requires some special stains. Common histochemical and cytochemical stains useful in diagnosis of tumors are listed in **Table 30**.

Table 30: Common histochemical and cytochemical stains useful in diagnosis of tumors.

Chemical substance	*Name of the stain*
Basement membrane/collagen	• Periodic acid Schiff (PAS) • Reticulin • Masson trichrome • Van Gieson
Glycogen	PAS with diastase
Mucin	Combined Alcian blue-PAS Mucicarmine
Cross-striation	Phosphotungstic acid hematoxylin (PTAH)
Enzymes	• Myeloperoxidase • Acid phosphatase • Alkaline phosphatase

Immunohistochemistry

Q. Write short note on immunohistochemistry and its role in the diagnosis of tumors.

Q. Discuss role of immunohistochemistry in diagnostic histopathology.

Q. List tumors in which immunohistochemistry has diagnostic role.

It is an immunological method of identifying the antigenic component in the cell or one of its components by using specific antibodies. It is widely used as a powerful adjunct to routine histologic examination in the diagnosis or management of malignant neoplasms.

Uses of immunohistochemistry

To categorize undifferentiated cancers Many malignant tumors of diverse origin resemble each other and are difficult to distinguish on routine hematoxylin and eosin (H&E) sections.

Neuroendocrine tumors: They show positivity for cytokeratins like carcinomas, but they can be identified by their contents (**Table 31**).

Table 31: Neuroendocrine and neuronal markers.

Marker	*Tumors*
Neuroendocrine markers	
Neuron-specific enolase (NSE)	Neuroendocrinal tumors, melanoma, neuroblastomas
Synaptophysin	Neuroendocrinal tumors
Chromogranin (proteins found in neurosecretory granules)	Neuroendocrinal tumors
Leu-7 (CD57)	MPNST, carcinoids, pheochromocytoma, small cell carcinoma of lung, follicular variant of papillary thyroid carcinoma
Neuronal markers	
Neurofilament protein	Small round cell tumors, neuroblastoma, ganglioneuroma, medulloblastoma, retinoblastoma, peripheral neuroepithelioma, Merkel cell tumors, carcinoid tumors, parathyroid tumors
Glial fibrillary acidic protein (GFAP) is an intermediate filament	Glial cell neoplasms of CNS, schwannoma

(MPNST: malignant peripheral nerve sheath tumor)

Soft tissue sarcomas (Table 32): They show intermediate filament positivity

- Vimentin
- Desmin is positive in smooth or striated muscle fibers
- Muscle-specific actin marker for muscle tissue.

Table 32: Muscle markers.

Marker	*Tumors*
Desmin	• Leiomyoma, rhabdomyoma, rhabdomyosarcoma, desmoplastic round cell tumor • Endometrial stromal sarcoma, peripheral neuroectodermal tumor (PNET)
Actin (SMA)	• Rhabdomyosarcoma, leiomyosarcoma, fibromatosis, myoepithelioma, angiomyolipoma, inflammatory myofibroblastic tumor • Adenoid cystic carcinoma
Myogenin	Rhabdomyosarcoma

Malignant lymphomas: They are generally positive for leukocyte common antigen (LCA, CD45). Markers for lymphomas and leukemias are called cluster designations (CDs) and useful to differentiate T and B lymphocytes, monocytes, and granulocytes and the mature and immature variants of these cells. Antigens useful for subclassification of hematolymphoid malignancy are presented in **Table 33**.

Vascular tumors: They are derived from endothelial cells, include benign hemangiomas, and malignant hemangiosarcomas and are positive for factor VIII-related antigen or certain lectins. Endothelial markers are presented in **Table 34**.

Melanocytic markers are presented in **Table 35**.

Proliferating cells: Cells in cell cycle show positivity for Ki-67 and proliferating cell nuclear antigen (PCNA).

Intermediate filaments and their use in diagnosis of neoplasms is presented in **Table 36**.

Table 33: Antigens useful for subclassification of hematolymphoid malignancy.

Antigen (predominant distribution)	*Diagnostic use*
CD45/LCA (lymphocytes)	To distinguish lymphoma from carcinoma or melanoma
CD3 (all T cells), CD4 (helper T cells), and CD8 (cytotoxic T cells)	Characterization of lymphoid infiltrate
CD19 and CD20 (B cells)	
CD15, L26, BLA36, CD30	Hodgkin lymphoma
CD34, TdT (blasts)	To detect acute leukemias
Myeloperoxidase, lysozyme (myeloid, monocytic cells)	Characterization of myeloid neoplasms
CD138, and kappa and lambda cytoplasmic light chains (plasma cells)	Characterization of plasma cell neoplasms

Table 34: Endothelial markers.

Marker	*Tumor*
VWF, Ulex Europeus 1	Vascular tumors
CD34	Angiosarcoma, Kaposi's sarcoma, dermatofibrosarcoma protruberans (DFSP), spindle cell lipoma, solitary fibrous tumor
CD31	Angiosarcoma, hemangioma, hemangioendothelioma
Thrombomodulin	Poorly differentiated malignant vascular tumors

Table 35: Melanocytic markers.

Marker	*Tumor*
HMB 45	• Melanoma, spitz nevus, pigmented nerve sheath tumor • Angiomyolipoma
S100	Melanoma, schwannoma, gliomas
Melan-A	Melanoma, adrenal cortical tumors

Table 36: Intermediate filaments and their use in diagnosis of neoplasms.

Type of intermediate filament	*Normal issue expression*	*Diagnostic usefulness*
1. Cytokeratin	All epithelial cells	Carcinoma
2. Vimentin	Mesenchymal cells	Sarcoma
3. Desmin	Muscle cells	Tumors of muscle (e.g., rhabdomyosarcoma)
4. Glial fibrillary acid protein (GFAP)	Glial cells	Glial tumors (e.g., astrocytoma)
5. Neurofilament (NF)	Neurons and neural crest derivatives	Neural tumors (e.g., neuroblastoma)

Table 37: Cellular antigens useful in classifying neoplasms.

Antigen (predominant distribution)	*Diagnostic uses*
Epithelial antigens	
• Cytokeratin (epithelial cells)	To distinguish carcinoma from lymphoma or melanoma
• Epithelial membrane antigen (epithelial cells)	To distinguish of carcinoma from melanoma
• Cytokeratin isoforms (epithelial cells)	To determine the primary site of metastatic carcinoma (pattern of expression of various isoforms is related to the site of origin)
Myogenous antigens	
• Desmin (myogenous cells)	To identify tumors of smooth muscle or skeletal muscle
• Muscle-specific actin (myogenous cells)	
Prostate-specific antigen (prostatic epithelium)	To identify metastatic prostatic carcinoma
Calcitonin (parafollicular epithelium of thyroid)	To distinguish medullary thyroid carcinoma from other tumors of thyroid
Alpha-fetoprotein (neoplastic hepatocytes and selected germ cell tumors)	To identify hepatocellular carcinoma, endodermal sinus tumor, and other germ cell tumors
β-human chorionic gonadotropin (placental tissue; trophoblastic and germ cell tumors)	To identify trophoblastic differentiation in germ cell tumors
HMB-45 (melanocytic cells)	To identify melanoma
CD31 (vascular endothelium)	To identify vascular neoplasms
CD34 (vascular endothelium and few tumors of soft tissue)	To identify vascular neoplasms, solitary fibrous tumors, dermatofibrosarcoma protuberans

Cellular antigens useful in classifying neoplasms is presented in **Table 37**.

Antigens useful for identification of infectious agents that helps to classify a neoplasm is presented in **Table 38**.

- *Example*: Few anaplastic carcinomas, lymphomas, melanomas and sarcomas may look almost similar under routine H&E sections. They should be accurately diagnosed because of their different modes of treatment and prognosis.
  - In poorly differentiated carcinoma intermediate filaments (e.g., cytokeratins) shows positivity (see **Table 36**).
  - Malignant melanomas when unpigmented (amelanotic melanoma) appear similar to other poorly differentiated carcinomas. They express HMB-45 and S-100 protein, but negative for cytokeratins.
  - Desmin is found in neoplasms of muscle cell origin.
  - Lineage-specific membrane proteins marker such as CD20 for tumors of B-cells.

To determine the origin of poorly differentiated metastatic tumors Cancer patients may present with metastases. In some of them, primary site is either obvious or can be detected by of clinical or radiologic findings. In patients with metastases cases in which the origin of the tumor is obscure. In such situations primary source of tumor can be determined by using tissue-specific or organ-specific antigens. Example include prostate-specific antigen (PSA) for prostatic carcinoma and thyroglobulin marker for carcinoma of the thyroid (**Table 39**).

Table 38: Antigens useful for identification of infectious agents that helps to classify a neoplasm.

Antigen	*Predominant distribution*	*Diagnostic use*
Epstein–Barr virus latent membrane protein 1	Lymphocytes	To identify EBV-associated lymphomas
Human herpesvirus 8	Vascular endothelium	To identify Kaposi's sarcoma
Merkel cell polyomavirus	Neuroendocrine cells	To identify Merkel cell carcinoma
p16	Epithelium	Surrogate marker for HPV infection
*Helicobacter pylori**	Stomach	To identify *Helicobacter pylori* in gastric biopsies

* Seen usually in gastritis rather than carcinoma

Table 39: Lineage-associated immunohistochemical markers useful in establishing the origin of a poorly carcinoma.

Lineage-associated markers	*Associated cancer*
Prostate-specific antigen (PSA) and prostate-specific acid phosphatase (PSAP)	Prostatic carcinoma
Carcinoembryonic antigen (CEA)	Colonic carcinoma
Thyroglobulin	Thyroid carcinoma
CA-125	Ovarian cancers
Nuclear receptors for estrogen and progesterone	Carcinoma of breast

Lineage-associated immunohistochemical markers useful in establishing the origin of a poorly carcinoma is presented in **Table 39**.

For prognosis or to select the mode of treatment:

- **Breast cancer (Fig. 105A to C):** Immunohistochemical detection of hormone (estrogen/progesterone) receptors in cancer cells of breast is having both prognostic and therapeutic significance. These receptor-positive cancers respond to antiestrogen therapy and have a better prognosis than receptor-negative breast cancers. Protein products of oncogenes such as ERBB2 (HER2/neu) can also be detected by immunostaining. Breast cancers with strong immunohistochemical positivity for the protein product of the ERBB2 gene product, HER2, have usually a poor prognosis. But these HER2/neu positive tumors respond to treatment with antibodies that block the activity of the HER2 receptor. The high-level expression of HER2 is due to amplification of the ERBB2 gene. Fluorescent in situ hybridization (FISH) can be used to confirm ERBB2 gene amplification and is sometimes used as an adjunct to immunohistochemical studies especially when the immunohistochemical stain gives an equivocal result.
- **Lung cancer and lymphoma:** Immunohistochemical stains for ALK protein can be used in lung cancers and lymphomas. In these tumors, presence of ALK expressing constitutively active ALK fusion proteins is an indication for treatment with drugs that inhibit the ALK tyrosine kinase.

Antigens that provide prognostic or predictive information in malignancy is presented in **Table 40**.

Antigens that helps to identify an inherited cancer syndrome is presented in **Table 41**.

Other markers useful in the diagnosis of neoplasms are presented in **Table 42**.

Electron Microscopy

It helps in the diagnosis of poorly differentiated/undifferentiated cancers, which cannot identify the origin by light microscopy, e.g., carcinomas show desmosomes and specialized junctional complexes, structures which are not seen in sarcomas or lymphomas.

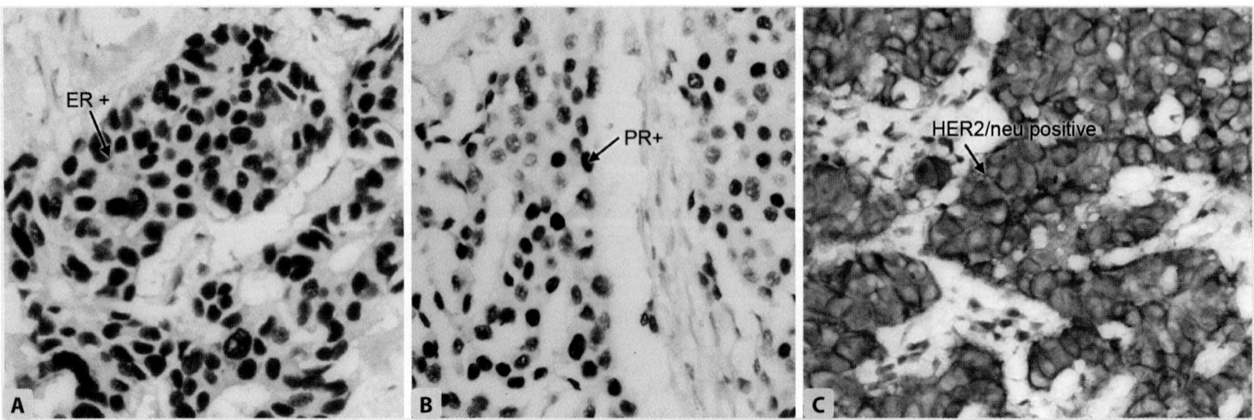

FIGS. 105A TO C: Immunohistochemistry in breast carcinoma: (A) ER positive; (B) PR positive and (C) HER2/neu positive.

Table 40: Antigens that provide prognostic or predictive information in malignancy.		
Antigen	**Predominant distribution**	**Diagnostic use**
Estrogen receptor and progesterone receptor	Breast epithelium and endometrium	For prediction of clinical response to hormonal therapy
HER2	Epithelium	Level of expression provides prognostic information and response to therapy
PD-L1	Many types of tumors	Level of expression predicts response to therapy
BRAF V600E mutation	Many types of tumors	Presence of V600E-activating mutation provides prognostic information and response to therapy in melanoma and thyroid carcinoma

Table 41: Antigens that helps to identify an inherited cancer syndrome.	
Antigen (distribution)	**Diagnostic use**
MLH1, PMS2, MSH2, and MSH6 (all types of cells)	Absence of staining indicates a defect in DNA mismatch repair (MMR). This may suggest the presence of Lynch syndrome

Table 42: Other markers useful in the diagnosis of neoplasms.	
Marker	**Tumor**
AFP	Hepatocellular carcinoma, yolk sac tumor, nonseminomatous germ cell tumors
hCG	Choriocarcinoma, syncytiotrophoblast cells in seminomas, embryonal/yok sac tumors
PLAP	Seminoma
PSA	Prostatic tumors, nodular hyperplasia of prostate, carcinoma of salivary gland, breast and urinary bladder
GCDFP-15	Carcinoma of breast, Paget's disease of skin, vulva, carcinoma of salivary gland and prostate

Flow Cytometry

Q. Write short note on modern techniques in tumor diagnosis.

It rapidly and quantitatively measures various individual cell characteristics, such as membrane antigens and the DNA content of tumor cells. However, it needs viable cells in suspension. This method uses fluorescently labeled antibodies against cell surface molecules and differentiation antigens are used to identify the nature of malignant cells. It is mainly used for identification of cellular antigens expressed by "liquid" tumors, especially those arising from blood forming tissues. Thus, flow cytometry is useful for identification and classification of tumors of T and B lymphocytes (leukemias and lymphomas), myeloid neoplasms and mononuclear-phagocytic cells. In contrast to immunohistochemistry, flow cytometry has an advantage in which multiple antigens are assessed simultaneously on individual cells. This is achieved by using combinations of specific antibodies linked to different fluorescent dyes.

Circulating Tumor Cells

Detection, quantification, and characterization of rare solid tumors cells (e.g., carcinoma, melanoma) circulating in the blood is emerging as a diagnostic modality though presently in research stage. Few latest devices detect three-dimensional flow cells coated with antibodies specific for tumor cells of interest (e.g., carcinoma cells) in the blood. It will be useful for early diagnosis, to assess the risk of metastasis and assess the response of tumor cells to therapy. Discussed in detail on pages 564 and 565.

Molecular Diagnosis Cytogenetics

Q. Describe the molecular techniques in diagnosis of neoplasia.

Many molecular or *cytogenetic* techniques are available for the diagnosis of tumors and for predicting their behavior. Commonly used are fluorescence in situ hybridization (FISH) technique and polymerase chain reaction (PCR) analysis.

a. **Diagnosis of cancer:** Though molecular techniques are not the primary method for diagnosis of cancer, they are useful in certain situations.
   - *Monoclonal (malignant) versus polyclonal (benign)*: T cell and B cell have unique antigen receptor gene rearrangements. Reactive lymphoid proliferations contain many different lymphocyte clones. Each of these clones have a different set rearrangements antigen receptor genes. PCR-based detection of rearranged T-cell receptor or immunoglobulin genes helps in differentiating monoclonal (neoplastic) and polyclonal (benign reactive) proliferations of T-or B-cells.
   - *Chromosomal alterations*: Many hematopoietic neoplasms (leukemias and lymphomas) and few solid tumors (e.g., Ewing's sarcoma) are characterized by particular translocations. These can be usually detected by routine cytogenetic analysis or FISH technique or by PCR analysis. For example, PCR-based detection of BCR-ABL transcripts will confirm the diagnosis of chronic myeloid leukemia. Some hematological malignancies are characterized by the presence of point mutations in particular oncogenes. For example, the diagnosis of polycythemia vera needs the identification of specific mutations in JAK2 (gene encodes a nonreceptor tyrosine kinase). Molecular techniques can be useful for the diagnosis of sarcomas with characteristic translocations. This is partly because the chromosome preparations are generally difficult to obtain from solid tumors. For example, many sarcomas of childhood (round blue cell tumors) may be difficult to distinguish from each other based on the their morphologic features. However, the detection of presence of the characteristic (11;22)

(q24;q12) translocation by PCR can help to confirm the diagnosis of Ewing sarcoma.

- *DNA microarrays*: This may used as either tiling arrays (cover the entire human genome), or SNP arrays (SNP chips). They allow high-resolution mapping of copy number changes (either deletions or amplifications) genome-wide and useful for diagnosis of cancer.

b. **Prognosis of cancer:** Few genetic alterations are of prognostic value and may be associated with a poor prognosis. These alterations determine the patient's subsequent therapy. They can be detected by routine cytogenetics and also by FISH or PCR assays. Example of poor prognostic feature is amplification of the *N-MYC* gene and deletions of 1p in neuroblastoma. In oligodendrogliomas the only genomic abnormality is the loss of chromosomes 1p and 19q. These patients respond better to therapy and survive longer when compared to tumors without 1p and 19q deletion and with EGF receptor amplification. Presence of point mutations in cancer genes such as *TP53* indicates poor outcome in many types of cancer. Assessment of the host immune response to tumors may also be helpful in assessing the prognosis. For example, by quantification of the number of infiltrating cytotoxic T cells.

c. **Detection of minimal residual disease:** PCR-based amplification of nucleic acid sequences unique to the malignant clone can detect minimal (measurable) residual disease or the onset of relapse in patients who are treated for leukemia or lymphoma. For example, detection of breakpoint cluster region (BCR)-ABL transcripts in treated patients with chronic myeloid leukemia (CML) by PCR gives the measure of residual leukemic cells in treated patients. The prognostic importance of minimal residual disease is well known in acute leukemia. Almost all advanced cancers are associated with both intact circulating tumor cells (CTCs) and products derived from tumors (e.g., cell-free circulating tumor DNA). Identification of tumor-specific nucleic acid sequences through sensitive blood tests may be useful in following tumor burden. Discussed in detail below on page 564.

d. **Detection of hereditary predisposition to cancer:** Germline mutations in many tumor suppressor genes are associated with increased risk for specific cancers. This will help in prophylactic surgery, and counselling of relatives at risk, e.g., *BRCA1, BRCA2* and the *RET* proto-oncogene. Detection of these mutated alleles requires an aggressive screening protocol, as well as provide an opportunity for prophylactic surgery. It also useful for genetic counselling of relatives who are at risk.

e. **Guiding therapy with oncoprotein-directed drugs:** It is useful in target therapy. Detection of mutations in a tumor can helps in selecting the therapies that directly target specific mutations. Many chemotherapeutic agents target oncoproteins that are present only in a subset of cancers of a particular type. Thus the molecular identification of genetic lesions that produce these oncoproteins is necessary for treatment of patients. Examples of therapy based on genetic lesions that guide therapy include the (i) *PML-RARA* fusion gene in acute promyelocytic leukemia, (ii) the *BCR-ABL* fusion gene in chronic myeloid leukemia and (iii) acute lymphoblastic leukemia, (iv) *ERBB1* (EGFR) mutations and *ALK* gene rearrangements in lung cancer, and (v) *BRAF* mutations in melanoma.

f. **Identifying mechanisms of drug resistance:** liquid biopsies. These tests depend on circulating tumor cells or cell-free DNA that is yielded from dying tumor cells into the blood. The most advanced tests of analyze cell-free tumor DNA for the presence of specific driver mutations that produce targetable oncoproteins (e.g., lung cancers). PCR based tests can be performed on peripheral blood at many times after treatment has begun. This avoids the need for repeat tissue biopsies. Liquid biopsies are discussed in detail on pages 564 and 564.

Molecular Profiling of Tumors

Q. Describe the various molecular techniques in diagnosis of neoplasia.

Q. Discuss the recent diagnostic approach to neoplasia.

Traditional Cancer Typing

Traditionally cancer is diagnosed and classified according to the morphological (histopathology/cytopathology) appearance of the cells and its surrounding tissue. It has limitations such as (i) it relies on a subjective review of the tissue which is dependent on the knowledge and experience of a pathologist, and therefore may not be reproducible, (ii) limited ability to determine the individual recurrence risk of cancer, (iii) insufficient to reflect the complicated underlying molecular events that drive the neoplastic process and (iv) histopathology reports lack or offer very little information regarding the potential drug treatment regime to which a cancer will respond. Traditional pathology reports help to determine treatment that leads to better outcomes. However, tumors with identical pathology may have different origins and respond differently to treatment.

Newer Cancer Diagnostics

Molecular profiling of tumors is the identification and documentation of the structure of a specific DNA, RNA, or protein molecule. Till recently, molecular studies of tumors consisted of analyzing individual genes. However, the revolutionary technologies which have achieved completion of the human genome sequence and more reliable methods of gene expression analysis have revolutionized cancer diagnosis and treatment. At present technology can provide several new useful information. They can rapidly sequence an entire genome and assess epigenetic modifications genome-wide (the epigenome). They are also useful to quantify all of the RNAs expressed in a cells (the transcriptome) and measure many proteins simultaneously expressed (the proteome). Thus, they provide all of the cell's metabolites (the metabolome). Present methods like DNA microarray technology can measure the expression *single gene to all genes* in the genome instead of only one gene at a time. By providing a molecular portrait of an individual cancer, this technology will help the clinicians to determine the origin of the cancer, its potential for metastasis, its specific drug responsiveness, and the probability of its recurrence. Classification of cancer typing by molecular profile overcomes the limitations of traditional cancer typing. A molecular profile determines the level of gene expression within the cancer by hybridizing the cellular RNA with known genes. However, RNA is prone to degradation and is a more difficult analyte to work with than DNA in clinical practice.

DNA Microarray

Currently, the most common method for large-scale analysis of RNA expression is based on DNA microarrays. A DNA microarray (also known as DNA chip or biochip) is a collection of microscopic DNA spots attached to a solid surface. This provides information on thousands of genes simultaneously. Once the gene expression pattern is determined, this information is compared to the expression profiles of cancers with known outcomes using a predetermined algorithm.

DNA Sequencing

It is the process of determining the precise order of nucleotides within a DNA molecule and is technically simpler than RNA sequencing. Next-generation sequencing refers to non-Sanger-based high-throughput DNA sequencing technologies. Millions or billions of DNA strands can be sequenced in parallel, yielding substantially more throughput and minimizing the need for the fragment-cloning methods that are often used in "Next-generation [NextGen] sequencing" which can be readily performed on virtually any tissue specimen. By nextGen sequencing, the process of whole-genome of individual tumors can be completed in as little as a few weeks. The cancer genome sequencing can identify new mutations in various cancers; describe the full, extensive collection of genetic lesions in individual cancers; and a presence of genetic heterogeneity in individual cancers from area to area. It is particularly useful to tumors, such as lung carcinomas, that are genetically diverse and require a "personalized" approach for successful targeted therapy. However, histopathological examination of tumors provides information about important characteristics of cancers, such as anaplasia, invasiveness, and tumor heterogeneity. These cannot be obtained from DNA sequences. Thus, the most accurate diagnosis and assessment of prognosis in cancer can be arrived by a combination of morphologic and molecular techniques (i.e., molecular profiling of tumors by RNA expression profiling, DNA sequencing, and DNA copy number arrays).

Tumor Markers

Q. Write short essay on tumor markers.
Q. Write short essay on CEA and AFP.

Tumor markers are products of malignant tumors that can be detected in the cells themselves or in blood and body fluids.

Usefulness

Tumor markers lack the sensitivity and specificity needed for the diagnosis of cancer. Hence, they cannot be used for definitive diagnosis of cancer. Their used are as follows:

- *Screening test for detection of cancer*: Tumor markers are used as screening tests. For example, PSA is the most common and useful tumor markers used to screen prostatic adenocarcinoma. High levels of PSA are found in the blood of prostatic carcinoma patients but it also may be elevated in benign prostatic hyperplasia. PSA test has low sensitivity and low specificity.
- *Determine the effectiveness of therapy*: Helps in monitoring the response to therapy
- *Detection of recurrence*: For example, PSA assay is very useful for detecting residual disease or recurrence following treatment for prostate cancer.

Tumor markers used in clinical practice: Many tumor markers have been identified and new markers are identified every year. Only a few of these markers are clinically useful. Tumor markers commonly used in clinical practice are:

- *Prostate-specific antigen (PSA)*: It is estimated in blood and is useful marker for prostatic adenocarcinoma. Prostatic carcinoma can be suspected when the blood PSA levels are elevated. Though PSA levels are usually elevated in prostatic cancer, PSA levels also may be elevated by benign prostatic hyperplasia. If there is no PSA level, it does not indicate the absence of prostate cancer. Thus PSA is specific for prostate and not specific for prostate cancer.
- *Carcinoembryonic antigen (CEA)*: It is secreted by carcinomas of the colon, pancreas, stomach, and breast
- *Alpha fetoprotein (AFP)*: It is produced by hepatocellular carcinomas, yolk sac tumors in the gonads, and occasionally teratocarcinomas and embryonal cell carcinomas.

Note: Similar to PSA, CEA and AFP levels can be raised in many nonneoplastic conditions. They lack the specificity and sensitivity needed for the early detection of cancers, but they may be useful in monitoring disease once the diagnosis is made. After the successful resection of the tumor, these markers disappear from the serum and their reappearance usually indicates recurrence. Other commonly used tumor markers include *human chorionic gonadotropin* (HCG) for testicular tumors, *CA-125* for ovarian tumors, and monoclonal *immunoglobulin* in multiple myeloma.

Types of markers (**Table 43**): These may be tumor-associated enzymes, hormones, oncofetal antigens, specific proteins, mucin and glycoproteins, enzymes and other molecular markers.

Methods for Early Diagnosis of Neoplasia

Q. Describe methods for early diagnosis of neoplasia.

Transformation of a normal cell into a cancerous state is a complex process. It is necessary to develop a measurable characteristic **to detect cancer at the early-stage before it is palpable or detectable by presently available sensitive screening technologies. Early-stage detection of cancer will provide a better outcome for therapeutic intervention.** Correct detection of cancer at an early stage has markedly increased the success of treatment, thereby decreasing the mortality due to cancer.

Screening Tests

One of the method of early detection of cancer is by screening test. Cancer screening aims to detect cancer early, before symptoms appear or progression beyond a treatable stage. Screening tests must be effective, safe, well-tolerated with acceptably low rate of false-positive and false-negative results. **Most routine screening tools for cancer detection are mainly based on examination of cell morphology, tissue histology, and measurement of serum markers.** Existing screening techniques **lack sufficient sensitivity and/or specificity for early detection of cancer**. They are not capable of distinguishing benign and indolent cancers from aggressive ones. Even the histopathological criteria are not sufficient for this distinction. For example, colonoscopy is a diagnostic screening method. It can detect precancerous polyps and early-stage colon cancer in only about 40% of colon cancers. The cancers may be missed by colonoscopy due to technical

Table 43: Common tumor markers.

Tumor marker	*Associated tumors*
1. Hormones	
• Human chorionic gonadotropin (hCG)	Trophoblastic tumors, nonseminomatous tumors of testis
• Calcitonin	Medullary carcinoma of thyroid
• Catecholamine and its metabolites	Pheochromocytoma and related tumors
• Ectopic hormones	Paraneoplastic syndromes (Table 29 of 10.6)
2. Oncofetal antigens	
• α-fetoprotein (AFP)	Cancer of liver, nonseminomatous germ cell tumors of testis
• Carcinoembryonic antigen (CEA)	Carcinomas of the colon, pancreas, lung and stomach and heart
3. Mucins and other glycoproteins	
• CA-125 • CA-19-9 • CA-15-3	• Ovarian cancer • Colon cancer, pancreatic cancer • Breast cancer
4. Isoenzymes	
• Prostatic acid phosphatase (PAP)	Prostate carcinoma
• Neuron-specific enolase (NSE)	Small-cell carcinoma of lung, neuroblastoma
5. Linage-specific proteins	
• Immunoglobulins	Multiple myeloma and other gammapathies
• Prostate-specific antigen (PSA) and prostate-specific membrane antigen	Prostate carcinoma
Serum: *EGFR* mutants	Lung cancer
Stool and serum	
• *TP53, APC, RAS* mutants	Colon cancer
• *TP53, RAS* mutants	Pancreatic cancer
Sputum and serum: *TP53, RAS* mutants	Lung cancer
Urine: *TP53* mutants	Bladder cancer

or other reasons. Among asymptomatic patients, 2–6% are missed cancers (especially cancers of the right side of the colon) even in the hands of experienced operators.

Tumor markers (refer pages 556–558 for immunohistochemical markers): Tumor markers are products of malignant tumors that can be detected in the cells themselves or in blood and body fluids. **Most secreted proteins studied as cancer screening tumor markers have low sensitivity and/or low specificity. This may be due to the use of non-sensitive techniques or several of these tumor markers are also produced by normal tissues.**

Biomarker

Definition of biomarker: National Cancer Institute (NCI) of the National Institutes of Health (NIH) defines biomarker as: **"A biological molecule found in blood, other body fluids, or tissues that is a sign of a normal or abnormal process, or of a condition or disease."**

A cancer biomarker is a substance or process that indicates the presence of cancer. A biomarker may be a molecule secreted by a tumor or a specific response of the body to the presence of cancer. **Biomarkers are also termed as molecular markers and signature molecules.** Biomarkers are measurable indicators of disease, and can be useful as early indicators of cancer. **Most of the screening tests and tumor markers have certain disadvantages. Hence, there is urgent need for the discovery of innovative (new) tools and novel molecular biomarker** to detect early occurrence of carcinogenesis at molecular levels; to predict the aggressiveness of pre-cancerous lesions; and to incorporate this information into existing screening methods. Thus, it should be useful for **cancer screening, diagnosis, and prognosis. Features of ideal biomarker is presented in Box 19.** The clinical value of a biomarker test is based on its positive predictive value (PPV), or how likely it is for test positive individuals to actually have neoplasia, and its negative predictive value (NPV), or how likely it is for test-negative individuals to not have neoplasia.

Biomarker (molecular marker) may be useful for early diagnosis of neoplasia. Biomarkers, along with existing screening and imaging techniques, can become very important diagnostic tools. **However, only a few biomarkers are useful in clinical practice especially in the field of carcinogenesis.**

With recent advances in genomics, epigenomics, and proteomics and availability of innovative (new) advanced techniques, new biomarkers are developed to identify and characterize biomarkers that drive the development and progression of cancer and to discover upstream genes/proteins. Biomarkers have gained great clinical importance because of their usefulness (**Box 20**) in early detection, diagnosis, prevention, treatment and prognosis of cancer.

Box 19: Features of ideal biomarker.

- Should indicate a reliable positive or negative correlation with the presence of neoplasia/disease
- Should have high sensitivity (true positive rate i.e., the ability to correctly identify individuals with neoplasia) and specificity (true negative rate i.e., the ability to correctly identify individuals without neoplasia)
- Should be easily accessible (e.g., by noninvasive methods for screening purposes), quantifiable, analyzable, and interpretable

Box 20: Various usefulness of biomarker in cancer.

- Before diagnosis: Used to detect early stage cancer, for risk assessment, screening, and follow-up prevention
- During diagnosis: Used for staging and grading of tumor/cancer
- During prognosis: To predict prognosis and the course of treatment
- Treatment: Determination of initial therapy, treatment response, and clinical outcome and determine therapy efficacy and or to be novel drug targets

Several genes, proteins, enzymes, hormones, carbohydrate moieties and a few oncofetal antigens have been identified as potential biomarkers. Few specific genomic biomarkers have been also proposed (e.g., TP53 protein that suppresses the growth of tumors). Increased lifetime risk of hereditary breast and ovarian cancer syndrome in women is associated with inherited mutations in the *BRCA1* and *BRCA2* genes. Mutations in *PTEN* are associated with Cowden syndrome (inherited disorder with increased risk of breast, thyroid, endometrial, and other types of cancers).

Reverse transcriptase polymerase chain reaction (RT-PCR), mass spectrometry (MS) technique and surface plasmon resonance (SPR) technique are used for molecular genetics, proteomics, and to detect bimolecular interaction respectively. Since biomarkers play an important role in at all stages of disease, it is important that before using them for clinical care, they must undergo rigorous evaluation, including analytical validation, clinical validation, and assessment of clinical utility.

Presently, recommendations for early detection of cancer in average-risk individuals are available for colorectal, cervical, breast, endometrial (in menopausal women) and prostate cancers, and in high-risk individuals in the case of lung cancer. Examples of biomarkers facilitating diagnosis and treatment of tumors is presented in **Table 44**. Protein-based biomarkers and their significance is presented in **Table 45**.

Epigenetic alterations (e.g., DNA methylation and histone modifications) are most common known molecular alterations in human neoplasia.

- DNA methylation as cancer biomarker: The altered DNA methylation can be detected by gene-specific and genome wide biomarker. They appear as promising tool, for assessing cancer risk, early diagnosis, molecular staging of tumors, and monitoring drug response.

Imaging Techniques in Cancer Diagnosis

Q. Describe value of imaging and molecular techniques in diagnosis of neoplasia.

Imaging modalities constitute an important part of cancer care and management. They operate over a wide range of size and time scales and permit real-time monitoring. They are highly convenience without tissue destruction, and are minimally invasive or non-invasive. Combined imaging modalities providescomplementary information and helps in the early diagnosis and prognosis of cancer. Recently metabolic, molecular (genetic, epigenetic, transcriptomic, and proteomic) markers and nanoprobes have been integrated to various imaging modalities.

Table 44: Examples of biomarkers facilitating diagnosis and treatment of tumors.

Biomarker	*Associated tumor*
Germline mutations in the high-penetrance genes breast cancer 1 (BRCA1) and breast cancer 2 (BRCA2)	Hereditary susceptibility to breast and ovarian cancers
Somatic mutations in phosphatidylinositol-4,5-bisphosphate 3-kinase catalytic subunit alpha (*PIK3CA*) gene	Colorectal tumors (predictive biomarker for adjuvant aspirin therapy)
v-raf murine sarcoma viral oncogene homolog B (BRAF) V600E mutations	Metastatic melanoma (can be treated with the BRAF inhibitor)
Translocation between the breakpoint cluster region (BCR) gene on chromosome 22 and the Abelson (ABL) tyrosine kinase gene on chromosome 9	Chronic myelogenous leukemia (CML). Imatinib against the BCR-ABL fusion product

Table 45: Protein-based biomarkers and their significance.

Biomarker	*Significance*
Overexpression of human epidermal growth factor receptor 2 (HER2; also known as ERBB2) in breast tumors	Marker for prognosis of breast cancer, as well as an effective target for treatment with trastuzumab, a HER2-specific monoclonal antibody
Levels of cancer antigen 25 (CA-125) in serum	Indicative of disease progression and treatment response in ovarian cancer (but has high false-positive rate)
Fibulin-3, in plasma and effusions of mesothelioma patients	For early detection, diagnosis and prognosis of pleural mesothelioma
Prostate-specific antigen (PSA)	Prostate cancer screening marker. PSA is a good biomarker for the monitoring and management of patients with advanced prostate cancer

Medical Imaging

This includes diagnostic and therapeutic imaging applications.

- Therapeutic imaging: It plays role in treatment planning, guidance, assessment of tumor treatment response, palliation, and expansion of new therapeutics.
- Diagnostic imaging: It plays role in prediction, screening, detection, localization, differential diagnosis, staging, and prognosis of cancer. It includes invasive and non-invasive techniques.

Positron emission tomography (PET): It has become an essential functional imaging tool in oncology clinical practice. It is useful for cancer staging, restaging, therapy response assessment, and follow-up. The high diagnostic accuracy of PET imaging depends on its molecular nature. Using different radiotracers, PET can detect early functional and biochemical alterations that occur at the molecular and cellular levels in cancer tissue. These alterations include alterations in metabolism, proliferation, and angiogenesis or distinctive biological features of cancer cells (e.g., specific receptor expression or tumor hypoxia). Future research can allow PET to be a more relevant and can play a leading role in the "personalized" management of oncologic patients.

Nanotechnology: The size of the tumor at the time of diagnosis is the most reliable factor in predicting cancer survival. Hence, early diagnosis of cancer is important for determining the prognosis. Presently available diagnostic methods can detect tumors only when they contain a minimum of one billion cells. However, with nanotechnology, it is possible to detect tumors 1000 times smaller than the usual detectable size and also earlier than the currently available diagnostic methods.

Box 21: Cancer screening methods for few common cancers

Breast cancer
- Clinical and self-breast examination
- Mammography, ultrasound, and magnetic resonance imaging
- Genetic screening,

Cancer of uterine cervix
- Screening of cervical smear by the Pap test or other methods

Colorectal cancer
- Fecal occult blood testing
- Colonoscopy, sigmoidoscopy

Prostate cancer
- Prostate specific antigen (PSA) test

Carcinoma lung
- Low-dose computed tomography (CT) in heavy smokers

Pancreatic cancer
- Regular screening with endoscopic ultrasound and MRI/CT imaging for high risk individuals with inherited genetics

Another advantage of nanoparticles is that it can be designed to cross the biological barriers. Hence, they can also be used to detect tumors not accessible to conventional diagnostic methods. In nanotechnology, inexpensive radioisotopes with short half-life can be combined with nanocarriers to target the specific tumor cells. The use of nanotechnology for clinical diagnosis with increased sensitivity and earlier detection of disease is known as nanodiagnostics. The novel nanodiagnostic tools used for the early diagnosis of cancer are (i) quantum dots (QDs), (ii) gold nanoparticles, and (iii) cantilevers. These may be future alternative to the PCR. Magnetic nanoparticles can be used to capture CTCs in the circulating bloodstream and these are detected by rapid photoacoustic method. The increased sensitivity depends on the interaction between analyte molecules and signal-generating particles. In nanotechnology there is one-to-one interaction between analytes and signal-generating particles and it detects a single analyte molecule (e.g., proteins and other biomolecules). Thus, nanotechnology has improved sensitivity for the early diagnosis of cancer, and can detect multiple protein biomarkers using nanobiosensors. Nanoparticles can be used for targeted drug delivery in cancer and this helps the combination of both diagnostics and therapeutics known as theranostics.

- Applications of nanotechnology in surgical oncology: Nanoparticles can be used to visualize tumor during surgery that helps proper removal and nanorobotics for remotely controlled diagnostics combined with therapeutics.

Cancer screening methods for few common cancers are presented in **Box 21**.

Liquid Biopsies as a Diagnostic Tool

Q. Discuss on liquid biopsies as a diagnostic tool in neoplasia.

Introduction: One of the main role of pathologists is to determine the presence or absence of tumor in clinical samples. It is needed for staging, monitoring response to treatment, and detecting relapse of neoplasia. This is critical step in determining the course of patient management. There are variety of methods and includes routine, histopathology and cytology along with immunohistochemistry (IHC) and flow cytometry. More recent approach is the detection of tumor cells and nucleic acids in blood and bone marrow samples. Main goal is the more accurate detection of disease spread and better patient care.

Circulating Tumor Cells (CTCs)

Cancer metastasis is a multistep process and occurs when cancer cells acquire the ability to escape their local environment. These cancer cells then enter the circulation to reach distant sites, attach at the distant site, and proliferate to form a metastatic deposit. Depending on the type of malignant tumor, cancer cells can enter either the lymphatic or venous circulation (or both). By lymphatic spread cancer involves local lymph nodes and through venous spread they involve lung, liver, or bone marrow. It was found that significant proportions of patients who undergo theoretically curative surgery for organ-confined tumors

Later develop recurrence of malignant disease. This points out that the current approaches of staging cancer are to some extent, inadequate. Sensitive detection of CTCs can be useful for improved staging and monitoring of cancer patients. Such techniques can also be used to the study of stem cell harvests and assessment of body fluids. Methods for detection of CTCs include immunohistochemistry, reverse transcription-PCR, antibody capture and size-based selection.

Cell-free Circulating DNA

Circulating tumor nucleic acids have multiple origins. They can present as cell-free nucleic acids (cfNA) or be extracted from intact CTCs. Three main categories of cfNA are being utilized in patients with cancer: DNA (cell-free DNA [cfDNA], mRNA (cell-free mRNA[cfmRNA]), and microRNA (cell-free microRNA[cfmiRNA]). Cell-free circulating DNA (cfDNA) in the blood of humans was discovered in 1948. Recently, this critical discovery has been utilized. It was observed that analysis of circulating tumor DNA can provide the same genetic information obtained from tumor tissue. It was found that the levels of cfDNA are usually higher in cancer patients than healthy individuals. Thus, it is possible to screen for the presence of disease through a simple blood test for cfDNA). The tumor-derived cfDNA has been shown to correlate with tumor burden, which changes in response to treatment or surgery.

Challenges faced: Though cfDNA has several benefits, it has certain challenges. These include

- Necessary to discriminate DNA released from tumor cells (ctDNA) from circulating normal DNA. The difference is that tumor DNA is associated with mutations. These somatic mutations (commonly single base pair substitutions), are present only in the genomes of cancer cells or precancerous cells and are not present in the DNA of normal cells of the same patient. This specificity helps using ctDNA as a biomarker.
- The cfDNA derived from tumor cells constitute only a very small fraction (<1%) of the total cfDNA. This limits the applicability of the cfDNA.

***Detection cfDNA*: The detection of tumor-specific genetic alterations in patients' blood is often called as liquid biopsies.** Various method used are:

- By use of next-generation sequencing and digital PCR techniques, it possible to define rare mutant variants in complex mixtures of DNA. By these techniques it is possible to detect point mutations, rearrangements, and gene copy number changes in individual genes in small quantities (few millilitres) of plasma.
- Whole-exome analyses can also be performed using circulating DNA extracted from the blood of cancer patients.

Applications: Detection of tumor-specific genetic alterations (liquid biopsies) has several applications in oncology.

- *To genotype tumors*: Analyses of cfDNA can be used to genotype tumors when there is no availability of tissue sample or is difficult to obtain tissue sample. Circulating tumor DNA fragments contain the identical genetic defects as that of tumor. Thus blood can reveal point mutations (EGFR, KRAS, BRAF, PIK3CA), rearrangements (e.g., EML4-ALK), and gene amplifications (MET) in tumors.
- *Monitor tumor burden*: Liquid biopsies are useful in monitoring tumor burden. This is very useful in the management of patients with cancer assessed with imaging. The ctDNA can be used as a surrogate for tumor burden like viral load (e.g., HIV viral load).
- *To monitor the genomic drift*: Liquid biopsies can also be used to monitor the genomic drift (clonal evolution) that occurs in tumors on treatment. Thus, analysis of ctDNA in plasma samples obtained pretreatment, during, and post treatment can be used for understanding of the mechanisms of primary and, especially, those tumors which acquired resistance to therapies.

Clinical Applications of Liquid Biopsies

- *Diagnosis*: ctDNA can be used to detect the presence of cancer and circulating viral DNA can be used to identify virus related cancers. After diagnosis, ctDNA allows patients' stratification and can help guiding therapeutic intervention. If early diagnosis is made in cancer patients, survival rates are 5–10 times higher compared with late-stage disease. However, there is no circulating biomarkers available at present for early detection of cancer. It is necessary to develop a method capable of identifying cancer beyond the limit of detection by radiologic imaging. ctDNA analyses is useful for disease monitoring in patients with metastatic disease but it is not effectiveness to identify cancers at early stage.
- *Screening*: Useful for identification of predictive biomarkers for early detection of cancer
- *Monitor response*: During therapy, ctDNA can be used to monitor therapeutic response and resistance to therapy.
- *Additional targets*: When a tumor progresses, ctDNA analysis can be used to know the tumor molecular heterogeneity and their targets for further guide effective therapeutic interventions.
- *Immunotherapy*: ctDNA analysis can be used to monitor microsatellite instability (MSI) status and tumor mutational loads. These are useful parameters for immunotherapy. The peripheral blood mononuclear cells can be used to profile T-cell receptors (TCRs). Liquid biopsies can be used to monitor cancer patients receiving immunotherapies based on checkpoint blockade with anti-PD-1 and anticytotoxic T-lymphocyte antigen-4 (anti-CTLA-4) antibodies (refer page 499). It was found that immune checkpoint inhibitors were significantly effective against tumors containing increased mutation load (tumor mutational burden).
- *Detection of minimal residual disease*: Liquid biopsies based on ctDNA can be used to detect minimal residual disease the following surgery or therapy. Minimal residual disease (measurable minimal disease) is a marker for prognosis and risk of relapse.

Cell Proliferation Markers

Q. Write short essay on cell proliferation markers.

Assessment of cell proliferation (proliferation index) is an important biological marker useful for predicting tumor behavior, likelihood of recurrence and malignant potential.

Methods: There are different cell proliferative markers. One of the oldest and most reliable method of assessing cell proliferation activity is counting of mitosis. The other methods include (i) DNA flow cytometry (FCM) to assess the S phase, (ii) bromodeoxy- uridine incorporation techniques, (iii) immunocytochemistry of various cell proliferation-related antigens, (iv) nucleolar organizer regions (NORs) counting, etc. Comparison of these techniques is presented in **Table 46**.

Mitotic Index

Mitosis is seen as dark clumps of chromosomes having extension in a basophilic cytoplasm on light microscope (see Fig. 13A), and it can be measured easily. Mitosis count is more predictable and reliable on histology section than on cytology smear.

Expression of mitotic figures: Number of mitosis in tumor is usually counted and expressed as number of mitotic figures per ten high power fields (/10HPF) or /HPF. Since it is highly subjective, there is no reproducibility and the field of vision may vary from microscope to microscope.

Mitotic index: To overcome the disadvantage of expressing mitotic figures/10HPF, it can be expressed number of mitotic figures per 1,000 cells. This is termed mitotic index.

Morphological features of ideal mitotic figures are presented in **Box 22**.

Advantage

Easy and reasonably reliable.

Disadvantages

- *Time of fixation*: Mitotic activity depends on the time of fixation of the tissue and tissues should be fixed immediately after excision. If the tissue fixation is delayed, the cell may complete its mitosis and the mitotic count may be lower.
- *Simulators of mitosis*: Many structures may simulate mitotic figures. These include apoptotic cell, mast cells, degenerated lymphocytes, etc. Hence, mitotic count should be carefully performed.

Table 46: Different methods to assess cell proliferation.

Technique	*Principle*	*Component of cell cycle detected*	*Advantages*	*Disadvantages*
Mitotic count: Mitotic figures are counted on light microscopy	Counting and estimation of mitotic figures on light microscopy	Cells in M phase of cell cycle	• Easy • Reproducible • Can be performed on archived material and routine sections or smear	• Mitotic count may vary depending on tissue fixation • Mitotic score may show subjective variation • Apoptotic body and mast cells may simulate mitotic figures
DNA precursor base incorporation	Labeled nucleotide analogs is picked up by proliferating cells in S phase. These can be stained by immunohistochemistry	Measures S phase of cell cycle	Gold standard because it is very accurate and reliable	Not useful for routine clinical use
DNA flow cytometry	DNA stochiometric dye stains DNA of single cells. relative DNA. These cells run through flow cytometer. Different fractions of cells in various stages can be calculated	Measure G_0/G_1, S and G_2/M phase cells separately. Results are expressed as percentage of cells in 5 phases	• Rapid method • Can analyse large number of cells • Reproducible	• Sophisticated technique • Target cells cannot be visualized • Expensive
Image cytometry	DNA stochiometric dye stains DNA and relative DNA content is measured on section or smear	Measure G_0/G_1, S and G_2/M phase cells separately	Target cells can be visualized by light microscopy and manual selection can be done	Slow technique Resolution of the Histogram is low
Immunohistochemistry (IHC) for proliferation associated antigens				
Proliferating cell nuclear antigen (PCNA)	PCNA is found in the nuclei of cells that undergo cell division	Progressive increase of PCNA in advanced G_1 and S phase cells	Immunostaining and can be done in paraffin embedded tissue	Not reliable as it is overexpressed even during DNA repair
Ki67 scoring	Ki67 antigen is expressed in proliferating cells	G_1, S and G_2 phase of cell cycle	• Easy method • Reproducible • Short half-life of the antigen and is very accurate with increased sensitivity • Correlates well with other markers	Strict scoring criteria is needed
Minichromosome maintenance proteins (MCM)	Initiating protein complex of DNA and initiates DNA replication	Proliferating cells	• Easy method • Reliable marker because the protein is stable throughout the cell proliferation • Better marker than Ki67	No major disadvantages
Nucleolar organizing regions (AgNOR)	NOR-related-associated proteins are argyrophilic. They can be stained with silver. AgNOR is closely related with cell proliferation	All proliferating cells	• Easy method • Can be performed on archival tissue	• Counting is subjective • Difficult to adopt for routine use

Box 22: Morphological features of ideal mitotic figures.

- Absence of nuclear membrane
- No clear zone in the center
- Shows hairy extension from the side
- Surrounding cytoplasm is basophilic instead of eosinophilia

DNA Precursor Base Incorporation Technique

In this technique, labeled nucleotide analogs (compound with a molecular structure closely similar to nucleotide) is used. Commonly used nucleotide analogs are tritiated thymidine or bromodeoxyuridine The proliferating cells (cells in S phase) incorporate the labeled nucleotide analogue during DNA synthesis of cell cycle. This can be demonstrated by autoradiography in case of radioactive thymidine and immunohistochemistry in case of bromodeoxyuridine. IHC is risky due to radioactive substrates used.

Disadvantages

Clinicalutilityofincorporationtechniquesislimited.Radioactive thymidine is radioactive hazards. Hence, radioactive thymidine is not used. Presently, bromodeoxyuridine is used and can be demonstrate by immunohistochemistry.

DNA Flow Cytometry and Image Cytometry

Normally, most cells are in a resting, or nonproliferating, phase of the cell cycle. During G_0/G_1 phase of cell cycle, the cells are diploid (2n i.e., they have two copies of each chromosome) and contain diploid amount (2n) of DNA. Cells duplicate their DNA during what is called S-phase and have four copies (tetraploid [4N]) of each chromosome. S phase cells contain diploid to tetraploid amount of DNA (2n–4n). Normal DNA flow cytometry and image cytometry (FCM) results will show that most of the cells are resting phase and contain only two copies of each chromosome. Only less than 10% of the cells will be in S-phase.

Principle: In both DNA FCM and image cytometry (ICM), a stoichiometric (meaning relating to or denoting quantities of reactants in simple integral ratios) dye is used. This dye binds with DNA of the nucleus of a cell depending on DNA amount. The amount of staining is measured, which indicates relative DNA content of the DNA in a nucleus.

DNA flow cytometry

It is a method of measuring the amount of deoxyribonucleic acid (DNA) in tumor cells and the percentage of cells actively replicating. It is performed on tissue and the cells from the solid tissue are separated from each other. These cells are mixed with a dye called propidium iodide that binds to DNA. This dye emits fluorescent light as the cells pass through the laser beam of the cytometer. The cytometer can also measure the size of cells. By analyzing the amount of fluorescence emitted by the cell's DNA content can be evaluated (termed as DNA index or ploidy analysis). It also helps identification of the population of cells in G_0/G_1, S phase and G_2/M phase of cell cycle. This helps in determining whether the cancer cells are dividing or not. This is called as S-phase analysis.

Interpretation

- DNA flow cytometry results are usually presented in graphical form (histogram). A normal histogram will show one large peak of resting cells, followed by a flat area and another smaller peak of cells about to divide.
- Abnormal results: Abnormal results will show as several peaks of differing sizes. An abnormal result does not always indicate malignancy. Hence, DNA flow cytometry results must be interpreted along with other tests to diagnose malignancy.

Image cytometry

It also provides a histogram and can help to assess the different population of cells in a cell cycle.

Advantages

DNA flow cytometry can rapidly analyze large population of cells. Hence, it provides better resolution of the histogram and reliable result.

Disadvantages

- Lack of specificity: It gives the result of all cells including, tumor cells, vascular endothelial cells and stromal cells. This is not specific only to tumor cells.
- More sophisticated and expensive technique.

Immunohistochemistry for Proliferation Associated Antigens

There are different antigens that measure cell proliferation.

Proliferating cell nuclear antigen

Proliferating cell nuclear antigen (PCNA) was popular cell proliferation marker.

Principle: PCNA is found in the nuclei of cells that undergo cell division. PCNA is related with the initiation of DNA replication and cell proliferation. The concentration of PCNA within the cell is transcriptionally regulated. Its concentration increases from resting cell to proliferating cell. There is a progressive increase of PCNA in advanced G_1 and S phase cells. This is followed by decreased level of PCNA in G_2 and M phase of cells. PCNA has a prolonged half-life and therefore it can be demonstrated even the cells enter into the G_0 phase. Three important functions of PCNA are listed in **Box 23.**

Advantage

Proliferation cell nuclear antigen immunostaining and can be done in paraffin embedded tissue.

Box 23: Important functions of proliferating cell nuclear antigen (PCNA).

- *Replication of DNA*: Coordinates the synthesis of leading and lagging strand of DNA. Recruits DNA replicating enzymes
- *Repair of DNA*: Helps to repair DNA through nucleotide excision repair (NER) and mismatch repair (MMR) process
- *Control of cell cycle*: PCNA binds with S phase specific cyclin-CDK complex and promotes cell proliferation

Disadvantages

- Poor correlation between PCNA score and Ki67 labeling index.
- PCNA is not specific to cell proliferation. It is also involved in DNA repair. Hence, PCNA is not advisable to use as a cell proliferation marker in cytology/histology.

Ki67

The name Ki67 is derived from Kiel University, Germany, and the number 67 refers to the clone number on the 96-well plate. Ki67 antigen is the most potent antigen only expressed by proliferating/dividing cells (cells in G_1, S and G_2 phase of the cell cycle. Ki67 is absent (not expressed) in resting cells (G_0 and early G_1 phase). It is widely used in routine pathological investigation as a proliferation marker. The gene of Ki67 antigen is located in chromosome 10 and its product is nuclear protein Ki67 (pKi67). The exact function of Ki67 is still unknown. Probably, it helps in ribosomal RNA (rRNA) synthesis and also maintenance of the mitotic spindle. Originally Ki67 immunostaining was only possible in frozen sections. Presently, other Ki67 monoclonal antibody (Ki67/MIB-1) is used on formalin fixed paraffin section. This gives results that are reproducible and reliable. Percentage of nuclei with positive staining in tumor cells are scored <10% (low), 10–20% (borderline) and >20% (high).

Advantages

- Gold standard: Evaluation of expression of Ki67 by immunostaining is considered as the best proliferation markers for routine use.
- Prognostic marker: It is also an important prognostic marker of many malignant tumors. Ki67 cutoff level above 10–14% indicates high-risk group in term of prognosis.

Disadvantage

Scoring systems for Ki67 are based on the percentage of tumor cells stained by an antibody. Proper Ki67 scoring (percentage of Ki67 Positive cell) is important for exact evaluation of cell proliferation.

Minichromosome maintenance proteins 2–7 (MCM2–7)

Minichromosome maintenance proteins are group of proteins that are involved in maintenance of minichromosome. MCM proteins are essential in the initiation of DNA replication and elongation of replication. MCM 2–7 family consists of total six proteins namely MCM 2–7. They combine with each other and make a heterohexameric structure. MCM proteins form complex with ORC, Cdt1 and Cdc6 and this complex initiates DNA replication.

Advantages

- Reliable marker: MCM 2–7 proteins are the reliable markers of proliferating cells. This is because the quiescent cells do not express MCM 2–7.
- Prognostic marker: MCM is a good prognostic marker. It correlates well with histological grade and lymph node metastasis of cancer.

Nucleolar organizing regions

Nucleolus also plays a role in proliferation because of nucleolar organizing regions (NORs). NORs are the segments of DNA closely associated with nucleoli. They are present on the short arm of acrocentric chromosomes 13, 14, 15, 21 and 22. NOR encode genes for r-RNA (ribosomal RNA) and various protein involved in the synthesis required for cell proliferation. The transcriptionally active NORs have argyrophilic proteins. Hence, they can be demonstrated by using silver (Ag) staining technique. So the term AgNOR has been developed. AgNOR assessment is closely related with rate of cell proliferation.

Advantages

Easy technique to assess cell proliferation.

Disadvantages

- Noncycling cell may also produce protein and may show AgNORs. Hence, it is necessary to measure baseline AgNOR score.
- AgNORs scoring may vary depending on thickness of the tissue section.

MICROVASCULAR DENSITY

Q. Write short essay on microvascular density in neoplasia.

Angiogenesis is one of hallmark of malignant tumor and is an essential step for local tumor growth and distant metastasis formation. The quantity of angiogenesis can be measured by microvascular density (MVD). Microvascular density is the concentration of small blood vessels in a malignant tumor.

Evaluation of Microvascular Density

In 1972, Brem reported the first quantitative method for histological grading of tumor angiogenesis. He correlated neovascularization with tumor grade in brain tumors. In the early 1990s, Weidner and co-workers developed a new method for measurement of MVD within isolated regions of high vessel concentration. They showed that MVD was a prognostic indicator for human breast and prostate carcinomas.

Standard method for quantifying tumor angiogenesis is to assess MVD based on immunohistochemistry (IHC) by light microscopy. This requires the use of specific markers to vascular endothelium and immunohistochemical procedures to visualize microvessels. Commonly used markers are CD31, CD34 and, antifactor VIII-related antigen. Variation in the estimation of MVD may be due to use of different pan endothelial cell markers. Antifactor VIII-related antigen is the most specific endothelial marker.

- First examine the whole tumor section at low magnification (40×). Identify the area with the highest density of vessels (hot spots).
- Next, count the individual microvessel at a high magnification (200×) in an adequate area. Count CD31-positive or CD34-positive vessels in three or five hot spots, respectively. Only continuous, membranous staining should be considered as positive.
- Give a count of one for any large microvessel with a lumen or any single, separated endothelial cell.
- The vessels should be counted within the epithelium and at the epithelium/stroma edge.
- Each single count is expressed as the highest number of microvessels identified at the hot spot.

Chalkley counting procedure: This is another method of counting microvascular density.

- Three most vascular areas (hot spots) with the highest number of microvessel profiles were chosen from tumor section.
- A 25-point Chalkley eyepiece graticule (a network of lines representing meridians and parallels) was applied to each hot-spot area. It is oriented in such a way that the maximum number of points to hit on, or within the areas of immunohistochemically highlighted microvessel profiles.
- The Chalkley count for a tumor was taken as the mean value of the three graticule counts.
- This technique is a simple and acceptable procedure for daily clinical use.

It was observed that in invasive breast carcinomas there was significant correlation between high Chalkley counts and axillary lymph node metastasis, large tumor size, and high histological grade.

Prognostic Significance of Tumor Vascularity

Microvascular density reflects the amount of angiogenesis within the primary tumor and correlates with the ability of tumor to grow and spread. Hence, counting of MVD is the morphological gold standard to assess the neovasculature in some human tumors. It is most predictive in tumors that induce significant angiogenesis such as carcinomas of breast, prostate and hematological malignancies.

LYMPHANGIOGENESIS

Q. Describe the process of lymphangiogenesis. Enumerate immuno/IHC markers of lymph-angiogenesis

Definition: The process of forming new lymphatic vessels (growth of new lymphatic vessels) from preexisting lymphatic vessels is termed as lymphangiogenesis. It is similar to angiogenesis (blood vessel development).

Role of Lymphatic Vessels

Lymphatic vasculature: It begins as thin-walled lymphatic capillaries that start blind ended in the peripheral tissues. These lymphatics have structure that is favorable for the absorption or uptake of fluids, proteins, and cells.

Structure of lymphatics: Lymphatic capillaries are lined by a continuous single-cell layer of endothelial cells having a discontinuous basement membrane. In contrast to blood vessels, they are not encircled by pericytes or smooth muscle cells. Usually, there is tight and adherens junctions between lymphatic endothelial cells and the majority of interendothelial cell interactions are maintained by "button-like" junctions. These overlapping junctions are responsible for the high permeability of peripheral lymphatic capillaries to interstitial fluids and proteins and it also helps for transmigration of immune cells. The structure of the lymphatic vasculature facilitates both the absorption of tissue fluids and trafficking of immune cells.

Lymphatic circulation: The lymphatic vascular network is a unidirectional transport system. In contrast to the blood vascular (circulatory) system, it does not have a central pump (heart is a central pump in case of blood circulation). Hence, the transport of lymph depends on skeletal muscle contraction and respiratory movement.

Lymphatic capillaries are connected to surrounding tissue by anchoring filaments. These filaments extend from the lymphatic deep into the adjoining tissue and firmly attach lymphatic endothelial cells to extracellular matrix fibers. Usually, lymphatic capillaries are closed. When the tissue pressure increases, the anchoring fibers open the lymphatic capillaries and allow the entry of protein-rich lymph fluid and immune cells into the lymphatic vascular system. Lymph that has entered the peripheral lymphatic capillaries initially drains to precollecting lymphatic vessels. Then the lymph flows into larger lymphatic vessels. These larger lymphatic vessels are surrounded by a basement membrane and lymph flow-promoting smooth muscle cells. These also have one-way valves that prevent retrograde lymph flow. All lymph from the collecting lymphatic vessels passes through several sequential lymph nodes and enter into the thoracic duct. From thoracic duct lymph enters the venous circulation at the junction of the jugular and subclavian veins.

Functions of lymphatics: Main function of lymphatics in normal physiology are:

- To regulate tissue fluid homeostasis: Lymphatics drain fluid from the interstices between cells and empty this fluid into the venous circulation.
- Immune cell trafficking in immunity: Lymphatics collect antigens and other macromolecules from various peripheral tissues, and transport immune cells (e.g., antigen-presenting dendritic cells) of the immune system from the periphery to lymph nodes. In the lymph nodes immune responses are initiated.
- Metabolism such as absorption of dietary fats.

The absence of lymphatic vessels is incompatible with life. Individuals with dysfunctional lymphatic vessels usually suffer from chronic edema and impaired immune responses.

Role of Lymphangiogenesis

Molecular mechanisms of angiogenesis (refer pages 474–477) has received considerable attention and the antiangiogenic therapeutic agents are being used in clinical practice. However, the molecular mechanisms regulating lymphangiogenesis were less studied. Over the past few years, progress has been achieved in the identification of regulatory molecules and markers specific to the lymphatic endothelium. Lymphangiogenesis plays an important role both in physiological and pathological processes.

- Physiological role: It was observed that the lymph ducts are assembled from endothelial cells originating in the same embryonic stem cell population that yields the endothelial cells of capillaries and larger blood vessels. During embryogenesis, the process of formation of a lymphatic vascular system is a dynamic process. The blood circulatory system is the first to evolve in embryos. This is followed by differentiation of blood vascular endothelial into lymphatic endothelial progenitor cells and they form cardinal vein. During embryonic development, lymphatic vessels often bud from developing capillaries before they separate and construct their own parallel network of interconnecting vessels. During embryogenesis the development of lymphatic system is controlled by the sequential activation of transcription factors. These include prosper-related homeodomain transcription factor (PROX1), Sox18 and COUP-TFII. Under normal physiological postnatal conditions, however, lymphangiogenesis (the formation of new lymphatic vessels) rarely.

- Pathological process: Lymphangiogenesis in adults, only occurs during certain pathological conditions such as inflammation, tissue repair, and tumor growth/ dissemination. Probably, postnatal lymphatic vessel formations occur mainly by hyperplasia of lymphatic vessels themselves, or sprouting from pre-existing lymphatics. Under pathological conditions, lymphangiogenesis occurs by the proliferation and sprouting of new vessels from preexisting lymphatic vessels.

Following discussion is restricted to lymphangiogenesis in cancer.

Lymphangiogenesis in Cancer

Metastatic to distant organs is the leading cause of mortality from cancer. Metastasis can occur by both the blood (circulatory) and lymphatic vascular systems, but the most common pathway of initial metastasis is through the lymphatic system. Tumor cells penetrate more easily into lymphatic capillaries than blood capillaries and the factors favouring this are listed in **Box 24**. The detection of tumor metastases in the tumor-draining lymph node (LN) is the first step in tumor dissemination. Lymph node status in cancer is one of the most important prognostic marker and therapeutic strategy decisions. Invasive tumor cells take the advantage of the loose, overlapping endothelial cell junctions and incomplete basement membrane of lymphatic capillaries to transport and survival of cancer cells.

Lymphatic vascular system plays a major role in cancer metastasis. Historically, lymphatic vessels were believed to be passive participants in tumor metastasis by simply allowing the passage of tumor cells through it. However, the discovery of several key lymphatic-specific molecular markers have highlighted the active role of the lymphatic vasculature in metastatic tumor spread. Induction of tumor lymphangiogenesis in the tumor enhances the metastatic spread of cancer cells to lymph nodes. This suggests that the therapeutic manipulation of lymphangiogenesis may be potentially beneficial.

Lymphangiogenesis occurs in the tumor as well as lymph nodes. The sentinel lymph node is the first node receiving lymph from the primary tumor, potentially containing metastatic cells. The sentinel lymph node shows active lymphangiogenesis.

Box 24: Factors that favor lymphatic spread of malignant tumors.

- Absence of a basal membrane in peritumoral lymphatic capillaries
- Structural changes developing in lymphatic vessels during lymphangiogenesis
- Facilitates the entry of tumor cells into lymphatic vessels and their migration ability by chemotaxis
- Lymphatic endothelial cells play a immunomodulatory role which may facilitate the survival of tumor cells

Molecular Mechanism of Tumor Lymphangiogenesis

Under pathological conditions, lymphangiogenesis occurs by the proliferation and sprouting of new vessels from pre-existing lymphatic vessels. The relative contribution from circulating endothelial progenitor cells to the formation of new lymphatic vessels not clearly understood. Recently identified lymphatic endothelial specific markers, such as hyaluronic acid receptor-1 (LYVE-1) and podoplanin, has helped to understand the mechanism of growth of lymphatic vessels (lymphangiogenesis) in the tumor microenvironment. Bone marrow-derived lymphatic progenitor cells as well as growth factors involved in lymphatic endothelial cell growth and migration may be involved in tumor lymphangiogenesis.

Lymphangiogenic factors: Several lymphatic-specific molecular markers and factors that promote lymphatic vessel growth have helped to understand the lymphatic vasculature in both physiological and pathological situations.

- *Vascular endothelial growth factor (VEGF)*: VEGF-C and –D (VEGF-C and VEGF-D) are prolymphangiogenic factors. These two are homologous to VEGF-A and -B, which play a major role in angiogenesis that creates the blood vasculature. VEGF-C and –D that bind to a tyrosine kinase receptor, VEGF receptor -3 (VEGF-R3) expressed on the lymphatic endothelial cells. Downstream of these receptor tyrosine kinases, protein kinases Akt and ERK1/ ERK2 are activated. VEGF-R3 is structurally related to the dominant VEGF receptor of blood capillaries namely VEGF-R2. VEGF-C is needed for lymphatic development during embryogenesis. VEGF-D not only stimulate lymphangiogenesis but also may stimulate angiogenesis by binding and activating VEGF-R2. Thus, both the blood and lymphatic networks seems to be derived from common evolutionary roots and develop from common precursors in the embryo. They continue to interact with one another in complex ways within adult tissues also.
- *Neuropilin receptor-2 (NRP2)*: It was originally identified in nervous system development, and acts as a coreceptor for VEGF-A, -C, and -D. It is normally expressed in lymphatic vessels during embryogenesis. Neuropilin receptors (NRPs) may function independently of VEGF receptors and act as modulators of endothelial cell migration. Neuropilin receptor-2 may be expressed in tumor-associated lymphatic vessels and indicates its involvement in tumoral lymphangiogenesis and metastasis. Blocking of neuropilin-2 using a neutralizing antibody reduced tumoral lymphangiogenesis, delayed metastasis to sentinel lymph nodes. It blocks the migration of lymphatic endothelial cell but not proliferation. It was observed that the expression of neuropilin-2 is localized on tumor-associated but not on normal preformed lymphatic vessels. Thus, this receptor may be an alternative target to prevent lymph node metastasis via the lymphatic vessels.
- *Other factors with prolymphangiogenic activity*: These include hepatocyte growth factor (binds to the c-met receptor), angiopoietin-1 and its endothelial cell–specific receptor Tie-2, fibroblast growth factor-1 and -2, platelet-derived growth factors, insulin-like growth factor-1 and -2, adrenomedullin, and endothelin-1.

Antilymphangiogenic factors: Transforming growth factor-β1 acts as a negative regulator of lymphangiogenesis.

Tumor lymphangiogenesis (Fig. 106)

Tumor-induced lymphangiogenesis is mediated by lymphangiogenic growth factors. These growth factors can be produced and secreted by the tumor cells themselves, stromal cells, tumor-infiltrating macrophages, or activated platelets. Important are VEGF-C and VEGF-D. Overexpression of either VEGF-C or VEGF-D in tumors significantly increases tumor-associated lymphatic vessel growth (mainly at the tumor margin). This is also associated with increased incidence of lymph node metastasis. It was observed that blockade of signaling via VEGFR-3 reduces the tumor lymphangiogenesis and lymphatic metastasis. VEGF-A also may be involved in tumor-mediated lymphangiogenesis and metastasis.

Apart from increasing lymphatic vessel density, lymphangiogenic growth factors also increase the size, enlarge and dilate the lymphatic vessel. VEGFR-2 activation is involved in vessel enlargement, whereas activation of VEGFR-3 is involved in lymphangiogenic sprouting. Enlarged lymphatic vessels that drain the tumor enhance the delivery of tumor cells to the lymph node. This is probably by increasing lymphatic flow rates and facilitation of metastatic tumor cell cluster dissemination.

Lymphangiogenesis and tumor progression

It is necessary to distinguish tumor lymphangiogenesis from angiogenesis. This needs specific molecular markers to discriminate between blood and lymphatic vessels. The role of lymphangiogenic factors in human cancer metastasis was studied mainly through immunohistochemical analysis of tumor tissue samples and retrospective comparison to patient outcomes. Several proteins have been identified which are expressed in lymphatic endothelial cells. These include D2-40 (podoplanin), CD 31, hyaluronic acid receptor-1 (LYVE-1), PROX1, NRP2 and VEGFR3. It was observed that increased lymphatic vessel invasion significantly increases the risk of lymph node metastasis, distant metastasis, and death. Majority of clinical studies have found a correlative relationship between the expression of lymphangiogenic factors and overall poor patient prognosis.

- *Breast cancer*: Lymphatic vessel invasion (LVI) was positively correlated with metastasis to sentinel nodes. This was specifically related to the presence of peritumoral LVI and was considered as a main prognostic indicator for the survival outcomes of patients with breast cancer. Increased lymphatic expression of VEGFR-3 in breast cancer also correlated with increased metastasis-containing lymph nodes and reduced patient disease-free and overall survival.
- *Other cancers*: Many diverse tumors show elevated expression of VEGF-C and/or VEGF-D. Their expression has been correlated with lymphatic vessel density (LVD), lymphatic metastasis, and disease outcome.

Uses of immunomarkers for lymphatics

Presence of tumor emboli in lymphatics (lymphatic vascular invasion [LVI]) or blood vessels (blood vascular invasion [BVI]) is a positive predictor of the occurrence of lymph node metastasis. The assessment of vascular or lymphatic invasion is usually carried out by routine hematoxylin and eosin staining (H&E). This may give rise to both false-positive and false-negative results. Hence, IHC identification may be more accurate method for identifying lymphatic vascular invasion (LVI). Immunomarkers for lymphatics is presented in **Box 25**.

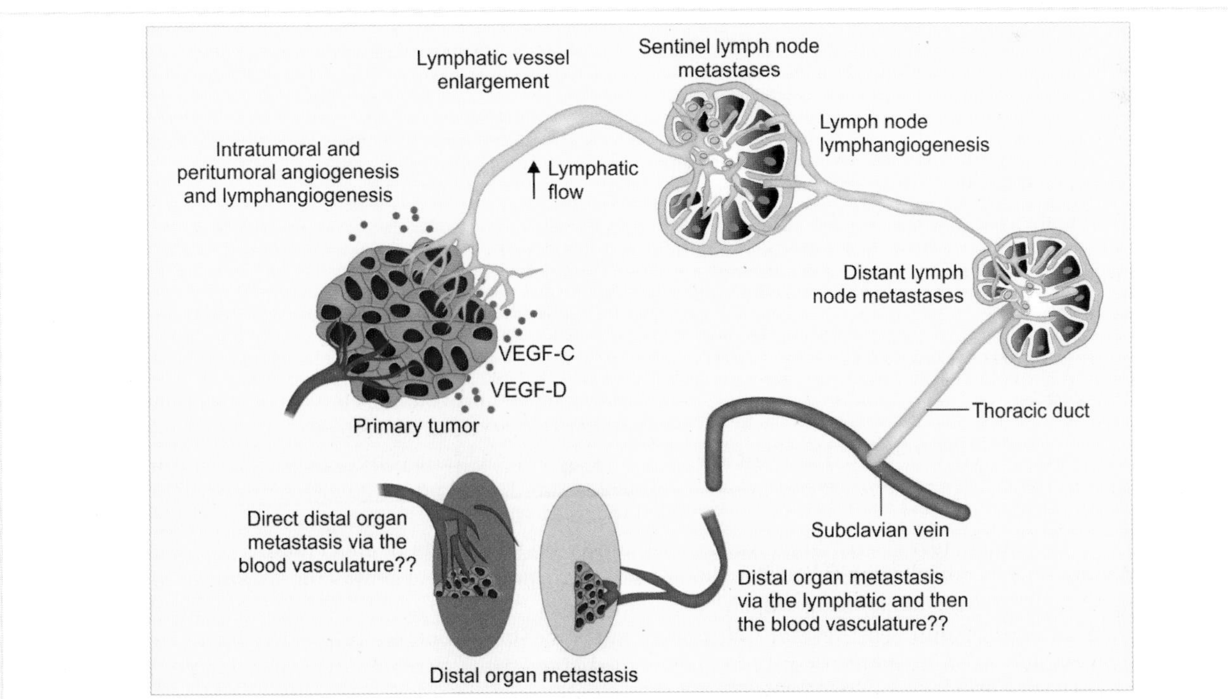

FIG. 106: Tumor-induced lymphangiogenesis. Lymphangiogenic growth factors such as VEGF-C and VEGF-D induce tumoral lymphangiogenesis mainly at the margin of the tumor and also within the tumor-draining lymph node prior to metastatic tumor dissemination. This is further enhanced upon arrival of metastatic cells. VEGF-induced lymphangiogenesis and the associated increase in lymphatic flow enhance metastatic spread to the lymph nodes and also to distal organs, probably via the thoracic duct. It is not clear whether metastatic cells can enter the blood circulation within metastatic lymph nodes.

Box 25: Immunomarkers for lymphatics.

Specific for lymphatics

- D2-40 (Podoplanin): Podoplanin is a mucin-type transmembrane glycoprotein expressed in lymphatic endothelial cells and is needed for development of lymphatics. This glycoprotein is not expressed in blood vessels, hence, is a useful marker of lymphatics
- CD 31 (also known as platelet endothelial cell adhesion molecule [PECAM1])
- LYVE-1 (lymphatic vessel hyaluronic acid receptor-1): It is a CD44 homolog is involved in hyaluronic acid transport and is expressed in embryonic and adult lymphatic endothelial cells
- Neuropilin receptor-2 (NRP2)

Endothelial cells of both blood vessels and lymphatics

- Vascular endothelial growth factor receptor -3 (VEGFR3): This receptor is mainly expressed on lymphatic endothelial cells. However, it can also be expressed on some fenestrated blood vessels and on some blood endothelial cells during tumor angiogenesis. Therefore, it is not an adequate marker to study tumor lymphangiogenesis
- Prospero-related homeobox (PROX1)

Determination of lymphatic vessel density

Sections are stained by immunohistochemical markers (e.g., D2-40, CD31).

- *Low power*: Stained slides are scanned under low power (10x).
  - Select six fields with the highest number of stained lymphatic vessels. They are considered as 'hotspots' areas having the greatest number of highlighted lymphatic vessels.
  - Lymphatic vessel density is counted in the intratumoral and peritumoral (within an area of 1mm from the invasion front) region. LVD is counted as the number of stained vessels per optical field and the number of D2-40.
- *High power*: Positive lymphatic vessels in each hotspot are calculated at a higher magnification (40x). The average of them is given as total LVD.
- Patients with tumors showing high peritumoral LVD and lymph node metastasis have a poor prognosis.

ROSSETTE AND PSEUDOROSETTE FORMING TUMORS

Q. Write short essay on rosette and pseudorosette forming tumors.

In pathology, a rosette (arrangement resembling a rose) is round arrangement of cells forming a central halo (a cellular lumen) or arrangement in a spoke circle (spoke-and-wheel) surrounding a central core or hub. The central hub may either consist of an empty-appearing lumen or a space filled with cytoplasmic processes. Rosettes are so named for their similarity to the rose casement (belt) found in gothic cathedrals (religious buildings in Europe). Most of rosettes are found in tumors of the nervous system in neoplasms of neuroblastic or neuroectodermal origin. Their detection helps in diagnosis of different tumors.

Table 47: Various types of rosettes and their associated tumors.

Type of rosette	*Associated tumors*
True Rosette	
• True ependymal rosette (tumor cells form gland like round or elongated structures that resemble the embryologic ependymal canal)	• Well differentiated ependymoma (minority of cases) • Ependymoblastoma (rare form of PNET)
• Flexner-Wintersteiner rosettes/ true neural rosettes (radial arrangements of a single layer of tumor cells around an apparent central cavity/lumen)	• Retinoblastoma • Pineoblastoma • Medulloepithelioma
Pseudo-Rosette	
• Homer Wright (neuroblastic) rosettes with central neuropil (meshwork of fibers)	• Medulloblastoma • Neuroblastoma • Pineoblastoma • Retinoblastoma • Supratentorial PNETs • Ewing's sarcoma
• Neurocytic rosette (irregular large lumen with neuropil [similar to Homer- Wright rosette])	Central neurocytoma
• Perivascular pseudorosettes (cuffs of radiating tumor cell, the cytoplasmic processes of which form nuclear-free zone composed of fibrillary processes that radiate toward a central blood vessel)	• Medulloblastoma • Ependymoma • Primitive neuroectodermal tumors (PNETs) • Central neurocytoma • Pilomyxoid astrocytoma • Glioblastoma

Various types of rosettes and their associated tumors are presented in **Table 47** and **Figure 107**.

TARGETED THERAPY IN CANCER

Q. Write short essay on targeted therapy in cancer.

Conventional therapies not only attack the cancer cell but also damage normal cells. One of the most important goals of modern cancer treatment is to develop more effective therapies that specifically target the cancer cell while sparing normal cells from the attendant damage. Targeted therapy is a type of cancer treatment, in which drugs are designed to "target" cancer cells that will not affect normal cells. Targets for these drugs are proteins that control the growth, division and spread of cancer cells. Targeted therapy **is personalized therapy** and is the foundation of precision medicine. In personalized medicine, specific treatments and therapies best suited to an individual's genotype are selected. It is safer and more effective therapy. Cancer therapy is no longer a "one size fits all" approach. Presently, the treatment of cancer is based on an understanding of underlying biologic mechanisms. Therapy is increasingly being tailored to the molecular specificity of a tumor.

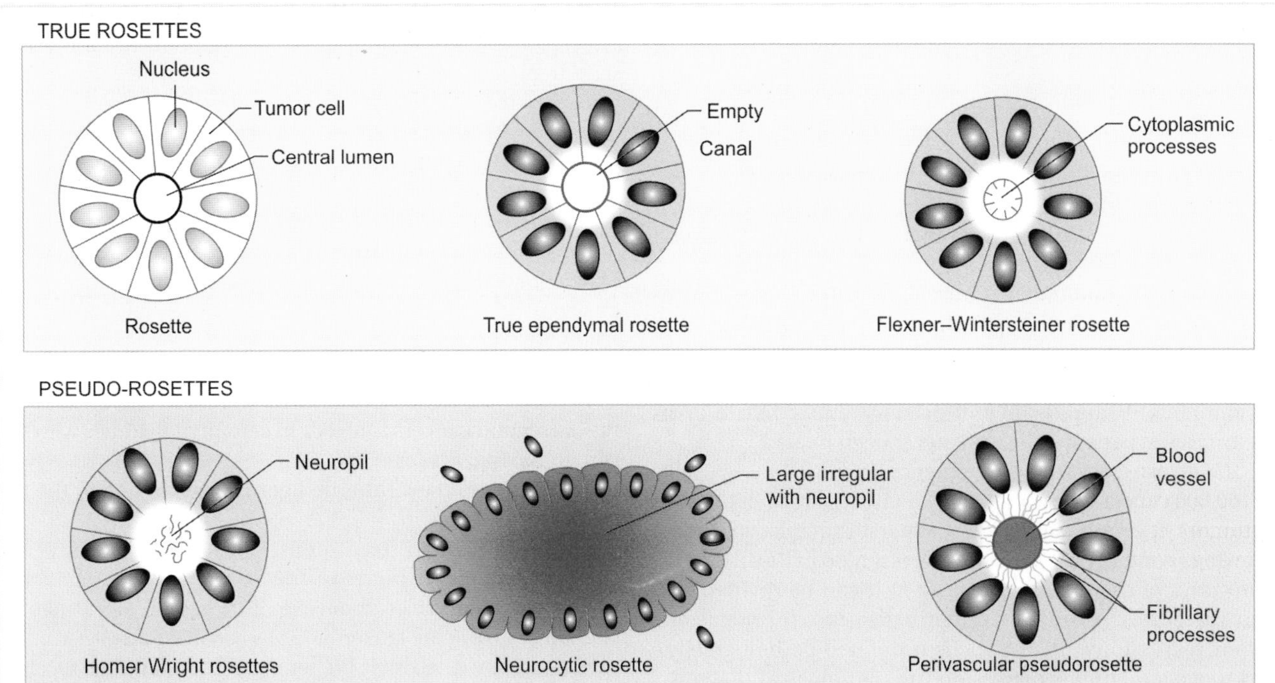

FIG. 107: Various types of rosettes.

Types

There are many different types of targeted therapies:

1. ***Hormone therapies*:** The growth of certain tumors depends on hormones. Hormone therapies act by preventing the producing the hormones by the body or by interfering with the action of the hormones. Hormone therapies are mainly used for breast cancer and prostate cancer.
2. ***Signal transduction inhibitors*:** When a cell receives a specific signal from its environment, signal is relayed within the cell through a series of molecules that ultimately produce the appropriate response. Contrary to conventional chemotherapy, therapies can be used to target signaling elements ("targeted signaling therapies" or "signaling therapies"). They have the advantage of being more selective against the cancer cells and to some extent have decreased toxicities towards normal cells. Signal transduction is one the molecules involved in this signalling process. Signal transduction inhibitors block the activities of molecules that participate in signal transduction. This prevents proliferation of cancerous cell. Example: imatinib (certain chronic leukemias).
3. ***Angiogenesis inhibitors*:** Tumor angiogenesis is one of the hallmark of cancer. Blood supplies oxygen and nutrients is required for the growth of tumors. Angiogenesis inhibitors block the formation of new blood vessels that feed and nourish the cancer cells. Some targeted therapies inhibit angiogenesis by interfering the action of vascular endothelial growth factor (VGEF) and other angiogenesis inhibitors target other molecules that stimulate new blood vessel growth. Example: bevacizumab (many different cancers).
4. ***Gene expression modulators*:** They modify the function of proteins involved in controlling gene expression.
5. ***Apoptosis inducers*:** Some cancer cells have strategies to avoid apoptosis. Apoptosis inducers cause cancer cells to undergo apoptosis.
6. ***Proteasome inhibitors*:** These disrupt normal cell functions so the cancer cells die. Example: bortezomib (multiple myeloma)
7. ***Immunotherapies*:** These trigger the immune system to destroy cancer cells. In immunotherapy monoclonal antibodies that recognize specific molecules on the surface of cancer cells are used. Some monoclonal antibodies are termed as targeted therapy because they have a specific target on a cancer cell. They find, attach to, and attack the target on the cancer cell. But other monoclonal antibodies act like immunotherapy. They are termed so because they make the immune system to respond better and thereby attack cancer cells more effectively. These **monoclonal antibodies** might deliver molecules by themselves or molecules with drugs into or onto the cancer cell to kill it. Examples: alemtuzumab (chronic leukemias), trastuzumab (breast cancers), cetuximab (colorectal, lung, head and neck cancers). Cancer immunotherapy is discussed in detail on pages 501–504.
    - **Monoclonal antibodies:** Binding of the monoclonal antibody to the target molecule leads to immune destruction of cancer cells that express that target molecule. Other monoclonal antibodies bind to certain immune cells and help these cells to destroy cancer cells.
    - **Monoclonal antibodies that deliver toxic molecules:** In this, a toxic molecule (e.g., radioactive substance, a chemical toxin or drug) is linked to the antibody. Once the antibody has bound to its target cancer cell, toxic molecules in the antibody is taken up by the cell

and ultimately the cancerous cell is killed. The toxin will not affect normal cells that lack the target for the antibody.

Epigenetic modification in cancer is discussed on pages 433–438.

Spontaneous Tumor Regression

Q. Write short essay on spontaneous tumor regression.

Definition: Spontaneous tumor regression is defined as spontaneous remission or partial/complete disappearance of a malignant tumor in the absence of any treatment.

According to some, spontaneous regression is partial or complete disappearance of primary tumor tissue or its metastases in patients who have never been treated.

It is an extremely rare phenomenon and may be 1 in 60,000 to 100,000 cancer cases. Though it can be observed in all types of tumors, it is frequent in some tumors. Examples of tumors showing spontaneous regression is presented in **Box 26**.

Categories of spontaneous regression: It can be divided into four categories: (i) primary tumor regression, (ii) metastatic tumor regression (primary focus is defined pathologically), (iii) metastatic tumor regression (no pathological diagnosis of primary tumor), (iv) radiologically-considered-metastasis tumor regression.

Pathogenesis of Spontaneous Regression

Activation of immune system has been found important in its pathogenesis. Various pathogenetic mechanism are listed in **Box 27**.

Box 26: Examples of malignant tumors that can undergo spontaneous regression.

- Neuroblastoma
- Renal cell carcinoma
- Germ cell tumors
- Malignant melanoma
- Lymphoma and leukemia
- Genitourinary cancer

Box 27: Various pathogenetic mechanism of spontaneous tumor regression.

- Apoptosis
- Tumor microenvironment
- DNA oncogenic suppression
- Immune modulation: tumor immunity
- Antiangiogenesis
- Genomic crisis resulting from telomerase exhaustion
- Infection
- Natural killer activity

Second Malignant Neoplasms

Q. Write short essay on second malignant neoplasms.

With increased survival from primary cancer, survivors of cancers are at an increased risk of developing second malignant neoplasm (SMN). A second cancer is a new cancer that develops in an individual who had cancer before and develop after the treatment of the primary neoplasm. Second cancer is a completely new and a different type of cancer than the first one and is not the same as a cancer recurrence. Second cancers are not uncommon. Regardless of their cause, second malignant neoplasms comprise the sixth most common group of malignancies after skin, prostate, breast, lung, and colorectal cancers. Second malignant neoplasms can develop both in childhood and adult-onset cancers.

Risk Factors

Risk of second cancers is higher in certain individuals who had certain types of first cancers.

Inherited genes: Few inherited genes may be one of the risk factor.

Type of cancer treatment. Both radiotherapy and chemotherapy can increase the risk of SMN later in life. Second malignancies can develop 20 years after treatment or later. In case of acute leukemia, SMN can occurs 2–4 years after chemotherapy. The risk is higher if the treatment was received for malignant tumors during childhood or young adult days.

Radiation therapy

The general criteria (**Box 28**) for attributing a second malignant neoplasm to the effects of radiation was defined by Goolden (1951).

Radiation-sensitive solid tissues and organs: Most important are the bone marrow, thyroid and female breast.

Susceptibility factors that increase the risk of second malignant neoplasm after radiation therapy includes:

- Individual susceptibility
- Directly depends on the total dose of radiation delivered during the course of treatment, type and energy of the radiation
- Type of dose delivery (protracted or instantaneous)
  - It was observed that, if the exposure time for a given total dose of radiation is extended, the biologic effect is reduced.
  - Protracted delivery of a dose over hours or days, usually result in less severe consequence. This is due to the reduced tumorigenic effect as compared to the instantaneous delivery of the total dose.

Primary tumor treated with radiation and associated secondary malignant neoplasms is presented in **Table 48**.

Box 28: Criteria for attributing a second malignant neoplasm to the effects of radiation.

- History of prior irradiation*
- Second malignant neoplasm occurring within the field of prior irradiation*
- Gross or microscopic evidence of radiation damage in the surrounding tissue
- A long, latent interval between the irradiation and the development of the malignancy

*Only these two criteria are considered essential.

Table 48: Primary tumor treated with radiation and associated secondary malignant neoplasms.

Primary tumor treated with radiation	*Type of secondary malignant neoplasms*
Hodgkin lymphoma	Cancer of breast, stomach, pancreas and intestine
Ovarian cancer	Leukemia, cancer of bladder and pancreas
Testicular cancer	Leukemia, cancer of stomach, bladder and pancreas
Lung cancer	Esophageal cancer, leukemia

Table 49: Primary tumor treated with chemotherapy and associated secondary malignant neoplasms.

Primary tumor treated with chemotherapy	*Type of secondary malignant neoplasms*
Hodgkin lymphoma	Carcinoma of thyroid, breast, and skin; melanoma of skin
Sarcomas	Myelodysplastic syndrome (MDS); acute myeloid leukemia (AML) and acute lymphoblastic leukemia (ALL)
Testicular cancer	AML, non-Hodgkin's lymphoma (NHL)
Lung cancer	Cancer of esophagus, leukemia, second primary lung cancers

Chemotherapy

Secondary malignant neoplasms occur only in a small percentage of individuals receiving chemotherapeutic regimen. It depends on environmental factors like smoking or cancer treatment therapies. Primary tumor treated with chemotherapy and associated secondary malignant neoplasms is presented in **Table 49**.

BIBLIOGRAPHY

1. Anastasiadou E, Jacob LS, Slack FJ. Non-coding RNA networks in cancer. *Nat Rev Cancer.* 2018;18(1):5-18.
2. Bailey MH, Tokheim C, Porta-Pardo E, Sengupta S, Bertrand D, Weerasinghe A, et al. Comprehensive characterization of cancer driver genes and mutations. *Cell.* 2018;173(2):371-85.e18.
3. Batlle E, Clevers H. Cancer stem cells revisited. *Nat Med.* 2017;23(10):1124-34.
4. Brabletz T, Kalluri R, Nieto MA, Weinberg RA. EMT in cancer. *Nat Rev Cancer.* 2018;18(2):128-34.
5. Brahmer JR, Tykodi SS, Chow LQ, et al. Safety and activity of anti-PD-L1 antibody in patients with advanced cancer. *N Engl J Med.* 2012;366(26):2455-65.
6. Butterfield LH, Kaufman HL, Marincola FM. Cancer Immunotherapy Principles and Practice. New York: Demos Medical Publishing; 2017.
7. Chabner BA, Longo DL. Cancer Chemotherapy, Immunotherapy and Biotherapy, 6th edition. Philadelphia: Wolters Kluwer; 2019.
8. Chen C-C, Feng W, Lim PX, et al. Homology-directed repair and the role of BRCA1, BRCA2, and related proteins in genome integrity and cancer. *Annu Rev Cancer Biol.* 2018;2:313-36.
9. Cilloni D, Saglio G. Molecular pathways: BCR-ABL. *Clin Cancer Res.* 2012;18(4):930-7.
10. Colditz G, Peterson LL. Obesity and cancer: evidence, impact, and future directions. *Clin Chem.* 2018;64(1):154-62.
11. Coleman WB, Tsongalis G J. The Molecular Basis of Human Cancer. New York: Springer Verlag_Humana Press_Springer: 2017.
12. DeBerardnis RJ, Chandel NS. Fundamentals of cancer metabolism. *Sci Adv.* 2016;2(5):e1600200.
13. De Palma M, Biziato D, Petrova TV. Microenvironmental regulation of tumour angiogenesis. *Nat Rev Cancer.* 2017;17(8):457-74.
14. DeVita VT, Lawrence TS, Rosenberg SA. DeVita, Hellman, and Rosenberg's Cancer Principles & Practice of Oncology, 11th edition. Philadelphia: Wolters Kluwer; 2019.
15. Dong H, Markovic SN. The Basics of Cancer Immunotherapy. Switzerland: Springer; 2018.
16. Dyson NJ. RB1: a prototype tumour suppressor and an enigma. *Genes Dev.* 2016;30(13):1492-502.
17. Fior R, Zilhão R. Molecular and Cell Biology of Cancer -When Cells Break the Rules and Hijack Their Own Planet. Switzerland: Springer Nature; 2019.
18. Flavahan WA, Gaskell E, Bernstein BE. Epigenetic plasticity and the hallmarks of cancer. *Science.* 2017;357(6348):eaal2380.
19. Gantsev S, Gantsev K, Kzyrgalin S. Atlas of Lymphatic System in Cancer Sentinel Lymph Node, Lymphangiogenesis and Neolymphogenesis. Switzerland: Springer Nature; 2020.
20. Gostissa M, Alt FW, Chiarle R. Mechanisms that promote and suppress chromosomal translocations in lymphocytes. *Annu Rev Immunol.* 2011;29:319-50.
21. Greaves M, Maley CC. Clonal evolution in cancer. *Nature.* 2012;481(7381):306-13.
22. Haanen JBAG, Lugowska I, Garassino MC, Califano R. ESMO handbook of immuno-oncology, 1st ed. Switzerland: ESMO Press; 2018.
23. Hanahan D, Weinberg RA. Hallmarks of cancer: the next generation. *Cell.* 2011;144(5):646-74.
24. Havel JJ, Chowell D, Chan TA. The evolving landscape of biomarkers for checkpoint inhibitor immunotherapy. *Nat Rev Cancer.* 2019;19(3):133-50.
25. Joerger AC, Fersht AR. The p53 pathway: origins, inactivation in cancer, and emerging therapeutic opportunities. *Annu Rev Biochem.* 2016;85:375-404.
26. Kerr DJ, Haller D G, van de Velde C J.H, Baumann M. Oxford Textbook of Oncology, 3rd edition. Oxford: Oxford University press; 2016.
27. Kumar V, Abbas AK, Aster JC, Deyrup AT. Robbins essential pathology, 1st edition. Philadelphia: Elsevier; 2021.
28. Kumar V, Abbas AK, Aster JC. Robbins basic pathology, 10th edition. Philadelphia: Saunders Elsevier; 2018
29. Kumar V, Abbas AK, Fausto N, et al. Robbins and Cotran pathologic basis of disease, 10th edition. Philadelphia: WB Saunders; 2021.
30. Lakhani SR. Dilly SA, Finlayson CJ, Gandhi M. Basic Pathology-An introduction to the mechanisms of disease,5th edition. Boca Raton: CRC Press; 2016.
31. Letai A. Apoptosis and cancer. *Annu Rev Cancer Biol.* 2017; 1:275094.
32. Liang J, Shang Y. Estrogen and cancer. *Annu Rev Physiol.* 2013;75:225-40.
33. Link. Principles of Cancer Treatment and Anticancer Drug Development. Switzerland: Springer; 2018.
34. Ly P, Cleveland D. Rebuilding chromosomes after catastrophe: emerging mechanisms of chromothripsis. *Trends Cell Biol.* 2017;27(12):917-30.
35. Maciejowski J, de Lange T. Telomeres in cancer: tumour suppression and genome instability. *Nat Rev Mol Cell Biol.* 2017;18(3): 175-86.

36. McGranahan N, Swanton C. Clonal heterogeneity and tumor evolution: past, present, and the future. *Cell*. 2017;168(4):613-28.
37. Mendelsohn J, Gray JW, Howley PM, Israel MA, Thompson CB. The Molecular Basis of Cancer. Philadelphia: Saunders; 2015.
38. Nebbioso A, Tambaro FP, Dell' Aversana C, et al. Cancer epigenetics: moving forward. *PLoS* Genet. 2018;14(6):e1007362.
39. Pakkala S, Ramalingam SS. Personalized therapy for lung cancer: striking a moving target. *JCI Insight*. 2018;3(15):e120858.
40. Pathria P, Louis TL, Varner JA. Targeting tumor-associated macrophages in cancer. *Trends Immunol*. 2019;40(4):310-27.
41. Plummer M, de Martel C, Vignat J, et al. Global burden of cancers attributable to infections in 2012: a synthetic analysis. *Lancet Glob Health*. 2016;4(9):e609-16..
42. Ramirez C. The Lymphatic System Components, Functions and Diseases. New York: Nova Science Publishers; 2016.
43. Riggi N, Aguet M, Stamenkovic I. Cancer metastasis: a reappraisal of its underlying mechanisms and their relevance to treatment. *Annu Rev Pathol*. 2018;13:117-40.
44. Roy M, Datta A. Cancer Genetics and Therapeutics. Singapore: Springer, 2019.
45. Santana-Codina N, Mancias JD, Kimmelman AC. The role of autophagy in cancer. *Annu Rev Cancer Biol*. 2017;1:19-39.
46. Shukla KK, Sharma P, Misra S. Molecular Diagnostics in Cancer Patients. Singapore: Springer Nature; 2019.
47. Simanshu DK, Nissley DV, McCormick F. RAS proteins and their regulators in human disease. *Cell*. 2017;170(1):17-33.
48. Spranger S, Gajewski TF. Mechanisms of tumor cell-intrinsic immune evasion. *Annu Rev Cancer Biol*. 2017;2:213-28.
49. Srivastava S. Biomarkers in Cancer Screening and Early Detection. Chichester: Wiley Blackwell; 2017.
50. Stine ZE, Walton ZE, Altman BJ, et al. MYC, metabolism, and cancer. *Cancer Discov*. 2015;5(10):1024-39.
51. Strayer DS, Saffitz JE. Rubin's Pathology: Mechanism of Human Disease, 8th edition. Philadelphia: Wolters Kluwer; 2020.
52. Thurin M, Cesano A, Marincola F M. Biomarkers for Immunotherapy of Cancer. New York: Springer Science; 2020.
53. Topalian SL, Hodi FS, Brahmer JR, et al. Safety, activity, and immune correlates of anti-PD-1 antibody in cancer. *N Engl J Med*. 2012;366(26):2443-54.
54. Wagener C, Stocking C, Müller O. Cancer Signaling from Molecular Biology to Targeted Therapy. Germany: Wiley-VCH; 2017.
55. Weinberg RA. The Biology of Cancer, 2nd edition. New York: Garland Science; 2014.
56. Worby CA, Dixon JE. PTEN. *Annu Rev Biochem*. 2014;83:641-69.
57. Zitvogel L, Kroemer G. Oncoimmunology A Practical Guide for Cancer Immunotherapy. Switzerland: Springer; 2018.

CHAPTER 11

Infections and Infestations

11.1 General Features of Microbial Pathogenesis

CHAPTER OUTLINE

- Introduction
- Host–microbe relationship
  - Microbial pathogenesis
- Host-pathogen interactions
  - Immune evasion by microbes
  - Host immunity causing injury
  - Infections in individuals with immunodeficiencies
  - Host damage by microbes
- Spectrum of inflammatory responses to infection
  - Major histologic patterns

INTRODUCTION

The term "infestation" refers to parasitic diseases caused by animals such as arthropods (i.e., mites, ticks, and lice) and worms. The term "infections" refers to diseases caused by protozoa, fungi, bacteria, and viruses.

Probably the greatest curse to mankind is the diverse group of disorders collectively called **infectious diseases**. Though there are effective vaccines and antibiotics available, infectious diseases remain a major health problem throughout the world. The infectious diseases cause more pain, suffering, disability and premature death than any other type of diseases in history. The marked effect of infectious diseases is greatest in less developed countries where there is inadequate access to medical care, malnutrition and is mostly seen in children younger than 5 years of age (e.g., respiratory infections, infectious diarrhea, and malaria). In developed countries it mainly affects older adults and immunosuppressed individuals or those with debilitating chronic diseases.

During the 20th century alone, it was observed that smallpox claimed between 300 million and 500 million human lives. Though smallpox has been eradicated due to vaccination, many other infectious agents continue to claim millions of human-lives each year. Examples of these infectious diseases include tuberculosis, malaria, childhood diarrhea, and acquired immunodeficiency syndrome (AIDS). In advance countries sepsis alone is responsible for considerable mortality each year. Many other infections have emerged for which there is little treatment and no cures. These include Ebola virus, severe acute respiratory syndrome (SARS), drug-resistant tuberculosis, pandemic strains of influenza virus, carbapenem-resistant Enterobacteriaceae (CRE), etc. Recent pandemic of virus—coronavirus disease 2019 (Covid-19) has caused infections throughout the world and claiming many human-lives (especially with comorbidity) from end of year 2019. It is continuing in 2020, even as this chapter is being written. The recent concern over these and other infectious diseases is animal reservoirs of microbes and thereby it can be transmitted to humans. Finally, the possibility that cruel people worser than the infectious agents may use infectious agents as weapons of warfare.

It is necessary to remember the past achievements of individuals **(Table 1)** who have helped to ease the human suffering in certain diseases.

Table 1: Achievements in infectious diseases.

Name of the scientist	*Discovery*
Edward Jenner (1798)	Use of cowpox (vaccinia) virus to immunize against smallpox
Oliver Wendell Holmes, Sr (1843)	Simple washing of hands between patients could dramatically reduce the incidence of puerperal postpartum fever
Ignaz Semmelweis (1846) in Vienna	Concluded that puerperal sepsis was contagious
Louis Pasteur (1822–1895)	Introduced techniques of sterilization Coined the term *vaccine* for prophylactic preparations
John Snow (1854)	Removal of the Broad Street pump handle, which ended the 1854 cholera outbreak in London
Joseph Lister (1867)	Antiseptic techniques in surgery
Robert Koch (1843–1910) in Germany	Perfected bacteriological techniques for the culture Life cycle of the anthrax bacillus (1876). Discovered the bacillus of tuberculosis (1882) and the cholera vibrio (1883)
Roux and Yersin (1888)	Identified a new mechanism of pathogenesis Discovered the diphtheria toxin
Paul Ehrlich (1854–1915)	Studied toxins and antitoxins in quantitative terms and laid the foundations of biological standardization
Ernst Ruska (1934)	Developed the electron microscope, and visualization of the viruses
Karl Landsteiner (1868–1943)	Foundations of immunochemistry
Alexander Fleming (1929)	Accidental discovery that the fungus *Penicillium* produces a substance (Penicillin) that destroys staphylococci

HOST–MICROBE RELATIONSHIP

Microorganisms interact with human hosts in different ways and this depends on characteristics of host and microorganism.

- **Transient microorganisms:** These **microorganisms are present in food or water or elsewhere in our environment** and are of little consequence**.** In general, they pass through the host without causing harm and without establishing residence in the host.
- **Commensal: These microorganisms are normal inhabitant of the human body.** They form normal flora coexist peacefully with their human hosts without any harm to humans. Most of these commensal organisms occupy microenvironmental niches that might otherwise be filled by potential pathogens. Thus, they help to prevent infectious disease. **In commensal relationships, either the microbe or host derives benefit; or both may benefit.** Literally, commensal means those that "eat at the same table". Humans and other animals harbor a complex ecosystem of commensal microbes (the ***microbiome***) and play important roles in health and disease.
- **Opportunistic pathogen:** A microbe that **causes disease *only* in humans who have depressed/compromised normal defense mechanisms**. One of the important consequences of the existence of the normal microbial flora is opportunistic infections. Microorganisms present as commensals are normally well behaved. Sometimes harmless commensal organisms may cause opportunistic infections, when the host's immune system is depressed (i.e., defenses are breached or attenuated). These organisms are generally the first to take advantage of this and gain access to parts of the body where they are normally not present. They may cause symptomatic infections and can even be fatal. Some opportunists may be low-virulence and universal. They do not cause disease in humans with normal immune systems and only occur in the immunosuppressed.
- **Pathogens:** Term pathogen is derived from the Greek, *pathos,* meaning the "birth of suffering." These are microorganisms that **regularly or frequently cause diseases in humans with normal immune defenses**. Human pathogens are transmitted from one human reservoir to another human. Mode of transmission may be either directly or through a fomite (e.g., contaminated instruments, contaminated food).
- **Accidental pathogens:** These are pathogens that do not usually affect humans, but cause disease in human by transmission through accidental contact with animals, insects, or the environment. These microorganisms are usually cause severe or deadly disease in humans and sometimes the causative agent of disease in other animals. These microbes are usually not directly or readily transmissible from human to human (e.g., rabies by rabid dog bite).

Microbial Pathogenesis

Microorganisms can be found in close association with every type of multicellular organism. Healthy human body is packed with billions of varied microorganisms that constitute about 10 times more than the number cells in the human body! This so-called *microbiome* is important for protection against transient pathogens. However, these are ready source of *opportunistic* organisms when the immune system of the individual is suppressed.

Virulence: Virulence is the **property of an organism that allows it to establish infection and to cause disease or death.** Virulence reflects both the inherent features of the offending microbe and the interplay of factors involved in host defense mechanisms. Most infectious diseases are caused by pathogenic organisms and they have a wide range of virulence.

Source of pathogens: The various sources of pathogenic organisms include **humans, animals, insect vectors, and the environment**. The pathogenic microbes are not found in the normal microbiota of healthy individuals. Thus, their presence in humans is diagnostic of an infection.

Routes of Entry of Microbes

Various routes by which microbes can enter the host are: **(1) by breaching epithelial surfaces, (2) inhalation, (3) ingestion, or (4) sexual transmission.** Generally, infections of respiratory, gastrointestinal, and genitourinary tract in healthy individuals are caused by virulent microorganisms. These microbes are capable of damaging or penetrating the mucosal epithelium. Skin infections in healthy individuals are mainly due to organisms which enter the skin through superficial injuries.

Skin

Normal defense mechanism: The intact keratinized epidermis of skin protects against infection by various ways. These include: (1) by acting as a mechanical barrier, (2) presence of a low pH, and (3) by producing substances toxic to bacteria (e.g., antimicrobial fatty acids and defensins, small peptides).

Mode of entry of microbes: Various modes are as follows:

- **Most skin infections are due to mechanical injury of the epidermis.** The injury may be minor trauma, large wounds, burns, and pressure-related ulcers. Infections may also enter through intravenous catheters in hospitalized patients or needle sticks in healthcare workers.
- **Through bite of insect or animal:** Some pathogens may penetrate the skin through an insect *(vector)* or animal bite. Various vectors include fleas, ticks, mosquitoes, and lice.
- **Release of enzymes:** For example, the larvae of *Schistosoma* release enzymes that dissolve the adhesive proteins that hold keratinocytes together. Then they can enter through unbroken skin.
- **Infection of intact epidermis:** Some fungi *(dermatophytes)* cause superficial infections of the intact stratum corneum, hair, and nails.

Gastrointestinal tract

Infection of gastrointestinal tract may occur when local defenses are evaded or overcome by a pathogen, or when local defenses are weakened so much that even normal flora produce disease.

Normal defense mechanism: The gastrointestinal tract has several local defenses. Various mechanisms are as follows:

- **Acidic gastric secretions:** They are very effective at killing certain organisms (e.g., *Vibrio cholerae*).
- **Mucus layer:** A layer of mucus covers the entire length of gastrointestinal tract and it prevents entry of luminal pathogens to the surface epithelium.
- **Pancreatic enzymes and bile detergents:** They can destroy organisms with lipid envelopes.
- **Production of antimicrobial defensins by epithelial cells** of gastrointestinal tract.
- **Production of IgA antibodies** in mucosal lymphoid tissues such as Peyer's patches are secreted into the lumen of the gut. This can neutralize potential pathogens.
- **Peristalsis** can clear as well prevent the local overgrowth of organisms.
- Normal gut microbiota can competitively inhibit colonization and overgrowth by potential pathogens, such as *Clostridioides difficile*.

Mode of entry of microbes: Most gastrointestinal pathogens are transmitted **by food or drink contaminated with fecal material**. These can enter due to bad hygiene and they produce diarrhea.

Mechanism of infection: Pathogens causing symptomatic gastrointestinal disease act through several distinct mechanisms.

- **Bacterial colonization and toxin production:** Some bacteria establish an infection and produce damaging toxins. Examples include *V. cholerae* and enterotoxigenic *Escherichia coli*. These bacteria attack the intestinal epithelium and multiply in the covering mucous layer. These organisms produce powerful exotoxins and produce symptomatic disease.
- **Adhesion and invasion of mucosa:** Some bacteria invade the intestinal mucosa and lamina propria leading to ulceration, inflammation, and hemorrhage. They manifest clinically as dysentery. Examples include *Shigella* species, *Salmonella enterica, Campylobacter jejuni,* and *Entamoeba histolytica*. Some invade superficially into oral and esophageal squamous mucosa in immunocompromised patients (e.g., *Candida albicans* causes thrush).
- **Producing toxin:** Some organisms can cause gastro-intestinal disease without establishing an infection in the host. They contaminate the food and produce toxins without bacterial colonization of gastrointestinal tract. For example, *Staphylococcus aureus* produces a powerful exotoxin during its growth in contaminated food. This causes acute food poisoning.
- **Resist normal defense mechanism:** Many common pathogens causing infections of gastrointestinal tract are resistant to local antimicrobial defensins secreted by epithelial cells.
  - **Acid-resistant protective outer coat:** Intestinal protozoa and helminths transmitted as cysts or eggs, respectively and they have outer coats that are resistant to acid.
  - **Disturbed peristalsis:** It can occur with intestinal obstruction, ileus and postsurgical adhesions.
  - **Resist defenses of bile and pancreatic enzymes:** For example, norovirus (the scourge of the cruise ship industry) is a nonenveloped virus is not inactivated by acid, bile, and pancreatic enzymes.
  - **Altering the normal gut microbiota:** Normal intestinal flora can competitively inhibit colonization and over-growth of potential pathogens, such as *C.difficile*.

Common routes of microbial infection are presented in **Table 2**.

Respiratory tract

Numerous microorganisms (e.g., viruses, bacteria, and fungi) are inhaled mainly in dust or aerosol particles.

Table 2: Common routes of microbial infection.

Major local defense/s	*Mechanism of loss of local defense*	*Examples of pathogens*
Skin		
Epidermal barrier	Mechanical injury	
	• Punctures, burns, ulcers	*Staphylococcus aureus, Candida albicans, Pseudomonas aeruginosa*
	• Needle sticks	Human immunodeficiency virus, hepatitis viruses (B, C and D)
	Bite of insects and animal	Malaria, rabies, yellow fever, plague, Lyme disease
	Direct penetration by release of enzymes	*Schistosoma species*
	Intact epidermis	*Dermatophytes*
Gastrointestinal tract		
Epithelial barrier	Microbes adhere and proliferate locally	*Vibrio cholerae, Escherichia coli, Giardia duodenalis*
	Microbes adhere and invade locally	*Shigella* species, *Salmonella* species, *Campylobacter* species
	Uptake through M (microfold) cells	Poliovirus, *Shigella* species, *Salmonella* species
	Producing toxins	Staphylococcus aureus
Resist normal defense		
• Acidic secretions	Acid-resistant outer coat of cysts and eggs	Many protozoa and helminths
• Peristalsis	Disturbed peristalsis: Intestinal obstruction, ileus, postsurgical adhesions	Mixed aerobic and anaerobic bacteria (*Escherichia coli, Bacteroides* species)
• Bile and pancreatic enzymes	Resistant microbial external coats	Hepatitis A, rotavirus, norovirus
• Normal protective microbiota	Broad-spectrum antibiotic use	*Clostridioides difficile*
Respiratory tract		
Mucociliary clearance	Direct attachment and local proliferation of microbes	Influenza viruses
	Paralysis of ciliary activity by toxins	*Haemophilus influenzae, Mycoplasma pneumoniae, Bordetella pertussis*
Resident alveolar macrophages	Resistance to killing by phagocytes	*Mycobacterium tuberculosis*
Urogenital tract		
Regular urination	Obstruction, microbial attachment, and local proliferation	*Escherichia coli*
Normal vaginal microbiota	Use of antibiotics	*Candida albicans*
Intact epidermal/epithelial barrier	Microbial attachment and local proliferation	*Neisseria gonorrhoeae*
	Direct infection/local invasion	Herpes viruses, syphilis
	Local trauma	Sexually transmitted infections (e.g., human papillomavirus

- **Microorganisms in large particles:** They are trapped in the mucociliary lining of the nose and the upper respiratory tract and these are carried to the back of the throat by ciliary action, where they are swallowed and cleared.
- **Microorganisms in smaller particles:** Those particles containing organisms smaller than 5 μm are carried into the alveoli. In the alveoli they are phagocytosed by leukocytes.

Mechanism of infection The mechanisms of respiratory infection can be studied in two categories: (1) on healthy individuals, and (2) in those with impaired local or systemic defenses.

In healthy individuals: The microorganisms infecting the respiratory tract of healthy individuals escape local defenses through several different mechanisms.

- **Direct attachment and local proliferation:** Some respiratory viruses enter and attach to epithelial cells in the lower respiratory tract and pharynx. For example, influenza viruses contain envelope proteins called *hemagglutinins*. These attach to sialic acid on the surface of epithelial cells and undergo endocytosis in the epithelial cells. This leads to viral entry and replication inside the epithelial cells.
- **Paralysis of ciliary activity by releasing toxins:** Some bacterial respiratory pathogens (e.g., *Mycoplasma pneumoniae* and *Bordetella pertussis*) release toxins that impair the ciliary activity of epithelial cells and increase their ability to produce infection.
- **Resistance to killing following phagocytosis:** Some organism produces respiratory infection by their capacity to resist killing following phagocytosis. For

example, *Mycobacterium tuberculosis* reach the alveoli are phagocytosed by alveolar macrophages. They survive within the phagolysosomes of macrophages by resisting their destruction.

In individuals with impaired local or systemic defenses: Some organisms produce disease when there are local or systemic impairment of defenses in the host.

- **Impaired local defense mechanism:** Respiratory mucociliary clearance may be damaged to by influenza, mechanical ventilation, smoking or cystic fibrosis. This favors for superinfection by bacteria.
- **Impaired systemic defense mechanism:** Many infectious agents cause respiratory infections primarily in patients with systemic immunodeficiency. Examples include opportunistic fungal infections in AIDS patients by *Pneumocystis jirovecii* and by *Aspergillus* species in patients with neutropenia.

Urogenital tract

Normal defense mechanism: Normally, urine contains small numbers of low-virulence bacteria. Various protective mechanisms include:

- **Urination:** By regular emptying of urine from the bladder during micturition expels and eliminates microbes. Thus, urinary tract is protected from infection.
- **Normal vaginal microbiota:** In females, from puberty until menopause the vagina contains lactobacilli. These lactobacilli ferment glucose to lactic acid and produce a low pH in the vagina. The acidic pH suppresses the growth of pathogens and there by protect pathogens entering urethra.
- **Intact epidermal/epithelial barrier:** It prevents invasion by microbes.

Mechanism of infection Obstruction of urinary flow and/or reflux of urine are major factors that predisposes to urinary tract infections.

- **Microbial attachment and local proliferation:** Presence of any obstruction to the urinary tract favors urinary tract infection. Pathogens causing urinary tract infections (e.g., *E. coli*) usually enter the urinary tract through the urethra. They attach or adhere to urothelium so that they are prevented from being washed away during urination.
- **Altered vaginal microbiota:** Females are more prone (about 10 times more) to urinary tract infections compared to males. It is because of short urethra (length is 5 cm in females compared to 20 cm in male) and close proximity of urethra with rectum that makes females more susceptible to entry of bacteria from the rectum. Use of antibiotics can kill the protective lactobacilli in the vagina. This allows overgrowth of yeast and can cause vaginal candidiasis.
- **Damage to epidermal/epithelial barrier**
    - **Microbial attachment and local proliferation:** *Neisseria gonorrhoeae* can attach and proliferate.
    - **Direct infection/local invasion:** For example herpes viruses and syphilis.
    - **Local trauma:** Various sexually transmitted infections [e.g., human papillomavirus (HPV)] may develop infection due to local trauma.

Spread of Microbes through the Body

Some pathogenic microorganisms remain localized to the initial site of infection and produce disease. Other pathogens are capable of invading tissues and spread to distant sites through the lymphatics, the blood, or the nerves **(Fig. 1)**. Pathogenic microbes can spread within the body in several ways and these are discussed here.

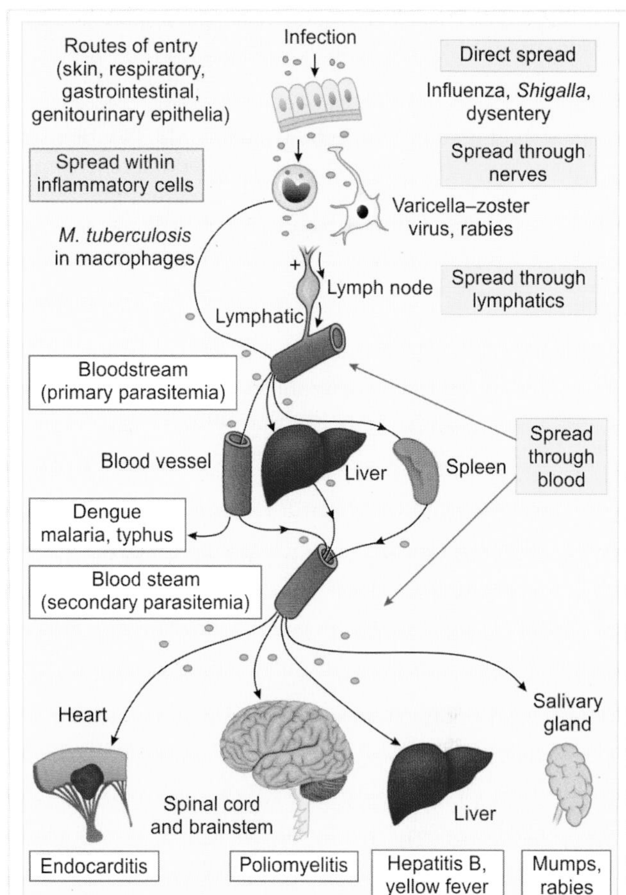

FIG. 1: Various routes of entry of microbes and spread of infection through the body. Microbes enter the body, through epithelial or mucosa l surface. Infection may remain localized to the site of entry and multiply or may spread to other sites of the body. The microbes may penetrate the epithelial or mucosal barriers to enter the body. Most common microbes spread through the lymphatics or bloodstream (either freely or within inflammatory cells). Few viruses and bacterial toxins may travel through nerves (e.g., rabies).

Direct spread: Some microorganisms may be confined to the site of initial entry into the body. They may locally extend the infection into neighboring tissues. Some pathogens may secrete enzymes. They may break down tissues and allow the organisms to spread contiguously in tissue. Certain bacteria can dramatically spread through tissues and cause rapidly fatal disease (e.g., necrotizing fasciitis caused by some strains of group A streptococci).

Lymphatic spread: After the organisms attach to the surface of skin or mucosa, they can travel through the lymphatics to regional lymph nodes. From lymph nodes they may reach the bloodstream.

Blood spread: This is the most common and efficient mode of microbial dissemination. Through this route organism can reach all organs. The consequences of blood-borne spread of pathogens depend on several factors: (1) the virulence of the organism, (2) the severity of the infection, (3) the pattern of microbial seeding, and (4) host factors (e.g., immune status). The spread of the infection may produce a single infectious nidus (an abscess or tuberculoma); multiple small sites of infection (e.g., miliary tuberculosis or *Candida* microabscesses) or infection of the heart [infectious endocarditis and vessels (mycotic aneurysm)]. However, disseminated pathogens may produce a systemic inflammatory response syndrome (SIRS) called *sepsis*. This is characterized by fever, low blood pressure, and coagulopathies. If not corrected, these may progress to multiorgan failure and death, even in previously healthy individuals.

Spread though nerves: Peripheral nerve is an important pathway for the spread of certain viruses and toxins from peripheral parts of the body to the central nervous system (CNS). Viruses, such as **rabies virus, poliovirus, and varicella zoster virus** infect the peripheral nerves and then travel along axons and spread to the CNS.

Release from the Body and Transmission of Microbes

Microbes have different way to ensure their transmission from one host to the next. They may be released from one host to infect the new host. Microbes may exit from the infected host by skin shedding, coughing, sneezing, voiding of urine or feces, during sexual contact, or through insect vectors. Most of the pathogens are released for only brief periods of time. Some may periodically be released during disease flares and few may be shed for long periods by asymptomatic carrier hosts. Majority of pathogens persist outside of the body for only short periods of time and they must be passed quickly from infected host to new host usually by direct contact.

Routes of transmission: The pathogens can be directly or indirectly transmitted. Indirect transmission occurs as vehicle-borne, vector-borne, or airborne transfers. **Most pathogens are directly transmitted from individual to individual by droplets, fecal-oral, sexual routes or vertical transmission.**

- **Through droplets:** It is the most common mode for microbes infecting respiratory tract. Infections by viruses and bacteria spread through aerosol and droplets released into the air and infect the respiratory tract. Some respiratory pathogens (e.g., influenza viruses) spread in large droplets and travel >3 feet from the source. Some including *M. tuberculosis* and varicella-zoster virus, spread in small particles and can travel longer distances.
- **Fecal-oral route:** Most enteric pathogens spread by the fecal-oral route. This is through ingestion of stool-contaminated water or food. Water-borne pathogens especially causing epidemic outbreaks are spread in this fashion. Examples include hepatitis A and E viruses (HAV and HEV), poliovirus, rotavirus, *V. cholerae, Shigella* species, *C. jejuni,* and *S. enterica*. Some parasitic helminths (e.g., hookworms, schistosomes) shed eggs in stool and they hatch as larvae. These larvae can penetrate the skin of the new host and produce infestation.
- **Sexual transmission:** It usually requires prolonged intimate or mucosal contact. Examples of sexually transmitted causative microbes are viruses [e.g., herpes simplex virus (HSV), HIV, HPV]; bacteria (*Treponema pallidum, Neisseria gonorrhoeae*); protozoa (*Trichomonas vaginalis);* and arthropods (*Phthirus pubis,* lice).
- **Other routes of transmission:** There are several other routes of transmission of disease.
    - **Through saliva:** Some viruses replicate in the salivary glands or the oropharynx and can be transmitted through saliva [e.g., Epstein–Barr virus (EBV)].
    - **Blood meal:** Some human pathogens such as protozoa (e.g., *Plasmodium* causing malaria) are spread through blood meals taken by arthropod vectors (mosquitoes, ticks, mites).
    - **Other routes: Zoonotic infections** are transmitted **from animals to humans**. They may be transmitted either by direct contact (including animal bites), use of animal products, or via an invertebrate vector.
- **Vertical transmission:** Vertical transmission is mode of transmission in which **infectious agents are passed from mother to fetus or new-born child**. This is a common mode of transmission for some pathogens. Various routes of vertical transmission are as follows:
    - **Placental-fetal transmission:** This route of transmission mostly occurs when the mother gets infected with a pathogen during pregnancy. Some infections interfere with development of fetus and the severity and type of damage depend on the age of the fetus at the time of infection. For example, rubella virus infection during the first trimester can produce malformations of heart, intellectual disability, cataracts, or deafness whereas rubella virus infection during the third trimester has little effect.
    - **Transmission during birth:** It is transmission of infection from infected mother to fetus during delivery of the child. This is caused by contact with infectious agents during passage through the birth canal. For example, gonococcal and chlamydial conjunctivitis.
    - **Postnatal transmission in maternal milk:** After delivery, infected mother can transmit the infection to the child through breast milk. Examples include cytomegalovirus (CMV), human immunodeficiency virus (HIV), and hepatitis B virus (HBV).

HOST-PATHOGEN INTERACTIONS

The outcome of infection depends on the virulence of the microbe and the nature of the host immune response. The host response may eliminate the infection or, in some cases, exacerbate or cause tissue damage. The mechanisms by which the body prevents or controls infections are called defense mechanisms. The host has many complex defense mechanisms against pathogens (e.g., physical barriers, innate and adaptive immune systems). Microbes are intelligent enough to undergo continuous evolution to fight against host defenses. Few specific features of microbes by which microbes evade host immune response are discussed here.

Immune Evasion by Microbes

Most of pathogenic microbes have evolved one or more methods to evade host defenses (**Fig. 2**).

- **Antigenic variation:** Normally, antibodies are produced against microbial antigens. Their functions include: (1) prevention of microbial adhesion and uptake into cells, (2) act as opsonins and promote phagocytosis, and (3) fix complement. This host defense mechanism is evaded by microbes by expressing a different surface antigen. This new antigen escapes recognition of microbes (e.g., *Borrelia*

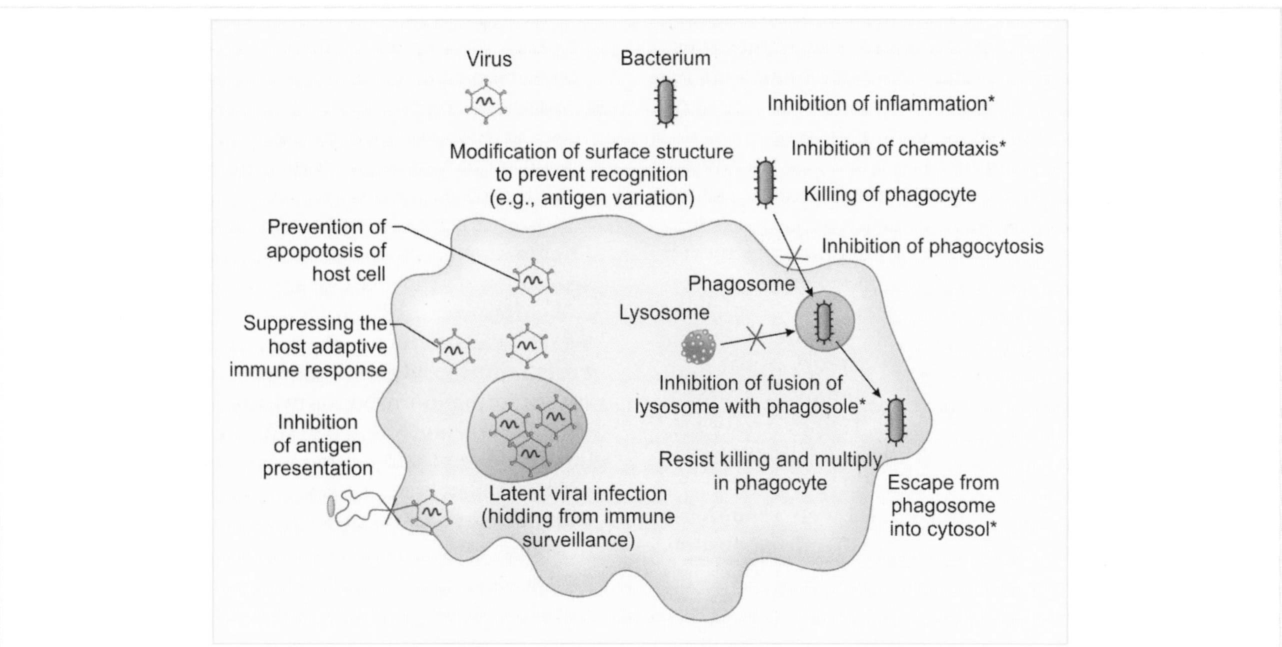

*Minor mechanism.

FIG. 2: Major mechanisms or strategies used by viral and bacterial microorganisms (pathogens) to escape recognition by innate and adaptive immunity.

species and trypanosomes). Influenza viruses contain a segmented ribonucleic acid (RNA) genome that can undergo frequent recombination events. This produces antigenic drift (alteration in antibody-binding sites of major viral envelope glycoproteins) and antigenic shift (formation of a hybrid a new strain virus from two viral strains). Some microbes undergo mutation to produce several genetic variants (e.g., >95 capsular polysaccharides present in different strains of *Streptococcus pneumoniae*).

- **Inactivating antibodies or complement:** Pathogen may inactivate antibodies or complements.
- **Microbial strategy in relation to phagocytes**
  - **Inhibition of chemotaxis or the mobilization of phagocytic cells:** Various substances from bacteria attract phagocytes and some substances react with complement and generate powerful chemotactic factors (e.g., C5a). Microorganisms can inhibit chemotaxis and thereby limiting the accumulation of neutrophils and macrophages to the exact site of infection. Some bacterial toxins can inhibit the mobilization of neutrophils and macrophages. For example, streptococcal streptolysins kill phagocytes and suppress neutrophil chemotaxis in even lower concentrations.
  - **Inhibition of phagocytosis:** Some pathogens develop strategies to avoid phagocytosis. The carbohydrate capsule present on the surface of many bacteria (*e.g., S. pneumoniae, Neisseria meningitidis, Haemophilus influenzae*) can prevent their phagocytosis by neutrophils. For example, *S. aureus* expresses protein A, which attached to the Fc portion of antibodies. This competitively reduces the binding of the antibodies to Fc receptors on phagocyte and thereby prevents phagocytosis. Some bacteria produce an outside coating on their surface to prevent phagocytosis. The coating may be composed of host cell components or a polysaccharide capsule.
  - **Prevention of killing by phagocytes:** Some pathogens inhibit intracellular killing of microbes in phagocytes. Examples include:
    - Inhibition of fusion of lysosome with phagocytic vacuole: Mycobacteria **inhibit phagosome-lysosome fusion.**
    - Escape from the phagosome: *Listeria monocytogenes* causes **disruption of phagosome membrane and escapes onto the cytosol of phagocyte**.
    - Resistance to killing and digestion in the phagolysosomes: Other pathogens that avoid killing by phagocytes include *Cryptococcus neoformans,* and certain protozoa (e.g., *Leishmania* species, *Trypanosoma* species, *Toxoplasma gondii*).
- **Evasion of apoptosis and control of host cell metabolism:** Some viruses synthesize proteins that prevent apoptosis of the host cell. This allows time for replication, enter latency, or to transform infected host cells. Microbes that are capable of intracellular replication (viruses, some bacteria, fungi, and protozoa) also express factors that modify autophagy and thereby prevent degradation.
- **Suppressing the host adaptive immune response:** Interferons (IFNs) inhibit viral replication and various mechanisms may interfere with INF and include:
  - **Interfering with IFNs:** INFs are the group of signaling proteins synthesized and released by host cells in response to the presence of several viruses. Some viruses may interfere with function of IFN by producing soluble homologs of IFN-α/β or IFN-γ receptors. They inhibit the actions of secreted IFNs.

- ○ **Inhibition of JAK/STAT cytokine receptor signaling pathway:** This pathway is involved in immune cell division, survival, activation and recruitment. Some viruses produce proteins that inhibit the JAK/STAT cytokine receptor signaling pathway.
- ○ **Production of proteins** that inactivate or inhibit double-stranded RNA-dependent protein kinase [protein kinase R (PKR)].

- **Evasion of recognition by CD8+ cytotoxic T lymphocytes (CTLs) and CD4+ helper T cells:** T cells recognize antigens present in pathogens presented by MHC molecules, class I for CTLs and class II for CD4+ cells. Many deoxyribonucleic acid (DNA) viruses (e.g., HSV, CMV, EBV) attach to or change location of MHC class I proteins and impair peptide presentation to CD8+ T cells. Herpes viruses also can degrade MHC class II molecules and impair antigen presentation to CD4+ T-helper cells.
- **Downregulation of antimicrobial T cell responses:** Gradual loss of T cell potency is called as **T-cell exhaustion.** It is observed in chronic infections by HIV, hepatitis C virus (HCV), and HBV.
    - ○ **Programmed cell death protein 1 (PD-1):** It is an immune checkpoint cell surface receptor and normally maintains T-cell tolerance to self-antigens. It is an important mediator of T-cell exhaustion during chronic viral infection. Cancers utilize the same mechanisms to suppress destructive immune responses (refer pages 496 and 497 Fig. 77 of Chapter 10). Anti–PD-1 immunotherapy is used for the treatment of cancers and probably may be useful as an adjunctive therapy for chronic infections that are resistant to antimicrobial therapy.
- **Establishing a state of latent infection:** It is another method of avoiding the recognition by immune system. During latent infection viruses survive in a silent state in infected cells. There is few, if any, expression of viral genes during latent infection and there are hidden from immune surveillance (e.g., latent infections of neurons by HSV and varicella-zoster virus, and of B lymphocytes by EBV).
- **Disabling or killing of cells of the immune system:** Pathogens can infect cells of the immune system and interfere with their function (e.g., HIV infects and destroys CD4+ T cells). **Some bacteria form interactive colonies and form a polysaccharide matrix called biofilm.** This slimy coating on solid surfaces may be composed of a single species or several species. These bacteria may be hidden and protected from the host's immune mechanisms. Example for the biofilm is plaque that forms on tooth enamel.
- **Endospore formation:** Some bacteria can create endospores. These spores are in a resting state and are resistant to heat, chemical agents, and desiccation. When the environment is more favorable, these spores get reactivated. Examples include *Bacillus* and *Clostridium.*

Host Immunity Causing Injury

Immune response by the host against microbes is usually protective. But at times the **host immune response to microbes may be responsible for the tissue injury.** Various examples in which immune response causes injury are given here:

- **Tuberculosis:** It is a chronic granulomatous inflammatory disease caused by *M. tuberculosis.* The granulomatous reaction against *M. tuberculosis* segregates the bacilli and prevents their spread. But it can also cause damage to tissue and produce fibrosis.
- **Hepatitis B and C:** Damage to hepatocytes in infection by HBV and HCV is mainly due to the effects of the immune response on infected liver cells. This response is produced as a protective response to clear the virus, but host T cells and, probably natural killer (NK) cells kill the hepatocytes.
- **Rheumatic heart disease:** In this, antibodies are produced against the streptococcal M protein. These antibodies can cross-react with cardiac proteins and damage the heart and lead to rheumatic heart disease.
- **Poststreptococcal glomerulonephritis:** It is characterized by the formation of immune complexes between anti-streptococcal antibodies and streptococcal antigens. These immune complexes get deposited in the renal glomeruli, produce inflammation and glomerulonephritis.
- **Inflammatory bowel disease:** It is characterized by cycle of inflammation and epithelial injury and microbes play a role.
- **Cancers associated with microbes:** Viruses (HBV, HCV) and bacteria *(Helicobacter pylori)* are associated with cancers. Probably these microbes trigger chronic inflammation and provide a fertile ground for the development of cancer.

Infections in Individuals with Immunodeficiencies

Impaired function of the immune system is an important risk factor for the development of infections. **Impaired immune system may be inherited or acquired defects in innate and adaptive immunity.** Impaired immune system renders the affected individual susceptible to both opportunistic and pathogenic infections. Organisms that cause disease in immunodeficient individuals but not in individual with intact immune systems are called opportunistic and infections are termed as **opportunistic infections.**

Acquired causes of immunodeficiencies

Opportunistic organisms (e.g., *Aspergillus* species and *Pseudomonas* species) cause infections in patients with immune deficiency. Decreased immune responses can reactivate latent infection (e.g., herpes viruses and *M. tuberculosis*). Severely immunocompromised individuals may need isolation till their immune status improves. Various acquired causes of immunodeficiency are as follows:

- Most often immunodeficiency is caused by infection with HIV, the cause of AIDS.
- Infiltrative processes that suppress bone marrow function, e.g., leukemia.
- Immunosuppressive drugs used in the treatment of cancer, autoimmune diseases, organ transplant recipients and hematopoietic stem cell transplantation.
- Many other factors can reduce ability to resist infection. These include poor nutritional status (e.g., malnutrition), young or old age, and chronic illness.
- Nonimmune diseases or injuries can also increase the susceptibility to infection. Examples include:
    - ○ *Pseudomonas aeruginosa* and *Burkholderia cepacia* in cystic fibrosis due to a defective transmembrane conductance regulator.

- *S. pneumoniae* in patient with sickle cell disease due to loss of splenic macrophages.
- *P. aeruginosa* in patients with burns due to barrier disruption.

Inherited Causes of Immunodeficiencies

Inherited (primary) immunodeficiency diseases are rare. They involve the specific components of host defense, and have the exclusive vulnerabilities to certain pathogens.

- **Antibody deficiencies:** It is observed in patients with X-linked agammaglobulinemia. It is associated with increased susceptibility to infections by extracellular bacteria (e.g., *S. pneumoniae, H. influenzae,* and *S. aureus*) and few viruses (e.g., rotavirus and enteroviruses).
- **Defects in complement:** It usually involves the early components of the complement cascade (C1, C2, C3 or C4). These individuals are susceptible to infections by encapsulated bacteria (e.g., *S. pneumonia*). Deficiencies of the late membrane attack complex components (C5 to C9) are associated with infections due to *Neisseria* species.
- **Defects in neutrophil function:** One of the examples is chronic granulomatous disease. This lead to increased susceptibility to infections with *S. aureus,* some gram-negative bacteria, and fungi.
- **Defects in toll-like receptor (TLR) signaling pathways:** It produces variable effects. MyD88 and IRAK4 are downstream signaling proteins of many TLRs. Mutations in these, predispose to pyogenic bacterial infections *(S. pneumoniae)*. Impaired TLR3 responses are associated with childhood HSV (*herpes simplex virus*) encephalitis.
- **T-cell defects:** These defects are associated with susceptibility to intracellular pathogens (e.g., viruses and few parasites). Inherited mutations that causes impaired production of T-helper 1 (Th1) cells (e.g., mutations in IL-12 or IFN-γ receptors, or the transcription factor STAT1) are associated with infection by atypical mycobacteria. Defects that impair the production of Th17 cells (e.g., mutations in STAT3) are associated with chronic mucocutaneous candidiasis.

Host Damage by Microbes

Pathogen agents produce infection and cause damage to tissues. The mechanisms of tissue damage are as follows:

- **Direct damage or transformation of host cell:** Pathogens can contact or enter host cells and can directly cause **cell death**. Otherwise, pathogens may cause changes in cellular metabolism and proliferation producing transformation.
- **Damage by toxins, enzymes or blood vessels***:* Pathogens may produce—(2) *toxins* that kill cells at a distance or (2) release *enzymes* that degrade tissue components, or (3) damage blood vessels and cause ischemic necrosis.
- **Damage by immune responses***:* Pathogens can elicit immune responses in host. Even though they are against the invading pathogens they can cause damage to host tissue.

Mechanisms of Viral Injury

The size of viruses ranges from 20 to 300 nm. Viruses may be divided into RNA or DNA depending on their nucleic acid content. These DNAs or RNA are surrounded by a protein envelope or shell. Some viruses also have lipid membranes. **Viruses do not metabolize or do not have the capacity to reproduce independently. They are intracellular parasites and need living cells for their replication.**

Tropism

Viruses can damage host cells directly by entering into host cells and replicating inside the cell at the cell's expense. The **property of viruses to infect certain cells and not others** is termed as *tropism.* **A major factor for tissue tropism is the presence of viral receptors on host cells.** Host cells normally have proteins on the cell surface that act as receptors for host factors. Viruses attach these proteins on the surface of host cells. This is one of the methods by which viruses infect cells, survive within cells, and spread. Examples include:

- HIV glycoprotein gp120 attaches to CD4+ on T cells and to the chemokine coreceptors CXCR4 (present on T cells) and CCR5 (mainly on macrophages).
- EBV attaches to complement receptor 2 (also called as CR2 or CD21) on B cells.
- John Cunningham (JC) virus infection produces leuko-encephalopathy and involves oligodendroglial cells in the CNS. This is because JC viral genes need glial-specific host transcription factors for their expression.

Physical barriers and tropism: Physical barriers may be responsible for tissue tropism of virus. Examples include:

- **Enteroviruses** multiply in the intestine partly because they are **not inactivated by acids, bile, and digestive enzymes.**
- **Rhinoviruses** infect the cells of upper respiratory tract because they **need low temperature of upper respiratory tract for their replication**.

Methods of damage by viruses

Once viruses are inside host cells, there are different mechanisms by which viruses can damage or kill the cells **(Fig. 3)**.

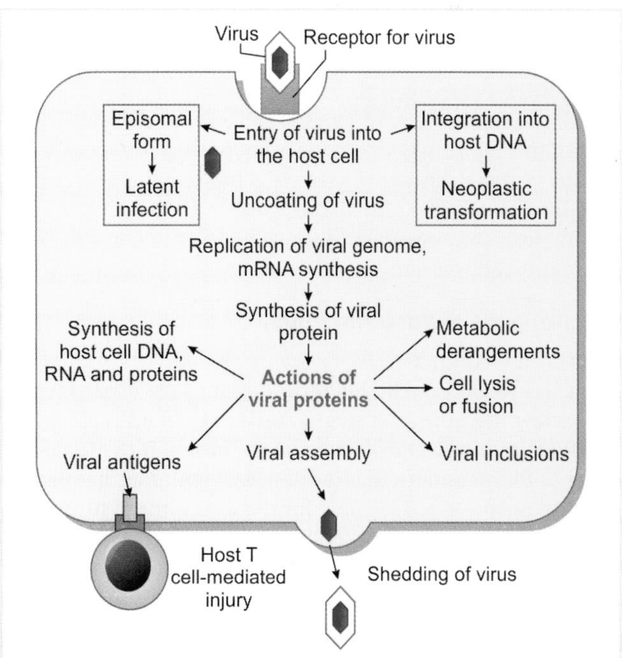

FIG. 3: Various mechanisms of cellular alterations and damage by viruses.

Direct cytopathic effects: Viruses can kill the infected host cells. Various mechanisms of cytopathic effect are as follows:

- Some viruses kill cells by **preventing production of important macromolecules by host cells** (e.g., host cell DNA, RNA, or proteins), or viruses **may produce degradative enzymes and toxic proteins**. For example, poliovirus inactivates cap binding protein required for translation of host cell mRNAs. But it does not affect the translation of poliovirus mRNAs.
- Viruses can produce host cell death by **activation of so-called *death receptors*** [belonging to tumor necrosis factor (TNF) receptor family] present on the plasma membrane. This leads to activation of apoptosis.
- After invading the host cells, virus diverts intracellular biosynthetic and metabolic pathways of infected host cells to **synthesize large amounts of** virus-encoded nucleic acids and **viral proteins**. These proteins include unfolded or misfolded proteins and they **stimulate the ER stress response**. This in turn may activate proapoptotic pathways.
- Some viruses **encode proteins that are proapoptotic** [e.g., HIV viral protein R (Vpr)].

Antiviral immune responses: Viruses promote release of chemical mediators that elicit inflammatory or immunologic responses. Host lymphocytes can recognize and destroy virus-infected cells. However, CTLs can also cause tissue injury.

Transformation of infected cells: Some viruses may remain within cells, either by integrating into the host genomes or by remaining episomal form (without integration into the genome of host cells). Oncogenic viruses can cause cell proliferation and survival resulting in tumor formation. Various mechanisms of transformation include by virus-encoded oncogenes, expression of viral proteins that inactivate tumor suppressors, and insertional mutagenesis. For example, HPVs cause squamous cell proliferative and may cause common warts or cervical cancer. EBV causes endemic Burkitt lymphoma in Africa and other tumors. Human T-cell leukemia virus-1 (HTLV-1) causes a form of T-cell leukemia/lymphoma.

Latent infection: Some viruses infect and **remain in cells without interfering with cellular functions**. This process is called **latency**. Latent viruses can produce disease years after a primary infection. Opportunistic viral infections may be due to reactivation of latent virus infections. For example, CMV and herpes simplex viruses commonly present as latent agents and they produce disease when the cell-mediated immunity is impaired.

Mechanisms of Bacterial Injury

Bacterial virulence

Host tissue damage by bacteria depends on three factors. These are the ability of the bacteria: (1) to adhere to host cells, (2) to invade host cells and tissues, and (3) to deliver toxins. Pathogenic bacteria contain **virulence genes and encode proteins** responsible for the above three properties. The virulence genes are usually grouped together in clusters called *pathogenicity islands*. An example of the importance of virulence genes is observed in the various strains of *S. enterica*. All *S. enterica* strains that infect humans are closely related and form a single species (i.e., they have many housekeeping genes). Presence of virulence genes determine whether particular *S. enterica* causes life-threatening typhoid fever or self-limited enteritis.

Mobile genetic elements (MGEs) and gene transmission: MGEs are a type of genetic material that can move around within a genome, or that can be transferred from one species or replicate to another. Examples of mobile genetic elements are plasmids and bacteriophages. MGEs can transmit functionally important genes to bacteria. These genes include genes involved in pathogenicity and drug resistance. Genes for toxins usually found in the genomes of bacteriophages and sometimes in plasmids. These genes of toxins include genes that encode the toxins involved in the pathogenesis of the infections (e.g., cholera, diphtheria, and botulism). Genes for acquired antibiotic resistance traits are more commonly observed on plasmids, and these can spread within bacterial species and other distantly related organisms. For example, a plasmid with genes for vancomycin resistance can spread to *Enterococcus* species, and also to more distantly related (and virulent) *S. aureus*.

Quorum sensing and autoinducers: It is the process of regulation of gene expression in response to fluctuations in cell-population density. Many bacteria coordinately regulate gene expression by *quorum sensing*. Quorum sensing permits bacteria to express gene only when they grow to reach a high concentration. Growing of bacteria is achieved by secreting small autoinducer molecules by bacteria. Autoinducers when present at high levels induce expression of genes. These genes may be for toxin production *(S. aureus),* for genetic transformation *(S. pneumoniae),* or production of biofilms *(P. aeruginosa).* The various autoinducers are N-acyl-homoserine lactones in gram-negative bacteria, peptides in gram-positive bacteria. If there is coordinated expression of virulence factors by bacteria, they may allow bacteria to grow in various sites in the host (e.g., abscess, pneumonia) and thereby protect from host defenses.

Biofilms: Some bacteria form interactive colonies and form a **viscous layer of extracellular polysaccharide matrix** called biofilm. This slimy coating on solid surfaces **may be composed of a single species or several species**. These bacteria may be hidden and protected from the host's immune mechanisms. These biofilms highly adhere to host tissues (plaque that forms on tooth enamel) or devices such as intravascular catheters and artificial joints. **Biofilms increase the virulence of bacteria** by protecting the microbes from immune mechanisms as well as increase their resistance to antimicrobial drugs. Biofilm formation appears to be significant in the persistence and relapse of bacterial endocarditis, artificial joint infections, and respiratory infections in individuals with cystic fibrosis.

Bacterial adherence to host cells

Bacteria attach to host cells and tissues by using various structures on their surface.

Adhesins: These are adhesive structure proteins present on the surface of bacteria. They attach the bacteria to host cells or extracellular matrix. **Adhesion is a specific reaction between surface receptors on the host cells and ligands on the surface of bacteria**. Adhesins have a wide range of host cell specificity. For example, *Streptococcus pyogenes* attaches to host tissues by adhesins protein F and teichoic acid. These adhesins present on the surface of the bacterial cell wall and attach to fibronectin present on the surface of host cells and in the extracellular matrix. Adhesins serve as virulence factors and loss of adhesins usually results in converting the bacteria into avirulent form.

Pili (fimbria): These are filamentous (hair-like) structures that project from the surface of bacteria and they act as adhesins. They act as virulence factor and promote attachment to host cells and inhibit phagocytosis. The stalks of pili are consisting of repeating protein (peptide) subunits (pilins) consisting of conserved (constant) and variable regions in tip. The tip consists of variable fibrillum and undergo antigenic and phase variation. This tip is responsible for the tissue-binding specificity of the bacteria. For example, *E. coli* that causes urinary tract infections expresses tip fibrillum that has tissue-tropism for urinary tract epithelium. In the urinary bladder, its tip fibrillum binds to d-mannosylated receptors on bladder epithelium, and in the renal epithelium it binds to galabiose-containing glycosphingolipids. Pili can act as targets of the host antibody response. Some bacteria (e.g., *N. gonorrhoeae*) vary their pili so that they can avoid the attack by host immune system.

Intracellular bacteria

Mechanism of entry of bacteria into host cells: Bacteria have developed many mechanisms to enter the host cells. Some bacteria use receptors on cells such as macrophages that are important in the host immune response and through these receptors they gain entry. *M. tuberculosis* enters macrophages by using receptors for opsonins (antibodies and C3b) and other poorly defined nonopsonic receptors. Few gram-negative bacteria enter epithelial cells through type III secretion system. This secretion system consists of needle-like structures projecting from the surface of bacteria and they attach to host cells. Then these proteins create pores in the membrane of host cell and inject bacterial proteins into the cell. These bacterial proteins cause rearrangement of the cytoskeleton of host cell in a manner that favors entry of bacteria into the host cell.

Consequences of entry of bacteria into host cells: After bacteria enter into the host cell, the fate of bacteria as well as the infected host cell varies and it mainly depends on the type of organism.

- **Lysis of host cells:** *Shigella* species and *E. coli*—they inhibit the synthesis of host protein, replicate rapidly, and lyse the host cell within hours.
- **Killing of bacteria:** Most bacteria are phagocytosed (ingested) and forms the phagosome within the phagocytic cells (e.g., macrophage). Phagosome fuses with an acidic lysosome to form a phagolysosome. The lytic enzymes of lysosomes kill the bacteria within macrophages.
- **Blockage of phagolysosome formation:** Some bacteria escape the destruction by phagocytosis. For example, *M. tuberculosis* blocks fusion of the lysosome with the phagosome. This leads to their continuous proliferation within the macrophage.
- **Exit from phagosome into cytosol:** Some bacteria prevent their destruction in macrophages by leaving the phagosome and entering the cytoplasm of macrophage. For example, *L. monocytogenes* (refer page 635) produces a pore-forming protein called listeriolysin O and two phospholipases. They destroy the membrane of phagosome and allow the bacterium to enter into the cytoplasm. Thus, they are protected from the killing mechanisms of macrophages. In the cytoplasm of macrophages, *L. monocytogenes* alters the actin cytoskeleton so that it promotes direct spreading of the bacteria into neighboring healthy cells.

Advantages of intracellular bacteria: The growth of bacteria inside cells has certain advantages.

- **Escape from immune system:** These bacteria can escape from certain effector mechanisms of the immune response (e.g., antibodies and complement).
- **Spread of bacteria:** This also helps the spread of the bacteria. For example, spread can occur by the transport of infected macrophages carrying *M. tuberculosis* from the lung to draining regional lymph nodes and other more distant sites.

Bacterial toxins

Toxin Toxin is **bacterial substance that produces illness**. Toxins are classified as endotoxin and exotoxins. Endotoxin is a component of the gram-negative bacterial cell whereas exotoxins are proteins that are secreted by bacteria.

Bacterial endotoxin: It is a **heat stable lipopolysaccharide (LPS) or endotoxins present in the outer membrane of cell wall of gram-negative bacteria. These toxins can stimulate host immune responses as well as cause injury to the host.**

- **Lipid A:** It is the core of LPS. Toxicity of endotoxin of LPS depends on lipid component namely lipid A. It is the part of LPS that attaches the molecule in the host cell membrane. They are not secreted outside the wall of bacteria and are released only by disintegration of cell wall.
- **Binding:** LPS attaches to the cell-surface receptor CD14. They form LPS/CD14 complex and then binds to TLR4.
- **Other molecules** present in the outer surface of gram-positive bacteria can have similar effects to that of LPS (e.g., lipoteichoic acid binds to TLR2).
- **Beneficial effects of lipid A or lipoteichoic acid:** The response by the host to lipid A or lipoteichoic acid of bacteria is beneficial to the host. It activates protective immunity in many ways:
    - Stimulates the production of important cytokines and chemoattractants (chemokines) by immune cells.
    - Increases the expression of costimulatory molecules. This increases activation of T-lymphocyte.
- **Role in septic shock:** High levels of endotoxin play role in the pathogenesis of septic shock, disseminated intravascular coagulation (DIC), and acute respiratory distress syndrome. This is mainly by release of primary inflammatory mediators namely cytokines [e.g., TNF, interleukin-1 (IL-1), IL-6, and IL-12]. LPS activates complement, coagulation, fibrinolysis and bradykinin systems.

Exotoxins: These are **proteins secreted by bacteria and cause cellular injury and disease**. Exotoxins can damage human cells, either at the site of bacterial growth or at distant sites. Exotoxins are usually named according to their site or mechanism of activity. Thus, toxins that act on the nervous system are **neurotoxins;** those that affect intestinal cells are **enterotoxins**. Some toxins that kill target cells, such as diphtheria toxin or some of the *Clostridium perfringens* toxins, and are termed as **cytotoxins.** According to their mechanism of action, they can be classified into mainly three categories.

1. **Enzymes:** Bacteria secrete many different enzymes such as proteases, hyaluronidases, coagulases, and fibrinolysins. These enzymes act on substrates in host tissues or on host cells. These enzymes can cause destruction of tissue and lead to formation of abscess. For example, *S. aureus*

produce an exfoliative toxin and causes a disease known as staphylococcal scalded skin syndrome. In this the toxin degrades proteins that hold keratinocytes together and causes detachment of the epidermis from the deeper skin.

2. **Toxins that alter intracellular signaling or regulatory pathways:** These types of exotoxins are caked A-B toxins. They usually consist of two subunits namely—an active (A) subunit with enzymatic activity and a binding (B) subunit that binds to receptors on the cell surface. The binding (B) subunit transports the A subunit into the cell cytoplasm. The effects of these toxins depend on the binding specificity of the subunit B and the cellular pathways affected by the subunit A. This type of A-B toxins is produced by many bacteria such as *Bacillus anthracis, V. cholerae,* and some strains of *E. coli.*
3. **Neurotoxins:** These are A-B toxins produced by *Clostridium botulinum, Clostridium perfringens,* and *Clostridium tetani.* They prevent the release of neurotransmitters and causes paralysis. The A subunit binds specifically with proteins involved in secretion of neurotransmitters at the synaptic junction. They do not damage neurons. Tetanus and botulism are deadliest diseases that can produce death from respiratory failure by paralyzing the muscles of the chest and diaphragm.

Superantigens: These are the type of bacterial toxins that have an affinity for the T-cell receptor of T cells. This stimulates a large number of T lymphocytes leading to massive (enhanced) proliferation of T-lymphocyte (as many as 20% of T cells respond, compared with 0.01% responding to the usual processed antigens). This difference is due to their ability of superantigens to recognize a relatively conserved region of the T-cell receptor. Activated T cells release inordinately large amounts of T-cell cytokines, such as IL-2, IFN-γ, and TNF-α. These cytokines can lead to SIRS.

SPECTRUM OF INFLAMMATORY RESPONSES TO INFECTION

Limited morphological patterns: Microbes infecting humans have numerous molecular diversity. However, the tissue responses produced by host to these microbes show limited number of morphological patterns as well as mechanisms producing these responses. Many pathogens produce similar morphological patterns of reaction and only few microorganisms show unique or pathognomonic features.

Immune status and morphological response: Sometimes the immune status of the host decides the histopathological changes of the inflammatory response to microbes. For example, pyogenic bacteria in a normal host cause intense leukocyte responses, whereas it may produce necrosis of tissue with minimal leukocyte exudation in a patient with severe neutropenia. *M. tuberculosis* in a patient without immunocompromise produces a well-formed granuloma with few mycobacteria, whereas in a patient with AIDS, it multiplies in large numbers inside the macrophages without producing granulomas.

Major Histologic Patterns

There are five major histologic patterns of tissue reaction in infections **(Table 3)**.

Table 3: Summary of spectrum of inflammatory responses to infection.

Type of tissue response	*Pathogenesis*	*Examples*
Suppurative (purulent) infection	• Increased vascular permeability • Chemoattractants from bacteria lead to leukocyte infiltration (mainly neutrophils) • Formation of "pus	Pneumonia *(Staphylococcus aureus)* Abscesses (*Staphylococcus* species, anaerobic and other bacteria)
Mononuclear and granulomatous inflammation		
Mononuclear Inflammation	Mononuclear infiltrates (monocytes, macrophages, plasma cells, lymphocytes)	Syphilis
Granulomatous Inflammation	Cell-mediated immune response to pathogens ("persistent antigen") and formation of granulomata	Tuberculosis, tuberculoid leprosy
Cytopathic-cytoproliferative reactions		
Cytopathic reactions	Necrosis or proliferation (including multinucleation) of host cells	Chicken pox, shingles
Cytoproliferative reactions	Viral transformation of cells	Cervical cancer (human papillomavirus)
Tissue necrosis	• Toxin mediated tissue destruction • Lack of inflammatory cells • Rapid progression	• Gangrene *(Clostridium perfringens)* • Hepatitis (hepatitis B virus)
Chronic inflammation or scarring	• Repetitive injury leads to fibrosis • Loss of normal parenchyma	Chronic hepatitis with cirrhosis (hepatitis B and C viruses)
No inflammatory reaction	Severe immune compromised individuals	• *Mycobacterium avium* in untreated AIDS (T-cell deficiency) • Mucormycosis in bone marrow transplant patients (neutropenia)

Suppurative (Purulent) Inflammation

- **Features:** Suppurative inflammation is characterized by **increased vascular permeability and leukocytic infiltration, predominantly of neutrophils**.
- **Pyogenic bacteria:** Chemoattractants released from the "pyogenic" (pus-forming) bacteria attract numerous neutrophils to the site of infection. The pyogenic bacteria include mainly **gram-positive cocci and gram-negative rods**.
- **Morphology:** It shows **pus consisting of collections of numerous dying and dead neutrophils and liquefactive necrosis** of the tissue involved. The sizes of suppurative or purulent lesions range from tiny multiple microabscesses to diffuse involvement. Microabscess may form in multiple organs during bacterial dissemination secondary to an infected vegetation in heart valve. Diffuse involvement may involve of large portion of the organs such as entire lobes of the lung in pneumonia.
- **Pattern of damage:** The degree of tissue destruction depends on the location of infection and the infective organism. Examples are as follows:
    - **Type of infective organism:** *S. pneumoniae* causes lobar pneumonia that can completely resolve without involving the alveolar walls, whereas *S. aureus* and *Klebsiella pneumoniae* damage alveolar walls and form abscesses which may heal with formation of scar.
    - **Location of infection:** Bacterial pharyngitis *(S. pyogenes)* can resolve without sequelae, whereas acute bacterial inflammation of a joint if not treated immediately can cause destruction of the joint.

Mononuclear and Granulomatous Inflammation

- **Features:** It is characterized by **diffuse, interstitial infiltrates mainly mononuclear cells**. They are a common feature of all chronic inflammatory processes. They usually occur as acute response to viruses, intracellular bacteria, or intracellular parasites and as chronic inflammatory response to spirochetes and helminths.
- **Type of mononuclear cells:** The type of predominant mononuclear cell in the inflammatory lesion depends on the host immune response to the organism. Examples are as follows:
    - **Plasma cells** are predominant cells in the lesions of **primary and secondary syphilis**.
    - **Lymphocytes** predominate in **HBV infection or viral infections of the brain**. These lymphocytes reflect cell-mediated immune responses against the pathogen or pathogen-infected cells.
    - **Macrophages:** In some infections macrophages may become filled with organisms. For example, in *M. avium* complex infections in AIDS patients, they cannot mount an effective immune response to the organisms and the organisms fill the macrophages.

Granulomatous inflammation

It is a distinctive form of mononuclear inflammation characterized by formation of granulomas. Granulomatous inflammation is characterized by circumscribed accumulation and aggregation of activated modified macrophages called "epithelioid" (called so because morphologically they resemble epithelial cells). Some of the macrophages may fuse to form giant cells. Granulomas may show a central area of caseous necrosis. Granulomatous inflammation usually occurs in response to infectious agents that resist eradication and are capable of stimulating strong T cell-mediated immunity (e.g., *M. tuberculosis, Histoplasma capsulatum*, schistosome eggs).

Cytopathic-cytoproliferative Reaction

Features: These morphological reactions are characterized by **necrosis of cells** (cytopathic) **or proliferation of cells** (cytoproliferative). It usually has scanty inflammatory cells. These morphological reactions are usually found in infection by viruses.

- **Inclusion bodies or multinucleated cells:** Some viruses replicate within host cells and form viral aggregates that may be seen as inclusion bodies (e.g., herpes viruses or adenovirus) or the viruses may induce the host cells to fuse and form multinucleated cells called *polykaryons* (e.g., measles virus or herpes viruses).
- **Formation of blisters:** Some viruses may produce focal cell damage in the skin resulting in detachment of epithelial cells to form blisters.
- **Cytoproliferation:** Some viruses can stimulate epithelial cells to proliferate (e.g., venereal warts caused by HPV or the umbilicated papules of molluscum contagiosum caused by poxviruses).
- **Neoplastic transformation:** Some viruses can lead to formation of malignant neoplasms.

Tissue Necrosis

- **Features:** It is characterized by severe necrosis (gangrenous necrosis) and tissue damage.
- **Causes:** It is usually observed in infections due to *C. perfringens* and other organisms such as *Corynebacterium diphtheriae* that secrete powerful toxins. The parasite *E. histolytica* causes ulcers in the colon and liver abscesses. These are characterized by extensive tissue destruction with liquefactive necrosis and little inflammatory infiltrate. Some viruses can cause widespread and severe necrosis of host cells associated with inflammation (e.g., total destruction of the temporal lobes of the brain by HSV or the massive necrosis liver by HBV).

Chronic Inflammation and Scarring

Features: Many infections can produce chronic inflammation. These inflammations can either heal completely or produce extensive scarring.

Examples: These include the following:

- Chronic HBV infection of liver may cause extensive scarring leading to **cirrhosis of the liver**. Cirrhosis is characterized by complete loss of normal liver architecture in which dense fibrous tissue surrounds the nodules of regenerating hepatocytes.
- **Fibrosis of the liver or fibrosis of the urinary bladder** wall may be rarely caused by eggs of *Schistosoma haematobium.*
- **Constrictive fibrous pericarditis** may occur in tuberculosis.
- **Lung in patients with AIDS:** *Pneumocystis* species, causes interstitial inflammation whereas infection with CMV causes cytolytic changes.
- Physical or chemical agents.

Spectrum of inflammatory responses to infection is summarized in **Table 3**.

11.2 Viral Infections

CHAPTER OUTLINE

General Features

Viruses can be divided into ribonucleic acid (RNA) or deoxyribonucleic acid (DNA) virus depending on the presence of RNA or DNA. They range from 20 to 300 nm. Depending on the type, they consist of either RNA or DNA that is surrounded by a protein shell. Some also have envelope of lipid membranes. **Viruses do not metabolize or reproduce independently. Thus, they are obligate intracellular parasites and need living cells for their replication.** Once they invade the cells, they divert or hijack the intracellular biosynthetic and metabolic pathways and synthesize virus-encoded nucleic acids and proteins.

Killing or interfering with the function of infected cells: Viruses usually produce disease by killing infected host cells. However, it may produce disease without destroying cells. For example, rotavirus is a common cause of diarrhea. It interferes with the function of infected enterocytes by preventing enterocytes from synthesizing proteins that transport molecules from the intestinal lumen. Thus, it produces diarrhea without immediately killing the enterocytes.

Release of mediators: Viruses may promote release of chemical mediators thereby eliciting inflammatory or immunologic responses. For example, the symptoms of the common cold are due to release of bradykinin from infected cells.

Cell proliferation: Some viruses may cause proliferation of cells to form tumors. For example, human papillomaviruses (HPVs) can cause proliferative lesions squamous cell (e.g., common warts and cervical carcinoma).

Latency: Some viruses infect and persist within the cells without interfering with cellular functions. This process is termed as **latency**. These latent viruses may produce disease years after a primary infection. Opportunistic infections may be due to reactivation of latent virus infections. Cytomegalovirus (CMV) and herpes simplex viruses (HSVs) are commonly present as latent agents. They produce disease when the individuals develop impairment in the cell-mediated immunity.

Episomal form or integration into genome of host cell: Some viruses may be present within host cells and they may be either integrated into host genomes or may remain in an episomal form. Viruses that get integrated into the genome of host cell can produce tumors in such host cells. For example, Epstein–Barr virus (EBV) causes endemic Burkitt lymphoma in Africa and other tumors. Human T-cell leukemia virus-1 (HTLV-1) causes a form of T-cell leukemia/lymphoma.

Viruses can cause many clinically important acute and chronic infections. They may affect almost every organ system and few selected human viruses and the disease produced is presented in **Table 4**.

Classification of viruses: Viruses may be classified as RNA viruses or DNA viruses depending on the nucleic acid content. RNA viruses usually follow different paths to cause disease than most of the DNA viruses. RNA viruses require different enzymes for their infectious cycles, and differ in their biology than DNA viruses. One of the main differences between some RNA viruses and many DNA viruses is that the polymerases present in some important pathogenic RNA viruses [e.g., human immunodeficiency virus-1 (HIV-1), hepatitis C virus (HCV)] and they do not proofread the strand being synthesized. Two important consequences of this are: (1) the mutation rate is very high and (2) major proportion of daughter virions is inactive. Examples of RNA and DNA viruses causing infectious disease in humans are presented in **Table 5**. Sizes of various human DNA and RNA viruses in comparison with *Escherichia Coli* are shown in **Figure 4**.

ACUTE (TRANSIENT) INFECTIONS

The viruses causing acute transient infections elicit effective immune responses. This response destroys the virus and thereby limits the durations of these viral infections. These viruses are structurally heterogeneous. They may show widely different degrees of genetic diversity. This is responsible for

Table 4: Examples of viruses and viral diseases in human.

Species	*Disease*
Systemic with skin eruptions	
• Measles virus	Measles (rubella)
• Rubella virus	German measles (rubella)
• Varicella-zoster virus	Chickenpox, shingles
• Herpes simplex virus 1	Oral herpes ("cold sore")
• Herpes simplex virus 2	Genital herpes
Systemic with hematologic disorders	
• Cytomegalovirus	Cytomegalic inclusion disease
• Epstein–Barr virus	Infectious mononucleosis
• Human immunodeficiency viruses 1 and 2	Acquired immunodeficiency syndrome
Arboviral and hemorrhagic fevers	
• Dengue viruses 1 to 4	Dengue hemorrhagic fever
• Yellow fever virus	Yellow fever
• Skin/genital warts	Human papillomavirus condyloma; cervical carcinoma
Central nervous system	
• Poliovirus	Poliomyelitis
• JC virus	Progressive multifocal leuko-encephalopathy (opportunistic)
Respiratory System	
• Adenovirus	Upper and lower respiratory tract infections Conjunctivitis Diarrhea
• Rhinovirus	Upper respiratory tract infection
• Influenza viruses A, B	Influenza
• Respiratory syncytial virus	Bronchiolitis Pneumonia
Digestive tract	
• Mumps virus	Mumps Pancreatitis Orchitis
• Rotavirus	Childhood gastroenteritis
• Norovirus	Gastroenteritis
Liver	
• Hepatitis A virus (HAV)	Acute viral hepatitis
• Hepatitis B virus (HBV)	Acute or chronic hepatitis
• Hepatitis D virus (HDV)	With hepatitis B virus, acute or chronic hepatitis
• Hepatitis C virus (HCV)	Acute or chronic hepatitis
• Hepatitis E virus (HEV)	Acute viral hepatitis

Table 5: Examples of RNA and DNA viruses causing infectious disease in humans.

RNA viruses	*DNA viruses*
• **Respiratory viruses** ○ The common cold ○ Influenza ○ Parainfluenza virus ○ Respiratory syncytial virus ○ Severe acute respiratory syndrome (SARS) ○ Associated coronavirus • **Viral exanthems** ○ Measles (Rubella) ○ Rubella • **Mumps** • **Intestinal virus infections** ○ Rotavirus infection ○ Norwalk virus and other viral diarrheas • **Viral hemorrhagic fevers** ○ Yellow fever ○ Ebola hemorrhagic fever ○ West Nile virus	**Adenovirus** • **Human parvovirus (erythrovirus) B19** • **Smallpox (variola)** • **Monkeypox** • **Herpesviruses** ○ Varicella-zoster virus ○ Herpes simplex virus • **Epstein–Barr virus** • **Cytomegalovirus** • **Human papillomavirus**

(DNA: deoxyribonucleic acid; RNA: ribonucleic acid)

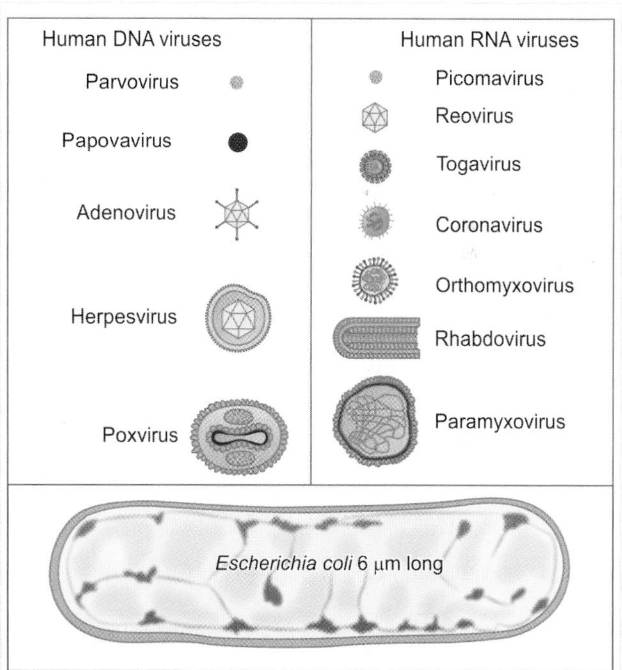

(DNA: deoxyribonucleic acid; RNA: ribonucleic acid)

FIG. 4: Sizes of various human DNA and RNA viruses in comparison with *Escherichia Coli* (bacteria).

the susceptibility of the host to reinfection by viruses of the same type but with different genetic subtype. For example, the mumps virus has only one genetic subtype and infects an individual only once. Influenza viruses can repeatedly infect the same individual because of periodic development of new genetic variants. Immunity to some viruses (e.g., viruses infecting respiratory and gastrointestinal tract) wanes with time. This also allows the same virus to infect the host repeatedly.

A viral exanthema is an eruptive skin rash and usually due to a viral infection. Examples include measles, mumps, rubella, and chickenpox.

Measles (Rubella)

Measles is an **acute viral infection** caused by measles (rubella) virus. Measles virus is an enveloped, single-stranded RNA virus of the paramyxovirus family. Paramyxoviridae family also includes respiratory syncytial virus (RSV), parainfluenza virus (a cause of croup), and *Human metapneumovirus*. There is only one serotype of measles virus.

- **Mode of transmission:** Measles virus is transmitted by the airborne route via respiratory droplets (aerosols) and secretions.
- Measles can be prevented by currently available live, attenuated vaccine. It is highly effective in both preventing and eliminating spread of virus spread. Epidemics of measles occur among unvaccinated individuals. Among nonimmunized individuals, it primarily affects children. C vaccines.
- **Incubation period:** 9–11 days.

Pathogenesis

Cell-surface receptors: There are three cell-surface receptors for measles hemagglutinin protein.

1. **Signaling lymphocytic activation molecule family member 1 (SLAMF1):** It is expressed on activated lymphocytes, dendritic cells, and monocytes. It is the initial receptor for viral infection.
2. **Nectin-4:** It is expressed on the basal surface of epithelial cells. It is needed for replication of the virus within the respiratory tract, before the virus spreads in respiratory secretions.
3. **CD46:** It was used only by culture-adapted virus (including the vaccine strain), and not wild-type virus.

The initial site of infection by measles virus is the mucous membranes of the nasopharynx and bronchi.

- Measles can replicate in many cell types such as epithelial cells and leukocytes. Initially, virus replicates (multiplies) within the respiratory tract. Then it spreads to local lymphoid tissues of the respiratory tract. It is followed by viremia and systemic dissemination of virus to many tissues. Main tissues involved are conjunctiva, skin, respiratory tract, urinary tract, small blood vessels, lymphatic system, and central nervous system (CNS).

Diseases produced: Measles virus causes a wide range of disease ranging from mild, acute, self-limited infections to severe systemic manifestations. It can produce severe disease in patients with defects in cellular immunity (e.g., with HIV or hematologic malignancy), in the very young, the sick or the malnourished individuals.

- Majority of children develop T-cell–mediated immunity to the virus. This helps to control the viral infection and is responsible for the production of the measles rash. Therefore, the measles rash is less common in patients with deficiencies in cell-mediated immunity. Measles rash is due to the action of T lymphocytes on virally infected vascular endothelium.
- In malnourished children, it may cause croup, pneumonia, diarrhea and protein-losing enteropathy, keratitis (producing scarring and blindness), encephalitis, and hemorrhagic rashes ("black measles").
- Antibody-mediated immunity against measles virus protects against reinfection.

Immunosuppression: Measles can produce transient but severe immunosuppression. This can lead to secondary bacterial and viral infections. This is responsible for morbidity and mortality that are associated with measles. There may be reduced delayed-type hypersensitivity responses and reduction in lymphocyte responses. This may be due to inhibition of the ability of infected dendritic cells to stimulate lymphocytes.

MORPHOLOGY

Measles virus causes an acute disease, characterized by upper respiratory tract symptoms, fever, and rash.

Organs affected: Measles **affects multiple organs.**

- **Measles skin rash (Fig. 5B):** It is blotchy, reddish-brown. Skin lesions begin on the face which usually spreads to trunk, and proximal extremities. It is produced by dilated blood vessels of skin, edema, and a mononuclear (lymphocytic) perivascular infiltrate.
- **Koplik spots (Fig. 5A):** These are **pathognomonic mucosal lesions of measles**. It consists of ulcerated mucosal lesions in the oral cavity on the posterior buccal mucosa near the opening of the Stensen (parotid) ducts. They appear as small, irregular, bluish-white dots on a red base measuring 1 mm in diameter surrounded by erythema. It shows **necrosis, neutrophilic exudate, and neovascularization**.

Continued

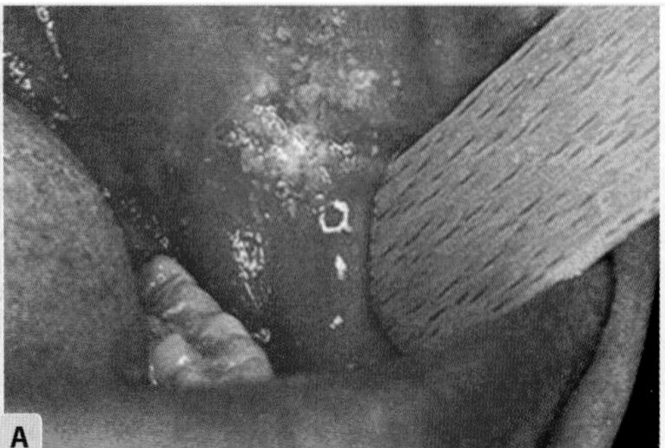

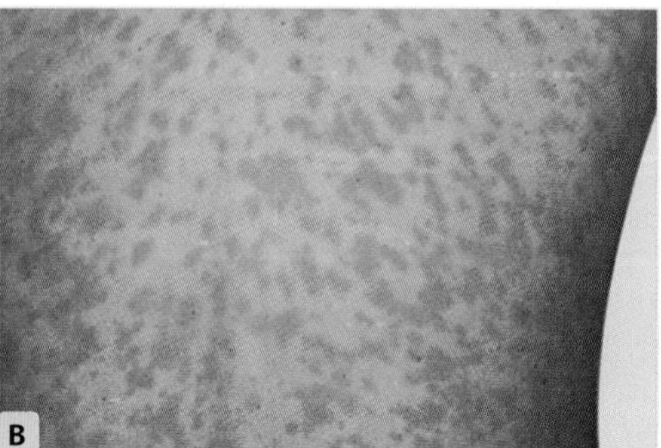

FIGS. 5A AND B: (A) Koplik spots—pathognomonic of measles which appears as greyish white dots on the buccal mucosa; (B) maculopapular rashes in measles.

Continued

- **Lymphoid organs-Warthin-Finkeldey cells:** Lymphoid organs (e.g., cervical and mesenteric lymph nodes, spleen, and appendix) show marked follicular hyperplasia, with prominent enlarged germinal centers. There are **randomly distributed multinucleate giant cells** containing up to 100 nuclei, called **Warthin-Finkeldey giant cells (pathognomonic of measles)**. These giant cells are **formed due to fusion of infected cells** and have eosinophilic both intranuclear and intracytoplasmic inclusion bodies. These are also seen in the lung and sputum.
- **Pneumonia:** Mild types of measles pneumonia show peribronchial and interstitial mononuclear cell infiltration. It is similar to other nonlethal viral infections.

Clinical Features

Measles presents with fever, rhinorrhea, cough, and conjunctivitis. It progresses to produce characteristic lesions in mucosa and skin. The rash fades within 3–5 days, and symptoms gradually resolve.

Complications: Its clinical course may be much more severe in very young, malnourished, or immunocompromised individuals.

- **Secondary bacterial infections:** For example, otitis media and pneumonia.
- **Late complications:** In immunocompromised patients, rare late complications years after a measles infection and include:
    - Subacute sclerosing panencephalitis (SSPE): It is slow, chronic neurodegenerative disorder. The exact pathophysiology of SSPE is not known.
    - Measles inclusion body encephalitis.

Diagnosis: It is by clinical features, by serology, or by detection of viral antigen in nasal exudates or by detection of viral RNA in respiratory secretions or urinary sediments.

Mumps

Mumps virus: Mumps is an acute systemic viral infection causes by mumps virus. Like measles virus, mumps virus is a member of the Paramyxoviridae family. Mumps virus is an enveloped, single-stranded RNA virus. Mumps virus contains two types of surface glycoproteins with following activities namely:

1. Hemagglutinin and neuraminidase activities
2. Cell fusion and cytolytic activities.

Mumps virus is **highly contagious and primarily infects children**. It causes an **acute, self-limited systemic illness**, characterized by **pain and swelling of the salivary glands** (mainly parotid gland) and meningoencephalitis.

Mode of spread: The virus is transmitted by the respiratory route (1) by droplet infection (through inhalation), (2) by direct contact with respiratory droplets, or (3) through saliva and fomites. **Humans are the only natural hosts** of the mumps virus. The peak infectivity is 2–3 days before the onset of the parotitis and for 3 days afterwards. Mumps viruses enter the upper respiratory tract of or contact. About 90% of the exposed individuals become infected, though only about 65% develop symptoms. Vaccination by a live attenuated mumps vaccine prevents mumps, and it has been eliminated from most developed countries.

Incubation period is about 15–20 days (average 18 days).

Pathogenesis

After inhalation of mumps virus or contact with respiratory droplets containing mumps virus, it enters the upper respiratory tract and infects the respiratory tract epithelium. From there, it spread to draining lymph nodes. In the lymph node, the virus replicates in lymphocytes (preferentially in activated T cells), and then spreads through the blood to other sites. The most commonly involved sites are the salivary glands (especially parotids), CNS, pancreas, testes, and ovary. Epididymo-orchitis develops in 20% of males infected after puberty. Aseptic meningitis is the most common extrasalivary gland complication of mumps and occurs in about 10–15 % of cases.

MORPHOLOGY

Mumps parotitis: Mumps involves mainly parotid salivary glands. It is bilateral in about 70% of patients. This produces pain and swelling of salivary glands.

- **Gross:** The involved glands are enlarged, moist, glistening, and have a doughy consistency. On cut section, they are reddish-brown in color.
- **Microscopy:** The interstitium of salivary gland shows edema and diffuses infiltration by macrophages, lymphocytes, and plasma cells. The edema and inflammation compress the acini and ducts. Neutrophils and necrotic debris may fill the lumen of the salivary duct and cause focal necrosis and desquamation of involved lining epithelium.

Mumps orchitis/epididymo-orchitis: Mumps orchitis is usually unilateral. Testis may be markedly swollen (about three times of the normal size) due to edema, mononuclear cell infiltration, and focal hemorrhages. Because the testicular parenchyma is tightly confined within the tunica albuginea, swelling of testicular parenchyma may compromise the blood supply and produce focal areas of infarction. The testicular damage can produce scarring, atrophy, and, rarely if severe causes sterility.

Mumps pancreatitis: Mumps infection can damage of acinar cells of the pancreas. This may release digestive enzymes and produce parenchymal and fat necrosis and neutrophil-rich inflammation.

Mumps encephalitis: Mumps infection may produce perivenous demyelination and perivascular mononuclear cuffing.

Clinical Features

Primarily affects school-aged children and young adults (peaks at 5–9 years of age) and is uncommon before 2 years of age.

- **Prodromal symptoms:** Nonspecific and includes malaise, low-grade fever, myalgia, anorexia, headache, anorexia, and tenderness at the angle of the jaw.
- **Parotid gland enlargement:** Prodromal symptoms are followed by severe pain over the parotid glands due to parotitis. Parotitis produces either unilateral or bilateral

parotid swelling (75% of cases). It is accompanied by obliteration of the space between the earlobe and the angle of the mandible. The chief complaints at this stage are difficulty in eating, swallowing, and talking. Submandibular gland involvement is less frequent.

- **Mumps encephalitis/meningitis:** Symptomatic meningeal involvement usually presents with headache, stiff neck, and vomiting.
- **Mumps pancreatitis:** Severe pancreatitis is rare in mumps and some may develop type 1 diabetes mellitus. Patients show elevated serum amylase.

Diagnosis

The diagnosis is usually made on the basis of the clinical features. In atypical cases, diagnosis is confirmed by following investigations:

- **Serological test:** Demonstration of a mumps-specific immunoglobulin M (IgM) response in a blood or oral fluid during infection is diagnostic.
- **Demonstration virus:** Culture of virus or identification of viral RNA by genome polymerase chain reaction (PCR) or antigen detection assays, from saliva, throat swab, urine, and cerebrospinal fluid (CSF).

Poliomyelitis

Poliomyelitis is more **commonly known as polio**. The term poliomyelitis is used to describe **inflammation of the gray matter of the spinal cord** produced by an infection by poliovirus.

- **Poliovirus** is a small, spherical and has only a protein capsid without an envelope (unencapsulated/nonenveloped) single-stranded **RNA virus** belonging to the *Enterovirus* genus of *Picornaviridae* family. The term *Picornaviridae* comes from *pico* ("small" in Latin) and *RNA*. There are three serotypes of poliovirus and most infections are caused by type 1.
- **Polio vaccines:** There are two polio vaccines. The vaccines have eradicated polio in India.
    i. **Salk vaccine:** It is made of inactivated poliovirus (formalin fixed/killed) particles and Salk vaccine is also known as the inactivated polio vaccine (IPV). It is injected into muscle.
    ii. **Sabin or oral polio vaccine (OPV):** Sabin vaccine is made of live, but weakened (attenuated) poliovirus.
- Polio eradication was possible because (1) poliovirus infects only humans, (2) shows limited genetic variation, and (3) is effectively neutralized by antibodies produced by immunization. The inactivated (injected) poliovirus vaccine protects against all three serotypes. The attenuated (oral) poliovirus vaccine is available in various combinations of one, two, or all three serotypes. Currently used vaccine contains one or two serotypes.
- **Mode of infection:** Poliovirus infects only humans and is transmitted by the **fecal-oral route** (like other enteroviruses).
- **Incubation period:** About 10 days.

Pathogenesis

- The tough protein coat of polio virus protects it from stomach acid and allows it to reach and bind to intestinal cells. The polio virus infects human cells by binding to CD155, a molecule expressed on different cell types such as epithelial cells, lymphocytes, and neurons.
- The polio virus is ingested and replicates in the mucosa of the pharynx, tonsils, and gut (Peyer patches in the ileum).
- From the mucosa, it spreads through lymphatics to lymph nodes and to the blood. This produces transient viremia and fever. In nonimmunized patient, poliovirus infection causes a subclinical or mild gastroenteritis. Most poliovirus infections are asymptomatic and in about 1% of infected individuals poliovirus invades the CNS and enters motor neurons via binding sites on their plasma membranes and replicates in motor neurons of the spinal cord (spinal poliomyelitis) or brain stem (bulbar poliomyelitis).
- In most of the individuals, antiviral antibodies control the disease and it is not clear whether they fail to contain the virus in some individuals.
- Spread of virus to the nervous system may occur by any one of the two routes namely (1) through the blood or (2) by retrograde transport of the virus along axons of motor neurons.
- Rarely, poliomyelitis may develop after vaccination. This may be due to mutations in the attenuated viruses to revert to wild-type, virulent, and forms.

MORPHOLOGY

Spinal cord: Poliovirus is **cytolytic** and **causes rapid rupture of infected cell**. This lysis of infected neurons causes severe inflammation of the myelin, or myelitis. Hence, the disease is termed poliomyelitis.

Infected motor neuron cells may undergo chromatolysis. The chromatolysis is the dissolution of Nissl bodies in the neurons cell. After chromatolysis, these neuronal cells are phagocytosed by macrophages (neuronophagia). Acute cases of poliomyelitis show mononuclear cell (mainly lymphocyte) surround blood vessels forming perivascular cuffs in the spinal cord and brainstem. There is also neuronophagia in the anterior horn motor neurons of the spinal cord. The inflammatory reaction is usually found in the anterior horns and may extend into the posterior horns. Sometimes, the damage may be severe and produce cavitation. The motor cortex usually does not show inflammation but may contain microglial nodules. These nodules consist of focal collections of microglia and lymphocytes. In long-term survivors of symptomatic poliomyelitis and in cases of healed poliomyelitis, postmortem examination shows following changes:

1. Loss of neurons with secondary degeneration of corresponding ventral roots and peripheral nerves.
2. Gliosis in the affected anterior horns of the spinal cord.
3. Atrophy of the anterior (motor) spinal roots.
4. Neurogenic atrophy of denervated muscle.

Clinical Features

Poliovirus causes an acute systemic viral infection. It can produce a wide range of clinical manifestations ranging from mild, self-limited infections to paralysis of limb muscles and respiratory muscles.

- **Nonspecific symptoms:** These include fever and malaise.
- **Central nervous system infection:** It causes meningeal irritation and shows CSF features of aseptic meningitis.

The disease may not progress further or may progress to involve the spinal cord.

- **Spinal cord involvement:** When polio affects the motor neurons of the spinal cord, it destroys motor neurons and leads to flaccid (lacking in strength) paralysis. This is associated with wasting of muscle and hyporeflexia in the corresponding region of the body. This is the characteristic permanent neurologic residue of poliomyelitis. Patients with milder disease may show asymmetric and patchy paralysis, mainly involving the legs. Usually about a week after infection, improvement begins and only some of the muscles affected at the beginning may remain permanently paralyzed. When the destruction of motor neurons, paresis, or paralysis affects the diaphragm and intercostal muscles, it may produce severe paralysis of the respiratory muscles (with respiratory failure) and may be life-threatening. In severe cases, the muscles of the neck, trunk, and all four limbs may become powerless.
- **Postpolio syndrome:** It can occur in patients 25–35 years after resolution of the initial illness. Postpolio syndrome is progressive but is not usually life threatening. It is characterized by progressive weakness due to deterioration of muscle function and is associated with decreased mass of the muscle and serious pain in the body region where infection originally took place. This is due to superimposed loss of remaining motor neurons, without any viral reactivation. Postpolio syndrome is not infectious.
- **Myocarditis:** Sometimes myocarditis may develop as complication of the acute infection.

Diagnosis: It can be by viral culture or identification of viral RNA in throat secretions or, more usually in stool, or by serology. Reverse transcriptase PCR (RT-PCR) is used to detect the viral mRNA. Poliovirus RNA can also be detected in anterior horn cell motor neurons.

Various enteroviruses and diseases produced are presented in **Table 6**.

Table 6: Various enteroviruses and diseases produced.

Enterovirus	*Diseases produced*
Coxsackie virus A	Childhood diarrhea and rashes
Enterovirus 70	Conjunctivitis
Coxsackie viruses and echovirus	Viral meningitis
Coxsackie virus B	Myopericarditis

Rabies

Rabies is a viral disease causing **severe encephalitis.** Rabies virus is an enveloped, single-stranded RNA virus belonging to the rhabdovirus (Greek for "rod-shaped") group. **Rabies virus is sensitive to and killed by ethanol, iodine preparations, and soap detergents**.

Natural reservoirs: The main reservoirs of rabies virus include dogs, and various wild mammals such as wolves, foxes, and skunks. Bats and domestic animals, including cattle, goats and swine, also carry the disease.

Mode of transmission: Rabies is a classical **zoonosis,** i.e., a disease passed from animals to humans. It is transmitted to humans via contaminated saliva, introduced by the **bite of a rabid animal (usually a dog)**. It has also been noticed that exposure to certain species of bats can also cause rabies even without a known bite. Iatrogenic transmission has been reported via corneal, solid organ, and tendon transplants.

Incubation period usually ranges from **1 to 3 months** and it depends on the distance between the wound and the brain. It may be extremely short as 10 days or long as 18 months.

Pathogenesis

- At first, the rabies virus slowly replicates in the muscle cells at the wound site (bite of a rabid animal) and then enters a peripheral nerve. Once it reaches the peripheral nervous system (PNS), it is rapidly transported through neurons by retrograde axoplasmic flow to the spinal cord and brain. Rabies virus hijacks a cellular transport system down the axon that usually carries neurotransmitters. This helps in speeding its spread from neuron to neuron. After invading brain cells, rabies virus spreads back out into the PNS to reach the salivary glands and other organs.
- Unlike poliovirus, rabies virus does not produce lysis of host cells.
- Symptoms of rabies, symptoms are due to the ability of the virus to shut down normal neuron functioning. Apoptosis, is seen very late in the disease, indicating that the immune system cannot react in time to stop the virus.
- Virus replicates and is shed from tissues that are well supplied with nerves, including the salivary glands. This is responsible for so easy transmission of rabies through bites.

MORPHOLOGY

Gross

External examination of the brain shows edema and vascular congestion.

Microscopy

- It shows widespread neuronal degeneration and an inflammatory reaction. Inflammation is most severe mainly in the brainstem and can also be seen in the cerebellum and hypothalamus. Also there is perivascular collection of lymphocytes, scattered neurons with chromatolysis, and neuronophagia and microglial nodules.
- **Negri bodies:** These are the **pathognomonic microscopic features and confirm the diagnosis of rabies.** These Negri bodies are cytoplasmic, round to oval, eosinophilic inclusions (**Figs. 6A and C**), and represent small clusters of virus inside the neurons. They can be found in pyramidal neurons of the hippocampus and Purkinje cells of the cerebellum. Rabies virus can be identified within the Negri bodies by ultrastructural and immunohistochemical methods (**Fig. 6B**).

Clinical Features

- **Nonspecific symptoms:** Rabies presents with nonspecific symptoms such as malaise, headache, and fever. **Local paresthesia around the wound** along with above symptoms is diagnostic of rabies.

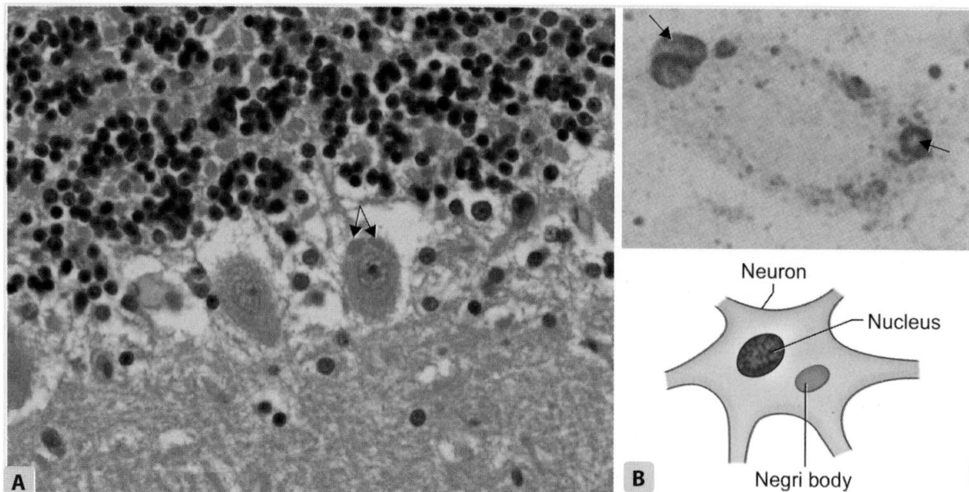

FIGS. 6A TO C: (A) Neuron with cytoplasmic inclusions (Negri bodies) in rabies (H&E); (B) immunohistochemistry showing rabies-infected neuronal cell with rabies virus antigen and intracytoplasmic inclusion; and (C) diagrammatic appearance of neuron with Negri body in rabies.

- **Central nervous system excitability:** As the infection progresses, patient develops severe CNS excitability. The slightest touch is painful and causes violent motor responses or produce convulsions. Signs of meningeal irritation and flaccid paralysis may develop as the disease progresses.
- **Hydrophobia:** Destruction of neurons of the brainstem by rabies virus causes painful spasms of the throat, contracture of the pharyngeal muscles on swallowing causing difficulty in swallowing and produces foaming at the mouth with a tendency to aspirate fluids. This causes aversion/fear to swallow even water (original name, hydrophobia).
- After the development of symptoms, the disease relentlessly progresses and produces coma and death from respiratory failure within 1 to several weeks.
- **Postexposure prophylaxis:** Patients who suspect exposure to rabies are injected with both antirabies antibodies (hyperimmune globulin) and the inactivated (killed-virus) rabies vaccine for rabies.
- **Cerebrospinal fluid findings:** These include (1) a moderate increase in lymphocytes, (2) a moderate rise in protein level, and (3) unaltered level of glucose and CSF pressure.
- **Diagnosis:**
  - Infected animals: Tested using direct antibody fluorescence after a human is bitten.
  - Diagnosis in humans: It is done by RT-PCR.
  - Postmortem diagnosis: By demonstration of Negri bodies in brain tissue.

West Nile Virus Infections

West Nile virus (WNV) is an enveloped, single-stranded RNA, arbovirus (named for arthropod-borne) and is a member of Flaviviridae family. *Flavivirus* group also includes viruses that cause dengue fever and yellow fever.

Arboviruses: They belong to different families and different arboviruses have different reservoir species and geographic distribution. But they share key similarities namely, all arboviruses are:
- Enveloped, single-stranded RNA viruses
- Transmitted by arthropods such as mosquitoes or ticks.

Mode of transmission: WNV is transmitted by mosquitoes. The mosquitoes become infected with the WNV upon taking a blood meal from an infected reservoir, usually an infected bird. Infected birds develop prolonged viremia and are the main reservoir for the WNV. When infected mosquitoes feed on animals/mammals, some of the viruses already present in their stomachs regurgitate into the bite of the latest victim. Thus the virus is passed from one animal to another.

Humans are considered a "dead-end host" or incidental hosts. This is because the humans have low number of virus particles in the blood and are unlikely that a mosquito would become infected from a human blood meal. Most affected patients develop infection following a mosquito bite. Less commonly, human-to-human transmission may occur following blood transfusion, organ transplantation, breastfeeding, or transplacental spread.

Incubation period: It ranges from 3 to 15 days.

Pathogenesis

After inoculation of WNV into human by a mosquito, the virus replicates in dendritic cells of the skin and then carried to lymph nodes. In the lymph node, the virus further undergoes replication and then carried into the bloodstream. In some individuals, the viruses cross the blood-brain barrier and infect neurons in the CNS. After replication or by triggering apoptosis, WNV lyses and damages neurons

MORPHOLOGY

Brain shows mononuclear meningoencephalitis or encephalitis. The brainstem, mainly the medulla may show extensive involvement.

Microscopically, it shows perivascular and leptomeningeal chronic inflammation, varying degrees of neuronal necrosis in gray matter, neuronal degeneration, microglial nodules (consisting of microglial forming aggregates around small foci of tissue necrosis), and neuronophagia. These are mainly observed in the temporal lobes and brainstem of patients who died due to infection by WNV. In some patients, there may be endoneurial mononuclear inflammation of the root of cranial nerves.

Clinical Features

- West Nile Virus produces an acute systemic infection and can have two very different types of presentations:
  i. Mild and self-limited infection or
  ii. Neuroinvasive disease
- Most human WNV infections are subclinical and are usually asymptomatic. In about 20% of infected patients, it may present with fever, headache, maculopapular rash, myalgia, fatigue, lymphadenopathy, polyarthropathy, anorexia, and nausea.

Complications

- **Central nervous system complications:** Patients with severe disease may develop acute aseptic meningitis, encephalitis, or meningoencephalitis. This may produce convulsions and coma. About 10% of patient with meningoencephalitis may be associated with long-term neurologic sequelae (cognitive and neurologic impairment). Immunosuppressed and older individuals have increased risk of severe disease.
- **Other complications:** These are rare and include hepatitis, hepatosplenomegaly, myocarditis, anterior myelitis, and pancreatitis.

Diagnosis: WNV can be found in the blood for up to 10 days in immunocompetent febrile patients, and as late as 22–28 days after infection in immunocompromised patients. The diagnosis is usually made by serology, but viral culture and PCR-based tests are also used.

- **Cerebrospinal fluid findings:** It shows moderate pleocytosis and raised protein levels in the CSF.

Viral Hemorrhagic Fever

Q. Classify viral hemorrhagic fevers (VHFs) and discuss the laboratory diagnosis.

Viral hemorrhagic fever (VHF) is a **group of severe life-threatening multisystem syndrome** caused by different viral infections. They are **characterized by vascular damage, leading to varying degrees of widespread hemorrhage (bleeding from the eyes, mouth, ears, skin pores, and internal organs), shock, and sometimes death**. VHFs are zoonotic diseases caused by viruses that reside in either animal reservoirs or arthropod vectors. These are usually named for the area where they were first described. VHF is caused by enveloped RNA viruses belonging to four different major groups/families of viruses namely (1) Arenaviridae (e.g., Lassa fever in Africa), (2) Filoviridae (e.g., Ebola and Marburg virus infections in Africa), (3) Bunyaviridae [e.g., Rift Valley fever in Africa; hantavirus hemorrhagic fever with renal syndrome in Asia; and Crimean-Congo hemorrhagic fever (CCHF), which has an extensive geographic distribution], and (4) Flaviviridae e.g., yellow fever in Africa and South America and dengue in Asia, Africa, and the Americas). VHFs can be classified into four epidemiologic groups depending on the differences in routes of transmission, vectors, and other epidemiological features (**Table 7**). Lassa fever and Ebola and Marburg virus infections are also transmitted from person to person.

Table 7: Classification of viral hemorrhagic fevers according to vectors transmitting them.
Mosquito-borne
• Yellow fever • Rift valley fever • Dengue hemorrhagic fever • Chikungunya hemorrhagic fever
Tick-borne
• Omsk hemorrhagic fever • Crimean hemorrhagic fever • Kyasanur forest disease
Zoonotic (rodents)
• Lassa fever • Bolivian hemorrhagic fever • Argentine hemorrhagic fever • Korean hemorrhagic fever
Fruit bats (filoviruses)
• Ebola virus disease

General Features

Disease spectrum: Various viruses causing VHFs can produce a spectrum of illnesses that may range from a mild acute disease to severe, life-threatening disease.

- **Mild disease:** It is characterized by fever, headache, myalgia, rash, neutropenia, and thrombocytopenia.
- **Severe life-threatening disease:** This is characterized by a sudden hemodynamic deterioration and shock.

Mode of transmission: These viruses pass through an animal or insect host during their life cycles, and these are restricted to areas in which the corresponding hosts reside.

- Humans are incidental hosts. They get infected when they come into contact with infected hosts (usually rodents) or insect vectors (mosquitoes and ticks).
- Some viruses such as Ebola, Marburg, and Lassa can also spread from person to person.
- Occasionally, infected humans transfer the viruses through blood or semen.

Pathogenesis: The pathogenesis of the infection varies, but some common feature is damage to blood vessels.

- **Damage to blood vessels:** It is usually prominent. It may be either due to direct infection and damage of the endothelial cells, or indirectly by inflammatory cytokines liberated by viral infected macrophages and dendritic cells.

MORPHOLOGY

Hemorrhagic manifestations: This usually manifest as **petechiae**.

- They may be caused due to combination of thrombocytopenia or platelet dysfunction, endothelial injury, cytokine-induced disseminated intravascular coagulation (DIC), and deficiency of clotting factors (due to liver injury).
- Hemorrhages may be prominent in some viral infections (e.g., Congo-Crimean fever) and rarely may be life-threatening.

Continued

Continued

Necrosis of tissues: It may develop secondary to the vascular lesions and hemorrhages. It may vary from mild and focal to massive necrosis. Usually there is minimal inflammatory response.

Ebola Virus Disease

Q. Write short essay on Ebola.

Ebola virus is a single-stranded ***RNA virus belonging to the Filoviridae family***. Ebola virus disease (EVD), earlier known as **Ebola hemorrhagic fever**, is a severe, often **fatal disease** in humans. EVD outbreaks have a very high fatality rate of around 90%. EVD outbreaks occurred primarily in remote villages in several regions of Africa (Central and West Africa), near tropical rainforests. The virus infects humans, gorillas, chimpanzees, and monkeys. The only other filovirus pathogenic to humans is Marburg virus, which produces Marburg hemorrhagic fever.

Source of infection: The natural host of the Ebola virus is the fruit bats of the Pteropodidae family. Humans recovered from the disease can transmit the virus through semen for up to 7 weeks after recovery from illness. Several species of fruit bats of the Pteropodidae family, apes, or monkeys have been identified as the natural reservoir of Ebola virus.

Mode of transmission: The virus spreads in the human population through human-to-human transmission by the following modes:

- **Direct (close) contact (through broken skin or mucous membranes) with the blood, secretions,** used needles, **organs or other bodily fluids of infected people or animals.**
- **Indirect contact with environments contaminated with such fluids.** Healthcare workers and family members may be infected due to exposure of virus while treating patients with EVD or during funerary preparation of the bodies of deceased victims.

Incubation period: 2–21 days.

Pathogenesis

The Ebola virus after its entry into the host attacks macrophages and dendritic cells. There will a massive inflammatory response due to an influx of cytokines.

Ebola virus can infect almost every cell in the body. Thus, it can involve organs such as the spleen, kidneys, liver, and lungs. The virus massively replicates in endothelial cells, mononuclear phagocytes, and hepatocytes.

Evasion of adaptive immunity: The virus targets antigen-presenting cells and thus prevents the adaptive immune response from fighting against the infection. The virus has a specific mechanism by which it evades the adaptive immune response and allows the virus to rapidly replicate thereby producing high levels of viral particles. This mechanism is brought out by two viral proteins namely VP24 and VP35. Both these viral proteins inhibit the action of type I IFN.

- **VP24:** It blocks type I interferon (IFN) signaling by preventing dimerization of tyrosine kinase and nuclear translocation of signal transducers and activators of transcription-1 (STAT-1).
- **VP35:** It binds to double-stranded viral RNA in infected host cells. Thus, it prevents detection of the viral RNA by cytoplasmic receptors that stimulate type I IFN production.
- **Viral surface protein GP:** This is found in nonvirus-associated soluble form, probably, they block the host antibodies from neutralizing intact virus. Antibodies are not detected during Ebola infection.

MORPHOLOGY

Ebola virus produces widespread destructive tissue lesions.

- **Necrosis:** Severe necrosis is seen in the liver, kidneys, gonads, spleen, and lymph nodes. Liver shows hepatocellular necrosis, Kupffer cell hyperplasia, Councilman bodies, and microsteatosis.
- **Hemorrhage**
  - Lungs: Usually hemorrhagic
  - Petechial hemorrhages: They are found in the skin, mucous membranes, and internal organs.
- **Shock:** It is produced because of injury to the microvasculature and increased endothelial permeability.

Clinical Features

- Acute EVD is characterized by **sudden onset of high-grade fever**, associated with **severe weakness,** sore throat, **muscle pain, and headache.** This is termed as "dry phase."
- The **hallmark of next "wet phase" is blood-tinged coughing, bloody diarrhea, and/or blood-laden vomit;** a **skin rash** may also appear.
- Some patients may develop severe internal and external bleeding/hemorrhage. These may in the form of bleeding from injection sites, petechiae, gastrointestinal tract, and gingiva. Patients who survive Ebola infection develop lifelong immunity to the strain that infected them.

Complications include acute renal failure, hemorrhagic manifestations, DIC, hepatitis, and MODS (multiple organ dysfunction syndrome). Death occurs in half of infected patients.

Diagnosis is by clinical and serological tests.

Yellow Fever

Yellow fever is an acute hemorrhagic fever caused by an insect-borne *Flavivirus*. Other pathogenic flaviviruses cause Omsk hemorrhagic fever and Kyasanur Forest disease. Yellow fever virus is an enveloped, single-stranded RNA virus.

Sometimes yellow fever is associated with extensive hepatic necrosis and jaundice and may lead to fulminant hepatic failure.

Epidemiology: Yellow fever virus is restricted to parts of Africa and South America, including both jungle and urban areas.

Reservoir of infection: It is usually tree dwelling (place of residence) monkeys. These are not affected by the virus.

Mode of infection: The virus is passed among tree dwelling monkeys in the forest canopy (uppermost branches of the trees in a fores) by mosquitoes. Humans develop jungle yellow fever due to bite by infected ***Aedes mosquitoes***. Felling trees increases the risk of viral infection, because mosquitoes are brought down with the tree. The infected human on return from the forest to the village or city, becomes a reservoir for epidemic yellow fever **in the urban setting**, where the **vector is *Aedes aegypti***.

Pathogenesis

Virus is inoculated into the human through the mosquito bite and the virus is deposited into tissue. The virus is taken up by dendritic cells and is then carried to the lymph nodes where the virus can kill dendritic cells. They release more viruses to infect macrophages; once the virus enters a host cell, infected macrophages migrate through blood and lymph, where they die and release more viruses to the patient's organs. The virus replicates within the human tissue and vascular endothelium. Then it spreads through the bloodstream. The virus has a tropism for liver cells. Sometimes, it produces extensive acute destruction of hepatocytes. Severe damage to the endothelium of small blood vessels may cause loss of vascular integrity, hemorrhages, and shock.

MORPHOLOGY

Liver: Yellow fever virus causes **coagulative necrosis** of hepatocytes. Necrosis begins in the middle of hepatic lobules and spreads toward the central veins and portal tracts. Sometimes the viral infection produces confluent midzonal necrosis (i.e., necrosis in the middle of the hepatic lobules). In the most severe cases, entire hepatic lobule undergoes necrosis. Some necrotic hepatocytes become intensely eosinophilic with loss of nuclei. These hepatocytes may be dislodged from adjacent hepatocytes and are termed as **Councilman bodies** (apoptotic bodies).

Clinical Features

Yellow fever is characterized manifests as sudden onset of fever, chills, headache, myalgias, nausea, and vomiting. Some patients may develop jaundice with signs of hepatic failure after 3–5 days. Hence, it termed as "yellow" fever. This can lead to deficiencies of clotting factors and diffuse hemorrhages. In severe disease, classical feature is vomiting of clotted blood ("black vomit"). Patients with massive hepatic failure may progress to coma and death usually within 10 days of onset of disease. Overall mortality of yellow fever is about 5%, but in patients with jaundice, it may be up to 30%.

Zika Virus Infections

Q. Write short essay on Zika virus (ZIKV).

- Zika virus is an arbovirus, belongs to the Flaviviridae family.
- It is enveloped and icosahedral with a nonsegmented, single-stranded, positive-sense RNA genome. It was first identified in Zika forest of Uganda in 1947. Over the decades, it spread to Pakistan, India, and the Pacific Islands.

Mode of Spread

- **Through *Aedes* mosquito:** ZIKV is transmitted by ***Aedes* mosquito** species primarily *A. aegypti*. The extrinsic incubation period in mosquitoes is about 10 days. Rarely, mother to child transmission and one case of sexual transmission has been reported. Probably, there is an animal reservoir for the virus, although none has been demonstrated to be a source of human infection. The vertebrate hosts of the disease are monkeys and humans. The virus infects dendritic cells near the site of inoculation, and later spreads to lymph nodes, and produces viremia.
- **Other modes of transmission:** It may also develop through perinatal transmission, blood transfusion, and sexual contact. The virus is detectable in semen, vaginal secretions, breast milk, and urine for up to several months after infection.

Incubation period: 10 days.

MORPHOLOGY

Brain abnormalities: Common adverse outcomes associated with ZIKV infection are—cerebral calcifications, cerebral atrophy, ventricular enlargements, and hypoplastic cerebral structures. Microcephaly occurred in a small number of infants born to infected women.

Ocular abnormalities: These include pigment mottling, chorioretinal atrophy, and optic nerve abnormalities.

Autopsy findings:
- Common findings in new-born children include microcephaly, ventriculomegaly, and congenital joint contractures (arthrogryposis), and pulmonary hypoplasia.
- Other findings include severe depletion of neurons, thinning of the brain parenchyma, with microcalcifications and microglial nodules.
- Viral proteins were detected in degenerating neurons and glial cells, and in chorionic villi of the placenta in some cases. These findings indicate replication of virus with associated necrosis in these cells. ZIKV replicates in and kills human neurons.
- Viral RNA can be detected in brain tissues in all cases, but virus is absent or present in small amount in other tissues.

Clinical Features

It produces usually mild and nonspecific symptoms similar to a mild form of dengue fever with mild headaches, maculopapular rash, fever, malaise, conjunctivitis, myalgia, and arthralgia lasting a few days to 1 week. Within 2–4 days, the rash starts fading, and fever resolves within 3 days.

- **Neurological complications:** In a small number of adult patients, the infection may produce neurologic complications, primarily Guillain–Barré syndrome. In such cases, the infection damages the myelin sheath that surrounds nerves, resulting in muscle weakness, and paralysis.
- **Congenital infection due to perinatal transmission** leads to fetal death or moderate-to-severe brain defects in the fetus and new-born child. These are more frequent following infection during the first and second trimesters. Defects in the child include microcephaly, chorioretinal atrophy, hydranencephaly, intrauterine growth restriction (IUGR), and hydrops fetalis. Most dangerous time is during first trimester of pregnancy and during this period, it can damage the brain of fetus.

Diagnosis
- **Sample to be tested:** Blood saliva and urine.
- **Polymerase chain reaction:** Useful in the first 3–5 days after the onset of symptoms. It directly detects the virus or specific viral antigens in the clinical specimen.
- **Serology test:** Detects the presence of antibodies and useful only after 5 days.

Dengue

Q. Write short essay on dengue fever.

Dengue fever is caused by dengue virus (arbovirus) that are of four serotypes types namely 1, 2, 3, or 4. Dengue virus is enveloped, single-stranded RNA genome, belongs to Flaviviridae family. It is the **most common arthropod-borne viral infection in humans in the world**.

Source of Infection

Humans suffering from dengue are main amplifying host of the virus and infective during the first 3 days of the illness (the viremic stage). About 2 weeks after feeding (day time) on an infected individual, mosquitoes become infective and remain so for life. Dengue is usually endemic.

Mode of Transmission

All are **transmitted by the day time *Aedes* mosquito biting in tropical and subtropical regions**. *A. aegypti* is the most common mosquito involved in transmission which breeds in stagnant water (e.g., collections of water in containers, water-based air coolers, and tire dumps). Cases usually increase with the onset of the rainy season, when mosquitoes proliferate.

Incubation period: 4–10 days following the mosquito bite.

Pathogenesis

Probably, the immune response against dengue virus partly determines the severity of the infection.
- **First infection with dengue virus:** As mentioned earlier, there are four serotypes of dengue virus. Infection with each of the four serotypes stimulates lifelong protective immunity against reinfection with the same serotype. But patients get only a fleeting immune protection against other dengue serotypes. Infection with one serotype also stimulates a cross-reactive antibody response for other serotypes of the virus. These antibodies are weak and nonprotective.
- **Second infection with dengue virus of different serotype:** Subsequent infection with a different serotype in an individual is probably linked to a greater risk of developing a more severe dengue.
  - In these patients, who have cross-reactive antibodies due to previous infection by dengue virus of different serotype, increases the uptake of virus into macrophages via Fc receptors.
  - This antibody-dependent enhancement of uptake of virus into macrophages probably increases the infectivity of the virus and contributes to severe dengue. **Two most severe manifestations of the disease—dengue hemorrhagic fever (DHF) and dengue shock syndrome (DSS)**.
  - The same phenomenon may be responsible for severe dengue developing in infants who having maternal derived antibodies against dengue virus.

Clinical Features

Dengue is a systemic, dynamic, and tropical disease. It has a wide clinical spectrum and includes both severe and nonsevere clinical manifestations. Asymptomatic infections are common (especially in children), but it is more severe in infants and the elderly. **Triad of symptoms** include—**hemorrhagic manifestations, evidence of plasma leakage, and platelet counts of <100,000/μL**.

Phases of Dengue

After the incubation period, dengue begins abruptly and is followed by the three phases—(1) febrile, (2) critical, and (3) recovery.

1. Febrile phase
- Characterized by the abrupt onset of **high-grade fever** and this phase last for 2–7 days. Fever may be continuous or saddle-back (see below).
- It often accompanied by **facial flushing, skin erythema,** severe **generalized body ache ("break-bone fever"/** Dandy fever**), myalgia, arthralgia, malaise, headache retrobulbar pain** (worsens on eye movements), **severe backache** (which is a prominent symptom), **anorexia, nausea, and vomiting.**
- **Saddle-back fever:** In few cases fever subsides and other symptoms disappear after 3–4 days. This remission may last for 2 days and then the fever returns together with others symptoms but milder. This biphasic or "saddle-back" pattern is **considered characteristic of dengue**.
- **Mild hemorrhagic manifestations** such as petechiae and mucosal membrane bleeding (e.g., nose and gums) may be found.

2. Critical phase
- Around the time of falling (defervescence = the period of abatement of fever) of fever (usually on days 3–7 of illness), an **increase in capillary permeability** along with **increase of hematocrit** levels may occur. This marks beginning of critical phases.
- In severe dengue (DHF), there will be **widespread hemorrhages** throughout the body, **hepatic necrosis with liver failure, reduced consciousness, organ failure, hyaline membrane formation in the lung, and plasma leakage leading to shock and respiratory distress**.

3. Recovery phase
- If the patient survives the 24–48 hours critical phase, a **gradual reabsorption of extravascular compartment fluid** takes place during the subsequent 48–72 hours.
- It is characterized by **improvement** in the general well-being, return of appetite, disappearance of gastrointestinal symptoms, and stabilization of hemodynamic status and diuresis.

Laboratory diagnosis of dengue
- Increased hematocrit (hemoconcentration) and metabolic acidosis.

- Virus isolation (within 3 days after onset).
- Immunoglobulin M enzyme-linked immunosorbent assay (IgM ELISA) (after 1 week of onset).
- Hemagglutination inhibition assay (HAI).

Crimean–Congo Hemorrhagic Fever

Q. Write short essay on Crimean Congo Fever.

Crimean-Congo hemorrhagic fever (CCHF) is a widespread, severe VHF caused by a tick-borne virus (Nairovirus) belonging to the Bunyaviridae family. CCHF is endemic in Africa, the Balkans, and the Middle East and Asian countries

Source of infection: The hosts of the CCHF virus include a **wide range of wild and domestic animals such as cattle, sheep, and goats**. Animals become infected by the bite of infected ticks and the virus remains in the bloodstream of infected animal for about 1 week after infection. This allows the tick-animal-tick cycle to continue when another tick bites. The principal tick vector belongs to the genus *Hyalomma*.

Mode of transmission: The CCHF virus is **transmitted to humans either by tick bites or through contact with infected animal blood or tissues during and immediately after slaughter**. Human-to-human transmission can occur from close contact with the blood, secretions, organs, or other bodily fluids of infected persons. Hospital-acquired infections can also occur due to improper sterilization of medical equipment and reuse of needles.

Incubation period: It depends on the mode of acquisition of the virus. Following tick bite, the incubation period is usually 1–3 days and following contact with infected blood or tissues, it is usually 5–6 days.

Clinical features: It presents with sudden onset fever, myalgia, (muscle ache), dizziness, neck pain and stiffness, backache, headache, sore eyes, and photophobia (sensitivity to light). Other symptoms include nausea, vomiting, diarrhea, abdominal pain, and sore throat followed by sharp mood swings and confusion. Signs include liver enlargement, tachycardia, lymphadenopathy and a petechial rash, ecchymoses, and other hemorrhagic phenomena.

Diagnosis: Various laboratory tests used for the diagnosis of CCHF virus infection are—ELISA, antigen detection, serum neutralization, RT-PCR assay and virus isolation by cell culture.

Summary of VHFs is presented in **Table 8**.

Table 8: Summary of viral hemorrhagic fevers.

Virus/disease (vector)	*Clinical features*	*Lab diagnosis*
Flaviviridae family		
Kyasanur Forest disease (Tick)	Fever, myalgia, gastrointestinal disturbance, hemorrhage, and meningoencephalitis	• High RBC count • Serological: IgM ELISA • Virus isolation
Yellow fever (mosquito)	Fever, myalgia, jaundice liver and kidney failure hemorrhages, delirium	• RBC high • WBC low • High AST/ALT • Antigen detection: Antigen-capture ELISA serology: IgM positive from the 5th day, RT-PCR for yellow fever virus • Virus isolation
Dengue (mosquito)	Described on page 600 above	
Arenaviridae family		
Lassa fever (rodent)	Fever, prostration, rash, effusions, and hemorrhages	• High RBC • High WBC • Low platelet count • Proteinuria • High AST • Serological tests
• Argentine • Bolivian • Brazilian • Venezuelan hemorrhagic fever	Cerebellar signs	• High RBC • Low WBC • Low platelet count • Proteinuria • Antibody detection
Bunyaviridae family		
Phlebovirus: Rift valley fever (mosquito)	Febrile myalgia, hepatitis, retinitis, encephalitis	High RBC, low WBC, high AST/ALT serological
Nairovirus: Crimean Congo (Tick)	Fever, myalgia	High AST ELISA

Continued

Continued

Virus/disease (vector)	*Clinical features*	*Lab diagnosis*
Hantavirus: Hemorrhagic fever with renal failure (Rodent)	Fever, myalgia, hypotensive stage, oliguric stage, and polyuric stage	High hematocrit, leukocytosis, thrombocytopenia, high creatinine IG, ELISA, RT-PCR
Hantavirus pulmonary syndrome (rodent)	Fever, pulmonary edema, hypoxemia, and respiratory failure	• High hematocrit • Leukocytosis • Thrombocytopenia • High creatinine • ELISA • RT-PCR
Filoviridae family		
Ebola (not known)	Fever, headache, myalgia, hemorrhage, GI symptom, chest pain, delirium	• Serology • Culture in cell lines
Marburg (not known)	Headache, fever, vomiting, chest pain, muscle aches, red eyes, and bleeding	Electron microscopy: Filamentous virus in blood

(ALT: alanine aminotransferase; AST: aspartate aminotransferase; ELISA: enzyme-linked immunosorbent assay; IgM: immunoglobulin M; RBC: red blood cell; WBC: white blood cell; RT-PCR: reverse transcriptase polymerase chain reaction)

Laboratory Diagnosis of Viral Hemorrhagic Fevers

Q. Write short essay on laboratory diagnosis of VHFs.

Viral infections in tropical regions are usually transmitted to humans by arthropods or rodent. In patients with suspected viral infection, a recognized history of mosquito bite(s) has not diagnostically useful. However, a history of tick bite(s) is more diagnostically useful.

Laboratory diagnosis is needed in all cases, though epidemics may occasionally provide enough clinical and epidemiologic clues for a presumptive etiologic diagnosis.

- For most arthropod-borne and rodent-borne viruses, **acute-phase serum samples** (collected within 3 or 4 days of onset). They will usually be positive.
- **Demonstration of rising antibody titers** is also useful. Rapid tests for VHFs are available which reliably detect antigen by ELISAs, IgM capture ELISAs, and multiplex PCR assays. These tests can diagnose on a single serum sample within a few hours and are very useful in patients with severe disease.
- More sensitive is RT-PCR assay. It may be used for diagnoses on samples without detectable antigen. PCR (RT-PCR) assay may also useful for providing genetic information about the etiologic agent.

Novel Coronavirus SARS-CoV-2 (COVID-19)

Highly contagious and infectious severe acute respiratory syndrome coronavirus-2 (SARS CoV-2) is a novel strain of coronavirus that has not been previously identified in humans. The virus was named SARS-CoV-2. The term "coronavirus" was first coined by June Almeida and David Tyrrell who first observed and studied human coronaviruses. The diseases caused by this novel coronavirus are called COVID-19. SARS-CoV-2 is a single-stranded RNA virus of ~30 kb genome size and belongs to genus *Coronavirus* and family Coronaviridae. The COVID-19 virus is an enveloped single-stranded RNA virus with surface spike proteins. Similar to other coronaviruses, this group has distinctive contour under electron microscope. Hence, its name "coronavirus" ("corona" means crown). During early December, 2019, cases of pneumonia of unknown cause were identified in the city of Wuhan, capital city of Hubei province, China. Many of these initial cases had close contact with wet markets that sell fresh meat, fish, and other perishable produce. The outbreak increased during December, and on December 31st the WHO was informed of an outbreak of a new cause of pneumonia. Cases of COVID-19 were reported outside of China as early as January 13th in individuals who had traveled from Wuhan. The infection had become a worldwide pandemic. By May, 2021, there were 165 million cases and about 3.43 million deaths. Apart from severe health consequences, this devastating pandemic of COVID-19 has caused major social and economic disruptions world over.

Severe Acute Respiratory Syndrome Coronavirus-2

Sequencing of the full viral genome has been achieved. This has resulted in development of a rapid molecular diagnostic assay during the evolving outbreak. The study of genomic sequence shows that COVID-19 is related to bat coronaviruses and the SARS coronavirus. The genome of SARS-CoV-2 is similar to other coronaviruses and consists of 10 open reading frames (ORFs). SARS-CoV-2 spike protein has higher affinity to angiotensin-converting enzyme 2 (ACE2) receptor when compared to SARS-CoV.

Mode of Transmission

Epidemiological studies suggest that the origin of this novel strain of virus was a seafood and animal market in Wuhan. Thus, it was initially transmitted from animal to human followed by person-to-person transmission. Transmission among humans occurs via close contact with an infected individual through respiratory droplets. Infected individuals appear to be most infectious just before or for several days after the beginning of symptoms when viral loads peak. However, patients who remain asymptomatic can also transmit the infection. In the majority of cases, the viable virus disappears 8 days after the onset of symptoms. Thus, in most protocols, the quarantine is stopped 10 to 14 days after the onset of symptoms. Airborne transmission occurs when viable virus becomes airborne.

This may occur after an infected individual exhales, speaks, particularly in a loud voice, sings, coughs or sneezes.

Infectious particles: They can be classified as either large droplets (larger than 5 micrometers), or aerosols (<5 micrometers). A mixture of large particles and aerosols are generated when infected patient coughs or sneezes. Certain medical procedures (e.g., intubation, noninvasive positive-pressure ventilation) cause aerosol formation.

- **Large droplets:** Large droplets, after leaving the respiratory tract of patients, rapidly fall to the ground-usually within 6 feet of an infected patient. The CDC has defined a close contact as "someone who was within six feet of an infected person for a cumulative time of 15 minutes or more over a 24-hour period starting from 2 days before illness onset (or for asymptomatic patients, 2 days prior to test specimen collection) until the time the patient is isolated." Large droplet transmission seems to be the major route of transmission of Covid-19. Nonetheless, some data do support the possibility of aerosol transmission of COVID-19 during the pandemic.
- **Aerosols:** They evaporate quickly, leaving infectious particles suspended in the air for a considerable period of time (usually hours)-in closed and particularly in poorly ventilated spaces.

Risk of transmission: Average number of people who are infected by an index case is termed as the reproduction number. For COVID-19 the average reproduction number is 2 to 3. Risk of transmission of Covid-19 varies depending on the type of exposure. For example, with close contact exposure, the risk is probably 5% whereas household contact it can be as high as 40%. But brief interactions (e.g., shopping) have a risk of <1%. Because the reproduction number for COVID-19 is low, masks and social distancing of 6 feet reduces the risk of transmission and incidence of disease. N-95 masks provide protection for both aerosols and large droplets. There is little epidemiologic or clinical data to suggest significant transmission through fomites, although it is reasonable to keep open the possibility and act on that assumption. COVID-19 is much less likely to be transmitted in outside venues. This is because of rapid dispersal of droplets and aerosols. Sunlight and ultraviolet light rapidly inactivate the virus.

Incubation period for COVID-19: Average 5 days but can range from 2 to 11 days. Rarely, the incubation period can extend to 14 days or even longer.

Pathogenesis

The 180-kDa spike (S) protein of the virus binds to the peptidase angiotensin-converting enzyme 2 receptor (ACE2) on cell surfaces. This causes fusion of viral and cell membrane fusion and virus enters into the cells. Membrane fusion also needs the interaction of other proteases, particularly transmembrane protease serine 2 (TMPRSS2), on cell surfaces. The presence of ACE2 determines cell tropism of COVID-19 and AGE2 is mainly found on epithelial cells of both the upper and lower respiratory tract. ACE2 also observed in other tissues including vascular endothelial cells, the gastrointestinal tract, and kidney. SARS-CoV-2 virus enters cells by endocytosis. The virus uses the cells' own machinery to reproduce. These viruses are released and infect other cells. Infection of nasal epithelial cells during early infection may produce initial upper respiratory symptoms and anosmia. Virus also infects bronchial, alveolar, and endovascular epithelial cells early and causes an inflammatory response. The inflammatory response consists of neutrophils, T lymphocytes, macrophage. They release cytokines including TNF-α, and IL-6. In the lungs, as the infection and inflammatory reaction progresses, it produces interstitial thickening, pulmonary edema, activation of the coagulation pathway, and lymphocyte depletion. Inflammation can result in fibrosis with marked compromise of pulmonary function.

Host defenses against coronaviruses consist of innate and specific immunity. But the specific immune mechanisms and their relative importance is not known. At the sites of infection (particularly the lung with endothelial damage), immune cells including T and B lymphocytes, macrophages, and neutrophils are attracted. They release cytokines and inflammatory molecules such as interleukins 1 and 6, interferons, TNF-α. There is also production of IgM and IgG antibody and activation of the coagulation system with increases in D-dimer and micro- and macro-thrombosis. Inflammatory markers such as erythrocyte sedimentation rate (ESR), C-reactive protein (CRP), ferritin, and lactic dehydrogenase (LDH) levels are raised. One of the characteristic features of the inflammatory process is the destruction of both CD4 and CD8 T lymphocytes by apoptosis. This leads to lymphopenia. It is found experimentally that neutralizing antibodies directed toward the S protein provide protection after infection. This is the basis of vaccine development that targets the response against this S protein. Recently it was found that the specific immune response to SARS-CoV-2 consists of CD4, CD8, and antibody in a coordinated response. Absence of such a response and reduced number of T cells are observed in individuals over 65 and this may be responsible for increased susceptibility to the virus.

MORPHOLOGY

High SARS-CoV-19 titers are found during autopsy particularly in the lung, but also in blood, liver, kidney, brain, and heart.

Lung: Autopsy of patients who died of COVID-19, shows diffuse alveolar damage in all lobes but more severe in the lower lobes. During the early phase of acute alveolar damage, it shows edema, formation of hyaline membrane, and thickened alveolar septa with perivascular lymphocytic infiltration. Severe injury to endothelial cells is associated with disrupted cell membranes and the presence of virus. Pulmonary vessels including alveolar capillaries show widespread microthrombi and vascular angiogenesis. Both these vascular changes distinguish it from the pathology of severe influenza infection. In later stages, lung shows diffuse alveolar damage, proliferation of fibroblast leading to fibrosis, hyperplasia of pneumocyte and thickening of interstitium and collapse of the alveoli. In some areas of diffuse alveolar damage, metaplasia or widespread fibrosis or bronchopneumonia may occur.

Continued

Continued

Other organs: These are as follows:

- Heart: Lymphocytic myocarditis and epicarditis
- Liver: Periportal lymphocytic infiltration, hepatic congestion, steatosis, hepatic cell necrosis, and central vein thrombosis.
- Kidney: Acute tubular injury
- Brain: Extensive inflammation in the olfactory bulbs and medulla oblongata.
- Focal pancreatitis, adrenocortical hyperplasia, and lymphocyte depletion in spleen and lymph nodes.
- Thrombotic features in multiple organs including lung, heart, and kidney.

Diffuse intravascular coagulation (DIC): Severe COVID-19 can activate coagulation and consumption of clotting factors resulting in DIC. Increased coagulation can produce deep venous thrombosis and lead to pulmonary embolism, myocardial infarction, stroke, and vascular compromise in other organs. Thrombosis of small and mid-sized pulmonary arteries with associated infarction can also occur. Neutrophilic plugs composed of neutrophil extracellular traps (NETS) may also be seen. NETS are composed of extracellular strands of DNA from neutrophils that trap pathogens. NETS may also found with platelets, which may induce thrombus formation.

Clinical Features

Data available suggests that a significant percentage of infected people remain asymptomatic. Its manifestations vary from mild-to-severe respiratory illness. Majority of patients (probably about 81%) who contract the virus recover after a flu-like disease. It can produce severe and sometimes fatal illness with acute respiratory distress syndrome (in about 14%), which is defined as cytokine storm. About 5% may become critically ill.

Presenting symptoms: Early in the disease, it frequently produces upper respiratory tract symptoms including rhinorrhea and nasal congestion. Other common symptoms include fever, dry cough and dyspnea, fatigue, myalgias, and headache. Some patients initially may develop gastrointestinal symptoms such as nausea and vomiting and/or diarrhea. Similar to other respiratory viruses, anosmia is frequently reported by patients with COVID-19 (up to 64%), although it is not often the presenting symptom.

Respiratory symptoms

They predominate in most patients with COVID-19. These include nonproductive cough, dyspnea, and at times chest pain predominate. The degree of pulmonary involvement and the need for hospitalization is determined by peripheral pulse oxygen levels. Some patients do not present with dyspnea despite low peripheral oxygen levels (<90). The respiratory symptoms are progressive in about 17% to 35% of patients and requires hospitalized and ICU care. Severe cases of hypoxemia may require sequentially supplemental oxygen, noninvasive respiratory support (e.g., noninvasive high-flow nasal cannulas), invasive respiratory support with intubation, and in extreme cases extracorporeal membrane oxygenation (ECMO). It is usually associated with bilateral ground-glass opacities, consolidation, and peripheral distribution in the lower lobes on chest imaging by plain radiographs and particularly chest CT. This is observed especially in elderly patients and those with comorbidities such as diabetes, chronic obstructive pulmonary disease (COPD), and heart failure. It is to be noted that, even patients with no symptoms but positive COVID-19 testing may have characteristic findings on chest CT.

Extrapulmonary manifestations

In severely ill patients, COVID-19 infection may produce various extrapulmonary manifestations. These includes cardiovascular, renal, gastrointestinal, neurologic, thromboembolic, and endocrine.

Cardiovascular system: Myocarditis, cardiomyopathy, and acute coronary syndrome with elevated troponin levels can develop in 20% to 30% of hospitalized patients, particularly critically ill patients. Cardiac injury may be due to direct infection of cardiac myocytes by the virus or indirectly by the inflammatory response. Inflammation can cause thrombosis and endothelialitis. Cardiac arrhythmias (e.g., atrial fibrillation, heart block) may develop in up to 17% of hospitalized patients. Congestive heart failure occurs frequently in critically ill patients.

Thromboembolic manifestations: In ICU patients, vascular instability, sepsis-like picture, and bleeding and coagulation abnormalities are common. Thrombosis of both the venous and arterial systems develops in about 25% of hospitalized patients and >50% in ICU patients.

Renal system: Acute kidney injury (AKI) develops in about 37% of severely ill hospitalized patients and up to 14% may require dialysis. Hematuria and proteinuria are common in severely ill patients.

Gastrointestinal system: Its involvement produces symptoms such as anorexia, diarrhea, and nausea in up to one-third of patients. In some patients, gastrointestinal symptoms may be the initial indications of COVID-19.

Hepatocellular injury: Severe COVID-19 may produce liver injury in up to 20% of patients.

Neurologic manifestations: These include headache, dizziness, and anosmia. The nasal epithelium has a high frequency of ACE2 and is an early target for COVID-19. This is probable responsible anosmia. Delirium, acute vascular stroke, encephalopathy, and encephalitis may also occur.

Endocrine abnormalities: Hyperglycemia is common in hospitalized patients. Patients with preexisting diabetes mellitus or obesity are at greater risk for severe disease.

Long COVID: Many patients continue to have symptoms for 2 to 3 months after acute infection and is described as "long COVID". Recently, post-acute COVID-19 is defined as symptoms extending beyond 3 weeks and chronic COVID-19 beyond 12 weeks.

Risk factors for severe disease and mortality: The most common risk factors for severity and hospitalization are diabetes mellitus and obesity, cardiovascular disease (including hypertension), and chronic lung disease. Other chronic diseases include immunocompromised conditions, chronic renal disease, and chronic neurologic and psychiatric disorders.

Personal protective measures are necessary to prevent SARS-CoV-2 infection.

Laboratory Diagnosis

The diagnosis depends on detection of nucleic acid, IgG/IgM antibodies, and a chest radiograph of the suspected individuals.

RT-PCR testing for COVID-19: It is the method of choice for detection of the viral RNA genome in nasopharyngeal swabs or nasal swabs is the most common diagnostic test. It can also be performed on respiratory (e.g., bronchoalveolar lavage) and stool samples. Viral RNA is measured by the number of polymerase chain reproductive cycles and expressed as threshold (Ct). Ct values <40 cycles indicate that a higher number of RNA copies are in the original sample and are regarded as positive. RT-PCR positivity is highest for bronchoalveolar lavage specimens followed by nasopharyngeal, nasal, and oral specimens. In some patients, RT-PCR may remain positive for 6 weeks or more. However, viable SARS-CoV-2 can be found only for the first 8 days after symptoms begin. False-negative results may be due to improper collection of specimen or due to collection too long before or after the onset of symptoms.

Other diagnostic tests: These include assays based on the following technology: antigen based, isothermal amplification (LAMP), sequencing, and CRISPR/Cas. Advantages of these include reduced time for results, reduced resources necessary for the test, use of saliva rather than nasopharyngeal or nasal specimens, and more accuracy.

Antibody response: The antibody response of infected persons is usually measured by an ELISA (enzyme-linked immunoassay) test. It detects the host's specific IgM and IgG antibodies to COVID-19 virus. Antibody testing include helps in diagnosis of acute disease and to determine immunity after infection. IgM and IgG antibodies are usually not detected until the second or third week of illness, and conversion for most patients occurs by the third to fourth week. After that IgM antibodies begin to decline and usually disappears by week 7, whereas IgG antibodies persist. Whether the persistence of the neutralizing antibodies protect and if so for how long are not known known at present.

Other laboratory investigations: Blood shows lymphopenia and elevated erythrocyte sedimentation rate, C-reactive protein, D-dimer, lactate dehydrogenase, and ferritin. Elevated blood sugar, creatinine, and hepatic enzymes are common

Vaccines

Development of vaccine is one of the highest priorities in COVID-19 research.

Traditional vaccine development: It usually takes more than a decade to complete. The traditional process includes: discovery (2 to 5 years); preclinical including animal studies (2 years); clinical (phase I: 2 years involving 10 to 50 individuals, phase II: 2 to 3 years involving hundreds of individuals, and phase III: protection studies involving thousands of individuals taking years); regulatory phase of 2 years; and manufacturing and delivery, which takes 1 to 2 years.

Covid-19 vaccine: Vaccines have in general targeted the spike protein, but it is not known what site on the molecule will be the most effective target. Types of vaccines include RNA/DNA, inactivated virus, live attenuated virus, nonreplicating vector, protein subunit, and replicating viral vector. Most of the vaccines have focused on mRNA. There are about eight potential vaccines in phase III trials in various countries. Two vaccines presently used in India are:

1. **Covishield or AZD-1222:** It makes use of a viral vector made using a weakened strain of the common cold virus (adenovirus), which contains genetic material similar to that of SARS-COV-2. Upon administration, the body's defences recognize the spike protein and prepare antibodies to evade out the infection.
2. **Covaxin:** It is prepared by using an inactive version of the virus. That is, the vaccine inactivates the virus's ability to replicate but sustains its life so that the immune system could mount a sufficient response when it comes in contact or recognizes an attack on the body in the future. Inactive vaccines are safer and reliable.

Respiratory Viruses

Common Cold

The common cold (coryza) is the most common and frequent viral disease. It is an acute, self-limited upper respiratory tract disorder caused by infection with a variety of RNA viruses. It is common to suffer usually six to eight colds per year in children and two to three in adults.

Causative RNA viruses: These include over 110 distinct rhinoviruses and several coronaviruses. About 40% of all colds are caused rhinoviruses, about 20% by coronaviruses and 10% by RSV.

Mode of spread: They spread from person to person through infected secretions. Infection is more common during winter months and during the rainy seasons. The spread is facilitated by indoor crowding.

Pathogenesis:

- Rhinoviruses and coronaviruses have an **affinity for respiratory epithelium** and usually reproduce at temperatures below 37°C (98.6°F). Thus, infection is **restricted to the cooler passages of the upper airway**. These viruses do not destroy respiratory epithelium and there are no visible alterations seen.
- After inhalation, the viruses infect the nasal respiratory epithelial cells. The infected epithelial cells produce increased production of mucus and edema. **Infected cells release chemical mediators**, such as **bradykinin** and are responsible for most of the symptoms associated with colds. These symptoms include increased production of mucus, congestion of nasal mucosa, and obstruction of eustachian tube.
- The stasis of mucus may predispose to secondary infection by bacteria. This in turn can produce bacterial sinusitis and otitis media.

Clinical features: Common cold presents with rhinorrhea, pharyngitis, cough, and low-grade fever. Symptoms usually last for about a week.

Influenza

Influenza is an acute, usually self-limited, infection of upper and lower airways caused by influenza virus.

Influenza virus: It is enveloped virus and contains single-stranded RNA. There are three distinct types of influenza virus that cause human disease namely A, B, and C. Influenza A is the most common and causes the most severe disease. Influenza D viruses primarily affect cattle and are not known to infect or cause illness in humans. Influenza strains are identified by their type (A, B, and C), serotype of their hemagglutinin (H) and neuraminidase (virus subtype), geographic origin, strain number, and year of identification. Epidemic influenza virus antigens frequently change. Hence, herd immunity that develops during one epidemic rarely protects against the next one.

Nomenclature of influenza viruses (Fig. 7): According to centres for disease control and prevention (CDC), the influenza viruses are named as follows:

- **Virus (antigenic) type (e.g., A, B, C):** This depends on the nucleoprotein (*NP*) gene of the virus.
- **Host of origin** (e.g., swine, equine, chicken, etc.). For human-origin viruses, no host of origin designation is given. Examples are as follows:
  - Duck: Avian influenza A (H1N1), A/duck/Alberta/35/76
  - Human: Seasonal influenza A (H3N2), A/Perth/16/2019
- **Geographical origin** (e.g., Denver, Taiwan, Johannesburg, etc.)
- **Strain number** (e.g., 7, 15, 33, etc.)
- **Year of isolation or collection** (e.g., 57, 1995, 2009, etc.)

Virus subtype: Influenza A viruses are divided into subtypes depending on two proteins on the surface of the virus namely hemagglutinin (H) and neuraminidase (N). There are 18 different hemagglutinin subtypes (H1 through H18) and 11 different neuraminidase subtypes (N1 through N11). There are about 198 different influenza A subtype combinations and only 131 subtypes have been detected in nature. H classification is based on the hemagglutinin encoded by the hemagglutinin (*HA*) gene. Most commonly H1, H2, or H3, also H5. The N classification depends on the type of neuraminidase encoded by neuraminidase (*NA*) gene. Most common is N1 or N2. Few examples of nomenclatures are as follows:

- Influenza A viruses: The hemagglutinin and neuraminidase antigen description are mentioned in parentheses [e.g., influenza A (H1N1) virus, influenza A (H5N1) virus]
- The 2009 pandemic virus: It was given a distinct name: A (H1N1) pdm09 so that it can be distinguished from the seasonal influenza A (H1N1) viruses that are prevalent before the pandemic.
- When humans are infected with influenza viruses that normally circulate in swine (pigs), these viruses are termed as variant viruses. Thus, they are designated with a letter 'v' [e.g., an A (H3N2) v virus].
- **Avian influenza virus ("bird flu") strain:** It emerged in 2003 and still continues to spread around the globe is designated **A (H5N1).**
- **Swine flu:** In 2009, a novel influenza A virus identified and is designated H1N1 ("swine flu") and produced pandemic infection. This strain of influenza A virus produced significant mortality in infected children and pregnant women.
- **Avian flu:** In 2013, another new virulent strain of avian flu virus, H7N9, was identified in China.

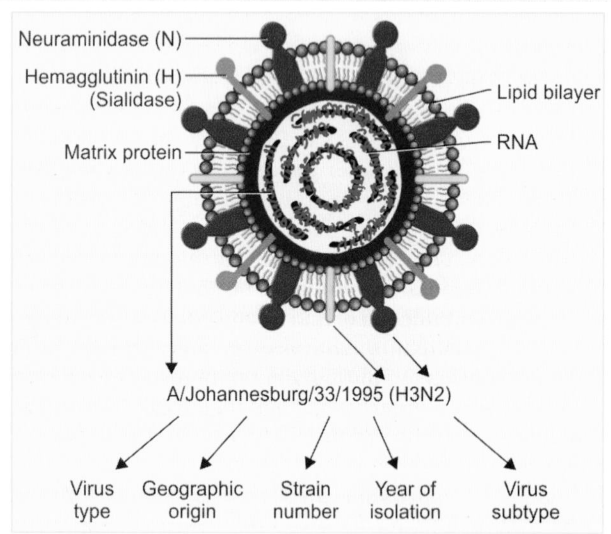

FIG. 7: Naming influenza viruses. The virus type (A, B, or C) is based on nucleoprotein characteristics encoded by the nucleoprotein (*NP*) gene of the virus. The H classification depends on the hemagglutinin encoded by the *HA* gene. Most common H types are H1, H2 or H3, also H5. The N classification depends on the type of neuraminidase encoded by the *NA* gene. Common are N1 or N2. The name starts with the virus type, followed by the place the virus was isolated (geographic origin), followed by the virus strain number, the year isolated, and finally, the virus subtype.

Mode of spread: Influenza is highly contagious and spreads from person to person by virus-containing respiratory droplets and secretions. It occurs in epidemics. Regularly, new strains develop, usually from animal hosts, where humans and animals, especially fowl, live in close contact.

Molecular pathogenesis: After inhalation, influenza virus reaches the surface of respiratory epithelial cell. A viral glycoprotein (hemagglutinin) binds to sialic acid residues on respiratory epithelium and gain entry into the cell. Once inside the infected cell, the virus directs the cell to produce its progeny viruses and produced death of the infected cell. Infection usually involves both the upper and lower airways. Destruction of ciliated epithelium paralyses the normal mucociliary clearance and predisposes to bacterial infection (e.g., *Staphylococcus aureus* and *Streptococcus pneumonia*) leading to bacterial pneumonia.

MORPHOLOGY

Influenza virus produces necrosis and desquamation of ciliated respiratory tract epithelium. This is accompanied by a predominantly lymphocytic inflammatory infiltrate. The infection may extend to the lungs and can lead to necrosis and sloughing of cells lining the alveoli. It may produce viral pneumonitis.

Clinical features: The characteristic clinical features include rapid onset of fever, chills, myalgia, headaches, weakness, and nonproductive cough. Symptoms may be due to an upper respiratory infection or those of tracheitis, bronchitis, and pneumonia. Epidemics are usually associated with deaths due to both influenza and its complications. These are especially seen in the elderly and individuals with underlying cardiopulmonary disease.

Swine flu (H1N1-novel influenza A)

Q. Write short essay Swine Flu.

Swine influenza virus (SIV) refers to influenza cases that are caused by Orthomyxovirus endemic to pig populations. SIV strains have been classified either as influenza virus C or one of the various subtypes of the genus influenza virus A. In late March and early April 2009, cases of human infection with swine influenza A (H1N1) viruses were first reported in Southern California and near San Antonio, Texas.

Swine influenza is a respiratory disease of pigs caused by type A influenza virus that regularly causes outbreaks of influenza in pigs that cause high levels of illness but low death rates in pigs. SIVs may circulate among swine throughout the year, but most outbreaks occur during the late fall and winter months similar to outbreaks in humans. The classical swine flu virus (an influenza type A H1N1 virus) was first isolated from a pig in 1930.The disease originally was nicknamed swine flu because the virus that causes the disease originally jumped to humans from the live pigs in which it evolved. The virus is a "reassortant"—a mix of genes from swine, bird, and human flu viruses.

Source of infection

- Droplets from cough or sneeze of an infected individual.
- Object contaminated by the cough or touch of an infected person.

Infected individual sheds the virus from the day prior to illness onset until resolution of fever. Hence infected individuals should be considered to be contagious up to 7 days from the onset of illness.

Signs and symptoms: Patients aged above 65, children below 5 years, pregnant women (especially during the third trimester) and those with underlying medical conditions (e.g., asthma, diabetes, obesity, and heart disease), or those with weakened immune system (e.g., on immunosuppressive medications or infected with HIV) are at high risk of serious complications. Various symptoms include—high grade fever, unusual tiredness, headache, running nose, sore throat, shortness of breath or cough, loss of appetite, aching muscles, and diarrhea or vomiting.

Complications: ARDS (acute respiratory distress syndrome) and MODS (multiple organ dysfunction syndrome).

Diagnosis

A confirmed case of novel influenza A (H1N1) virus infection is defined as a person with an influenza-like illness with laboratory confirmed novel influenza A (H1N1) virus infection by one or more of the following tests:

- Real-time RT-PCR.
- Viral culture from swabs (nasal, oral, and secretions of respiratory tract) can be used for virus isolation.

Parainfluenza Virus

The parainfluenza viruses cause acute, highly contagious upper and lower respiratory tract infections. These viruses are the most common cause of croup (laryngotracheobronchitis), which is characterized by stridor on inspiration and a "barking" cough. In croup there is subglottic swelling, airway compression and respiratory distress. Croup is common in children below the age of 3 years.

Parainfluenza viruses: These are enveloped, single-stranded RNA viruses that belong to the paramyxovirus family. There are four serotypes.

Mode of spread: The virus spreads from person to person through infectious respiratory aerosols and secretions.

MORPHOLOGY

Parainfluenza viruses infect and kill ciliated epithelial cells of respiratory tract and produce an inflammatory response. In very young children, it frequently extends into the lower respiratory tract and produces bronchiolitis and pneumonitis. In young children, the trachea is narrow and the larynx is small. Hence, the local edema of laryngotracheitis caused by parainfluenza viruses compresses the upper airway. This may obstruct breathing and cause croup.

Clinical features: Parainfluenza infection presents with fever, hoarseness, and cough. Characteristic feature is barking cough which is inspiratory stridor. The symptoms of parainfluenza infection are usually mild in older children and adults.

Respiratory Syncytial Virus

Respiratory syncytial virus belongs to the family Paramyxoviridae, same as that of as parainfluenza virus. The virus is highly contagious. The most common cause of bronchiolitis and pneumonia in infants (children younger than 1 year) is RSV.

Mode of spread: RSV spreads rapidly from child to child via respiratory aerosols and secretions. This is common in day-care centers, hospitals, and other settings where small children are confined.

MORPHOLOGY

Respiratory syncytial virus causes necrosis and produces sloughing of bronchial, bronchiolar, and alveolar epithelium. There is mainly lymphocytic inflammatory infiltrate. Sometimes the infected tissue may show multinucleated syncytial cells.

Clinical features: RSV infection in infants and young children produces bronchiolitis or pneumonitis. Clinically, it presents with wheezing, cough, and respiratory distress, sometimes associated with fever. It is usually self-limited and resolves within 1–2 weeks. RSV produces much milder disease in older children and adults. In healthy young children, mortality from RSV infection is very low. But it is significant in hospitalized children with congenital heart disease, chronic lung disease, prematurity, or immunosuppression.

Severe Acute Respiratory Syndrome

An epidemic of severe pneumonia occurred in China in early 2002. This has spread around the globe via international air travel. This emerging clinical disease is called **severe acute respiratory syndrome**.

SARS-CoV: The causative agent for SARS is a novel coronavirus, termed the SARS-associated coronavirus (SARS-CoV). SARS is a potentially fatal viral respiratory illness. SARS-CoV has not been eradicated and has the potential to re-emerge.

Source of infection: It is derived from a nonhuman host, most probably bats, with civets and other animals as likely intermediate hosts.

Incubation period: 2–7 days.

MORPHOLOGY

Lungs: Patients who died from SARS, the lungs showed diffuse alveolar damage. Microscopically, multinucleated syncytial cells without viral inclusions may be seen.

Clinical features: SARS presents with fever and headache. Soon it will be followed by cough and dyspnea. Coryza is usually not observed and it is quite common to develop diarrhea. Some patients develop ARDS and may develop complications and death. Most patients recover and symptoms last up to 10 days. Mortality rate may be as high as 15% in the elderly and in patients with other respiratory disorders.

Intestinal Virus Infections

Norovirus

Norovirus was **previously called as Norwalk-like virus**. Norovirus is a small icosahedral, nonenveloped virus with a single-stranded RNA genome. It is a **common cause of nonbacterial gastroenteritis** and about 50% of all gastroenteritis outbreaks worldwide are due to norovirus.

Source of infection: Humans are the only known reservoir.

Mode of transmission: It is transmitted from person to person mainly through fecal-oral transmission. Local norovirus outbreaks are usually initiated through contaminated food or water.

Incubation period: Up to 2 days.

Clinical features: It presents with vomiting, cramping abdominal pain, and watery diarrhea. Nonspecific symptoms include headache, chills, and myalgias. The symptoms usually resolve within 2–3 days in most cases.

MORPHOLOGY

Morphological features are nonspecific. These include mild shortening of villi, vacuolization of epithelial cells, hypertrophy of crypt, and infiltration of neutrophils, lymphocytes, and monocytes in the lamina propria.

Rotavirus

Rotavirus is an encapsulated virus with a segmented, double-stranded RNA genome and is a member of the family Reoviridae. There are five species (A–E) of rotavirus and type A, the most common.

Age group affected: Usually infects young children. **Most susceptible are children between 6 and 24 months of age.** Probably, the antibodies in breast milk provide protection during the first 6 months of life. Rotavirus produces severe watery diarrhea. It can lead to dehydration and death, if untreated. It is a **significant cause of diarrheal deaths.** Rotavirus outbreaks in hospitals and daycare centers are common.

Mode of infection: Rotavirus infection spreads from person to person by the oral-fecal route and infection spreads easily. Minimal infective inoculum requires is only 10 viral particles. Children shed huge amounts of virus in the stool. Siblings, playmates and parents, as well as food, water, and environmental surfaces become easily contaminated with virus. It has a short incubation period of up to 2 days.

Pathogenesis: Rotavirus selectively infects and destroys mature enterocytes in the upper small intestine. Enterocyte damage may be brought out by a viral factor called nonstructural protein 4 (NSP4). This can produce apoptosis of enterocytes. This disrupts the absorption of sugars, fats, and various ions from the lumen of the intestine. Factors causing diarrhea are—(1) loss of absorptive function, (2) net secretion of water and electrolytes, and (4) osmotic diarrhea caused by the incomplete absorption of nutrients. Infected enterocytes are shed from intestinal villi, and the regenerating epithelium initially lacks full absorptive capabilities.

MORPHOLOGY

Morphological changes in rotavirus infection are usually restricted to the duodenum and jejunum. There will be shortening of the intestinal villi and associated with mild infiltrate of neutrophils and lymphocytes.

Clinical features: Rotavirus infection presents with vomiting, fever, abdominal pain, and severe watery diarrhea. Vomiting usually lasts for 2–3 days, but diarrhea persists for 5–8 days. In young children, if adequate fluid is not replaced, diarrhea can lead to fatal dehydration.

Examples of arthropod-borne viruses (arboviruses) are presented in **Box 1**.

LATENT INFECTIONS

Q. Write short essay on latent viral infections and their laboratory diagnosis.

Definition of latency: It is defined as the **persistence of viral genomes in cells, but they do not produce infectious virus.**

Latent virus infections include *HSV infections, varicella-zoster virus (VZV) infections,* and *CMV infections.* Dissemination of the viral infection and tissue injury occurs when the latent

Box 1: Examples of arthropod-borne viruses (arboviruses).

- **Mosquito-borne**
  - Japanese encephalitis
  - West Nile encephalitis
  - Yellow fever
  - Dengue fever
  - Chikungunya disease
- **Tick borne**
  - Kyasanur Forest disease (KFD)
- **Direct contact**
  - Ebola disease

virus gets reactivated. Most frequent viruses that produce latent infections in humans are Herpesviruses.

Herpesvirus Infections

Herpesviruses: The virus family herpesviridae includes several large, encapsulated (enveloped), double-stranded DNA viruses.

The DNA genomes of these viruses encode approximately 70 proteins. Herpesviruses produce acute viral infection followed by latent viral infection. During latent infection, the viruses persist in a noninfectious form with periodic reactivation and shedding of infectious virus. Most of herpesviruses express some common antigenic determinants, and many produce type A nuclear inclusions (acidophilic bodies surrounded by a halo).

Types of human Herpesviruses (Table 9): There are over 80 types of herpesviruses and only eight of which infect humans (human herpesviruses). They are divided into three subgroups depending on the type of cell most frequently infected and the site of latency.

Herpes Simplex Virus Infections

Human herpes viruses 1 and 2 are also called HSVs (herpes simplex viruses), since they produce characteristic vesicular skin lesions. HSVs are common throughout the world and are common viral pathogens (**Table 10**) causing disease in human.

Table 9: Important pathogenic Human Herpesviruses (HHVs).

Group	*Viruses*	*Cells infected*	*Site of latency*
α-group	Herpes simplex virus 1 and 2 (HSV-1 and -2) and VZV (varicella-zoster virus or HHV-3)	Epithelial cells	Postmitotic neurons
β-group	CMV (HHV-5) and human herpesviruses 6 and 7 (HHV-6 and HHV-7)	Variety of cell types	Variety of cell types
γ-group	EBV (HHV-4) and Kaposi sarcoma–associated virus (KSHV/HHV-8)	Lymphoid cells	Lymphoid cells

Table 10: Various diseases caused by herpes simplex (HSV).

Viral type and common presentations	*Infrequent presentations*
HSV-1: Oral–labial herpes	• Conjunctivitis, keratitis • Encephalitis • Herpetic whitlow • Esophagitis* • Pneumonia* • Disseminated infection*
HSV-2: Genital herpes	• Perinatal infection • Disseminated infection*

*Usually occur in immunocompromised hosts.

HSV-1 and HSV-2 are antigenically (serologically) and epidemiologically **distinct HSVs**. But these **are closely related genetically and cause a similar set of primary and recurrent infections**.

Mode of infection: HSV spreads from person to person, mainly by **direct contact with infected secretions or open lesions**.

- **HSV-1:** It is **transmitted in oral secretions/saliva** (kissing or sharing eating utensils with an infected person) and usually **causes disease "above the waist."** The sites include oral, facial, and ocular regions. Infection frequently occurs in childhood.
- **HSV-2:** It is **transmitted by contact with genital lesions or secretions**. It usually **produces genital ulcers and neonatal herpes infection**. It is primarily a venereally transmitted pathogen. Neonatal herpes is acquired when a baby passes through an infected birth canal.

Primary HSV disease

Herpes simplex virus produces primary disease at a site of initial viral inoculation (usually oropharynx, genital mucosa, or skin).

MORPHOLOGY

Microscopy (Fig. 8): The cellular alterations induced by HSV include (1) nuclear homogenization, (2) **Cowdry type A intranuclear inclusions, and (3) multinucleated giant cells**. HSV-infected epithelial cells contain large, pink to purple intranuclear inclusions (Cowdry type A).

- **Cowdry bodies:** Cowdry bodies are named after the Canadian-American biologist **Edmund Vincent Cowdry** (1888–1975). These are eosinophilic or basophilic intranuclear inclusions composed of nucleic acid and protein and these cytopathic changes are considered a hallmark of viral infection (seen in cells infected with HSV, varicella-zoster virus, and CMV). Cowdry bodies are fixation artifacts and not due to direct result of the intracellular virus. These inclusions consist of viral replication proteins and virions at various stages of assembly. These intranuclear inclusions push the chromatin of host cell nucleus to the edges of the nucleus.

Continued

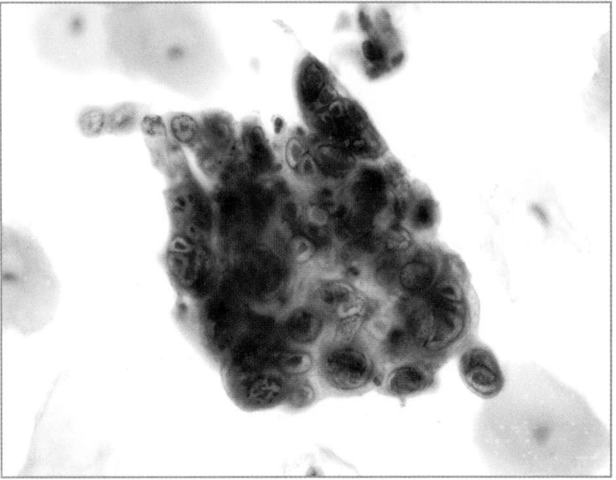

FIG. 8: Pap-stained smear showing multinucleated giant cells and intranuclear viral inclusion bodies typical of genital herpes simplex infection (HSV-2).

Continued

- There are two types of intranuclear Cowdry bodies.
  i. **Cowdry type A:** It is an acidophilic material of droplet-like masses surrounded by clear halos within nuclei. It is found in gingivostomatitis and conjunctivitis caused by HSV and also chicken pox caused by varicella zoster.
  ii. **Cowdry type B:** It is intranuclear eosinophilic without any nuclear change, seen in infection with poliovirus and cytomegalovirus (refer **Fig. 13**).

Herpes simplex virus also produces **inclusion-bearing multinucleated syncytia or giant cells**. Lesions produced by HSV-1 and HSV-2 range from self-limited cold sores and gingivostomatitis to life-threatening disseminated visceral infections and encephalitis.

Mucocutaneous lesions: Both viruses infect epithelial cells, replicate in the skin and the mucous membranes at the site of entry of the virus. They produce infectious virions at their entry site and destroy basal cells in the squamous epithelium, with resulting formation of vesicles in the epidermis. Necrosis of cells elicits an inflammatory response, initially consisting of neutrophils and then followed by lymphocytes. Primary infection resolves when humoral and cell-mediated immunity to the virus develop. HSV-1 and HSV-2 cause self-limited cold sores and gingivostomatitis.

- **Fever blisters or cold sores:** Both viruses replicate at the site of entry of the virus (namely-the skin and the mucous membranes usually oropharynx or genitals). They cause vesicular lesions of the epidermis. Fever **blisters or cold sores** are observed in the facial skin around mucosal orifices (lips and nose) where they are frequently bilateral and independent of skin dermatomes. Intraepithelial vesicles (blisters) are formed by intracellular edema and ballooning degeneration of epidermal cells. They may burst and crust over, but some may produce superficial ulcerations.
- **Gingivostomatitis:** It is usually observed in children and is mainly caused by HSV-1. It is characterized by a vesicular eruption extending from the tongue to the retropharynx. It is associated with cervical lymphadenopathy.
  - Herpetic whitlow: It is swollen, painful, and erythematous HSV lesions of the fingers or palm. It may develop in infants and, rarely, in healthcare workers due to occupational exposure to HSV.
- **Genital herpes** is more usually due to HSV-2 than by HSV-1. It is characterized by vesicles on the genital mucous membranes and external genitalia (see Fig. 13 of Chapter 17). These vesicles rapidly undergo superficial ulcerations and are surrounded by an inflammatory infiltrate.
  - **Neonatal herpes** is a serious complication that can follow maternal genital herpes (usually HSV-2). The virus is transmitted to the neonates during passage through the birth canal of the infected mothers, usually from th uterine cervix. Neonatal herpes begins 5–7 days after delivery. Neonate develops irritability, lethargy, and a mucocutaneous vesicular eruption. In the neonate, HSV-2 infection may be mild. More commonly in an unprotected new-born, the infection rapidly and easily spreads to involve multiple organs, including the brain. Dissemination produces generalized lymphadenopathy, splenomegaly, jaundice,

Continued

Continued

bleeding problems, respiratory distress, and necrotic foci throughout the lungs, liver, adrenals, and CNS. The infected new-born may develop seizures and coma.

Other lesions:

Apart from cutaneous and genital lesions, HSV can cause other lesions.

- **Ophthalmic lesions:** Two forms of corneal lesions may be produced
  i. **Herpes epithelial keratitis:** Corneal epithelial disease causing herpes epithelial keratitis may be due to direct viral damage. It shows virus-induced cytolysis of the superficial epithelium.
  ii. **Herpes stromal keratitis:** It is characterized by mononuclear cell infiltration around keratinocytes and endothelial cells. This leads to neovascularization, scarring, opacification of the cornea, and can lead to corneal blindness. This is due to the damage produced by an immunologic reaction to the HSV infection, rather than the cytopathic effects of the virus.
- **Nervous system**
  - **Herpes encephalitis:** HSV-1 can also produce rare but devastating herpes encephalitis. It develops when the virus that is latent in the trigeminal ganglion is reactivated. The virus travels retrograde to the brain. However, herpes encephalitis can also develop in individuals without and history of blister or "cold sores." Inherited mutations in TLR3 or components of its signaling pathway are likely to increase the risk of HSV encephalitis. When the infection retrogradely spreads to the brain, it usually involves the temporal lobes and orbital gyri of the frontal lobes.
  - **Aseptic meningitis:** It can develop due to HSV-2 infection in patients without genital involvement.
- **Disseminated herpesvirus infections:** Neonates and immunocompromised individuals (e.g., secondary to HIV infection, chemotherapy for underlying cancer or immunosuppression) may develop disseminated skin and visceral herpesvirus infections.
- **Herpes hepatitis:** It is very rare and may develop in immunocompromised patients and in previously healthy pregnant women and may lead to liver failure.
- **Increased risk of HIV:** Due to ulceration and suppression of the immune response, HSV-2 infection increases the risk of HIV transmission and increased risk of developing HIV infection.
- **Herpes esophagitis:** Patients with acquired immunodeficiency syndrome (AIDS) and other immunocompromised individuals are prone to develop herpes esophagitis. Early lesions consist of rounded 1–3-mm vesicles and mainly found in the mid to distal esophagus. As the lesion progresses, HSV-infected squamous cells slough from these lesions and produce sharply demarcated ulcers with elevated margins and they may coalesce. This can cause denudation of the esophageal mucosa. It may be complicated by superinfection with bacteria or fungi. Superimposed *Candida* infection is common. In immunocompromised patients, HSV may also infect the anal mucosa and produce painful blisters and ulcers.

Continued

Continued

- **Herpes bronchopneumonia:** It may develop due to intubation of a patient with active oral lesions and may produce necrotizing bronchopneumonia.

Latency and reactivation

The viruses spread from the primary sites of viral entry by invading the sensory neurons (nerve endings) that innervate the primary site in the oral or genital mucosa. Viral nucleocapsids ascend within axons and establish a latent infection in sensory neurons within corresponding ganglia.

- **Latency:** In immunocompetent individual, primary HSV infection resolves within few weeks. But, the virus DNA remains latent within the nucleus of the neuron and only latency-associated viral RNA transcripts (LATs) are synthesized. There is **no production of viral proteins during latency**. LATs may contribute to latency by (1) preventing apoptosis, (2) silencing lytic gene expression by forming heterochromatin, and (3) serving as precursors for micro-RNAs that downregulate expression of important HSV lytic genes.
- **Reactivation of HSV-1 and HSV-2:** From time to time, the virus awakens from latency and this may occur repeatedly with or without symptoms. During reactivation, the virus travels back down the nerve to the epithelial site served by the ganglion. Thus, the virus spreads from the neurons to the skin or to mucous membranes and again infects epithelial cells. Sometimes this secondary infection can produce ulcerating vesicular lesions. Mostly, the secondary infection does not cause visible tissue destruction, but contagious progeny viruses are shed from the site of infection. Probably during reactivation, release from epigenetic silencing occurs through a methylation/phosphorylation process. This is due to the cellular stress response pathways in neurons. Reactivation can occur even in the presence of normal immunity in host, because HSVs have developed methods to avoid immune recognition. For example, HSVs can escape killing by antiviral cytotoxic T lymphocytes (CTLs) by inhibiting the class I MHC recognition pathway. They can escape humoral immune defenses by generating "decoy" receptors that bind the Fc domain of immunoglobulin and inhibitors of complement. HSVs can infect multiple cell types, including dendritic cells (important for the antiviral immune response). Various factors can induce reactivation of latent HSV infection. These factors include intense sunlight, emotional stress, febrile illness and, in women, menstruation. In immunocompromised individuals both HSV-1 and HSV-2 can produce severe protracted and disseminated disease.

Clinical features

Clinical features of HSV infections vary depending on the host susceptibility (e.g., neonate, normal host, and compromised host), type of HSV, and site of infection. A prodromal "tingling" sensation develops at the site usually precedes the development of lesions in skin. Recurrent lesions appear weeks, months, or years later, at the initial site or at a region of nerve ganglion.

Laboratory diagnosis (Table 11)

Direct microscopic examination of a clinical sample Herpes simplex virus produces characteristic cytopathologic effects (CPEs). It can be identified in a **Tzanck smear** (a scraping of the base of a lesion), papanicolaou (Pap) smear (refer **Fig. 8**), or biopsy specimen. CPEs include multinucleated giant cells (syncytia), "ballooning" cytoplasm, and Cowdry type A intranuclear inclusions. A definitive diagnosis is by demonstrating viral antigen (using immunofluorescence or the immunoperoxidase method) or DNA (using in situ hybridization or PCR) in the tissue sample or vesicle fluid.

Table 11: Laboratory methods and test for viral infections.

Laboratory method or approach	*Test/Comment*
Direct microscopic examination of cells from base of lesion (Tzanck smear)	Multinucleated giant cells (syncytia),Cowdry type A inclusion bodies in cells and nuclear homogenization
Cell culture	Identification of cytopathological effect in cell cultures
Assay of tissue biopsy, smear, cerebrospinal fluid, or vesicular fluid for HSV antigen or genome	**Enzyme immunoassay, immunofluorescent stain, in situ DNA probe analysis, or PCR**
HSV type distinction (HSV-1 versus HSV-2)	Type-specific antibody, DNA probe analysis, and PCR
Serology	Serology is not useful except for epidemiological purpose

(DNA: deoxyribonucleic acid; HSV: herpes simplex virus; PCR: polymerase chain reaction)

Cell culture Virus can be obtained from vesicles but not crusted lesions. Specimens are obtained by aspiration of the lesion fluid or by application of a cotton swab to the vesicles. The sample is inoculated directly into cell cultures.

Genome detection Herpes simplex virus type-specific DNA probes, specific DNA primers for PCR, and quantitative PCR are useful for the detection and differentiation of HSV-1 and HSV-2. **PCR analysis** of the clinical sample or culture specimen is the method of choice for detection and distinction of HSV-1 and HSV-2 for most patients.

Serology Serologic procedures are used only for diagnosis of a primary HSV infection and for epidemiologic purpose. They are not useful for diagnosing recurrent disease because there is no significant rise in antibody titers during recurrent disease.

Varicella-zoster Virus Infections

Varicella-zoster virus **also called as human herpes virus 3** is a dermotropic and neurotropic virus and is a member of the family Herpesviridae. It causes two distinct clinical entities—(1) varicella (chickenpox) and (2) herpes zoster (shingles).

1. **Chickenpox:** Primary (first) **infection with VZV** produces ubiquitous (present worldwide), extremely/highly contagious, acute systemic illness called as chickenpox that is characterized by a generalized vesicular skin eruption. It usually occurs in childhood. It is mild in children but more severe in adults and in immunocompromised individuals.
2. **Herpes zoster (shingles):** The virus then remains latent, and its reactivation **of latent VZV** many years later in life giving rise to a localized vesicular skin eruption termed as herpes zoster ("shingles"). Shingles produces morbidity in older and immunosuppressed individuals.

Mode of Transmission

- Spreads from person to person mainly by the respiratory route through droplet infection.
- Direct contact with discharge from ruptured lesions on the skin.

Varicella-zoster virus is restricted to human hosts and humans are the only reservoirs of VZV. Chicken pox is contagious till pustules disappear.

Incubation period is about 10–21 days.

Pathogenesis (Fig. 9)

Initial infection: It produces **chicken pox**. VZV initially infects mucous membranes, skin, and neurons and produces a **self-limited primary infection in immunocompetent individuals**. There it replicates and disseminates through the blood and lymphatic systems. Many organs are infected during this viremic stage, but dominant clinical presentation is development of vesicular skin lesions. The virus spreads from the capillary endothelium to the epidermis, where its replication destroys the basal cells of epidermis. This causes separation of upper layers of the epidermis separate from the basal layer and form **vesicles (Fig. 10)**.

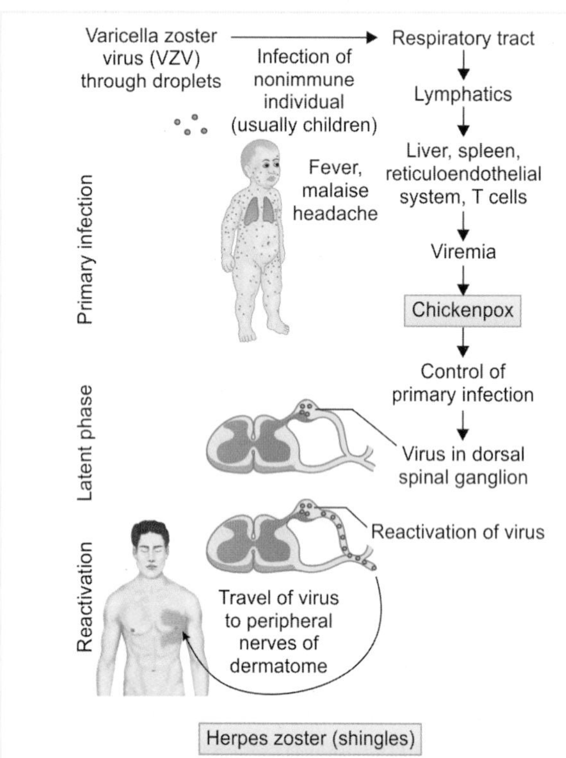

FIG. 9: Clinical entities produced by varicella-zoster virus (VZV) (chickenpox) and herpes zoster (shingles). Initial VZV in a nonimmune individual (usually a child) produces chickenpox. After the control of primary infection, VZV resides in a dorsal spinal ganglion, where it remains dormant for many years. Latent VZV is reactivated and spreads from ganglia along the sensory nerves to the peripheral nerves of sensory dermatomes. This causes herpes zoster (shingles).

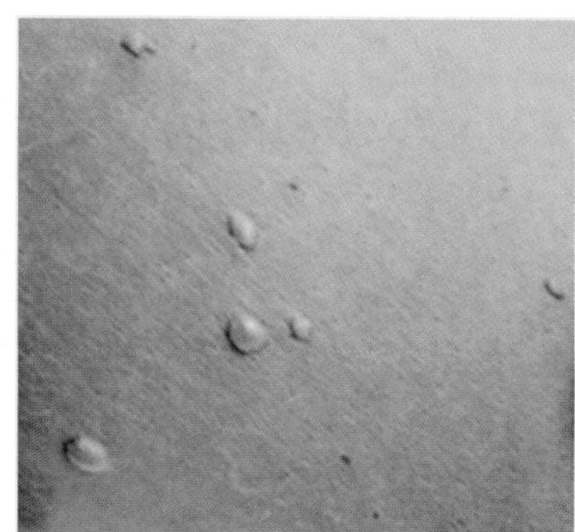

FIG. 10: Vesicles in chickenpox.

Latent infection: Like HSV, during primary infection, VZV evades immune responses and establishes a latent infection. Latent VZV infection is observed in neurons and/or perineuronal satellite cells around neurons in the dorsal nerve root sensory ganglia. During latency, transcription of viral genes continues, and viral DNA can be demonstrated years after the initial infection.

Reactivation and clinical recurrences: It produces **shingles (Fig. 11)** and these are uncommon but may occur many years after the primary infection. Shingles occurs when VZV replicates in ganglion cells and the virus travels down the sensory nerve from a single dermatome (area of skin that's supplied by a single spinal nerve). The virus then infects the corresponding epidermis and produces a localized, painful vesicular eruption. The virus is most likely to be latent in the trigeminal ganglia and localized recurrence of VZV is most common and painful in dermatomes innervated by trigeminal ganglia. Shingles rarely recurs in immunocompetent individuals, but risk of shingles increases with age and most cases occur among the elderly and in immunosuppressed individuals.

Diagnosis: VZV infection is diagnosed by (1) viral culture, (2) PCR, or (3) detection of viral antigens in cells scraped from superficial lesions.

MORPHOLOGY

Chickenpox

- **Gross:** Chicken pox presents with characteristic rash that develops about 2 weeks after respiratory infection. They appear in multiple waves centrifugally, first appear on the trunk followed by the face, and finally on the limbs. Rash appear first as **small pink macules** and **progress** rapidly **to papules and vesicles (Fig. 10) within 24 hours**. The vesicle resembles a dewdrop on a rose petal. Over several days, vesicles become pustules, which then rupture. Finally, these lesions dry up, heal, and form scabs. Vesicles may also develop on mucous membranes, especially the mouth.

Continued

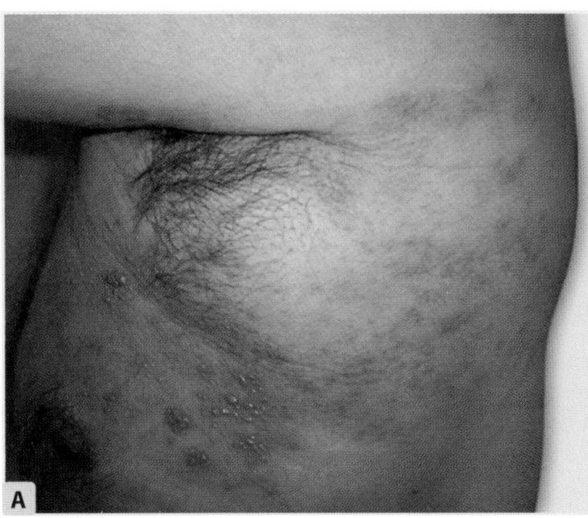

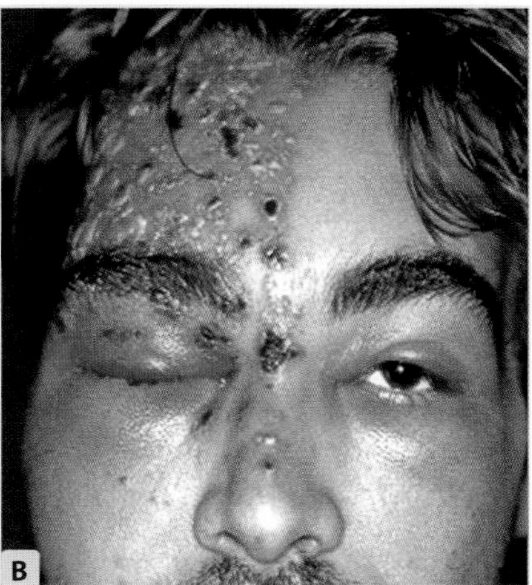

FIGS. 11A AND B: (A) Herpes zoster–dermatomal involvement; (B) Ramsay hunt syndrome.

Continued

- **Microscopy:** The lesions of chickenpox show intraepithelial vesicles with intranuclear inclusions in epithelial cells at the base of the vesicles. Vesicles may be filled with neutrophils and in few days, most vesicles rupture to produce shallow ulcers, crust over, and heal by regeneration. In infected cells, VZV causes a characteristic cytopathic effect and produces nuclear homogenization and intranuclear inclusions (Cowdry type A). Intranuclear inclusions are large and eosinophilic and are separated from the nuclear membrane by a clear zone (halo). Multinucleated cells are also common.
- **Scarring:** Usually, there will be no scar formation. However, if there is bacterial superinfection of vesicles ruptured by trauma, it may destroy the basal epidermal layer and produce scarring.

Shingles

- After this initial infection, VZV persists in latent form in the dorsal root ganglion of sensory nerves or cranial nerve ganglia. Shingles arises from the reactivation of his latent virus later in life. After reaching skin, the virus infects keratinocytes and causes vesicular lesions. These vesicles unlike chickenpox, are usually associated with intense itching, severe pain **(burning discomfort),** or sharp pain in the affected dermatome because of concomitant radiculoneuritis. Most commonly involves **thoracic dermatomes (Fig. 11A) or ophthalmic division of the trigeminal nerve** (vesicles may develop on the cornea and can produce corneal ulceration leading to blindness) (**Fig. 11B**). This pain is severe when the trigeminal nerves are involved; rarely, the geniculate nucleus is involved. This causes facial paralysis [Ramsay Hunt syndrome (**Fig. 11B**)]. Ramsay Hunt syndrome consists of triad of (1) ipsilateral facial paralysis/palsy (ipsilateral loss of taste and buccal ulceration), (2) ear pain, and (3) vesicles/rashes in the external auditory canal and auricle. Pain can persist for months after skin lesions resolve.
- **Microscopy:** The sensory ganglia show a dense, predominantly mononuclear infiltrate, and herpetic intranuclear inclusions within neurons and their supporting cells.

Continued

Continued

Other lesions

- Varicella-zoster virus can also produce interstitial pneumonia, encephalitis, transverse myelitis, vasculopathy, and necrotizing visceral lesions. This mainly develops in immunosuppressed individuals.
- Similar to HSV, patients with mutations in TLR3 have an increased risk of developing VZV encephalitis.

Laboratory Diagnosis

- **Isolation of VZV:** It is not done routinely. This is because the virus is labile during transport to the laboratory and replicates poorly in vitro.
- **Polymerase chain reaction and genome detection techniques:** These are useful for confirming a diagnosis.
- **Direct fluorescent antibody to membrane antigen (FAMA) test:** It can be performed on skin lesion scrapings or biopsy specimens.
- **Serologic tests:** The serological test to detect antibodies to VZV is used mainly to screen populations for immunity to VZV. However, because of normally low levels of antibody more sensitive tests such as immunofluorescence and ELISA are performed to detect the antibody. A significant increase in antibody level can be found in patient with herpes zoster.

Cytomegalovirus Infections

Cytomegalovirus is a congenital and opportunistic pathogen belonging to β-**group herpesvirus. CMV can cause a variety of disease manifestations.** It **depends on the age of the individuals and especially on the immune status of the host.**

Cytomegalovirus that usually produces asymptomatic or mononucleosis-like infection in healthy individuals. However, it produces devastating (destructive) systemic infections of the fetus, neonates, and immunocompromised patients. In these patients the virus may infect many different cell types and tissues.

Sources of CMV infection are presented in **Table 12**.

Table 12: Sources of cytomegalovirus infection.

Age group	*Source*
Neonate	Transplacental transmission, intrauterine infections, and cervical secretions
Infant or child	Body secretions: Breast milk, saliva, tears, and urine
Adult	Sexual transmission (semen), blood transfusion, and organ transplantation

Mode of transmission: CMV can be transmitted by several routes and depends on the age group affected. CMV spreads from individual to individual by contact with infected secretions and body fluids. These include the following:

- **Transplacental transmission (congenital CMV):** It is transmitted from mother who has a newly acquired or developed primary infection and who does not have protective antibodies.
- **Neonatal transmission (perinatal CMV):** It occurs through cervical or vaginal secretions during delivery of the child through birth canal or later through breast milk from a mother with active infection.
- **Transmission through saliva:** This may occur during preschool years, especially in day-care centers. Toddlers so infected can transmit the virus to their parents.
- **Transmission by the genital route (sexual contact):** This is the main mode of transmission after about 15 years of age. Spread can also occur through respiratory secretions and the fecal-oral route.
- **Iatrogenic transmission:** This mode of transmission can occur at any age via organ transplant or blood transfusion.

Pathogenesis

Cytomegalovirus can infect various cells in human. These include epithelial cells, lymphocytes, monocytes, and their bone marrow progenitors, dendritic cells and establish latency in white blood cells. Normal immune responses rapidly control infection, and prevent its bad effects. However, virus is periodically shed in body secretions. Similar to other herpesviruses, CMV may also remain latent for life. CMV can be reactivated when cellular immunity is depressed.

Acute CMV infection and immune suppression: Acute CMV causes transient but severe immunosuppression.

- Cytomegalovirus can infect dendritic cells and impair processing of antigen and their ability to stimulate T lymphocytes. Similar to other herpesviruses, CMV can evade immune defenses by down-regulating class I and II major histocompatibility complex (MHC) molecules and also by producing homologues of tumor necrosis factor (TNF) receptor superfamily members, interleukin-10 (IL-10), and class I MHC molecules. CMV can also evade NK cells by producing ligands that block activating receptors and class I-like proteins that engage inhibitory receptors. This knowledge is utilized for adoptive transfer of CMV-specific T cells to prevent CMV disease after bone marrow transplantation, and the CD8+ T cell response is probably the most important effector response. CD4+ T cells, γδ T cells, and NK cells are played an important role in immune control of the infection. CMV encodes many Fcγ-binding glycoproteins that operate as adversaries of host Fcγ receptors, inhibiting IgG-mediated immunity. Thus, CMV acts by both hiding from and actively suppressing the immune responses.
- Cytomegalovirus infection is usually produces symptoms in immunosuppressed individuals (e.g., organ transplant recipients). In such patients, the CMV infection usually due to reactivation of endogenous latent infection. The source may be either from the graft or in the recipient itself. Subsequent dissemination of CMV may lead to severe systemic disease.

Congenital Infections

Infected pregnant woman can transmit CMV to her fetus and the fetus is not protected by maternally derived antibodies. Hence, the virus invades cells of the fetal cells with only little initial immunologic response. This produces widespread necrosis and inflammation. CMV produces similar lesions in patients with suppressed cell-mediated immunity. CMV is the most common congenital pathogen.

In congenital CMV disease, infection is acquired in utero and has diverse clinical presentations.

- **Asymptomatic:** Majority (about 95%) of cases, it remains asymptomatic. Rarely, a totally asymptomatic infection may be followed months to years later by neurologic sequelae. These include delayed-onset intellectual disability and deafness.
- **Cytomegalic inclusion disease:** Sometimes, CMV produces classic cytomegalic inclusion disease. It develops when the virus is acquired from a mother with primary infection (who does not have protective antibodies). Cytomegalic inclusion disease resembles erythroblastosis fetalis. Affected infants may have intrauterine growth retardation and present with jaundice, hepatosplenomegaly, anemia, bleeding due to thrombocytopenia, and encephalitis. In severe fatal disease, the brain is usually smaller than normal (microcephaly) and may show foci of calcification. Diagnosis of neonatal CMV is by viral culture or PCR amplification of viral DNA in urine or saliva of the neonates. Infants, who survive CMV infection, usually develop permanent deficits such as intellectual disability, hearing loss, and other neurologic impairments.
- **Milder form of disease:** The congenital infection is not always devastating. It may produce milder form of disease such as interstitial pneumonitis, hepatitis, or a hematologic disorder. Most infants with milder form of cytomegalic inclusion disease recover, though some may develop intellectual disability later. Most congenital CMV infection may not be detected until later in life. This may manifest with minimal neurological or hearing defects without gross abnormalities.
- **Fetal death:** CMV may rarely cause fetal death in utero with conspicuous CNS lesions, liver disease and bleeding.

Perinatal Infections

Perinatal infection is acquired by the neonate during passage through the birth canal or from breast milk. It is usually asymptomatic because of protective maternal anti-CMV antibodies that are transmitted to the fetus. Though, these infants are asymptomatic, many of them continue to excrete CMV in their urine or saliva for months to years. Less commonly, infected infants may develop interstitial pneumonitis, failure to thrive, rash, or hepatitis. Rarely, it may produce mild effects on hearing and intelligence later in life.

Cytomegalovirus Mononucleosis

Cytomegalovirus infection in healthy young children and adults is usually asymptomatic. CMV infection in immunocompetent hosts beyond the neonatal period, most commonly manifest as an infectious mononucleosis-like illness, with fever, atypical lymphocytosis, lymphadenopathy, and hepatitis, marked by hepatomegaly and abnormal liver function tests. It is diagnosed by serological study. Most individuals recover without any sequelae. However, they may continue to excrete the virus in body fluids for months to years. Infected individuals, whether symptomatic or asymptomatic will remain seropositive for life. The virus is not cleared from the body and persists in latently infected leukocytes.

Cytomegalovirus in Immunosuppressed Individual

Severe CMV infection can occur in immunocompromised individuals (e.g., transplant recipients and HIV-infected individuals). The infection may be either new infections or reactivation of latent CMV.

- **Human immunodeficiency virus patients:** In the past, CMV was considered as the most common opportunistic viral pathogen in AIDS. At present, CMV infection in HIV patients is greatly reduced due to antiretroviral treatment.
- **Recipients of solid-organ transplants:** Patients who undergo transplantation such as heart, liver, and kidney may contract CMV from the donor organ. In such immunosuppressed individuals, serious, even life-threatening, disseminated CMV infections mainly affect the lungs (pneumonitis) and gastrointestinal tract (colitis).
    - **Pulmonary infection:** It shows an interstitial mononuclear infiltrate with foci of necrosis and the typical enlarged cells with inclusions. The pneumonitis can progress to acute respiratory distress syndrome.
    - **Infections of gastrointestinal tract:** It can cause intestinal necrosis, extensive ulceration, and typical enlarged cells with inclusions. There can be formation of pseudomembranes and debilitating diarrhea.
    - **Other features:** CMV can produce vasculopathy, neurocognitive impairment, and presence of immune markers. These markers include the accumulation of multifunctional terminally differentiated αβ T cells, γδ T cells, and NK cells.

Outcomes of cytomegalovirus (CMV) infections are shown in **Fig. 12**.

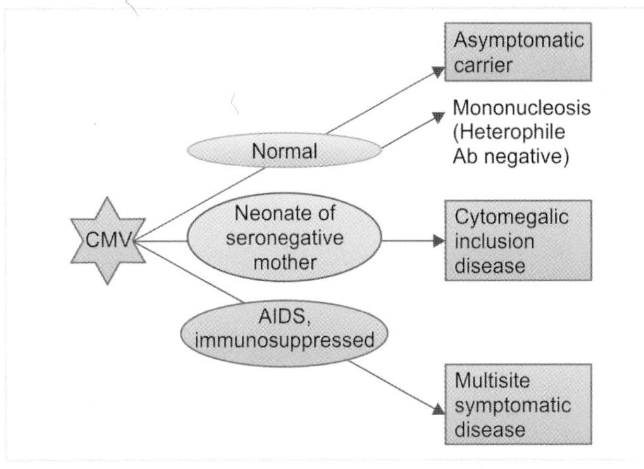

(Ab: antibody; AIDS: acquired immunodeficiency syndrome)

FIG. 12: Outcomes of cytomegalovirus (CMV) infections. The outcome of CMV infection depends mainly on the immune status of the patient.

MORPHOLOGY

In almost any organ, CMV causes focal necrosis with minimal inflammation.

Cells infected: These include

- **Glandular organs:** Parenchymal epithelial cells (**Fig. 13**) of glandular organs
- **Brain:** Neurons in the brain (13 B)
- **Lung:** Alveolar macrophages, epithelial cells, and endothelial cells
- **Kidney:** Tubular epithelial and glomerular endothelial cells.

Continued

Continued

Diagnostic features of CMV infection: (1) Cytomegaly, (2) intranuclear inclusions with characteristic Cowdry type B inclusions (**Figs. 13A and B**), and (3) ill-defined amphophilic intracytoplasmic inclusions. These are observed with hematoxylin and eosin (H and E), periodic acid–Schiff (PAS), and Grocott-Gomori methenamine silver (GMS) stains.

Features of infected cell: As its name implies, CMV-infected cells are strikingly enlarged (show gigantism of both the entire cell and its nucleus) and usually have a diameter of 40 µm. These cells show both cellular and nuclear pleomorphism.

- **Nuclei of infected cell:** The infected cells typically contain a giant nucleus, which is usually single. It contains **prominent, large, intranuclear basophilic inclusions** involving one-half of the nuclear diameters. These large inclusions are usually separated from the nuclear membrane by a clear halo/zone (i.e., surrounded by a clear halo) giving rise to "owl's eye" appearance (**Figs. 13A and B**). These intranuclear inclusions are Cowdry type B inclusions.
- **Cytoplasm of infected cell:** The cytoplasm of infected cells may also show smaller granular basophilic inclusions. They occur after formation of the intranuclear inclusion. Hence, not all CMV infected cells show them.

Laboratory Diagnosis

Diagnosis of CMV infection is by demonstration of characteristic morphologic alterations in tissue sections, viral culture, rising antiviral antibody titer, and detection of CMV DNA by PCR-method. Quantitative PCR-based assays help in monitoring CMV infection in individuals after transplantation.

Histopathology: The microscopic hallmark of CMV infection is the **cytomegalic cell,** which is an **enlarged cell** (25-35 mm in diameter) that contains a dense, **central, "owl's eye," basophilic intranuclear inclusion body** (**Fig. 13**). Such

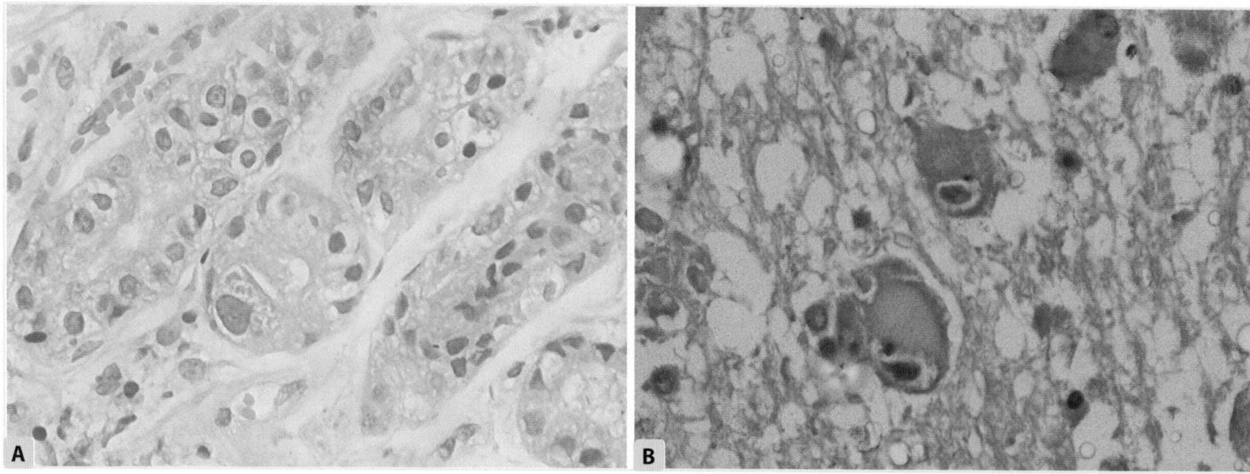

FIGS. 13A AND B: (A) Stomach shows glandular epithelium with one CMV infected cell. (B) CMV infection of brain. The infected cell shows prominent, large, and intranuclear inclusions surrounded by a clear halo giving rise to "owl's eye" appearance.

infected cells are thought to be epithelial in origin and may be found in any tissue and in urine. The inclusions are seen with Papanicolaou or hematoxylin-eosin staining.

Antigen and genome detection: A rapid, sensitive method of diagnosis is by detection of viral antigen. This may be by using immunofluorescence or an ELISA, or the viral genome, using PCR and related techniques in cells of a biopsy, blood, bronchoalveolar lavage, or urine sample. Distinction between active CMV from latent CMV needs detection of CMV mRNA or large amounts of DNA in blood.

Culture: Isolation of CMV is reliable in immunocompromised patients, who usually have high titers of virus in their secretions (e.g., semen of patients with AIDS).

Serology: Seroconversion is an excellent marker for primary CMV infection.

CHRONIC PRODUCTIVE INFECTIONS

In some of the viral infections, the immune system cannot destroy the virus, and these viruses continue to replicate and produce persistent viremia. This may be due to high mutation rate of viruses which escapes their control by the immune system. Examples include human deficiency virus (HIV—refer pages 1127–1152) and hepatitis B virus (HBV).

TRANSFORMING VIRAL INFECTIONS

Some viruses have capacity to transform infected cells into benign or malignant tumor cells. These are called as oncogenic viruses. They can stimulate cell growth and survival by different mechanisms. Various oncogenic viruses that can cause human cancer are EBV, HPV, HBV, and HTLV-1.

Epstein–Barr Virus Infections

Epstein–Barr virus causes infectious mononucleosis and is associated with the pathogenesis of several human tumors, (refer Box 18 of Chapter 10). Only infectious mononucleosis is discussed below.

Q. Write short essay on infectious mononucleosis.

Infectious mononucleosis **(glandular fever)** is an **acute, benign, self-limiting 13** lymphoproliferative disorder **caused by EBV**. It is characterized by fever, sore throat, generalized lymphadenopathy, splenomegaly, and the atypical activated T lymphocytes (mononucleosis cells). In the peripheral blood, some patient may develop hepatitis, meningoencephalitis, and pneumonitis.

Age group: Infectious mononucleosis occurs mainly in late adolescents or young adults.

Pathogenesis (Fig. 14)

- ***Mode of transmission***: It is transmitted by close human contact, mainly through the saliva during kissing (hence the nickname kissing disease).
- ***Incubation period***: It ranges from 4 to 8 weeks.

Epstein–Barr virus infects B lymphocytes and probably epithelial cells of the oropharynx or both. Probably, initially EBV infects oropharyngeal epithelial cells and then spreads to underlying lymphoid tissue (tonsils and adenoids) and infects mature B cells. Evidence for B cells as main reservoir of EBV infection comes from observation that individuals with X-linked agammaglobulinemia (they lack B cells), do not become latently infected with EBV or shed virus.

An EBV envelope glycoprotein binds to the receptor known as **CD21 (CR2)** present on B lymphocyte membrane. CD21 is the receptor for the C3d component of complement. The viral infection begins in the submucosal lymphoid tissues of nasopharynx and oropharynx, particularly the tonsils (**Fig. 14**). The infection of B cells may be either productive (lytic) or latent.

Productive infection: This type of infection is seen only in a **minority** of B cells. The infected B cells produce and **release virions accompanied by death** of these **B cells.** The released virions in turn infect other B cells.

Latent infection: In majority of B cells with EBV infection, the virus becomes latent inside the B cells. The virus remains as an extrachromosomal episomal form. There is **no viral replication** and the infected **B cells are not killed.** These latently infected B cells are transformed or **"immortalized"** so that they are capable of **proliferation indefinitely. Immortalization of B cell is the hallmark of EBV infection.**

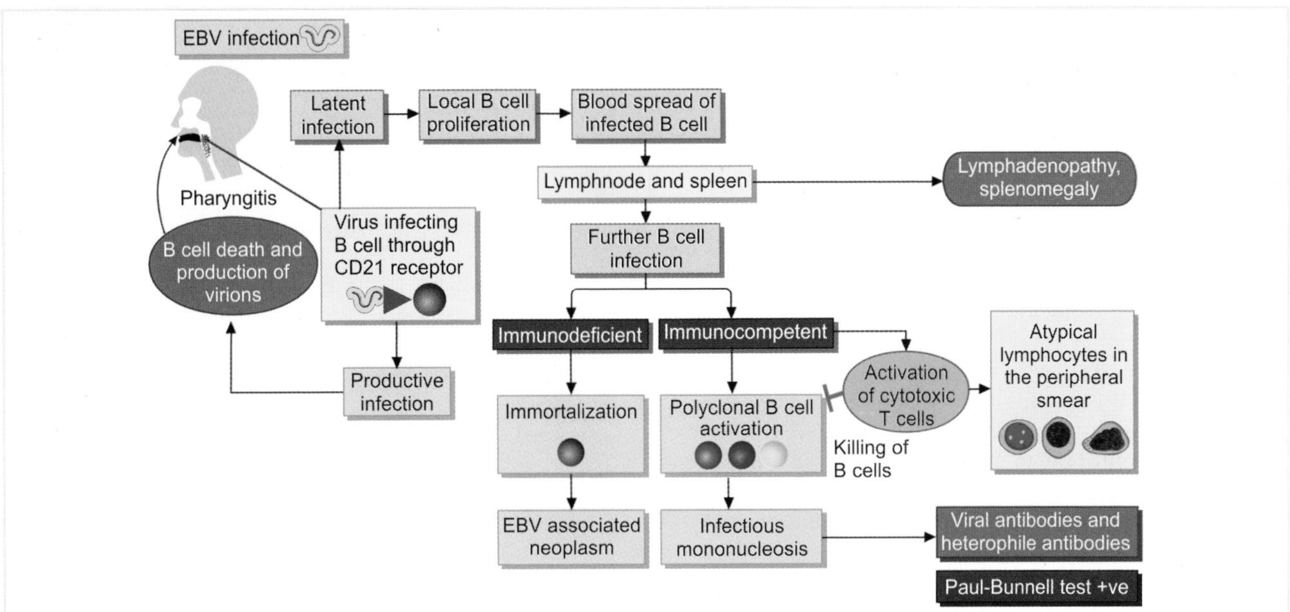

FIG. 14: Pathogenesis of Epstein–Barr virus (EBV) associated lesions.

Molecular basis of B cell proliferation During latent infection, few EBV genes are expressed which disturb the normal signaling pathways. The EBV gene products include:

Epstein–Barr nuclear antigen 1 (EBNA1): This gene product binds the EBV genome to chromosomes of B cells during mitosis. It mediates episomal persistence and maintenance of EBV in daughter cells when infected cells divide.

Latent membrane protein 1 (LMP1):

- It causes activation and proliferation of B-cells by mimicking a constitutively active form of CD40 (which is a B cell surface receptor). Similar to activated CD40, LMP1 binds to TNF receptor-associated factors (TRAFs), adaptor molecules which stimulate events that activate NF-κB and the JAK/STAT signaling pathway.
- Latent membrane protein 1 also prevents apoptosis by activating Bcl-2.

Epstein–Barr nuclear antigen 2 (EBNA2): It also causes activation and replication B-cell. It activates the transcription of many host cell genes, including genes that encode proteins that drive cell cycle (e.g., cyclin D).

Homologue of IL-10 (vIL-10): It is produced by EBV. It inhibits macrophages and dendritic cells and suppresses antiviral T cell responses.

Latently infected B cells multiply locally in the pharynx and subsequently circulate throughout the body producing a generalized infection of the lymphoid tissues (e.g., lymph nodes and spleen).

Immune responses to EBV infection

Epstein-Barr virus induces both humoral and cell-mediated immune response.

1. **Humoral immune response:** B cells latently infected with EBV are activated and begin to proliferate and to disseminate. EBV induces uncontrolled, polyclonal proliferation EBV-infected B cells, and the activated B cells produce various antibodies. They are subdivided into:
   - **Epstein–Barr virus-specific antibodies:** The most useful EBV-specific antibodies are against:
     - **Viral capsid antigens (VCAs)**
     - **Epstein–Barr virus nuclear antigen (EBNA)**

     Both VCA and EBNA antibodies are initially of IgM type followed by IgG type that persists for life. The presence of both VCA and EBNA antibodies in serum indicates that the individual had a previous infection. Production of antibody to EBNA requires lysis of the infected cell and usually indicates T-cell control of active disease and its presence indicates resolution of the disease. There are two early antigen (EA) namely EA-R (only cytoplasmic) and EA-D (diffuse in cytoplasm and nucleus) and the glycoproteins of the membrane antigen (MA) on the cell surface.
   - **Heterophile antibodies:**
     - Hetero and phile are derived from the Greek words meaning "different" and "affinity," respectively. An antibody formed in response to an antigen from one species but cross-reacts against antigens on the cells of other species is termed as **heterophile antibody.** These are produced against poorly defined antigens and are **nonspecific.**
     - Heterophile antibodies found in patients with infectious mononucleosis are capable of **agglutinating sheep/ox/horse red cells** but **not the human red cells.** This is the basis of diagnostic **Paul-Bunnell test** and other screening tests for infectious mononucleosis. They do not react with EBV antigens.
   - **Autoantibodies**, e.g., autoantibodies against platelets may cause transient immune-mediated thrombocytopenia in few patients with infectious mononucleosis. These are responsible for positive Wassermann reaction.
2. **Cell-mediated immune response:** Activated B cells also stimulate cell-mediated immune response and activate CD8+ cytotoxic T cells (CTLs) and NK cells. The latter two cells (i.e., CD8+ CTLs and NK cells) are **responsible for killing of the viral infected B cells** and also inhibit production of immunoglobulins by B cells. Though EBV

infects B cells, the characteristic **atypical lymphocytes** of this disease seen in the peripheral blood are mainly EBV-specific **CD8+ CTLs and NK cells.** The reactive proliferation of T cells is mainly seen in lymphoid tissues and causes lymphadenopathy and splenomegaly.

In healthy individuals, the fully developed humoral and cellular immune responses to EBV prevent viral shedding, and eliminate of B cells expressing the full complement of EBV latency-associated genes. In these individuals, the infection may either remain asymptomatic or develop self-limited infectious mononucleosis. In individuals with acquired deficiency in cellular immunity (e.g., AIDS and organ transplantation), reactivation of EBV can cause proliferation of B-cells. This proliferation can progress through a multistep process to EBV-associated B-cell lymphomas, and can also contribute to the development of some cases of Burkitt lymphoma. EBV associated Burkitt lymphoma shows a chromosomal translocation (most commonly an 8: 14 translocation) involving the *MYC* oncogene (refer Fig. 23 of Chapter 10).

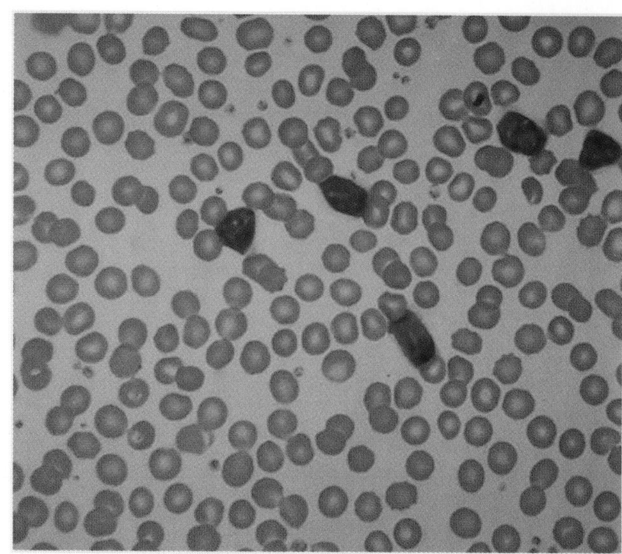

FIG. 15: Peripheral smear in infectious mononucleosis with atypical lymphocytes.

PERIPHERAL SMEAR

The smear findings provide important clues to the diagnosis and can be confirmed by serological tests.

- **RBCs:** Show normocytic normochromic picture.
- **WBCs:** The **total leukocyte count** is usually **increased** (12,000–25,000 cells/cu mm) and is due to **absolute lymphocytosis**, which constitutes >60% of the leukocytes. The characteristic finding is the presence of transformed lymphocytes (**Fig. 15**) in the smear. These cells, known as virocytes/**atypical** (activated) **lymphocytes (mononuclear cells)**; hence the disease is termed as infectious mononucleosis. These atypical lymphocytes constitute 5–80% of lymphocytes are **not pathognomonic** (strongly suggest the diagnosis) and are also observed in other viral fevers. These atypical lymphocytes represent transformed polyclonal **CD8+ subset (cytotoxic) of T cells** and not the virus-infected B cells. **Atypical features which help to identify atypical cells from normal lymphocytes include:**
  - **Size and shape:** Large in size (12–16 μm in diameter) and irregular in shape.
  - **Cytoplasm:**
    - Abundant with scattered azurophilic granules.
    - Increased cytoplasmic basophilia, more prominent at the edges.
    - Multiple clear cytoplasmic vacuoles and the cytoplasm shows scalloped margins at points of contact with other cells.
  - **Nucleus:**
    - Oval, indented, or folded nucleus.
    - Two to three times larger than those of normal lymphocytes.
    - Diffuse chromatin pattern with prominent nucleoli.

Platelets: Normal or mildly decreased.

MORPHOLOGY

The major morphological changes are observed in the lymph nodes, spleen, liver, CNS, and, occasionally, other organs.

Lymph Nodes

Gross: They are discrete and are enlarged throughout the body; mainly in the posterior cervical, axillary, and inguinal regions.

Microscopy

- **Paracortical T-cell proliferation:** Characteristically, it shows expansion of paracortical regions due to proliferation of activated T cells (immunoblasts). Sometimes, the proliferation of T-cell may be extensive and may be difficult to distinguish from that of non-Hodgkin lymphomas.
- **Immunohistochemistry:** By using specific antibodies, a minor population of EBV-infected B cells expressing Epstein–Barr nuclear antigen 2 *(EBNA2),* latent membrane protein 1 *(LMP1),* and other latency-specific genes can also be found in the paracortex.
- **Reed-Sternberg-like cells:** EBV-infected B cells resembling Reed-Sternberg cells (malignant cells of Hodgkin lymphoma) may be seen.
- **Mild follicular hyperplasia:** B-cell areas (follicles) may show mild hyperplasia.

Similar changes may be observed in the tonsils and lymphoid tissue of the oropharynx.

Spleen

Gross: It is enlarged in most of the patients. It weighs between 300 and 500 g. It is soft and fleshy, with a hyperemic cut surface. These spleens are susceptible to rupture, partly due to the rapid increase in size produces splenic capsule to become tense and fragile.

Continued

Continued

Microscopy: There are similar to that of the lymph nodes. They show an expansion of white pulp follicles and red pulp sinusoids due to the presence of numerous activated T cells.

Liver

Gross: Usually involved to some degree and produces moderate hepatomegaly.

Microscopy: It shows atypical lymphocytes in the portal areas and sinusoids. There may be foci of parenchymal necrosis. It is similar to that of other forms of viral hepatitis.

Clinical Features

Age: It is usually seen in young adults among upper socioeconomic classes in developed nations and children of low socioeconomic status.

Signs and symptoms: The symptoms of infectious mononucleosis develop after the initiation of the host immune response. Infectious mononucleosis usually presents with nonspecific prodromal symptoms followed by the **classical triad** of fever, pharyngitis, and lymphadenopathy.

- **Fever:** It is associated with headache, malaise, nausea, anorexia, and myalgia.
- **Pharyngitis:** Sore throat occurs in most of the patients.
- **Lymphadenopathy:** Usual lymph nodes enlarged are cervical, axillary, and inguinal. Mild-to-moderate splenomegaly is observed in about 50% of the patients.

Epstein–Barr virus also may be the cause of fever of unknown origin when there is no significant lymphadenopathy or other localized findings. Hepatitis may resemble that of hepatotropic viral syndromes, or a febrile rash may resemble rubella.

Serological tests

Demonstration of heterophile antibodies: The following tests will be useful for demonstration of heterophile antibodies:

- Paul-Bunnell test is characteristically positive.
- Monospot test is a sensitive slide test.

Demonstration specific antibodies against EBV antigens: These are demonstrated by ELISA. The EBV specific antibodies are:

- **Antibody against VCAs (anti-VCA):** These antibodies are initially of IgM type and later of IgG type (which persists for life).
- **Antibodies to EBNA:** This can be demonstrated by PCR.

Diagnosis of IM (Box 2)

Diagnosis of IM can be done with following findings (in increasing order of specificity):

- Lymphocytosis with the characteristic atypical lymphocytes in the peripheral blood.
- Positive heterophile antibody reaction (Monospot test).
- Rising titer of specific antibodies for EBV antigens (VCAs, EAs, or EBNA).

Usually, infectious mononucleosis resolves within 4–6 weeks in of the most patients.

Complications

Complications may occasionally occur and some of them are listed in **Box 3**.

Box 2: Diagnosis of Epstein–Barr virus (EBV).

- Symptoms: Triad-Fever, pharyngitis lymphadenopathy
- Complete blood cell count: Atypical lymphocytes (Downey cells and T cells)
- Heterophile antibody (transient)
- EBV–antigen-specific antibody
- Genome detection by PCR

(PCR: polymerase chain reaction)

Box 3: Complications of infectious mononucleosis.

- Hepatic dysfunction (most common): Jaundice, raised liver enzymes, disturbed appetite, and rarely liver failure
- Immunohemolytic anemia due to formation of IgM antibodies
- Immune thrombocytopenia
- Hemophagocytic syndrome
- Rupture of spleen with minor trauma (rare): Cause hemorrhage which may be fatal
- Nervous system involvement
- Other organs involvement: Kidneys, bone marrow, lungs, eyes, and heart
- Secondary bacterial infection of throat
- B cell lymphoma

B-cell lymphoma: Patients with absence of T-cell immunity (e.g., patients with HIV, or receiving immunosuppressive therapy) is uncontrolled proliferation of B-cells causing various neoplasms. It is usually initiated by an acute infection by EBV or reactivation of latent B-cell infection. It starts as polyclonal proliferation of B-cell which transforms to monoclonal B-cell lymphoma.

Inherited immunodeficiency: A rare inherited X-linked lymphoproliferation immunodeficiency disorder (also termed as *Duncan disease*) is caused by mutations in the *SH2D1A* gene. This gene encodes a signaling protein that participates in T-cell and NK-cell activation and production of antibody. In these individuals are usually normal until they are acutely infected with EBV usually during adolescence. These patients when get infected with EBV, there is an ineffective immune response to EBV. In >50% of patients, EBV causes an acute overwhelming infection that may be fatal. Others die due to EBV-positive B-cell lymphoma or infections related to hypogammaglobulinemia.

Other DNA Viruses

Adenovirus

Adenoviruses are nonenveloped DNA viruses.

Source: Respiratory and intestinal tracts of humans and animals.

Mode of spread: It spreads through direct contact, fecal–oral route, and occasionally water-borne transmission.

Incubation period is 1 week.

Clinical features

- Certain serotypes cause of acute respiratory disease and adenovirus pneumonia. Some adenoviruses cause chronic pulmonary disease in infants and young children.
- Certain adenovirus cause pediatric diarrhea. It usually affects immunocompromised individuals. The symptoms include diarrhea, vomiting, and abdominal pain. Usually, it resolves within 10 days.
- Patients with AIDS are susceptible to urinary tract infections and are caused by adenovirus type 35.
- In immunocompromised patients and transplant recipients, adenovirus can cause fulminant or disseminated disease. This may manifest as colitis, pneumonitis, pancreatitis, nephritis, meningoencephalitis, and hepatitis.

MORPHOLOGY

Lung

Necrotizing bronchitis and bronchiolitis: The changes include necrotizing bronchitis and bronchiolitis. This is characterized by sloughing of epithelial cells and filling of inflammatory infiltrate in the damaged bronchioles.

Interstitial pneumonitis: It is characterized by presence of areas of consolidation. There is also extensive necrosis, hemorrhage, and a mononuclear inflammatory infiltrate.

Intranuclear inclusions: Two distinctive types of intranuclear inclusions are observed namely (1) Cowdry type A inclusions and (2) smudge cells. They are seen in bronchiolar epithelial cells and alveolar lining cells. Infected cells may also show intranuclear inclusion bodies.

1. **Cowdry A inclusions:** Adenovirus produces cytopathic effects. In the early stages of adenovirus infection, it produces granular, slightly enlarged nuclei containing eosinophilic bodies intermixed with clumped basophilic chromatin. The eosinophilic bodies coalesce, to form larges masses and produce a central, granular, ill-defined mass surrounded by a halo. This is termed as Cowdry A inclusions.
2. **Smudge cells:** The second type of inclusion is the "smudge cell." It is more common and probably develops at a late-stage infected cell. The nucleus is round or ovoid, large and completely occupied by a granular amphophilic to deeply basophilic mass. There is no clear halo, and the nuclear membrane and nucleus are indistinct.

Small intestine

- Adenoviruses types 40 and 41 infect colonic and small intestinal epithelial cells. In patient with diarrhea due to adenovirus, biopsy may show epithelial degeneration but are usually nonspecific. These include villous atrophy and compensatory crypt hyperplasia. Viral nuclear inclusions are not common.

Human Parvovirus (Erythrovirus) B19

Human parvovirus B19 is **now known as erythrovirus**. It is a single-stranded DNA virus.

It causes a benign self-limited febrile illness in children known as **erythema infectiosum**. It can also produce systemic infections. This is characterized by rash, arthralgias, and transient interruption in red blood cell (RBC) production in nonimmune adults. Infection is common and usually occurs in outbreaks, mostly in children.

Mode of spread: It spreads from person to person by the respiratory route.

Pathogenesis: Human parvovirus B19 **infects erythroid precursor cells via the P-erythrocyte antigen**. It produces a characteristic cytopathic effect in these erythroid precursor cells. Nuclei of affected cells become enlarged. The chromatin of their nuclei is displaced peripherally by central, glassy, and eosinophilic inclusion bodies (giant pronormoblasts). It probably replicates in the respiratory tract before it spreads to erythropoietic cells.

Clinical features: Most individuals present with a mild exanthematous disease termed as **erythema infectiosum ("fifth disease")**. It is associated with an asymptomatic cessation in erythropoiesis (i.e., RBC production). However, in patients with chronic hemolytic anemias, this interruption in erythrocyte production causes severe, potentially fatal anemia. This is termed as **transient aplastic crisis**. When a fetus is infected by human parvovirus B19 through maternal infections. In fetus, cessation of erythropoiesis can lead to severe anemia, hydrops fetalis, and death in utero.

Smallpox (Variola)

Smallpox is a severe, highly contagious exanthematous viral infection produced by variola ("variola" from the Latin *varius,* meaning "pimple" or "spot") virus, a member of the family Poxviridae that belongs to the *Orthopoxvirus* genus. The virus is highly stable and remains infective for longtime outside its human host. It produces a disease with high mortality. There are two types of smallpox namely (1) *Variola major* (prototypical form of the infection) and (2) *Variola minor* (with mild systemic toxicity and smaller pox lesions).

Edward Jenner in 1796 performed the first successful vaccination by inoculating a child with exudate from the hand of a milkmaid infected with cowpox. Once the cowpox pustule had regressed in the child, Jenner challenged that child with smallpox and demonstrated that child was protected from the disease.

Smallpox was eradicated worldwide by a global vaccination program and the last case was reported in 1977. In 1980, World Health Organization (WHO) declared world free of smallpox. Two known repositories of variola virus remain: (1) at the CDC in the United States and (2) at the Institute for Virus Preparation in Russia. There has been vigilance to its re-emergence, either naturally or as a bioweapon. Interest in smallpox has re-emerged because of its potential as a bioweapon. Deliberate introduction of the smallpox virus through aerosolization can produce an epidemic in a few days.

Mode of transmission: Virus spread through the respiratory or oropharyngeal mucosa between victims and susceptible people. The virus is present in contaminated aerosols, droplets, lesional tissue, body fluids, or fomites. It may also spread through contact with lesions (which contains numerous viable virions). Viral titers in the saliva are highest during the first week of infection.

Incubation period: 12 days (range, 7–17 days) after exposure. During incubation period, the viral proliferate within the lymph nodes and subsequently disseminated and seed the other lymphoid tissues throughout the body.

Pathogenesis: The variola virus enters through the respiratory tract and is transported to regional lymph nodes. It replicates in lymph node and travels into blood stream to produce viremia.

MORPHOLOGY

Skin vesicles: They show cellular necrosis and areas of ballooning degeneration. They also show eosinophilic and intracytoplasmic inclusion bodies (Guarnieri bodies). These are not specific for smallpox because they can also occur in most poxviral infections.

Vesicles at other sites: Vesicles can also develop in the palate, pharynx, trachea, and esophagus.

In severe cases: There may involvement of stomach and intestine, hepatitis, and interstitial nephritis.

Clinical features: It develops abruptly with high fever, headache, backache, prostration, malaise, and vomiting. The characteristic rash follows in 2–3 days. It is most prominent on the face but also involves the hands and forearms. Subsequent eruptions develop on the lower extremities and the rash spreads centrally during the next week to the trunk. Lesions progress quickly from macules to papules, then to pustular vesicles. By 8–14 days after onset, the pustules form scabs. Sometimes, it may lead to scar formation or become hypopigmented on healing after 3–4 weeks. The disease is most contagious during the period from the development of the rash up to the 10th day. However, the patient remains contagious till scabs fall off.

Cause of death: May be due to DIC, hypotension, and multiorgan failure.

Monkeypox

Monkeypox is a rare viral zoonotic disease occurring mostly in Central and Western Africa. More recently, it is described in Sudan. It is the only remaining potentially fatal infection of humans caused by a member of the Poxviridae.

Epidemiology: The virus was first isolated from monkeys. Hence, its name is monkeypox. However, it is actually more prevalent in rodents in endemic areas. An outbreak of monkeypox occurred in United States in 2003 among individuals who either owned or had exposure to pet prairie dogs. Infected animals had been exposed to an infected Gambian pouched rat in an exotic pet store. Dormice and squirrels may also be natural reservoirs of the virus.

Mode of infection: Human acquires infection by a bite from an infected host or contact with its body fluids. Human-to-human transmission is uncommon.

Incubation period in humans is about 12 days.

Clinical features: Its clinical presentation closely resembles small pox, but it is milder. It presents with fever, headache, lymphadenopathy, malaise, muscle ache, and backache. Within 1–3 days after onset of fever, a papular rash develops on the face or other parts of the body. These skin lesions crusts and fall off. It usually lasts for 2 weeks. In Africa, mortality is high as 10%.

Chikungunya

Chikungunya is a viral fever caused by an *Alphavirus*. It is usually not fatal. However, during 2005–2006 outbreak occurred in India, where >200 deaths were reported mainly related to CNS involvement and fulminant hepatitis. Chikungunya (in Swahili of African dialect) means "that bends up." It was used in reference to the stooped posture developed due to the arthritic symptoms of the disease.

Mode of spread: By bites from *A. aegypti* mosquitoes.

Source of infection: Humans are the major reservoir of chikungunya virus.

Incubation period: 2–12 days.

Epidemiology: Observed in Tamil Nadu, Karnataka, Kerala, Andhra Pradesh, Rajasthan, Gujarat, and Madhya Pradesh. Significant numbers of cases have been reported from northern India including Delhi.

Clinical features: The fever usually lasts for 2–5 days and may be followed by an afebrile phase and then reappearance of fever **(saddleback pattern).** Skin involvement is more common in children and occurs about 40–50% of cases. It may appear at the beginning or several days (day 2 or 3 of the disease) of the illness. It is usually a pruritic maculopapular rash predominating on the trunk and limbs. Adults are more prone to migratory polyarthritis, which produces early morning pain and swelling, most often in the small joints of the ankles, feet, hands, and wrists. However, larger joints may also be affected. Arthritis may persist for months and may become chronic (6 months to several years) in patients who are positive for human leukocyte antigen (HLA)-B27.

Diagnosis

- **Blood:** Leukopenia and thrombocytopenia may occur but is uncommon.
- **Raised aspartate aminotransferases** and **C-reactive protein** may be found.
- **Demonstrating antibodies** using ELISA method for diagnosis.
- Molecular methods include **RT-PCR** to detect structural genes of virus in the blood sample.

Human Papillomavirus

Human papillomaviruses are nonenveloped, double-stranded DNA viruses.

Classification of HPV: There are >100 HPV types, different types causing different lesions (**Table 13**). They are classified as low and high oncogenic risk HPVs.

- **Low oncogenic risk:**
  - **HPV genome** is maintained in a **nonintegrated free episomal** (extrachromosomal) **form**.
  - **Virus freely replicates** and **causes the death of the host** cell and it is **known as productive infection**.
- **High oncogenic risk:**
  - **Integration into the host DNA:** In cancers, the HPV genome (viral DNA) is integrated into the genome of the host cell, which is important for malignant transformation. **Integration causes:**
    - **Overexpression of the oncoproteins E6 and E7.**
    - **Genomic instability** in the host cell.

Table 13: Classification of human papillomavirus.

Low-oncogenic risk HPV—benign lesions of squamous epithelium	
HPV types 1, 2, 4, and 7	Benign squamous papilloma (common warts and plantar warts)
HPV types 6, 10, 11, and 40 through 45	• Condylomata acuminata (anogenital warts) of the vulva, penis, and perianal region • Laryngeal papillomas
High-oncogenic risk HPV—malignant tumors	
HPV types 16 ,18, and 31	• Squamous cell carcinoma of the cervix and anogenital region • Oropharyngeal cancers (tonsil)

Mode of infection: HPV is transmitted by direct person-to-person contact. Most children infected with HPV develop common warts. The viruses that cause genital lesions are transmitted sexually.

Pathogenesis (Fig. 16)

Even though **HPV is a causative factor for cervical intraepithelial neoplasia (CIN) and cancer of the cervix, only few infected will develop cancer**. Most women infected with HPV clear the infection by immunological mechanisms.

- Human papillomavirus infection begins with inoculation of virus into a stratified squamous epithelium, where the virus enters the nuclei of **immature basal cells of the squamous epithelium, or immature metaplastic squamous cells** present at the squamocolumnar junction.
- **Infects only damaged surface epithelium** and **not the mature intact superficial squamous cells**. In areas of epithelial breaks or damage, the HPV can reach the immature cells in the basal layer of the epithelium.
- **Replication occurs in the maturing nonproliferating squamous cells which normally are arrested in the G1 phase of the cell cycle** (though the virus infects only the immature squamous cells). However, these mature cells actively progress through the cell cycle when infected with HPV by using the host cell DNA synthesis machinery to replicate its own genome. Infection stimulates proliferation of the squamous epithelium and produces the various HPV-associated lesions.
- **Human papillomavirus has to induce DNA synthesis** and must **reactivate the mitotic cycle** in such nonproliferating cells. Viral replication results in a cytopathic effect in HPV-infected cells. They show characteristic **"koilocytic atypia" (koilocytosis). This is characterized by** large squamous cells with shrunken nuclei with **nuclear atypia** enveloped in large cytoplasmic vacuoles (koilocytes) **forming a perinuclear halo (Figs. 17A to C).**

Molluscum Contagiosum

Molluscum contagiosum is a common, self-limited, highly contagious viral disease of the skin caused by a double-stranded DNA poxvirus.

Mode of infection: Usually spread by **direct contact**. Common among children and young adults.

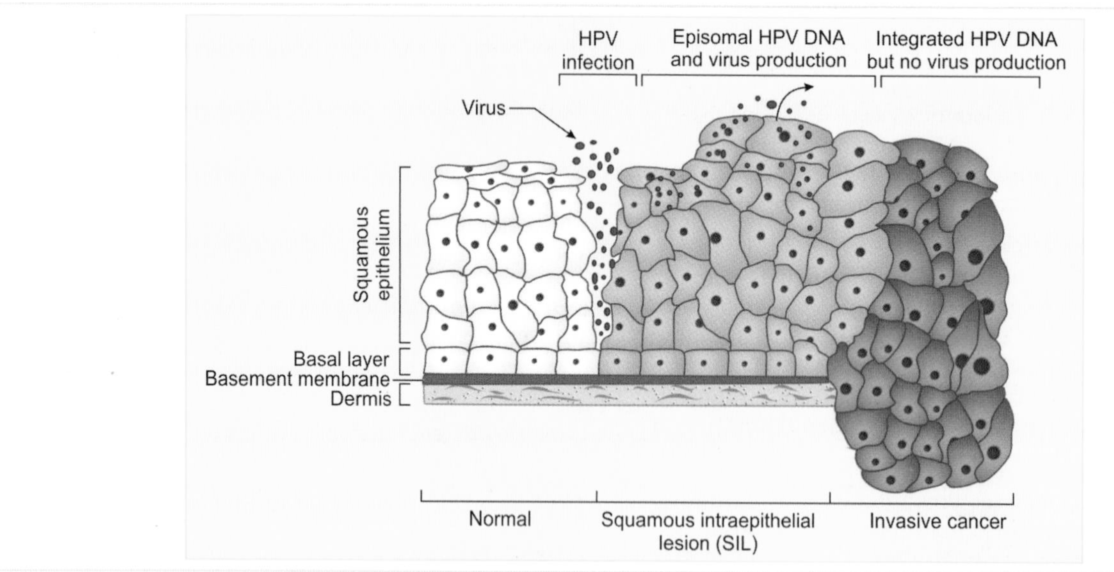

FIG. 16: Progression of human papillomavirus *(HPV)*–mediated cervical carcinoma. HPV infects and replicates in the epithelial cells of the cervix. As the epithelial cells mature and undergo differentiation, they release virus. Episomal HPV causes production of virus. In some epithelial cells, the circular genome integrates into host chromosomes, inactivating the E2 gene, which is necessary for replication. This stimulates growth of the cells and possible progression to neoplasia without virus production.

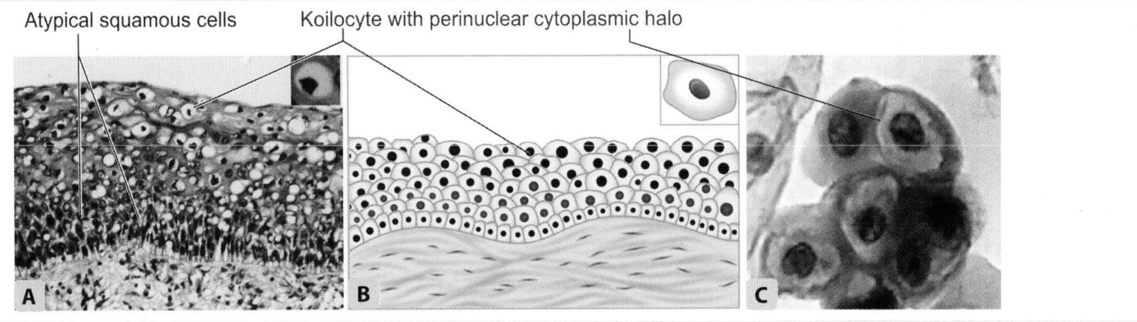

FIGS. 17A TO C: Squamous intraepithelial lesion due to human papillomavirus. (A) Hematoxylin and Eosin (H and E); (B) diagrammatic LSIL (low grade squamous intraepithelial lesion) with koilocyte; (C) Cervical cytology showing koilocytes.

MORPHOLOGY

Lesions

Infection leads to multiple lesions on the skin and mucous membranes, with a predilection for face, trunk, and anogenital areas. Individual lesions are small, firm, smooth, often pruritic, pink to skin-colored, and dome-shaped papules, generally ranging in diameter from 2 to 4 mm. Fully developed lesions have a characteristic central umbilication and in a fully-developed lesion, small amount of cheesy (curd/paste-like) keratinous material can be expressed on pressing from the central umbilication. This material if smeared onto a glass slide and stained with Giemsa may shows diagnostic molluscum bodies.

Microscopy (Fig. 18)

The microscopic picture is characteristic.

- **Infected epithelial cells:** Typical lesion consists of a sharply circumscribed (delimited) lobulated, cup-shaped mass of proliferating infected epithelial cells of epidermis growing down into the dermis.
- **Molluscum body:** As the infected epithelial cells differentiate within the mass, their cytoplasm is gradually filled by viral inclusion. These inclusions enlarge the epithelial cells and displace the nucleus. The **viral inclusions are diagnostically specific structures** (which appear ellipsoid) and are **termed as molluscum bodies**. The viral inclusions are found in cells of the stratum granulosum and the stratum corneum. Under hematoxylin and eosin stain, these **inclusions appear faintly granular eosinophilic in the blue-purple stratum granulosum and pale blue in the red stratum corneum**. These molluscum bodies contain numerous viral particles. Most lesions spontaneously regress.

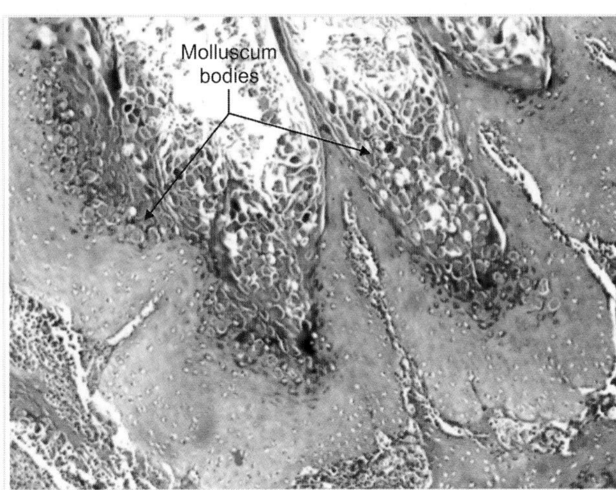

FIG. 18: Molluscum contagiosum. Epithelial cells of epidermis show ellipsoid cytoplasmic inclusions.

Japanese Encephalitis

Japanese encephalitis is a mosquito borne encephalitis caused by a *Flavivirus*.

Mode of transmission: It is a viral infection transmitted by infected *Culex tritaeniorhynchus* mosquitoes.

Source of infection: It is a zoonotic disease maintaining Japanese encephalitis virus in nature by pig-mosquito-pig and bird-mosquito-bird cycles. *C. tritaeniorhynchus* feeds mainly on the infected pigs and birds (e.g., herons and sparrows) and transmit the disease. Humans are accidental hosts.

Incubation period: 5–15 days after the mosquito bite.

Epidemiology: It is endemic in Bihar, Uttar Pradesh, Assam, Andhra Pradesh, Karnataka, Tamil Nadu, West Bengal, and Odisha states of India. It is most frequent in the rice growing countries (where irrigated rice fields are present).

Clinical Features

Age group: In endemic regions, the infection occurs in children between 3 and 15 years of age because of high background immunity in older individuals.

Presenting features

- **Prodromal period:** Following incubation period, the illness starts with fever, severe rigors, headache, malaise nausea, diarrhea, vomiting, cough, and myalgia that last for 1-6 days. Weight loss is prominent.
- **Acute encephalitic stage:** During this stage, fever is high, there is neck rigidity, and neurological signs such as irritability, altered consciousness/behavior, hemiparesis, and convulsions develop. Mental deterioration occurs over a period of 3–4 days and may terminate in coma.
- **Residual neurological defects feature** such as cognitive and speech impairment, emotional liability, cranial nerve palsies (e.g., ocular palsies-deafness), hemiplegia, quadriplegia, and Parkinsonian presentation

(extrapyramidal signs in the form of rigidity, dystonia, choreoathetosis, and coarse tremors) occur in about 70% of patients who have had CNS involvement.

Mortality ranges from 7% to 40% and is higher in children.

Diagnosis

- **Blood:** Leukocytosis with neutrophilia.
- **Cerebrospinal fluid examination:**
  - It shows **raised pressure and cell count**. During early stages, neutrophils may predominate but a lymphocytic pleocytosis is typical. CSF **protein is moderately raised** in about 50% of case.
  - **Virus isolation** from CSF.
  - **Detection of viral antigens** in CSF by indirect immunofluorescence assay (IFA).
- **Serological tests:** Detect antibodies to viral antigens. The various tests include virus neutralization test, hemagglutination inhibition, and complement fixation. **Antibody detection** in serum and CSF by IgM capture ELISA is a rapid diagnostic test.
- **Electroencephalogram (EEG):** Persistent abnormalities are common (particularly in children).
- **Imaging studies** by CT scan may show low-density areas in the temporal lobes. MRI scan is more sensitive in detecting early abnormalities.

Laboratory Diagnosis of Viral Infections

Q. Write short essay on laboratory diagnosis of viral infections.

Viral laboratory studies are mainly performed to confirm the diagnosis of viral agent of infection.

Specimen Collection, Transport and Storage

- **Type of specimen:** Selection of the appropriate specimen is dependent on the differential diagnosis and the laboratory tests to be performed (**Table 14**). However, the selection may be complicated because several viruses may cause the same clinical disease.
- **Time of collection:** Specimens should be collected early in the acute phase of the viral infection, before the virus ceases to be shed. For example, HSV and VZV or viral DNA may not be detected from lesions >5 days after the onset of symptoms. Hence, obtain specimen during acute illness for culture, antigen (Ag) detection and nucleic acid testing (NAT).
- **Transport to laboratory:** Specimen should be delivered to the laboratory as early as possible. This because many viruses are labile, and the samples are susceptible to bacterial and fungal overgrowth. Use appropriate viral

Table 14: Common pathogens, specimens to be collected and laboratory tests to be performed for diagnosis of viral infections.

Common pathogenic viruses	*Specimens to be collected*	*Laboratory test to be performed*
Blood		
HIV, hepatitis B, C, and D viruses, EBV, CMV, human T-cell leukemia virus, and HHV-6	Blood	ELISA for antigen or antibody, PCR, RT-PCR, and multiplex assays
Maculopapular rash		
Adenovirus, *Enterovirus* (Picornavirus)	Throat swab, rectal swab	PCR, RT-PCR
Rubella virus, measles virus	Urine	RT-PCR, ELISA
Vesicular rash		
Coxsackievirus, echovirus, HSV, and VZV	Vesicle fluid, scraping, or swab, *Enterovirus* in stool	HSV and VZV: Vesicle scraping (Tzanck smear), cell culture, PCR, and IF; *Enterovirus*: RT-PCR
Respiratory tract		
Influenza virus, paramyxoviruses, coronavirus, rhinovirus, and *Enterovirus* (Picornavirus)	Nasal washing, throat swab, nasal swab, and sputum	RT-PCR, ELISA, and multiplex assays; cell culture
Gastrointestinal tract		
Rotavirus, adenovirus, Norwalk virus, and reovirus	Stool, rectal swab	PCR, RT-PCR, and ELISA
Central nervous system (aseptic meningitis, encephalitis)		
Rabies virus	Tissue, saliva, brain biopsy, and CSF	IF of biopsy, RT-PCR
HSV, CMV, mumps virus, and measles virus	CSF	PCR or RT-PCR, virus isolation, and antigen assay
Enterovirus (Picornavirus)	Stool, CSF	RT-PCR
Arboviruses (e.g., togaviruses and bunyavirus)	Blood, CSF; rarely cultured	RT-PCR, serology; multiplex assays
Urinary tract		
Adenovirus, CMV	Urine	PCR (CMV may be shed without any apparent disease)

(CMV: cytomegalovirus; CSF: cerebrospinal fluid; EBV: Epstein–Barr virus; ELISA: enzyme-linked immunosorbent assay; HHV-6: human herpes virus 6; HIV: human immunodeficiency virus; HSV: herpes simplex virus; IF: immunofluorescence; PCR: polymerase chain reaction; RT-PCR: reverse transcriptase polymerase chain reaction; VZV: varicella-zoster virus)

Box 4: Various methods for laboratory diagnosis of viral infections.

- Cytological examination
- Electron microscopy
- Virus isolation and growth
- Detection of viral proteins (antigens and enzymes)
- Detection of viral genomes
- Serology

transport medium that contains antibiotics, proteins, such as serum albumin or gelatin and pH indicators.

- **Storage:** All specimens except blood should be stored at 4°C. Specimen should only be frozen a last resort.

Various methods for laboratory diagnosis of viral infections are listed in **Box 4**.

Cytological or Histopathological Examination

Q. Write short essay on viral inclusion bodies.

Cytological (morphologic study of cells) or histopathological (morphologic study of tissues) examinations are the readily available technique for detecting virus. Cytology and histopathology are less sensitive than culture. However, they are very helpful for viruses that are difficult or dangerous to isolate in the laboratory, such as parvovirus and rabies virus, respectively.

Many viruses produce a CPE in the tissue sample or in cell culture.

Cytopathologic effects (CPE): These include changes in morphology of cell, cell lysis, vacuolation, syncytia, and inclusion bodies. Pap- or Giemsa-stained cytological smears are examined for inclusions or syncytia.

- **Syncytia (syncytial cells):** Syncytial cells are aggregates of cells formed by fusion of individual cells. They form one large cell with multiple nuclei (i.e., multinucleated giant cells). Examples of viruses that cause formation of syncytia include, *Paramyxoviruses, HSV* (refer **Fig. 8**), *VZV, and HIV.*
- **Inclusion bodies (elementary bodies/viral inclusions):** Viral inclusions are intracellular structures either nuclear or cytoplasmic (**Table 15**) aggregates of stable substances, usually proteins. These may be produced due to either histologic changes in the cells caused by aggregates of virus or viral components in an infected cell or abnormal accumulations of cellular materials resulting from virus-induced metabolic changes in cell structures. For example, intranuclear inclusion in herpes simplex (refer **Fig. 8**) and intranuclear basophilic (owl's eye) inclusion bodies are found in large cells of tissues in infection due to CMV (refer **Fig. 13**), cytoplasmic Negri bodies (rabies virus inclusions **Fig. 6**) in brain tissue of patients with rabies. Inclusions in infection with CMV, adenovirus, parvovirus, papillomavirus, and molluscum contagiosum virus are detected by histopathological examination of tissue stained with hematoxylin and eosin.

  Note: Inclusion bodies apart from viral infection can also be characteristic of genetic diseases as in the case of neuronal inclusion bodies in disorders like frontotemporal dementia and Parkinson's disease.
- Examination of the cytological specimens for the specific viral antigens or viral genomes: This may be by in situ hybridization or processed for PCR for a rapid, definitive identification.

Electron Microscopy

In electron microscope (EM), a beam of electrons used instead of light, and magnets are used to focus the beam instead of the lenses used in a light microscope. The whole system is operated under a high vacuum. EM is not a standard routine clinical laboratory technique, because it is labor intensive and relatively insensitive. EM is most helpful for detecting viruses that do not grow readily in cell culture and to detect and identify some viruses if sufficient viral particles are present. In immune EM (immunoelectron microscopy), virus-specific antibody is added to the test suspension (sample). This causes clumping of viral particles to form antibody-bound aggregates. These aggregates allow more easy detection or visualization of virus particles than single virus particles. Thus, it is useful when virus particles are present in numbers too small for easy direct detection.

Uses

- Electron microscope is most useful for **detecting viruses that cause gastroenteritis** which cannot be detected by other methods (e.g., astroviruses) **and encephalitis-causing viruses** that are undetectable with cell culture (HSV, measles virus, and JC polyomavirus).
- For **rapid recognition and detect the etiology of newly recognized viral syndromes**. This is by identifying characteristic viral morphology by EM in infected tissue. For example, early recognition of Ebola virus as the cause of an outbreak of VHF (Ebola hemorrhagic fever) in Africa in the 1970s and Sin Nombre virus (hanta pulmonary syndrome) as the cause of fatal pneumonia in the four corners area of the southwest United States in the 1990s.

Viral Isolation and Growth

Isolation of the virus is useful for subsequent analysis but it may increase the risk for infection of the personnel involved.

Table 15: Various viral infection with inclusion bodies.

Intracytoplasmic eosinophilic (acidophilic)	*Intranuclear*		*Both intranuclear and intracytoplasmic*
	Eosinophilic (acidophilic)	*Basophilic*	
• Negri bodies (rabies) • Guarnieri bodies (vaccinia, variola) • Paschen bodies (fowlpox) • Henderson–Patterson bodies (molluscum contagiosum)	• Cowdry type A (herpes simplex virus, varicella zoster virus) • Torres bodies (yellow fever) • Cowdry type B (polio, adenovirus)	• Cowdry type B (adenovirus) • Owl's eye appearance (cytomegalovirus)	Warthin–Finkeldey bodies (measles)

A virus can be grown in tissue culture, embryonated eggs, and experimental animals. Only, tissue cell cultures are used for routine virus isolation in clinical laboratories.

Viral detection: A virus can be detected and initially identified by observing the virus-induced CPE in the cell monolayer, by immunofluorescence, or by genome analysis of the infected cell culture.

Detection of Viral Proteins

During viral replication, it produces viral enzymes and other proteins. These can be detected by biochemical, immunologic, and molecular biological techniques (**Box 5**). The viral proteins can be separated by electrophoresis and their patterns help to identify and distinguish different viruses.

Immunodiagnosis (antigen detection): Viral antigen in patient specimens can be detected by using high-quality, specific, sensitive, monoclonal, or monospecific viral antibody reagents. These antibodies are useful for detection, identification, and quantitation of the virus and viral antigen in clinical specimens. They form the basis of antigen detection by different techniques such as fluorescent antibody, enzyme immunoassay (EIA), latex agglutination, and immunoperoxidase (immunohistochemistry) tests.

- Viral antigens on the surface of a cell or within the cell can be detected by **immunofluorescence** (direct or indirect method) and **EIA.** Virus or antigen released from infected cells can be detected and quantitated by **ELISA, latex agglutination (LA).**

Enzyme activities: The detection and assay of characteristic enzymes can be used to identify and quantitate specific viruses. For example, the presence of RT (reverse transcripitase) in serum indicates the presence of a retrovirus or hepadnavirus.

Presently, test kits to detect single and multiple (multiplex) viral agents are commercially available. Rapid ELISA-like detection kits, similar to pregnancy tests, are also available for influenza and HIV.

Significance of virus detection

Detection of any virus in host tissues, CSF, blood, or vesicular fluid is a very significant finding. However, viral shedding may occur and may be not related to the disease symptoms. Some viruses can be intermittently shed without any symptoms in the affected individual. This shedding may be for periods that may range from weeks (enteroviruses in feces) to many months or years (examples include HSV or CMV in the oropharynx and vagina; adenoviruses in the oropharynx and intestinal tract). Also a negative result cannot exclude the diagnosis because it may be due to improper collection or handling, or contain neutralizing antibody, or sample obtained before or after viral shedding.

Box 5: Assays for viral proteins and nucleic acids.

Proteins
- Antigen detection (e.g., direct and indirect immunofluorescence, enzyme-linked immunosorbent assay, and Western blot)
- Protein patterns (electrophoresis)
- Enzyme activities (e.g., RT)
- Hemagglutination and hemadsorption

Nucleic Acids
- Polymerase chain reaction for DNA
- Reverse transcriptase PCR for RNA
- Real-time quantitative PCR
- Branched-chain DNA and related tests (DNA, RNA)
- Genome sequencing
- Restriction endonuclease cleavage patterns
- Size of RNA for segmented RNA viruses (electrophoresis)
- DNA genome hybridization in situ (cytochemistry)
- Southern, Northern, and dot blots

(DNA: deoxyribonucleic acid; PCR: polymerase chain reaction; RNA: ribonucleic acid)

Molecular Detection of Viral Genetic Material

During the past decade, the nucleic acid detection techniques are being used in virology laboratory. In this technique, both nucleic acid detection and genome amplification based systems are used in association with automated nucleic acid isolation techniques. By these molecular techniques, detection, identification, and quantitation are possible to generate results within 2–6 hours. Nucleic acid detection is by using sequence-specific nucleic acid probes. These probes are short segments of DNA that hybridize with complementary viral DNA or RNA segments. The probe is labeled with a fluorescent or chromogenic tag. This allows detection, if hybridization occurs. The probe reaction can occur in situ, such as in a thin tissue section; in liquid; or on a reaction vessel surface or membrane. Nucleic acid probes are most useful in situations such as (1) when the amount of virus is relatively abundant, (2) culture of virus is slow or not possible, and (3) immunoassays lack sensitivity or specificity.

The genetic sequence of a virus is a major feature that distinguishes the type, and strain of virus. These techniques have minimal risk from infectious virus.

Genome amplification

If the original specimen contains few number of the DNA target fragments that can be detected by probes, these DNA fragments can be amplified using molecular techniques such as PCR.

Methods: The method of choice for detection, quantification, and identification of viruses is by using genome amplification techniques.

- **Polymerase chain reaction for DNA**. PCR is used for genome amplification. In PCR method, short DNA targets are amplified to million times. By using appropriate primers for PCR, a million-fold amplification of a target sequence can be performed within a few hours. This technique is especially useful for detecting latent and integrated sequences of viruses (e.g., retroviruses, Herpesviruses, Papillomaviruses, and papovaviruses), when the viruses are present in low concentrations and viruses that are difficult or dangerous to isolate in cell culture. In conventional PCR, amplification and product detection take place separately. **Transcription-based amplification** uses RT and viral sequence-specific primers to make a complementary DNA (cDNA). The amplified genome is detected by hybridization of a luminescent DNA probe. ELISA can be used to detect the presence of the genome.

- **Reverse transcriptase-PCR for RNA**. It can be used to amplify and detect RNA viruses by enzyme RT. The first step in RT-PCR is to make a complementary DNA strand of the RNA segment of the virus. This is followed by usual PCR steps to multiply the DNA target leading to DNA amplicons. These signify the presence of the original RNA sequence.
- **Real-time PCR:** Rapid PCR testing is referred to as real-time PCR. It uses the same basic reagents and techniques as the original PCR method, but with the addition of fluorescently labeled sequence-specific probes. It is used for identification and quantification of RNA or DNA. In real-time PCR, **target amplification and detection occur simultaneously in the same tube**. Thus, it is a rapid method used for identification as well as to quantify the number of genomes (**virus load**).
- **Next generation sequencing:** Viral genomes can also be analyzed after genome amplification. Methods for sequencing DNA **(next generation sequencing)** have become rapid and inexpensive to be routine procedures. Once the sequence of a fragment or the entire genome has been obtained, it can be identified by computer.
- **Multiplex assays:** At present, automated commercial systems are available that are capable of **detecting multiple viruses in a single reaction–multiplexing**. These are termed as multiplex assays and microassays that analyze a panel of microbes from multiple samples. The PCR can be multiplexed by adding primers and probes for more than one pathogen. They reduce both costs and time to diagnosis. They process the sample, concentrate the genomic sequences, amplify the genomes for the different microbes (multiplex), and then rapidly detect the amplified DNA to indicate the presence of the viral genome. These assays are particularly useful for the diagnosis of respiratory pathogens. Isothermal amplification reactions are becoming more popular.

In situ analysis Like antibodies, virus-specific **DNA probes** can be used as sensitive and specific tools for detecting a virus. These DNA probes can detect the virus even in the absence of replication of virus.

Specific viral genetic sequences in fixed tissue biopsy specimens can be detected by **in situ hybridization** [e.g., **fluorescence in situ hybridization (FISH)**]. DNA probe analysis is especially useful for the detection of slowly replicating or nonproductive viruses (e.g., CMV and HPV), or when the viral antigen cannot be detected using immunologic tests.

Assays for viral proteins and nucleic acids are presented in **Box 5**.

Viral Serology

The humoral immune response provides a history of a patient's infections. Serology was the primary means of laboratory diagnosis of viral infections till the mid-1970s.

Uses: Viral serology is now used primarily–

- **For the identification of viruses that are difficult to isolate and grow in cell culture.**
- **For the identification of viruses that cause diseases of long duration** (e.g., EBV, HBV, and HIV).
- **For the identification of virus and its strain or serotype, whether it is an acute or chronic disease.**
- **To determine immune status**, whether it is a primary infection or a reinfection.
    - **Virus-specific immunoglobulin M antibody** is present during the first 2 or 3 weeks of a primary infection and generally indicates a recent primary infection. In most viral infections. IgM is undetectable 1–4 months after the acute infection resolves. But detectable levels of IgG remain for the life of the patient.
    - **Seroconversion** is indicated when there is at least **a fourfold increase in the antibody titer** between the serum obtained during the acute phase of disease and that obtained at least 2–3 weeks later during the convalescent phase.
    - **Reinfection or recurrence:** If a patient is infected with an antigenically similar virus or the original strain has remained latent and reactivates at a later time, it causes an anamnestic (secondary or booster) response. Then these virus-specific IgG and IgM antibody levels may again rise. The secondary IgM response may be difficult to detect. However, a significant (fourfold) rise of IgG titer is observed in immunocompetent patients.
- **To identify the stage of certain viral diseases:** The presence of antibodies and their titers to several main viral antigens can be utilized to identify the stage of disease caused by certain viruses. For example, for the diagnosis of viral diseases with slow courses (e.g., infectious mononucleosis caused by EBV, hepatitis B).
- **Serologic battery or panel:** This panel consists of assays for several viruses and may be used for the diagnosis of certain diseases.

Various serological assays are listed in **Box 6**. Various viral infections diagnosed by serology are listed in **Box 7**.

Box 6: Various serological assays (methods) to detect antiviral antibody.

- Complement fixation (CF)
- Hemagglutination inhibition
- Neutralization
- Immunofluorescence (direct and indirect)
- Anticomplement immunofluorescence (ACIF)
- Latex agglutination
- In situ enzyme immunoassay
- Enzyme-linked immunosorbent assay
- Radioimmunoassay
- Western immunoblotting

Box 7: Various viral infections diagnosed by serology.

- Epstein–Barr virus
- Rubella virus
- Hepatitis A, B, C, D, and E viruses
- Human immunodeficiency virus
- Human T-cell leukemia virus
- Arboviruses (encephalitis viruses)

11.3 Bacterial Diseases

CHAPTER OUTLINE

INTRODUCTION

Bacteria measure in the range of 0.1–10 μm and are the smallest living cells.

Basic Structure of Bacteria

Bacteria consists of three basic structural components**:** Nuclear body, cytosol, and cell envelope.

- **Nuclear body:** It consists of a single, coiled, circular molecule of double-stranded deoxyribonucleic acid (DNA) with associated ribonucleic acid (RNA) and proteins. In contrast to cells in humans, nuclear body is not separated from the cytoplasm by a special membrane.
- **Cytosol:** The cytosol is densely packed with ribosomes, proteins, and carbohydrates. It does not contain the structured organelles, such as mitochondria and Golgi apparatus found in human cells.
- **Cell envelope or outer layer:** The bacterial cell envelope consists of two components: (1) a **rigid cell wall and (2)** a **cytoplasmic** or **plasma membrane** (beneath the cell wall). Almost all bacteria, with the exception of the mycoplasma, have a rigid cell wall surrounding the cytoplasmic membrane. The rigid cell wall determines the shape of the bacteria. The envelope is a permeability barrier and is also actively involved in transport, protein synthesis, energy generation, DNA synthesis, and cell division.
- External to the cell wall, there may be flagella, pili, and/or a capsule.

Division: Bacterial cells divide by binary fission. However, many bacteria exchange genetic information carried on plasmids (small, specialized genetic elements capable of self-replication).

Classification of Bacteria

Bacteria can be classified in several different ways.

Depending on the Gram Staining

Bacteria can be classified according to the structural features of their envelope. The simplest envelope consists of only a phospholipid-protein bilayer membrane (e.g., mycoplasma). However, most bacteria have a rigid cell wall that surrounds the cell membrane. There are two types of bacterial cell walls as identified by their Gram stain properties:

- **Gram-positive bacteria:** Their cell walls contain teichoic acids and a thick peptidoglycan layer. These bacteria retain iodine–crystal violet complexes when decolorized. They **appear dark blue**.

- **Gram-negative bacteria:** These bacteria lose the iodine-crystal violet stain when decolorized. They **appear red with a counterstain.** Outer membranes of gram-negative bacteria contain a lipopolysaccharide component, known as endotoxin. This endotoxin is a powerful mediator of the shock that complicates infections with these organisms.

Depending on Presence or Absence of Capsule

Capsule

The cell walls of both gram-positive and gram-negative may be surrounded by an additional layer of polysaccharide or protein gel termed as a capsule. Capsule is formed by the viscid material secreted by bacteria on the cell surface (e.g., in *Streptococcus pneumoniae*). Capsule helps in bacterial attachment to the host cell and colonization as well it may protect bacteria from phagocytosis. Capsules are important in many infections.

Hence, bacteria may be classified as **encapsulated** or **unencapsulated**.

Depending on the Shape

Bacterial morphology is used for another classification. The cell wall of bacteria provides rigidity and provides shape. Depending on the shape of bacteria, they are classified into several types (**Fig. 19**).

- **Cocci** (from *kokkos* meaning berry): They are **round/ spherical or oval bacteria**. According to their growth in culture they can be subclassified. **Bacteria that grow in clusters** (resemble bunches of grapes) are called **staphylococci,** while **those that grow in chains** (align themselves in rows) are **streptococci**.
- **Bacilli** (from *baculus* meaning rod): These are **elongate rod-shaped bacteria** (e.g., *Bacillus anthracis*).
- **Vibrios:** These are **comma-shaped, curved rods** and derive their name from their characteristic vibratory motility.
- **Spirochetes** (from *speira* meaning coil and *chaite* meaning hair): These have **spiral curvaceous shape bacteria** (e.g., *Treponema pallidum*).

Depending on the Cultural Properties

This classification reflects the need of bacteria for oxygen. Most of the bacteria can be cultured on chemical media. According to their growth requirements on these media bacteria can be classified into different types.

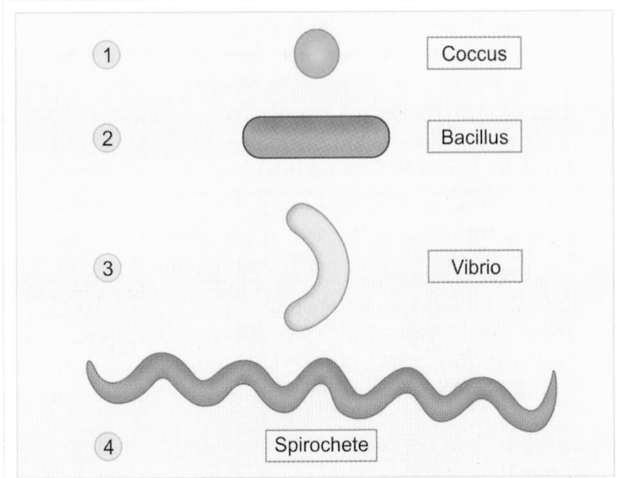

FIG. 19: Classification of bacteria depending on their shape.

- **Aerobes:** Bacteria that **require high levels of oxygen during culture** are termed **aerobic.** For example, *Pseudomonas aeruginosa* is an aerobic bacterium that requires an oxygen-rich environment to survive and multiply.
- **Facultative anaerobes:** Bacteria that **grow well with or without oxygen** are termed as **facultative anaerobes.** For example, *Escherichia coli* can survive in the presence or absence of oxygen, although they tend to prefer an oxygenated environment.
- **Obligate anaerobes:** They **grow without oxygen** and are **anaerobic.** For example, *Clostridium* species do not survive well in an oxygenated environment.
- **Microaerophilic:** These bacteria **survive with limited oxygen** and are **microaerophilic**.

Few examples of bacteria and associated diseases in human are presented in **Table 16**.

Table 16: Few examples of bacteria and associated diseases in human.

Bacteria	*Frequently-associated disease*
Respiratory system	
• *Streptococcus pyogenes*	Pharyngitis
• *Corynebacterium diphtheriae*	Diphtheria
• *Bordetella pertussis*	Pertussis (Whooping cough)
• *Streptococcus pneumonia*	Lobar pneumonia
• *Mycobacterium tuberculosis*	Tuberculosis
• *Legionella pneumophila*	Legionnaires' disease
Gastrointestinal system	
• *Helicobacter pylori*	Peptic ulcers
• *Vibrio cholerae,* enterotoxigenic *Escherichia coli*	Noninflammatory gastroenteritis
• *Shigella* species, *Salmonella* species, *Campylobacter jejuni,* enterohemorrhagic *Escherichia coli*	Inflammatory gastroenteritis
• *Salmonella* serotype *typhi*	Enteric (typhoid) fever
• *Clostridioides difficile*	Pseudomembranous colitis
Nervous system	
• *Neisseria meningitidis, Streptococcus pneumoniae, Haemophilus influenzae, Listeria monocytogenes*	Acute meningitis
• *Clostridium tetani, Clostridium botulinum*	Paralytic intoxications, tetanus, and botulism
Urogenital system	
• *Escherichia coli, Pseudomonas aeruginosa, Enterococcus* species	Urinary tract infections
• *Neisseria gonorrhoeae*	Gonorrhea
• *Chlamydia trachomatis*	Chlamydia
• *Treponema pallidum*	Syphilis

Continued

Continued

Bacteria	Frequently-associated disease
Skin and soft tissue	
• *Staphylococcus aureus*	Abscess, cellulitis
• *Streptococcus pyogenes*	Impetigo, erysipelas, and necrotizing fasciitis
• *Clostridium perfringens*	Gas gangrene
• *Bacillus anthracis*	Cutaneous anthrax
• *Pseudomonas aeruginosa*	Burn infections
• *Mycobacterium leprae*	Leprosy
Disseminated infections	
• *Yersinia pestis*	Plague
• *Borrelia burgdorferi*	Lyme disease
• *Brucella* species	Brucellosis (undulant fever)
Disseminated neonatal infection	
• *Streptococcus agalactiae, Listeria monocytogenes*	Neonatal bacteremia, meningitis
• *Treponema pallidum*	Congenital syphilis

GRAM-POSITIVE BACTERIAL INFECTIONS

Common gram-positive cocci infecting humans include *Staphylococcus* species, *Streptococcus* species, and *Enterococcus* species. Each of them cause many types of infections. Pyogenic inflammation is a type of inflammation characterized by increased vascular permeability and leukocytic infiltration, mainly of neutrophils. The neutrophils accumulate at the site of infection due to release of chemoattractants from the "pyogenic" (pus-forming) bacteria. These pyogenic bacteria are mostly extracellular gram-positive cocci and gram-negative rods.

Staphylococcal Infections

Staphylococcus aureus: *S. aureus* is a gram-positive pyogenic coccus and is the **most common bacterial pathogens in humans**. It usually grows in clusters resembling bunches of grapes. *S. aureus* is distinguished from other, less virulent staphylococci by the coagulase test. *S. aureus* is **coagulase positive** whereas other staphylococci are coagulase negative (e.g., *S. epidermidis*). It is normally present on the skin and can be readily inoculated into deeper tissues and produce suppurative infections. It is the **most common cause of suppurative infections** (pyogenic lesions) of the skin **lesions (boils, carbuncles, impetigo, wound infection, abscesses, and scalded-skin syndrome), abscesses, sepsis, osteomyelitis, pneumonia, *infective* endocarditis, food poisoning, septicemia and pyemia, and toxic shock syndrome (TSS)** (**Fig. 20**).

- ***Spread of S. aureus infection:*** It spreads by direct contact with colonized surfaces or persons. Most individuals are intermittently colonized with *S. aureus* and carry it on the skin, nares, or clothing. It can survive for long periods on inanimate surfaces.

Coagulase-negative staphylococci: Coagulase-negative staphylococci, such as *S. epidermidis,* **cause opportunistic infections** in catheterized patients, patients with prosthetic cardiac valves, intravenous (IV) drug users, and in continuous ambulatory peritoneal dialysis. *S. saprophyticus* commonly produces urinary tract infection in young females.

Pathogenesis

Virulence factors

S. aureus produces a many virulence factors. These include surface proteins (involved in adherence and evasion of the host immune response), secretion of enzymes (they degrade host structures), secretion of toxins (damage host cells), and proteins (responsible for development of antibiotic resistance).

Surface receptors: *S. aureus* expresses surface receptors for fibrinogen (called clumping factor), fibronectin, and vitronectin. These receptors molecules help pathogens to attach to endothelial cells of host.

Capsule: *S. aureus* produces a polysaccharide capsule. This helps in its attachment to artificial materials and is responsible for significant prosthetic valve and catheter-associated infection. It also helps in resisting phagocytosis by host cells.

Surface protein: *S. aureus* also expresses surface protein A. This protein attached to the Fc portion of immunoglobulins, thereby it can escape antibody-mediated killing.

S. aureus* toxins:** *S. aureus* produces many *(hemolytic)* toxins that **damage the host cell *membrane. These include:

- **α-toxin:** It is a protein that insert into the plasma membrane of host cells and forms pores. This allows toxic levels of calcium to leak into the host cells.
- **β-toxin:** It is a sphingomyelinase.
- **δ-toxin:** It is a detergent-like peptide.
- ***S. aureus* γ-toxin and leukocidin:** They lyse red blood cells (RBCs) and phagocytes, respectively.
- ***Exfoliative A and B toxins:*** These are serine proteases and cleave the desmosomal protein desmoglein 1. Desmoglein 1 tightly holds epidermal cells to each other. Exfoliative A and B toxins cause detachment of keratinocytes from one another as well as from the underlying basement membrane. This causes loss of barrier function and usually leads to secondary skin infections. Exfoliation may occur either locally at the site of infection (bullous impetigo) or may produce widespread loss of the superficial epidermis (staphylococcal scalded-skin syndrome).

Superantigens: *S. aureus* produces superantigens and they are responsible for food poisoning and TSS.

- **Toxic shock syndrome (TSS):** This syndrome is potentially fatal disorder. It most commonly occurs in menstruating women and present with high fever, nausea, vomiting,

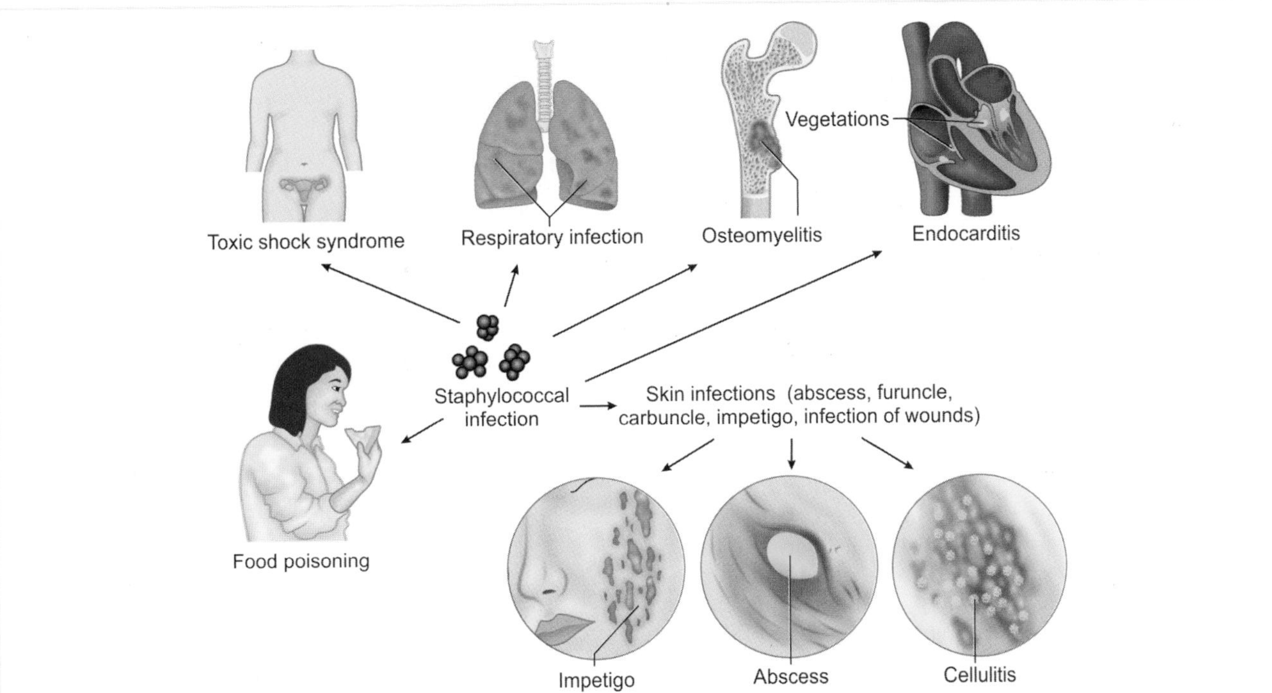

FIG. 20: Main effects of staphylococcal infection.

diarrhea, and myalgias. Subsequently, they go into hypotension (shock), renal failure, coagulopathy, liver disease, and respiratory distress. Within several days develop generalized erythematous (sunburn-like) rash, and soft-tissue necrosis at the site of infection. TSS was initially observed with use of tampons, particularly hyperabsorbent ones, which provide a site for *S. aureus* replication and toxin elaboration. Now it is known that TSS can be caused by growth of *S. aureus* at many sites, most common being in the vagina and infected surgical sites. TSS may rarely occur in children and men, and is then usually associated with an occult *S. aureus* infection. If not promptly treated, it can be fatal. TSS can also be produced by *S. pyogenes*. Bacterial superantigens cause polyclonal T-cell proliferation. This is achieved by its attachment to conserved portions of major histocompatibility complex (MHC) molecules and to relatively conserved portions of T-cell receptor β chains. Thus, superantigens stimulate up to 20% of T lymphocytes and release large amounts of cytokines such as tumor necrosis factor (TNF) and interleukin-1 (IL-1). This triggers the systemic inflammatory response syndrome (refer page 323). Superantigens produced by *S. aureus* also cause vomiting when ingested in food, probably by affecting the central nervous system (CNS) or the enteric nervous system.

***Antibiotic resistance S. aureus*:** It is one of the most important **clinical issues in treatment of *S. aureus* infections.** Methicillin-resistant *S. aureus* (MRSA) are resistant to almost all penicillin and cephalosporin antibiotics and are usually acquired in the hospital. Initially, MRSA was mainly observed in healthcare facilities, but now community-acquired MRSA infections are common. Hence, empirical treatment of *S. aureus* infections with cephalosporin antibiotics is not recommended.

MORPHOLOGY

Many *S. aureus* infections **begin as localized infections of skin and skin appendages**. They produce cellulitis (inflammation of subcutaneous connective tissue) and abscesses (local collection of pus). The destructive enzymes and toxins of *S. aureus* sometimes invade beyond the initial site. It can spread through blood or lymphatics to almost any location in the body. The most common sites of metastatic *S. aureus* infections are bones, joints, and heart valves. *S. aureus* also causes many distinct diseases by secreting toxins that are carried to distant sites.

Irrespective of the location of the lesion, ***S. aureus* causes pyogenic inflammation with local destruction of host tissue.** Except impetigo (it is limited to the superficial epidermis), staphylococcal skin infections begin around the hair follicles.

- **Furuncle (boil) and stye:** It is a focal suppurative inflammation of the skin and subcutaneous tissue. They may be single or multiple, or they may recur in successive crops. Furuncles usually localize on moist, hairy areas (e.g., face, eyelid, neck, axillae, groin, legs, pubic area, and submammary folds). Boils begin as nodules in and around the base of one hair follicle and grows and deepens. They remain painful and red for a few days. The abscess then produces thinning and yellow apices form and become necrotic and fluctuant. Rupture of overlying skin or incision relieves the pain. **Styes** are boils involving the sebaceous glands around the eyelid. **Paronychia** is the term used for staphylococcal infections of nail beds, and **felons** are the infections involving the palmar side of the fingertips and both produce severe pain. **Hidradenitis** is chronic suppurative infection of apocrine glands and is usually occur in the axilla.

Continued

Continued

- **Carbuncle:** It is a deeper suppurative infection and spreads laterally beneath the deep subcutaneous fascia. Then it superficially produces multiple adjacent draining skin sinuses. Carbuncles are usually seen beneath the skin of the upper back and posterior neck, where fascial planes favor their spread.
- **Staphylococcal scalded-skin syndrome (Fig. 21):** It is also termed as Ritter disease. It is most frequently observed in infants and children under 3 years with *S. aureus* infection of the nasopharynx or skin. It presents with a sunburn-like rash that begins on the face and spreads over the entire body. It produces fragile bullae and even gentle rubbing causes skin to desquamate (partial or total skin loss). In staphylococcal scalded-skin syndrome, the desquamation of the epidermis occurs at the level of the granulosa layer. It can be differentiated from toxic epidermal necrolysis, or Lyell disease, which is secondary to drug hypersensitivity and causes desquamation occurs at the epidermal–dermal junction. Desquamation is due to systemic effects of a specific exotoxin secreted by *S. aureus*. It begins to resolve in 1–2 weeks, as the skin regenerates.
- **Respiratory tract infections:** Staphylococcal infections of respiratory tract mostly occur in infants under 2 years, and especially under 2 months. It can produce ulcers of the upper airway, scattered foci of pneumonia, pleural effusion, empyema, and pneumothorax. In adults, staphylococcal pneumonia may occur in the setting of a predisposing condition such as viral influenza, which destroys the ciliated surface epithelium and leaves the bronchial surface vulnerable to secondary infection. Lung infections can also occur from a hematogenous source, such as an infected thrombus. *S. aureus* infections of lung show polymorphonuclear infiltrate similar to that of *S. pneumoniae* infections, but they cause more destruction of lung tissue.
- **Osteomyelitis:** Acute staphylococcal osteomyelitis usually develop in the leg bones and most often in boys between 3 and 10 years of age. Usually there is a history of infection or trauma. If not properly treated, acute may become chronic osteomyelitis. Adults above 50 years of age more frequently develop osteomyelitis of vertebra. It may complicate staphylococcal infections of the skin or urinary tract, prostatic surgery, or pinning of a fracture.
- **Bacterial arthritis:** *S. aureus* can cause septic arthritis, mostly between 50 and 70 years of age. Common predisposing conditions include rheumatoid arthritis and therapy with corticosteroids.
- **Septicemia:** Septicemia due to *S. aureus* occurs in patients with lowered resistance who are in the hospital for other diseases. They may be having underlying staphylococcal infections (e.g., septic arthritis, osteomyelitis), or some surgery (e.g., transurethral prostate resection) or infections from an indwelling IV catheter. It may produce serious complications such as miliary abscesses and endocarditis.
- **Bacterial endocarditis:** It may develop as a complication of *S. aureus* septicemia. It may involve normal valves, on valves damaged by rheumatic fever or on prosthetic valves. IV drug abuse predisposes to staphylococcal endocarditis.

Continued

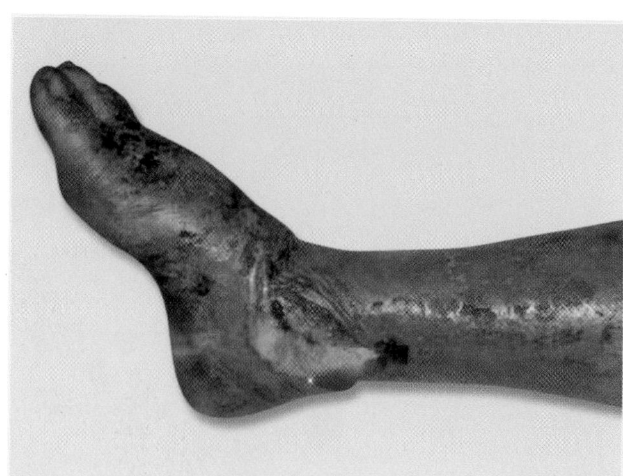

FIG. 21: Staphylococcal-scalded skin syndrome.

Continued

- **Staphylococcal food poisoning:** It usually begins <6 hours after a meal. It is characterized by sudden development of nausea and vomiting and usually resolve within 12 hours. This disease is caused by preformed toxin present in the food at the time it is consumed.
- **Infections of burns or surgical wounds:** The source of infections in these situations is from the patient's own nasal carriage or from medical personnel. Increased susceptibility is observed in newborns and elderly, malnourished, diabetic, and obese individuals.
- **Toxic shock syndrome** (described above on pages 630 and 631).

Streptococcal and Enterococcal Infections

Streptococcus is 1 μm in diameter, **nonmotile, and nonsporing gram-positive coccus**. It grows in pairs or chains (**Fig. 22**). It is frequently part of the endogenous flora of the skin and oropharynx. It has many strains and many strains are capsulated.

Classification: Based on hemolysis on blood agar, *aerobic, and facultative anaerobic streptococci are* classified into three varieties namely (1) alpha (α) hemolytic streptococci, (2) beta (β) hemolytic streptococci, and (3) nonhemolytic streptococci.

- **Alpha (α) hemolytic streptococci:** They produce a greenish discoloration with partial hemolysis around the colonies. The zone of lysis is small (1 or 2 mm wide) with indefinite margins. The unlysed erythrocytes can be found microscopically within this zone. Examples include viridans streptococcus and *S. pneumoniae* (pneumococcus). Most alpha hemolytic streptococci are normal commensals in the throat and may rarely cause opportunistic infections.
- **Beta (β) hemolytic streptococci:** They produce a sharply defined, clear, colorless zone of hemolysis, 2–4 mm wide, within which red cells are completely lysed. The **term "hemolytic streptococci" is strictly applied only to beta hemolytic strains**. Most pathogenic streptococci belong to this group.
    - **Subclassification: Based on carbohydrate antigen or Lancefield groups,** β-hemolytic streptococci are

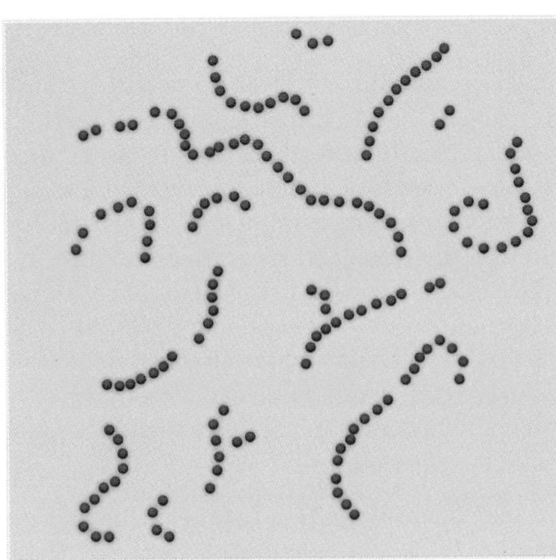

FIG. 22: Diagrammatic appearance of Streptococci (gram-positive cocci) growing in pairs or chains.

typed based on the nature of a surface carbohydrate (C) antigen on the cell wall. These are known as **Lancefield groups.** Twenty groups have been identified and named **A-H and K-V (without I and J).** Most important streptococcus is ***Streptococcus pyogenes,*** also called as ***group A streptococcus.***

- **Nonhemolytic streptococci:** They do not produce hemolysis in the medium and include mostly the fecal streptococci which are classified as the ***Enterococcus*** species. *Enterococci* are gram-positive cocci and similar to streptococci, they grow in pairs and chains. Hence, by morphology alone, they are difficult to distinguish from streptococci. They are usually resistant to commonly used antibiotics. They can cause endocarditis and urinary tract infection.

Streptococcus Pyogenes (group A)

It is one of the most common human pathogens, causing diseases of variety of organ systems. Diseases produced by *S. pyogenes* may be suppurative or nonsuppurative.

- **Suppurative infections:** It occurs at sites of bacterial invasion and characterized by tissue necrosis and usually involve acute inflammatory responses. They involve **skin, oropharynx, lungs, and heart valves.** Thus, they **cause pharyngitis, scarlet fever, erysipelas, impetigo cellulitis, myositis, pneumonia, and puerperal sepsis**.
- **Nonsuppurative diseases:** The locations of nonsuppurative diseases are far away (remote) from the site of streptococcal invasion. These are characterized by involvement of (1) organs far from the sites of invasion, (2) a time delay between the initial acute infection and development of disease, and (3) immune reactions. *S. pyogenes* are responsible for a number of postinfectious syndromes and three of these are major nonsuppurative complications. These includes (1) rheumatic fever, (2) acute poststreptococcal glomerulonephritis, and (3) erythema nodosum.

Pathogenesis

The different species of streptococci produce many virulence factors and toxins. *S. pyogenes, S. agalactiae,* and *S. pneumoniae* contain capsules and these resist their phagocytosis.

Toxins produced by S. pyogenes They secrete several exotoxins and include erythrogenic toxins and cytolytic toxins **(streptolysins S and O)**. Virulent *S. pyogenes* can cause rapidly progressive necrotizing fasciitis and are termed as flesh-eating bacteria.

- **Erythrogenic toxins:** *S. pyogenes* secretes a phage-encoded pyrogenic exotoxin and is responsible for fever and the rash of scarlet fever.
- **Cytolytic toxins:** Streptolysin S destroys neutrophils after they ingest *S. pyogenes.* Streptolysin O induces production of a continuously high titer of antibody [i.e., antistreptolysin O (ASLO)] and this is used as marker for the diagnosis of *S. pyogenes* infections and their nonsuppurative complications.

Enzymes produced It produces **hemolysins, DNAase, hyaluronidase, and streptokinase**. They are responsible for damage and invasion of human tissues.

Components of cell wall *S. pyogenes* has cell wall components that protect it from the inflammatory response. One of them is a surface protein called as **M protein** that protrudes from cell walls of virulent strains. This prevents complement deposition, thereby protecting bacteria from being phagocytosed. It also contains another surface protein called **complement C5a peptidase** that destroys chemotactic peptide C5a. This blocks its opsonizing effect and inhibit phagocytosis. *S. pyogenes* attaches to host epithelial cells by binding to fibronectin on their surface.

Rheumatic fever It is postinfectious disease probably caused by antistreptococcal M protein antibodies and T cells that cross-react with cardiac proteins.

Other Streptococci

Streptococcus agalactiae (group B)

It colonizes the female genital tract. This is a major pathogen found in the female genital tract, rectum, and also throat. **Chorioamnionitis, septic abortion,** and **puerperal sepsis** may occur due to this pathogen during pregnancy. Urinary tract infection may occur in both sexes. Hematogenous spread may result in endocarditis, pneumonia, empyema, meningitis, and peritonitis. Immunocompromised hosts and elderly subjects are more susceptible.

Streptococcus pneumoniae (often called pneumococcus)

It is the most important **α-hemolytic streptococcus** and one of the most common human bacterial pathogens. *S. pneumoniae* is an **aerobic, gram-positive diplococcus**. Most strains that produce clinical disease have an antiphagocytic capsule and is the most important virulence factor of *S. pneumonia.* It also produces a toxin called pneumolysin. This toxin inserts into host cell membranes and lyses the host cells, thereby increases the damage to tissue. It is a **common cause of community-acquired pneumonia in older adults and meningitis in children and adults**. *S. pneumonia* may also cause infections of middle ear **(otitis media)**, sinuses (**sinusitis**), and meninges **(meningitis)**.

Viridans-group streptococci

These include α-hemolytic and nonhemolytic streptococci found in normal oral microbiota. They are commonly responsible for endocarditis.

Streptococcus mutants

It is the major bacteria causing dental caries. It produces caries by metabolizing sucrose to lactic acid. This in turn causes demineralization of tooth enamel. It also secretes high-molecular weight glucans that promote aggregation of bacteria and dental plaque formation.

Diagnosis of streptococcal infections

They are diagnosed by culture and, in patient with pharyngitis, by the rapid streptococcal antigen test.

Enterococci

These are **low-virulence bacteria**. They have an antiphagocytic capsule but they injure host cells by producing enzymes. The enterococci are resistance to antibiotics and they are pathogenic mainly in immunosuppressed patient populations (e.g., individuals undergoing organ or stem cell transplantation) and who are frequently given antimicrobial agents that alters the commensal microbiota. Causes are urinary tract infections, biliary tract infections, septicemia, peritonitis, infective endocarditis, and abdominal suppuration.

MORPHOLOGY

Streptococcal infections are characterized by diffuse interstitial neutrophilic infiltrates and the destruction of host tissues is minimal. The skin lesions produced by streptococci (furuncles, carbuncles, and impetigo) resemble those due to staphylococci.

Streptococcal pharyngitis: *S. pyogenes* is the common bacterial cause of pharyngitis. It spreads through direct contact with oral or respiratory secretions. It is characterized by edema, epiglottic swelling, and punctate abscesses of the tonsillar crypts. It may be accompanied by cervical lymphadenopathy. Severe pharyngeal infection if associated with peritonsillar or retropharyngeal abscess may encroach on the airways.

- **Complications: Rheumatic fever** and **poststreptococcal glomerulonephritis** are two major immunologically triggered complications of streptococcal infection of the upper oropharyngeal regions.

Erysipelas: It is caused by exotoxins from superficial infection with *S. pyogenes*. It is characterized by rapidly spreading erythematous swelling of the skin. It is common in warm climates. It usually begins on the face or less frequently, on the body or an extremity. It spreads rapidly. The rash has a sharp, well-demarcated, clear advancing margins, serpiginous border. On the face they may show a "butterfly distribution." Microscopic examination shows a diffuse, edematous, neutrophilic inflammatory reaction in the dermis and epidermis extending into the subcutaneous tissues. The inflammatory infiltrate is most severe around vessels and adnexa of the skin. Cutaneous microabscesses and small foci of necrosis may be formed, but tissue necrosis is usually minor component.

Continued

Continued

Scarlet fever (scarlatina): It is associated with pharyngitis due to *S. pyogenes,* and is most common between 3 and 15 years of age. Scarlet fever is caused by an erythrogenic toxin. It is manifested by a punctate erythematous (red) rash on the skin and mucous membranes. In the skin rash is most prominent over the trunk and inner aspects of the arms and legs. The face is also involved. In the face usually a small area around the mouth remains unaffected and this produces circumoral pallor. In the tongue, there may be a yellow-white coating, which sheds to reveal a "beefy-red" surface. The skin usually becomes hyperkeratotic and scaly during the convalescence period.

Impetigo (pyoderma): It is a localized, intraepidermal infection due to *S. pyogenes* or *S. aureus*. Strains of *S. pyogenes* that produce impetigo are antigenically and epidemiologically distinct from those that produce pharyngitis. It spreads by direct contact and mostly develop children between 2 and 5 years of age. Infection begins with colonization of bacteria in the skin. Minor trauma or an insect bite then inoculates the bacteria into the skin. These bacteria form an intraepidermal pustule, which ruptures and leaks a purulent exudate. Lesions begin as localized erythematous papules on the exposed body surfaces. These papules become pustules, which erode to form a thick honey colored crust. Impetigo sometimes may complicate to produce acute poststreptococcal glomerulonephritis, but it does not lead to rheumatic fever.

Streptococcal cellulitis: This is an acute spreading inflammation of the loose connective tissue of the deeper layers of the dermis and the subcutaneous tissue due to entry of the organism through the abrasions of the skin. Cellulitis usually begins at sites of unnoticed injury. It appears as spreading areas of redness, warmth, and swelling.

Pneumonia and empyema: Streptococcal pneumonia usually follows a viral infection, and it manifests as bronchopneumonia. In many cases empyema develops as a complication.

Streptococcal TSS: Infection by group A *Streptococcus* may lead to vascular collapse and organ failure. M-protein which is a constituent of the cell wall is the virulence factor, which plays the major role in the pathogenesis of TSS. It forms large aggregates with fibrinogen, in blood and tissues. These activate polymorphonuclear leukocytes intravascularly and this leads to the production of TSS (refer page 630 and 631).

Puerperal sepsis: Puerperal sepsis is postpartum infection of the uterine cavity due to *S. pyogenes*. It develops due to the contaminated hands of attendants at delivery.

Diphtheria

- Diphtheria is caused by *Corynebacterium diphtheria.*
- *Corynebacterium diphtheria* is a slender gram-positive rod with clubbed ends.

- **Mode of spread:** From person-to-person in respiratory droplets (respiratory diphtheria) or skin exudate (cutaneous diphtheria).
- **Incubation period:** Commonly 3–4 days.
- **Immunization with diphtheria toxoid (formalin-fixed toxin):** It stimulates production of toxin-neutralizing antibodies which protect persons from the lethal effects of the toxin. Diphtheria is preventable by vaccination with inactivated *C. diphtheria* toxin (toxoid).

Pathogenesis

Produces toxins: *Corynebacterium diphtheriae* produces a diphtheria toxin which is one of the most potent toxin. It is a protein called A-B toxin composed of two peptides chains—the A and B subunits—held together by a disulfide bond. It blocks protein synthesis by host cell. The A subunit (fragment) of toxin acts within the cytoplasm and catalyzes the covalent transfer of adenosine diphosphate (ADP)-ribose to elongation factor-2 (EF-2). This inhibits EF-2 function, which is needed for the translation of mRNA into protein. The B subunit binds glycolipid receptors on target cells. A single molecule of diphtheria toxin can kill a cell by ADP-ribosylating. Thus, it can inactivate more than a million EF-2 molecules.

Pathogenesis Inhaled *C. diphtheria* is carried in respiratory droplets, enters the pharynx and usually proliferates at the site of attachment on the mucosa (tonsils, nasopharynx, oropharynx, larynx, or trachea). The diphtheria toxin produced is absorbed systemically and acts on many tissues, with the heart, nerves, and kidneys being most susceptible to damage.

MORPHOLOGY

Types of diphtheria: Common types include:

Respiratory diphtheria: It causes **pharyngeal infection or less often infection of nose or larynx**. It produces exotoxin which causes necrosis of the epithelium and formation of a dense fibrinosuppurative exudate. The coagulation of this exudate on the ulcerated necrotic surface creates a tough, thick, dirty gray to black, superficial membrane ("wash-leather") known as **pseudomembrane** (because it is not formed by viable tissue). The pseudomembrane is **diagnostic pathologic feature of diphtheria** (from the Greek, *diphtheria,* "pair of leather scrolls"). **Pseudomembrane is composed of sloughed epithelium, necrotic debris, neutrophils, fibrin, and bacteria that line affected respiratory passages.** The epithelial surface beneath the pseudomembrane is denuded, and the submucosa appears acutely inflamed (with intense neutrophilic infiltrate) and hemorrhagic. When the membrane sloughs off, there is bleeding. The inflammation causes swelling in surrounding soft tissues, which can be severe enough to cause respiratory compromise leading to asphyxia. With control of the infection, the pseudomembrane is either coughed-up or dissolved by enzymatic digestion.

- The **exotoxin can also damage the heart, nerves, and other organs**. When the heart is involved, the myocardium shows droplets of fat in the myocytes (fatty change) and focal necrosis of myofibers. In the case of neural involvement, affected peripheral nerves show polyneuritis with degeneration of the myelin sheaths and axis cylinders (demyelination).

Cutaneous diphtheria: It results from inoculation of the organism into a break in the skin. It manifests as a pustule or ulcer. The chronic ulcers are covered by a dirty gray membrane without any systemic damage.

Listeriosis

Listeriosis is caused by *Listeria monocytogenes,* a small, motile, **gram-positive** coccobacillus. It is a facultative intracellular pathogen.

Epidemiology: Listeriosis is usually sporadic but may be epidemic.

- **Source of infection:** *L. monocytogenes* can be found on surface water, soil, vegetation, and feces of healthy individuals. Most human infections usually occur in the summer in urban region. *L. monocytogenes* grows at refrigerator temperatures. Outbreaks of *L. monocytogenes* infection most often associated with use of unpasteurized milk, contaminated cheese, and dairy products or processed fruits and vegetables.

Diseases produced: In most individuals, it causes gastroenteritis after ingestion of sufficient quantity of *L. monocytogenes* and it **causes severe food-borne infections in vulnerable hosts.** Particularly more susceptible to severe *L. monocytogenes* infection are pregnant women, neonates, older adults, chronic alcoholics, patients with cancer or receiving immunosuppressive therapy and those with acquired immune deficiency syndrome (AIDS). In pregnant women, it can cause amnionitis that may result in abortion, stillbirth, or neonatal sepsis. In neonates and immunosuppressed adults, it can produce disseminated disease (granulomatosis infantiseptica of the newborn) and an exudative meningitis.

Pathogenesis: *L. monocytogenes* has an unusual life cycle and thereby able to evade intracellular and extracellular host antibacterial defenses. The bacteria attach to receptors on host epithelial cells and macrophages and they are phagocytosed. After phagocytosis by host cells, the bacteria enter phagolysosomes, where acidic pH activates a pore-forming protein called listeriolysin *O* and two phospholipases. Listeriolysin O is an exotoxin that disrupts the vesicular membrane of phagolysosomes and allows bacteria to escape into the cytoplasm of host cell. After replicating in the host cell cytoplasm, a bacterial surface protein called Act A binds to an actin nucleating complex called the Arp2/3 complex. This induces actin polymerization and generates force to propel the bacteria from infected host cell into the adjacent, uninfected host cells. Thus, *Listeria* spread from one cell to another without exposure to the extracellular environment. Resting macrophages cannot kill the intracellular bacteria, whereas macrophages that are activated by interferon-γ (IFN-γ) can. Thus, an effective host response to *L. monocytogenes* depends on production of IFN-γ by NK cells during early infection and Th1 and CD8+ T cells in chronic infection. Increased risk for listeriosis is observed in patients with defects in cell-mediated immunity (e.g., with decreased CD4+ lymphocytes).

MORPHOLOGY

Acute infections by *L. monocytogenes* produce an exudative inflammation with numerous neutrophils.

Meningitis due to *L. monocytogenes*: It is macroscopically as well as microscopically indistinguishable from meningitis due to other pyogenic bacteria. **Detection of gram-positive bacilli in the cerebrospinal fluid (CSF) is diagnostic.** **Focal abscesses:** They may alternate with grayish or yellow nodules of necrotic amorphous tissue debris. They can develop in any organ, including the lung, liver, spleen, and lymph nodes.

Chronic infections: When infections are present for longer periods, large numbers of macrophages may appear in the lesions. However, granulomas are rare.

Infection in infants: Infants born with *L. monocytogenes* sepsis usually develop a papular red rash over the extremities. The placenta may show listerial abscesses. A smear prepared from the meconium will show gram-positive bacilli.

Septicemic listeriosis: It is a severe febrile disease most commonly observed in immunodeficient patients. It may lead to shock and disseminated intravascular coagulation and may be misdiagnosed as gram-negative sepsis.

Anthrax

- Anthrax is a **necrotizing, zoonotic disease caused by *B. anthracis*.** It is a large, spore-forming (central spore) gram-positive rod-shaped and one of the largest of pathogenic bacterium found in environmental sources.
- It produces toxins and is responsible for the clinical features of disease that most closely correlated with its virulence.

Epidemiology

Source of infection: Major reservoirs for *B. anthracis* are goats, sheep, cattle, horses, pigs, and dogs. Spores form in the soil and dead animals. These spores are resistant to heat, desiccation, and chemical disinfection for years.

Mode of transmission: Humans are infected when spores enter the body through breaks in the skin. It occurs through direct contact (inoculation of the spores) with an infected animal particularly herbivores. Infection is most frequent as an occupational disease in farmers, butchers, and dealers in wool and animal hides (hide or skin is an animal skin treated for human use). Spores of *B. anthracis* can also be ingested (by eating meat or products from infected animals) or inhaled. Humans may develop disease also from handling meat or exposure to contaminated (infected) animal byproducts (e.g., hides, wool (fine, soft curly or wavy hair forming the coat of a sheep, goat, or similar animal), brushes, or bone meal). Deliberate release of anthrax spores is an important bioterrorist weapon. Anthrax spores can be made into a fine powder and can be used as a potent biological weapon. Recent domestic bioterrorism episode involved transport of organisms by the postal system (delivered in the mail).

Incubation period: Up to 1–10 days.

Major Forms of Anthrax

Anthrax is characterized by necrotizing inflammatory lesions in the skin or gastrointestinal (GI) tract or systemically. There are three major forms of anthrax depending on the route of entry of the anthrax spores.

Cutaneous anthrax

- It is the **most common type** of anthrax (up to 95% of naturally occurring all anthrax infections). It follows inoculation of spores into the subcutaneous of the exposed skin. Occupational exposure to anthrax spores during processing of hides and bone products results in cutaneous anthrax.
- **Skin lesions (Hide porter's disease):** It begins as a small, painless, itching (pruritic), erythematous, maculopapule. The base is edematous and hemorrhagic. The lesion is initially painless despite edema. It enlarges within 2 days to form a vesicle filled with serosanguinous fluid, and is surrounded by gross edema ("**malignant pustule**"). As the vesicle enlarges, there may be marked edema around it and may be accompanied by regional lymphadenopathy (poor prognosis). The vesicle ruptures and forms ulcer. Bloody purulent exudate accumulates and gradually darkens to purple or black. The ulcer dries and forms a central depressed characteristic thick black "**eschar**" surrounded by blebs. The eschar dries and falls off as the person recovers. Despite marked edema, pain is infrequent. Bacteremia is rare. It is self-limiting illness in the majority of patients, but occasionally perivascular edema and regional lymphadenopathy (lymphatic invasion precedes septicemia) may be associated with marked toxemia.

Pulmonary, or inhalational anthrax

It is **extremely rare** and follows inhalation of airborne spores of *B. anthracis*. It is sometimes called **"wool sorters' disease"** because it is a hazard of handling raw wool. Bioterrorism-related anthrax is also due to inhalation of spores. After inhalation, the spores are phagocytosed in the alveoli and are carried by these phagocytes to lymph nodes. In the lymph node they germinate and produce bacilli. They release toxins which produce hemorrhagic mediastinitis.

Clinical features It begins as prodromal a flu-like illness of 1–6 days characterized by fever, nonproductive cough, dyspnea, headache, and chest or retrosternal discomfort. Then there is abrupt onset of increased fever, bronchopneumonia causing hypoxia, sweating, and rapidly progresses to respiratory failure and shock. Death may occur within 1–2 days. Symptoms of septicemia may develop 3–14 days following exposure. Frequently, meningitis may occur during bacteremia. Without rapid and aggressive treatment at the onset of symptoms, the mortality ranges from 50 to 90%.

Septicemic anthrax It is more common in pulmonary anthrax than cutaneous anthrax. Septicemia may lead to disseminated intravascular coagulation. Bacterial toxin can depress the respiratory center.

Gastrointestinal anthrax

It is rare and is usually associated with eating of undercooked meat products contaminated with *B. anthracis*. The cecum

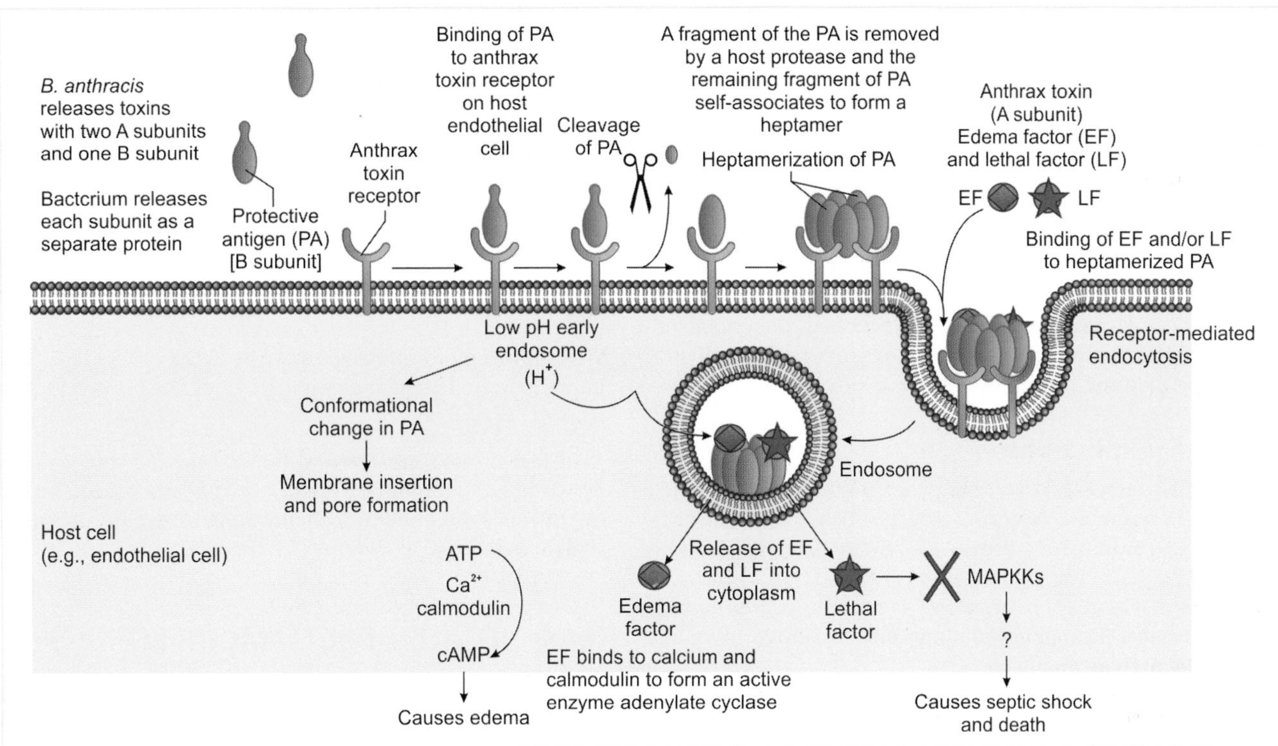

FIG. 23: Mechanism of action of anthrax toxins (read text for description).

is involved and initially it manifests with nausea, abdominal pain, and vomiting, followed by severe bloody diarrhea (severe gastroenteritis) and, sometimes, bacteremia/toxemia. Mortality is about 40%. Death may develop rapidly due to fulminant diarrhea and massive ascites.

Pathogenesis

The spores of *B. anthracis* germinate in the human body and give rise to vegetative bacteria. They multiply and produce powerful toxins and contain an antiphagocytic polyglutamyl capsule. The mechanisms of action of anthrax toxins are presented in **Figure 23**.

- **Release of anthrax toxin:** It contains two A subunits and one B subunit. Each subunit is released as a separate protein.
  - The two A subunits are (1) *edema factor* (EF) and (2) *lethal factor* (LF).
  - The B subunit is called as the *protective antigen* (PA). This is named so because antibodies against it protect the host against the effects of the toxins. PA is not toxic, but it helps to transfer the toxic EF and LF into cells.
- **Binding of PA to host endothelial cell:** PA (B subunit) binds to host cell surface receptor that is highly expressed on endothelial cells.
- **Removal of fragment of PA:** A fragment of the PA is then removed by a host protease and the remaining fragment of PA self-associates to form a heptamer (molecule formed from seven monomers).
- **Binding of EF or LF to PA and endocytosis:** One to three molecules of the EF or LF attach to a PA heptamer and forms a complex. This complex is then endocytosed into the host cell.
- **Movement of EF or LF into cytoplasm:** The low pH inside the endosome produces a conformational change in the PA heptamer. This creates a channel in the membrane of the endosome and/through this channel EF or LF moves into the cytoplasm.
- **In the cytoplasm:** Actions of EF and LF in the cytoplasm are as follows:
  - EF binds to calcium and calmodulin to form an active enzyme adenylate cyclase. This enzyme converts adenosine triphosphate (ATP) to intracellular cyclic adenosine monophosphate (cAMP) and alters the function of cell. This leads to edema.
  - LF is a protease that destroys mitogen-activated protein kinase kinases (MAPKKs). These kinases regulate the activity of MAPKs. These MAPKs are main regulators of cell growth and differentiation. The dysregulation of MAPKs leads to cell death. It may be responsible for septic shock.

MORPHOLOGY

Bacillus anthracis produces extensive tissue necrosis at the sites of infection. The **exudative inflammation is rich in neutrophils and macrophages.**

Demonstrating the organism: A stained smear of fluid taken from the edge of a skin lesion may demonstrate the organism. The organism may also be demonstrated in stools, laryngeal secretions, sputum, and CSF. They **appear as large, boxcar-shaped gram-positive extracellular bacteria in chains**. It is better appreciated using the **Brown and Brenn stain**.

Culture of blood and other body fluids: *B. anthracis* can be cultured in mice, rabbits, or guinea pigs.

Continued

Continued

Inhalational anthrax: It is characterized by numerous foci of hemorrhage in the mediastinum and hemorrhagic lymphadenitis of hilar and peribronchial lymph nodes. The lungs usually show a perihilar interstitial pneumonia with infiltration of macrophages and neutrophils and pulmonary vasculitis. In about 50% of cases, hemorrhagic lung lesions are associated with vasculitis. Mediastinal lymph nodes show edema and macrophages containing phagocytosed apoptotic lymphocytes. *B. anthracis* is usually found in the alveolar capillaries and venules. In fatal cases, the organism can be demonstrated in multiple organs (spleen, liver, intestines, kidneys, adrenal glands, and meninges).

Nocardial Infections

***Nocardia* species are aerobic gram-positive** filamentous, branching **bacteria.** *Nocardia* species grows in distinctive branched chains. In culture, *Nocardia* form thin aerial filaments resembling hyphae. They are weakly acid-fast and must be distinguished from the morphologically similar actinomycetes. Though morphologically it is similar to molds, ***Nocardia* are true bacteria.**

Epidemiology: *Nocardia* species are widely distributed in soil. In humans, disease is caused by inhaling or inoculating soil-borne organisms. It is not transmitted from person to person. It is most common in patients with impaired or defective immunity, particularly cell-mediated immunity and develops as **opportunistic infections**. Thus, predisposing factors include organ transplantation, long-term (prolonged) corticosteroid therapy, human immunodeficiency virus (HIV) infection, lymphomas, leukemias, diabetes, and other debilitating diseases.

Species: *Nocardia* species cause respiratory infections. *N. asteroides* is the most common pathogenic species causing disease (respiratory tract) in humans. Two other pathogenic species of *Nocardia,* namely *N. brasiliensis* and *N. caviae,* may cause pulmonary nocardiosis similar to *N. asteroides.* They are usually found in underdeveloped countries as a cause of mycetomas. The organism elicits a quick infiltrate of neutrophils. If an infected individual mounts an efficient cell-mediated immune response, the infection may be eliminated. Various diseases produced are as follows:

- **Respiratory infection:** The respiratory tract is the usual portal of entry. *Nocardia* species infection begins as an indolent slowly progressive disease. It presents with fever, weight loss, and cough, which may be mistaken for tuberculosis or malignancy. It may progress to pyogenic pneumonia. In immunocompromised individuals *Nocardia* produces pulmonary abscesses, which are usually multiple and confluent. Direct extension to the pleura, trachea, and heart and blood-borne metastases to the brain (CNS) or skin carry a grave prognosis.
- **CNS infection:** Infections of the CNS are also indolent. They cause varying neurologic deficits depending on the site of the lesions.
- ***N. brasiliensis*:** It produces infections of skin following injuries contaminated with soil. It manifests as cellulitis, lymphocutaneous disease, and actinomycetoma with formation of nodules that progress to form chronic draining fistulae.

MORPHOLOGY

Microscopy

Nocardia species produce a suppurative inflammation with neutrophils, central **liquefactive necrosis** and surrounded by granulation tissue and fibrosis. Nocardial abscesses show scattered organisms. Granulomas do not form.

Gram stain: In tissue sections, *Nocardia* species appear as slender, beaded, gram-positive rods arranged in branching filaments.

Silver impregnation: Bacteria can be demonstrated by silver impregnation. Irregular staining of the filaments produces a beaded appearance.

Acid-fast stains (Fite-Faraco stain): *Nocardia* species stain positively with modified acid-fast stains (Fite-Faraco stain). In contrast, *Actinomyces* species, appear similar on Gram stain of tissue.

GRAM-NEGATIVE BACTERIAL INFECTIONS

Many gram-negative bacteria are pathogenic to humans and they are increasingly becoming resistant to antibiotics, including carbapenem-resistant *Klebsiella pneumonia,* and cephalosporin-resistant *N. gonorrhoeae.*

Gram-negative bacterial infections are diagnosed by culture.

Neisserial Infections

Neisseria species are gram-negative, aerobic, nonsporulating, nonmotile and are arranged typically in pairs (**diplococci**) (**Fig. 24**). These diplococci are flattened on the adjoining sides and give rise the pair the shape of a coffee bean.

Growth characteristics: These aerobic bacteria have strict nutritional requirements. They do not grow on ordinary media. They grow best on enriched media such as lysed sheep's blood (chocolate) agar.

Pathogenic versus commensal: Pathogenic *Neisseria* species usually are capable of secreting single-stranded DNA for transformation of other *Neisseria* species, whereas this ability is not seen in commensal *Neisseria* species.

Genus: The genus contains two clinically important *Neisseria* species Namely *N. meningitidis* and *N. gonorrhoeae.*

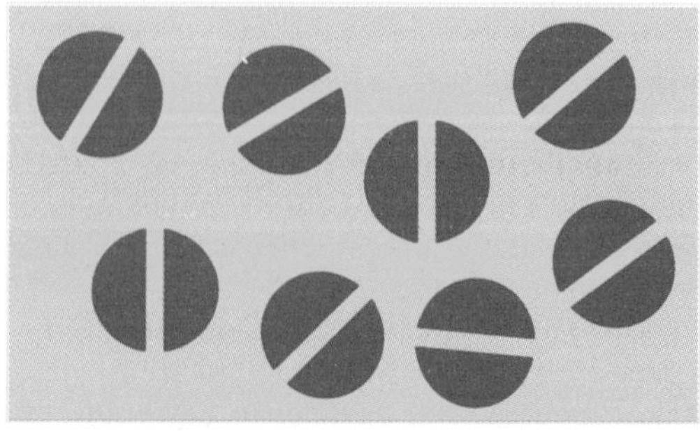

FIG. 24: Diagrammatic appearance of *Neisseria* showing flat adjacent sides of gram-negative diplococci.

Neisseria meningitides

It **causes bacterial** (meningococcal) **meningitis, particularly in adolescents and young adults.** This commonly colonizes the oropharynx and spreads by the respiratory route. In most of the normal individuals, an immune response eliminates the colonizing organism. This immune response also protects against subsequent infection with the same serotype of bacteria.

Subtypes: Meningococci (*N. meningitides)* are capsulated and depending on their capsular polysaccharide antigens, they are classified into several capsular serotypes. Only five of these serotypes cause most cases of meningitis in humans. Invasive disease develops when individuals come across new strains to which they are not immune. This happens in young children or young adults living in crowded places [e.g., military barracks (buildings used to house soldiers.) or college dormitories].

Even in the absence of pre-existing immunity, only a small percentage of individuals infected with *N. meningitidis* develop meningitis. To produce infection, the bacteria must invade cells of respiratory epitheliums and enter the blood. In the circulating blood, the bacterial capsule prevents the opsonization and destruction of the bacteria by complement proteins. The complement acts as a first-line defense against *N. meningitides*. Therefore, increased rates of serious infection are observed in individuals with inherited defects in the complement proteins (C5 to C9) that form the membrane attack complex, or patients with paroxysmal nocturnal hemoglobinuria who receive treatment with an antibody inhibitor of the membrane attack complex. *N. meningitidis* can be endemic or epidemics.

Pathogenesis: Meningococcal capsule has antiphagocytic properties and this helps in the maintenance of infection. Endotoxin lipopolysaccharide released during autolysis is responsible for the toxic effects found in disseminated meningococcal disease. The vascular endothelium is particularly very sensitive to the endotoxin. There is triggering and upregulation of inflammatory cascade systems, cytokines, and nitric oxide (NO). Meningococci (also gonococci) secrete IgA protease which cleaves IgA. This helps the *Neisseriae* to evade immunoglobulins of this subclass.

Prophylaxis: Highly effective conjugate vaccines for *N. meningitidis* are available. They are composed of capsular polysaccharides conjugated to antigenic proteins. The vaccines induce good immunity after a single dose in older children and adults.

Neisseria gonorrhoeae

Neisseria gonorrhoeae, also called **gonococcus, is an important cause of sexually transmitted infection (STI)**. It is second most common cause of bacterial STIs (first being *C. trachomatis*). *N. gonorrhoeae* is an **unencapsulated, aerobic, bean-shaped, piliated, gram-negative diplococcus**. It causes an acute suppurative genital tract infection known as **gonorrhoea**. *N. gonorrhoeae* infection usually manifests locally in the genital or cervical mucosa, pharynx, or anorectum. However, disseminated infections may occur.

Definition: Gonorrhea is an STI due to the gram-negative diplococcus, *N. gonorrhea*. It commonly infects columnar epithelium in the lower genital tract (cervicitis, urethritis), rectum (proctitis), and eye (conjunctivitis).

Structure

Pili: *Neisseria* species have long hair-like surface appendages (extensions), termed "pili," that project from the cell wall. The pili are composed of polypeptides (repeating peptide subunits) called pilin. Pili enhance attachment of the organism to host epithelial and mucosal cell surfaces. Hence, pili are important virulence factors. Pili are also antigenic.

- **Antigenic variation (Fig. 25):** Pili are encoded by the pilin gene. There are about many gonococcal pili genes that code for pilin protein. These genes have a promoter and coding sequences for 10–15 pili protein variants. Most of the pili genes are not expressed at any given time because they lack promoters (that is, they are "silent"). At any point in time, only one of the coding sequences is adjacent to the promoter, and this allows it to be expressed. By shuffling and homologous recombining chromosomal regions one of the pilin coding sequences is inserted next to the promoter. Thus, a single strain of *N. gonorrhoeae* can, at different times, synthesize ("express") multiple pilins that have different amino acid sequences. This leads to expression of a different pilin variant. This process is known as antigenic variation by gene conversion. This is responsible for the organism to produce antigenically different pilin molecules at high frequency.

Opacity proteins: Opacity (Opa/OPA) proteins are so named because of their tendency to make gonococcal colonies opaque. They present in the outer membrane of the bacteria. They are also involved in pathogenesis (refer below).

Portal of entry: These include nasopharynx, urethra, cervix, or rectum. Gonococcal pharyngitis and proctitis are also sexually transmitted.

Incubation period: Usually 2–10 days following exposure.

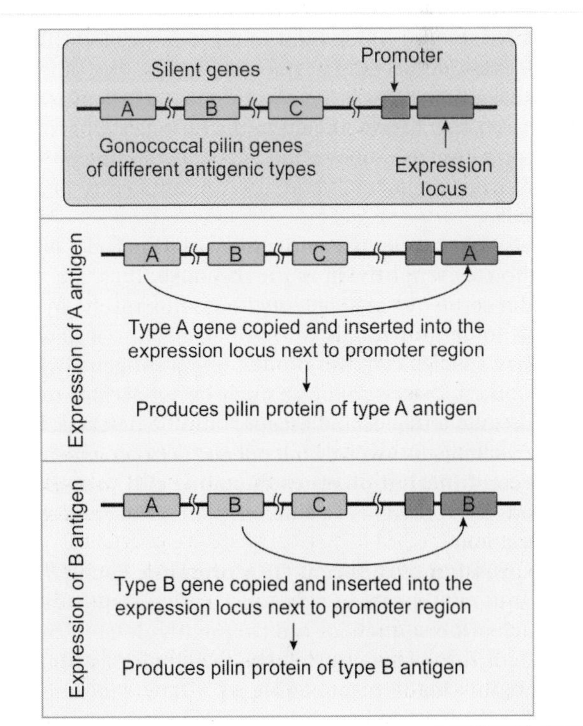

FIG. 25: Diagrammatic representation of antigenic variation in the gonococcus.

Mode of transmission: It spreads directly from person to person. Except for perinatal transmission, spread is by sexual intercourse. Genital-genital, genital-anorectal, or oro-genital or oro-anal contact or from mother-to-child transmission during delivery. Infected people who are asymptomatic are a major reservoir of infection.

- **Males:** Infection in men manifests as urethritis. Ascending spread in men is less common and can lead to epididymitis.
- **Females:** In women, *N. gonorrhoeae* infection causes endocervicitis. Usually it is asymptomatic and may go unnoticed. In women with untreated gonorrhoea, infection often ascends the genital tract, producing endometritis, salpingitis, and can lead to pelvic inflammatory disease (PID). This can lead to infertility or ectopic pregnancy.
- **Ophthalmia neonatorum:** Nonvenereal, direct neonatal infection by *N. gonorrhoeae* occurs during delivery from the passage of child through birth canal of a mother with gonorrhea. It usually manifests as conjunctivitis and may lead to blindness and, rarely, sepsis. The infection of eye can be prevented by instillation of silver nitrate or antibiotics in the newborn's eyes at birth.
- **Dissemination:** Similar to *N. meningitidis, N. gonorrhoeae* can disseminate and produce bacteremia. This occurs rarely and usually in patients who are deficient in the complement proteins that form the membrane attack complex. Disseminated infection of adults and adolescents usually results in septic arthritis. This may be associated with skin lesions namely rash of hemorrhagic papules and pustules.

Diagnosis: Infection is diagnosed by culture and polymerase chain reaction (PCR) tests.

Pathogenesis (Fig. 26)

At the site of entry, *Neisseria* species adhere to and invade nonciliated epithelial cells of mucous membranes. Initially, *Neisseria* species attach to surface epithelial cells through pili (refer above), which bind to a protein called CD46 that is expressed on all human nucleated cells. The pili contain a protease that digests IgA on the mucous membrane and facilitate bacterial attachment to the host cell. Opacity (Opa/ **OPA**) proteins (refer above) increases the binding of *Neisseria* species to epithelial cells and also promote entry of bacteria into cells.

***Neisseria* species use antigenic variation** (refer above) **as a method to escape the immune response.** There are multiple capsular serotypes of *N. meningitidis.* This results in meningitis in some individuals who are exposed to a new strain. *Neisseria* species can also produce new antigens by genetic mechanisms. This also allows a single bacterial clone to change its expressed antigens and escape immune defences by host. Such mechanisms involve both pili and OPA proteins:

- **Recombination of genes encoding pili proteins:** This leads to expression of a different pilin variant and antigenic variation.
- **Expression of different OPA proteins:** Each *OPA* gene has many repeats of a five-nucleotide sequence. These nucleotide sequences are frequently deleted or duplicated. These changes shift the reading frame of the gene and this leads to encoding of a new sequence. Stop codons may also have introduced either by the additions and deletions. This determines whether each *OPA* gene is expressed or silent. Thus, at any time *Neisseria* species can express either one, none, or multiple OPA proteins.

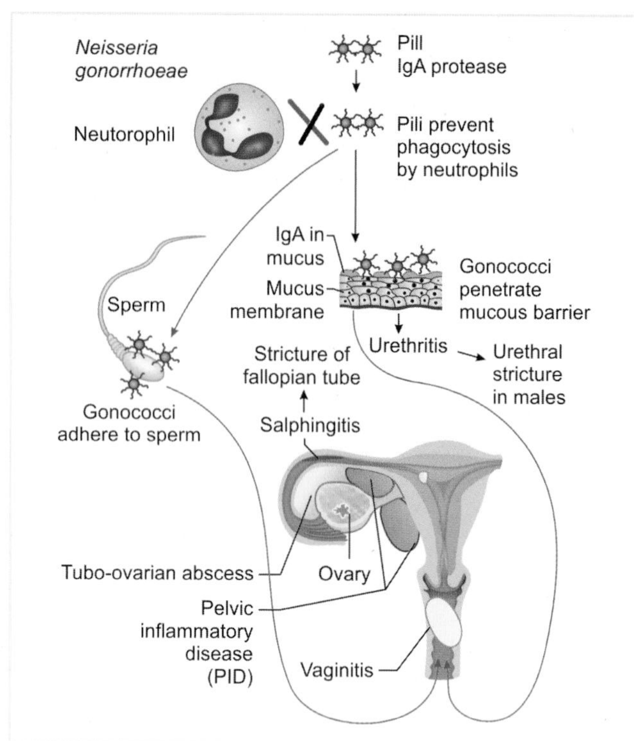

FIG. 26: Pathogenesis of gonococcal infections. *Neisseria gonorrhoeae* has surface pili which prevents against phagocytosis by neutrophils. The pili contain an immunoglobulin A (IgA) protease that digests IgA on the luminal surface of the mucous membranes of the urethra, endocervix, and fallopian tube. This further facilitates the attachment of gonococci. Gonococci can produce endocervicitis, vaginitis, and salpingitis in females. In males, gonococci can cause urethritis and, sometimes, urethral stricture. Gonococci may also get attached to sperm heads and can be carried into the fallopian tube. It can produce stricture of the fallopian tube, pelvic inflammatory disease (PID) or tubo-ovarian abscess.

MORPHOLOGY

Gonorrhea is a suppurative infection and elicit a severe acute inflammatory response. This produces great amount of pus and usually forms submucosal abscesses. Smears prepared from pus show numerous neutrophils, often containing phagocytosed bacteria. If untreated, the inflammation becomes chronic and shows predominant of macrophages and lymphocytes.

Diagnosis

- **Gram's staining and culture** of urethral exudates, genital, rectal, pharyngeal, or ocular secretions show gram-negative intracellular monococci and diplococci.
- **Sterile pyuria:** Urine may show polymorphonuclear leukocytes with a negative urine culture report.
- **Nucleic acid probe tests:** Nucleic acid amplification tests (NAATs) are more sensitive than culture. They can be performed on urine samples, swabs from endocervix, urethra, rectum, and pharynx.

- Direct antigen detection by fluorescein-conjugated monoclonal antibodies and direct fluorescence microscopy.
- Enzyme-linked immunoassays for the detection of gonococcal antigen.
- Blood cultures in disseminated disease.

Complications: If untreated infections can develop following complications:

- **In females:** In 50% of infected women, gonorrhea remains asymptomatic. It can cause PID. Local complications includes endometritis, salpingitis, tubo-ovarian abscess, bartholinitis, peritonitis, and perihepatitis. Fallopian tubes may get distended with pus causing acute abdominal pain. Infertility occurs when inflammatory adhesions block the tubes. From the fallopian tubes, gonorrhea may spread to the peritoneum; when it heals fine "violin string" adhesions may develop between the liver and the parietal peritoneum (Fitz-Hugh-Curtis syndrome). Chronic endometritis is a complication of gonococcal infection and is usually the consequence of chronic gonococcal salpingitis.
- **In male patients:** Periurethritis, epididymitis epididymo-orchitis, and prostatitis. It may result in infertility.
- **Newborns:** Ophthalmia neonatorum in newborns.

Whooping Cough or Pertussis

Pertussis or whooping cough is a highly communicable acute bacterial disease of childhood, caused by the gram-negative coccobacillus ***Bordetella pertussis***. The wide use of DPT (**D**iphtheria, **P**ertussis and **T**etanus) vaccine has reduced the prevalence of whooping cough.

Incubation period: About 1–2 weeks.

Mode of spread: *B. pertussis* is a highly contagious disease. It spreads from person to person, mainly by respiratory aerosols. Humans are the only reservoir of infection.

Age group: Classic case is seen in childhood, with 90% occurring below 5 years of age.

Pathogenesis

- *Bordetella pertussis* has strong affinity for the brush border of the bronchial epithelium and also invades macrophages. It contains a filamentous hemagglutinin that attaches to carbohydrates present on the surface of respiratory epithelial cells and also attaches to CR3 (Mac-1) integrins on macrophages.
- **Virulence factors of *B. pertussis*:** These include pertussis toxin, adenylate cyclase toxin, dermonecrotic toxin, and tracheal cytotoxin. Pertussis toxin is an **A-B toxin** and consists of five subunits.
    - **A unit:** Like cholera toxin, ADP-ribosylates inactivates guanine nucleotide-binding proteins. This results in inability of G proteins to transduce signals and interrupts the effect of chemokines that use G protein-coupled receptors.
    - **B component:** It has four subunits that attaches to extracellular molecules and allow the A subunit to enter the cells. The B subunit can also attach to cell surface molecules such as toll-like receptors-4 (TLR4), and thereby it can initiate signaling events in cells. Pertussis toxin subunits impair host defenses mainly by (1) inhibiting recruitment of neutrophil and macrophage and (2) activation and paralyzing cilia.
    - ***Bordetella pertussis* also produces adenylate cyclase toxin**. This toxin enters host cells and converts ATP to supraphysiologic levels of cAMP. The increased levels of cAMP inhibit phagocytosis, the oxidative burst, and NO-mediated killing in neutrophils and macrophages, and forms neutrophil extracellular traps (NETs).
- The toxin produced by the organism inhibits neutrophils and macrophages and paralyze cilia. Within 7–10 days after exposure, catarrhal stage of whooping cough begins and is the most infectious stage.

MORPHOLOGY

- *Bordetella pertussis* proliferates and stimulates the bronchial epithelium to produce abundant tenacious mucus causing **laryngotracheobronchitis**.
- In severe cases, it causes erosion of bronchial mucosal, hyperemia, and copious mucopurulent exudate. Tracheobronchitis is associated with necrosis of ciliated respiratory epithelium and an acute inflammatory response. Because of the loss of the protective mucociliary action, patients have increased susceptibility to develop pneumonia from aspirated oral bacteria. Coughing paroxysms and vomiting make aspiration likely. Most common cause of death is due to secondary bacterial pneumonia.
- Enlargement of lymphoid follicles in the bronchial mucosa and peribronchial region is also seen.
- Peripheral blood shows **marked lymphocytosis** (up to 90%).

Clinical Features

Whooping cough is a prolonged upper respiratory tract disease that usually lasts for 4–5 weeks. It passes through three stages:

1. **Catarrhal stage:** This first stage is highly infectious. It resembles a common viral upper respiratory tract illness characterized by upper respiratory catarrh with rhinitis (runny nose), lacrimation (conjunctivitis), low-grade fever, and an unproductive cough. This stage lasts about 1–2 weeks.
2. **Paroxysmal stage:** It is called so because of the characteristic paroxysms of coughing.
    - **Whoop:** During this stage, the cough becomes spasmodic, more frequent and severe with repetitive bouts of 5–10 coughs. It is characterized by **paroxysms** episode **of violent coughing** followed by a characteristic **classic,** long, **loud** (high-pitched) **inspiratory audible "whoop."** This gives the disease its name, "whooping cough." The whoop is due to rapid inspiration against a closed glottis at the end of a paroxysm. It is observed only in younger patients in whom the lumen of the respiratory tract is narrowed due to mucus secretion and mucosal edema. These paroxysms usually terminate in vomiting. Early paroxysmal stage is also infectious. The paroxysms persist for 2–3 weeks.
    - **Other features** include conjunctival suffusion and petechiae and ulceration of the frenulum of the tongue. Patients have marked lymphocytosis; total leukocyte counts often exceed 40,000 cells/μL.

3. **Convalescence stage:** It follows the paroxysmal phase during which slow resolution of whoop occurs. This phase can last 1–3 months, and cough may persist for several weeks to months. The condition is self-limiting but may cause death due to asphyxia especially in infants younger than 1 year of age. Children with pertussis may have coughing spells for up to 10 weeks.

Diagnosis: PCR is more sensitive than culture.

Pseudomonal Infections

***Pseudomonas aeruginosa* is an opportunistic, widely distributed, aerobic,** motile (it has polar flagella) **gram-negative bacillus.** It requires moisture and only minimal nutrients. It is found in soil, water, plants, and animals and thrives on moist environmental surfaces. Though it may colonize healthy humans without causing disease, it is responsible for significant opportunistic pathogen and a major cause of nosocomial (hospital-acquired) infections. It is highly antibiotic-resistant opportunistic pathogen and only infrequently infects humans.

Predisposing factors: It is a frequent, deadly pathogen in individuals with cystic fibrosis (CF), severe burns, or neutropenia. Many patients with CF die of pulmonary failure secondary to chronic infection with *P. aeruginosa.* Other predisposing factors include urinary catheterization, diabetes debilitated, and immunosuppressed individuals. *P. aeruginosa* may cause nosocomial pneumonia, nosocomial urinary tract infections, wound (surgical site) infections, infections of severe burns, and infections of patients undergoing either chemotherapy for neoplastic disease (immunosuppressed) or antibiotic therapy. *P. aeruginosa* is a common cause of **hospital-acquired** nosocomial **infections** and it can grow in washbasins, IV tubing, respirator tubing, nursery cribs, etc. It can cause corneal keratitis in individuals wearing contact lenses, endocarditis and osteomyelitis in IV drug abusers, external otitis (swimmer's ear) in healthy individuals, and severe external otitis in diabetic individuals.

Significance: *Pseudomonas aeruginosa* can be very resistant to most antibiotics. This make these infections difficult to treat. It may infect extensive skin burns and can lead to sepsis.

Pathogenesis

Pseudomonas aeruginosa **produces numerous toxins** (proteins) **and extracellular products** (extracellular enzymes such as elastase, alkaline protease) that promote local tissue invasion (necrotizing lesions) and dissemination of the organism. This allows it to attach, invade, and destroy host tissues (causing local tissue damage) as well avoid host inflammatory and immune defences. The organism produces extracellular enzymes such as elastase, alkaline protease, and cytotoxin. They facilitate tissue invasion and are partly responsible for the necrotizing lesions of *Pseudomonas* infections. The elastase secreted by *P. aeruginosa* helps them to invade blood vessel walls.

- *Pseudomonas aeruginosa* infection begins with attachment to and colonization of host tissue. Injury to epithelial cells exposes surface molecules that serve as binding sites for the pili of *P. aeruginosa.* Pili mediate adherence to host cells. Many strains of *P. aeruginosa* secrete a proteoglycan that surrounds and protects these organisms from mucociliary action, complement, and phagocytes.
- **Infection in lung:** Mucoid strains predominate in patients with CF. The mucoid capsule is composed of alginate. Alginate expression is responsible for resistance to phagocytosis and clearing in the CF lung.
    - **Early during infection** of the lungs in patients with CF, the organism secretes an A-B exotoxin called exotoxin A. This toxin, similar to diphtheria toxin, inhibits protein synthesis by ADP-ribosylating the ribosomal protein EF-2 and leads to the death of host cells. During early stage, the *P. aeruginosa* uses a type III secretion system (T3SS) to transport effector proteins into host cells. T3SSs are complex bacterial structures that enable *P. aeruginosa* to inject bacterial effector proteins directly into the host cell cytoplasm, bypassing the extracellular milieu. This reduces the ability of host cells to generate antibacterial reactive oxygen species and also induces apoptosis of the host cells.
    - **Later in chronic infection** in the lungs of patients with CF, *P. aeruginosa* become organized into biofilms. Biofilm partly composed of alginate secreted by bacteria and within the biofilm, the bacteria are protected from antibodies, complement, phagocytes, and antibiotics. At this stage, there is reduction in the release of exotoxin A and the expression of the T3SS. This in turn somewhat lowers the virulence of become, but it continues to damage the host tissue by stimulating inflammation and by releasing enzymes (proteases and elastases). During chronic infection, *P. aeruginosa* develops antibiotic resistance making its treatment difficult. This is due to production of biofilm and genetic changes.

MORPHOLOGY

Pseudomonas infection produces an acute inflammatory response. The bacterium often invades small arteries and veins (due to elastase produced by bacteria). This causes thrombosis and hemorrhagic necrosis, particularly in the lungs and skin.

Lung: Blood vessel invasion by *Pseudomonas* species predisposes to dissemination and sepsis and causes multiple nodular lesions in the lungs namely **necrotizing pneumonia.** This **necrotizing lesion** is distributed through the terminal airways in a fleur-de-lis pattern (symbol of a stylized lily or iris used for decorative purposes). This consists of striking pale necrotic centers and red, hemorrhagic peripheral areas.

- **Microscopic appearance:** Gram stains of necrotic tissue infected with *Pseudomonas* commonly shows masses of organisms, often concentrated in the walls of blood vessels. The surrounding host cells show coagulative necrosis. This gram-negative **bacterial vasculitis** along with thrombosis and hemorrhage is highly suggestive (not pathognomonic) of *P. aeruginosa* infection.
- **Complications:** Bronchial obstruction caused by mucus plugging and subsequent *P. aeruginosa* infection is usual complication in patients with CF. Chronic *P. aeruginosa* infection may lead to bronchiectasis and pulmonary fibrosis.

Continued

Continued

Skin: In skin burns, *P. aeruginosa* proliferates extensively, penetrates deeply into the veins, and spreads through blood. Sometimes disseminated infection may produce well-demarcated nodular, necrotic, and hemorrhagic oval skin lesions called **ecthyma gangrenosum**. These necrotic lesions represent sites where the organism has disseminated to the skin, invaded blood vessels, and produced localized hemorrhagic infarcts.

DIC: *P. aeruginosa* bacteremia may lead to DIC.

Clinical features: *Pseudomonas* infections are among the most aggressive bacterial diseases in human, often progressing rapidly to sepsis.

Melioidosis

Melioidosis (Rangoon beggars disease) is an uncommon disease caused by *Burkholderia* (formerly *Pseudomonas*) *pseudomallei.*

Source of infection: *Burkholderia pseudomallei* is a small gram-negative bacillus in the soil and surface water of tropical areas. It flourishes in wet environments, such as rice paddies and marshes.

Mode of infection: The skin is the usual portal of entry. The organisms enter through pre-existing skin lesions such as penetrating wounds and burns. It may also be acquired by inhalation of contaminated dust or aerosolized droplets.

Incubation period: It may last months to years, and the clinical course is variable.

Pathology and Clinical Features

Acute melioidosis: It produces pulmonary infection that may range from a mild tracheobronchitis to an overwhelming cavitary pneumonia. In severe cases, it presents with the sudden onset of high fever, constitutional symptoms, and a cough (may be with blood-stained sputum). Sometimes, there may be splenomegaly, hepatomegaly, and jaundice. Diarrhea may be as severe as in cholera. In spite of antibiotic therapy, fulminating septicaemia shock, coma, and death may occur. Acute septicemic melioidosis causes discrete abscesses in many organs throughout the body, especially in the lungs, liver, spleen, and lymph nodes.

Chronic melioidosis: It is characterized by a persistent localized infection of the lungs, skin, bones, or other organs. Lesions may be either suppurative or granulomatous abscesses. In the lung, it may be mistaken for tuberculosis. In some patients, chronic melioidosis may remain dormant for months or years, only to appear suddenly.

Plague

Yersinia pestis* is a small, gram-negative, nonmotile facultative intracellular bacterium that causes an invasive, frequently fatal infection called plague.** It can be used for biological warfare. Three human pathogens of ***Yersinia species are *Y. pestis, Y. enterocolitica,* and *Y. pseudotuberculosis. Y. enterocolitica* and *Y. pseudotuberculosis* are genetically similar to *Y. pestis* and they cause fecal-orally transmitted ileitis and mesenteric lymphadenitis. Plague is also called as **"black death."**

Epidemics: Historically, plague caused massive epidemics that killed many human beings. In major plague epidemics *Y. pestis* was first introduced into large urban rat populations. Infection spread first among rats and killed the rats. Flies were infected when fed on these dead rats and they spread it to human population, causing widespread disease. In mid-14th century (1347–1350), the Black Death pandemic in Europe killed 30–60% of Europe's population.

Features of *Y. pestis*: It contains a plasmid-borne complex of genes and secretes many virulence factors that are immunosuppressive or antiphagocytic. These virulence factors include the Yop virulon/proteins (secreted by a T3SS), the Pla protease (plasminogen activator that prevents blood clotting), and a proteinaceous capsule (F1 antigen), which is antiphagocytic. A hollow syringe-like structure projects from the bacterial surface, binds to host cells, and injects bacterial proteins called *Yops* (*Yersinia* outercoat proteins) into the host cell. YopE, YopH, and YopT inactivate molecules that regulate actin polymerization and thereby prevent phagocytosis of bacteria. YopJ inhibits the signaling pathways that are activated by LPS. This prevents the production of inflammatory cytokines. *Y. pestis* stains more heavily at the ends (i.e., bipolar staining), particularly with Giemsa stains.

Mode of transmission: It is transmitted from rodents to humans by flea bites or, less often, from one human to another by aerosols.

Source of infection: *Y. pestis* infection is an endemic zoonosis in many parts of the world. The main reservoirs are wild rodents (sylvatic rats, squirrels) that spread infection to the domestic rat species *(Rattus rattus)* and finally infected rat fleas (*Xenopsylla cheopis*). These fleas bite humans when there is a sudden reduction in the rat population.

Route of Infection

- **Rat flea bite:** Fleas transmit it from animal to animal, and most common route of human infections is from bite of a plague-infected rat flea.
- **Direct contact with infected tissues or fluids from sick or dead plague-infected animals**. Hunters and trappers can develop plague from handling rodents.
- **Droplet infection** from plague pneumonia or by laboratory exposure. Some infected humans develop plague pneumonia and shed large numbers of organisms in aerosolized respiratory secretions. This can cause person-to-person transmission.

Incubation period: Up to 3–6 days (shorter in pneumonic plague).

Pandemics: Historically, three great plague pandemics have caused >200 million deaths, including the dramatic name Black Death epidemic in 14th century Europe (Justinian 541 AD, Black Death 1346, China 1855). An outbreak in Madagascar during 2017 resulted in over 2,400 cases and >200 deaths.

Pathogenesis

In the flea

Yersinia pestis has two growth phases in the flea. The infectious cycle begins when a flea ingests a blood meal from an animal that is infected and bacteremic. In the early phase bacteria aggregate in the proventriculus but do not block blood flow completely. In the late phase, *Y. pestis* produces a biofilm that blocks (obstructs) the infected flea's midgut. This blockage prevents the flea from digesting the blood meal so it is consequently starved and hungry. It searches for a productive meal. When the starving flea next attempts to feed, before it feeds it bites and regurgitates these bacteria from its foregut into the new animal's skin. Thus flea infects the rodent or human by biting.

In humans

- After inoculation into the skin, *Y. pestis* is phagocytosed by neutrophils and macrophages. *Y. pestis* ingested by neutrophils are killed whereas those engulfed by macrophages survive and replicate intracellularly within macrophages. The macrophage carries bacteria from the site of inoculation to regional lymph nodes. In the lymph node bacteria continue to multiply and inhibit the host from mounting an effective response. It produces extensive hemorrhagic necrosis.
- **Dissemination:** From regional lymph nodes, bacteria disseminate via the bloodstream and lymphatics. Hematogenous spread of bacteria to other organs or tissues results in additional hemorrhagic lesions at these sites.

MORPHOLOGY

Yersinia pestis infection causes enlargement of lymph node (buboes), pneumonia, or sepsis with a marked neutrophilia.

Microscopy: It shows (1) massive proliferation of the *Y. pestis,* (2) presence of protein-rich and polysaccharide-rich effusions with few inflammatory cells, (3) necrosis of tissues and blood vessels associated with hemorrhage, thrombosis, and marked swelling of tissue, and (4) as healing begins, infiltration of neutrophils adjacent to necrotic areas. *Y. pestis* stains more densely at two ends (i.e., bipolar staining with safety pin appearance) and a clear central area (**Fig. 27**), particularly with Giemsa or methylene blue stains.

Three clinical presentations of *Y. pestis* infection are as follows:

- **Bubonic plague:** As the infected flea bite (usually on the legs), a small pustule or ulcer is formed. There is dramatic enlargement of draining lymph nodes within a few days. The lymph node becomes soft, fluctuant (due to extensive hemorrhagic necrosis), pulpy, and plum colored, and may infarct or rupture through the skin. Affected lymph nodes were called *buboes,* from the Greek word for "groin," giving rise to the name for this form of plague. Infected patients often develop necrotic, hemorrhagic skin lesions. Hence this is also named "black death."
- **Septicemic plague:** In this form, foci of necrosis develop in lymph nodes throughout the body and also in organs rich in mononuclear phagocytes. Fulminant bacteremia can produce DIC with widespread hemorrhages and thrombi.
- **Pneumonic plague:** It is characterized by severe, confluent, hemorrhagic, and necrotizing broncho-pneumonia. It releases organisms into the alveoli and airways. These are expelled by coughing, and can spread of the disease. Lung involvement may be accompanied by fibrinous pleuritis.

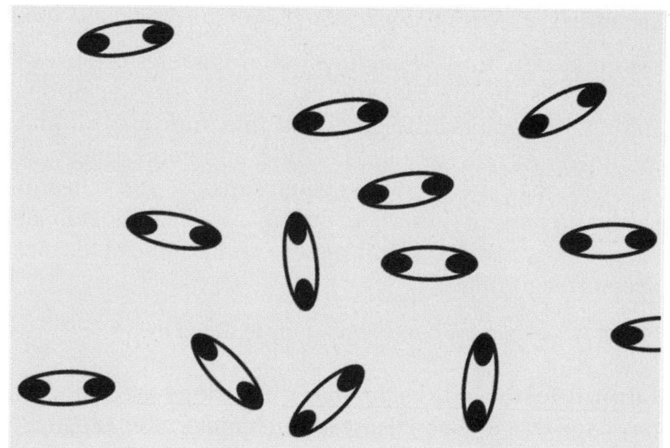

FIG. 27: Schematic appearance of *Y. pestis* with bipolar staining.

Clinical Features

Type of plague: Three clinical forms are recognized: bubonic, septicemic, and pneumonic.

- **Bubonic plague:** Onset is usually **acute/sudden** and begins 2–8 days after the flea bite. Symptoms include severe headache, high fever, rigor, chills, and myalgias. This is followed by painful enlargement of regional lymph nodes. Mostly lymph nodes in the groin are involved because flea bites usually occur in the lower extremities. Without treatment, disease progresses to septic shock within hours to days after appearance of the bubo (called so because they are rarely fluctuant).
- **Septicemic plague** (10% of cases): It occurs when bacteria directly enter into the blood and do not produce lymph node enlargement (no buboes). Patients die due to extensive growth of bacteria in the bloodstream. The patient is toxic and present with fever, prostration and meningitis occur suddenly, and death may occur within 48 hours. All blood vessels contain bacilli, and fibrin casts surround the bacteria in renal glomeruli and dermal vessels. Gangrene of acral regions (tip of the nose or the fingers and toes) may develop due to thrombosis of small artery in advanced stages (hence named Black Death).
- **Pneumonic plague:** It may occur as a primary infection in the lung due to inhalation of airborne particles from carcasses of animals or the cough of infected people. It may also develop as a secondary infection (as a complication of the bubonic and septicemic plague—secondary pneumonia). Primary form develops within 1–6 days after infection with high fever, cough and dyspnea begin suddenly. There is copious blood-stained, frothy, highly infective sputum and it shows plenty of bacilli. Respiratory distress/failure and endotoxic shock kill patients within 1–2 days.

Investigations and Diagnoses

Diagnosis is based on clinical, epidemiological, and laboratory findings.

- **Demonstration of organism:** For rapid diagnosis, smears are prepared from blood, sputum, bubo aspirate (lymph node aspirate), and CSF. They are stained with Gram, Giemsa, or Wayson's stains (contains methylene blue) and examined under microscopy. *Y. pestis* is seen as bipolar staining coccobacilli, giving a "safety pin" appearance.

- **Culture of organism:** From blood, sputum, and bubo aspirates.
- **Serological diagnosis:** A presumptive diagnosis in an appropriate clinical setting is possible by a rapid antigen detection test (by immunofluorescence, using *Y. pestis* F1 antigen-specific antibodies).
- **Blood:** White blood cell (WBC) count 20,000/mm^2 and/or thrombocytopenia in about 50% of patients

Chancroid (Soft Chancre)

Chancroid is an acute, ulcerative STI caused by *Haemophilus ducreyi*.

***Haemophilus ducreyi*:** It is a small, gram-negative bacillus. It appears in tissue as clusters of parallel bacilli and as chains, resembling schools of fish. **Infections lead to painful genital ulcers and lymphadenopathy**. It grows poorly in culture and need uncommon and highly-enriched media. Because PCR-based tests are not widely available, it may be underdiagnosed.

- **Incubation period:** Usually 3–10 days.
- **Infection is acquired** due to a break in the epithelium **during sexual contact with an infected individual**.

Chancroid is most common in tropical and subtropical areas especially in low socioeconomic groups. It is one of the most common causes of genital ulcers in less developed countries (especially Africa, Southeast Asia, and the Caribbean) where it serves as an important cofactor in the transmission of HIV infection. It has been suggested that open genital ulcers facilitate spread of HIV. The disease occurs in men who have frequent sex with prostitutes.

MORPHOLOGY

Lesion in the external genitalia: *H. ducreyi* enters through breaks in the skin and it multiplies there.

- **Sites of lesions:** In males, the primary lesion is usually seen on the **penis** (prepuce and frenulum); in females, lesions occur in the **vagina** (vaginal entrance) or the periurethral/perineal region.
- **Lesion:** Four to seven days after inoculation, a **tender erythematous papule** (raised lesion) develops at the site of inoculation in the external genitalia. After another 2–3 days, the surface of the **primary erythematous papule breaks down and produces a classic chancroidal ulcer**.
- **Characteristics of ulcer:** This chancroid ulcer is superficial, irregular, circumscribed, and painful. Ulcers may range from 0.1 to 2 cm in diameter and bleeds easily. Ulcers have ragged and undermined edges, and base of the ulcer shows a shaggy, yellow-gray exudate. **In contrast to the primary chancre of syphilis, the ulcer of chancroid is not indurated**. Ulcer may be single. If multiple, they may merge to form giant serpiginous ulcer.

Lymphadenopathy: Organisms are carried within macrophages to regional lymph nodes. About 7–10 days after the appearance of primary lesion, patients develop **unilateral, painful, suppurative, tender inguinal lymph nodes** (usually unilateral) in about 50% of cases. If the infection is not treated, the **enlarged nodes become matted and progress to form large unilocular buboes which suppurate**. Overlying skin becomes inflamed, breaks down, and drains pus from the underlying node. This produces a chronic, draining ulcer.

Continued

Continued

Microscopy: The ulcer of chancroid consists of superficial zone of neutrophilic debris and fibrin. The underlying zone shows granulation tissue containing necrotic areas and thrombosed vessels. Below the layer of granulation tissue, a dense, lymphoplasmacytic inflammatory infiltrate is observed. Coccobacilli can be sometimes demonstrated in tissue sections or in smears from the ulcers stained by Gram or silver stains. Usually these bacteria are obscured by other bacteria that colonize the ulcer base.

Diagnosis: It is based on the microscopic identification and culture isolation of *H. ducreyi* in scrapings from ulcer or pus from bubo. PCR technique not commercially available. Detection of antibody to *H. ducreyi* using enzyme immunoassay (EIA) may be useful.

Granuloma Inguinale

Granuloma inguinale, or donovanosis, is a chronic inflammatory STI caused by *Klebsiella granulomatis*. It was formerly called *Calymmatobacterium donovani*. ***K. granulomatis*** is a minute (small), **encapsulated, nonmotile, gram-negative coccobacillus.**

Source of infection: Humans are the only hosts of *K. granulomatis.*

Incubation period: 3–40 days.

Epidemiology: Granuloma inguinale is rare in temperate climates but is common and endemic in some rural tropical and subtropical areas and some lower-income countries. Highest incidence has been observed in Papua New Guinea, central Australia, and India. Most patients are in the group of 15–40 years.

MORPHOLOGY

Sites: Granuloma inguinale occurs on the moist stratified squamous epithelium of the genitalia or, rarely, the oral mucosa or pharynx.

Lesion: It begins as a **raised papular lesion which eventually ulcerates to produce a characteristic lesion** that appears as **raised, soft, beefy-red, superficial ulcer**. It contains abundant (exuberant) granulation tissue, which manifests grossly as a protuberant, soft, painless mass. It resembles a fleshy mass herniating through the skin. As the lesion progresses, its borders become raised and indurated. Untreated cases are characterized by the development of extensive disfiguring scarring. These **may be associated with urethral, vulvar, or anal strictures.** Rarely lymphatic obstruction and lymphedema (elephantiasis) of the external genitalia may occur.

Regional lymph nodes are usually not involved or may show only nonspecific reactive changes. This is in contrast to chancroid which shows prominent enlargement of regional lymph nodes.

Microscopy: Active lesions show marked hyperplasia of epithelium at the borders of the ulcer and sometimes may mimic carcinoma (pseudoepitheliomatous hyperplasia). The base of the ulcer and below the surrounding epithelium, a mixture of neutrophils and mononuclear inflammatory cells

Continued

Continued

is observed. The **organisms can be demonstrated in Giemsa-stained smears prepared from the exudate**. They **appear as minute, encapsulated coccobacilli (Donovan bodies) in macrophages**. They show bipolar chromatin condensation giving safety pin appearance. Silver stains (e.g., the Warthin-Starry stain) may also demonstrate the organism.

Diagnosis: The causative organism is difficult to culture and PCR assays are not widely available. Hence, it is diagnosed by microscopic examination of material from the lesion (tissue crush preparation or biopsy of the ulcer). Microscopy examination shows dark staining intracellular bipolar-staining Donovan bodies.

SEXUALLY TRANSMITTED INFECTIONS

Q. Write short essay on approach to diagnosis of sexually transmitted infection/disease.

A variety of organisms can be transmitted through sexual contact and are termed as STI. Sexually transmitted disease (STD) are a **group of communicable diseases that are transmitted predominantly by sexual contact and caused by a wide range of bacterial, viral, protozoal, and fungal agents and ectoparasites** (**Table 17**). If STI is present in a child, unless acquired during birth, strongly suggests sexual abuse.

Mode of spread: Some pathogens (e.g., *Chlamydia trachomatis, N. gonorrhoeae*) almost always spread by sexual intercourse. Some (e.g., *Shigella* species, *E. histolytica*) typically spread by other means, but are also occasionally spread by oral-anal sex.

Table 17: Classification of important sexually transmitted infections.

Pathogens	*Disease produced*
Viruses	
Herpes simplex virus	Primary and recurrent herpes, neonatal herpes
Hepatitis B virus	Hepatitis
Human papillomavirus	• Males: Cancer of penis • Females: Cervical dysplasia and cancer, vulvar cancer Condyloma acuminatum
Human immunodeficiency Virus	Acquired immunodeficiency syndrome
Chlamydiae	
Chlamydia trachomatis	• Males: Urethritis, epididymitis, and proctitis • Females: Urethral syndrome, cervicitis, bartholinitis, salpingitis, and sequelae • Both sexes: Lymphogranuloma venereum
Mycoplasmas	
Ureaplasma urealyticum	Urethritis
Bacteria	
Neisseria gonorrhoeae	• Males: Epididymitis, prostatitis, and urethral stricture • Females: Cervicitis, endometritis, bartholinitis, salpingitis, and sequelae (infertility, ectopic pregnancy, recurrent salpingitis) • Both sexes: Urethritis, proctitis, pharyngitis, and disseminated gonococcal infection
Treponema pallidum	Syphilis
Haemophilus ducreyi	Chancroid
Klebsiella granulomatis	Granuloma inguinale (donovanosis)
Fungus	
Candida albicans	Females: Vaginal thrush
Protozoa	
Trichomonas vaginalis	• Males: Urethritis and balanitis • Females: Vaginitis
Entamoeba histolytica	
Giardia lamblia	
Ectoparasites	
Sarcoptes scabiei (Mite)	Genital scabies
Phthirus pubis (Lice)	Pubic lice

General Features of STI

- **Infection and spread:** The organisms causing STIs first become established locally and then spread from the urethra, vagina, cervix, rectum, or oral pharynx. The development of STIs depends on direct contact for person-to-person spread. This is because these pathogens cannot survive in the environment. Transmission of STIs usually occurs from asymptomatic individuals who do not know that they have an infection.
- **Infection with one STI-associated organism increases the risk of another STI:** This is because the risk factors are the same for all STIs. Also the epithelial injury caused by *N. gonorrhoeae* or *C. trachomatis* predisposes the chance of coinfection with the other, as well as the risk of HIV infection if there is concomitant exposure.
- **Spread from mother to fetus:** The organisms causing STIs can spread from a pregnant woman to the fetus. This can produce severe damage to the fetus or child. For example, perinatal infection by *C. trachomatis* causes conjunctivitis, and neonatal HSV infection is more likely to cause visceral and CNS disease than is infection acquired later in life. Syphilis frequently causes miscarriage.

Features and diagnosis of STI/disease is discussed under individual diseases.

MYCOBACTERIAL INFECTIONS

Mycobacteria are long (2–10 μm in length), slender, aerobic rods that are nonmotile and do not form spores. Mycobacteria are distinctive organisms with cell wall architecture like that of gram-positive bacteria, but have a **unique waxy cell wall.** The waxy cell wall is unusual in that it is **composed of large amounts (approximately 60 percent) of lipid**. This lipid includes **unusual glycolipids and lipids including mycolic acid** (β-hydroxylated fatty acid). These lipid form complex with a variety of polysaccharides and peptides, creating a waxy cell surface that makes mycobacteria strongly hydrophobic. The lipid-rich content of cell wall makes them resistant to penetration by aniline/chemical dyes including crystal violet used in the Gram stain, interferes with staining by dyes. Thus, although mycobacteria are structurally gram-positive, this property is difficult to demonstrate by routine staining. Thus, they appear as weakly gram-positive. The unusual **waxy lipids of the cell wall make mycobacteria to stain poorly** but, once stained, they cannot be easily decolorized by treatment with acidified organic solvents. Therefore, the **mycobacteria** are termed **"acid-fast" (i.e., they retain carbol fuchsin even on treatment with a mixture of acid alcohol).** Their cell walls make resistant to many chemical disinfectants and convey resistance to the corrosive action of strong acids or alkalis. This property is made for decontaminating clinical specimens, such as sputum, in which nonmycobacterial organisms are digested by such treatments. Mycobacteria are also resistant to drying but not to heat or ultraviolet (UV) irradiation. **Mycobacteria are strictly aerobic**. Most species of mycobacteria grow more slowly (with generation times of 8–24 hours) than other pathogenic bacteria. They grow in straight or branching chains.

Mycobacteria produce no known toxins but damage human tissues by inducing inflammatory and immune responses. They produce diseases that are chronic and slowly progressive. Most mycobacterial pathogens survive and replicate within cells (intracellularly) of the monocyte/macrophage lineage. Mycobacterial infections usually form slow-growing granulomatous inflammation (lesions) that are responsible for major tissue destruction. The two main mycobacterial pathogens namely *Mycobacterium tuberculosis* (MTB) and *Mycobacterium leprae,* only infect humans and they have no environmental reservoir. Other pathogenic mycobacteria are environmental organisms and they only occasionally cause disease in humans.

TUBERCULOSIS

Definition: Tuberculosis (also called Koch's disease) is a **communicable, chronic granulomatous disease** caused by ***Mycobacterium tuberculosis***.

- **Lungs are the prime target and produces chronic pulmonary disease.** But it can be systemic disease and can infect any organ. Disease is mainly caused by *M. tuberculosis hominis* (Koch bacillus) but also occasionally by *M. tuberculosis bovis.* **It is the leading infectious cause of death worldwide.** Presently it has increasingly become a cause for special concern in immunocompromised patients.
- Most cases of tuberculosis are caused by ***Mycobacterium tuberculosis hominis*** (human strain). The **source of infection is patients with active open case of tuberculosis**. Open case of tuberculosis is a patient with tuberculosis in which cavitatory lung lesion is communicated to the external environment through the patient's airways.
- **Oropharyngeal and intestinal tuberculosis** can be caused by drinking milk contaminated with ***M. bovis*** (bovine strain) from infected cows. Routine pasteurization has almost eliminated this source of infection.
- ***Mycobacterium avium*** **and intracellulare**, which are nonpathogenic to normal individuals but cause infection **in patients with AIDS**.

Characteristics of Mycobacteria

- *Mycobacterium tuberculosis* is an aerobic, slender, nonmotile, rod-shaped, acid-fast bacillus, measuring 2–10 µm in length.
- It has a lipid coat which makes it **difficult to stain**, but **once stained resists decolorization by acids and alcohol.** Hence, it is termed as acid-fast bacilli (AFB), because once stained by carbol fuchsin [present in **Ziehl–Neelsen (ZN) stain**], it is not decolorized by acid and alcohol.
- It grows slowly in culture, with a doubling time of 24 hours. About 3–6 weeks are commonly needed to produce visible growth in culture.
- Various acid fast organisms include (1) *Mycobacterium tuberculosis,* (2) *M. leprae,* (3) *M. smegmatis,* (4) Atypical *Mycobacterium,* (5) *Nocardia, (6) Rhodococcus,* (6) Legionella *micdadei,* (7) Protozoa (e.g., Isospora, *Crytosporidium parvum*). Various acid fast structures includes (1) Head of human sperm, (2) Embryophora of *T. saginata,* (3) Hooklets of *E. granulosus* and (4) Keratin.

Epidemiology

- Tuberculosis is common in India. Incidence of tuberculosis is high wherever there is **poverty**, **overcrowding, and chronic debilitating illness**. Rates of infection are now low in developed countries.
- **Diseases that are associated with increased risk:** Diabetes mellitus, Hodgkin lymphoma, malnutrition, immunosuppression, alcoholism, chronic lung disease (e.g., silicosis), and chronic renal failure.
- **HIV is the most important risk factor.**

Infection versus Disease

Exposure of an individual to *M. tuberculosis* does not necessarily equate to infection and clinical tuberculosis. The course of tuberculosis depends on age and immune competence of the individual as well as total burden of mycobacteria. Some patients may have only asymptomatic infection, while in others, tuberculosis may be a destructive, disseminated disease. Thus, **infection with *M. tuberculosis* has to be differentiated from active disease**.

- **Infection:** Tuberculous infection **indicates the presence of bacteria and it is growing in the body,** which **may be symptomatic (active disease) or may not be symptomatic** (latent infection). Most of the healthy individuals with primary tuberculosis are asymptomatic, though there may be fever and pleural effusion. Only evidence of infection in these individuals may be the presence of a tiny, fibrocalcific pulmonary nodule at the site of the infection. Bacteria may remain dormant in such lesions for decades.
- **Disease:** Active tuberculosis is a subset of **tuberculous infections manifested by destructive, symptomatic disease**. If immune defenses in an individual with dormant infection are lowered, the infection may become reactivated. This can produce communicable and potentially life-threatening disease. Secondary tuberculosis is always an active disease.

Immunity and hypersensitivity: *M. tuberculosis* stimulates both a humoral and a cell-mediated immune response. Though circulating antibodies appear, they do not bring out resistance to the organism. Instead, cell-mediated immunity and the accompanying delayed hypersensitivity (Type IV) directed against a number of bacterial protein antigens (tuberculoproteins), develop in the course of infection. Both not only confer an enhanced ability to localize the mycobacterial infection and restrict growth of the organism, but also cause a greater capacity to damage the host. Thus, they contribute to both the pathology of and immunity to the disease. The effector cells for both cell-mediated immunity and hypersensitivity reaction are CD4+ T cells (also called Th1 cells or T helper cells).

- **Cell-mediated immunity:** Tuberculosis developing first time in an immunocompetent individual depends on the cell-mediated immunity.
- **Type IV hypersensitivity reactions:** Develop to mycobacterial antigens and are **responsible for the tissue destruction, such as caseating granulomas and cavitation**. Appearance of type IV hypersensitivity reaction also signals the development of protective immunity.

Mode of Transmission

Inhalation

It is the **most common mode** of transmission.

- **Source of organisms** is from humans with an **active open case of pulmonary tuberculosis** to a susceptible host.
- Patients with active open pulmonary tuberculosis, shed large numbers of mycobacteria into the sputum. *M. tuberculosis* is transmitted from one individual to the other by aerosol. The aerosol droplets containing tubercle bacilli are created and expelled while coughing, sneezing, and talking that creates aerosolized respiratory droplets. Droplets usually evaporate, leaving an organism (droplet nucleus). Because of resistance to desiccation, the mycobacteria can remain viable as droplet nuclei suspended in room air for at least 30 minutes. These are readily carried in the air. Main mode of transmission from person-to-person is by inhalation of the aerosol. A single infected patient can transmit the organism to numerous people in an exposed group, such as a family, classroom, or hospital ward without proper isolation. When an individual inhales the droplets, these lodge in the lung and cause infection.

Ingestion

- **Source of organisms:** Tuberculosis may be transmitted by drinking nonpasteurized milk contaminated with *Mycobacterium bovis* from infected cows.
- **Site of infection:** *M. bovis* causes oropharyngeal and intestinal tuberculosis.
- Eradication of tuberculous herds with tuberculosis and **pasteurization** has almost **eliminated this mode of transmission** of tuberculosis. It can be seen in countries that have tuberculous dairy cows and unpasteurized milk. Nowadays, the ingestion mode of transmission occurs when a patient with open case of tuberculosis swallows the infected sputum which results in tuberculosis of intestine.

Inoculation

It is extremely rare mode of transmission. It may develop during postmortem examination, while cuts resulting from handling tuberculous infected organs.

Pathogenesis

Initial infection in a previously unexposed, immunocompetent individual stimulates both a humoral and a cell-mediated immune response. However, the circulating antibodies do not play a significant role. **The outcome of initial depends on the development of antimycobacterial T cell-mediated immunity.** The T cell-mediated immunity controls the host response to the mycobacteria and also responsible for development of pathologic lesions (e.g., caseating granulomas and cavitation). Lung being commonly involved in tuberculosis; the pathogenesis is considered with respect to pulmonary tuberculosis.

Sequence of Events in Primary Pulmonary Tuberculosis (Figs. 28A and B)

Various steps involved in infection by *M. tuberculosis* are discussed below.

Infection before activation of cell-mediated immunity

Initial infection with *MTB* **in a nonsensitized individual** is called **primary tuberculosis.** The following sequence of events occur.

Entry of mycobacteria into macrophages **First time**, when the **virulent tubercle bacilli** are deposited in the tissue, they primarily **infect macrophages**. In the lung, MTB undergo **phagocytosis and enter** into the alveolar macrophages mediated by several receptors expressed on the phagocytic **macrophage.** These receptors include:

- **Mannose-binding lectin receptors:** They bind lipoarabinomannan (LAM), a glycolipid in the cell wall of tubercle bacilli.
- **Type 3 complement receptor (CR3):** It binds mycobacteria opsonized by C3b.

Replication of mycobacteria within macrophages:

- **Blocks the formation of phagolysosome:** Normally, the phagosome fuses with lysosome inside the phagocytic cell and destroy the organism. But *M. tuberculosis* inhibits maturation of the phagosome and **blocks fusion of the phagosome and lysosome** inside the macrophages. The blockage is achieved by recruiting a host protein called coronin to the membrane of the phagosome. Coronin is an actin-binding plasma membrane-associated protein that retains on the phagosomal membrane. Coronin in turn activates the phosphatase calcineurin that inhibits phagosome-lysosome fusion and prevents formation of phagolysosome.
- **Replication of mycobacteria in the macrophage:** Inhibition of phagolysosome formation protects *M. tuberculosis* from the microbicidal mechanisms of lysosomes and they replicate unchecked within the phagosome of the macrophage. Thus, in the nonsensitized individual, during the earliest stage of primary tuberculosis (<3 weeks), *M. tuberculosis* proliferate in the pulmonary alveolar macrophages in alveoli.
- **Bacteremia: Replicated mycobacteria may be released from macrophages and may produce bacteremia** and seeding of tubercle bacilli at many sites. This bacteremia may be either asymptomatic or may have a mild flu-like illness.

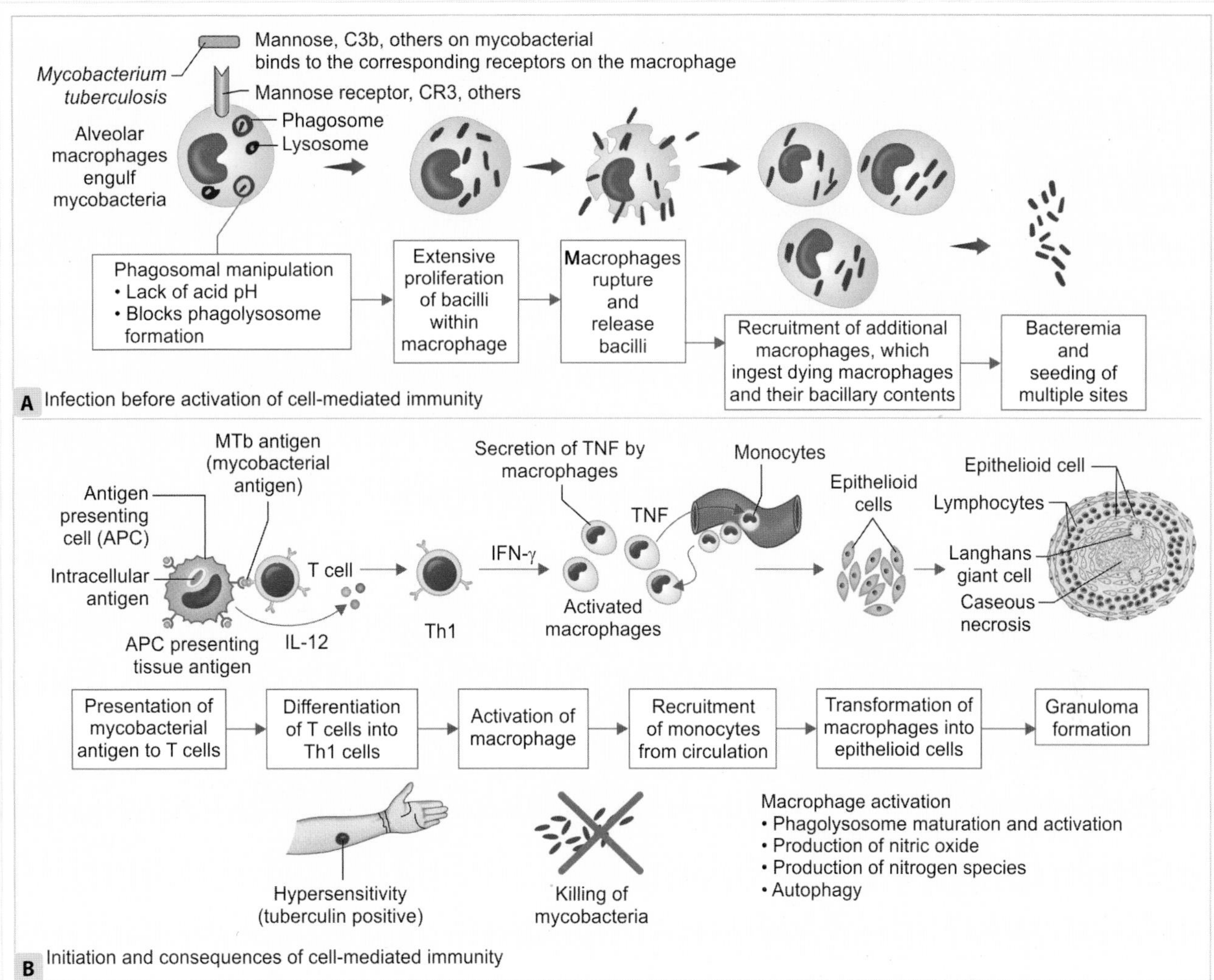

(IFN-γ: interferon-gamma; IL: interleukin; TNF: tumor necrosis factor)

FIGS. 28A AND B: Sequence of events in primary tuberculosis of lung. (A) Infection before activation of cellmediated immunity; (B) Initiation and consequences of cellmediated immunity.

Innate immunity Many pathogens-associated molecular patterns (PAMPs) in the *M. tuberculosis* are recognized by innate immune receptors. For example, mycobacterial LAM binds TLR2, and unmethylated CpG nucleotides bind to TLR9. These interactions initiate and increase the innate and adaptive immune responses.

- **Genetic factor: NRAMP1 is a transmembrane protein** (a product of *SLC11A1* gene formerly called *NRAMP1* gene) **inhibits microbial growth**. In individuals with **polymorphisms in the *NRAMP1*** (**n**atural **r**esistance-**a**ssociated **m**acrophage **p**rotein 1) **gene, tuberculosis may progress due to the absence of an effective immune response**.

Initiation and consequences of cell-mediated immunity:

Cell-mediated immunity develops about 3 weeks after exposure.

The Th1 response:

- **Presentation of mycobacterial antigen to T cells:** About 3 weeks after infection, the macrophages (containing bacilli) degrade some mycobacteria and process the mycobacterial (MTb) antigen. Infected macrophages [which is also an antigen-presenting cell (APC)] carry mycobacterial antigens to the draining lymph nodes and present antigens to T lymphocytes.
- **Differentiation of T cells into Th1 cells:** After the mycobacterial antigen is presented to T cells, they differentiate into T-helper 1 (Th1) cell and a Th1 response is mounted. **Immunity to *M. tuberculosis* is mainly mediated by Th1 cells.** Differentiation of T cells into Th1 cells depends on IL-12 and IL-18. These interleukins are produced by APCs that have encountered the mycobacteria. Stimulation of TLR2 by mycobacterial ligands stimulates the production of IL-12 by dendritic cells (DCs). Development of Th1 responsive to *M. tuberculosis* antigen is the hypersensitivity response to the organism.

Th1-mediated macrophage activation and killing of mycobacteria:

Role of Th1 cells: Th1 cells, both in lymph nodes and in the lung, produce IFN-γ. **IFN-γ has several functions.**

- **Activation of macrophage:** The macrophages that first ingest *M. tuberculosis* cannot kill it. But later the hypersensitivity and cell-mediated immunologic responses eventually contain the infection. IFN-γ is the important mediator that activates macrophages and facilitates them to become bactericidal to *M. tuberculosis*. Activation of macrophages that can ingest and destroy the bacilli accounts for the cell-mediated immune response. Thus, **Th1 cells stimulate macrophages to kill the mycobacteria.** These responses together fight against the bacilli, a process that requires 3–6 weeks to come into play.
- **Stimulates formation of the phagolysosome in infected macrophages:** IFN-γ stimulates maturation and activation of the phagolysosome in infected macrophages. This exposes the mycobacteria to a harmful acidic, oxidizing environment.
- **Generation of reactive nitrogen intermediates:** IFN-γ stimulates expression of inducible NO synthase in the macrophages and produces NO. NO combines with other oxidants to generate reactive nitrogen intermediates, which are important for killing of mycobacteria.
- **Mobilization of antimicrobial peptides** (defensins): IFN-γ mobilizes cationic antimicrobial peptides (defensins) against the bacteria.
- **Stimulates autophagy:** IFN-γ stimulates autophagy. This process of autophagy sequesters and destroys damaged organelles and intracellular bacteria such as *M. tuberculosis*.

Activated macrophages also secrete TNF and chemokines. They recruit more monocytes from the blood circulation. This monocytic recruitment may be affected if the patient is on treatment with a TNF antagonist (e.g., rheumatoid arthritis) and these individuals have an increased risk of tuberculosis reactivation.

Granulomatous inflammation and tissue damage Apart from activation of macrophages to kill mycobacteria, the Th1 is also responsible for the **formation of granulomas and caseous necrosis.** If an infected individual is immunologically competent and the burden of mycobacteria is small, an intense granulomatous reaction is produced. Tubercle bacilli are ingested and killed by activated macrophages and infection is successfully contained.

- **Transformation of macrophages into epithelioid cells:** Macrophages activated by IFN-γ are transformed into "epithelioid histiocytes" ("epithelioid cells").
- **Granuloma formation:** Epithelioid cells form a microscopic aggregates surrounded by a rim of lymphocytes, is referred as a granuloma. Some of these "epithelioid cells" may fuse to form giant cells, and this pattern of inflammation is known as **granulomatous inflammation**. Many of the individuals infected with *M. tuberculosis*, the response to the infection may halt at this stage without any significant tissue destruction or illness.
- **Caseous necrosis:** In some individuals the infection may progresses especially in individuals who are older or immunosuppressed. When the number of bacilli is high, in these individuals the hypersensitivity reaction produces significant tissue necrosis in the center of granuloma. This necrotic material has a characteristic cheese-like (caseous) consistency. Hence, this necrosis is termed caseous necrosis.

Host susceptibility to disease Host factors may predispose to increased susceptibility to tuberculosis.

- **AIDS:** It is the major risk factor for progression of infection to active disease (refer infection versus disease on page 647). It is due to the immunological deficiency that fails to control the mycobacteria.
- **Other factors:** Host susceptibility to tuberculosis is increased in immunosuppressed (or immunocompromised) individuals (e.g., glucocorticoids, cancer therapy), individuals on treatment with TNF inhibitors, transplant recipients (solid organ and stem cell), renal failure, and malnutrition.
- **Defects in lymphocyte activation:** Rarely individuals may have inherited mutations that affect or interfere with the Th1 response (e.g., loss of the IL-12 receptor β1 protein). They are increasingly susceptible to severe tuberculosis. They also develop symptomatic infection even with normally avirulent (so-called "atypical") mycobacteria, such as the *Mycobacterium asvium* complex (MAC) or with the attenuated BCG (Bacillus Calmette–Guérin) vaccine strain. This group of genetic disorders is called **Mendelian susceptibility to mycobacterial disease.**

Types of Tuberculosis

Clinical tuberculosis can be divided into two important types and these have different pathophysiology. These two types are: (1) primary tuberculosis and (2) secondary tuberculosis.

Primary Tuberculosis

Definition: Primary tuberculosis is initial (first) infection that occurs on first exposure to the organism **in an unsensitized** (previously unexposed) **individual**.

- About 5% of newly infected individuals develop clinically significant disease.
- **Source of the infection:** It is always **exogenous**.
- In most individuals, the primary tuberculous infection is controlled, but in others it may progress (termed as progressive primary tuberculosis).

MORPHOLOGY

Sites of primary tuberculosis: Lung, intestine, tonsil, and skin (very rare).

Lung

It is the **most common site** of primary tuberculosis and almost always infection begins in the lungs.

Ghon Lesion

Following inhalation, tubercle bacilli gets deposited in the distal airspaces.

- **Site of deposit:** Usually tubercle bacilli get deposited in the **lower part of the upper lobe or upper part of the lower lobe near the pleural surface** (subpleural).
- **Ghon focus (Figs. 29A and B):** About 2–4 weeks after the infection sensitization develops in the host. It produces a circumscribed **gray-white area of** inflammation with consolidation measuring about **1–1.5 cm in the lung.** This lesion is known as the Ghon focus. In most of the patients, the center of Ghon focus undergoes caseous necrosis.
- **Regional lymphadenitis:** Tubercle bacilli (free or within macrophages) are carried along the lymphatics to the regional draining nodes. The involved lymph nodes often show caseous necrosis.

Continued

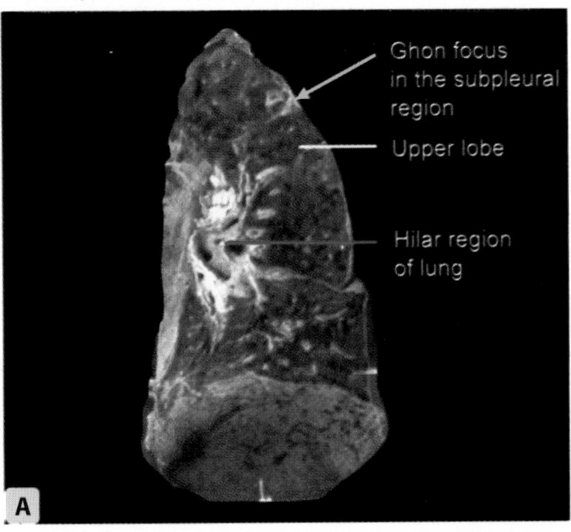

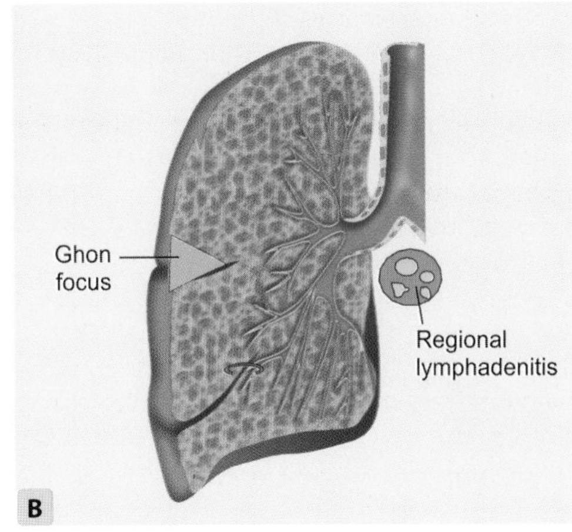

FIGS. 29A AND B: Gross appearance of primary pulmonary tuberculosis; (A) cut section of lung with Ghon focus. (B) Diagrammatic. Ghon complex consists of gray-white parenchymal focus under the pleura and enlarged hilar lymph nodes with caseation.

Continued

Ghon Complex

The combination of subpleural parenchymal lung lesion (**Ghon focus**) and **regional lymph node** involvement is called as ***Ghon complex.***

Fate of Ghon Complex

During the first few weeks of infection, mycobacteria disseminate through lymphatics and blood vessels to other parts of the body. Primary tuberculosis follows one of two courses: (1) healing and (2) progression or spread.

- **Healing:** In **majority** (about 95%) of individuals, cell mediated immunity controls the infection and primary tuberculosis is self-limited. If the lesion arrests, the tubercle **heals** (both in lungs and lymph nodes). The **hallmark of healing is fibrosis** (and shrinkage) and Ghon complex undergoes progressive fibrosis, followed by radiologically detectable **dystrophic calcification** (Ranke complex), and very **rarely ossification**. Small numbers of viable but nonproliferating mycobacteria may remain for years in healed lesions (pulmonary or extrapulmonary). Later, if immune mechanisms wane or fail, these resting bacilli may proliferate and produce serious secondary tuberculosis.
- **Spread:** During the first few weeks **lymphatic and hematogenous dissemination** occurs to other organs or parts of the body. In spite of seeding of other organs, no lesions develop in other organs. But in immunologically immature subjects (young children or immunosuppressed patients), infection may progress at the primary site in the lung, in the regional lymph nodes, or in multiple sites of dissemination. This process produces **progressive primary tuberculosis.** Progressive primary tuberculosis in immunosuppressed individuals spreads in a similar manner as spread of secondary tuberculosis. It is discussed on pages 653–655.

Other Sites of Primary Complex

- **Intestine:** Primary focus in the small intestine (usually ileal region) along with mesenteric lymphadenitis. Consumption of pasteurized milk has eliminated primary tuberculosis of intestine.

Continued

Continued

- **Tonsils:** Primary focus in the pharynx and tonsil with cervical lymph node enlargement.
- **Skin:** Primary focus in the skin along with regional lymph node involvement.

Microscopy (Figs. 30A and B)

The lesion at the sites of active involvement shows characteristic granulomatous inflammatory reaction. These granulomas may be both caseating and noncaseating tubercles. **Granuloma in tuberculosis is called as tubercle** (tuberculoid granuloma). Tubercle may show central area of caseous necrosis (caseating granuloma/soft tubercle) or may not show caseation (noncaseating tubercles/hard tubercle). In practice, it is better to term tuberculous lesions as either "necrotizing" or "nonnecrotizing," and to avoid the terms "caseating" versus "noncaseating. ***The characteristic lesion of tuberculosis is a spherical granuloma with central caseous necrosis.*** Individual tubercles are identified only by microscopic examination. When multiple granulomas coalesce they may be grossly identified.

Caseating (necrotizing) granuloma consists of:

- **Central area/zone of caseous necrosis:** The center of the granuloma (tubercle) undergoes a characteristic expanding, caseous (cheesy) necrosis. Tissue damage is produced by the destruction of both bacilli and phagocytes. They release of degradative enzymes and reactive nitrogen and oxygen species (e.g., superoxide radicals).
- **Surrounded by midzone of epithelioid cells** (modified macrophages), some of which may fuse to form multinucleate giant cells. The **giant cells may be Langhans** type (nuclei arranged in horseshoe pattern) **or foreign body type** (nuclei in the center). The epithelioid cells are **surrounded by rim of lymphocytes.**
- These granulomas are usually enclosed in the **peripheral collar** fibroblasts.

Note: Before the development of effective cell-mediated immunity, many giant cells in the lesions show nuclei that have aggregate toward one pole of the giant cell (polarization). When infection is effectively controlled, Langhans giant cells

Continued

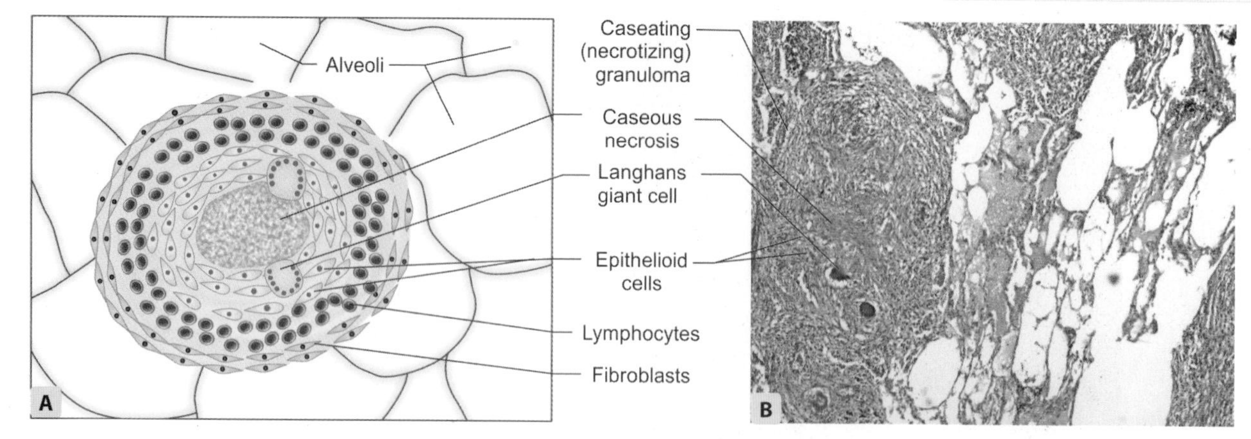

FIGS. 30A AND B: Microscopic appearance of tuberculous lung. (A) Diagrammatic; (B) Photomicrograph. Central area of caseation surrounded by epithelioid and multinucleated giant cells.

Continued

with peripheral nuclei arranged in horse-shoe pattern or giant cells with centrally placed nuclei predominate. If cell-mediated immunity is profoundly diminished (immunocompromised individuals), granulomas may be poorly formed or absent and their macrophages show abundant bacilli.

- In tuberculosis, there is correlation between T cell-mediated immunity and resistance. In a sensitized individual T-cell-mediated immunity produces a positive tuberculin test. If there is loss of T cell immunity, a previously tuberculin-positive individual may become tuberculin negative. This may be a dangerous sign that resistance to the mycobacteria in the host has faded.

Secondary Tuberculosis

Synonyms: Postprimary tuberculosis, reactivation tuberculosis.

Definition: Secondary tuberculosis is the type of tuberculosis that arises (develops) in a previously sensitized host (individual).

- It may follow shortly or more commonly months to years after initial infection (i.e., primary tuberculosis), usually when the resistance of the host is weakened.
- **Source of infection:**
  - **Most common source** of mycobacteria in secondary tuberculosis is **reactivation of a latent infection (i.e.,** dormant mycobacteria from old granulomas) **of primary tuberculosis** (in a previously sensitized individual). Reactivation is apparently caused when the immune status of host is weakened/impaired in various conditions that predispose to re-emergence of latent/dormant *M. tuberculosis.* These conditions include cancer, anticancer chemotherapy, immunosuppressive therapy, malnutrition, alcoholism, advanced age, severe stress, immunosuppressive medication or diseases (such as diabetes and, particularly, AIDS). It may also occur when a large dose of virulent mycobacteria overcomes the host immune system.
  - Rarely it may be exogenous reinfection (i.e., newly acquired second infection by mycobacteria).
- Reactivation of the infection or re-exposure to the mycobacteria is characterized by rapid mobilization of a defensive reaction but also associated with increased necrosis of tissue.
- Reactivation is more common in low-prevalence regions, and reinfection plays an important role in regions where there is high illness.

MORPHOLOGY

Organ involved: Any organ or location may be involved in secondary tuberculosis, but the **lungs are the most common site of involvement.**

Gross (Figs. 31A and B)

Lesions in lung

- **Site:** In the lungs, secondary tuberculosis classically usually begins in the **apex of the upper lobes** (apical–posterior segments) of one or both lungs, **within 1–2 cm of the apical pleura**. The affinity to affect the apex of lung is **because lung apices have higher mean oxygen tension** (ventilation/perfusion ratios are high) compared with that in the lower zones that favors mycobacterial growth.
- **Appearance: Initially-small focus (<2 cm in diameter) of consolidation**, sharply circumscribed, firm and **gray-white to yellow** in color. They show variable degrees of central caseation and peripheral fibrosis.
- **Cavitation:** T-cell-mediated immune responses to the tuberculous antigens lead to tissue necrosis and production of tuberculous cavities. Destruction of the lung tissue leads to air-filled cavities where mycobacteria replicate actively. In contrast to primary tuberculosis, cavitation occurs readily in the secondary tuberculosis. Cavitation in the lung is almost inevitable in neglected case of secondary tuberculosis. When first detected clinically, the cavities are usually 2–4 cm but they can exceed 10 cm. Apical cavities are optimal sites for multiplication of *M. tuberculosis* and large numbers of mycobacteria are produced in this cavity. The cavities contain necrotic material teeming with mycobacteria and are surrounded by a granulomatous response. Mycobacterial populations in cavity often

Continued

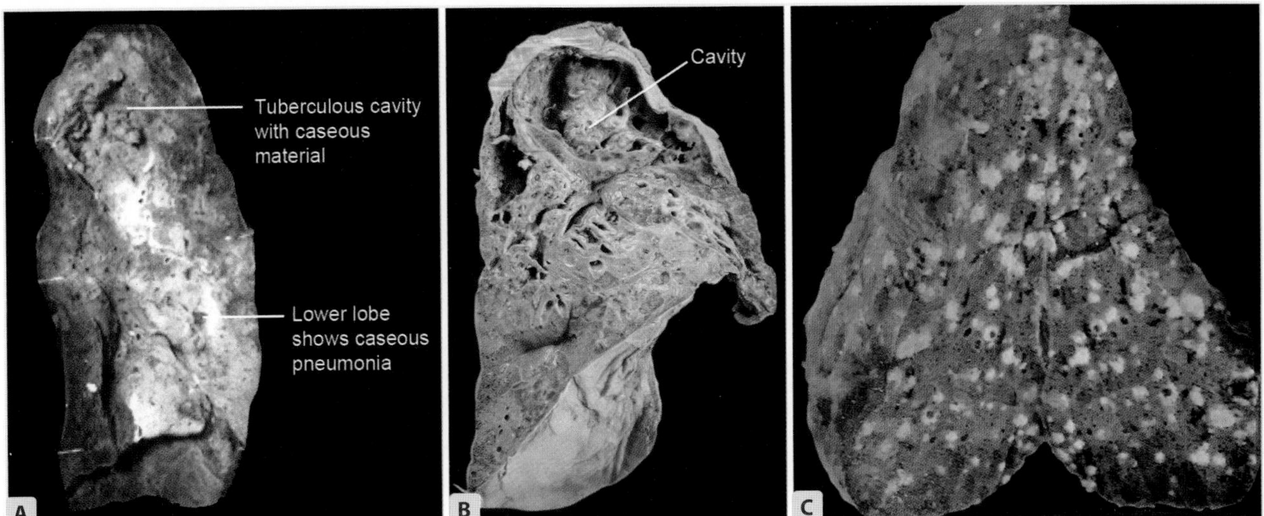

FIGS. 31A TO C: Secondary pulmonary tuberculosis. (A) Early; (B) Advanced. The lung shows gray-white areas of caseation with a cavity in the upper lobe; (C) Miliary tuberculosis of the lung. The cut surface shows numerous gray-white granulomas.

Continued

become quite large. The erosion of the cavities into an airway produces a communication between airways and infective focus of mycobacteria. Many of mycobacteria are shed (for example, in sputum). This is an important source of infection, because sputum contains bacteria and when the patient coughs it forms infected aerosol.

- **Regional lymph nodes involvement:** In secondary tuberculosis, the patients have hypersensitivity developed during primary tuberculosis. Hence, the mycobacteria elicit a prompt and marked tissue response that tends to wall off the focus of infection. Because of this, the **involvement of regional lymph nodes is less prominent** during secondary tuberculosis than in primary tuberculosis.

Microscopy (refer microscopy of primary tuberculosis above on page 651)

- Active lesions of secondary tuberculosis show characteristic coalescent tubercles with central caseation [caseating (necrotizing) **granulomas**].
- **Acid-fast stain:** Tubercle bacilli can usually be demonstrated with acid-fast stains in early exudative and caseous phases of granuloma formation. But in the late fibrocalcific stages, they are usually too few to be found.

Fate of Secondary Tuberculosis (Fig. 32)

Localized, apical, secondary pulmonary tuberculosis may **heal or the disease may progress**.

Healing

Healing may occur either spontaneously or after therapy. In immunocompetent individuals, the initial localized, apical, **parenchymal focus of secondary pulmonary tuberculosis may progressively heal with fibrous encapsulation.** This produces a localized, apical focus with **fibrosis and calcification** (producing fibrocalcific scars), rarely ossification.

Progress

Secondary tuberculosis of lung may progress and extend along several different pathways.

Continued

Continued

Progressive pulmonary secondary tuberculosis

It occurs mainly in the elderly and immunosuppressed individuals. Apical lesion may expand into surrounding lung tissue and may later erode into bronchi and vessels.

- **Erosion into bronchi:** It empties the central area of caseous necrosis into the bronchi. This results in a **ragged, irregular apical cavity (Figs. 31A and B) in the lung** surrounded by fibrous tissue. This produces an **important source of infection**, because when the patient coughs, sputum-containing mycobacteria are released into the atmosphere as infected aerosol.
- **Erosion of blood vessels:** It may result in **hemoptysis**.

Healing by fibrosis: With prompt and adequate treatment, **the progress of lung lesions may be arrested. However, healing** by fibrosis usually distorts the pulmonary architecture. These healed tuberculous cavities are now free of inflammation and they may persist or become fibrotic.

Spread of infection

If a patient with progressive pulmonary tuberculosis who had inadequate treatment or developed impairment in the defense mechanisms, the tuberculous infection may spread through different routes. Progressive primary tuberculosis in immunosuppressed individuals also spreads in a similar manner. The spread may be (1) local/direct, (2) via airways/mucosa, (3) through lymphatic channels or (4) through blood vessels (vascular system).

Local/direct spread: Tuberculosis can directly spread to the surrounding tissue. In the lung with progressive pulmonary tuberculosis, the pleural cavity is invariably involved. The local spread to the pleura may lead to serous **pleural effusions**, **tuberculous empyema** (due to rupture of a caseous lesion and spilling bacilli into the pleural cavity), or **obliterative fibrous pleuritis**. It may lead to pleural fibrosis and adhesions. If the cavitary disease of lung involves nearby pulmonary artery, it may produce a Rasmussen aneurysm and there will risk of rupture of vessel; leading to fatal hemoptysis.

Continued

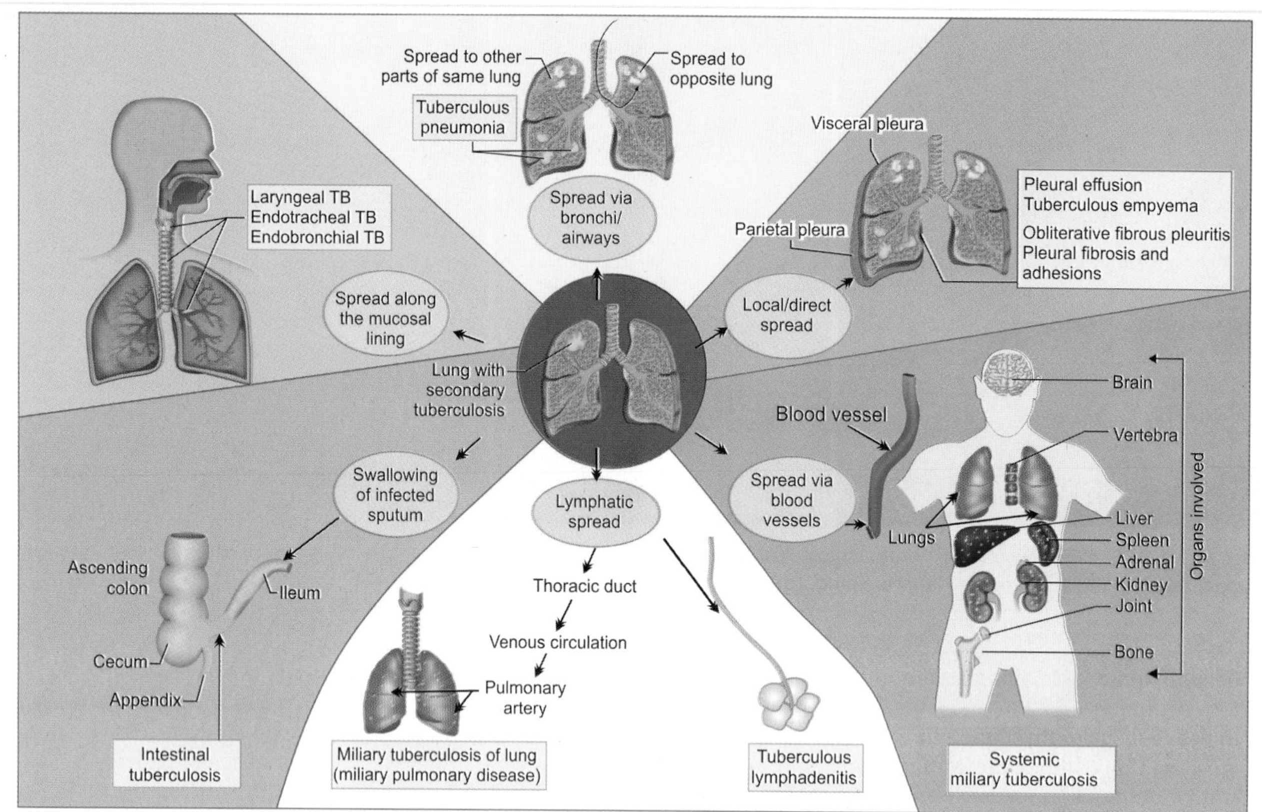

FIG. 32: Various ways of spread and complications of secondary tuberculosis of lung.

Continued

Spread through bronchi/airways: Liquefaction in the center of granuloma continues until the tubercle ruptures into nearby bronchiole. This allows mycobacteria to spill into the bronchiole (Fig. 33) and be disseminated throughout the respiratory system and other systems of the body. Spread through bronchi or airways may produce tuberculous pneumonia. It can spread to other parts of same lung as well as opposite lung. Erosion into a bronchus causes seeding of mycobacteria into the bronchioles, bronchi, and trachea.

Spread along mucosal lining: Spread through lymphatic channels or along the mucosal lining from mycobacteria present in the expectorated infectious material may lead to **endobronchial**, **endotracheal,** and **laryngeal tuberculosis**. Mycobacterial spread along the mucosal surfaces of the airways to produce ulcerated lesions in the larynx and tracheobronchial tree. In the larynx, it causes hoarseness and pain on swallowing. The mucosal lining may show tiny granulomatous lesions that may only be identified microscopically.

Intestinal tuberculosis (Fig. 34): In the past, intestinal tuberculosis resulted by the drinking of unpasteurized milk contaminated with bovine tuberculosis, now it is rare. Nowadays intestinal tuberculosis is caused by the **swallowing of coughed-up infective material** in patients with open case of advanced pulmonary tuberculosis.

Usually the mycobacteria are seeded to mucosal lymphoid aggregates of the small and large bowel. They produce granulomatous inflammation (**Fig. 30**) and may cause ulceration of the overlying mucosa, particularly in the ileum. Healing may produce strictures causing intestinal obstruction.

Continued

Continued

Lymphatic spread: Spread through lymphatic channels mainly reach regional lymph nodes. From lymph nodes mycobacteria can enter the systemic circulation to spread (disseminate) to other organs.

- **Miliary pulmonary disease:** It is the disseminated form of tuberculosis. When the **dissemination occurs only to the lungs**, it is called miliary pulmonary disease (**Fig. 31C**).
  - **Mechanism of development:** Tubercle bacilli draining through lymphatics enter the venous blood. The venous blood enters to the right venous side of the heart. From right ventricle, bacilli enter to the lungs through pulmonary artery.
  - **Lesions:** Miliary pulmonary disease produces multiple, small, yellow, nodular lesions scattered throughout the parenchyma of both the lungs (**Fig. 30C**). Each lesion may be either microscopic or small, grossly visible (2 mm) foci of yellow-white consolidation. These foci of lesions resemble millet seeds (cereal composed of small seeds), hence named **"military."** Miliary lesions may expand and fuse with other miliary lesions. This may result in consolidation of large regions or even whole lobes of the lung.
- **Lymphadenitis:** It is most frequent presentation of extra-pulmonary tuberculosis. Tuberculous lymphadenitis usually occurs in the cervical region (scrofula = glandular swelling produced by tuberculosis). The nature of tuberculous lymphadenitis in HIV positive and negative is different.

Continued

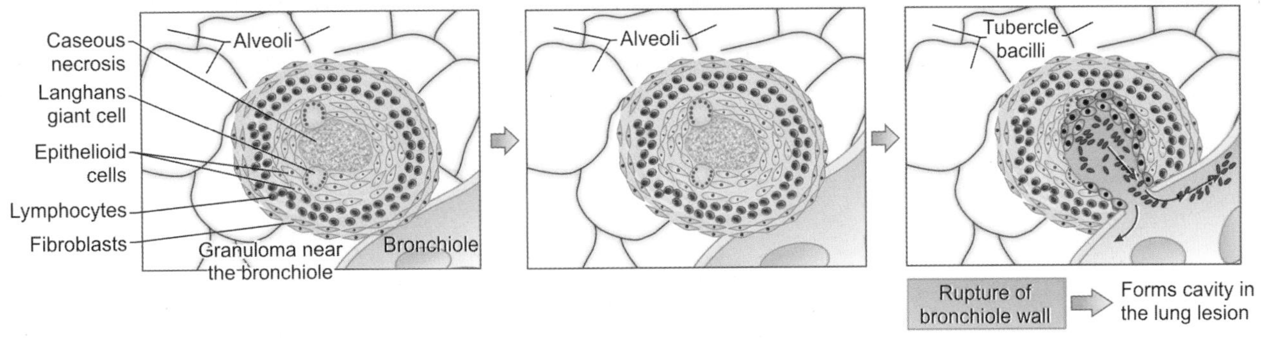

FIG. 33: Progression of active tuberculosis in lung and erosion of bronchiole.

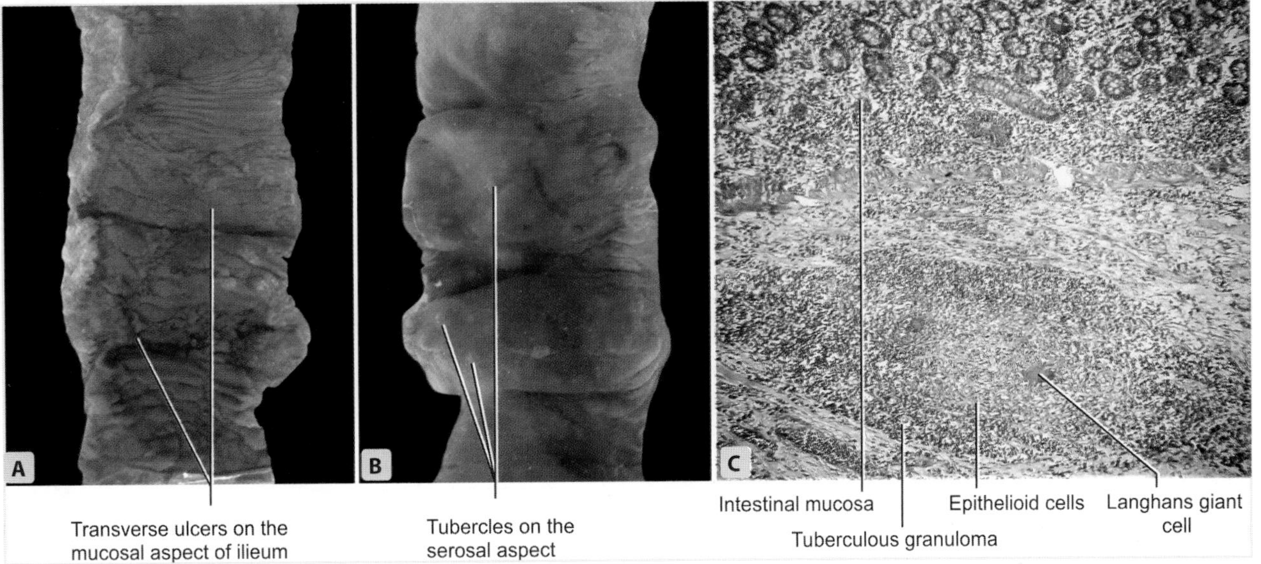

FIGS. 34A TO C: Ileum with tuberculous ulcer on the mucosal aspect. (A) Specimen; (B) Serosal aspect shows tubercles; (C) Microscopy of tuberculosis of intestine.

Continued

- HIV-negative individuals: Lymphadenitis is frequently unifocal and localized.
- HIV-positive individuals: Lymphadenitis almost always is multifocal with systemic symptoms. There is active tuberculosis either involving lung or other organs.

Spread via blood vessels (hematogenous spread): Tubercle bacilli may enter into blood through blood vessels. It may produce either systemic miliary tuberculosis or isolated organ tuberculosis.

- **Systemic miliary tuberculosis (Figs. 35A to D):** Tubercle bacilli may also spread throughout the body through the bloodstream and cause military tuberculosis. Miliary pulmonary disease involves only lungs whereas systemic miliary tuberculosis **can involve any organ**. Systemic miliary tuberculosis occurs when tubercle bacilli disseminate through the systemic arterial system. Most commonly involved organs are liver, bone marrow, spleen, adrenals, meninges, kidneys, fallopian tubes, and epididymis. But no organ is exempt.

Continued

Continued

- **Isolated-organ tuberculosis:** Dissemination of tubercle bacilli through blood may seed and **produce tuberculosis in any organ or tissue**. This results in isolated organ tuberculosis and may be the presenting manifestation. Commonly involved organs in isolated organ tuberculosis are presented in **Box 8**.

Various ways of spread and complications of secondary tuberculosis of lung are presented in **Figure 32**.

Natural history and various stages of tuberculosis are depicted in **Figure 36**.

Various terms used and lesions in tuberculosis are presented in **Box 9**.

Main difference between primary and secondary tuberculosis of lung is presented in **Table 18**.

Clinical Features

Clinical features of primary tuberculosis

In most individuals (about 90%), primary infection is successfully arrested and primary tuberculosis is generally

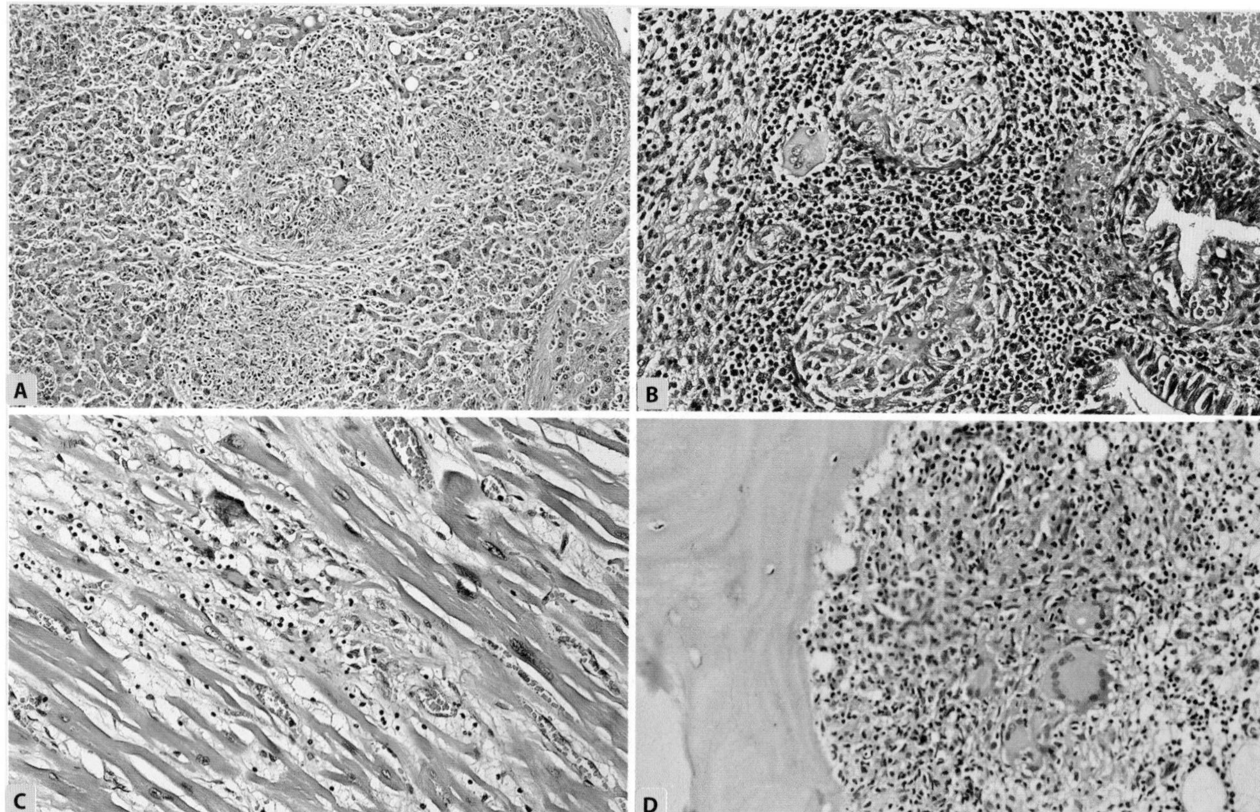

FIGS. 35A TO C: (A) Miliary tuberculosis of liver. (B) Tuberculosis of endometrium. (C) Tuberculosis of myocardium; and (D) tuberculosis of bone marrow.

Box 8: Commonly involved organs in isolated organ tuberculosis.

- Meninges (tuberculous meningitis)
- Kidneys (renal tuberculosis)
- Adrenals (formerly an important cause of Addison disease)
- Bones (osteomyelitis):
  - **Pott disease:** When tuberculosis involves the vertebrae, the disease is called as **Pott disease**. In these patients, paraspinal "cold" abscesses may track along tissue planes and may clinically present as an abdominal or pelvic mass
- Fallopian tubes (salpingitis)
- Epididymis (epididymitis)

asymptomatic. Most people are unaware of this initial encounter and the only evidence of primary tuberculosis may be a positive tuberculin test. A chest radiograph sometimes may show the initial pulmonary nodule (a healing tubercle), and some fibrosis.

Progressive primary tuberculosis: About 10% of individuals with an arrested primary infection develop clinical tuberculosis at some later time in their lives. This tuberculosis is called progressive primary tuberculosis. In these patients, symptoms are usually insidious and nonspecific. These include fever, weight loss, fatigue, and night sweats. Sometimes, symptoms may develop abruptly with high fever. It may resemble an acute bacterial pneumonia with consolidation of the lobe, hilar adenopathy, pleurisy, and pleural effusion. Cough and hemoptysis develop only when there is well-established active pulmonary disease.

Miliary tuberculosis: Lymphatic and hematogenous dissemination following primary infection may result in the development of military tuberculosis. Symptoms in military tuberculosis vary depending on the organs affected (e.g., tuberculous meningitis, if meninges are involved) and tend to occur late in the course of disease.

Clinical features of secondary tuberculosis

Secondary pulmonary tuberculosis Localized secondary tuberculosis may be without any symptoms (asymptomatic). If clinical manifestations appear, they are usually slow (insidious) in onset.

Systemic symptoms: These are produced due to cytokines released by activated macrophages (e.g., TNF and IL-1).

- **General symptoms:** Systemic symptoms commonly develop early in the disease.
  - **Nonspecific:** These include general malaise, fatigue, anorexia, and weight loss.
  - **Low-grade fever:** Usually, the **fever is low grade and remittent** (appearing late each afternoon and then subsiding—commonly known as **evening rise of temperature**), associated with night sweats.
- **Sputum:** As the disease progressively involves the lung, cough (may be mistaken due to smoking or a cold) with increasing amounts of sputum is produced. At first sputum

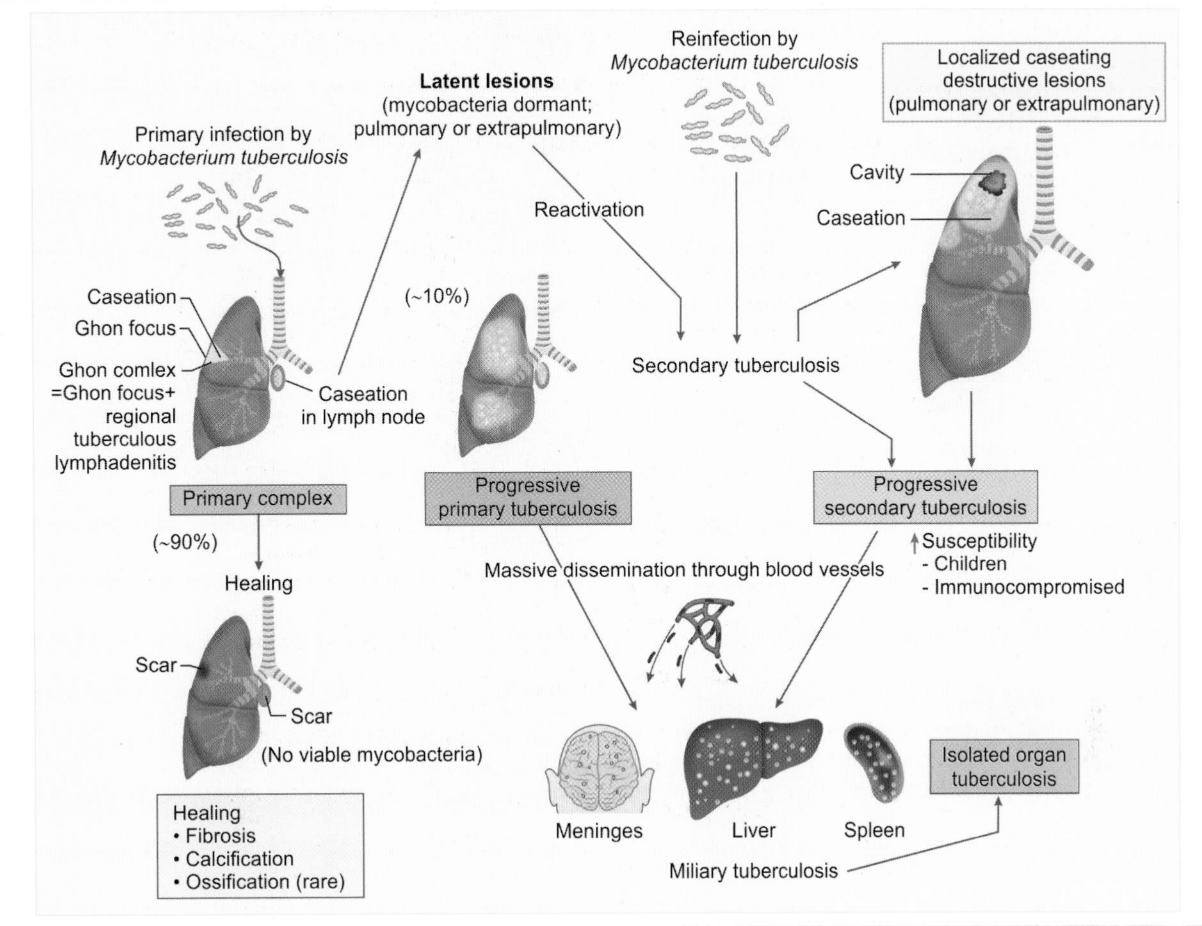

FIG. 36: Natural history and various stages of tuberculosis.

Box 9: Various terms used and lesions in tuberculosis.

- Assman focus: Infraclavicular lesion of tuberculosis
- Rich focus: Tuberculous granuloma occurring on the cortex of the brain that ruptures into the subarachnoid space
- Weigert (Wigard) focus: Healed foci of TB in the intima of blood vessels
- Simon focus: Healed calcified caseous nodule of tuberculosis at the apex of lung
- Simmond focus: Healed foci of TB in the liver
- Puhl's lesion: Isolated lesion of chronic tuberculosis in the lung apex (without lymph node involvement). The lesion is also referred to as "Aschoff-Puhl reinfection".
- Ranke complex: Healed primary complex consisting of calcified peripheral and calcified hilar nodes
- Rasmussen aneurysm: Aneurysm of pulmonary artery within the tuberculous cavity. May rupture and cause hemoptysis

is mucoid and later becomes purulent. Cavitation may be accompanied by hemoptysis and some amount of hemoptysis is observed in about 50% of patients with secondary pulmonary tuberculosis. Sometimes hemoptysis is severe.

- **Pleuritic pain:** It may develop if the pulmonary infection extends into the pleural surfaces.

Table 18: Main difference between primary and secondary tuberculosis (TB) of lung.

Characteristics	*Primary TB*	*Secondary TB*
Type of infection	Initial infection in an unsensitized individual	Infection in a previously sensitized individual
Source of infection	Exogenous	Usually endogenous activation of latent infection
Site of lung involved	Lower part of upper lobe or upper part of lower lobe. It is subpleural in location.	Apex and posterior segments of the upper lobe and superior segments of lower lobe
Regional lymph node involvement	Significant and prominent	Not prominent
Sputum for AFB	Rarely positive	Commonly positive
Cavity formation	Rare	Common
Healing	Mainly by calcification	By fibrosis
Extrapulmonary complications	Very common	Lesion usually localized to lung

(AFB: acid-fast bacilli)

Complications of secondary pulmonary tuberculosis These are as follows:

- **Hemoptysis** due to erosion into small pulmonary arteries adjacent to the tuberculous cavity.
- **Bronchopleural fistula:** It may develop when a tuberculous cavity in the subpleural region ruptures into the pleural space. It may lead to tuberculous empyema and pneumothorax.
- **Aspergilloma:** It is a fungal mass produced due to superinfection of a persistent open cavity with *Aspergillus*. It may fill the entire cavity and form a fungal ball.

Extrapulmonary tuberculosis The extrapulmonary disease occurs after the disease is disseminated. The signs and symptoms depend on the particular organ system involved.

Multidrug-resistant tuberculosis (MDR-TB): Presently all newly diagnosed cases of tuberculosis are treated with prolonged courses of four antituberculous antibiotics, including isoniazid, pyrazinamide, rifampin, and ethambutol. Strains of *M. tuberculosis* resistant to these antibiotics are now seen more commonly than it was in past years. It is usually as a consequence of poor compliance with the full regimen of antibiotic therapy.

Prognosis: It is usually good when infections are localized to the lungs, except when they are caused by drug-resistant strains of mycobacteria or tuberculosis occurring in debilitated individuals. Untreated secondary tuberculosis is a wasting disease that is eventually fatal. In the past, chronic cavitary tuberculosis was a common cause of secondary amyloidosis. All stages of HIV infection are associated with an increased risk of tuberculosis.

Diagnosis and Laboratory Identification

Q. Write short essay on recent advances in diagnosis of tuberculosis.

Chest radiographs: It shows unilateral or bilateral apical cavities and suggests the diagnosis of secondary tuberculosis.

Diagnosis of active pulmonary tuberculosis includes **history**, clinical symptoms, abnormal chest radiographs, **and** confirmation by **laboratory** findings. Routine laboratory tests in tuberculosis are listed in **Box 10**.

Tests for laboratory identification of tuberculosis can be mainly divided into (1) bacteriological diagnosis and (2) molecular diagnosis. Various investigations in the laboratory diagnosis of tuberculosis are listed in **Box 11**.

Box 10: Routine laboratory tests in tuberculosis.

- Hematological investigations: ESR, hemoglobin estimation, peripheral blood smear shows moderately elevated total WBC count with lymphocytosis (~80% lymphocytes)
- Sputum examination: For microscopy and acid-fast bacilli; and culture of sputum
- Cytological examination: Analysis of body fluids depending on the organ involved (e.g., CSF, pleural, pericardial, and ascitic fluid)

(CSF: cerebrospinal fluid; ESR: erythrocyte sedimentation rate; WBC: white blood cell)

Box 11: Various investigations in the laboratory diagnosis of tuberculosis.

Bacteriological diagnosis

Smear microscopy with acid-fast stain:
- Histopathology
- Mycobacterial culture

Identification of *Mycobacterium tuberculosis* complex (MTC or MTBC)
- Chromatographic immunoassay
- Serological or immunological methods

Diagnosis of latent *M. Tuberculosis* infection
- Tuberculin test
- Interferon-gamma (γ) release assay test

Molecular diagnosis

Nucleic acid amplification technology:
- PCR-based assays
- Line probe assays (LPAs)
    - INNO-LiPA
    - Genotype LPA
    - Cartridge-based nucleic acid amplification test (CBNAAT)
    - TrueNat
    - Loop-mediated isothermal amplification (LAMP)
    - Genedrive

Molecular typing of *M. tuberculosis*

DNA sequencing
- Pyrosequencing
- Whole genome sequencing (WGS)

Future prospects in diagnostics of tuberculosis

Drug susceptibility testing (DST)

Bacteriological Diagnosis

Identification of mycobacteria in clinical specimens: Examination of clinical specimens (e.g., sputum, urine, or CSF) is of critical diagnostic importance. There are many tests to detect *M. tuberculosis* in patients with active disease. These tests are performed in patients suspected of having tuberculosis. The bacteriological examination consists of (1) AFB smear examination, (2) specimen culture and identification, (3) direct detection of MTB in the clinical specimen with a NAAT, and (4) drug susceptibility testing (DST). Other tests include measurement of ADA activity in pleural fluids and histopathological examination of specimens.

Smear microscopy with acid-fast stain

AFB microscopy: A microscopic identification of **acid-fast tubercle bacilli in the** clinical **specimen (e.g., sputum)** using techniques such as the **Ziehl–Neelsen stain** is the **most rapid test and easiest procedure** for acid-fast mycobacteria. Its cost is less.

Identification: Mycobacteria are best identified by their red color in acid-fast bacillus-stained sections. Mycobacteria can show significant morphologic variability. They are curvilinear, vary in length, and exhibit a characteristic "beaded" appearance owing to nonhomogeneous uptake of the AFB stain. Various acid-fast organisms and structures are presented in **Table 19**.

Table 19: Various acid-fast organisms and structures.

Acid-fast organisms	Acid-fast structures

• *Mycobacterium tuberculosis*
• *M. leprae*
• *M. smegmatis*
• Atypical *Mycobacterium*
• *Nocardia*
• *Rhodococcus*
• *Legionella micdadei*
• Protozoa:
  ○ Isospora
  ○ *Cryptosporidium parvum*
	• Head of human sperm
	• Embryophore of *Taenia saginata*
	• Hooklets of *Echinococcus granulosus*
	• Keratin

Apart from carbolfuchsin methods [includes the ZN and Kinyoun methods (direct microscopy)], most modern laboratories use the fluorochrome procedure using **auramine-O or auramine-rhodamine dyes and examined under fluorescence microscopy.** It is **more sensitive than the ZN method.** However, it is expensive because it needs expensive mercury vapor light sources and a dark room. Less expensive light-emitting diode (LED) fluorescence microscopes are now tool of choice. They are as sensitive as—or more sensitive than—traditional fluorescence microscopes and are used in developing countries.

- **Advantages:** Sputum smear microscopy is an easy, inexpensive, and rapid method for detecting infectious cases of pulmonary TB.
- **Disadvantage:** Many patients with TB have negative AFB smears and a subsequent positive culture. Negative smears do *not* exclude TB. It has a low specificity. *M. tuberculosis* cannot be accurately distinguished on morphological appearance from other pathogens in the genus, from some saprophytic mycobacterial species [i.e., nontuberculous mycobacteria (NTM)] that may contaminate in the laboratory, or from those mycobacteria that may be part of the normal flora. Dead and viable mycobacteria are also not distinguished. Hence, definitive identification of *M. tuberculosis* can only possible by culturing the mycobacteria in or by using one of the newer molecular methods. Moreover, drug-resistant forms cannot be differentiated from susceptible strains.

For patients with signs or symptoms of pulmonary TB, for AFB smear and mycobacterial culture, it is recommended to obtain one or two sputum specimens, preferably collected early in the morning. If tissue is obtained for culture, it is important that the portion of the specimen intended for culture should not be put in preservation fluid such as formaldehyde.

Histopathology: Laboratory diagnosis of extrapulmonary tuberculosis is done through histopathological examination of tissue specimens. The sensitivity depends on sampling and reduced granuloma formation in patients with HIV infection reduces the specificity.

- Types of samples: These include (1) aspiration of the lymph nodes and (2) tissue biopsy (without surgery, during surgery and postmortem).

Mycobacterial culture

Definitive diagnosis of tuberculosis depends on the isolation and identification of *M. tuberculosis* from a clinical specimen or the identification of specific DNA sequences in a NAAT. Conventional cultures require 2–8 weeks to culture the tubercle bacillus because of its slow growth on laboratory media. However, **culture is the gold standard (mainstay) for the definitive diagnosis of TB**, because they can detect small numbers of organisms the original sample. At present, mycobacterial culture can be performed on solid media or liquid media. Culture on solid agar media need 3–6 weeks for growth, whereas culture in liquid media can provide the results within 2 weeks.

Solid media Specimen is inoculated into conventional egg-based solid media [e.g., Lowenstein-Jensen (LJ)] or agar-based solid medium (Middlebrook 7H10 or 7H11) and incubated at 37°C (under 5% CO_2 for Middlebrook medium). Mycobacteria, including *M. tuberculosis*, grow slowly and 4–8 weeks may be needed before growth is detected on these conventional culture media. They are especially used for sputum culture. Newer solid cultures are available and include nitrate reductase assay (NRA), thin layer agar (TLA) culture, and colorimetric redox indicator (CRI).

Liquid media Currently used liquid media (e.g., Middle brook 7H9 broth) support rapid growth than solid media. During the last four decades, numerous diagnostic methods and modifications have been developed for the early growth of *M. tuberculosis*. During 1980s, **semiautomated and automated liquid culture systems** became available, which facilitated rapid growth and detection of *M. tuberculosis* with a turnaround time (TAT) of about 10 days.

Newer rapid methods Although a combination of solid and liquid media is currently the gold standard for the primary isolation of mycobacteria, there are few new (modern), rapid methods of culture available. These include the **BACTEC-TB460 radiometric system, and the Mycobacteria Growth Indicator Tube (MGIT), ESP culture system II,** and **microscopic observation drug susceptibility (MODS).**

1. **BACTEC radiometric system:** In this assay, to the liquid culture media radiolabeled (14 C labeled) substrate (palmitic acid) is inoculated. If the inoculum contains live TB bacilli, they utilize the 14 C labeled substrate (palmitic acid) and release radioactive labeled carbon dioxide (14 CO_2). *BACTEC-TB460* radiometric system measures the radioactive CO_2 released during decarboxylation of 14 C labeled substrates. BACTEC instrument quantitatively measures the amount of radioactivity. The daily increase in the growth index is directly proportional to the rate and amount of growth of mycobacteria in the medium. TAT is 5–10 days. By adding inhibitory substances to the medium, DST (drug susceptibility testing) can also be performed.
2. **MGIT (mycobacteria growth indicator tube):** It is a liquid-culture system commercially available as an automated BACTEC MGIT-960 system. This system uses tubes containing enriched Middlebrook 7H9 broth with an oxygen-sensitive fluorescence sensor dissolved in the liquid medium. These are embedded in silicone at the bottom of the tube. If mycobacteria grow in the culture medium, it consumes oxygen and it fluoresces orange when probed with UV light. Thus, the appearance of fluorescence indicates active growth of mycobacteria. It detects early growth (7–12 days) and is useful for rapid phenotypic drug susceptibility. The tubes are read weekly until the eighth

week of incubation before the result is declared to be negative.

3. **ESP culture system II:** In this method, growth of *M. tuberculosis* is detected by estimation of rate of oxygen (due to the metabolic activity) of microorganism's consumption which is present within the upper headspace of the culture vials.
4. **MODS:** It is a noncommercial culture method. It uses a liquid medium that favors faster growth of the TB bacillus and thereby helps in the early microscopic visualization of characteristic cord formations with an inverted light microscope. It also helps in assessing drug sensitivity or resistance.

Advantages of identification of *M. tuberculosis* from culture: (1) confirms the diagnosis, (2) isolation of the mycobacteria is essential for determining its antibiotic sensitivity (susceptibility), and (3) also confirms the specific identity of the mycobacteria by growth and biochemical characteristics. Due to its high sensitivity, it can detect tuberculosis even in cases where smear was negative for acid fast bacillus.

Disadvantages: Culture medium is highly prone to contamination and expensive. Needs dedicated facilities and infrastructure for media preparation, specimen processing, and growth of organisms. It also requires skilled laboratory personnel and specialized biosafety conditions.

Cultures should be performed in all diagnostic specimens, regardless of the results of AFB smear or NAAT.

Extrapulmonary tuberculosis: For nonrespiratory TB part or all of any of the following samples should be placed in a dry container (and not in formalin) and submitted for TB culture:

- Lymph node biopsy
- Pus aspirated from lymph nodes.
- Pleural biopsy
- Any surgical or radiologically obtained sample submitted for routine culture.
- Histopathology sample
- Aspiration sample
- Autopsy sample

Identification of *Mycobacterium tuberculosis* complex

The mycobacteria comprising the **MTC** or **MTBC** are a genetically related group of ***Mycobacterium*** species that can cause tuberculosis in humans.

Biochemical tests MTB complex can easily be differentiated with a set of biochemical tests. MTB complex are niacin positive, reduce nitrates to nitrites, and possess pyrazinamidase (helps the distinction between MTB and *M. bovis*) as well as a heat-sensitive (thermolabile) catalase. These biochemical tests for identifying MTC or MTBC are time-consuming. Hence, in 2007, WHO recommended assays for confirmation of MTC or MTBC based on the detection of a TB-specific antigen from positive cultures. These include liquid culture assays, DST (drug susceptibility testing), and rapid speciation (strip speciation) tests that help in rapid diagnosis of TB and MDR-TB.

Chromatographic immunoassay If culture is positive in solid or liquid media, it is necessary **to differentiate MTC** or **MTBC from other NTM (nontuberculous mycobacteria).** Chromatographic immunoassay is a qualitative method of identification to differentiate **MTC** or **MTBC** from positive cultures. MTC or MTBC strains (except some substrains of *M. bovis* BCG and NTM) predominantly secrete MPB64 protein. This can be used as diagnostic discriminator between MTC or MTBC and NTM. In this method, monoclonal antibodies against MPB64 are used for the assays.

Q. Write short essay on recent advances in serodiagnosis of tuberculosis.

Serological or immunological methods in serological methods blood serum is used and this can be easily Performed in resource-limited settings. Serologic tests are based on detection of antibodies to a variety of mycobacterial antigens. These immunodiagnostic tests can provide indirect evidence current or past infections of MTB. Exception of tuberculin skin test (TST), they have been found to be of limited application as diagnostic use because of their cross reactivity, poor sensitivity, low specificity, and their poor reproducibility. Hence, it is not an attractive choice as a diagnostic tool. False positivity is a major limitation in antibody detection. Determinations of adenosine deaminase and IFN-γ levels in pleural fluid may be used as adjunctive tests in the diagnosis of pleural TB.

Diagnosis of latent *M. tuberculosis* infection

Screening of individuals having latent TB infection (LTBI) requires the development of new diagnostic tools. Two tests currently exist for identification of LTBI: the TST and IGRAs. Interferon-gamma release assays (IGRAs) were developed to diagnose LTBI; however, tuberculin (Mantoux) test (tuberculin skin test) is the least expensive test. The TST and IGRA are based on the principle of capturing the interaction of T cells to TB antigens.

Tuberculin (Mantoux) test: Infection by mycobacteria leads to development of delayed hypersensitivity to protein antigens of *M. tuberculosis* which is detected by the TST (tuberculin skin/reaction test). This test is being used in diagnostic algorithm for pediatric age group as a **supportive evidence**. It is most widely used in screening for LTBI. For details refer page 1082 and Fig. 38 of Chapter 15.

- In the Mantoux test, purified protein derivative (PPD) is prepared from culture filtrates of the mycobacteria and biologically standardized. Activity is expressed in tuberculin units.
- In the routine procedure (Mantoux test), measured amount **(0.1 mL) of PPD** is injected **intradermally** in the forearm. The greatest limitation of PPD is its lack of mycobacterial species specificity.
- It is read 48–72 hours after the injection for presence and size of an area of induration. If it produces a **visible and palpable induration** (hardening) **of 10 mm diameter or more** at the site of injection of PPD, the test is considered as positive. Skin reaction occurs due to type IV delayed hypersensitivity as an immunologic response.
- **Significance:** Although tuberculin tests can be used to document contact with the tubercle bacillus, they do not confirm that the patient currently has active disease.
    - **Positive tuberculin test: It indicates T cell-mediated immunity** to mycobacterial antigens. A positive reaction usually develops 4–6 weeks after initial exposure to the mycobacteria. Test remains positive

for life, though it may wane after some years or when immunosuppression occurs either due to medications or disease. Positive Mantoux test indicates that the individual is exposed to mycobacterial antigen. It does not differentiate between infection and disease.

- **False-negative reactions:** It is seen in certain viral infections, sarcoidosis, malnutrition, Hodgkin lymphoma, immunosuppression, and overwhelming active tuberculous disease.
- **False-positive reactions:** It is seen in infection by **atypical mycobacteria** or prior **vaccination with BCG.**

Interferon-gamma release assay test: It was developed because of high percentage of false reporting in interpretation of tuberculin test. The IGRA assay detects MTB antigens. These MTB antigens include the early secretory antigen target 6 (ESAT-6) and culture filtrate protein 10 (CFP-10). Both of these MTB antigens stimulate production of interferon-gamma in the host. The IGRAs are more sensitive (81%) and specific (88%). The IFN-γ is measured in the blood sample from the suspected patient.

Disadvantages of immunodiagnostic tests: Due to their cross reactivity, poor sensitivity, and high false reports especially in high-TB-burden countries (with exception of TST), Government of India has banned the use and also the sale of these diagnostic tests.

Molecular Diagnosis

Nucleic acid amplification technology

Molecular techniques are used for amplification of mycobacterial nucleic acid and are used as the analyte. Molecular techniques are used for the detection and identification of MTB. PCR is the most common method of NAAT. Other methods include ligase chain reaction, strain displacement amplification, LAMP, and transcription-mediated amplification. Recently, real-time (RT) PCR technique depending on fluorescent-probe detection or melting-curve analysis is available. The use of molecular biology is essential in the rapid diagnosis of mycobacteria. Molecular methods based on capturing nucleic acids are emerged as a rapid screening tool.

Advantages: These include: (1) they can be directly used on the sample material, or culture, (2) can be used as a rapid (within few hours), screening method and also for straight forward differentiation of species assay from culture material, and (3) can have a high specificity and sensitivity.

Disadvantages: Molecular tests are expensive, require expertise, and may not differentiate active infection as DNA from a dead *Mycobacterium* due to antibiotic treatment can be detected and amplified by PCR.

Molecular techniques can also detect resistance genes such as catalase (katG) or RNA polymerase (rpoB). Mutations in these genes have been associated with resistance to isoniazid and rifampicin, respectively. By use of molecular primers in RT-PCR reaction, it is possible to differentiate between the presence of the wild-type sequence and mutated sequence associated with drug resistance.

PCR-based assays Traditional biochemical tests mostly used for identification of mycobacteria have longer TAT, the results are uncertain. Therefore, PCR-based assays have been implemented in the more rapid, sensitive, specific diagnosis of tuberculosis. PCR can detect as few as 10 organisms in clinical specimens. PCR amplification of *M. tuberculosis* DNA is a specific gene amplification assays and requires careful interpretation. Hence, it must be strongly correlated with other parameters (e.g., clinical, histological, cytological, biochemical, imaging, and therapeutic specifications) while making final conclusion, especially in the diagnosis of drug-resistant TB. In acid-fast smear positive samples, PCR assays are as sensitive as culture, but in smear-negative tuberculosis PCR is slightly less sensitive, and substantially less sensitive in children. It can differentiate *M. Tuberculosis* from atypical mycobacteria. Culture remains the gold standard, but PCR should also be performed if active tuberculosis is suspected because of the quick availability results.

Q. Write short essay on concept of point-of-care (POC) testing in tuberculosis.

Line probe assays Line probe assay is a PCR-based multiplex **genotypic DST** assay. If simultaneously it directly **detects the presence of MTC** or **MTBC** in the patient sample and if *M. tuberculosis* are present it is also useful to identify whether it is resistant to drugs rifampin and isoniazid (i.e., drug resistance mycobacteria).

1. **INNO-LiPA:** INNO-LiPAs are two different LPA kits. They are **used for the detection of drug resistance and identification of the genus *Mycobacterium*** and 16 distinct mycobacterial species, respectively. It can be done on either liquid or solid cultures. The INNO-LiPA test consists of three major steps: DNA extraction, DNA amplification, and hybridization.
2. **Genotype LPA:** It is based on the patented DNA strip technology. It can genetically differentiate the genus *Mycobacterium* from other different species.
3. **Cartridge-based nucleic acid amplification test (CBNAAT** or CB-NAAT, GeneXpert): Majority of RT-PCR assays are used in rapid and specific detection of *M. tuberculosis* in the clinical specimens. CBNAAT assay is an automated cartridge-based molecular technique which not only detects *MTB* but also (simultaneously detect) rifampicin resistance within less than 2 hours. It has high sensitivity unlike smear microscopy particularly in HIV-positive individual and is also less time-consuming compared to sputum culture (which takes several weeks). This has been endorsed by WHO as an initial diagnostic test for tuberculosis. The Xpert MTB/RIF is a real-time fully automated NAAT for rapid diagnosis of TB with high specificity and sensitivity (approaching that of liquid culture). Xpert MTB/RIF has biosafety and training requirements is minimal. Xpert MTB/RIF is also recommended as a stand-alone diagnostic screening test in individuals at risk of MDR-TB. Recently, the new Xpert MTB/RIF Ultra assay (Ultra) is available and has higher sensitivity. However, this new Ultra cartridge, because of this greater sensitivity, also detects nonviable bacilli and consequently has lower specificity than Xpert MTB/RIF.
   - **TrueNat:** The TrueNat TB test (in-house product from India) is a **new molecular test that can diagnose TB in 1 hour** and **simultaneously detect drug resistance** to rifampicin. It is semiautomated and battery operated method and can be performed in outdoor without electricity. It fulfils the objective of maximum conclusion on minimum prerequisites.

Box 12: Ideal characteristics of a point-of-care (POC) assay for diagnosing tuberculosis.

- Detect both pulmonary or extrapulmonary tuberculosis (TB)
- Useful in children and adults, HIV-positive or HIV-negative TB presumptive cases
- Can be used in many easily accessible body samples
- Can be used by healthcare workers with minimal training
- Can be used in peripheral health facilities or community and operable in broad ranges of temperature and humidity
- Should deliver results in <20 minutes
- No or minimal maintenance needed
- Economical
- High sensitivity and high specificity

Box 13: Point-of-care diagnostic testing in tuberculosis.

- Xpert MTB/RIF (real-time automated nucleic acid amplification technology) and Xpert MTB/RIF Ultra
- Loop-mediated isothermal amplification (TB-LAMP)
- Lateral flow lipoarabinomannan (LAM)

Point-of-care testing (POCT) refers to testing in close proximity to the patient where a medical decision can be made immediately based on the result. The TrueNat machine is designed as a **POC machine** and testing of sample can be performed as soon as a suspected TB patient with symptoms is seen. The procedure consists of DNA extraction that requires 25 minutes and another 35 minutes to diagnose TB. Another 1 hour is needed for testing of rifampicin drug resistance. Ideal characteristics of a POC assay for diagnosing tuberculosis is presented in **Box 12** and POC diagnostic testing in tuberculosis is listed in **Box 13**.

- **Loop-mediated isothermal amplification:** TB-LAMP is a manual NAAT in which DNA amplification along with gene detection is performed in a single step. It is one of the **POC tests** that can be used at outreach centers as a near-patient assay. It does not need sophisticated instruments and laboratory infrastructure.
- **Advantages:** LAMP is rapid with TAT of 40 minutes. It is relatively simple to use and gives result usually observed through the naked eye under UV light (interpreted through a visual display). It has increased sensitivity than smear microscopy and additional 40% more patients can be detected than smears. Once smear microscopy results are known and documented, this can also be implemented as an add-on test.
- **Limitations:** It cannot differentiate drug-resistant TB and drug-sensitive TB. It has less specificity than smear microscopy and can produce increase in false-positive results.

  The new TB-LAMP assay is a newer assay that requires minimal laboratory infrastructure and has few biosafety requirements.
- **Genedrive:** This is new assay based on NAAT for detection of TB and rifampin-resistant TB. It has low accuracy and is considered suboptimal compared to smear microscopy. Hence, it is not supported by the WHO requirements.

Molecular typing of MTB

Molecular typing involves DNA fingerprinting (shows the genetic makeup) of *M. tuberculosis* strains, and this improves the understanding in complexity of TB transmission. There are several molecular typing assays for MTB now available.

Spoligotyping (Spacer Oligonucleotide Typing): Spoligotyping is a direct, less expensive, quick, and reproducible assay to aim the phylogeny (relationships among different groups) of MTC or MTBC strains. Spoligotyping is more commonly applied to identify the genotype family; and this technique is not useful for typing of strain.

MIRU-VNTR (*Mycobacterium* Interspersed Repetitive Units—Variable Number Tandem Repeats typing): This helps to identify the genetic polymorphisms within bacterial species. It is more suitable as a high-discrimination typing method for highly conserved genotypes.

RFLP typing: Restriction fragment length polymorphism (RFLP typing) is most largely used method for typing bacterial strains. Though it needs highly experienced manpower and sophistication, RFLP is still superior and is also used for strain typing.

DNA sequencing

DNA sequencing is the **process of determining the sequence of nucleotides in the DNA**. This technique involves the amplification and identification of genetic mutations in different genomic regions. It simultaneously provides fast and specific identification of mycobacterial species as well as drug resistance strains. DNA sequencing mostly involves pyrosequencing, next-generation sequencing (NGS), and/or whole genome sequencing (WGS).

Pyrosequencing Pyrosequencing uses sequencing by synthesis approach. In this modified nucleotides are added and removed one at a time, with chemiluminescent signals produced after the addition of each nucleotide. It determines the nucleic acid sequence of short segments without electrophoresis. It is useful for diagnosis of mycobacteria with positive cultures as well as smear-positive sputum examples. This is more economical than conventional sequencing and with automated sequencers results can be obtained within 1–3 days.

Whole genome sequencing Whole genome sequencing (WGS) provides complete data on resistance mutations and strain typing for monitoring transmission. Detection of resistance mutations helps in a personalized treatment of drug-resistant tuberculosis and improves the outcomes. WGS is expensive and requires dedicated infrastructure, and requirement of skilled manpower with analysis expertise. Hence, it is used most commonly in high-income countries.

Future Prospects in TB Diagnostics

Evolution in laboratory diagnosis of MTB has reduced the time of identification and drug susceptibility results. Continuous efforts are going on for increasing reproducibility, improvement of performance, and reducing the cost and need for infrastructure. Some of the future projections in TB diagnostics are as follows:

Alere determine TM LAM assay: It is a lateral flow (LF)-based immunodiagnostic strip test used for the detection of LAM antigen in urine. LF-LAM is useful in the diagnosis of TB in HIV-positive adult patients. It is also useful in patients who are not able to expectorate sputum, with other immunocompromised condition, and patients who cannot move out will be benefitted with LF-LAM assay. It is also one of the POC test used in tuberculosis.

Cepheid gene Xpert ultra: It works on the same principle of CBNAAT, but has greater sensitivity in direct smear-negative rather culture-positive specimens, pediatric specimens, extra pulmonary specimens (such as CSF), and paucibacillary specimens mostly from HIV-positive patients.

RCReady® 80: It is a molecular diagnostic tool, developed by Tosoh Bioscience (Japan). It is a stand-alone assay that can process up to eight samples, and need a computer platform for its operation. Amplification of MTBC specific target is performed by utilizing transcription-reverse transcription concerted reaction (TRCR) amplification technology. Results are obtained within 30 minutes.

Volatile Organic Compounds (VOCs): The VOCs in breath are mycobacterial metabolites and can be used as biomarkers of active pulmonary tuberculosis. These metabolites are products of oxidative stress (reaction to the mycobacterial disease), or from the bacteria per se (metabolites of MTB). These devices have been recently proposed for the rapid screening and diagnosis of TB. The devices are portable and handheld. In this, a patient suspected (potentially infected) of TB inhales into the device tube, VOCs produced by MTB in the lungs. It binds with titanium oxide nanotubes immobilized in the gadget. Upon binding, it produces an electrical impulse and this impulse is captured and read by applications in smartphones.

Assays for diagnosing LTBI: C-Tb is a novel skin test for differentiating LTBI. The test determines the body's resistant reaction to two definitive MTB antigens namely: ESAT-6 and CFP10.

Automated microscopy platforms: Conventional visual examination for AFB is by direct microscopic examination of sputum smear. With the advent of automated imaging, advances also developed in this visual technique and examples are briefly described below.

- **The TBDx system:** It is a mechanized computerized automated microscopy platform. Its stage consists of a great magnifying lens (with higher resolution power) in the microscope. It has an imaging framework with a slide holding adjustment. In a single run, it can analyze up to 200 arranged smears by using fluorescent microscopy.
- **Capture-XT™:** This is an MTB cell advancement gadget in development stage. It can enhance the sensitivity of concentration techniques, for example, sputum sedimentation. It is battery operated and most likely work for 8 hours on a single charge.

Surface plasmon resonance (SPR) sensing: SPR-based biosensors systems have several ultrasensitive detectors and are expected to be in the market as a fully integrated POC SPR imaging-based diagnostic system.

Use of nanoparticles: Quantum (minimum amount of any physical entity) dots 1–6 nm nanoparticles can be made to function using capture probe or antibodies coated with capture probe. Nanotechnology-based technology can identify protein and nucleic acids utilizing a sandwich of standardized magnetic and bar-code probes tag tests.

Lab-on-a-chip: A lab-on-a-chip is a class of miniaturized device that combine and automate multiple laboratory technique into a system that fits on a chip. The chip is a single-board computer that can be up to a maximum of few square centimeters in size. Lab-on-a-chip frameworks can be used for the identification of appropriate biomolecules. It is now possible to single molecule from minute amounts of genetic materials.

Future NGS platforms: Presently smaller, powerful, and user-friendly, innovative devices for use in regions with comparatively smaller research facilities are being developed. The combination of interdisciplinary sciences such as molecular biophysics, nanobiotechnology, immunology, biochemistry, genomics, biomedical sciences, and bioinformatics are undergoing research for diagnostic development from the biological to the molecular level. These advancements promise future diagnosis tuberculosis to be rapid, accurate, and cost-effective and help in identifying multiple drug-resistant TB strains.

WHO-approved microbiological tests for active tuberculosis are presented in **Table 20**.

Drug Susceptibility Testing

Q. Write short essay on multidrug resistant (MDR) tuberculosis.

In all patients, the initial MTB isolate should be tested for resistance to first-line anti-TB drugs, namely isoniazid, rifampin, ethambutol, and pyrazinamide. The results obtained guide clinicians in choosing the appropriate drugs for every patient. Drug-resistant TB, includes MDR-TB, is defined as resistance to at least isoniazid and rifampicin (the two most important anti-TB first-line drugs) and extensively drug-resistant TB (XDR-TB) is defined as MDR-TB plus resistance to any fluoroquinolone such as moxifloxacin and at least one of three injectable second-line drugs (amikacin, capreomycin, or kanamycin). As per WHO all TB patients should have DST to at least rifampin for all initial isolates of *M. tuberculosis* because rifampin resistance probably precedes MDR-TB. Indications for DST are listed in **Box 14**. In a bacteriologically confirmed case, rapid reporting of DST to first-line drugs and/or second-line drugs and also detection of drug resistance plays a key role in the early implementation of treatment. It can be by **phenotypic methods or genotyping method**.

Drug resistance detection using phenotypic methods

phenotypic DST methods are done in solid or liquid media as direct or indirect tests. Phenotypic methods such as indirect testing assays are considered as the gold standard.

- **Direct testing:** In this, susceptibility testing is conducted directly with the clinical specimen to a batch of drug-containing and a drug-free media. A concentrated specimen is inoculated directly. Results are obtained rapidly on liquid medium, with an average reporting time of 3 weeks.
- **Indirect testing:** In this method, susceptibility testing is conducted indirectly with mycobacterial cultures on solid or liquid medium. A pure culture prepared from the original specimen is inoculated on the drug-containing culture media. With indirect testing on solid medium, results may not be available for ≥8 weeks.

Drug resistance detection using genotypic methods

Genotypic methods are **not routinely used** in the mycobacterium laboratory and they are mainly used for research purposes. Highly reliable genotypic methods are available for screening of patients at increased risk of drug-resistant tuberculosis. These methods rapidly identify genetic mutations in gene regions known to be associated with resistance to rifampin (such as those in *rpo*B) and isoniazid (such as those in *kat*G and *inh*A). These methods include the Xpert MTB/RIF, Xpert MTB/RIF Ultra assays and molecular LPAs. First, DNA is extracted from *M. tuberculosis* isolates or from clinical specimens. Then the resistance gene regions are amplified by PCR, and labeled. Finally, probe-hybridized PCR products are detected by colorimetry. There are also few noncommercial, inexpensive culture and susceptibility testing methods (e.g., microscopically observed drug susceptibility, nitrate reductase, and CRI assays) that can be used in resource-limited settings.

Nontuberculous Mycobacterial Infections

Q. Write short essay on nontuberculous mycobacterial infections.

Nontuberculous mycobacteria (NTM) are also termed as atypical mycobacteria (in contrast to *M. tuberculosis*, regarded as the "typical" mycobacterium), mycobacteria other than tuberculosis, and environmental mycobacteria. NTM refer to mycobacteria other than *M. tuberculosis,* its close relatives (*M. bovis, M. caprae, M. africanum, M. pinnipedii, M. canetti*), and *M. leprae.*

Epidemiology

Nontuberculous mycobacteria are highly adaptable and ubiquitous in the environment, water, and soil. Specific NTM have recurring shallow recess (niches). For example, *M. simiae* in certain aquifers (underground layer of water-bearing permeable rock), *M. fortuitum* in pedicure (cosmetic treatment of the feet and toenails) baths, and *M. immunogenum* in metal working fluids.

Table 20: WHO-approved microbiological tests for active tuberculosis.

Type of test	*Site of tuberculosis*
Sputum smear microscopy	Pulmonary tuberculosis (TB)
Nucleic acid amplification tests (NAAT) [no-MTB Xpert/RIF]	Pulmonary TB and extra-pulmonary tuberculosis (EPTB)
Xpert MTB/RIF	PTB, EPTB, and rifampicin (RIF) resistance TB
Automated liquid culture and species identification based on MPT64	PTB, EPTB; speciation (formation of new and distinct species in the course of evolution)

Box 14: Indications for drug susceptibility testing.

- One or more risk factors for drug resistance are identified
- If the patient either fails to respond to initial therapy
- Treatment failure: Relapse after the completion of treatment

Prevalence: NTM disease prevalence has increased worldwide. The number of identified species of NTM is growing because of the use of DNA sequence typing for speciation. Currently, the number of known species is 170. The prevalence of specific species of NTM varies and depends on geographic regions. The most frequent human pathogens are MAC (*Mycobacterium avium* complex), *M. abscessus* complex, and *M. kansasii.* Identification of the specific species is important because of the difference in treatment. Using traditional physical and biochemical tests, it is difficult to distinguish *M. avium* and *M. intracellulare*, and also they have similar clinical features. Hence, these two are grouped into MAC. Newer molecular techniques can distinguish these two species, as well as *M. chimaera* in the same complex. *M. marinum* is a common cause of cutaneous and tendon infections in coastal regions and it develops in individuals exposed to fish tanks or swimming pools.

The true epidemiology of infections due to NTM is difficult to determine because its isolation often is not reported and its differentiation from *M. tuberculosis* is usually not performed. It is problematic especially during therapy for tuberculosis when smears positive for AFB are considered evidence of treatment failure. Thus NTM are identified these will be treated as tuberculosis and reported as treatment failure because NTM do not respond to antituberculous treatment.

Predisposing factors: Normal host defense mechanisms can usually prevent infection by NTM. NTM cause disease only rarely in normal healthy individuals except in vulnerable individuals. These vulnerable group includes those with impairment of host defense, as in bronchiectasis, or breached, as by inoculation with postsurgical or post-traumatic infections (e.g., liposuction, trauma, and cardiac surgery). Disseminated disease can develop when there is significant immune dysfunction. The immune dysfunction may be due to immunosuppression from advanced HIV, transplantation, treatment with TNF inhibitors, and rare cases of anti-IFN-γ autoantibodies or inherited defects in the IL-12/IFN-γ pathways. NTM causing pulmonary disease is much more common and is predominantly associated with structural lung damage (e.g., CF, bronchiectasis, primary ciliary dyskinesia, chronic obstructive pulmonary disease, or pneumoconiosis) but not associated with systemic immunodeficiency.

Transmission: There is little human-to-human transmission of NTM. Occasionally, human-to-human transmission of NTM can occur in small number of patients with CF.

Clinical presentations: These include chronic pulmonary disease (most common), lymphadenitis, cutaneous disease, and disseminated disease. MAC causes widely disseminated infections in patients with severe T-cell immunodeficiency and MAC proliferate abundantly in many organs, including the lungs and GI system. Patients develop fever, with immense night sweats and weight loss. MAC infection in an individual without HIV or another severe immunodeficiency, primarily infects the lung. This causes a productive cough and sometimes fever and weight loss. Radiographically, there may be fibrocavitary lesions primarily in the upper lobes or nodular bronchiectasis with multifocal clusters of small nodules. NTM biofilm development on medical devices has been observed as a source of MAC in many recent cases.

Pathobiology

CD4+ T lymphocytes were considered as main effector cells against NTM. Disseminated MAC disease was highly correlated with a decline in numbers CD4+ T lymphocyte. It was observed that TNF-α is essential in mycobacterial control. Powerful inhibitors of cytokine, namely TNF-α, neutralize this cytokine and inhibit the formation of granuloma.

Genetic factors: In individuals without the predisposing/risk factors, susceptibility to disseminated infection with NTM may have genetic basis such as specific mutations in the IFN-γ/IL-12 synthesis and response pathways.

Pathogenesis (Fig. 37)

- Mycobacteria are phagocytosed by macrophages and produce IL-12.
- Interleukin-12 activates T lymphocytes and natural killer (NK) cells through binding to its receptor IL-12R. IL-12 stimulates T lymphocytes and NK cells to secretion of IFN-γ.
- Interferon-γ produces following effects (1) activation of neutrophils and macrophages to produce reactive oxidants and Fc receptors, and (2) concentration of certain antibiotics intracellularly.
- Signaling by IFN-γ through its receptor (IFN-γR) leads to phosphorylation of STAT1. This in turn regulates IFN-γ-responsive genes, such as those coding TNF-α and stimulates the production of TNF-α. TNF-α leads to the killing of intracellular organisms such as mycobacteria, salmonellae (*Salm.*), and some fungi.
- Tumor necrosis factor-α signals through its own receptor (TNF-αR) via a downstream complex containing the nuclear factor κB (NF-κB) essential modulator (NEMO). This also contributes to the killing of intracellular bacteria. Hence, the positive feedback loop between IFN-γ and IL-12 drives the immune response to mycobacteria and other intracellular infections. These genes are important in the pathway of mycobacterial control. Specific Mendelian mutations in these genes may be associated with disseminated disease.

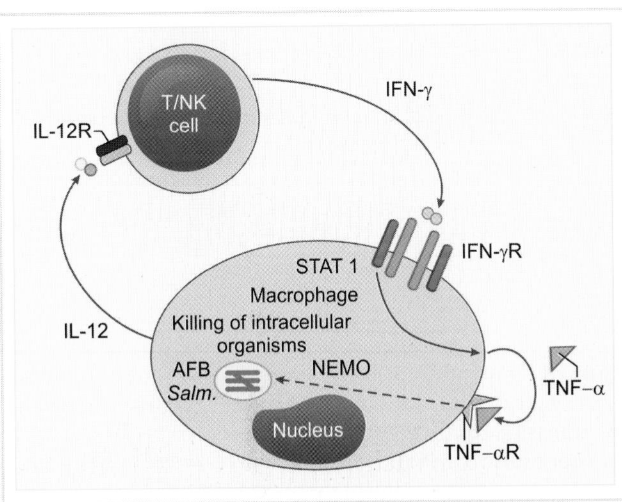

FIG. 37: Cytokine interactions of infected macrophages with T and natural killer (NK) lymphocytes. Infection of macrophages by mycobacteria [acid-fast bacilli (AFB)] leads to the release of interleukin-12 (IL-12). IL-12 acts on its receptor complex (IL-12) and produces interferon-γ (IFN-γ). Through its receptor (IFN-γR), IFN-γ activates STAT1, stimulating the production of tumor necrosis factor-α (TNF-α) and leads to the killing of intracellular organisms such as mycobacteria, salmonellae (Salm.), and some fungi. TNF-α acts through its receptor (TNF-αR) and via a downstream complex containing the nuclear factor κB (NF-κB) essential modulator (NEMO) to activate NF-κB. This also contributes to the killing of intracellular bacteria.

MORPHOLOGY

Hallmark of MAC infections in patients with HIV is the presence of numerous AFB within macrophages (Figs. 38A and B). Depending on the severity of immunodeficiency, MAC infections may be localized to the lungs or can disseminate throughout the mononuclear phagocyte system. Dissemination can cause enlargement of involved lymph nodes, liver, and spleen. Large number of organisms in swollen macrophages may produce a yellow pigmentation of the affected organ. Microscopically, granulomas, lymphocytes, and tissue destruction are rare.

Source and pathology of nontuberculous mycobacterial infections are presented in **Table 21**.

LEPROSY

Leprosy (Hansen disease—after the discovery of the causative organism by Hansen), is a **chronic**, **granulomatous**, slowly progressive, nonfatal, destructive infection **caused by *M. leprae*.**

Sites of involvement: Mainly involves the **peripheral nerves** (from large nerve trunks to microscopic dermal nerves), **skin and mucous membranes** (nasal) and results in disabling deformities. Its clinical manifestations are largely confined to the skin, peripheral nervous system, upper respiratory tract, eyes, and testes.

Epidemiology

Leprosy is one of the oldest human diseases and lepers were isolated from the community in the olden days. Leprosy was first described in ancient Indian texts from the sixth century BC. Leprosy is now rare in developed countries. Leprosy is associated with poverty (low income) and rural residence. Though it has low communicability, leprosy remains endemic in several tropical nations, such as India, Papua New Guinea, Southeast Asia, and tropical Africa. It is also common in China, Myanmar, Indonesia, Brazil, Nigeria, Madagascar, and Nepal. Its onset is usually in the second and third decades of life. It is usually not associated with AIDS, perhaps because of leprosy's long incubation period.

Mycobacterium leprae

- It is slender, **weakly acid-fast**, obligate, intracellular bacillus (0.3–1 μm wide and 1–8 μm long). It **closely resembles *MTB* but is less acid-fast.** It is indistinguishable microscopically from other mycobacteria, and usually **detected in tissue sections by Fite-Faraco stain.**
- **Proliferates at low temperature** of the human skin.
- **Cannot be cultured** on artificial media or in cell culture.

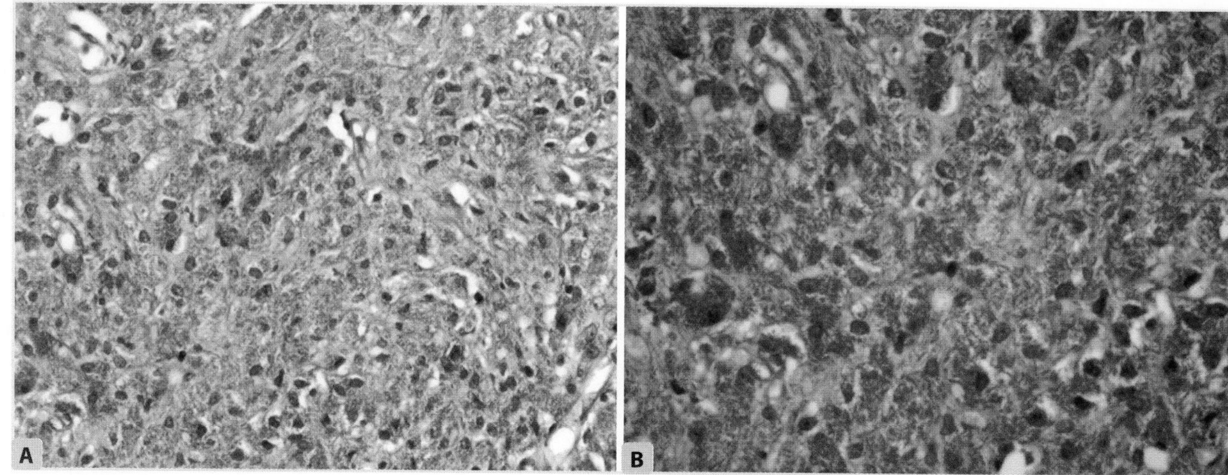

FIGS. 38A AND B: *Mycobacterium avium* complex showing numerous acid-fast bacilli within macrophages (A: low magnification and B: high magnification).

Table 21: Source and pathology of nontuberculous mycobacterial infections.

Organism (age group affected)	*Source of infection*	*Pathology*
Mycobacterium kansasii (50–70 years)	Inhalation of organisms from soil, dust, or water	Slowly progressive chronic granulomatous pulmonary disease (similar to that caused by *M. avium intracellulare*)
M. scrofulaceum (1–5 years)	It is a common soil inhabitant and probably ingested from soil or dust by toddlers playing in soil	Granulomatous cervical lymphadenitis; affects the submandibular lymph nodes. Disease is localized, and surgical excision of affected lymph nodes is curative
M. marinum (any age)	• Direct inoculation of organisms from fish or underwater surfaces • Infection is acquired by traumatic inoculation, such as abrading an elbow on a swimming pool ladder or cutting a finger on a fish spine	Localized nodular skin lesions; tissue reactions may be pyogenic or granulomatous inflammation (swimming pool granuloma)
M. ulcerans (usually 5–25 years)	Probably inoculation of environmental organisms	Large, solitary, severe ulcer of skin and subcutaneous tissue of extremities; coagulative necrosis
M. fortuitum and *M. chelonae* (any age)	Ubiquitous in the environment. Infection follows traumatic or iatrogenic inoculation material contaminated with environmental organisms	Tissue reaction can be pyogenic or granulomatous; painless, pyogenic inflammation (fluctuant abscesses) at the site of inoculation; ulcerate and gradually heal spontaneously

- **Experimental animals:** Lepra bacilli grow at sites where the temperature is below that of the internal organs. Examples: **Foot pads of mice**, ear lobes of hamsters, rats, and other rodents.
- **Experimentally transmitted to nine branded armadillos [they have low body temperature ranging from 32 to 35°C (89.6°F–95°F)].**
- **Antigen in lepra bacilli: The bacterial cell wall contains mainly 2 antigens namely *M. leprae*-specific phenolic glycolipid (PGL-1) and LAM (lipoarabinomannan).**

Source of infection: *M. leprae* may be present in human respiratory (nasal) secretions, ulcerated lesions of infected persons, or soil.

Mode of transmission: It has comparatively low communicability and the mode of infection remains uncertain. Transmission routes may be multiple.

1. **Inoculation/inhalation:** Likely to be transmitted from person to person through aerosols from asymptomatic lesions in the upper respiratory tract or open wounds. Inhaled *M. leprae* is taken up by alveolar macrophages and disseminates through the blood, but replicates only in relatively cool tissues of the skin and extremities.
2. **Intimate contact:** Intimate contact for many years with untreated leprosy patients is another mode of transmission. They shed many bacilli from damaged skin, nasal secretions, mucous membrane of mouth, and hair follicles.

Incubation period: Generally, 5–7 years (may range from 2 to 40 years).

Classification

Q. Write short essay on classification of leprosy.

A. Ridley and Jopling (1966) Classification

It depends on the clinicopathological spectrum of the disease, which is **determined by the immune resistance of the host (Flowchart 1)**. Leprosy is classified into five groups with two extremes or polar forms, namely—tuberculoid and lepromatous types.

1. **Tuberculoid leprosy (TT):** It is the polar form that has maximal immune response.
2. **Borderline tuberculoid (BT):** In this type, the immune response falls between BB and TT.
3. **Borderline leprosy (BB):** It exactly falls between two polar forms of leprosy.
4. **Borderline lepromatous (BL):** It has the immune response that falls between BB and LL.
5. **Lepromatous leprosy (LL):** It is the other polar form with least immune response.

Variants of leprosy

- **Indeterminate leprosy:** It is an initial nonspecific stage of any type of leprosy. Pure neural leprosy with neurologic involvement is the main feature. The skin lesions of leprosy are not seen. Indeterminate leprosy and tuberculoid lesions are paucibacillary and their diagnosis is made together with clinical evidence (for microscopy refer page 674).
- **Histoid leprosy:** It is a variant of LL in which the skin lesions grossly resemble nodules of dermatofibroma (a soft tissue tumor involving skin) and microscopically (refer page 673) shows numerous lepra bacilli.

B. WHO Classification

- **Paucibacillary:** It includes only smear negative cases belonging to: Indeterminate (I), tuberculoid (TT), and borderline tuberculoid (BT) cases classified under Ridley–Jopling classification.
- **Multibacillary:** It includes all mid-borderline (BB), borderline lepromatous (BL), and lepromatous (LL) under Ridley–Jopling classification. It also includes any other smear positive case.

Pathogenesis

- *Mycobacterium leprae* is phagocytosed by macrophages and disseminates in the blood. However, it proliferates mainly in relatively cool tissues of the skin and extremities. It replicates best at 32–34°C (temperature of the human skin) and lesions tend to occur in cooler parts of the body (e.g., hands and face).
- *Mycobacterium leprae* does not secrete any toxins, and its virulence depends on properties of its cell wall (similar to that of *M. tuberculosis*) and immunization with BCG may provide some protection against *M. leprae* infection.
- Cell-mediated immunity is reflected by **delayed-type hypersensitivity reactions to dermal injections of a bacterial extract called lepromin.**
- Leprosy produces a confusing variety of clinical and pathologic features. Lesions may vary from the small, insignificant macules of TT to the diffuse, disfiguring of LL. This extreme variation of presentation is probably due to differences in immune reactivity.
- Most (95%) individuals have a natural protective immunity to *M. leprae* and do not get infected, in spite of intimate and prolonged exposure to *M. leprae*. Susceptible individuals (5%) may develop symptomatic infection.
- ***M. leprae*** causes two remarkably different (extremes) patterns of disease, called tuberculoid (with high resistance) or lepromatous (with little or no resistance) type of leprosy. Most patients, in between these extremes, have **borderline leprosy**. They are associated with different T-cell responses. The T-helper (Th1) lymphocyte response to *M. leprae* determines which of the pattern an individual develops. Some leprosy patients may show a mixed Th1/Th2 cytokine pattern.
    - **Tuberculoid leprosy:** This is less severe form and patients have a Th1 response associated with secretion of IL-2, IFN-γ, and IL-12 as well as a Th17 response. In contrast, IL-4, IL-5, and IL-10 mRNAs are scarce. The ratio between helper CD4+ over CD8+ T lymphocytes is 2:1. As with *M. tuberculosis*, IFN-γ is essential for an effective host macrophage response. This is responsible for low microbial burden. Also, the production of antibody is low. These patients present with dry, scaly skin lesions that lack sensation. They usually have **asymmetric involvement of large peripheral nerves.** In India 90% of cases are tuberculoid type. Strong T cell and macrophage activation results in a localized infection.
    - **Lepromatous leprosy:** It is a more severe form and patients have a weak Th1 response and, in some patients there may be a relative increase in the Th2 response (predominant Th2 response). In LL tissues, the ratio of CD8+ to CD4+ T lymphocytes is a 2:1. LL patients also have hyperglobulinemia, and LL tissues demonstrate a Th2 cytokine profile (i.e., rich in mRNAs for IL-4, IL-5, and IL-10 and poor in those for IL-2, IFN-γ, and IL-12). It appears that IL-2 and IFN-γ cytokines mediate a protective tissue response in leprosy. There is a poor cell-mediated immunity and an inability to control the bacteria. This results in proliferation of lepra bacilli. Occasionally (most often in the LL) antibodies are produced against *M. leprae* antigens. Paradoxically, these antibodies are usually not protective. Instead these antibodies can form immune complexes with free *M. leprae* antigens and its consequences. Thus, they can lead to erythema nodosum, vasculitis, and glomerulonephritis. It is characterized by symmetric thickening of skin and formation of nodules. There is widespread **invasion** of the mycobacteria into Schwann cells (SCs) and into **endoneural and perineural** macrophages. This results in damage to the peripheral nervous system. In advanced cases, *M. leprae* is present in sputum and blood.
    - Apart from above two forms individuals can also develop an intermediate form of disease, called **borderline leprosy**.

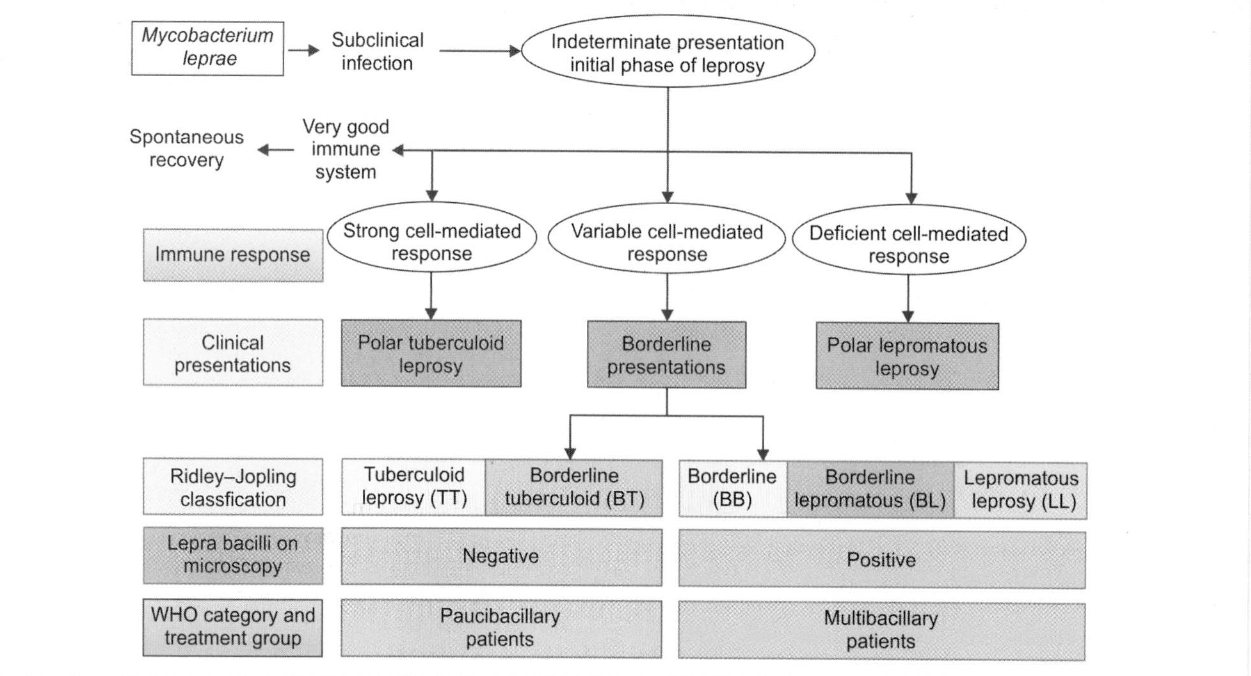

FLOWCHART 1: Ridley–Jopling classification of leprosy.

Immunology of Leprosy

Q. Discuss immunopathology/immunology/immunity in leprosy.

Clinical manifestation of leprosy is highly influenced by the immune response of the host. It is a classical model of disease for understanding human host defenses against intracellular pathogens. The spectrum in leprosy is one of the classical examples of the same pathogen leading to varied clinicopathological presentations. The genome of *M. leprae* has been fully sequenced and found that it is conserved (99.99% identity) between different strains. Thus the diverse clinical manifestations of leprosy are due to the variable responses by the infected host. Leprosy is a unique infection with spectrum of immune response by the host. The tuberculoid polar form (TT) is the one end of the spectrum in which there is intense cellular immunity, with few bacilli and a limited number of lesions. The lepromatous polar form (LL) represents the other end of pole in which there is least cellular immunity with extensive lesions and intense growth of the bacillus in macrophages (an infection specific immunological anergy; "split anergy"). The intermediate borderline forms are immunologically dynamic. They have immunological features between the two polar forms and progressive reduction of the cell-mediated response from the BT to the BB and BL forms.

The defense against leprosy similar to any pathogen/external agent is first initiated by the innate immune response and subsequently after a lag period by the acquired immune response. Both innate and acquired immune response function through cells as well as soluble factors.

Innate Immunity

The initial or immediate host response to a pathogen is called the innate immune response. Cells of the innate immunity (macrophages, DCs, and NK cells) and the mediators secreted by them (e.g., cytokines) contribute to clearance as well as in shaping the adaptive immune response against *M. leprae* (**Table 22**).

Table 22: Important role of various cells of the innate immunity.

Cell	*Role in immune response to Mycobacterium leprae*
Macrophages	• Phagocytic and antimicrobial function. Macrophages can assume proinflammatory (M1) or anti-inflammatory (M2) phenotypes • M1 is increased in TT spectrum and has antimicrobial property • M2 is increased in LL spectrum and has phagocytic function • Cytokine release modulates the adaptive Th response
Dendritic cells (DC)	• These are professional antigen-presenting cells and release proinflammatory cytokines • Marked decreased in LL • *M. leprae* inhibit activation and maturation of DCs • Phenolic glycolipid-1 (PGL-1) also impairs DC maturation and activation
Schwann cells	Interact with PGL-1 of the bacillus for interiorization
Keratinocytes	• Increases expression of Intercellular adhesion molecule (ICAM) in TT • Upregulates human beta-defensins 2 and 3 on stimulation with *M. leprae* • Major producer of C–X–C motif chemokine 10 (CXCL10 also known as interferon-γ) in TT • They present *M. leprae* to CD4+ T cells

(TT: tuberculoid leprosy; LL: lepromatous leprosy)s

Table 23: Role of toll-like receptors (TLRs) in innate immune response to *Mycobacterium leprae*.

Toll-like receptors	*Role in innate immune response*
TLR1/2	• Most important for recognition of *M. leprae* by innate immune cells • Involved in apoptosis of Schwann cell
TLR4	• Role and ligands not well known • Neutralizing antibodies to TLR4 leading to decreased TNF, IL-6, CXCL-10 production by macrophages stimulated with *M. leprae*

(CXCL-10: C–X–C motif chemokine 10; IL: interleukin; TNF: tumor necrosis factor)

Pattern recognition receptors: Cells of innate immunity recognize many pathogens via general molecular pattern recognition. There is various pattern recognition receptors (PRRs) that recognize *M. leprae*. Most prominent are the TLRs (toll-like receptors). TLRs are a highly conserved family of proteins present on macrophages and DCs. They are crucial for recognition of microbial pathogens and play a role both in innate and acquired immune responses. *M. leprae* mainly activates the TLR2/1 heterodimer and TLR4 (**Table 23**). These receptors are mainly expressed on macrophages and DCs. Of the various types of leprosy, TLR1 and TLR2 are more strongly expressed in skin lesions of TT than LL. TLR2 and TLR4 recognize mycobacteria and release IL-12, a cytokine that induces proinflammatory cytokines such as IFN-γ.

Role of cytokines: In innate immune responses, cytokines are produced rapidly after encounter with microbes and other stimuli. These cytokines induce inflammation. The local cytokine milieu influences the expression and activation of these TLRs. These cytokines include TNF, IL-1, IL-12, type I IFNs, IFN-γ, and chemokines. Their main sources are macrophages, DCs, and NK cells. This indicates the role of adaptive immune response on innate immunity.

Activation of TLR1 in response to *M. leprae* leads to an inflammatory response through the production of TNF-α. Th2 cytokines seem to inhibit activation of the TLRs. *M. leprae* has about 31 lipoproteins that can serve as pathogen-associated molecular patterns (PAMP) which can be recognized by TLR2-TLR1 heterodimers.

Consequences of activation of the TLR 2/1 heterodimer: TLRs are transmembrane molecules, and they also play a role in signaling following their engagement. The cytoplasmic tail of TLR is linked to transcription factors such as nuclear factor kappa-light-chain-enhancer of activated B-cells (NF-kB). The activation of the TLR 2/1 heterodimer by PAMP of *M. leprae* in turn activates downstream transcription factors, mainly NF-kB and vitamin D receptor (VDR). This triggers the macrophages to produce proinflammatory cytokines and antimicrobial peptides.

Schwann cells (SCs): These are another group of cells of the macrophage lineage. They are present in peripheral nerves. *M. leprae* is the only bacterium that infects them. SC dystroglycans interact with PGL-1 of the bacillus for interiorization.

Phenolic glycolipid-1 (PGL-1): It is the specific glycolipids expressed by *M. leprae*. Various functions of PGL-1 are as follows:

- It plays an important role in pathogenesis of leprosy.
- It is used for serological diagnosis of leprosy.
- It increases the survival of intracellular bacilli: PGL-1 plays an important role in downregulating the inflammatory immune response. It inhibits DC maturation and activation, facilitates entry of bacilli into macrophages and SCs, and scavenges potentially cytocidal oxygen metabolites. All these functions increase the survival of intracellular lepra bacilli.
- PGL-1 plays a crucial role to the ability of *M. leprae* to invade, survive, and proliferate in the hostile intracellular environment.

Macrophages: Macrophages can assume proinflammatory (M1) or anti-inflammatory (M2) phenotypes. They play main role and are preferentially infected by *M. leprae*. They perform antimicrobial and phagocytic functions.

- **M2 macrophages:** The M2 macrophages are highly phagocytic, and are involved in clearing of debris for tissue repair.
    - In *M. leprae* infection, M2 macrophages phagocytose the bacteria, but are not able to mount an antimicrobial response.
    - M2 macrophages also take up host-derived lipids, providing necessary nutrients for sustaining mycobacterial growth.
    - They also produce anti-inflammatory cytokines (IL-4, IL-10, and IL-13), growth factors [TGF-β and basic fibroblast growth factor (bFGF)], and enzymes (e.g., arginase 1). They contribute to the immunosuppressive mechanisms as well as tissue repair.
- **M1 macrophages:** These are proinflammatory, weakly phagocytic cells, but show a strong antimicrobial response. Therefore, the induction of M1 macrophages is required for host defense. The antimicrobial response of M1 macrophages is by producing free radicals via inducible NO synthase (iNOS) pathway.

Apart from the major pathways of innate immunity discussed above, there are few minor/less defined components. These are as follows:

Complement system: The complement cascade is activated by mannose-capped LAM (lipoarabinomannan) present in the *M. leprae*. This causes damage to the infected nerves and plays an important role in erythema nodosum leprosum (ENL).

Apoptosis: Apoptotic cells are more frequent in TT and reversal reaction (RR).

Adaptive Immunity

T cell response

The Th1/Th2 paradigm (pattern): The two distinctive CD4 T cell subsets are Th1 and Th2. They differ in cytokine secretion pattern and other functions. Each of these T cell subsets produces cytokines. These cytokines promote their own growth factors, thus forming a feed forward loop. This in turn promotes further differentiation of the subsets of Th1 and Th2. This is termed as Th1/Th2 balance hypothesis.

Immature effector CD4 T cells can differentiate into either Th1 or Th2 cells and depends on the cytokines present. An increased expression of cytokines such as INF-γ and IL-2 is observed in the tuberculoid spectrum. The cytokines such as IL-4, IL-5, and IL-10 are found in the lepromatous spectrum. The decision as to which pathway a naïve. T cell will follow is taken during its first encounter with antigen. An antigen that interacts strongly with the T-cell receptor leads to formation of Th1 cell, whereas a weak interaction leads to Th2. IL-2 and IL-12 induce differentiation into Th1 cells from CD4+ T cell (naïve T cell) whereas IL-4 induces differentiation of CD4+ T cell into Th2 cells. IL-4 is also secreted by Th2 cells and inhibits development of Th1 cells. Similarly, cytokines produced by Th1 cells (e.g., IFN-γ) inhibit Th2 differentiation (not shown in **Fig. 39**). Th1 or Th2 development is driven by transcription factors induced by the cytokines. There is reciprocal relationship between Th17 and Treg (T regulatory) cells (**Fig. 39**).

Th1 response pattern is seen in the tuberculoid spectrum. Th1 cells enable the immune response to activate macrophages and cell-mediated immunity. This is via production of IFN-γ and TNF-α. This activates macrophages and induces the production of iNOS. This in turn destroys the bacillus by means of free radical release. IFN-γ is a very important cytokine required for protection against mycobacterial infections including leprosy.

The Th2 (often called helper T cells) predominance is observed in the lepromatous pole. It leads to production of IL-4, IL-10, and TGF-β that facilitates survival of the bacillus as well as the elevated selective production anti-*M. leprae* antibodies seen in lepromatous patients.

Th17 cells: In addition to the Th1 and Th2 subsets, Th17 cells may form the third effector T helper cell subset in leprosy. IL-17 is the cytokine associated with this subtype and has proinflammatory functions. IL-17 is also an important component of the innate immune response. The production of IL-17 is induced by interaction of pathogens with the PRRs present on certain innate immune cells.

T regulatory cells (Treg): These are class of T cells essential for maintaining peripheral tolerance and preventing autoimmune diseases. Tregs are the most potent cell type that suppresses effector T cell response in intracellular infections such as tuberculosis, leprosy, and leishmaniasis.

Antibody response

Antibody response is enhanced in lepromatous and reduced in TT. In the lepromatous type, there is a polyclonal B-cell response as even autoantibodies are observed in circulation. However, it is to be noted that the presence of autoantibodies is not associated with manifestations of autoimmune disease in leprosy. Thus, there is inverted relationship between humoral and T-cell-mediated immunity. Also the presence of antibodies is associated with presence of bacilli in LL indicating thereby that protection in leprosy is not mediated by antibodies. This is because these antibodies do not penetrate living cell membrane and thus have no effect on *M. leprae* which is an intracellular pathogen. However, these antibodies may play a role in capturing bacilli or their products when they are released in tissues or circulation. These antibodies may also form antigen-antibody (immune) complexes.

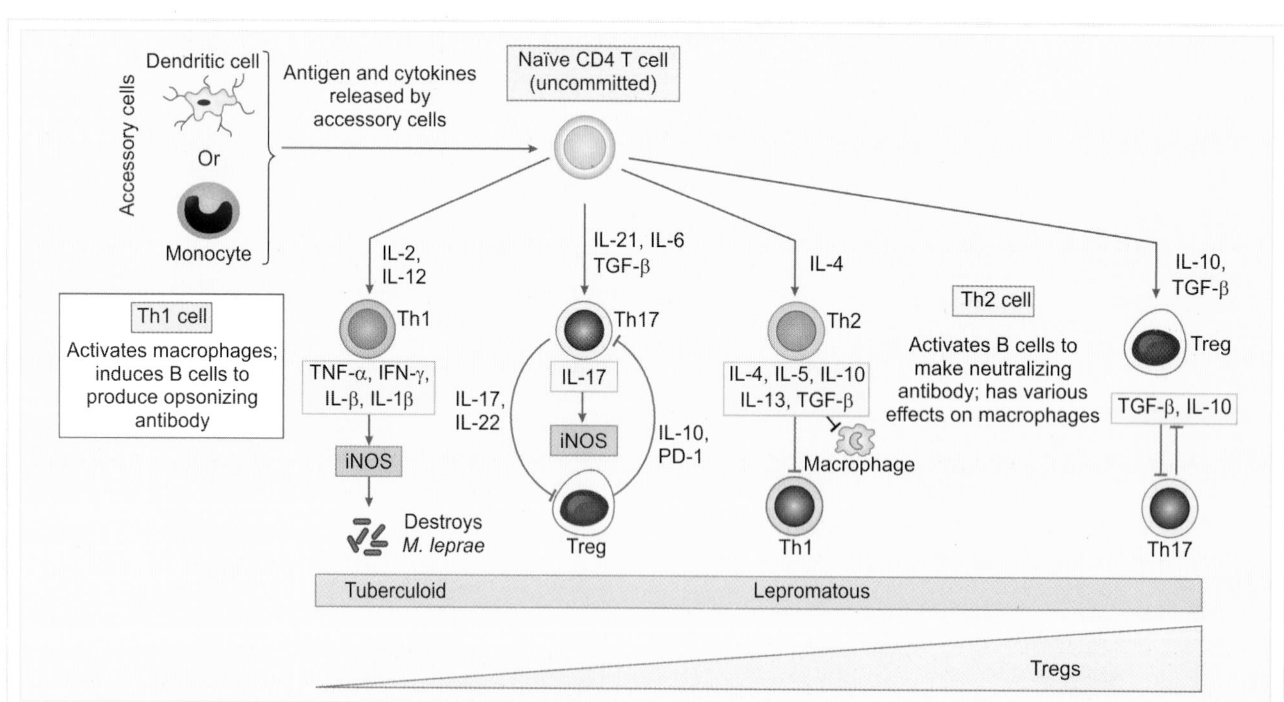

(iNOS: inducible nitric oxide synthase; IL: interleukin; TGF: transforming growth factor; *M. leprae*: *Mycobacterium leprae*; PD-1: programmed cell death protein 1)

FIG. 39: Role of T helper cells across the spectrum of leprosy. Immature effector CD4 T cells can differentiate into either Th1 or Th2 cells and depends on the cytokines present. IL-2 and IL-12 induce differentiation into Th1 cells whereas IL-4 induces Th2 differentiation. IL-4 is also secreted by Th2 cells and inhibits development of Th1 cells. Similarly, cytokines produced by Th1 cells (e.g., IFN-γ) inhibit Th2 differentiation (not shown in Figure). Th1 or Th2 development is driven by transcription factors induced by the cytokines. There is reciprocal relationship between Th17 and Treg (T regulatory) cells.

Q. Write short essay on neuritic leprosy.
Q. Write short essay on nondermatological leprosy.
Q. Write short essay on visceral leprosy.
Q. Write short essay on lymph node changes in leprosy.

MORPHOLOGY

Two extremes or polar forms of the diseases are the tuberculoid and lepromatous types.

1. Tuberculoid Leprosy

It is the less severe form of leprosy. It is very slow in its course and most patients die with leprosy.

Lesion in Skin

- **Number of lesions:** Single or very few lesions.
- **Site:** Usually on the face, extremities, or trunk.
- **Type:** Localized, well-demarcated, red or hypopigmented, dry, elevated, skin patches (**Fig. 40A**) having raised outer edges and depressed pale centers (central healing). As they progress they develop irregular shapes with indurated, elevated, hyperpigmented margins and depressed pale centers (central healing). These lesions are devoid of the normal skin organs (sweat glands and hair follicles) and thereby appear dry, scaly, and anhidrotic.

Nerve Involvement (Fig. 40B)

- Dominating feature in TT.
- Nerves are surrounded by granulomatous inflammatory reactions and may destroy small (e.g., the peripheral twigs) nerves.
- Nerve involvement produces degeneration of nerves and causes loss of sensation in the skin leading to atrophy of skin and muscle. These affected parts are liable to trauma, and lead to the development of chronic skin ulcers.
- **Consequences:** It may lead to contractures, paralyses, and autoamputation of fingers or toes. Involvement of facial nerve can lead to paralysis of the eyelids, keratitis, and corneal ulcerations.

Continued

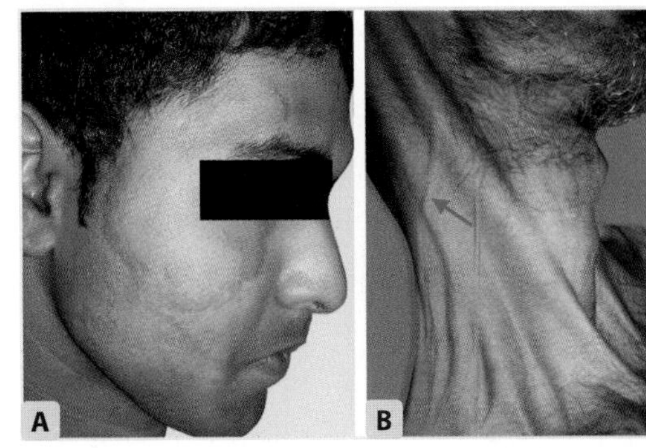

FIGS. 40A AND B: (A) Localized, well-demarcated, red or hypopigmented skin patches on the face; (B) Visible greater auricular nerve thickening.

Continued

Microscopy (Figs. 41A and B)

- **Granuloma:** All the sites involved show granulomatous lesions that closely resemble granulomas observed in tuberculosis. These granulomas are well-formed, circumscribed and noncaseating (no caseation). Termed TT because the granulomas resemble those found in tuberculosis. Granulomas are composed of epithelioid cells (modified macrophages), Langhans giant cells, and lymphocytes.
- **Absence of Grenz zone:** Granulomas in the dermis extend to the basal layer of the epidermis (without a clear/Grenz zone).
- **Fite-Faraco (modified Z-N stain for demonstration of lepra bacillus) stain** generally does not show lepra bacillus, hence the name "paucibacillary" leprosy.
- **Nerve fibers are swollen and there is perineural** (surrounding nerve fibers) **inflammation** by lymphocytes (**Fig. 42**). In TT, T cells breach the perineurium, and destroy SCs (Schwann cells) and axons. This may result in fibrosis of the epineurium, replacement of the endoneurium with epithelial granulomas. Such invasion and destruction of nerves in the dermis by T cells are pathognomonic for leprosy.

Continued

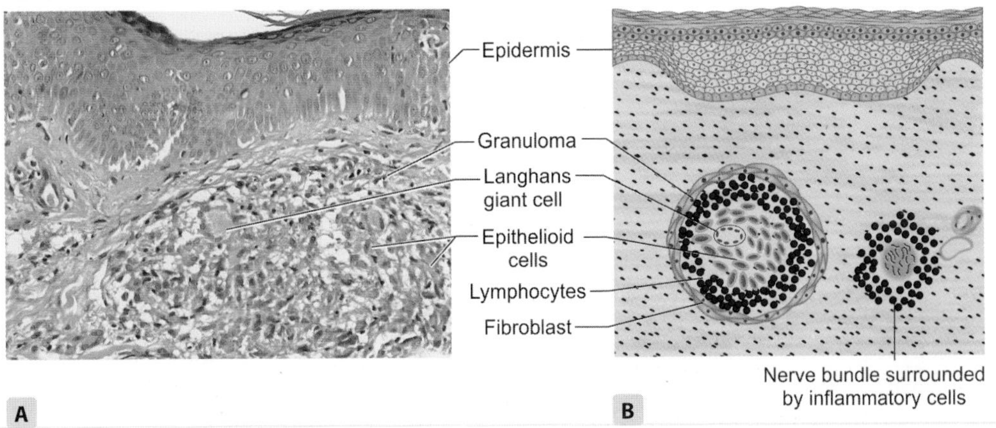

FIGS. 41A AND B: Microscopy of tuberculoid leprosy with circumscribed noncaseating granulomas photomicrograph (A); Diagrammatic (B).

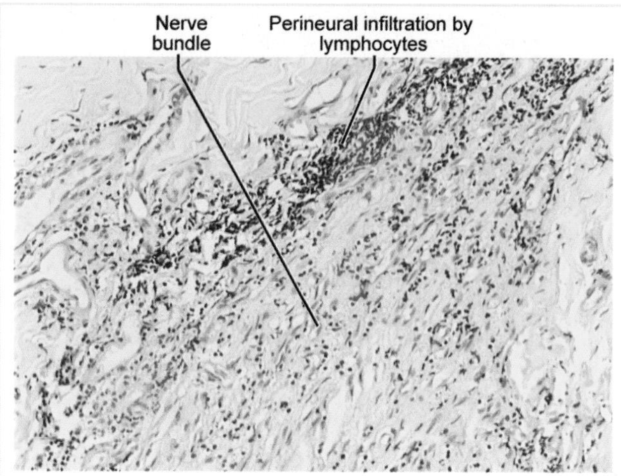

FIG. 42: Nerve involvement in tuberculoid leprosy.

Continued

- **Strong T-cell immunity:** It is responsible for granulomas formation, without lepra bacilli. The lesions cause minimal disfigurement and are not infectious.

Lymph node: In TT, the involved lymph nodes are generally smaller and the germinal centers inconspicuous. Non-necrotizing granulomas, similar to that sarcoidosis, are scattered throughout the parenchyma of lymph node. The macrophages appear as epithelioid cells and are arranged concentrically. Multinucleated giant cells of the Langhans type are also seen in the granulomas. No lepra cells are seen.

2. Lepromatous Leprosy

It is the more severe form and is also called anergic leprosy, because of the unresponsiveness (anergy) of the host immune system.

Sites involved: It involves the skin, peripheral nerves, anterior eye chamber, upper airways (down to the larynx), testes, hands, and feet. The vital organs and CNS are rarely affected, probably because *M. leprae* cannot grow due to too high core temperature at these sites.

Continued

Continued

Lesion in skin

- Thickening of skin and multiple, symmetric, **macular, papular, or nodular** (tumor-like) lesions. The nodular skin lesions may ulcerate. Most lesions of skin are hypoesthetic or anesthetic.
- More severe involvement of the cooler areas of skin [e.g., face (**Fig. 43A**), earlobes (**Fig. 43B**), wrists, elbows, knees, and feet], than warmer areas (e.g., axilla and groin). Lesions in the nose may cause persistent inflammation and produce bacilli-laden discharge. These may be source of infection.
- As the disease progresses, the nodular lesions in the face and earlobes may coalesce to produce a lion-like appearance known as **leonine facies** (**Fig. 43C**). This may be accompanied by loss of eyebrows and eyelashes.
- A form of LL without visible skin lesions but with diffuse dermal infiltration and a demonstrably thickened dermis is called *diffuse lepromatosis*.

Peripheral nerves

- It symmetrically involves particularly the ulnar and peroneal nerves and these nerves may approach the skin surface resulting palpable nerves. These nerves are invaded by mycobacteria with minimal inflammation.
- Damage to the nerves causes loss of sensation. Hence, the, patient is likely to liable for trophic changes in the hands and feet.
- Sometimes, TT may present with only nerve involvement without any skin lesions (**neural leprosy or pure neuritic leprosy).**

Testes

- Usually, severely involved, leading to destruction of the seminiferous tubules and may produce sterility.

Other sites

- **Anterior chamber of the eye:** Blindness.
- **Upper airways:** Chronic nasal discharge and voice change.

Microscopy of Skin Lesion (Figs. 44A to D)

- **Flattened epidermis:** Epidermis is thinned and flattened (loss of rete ridges) over the nodules.

Continued

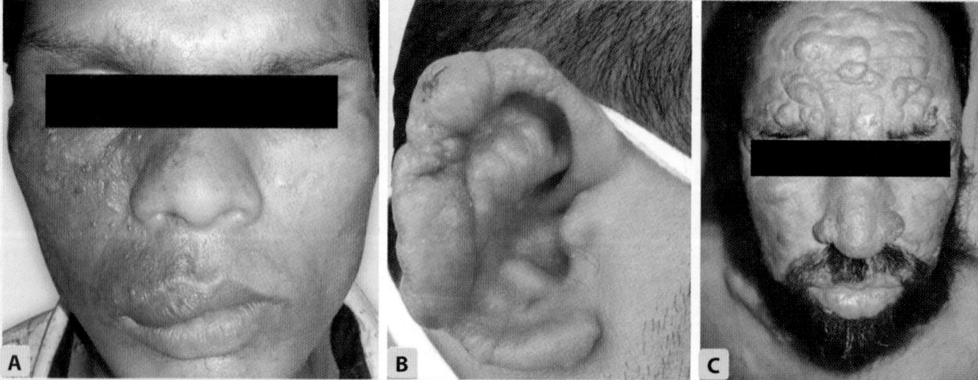

FIGS. 43A TO C: Lesions of lepromatous leprosy. (A) Facial involvement; (B) Nodular lesions on ear; (C) Leonine facies.

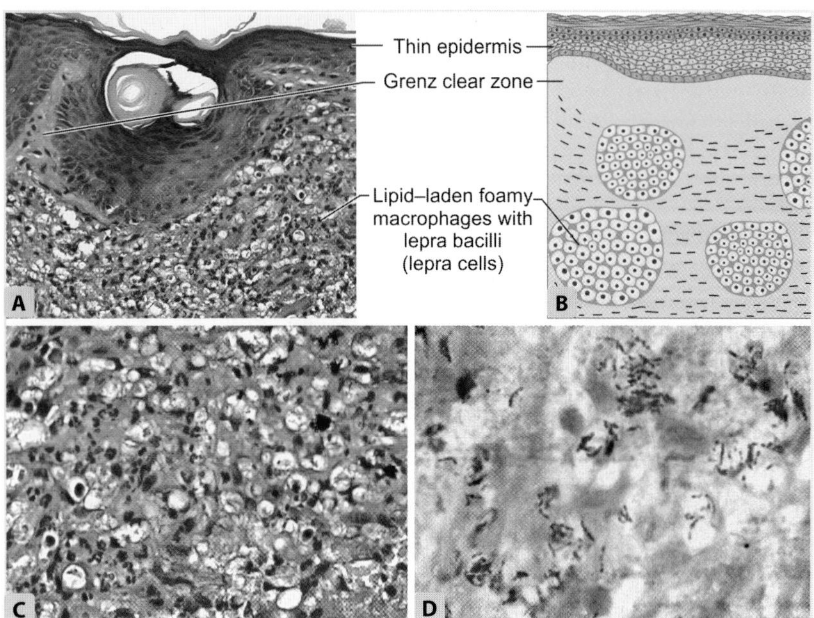

FIGS. 44A TO D: Microscopic appearance of lepromatous leprosy. (A) Photomicrograph; (B) Diagrammatic. The epidermis is thinned and the dermis shows dense collections of lepra cells. The epidermis is separated from the collections of lepra cells by an uninvolved Grenz zone; (C) Photomicrograph. High power view showing foamy macrophages; (D) Acid-fast lepra bacilli within macrophages (Fite-Faraco stain).

Continued

- **Grenz (clear) zone:** It is a characteristic, narrow, uninvolved "clear zone" of the dermis (normal collagen) which separates the epidermis from nodular accumulations of macrophages.
- **Lepra cells:** The nodular or diffuse lesions contain large aggregates of lipid-laden foamy macrophages filled with large clumps ("globi") of acid-fast lepra bacilli (*M. leprae*). These lipid-laden macrophages are termed as lepra cells or Virchow cells. Macrophages do not destroy the bacilli, but probably act as microincubators.
- **Fite-Faraco (acid-fast) stain:** It shows numerous lepra bacilli ("red snappers") within the foamy macrophages. They may be arranged in a parallel fashion like cigarettes in a pack.
- **Multibacillary:** Due to the presence of numerous bacteria, LL is also referred to as "multibacillary."
- **Disfigurement and destruction:** As the infiltration in the dermis slowly expand, they distort and disfigure the face, ears, and upper airway and to destroy the eyes, eyebrows and eyelashes, nerves, and testis. It is common to find claw-shaped hands, hammer toes, saddle nose, and pendulous ear lobes.

Histoid leprosy: It is a variant of LL and was first described in 1963 by Wade. It clinically presents as localized crops of shiny nodules of different sizes. The nodules are sometimes large and pedunculate. Microscopically, it is characterized by the presence of hypercellular granuloma, predominantly composed of spindle-shaped cells. These cells give an impression of expanding centrifugal growth. The centrifugal growth of these spindle-shaped cells compresses the fibrous tissue to form a clear pseudo capsule. Uniform arrangement of these cells in whorls appear similar to histiocytoma. Hence, it is the term "histoid" used to describe this entity.

Continued

Continued

The cells have numerous bacilli. Some of the cases show areas with predominately polygonal cells which resemble conventional macrophages. Some lesions of histoid leprosy may show nests or islands of epithelioid cells without any lepra bacilli in them and are known as "epithelioid contaminants." Grenz zone is mostly present.

Lymph nodes: The lymph nodes may be considerably enlarged and generalized lymphadenopathy is observed in LL. The germinal centers are prominent, and large aggregates of plasma cells are seen at the corticomedullary junction and in the medullary cords.

- **In LL**, there may be thickening and fibrosis of the capsule of lymph node. The **paracortical areas** (T-cell region) are largely depleted of lymphocytes, which are replaced by **sheets of foamy macrophages**. These macrophages show mycobacteria (lepra cells). In early lesions, only one or a few bacilli are present in the cytoplasm of macrophages. In advanced cases, typical foamy macrophages or lepra cells containing masses of AFB (globi) are common. Macrophages in the subcapsular region of the lymph nodes are more heavily parasitized with bacilli than do those in deeper areas. After the macrophages degenerate, the bacilli are released free in the tissues.
- **In tuberculoid and BB**, lymph nodes draining the skin lesions show **epithelioid cell granulomas throughout the cortex and medulla of involved lymph nodes**. Caseous necrosis is absent.

Advanced disease: It may show aggregates of macrophages in the splenic red pulp and the liver. *M. leprae* may be present in sputum and blood.

3. Borderline Leprosy

Some individuals may have with intermediate forms of disease, called borderline leprosy.

Continued

Continued

- Borderline tuberculoid shows epithelioid cells and numerous lymphocytes with a narrow clear subepidermal zone. Lepra bacilli are few and found in nerves.
- Borderline lepromatous shows predominantly histiocytes, few epithelioid cells, and lymphocytes. Numerous lepra bacilli are found.
- Mid-borderline (BB) or dimorphic form shows sheets of epithelioid cells without any giant cells. Few lymphocytes are found in the perineurium. Lepra bacilli are seen mostly in nerves.

4. Indeterminate Leprosy

Microscopically, features are nonspecific and few findings help in suspecting leprosy. These include: (1) local infiltration of lymphocytes or mononuclear cells surrounding the skin adnexa (e.g., hair follicles and sweat glands) or around blood vessels; (2) involvement of nerve (if seen strongly favors the diagnosis); and (3) finding of lepra bacilli (which confirms the diagnosis).

Morphologic index (MI): *M. leprae* appears bright pink under Ziehl–Neelsen staining in a smear. Usually *M. leprae* shows highly polymorphic morphology. Few are brightly and uniformly stained with parallel sides, rounded ends, length being five times the breadth. These mycobacteria are called "solid bacteria". Mostly *M. leprae* in smear appears irregularly stained and fragmented or granular. The transformation into granules is considered as degeneration and that the bacilli are altered dead. These findings are the basis for the morphological index (MI). MI gives an idea of solid, fragmented and granular forms in a smear (**Fig. 45**). MI is a measure of the number of AFB in skin scrapings that stain uniformly bright, correlates with viability of AFB.

Bacteriologic index (BI): It quantifies *M. leprae* in tissue or smears and thus measures of the density of *M. leprae* in the dermis. It scored from 1+ to 6+ (range from 1 to 10 bacilli per 100 fields to >1,000 per field) as multibacillary leprosy whereas BI of 0 + is termed paucibacillary. In untreated patients, it may be as high as 4–6+ and falls by 1 unit per year during effective antimicrobial therapy. The rate of decrease of BI is independent of the relative potency of therapy. **A rising MI or BI suggests relapse and perhaps if the patient is on treatment it suggests drug resistance**.

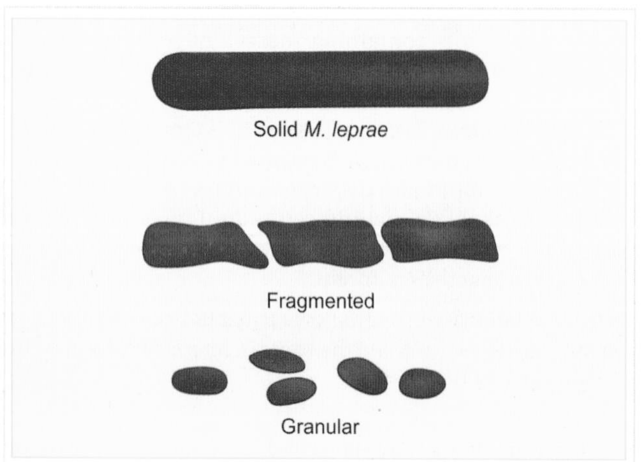

FIG. 45: Diagrammatic representation of solid and nonsolid lepra bacilli.

Mycobacterium lepromatosis: It is a recently discovered mycobacterial species that is genetically similar to *M. leprae* and evolved from a common mycobacterial ancestor.

Lepromin Test

It is **not a diagnostic test** for leprosy. It is **used for classifying** the leprosy based on the immune response.

- **Procedure:** An antigen extract of *M. leprae* called lepromin is intradermally injected.
- **Reaction:**
  - An **early positive reaction** appearing as an indurated area in 24–48 hours is called **Fernandez reaction**.
  - A **delayed granulomatous reaction** appearing after 3–4 weeks is known as **Mitsuda reaction**.
- **Interpretation:**
  - **Lepromatous leprosy:** It shows **negative lepromin test** due to suppression of cell-mediated immunity.
  - **Tuberculoid leprosy:** It show **positive lepromin test** because of delayed hypersensitivity reaction.

Reactions (Reactional States) in Leprosy

Q. Write short essay on reactions in leprosy.

The immunity in leprosy may change spontaneously or following treatment. Lepra reactions consist of several common immunologically mediated episodes of acute or subacute inflammatory states. They interrupt the relatively uneventful usual chronic course of disease. Some of these reactions precede diagnosis and the before starting antimicrobial therapy. These reactions may bring for medical attention and diagnosis. Other reactions follow after the appropriate chemotherapy is started. These reactions may make the patient to feel that their leprosy is worsening and they may lose confidence in conventional therapy. Reactions can occur in any type of leprosy except the indeterminate type. Unless promptly and adequately treated, they can lead to deformity and disability.

Type 1 Lepra Reactions

Type I lepra reaction (downgrading and RRs)

Borderline leprosy is the most unstable form of leprosy where immune status may shift up or down. Type 1 lepra reactions occur in almost 50% of patients with borderline forms of leprosy but not in patients with pure lepromatous disease.

Clinical manifestations: They **produce classic signs of inflammation within previously skin lesions** such as macules, papules, and plaques and, occasionally there may be appearance of new skin lesions, **neuritis**, and (less commonly) **low-grade fever**. Most frequently involved nerve trunk in this process is the ulnar nerve at the elbow. This may become painful and extremely tender. If patients with affected nerves are not treated promptly with glucocorticoids, it will lead to irreversible nerve damage within 24 hours. The most striking manifestation is foot drop and occurs when there is involvement of peroneal nerve.

Types of type 1 reaction: The type 1 reaction (T1R) is a delayed hypersensitivity reaction associated with sudden alteration of cell-mediated immunity. This is associated with a shift in the patient's position in the leprosy spectrum. T1R may be of two types:

1. **Downgrading reaction:** When type 1 lepra reactions develop before the appropriate antimicrobial therapy is started, they are called as *downgrading reactions.* In this situation, the **immunity decreases and the disease histologically moves more toward lepromatous type**.
2. **Reversal (upgrading) reactions:** When type 1 lepra reactions develop after the therapy is started, they are called reversal or upgrading *reactions.* The **immunity** improves and the disease may shift from borderline spectrum toward TT. RRs usually occur in the first months or years after the initiation of therapy but may develop several years after therapy. Without treatment, natural tendency of subpolar tuberculoid and borderline leprosy is to downgrade slowly toward the lepromatous pole. This reaction is termed `reversal reaction' because of natural tendency is reversed with treatment. RRs are associated with a Th1 cytokine profile, with an infiltration of CD4+ T helper cells and increased levels of IFN-γ and IL-2. A unique feature of leprosy in type 1 reactions is presence of large numbers of T cells bearing γ/d receptors.

Microscopically, the most characteristic feature of type 1 lepra lesions is edema. Its diagnosis is mainly made on clinical features.

Type 2 Lepra Reaction: Erythema Nodosum Leprosum

Type 2 reaction is commonly known as erythema nodosum leprosum (ENL). ENL is an immune complex syndrome (antigen-antibody reaction involving complement). It causes inflammation of skin, nerves and other organs, and generally malaise. It is an example of type III hypersensitivity reaction or Arthus phenomenon and immune complex formation is involved in the pathogenesis of type II lepra reaction (T2R). Erythema nodosum leprosum **occurs only in patients near the lepromatous end of the leprosy spectrum (BL/LL)**, and develops in nearly 50% of this group. Though ENL may develop before the diagnosis of leprosy and the initiation of therapy (sometimes, prompt the diagnosis), in **90% of patients it follows after the chemotherapy is started** and **usually within 2 years**.

Clinical features: The most common clinical features of ENL is development of crops of painful erythematous papules or nodules. These may resolve spontaneously in a few days to a week but may recur. There is associated malaise, high fever, and arthralgia. Other clinical features that may be observed include neuritis, lymphadenitis, uveitis, orchitis, and glomerulonephritis. There may be anemia and leukocytosis, and liver function tests may show increased aminotransferase levels. It may develop either a single episode or may become chronic and recurrent. Episodes may be either mild or severe and generalized.

Microscopy: Skin biopsy of papules shows **vasculitis or panniculitis**, sometimes with many lymphocytes and polymorphonuclear leukocytes. Lepra bacilli are seen in the foamy macrophages.

Circulating TNF is raised in ENL and they may play a central role in the pathobiology of this syndrome. ENL is probably due to deposition of immune complex.

Lucio's phenomenon: It is an unusual reaction seen exclusively in patients with the diffuse lepromatosis form of LL, usually those who are untreated. It is **characterized by development of recurrent crops of large, sharply marginated, ulcerative lesions, mainly on the lower extremities**. If they are generalized, they may be secondarily infected leading to septic bacteremia. Microscopically, it is characterized by ischemic necrosis of the epidermis and superficial dermis. The endothelial cells are loaded with AFB. There is endothelial cells proliferation and thrombus formation in the larger vessels of the deeper dermis. Lucio's phenomenon is **probably mediated by immune complexes**.

Complications

Nerve involvements: Complications of the extremities are mainly as a consequence of neuropathy leading to insensitivity and myopathy.

- **Sensory nerve involvement** produces sensory dysfunctions like glove and stocking anesthesia (more common in LL), chronic nonhealing plantar ulcers, and repeated injuries to hands and feet (leading to **autoamputation** of fingers or toes).
- **Motor nerve involvement** produces muscle weakness, wasting, and later paralysis followed by contractures. Nerve involved and their consequences are as follows:
  - **Ulnar nerve:** Most commonly involved and produces claw hand (**Fig. 46**)
  - **Median nerve:** Ape hand
  - **Lateral popliteal nerve:** Foot drop
  - **Posterior tibial nerve:** Claw toes or hammer toes
- **Autonomic involvement** produces anhidrosis or hyperhidrosis.
- **Cranial nerve involvement:** Facial nerve is commonly affected and results in facial paralysis, lagophthalmos, exposure keratitis, and corneal ulcerations (may lead to blindness). Trigeminal nerve involvement may develop early causing loss of corneal reflex. Greater auricular nerve (**Fig. 41B**), supraorbital, supratrochlear, and infraorbital nerves are also thickened.

Nose: In LL, there may be chronic nasal congestion and epistaxis. Long-untreated LL leprosy may produce destruction of the nasal cartilage leading to saddle-nose deformity or anosmia.

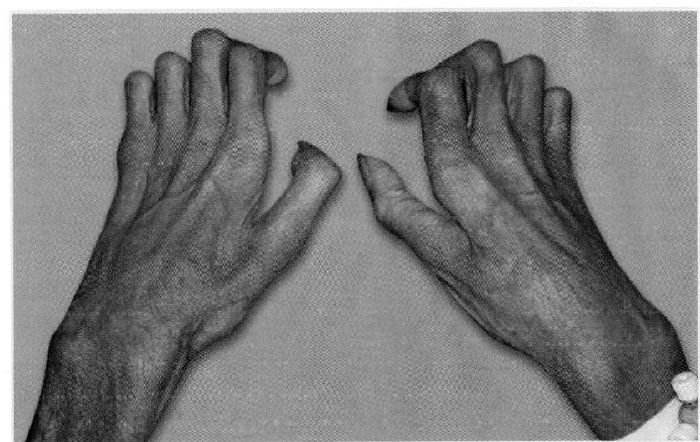

FIG. 46: Bilateral claw hand.

Table 24: Differences between lepromatous, tuberculoid leprosy, and borderline leprosy.

Characteristics	*Lepromatous leprosy (LL)*	*Tuberculoid leprosy (TT, BT)*	*Borderline (BB, BL) leprosy*
Clinical features			
Skin lesions	Symmetrical, multiple, ill-defined, macular, nodular	One or few asymmetrical, annular, hypopigmented, well-defined macular with a tendency toward central clearing, elevated borders	Intermediate between BT- and LL-type lesions; ill-defined plaques with an occasional sharp margin; few or many in number
Disfigurement	Leonine facies, loss of eyebrows, pendulous earlobes, claw-hands, saddle nose	Minimal disfigurement	Variable
Nerve involvement	Seen, but with less severe sensory loss than tuberculoid	Common with sensory disturbances. Skin lesions anesthetic early; nerve abscesses most common in BT	Hypoesthetic or anesthetic skin lesions; nerve trunk palsies, at times symmetric
Microscopy of skin lesions			
Type of lesion	Nodular or diffuse collections of lepra cells within dermis	Noncaseating granulomas composed of epithelioid cells and giant cells	Intermediate between BT- and LL-type lesions
Grenz/clear zone between inflammatory cells and epidermis	Present	Absent	Absent
Lepra bacilli	Plenty within the lepra cells as globular masses (globi)	Rare, if any	Present in macrophages
Acid-fast bacilli (Bacillary index)	4–6+	0–1+	3–5+
Lymphocytes	0–1+	2+	1+
Macrophage differentiation	Foamy changes is the rule	Epithelioid cell	Epithelioid in BB; usually undifferentiated but may have foamy changes in BL
Langerhans giant cells	Nil	1–3+	Nil
CD4+/CD8+ T cell ratio in lesions	0.50	1.2	BB: NT; BL: 0.48
Other features			
Immunity	Suppressed-low resistance	Good immunity-high resistance	Intermediate
Lepromin skin test	Negative	Positive (+++)	Negative
Infectivity	High	Low	Intermediate
Mycobacterium leprae PGL-1 antibodies	95%	50%	95%
Complications	Erythema nodosum leprosum (ENL) may cause vasculitis, glomerulonephritis and nerve damage	Nerve damage can lead to sensory disturbance, paralysis	

(BB: mid-borderline; BL: borderline lepromatous; BT: borderline tuberculoid; TT: polar tuberculoid; LL: polar lepromatous; BI: bacteriologic index; NT: not tested; PGL-1: phenolic glycolipid 1)

Eye: Cranial nerve palsies, lagophthalmos, corneal insensitivity corneal ulcerations, and opacities may complicate leprosy. In LL leprosy, the anterior chamber of the eye is invaded by bacilli. ENL may result in uveitis, cataracts, and glaucoma. Thus, leprosy is a major cause of blindness in the developing countries.

Testes: In LL it can cause aspermia or hypospermia, impotency, and infertility.

Amyloidosis: Secondary amyloidosis may occur as a complication of LL leprosy and ENL.

Nerve abscesses: Patients with leprosy, especially those with the BT form, may develop abscesses of nerves (most commonly the ulnar).

Differences between lepromatous and TT are presented in **Table 24.**

Diagnosis of Leprosy

1. **Clinical examination:**
   - **Sensory testing**
   - Examination of peripheral nerve.
2. **Demonstration of AFB:**
   - Skin smears prepared by slit and scrape method: The smears are made from skin lesions (earlobes and dorsum of the ring or middle finger) by scraped incision method and the dermal material (fluid obtained) onto a glass slide and stained for AFB. It is useful in BL and LL.

- ***Mycobacterium leprae* can be demonstrated in tissue sections, in split skin smears by splitting the skin, and in nasal smears by the following techniques:**
    - **Acid-fast (ZN) staining**.
    - **Fite-Faraco staining** procedure is a modification of ZN procedure and is considered better for more adequate staining of tissue sections **(Fig. 44D)**.
    - **Grocott-Gomori methenamine silver** (GMS) staining can also be employed.
- **Nasal swabs stained by ZN method:** The staining procedure is similar to that procedure employed for *M. tuberculosis* but can be decolorized by lower concentration (5%) of sulfuric acid (less acid-fast).

3. **Skin biopsy:** Involvement of peripheral nerves in a skin biopsy taken from the affected area is pathognomonic, even in the absence of bacilli. Lepra bacilli can be demonstrated in LL and BL types by Fite-Farraco stain.
4. **Lepromin test:** It is used for classifying the leprosy (refer page 674) based on the immune response.
5. **Nerve biopsy**
6. **Serological test is not sensitive or specific enough for diagnosis.**
    - Hypergammaglobulinemia is common in LL and can give false-positive serological tests [venereal disease research laboratory (VDRL), rheumatoid factor and antinuclear antibodies].
    - IgM antibodies to PGL-1 may be found in 95% of LL and in 60% of TT. However, these antibodies may also be present in normal individuals.
7. **PCR testing for *M. leprae* DNA:** Detection of *M. leprae* DNA is possible in all types of leprosy using the PCR, but not sensitive or specific enough for diagnosis. It can be used to assess the efficacy of treatment.

SPIROCHETE INFECTIONS

Spirochetes are long, slender, gram-negative, corkscrew-shaped helical bacteria. They have specialized cell envelopes that permit them to move by flexion and rotation. The membrane covering the bacteria is called an outer sheath, which mask bacterial antigens from the host immune response. Spirochetes have the basic cell wall structure of gram-negative bacteria but stain poorly with the Gram stain. The thinner organisms cannot be identified by routine microscope because they are below the resolving power of routine light microscopy. Hence, specialized techniques, such as dark field microscopy or silver impregnation, are required to visualize them. Three genera of spirochetes, namely (1) *Treponema,* (2) *Borrelia* and (3) *Leptospira,* cause disease in human (**Table 25**). Morphology of three different spirochetes is diagrammatically shown in **Figure 47**.

SYPHILIS

Syphilis (lues) is a **chronic, STI caused by spirochete *T. pallidum***.

It produces varied (multiple) clinical and pathologic manifestations.

Syphilis was first recognized in Europe in the 1490s and was related to Columbus's return from the New World. Probably sailors of Vasco da Gama brought it to India. Originally, syphilis was an acute disease that caused destructive skin lesions and caused early death. However, presently it has become milder, with a lengthier and insidious clinical course.

Epidemiology: Syphilis is a worldwide disease transmitted almost always by sexual contact. Infection may also spread

Table 25: Spirochete causing infections in humans.

Disease	*Organism*	*Mode of transmission*	*Clinical manifestation*
Treponemes			
Syphilis	*Treponema pallidum* (*T. pallidum* subspecies *pallidum)*	Sexual contact, congenital	Chronic sexually transmitted infection (STI) with multiple clinical presentations
Bejel	*Treponema endemicum* (*T. pallidum,* subspecies *endemicum)*	Mouth-to-mouth contact	Mucosal, skin, and bone lesions
Yaws	*Treponema pertenue* (*T. pallidum* subspecies *pertenue)*	Skin-to-skin contact	Skin and bone
Pinta	*Treponema carateum* (*T. pallidum* subspecies *carateum)*	Skin-to-skin contact	Skin lesions
Borrelia			
Lyme disease	*Borrelia burgdorferi*	Tick bite	Chronic systemic infection that involves multiple organ systems. Initially produces skin lesion and later produces cardiac, neurologic, or joint disturbances
Relapsing fever	*B. recurrentis*	Tick bite, louse bite, and related species	Relapsing flu-like illness
Leptospira			
Leptospirosis	*Leptospira interrogans*	Contact with animal urine	Flu-like illness, meningitis

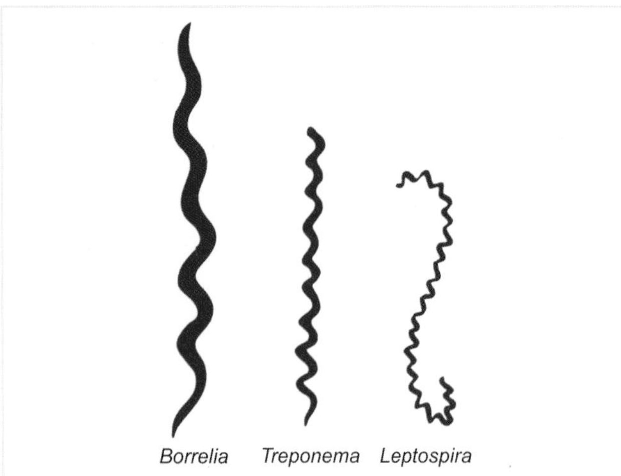

FIG. 47: Comparative morphology of different spirochetes (diagrammatic).

from an infected mother to her fetus **(congenital syphilis)**. Since the introduction of penicillin treatment, the incidence of primary and secondary syphilis has declined.

Transplacental transmission of *T. pallidum* occurs readily, and active disease during pregnancy results in congenital syphilis. However, in the past decade its incidence increased dramatically among homosexual men, particularly those with HIV infection.

Etiology

The causative spirochete, *T. pallidum* subspecies *pallidum*, hereafter simply referred as *T. pallidum*.

***T. pallidum* (Fig. 48A):**

- It is a **thin, delicate, corkscrew-shaped,** long **spirochete,** measures about 10 µm long with tapering ends and has about 10 regular spirals.
- Actively motile, showing rotation round the long axis, backward and forward motion.
- It is very fragile and is killed by soap, antiseptics, drying and cold.
- It cannot be grown in culture in artificial media.
- **Staining:** It does not stain with ordinary bacterial stains and is too slender to be seen in Gram stain. *T. pallidum* is so thin that it cannot be observed by conventional light microscopy. It requires **silver stains (silver impregnation), dark-field examination, and immunofluorescence techniques for** visualizing them. In **silver impregnation, Fontana's method** is useful for staining smears and **Levaditi's method for tissue sections.**
- **Antigenic structure:** The outer surface of the spirochete is sparse in proteins, and it is only weakly antigenic. The antigenic structure of *T. pallidum* is complex. Treponemal infection can induce at least three types of antibodies:
  i. **Reagin antibody:** It reacts in the standard or nonspecific tests for syphilis, such as Wassermann, Kahn, and VDRL. In these tests a hapten extracted from beef heart is used as the antigen. This lipid hapten is known as **cardiolipin.**
  ii. **Group antigen:** It is found in *T. pallidum* as well as in nonpathogenic cultivable treponemes like the Reiter treponeme.
  iii. **Species specific:** It is probably polysaccharide in nature. The antibody to this antigen is demonstrated by specific *T. pallidum* tests. These tests give positive results only with the sera of patients infected with pathogenic treponemes.
- **Source of infection:** An open lesion of **primary or secondary syphilis**. Lesions in the mucous membranes or skin of the genital organs, rectum, mouth, fingers, or nipples.

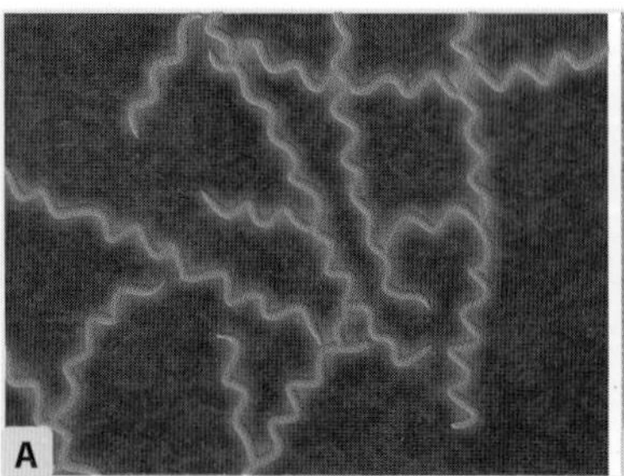

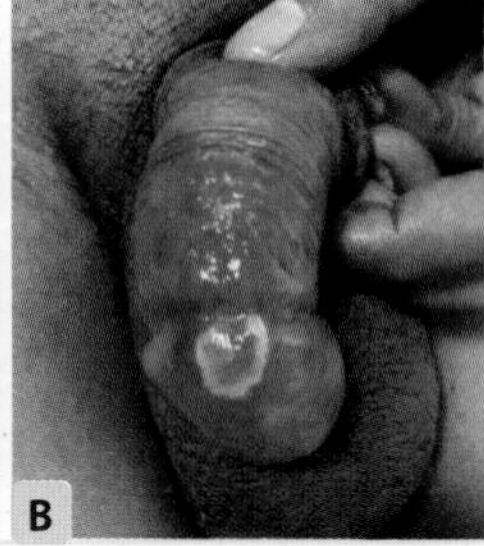

FIGS. 48A AND B: (A) Diagrammatic appearance of *Treponema pallidum* under Dark-field examination; (B) Primary chancre on glans penis.

Mode of Transmission

- **Sexual contact:** It is the usual mode of spread. Person-to-person transmission needs direct contact between a rich source of spirochetes (e.g., primary chancre) and mucous membranes or abraded skin of the genital organs, rectum, mouth, fingers, or nipples. It enters the body through a break in the skin or by penetrating mucous membranes (e.g., of the genitalia).
- **Transplacental transmission:** From mother with active disease, syphilis can be transmitted to the fetus (during pregnancy) and can produce congenital syphilis.
- **Blood transfusion.**
- **Direct contact:** With the open lesion is rare mode of transmission.

Pathogenesis

Basic microscopic lesion: Irrespective of stage, the basic microscopic lesion of syphilis consists of:

- **Mononuclear inflammatory infiltrate:** Predominantly of plasma cells and lymphocytes.
- **Proliferative endarteritis:** It affects small vessels (small arteries and arterioles) and is characterized by endothelial cell proliferation and swelling and vessel walls. These vessels are surrounded by plasma cell-rich infiltrate (**periarteritis**) which is characteristic of all stages of syphilis. There are also concentric layers of proliferating fibroblasts that produces vascular lesions with an "onion skin" appearance. Most of the pathology of syphilis is due to the ischemia produced by the vascular lesions. **Luetic vasculitis is** characteristic of syphilis.
- **Obliterative endarteritis: Lymphocytes and plasma cells infiltrate small arteries and arterioles**. It produces a characteristic obstructive vascular lesion termed as **endarteritis obliterans.** Its pathogenesis is unknown.

The immune response by host to *T. pallidum* reduces the burden of bacteria. It can resolve the local lesions but may not eliminate the systemic infection. Superficial sites of infection (chancres and rashes), *T. pallidum* induce an inflammatory response and show severe inflammatory infiltrate composed of T cells, plasma cells, and macrophages. These inflammatory cells surround *T. pallidum*. The infiltrating CD4+ T cells are Th1 cells may activate macrophages to kill *T. pallidum*. Tremayne-specific antibodies can activate complement in the lesion and opsonize the bacteria for phagocytosis by macrophages. Though it is phagocytosed, in many patients, the organism persists and proliferates despite these host responses. One of the mechanism that allows the organism to persist may be antigenic diversity. For example, a protein called TprK present in the outer membrane of *T. pallidum*, accumulates structural diversity during the course of infection through gene conversion (recombination) between silent donor sites and the *tprK* gene. The difficulty of in vitro culture of this organism has limited study of its pathogenesis. Chronic infection and inflammation cause destruction of tissue and may persist sometimes for decades.

Stages of Syphilis (Flowchart 2)

Treponema pallidum reproduces at the site of inoculation and passes to regional lymph nodes. Then it enters to the systemic circulation, and disseminates throughout the body. Syphilis can be **(1) congenital or (2) acquired**. The course of acquired syphilis is divided into three stages: (1) primary syphilis, (2) secondary syphilis, and (3) tertiary syphilis. These stages have distinct clinical and pathologic manifestations.

Primary Syphilis

This stage develops about **3 weeks** (week to 3 months) **after contact** with an infected individual and the lesion is primary chancre.

Primary chancre

It is the classical lesion of primary syphilis.

MORPHOLOGY

Sites: In primary syphilis the lesion is termed primary chancre and is located at the site of treponemal invasion. These include **penis (Fig. 48B) or scrotum** in men and **cervix, vulva,** and **vaginal wall** in women. It may also be seen in the anus or mouth in both sexes. These lesions are painless and may not be noticed by patients especially chancre in the uterine cervix, anal canal, and mouth.

Gross Features

- It is single, firm, **nontender (painless)**, slightly raised, **red papule** (chancre) up to several centimeters in diameter. As it progresses it erodes to create a clean-based shallow ulcer. The borders are firm and raised. Because of the induration adjoining (surrounding) the ulcer, it creates a button-like mass directly adjacent to the eroded skin. Induration produces little hardness; hence it is termed as **hard chancre** (**Fig. 48B**). It is **called hard chancre to distinguish it from the nonindurated lesions of "soft chancre" caused by *H. ducreyi*.** *T. pallidum* spread from these lesions throughout the body by hematologic and lymphatic dissemination.
- **Demonstration of *Treponema*:** Plenty of treponemes are present in hard chancre and can be demonstrated in the chancre by (1) silver stains (e.g., Warthin–Starry stain) or (2) immunofluorescence techniques, or (3) Dark-field examination.

Microscopy

- **Mononuclear infiltration:** Consisting of **plasma cells,** with scattered **macrophages and lymphocytes**. These cells are also seen surrounding the blood vessels (periarteritis).
- **Blood vessels with proliferative endarteritis:** It is characterized by endothelial cell proliferation and later progresses to produce intimal fibrosis. Spirochetes are concentrated in the vessel walls and in the epidermis around the ulcer.

Continued

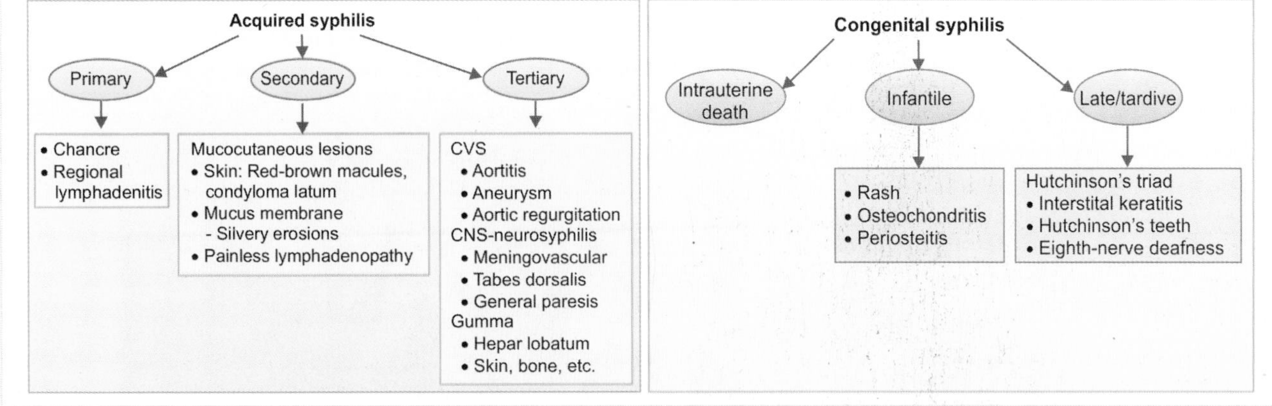

(CVS: cardiovascular system; CNS: central nervous system)

FLOWCHART 2: Various manifestations of syphilis.

Continued

Regional lymphadenitis

- It is due to nonspecific acute or chronic inflammation. Microscopically, they show plasma cell-rich infiltrates, or granulomas.
- Treponemes may spread throughout the body by blood and lymphatics even before the appearance of the chancre.

Symptoms: Usually, painless and often unnoticed.

Fate: It heals in 3–6 weeks without scarring with/without therapy.

Secondary Syphilis

This primary lesion heals spontaneously (even without treatment), but the spirochetes continues to spread throughout the body via the lymph and blood. After an asymptomatic period as long as 24 weeks, followed by the secondary stage. Thus, it develops 2–10 weeks after the primary chancre in about 75% of untreated patients. Secondary syphilis indicates dissemination of spirochetes. Its manifestations are due to systemic spread and proliferation of the spirochetes within the skin and mucocutaneous tissues. The secondary stage may be accompanied by multiorgan involvement with proliferation of organism in many organs and cause lesions. These include lymphadenitis, hepatitis, meningitis, nephritis, or chorioretinitis.

MORPHOLOGY OF SECONDARY SYPHILIS

Mucocutaneous Lesions

Secondary syphilis shows **widespread mucocutaneous lesions.** These lesions are **painless, superficial lesions, and contain spirochetes and are infectious** (similar to primary chancre). They involve mainly the **skin (palms of the hands, and soles of the feet) and mucosal surfaces (oral cavity)**.

Skin Lesions

Skin rashes: Consist of distinct (discrete) red-brown macules and measure <5 mm in diameter. However, they may be maculopapular, follicular, scaly, pustular, or annular.

Continued

Continued

Sites: They are more frequent on the palms of the hands (**Fig. 49A**), or soles of the feet and trunk.

Condylomata lata (Fig. 49B): These are broad-based, elevated exudative plaques with numerous spirochetes. They are seen in moist areas of the skin, such as the anogenital region (perineum, vulva, and scrotum), inner thighs, and axillae.

Other lesions: These include follicular syphilids (small papular lesions around hair follicles that cause loss of hair) and nummular syphilids (coin-like lesions of the face and perineum).

Mucosal Lesions

These usually occur in the mucous membranes of oral cavity or vagina or pharynx as silvery-gray superficial erosions. These lesions contain numerous *T. pallidum* and are highly infectious.

Microscopy: The mucocutaneous lesions of secondary syphilis show similar to basic microscopic lesion of syphilis (refer page 678 and 679). Thus it shows infiltration by plasma cells and endarteritis obliterans. Inflammation is usually less intense than in primary chancre.

Painless Lymphadenopathy

Characteristic changes may be observed in lymph nodes, especially epitrochlear nodes. The involved lymph nodes show thickening of the capsule, follicular hyperplasia, increased plasma cells and macrophages and luetic vasculitis. Spirochetes are plenty in the lymph nodes of secondary syphilis.

Meninges

Meninges are commonly seeded with *T. pallidum,* but it is usually asymptomatic.

Symptoms: Mild fever, malaise, and weight loss are common in secondary syphilis, which may last for several weeks. Asymptomatic neurosyphilis may develop in 8–40% of patients, and symptomatic neurosyphilis (meningitis, visual changes, or hearing changes) develops in 1–2%. The lesions of secondary syphilis last several weeks and subside (heals) even without treatment. Patient then enters the latent stage of the disease that can last for many years.

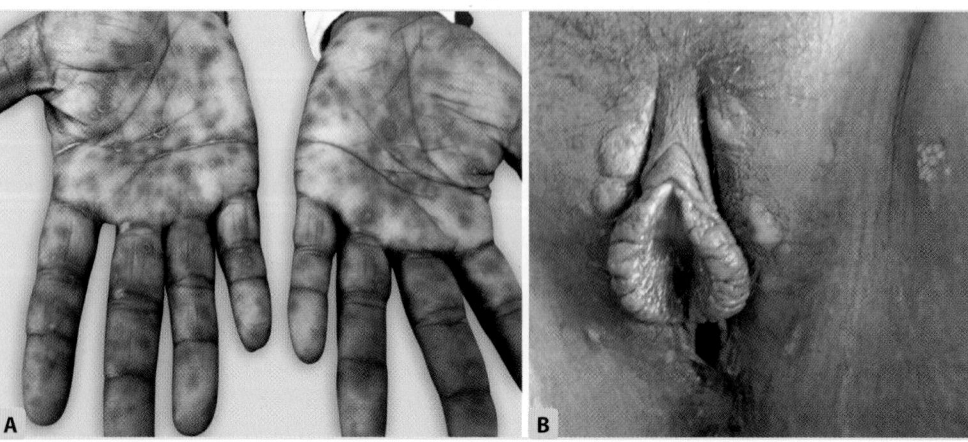

FIGS. 49A AND B: (A) Symmetrical skin rashes of secondary syphilis on palm; (B) Condyloma lata of vulva and perineum composed of broad-based elevated plaques.

Tertiary Syphilis

Q. Write short essay on tertiary syphilis.

Latent syphilis: After the lesions of secondary syphilis have subsided patients enter an asymptomatic latent phase of the disease.

- The latent period may last for 5 years or more (even decades), but spirochetes continue to multiply. During this period, the deep-seated lesions of tertiary syphilis gradually develop in one-third of untreated patients.
- This stage is rare if the patient gets adequate treatment, but can occur in about one-third of untreated patients.
- Tertiary syphilis: The fundamental vascular lesion of syphilis is obliterative endarteritis (refer basic microscopic lesion above on page 678 and 679). This is responsible for focal ischemic necrosis and for many of the processes associated with tertiary syphilis.

Manifestations: Three main manifestations of tertiary syphilis are: **cardiovascular syphilis, neurosyphilis, and so-called benign tertiary syphilis.** These three manifestations may occur alone or in combination. It usually manifests after a latent period of 5 years or more till here.

Cardiovascular syphilis

Q. Write short essay on syphilitic aneurysm.

Most **frequently involves the aorta** and known as **syphilitic aortitis.** Though exact pathogenesis of this vascular lesion is not known, the presence of intense inflammatory infiltrate along with scarcity of treponemes suggests that it may be an immune response. Obliterative endarteritis and periarteritis due to syphilis occurs in the vasa vasorum of the thoracic aorta. These vessels branch out in the adventitia and penetrate the outer and middle thirds of the aorta. They become surrounded by plasma cells, lymphocytes, and macrophages. Obliterative changes in the vasa vasorum cause focal ischemia of media. This produces focal necrosis of the media and scarring. There is loss of SMC (smooth muscle cell) and disruption and disorganization of elastic fibers. There is also inadequate or inappropriate synthesis of extracellular matrix (ECM). The aortitis (syphilitic mesoaortitis) and the intense pressure of the blood eventually forces the weakened wall of the ascending aorta and aortic arch to slowly progressively dilate to form a fusiform aneurysm. This in turn causes aortic valve insufficiency and aneurysms of the proximal (thoracic) aorta. Syphilis was once the most common cause of aortic aneurysms. Because syphilis has become less common, tertiary syphilis causing syphilitic vascular disease, including aortitis and aneurysms is rare.

MORPHOLOGY

Lesions of tertiary syphilis are most frequently observed in the aorta, the CNS, and the liver, bones, and testes.

Syphilitic aortitis (Fig. 50): It accounts for more than 80% of cases of tertiary syphilis, and affects the proximal aorta. Slowly progressive endarteritis obliterans of vasa vasorum causes occlusion of the vasa vasorum. This leads to necrosis of the aortic media associated with inflammation and is termed as syphilitic mesaortitis. The presence of adventitial lymphoplasmacytic infiltration on microscopy suggests syphilitic etiology.

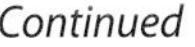

Continued

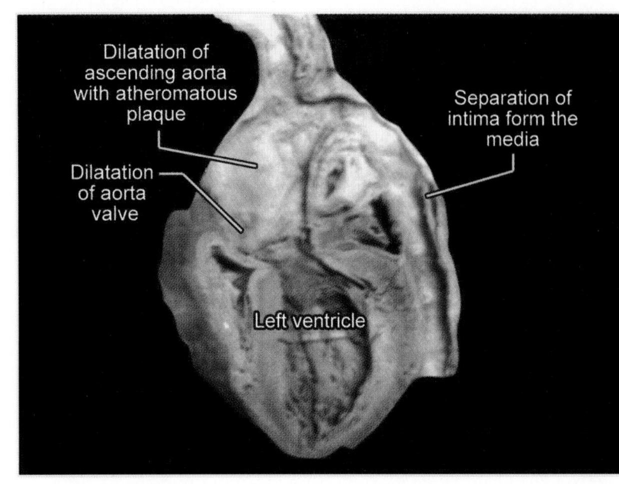

FIG. 50: Syphilitic mesoaortitis (inflammation of the tunica media), aortic aneurysm, aortic valve insufficiency (dilatation) with atherosclerosis of ascending aorta.

Continued

Saccular aneurysm and aortic valve insufficiency:

- As the syphilitic aortitis progress, there will be necrosis and scarring of the aortic media. The aortic media is gradually replaced by scar tissue. This causes loss of elasticity, strength, and flexibility (resilience) and produces gradual weakening and stretching of the aortic wall. The development of medial scarring is because the medial fibrosis inhibits development of the dissecting hematoma in aorta in syphilis.
- Gradual weakening and slow progressive dilation of the aortic root and arch. This dilates the aortic ring, separation of the valve cusps, and regurgitation of blood through the aortic valve (aortic insufficiency). The proximal aorta shows aneurysms (usually saccular). Syphilitic aneurysms develop in the ascending aorta, which is unusual site for the more common athero-sclerotic aneurysms.
- On gross examination, the depressed medial scars create a roughened intimal surface. The intima of the aorta appears rough and pitted (hollow or indentation) and it resemble a bark of tree (**tree-bark appearance**).

Myocardial ischemia: Narrowing of the coronary artery ostia (at the origin from aorta) caused by luetic vasculitis and subintimal scarring may lead to myocardial ischemia/ infarction.

Neurosyphilis

Q. Write short essay on neurosyphilis.

Neurosyphilis is another manifestation of the tertiary syphilis and occurs in only about 10% of patients with untreated infection. The slowly progressive syphilitic infection damages the **meninges, cerebral cortex, spinal cord, cranial nerves, or eyes**. Neurosyphilis **may be asymptomatic or symptomatic.**

Asymptomatic neurosyphilis It accounts for about one-third of cases of neurosyphilis. It is initially suspected on finding of CSF abnormalities. These abnormalities include pleocytosis (increased numbers of inflammatory cells namely lympho-cytes and plasma cells), raised levels of protein, or reduced glucose. These CSF changes reflect entry of bloodborne spirochetes into the meninges, leading to a transient and often asymptomatic meningitis. Antibodies stimulated by the spirochetes can also be detected in the CSF, which is the most specific test for neurosyphilis. It is necessary for all patients with tertiary syphilis to be tested for neurosyphilis even if they do not have neurologic symptoms.

Symptomatic disease Tertiary syphilis of the CNS can be subclassified according to the predominant tissue affected. Affected patients usually show an incomplete or mixed picture, most commonly the combination of tabes dorsalis and paretic disease (taboparesis). Patients with HIV are at increased risk for neurosyphilis because of impaired cell-mediated immunity. These patients particularly develop acute syphilitic meningitis or meningovascular disease and in these patients, disease progression and severity develops at an accelerated rate.

MORPHOLOGY

- **Meningovascular syphilis** (meninges): Chronic meningovascular disease is characterized by chronic meningitis and involves base of the brain, cerebral convexities, and spinal leptomeninges.
    - **Microscopy:** It may be associated with basic microscopic features of syphilis namely obliterative endarteritis (Heubner arteritis) and distinctive perivascular inflammatory reaction rich in plasma cells and lymphocytes. Cerebral gummas (plasma cell-rich mass lesions) may also develop in the meninges and extend into the adjoining parenchyma.
- **Paretic neurosyphilis (cerebral cortex):** It is caused due to invasion of the brain by *T. pallidum.* Clinically it manifests as insidious but progressive cognitive impairment associated with mood alterations (including delusions of grandeur). It may progress to severe dementia (hence called as **general paresis of the insane**). Parenchymal damage of the cerebral cortex is common in the frontal lobe, but can be observed in other areas of the cerebral cortex.
    - **Microscopy:** It is characterized by loss of neurons, proliferation of microglia, gliosis, and iron deposits. Iron deposits can be found in the perivascular region and in the neuropil, and are probably the sequelae of small bleeds resulting from microvascular damage. Iron can be demonstrated with the Prussian blue stain. **Sometimes, spirochetes can be demonstrated in tissue sections by Levaditi's method of silver** stain.
- **Tabes dorsalis (spinal cord):** It involves spinal cord and is the result of damage to the sensory axons in the dorsal roots. The impairment of spinal dorsal column function is manifested by loss of joint position sense and fine touch and ataxia (locomotor ataxia). There is also loss of pain sensation and this leads to damage to skin and joint (Charcot joints). The patient loses position sense in the legs and depends on visual cues for the position of their feet and legs in space. In darkness or when the patient's eyes are closed, they become unsteady and may even fall. This **inability to remain standing with eyes closed is called a positive Romberg sign** and indicates

Continued

Continued

severe dysfunction of posterior column of spinal cord. Other sensory disturbances include the characteristic "lightning pains"; and absence of deep tendon reflexes.
    - **Microscopy:** It shows loss of both axons and myelin in the dorsal roots (**demyelination of posterior column, dorsal root, and dorsal root ganglia).** The corresponding areas show pallor and atrophy in the dorsal columns of the spinal cord. Spirochetes are not demonstrable in the lesions of spinal cord.

Benign tertiary syphilis

Its hallmark or characteristic feature is formation of nodular lesions called **gummas**. Gummas reflect development of **delayed hypersensitivity to the spirochete**. Gummas are very rare because of the use of effective antibiotics and may be found in patients with AIDS. Gummas are usually localized lesions and do not produce any significant damage to the patient. Gumma in the bone may characteristically produce pain, tenderness, swelling, and pathologic fractures. Gummas in the skin and mucous membranes may produce nodular lesions or, rarely, destructive, ulcerative lesions.

MORPHOLOGY

Syphilitic gummas may be single or multiple.
- **White-gray and rubbery.**
- Vary in size from microscopic lesions (resembling tubercles seen in tuberculosis) to large tumor-like masses.

Site: They **can occur in any organ or tissue** but mainly involve.
- Skin, subcutaneous tissue, and the mucous membranes of the upper airway and mouth.
- Bone and joints
- In the liver, scarring as a consequence of gummas may cause a distinctive hepatic lesion known as hepar lobatum.

Microscopy: Gummas are **granulomatous lesions**. Center of the gummas shows coagulative necrosis, surrounded by plump, palisading epithelioid macrophages, occasional giant cells and fibroblasts. They are in turn surrounded by plenty of mononuclear leukocytes, mainly plasma cells. Treponemes are scant in gummas and are difficult to demonstrate.

Congenital Syphilis

Congenital syphilis is syphilis developing in the fetus and is transmitted from an infected mother to fetus.

Transplacental transmission: *T. pallidum* can cross placenta and spread from infected **mother to the fetus** (during pregnancy). Transmission occurs when **mother is suffering from primary or secondary syphilis** (when the spirochetes are abundant). It can also be transmitted by mother suffering from primary syphilis to child during delivery. Because routine serologic testing for syphilis is done in all pregnancies, congenital syphilis is rare.

In fetal infection can produce intrauterine death (stillbirth), neonatal illness or death, or progressive postnatal (tardive syphilis) disease.

Lesions of congenital syphilis: They are identical to those of acquired disease in adults. In the infected fetus, the treponeme disseminates in fetal tissues. The proliferating organisms in the infected tissues and accompanying inflammatory response injures the fetal tissues. The chronic inflammatory infiltrate shows basic microscopic features of syphilis namely infiltration of plasma cells and lymphocytes and endarteritis obliterans. Almost any tissue can be affected, but characteristically involved are the skin, bones, teeth, joints, liver, and CNS.

1. **Intrauterine death and perinatal death:** Congenital syphilis may result in intrauterine and perinatal death.
2. **Early (infantile) syphilis:** It occurs in the first 2 years of life.

MORPHOLOGY

Lesions are similar to that of acquired secondary syphilis in adults.

- **Nose:** It usually manifest in the first few months of life by a conspicuous mucopurulent **nasal discharge** and congestion (**snuffles**). The nasal mucosa appears edematous and may ulcerate, leading to nosebleeds.
- **Skin:** A maculopapular rash is common early in congenital syphilis. The rash is more severe than that of adult secondary syphilis. It produces a **desquamating or bullous eruption/rash** mainly in the hands, feet (palms and soles as in secondary syphilis of adults), and around the mouth and anus. It can lead to epidermal sloughing of the skin. However, it may cover the entire body or any part of it. Cracks and fissures **(rhagades)** may be seen around the mouth, anus, and vulva. Flat raised plaques **(condylomata lata)** may develop around the anus and female genitalia early or after a few years.
- **Skeletal abnormalities:** These are common and **affect all bones, but lesions of the nose and lower legs are most peculiar.**
  - **Syphilitic osteochondritis:** Inflammation of bone and cartilage is more distinctive in the nose. Destruction of the vomer causes collapse of the nasal bridge and later results in characteristic flattening of the nose, so-called **saddle nose deformity**.
  - **Syphilitic periostitis:** Periosteal inflammation with excessive formation of new bone **(periostitis)** is common. It involves the anterior tibia and causes distinctive anterior bowing or outward curving **(saber shins)**.
  - **Other changes:** Widespread disturbance in endochondral bone formation is also seen. There is widening of the epiphyses as the cartilage overgrows, and displaced islands of cartilage may be observed within the metaphysis.
- **Liver:** It is usually severely affected in congenital syphilis and produces neonatal hepatitis. There will be hepatomegaly and liver shows diffuse fibrosis portal tracts and around individual liver cells or groups of hepatocytes. It divides the hepatic cells into small nests. Occasionally hepatic gummas (i.e., focal lesions resembling granulomas) may occur and heal with dense scars. Retraction of fibrous tissue and scars produces deep clefts and a gross pseudolobation of the liver. This condition is called as **hepar lobatum.** It should not be confused with cirrhosis. This is accompanied by the

Continued

Continued

characteristic lymphoplasmacytic infiltrate and vascular changes of syphilis.

- **Lungs:** They show distinctive pneumonitis with diffuse interstitial fibrosis. In the syphilitic stillborn, the lungs appear pale, hypocrepitant/airless and is termed as **pneumonia alba**.
- **Nervous system:** It is commonly involved, with symptoms that may start during infancy or after 1 year. **Meningitis** may cause convulsions, mild hydrocephalus, and mental retardation.
- **Other organs:** The generalized spirochetemia similar to that of secondary syphilis may lead to diffuse interstitial inflammatory reactions in practically any other organ. These include the pancreas, kidneys, heart, spleen, thymus, endocrine organs, and CNS. Anemia and lymphadenopathy may also occur in early congenital syphilis.

3. **Late (tardive) syphilis: Manifests 2 years after birth, and about 50% of untreated children with neonatal syphilis will develop late manifestations.**

MORPHOLOGY

Distinctive late manifestations of congenital syphilis are **Hutchinson's triad.** It consists of:

1. **Interstitial keratitis:** Progressive corneal vascularization **(interstitial keratitis)** occurs as early as 4 years and as late as 20 years of age. The cornea finally scars and becomes opaque.
2. **Hutchinson's teeth:** The permanent incisors appear like small screwdrivers or small peg-shaped with notches in the enamel and molars malformed **(mulberry molars).**
3. **Eighth-nerve deafness**

Apart from interstitial keratitis, other ocular changes may also be present and include choroiditis and abnormal retinal pigmentation. **Meningovascular syphilis** is common and may lead to eighth-nerve deafness, optic nerve atrophy, mental retardation, paresis, and other complications.

Laboratory Diagnosis

Laboratory diagnosis consists of demonstration of the spirochetes under the microscope and serological test to demonstrate antibodies in serum or CSF.

Microscopic Demonstration

Spirochetes can be detected microscopically from primary and secondary lesions of acquired syphilis and superficial lesions in cases of congenital syphilis. Smears are prepared from exudate and are examined by following methods:

- **Dark-field illumination (dark ground examination):** Though it is useful, it has low sensitivity.
- **Silver impregnation:** Smears can be stained by Fontana's method and tissue sections by Levaditi's method.
- **Immunofluorescent stain: Direct fluorescent antibody test for *T. pallidum* (DFA-TP)** is a better and safer method for microscopic diagnosis. DFA-TP test is done using fluorescent tagged anti *T. pallidum* antiserum. The test is more reliable because of use of specific monoclonal antibody.

Serological Tests

Syphilis is usually diagnosed serologically and these tests form the mainstay (backbone) of laboratory diagnosis of syphilis. Infection with *T. pallidum* evoke two kinds of antibodies: (1) antitreponemal antibodies that are specific to the treponemal surface proteins and (2) nontreponemal antibodies (reagin), that are directed against normal phospholipid components of mammalian membranes, such as cardiolipin. Accordingly, serological tests for syphilis can be classified as nontreponemal antibody tests and antitreponemal antibody tests.

Nontreponemal antibody tests

- **Nature of antibody:** These tests measure antibody to **cardiolipin-cholesterol-lecithin antigen.** This antigen is present in both host tissues and *T. pallidum.*
- **Tests for detection:** These tests are called as standard tests for syphilis (STS). In these tests antibodies are detected by two methods namely (1) the rapid plasma reagin **(RPR)** and (2) VDRL tests.
- **Advantages:** They are routinely used because of low cost, easy method of testing, and quantifiable results that can be used to follow response to treatment.
- **Disadvantages:** Nontreponemal assays are nonspecific.
    - **False-positive VDRL test:** Because the cardiolipin antigen is present both in *T. pallidum* and in host tissues, the STS may give rise to **biological false positive (BFP) reactions.** It is the major disadvantage and false-positive reactions can be observed in certain acute infections, collagen vascular diseases (e.g., systemic lupus erythematosus), drug addiction, pregnancy, hypergammaglobulinemia of any cause, and LL.

Treponemal antibody tests

These measure antibodies that react specifically with *T. pallidum*. Automation of these complex tests is available in the market. These assays include:

- **Fluorescent treponemal antibody absorption test** (FTA): Currently used modification of FTA test is the PTA-absorption **(FTAABS) test.** It is accepted as a standard reference test.
- ***T. pallidum* enzyme immunoassays (EIA)** using *T. pallidum* antigens are commercially available. This is a rapid agglutination using latex particles coated with three immunodominant proteins of *T. pallidum,* obtained by recombinant technology. It is claimed to be as specific as TPHA, and more sensitive.
- ***T. pallidum* hemagglutination assay (TPHA):** This assay for *T. pallidum* antibodies uses tanned RBCs sensitized with a sonicated (ultrasonic vibration to fragment cells) extract of *T. pallidum* as antigen. The procedure currently in use is a **microhemagglutination test** (MHA-TP), which is capable of being automated.
- ***T. pallidum* immobilization (TPI)** was once considered the **gold standard** in syphilis serology. The TPI test has now been supplanted by specific and much simpler other tests such as FTA-ABS and TPHA.

Advantages: Antitreponemal antibody tests are **more specific than reagin-based tests**.

Disadvantages: These tests remain positive during and after successful treatment. Hence, they are not useful for monitoring therapy.

Rapid POC (point of care) tests: These can be done by using fingerstick blood (though serum shows higher sensitivity). These are inexpensive, and are simple and do not need highly trained technologists.

Rapid tests and PCR assays are not commonly used due to lower sensitivities and specificities.

Significance of serological tests

- **Sensitivity and stage of syphilis:**
    - Both treponemal and nontreponemal antibody tests are only moderately sensitive (~70–85%) for primary syphilis but are very sensitive (>95%) for secondary syphilis.
    - Treponemal tests are very sensitive for tertiary and latent syphilis. In contrast, nontreponemal antibody titers gradually fall. Hence, nontreponemal tests are less sensitive for tertiary or latent syphilis.
- **Monitoring the treatment:** The levels of nontreponemal antibody fall with successful treatment of syphilis. Hence, changes in their titers can be used to monitor therapy. Treponemal tests cannot be quantified and remain positive, even after successful therapy.
- **Screening and confirmation:** Both nontreponemal or treponemal tests can be used for initial screening for syphilis. However, positive results of one type of test should be confirmed by performing a test of the other type (e.g., if nontreponemal test is positive confirm it with a treponemal test and *vice versa*). Confirmatory testing is required due to occurrence of false-positive results in both nontreponemal and treponemal tests. Causes of false-positive results in the both types of tests include pregnancy, autoimmune diseases, and infections other than syphilis.

Jarisch–Herxheimer reaction: Treatment of syphilitic patients having a high bacterial load, by antibiotics can cause a massive release of endotoxins, and cytokine that may manifest with high fever, rigors, hypotension, and leukopenia. This syndrome is called the Jarisch–Herxheimer reaction, which can develop not only in syphilis but also in other spirochetal diseases, such as **Lyme disease**.

Examination of CSF: In latent and cardiovascular syphilis, CSF should be examined because of coexistence of asymptomatic neurological disease. CSF should be examined in neurosyphilis and in both early and late congenital syphilis.

NONVENEREAL TREPONEMATOSES

Treponemes, in tropical and subtropical regions, cause nonvenereal, chronic diseases similar to *T. pallidum.* Like syphilis, they develop following inoculation of the treponeme into mucocutaneous surfaces. They also develop well-defined clinical and pathologic stages, including a primary lesion at the site of inoculation, secondary skin eruptions, a latent period, and a tertiary late stage.

Yaws

Yaws is a tropical disease caused by *T. pertenue.* It occurs in poor rural populations in warm, humid areas of tropical region (e.g., Africa, South America, Southeast Asia, and Oceania). It mainly affects children and adolescents in tropical regions.

Mode of transmission: Skin-to-skin contact and enters through breaks or abrasions in skin.

Incubation period: 2–5 weeks after exposure.

MORPHOLOGY

A single "mother yaw" appears at the site of inoculation and usually observed on an exposed part. It starts as a papule and evolves to a 2–5 cm "raspberry-like" papilloma. In the secondary or disseminated stage, similar but smaller skin eruption of yaws appears on other parts of the skin. Painful papillomas on the soles of the feet make the patients to walk on the side of their feet like a crab. This condition is called as **"crab yaw."**

Microscopy: The mother yaw and secondary lesions in the skin show epidermis with hyperkeratosis and papillary acanthosis. It is accompanied by severe neutrophilic infiltrate in the epidermis. The epidermis at the apex of the papilloma undergoes lysis and form a shallow ulcer. This is accompanied by infiltration of plasma cells in the upper dermis. Numerous spirochetes can be demonstrated in the dermal papillae.

Treponemes are carried through the blood and disseminate to bones, lymph nodes, and skin. Treponemes grow in these sites during a latent period of 5 or more years. In tertiary stage, it can produce cutaneous gummas, which are destructive to the face and upper airway. Periostitis of the tibia can cause "saber shins" or "boomerang legs."

Bejel

Bejel (also known as "endemic syphilis") is found in Africa, western Asia, and Australia.

Causative agent: It is caused by *T. pallidum* subspecies *endemicum*. It is morphologically and serologically indistinguishable from *T. pallidum* causing syphilis.

Mode of transmission: It is transmitted from an infected infant to the breast of the mother. It may also be transmitted from mouth to mouth or from utensils to the mouth.

MORPHOLOGY

Primary lesions occur on the breast of nursing mother and it is rare in other sites. Secondary lesions in the mouth are similar to the mucosal lesions of secondary syphilis. It may spread from the upper airway to the larynx. Lesions may be seen in the perineum and bone, and gummas may develop in the breast, skin, airways, and bone.

Pinta

Pinta (term derived from the Spanish for "painted" or "blemish") is a tropical skin disease caused by *T. carateum*. It shows variably colored spots on the skin. Pinta has three stages and all the lesions are limited to the skin and tend to merge. Transmission is by skin-to-skin inoculation and usually requires a long intimate contact with an infected person.

Lyme Disease

Q. Write short essay on Lyme disease.

Lyme disease is an arthropod-borne infection caused by large, microaerophilic **spirochetes** belonging to **the genus *Borrelia*.** It **can be localized or disseminated with a tendency to cause persistent joint disturbances (chronic arthritis).**

Epidemiology: Lyme disease was first described in the mid-1970s in patients from the town Lyme, Connecticut, where there was an epidemic of arthritis associated with skin erythema. It is now recognized in many other areas.

Etiology: The three pathogenic genospecies of *Borrelia* that cause Lyme diseases are *B. burgdorferi* (major cause), *B. afzelii*, and *B. garinii*. *Borrelia* has few proteins with biosynthetic activity and is dependent on its host for most of its nutritional needs.

Mode of transmission: The spirochetes are **transmitted from its animal reservoir by the bite of the minute *Ixodes* tick.** This pinhead-sized tick is found in wooded areas, where it usually feeds on mice (rodents) and deer.

Clinical Features

At the site of inoculation, *B. burgdorferi* reproduces locally. Then it spreads to regional lymph nodes and disseminates throughout the body via the bloodstream. Like other spirochetal diseases, Lyme disease is a chronic systemic infection occurring in stages, with remissions and exacerbations. It involves multiple organ systems and begins with a characteristic skin lesion and later manifests as cardiac, neurologic, or joint disturbances. It can be divided into three clinical stages.

Stage 1 (early localized infection): It begins 3–35 days after the tick bite. In this stage, the disease is localized and spirochetes multiply and spread in the dermis at the site of a tick bite (site of inoculation). This causes an expanding area as **erythematous macule or papule** that grows into an erythematous patch 3–7 cm in diameter. It is usually extremely red at its periphery, with pale center (central clearing) and give an annular appearance. This early characteristic skin lesion is termed as **erythema migrans (erythema chronicum migrans)**. This may be accompanied by fever and lymphadenopathy. The rash disappears spontaneously within 4–12 weeks.

Microscopically, the skin and synovium shows a chronic inflammatory infiltrate, composed of lymphocytes and plasma cells. This stage manifests by fever, fatigue, headache, arthralgias, and regional lymphadenopathy.

Stage 2 (early disseminated infection): The second stage begins weeks to months after the skin lesion. During this stage, spirochetes spread hematogenously throughout the body. It causes **secondary annular skin lesions, lymphadenopathy, migratory joint and muscle** (musculoskeletal) **pain, cardiac arrhythmias** (particularly atrioventricular block), and **neurologic abnormalities** (most commonly meningitis and facial nerve palsies). *B. afzelii* is associated with borrelial lymphocytoma, characterized by blue to red swelling of the earlobe or nipple, with lymphocytic infiltration.

Stage 3 (late persistent infection): The third stage of Lyme disease manifests many months to years after the tick bite. It mainly produces **joint, skin, and neurologic abnormalities.** *B. burgdorferi* usually characterized by a chronic arthritis (arthralgia) sometimes with severe damage (severe arthritis) to large joints especially the knee. Less often, patients will have mild to debilitating polyneuropathy and encephalitis. In patients who die of the disease, *Borrelia* are seen at autopsy in almost all organs, including the skin, myocardium, liver, CNS, and musculoskeletal system.

Pathogenesis

Borrelia burgdorferi does not secrete endotoxin or exotoxins that can damage the host. Probably most of the pathological features of infection are **secondary to the immune response** against the *Borrelia* and the **accompanying inflammation**.

- **Immune response:** The bacterial lipoproteins bind to TLR2 on macrophages and stimulate the initial immune response. Macrophages release proinflammatory cytokines (IL-6 and TNF) and generate bactericidal reactive nitrogen intermediates. This reduces but usually does not eliminate the infection. Chronic manifestations of Lyme disease (e.g., late arthritis) may be caused by the immune response against some unknown, bacterial antigen that cross reacts with a self-antigen.
- **Inflammation:** T cells and cytokines trigger the inflammatory lesions.

Borrelia-specific antibodies develop 2–4 weeks after infection trigger complement-mediated phagocytosis and killing of the bacteria. Escape of destruction is achieved by the following ways:

- *Borrelia burgdorferi* escapes the antibody response and survive by undergoing antigenic variation.
- *Borrelia burgdorferi* has a plasmid with a single promoter sequence and multiple coding sequences for an antigenic surface protein, VlsE. One of the coding sequences of the multiple coding sequences of VlsE can move into position next to the promoter and be expressed. Thus, when an antibody response to one VlsE protein is mounted, bacteria express an alternate VlsE protein. Thus it can escape immune recognition.

MORPHOLOGY

Skin lesions caused by *B. burgdorferi*: They show edema and a lymphocytic-plasma cell infiltrate.

Synovium and joints:

- During early Lyme arthritis, the histopathological features of synovium are indistinguishable from that of early rheumatoid arthritis. These include villous hypertrophy, synovial hyperplasia, and abundant lymphocytes and plasma cells infiltrate in the subsynovium. A **distinctive feature of Lyme arthritis is an arteritis**. This characteristically produces **onion skin-like lesions** resembling those seen in lupus.
- In late Lyme disease, extensive erosion of the cartilage in large joints may occur.

CSF: In Lyme meningitis, the CSF shows increased cells due to a marked lymphoplasmacytic infiltrate, and it contains antispirochete IgGs.

Diagnosis: Main method of diagnosis is by serology. Antibody titers (initially IgM, later IgG) against the organism is the most important method to establish the diagnosis. PCR can also be performed on infected tissue.

Leptospirosis

Q. Write short essay on leptospirosis.

Leptospirosis is a globally important zoonotic disease caused by the spirochetes of the genus *Leptospira* namely *Leptospira interrogans*.

Synonyms: Autumn fever, seven-day fever, Canefield fever, Swamp fever, Weil disease, rice-field fever, Swineherd's disease.

Source of Infection

Leptospirosis is **ubiquitous in wildlife and in many domestic animals**. Reservoirs of organisms include **rodents** (most frequent), **foxes, skunks, dogs, and domestic livestock**. Many **animals shed the organism into the urine in massive numbers** for long period but infection is asymptomatic in these animals. Outbreaks of leptospirosis may occur with flooding.

Mode of Transmission

- **Direct contact:** Human infection occur either by direct contact (especially slaughterhouse workers and trappers) **with urine or tissue of an infected animal** (e.g., infected rats). Transmission may occur through cuts, abraded skin, and mucous membranes (nasopharynx, oral mucosa, conjunctiva, and vagina). Prolonged immersion in contaminated water or mud favors invasion, as the spirochete can survive in fresh water for months and for up to 24 hours in sea water. Warm and moist environments favor survival of the spirochetes, the incidence of leptospirosis is higher in the tropics.
- **Ingestion of contaminated water, soil, or vegetation**.

Incubation period: It is usually 1–2 weeks (7–14 days) but ranges from 1 to 30 days.

Pathogenesis (Fig. 51)

In more severe infections, typically illness of leptospirosis has two phases (biphasic disease).

1. **Leptospiremic** (initial/first) **phase:** It is named so because leptospirae are present in the blood and CSF during this phase. After entry of the organisms into the human, they proliferate and disseminate through blood into all organs (leptospiremic phase). The organisms can survive in the nonimmune host. They evade complement-mediated killing, resist ingestion and killing by neutrophils, monocytes, and macrophages. Patient present with an abrupt onset of fever, shaking chills, headache, and myalgias. Symptoms subside after 1–2 weeks, as the leptospires disappear from the blood and bodily fluids. **Conjunctival suffusion/congestion** (redness or hyperemia without exudate) without conjunctivitis (**Fig. 52**) is very helpful, notable sign for detecting the disease.
2. **Immune** (second) **phase:** It begins within 3 days of the end of the leptospiremic phase. During the immune phase, the IgM antibodies appear and leptospires disappear from the blood. However, the organism persists in various organs including liver, lung, kidney, heart, and brain. The earlier symptoms recur, and patient also develops signs of meningeal irritation. During this period, the CSF shows a prominent pleocytosis. In severe cases, jaundice

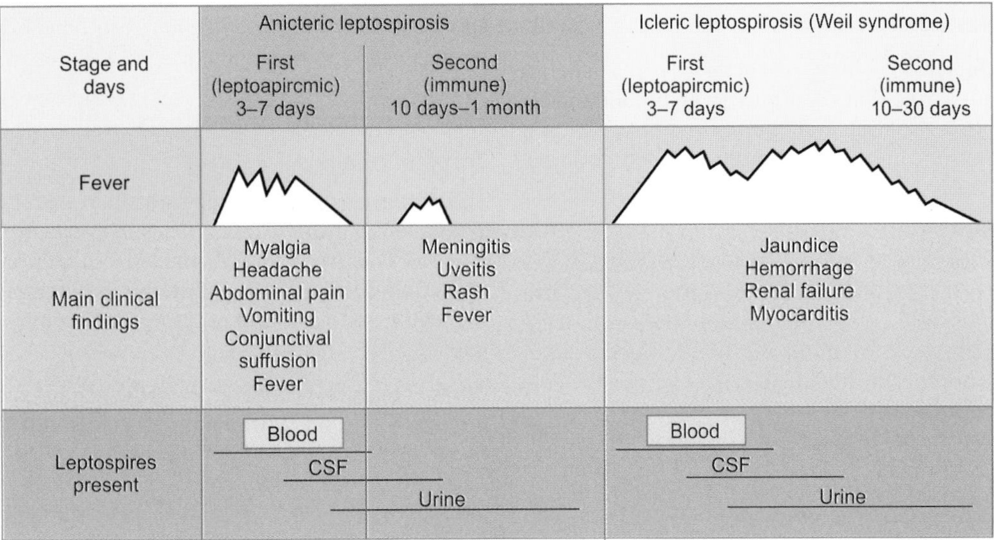

Anicteric leptospirosis
Icleric leptospirosis (Weil syndrome)
Stage and days
First (leptoapircmic) 3–7 days
Second (immune) 10 days–1 month
First (leptoapircmic) 3–7 days
Second (immune) 10–30 days
Fever
Main clinical findings
Myalgia
Headache
Abdominal pain
Vomiting
Conjunctival suffusion
Fever
Meningitis
Uveitis
Rash
Fever
Jaundice
Hemorrhage
Renal failure
Myocarditis
Leptospires present
Blood
CSF
Urine

(CSF: cerebrospinal fluid)

FIG. 51: Pathogenesis of leptospirosis.

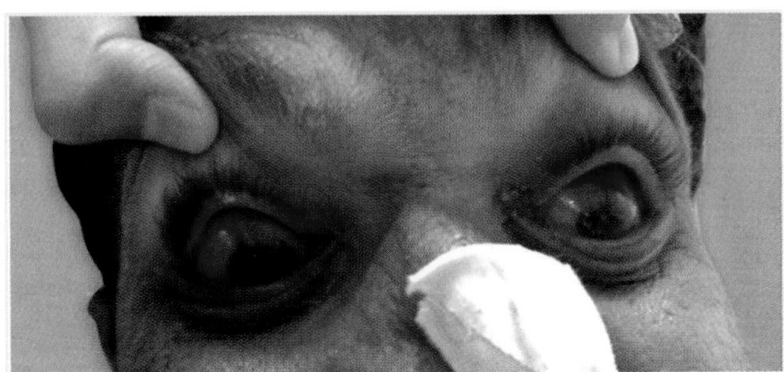

FIG. 52: Conjunctival suffusion and jaundice in leptospirosis.

may develop followed by hepatic and renal failure and there will be widespread hemorrhages and shock. This severe form of leptospirosis has historically been referred to as **Weil disease.** Weil disease or syndrome is not a specific subgroup of leptospirosis, but indicates severe leptospirosis. It can develop during the second (immune) phase of leptospirosis or as a progressive illness. It is dramatic life-threatening event characterized by jaundice, hemorrhagic manifestations, renal failure, and acute respiratory distress syndrome (ARDS), etc.

Prognosis: Most of the patients (90%) with leptospirosis have mild, self-limited, febrile disease and resolves within a week without sequelae. Untreated Weil disease has a mortality rate of 5–30%. More severe infections may result in hepatic and renal failure, which may be fatal.

MORPHOLOGY

Autopsy

General features: Many tissues show bile staining and many organs show hemorrhages. The main lesion is a **diffuse vasculitis and injury to the capillaries.**

Continued

Continued

Liver: It shows lobular disarray, erythrophagocytosis by Kupffer cells, minimal necrosis of hepatocytes, neutrophils in the sinusoids, and portal tracts with a mixed inflammatory cell infiltrate.

Kidney: Renal tubules are swollen and lining cells show necrosis. Numerous spirochetes are seen in the lumen of tubules particularly in bile-stained casts in the tubules.

Investigations

Urine examination: During early part of the illness shows microscopic hematuria, pyuria, and proteinuria. The tightly coiled spirochete may be visualized in the urine by phase contrast or dark field microscopy.

Blood:

- **Total leukocyte count** may vary, but polymorphonuclear leukocytosis (neutrophilia of >70%) with shift to left is very frequent.
- **Anemia** may develop due to intravascular hemolysis, azotemia, and blood loss caused by hemorrhage.
- **Thrombocytopenia** in severe infection.
- **Elevated markers of inflammation: Raised erythrocyte sedimentation rate** and **C-reactive protein** level.
- **Raised blood urea nitrogen (BUN) and hyperkalemia** occur with renal failure.
- **Coagulation studies** may show a prolonged prothrombin time which is reversible with vitamin K administration.
- **Creatinine phosphokinase (CPK)** are elevated in 50% of patients during the first week of illness. This helps in differentiating leptospirosis from viral hepatitis.
- **Liver function tests** show raised aspartate transaminase (AST) and alanine aminotransferase (ALT) (up to five times normal), conjugated hyperbilirubinemia, and raised alkaline phosphatase. Marked elevations of bilirubin and

mild elevated transaminases level are characteristically found in Weil syndrome.

CSF examination: It may be abnormal in up to 90% of patients. Cell counts are increased (but <500/mm^3) with predominance of neutrophils. Protein levels may be normal or raised and glucose level is normal. In severe jaundice, xanthochromia can be seen.

Serological tests:
- **IgM antibodies** may be detected in blood by microscopic agglutination test (MAT), during the immune (second) phase of illness. IgM ELISA and immunofluorescent techniques are easy to perform and rapid immunochromatographic tests are specific but are of moderate sensitivity in the first week of disease.
- **Demonstration of leptospiral antigen** by radioimmunoassay or ELISA.

Culture: Diagnosis can be confirmed by culture (on Fletcher's medium) of the blood or CSF during the first week (leptospiremic phase) of illness or of the urine from the second week onward. It may take several weeks.

Detection of leptospiral DNA by PCR in blood during early symptomatic disease and in urine from the eighth day of illness.

Relapsing Fever

Relapsing fever is an acute, febrile, septicemic illness caused by infection with any of several species of *Borrelia* spirochetes. Its characteristic clinical presentation is two or more episodes of fever separated by varying periods of well-being (hence termed relapsing fever). There are two main types of relapsing fever namely epidemic and endemic.
- **Epidemic relapsing fever:** It is caused by *B. recurrentis*. Humans are the only reservoir of this spirochete. It is transmitted by the bite of an infected louse namely *Pediculus humanus* (louse-borne relapsing fever).
- **Endemic relapsing fever:** It is produced by a number of *Borrelia* species. It is transferred from rodents and other animals by the bite of an infected tick (tick-borne relapsing fever).

MORPHOLOGY

Spleen: In severe and fatal infections, the spleen is enlarged. Spleen shows miliary microabscesses. Tangled aggregates of spirochetes are formed around the central necrotic material.

Liver: Central and mid zones of the liver show infiltration by lymphocytes and neutrophils. Spirochetes are found lying free in the sinusoids.
Focal hemorrhages develop in many organs.

Clinical features: It presents with arthralgias, lethargy, fever, headache, and myalgias within 1–2 weeks after a bite of an infected arthropod. The fever disappears suddenly within 3–9 days, only to begin after 7–10 days. During the afebrile period, spirochetes disappear from the blood. This episode of relapse continues and with each relapse, symptoms become milder and the duration of illness becomes shorter. In severe cases, the initial episode of fever may be associated with a rash, meningitis, myocarditis, liver failure, and coma. The liver and spleen show enlargement. There are petechiae in the skin, hemorrhages in the conjunctiva and abdominal tenderness.

Fusospirochetal Infections

Tropical Phagedenic Ulcer

Tropical phagedenic (rapid spreading and sloughing) ulcer also called as **tropical foot** is caused by two organisms namely *Bacillus fusiformis* and *T. vincentii*. It produces a painful, necrotizing lesion of the skin and subcutaneous tissues of the leg in tropical climates. Malnutrition may predispose to infection.

Clinical features: Tropical phagedenic ulcer usually starts on the skin at the site of trauma in the leg and develops rapidly. The surface sloughs and forms a painful ulcer. The ulcer has raised borders and a cup-shaped crater, which contains a gray, putrid exudate. The ulcer may be deep enough to expose the underlying bone and tendons. The margin of the ulcer may show fibrosis, but complete healing of ulcer may be delayed for years. Complications of ulcer include secondary infection, osteomyelitis of tibia and squamous cell carcinoma.

Noma

Noma (gangrenous stomatitis, cancrum oris) is characterized by rapid progressive necrosis of soft tissues and bones usually involving the mouth and face. Less commonly, it may involve other sites (e.g., chest, limbs, and genitalia). It is a destructive lesion that affects malnourished children in the tropical region and many of them are debilitated by recent infections (e.g., measles, malaria, and leishmaniasis). Organisms usually predominate in these lesions include *T. vincentii, B. fusiformis, Bacteroides* species, and *Corynebacterium* species.

Clinical features: Initially it starts as a small, unilateral, papule, usually on the cheek opposite the molars or premolars. This quickly progress to a large, painful destructive, disfiguring malodorous ulcer. The advanced ulcers show necrosis of skin, muscle, and adipose tissue. The underlying bone may be exposed. Without treatment, patients usually die.

ANAEROBIC BACTERIAL INFECTIONS

Many anaerobic bacteria constitute normal microbiota in sites of the body where the oxygen levels are low. These anaerobic microbiotas can cause disease (e.g., abscesses or peritonitis) when they gain entry into normally sterile sites or when the balance of individual is upset resulting in overgrowth of pathogenic anaerobes (e.g., *C. difficile* colitis with antibiotic treatment). Environmental anaerobes also can cause disease (tetanus, botulism, and gas gangrene).

Abscesses

Localized accumulation of pus is called abscess.

Causes: Usually abscess is caused by commensal bacteria from adjacent sites (oropharynx, intestine, and female genital tract). Hence, the species found in an abscess usually reflect the normal microbiota in that site. The infections causing abscesses are usually due to mixed anaerobic and facultative aerobic bacterial infections. Most anaerobes that produce abscesses are part of the normal microbiota. Hence, these organisms do not produce significant toxins.

- **Head and neck abscesses:** The bacteria found in head and neck abscesses originate from oral and pharyngeal microbiota. Common commensal anaerobes include the gram-negative bacilli *Prevotella* species and *Porphyromonas* species. These commensal organisms may be mixed with the facultative *S. aureus* and *S. pyogenes. Fusobacterium necrophorum* is an oral commensal that causes Lemierre syndrome (characterized by infection of the lateral pharyngeal space and septic thrombosis of jugular vein).
- **Abdominal abscesses:** These are caused by the commensal anaerobes of the GI tract. These include gram-positive *Peptostreptococcus* species and *Clostridium* species, as well as gram-negative *Bacteroides fragilis* and *Escherichia coli.*
- **Genital tract infections in women:** For example, Bartholin cyst abscesses and tubo-ovarian abscesses may be caused by anaerobic gram-negative bacilli, such as *Prevotella* species, often mixed with *E. coli* or *S. agalactiae.*

MORPHOLOGY

Abscesses resemble those of the common pyogenic infections. But abscess caused due to anaerobes contain discolored and foul-smelling pus. The abscess is usually poorly walled off.

- **Microscopy:** It consists of pus, which is formed by masses of dying and dead neutrophils and liquefactive necrosis of the involved tissue. Gram stain reveals mixed infection with gram-positive and gram-negative rods and gram-positive cocci mixed with neutrophils.

Clostridial Infections

Clostridium species are gram-positive bacilli that grow under anaerobic conditions (obligate anaerobic bacilli). They produce spores (spore-forming) and are present in the soil. Four types of disease are caused by *Clostridium* species. **The neurotoxins are produced by *C. botulinum* and *C. tetani*.** They **inhibit release of neurotransmitters and lead to paralysis.**

Gas Gangrene (Clostridial Myonecrosis)

Gas gangrene is a necrotizing, gas-forming infection that begins in contaminated wounds and spreads rapidly to adjacent tissues. It can be fatal within hours of onset. *C. perfringens* is the most common cause of gas gangrene, but other clostridial species (e.g., *C. septicum*) occasionally produce the disease. They cause cellulitis and myonecrosis of traumatic (penetrating wounds) and surgical wounds. Spontaneous gas gangrene due to *C. septicum* can develop with an underlying malignancy. Uterine myonecrosis is usually associated with illegal (criminal) abortions. Mild food poisoning and infection of the small bowel is associated with ischemia or neutropenia and this may lead to severe sepsis.

Incubation period: 2–4 days after injury.

Ingestion of food contaminated with *C. perfringens* causes a brief diarrhea. Spores, usually in contaminated meat, survive cooking, and the organism proliferates in cooling food. *C. perfringens* enterotoxin forms pores in the epithelial cell membranes, lysing the cells and disrupting tight junctions between epithelial cells.

Molecular pathogenesis: Gas gangrene develops following deposition of anaerobic *C. perfringens* into tissue. *C. perfringens* does not grow in the presence of oxygen. Hence, tissue death is essential for growth of the bacteria in the host. Growth of clostridial needs extensive devitalized tissue (e.g., severe penetrating trauma, injuries during war, and septic abortions). If wounds are debrided promptly, myonecrosis due to Clostridia rarely occurs. These bacteria release collagenase and hyaluronidase. These enzymes degrade ECM proteins and contribute to bacterial invasiveness. But the most powerful virulence factors are the many toxins produce by them. *C. perfringens* secretes 14 toxins, the most important being α-toxin. This toxin (myotoxin) has many actions. Clostridial myotoxin is a phospholipase and can destroy lecithin which is a major component of cell membranes. Thus, it destroys cell membranes of red cells, leukocytes, platelets, and muscle cells, causing myonecrosis (of previously healthy muscle). It has also a sphingomyelinase activity and this can damage nerve sheath.

MORPHOLOGY

Gross

Clostridial cellulitis

It originates in infected wounds. It can be differentiated from infection caused by pyogenic cocci because of its foul odor, thin, discolored exudate, and the relatively sudden and wide destruction of tissue.

Microscopy: The amount of tissue necrosis is disproportionate to the number of neutrophils and gram-positive bacteria present. Clostridial cellulitis usually has granulation tissue at its borders, is treatable by debridement and antibiotics.

Clostridial gas gangrene

It develops 1–3 days after injury and is life-threatening. It is characterized by severe edema (due to extensive fluid exudate causes swelling of the affected region), large bullous vesicles on the overlying skin that rupture and enzymatic necrosis of involved muscle cells. Involved tissues at the site of wound rapidly become mottled (marked with spots or smears of color) and becomes frankly necrotic. The muscle tissue in the site may even liquefy. Gas bubbles caused by bacterial fermentation appear within the gangrenous tissues. It expands the underlying soft tissues and the skin covering the site becomes tense. As the infection progresses, the inflamed muscles become soft, blue-black, friable, and semifluid. This is due to the massive proteolytic action of the released bacterial enzymes.

Microscopy: The involved region shows extensive necrosis of tissue (**myonecrosis**) with dissolution of the cells, hemolysis, and marked vascular injury with thrombosis. Characteristically, there is lack of inflammatory cells (e.g., neutrophils), because of their destruction by the myotoxin. Affected tissues usually contain typical, lozenge-shaped, gram-positive rods.

In individuals with neutropenia, *C. perfringens* is associated with dusk-colored, wedge-shaped infarcts in the small bowel. Regardless of the site of entry, when *C. perfringens* disseminates through blood, it forms widespread gas bubbles.

Clinical features: It presents with sudden, severe pain at the wound site. The affected region is tender and edematous. The skin darkens due to hemorrhage and cutaneous necrosis. The lesion shows a thick, smelly serosanguineous discharge that may contain gas bubbles. Complication such as hemolytic anemia, hypotension, and renal failure may develop. In the terminal stages, patient develops coma, jaundice, and shock.

Tetanus

It is also termed as "lockjaw" because of early involvement of the muscles of mastication. It is caused by *Clostridium tetani*.

Source of infection: *C. tetani* is found in the soil and in the lower intestine of many animals. The organism derived from animal and human excreta can contaminate the soil.

Mode of infection: *C. tetani* enters the body through a contaminated wound (injury may be trivial). It can also develop as complication in IV drug misusers. Neonatal tetanus may develop following contamination of the umbilical stump, often after dressing the area (unhygienic practices) with dung (e.g., in many developing countries) or site of circumcision, causing tetanus neonatorum.

Incubation period: Varies from 2 days to several weeks after injury. Shorter the incubation period, the more severe the attack and the worse the prognosis.

Pathogenesis: During circumstances unfavorable to the growth of *C. tetani*, it forms spores and remains dormant for years in the soil. Spores germinate and organism multiplies only in the anaerobic conditions. Necrotic tissue and suppuration create a fertile anaerobic environment for the spores to revert to vegetative bacteria. Thus, it multiply in areas of tissue necrosis or wherever the oxygen tension is reduced by the presence of other organisms (e.g., aerobic organism). *C. tetani* is not invasive and infection remains localized. Tetanus toxin is released from autolyzed vegetative cells. Its clinical manifestations are due to the **potent neurotoxin** (exotoxin) released by organism called **tetanospasmin**. Neurotoxin is transported retrograde through the ventral roots of peripheral nerves to the anterior horn cells of the spinal cord. It crosses the synapse and binds to ganglioside receptors on presynaptic terminals of motor neurons in the ventral horns. After it is internalized, its endopeptidase activity selectively cleaves a protein that mediates exocytosis of synaptic vesicles. Thus, release of inhibitory neurotransmitters (namely γ-aminobutyric acid) is blocked, permitting unopposed neural stimulation and sustained contraction (violent spastic paralysis) of skeletal muscles **(tetany)**. Neurotoxin increases the muscle tone and generalized spasms of skeletal muscles (lockjaw). The loss of inhibitory neurotransmitters also accelerates the heart rate and leads to hypertension and cardiovascular instability. Tetanus toxoid (formalin-fixed inactivated tetanus toxin) is part of the DPT (diphtheria, pertussis, and tetanus) immunization, and this has largely decreased the incidence of tetanus from developed countries. But, tetanus is still a common and lethal disease in some developing countries.

Morphology: Neurologic damage caused by tetanus toxins is severe, but the neuropathologic changes are subtle and nonspecific.

Clinical features: Tetanus begins subtly with fatigue, weakness, and muscle cramping that progress to rigidity.

- **Lockjaw:** General malaise is rapidly followed by the most important symptom namely trismus. It is due to spasm of the masseter (spastic rigidity) muscles, which causes difficulty in opening the mouth and in masticating.
- **Risus sardonicus:** When the tonic rigidity involves the muscles of the face, neck and trunk, contraction of the frontalis and the muscles at the angles of the mouth produces characteristic grinning expression known as "risus sardonicus." Facial expression in risus sardonicus is characterized by raised eyebrows and grinning distortion of the face resulting from spasm of facial muscles.
- **Opisthotonus:** Varying degree of rigidity develops in the muscles at the neck, trunk, and back. The back is usually slightly arched (backward arching "opisthotonos") and the abdominal wall appears board-like.

Painful generalized muscle spasms **can be spontaneous or may be induced by abrupt stimuli** such as movement or noise or by light or touch. Laryngeal spasm can impair respiration and can be fatal; esophageal and urethral spasm can produce dysphagia and urinary retention, respectively. Patients are mentally alert. Infants and older individuals have the highest mortality.

Death: Spasms gradually increase in frequency and severity and death may occur from exhaustion, hypoxia, cardiac arrest, asphyxia, respiratory failure, or aspiration pneumonia or exhaustion. Mild cases with rigidity usually recover.

Investigations/diagnosis:

- Diagnosis is usually made on clinical grounds.
- ***C. tetani*:** Rarely possible to isolate from wounds (original locus of entry).

Botulism

Botulism is caused by *Clostridium botulinum*.

Epidemiology: *C. botulinum* spores are widely distributed and are resistant to drying and boiling. It is usually present in inadequately cooked foods and improperly home canned foods that are stored without refrigeration. These circumstances provide suitable anaerobic conditions for growth of the vegetative cells and produces a potent neurotoxin. This toxin is the most potent poison known and cause disease after ingestion of even picogram (as low as 0.05 g) amounts.

Mode of infection

- **Ingestion:** It can contaminate many foodstuffs such as canned or bottled foodstuff, in which it can multiply. Most cases of botulism are due to consumption of contaminated food being served undercooked. Contaminated honey causes infant botulism, in which the organism colonizes the GI tract.
- **Inoculation:** Wound botulism can develop in injection drug-users.
- **Incubation period:** Up to 2 hours to 8 days.

Classification

- **Food-borne botulism:** It occurs due to ingestion of toxin present in the contaminated food (fish, canned food) and it is the most common type of botulism.

- **Infantile botulism:** It develops due to ingestion of spores, which germinate and proliferate in infants' intestines and produce toxin.
- **Wound botulism:** It follows the contamination of wounds, street heroin injection contaminated with *C. botulinum*. Other types are inhalational and iatrogenic botulism.

Pathophysiology: There are seven serotypes of neurotoxin with diverse mechanisms of action. They are labeled as A to G. Ingested botulinum neurotoxin resists gastric digestion and is absorbed in the proximal small intestine and transported into the blood. Circulating toxin reaches the cholinergic nerve endings at the myoneural junction. The most common toxin is serotype A. This toxin binds gangliosides at presynaptic nerve terminals on motor neurons and is transported into the cell. In the cytoplasm, the A fragment of botulism toxin cleaves a protein called synaptobrevin. The synaptobrevin protein normally mediates fusion of neurotransmitter-containing vesicles with the neuron membrane. By claving protein called synaptobrevin, the toxin blocks vesicle fusion with the neuron membrane. This in turn prevents the release of acetylcholine at the neuromuscular junction and results in flaccid (reduced muscle tone) paralysis of respiratory and skeletal muscles. When the respiratory muscles are affected, botulism can lead to death. The use of botulism toxin (Botox) has been recently found widespread popularity in cosmetic surgery because of its ability to cause paralysis of strategically chosen muscles on the face erase frown (furrow one's brows in an expression indicating disapproval, displeasure).

Morphology: Despite the severe neurologic damage caused by botulinum toxins, the neuropathologic changes are subtle and nonspecific.

Clinical features: Botulism is characterized by a descending paralysis, first affecting cranial nerves and causing blurred or double vision, photophobia, dry mouth, and difficulty in swallowing. It may progress to weakness of the neck muscles, **symmetrical descending limb weakness,** diaphragm and accessory muscles of breathing, respiratory paralysis, and death. Untreated botulism is usually lethal. Botulinum toxin can be used as treatment for many forms of dystonia.

Diagnosis

- Diagnosis of botulism is usually based on clinical features.
- **Detection of toxin:** In blood (foodborne) or stools (infant botulism) or in the contaminated food.
- Culture of organism from wound.

Pseudomembranous Colitis

Pseudomembranous colitis is usually caused by *Clostridioides* (formerly *Clostridium*) *difficile*. It is also referred to as antibiotic-associated colitis, *C. difficile* colitis or antibiotic-associated diarrhea. Other organisms such as *Salmonella, Clostridium perfringens* type A, or *S. aureus* may also produce diarrhea following antibiotic therapy, only *C. difficile* causes pseudomembranous colitis. It is an acute necrotizing infection of the terminal small bowel and colon and it can be lethal. It is responsible for 25–50% of antibiotic-associated diarrhea.

Risk factors: These include **antibiotic treatment, advanced age, hospitalization, and immunosuppression.**

Molecular pathogenesis: *C. difficile* resides in the colon in some healthy individuals. The growth of *C. difficile* is normally limited by the commensal bacteria in colon. When normal intestinal flora is disturbed or changed, it reduces the competition by normal commensal microbiota. The normal colonic commensal microbiota is usually disrupted due to antibiotic treatment (e.g., clindamycin). Almost any antibiotic may be responsible; and it mainly depends on the frequency of its use and the effect on colonic microbiota. This allows proliferation or overgrowth of *C. difficile* in the intestines. *C. difficile* does not invade, but secretes two exotoxins. Toxin A is an enterotoxin stimulates chemokine production and thus attracts leukocytes and causes fluid secretion; toxin B is a cytotoxin that causes distinctive direct cytopathic effects. Both toxins are glucosyltransferases. Toxins produced by *C. difficile* cause the ribosylation of small GTPases such as Rho. This disrupts the epithelial cytoskeleton, tight junction barrier loss, cytokine release, and apoptosis. The toxin damages the mucosal cells of colon thereby causing *pseudomembranous colitis*.

Other conditions that precipitate such colitis include bowel surgery, dietary changes, and chemotherapeutic agents. In hospitals many patients receive antibiotics and they may shed *C. difficile* in the stool and this may result in person-to-person spread.

MORPHOLOGY

Clostridioides difficile destroys mucosal cells of colon and produces denudation of surface epithelium. This triggers an acute inflammatory infiltrate and the superficial lamina propria contains a dense infiltrate of neutrophils and occasional fibrin thrombi within capillaries. Lesions in mucosa range from focal colitis limited to a few crypts and only detectable on biopsy, to massive merging mucosal ulceration. Initially, inflammation involves only the mucosa, but it can extend into the submucosa and muscularis propria. A "pseudomembrane" is made up of an adherent layer of inflammatory cells and debris. It is composed of inflammatory exudate, cellular debris, neutrophils and fibrin, usually forms over affected areas of the colon. It is not specific and may also be found in ischemia or necrotizing infections. However, **histopathological appearance of *C. difficile*-associated colitis is pathognomonic.** Specific features are the appearance of mucopurulent exudate that characteristically erupts from damaged crypts to form "volcano" lesions and coalesces to form pseudomembranes.

Clinical features: *C. difficile* colitis usually begins with very mild symptoms or with watery diarrhea, fever, and abdominal pain. Stools may be profuse and usually show neutrophils. The symptoms and signs are not specific and is not possible to distinguish *C. difficile* colitis from other acute inflammatory diarrheal diseases. Mild cases can be treated by discontinuing the precipitating antibiotic. More severe cases need administration of an antibiotic effective against *C. difficile*. Potentially fatal complication is the development of toxic megacolon, characterized by marked dilatation of the colon

Lab findings: (1) Leukocytosis, (2) Protein loss can lead to hypoalbuminemia, (3) Fecal leukocytes and occult blood may be present. Diagnosis is by detection of *C. difficile* toxin, rather than by culture, and characteristic histopathological findings.

OBLIGATE INTRACELLULAR BACTERIAL INFECTIONS

Obligate intracellular bacteria are adapted to the intracellular environment and proliferate only within host cells. However, some of may survive outside of host cells. They capture amino acids and ATP for energy from host cells. Some cannot synthesize own ATP (e.g., *Chlamydia* species), whereas others can synthesize some of their own ATP (e.g., the rickettsiae).

Chlamydial Infections

Q. Write short essay on Chlamydial infections.

Chlamydiae are obligate intracellular parasites. They are smaller than most other bacteria. They cannot synthesize their own ATP. Hence, they must parasitize the metabolic machinery of a host cell to reproduce. Chlamydial infections are widespread and affects birds and mammals including humans). Three species of Chlamydiae cause infection in human. These are (1) *Chlamydia trachomatis,* (2) *Chlamydia psittaci,* and (3) *Chlamydia pneumoniae.*

Chlamydia Trachomatis

Chlamydia trachomatis is a small gram-negative obligate intracellular bacterial pathogen.

Life cycle (Fig. 53): *C. trachomatis* has a unique life cycle and it exists in two morphologic forms:

- **Elementary body:** The infectious form is called the elementary body. It is the smaller, metabolically inactive form and survives extracellularly. It attaches to the host cell and elementary body use a T3SS to inject a protein, TARP, into host cells. It leads to actin remodeling at the site of bacterial entry. It undergoes phagocytosis and forms a vacuole in the host cell.
- **Reticulate body:** Inside the host cell, the elementary body differentiates into a larger, metabolically active form, called the reticulate body. This occurs within a membrane-bound inclusion derived from the endosome. The bacteria modify the inclusion and prevent it from forming phagolysosome. Host lipids, present in the Golgi apparatus, and GTPases typical of recycling endosomes and the Golgi apparatus are recruited to the inclusion. This marks the inclusion as a nonphagocytic compartment. The reticulate body hijacks the host cell metabolism and uses ATP and amino acids from the host cell to replicate. The reticulate body repeatedly divides and forms new infectious daughter elementary bodies. They lyse the harboring host cell or are extruded from the infected cell. The necrotic debris of host cell stimulates inflammatory and immunologic responses. This further damages the infected tissue.

Serotypes: There are different serotypes of the bacteria. The three distinct types of diseases caused by various serotypes of *C. trachomatis* are:

- **Urogenital epithelial infections and inclusion conjunctivitis:** These are caused by serotypes D to K.

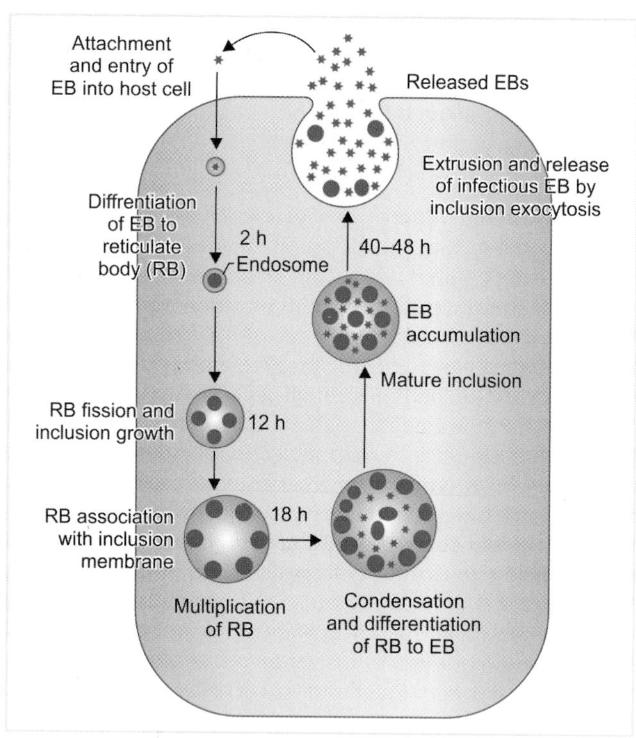

(EB: elementary body; RB: reticulate body)

FIG. 53: Life cycle of *Chlamydia trachomatis.*

- **Lymphogranuloma venereum (LGV):** Caused by serotypes L1, L2, and L3
- **Ocular infection of children (trachoma):** Caused by serotypes A, B, and C.

Genital infection by *Chlamydia trachomatis*

Infections with *Chlamydia trachomatis* are the most common bacterial STDs in the world.

Urogenital epithelial infections and inclusion conjunctivitis are caused by serotypes D to K. Genital *C. trachomatis* infections (except LGV) produce clinical features similar to that caused by *N. gonorrhoeae.*

- **In men:** They produce urethritis and sometimes epididymitis, prostatitis, or proctitis. Unlike *N. gonorrhoeae* urethritis, *C. trachomatis* urethritis may be asymptomatic and may go untreated. Diagnosis of *C. trachomatis* urethritis can be done using nucleic acid tests amplification performed on genital swabs or urine specimens.
- **In women:** Infection usually begins with cervicitis that can progress to endometritis, salpingitis, and generalized infection of the pelvic adnexal organs (PID). Repeated episodes of salpingitis produce scarring and can lead to **infertility or ectopic pregnancy**. In women, both *N. gonorrhoeae* and *C. trachomatis* frequently cause asymptomatic infections.
- **Perinatal transmission of *C. trachomatis*:** It causes neonatal conjunctivitis and pneumonia.

MORPHOLOGY

Features of *C. trachomatis* **urethritis** are essentially **similar to those of gonorrhea**. The primary infection is characterized by a mucopurulent discharge and it shows predominantly neutrophils. Organisms cannot be seen in Gram-stained smears or tissue sections.

Lymphogranuloma venereum

Genital infection with the L serotypes (types LGV 1, 2, and 3) of *C. trachomatis* causes a chronic, ulcerative STD called *lymphogranuloma venereum*.

Epidemiology: Lymphogranuloma venereum is not common in developed nations but is endemic in the tropical and subtropical regions. It constitutes about 5% of STD in India.

Incubation period: Up to 3–30 days.

Clinical features: Three characteristic stages are:

1. **Primary genital lesion:** *C. trachomatis* is introduced through a break in the skin. LGV starts as an asymptomatic small painless papule at the site of inoculation (external genitalia either on the genital mucosa or nearby skin of penis, vagina or cervix; lips, tongue and fingers may also be primary sites) and tends to ulcerate.
2. **Regional lymphadenopathy:** A few days to weeks, the ulcers heal. Growth of the organism occurs and organism is transported by lymphatics to regional (draining) lymph nodes and produces regional lymphadenopathy (usually unilateral). The lymph nodes are initially discrete, painful, and fixed.
3. **Buboes:** Later in the course, **necrotizing lymphadenitis** with abscesses develops. The coalescing abscesses often develop a stellate shape. The lymph nodes may become matted (coalesce), tender fluctuant (buboes), and frequently ulcerate and discharge pus. The skin covering it becomes thinned, inflamed, and fixed. Finally, multiple draining fistulae may occur. If not treated, the intense inflammation can cause severe scarring, fibrosis, and strictures in the anogenital tract. Rectal strictures are particularly common in women. It may also cause chronic lymphatic obstruction and ischemic necrosis of overlying structures.

Diagnosis:

- **Demonstration of the organism:** In active lesions, the diagnosis may be made by demonstration of the organism in biopsy sections or smears of exudate.
- **Detection of deoxyribose nucleic acid (DNA):** Direct immunofluorescent antibody and NAATs (nucleic acid amplification tests) are positive which should be confirmed by RT-PCR for LGV specific DNA.
- **Isolation of the LGV (L1–3 serotypes) strain of *Chlamydia*:** Tissue culture from swab obtained from ulcer aspirated bubo pus, rectum, urethra, endocervix, or from other infected tissue is the most specific test; however, sensitivity is only 75–85%.
- **Serological tests:** In more chronic cases, the diagnosis depends on the demonstration of antibodies to the appropriate chlamydial serotypes in the patient's serum microimmunofluorescence (micro IF) test; complement fixation (CF) test is used to detect antibodies.

MORPHOLOGY

Primary lesion of lymphogranuloma venereum: It shows a **mixed granulomatous and neutrophilic inflammatory response**. Chlamydial inclusions can be found in the cytoplasm of epithelial cells or inflammatory cells.

Continued

Continued

Regional lymphadenopathy: It is common. Lymph node shows a **granulomatous inflammatory reaction associated with irregularly shaped foci of necrosis containing neutrophils (stellate abscesses) in the center**. It is surrounded by palisading epithelioid cells, macrophages, and occasional giant cells. This in turn shows a rim of lymphocytes, plasma cells, and fibrous tissue. As the lesion advances, the inflammatory reaction is dominated by nonspecific chronic inflammatory infiltrates and extensive fibrosis. Fibrosis may lead to local lymphatic obstruction, lymphedema, and strictures.

Trachoma

Trachoma is a chronic infection that leads to progressive scars of the conjunctiva and cornea. It is a leading cause of blindness in many developing countries. *C. trachomatis* serotypes A, B, Ba, and C cause the disease.

Epidemiology: Trachoma is associated with poverty, poor personal hygiene, and inadequate public sanitation. It is most prevalent in dry or sandy regions. Trachoma remains a major problem in India.

Mode of transmission: It usually spreads by direct contact but it may also be transmitted by fomites, contaminated water and probably flies. Only humans are naturally infected. Important reservoir is subclinical infections. In endemic regions, infection occurs during early childhood, becomes chronic, and finally progresses to blindness.

MORPHOLOGY

Conjunctiva: *C. trachomatis* reproduces in the conjunctival epithelium.

Microscopy: It produces a mixed acute and chronic inflammatory infiltrate. In the conjunctiva, early lesions show chronic inflammation, lymphoid aggregates, focal degeneration, and chlamydial inclusions. As it progresses, lymphoid aggregates enlarge, and scarred develops in the conjunctiva along with focal hypertrophy.

Cornea: It is invaded by blood vessels and fibroblasts and forms a scar reminiscent of a cloth (*pannus* in Latin). Finally, it becomes opaque.

Clinical features: During early phase there is sudden onset of inflammation in the palpebra and conjunctiva. This is characterized by tearing, purulent conjunctivitis, and photophobia. Within 3–4 weeks, the lymphoid aggregates can be seen as small yellow grains beneath the palpebral conjunctivae. After months or years, deformities develop in eyelid and interfere with normal ocular function. Secondary bacterial infections and corneal ulcers can occur and finally blindness develops.

Psittacosis (Ornithosis)

Psittacosis is a self-limited pneumonia transmitted to humans from infected birds and is caused by *C. psittaci*. The resulting disease is known as both psittacosis (transmitted by infected parrots) and ornithosis (transmitted by infected birds in general).

Source of infection: In the infected birds, *C. psittaci* is present in the blood, tissues, excreta, and feathers.

Mode of infection: It is through inhalation and occurs when humans inhale infectious excreta or dust from feathers of infected birds.

Epidemiology: Infection is endemic in tropical birds, but *C. psittaci* can infect any bird and can spread to humans.

MORPHOLOGY

Lung: *C. psittaci* first infects pulmonary macrophages in the alveoli. They carry the organism to the phagocytes of the liver and spleen. Organisms are reproduced at these sites. They spread via the bloodstream and produce systemic infection and also cause diffuse involvement of the lungs. *C. psittaci* reproduces also in the lining cells of alveoli and destroys them. This produces an inflammatory response and causes predominantly interstitial pneumonia. Microscopically, interstitium shows inflammatory infiltrate of lymphocytes.

Disseminated infection: It is characterized by foci of necrosis in the liver and spleen. Diffuse mononuclear cell infiltrates are seen in the heart, kidneys, and brain.

Clinical features: It varies. Usually presents with persistent dry cough, high fever, headache, malaise, myalgias, and arthralgias. The disease is rarely fatal.

Chlamydia pneumoniae

Chlamydia pneumoniae infection is very common. It produces acute, self-limited, usually mild respiratory tract infections, including pneumonia.

Mode of transmission: It is transmitted from person to person.

Clinical features: It presents with fever, sore throat, and cough. Severe pneumonia develops only in individuals with an underlying pulmonary condition. Untreated disease usually resolves within 2–4 weeks.

ENTEROPATHOGENIC BACTERIAL INFECTIONS

Escherichia coli

Escherichia coli is the most frequent and important human bacterial pathogens, causing >90% of all urinary tract infections and many cases of diarrhea. It is also a major opportunistic pathogen that can produce pneumonia and sepsis in immunocompromised individuals and meningitis and sepsis in newborns.

Escherichia coli consists of a group of antigenically and biologically diverse, aerobic (facultatively anaerobic), gram-negative bacteria. Most strains of *E. coli* are present in the intestine of healthy individuals as commensals and most are nonpathogenic. They are well adapted to growth in the colon of humans without harming the host. However, a subset of *E. coli* can behave aggressively when it gains entry into usually sterile sites in the body sites (e.g., urinary tract, meninges, or peritoneum) and cause disease in humans.

Escherichia coli Diarrhea

Escherichia coli causing diarrhea have specialized virulence properties. They are usually plasmid-borne. There are distinct strains of *E. coli* that cause diarrhea. These are classified according to morphology, pathogenesis, and in vitro behavior. Subgroups of major clinical importance are enterotoxigenic *E. coli* (ETEC), enteropathogenic *E. coli* (EPEC), enterohemorrhagic *E. coli* (EHEC), enteroinvasive *E. coli* (EIEC), and enteroaggregative *E. coli* (EAEC).

Enterotoxigenic *Escherichia coli*

It produces diarrhea in poor tropical areas and is the main cause of "traveler's diarrhea" in visitors to such regions. It is usually transmitted through contaminated water and food. Children below 2 years of age are particularly susceptible. Many may be asymptomatic carriers of the infection.

Molecular pathogenesis: Diarrhea develops in nonimmune individuals (local children or travelers from abroad) when the organism ingested through water or food. Enterotoxigenic strains are noninvasive and adhere to the intestinal mucosa and produce heat-labile (LT) and heat-stable (ST) enterotoxins. These toxins produce diarrhea by causing secretory dysfunction of the small bowel. LT enterotoxins is similar to cholera toxin (both structurally and functionally), and acts on guanylyl cyclase resulting in increased intracellular cAMP and chloride secretion. ST enterotoxin binds to guanylate cyclase, and increases intracellular cyclic guanosine monophosphate (cGMP). Its actions are similar to those induced by LT enterotoxin. Like cholera, the secretory, noninflammatory diarrhea induced by ETEC does not produce any distinctive macroscopic or light-microscopic changes in the intestine. It causes an acute, self-limited diarrhea with watery stools. The stool does not contain any neutrophils or RBCs. In severe cases, fluid and electrolyte loss can lead to severe dehydration and death.

Enteropathogenic *Escherichia coli*

It causes diarrhea in poor especially in infants and young children in tropical areas. It is **an important cause of endemic diarrhea.** EPEC is transmitted by ingesting contaminated food or water.

Pathogenesis: It is not an invasive organism. EPEC is capable of attaching and effacing (A/E) lesions. It produces the disease by tightly attaching (adhering) to apical membranes of small intestinal epithelial cells and cause local loss (i.e., effacement or deformation) of the microvilli. The proteins needed for creating A/E lesions include Tir, which is inserted into the plasma membrane of intestinal epithelial cell. Tir acts as a receptor for the bacterial outer membrane protein intimin. EPEC presents with diarrhea, vomiting, fever, and malaise.

Enterohemorrhagic *Escherichia coli*

Enterohemorrhagic E. coli are divided into *E. coli* O157:H7 and non-O157:H7 serotypes. EHEC 0157:H7 causes a bloody diarrhea. It is usually transmitted by the ingestion of inadequately cooked ground beef, meat, or contaminated milk and vegetables. This may be followed by the **hemolytic-uremic syndrome (HUS).**

Pathogenesis: EHEC adheres to colonic mucosa. Both O157:H7 and non-O157:H7 serotypes secrete Shiga-like toxins. They destroy the epithelial cells of the intestine. Patients present with clinical symptoms similar to those resulting from *S. dysenteriae* infection and include cramping abdominal pain, low-grade fever, and sometimes bloody diarrhea. Microscopically, stool shows both leukocytes and RBCs. If antibiotics are used, they kill the bacteria and release of Shiga-like toxins. This can increase the risk of hemolytic uremic syndrome especially in children. Hence, antibiotics are not recommended.

Enteroinvasive *Escherichia coli*

Enteroinvasive *E. coli* causes dysentery that is clinically and pathologically indistinguishable from that caused by *Shigella.* EIEC shares extensive DNA homology and antigenic and biochemical characteristics with *Shigella.* It is usually transmitted by the ingestion of contaminated food or water or by person-to-person contact.

Pathogenesis: EIEC does not produce toxins. EIEC invades and destroys cells lining the mucosa of the distal ileum and colon. Similar to shigellosis, the mucosa of the distal ileum and colon shows acute inflammation. There are focal erosions and sometimes may covered by an inflammatory pseudomembrane. Patients present with abdominal pain, fever, tenesmus, and bloody diarrhea.

Enteroaggregative *Escherichia coli*

Enteroaggregative *E. coli* has a unique "stacked brick" morphology when attached to epithelial cells of the intestine. They cause diarrhea in children and adults including traveler's diarrhea. It causes nonbloody diarrhea that may be prolonged in patients with immunodeficiency.

Pathogenesis: The bacteria attach to enterocytes via adherence fimbriae. This is aided by a bacterial surface protein called dispersin. This protein neutralizes the negative surface charge of lipopolysaccharide. Microscopic changes are minimal.

Escherichia coli Urinary Tract Infection

Epidemiology: Urinary tract infections with *E. coli* are most common in sexually active females and in individuals of both sexes having structural or functional abnormalities of the urinary tract. They infect more than 10% of the human population, often repeatedly.

Source: *E. coli* in the urinary tract are usually derived from fecal contamination of the perineum and periurethral areas.

Pathophysiology: *E. coli* gain entry into the sterile proximal urinary tract by ascending through the distal urethra. Shorter urethra in female provides a less effective mechanical barrier to infection, hence are much more prone to urinary tract infections. Sexual intercourse drives the organisms into the female urethra. Uropathogenic *E. coli* (*E. coli* causing urinary tract infection) have specialized adherence factors (Gal-Gal) on the pili. This helps them to attach to galactopyranosyl-galactopyranoside residues present on the uroepithelium. Predisposing factors include structural abnormalities of the urinary tract (e.g., congenital deformities, prostatic hyperplasia, strictures) and instrumentation (catheterization), facilitate the development of urinary tract infections.

Pathology and clinical features: Urinary tract infections caused by *E. coli,* initially produce an acute inflammatory infiltrate at the site of infection (usually the mucosa of urinary bladder). Infections of the bladder or urethra clinically present as urinary urgency, burning on urination **(dysuria). Microscopic examination of urine shows** leukocytes (neutrophils). Infection from bladder may ascend to involve the kidney **(pyelonephritis).** With pyelonephritis, patient develops acute flank pain and fever with chills. Peripheral smear shows raised WBC count with neutrophilia. The neutrophils spill from the mucosa into the urine and microscopically it shows numerous neutrophils accompanied by WBC cast. Chronic infection of the kidney may lead to chronic pyelonephritis and renal failure.

Escherichia coli Pneumonia

Enteric gram-negative bacteria-causing pneumonia is due to opportunistic infection. Hence, it occurs mostly in debilitated persons. *E. coli* is the most common cause in such individuals. However, other bacteria present in the normal intestinal flora, such as *Klebsiella, Serratia,* and *Enterobacter* species, can also produce pneumonia.

Pathophysiology: In healthy individuals, enteric gram-negative bacteria are transiently introduced into the oral cavity. Gram-positive bacteria in the normal flora adhere to the fibronectin that coats mucosal cell surfaces. Enteric gram-negative bacteria cannot compete with these predominant gram-positive bacteria in the normal flora. However, chronically ill or severely stressed individuals secrete a salivary protease which can degrades fibronectin. This permits the gram-negative enteric bacteria to overcome the normal gram-positive flora and colonize the oropharynx. The contaminated droplets from the oral flora are aspirated into the respiratory tract. Debilitated patients have weak local defenses and cannot destroy organisms in these aspirated droplets. Further entry and survival of the aspirated organisms is facilitated due to decreased gag and cough reflexes, abnormality in neutrophil chemotaxis, injury to the epithelium of respiratory tract, and foreign bodies (e.g., endotracheal tubes). In the lung, *E. coli* in the aspirated material proliferates in terminal airways and produces pneumonia.

MORPHOLOGY

Escherichia coli pneumonia usually develops at multiple sites in the lung. Multifocal areas of consolidation occur in the terminal airways and surrounding alveoli.

Microscopy: The alveoli and terminal airways show proteinaceous fluid, fibrin, neutrophils, and macrophages.

Clinical features: Pneumonia due to *E. coli* and other enteric gram-negative organisms usually develops in patients who are already severely ill. Hence, the symptoms of pneumonia may be less obvious than in healthy individuals. It may present with malaise, fever, and dyspnea. If *E. coli* pneumonia is untreated, the organisms may invade the blood and can lead to fatal septicemia.

Escherichia coli Sepsis (Gram-negative Sepsis)

Escherichia coli is the most common cause of sepsis due to enteric gram-negative bacteria. Other gram-negative organisms, such as *Pseudomonas, Klebsiella,* and *Enterobacter* species, also can cause similar sepsis.

Pathophysiology: *E. coli* sepsis is usually occurring as an opportunistic infection, in individuals with predisposing conditions (e.g., neutropenia, pyelonephritis, and cirrhosis), and in patients who are hospitalized for some other illness. Occasionally, *E. coli* and other enteric gram-negative bacteria normally reside in the human colon can gain entry into the bloodstream. In healthy individuals, these bacteria are phagocytosed by macrophages and circulating neutrophils. Patients with neutropenia or cirrhosis develop *E. coli* sepsis due to impaired ability to eliminate these bacteria even when the bacteremia is mild. In patients with ruptured abdominal organs or acute pyelonephritis gram-negative sepsis develops because the entry of large numbers of bacteria into the circulation that overcomes the normal defenses. *E. coli* in the bloodstream produces septic shock due to the effects of TNF and other factors released from macrophages stimulated by bacterial endotoxin.

Neonatal E. Coli Meningitis and Sepsis

Meningitis and sepsis in the first month after birth are mainly caused by *E. coli* and group B streptococci. Both organisms colonize the vagina of the mother, and newborns acquire them when they pass through the birth canal during delivery. *E. coli* then colonizes the infant's GI tract. From GI tract organisms gain entry into the bloodstream and then seed the meninges. The pathology of *E. coli* meningitis is similar to that of other bacterial meningitides.

Typhoid Fever

Q. Write short essay on typhoid enteritis.

- Typhoid fever (enteric) is an **acute systemic disease** caused by infection with *Salmonella typhi.*
- Paratyphoid fever is clinically similar but milder disease caused by *Salmonella paratyphi.* **Enteric fever** is the general term, which includes **both typhoid and paratyphoid fever**.

Etiology

Causative agent: Enteric fevers are caused by ***Salmonella typhi* and *Salmonella paratyphi*.** *Salmonella* are gram-negative, flagellate, motile, nonsporulating, facultative anaerobic bacilli (rods). Boiling or chlorination of water and pasteurization of milk destroy the bacilli.

Source of infection: Humans are the only natural reservoir and includes:

- **Patients suffering from disease:** Infected urine, feces, or other secretions from patients.
- **Chronic carriers of typhoid fever:** *S. typhi* or *S. paratyphi* **colonizes in the gallbladder** or biliary tree may be associated with gallstones and the chronic carrier state. Mary Mallon during 19th century worked as a cook. She was a healthy carrier of Salmonella typhi. Her nickname of "Typhoid Mary" had become synonymous with the spread of disease. Many were infected due to her denial of being ill. Later she was forced into quarantine for a total of 26 years and died alone without friends.

Mode of transmission: From **person-to-person contact**.

- **Ingestion** of **contaminated food** (especially dairy products) and shellfish or **contaminated water**.
- **Direct spread:** Rare by **finger-to-mouth contact** with feces, urine, or other secretions.

Incubation period: Usually 7–14 days.

Pathogenesis (Fig. 54)

- The typhoid bacilli (*Salmonella*) are **ingested through contaminated food or water and** able to **survive in gastric acid of the stomach.** Then they reach mucosa of small intestine.
- **Events during incubation period:**
    - During the initial asymptomatic period (about 2 weeks), the *Salmonella* **attach to the microvilli** and penetrate the **ileal mucosa** of the small intestine**.** Invasion tends to be most prominent in the ileum in areas overlying Peyer's patches. They reach lamina propria and submucosa.
    - *Salmonella* are **phagocytosed by the macrophages** (mononuclear phagocytes) present in the lymphoid tissue and **Peyer's patches** in the submucosa of small intestine.
    - *Salmonella* block the respiratory burst of the phagocytes and **multiply within the macrophages.** The organisms are **carried to** the **mesenteric lymph node** via lymphatics. They multiply in the lymph nodes and **via** the **thoracic duct** enter the **bloodstream** causing **transient bacteremia**.
- **During bacteremia**, the bacilli are **seeded in many organs.** They colonize reticuloendothelial tissues (**liver, gallbladder, spleen, bone marrow,** and lymph nodes), where bacilli multiply further. This causes **massive bacteremia** (occurs toward the end of incubation period) and disease clinically manifests. Infection of macrophages stimulates production of IL-1 and TNF. They cause prolonged fever, malaise, and wasting characteristic of typhoid fever.
- **Bile is a good culture medium for the typhoid bacillus,** and bacilli **multiply in the gallbladder.** The bacilli are continuously shed through the bile into the intestine.
- The earliest change is degeneration of the intestinal epithelium brush border. In the intestine, the bacilli are localized to the **Peyer's patches and lymphoid follicles** of the terminal ileum. As bacteria invade, Peyer's patches become hypertrophic. They cause inflammation, plateau-like elevations of Peyer's patches and necrosis of overlying mucosa. This results in characteristic **oval typhoid ulcers** oriented along the long axis of the bowel.

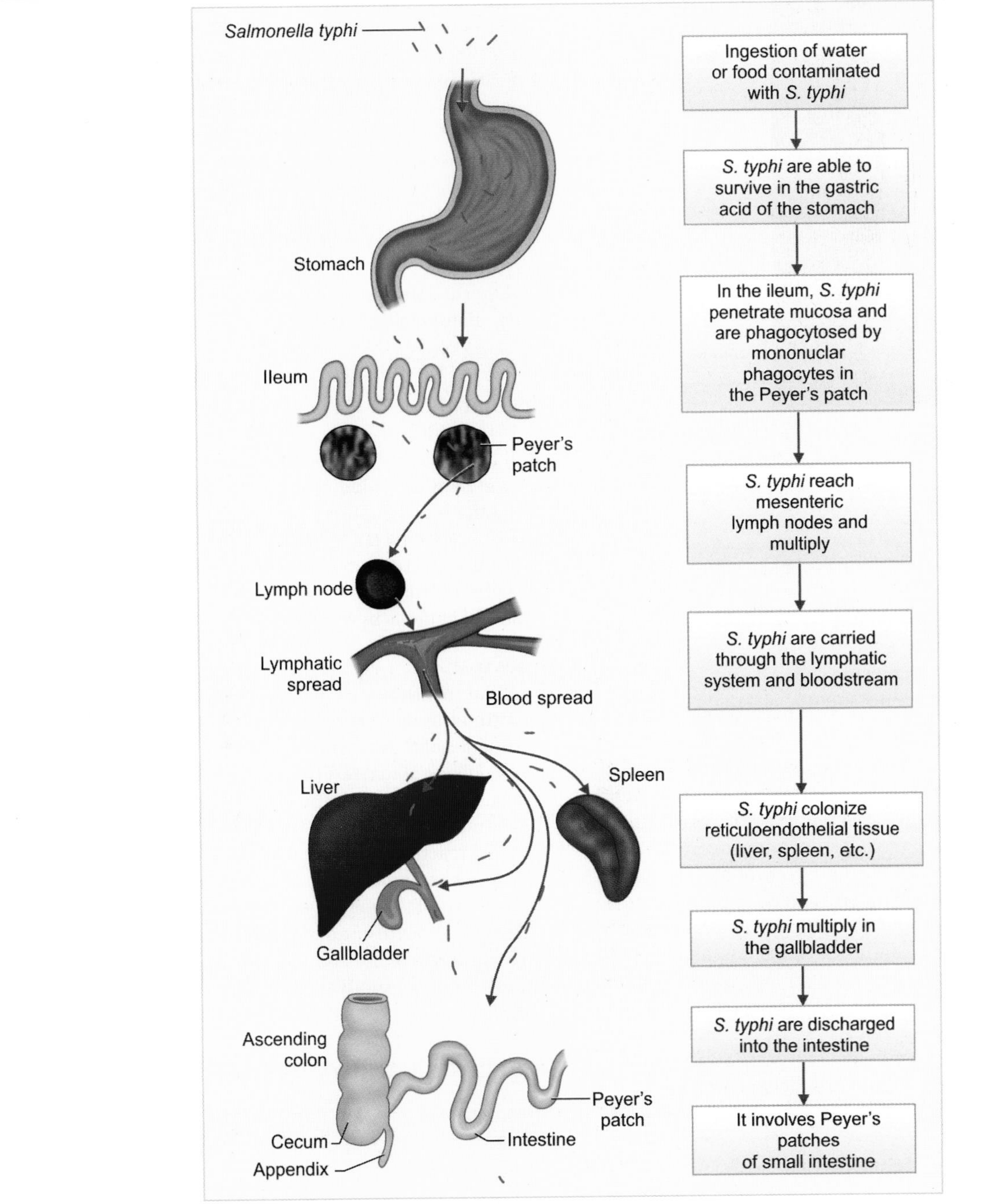

FIG. 54: Pathogenesis of typhoid fever.

MORPHOLOGY

Lesions may be (1) intestinal and (2) extraintestinal.

Intestinal Lesions

Gross (Fig. 55)

- **Site:** Most commonly involved is **terminal ileum**, but may be seen in the jejunum and colon.
- **Appearance:** Peyer's patches in the terminal ileum enlarge into sharply delineated, plateau-like elevations. The shedding of mucosa produces typhoid ulcers.

Continued

Continued

- **Characteristics of typhoid ulcer:**
  - **Number: Varies**
  - **Orientation: Oval ulcers oriented along the long axis of the bowel** (tuberculous ulcers of small intestine are transverse).
  - **Base of the ulcer:** It is **black** due to sloughed mucosa.
  - **Margins: Slightly raised** due to inflammatory edema and cellular proliferation.
  - **No fibrosis:** Hence, narrowing of the intestinal lumen seldom occur in healed typhoid lesions.

Continued

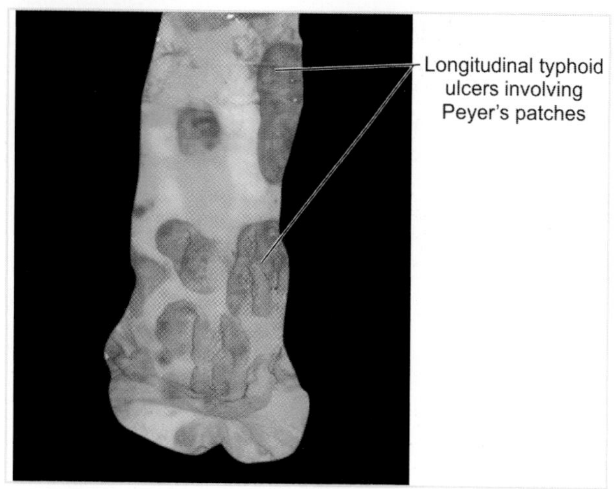

FIG. 55: Gross appearance of typhoid ulcers in the ileum of small intestine.

Continued

Microscopy

- **Mucosa: Oval ulcers** over the Peyer's patches.
- **Lamina propria:**
  - **Macrophages** containing bacteria, RBCs (erythrophagocytosis), and nuclear debris.
  - **Lymphocytes and plasma cells**
  - **Neutrophils** within the superficial lamina propria.

Extraintestinal Lesions

- **Typhoid nodules:** Systemic dissemination of the bacilli leads to **formation of focal granulomas** termed **typhoid nodules.** These nodules are composed of **aggregates of macrophages** (typhoid cells) containing ingested bacilli, RBCs, and lymphocytes. They are **common in the lymph node, liver, bone marrow, and spleen.**
- **Mesenteric lymph nodes:** They are enlarged due to accumulation of macrophages, which contains typhoid bacilli.
- **Liver:** It shows small, scattered foci of hepatocyte necrosis replaced by **typhoid nodules.**
- **Spleen:** It is enlarged and soft.
- **Abdominal muscles:** Zenker's degeneration (severe glassy or waxy hyaline degeneration or necrosis of skeletal muscles).
- **Gallbladder: Typhoid cholecystitis**

Clinical Features

- Onset is gradual and patients present with anorexia, abdominal pain, bloating, nausea, vomiting, and diarrhea.
- **Fever: Continuous rise in temperature** (step-ladder fever).
- **Rose spots:** These are small erythematous maculopapular lesions on the skin that fade on pressure, appear on the chest and abdomen, and occur during second or third week.
- **Spleen:** It is soft and palpable and may be accompanied by hepatomegaly.

Complications

- ***Intestinal complications***: It can be fatal. The most common intestinal complication is ileus. **Perforation** of typhoid ulcer and **hemorrhage from the ulcer** may occur at the end of the second week or during the third week of the illness.
- ***Extraintestinal complications*: Encephalopathy, meningitis, seizures, endocarditis, myocarditis, pneumonia, and cholecystitis. Sickle cell disease patients are susceptible to *Salmonella* osteomyelitis.**
- ***Carrier state***: Persistence of bacilli in the **gallbladder or urinary tract** may result in passage of bacilli in the feces or urine. It causes a '**carrier state and is** source of infection to others.
- **General complications:** Toxemia, dehydration, peripheral circulatory failure, and DIC.

Laboratory Diagnosis

Isolation of bacilli

- **Blood culture:** It is positive in **first week** of fever in 90% of patients and remains positive in second week till the fever subsides. Blood culture rapidly becomes negative on treatment with antibiotics.
- **Stool cultures:** It is almost as valuable as blood culture and becomes positive in the **second and third** weeks.
- **Urine culture:** It reveals the organism in approximately 25% of patients by **third week.**

Other tests

- **Widal reaction:** Classic Widal test **measures** agglutinating **antibodies against** *O, H,* and **Vi antigens** of *S. typhi* and H antigens of *S. paratyphi* A and B, but **lacks sensitivity and specificity**. Widal test (immunological reactions) becomes positive from end of the first week till fourth week. There are many false-positive and occasional false-negative Widal reactions.
- **Other serologic tests:** They are available for the rapid diagnosis of typhoid fever with a higher sensitivity.
- **Total leukocyte count:** It shows **leukopenia with relative lymphocytosis**. Eosinophils are usually absent.
- **Molecular methods:** PCR detects flagellin, *Somatic* gene, and *Vi* gene.

Shigellosis–Bacillary Dysentery

Bacillary dysentery is **a necrotizing infection** of the **distal small bowel and colon** caused by ***Shigella.***

Etiology

- *Shigella* causes bacillary dysentery and is one of the **most common causes of bloody diarrhea.**
- *Shigella* is an unencapsulated, nonmotile, facultative anaerobic gram-negative bacilli. It belongs to the Enterobacteriaceae and is closely related to *EIEC.*
- *Shigella* species that cause colitis are classified into four major subgroups, namely, *S. dysenteriae* (most virulent), *S. flexneri*, *S. boydii*, and *S. sonnei*.

Source of infection: Humans are the only natural reservoir.

Mode of transmission: By **ingestion** through fecal–oral route or via fecally contaminated water and food. It can be acquired by oral contact with any contaminated surface (e.g., clothing, towels, or skin surfaces).

Incubation period: It ranges from **1 to 3 days.**

Pathogenesis

- *Shigella* is the **most virulent** enteropathogens and ingestion of few (10–100 organisms) produces disease.
- After ingestion, *Shigella* reaches the stomach. It is **resistant to the action of acid in the stomach**. Small intestinal infections do not occur unless the patient has disturbance in motility of intestine.
- **In the colon**, the bacteria penetrate the intestinal mucous epithelium and are **taken up by M or microfold epithelial cells.** They proliferate inside the cytoplasm of these epithelial cells and penetrate into the lamina propria where they are phagocytosed by macrophages. *Shigella* induces apoptosis of macrophages and causes inflammatory reaction. It loosens the intercellular barriers and damages surface epithelium leading to superficial ulcers. These ulcers allow entry of *Shigella* in the intestinal lumen to the colonocyte basolateral membrane.
- *Shigella* **produces a toxin** that has cytotoxic, neurotoxic, and enterotoxic effects. When inflammation is severe, ileus, toxic megacolon, gross hemorrhage, and perforation may develop.

MORPHOLOGY

Gross (Fig. 56)

- **Site of lesions:** Most prominent in the **left (distal) colon** mainly in the **rectosigmoid area,** although the entire colon and distal ileum can be involved. Mostly, the **lesions are continuous and diffuse.**
- **Characteristics of ulcer:** Mucosa shows **edema, ulceration,** and appears **friable granular and hemorrhagic**. In severe infections, a gray mucopurulent exudate covers the mucosa. **Ulcers** appear first on the edges of mucosal folds, **perpendicular to the long axis of the colon**.

Microscopy

Changes are predominant in the **mucosa**.

- **Early stage:** It shows erosions and **small aphthous ulcers** (microulcers), with **infiltration by neutrophils** below the microulcers.
- **Advanced stage:**
  - **Necrosis of epithelial cells** and the damaged **mucosa is covered by purulent exudate** (composed of detached epithelial cells, neutrophils, and RBCs).

Clinical Features

- Presents as diarrhea, fever, and abdominal pain.
- The initial watery diarrhea progresses to a dysenteric phase.
- Stool culture is required for confirmation of *Shigella* infection.

Complications

Long-term complications of *Shigella* infection are **uncommon**.

- **Reiter syndrome:** A triad of sterile arthritis, urethritis, and conjunctivitis. It **mainly affects HLA-B27-positive men** between 20 and 40 years of age.
- **Hemolytic-uremic syndrome:** It is **due to toxin** secreted by *Shigella* organisms.

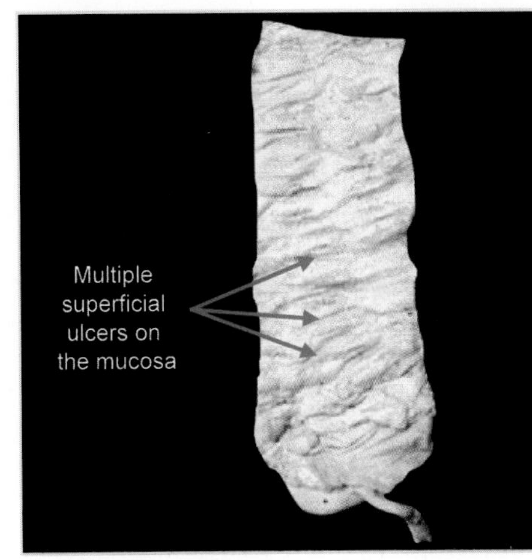

FIG. 56: Bacillary dysentery. Specimen of cecum and ascending colon (with appendix). Mucosa shows multiple superficial ulceration with intervening normal mucosa.

Cholera

Cholera is an acute severe diarrheal illness caused by the enterotoxin of curved (**comma-shaped)**, aerobic, flagellated, gram-negative bacillus, *Vibrio cholerae*. Since 1817 seven great pandemics have occurred.

- *Vibrio cholerae* colonizes in the small intestine. It causes explosive, severe watery diarrhea with rapid depletion of extracellular fluid and electrolytes.
- *Vibrio cholerae*: The incidence of cholera increases during summer, indicating that more rapid growth of *Vibrio* bacteria occurs at warm temperatures. It is killed by temperatures of 100°C in a few seconds but can survive in ice for up to 6 weeks. The **major pathogenic strain** has a **somatic antigen (O1)** and has **two biotypes: classical and El Tor. New classical toxigenic strain, serotype O139** (Bengal serogroup), is still major cause of cholera in India.

Mode of Transmission

By the fecal-oral route: Infection spreads via the stools or vomitus of symptomatic patients. Contaminated drinking water is the major source of the dissemination, although contaminated foodstuffs (shellfish and food contaminated by flies), and hands of contact carriers may contribute in epidemics. Epidemics spread in areas where human feces contaminate the water supply. Shell fish and plankton (small and microscopic organisms floating in the sea or fresh water) can be reservoirs of *V. cholerae*.

Incubation period is about **12–48 hours** (ranges from 1 to 5 days).

Pathogenesis (Fig. 57)

- **Entry into intestine:** After ingestion bacteria reach the stomach. In the stomach they survive and pass into the small intestine. *Vibrio* organisms are noninvasive and remain within the lumen of the intestine. In the small intestine *V. cholerae* proliferate in the lumen. For efficient colonization, proteins involved in motility and attachment

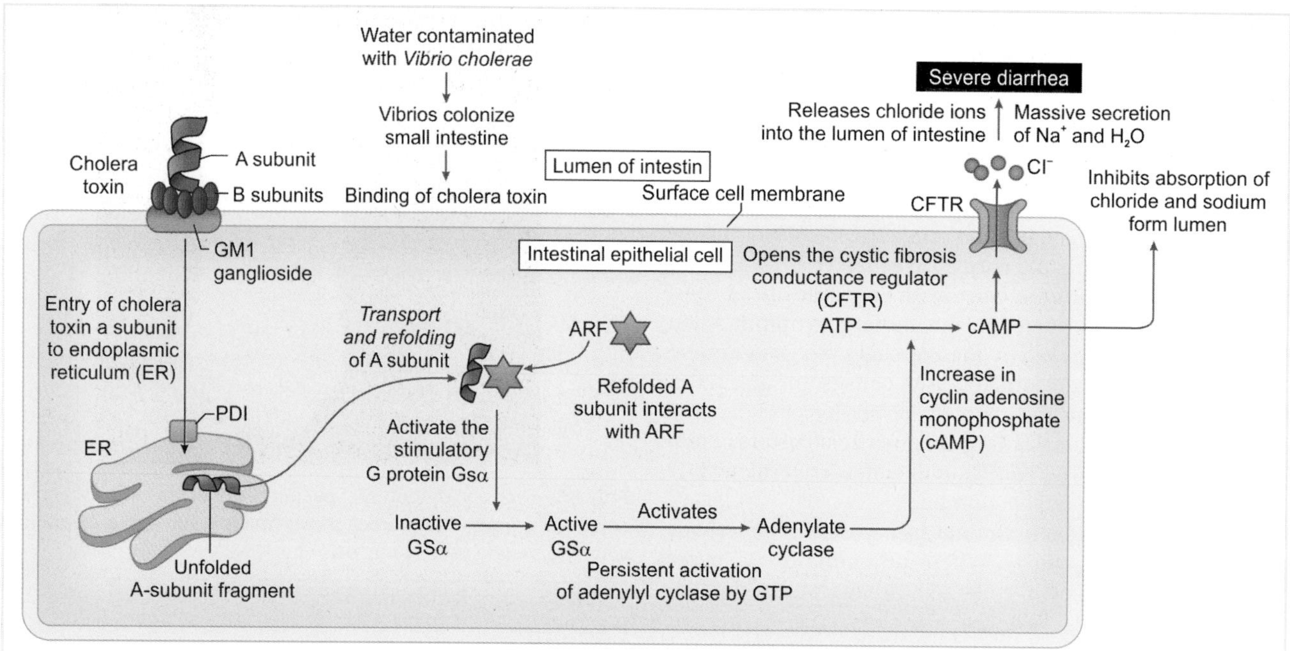

(ATP: adenosine triphosphate; PDI: protein disulphide isomerase)s

FIG. 57: Cholera toxin transport and various steps involved in the development of cholera. Infection comes from water contaminated with *Vibrio cholerae* or food prepared with contaminated water. Organism traverses the stomach and enters the small intestine and propagate. They do not invade the intestinal mucosa, but secretes a potent toxin. Cholera toxin has two subunits A and B. B subunit binds to GM1 ganglioside on the surface of intestinal epithelial cells and allows the transport of A subunits to the endoplasmic reticulum (ER). In the ER, protein disulfide isomerase reduces the A subunit of the toxin, and unfolds a fragment of the A subunit. This peptide fragment of the A subunit is then transported into the cytosol and gets refolded. Along with an ADP-ribosylation factor (ARF), the refolded A subunit then converts inactive Gsα to active form. This leads to activation of adenylate cyclase (AC) and the cyclic adenosine monophosphate (cAMP) produced. cAMP opens cystic fibrosis transmembrane conductance regulator (CFTR) to cause secretion of chloride into the lumen of intestine leading to diarrhea.

are necessary. Hemagglutinin, a metalloproteinase, helps for bacterial detachment and shedding into the stool. This is responsible for dissemination.

- **Choler toxin:** *V. cholerae* produces a powerful **exotoxin** called **cholera toxin**. Cholera toxin is encoded by a virulence phage. This toxin is composed of single A subunit and five B subunits.
- **Entry of toxin into the intestinal epithelial cells:** The B subunit binds to GM1 ganglioside on the surface cell membrane of intestinal epithelial cells. The A subunit of the toxin then enters the cell by endocytosis and carried to the endoplasmic reticulum (ER). In the ER, protein disulfide isomerase reduces the A subunit of the toxin, and unfolds a fragment of the A subunit. This peptide fragment of the A subunit is then transported into the cytosol. This transport is carried out using same host cell machinery that normally transport misfolded proteins from the ER to the cytosol.
- **Activation of adenylyl cyclase and increase in cAMP:** Once in the cytosol, the A subunit fragment refolds and interacts with cytosolic ADP-ribosylation factors (ARFs) to activate the stimulatory G protein Gsα. This activates (stimulates) adenylate cyclase. This results in consequent increase in intracellular cAMP.
- **Actions of cAMP:** The cAMP opens the CF conductance regulator (CFTR). This releases chloride ions into the lumen. The cAMP also inhibits absorption of chloride and sodium. The accumulated chloride, bicarbonate, and sodium within the intestinal lumen creates an osmotic force that draws water into the intestinal lumen. It occurs mainly in the small bowel and causes massive diarrhea.

MORPHOLOGY

Grossly, the intestine appears normal or only slightly hyperemic. *V. cholerae* show only minimal visible histological changes in the mucosal biopsies. The intestinal epithelium is intact with depletion of mucus.

Clinical Features

- Majority with cholera may have a mild illness that cannot be distinguished clinically from diarrhea due to other infective causes. Severe cases, present abruptly with severe, painless, watery diarrhea without pain or colic, followed by vomiting (vomiting may be absent).
- **Rice-water stool:** Following the evacuation of normal gut fecal contents, characteristic "rice-water" stool, and is sometimes described as having a fishy odor, is passed, consisting of clear fluid with flecks of mucus.
- **Loss of fluid and electrolytes:** Leading to intense dehydration with muscular cramps. Severe depletion of extracellular fluid produces hypotension, metabolic acidosis, and hypokalemia. In severe cases, massive fluid loss may lead to hypovolemic shock and acute tubular necrosis resulting in renal failure.

- **Cholera sicca:** Occasionally, a very **severe form of the cholera** occurs with **accumulation of fluid into the dilated bowel.** This **kills the patient before typical GI symptoms** appear. It is called as "cholera sicca."

Diagnosis

- **Clinical diagnosis** can be easily made during an epidemic. Otherwise, the diagnosis requires bacteriological confirmation.
- **Stool examination: "Hanging drop" preparation** of the freshly passed stool shows the characteristic of rapidly motile (shooting star motility) *V. cholerae* (this is not diagnostic, as *Campylobacter jejuni* may give a similar appearance).
- **Culture** of the stool or a rectal swab can isolate and identify the *V. cholerae* and also establish antibiotic sensitivity.

Campylobacter Enterocolitis

Campylobacter jejuni is the major human pathogen in the genus *Campylobacter.* ***Campylobacter jejuni* is the most common enteric pathogen causing bacterial diarrhea in the developed world. It is also an important cause of traveler's diarrhea and food poisoning.** It causes an acute, self-limited, inflammatory diarrhea.

Campylobacter jejuni is a microaerophilic, flagellated curved (comma-shaped) gram-negative organism. It is morphologically similar to the vibrios.

Source and mode of infection: Infections are usually acquired following ingestion of improperly cooked poultry chicken and meat and contaminated food. Outbreaks can be caused due to consumption of unpasteurized raw milk or contaminated water. The bacteria inhabit GI tracts of many animals (e.g., cows, sheep, chickens, and dogs) and constitute animal reservoir for infection. *C. jejuni* can also spread from person to person by the fecal–oral route. Ingestion of as few as 500 *C. jejuni* can cause disease.

Incubation period: It is up to 8 days.

Pathogenesis

Ingested *C. jejuni* survives in the acidity of stomach and multiplies in the alkaline environment of the upper small intestine. The pathogenesis of *Campylobacter* infection is poorly known. Four major properties that contribute to virulence are motility, adherence, toxin production, and invasion. Flagella makes *Campylobacter* to be motile and facilitates its adherence and colonization. Some *C. jejuni* secretes cytotoxins that produce direct damage to epithelium or a cholera toxin-like enterotoxin. Dysentery (i.e., bloody diarrhea) is usually seen when there is bacterial invasion and is found in only few *Campylobacter* strains. Enteric fever develops when bacteria proliferate within the lamina propria and mesenteric lymph nodes.

Extraintestinal manifestations: Reactive arthritis can result from *Campylobacter* infection, mainly in patients with HLA-B27 genotype. Other extraintestinal complications include erythema nodosum and Guillain–Barré syndrome. Guillain–Barré syndrome is an immunologically mediated inflammation of peripheral nerves and produces flaccid paralysis. Molecular mimicry may be responsible for the pathogenesis of Guillain–Barré syndrome. Probably the serum antibodies to *C. jejuni* lipopolysaccharide cross-react with peripheral and CNS gangliosides.

MORPHOLOGY

Campylobacter jejuni causes a superficial enterocolitis and mainly involves the terminal ileum and colon.

Microscopy: It shows focal necrosis of intestinal epithelium and acute inflammation. Biopsy findings are nonspecific. Mucosal and intraepithelial neutrophil infiltrates are prominent mainly in the superficial mucosa. Cryptitis (neutrophil infiltration of the crypt epithelium) and crypt abscesses (accumulations of neutrophils within lumens of epithelial crypts) may also be observed. The crypt architecture is preserved, though its assessment can be difficult whenever there is severe damage to the mucosa. These changes undergo resolution in 7–14 days.

Clinical Features

Main symptom is watery diarrhea (>10 stools per day), either acute or following an influenza-like prodrome. In 15% of adults and more than 50% of children it can cause dysentery (containing gross blood and mucus). Diagnosis is mainly by stool culture.

Yersinia

Three *Yersinia* species can cause disease in humans. *Y. enterocolitica* and *Y. pseudotuberculosis* cause GI disease and *Y. pestis causes* pulmonic and bubonic plague. *Y. enterocolitica* and *Y. pseudotuberculosis* are facultative anaerobes, gram-negative, coccoid or rod-shaped bacteria.

Source of infection: *Y. enterocolitica* and *Y. pseudotuberculosis* are found in feces of wild and domestic animals such as rodents, sheep, cattle, dogs, cats, and horses. *Y. pseudotuberculosis* is also seen in domestic birds (e.g., turkeys, ducks, geese, and canaries). Both organisms can contaminate drinking water and milk.

Mode of infection: Infections are mostly due to ingestion of pork, raw milk, and contaminated water. *Y. enterocolitica* is mostly acquired from consumption of contaminated meat, and *Y. pseudotuberculosis* from contact with infected animals.

Pathogenesis

Yersinia proliferates in the ileum and invades M cells of intestine. These organisms use specialized bacterial proteins, called adhesins. These adhesins bind to β1 integrins present on the epithelial cells of host intestine. A pathogenicity island encodes proteins that mediate iron capture and transport. It is similar iron transport systems and are also present in *E. coli, Klebsiella, Salmonella,* and enterobacteria. In *Yersinia,* **iron increases virulence and stimulates systemic dissemination. Thus, individuals with increased nonheme iron (e.g., certain chronic forms of anemia or hemochromatosis) have increased risk for sepsis and death due to *Yersinia*.**

MORPHOLOGY

Yersinia infections predominantly involve the ileum, appendix, and right colon. The organisms proliferate extracellularly in lymphoid tissue and cause enlargement of regional lymph node and hyperplasia of Peyer's patch. It produces thickening of bowel wall. The mucosa covering lymphoid tissue in the intestine may become hemorrhagic, and produce aphthous erosions and ulcers. They show infiltration by neutrophils and also granulomas. *Y. pseudotuberculosis* localizes in ileal-cecal lymph nodes and produces abscesses and granulomas in the lymph nodes, spleen, and liver. Similar to *Shigella,* these lesions may cause diagnostic confusion with Crohn disease.

Clinical Features

Yersinia infection commonly presents with abdominal pain, nausea, vomiting, and abdominal tenderness. Fever, diarrhea is less common. Invasion of Peyer's patch with involvement of regional lymphatics and abdominal pain in the right lower quadrant can mimic acute appendicitis.

Extraintestinal symptoms: These include **pharyngitis, arthralgia, and erythema nodosum.**

Diagnosis: *Yersinia* can be detected by stool culture on *Yersinia*-selective agar. In patients with extraintestinal disease, lymph nodes or blood cultures may also be positive.

Complications: These include reactive arthritis with urethritis and conjunctivitis, myocarditis, erythema nodosum, and kidney disease.

BACTERIAL INFECTIONS WITH ANIMAL RESERVOIRS OR INSECT VECTORS

Brucellosis

- Brucellosis (Malta fever, undulant fever, Mediterranean fever, Rock fever of Gibraltar) is a zoonotic (acquired from domestic animals) infection caused by *Brucella* species.
- *Brucella* are small, aerobic, gram-negative rods. They primarily infect monocytes/macrophages in humans.
- **Species:** There are four *Brucella* species and each species of *Brucella* has its own animal reservoir. Four species of *Brucella* are: *B. melitensis* (goats, sheep and camels), *B. abortus* (cattle), *B. suis* (swine, pigs), and *B. canis* (dogs).
- Natural reservoir of brucellosis is animals. Almost every type of domesticated animal and many wild ones are infected by *Brucella*. The organisms reside in the genitourinary systems of animals', and infection is usually endemic in animal herds.

Mode of Infection

- **Ingestion:** Infected animals may excrete *Brucella* in their milk, and human infection is acquired by ingesting contaminated dairy products (especially unpasteurized raw milk) and uncooked meat.
- **Direct infection:** Direct contact with infected animal urine, feces, vaginal discharge, and uterine products may act as sources of infection and they may enter humans through abraded skin. Brucellosis can occur as an occupational hazard in ranchers (who owns or manages a large farm), herders (person who takes care of a large group of animals of the same type), veterinarians (a person qualified to treat diseased or injured animals), and slaughterhouse (place where animals are killed for their meat) workers.
- **Inhalation of infectious aerosols:**
  - Pens, tables, slaughter houses
  - Conjunctival splashes, injection
- **Person-to-person transmission is very rare,** particularly mother-to-child.

Pathogenesis

Brucella gain entry into the blood circulation through skin abrasions, lungs, conjunctiva, or oropharynx.

From the blood stream, they spread to the liver, spleen, lymph nodes, and bone marrow, where they multiply in macrophages. Generalized hyperplasia of macrophages occurs and may cause lymphadenopathy and hepatosplenomegaly. Organisms are periodically released from infected phagocytic cells and may be responsible for the febrile episodes of the brucellosis. *Brucella* usually cannot be demonstrated histologically.

MORPHOLOGY

Infection with *B. abortus* produces noncaseating granulomas in the liver, spleen, lymph nodes, and bone marrow. By contrast, infection with *B. melitensis* do not produce classic granulomas, instead only small aggregates of mononuclear inflammatory cells are seen scattered throughout the liver. Infection with B. suis may cause suppurative liver abscesses.

Clinical Features

Brucellosis is a systemic infection and can involve any organ or systems. It has a very insidious onset with varying clinical signs in 50% of cases. The most common sign in all patients at some time during the illness, is an intermittent/irregular fever. It can wax and wane with variable duration (over weeks to months if untreated). Hence termed as *undulant fever.* Human brucellosis may manifest as an acute systemic disease or as a chronic infection.

Complications: Most common complications of brucellosis are seen involving the bones and joints. This may be spondylitis of the lumbar spine, sacroiliitis, arthritis, and suppuration in large joints. Others include peripheral neuritis, meningitis, orchitis, endocarditis, myocarditis, and pneumonia.

Diagnosis

- **Culture:** Definitive diagnosis depends on the isolation of the *Brucella.*
- **Serological tests** may also aid diagnosis and are of greater value in chronic disease. In ***Brucella* agglutination test,** a fourfold or greater rise in titer of agglutination antibody (IgM) is highly suggestive of brucellosis. Raised serum IgG level indicates current or recent infection; a negative test excludes chronic brucellosis.
- Species-specific PCR tests.

Cat-scratch Disease

Cat-scratch disease is a self-limited infection. It is usually caused by *Bartonella* strain *Bartonella henselae* and, more rarely, *Bartonella quintana. Bartonella* are small (0.2–0.6 µm) gram-negative bacterial rods. Cat-scratch disease is more common in children (80%) than in adults. *Bartonella* are difficult to culture. But can be easily seen in tissue sections of the skin, lymph nodes, and conjunctiva when stained with a silver impregnation technique.

Source of infection: The animal reservoir is cats.

Mode of infection: Infection develops by inoculation of bacillus into the skin by the claws of cats (or rarely other animals) or by thorns or splinters. Sometimes the conjunctiva can become contaminated by close contact with a cat, probably by licking by the cat around the human eye.

Pathology

After inoculation, *Bartonella* multiply in the walls of small vessels and about collagen fibers at the site of inoculation. They are carried to regional lymph nodes and they produce **suppurative** and **granulomatous lymphadenitis (Figs. 58A and B)**. During early stages, clusters of bacteria fill and expand lumen of small blood vessels. In late lesions, bacteria are usually not seen.

Clinical Features

A papule develops at the site of inoculation. This is followed by enlargement of regional lymph nodes. Lymph nodes are tender and enlarged for 3–4 months and may drain through the skin. About 50% of patients may have symptoms such as fever and malaise, rash, a brief encephalitis, and erythema nodosum. Other clinical presentations are as follows:

- **Parinaud oculoglandular syndrome** (preauricular adenopathy secondary to conjunctival infection).
- **Bacillary angiomatosis:** It is a vascular skin disease and can extend to involve other organs. It is mostly seen in immunocompromised patients.
- **Bacillary peliosis:** It affects the liver and spleen and they show blood-filled cystic spaces. It also occurs in patients with severe immunologic compromise.

PULMONARY INFECTIONS WITH GRAM-NEGATIVE BACTERIA

Klebsiella and *Enterobacter*

Klebsiella and *Enterobacter* species are short, encapsulated, gram-negative bacilli. They **produce nosocomial infections that cause necrotizing lobar pneumonia.** A **nosocomial infection** is an infection that originate or takes place in a hospital (i.e., acquired in a hospital). **Nosocomial infections can also be termed as healthcare-associated infections** (HAIs) and **hospital-acquired infections.**

Epidemiology: *Klebsiella* and *Enterobacter* are responsible for about 10% of all hospital-acquired (nosocomial) infections. These infections may involve the lungs, urinary tract, biliary tract, and surgical wounds. In hospital it can transmit infection from person-to-person. **Mode of infection is inhalation**.

Predisposing factors: These include patient with obstructive pulmonary disease in endotracheal tubes, indwelling catheters, chronic debilitating diseases, malnourishment, chronic alcoholism, and immunosuppression. These organisms may produce secondary pneumonia as a complication of influenza or other respiratory viral infections.

MORPHOLOGY

After inhalation, these bacteria multiply in the alveolar spaces of lung. This produces consolidation of lung parenchyma and alveoli get filled with a mucoid exudate with macrophages and fibrin. The accumulated exudate compresses the alveolar walls. This can lead to necrosis and formation of small abscess. Numerous small abscesses may coalesce and may form cavity.

Clinical features: They clinically present with sudden onset of pneumonia, fever, pleuritic pain, and productive cough. The characteristic feature is **thick mucoid** (often blood-tinged) **sputum**. The sputum is mucoid **because the organism produces an abundant viscid capsular polysaccharide**. The patient may find difficult to expectorate the sputum due to its thick nature. If the infection is severe, patient may develop dyspnea, cyanosis, and death may occur within 2–3 days.

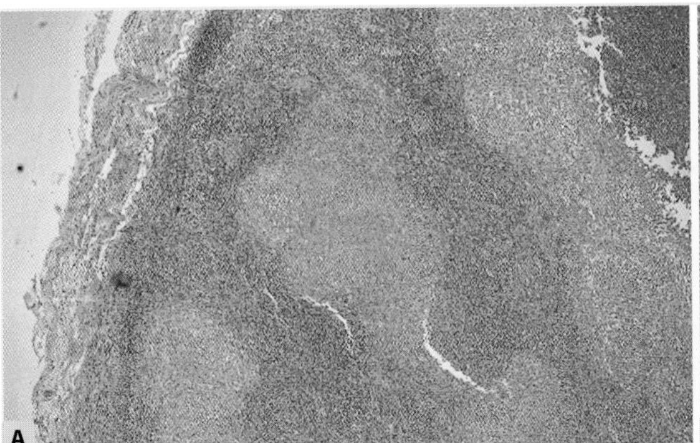

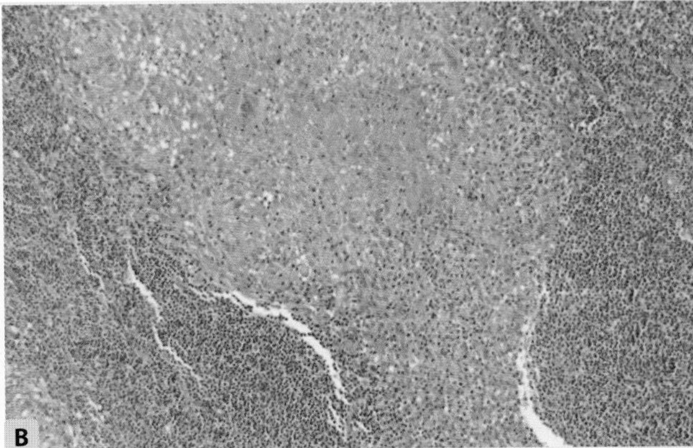

FIGS. 58A AND B: Cat-scratch disease showing lymph nodes with suppurative and granulomatous lymphadenitis.

Complications: *Klebsiella* and *Enterobacter* infections may lead to fulminating, often fatal, septicemia. Recently, there is emergence of a group of highly drug-resistant members of the Enterobacteriaceae, including *Klebsiella* and *Enterobacter*. These are called as carbapenem-resistant Enterobacteriaceae (CRE). They are resistant to the carbapenem class of antibiotics. Carbapenem are considered to be the "drugs of last resort" for such infections. These carbapenem-resistant *Klebsiella pneumoniae* (CRKP) produces an enzyme, or a β-metallo-lactamase 1(NDM-1). These strains are resistant to almost all *presently* available antibiotics.

Legionella

Legionella pneumophila is a minute aerobic bacillus. It has the cell wall structure of a gram-negative organism but stains poorly with Gram stains. It was first identified at the 1976 American Legion convention in Philadelphia.

Source of infection: *Legionella* are present as natural bodies of fresh water in small numbers. They survive chlorination. They proliferate in artificial aquatic environments [e.g., water-cooling towers, water heaters, humidifiers, tubing systems of domestic (potable) water supplies and evaporative condensers].

Mode of infection: It is transmitted by either inhalation of aerosolized organisms or aspiration of contaminated drinking water.

Predisposing factors: This organism is not part of normal human flora and it is not contagious. Respiratory tract defences (e.g., mucociliary mechanism of the airway) are the first line of defense against *Legionella* infection. Conditions that interfere with these respiratory defense mechanism (e.g., smoking, alcoholism, and chronic lung diseases) increase the risk of developing *Legionella* pneumonia. Other predisposing conditions include cardiac, renal, immunologic, or hematologic disease. Organ transplant recipients and immunosuppressed patients are particularly at increased risk.

Incubation period: Up to 2–10 days

Diseases produced: *Legionella* cause two distinct diseases: (1) **Pneumonia** and (2) **Pontiac fever**.

Pathogenesis

The pathogenesis of *Legionella* pneumonia (Legionnaires disease) is known whereas that of Pontiac fever is not clearly understood.

***Legionella* pneumonia:** *Legionella* after inhalation reach the terminal bronchioles or alveoli. They are phagocytosed by alveolar macrophages. They replicate within phagosomes of macrophages and blocks the fusion of lysosomes with the phagosomes. Thus, it protects itself from destruction by lysosomal enzymes. The multiplying *Legionella* are released from macrophages. The released *Legionella* infect new macrophages. When host develops immunity, macrophages gets activated and prevent the intracellular growth of organisms.

MORPHOLOGY

Legionnaires disease is an acute bronchopneumonia. It is usually patchy.

Microscopy: Alveoli and bronchioles are filled with an exudate composed of proteinaceous fluid, fibrin, macrophages, and neutrophils. Alveolar walls undergo destruction and produce necrosis. This leads to formation of microabscesses. Many macrophages show cytoplasmic vacuoles containing *L. pneumophila* causing pushing of the nuclei to the periphery (eccentric nuclei).

When pneumonia resolves, the lungs heal with little permanent damage.

Clinical features: It usually presents with rapidly progressive pneumonia, fever, nonproductive cough, and myalgia. Pneumonia may be mild to life-threatening. Chest X-ray shows unilateral, diffuse, and patchy consolidation. It may progress to widespread nodular consolidation. Toxic symptoms, hypoxia, and lack of interest may be prominent. Death may occur within a few days. In patients who survive, convalescence is prolonged.

Pontiac Fever

It is a self-limited, flu-like upper respiratory tract infection. It clinically manifests as fever, malaise, myalgias, and headache. In contrast to Legionnaires disease, it does not produce pulmonary consolidation and resolves spontaneously in 3–5 days.

Diagnosis: It is diagnosed by detecting *Legionella* DNA in sputum using a PCR-based test or by identification of *Legionella* antigens in the urine. Though culture is considered as diagnostic gold standard, it takes 3–5 days for the result.

Melioidosis

Melioidosis (Whitmore disease, Rangoon beggars disease) is an uncommon disease caused by *Burkholderia* (formerly *Pseudomonas*) *pseudomallei*. It is an aerobic, small gram-negative motile bacillus, with "safety pin" appearance. The organism grows in wet environments, such as rice paddies and marshes (an area of low, wet land, usually covered with tall grasses). It is an opportunistic pathogen found in surface water and moist soil and produces exotoxin.

Mode of transmission:

- **Contact with contaminated soil or water:** It is the most common route of acquiring the disease. The skin is the usual portal of entry. The organisms enter through pre-existing lesions (e.g., penetrating wounds, burns).
- **Other routes:** These include aspiration or ingestion of contaminated water and inhalation of dust or aerosolized droplets from soil. Transmission between infected animals and/or infected individual is very rare. Person-to-person transmission may rarely occur through sexual contact with an individual with prostatic infection.

Incubation period: It varies from 2 days to months to many years. *B. pseudomallei* can survive in phagocytic cells. Hence, melioidosis can result after a latent period.

Risk factors: Immunosuppressive events or chronic diseases such as diabetes, chronic alcohol use, chronic renal disease, and chronic lung disease.

Pathology and Clinical Features

Most infections are asymptomatic and its clinical course is variable. It may produce acute or chronic melioidosis.

Acute melioidosis: It is a pulmonary infection and is the most common form. It ranges from a mild tracheobronchitis to an overwhelming cavitary pneumonia. In severe cases, patient presents with the sudden onset of high fever, constitutional symptoms, and a cough with blood-stained sputum. Acute septicemic melioidosis **is characterized by distinct abscesses in many organs** throughout the body (e.g., lungs, liver, spleen, and lymph nodes).

Chronic melioidosis: It is a persistent localized infection that may involve the lungs, skin, bones, or other organs. Lesions appear as suppurative or granulomatous abscesses. In the lung, it may be mistaken for tuberculosis.

Diagnosis

- It is **difficult** and has been called the great imitator (especially tuberculosis) because there are no pathognomonic lesions. Any organ can be affected and the lesions have no distinguishing characteristics.
- **Isolation of the organism** from blood, sputum, tissues, or wound exudates by culture can help to diagnose the disease.
- **Serological tests** for titers may also be used for diagnosis. Serological tests available include agglutination tests, indirect hemagglutination, complement fixation, immunofluorescence, and enzyme assays. Improved methods for rapid diagnosis are being evaluated.

11.4 Rickettsial Infections

CHAPTER OUTLINE

- Rocky mountain spotted fever
- Epidemic (Louse-borne) typhus
- Endemic (murine) typhus
- Scrub typhus
- Q fever
- Ehrlichiosis and anaplasmosis

Q. Write short essay on rickettsial infection.

Rickettsiae are a heterogeneous group of small, obligatory intracellular, gram-negative coccobacilli and short bacilli. Most of rickettsiae are vector-borne and transmitted by a tick, mite, flea, or louse vector. Four important members of *Rickettsia* group are *Rickettsia* species, *Orientia* species, *Ehrlichia* species, and *Anaplasma* species obligate intracellular bacteria.

Features: The rickettsiae pathogens cannot replicate outside a host. Unlike chlamydiae, rickettsiae replicate by binary fission (asexual reproduction by a separation of the body into two new bodies). They synthesize their own adenosine triphosphate (ATP) and can obtain ATP from the host. The organisms induce endocytosis by host target cells and replicate in the cytoplasm of host cells.

Except in the case of louse-borne typhus, humans are accidental hosts. Human infections result from insect bites. Several species of *Rickettsia* cause different diseases in human. Among the major group of rickettsioses, the **commonly** reported diseases (**Table 26**) in India are: (1) *Scrub typhus,* (2) *Murine (endemic) typhus,* (3) *Indian tick typhus, and* (4) *Q fever*. Human rickettsial infections are traditionally divided into the **"typhus group" and the "spotted fever group."** Most are febrile infections with a characteristic rash. An ***eschar*** is the characteristic lesion that develops at the site of inoculation.

Pathogenesis: The target cells for all rickettsiae in humans are endothelial cells of capillaries and small vessel. The organisms reproduce within the cytoplasm of endothelial cells and kill them. This produces a necrotizing vasculitis. The **severe manifestations of rickettsial infections are mainly due to infection of endothelial cells, causing endothelial dysfunction and injury.** The rickettsiae that cause typhus and spotted fevers mainly infect vascular endothelial cells, especially those in the lungs and brain. The rickettsiae enter endothelial cells by endocytosis. Using hemolysins, they escape from the endosome into the cytoplasm and disrupt phagosomal membranes. Rickettsiae proliferate in the cytoplasm of endothelial cell. They may either lyse the cell (typhus group) or spread from cell to cell using actin-based motility (spotted fever group). The widespread dysfunction of endothelial cells can lead to shock, peripheral and pulmonary edema, and disseminated intravascular coagulation (DIC), renal failure, and central nervous system (CNS) manifestations (including coma). The innate immune response to rickettsial infection includes natural killer (NK) cells, which produce IFN-γ. Subsequent cytotoxic T lymphocyte (CTL) responses are extremely important for eradication of rickettsial infections. Activated NK cells and T cells produce interferon (IFN)-γ and tumor necrosis factor (TNF) and they stimulate the production of bactericidal nitric oxide derivatives. CTLs lyse infected cells and reduce the proliferation of rickettsiae.

Staining: Rickettsiae have cell wall structures like that of gram-negative, rod-shaped bacteria. However, they do not stain well (poorly stained) with Gram stain. They are best demonstrated by the Gimenez method or with acridine orange.

Rocky Mountain Spotted Fever

Rocky Mountain spotted fever (RMSF) is an acute, potentially fatal, systemic vasculitis caused by *Rickettsia rickettsii*. Its name is derived from its discovery in Idaho, but the disease is uncommon in the Rocky.

It is transmitted to humans by bites of infected ticks (vectors for *R. rickettsia*). *R. rickettsia* is transmitted from mother to progeny ticks, thereby maintaining a natural reservoir for human infection.

Pathogenesis: *R. rickettsii* organisms in salivary glands of ticks are inoculated into the dermis of skin of the host as the ticks feed. Organisms spread lymphohematogenously throughout the body of the human host and infect endothelial cells of small blood vessels. They enter into the cytoplasm of vascular endothelial cells and reproduce. Then, they are shed into the vascular and lymphatic systems. They further infect and destroy the vascular endothelium, which causes a systemic vasculitis. The inflammatory damage to blood vessels of skin produces hemorrhagic rash and is the most visible manifestation of the generalized vascular injury. This rash extends over the entire body, including the palms of the hands and soles of the feet. This is the hallmark of Rocky Mountain spotted fever. In contrast to other rickettsiae that infect only endothelial cells of capillaries, *R. rickettsii* spreads also to vascular smooth muscle and endothelium of larger vessels. Extensive damage to blood vessel walls causes increased vascular permeability and fluid exudation (edema) and ischemia. Fluid loss can be so extensive as to lead to hypovolemia and shock. Damage to pulmonary capillaries can produce pulmonary edema and acute alveolar injury.

Table 26: Common rickettsial infections.

Diseases	*Rickettsial agent*	*Insect vector*	*Mammalian reservoir*	*Clinical features*
Typhus group				
Louse-borne typhus (Epidemic typhus)	*Rickettsia prowazekii*	Louse	Human	Fever/chills, myalgia, headache, rash (no eschar) all over body except palm, sole, and face
Murine typhus (Endemic typhus)	*Rickettsia typhi*	Flea	Rodents	Fever, myalgia, headache, rash (no eschar), trunk, extremities, and milder form of illness
Scrub typhus	*Orientia tsutsugamushi*	Mite	Rodents	Fever, headache, rash with eschar* cigarette burn sign, and lymphadenopathy
Spotted fever group (genus *Rickettsia*)				
Indian tick typhus	*Rickettsia conorii*	Tick	Rodent and dog	Fever, headache, and rash with eschar, first appear on wrist and ankle
Rocky mountain spotted fever	*Rickettsia rickettsii*	Tick	Rodents and dogs	Fever, headache, rash (no eschar)—first appear on wrist and ankle, palms and soles involved, systemic complications—respiratory, cardiovascular, central nervous, renal, and hepatic system
Rickettsial pox	*Rickettsia akari*	Mite	Mice	Mild illness, fever, headache, vesicular rash with eschar, lymphadenopathy, and resemblance to chicken pox
Others				
Q fever	*Coxiella burnetii*	Nil (by inhalation)	Cattle, sheep, and goats	Fever, headache, fatigue, pneumonia, endocarditis, and no rash
Trench fever Rochalimaea	*Bartonella quintana*	Louse	Human	Fever, splenomegaly, bone pains, and maculopapular rash

*In scrub typhus, the eschar begins as a small papule, then enlarges, undergoes central necrosis, and eventually acquires a blackened crust with an erythematous halo that resembles a cigarette burn. The eschar resembling "**cigarette burn mark**" is seen in 95% of cases and is most important diagnostic clue of scrub typhus.

MORPHOLOGY

Rocky Mountain spotted fever is characterized by **vascular lesions throughout the body and responsible for the rash.** They affect capillaries, venules, arterioles, and, sometimes, larger vessels. The vascular lesions often lead to acute necrosis, reactive hyperplasia of vascular endothelial cells, fibrin extravasation, and occasionally thrombosis of the small blood vessels, including arterioles. In severe Rocky Mountain spotted fever, foci of necrotic skin appear and are prominent over the fingers, toes, elbows, ears, and scrotum. The perivascular inflammatory response is initially by neutrophils and macrophages and later by lymphocytes and plasma cells. They are seen in the brain, skeletal muscle, lungs, kidneys, testes, and heart muscle. The vascular lesions in the brain may involve larger vessels and produce microinfarcts and extravasation of blood into surrounding tissues. The intracellular bacilli are oriented in parallel rows and in an end-to-end pattern produces an appearance of a "flotilla at anchor facing the wind." Development of a noncardiogenic pulmonary edema causing acute respiratory distress syndrome is the major cause of death.

Clinical features: Rocky Mountain spotted fever manifests with fever, headache, and myalgias, followed by a hemorrhagic skin rash. If untreated, 20–50% of infected patients die within 8–15 days.

Epidemic (Louse-borne) Typhus

Epidemic typhus is a severe systemic vasculitis transmitted from person to person by bites of infected body lice. It is caused by *Rickettsia prowazekii,* an organism that has a human–louse–human life cycle (**Fig. 59**). The human body louse (*Pediculus humanus corporis*) lives in clothing under poor hygienic conditions.

Epidemiology: Devastating epidemics of typhus were associated with poverty and poor sanitation, when individuals live in close contact during natural disasters, famine, or war.

MORPHOLOGY

The pathologic findings in infection by *R. prowazekii* are similar to those in Rocky Mountain spotted fever and other rickettsial diseases. At autopsy, except for splenomegaly and occasional areas of necrosis, there is no significant finding.

Microscopy: It shows mononuclear cell collections in various organs (e.g., skin, brain, and heart). These mononuclear cells include mast cells, lymphocytes, plasma cells, and macrophages. They are frequently arranged as **typhus nodules** around arterioles and capillaries. Throughout the body, the endothelium of small blood vessels shows focal necrosis and hyperplasia and inflammatory cells in the wall. Rickettsiae can be demonstrated within the cytoplasm of endothelial cells.

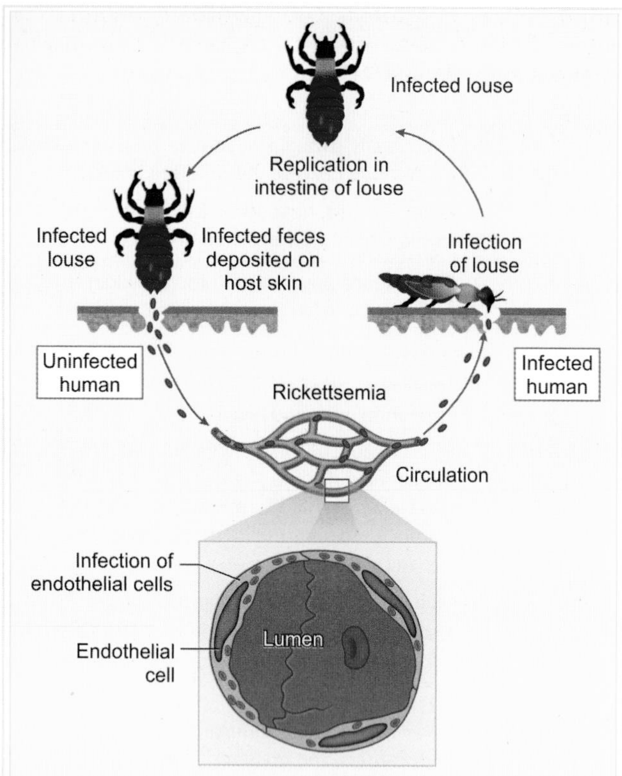

FIG. 59: Epidemic typhus (louse-borne typhus). Man–louse–man life cycle of *Rickettsia prowazekii*. Epidemic typhus begins as a localized infection of capillary endothelium and progresses to a systemic vasculitis. This organism multiplies in endothelial cells, which detach, rupture, and release organisms into the circulation (rickettsemia). When a louse takes a blood meal from a rickettsemic patient (infected patient with rickettsemia), it becomes infected with rickettsiae. The organisms enter the midgut epithelial cells of louse. It multiplies and ruptures these epithelial cells and released rickettsiae into the lumen of the louse intestine are shed in its feces in large numbers. The infected louse leaves a febrile infected person and deposits infected feces on the skin or clothing of its subsequent host during its blood meal. Contaminated feces of infected louse get deposited uninfected host, penetrate an abrasion (autoinoculation of the organisms by scratching), or are inhaled (when the person inhales airborne rickettsiae from clothing containing louse feces). The rickettsiae then enter endothelial cells of vessels and multiply there. Rupture of endothelial cells release organisms into the circulation (rickettsemia) and thus completing the cycle. The infected louse gets killed by the rickettsiae and does not pass *R. prowazekii* to its offspring.

Clinical features: Symptoms of louse-borne typhus are fever, headache, and myalgias. This is followed by a rash. The rash is initially macular, which progresses to a petechial, maculopapular rash on the entire body except the face, palms, and soles. In fatal cases, the rash may become confluent and purpuric.

Endemic (Murine) Typhus

Endemic typhus is caused by *Rickettsia typhi* and is similar to epidemic typhus but tends to be milder.

Rickettsia typhi consists of rat–flea–rat cycle of transmission. However, humans get infected with *R. typhi*, interrupting this rat–flea–rat cycle of transmission and *R. typhi* is maintained in mammalian host–flea cycles with rats. Fleas acquire *R. typhi* from rickettsemic rats and these rats carry the *R. typhi* throughout their life span. Nonimmune rats and humans are infected when *Rickettsia*-laden flea feces contaminate pruritic bite lesions on the skin. They may enter the body via the small wound made by the bite. *R. typhi* may also contaminate clothes and transmission can occur via inhalation of aerosolized rickettsiae from flea feces. If inhaled, they cause pulmonary infection. Infected rats appear healthy, though they are rickettsemic for ~2 weeks.

Scrub Typhus

Scrub typhus **(Tsutsugamushi fever)** is mite-borne, acute, febrile illness of humans caused by *Orientia tsutsugamushi* (previously known as *Rickettsia tsutsugamushi*), the only member of its genus. *O. tsutsugamushi* differs considerably from *Rickettsia* species both genetically and in cell wall composition (i.e., it lacks lipopolysaccharide). Rodents are the natural mammalian reservoir. From rodents, the organism is transmitted to human by trombiculid-infected larval mites known as chiggers (the only stage that feeds on a host). These mites transmit infection to their larvae, which crawl to the tips of vegetation and attach to passers-by. While feeding, mites inoculate *O. tsutsugamushi* into the skin. Rickettsemia and lymphadenopathy develop shortly.

A multiloculated vesicle develops at the site of inoculation and it ulcerates and forms a characteristic eschar (dry, dark scab or falling away of dead skin). As the lesion in the skin heals, patient suddenly develops headache, fever myalgia, and cough. This is followed by pneumonia, a macular rash, prominent inflammatory lymphadenopathy, and hepatosplenomegaly. Severe infections may be associated with complications such as myocarditis, meningoencephalitis, and shock. In untreated patients, mortality rates may be up to 30%.

Q Fever

Q fever is a self-limited, systemic infection caused by *Coxiella burnetii. Coxiella burnetii* is a small pleomorphic coccobacillus with a gram-negative cell wall. Unlike true rickettsiae, *C. burnetii* enters cells passively upon phagocytosis by macrophages. It does not produce a vasculitis. Hence, there is no rash.

Source of infection: Infection is endemic in many wild and domesticated animals. The usual sources of human infection are cattle, sheep, and goats. These animals shed numerous organisms in urine, feces, milk, and bodily fluids. Q fever is more common in herders, slaughterhouse workers, veterinarians, dairy workers, and others with occupational exposure to infected domesticated animals.

Mode of infection: Q fever in humans occurs due to exposure to infected animals or animal products. Infection can also spread from person to person by aerosol droplets.

Pathogenesis: *Coxiella burnetii* is inhaled and is phagocytosed by alveolar macrophages. They escape intracellular killing in macrophages by inhibiting the phagosome maturation (cathepsin fusion) and has adapted to the acidic phagolysosome by producing superoxide dismutase. Thus, they replicate in the phagolysosomes. Recruitment of neutrophils and macrophages leads to formation of focal bronchopneumonia. The organism disseminates through the body, mainly infecting monocytes/macrophages. Majority of infections resolve with the development of specific cell-mediated immunity. Occasionally, it may persist as chronic infections.

MORPHOLOGY

The lungs and liver are most prominently involved organs in Q fever:

Lungs: It shows single or multiple irregular areas of consolidation. Microscopically, it shows alveoli filled with neutrophils and macrophages. Giemsa stain may demonstrate organisms in macrophages.

Liver: It shows multiple **microscopic granulomas with a distinctive "fibrin ring."** In these granulomas, epithelioid macrophages encircle a ring of fibrin.

Clinical features: It may be acute or chronic. Usually, Q fever presents as a self-limited mildly symptomatic febrile disease. More severe cases may present with headache, fever, fatigue, and myalgias, with no rash. Pulmonary infection is almost always present. It usually resolves spontaneously within 2–14 days. Chronic Q fever usually manifests as endocarditis in patients with previous valvular heart disease, immunosuppression, or chronic renal insufficiency.

Ehrlichiosis and Anaplasmosis

- Ehrlichiosis is caused mainly by *Ehrlichia chaffeensis* transmitted by the lone star tick. They predominantly infect monocytes.
- *Anaplasmosis* is caused by *Anaplasma phagocytophilum* and is transmitted by deer tick. It predominantly infects neutrophils.
- **Ehrlichiosis** and **anaplasmosis** have similar clinical presentations. They usually manifest with abrupt onset of fever, headache, and malaise. It may progress to respiratory insufficiency, renal failure, and shock. Rash may be found in about 40% of patients with *E. chaffeensis* infections. The rash is nonspecific and can be macular, maculopapular, or petechial. Characteristic cytoplasmic inclusions (morulae) composed of masses of bacteria are present in leukocytes. These bacteria occasionally form the shape of a mulberry.

Diagnosis: Rickettsial diseases are usually diagnosed depending on clinical features. Diagnosis is confirmed by serology or immunostaining of the organisms.

11.5 Fungal Infections and Opportunistic Infections

CHAPTER OUTLINE

- Introduction
  - Major types of fungal infections
- Yeast infections
  - Candidiasis
  - *Candida auris* infections
  - Cryptococcosis
  - Pneumocystis infections
- Molds
  - Aspergillosis
  - Mucormycosis (zygomycosis)
  - Entomophthoramycosis
- Dimorphic fungi
  - Histoplasmosis
  - Blastomycosis
  - Coccidioidomycosis
  - Paracoccidioidomycosis (south american blastomycosis)
  - Sporotrichosis
  - Phaeohyphomycoses
  - Mycetoma
  - Rhinosporidiosis
  - Laboratory diagnosis of fungal infection

INTRODUCTION

Mycology is the study of fungi. Fungi are eukaryotes (organism with complex cells or a single cell with a complex structure). Thus, they possess nuclear membranes and cytoplasmic organelles (e.g., mitochondria and endoplasmic reticulum). They are larger and more complex than bacteria and vary in size from 2 to 100 μm. They grow as multicellular filaments (mold) or individual cell alone or in chains (yeast).

Morphological types: Fungi have cell wall, which gives them a shape. There are two morphologic types of fungi namely yeasts and molds.

- **Yeasts (Fig. 60A):** They are **unicellular forms of fungi**. They are round to oval. They reproduce by budding, a process by which daughter organisms pinch off from a parent. Some yeasts (e.g., *Candida albicans*) produce buds that fail to detach, but instead become elongated, producing a chain of elongated yeast cells called **pseudohyphae** (i.e., chains of elongated yeast cells that resemble hyphae). Budding is a common mode of asexual reproduction, typical of yeasts. A fungal cell may produce single or multiple buds.
- **Molds (Fig. 60B):** These are multicellular, thread-like filamentous fungal colonies with branching tubules, or **hyphae** measuring 2–10 μm in diameter. Hyphae are tubular, branching filaments of fungal cells, the mold form of growth. Most hyphal cells are separated by porous cross-walls or septa. Pseudohyphae are chains of elongated buds or blastoconidia and the septations between cells are constricted. The mass of tangled hyphae in the mold form is called a **mycelium.** They grow and divide at their tips. Some hyphae are separated by septa that are located at regular intervals and others are nonseptate. They can produce round cells known as **conidia**, which can easily become airborne, disseminating the fungus. Conidia is asexual reproductive structures (mitospores) produced either from the transformation of a vegetative yeast or hyphal cell or from a specialized conidiogenous cell. Conidia may be formed on specialized hyphae, termed conidiophores. Microconidia are small, and macroconidia are large or multicellular.
- **Dimorphic fungi:** Many fungi are dimorphic, i.e., they grow and exist as yeast or molds, depending on environmental conditions (yeast form at human body temperature and a mold form at room temperature).
  - Grow as filamentous (mold/mycelia) forms at room temperature (or culture at 22–25°C).
  - Grow as yeast form at human body temperature (or culture at 37°C).

Spore is a specialized propagule and can form can give rise to new fungi. They have enhanced survival value, such as resistance to adverse conditions or structural features that promote dispersion. Spores may result from asexual (e.g., conidia or sporangiospores) or sexual reproduction.

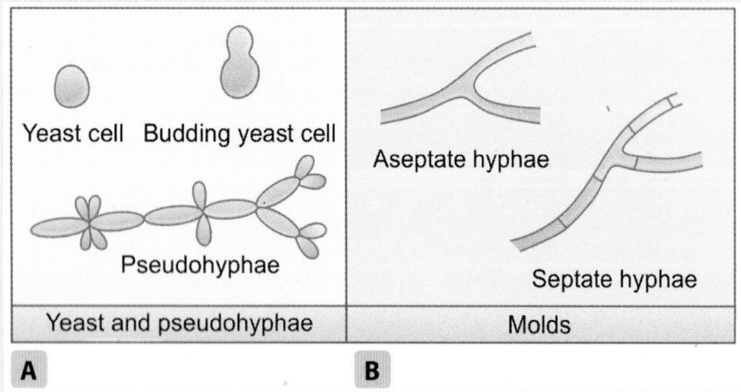

FIGS. 60A AND B: Morphological types of fungi.

Major Types of Fungal Infections (Table 27)

There are >100,000 known fungi and only a few cause diseases in humans. Fungal infections are also known as mycoses. Human fungal infections are divided into four major types:

1. **Superficial and cutaneous mycoses:** Common and limited to the skin, hair, and nails.
2. **Subcutaneous mycoses:** Involve the skin, subcutaneous tissues, and lymphatics.
3. **Endemic mycoses:** Caused by dimorphic fungi (e.g., coccidioidomycosis) that are not a part of the normal human microbiota, but rather are acquired from

Table 27: Examples of major mycoses and causative fungi.

Category and mycosis	Causative fungal agents
Superficial mycoses	
• Pityriasis versicolor	*Malassezia* species
Cutaneous mycoses	
• Dermatophytosis	*Microsporum* species, *Trichophyton* species, and *Epidermophyton floccosum*
• Candidiasis of skin, mucosa, or nails	*Candida albicans* and other *Candida* species
Subcutaneous mycoses	
• Chromoblastomycosis	*Phialophora verrucosa, Fonsecaea pedrosoi*, and others
• Mycetoma	*Pseudallescheria boydii, Madurella mycetomatis*, and others
• Sporotrichosis	*Sporothrix schenckii*
• Phaeohyphomycosis	*Exophiala, Bipolaris, Exserohilum*, and other dematiaceous molds
Endemic (primary, systemic)* mycoses	
• Coccidioidomycosis	*Coccidioides posadasii* and *Coccidioides immitis*
• Histoplasmosis	*Histoplasma capsulatum*
• Blastomycosis	*Blastomyces dermatitidis*
• Paracoccidioidomycosis	*Paracoccidioides brasiliensis*
Opportunistic mycoses	
• Systemic candidiasis	*C. albicans* and many other *Candida* species
• Cryptococcosis	*Cryptococcus neoformans* and *Cryptococcus gattii*
• Aspergillosis	*Aspergillus fumigatus* and other *Aspergillus* species
• Phaeohyphomycosis	*Cladophialophora bantiana*; species of *Alternaria, Cladosporium, Bipolaris, Exserohilum*, and numerous other dematiaceous molds
• Mucormycosis (zygomycosis)	Species of *Rhizopus, Lichtheimia, Cunninghamella*, and other members of the order Mucorales
• Hyalohyphomycosis	Species of *Fusarium, Paecilomyces, Trichosporon*, and other hyaline molds
• Pneumocystis pneumonia	*Pneumocystis jiroveci*
• Penicilliosis	*Talaromyces marneffei*

*The endemic mycoses can also produce opportunistic infections

environmental sources. They can produce serious systemic illness in healthy individuals.

4. **Opportunistic mycoses:** These are caused by organisms (e.g., *Candida* and *Aspergillus*) that commonly are components of the normal human microbiota. These are universally present in nature and they only infect individuals who are immunocompromised. Most fungi are "opportunists." **Impaired defenses or immunosuppression** can be due to administration of corticosteroids, antineoplastic therapy, and congenital or acquired T-cell deficiencies. These **conditions predispose to mycotic infections.** They can cause life-threatening systemic diseases in individuals who are immunosuppressed.

YEAST INFECTIONS

Candidiasis

Q. Write short essay on candidiasis.

The genus *Candida* consists of >200 species of which about 15–20 species are frequently seen in human infections. More frequent in human are *C. albicans, C. glabrata, C. tropicalis, C. parapsilosis,* and *C. krusei*. ***C. albicans* is the most common fungal pathogen of humans.**

Many are present in endogenous human flora and they **live as** benign **commensals.** *Candida* species reside normally in the skin, mouth, gastrointestinal tract, and vagina. They are well adapted to life on or in the human body. They seldom produce disease in healthy individuals. However, they can produce disease when host defenses are compromised.

Infection: Most *Candida* infections occur when the normal commensal flora breaches the skin or mucosal barriers. These infections may be either restricted to the skin or mucous membranes or may disseminate widely.

Pathogenesis

A single strain of *Candida* can live as commensal or may become pathogenic. There is no environmental reservoir for *C. albicans*. *Candida* can shift between different phenotypes. Phenotypic switching is the mechanism by which *Candida* adapts to changes in the host environment (e.g., produced by antibiotic therapy, the immune response, or altered host physiology). *C. albicans* is capable of shifting between nine distinct cell shapes.

Protective mechanisms: Mechanical barriers, inflammatory cells, humoral immunity, and cell-mediated immunity prevent the invasion by *Candida*.

- **Cells involved in protection against *Candida* infection: These include neutrophils, macrophages and Th17 cells.**
  - **Neutrophils and macrophages:** These are phagocytes that phagocytose *C. albicans*. Oxidative killing by these phagocytes is a first line of host defense. Thus, individuals with neutropenia or defects in NADPH oxidase or myeloperoxidase (involved in oxidative killing) increase the risk of *C. albicans* infection. Filamentous forms of *C. albicans*, but not yeast, can escape from phagosomes formed during phagocytosis and these *C. albicans* enter the cytoplasm and proliferate.
  - **Th17 cells:** The yeast forms of *C. albicans* can activate dendritic cells by different pathways, more than that by the filamentous forms of the fungi. For example, yeast form expresses β-1,3-glucan and engages dectin on dendritic cells. This causes production of interleukin (IL)-6 and IL-23 and promotes Th17 responses. The Th17 responses by *C. albicans* in turn promote the recruitment of neutrophils and monocytes. These

responses are important for the protection against *C. albicans* infection. Thus, recurrent mucocutaneous candidiasis develops in individuals with either low T-cell counts due to HIV infection or inherited defects in the development Th17 cell.

- **Resident bacterial flora:** This normally limits the number of fungal organisms. These may be achieved by following mechanisms:
  - Bacteria block attachment of *Candida* to epithelial cells.
  - Bacteria compete with of *Candida* for their nutrients.
  - Bacteria prevent conversion of the fungus to tissue-invasive forms.

When any of these defenses is compromised, *Candida* can produce infections. Use of **antibiotics suppresses competing bacterial flora. This is the most common precipitating factor for candidiasis.** Under such conditions there will be growth of *Candida*, and the yeast form gets converted to its invasive form (hyphae or pseudohyphae). *Candida* invades superficially and elicits an inflammatory or immunologic response.

Mechanism of production of infection

- **Production of adhesins:** *C. albicans* produces many functionally different adhesins (e.g., integrin-like protein) that can bind to fibrinogen, fibronectin, laminin, epithelial cells, and endothelial cells. This helps them to adhere to host cells and is important determinant of virulence.
- **Production of enzymes:** *C. albicans* also produces many enzymes that help for invasion (e.g., nine secreted aspartyl proteinases). They help for invasion by degrading extracellular matrix proteins. The enzyme catalases prevent the oxidative killing of *C. albicans* within the phagocytic cells.
- **Various other factors:** *C. albicans* is **capable of growing as biofilms**. Biofilm is a thin usually resistant layer of microorganisms (microbial communities) that form on and coat various surfaces. Biofilms are irreversibly associated and are not removed by gentle rinsing. They reduce the organism's susceptibility to immune responses and antifungal drug therapy. Formation of biofilm by *C. albicans* contributes to its capability to cause disease. About 30 factors help in adhesion, maturation, and dispersion of *C. albicans* in the formation of biofilm. The biofilm of *C. albicans* consists of mixtures of yeast, filamentous forms, and fungal-derived extracellular matrix. *C. albicans* can form biofilms on implanted medical devices.
- **Predisposing skin lesion for superficial Candidiasis:** *Candida* normally inhabits skin surfaces. But, it does not produce disease in the skin without a predisposing lesion in the skin. The most common factor or skin lesion is maceration, or softening and destruction of the skin. Chronically warm and moist areas (e.g., between fingers and toes, between skinfolds, and under diapers) are susceptible to maceration and superficial Candidiasis.
- **Invasive Candidiasis:** Use of potent broad-spectrum antibiotics destroys bacteria that otherwise limit colonization of *Candida*. Use of medical devices (e.g., intravascular catheters, monitoring devices, endotracheal tubes, and urinary catheters) provides access of *Candida* to sterile sites. Individuals with AIDS and iatrogenic neutropenias are susceptible to even weak pathogens, such as *Candida*. Intravenous drug users develop invasive candidiasis due to direct inoculation of the fungi into the bloodstream.

MORPHOLOGY

General microscopic features: In tissue section, all forms (yeast, pseudohyphae, and true hyphae) of *C. albicans* may be present together in the same tissue (**Fig. 61**). But usually, yeast and pseudohyphae are more frequent and true hyphae are less common.

- Yeast is a unicellular (single-cell) form of fungi. They are round and measure 3–4 μm in diameter.
- **True hyphae** show the presence of septae and develop under reduced oxygen tension.
- The **pseudohyphae** form consists of chain of budding yeast cells joined end-to-end at constrictions (**Fig. 62** Inset). They represent an important diagnostic clue.

Superficial Candidiasis

Though the various forms of candidiasis vary in clinical severity, most are localized and produce superficial diseases, limited to a particular mucocutaneous site. Diabetic and burn patients are susceptible to superficial candidiasis. Various sites are as follows:

Thrush: Most common mucocutaneous candidiasis develops as a superficial infection on mucosal surfaces of the **oral cavity (thrush) (Fig. 61)**. It involves the tongue and mucous membranes of the mouth. This form of candidiasis is found in newborns, debilitated individuals, children receiving oral steroids for asthma, after a course of broad-spectrum antibiotics (destroy competing normal bacterial flora), and HIV-positive patients.

Florid proliferation of the fungi **produces a gray-white, friable, dirty-looking, and curd-like pseudomembrane** and is adherent to affected surface. This is composed of matted fungi, necrotic debris, neutrophils, and bacteria. Deep under

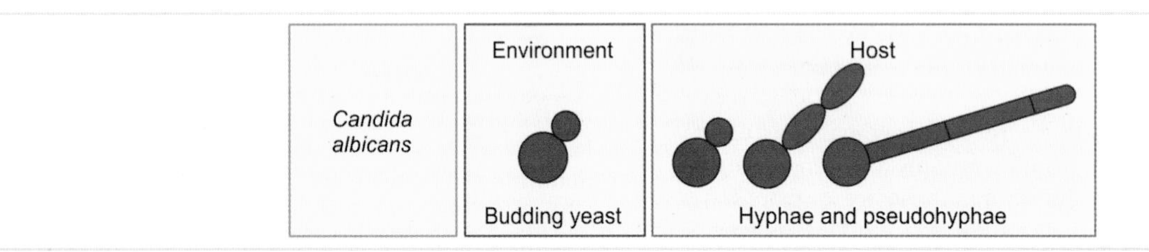

FIG. 61: Diagrammatic appearance of *Candida albicans*.

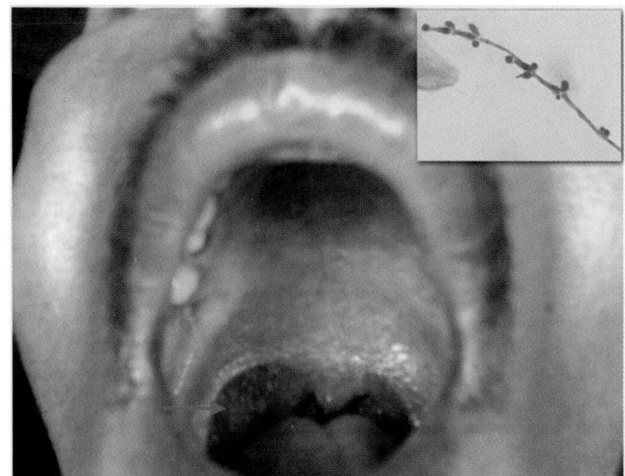

FIG. 62: Candidiasis (arrow) in a patient with acquired immunodeficiency syndrome (AIDS). Inset shows pseudohyphae of *Candida*.

the surface of pseudomembrane, it shows mucosal hyperemia and inflammation. They can be dislodged by scraping. Removal of the membranes leaves a painful, bleeding surface.

***C. albicans* esophagitis:** It occurs commonly in AIDS patients and in patients with hematolymphoid malignancies. Clinically, it presents with dysphagia (painful swallowing) and retrosternal pain. Endoscopic examination shows white plaques and pseudomembranes resembling oral thrush on the esophageal mucosa.

***C. albicans* vaginitis/vulvovaginitis (Fig. 63):** Candidal vaginitis is common and is most intense when vaginal pH is low. It develops in women who are diabetic, pregnant, or on corticosteroids or oral contraceptive pills or on antibacterial agents (which alter the vaginal flora). It is associated with intense vaginal and/or vulvar itching and a thick, curd-like discharge from vagina. Involved areas of the vulva are erythematous and tender. Candidal vaginitis is characterized by superficial invasion of the squamous epithelium, but inflammation is usually scanty.

Cutaneous candidiasis: It may present in many different forms. These include infection of the nail proper (onychomycosis), nail folds (paronychia), hair follicles (folliculitis), moist, intertriginous skin (infection of opposed skin surfaces), such as armpits or webs of the fingers and toes (intertrigo), and penile skin (balanitis).

- **In healthy** individual, *Candida* can cause **vaginitis/ vulvovaginitis** and **diaper rash** (cutaneous candidal infection in the perineum of infants, the region in contact with wet diapers).
- **Paronychia:** Infection of the nail bed.

Invasive/Disseminated Candidiasis

Candidal sepsis and disseminated candidiasis: Systemic candidiasis is rare. It can be caused by dissemination of *Candida* into the bloodstream and thereby spreading into various tissues or organs. *Candida* may enter through ulcerated skin or mucous membrane lesions. It can develop especially in patients with indwelling intravenous lines or catheters, or undergoing peritoneal dialysis. Severe disseminated candidiasis develops mostly in patients with neutropenia (e.g., due to acute leukemia, after chemotherapy, or hematopoietic

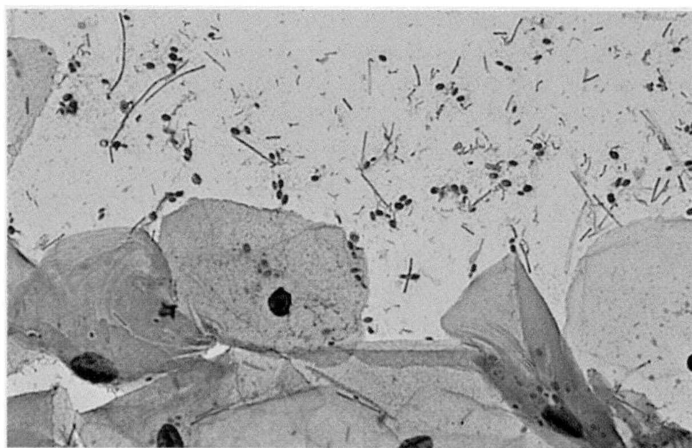

FIG. 63: Vaginal smear showing numerous unicellular yeast cells and few pseudohyphae.

stem cell transplantation). Various invasive types of Candidiasis include—(1) renal abscesses, (2) myocardial abscesses and endocarditis, (3) brain microabscesses and meningitis, (4) endophthalmitis (any eye structure can be involved), and (5) hepatic abscesses. In these locations, depending on the immune status of the infected individual, it may either produce little inflammation or suppurative process, or occasionally produce granulomas. It may lead to disseminated intravascular coagulation (DIC) and shock.

- **Candidal endocarditis:** *Candida* species endocarditis is the most common fungal endocarditis that occurs in patients with prosthetic heart valves, in intravenous drug abusers (drug users)

Laboratory Diagnosis of Candidiasis

- **Superficial candidiasis:** Gram stain, KOH preparation on suspected skin lesions
- **Systemic infections**
    - Histopathology
    - Culture
    - Serological tests: Immunodiffusion

Candida Auris Infections

Candida auris is an emerging pathogen. It is associated with multiple nosocomial infections. It is resistant to antifungal agents and is difficult to identify them with traditional laboratory diagnostics. Increased colonization and infection with non-*albicans Candida* species may be partly due to increased use of prophylactic antifungal agents. *C. auris* infection occurs in intensive care units and central venous or urinary catheters. Probably formation of biofilm formation is responsible for its virulence. *C. auris* colonizes in nares, groin, axilla, and rectum. *C. auris* can on survive on dry and moist surfaces up to 14 days.

Cryptococcosis

Q. Write short essay on cryptococcoma/pathological feature of cryptococcal infection and its lab diagnosis.

Species

Cryptococcosis is a systemic mycosis. Two species of *Cryptococcus* namely—*C. neoformans* and *C. gattii* can cause disease in humans. Both of them grow as encapsulated yeasts.

1. ***Cryptococcus neoformans***
   - **Source:** *Cryptococcus neoformans* is present in the soil and in bird (particularly pigeon) droppings which are alkaline and hyperosmolar. These conditions keep cryptococci small, thereby allowing inhaled organisms to reach the terminal bronchioles.
   - **Appearance:** They appear as faintly basophilic yeasts with a clear, 3–5-μm-thick, mucinous capsule (see **Fig. 65**). *C. neoformans* is unique among pathogenic fungi in that it has a proteoglycan capsule. This is responsible for its pathogenicity.
   - **Mode of infection** in human is through inhalation.
   - **Susceptibility:** Mainly affects the meninges and lungs. Though *C. neoformans* can cause meningoencephalitis in healthy individuals, more frequently it causes an opportunistic infection in patient with impaired cell mediated immunity**.** These conditions include AIDS, leukemia, lymphoma, systemic lupus erythematosus, or sarcoidosis, and in immunosuppressed transplant recipients. Many of these patients receive high-dose corticosteroids and is a major risk factor for *C. neoformans* infection.
2. *Cryptococcus gattii*
   - **Source and mode of infection:** *Cryptococcus gattii* is found in soil, and is acquired by inhalation. It causes disease in immunologically normal individuals and usually present as large lesions producing mass effects or may mimic the radiologic appearance of a neoplasm.

   Natural history of Cryptococcosis is presented in **Fig. 64**.

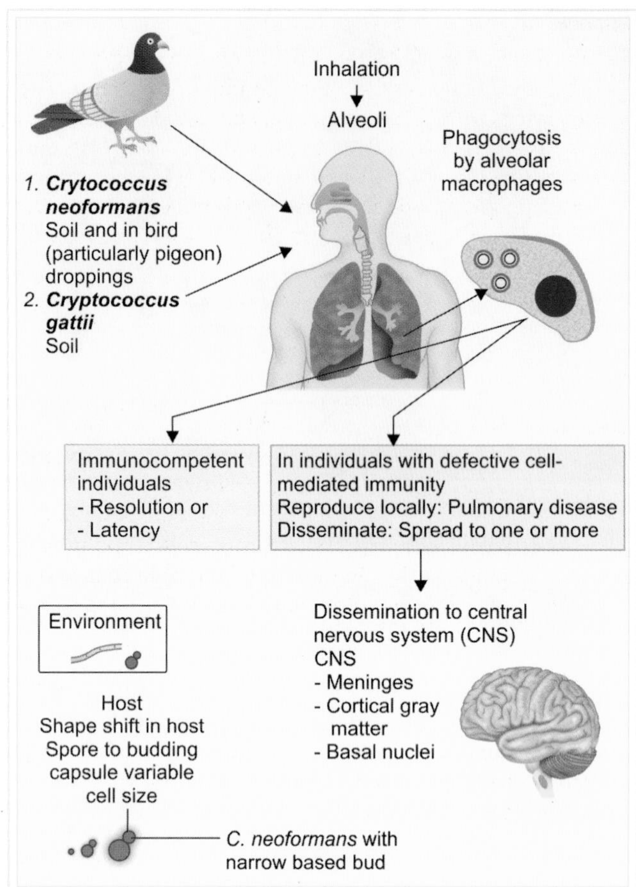

(*C. neoformans: Cryptococcus neoformans*)

FIG. 64: Natural history of Cryptococcosis.

Pathogenesis

In immunocompetent individuals, neutrophils and alveolar macrophages kill *C. neoformans,* and there is no development of clinical disease. By contrast, in a patient with defective cell-mediated immunity, the Cryptococci survive, reproduce locally and then disseminate. Various virulent factors of *Cryptococcus* which helps it in evasion of host defenses are:

Polysaccharide capsule: Glucuronoxylomannan present in the capsule of Cryptococci prevents its phagocytosis by alveolar macrophages, and also leukocyte migration, and recruitment of inflammatory cells.

- **Blocking of dendritic cell maturation:** *Cryptococcus species* can block dendritic cell maturation. This is achieved by reducing MHC class II-dependent antigen presentation and inhibiting the production of IL-12 and IL-23.
- **Production of large Titan cells with thickened cell wall:** *Cryptococcus* species can produce large cells greater than 12 μm and having a thick cell wall. These cells are called *Titan cells.*
- **Production of small cells:** *Cryptococcu*s species can also produce small (micro) cells of 2 to 4 μm. These may be adapted for growth in macrophages.

Melanin production: Laccase in the Cryptococci catalyzes melanin formation. Melanin has following features: (i) antioxidant properties, (ii) reduces its phagocytosis, (iii) counteracts the effects of antifungal agents, (iv) binds iron, and (v) provides cell wall integrity.

Enzymes: Phospholipases present in Cryptococci degrade host cell wall components and may help in invasion of tissue. Urease helps neutralize the reactive oxygen species and pH of the phagocytic cell and inhibits killing of the yeast by neutrophils and reactive oxygen species.

Differential cellular response to phagocytes: After phagocytosis of *C. gattii,* the reactive oxygen species in the phagocyte may stop growing of some cells and acquire an unusual morphology with tubularization of mitochondria, whereas other cells rapidly divide.

MORPHOLOGY

Cryptococcus has yeast form and there are no pseudohyphal or hyphal forms.

- The cryptococcal yeast measures 5–10 μm and has a highly characteristic thick gelatinous capsule containing a polysaccharide (**Fig. 65**).
- **Special stains: Because of the thick capsule, *Cryptococcus neoformans* stains poorly with the routine hematoxylin and eosin stain**. It appears as bubbles or holes. Fungal stains [periodic acid–Schiff (PAS) and Grocott methenamine silver (also known as Grocott-Gomori's Methenamine Silver and commonly

Continued

Continued

abbreviated as GMS **Fig. 66**)] demonstrate the yeasts well and it appears to be surrounded by a halo. The polysaccharide present in the capsule of the *Cryptococcus* stains intensely red with periodic acid-Schiff and mucicarmine stain. It is detected with antibody-coated beads in an agglutination assay. **India ink preparations** produce a negative image and the thick capsule as a clear halo within a dark background.

- *Cryptococcus* can be detected in blood or cerebrospinal fluid (CSF) with various immunoassays.

Sites Involved

Lungs

Lung is the primary site of infection and it is **usually mild and asymptomatic.** Lesions in the lungs can be seen in 50% of patients. In infection by *C. gattii,* even if the fungus spreads to the central nervous system (CNS), it forms a solitary pulmonary granuloma similar to the circumscribed (coin) lesions known as *cryptococcomas* (granulomas surrounded by fibrosis). It is similar to those caused by *Histoplasma.*

MORPHOLOGY

Lung: Lesions may be diffuse or show focal areas of consolidation. Affected alveoli are distended by clusters of cryptococci, usually with minimal inflammation.

Central nervous system

Though the lung is the portal of entry, the CNS is the most common site (95% of cryptococcal infections) of disease. It is due to the nourishing environment provided by the CSF.

- Major lesions of ***Cryptococcus*** occur in the CNS, mainly involving the meninges, cortical gray matter, and basal nuclei.
- **Host response** to cryptococci varies and depends on the immunity of the host.
  - ***Immunosuppressed patients:*** There may not be any inflammatory reaction and gelatinous masses of fungi can grow in the meninges or expand the perivascular Virchow–Robin spaces within the gray matter. This produces soap-bubble lesions within Virchow–Robin spaces (**Fig. 65A** and **B**).
  - ***Severely immunosuppressed patients:*** *C. neoformans* may widely spread or disseminate to the skin, liver, spleen, adrenals, and bones.
  - In **nonimmunosuppressed individual** or in those with protracted disease, the fungi produce a chronic granulomatous reaction. Granulomatous reaction consists of macrophages, lymphocytes, and foreign body-type giant cells. There may be suppuration and rarely granulomatous arteritis of the circle of Willis may occur.

Cryptococcoma: Cryptococcomas are a rare complication of infection by the *Cryptococcus*. It produces a discreet, encapsulated lesion of immune infiltrates and pathogen forms. The clinical presentation of cryptococcoma depends on

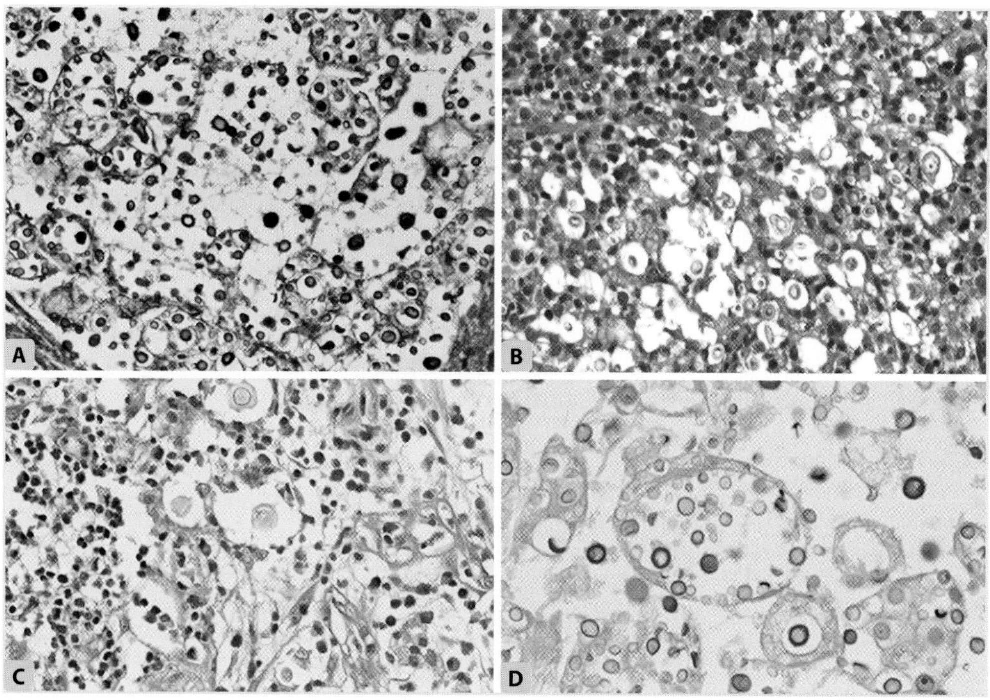

FIGS. 65A TO D: (A and B) Cryptococci forming gelatinous masses expanding the perivascular Virchow–Robin spaces within the gray matter of cerebral cortex producing the soap-bubble lesions in a patient with AIDS. Cryptococci appear as bubbles or holes under hematoxylin and eosin (H&E), (C) Cryptococcoma composed of Cryptocooci surrounded by lymphocytic infiltrate (H&E); (D) periodic acid–Schiff (PAS) stains capsule intensely red and it appears to be surrounded by a halo.

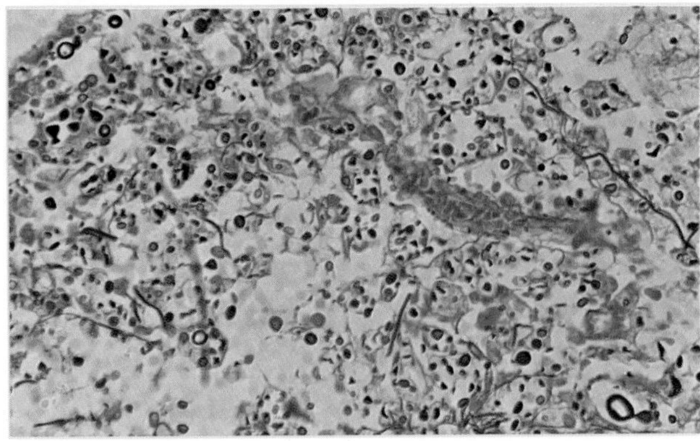

FIG. 66: Cytococci stained by Grocott–Gomori's methenamine silver (GMS) stain.

the organ affected. Usually, it involves CNS or lung, but there may be multiorgan involvement. Occasionally, *C. neoformans* in the CNS may cause localized neuroparenchymal or choroid plexus-based proliferation and may produce intraventricular masses known as cryptococcomas. It may cause hydrocephalus and symptoms of raised intracranial pressure are common and pulmonary infection may present with pleuritic chest pain and fever.

MORPHOLOGY

Cryptococcal meningoencephalitis: The entire brain is swollen and soft, and leptomeninges are thickened and gelatinous. This is due to infiltration by the large numbers of thickly encapsulated cryptococci. Inflammatory responses vary and are usually minimal. Inflammation, if found, is neutrophilic, lymphocytic, or granulomatous.

Clinical features: Cryptococcal CNS disease begins insidiously and presents with headache, dizziness, sleepiness, and loss of coordination. Without treatment, cryptococcal meningitis is invariably fatal.

Rare sites: Rarely, it may involve skin, liver, and other sites.

Laboratory Diagnosis

Following methods are used for the diagnosis of cryptococcosis:

- ***Histopathology:*** Demonstration of yeast cells in tissues by using hematoxylin and eosin (H and E), Grocott-Gomori's methenamine silver (GMS), and mucicarmine stains
- ***Cerebrospinal fluid examination for fungal cells:*** *Cryptococcus* can be visualized in the CSF by mixing CSF with India ink. It stains the capsule of fungal cells and is a useful rapid diagnostic technique. Cryptococcal cells in India ink have a distinctive appearance because their capsules exclude ink particles. However, in patients with a low-fungal burden, the CSF India ink examination may yield negative results. This examination should be performed by a trained individual, because leukocytes and fat globules can sometimes be mistaken for fungal cells.
- ***Cultures of CSF and blood:*** Positive culture for cryptococcal cells is diagnostic for cryptococcosis.
- ***CSF in cryptococcal meningitis:*** CSF examination usually shows features of chronic meningitis with mononuclear cell pleocytosis and increased protein levels.
- ***Cryptococcal antigen (CRAg):*** Its detection in CSF and blood is useful test. The assay is based on serologic detection of cryptococcal polysaccharide and is both sensitive and specific. A positive CRAg test strongly indicates cryptococcosis. Fluorescein-labeled anti-Cr can be used. It may be negative in pulmonary cryptococcosis. Hence, the test is less useful in the diagnosis of pulmonary disease and is of only limited use in monitoring the response to therapy.
- Serology does not distinguish between recent or past infection.
- Latex agglutination test for Ag is more sensitive and specific.

Pneumocystis Infections

Pneumocystis jirovecii *(P. jirovecii)* is a **yeast-like fungus**. It primarily causes lung infections and is a common and significant opportunistic infection in AIDS patients, in spite of significant improvements with antiretroviral therapy. The organism can cause a **rapidly progressive, often fatal bilateral pneumonia in individuals with impaired cell-mediated immunity**. ***Pneumocystis jirovecii*** was **formerly called as *Pneumocystis carinii*** and was originally classified as a protozoal parasite. It is recently reclassified with the fungi. There are many *Pneumocystis* species and each species is host specific. There are three forms of the organism namely—(1) trophozoites, (2) sporocytes, and (3) cysts.

- **Trophozoites** are of 1–4-μm long, pleomorphic, intracystic, or extracystic, and have a nucleus, cytoplasm, and extensively folded plasmalemmas. The trophozoites forms are not visible with a cell wall stain (e.g., methenamine silver).
- **Sporocytes** of 5–6 μm.
- **Cysts** measure 5–8 μm and have a characteristic cup-shaped (crescentic) appearance, or they are oval with a central dot.

Source of infection: No environmental source or external reservoir outside of humans has been identified for *P. jirovecii*. Probably, most cases of pneumocystosis are due to activation of latent endogenous infection. However, Pneumocystis pneumonia can occur among severely malnourished (and thus immunosuppressed) infants in nurseries. In such cases, it may be due to primary infection.

Mode of transmission: It is through airborne route and probably healthy individuals act as the reservoir.

Pathogenesis: Infection with *P. jirovecii* induces both humoral and cellular immune response. *P. jirovecii* reproduces in alveolar type 1 lining cells, and active disease is observed in the lungs. After reaching the alveoli, *Pneumocystis* trophozoites attach to alveolar lining cells. Trophozoites feed on host cells and enlarge and transform into the cyst form. These cysts contain daughter organisms. The cyst ruptures to release new trophozoites. These trophozoites attach additional alveolar lining cells. If the process is not halted by the host immune system or antibiotics, infected alveoli become filled with organisms and proteinaceous fluid. This progressive filling of alveoli with organism proteinaceous fluid prevents adequate gas exchange. This produces slow suffocation.

MORPHOLOGY

Pneumocystis jirovecii causes progressive consolidation of the lungs. *P. jirovecii* may be detected in cytological specimen obtained from induced sputum or specimens obtained by bronchoscopy.

Microscopy of lung: The lumen of alveoli shows a frothy, eosinophilic, and honeycombed exudate material composed of alveolar macrophages and cysts and *P. jirovecii* trophozoites. The interstitium shows thickening. Hyaline membranes and type-2 pneumocytes are prominent. In newborns, alveolar septa are thickened by lymphoid cells and macrophages. The various forms of *P. jirovecii* are best seen with methenamine silver stains. In bronchoalveolar lavage fluid, the clusters of organisms may be 200 µm in diameter. The cysts may be stained with Grocott–Gomori's methenamine silver (GMS) stain (**Fig. 67**) or by a fluorescent monoclonal antibody, and the trophic and intracystic forms are stained with the Wright–Giemsa stain. Wright–Giemsa stain shows nucleus and mitochondria.

Extrapulmonary involvement: It is not common. It can rarely involve lymph nodes, spleen, bone marrow, liver, etc.

Clinical features: *P. jirovecii* pneumonia presents with fever and progressive shortness of breath, often exacerbated by exertion and accompanied by a nonproductive cough. Dyspnea may be subtle in onset and slowly progresses over many weeks. Untreated disease is fatal.

Diagnosis: Chest radiographs show a diffuse pulmonary process.

- The diagnosis requires **alveolar material** obtained by bronchoscopy, endobronchial washing, or sputum induction for staining.
- ***Histopathology:*** Lung biopsy shows typical granular foaming honeycomb material in the alveolar lumen seen under H and E stain and GMS stain shows crescent or cup-shaped cysts of *P. jirovecii* (**Fig. 67**).
- **Fluorescein-conjugated antibody stains** are commonly used for the diagnosis.
- **Beta-D-glucan will be raised** but is not specific for *Pneumocystis* species.
- **Polymerase chain reaction** (PCR) tests are sensitive and specific for their diagnosis.
- **Culture:** Not successful.
- **Serum antibodies** to *P. carinii* measured by complement fixation test (CFT) and enzyme-linked immunosorbent assay (ELISA).

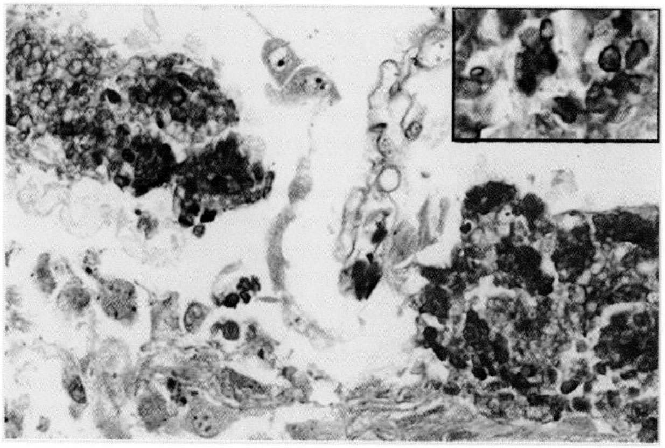

FIG. 67: *Pneumocystis jirovecii* pneumonia. Grocott–Gomori methenamine silver (GMS) stain shows showing crescent or cup-shaped cysts (inset) of *P. jirovecii* stained black.

MOLDS

The medically important dimorphic fungi include *Blastomyces dermatitidis, H. capsulatum,* and *Coccidioides immitis.*

Aspergillosis

Q. Write short essay on aspergillosis.

Aspergillus is a common **ubiquitous** environmental fungus (**mold).** In about >200 identified species of *Aspergillus,* about 20 cause human disease. *Aspergillus* is a saprophyte (lives on dead or decaying organic matter) found in soil, decaying plant matter and dung. ***Aspergillus fumigatus* is the most common pathogenic human species of the fungus.** It causes opportunistic infections in immunocompromised individuals, usually involving the lungs. It may also produce serious sinusitis and invasive disease.

There are three types of pulmonary aspergillosis:

- **Allergic bronchopulmonary aspergillosis** in healthy individuals.
- **Colonization of a pre-existing pulmonary cavity** (**aspergilloma** or **fungus ball**).
- **Invasive aspergillosis.**

Predisposing factors: These include conditions causing neutropenia and immunosuppression (e.g., use of corticosteroids).

Pathogenesis

Mode of transmission: Lung is the major portal of entry. Pulmonary aspergillosis is transmitted by inhaling small sized (about 2–3 µm) airborne spores of *A. fumigatus*, termed **conidia (Fig. 68)**, that are present in the air in almost all environment.

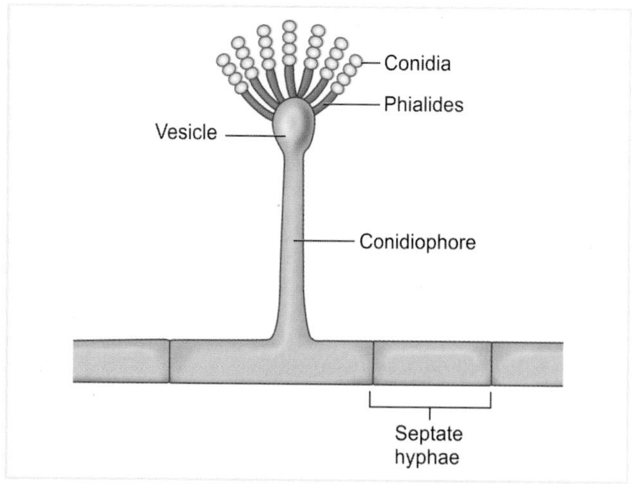

FIG. 68: Conidia of *Aspergillus*.

After inhalation, the small spores (conida) can easily reach the alveoli. Chances of exposure are more when the habitat of the fungus is disturbed. This may occur during soil excavations or handling decaying organic matter. Conidia are coated in hydrophobic proteins. This masks the recognition of microbial molecules from innate immune system. As conidia grow and form hyphae, these molecules are exposed.

Alveolar macrophages recognize conidia through TLR2 and the lectin dectin-1 receptors. Both receptors recognize β-1, 3-glucan present in the fungal cell wall and activate phagocytes to ingest and kill the conidia.

In immunosuppressed individuals, conidia can produce hyphae and these hyphae invade tissues. TLRs can recognize products of the fungal hyphae and release pro-inflammatory mediators (e.g., TNF, IL-1, and chemokines). Neutrophils produce reactive oxygen intermediates and kill hyphae. Invasive aspergillosis is usually associated with neutropenia and impaired neutrophil defenses.

The life cycle of *Aspergillus* is presented in **Fig. 69**.

Virulence factors: *Aspergillus* produces many virulence factors. These include **adhesins, antioxidants** (e.g., melanin pigment, mannitol, catalases, and superoxide dismutases), **enzymes** (phospholipases and proteases), **and toxins.** The antioxidant defenses are mediated by melanin pigment, mannitol, catalases, and superoxide dismutases. This fungus also produces enzymes such as phospholipases, proteases, and toxins. Their roles are not known.

Aflatoxin: It is produced by *Aspergillus* species that grow on the surface of improperly stored some crops, including corn and peanuts. This particularly grows in warm regions. Aflatoxin is a hepatotoxic as well carcinogen and causes acute and chronic toxicity in liver and is associated with increased risk of liver cancer.

Lesions

Sensitization to *Aspergillus* spores can cause **allergic alveolitis.**

Allergic bronchopulmonary aspergillosis

After inhalation of *Aspergillus* spores (conida), it delivers fungal antigens to airways and alveoli. It is associated with sensitization and development of type I hypersensitivity in susceptible individual with asthma (20% of asthmatic eventually develop this disorder). Subsequent exposure produces an allergic response. This is aggravated, if spores can germinate and grow in the airways. Because, this causes long-term exposure to the antigen.

Colonizing aspergillosis (*aspergilloma*)

Inhaled spores germinate in **pulmonary cavities or bronchiectasis.** These hollows provide the warm humid atmosphere for their germination and they fill these cavities with masses of hyphae. This mass is called aspergilloma.

Clinical features: Aspergillomas occur most commonly in old tuberculous cavities. Patients with aspergillomas usually present with recurrent hemoptysis. Radiologically, a dense round ball in a cavity is characteristically seen.

Invasive Aspergillosis

Invasive aspergillosis is an opportunistic infection, which develops in patients with neutropenia or immunosuppression (e.g., high-dose steroid or cytotoxic therapy or acute leukemia). Usually, the primary lesions are observed in the lung. However, widespread hematogenous dissemination may lead to involvement of the heart valves and brain. In patients with severe neutropenia, inhaled spores germinate to produce hyphae. They invade through bronchi into the lung parenchyma and then may spread widely. Acute aspergillosis may also start in a nasal sinus and spread to the face, orbit, and brain.

Clinical features: Invasive aspergillosis clinically presents with fever and multifocal pulmonary infiltrates in an immunocompromised patient. It is usually fatal.

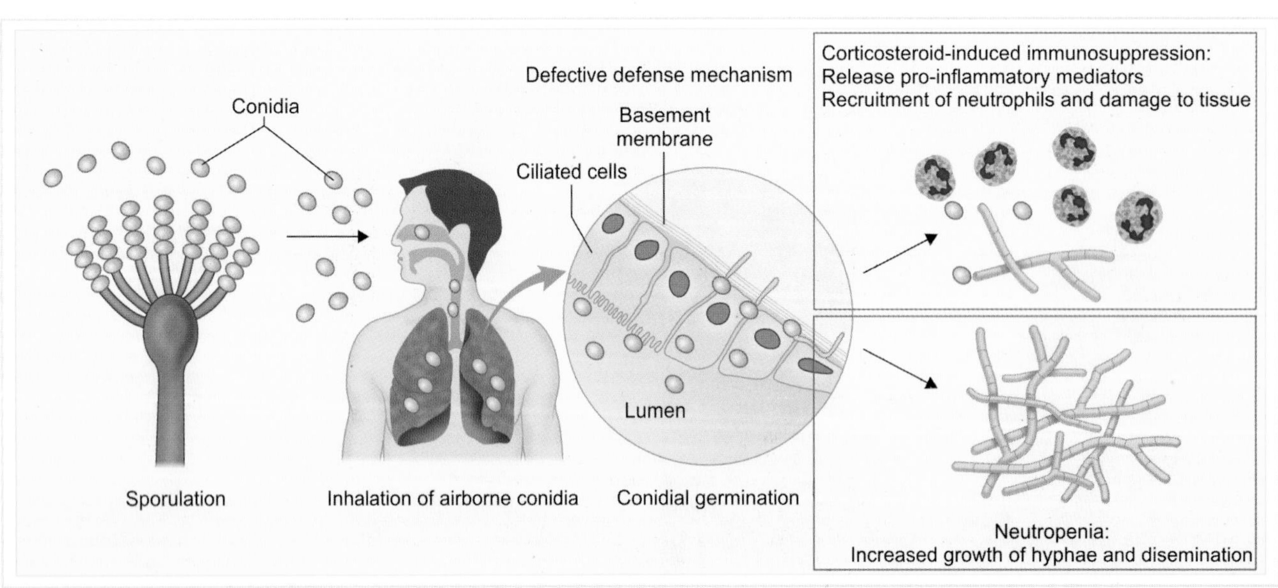

FIG. 69: The life cycle of *Aspergillus*.

MORPHOLOGY

In tissues, *Aspergillus* species appear as septate hyphae and measure 2–7 µm in diameter. It **branches progressively at acute angles**. *Aspergillus* produces **multiple dichotomous branching**. The term *Aspergillus* is derived from a fancied resemblance of this organism to the aspergillum, a device used to sprinkle holy water during Catholic religious ceremonies.

Allergic bronchopulmonary aspergillosis: Bronchi and bronchioles show infiltrates of lymphocytes, plasma cells, and variable numbers of eosinophils. Sometimes, airways may be impacted with mucous and fungal hyphae. Exacerbations of asthma in these patients are usually accompanied by pulmonary infiltrates and eosinophilia.

Colonizing aspergillosis (aspergilloma) (Figs. 70A to D): An aspergilloma refers to growth of the fungus within the cavities of lung with minimal or no invasion of the tissues (the nose also is usually colonized). Lung cavities are usually the result of prior tuberculosis, bronchiectasis, old infarcts, or abscesses. Proliferating masses of tangled hyphae form dense, round brownish "fungus balls" measuring 1–7 cm in diameter are seen lying free within the fibrous cavity of lung. The cavity wall consists of collagenous connective tissue infiltrated by lymphocytes and plasma cells.

Invasive aspergillosis: The primary lesions usually occur in the lung and produce necrotizing pneumonia. They appear

Continued

Continued

as sharply delineated, rounded, gray foci (**Fig. 71**) with hemorrhagic borders. These lesions are called as target lesions. *Aspergillus* invades blood vessels and produces thrombosis. It produces multiple nodular infarcts throughout both lungs. When larger pulmonary arteries are involved, it results in formation of large, wedge-shaped, pleural-based infarcts. Vascular invasion can also lead to dissemination of fungus to other organs.

Aspergillus forms fruiting bodies (usually in lung cavities) and septate filaments, 5–10 µm thick, branching (**Fig. 70**) at acute angles (40°).

***Aspergillus* forms fruiting bodies (usually in lung cavities).** Fruiting body is multicellular structure on which spore-producing structures are formed. ***Aspergillus* appears as septate filaments, 5–10 µm thick, branching at acute angles (40°)** (see **Fig. 70**). By morphology alone, *Aspergillus* hyphae without the distinct fruiting body cannot be differentiated from *Pseudallescheria boydii* and *Fusarium* species. ***Aspergillus* has a tendency to invade blood vessels**. Hence, areas of hemorrhage and infarction are usually superimposed on the necrotizing, inflammatory tissue reactions. Rhinocerebral *Aspergillus* infection in immunosuppressed patients resembles that infection is caused by mucormycoses (e.g., *Mucor* species and *Rhizopus* species).

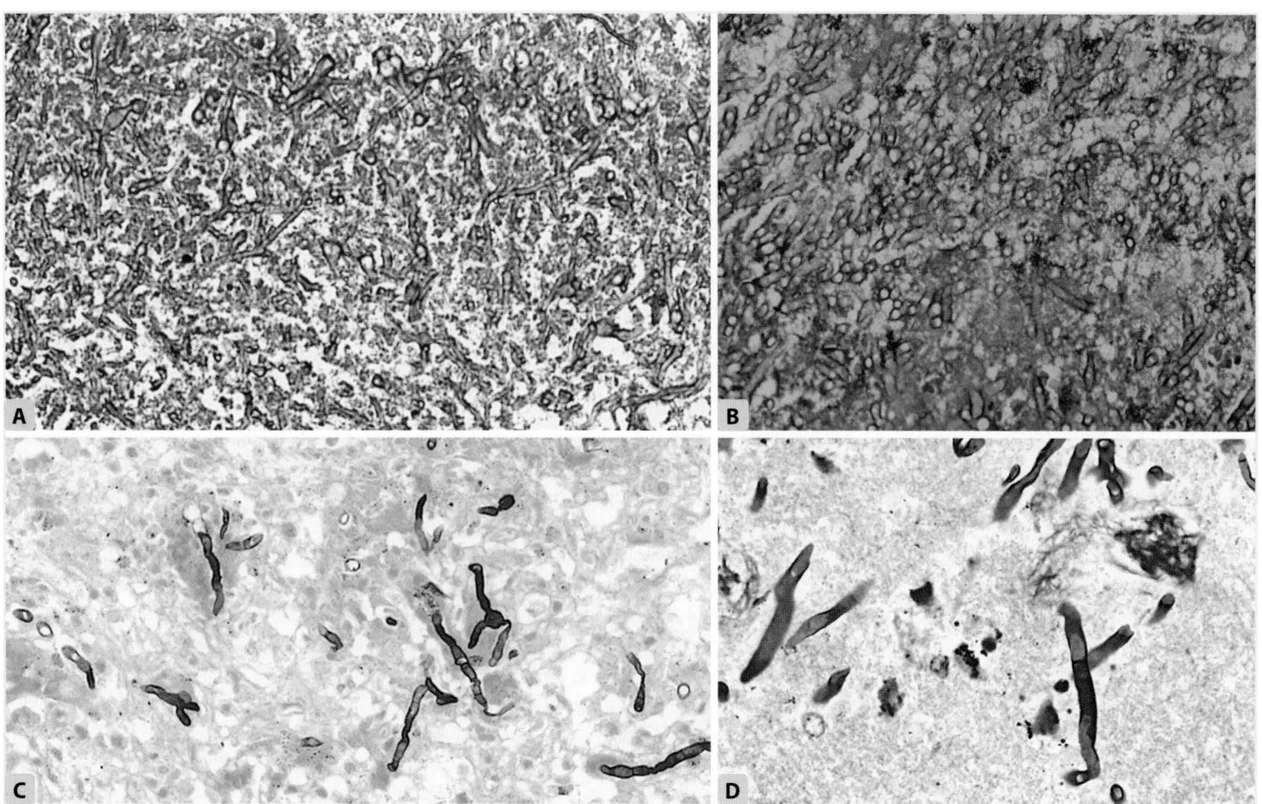

FIGS. 70A TO D: *Aspergillus* consisting of septate hyphae with acute-angle branching. (A and B) Hematoxylin and eosin (H and E); (C) Aspergilloma (GMS); (D) Invasive aspergillosis (GMS).

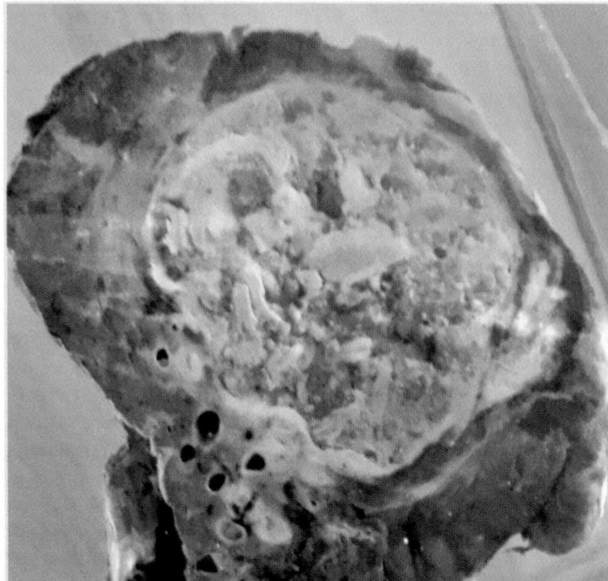

FIG. 71: Invasive aspergillosis showing sharply delineated, rounded, gray foci in the lung.

Laboratory Diagnosis of Aspergillosis

- **Direct examination:** With 10% potassium hydroxide (KOH).
- **Histopathological examination:** H and E and GMS stain
- **Culture**
- **Immunology/serology:** Immunodiffusion
- **DNA probes:** Efficient and rapid diagnostic method

Mucormycosis (Zygomycosis)

Q. Write short essay on Zygomycetes.

Mucormycosis (formerly zygomycosis) is a group of life-threatening, severe, necrotizing, invasive, and opportunistic infections caused by fungi of the order Mucorales of the subphylum Mucoromycotina (formerly known as the class Zygomycetes). *Mucormycotina* is bread mold environmental fungus that includes *Mucor, Rhizopus, Rhizomucor, Lichtheimia* (formerly *Absidia*), and *Cunninghamella*. **Mucormycosis is highly invasive and constantly progressive infection** that results in higher rates of morbidity and mortality. They produce infections that begin in the nasal sinuses or lungs. Mucoromycotina is widely found in nature and does not infect immunocompetent individuals. But, they can infect immunosuppressed individuals and cause mucormycosis.

Source of infection: Zygomycetes are universally present in soil, food, and decaying vegetable matter.

Mode of transmission: They are transmitted by airborne asexual spores. Inhalation of spores is the most common route of entry into the body. When these spores are inhaled, in susceptible individuals, disease begins in the lungs. However, infection can occur through skin (percutaneous exposure) in immunologically normal individuals after traumatic implantation of soil or vegetation or ingestion.

Predisposing factors: These fungi cause infection exclusively in patients with diabetes, defects in phagocytic function (e.g., neutropenia after treatment for leukemia or use of high-dose corticosteroids), solid organ or hematopoietic stem cell transplantation (HSCT), and/or iron overload (elevated levels of free iron), and breakdown of the skin barrier (e.g., in burns, surgical wounds, or trauma). These predisposing factors support fungal growth in serum and tissues.

Pathogenesis

After inhalation of spores, macrophages phagocytose them and kill the germinating sporangiospores by nonoxidative mechanism. *Mucormycotina* hyphal components are recognized by TLR2. They produce a proinflammatory cascade of cytokines including IL-6 and TNF. Neutrophils play main role in killing hyphae after germination by damaging the walls of hyphae directly. If there is diminished number or function of macrophages or neutrophils, the infection becomes established and there is increased possibility of invasive infection. Different *Mucor* species vary in resistance to phagocytosis of spores and in neutrophil damage to hyphae. Free iron acts as a promoter of *Mucormycotina* growth and if there is increased availability of free iron, there is increased probability of infection. Increased free iron is observed in diabetic patients due to ketoacidosis and/or glycosylation-induced poor iron affinity. In patients on chronic iron chelation treatment, deferoxamine (iron-chelating agent) acts as a fungal siderophore that directly deliver iron to the Mucorales.

MORPHOLOGY

Mucormycetes form broad, ribbon-like, nonseptate large (8–15 μm across) hyphae of variable width (ranging from 6–50 μm) with uneven thickness. These hyphae exhibit frequent right-angle branching (branch at right angles), have thin walls, and lack septa (**Fig. 72**). In tissue sections, they appear as hollow tubes. The right-angle branching is distinct from *Aspergillus* hyphae and this can be readily observed in hematoxylin and eosin or special fungal stains (**Figs. 73A to D**). Since there is no cross-wall, their liquid contents flow, leaving long empty segments. The collapsed hyphae may resemble "twisted ribbons."

Lesions:

Sites involved: Mucormycosis can be divided into six clinical syndromes—(1) rhino-orbital-cerebral (rhinocerebral), (2) pulmonary, (3) cutaneous, (4) gastro-intestinal, (5) disseminated, and (6) miscellaneous. It depends on whether the spores (which are widespread in dust and air) are inhaled or ingested.

1. **Rhino-orbital-cerebral (rhinocerebral) mucormycosis:** It is most common in patients with diabetes.

   It results from germination of the sporangiospores in the nasal passages. Fungi proliferate in nasal sinuses. Then, hyphae may spread from nasal sinuses and invade surrounding tissues and extend into facial soft tissues, nerves, and blood vessels. Involvement of blood vessels causes thrombosis, infarction, and necrosis. The

Continued

Continued

Mucormycotina cause local tissue necrosis. The palate or nasal turbinates are covered by a black crust, and underlying tissue become friable and hemorrhagic. Fungal hyphae grow into the arteries and cause destructive, rapidly progressive, septic infarction of affected tissues. Then, it may invade arterial walls **(Figs. 69B** and **C)** spread to the orbit and penetrate the periorbital tissues and cranial vault. In the brain, it gives rise to **rhinocerebral mucormycosis.** Extension of infection into the brain leads to fatal, necrotizing, and hemorrhagic meningoencephalitis. Sometimes, fungi may invade arteries and induce thrombosis in the brain leading to cerebral infarctions.

2. **Pulmonary mucormycosis: Lung involvement** with *Mucormycotina* may be primary (in individuals with severe immunodeficiency) or secondary to rhinocerebral disease. This infection resembles invasive pulmonary aspergillosis. The lung lesions show combination of areas of hemorrhagic pneumonia with vascular invasion/thrombi and distal multiple areas of septic infarction. Both rhinocerebral and pulmonary mucormycosis are usually fatal.
3. **Cutaneous disease:** This infection may result from external implantation of the fungus or from hematogenous dissemination. External implantation may occur due to the exposure to soil during trauma (e.g., in a motor vehicle accident), penetrating injury with plant material (e.g., a thorn), injections of medications (e.g., insulin), catheter insertion, and contamination of surgical dressings. Cutaneous disease can be highly invasive, penetrating into muscle, fascia, and even bone.
4. **Gastrointestinal disease:** It may occur in association with disseminated disease, or in immunocompromised individuals or as a nosocomial process following administration of medications mixed with contaminated wooden applicator sticks.
5. **Disseminated disease:** Hematogenous dissemination may occur from any primary site of infection. The most common site of dissemination is the brain, but any other organ may be involved.
6. **Miscellaneous forms of disease:** Miscellaneous forms of mucormycosis may affect any body site (e.g., bones, mediastinum, trachea, kidneys, and peritoneum).

Diagnosis

- **Direct microscopy**: With 10–20% KOH (potassium hydroxide) shows characteristic broad, branched, occasionally distorted hyphae.
- **Histopathological examination:** H and E and GMS stain (refer text above on page 720 and **Fig. 73D**).
- Culture
- *Immunology and serology*: Not satisfactory.

Entomophthoramycosis

Entomophthoromycota comprise members in the genera *Basidiobolus* and *Conidiobolus*. The species of these genera cause entomophthoramycosis. This infection is restricted to the subcutaneous tissues and rarely involves other organs.

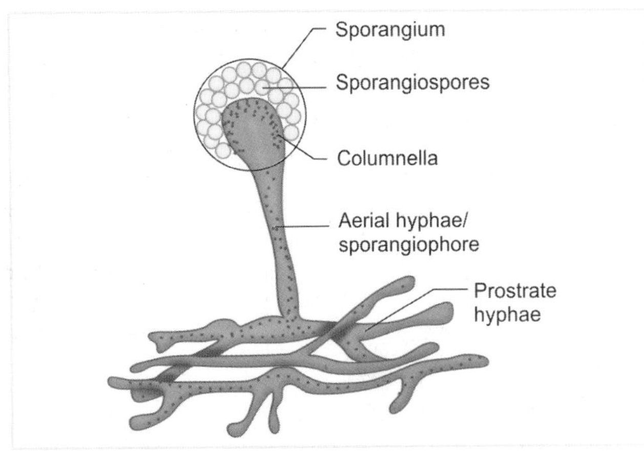

FIG. 72: Diagrammatic appearance of mucormycetes.

They are characterized by the production of a variety of spores. Entomophthoromycota are characterized by the production of slow-growing tumoral-like masses in the infected tissues that in some cases remain indolent for years. The area most commonly affected by *Conidiobolus* species is the face (generally around the nose), whereas *Basidiobolus* species are frequently found on limbs, the intestinal tract, and rarely in other body areas. Both *Conidiobolus* species and *Basidiobolus* species are thermophilic fungi. Thus, these species are more commonly found in tropical and subtropical humid areas. The majority of the fungi causing entomophthoramycosis develop short or long, broad (ribbon-type), sparsely septate hyphae in the infected host tissues (**Fig. 74**). These **pathogens produce a red-colored reaction around the invading hyphae in the infected tissue**. This is **termed as the Splendore–Hoeppli phenomenon**.

DIMORPHIC FUNGI

Dimorphic fungi exist in distinct environmental niches as molds that produce conidia and they represent their infectious form. In tissues and at temperatures of >35°C, the mold gets converted to the yeast form. The important dimorphic fungi include blastomyces, histoplasma, and coccidioidomycosis. **Figure 75** shows diagrammatic appearance of dimorphic fungi in environment and host.

Histoplasmosis

Histoplasmosis is an infection caused by *Histoplasma capsulatum.*

Histoplasma capsulatum: It is the thermal dimorphic fungus. The two forms of *Histoplasma* are mycelia and yeast.

1. **Mycelia:** These are the naturally infectious form of *Histoplasma.* They have a characteristic appearance, with microconidial and macroconidial forms. Microconidia are oval and small (2–4 µm) and can easily reach the terminal bronchioles and alveoli.
2. **Yeast (Figs. 75 and 76):** The yeast forms are characteristically small (2–5 µm), round, and has a central basophilic

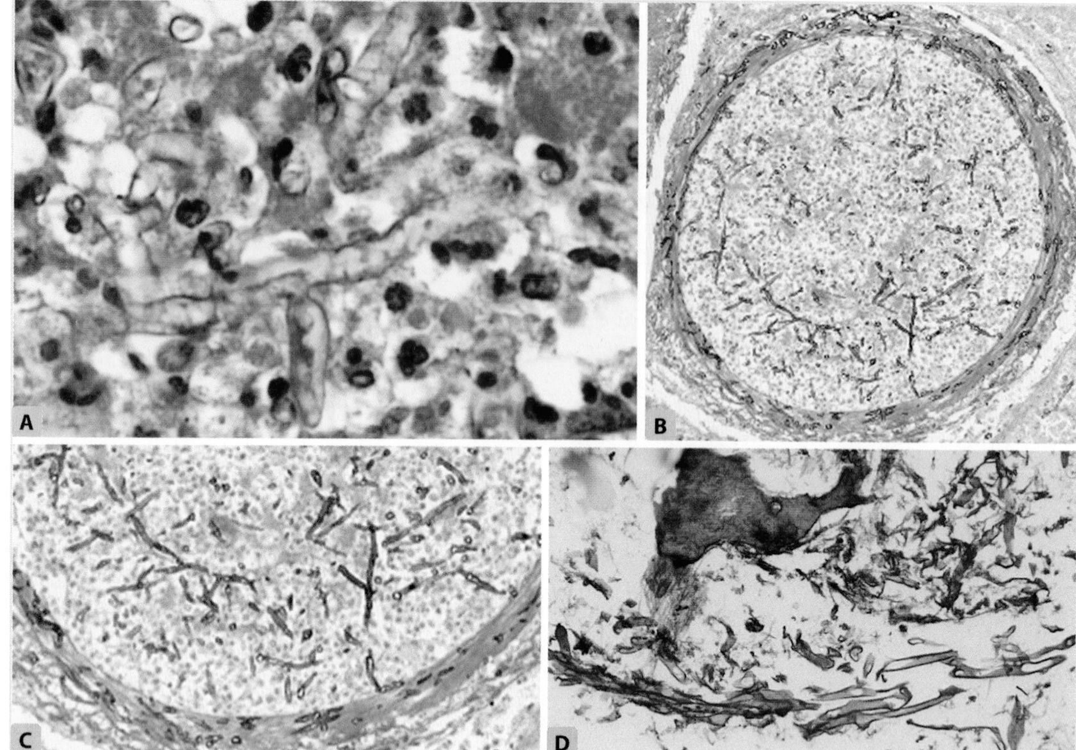

FIGS. 73A TO D: Mucormycosis. Broad, ribbon-like nonseptate hyphae (10–15 µm in width) with right angle branching. (A to C) Meningeal blood vessels with angioinvasive *Mucor* species. (A) Hematoxylin and eosin; (B and C) Silver stain shows angioinvasive *Mucor* species both inside the lumen and wall of the vessel. Note the irregular width and near right-angle branching of the hyphae. (D) Mucormycosis in nasal sinuses [periodic acid–Schiff (PAS)].

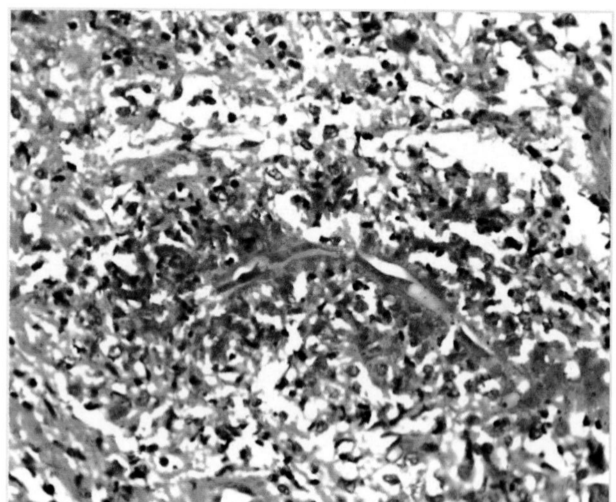

FIG. 74: Entomophthoramycosis of nose showing broad (ribbon-type), sparsely septate hyphae surrounded by Splendore–Hoeppli phenomenon.

body surrounded by a clear zone or halo, which in turn is encircled by a rigid cell wall. It may show occasional narrow budding. After infecting the host, mycelia transform into the yeasts. These yeast forms are found inside macrophages and other phagocytes. In caseous lesions, silver impregnation can identify the remains of degenerating yeast forms.

In the laboratory, *H. capsulatum* mycelia are best grown at room temperature (i.e., hyaline mold at ambient temperature), whereas yeasts are grown in the body [37°C (98.6°F)] temperature on enriched media.

Source of infection: Soil contaminated with bird or bat droppings and it promotes the growth and sporulation of *Histoplasma.* Bat nests, caves, and soil beneath trees are foci of exposure in the tropical regions.

Mode of infection: Small spores (microconidia) are the infectious form of the fungus. *H. capsulatum* infection is acquired by inhalation of dust particles from soil contaminated with bird or bat droppings that contain these small infectious spores (microconidia). Disruption of soil (e.g., excavation, cleaning of chicken coops, demolition and remodeling of old buildings, and cutting of dead trees) containing the organism leads to aerosolization of the microconidia and infection of nearby humans. The portal of entry is almost always the lung through inhalation.

Pathogenesis

The pathogenesis of histoplasmosis is not completely known.

Before the development of cellular immunity: Following inhalation, microconidia of *Histoplasma* reach the alveolar spaces. In the alveoli, microconidia are rapidly recognized and engulfed by alveolar macrophages. The microconidia then transform into budding yeasts. This process of transformation

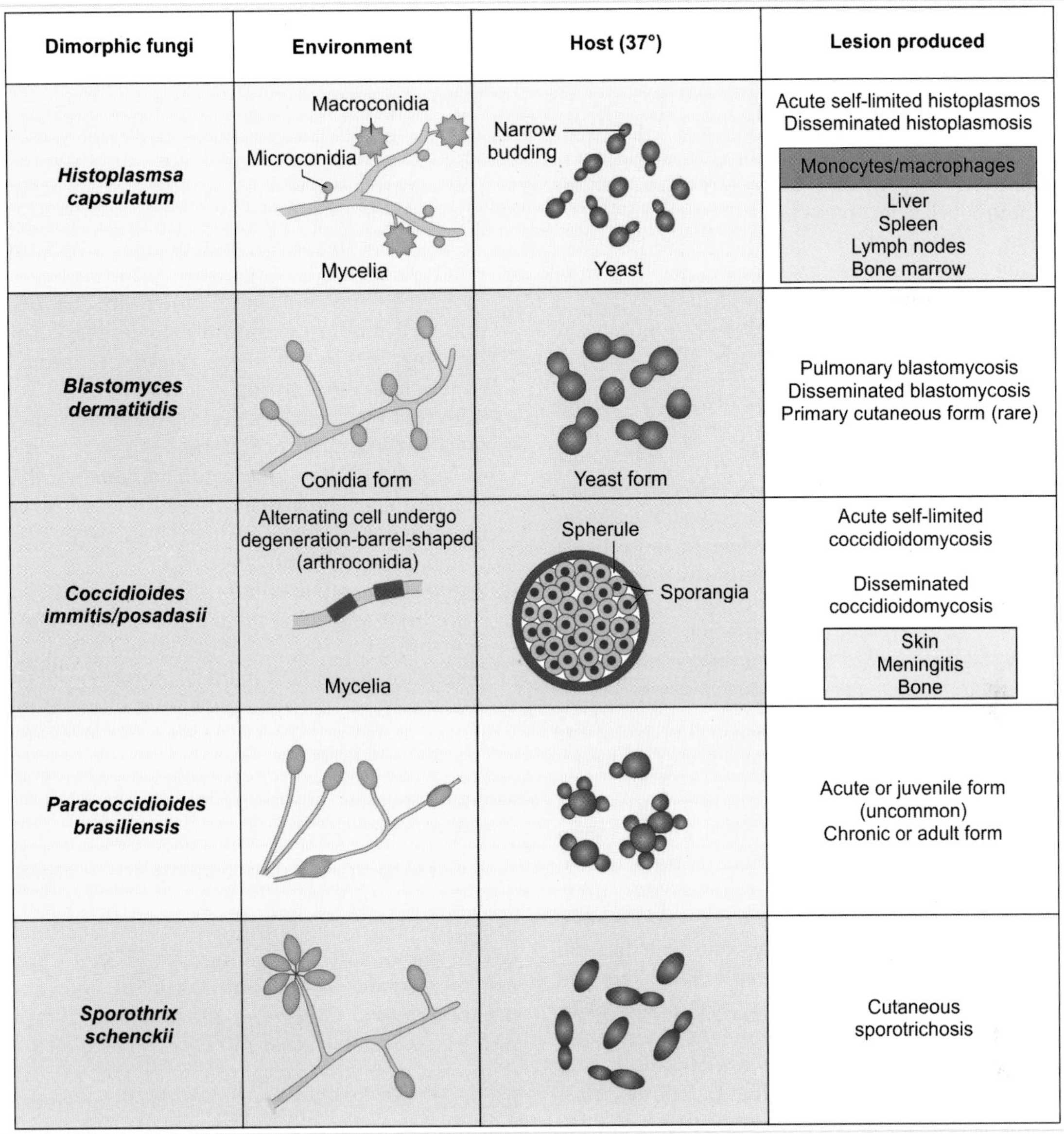

Dimorphic fungi	Environment	Host (37°)	Lesion produced
Histoplasmsa capsulatum	Macroconidia Microconidia Mycelia	Narrow budding Yeast	Acute self-limited histoplasmos Disseminated histoplasmosis Monocytes/macrophages Liver Spleen Lymph nodes Bone marrow
Blastomyces dermatitidis	Conidia form	Yeast form	Pulmonary blastomycosis Disseminated blastomycosis Primary cutaneous form (rare)
Coccidioides immitis/posadasii	Alternating cell undergo degeneration-barrel-shaped (arthroconidia) Mycelia	Spherule Sporangia	Acute self-limited coccidioidomycosis Disseminated coccidioidomycosis Skin Meningitis Bone
Paracoccidioides brasiliensis			Acute or juvenile form (uncommon) Chronic or adult form
Sporothrix schenckii			Cutaneous sporotrichosis

FIG. 75: Diagrammatic appearance of dimorphic fungi in environment and host. Diagrammatic appearance of dimorphic fungal pathogens.

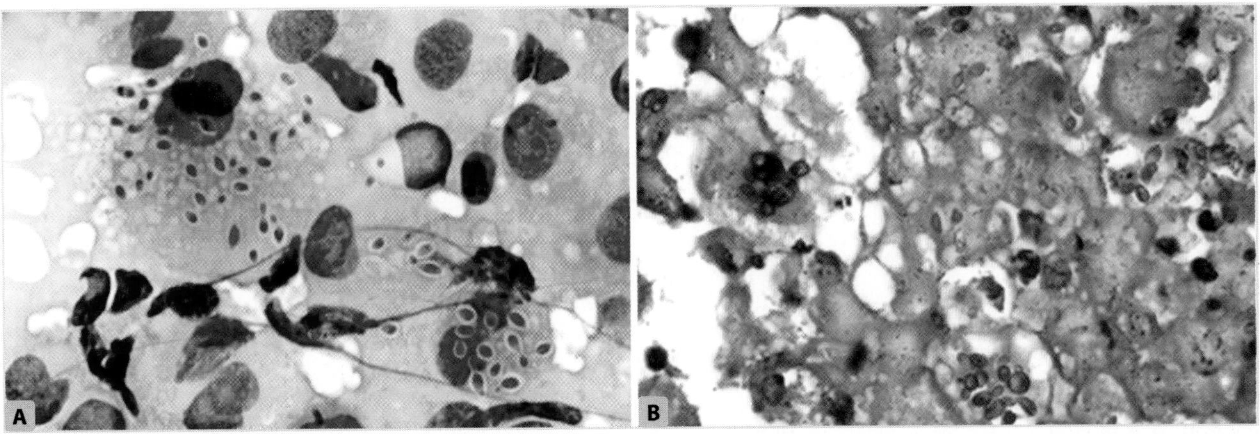

FIGS. 76A AND B: Histoplasmosis of lung. Bronchoalveolar lavage fluid shows numerous intracellular yeasts of *Histoplasma capsulatum* within an alveolar macrophage. They appear as small round with a central basophilic body surrounded by a clear zone or halo, which in turn is encircled by a rigid cell wall. (A) May–Grünwald–Giemsa (MGG) stain. (B) Grocott's–Gomori'smethenamine silver stain (GMS).

is essential for the pathogenesis of histoplasmosis and is dependent on the availability of calcium and iron inside the phagocytes. The yeasts are capable of multiplying inside resting macrophages. Neutrophils and then lymphocytes are attracted to the site of infection. The development of T-cell immunity takes about 1–2 weeks after infection. Before the development of cellular immunity, macrophages ingest but cannot kill the organism without T-cell help. Thus, before the development of T-cell immunity, organism multiplies within phagolysosomes and disseminate. The yeasts use the phagosomes for their transportation to regional draining lymph nodes. This is followed by hematogenous dissemination throughout the reticuloendothelial system.

After the development of cellular immunity: In individuals with adequate cell-mediated immunity, cellular immunity usually develops about 2 weeks after infection. The infection is controlled by Th1 helper T cells that recognize fungal antigens. T cells secrete interferon-γ (IFN-γ), which activates macrophages and enables the macrophages in the process of killing the intracellular yeasts and control the progression of disease. In addition, *Histoplasma* induces macrophages to secrete interleukin-12 and tumor necrosis factor-α (TNF-α) is involved in cellular immunity to *H. capsulatum*. TNF recruits and stimulates other macrophages to kill *Histoplasma*.

Course of infection: It varies depending on the size of the infecting inoculum and the immunological status of the host.

In immunocompetent host: Like *Mycobacterium tuberculosis, H. capsulatum* is an intracellular pathogen and is found mainly in phagocytes. The macrophages are transformed into epithelioid cells and surrounded by lymphocytes. These form granulomas to contain the organisms. These granulomas usually undergo fibrosis and calcification. Thus, calcification in the lung nodules, mediastinal lymph nodes, and liver and spleen are frequent in healthy individuals from endemic areas. Histoplasmosis can occur in immunocompetent individuals but is usually more severe in individuals with deranged cell-mediated immunity. In immunocompetent individual, most infections (95%) involve small inocula of organisms. They affect small areas of the lung and regional lymph nodes and usually remain unnoticed. Exposure to a large inoculum (e.g., as in an excavated bird roost), it may produce rapidly evolving disease of lung. It produces large areas of consolidation in the lung, prominent mediastinal and hilar nodal involvement, and spread of the infection to the liver, spleen, and bone marrow.

In immunocompromised hosts: Infection with *H. capsulatum* produces some immunity to reinfection. In individuals with impaired cellular immunity, the infection is not controlled properly and can disseminate throughout the reticuloendothelial system. Progressive disseminated histoplasmosis (PDH) can involve many organs such as the lungs, bone marrow, spleen, liver, adrenal glands, and mucocutaneous membranes. Unlike latent tuberculosis, latent histoplasmosis usually does not undergo reactivation. Disseminated histoplasmosis can develop in infants, patients with AIDS and on long-term corticosteroids.

Resemblance between histoplasmosis and tuberculosis: Histoplasmosis resembles tuberculosis in many ways and includes both clinical and morphological features. These are as follows:

- Primary infection begins with phagocytosis of microconidia/mycobacteria by alveolar macrophages.
- Like *M. tuberculosis, H. capsulatum* reproduces in immunologically naïve macrophages. As organisms grow, more macrophages are recruited to the site of infection. This produces an area of consolidation in the lung parenchyma. A few macrophages carry organisms first to hilar and mediastinal lymph nodes. Then they disseminate throughout the body and further infect monocytes/macrophages. The organisms proliferate within these monocytes/macrophages till the onset of hypersensitivity and cell-mediated immune responses. This usually develops within 1–3 weeks. Normal immune responses usually limit the infection.
- Activated macrophages destroy the phagocytosed yeasts/mycobacteria and form necrotizing granulomas at sites of infection. They may result in coin lesions on chest radiography. It is chronic, progressive, and secondary lung disease, which is localized to the lung apices. They produce cough, fever, and night sweats.
- **Spread to extrapulmonary sites**: Various sites involved in both diseases include mediastinum, adrenal glands, liver, or meninges.
- Wide dissemination in immunocompromised patients.

MORPHOLOGY

Lung: It causes usually a self-limited disease but may lead to a systemic granulomatous disease.

Acute self-limited histoplasmosis: In otherwise healthy adults, *Histoplasma* infections produce necrotizing **granulomas** in the lung, mediastinal and hilar lymph nodes, spleen, and liver. During early infection, **granulomas are composed of caseous material, surrounded by macrophages, Langhans giant cells, lymphocytes, and plasma cells**. Yeast forms of *H. capsulatum* can be demonstrated within macrophages and in the caseous material. The lesions may coalesce to produce areas of consolidation. With spontaneous resolution or effective treatment, the cellular components of the granuloma largely disappear and it undergoes fibrosis, calcification, and forms "fibrocaseous nodule". The concentric calcification produces tree-bark appearance. Microscopic differentiation of histoplasmosis from tuberculosis, sarcoidosis, and coccidioidomycosis needs identification of the 3–5-μm thin-walled yeast forms. These yeast forms may persist in tissues for years.

These are the naturally infectious form of *Histoplasma*. They have a characteristic appearance, with microconidial and macroconidial forms. Microconidia are oval and small (2–4 μm) and can easily reach the terminal bronchioles and alveoli.

Disseminated histoplasmosis: It is characterized by progressive organ infiltration with macrophages containing *H. capsulatum*.

- **Mild cases:** The immune responses can control the organism, but cannot eliminate it. Disease remains restricted to macrophages in infected organs for long periods.

Continued

Continued

- **Fulminant disseminated histoplasmosis:** It occurs in immunosuppressed individuals, there is no granuloma formation. There will be focal accumulations of clusters of macrophages (mononuclear phagocytes) filled with yeast forms of *H. capsulatum*. These are found throughout the body in organs such as liver, spleen, lungs, intestine, adrenals, and meninges.

Clinical features: Most infections are self-limited and asymptomatic. The majority of cases resolve spontaneously. In patients with impaired cell-mediated immunity, disseminated histoplasmosis presents with fever, headache, weakness, and cough. The disease may persist and progress for years, even decades. With more severe immunodeficiency, dissemination may progress rapidly and present with high fever, cough, and pancytopenia.

Laboratory Diagnosis

The diagnosis of histoplasmosis may be by the following methods:

- Serologic tests for antibodies and fungal antigens:
  - *Latex agglutination test*: Latex particle coated with antigenic fungal extract detects IgM antibodies in first 2 weeks.
  - *Complement fixation test*: Performed with antigens prepared from both yeast and mycelial fungus.
  - *Immunodiffusion test*
- Culture
- Identification of the fungus in tissue biopsies or by cytology (**Fig. 77**).

Blastomycosis

Blastomyces dermatitidis is dimorphic fungus that is inhabitant of soil. It grows as a mold in warm moist soil, rich in decaying vegetable matter. *B. dermatitidis* is the asexual state of *Ajellomyces dermatitidis* and two serotypes have been identified. *B. dermatitidis* shows thermal dimorphism, i.e., it grows as the mycelial phase at room temperature and as the yeast phase at 37°C. Under the light microscope, the yeast cells are usually 8–15 μm in diameter, have thick refractile cell walls, are multinucleated, and show a single, large, and broad-based bud (refer **Fig. 75**).

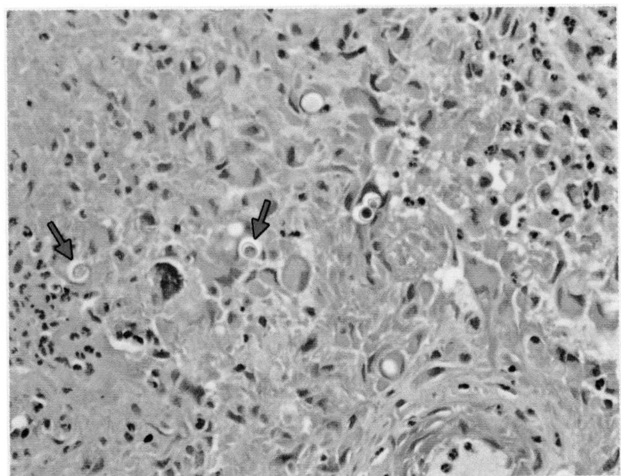

FIG. 77: Pulmonary blastomycosis showing yeast with thick sharply defined wall (arrow).

Mode of infection: Blastomycosis is acquired by inhalation of infectious spores (conidia) of *Blastomyces dermatitidis* from the soil. Disturbance of the soil, either by construction or by recreation activities (e.g., hunting or camping), leads to formation of aerosols containing fungal spores. Rarely, primary cutaneous form results from direct inoculation of organisms into the skin.

Pathogenesis

After inhalation of the conidia of *B. dermatitidis,* alveolar macrophages and polymorphonuclear leukocytes play an important role in phagocytosis and killing of the inhaled conidia of *B. dermatitidis*. The interaction of mediators of the innate immune response with local host factors (e.g., lung surfactant) plays a critical role in inhibiting conversion conidia form to the pathogenic yeast form (which reproduce by budding). This inhibition prevents the development of symptomatic disease. If conidia are converted into the thick-walled yeast form, phagocytosis and killing become difficult, and there is likely development of clinically apparent infection. T lymphocyte (mainly Th1) response is responsible for limiting the infection and dissemination. The host responds to the proliferating organisms by recruiting neutrophils and macrophages. This produces a focal bronchopneumonia. However, organisms persist until the onset of specific hypersensitivity and cell-mediated immunity. After this, the activated neutrophils and macrophages kill organism.

MORPHOLOGY

Blastomyces dermatitidis causes a chronic granulomatous and suppurative pulmonary disease called as blastomycosis. It usually followed by dissemination to other body sites, mainly the skin and bone. There are three clinical forms of blastomycosis—**(1) pulmonary blastomycosis, (2) disseminated blastomycosis, and a rare (3) primary cutaneous form.**

1. **Pulmonary blastomycosis:** Blastomycosis is usually confined to the lungs, where infection mostly produces small areas of consolidation (pneumonia). The pneumonia usually resolves spontaneously, but may persist or progress to a chronic lesion. In the normal individual, the lung lesions of blastomycosis produce suppurative granulomas. Pulmonary disease usually resolves by scarring. Some may progress to produce miliary lesions or cavities. Macrophages have a limited capacity to ingest and kill *B. dermatitidis*. The persistence of the yeast cells *B. dermatitidis* causes recruitment of neutrophils.
2. **Disseminated blastomycosis:** It may occur in immunocompromised individuals.
3. **Primary cutaneous form:** It is very rare and occurs due to direct inoculation. The skin (>50%) and bones (>10%) are the common sites of extrapulmonary blastomycosis. Skin infection usually produces marked pseudoepitheliomatous hyperplasia, and gives a warty appearance to the lesions. This may be mistaken for squamous cell carcinoma.

Continued

Continued

Microscopy: In tissue sections from infected area, *B. dermatitidis* appears as a round, 5–15 µm yeast cell that divides by broad-based budding. With hematoxylin and eosin stains, the yeasts are rings with thick, sharply defined cell walls (**Fig. 77**). It has a thick, double-contoured cell wall and visible nuclei in a central body. They may be found in epithelioid cells, macrophages or giant cells, or they may be seen lying free in microabscesses.

Clinical features: Pulmonary blastomycosis is self-limited in about one-third of patients. Symptomatic acute infection present with a flu-like illness, with fever, arthralgias, and myalgias. Progressive pulmonary disease presents with low-grade fever, weight loss, and cough. Skin lesions may resemble squamous cell carcinomas of the skin. Lung infection though resolves completely, in some patients, it may produce lesions at distant sites months to years later.

Coccidioidomycosis

Coccidioidomycosis (commonly known as Valley fever) is caused by dimorphic soil-dwelling fungi of the genus *Coccidioides*. There are two species, *C. immitis* and *C. posadasii*.

Source of infection: *C. immitis* is a dimorphic fungus that grows as a mold in the soil, where it forms spores. *C. immitis* is found in the soil. Coccidioidomycosis is particularly common in California's San Joaquin Valley, where it is called **"valley fever."** Dry and windy weather, which lifts spores into the air, favors infection. The disease is not contagious. *Coccidioides* organisms exist as filamentous molds in the soil. Within this mycelial structure, individual filaments (*hyphae*) elongate and branch (some grow upward). Alternating cells within the hyphae undergo degeneration and leave barrel-shaped viable elements called *arthroconidia* (refer **Fig. 75**).

The course of coccidioidomycosis varies from acute, self-limited disease to disseminated infection. It depends on the size of the infecting dose of the organism and the immune status of the host.

Pathogenesis

After inhalation in a susceptible host, the arthroconidia reach the alveoli and terminal bronchioles. The arthroconidia enlarge, become rounded, and develop internal septations. The resulting structures, called *spherules*, may become as large as 200 µm in size and these are unique to *Coccidioides*. The spherules then mature to form sporangia (measuring 30–60 µm in diameter). These sporangia gradually fill with 1–5 µm, uninuclear elements called endospores. These accumulate by endosporulation, a process unique among pathogenic fungi. Finally, the spherules may rupture and release endospores, which then repeat the cycle.

Almost all who inhale the arthroconidia/spores of *C. immitis* become infected and develop a delayed-type hypersensitivity reaction to the fungus. But, most of these individuals remain asymptomatic. Infectivity of *C. immitis* is partly because infective arthroconidia, when ingested by alveolar macrophages, block fusion of the phagosome and lysosome. Thereby, they resist intracellular killing. About 10% of infected individuals develop lung lesions, and <1% of individuals develop disseminated *C. immitis* infection. Disseminated form frequently involves the skin and meninges. Immunosuppressed individuals are at high risk for disseminated disease.

Coccidioidomycosis begins as focal bronchopneumonia at the site of deposition of arthroconidia/spores. It produces a mixed inflammatory infiltrate composed of neutrophils and macrophages. However, the spores survive inside these immunologically naïve inflammatory cells. As in tuberculosis and histoplasmosis, the host can control infection by *C. immitis* only when inflammatory cells become immunologically activated. With the onset of specific hypersensitivity and cell-mediated immune responses, necrotizing granulomas form and phagocytes kill or contain the fungi. This results in an acute and self-limited disease. Exposure to large numbers of organisms may result in extensive pulmonary involvement and fulminant disease.

Disseminated coccidioidomycosis occurs in immunocompromised individual. It may follow primary infection or reactivation of old disease. Pregnant women are also susceptible to spread of the disease, if they develop primary infection during the latter half of pregnancy.

MORPHOLOGY

Coccidioidomycosis is a chronic, necrotizing mycotic infection. It resembles tuberculosis both clinically and pathologically.

Acute self-limited coccidioidomycosis: It produces solitary lesions or patchy pulmonary consolidation. Microscopically, the involved alveoli are infiltrated by neutrophils and macrophages. *C. immitis* spherules attract an infiltrate of macrophages, whereas endospores mainly elicit neutrophil response. Once the host develops an immune reaction, necrotizing, caseous granulomas develop. Successful immune responses result in healing of the granulomas. Sometimes, healing may form a fibrocaseous nodule composed of caseous material surrounded by residual macrophages and a thin capsule. In contrast to histoplasmosis, calcification of old granulomas in coccidioidomycosis is rare.

Disseminated coccidioidomycosis: It may involve almost any site in the body and may manifest as a single lesion in the extrathoracic site or as widespread disease, involving the lungs, skin, bones, meninges, adrenals, lymph nodes, liver, spleen, and genitourinary tract. Inflammatory responses at sites of dissemination are highly variable. It may be purely granulomatous, pyogenic, or mixed.

Microscopy: *C. immitis* within macrophages or giant cells appears as thick-walled, nonbudding spherules 20–60 µm in diameter, often filled with small endospores. Both the spherules and endospores of *C. immitis* stain with hematoxylin and eosin. Spherules in various stages of development appear as basophilic rings. Mature spherules (sporangia) containing endospores appear as smaller basophilic rings. Similar to other fungi, PAS and GMS stains can be used to enhance the staining of *C. immitis*.
When the spherules rupture to release the endospores, superimposed pyogenic reaction develops.

Clinical features: Coccidioidomycosis produces protean manifestations. This may vary from a subclinical respiratory infection to a rapidly fatal disseminated disease. Like syphilis and typhoid fever, this disease is also a great imitator. Almost any complaint or syndrome may be its initial presentation.

Most individuals with coccidioidomycosis (>60%) are asymptomatic. Symptoms in symptomatic patients include a flu-like syndrome, with fever, cough, chest pain, and malaise. Infection usually resolves spontaneously. Cavitation in the lung is the most usual but rare (<5%) complication of pulmonary coccidioidomycosis. The cavity is usually solitary and may persist for years. This may be mistaken for cavity of tuberculosis.

Progression or reactivation of coccidioidomycosis may produce destructive lesions in the lungs or disseminated lesions in other organs. *C. immitis* infections outside the lungs produce life-threatening disease. The signs and symptoms of disseminated coccidioidomycosis depend on the site involved. Coccidioidal meningitis presents with headache, fever, alteration in mental status or seizures, and is often fatal if untreated. Skin lesions in disseminated disease usually have a warty gross appearance.

Laboratory Diagnosis of Coccidioidomycosis

- Direct examination: 10–20% KOH (potassium hydroxide)
- Culture
- Histopathology: Spherules and endospores are diagnostic.
- Serology: Complement fixation test (CFT) and latex agglutination test.

Paracoccidioidomycosis (South American Blastomycosis)

Paracoccidioidomycosis is a chronic granulomatous infection caused by *Paracoccidioides brasiliensis*. *P. brasiliensis* is a thermally dimorphic fungus (refer **Fig. 75**) and its mold form is present in the soil. Paracoccidioidomycosis primarily involves lung and may disseminate to involve skin, oropharynx, adrenals, and the macrophages of the liver, spleen, and lymph nodes.

Mode of infection: Paracoccidioidomycosis is acquired by inhaling spores.

Disease: Two major syndromes are associated with paracoccidioidomycosis—(1) the acute or juvenile form (uncommon) and (2) the chronic or adult form.

- *Acute form*: It occurs mostly in individuals <30 years old, and manifests as disseminated infection of the reticuloendothelial system. It also develops in immunocompromised persons.
- *Chronic form*: It constitutes ~90% of cases and predominantly observed in older men.
- Most infections are asymptomatic. Reactivation of latent infection occurs and active disease can develop many years after someone leaves an endemic region. Interestingly, men develop symptomatic infections 15 times more often than women.

MORPHOLOGY

Paracoccidioidomycosis may involve either the lungs alone or multiple extrapulmonary sites (e.g., skin, mucosal surfaces, and lymph nodes). *P. brasiliensis* produces a mixed suppurative and granulomatous response. The lesions are similar to those seen in blastomycosis and coccidioidomycosis.

Clinical features: Acute paracoccidioidomycosis usually produces an acute, self-limited, and mild disease. Progressive pulmonary diseases produce symptoms similar to those of tuberculosis. Chronic mucocutaneous ulcers may be one of the manifestations of extrapulmonary disease.

Sporotrichosis

Sporothrix schenckii is a thermally dimorphic fungus and is found in sphagnum moss (nonflowering plant), decaying vegetation, and soil. This dimorphic fungus (refer **Fig. 75**) grows as a mold in soil and decaying plant matter and as yeast in the body. It causes sporotrichosis that is a chronic infection of the skin, subcutaneous tissues, and regional lymph nodes.

Mode of infection: Cutaneous sporotrichosis develops by accidental inoculation of the fungus from thorns (especially rose thorns) or splinters, or by handling reeds or grasses. It affects individuals who are involved in outdoor activities such as landscaping, gardening, botanical nursery workers, and tree farming and others who develop abrasions while working with soil, moss, hay, or timbers. Infected animals (e.g., cats) can also transmit *S. schenckii* to humans.

Pathogenesis

By inoculation, *S. schenckii* enters into the skin and proliferates locally. There will be an inflammatory response at that site and it will produce an ulceronodular lesion. The infection usually spreads along subcutaneous lymphatic channels and results in a chain of similar nodular skin lesions. Extracutaneous disease (e.g., joint and bone) is usually less common than skin disease.

MORPHOLOGY

Cutaneous sporotrichosis: The lesions usually develop in the dermis or subcutaneous tissue. The periphery of the nodules of ulceronodular lesion shows granulomatous reaction and the center shows suppuration. The epithelium surrounding skin lesion shows exuberant pseudo-epitheliomatous hyperplasia. Some yeasts are surrounded by an eosinophilic, spiculated zone and are caked as "asteroid bodies". The material surrounding the yeasts ("Splendore-Hoeppli substance") probably represents antigen-antibody complexes.

Clinical features: Cutaneous sporotrichosis starts as a single nodular lesion at the site of inoculation. The usual site includes hand, arm, or leg. Weeks after the infection, additional nodules may develop along with the lymphatic drainage of the primary lesion. Nodules usually ulcerate and discharge serosanguineous fluid. Joint involvement may produce pain and swelling of the affected joint, without involvement of the covering skin.

Phaeohyphomycoses

The term *phaeohyphomycosis* is used to describe any infection with a pigmented mold. Dematiaceous or brown-black fungi are the common organisms in the soil. These fungi contain melanin, which produces dark pigmentation of their hyphae and conidia. They cause phaeohyphomycoses and includes two specific syndromes namely—(1) chromoblastomycosis and (2) eumycetoma as well as all other types of infections caused by these organisms.

Etiologic agents: Many pigmented molds can cause human infection. Most are found in the soil or on plants. Disseminated infection and focal visceral infections are caused by different dematiaceous fungi. Examples include *Alternaria*, *Exophiala*, *Curvularia*, and *Wangiella* species. *Fonsecaea* and *Cladophialophora* species are responsible for most cases of chromoblastomycosis. The most common cause of eumycetoma is *Madurella* species.

Mode of infection: Most dematiaceous fungi are directly inoculated. They cause localized subcutaneous infections. However, disseminated infections and serious focal visceral infections can occur, especially in immunocompromised patients. **Chromoblastomycosis and eumycetoma are acquired by inoculation through the skin**. These two syndromes are seen in tropical and subtropical areas and develop mostly in rural laborers who are frequently exposed to the organisms.

Chromoblastomycosis

Chromoblastomycosis is also known as chromomycosis. It is an indolent **chronic skin infection of subcutaneous tissue characterized by nodular, verrucous, or plaque-like painless lesions**. The lesions usually begin as papules and over the years become verrucous crusted and sometimes ulcerated. These lesions predominantly develop on the lower extremities and slowly grow over months to years. This may be caused by several species of fungi that live as saprophytes in soil and decaying vegetable matter. The **fungi are brown, round**, thick walled, and measure 8 µm across. They have been **likened to "copper pennies" (Figs. 78A and B)**. The infection is most common in barefooted agricultural workers in the tropics. The fungus is inoculated by trauma, usually below the knee. The infection spreads by contiguous growth and through lymphatics. Eventually, it may involve an entire limb. There is usually no extension of infection to adjacent structures, as is observed with eumycetoma. Long-term complications include bacterial superinfection, chronic lymphedema, and (rarely) the development of squamous cell carcinoma.

Mycetoma

Definition: Mycetoma is defined as a **chronic suppurative infection involving a limb, shoulder, or other tissues** and is **characterized by draining/discharging sinuses**. The discharging grains (material) consist of colonies of fungi or bacteria.

Types: Mycetomas can be divided into two main types depending on the causative agent namely—(1) **eumycetoma** (fungal disease and comprises about 40–50% of cases) and (2) **actinomycetoma** (higher bacteria and comprises about 50% of cases). The fungi causing eumycetoma include both hyaline molds and by brown-black molds.

Eumycetoma

- **Etiology:** It is a chronic granulomatous fungal disease caused by true fungi, *Madurella mycetomatis*, or *Madurella grisea*.
- **Mode of infection:** The organisms are inoculated directly from soil into bare feet during agricultural work, from carrying of contaminated sacks on the shoulders, and into the hands from infected vegetation.

MORPHOLOGY

It involves skin and subcutaneous tissue. After several months of infection, the affected site, most commonly foot, manifests as an open area or break in the skin. The affected part is swollen and when foot is affected, it is termed as mycetoma pedis (mycetoma of the foot) or "Madura foot" (**Fig. 79**). This was initially named Madura foot, after its discovery in the region called Madura in India. The infection extends deeply into the subcutaneous tissues along the fascia and eventually invades the bones. They drain serosanguinous fluid containing granules through sinus tracts. The size, color, and degree of hardness of granules depend on the etiologic species and are characteristic of mycetoma. The surrounding tissue shows granulomatous reaction. The fungi stain positively with Grocott-Gomori's methenamine silver (GMS) stain.

Actinomycosis

- It is a chronic suppurative disease caused by anaerobic bacteria, *Actinomyces israelii*. It is not a fungus.
- The organisms are commensals in the oral cavity, gastrointestinal (GI) tract, and vagina.

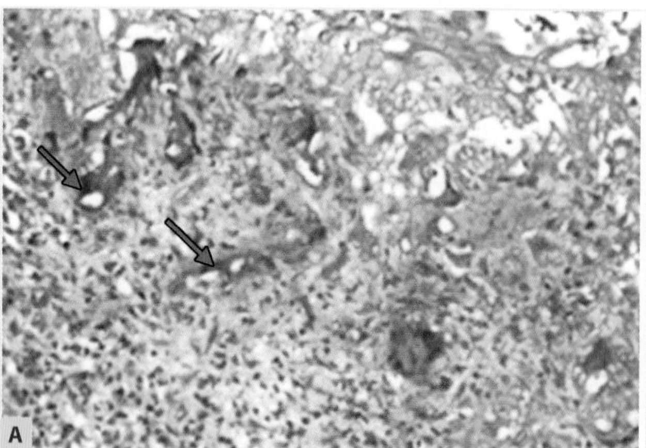

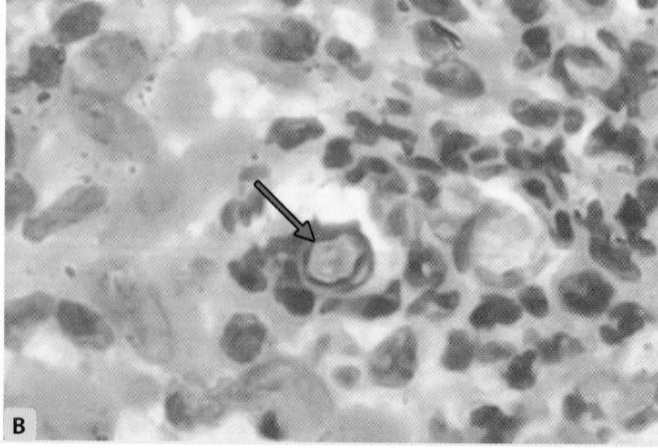

FIGS. 78A AND B: Chromoblastomycosis involving subcutaneous tissue. The fungi are brown, round, thick walled, and have been likened to "copper pennies".

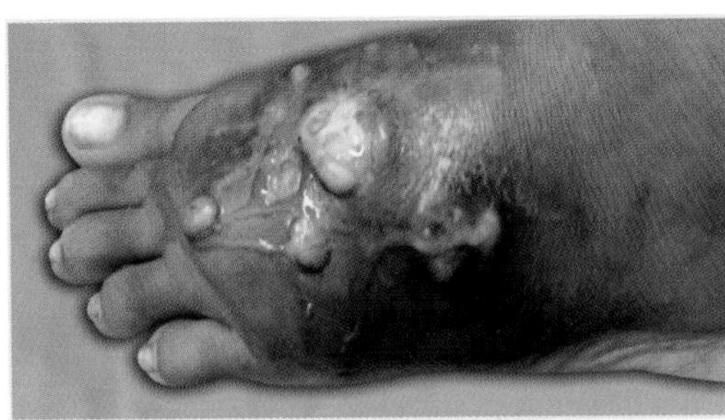

FIG. 79: Mycetoma (Madura foot) showing numerous sinuses discharging serosanguinous fluid.

Mode of infection: Infection is always endogenous in origin and not due to personal contact. Break in mucocutaneous continuity, diminished immunity due to some underlying disease favors the organism to invade, proliferate, and disseminate.

MORPHOLOGY

Depending on the anatomic location of lesions, actinomycosis is divided into four types:

1. **Cervicofacial actinomycosis:**
   - It is the most common form (60%) and has best prognosis.
   - Infections gain through tonsils, carries teeth, periodontal diseases, or trauma following extraction of tooth.
   - In the beginning, a firm swelling develops in the lower jaw (i.e., lumpy jaw). Later, the mass breaks down and forms abscess and sinuses. Typically, the sinus discharges yellow sulfur granules. The infection may spread into the adjacent soft tissues and may destroy the bone.
2. **Thoracic actinomycosis:**
   - The infection of lung is a result of aspiration of organism from the oral cavity or extension of infection from abdominal or hepatic lesions.
   - Initially, lung lesions resemble pneumonia but as the disease progresses, these spread to the whole lung, pleura, ribs, and vertebrae.
3. **Abdominal actinomycosis:**
   - The common sites are appendix, cecum, and liver.
   - The infection occurs as a result of swallowing of organism from oral cavity or as an extension from thoracic cavity.
4. **Pelvic actinomycosis (Fig. 80):**
   - It develops as a complication of intrauterine contraceptive devices (IUCDs).

Microscopy (Figs. 81A and B)

Following features are seen irrespective of the location of actinomycosis:

- *Granulomatous reaction with central suppuration*: There is formation of abscesses in the center of lesions and the periphery of the lesions shows chronic inflammatory cells, giant cells, and fibroblasts.
- The central abscess contains bacterial colony (sulfur granule) characterized by radiating filaments (was called

Continued

Continued

as ray fungus) surrounded by hyaline, eosinophilic, and club-like ends, which represent immunoglobulins.
- *Special stains for bacteria*: The organisms are gram-positive filaments and nonacid-fast (except nocardia). They stain negatively with Grocott-Gomori's methenamine silver (GMS) stain.

Rhinosporidiosis

Rhinosporidiosis is an inflammatory disease caused by eukaryotic fungal pathogen *Rhinosporidium seeberi*. Usually, it occurs in nasopharynx as polyp but may also be observed in larynx and conjunctiva. It is endemic in India and Sri Lanka and sporadic in other parts of the world.

MORPHOLOGY

Microscopy (Figs. 82A and B):

- Structure of nasal mucosa.
- Many spherical cysts called as sporangia measuring up to 200 nm in diameter having thick wall (chitinous wall) are seen. Each of these cysts (i.e., sporangium) contains numerous small basophilic round spores of the size of erythrocytes. On rupture of a sporangium, the spores may be discharged into the submucosa or on to the surface of the mucosa.
- Chronic inflammatory cells (plasma cells, lymphocytes, histiocytes, and neutrophils) infiltrate in the intervening and subepithelial layer.

Laboratory Diagnosis of Fungal Infection

Q. Discuss laboratory diagnosis of fungal infection.
Q. Write short essay on demonstration of fungus in tissues.

Specimen collection and processing: As with all types of infectious diseases, the laboratory diagnosis of fungal infection directly depends on the proper collection of appropriate clinical material. It should be promptly delivered to the clinical laboratory. Normally, the specimen is collected from the

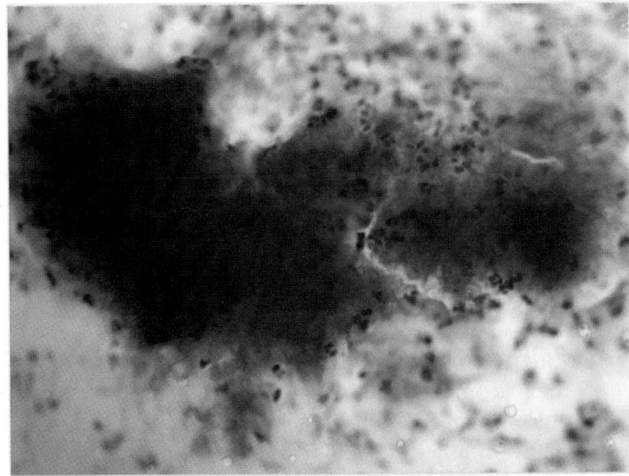

FIG. 80: Actinomycosis in vaginal smear.

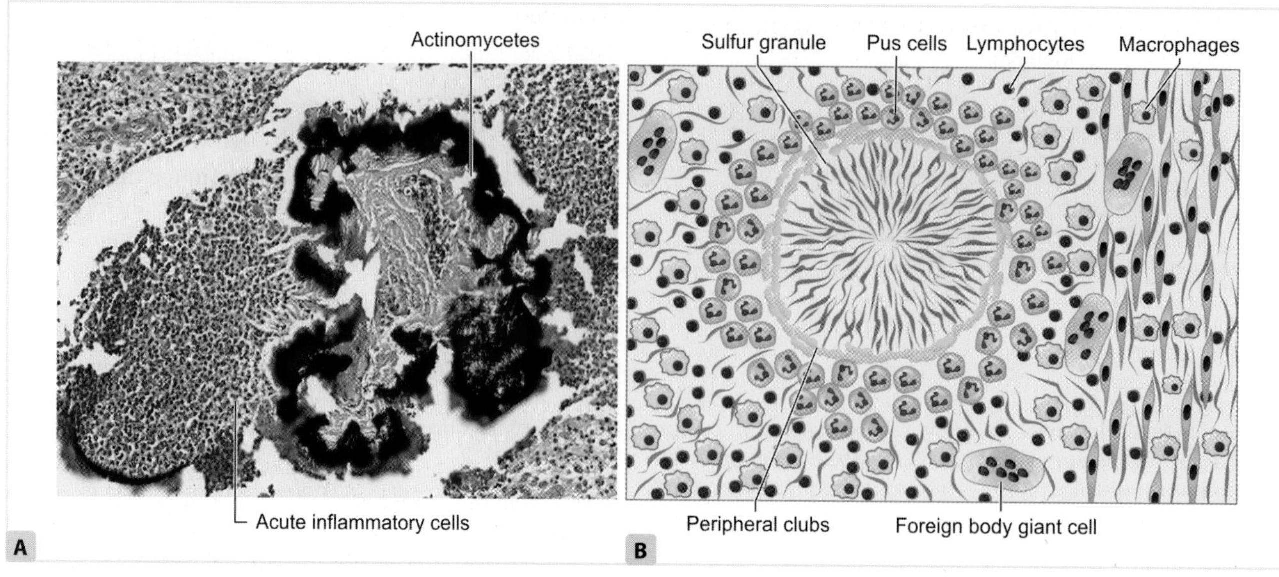

FIGS. 81A AND B: Microscopy of actinomycosis showing central bacterial colony surrounded inflammatory cells. (A) Hematoxylin and eosin and (B) Diagrammatic representation.

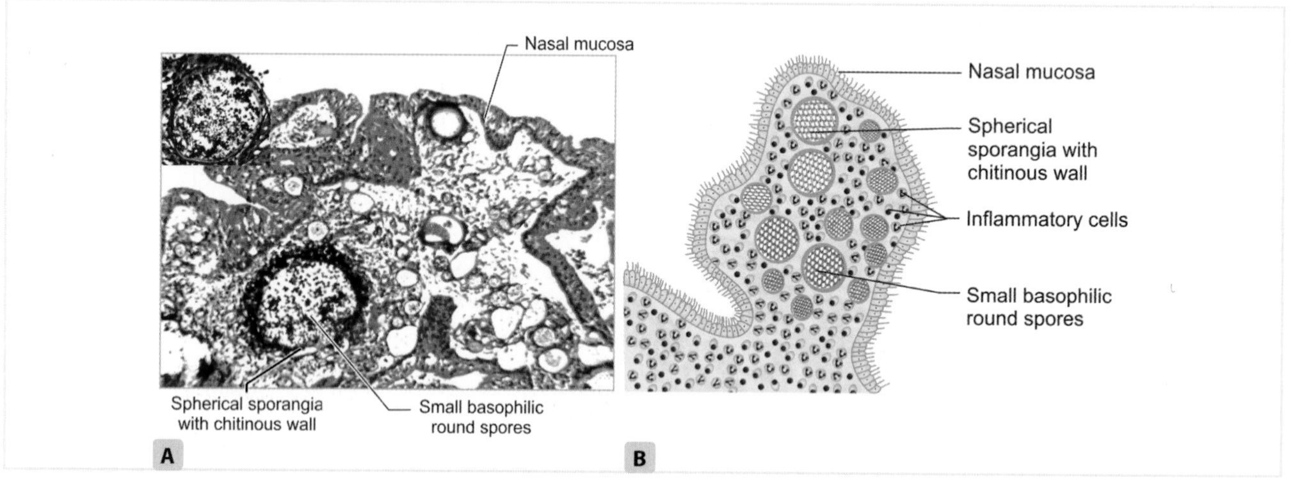

FIGS. 82A AND B: Rhinosporidiosis of nasopharynx showing spherical sporangia: (A) Hematoxylin and eosin (H&E); (B) Diagrammatic representation.

affected site. In the case of suspected disseminated (spreading) infections, it needs collection of blood samples.

- *Superficial mycoses*: Skin scrapping, infected hairs and nails, mucosal scrapping, or swabs.
- *Subcutaneous mycoses*: Pus, discharge, crust, biopsy, and swabs from the lesion.
- *Systemic mycosis*: Sputum, urine, pus, feces, CSF, blood, biopsy, etc.

Various laboratory methods for the diagnosis of fungal disease are listed in **Box 15.**

Conventional Microbiologic Methods

Direct microscopic examination

Direct microscopic examination of tissue sections and clinical specimens of material from the lesion is the most rapid and cost-effective method for the diagnosis of fungal infections. Direct microscopic examination is also performed on fungal isolates.

Advantages: Yeasts or hyphal structures of fungus in tissue can be microscopically detected within an hour, whereas culture results may take days or weeks. Certain fungus may be detected and identified by microscopy because of its distinctive morphology. For example, detection of characteristic cysts, yeast cells, or spherules can confirm an etiological diagnosis of infections caused by *P. jirovecii, H. capsulatum, B. dermatitidis*, or *C. immitis/posadasii*, respectively. Although the morphological appearance of *Candida*, a mucoromycete, or *Trichosporon* in tissue may be helpful for the diagnosis of the type of infection (i.e., candidiasis, mucormycosis, and trichosporonosis), the actual species of fungus causing the infection may not be known without culture. Microscopical detection of fungi in tissue in the laboratory is useful in selecting the most appropriate means to culture the specimen and is also helpful in determining the significance of culture results.

Box 15: Various laboratory methods for the diagnosis of fungal disease.

Conventional microbiologic methods:
- Direct microscopy (Gram, Giemsa, and calcofluor white stains)
- Culture
- Identification
- Susceptibility testing

Histopathological and/or cytological methods:
- Light microscopy:
  - Routine stains (H and E)
  - Special stains (GMS, PAS, and mucicarmine)
- Direct immunofluorescence
- In situ hybridization

Immunologic (serological) methods: Antibody or antigen detection—
- Latex agglutination test
- Compliment fixation test
- Immunodiffusion
- Counter current immunoelectrophoresis
- Enzyme-linked immunosorbent assay (ELISA)
- Radioimmunological assay
- Immunofluorescence test
- Exoantigen test

Molecular methods:
- Direct detection (nucleic acid amplification)
- Identification
- Strain typing

Biochemical methods:
- Metabolites
- Cell wall components
- Enzymes

(GMS: Grocott–Gomori's methenamine silver; H and E: hematoxylin and eosin; PAS: periodic acid–Schif)

Disadvantages: Though direct microscopy is useful in diagnosing fungal infection, **both false-negative and false-positive results may occur**. Microscopy is less sensitive than culture, and a negative result does not rule out a fungal infection.

Stains: Different stains and microscopic techniques may be used to detect and characterize fungi directly in clinical material (**Table 28**). Most often used include staining of smears and touch preparations with either Gram or Giemsa stains and the fluorescent reagent calcofluor white.

- **Gram stain:** It is useful for detection of yeasts (e.g., *Candida* or *Cryptococcus*), and filamentous fungi (e.g., *Aspergillus*). Fungi are usually gram positive but may appear speckled or gram negative.
- **Giemsa stain:** It is especially useful for detecting the intracellular yeast forms of *H. capsulatum* in peripheral blood smears, bone marrow, or touch preparations of tissue.
- **Calcofluor white staining coupled with fluorescent microscopy:** Calcofluor white stains fluoresce the cell walls of fungi and make it easier and faster to detect the fungus. It is used for identification of fungi in fluid specimens.

Selected methods and stains commonly used for direct microscopic detection of fungal elements in clinical specimens are presented in **Table 28**.

Culture

Definitive identification of some requires isolation of the fungus in culture. It is the most sensitive means of diagnosing a fungal infection. Culture is also needed to identify the etiologic agents.

Histopathological and/or Cytological Methods

Light microscopy

In the cytology and/or histopathology laboratory, stains such as hematoxylin and eosin (H and E), GMS, and PAS are used for detection of fungi in cytologic preparations, fine-needle

Table 28: Selected methods and stains commonly used for direct microscopic detection of fungal elements in clinical specimens.

Method/Stain	*Use*	*Comments*
Gram stain	Detection of fungi	• Commonly performed • Stains most yeasts and hyphal elements • Most fungi stain gram positive, but some (e.g., *Cryptococcus neoformans*) show stippling or appear gram negative
Giemsa stain	Examination of bone marrow, peripheral blood smears, touch preparations of tissue, and respiratory specimens	• Detect intracellular *Histoplasma capsulatum* and both intracystic and trophic forms of *P. jirovecii* • Does not stain the cyst wall of *Pneumocystis* • Does stain organisms other than *Histoplasma* and *Pneumocystis*
Calcofluor white stain coupled with fluorescent microscopy	Detection of all fungi (including *Pneumocystis jirovecii*) in fluid specimens	• Rapid (1–2 min); detects fungal cell wall chitin by bright fluorescence • Used in combination with potassium hydroxide • Needs fluorescent microscope
Fluorescent monoclonal antibody treatment	Examination of respiratory specimen for *P. jirovecii*	• Sensitive and specific method for detection the cysts of *P. jirovecii* • Does not stain the extracystic (trophic) forms

aspirates, tissues, body fluids, and exudates (**Table 29**). These stains can detect fungi such as *B. dermatitidis, H. capsulatum, C. immitis/posadasii, Candida* species, *C. neoformans,* and the hyphae of mucormycetes, *Aspergillus,* and other molds. **India ink preparation** is used for negative staining of capsulated yeast (e.g., *Cryptococcus*). When positive, an India ink preparation of CSF is diagnostic for cryptococcosis.

Histopathological examination: The definitive diagnosis of any fungal infection needs histopathological identification of the fungus invading tissue and accompanying evidence of an inflammatory response. Histopathological examination of fixed tissue is useful for determination whether the fungus is invading the tissue or merely present superficially. This information is helpful in distinguishing between actual infection and colonization. Most fungi can be identified on tissue sections stained with hematoxylin and eosin (H and E stain), but small numbers of organisms may be missed. The microscopic features of the more common fungal pathogens are presented in **Table 29**.

Special stains (Table 29): The more fungus-specific stains are the GMS and PAS stains. They outline fungal cell walls and are commonly used to detect fungal infection in tissues. These stains are useful when fungi are present in small numbers and for clearly defining characteristic features of fungal morphology.

- **Periodic acid-Schiff stain:** Fungal elements are stained magenta against pink-green background. It stains polysaccharide present in fungi.
- **Grocott-Gomori's methenamine silver stain**: Fungal elements are stained black against green background. It is best for screening purpose and to demonstrate actinomycete.
- **Gram stain**: *Candida* (unlike other fungi) is better seen on gram stained tissue smears. Gram-positive are actinomycetes and nonfilamentous bacteria of Botryomycoses. Hematoxylin and eosin stain is not sufficient to identify *Candida* in tissue specimens.
- **Mucicarmine:** Stains mucoid capsule of *Cryptococci.*
- **Modified acid-fast stain**: Stains *Nocardia* species.
- **Melanin stain (e.g., Fontana Mason)**: For demonstration of melanin and melanin-like substances in certain fungi (e.g., *Cryptococcus*).

Stains used in histopathology for detection of fungal elements are presented in **Table 30**.

Table 29: Microscopic features of the more common fungal pathogens.

Fungus	*Microscopic features in clinical specimens*
Candida	• Oval budding yeasts measuring 2–6 μm in diameter • Hyphae and pseudohyphae may be present
Cryptococcus neoformans	• Spherical budding yeasts of variable size, 2–15 μm • Capsule may be present • No hyphae or pseudohyphae
Aspergillus	• Septate, dichotomously branched hyphae of uniform width (3–6 μm)
Mucormycetes	• Broad, thin-walled, pauciseptate hyphae, 6–25 μm with nonparallel sides and random branches • Hyphae usually stain well with H and E stain but stain poorly with GMS stain
Histoplasma capsulatum	Small (2–4 μm) budding yeasts within macrophages
Blastomyces dermatitidis	Large (8–15 μm), thick-walled, and broad-based budding yeast
Dematiaceous molds	• Pigmented (brown, tan, or black) hyphae, 2–6 μm wide • May be branched or unbranched • Usually constricted at point of septation
Coccidioides immitis/posadasii	• Spherical, thick-walled spherules, 20–200 μm • Mature spherules contain small, 2–5 μm endospores
Pneumocystis jirovecii	• Cysts are round, collapsed, or crescent shaped • Trophic forms seen on special stains

(GMS: Grocott-Gomori's methenamine silver; H and E: hematoxylin and eosin)

Table 30: Stains used in histopathology for detection of fungal elements.

Method/Stain	*Use*	*Comments*
Hematoxylin and eosin (H and E) stain	Usual histopathological stain	• Best stain to demonstrate host reaction in infected tissue • Stains most fungi • Useful in demonstrating natural pigment in dematiaceous fungi
GMS stain	Detection of fungi in histologic sections and *Pneumocystis jirovecii* cysts in respiratory specimens	• Best stain for detecting all fungi • Stains hyphae and yeast forms black against a green background • Usually performed in histopathology laboratory
Mucicarmine stain	Histopathological stain for mucin	• Useful for demonstrating capsular material of *Cryptococcus neoformans* • May also stain the cell walls of *Blastomyces dermatitidis* and *Rhinosporidium seeberi*
PAS stain	Histological stain for fungi	• Stains both yeasts and hyphae in tissue • PAS-positive artifacts may resemble yeast cells

(GMS: Grocott-Gomori's methenamine silver; PAS: periodic acid-Schiff)

Matrix-assisted laser desorption ionization time-of-flight mass spectrometry (MALDI-TOF MS): It may be used for detection and speciation. Point-of-care and lateral-flow testing techniques are under development for many fungal infections.

Direct immunofluorescence stain

It is used for demonstration of fungi in tissues and smears by using antibodies, combined with fluorescence dye.

Immunologic (serological) methods Determination of antibody (Ab) and/or antigen (Ag) titers in serum may be useful for the diagnosis of fungal infections. Various methods available for detection of antibody or antigen are listed in **Box 15**. When serological tests are performed in a serial fashion, Ab/Ag titers are also useful for monitoring the progression of disease and the patient's response to therapy. However, most tests for antibodies lack both sensitivity and specificity for diagnosis of invasive fungal infections (exception of antibody tests for histoplasmosis and coccidioidomycosis).

Molecular Methods

Polymerase chain reaction to directly detect fungal-specific nucleic acids in clinical material is used for the rapid diagnosis of fungal infections. Recent developments, such as real-time, gene chip technology, and the coupling of nanotechnology with magnetic resonance detection, although not yet available in most mycology laboratories, will be useful in the prompt diagnosis of fungal infection.

Biochemical Methods

Metabolites: Detection of fungal metabolites in serum or other body fluids may be useful for the diagnosis of invasive fungal infection. The detection of fungal metabolites is useful for the rapid diagnosis of both candidiasis and aspergillosis. For example, detection of D-arabinitol in serum indicates hematogenously disseminated candidiasis and detection of elevated levels of D-mannitol in bronchoalveolar lavage fluid is useful in the diagnosis of pulmonary aspergillosis. However, due to the lack of a commercially available test and variability in sensitivity and specificity, the diagnostic utility of metabolite detection remains uncertain.

Cell wall components: These include immunoassays for detection of *Aspergillus* galactomannan and *Candida* mannan and anti-mannan. Another fungal-specific cell wall component namely 1,3-β-glucan may be detected in the serum of patients infected with *Candida, Aspergillus,* and *P. jirovecii*. This is detected by the limulus lysate assay.

Skin tests were commonly used in earlier days, but not useful for diagnosis.

11.6 Parasitic Diseases

CHAPTER OUTLINE

- Introduction
- Protozoa
  - Malaria
  - Babesiosis
  - Amebiasis
  - Leishmaniasis
  - African trypanosomiasis
  - Chagas disease (american trypanosomiasis)
  - Toxoplasmosis
  - Cryptosporidiosis
  - Giardiasis
  - Trichomonas vaginalis
- Metazoal infections
  - Cestodes: Intestinal tapeworms
  - Tissue nematodes
  - Trematodes (flukes)
  - Intestinal nematodes
  - Filarial nematodes
- Techniques for diagnosis of infectious agents

INTRODUCTION

Parasitism is the mode of existence of organisms called as parasite. **Parasite** is an organism which infects another called as the **host.** The parasites **live in or on their hosts and cause them harm** while itself deriving a benefit. **The residence time for a parasite in or on a host is variable.**

Ectoparasites and endoparasites: Parasites that live on the external surface of their hosts and are termed as **ectoparasites (e.g.,** human body louse *Pediculus humanus humanus).* They are said to cause **infestations.** In contrast, **endoparasites (e.g.,** adult tapeworm *Taenia solium* or the trematode *Schistosoma mansoni)* **live inside their host's body** and are said to cause **infections.**

Obligatory, facultative, and opportunistic parasites: They are described here.

- An **obligatory parasite needs** a **suitable host to complete its life cycle**. Without such a host, obligate parasites cannot exist. Example is intestinal roundworm *Ascaris lumbricoides*. It can develop to adulthood in the small intestine of humans. Its eggs are passed in the host's feces and survive outside the host for a time. But if another human does not ingest these eggs, the parasite could not persist.
- **Facultative parasites** are **usually free-living**. But, **if they are given the opportunity, they can adopt a parasitic existence**. For example, *Naegleria fowleri*, normally a free-living ameba living in the muddy bottoms of aquatic environments. This is capable of colonizing and multiplying in the human brain if it is inhaled through the nasal passages.
- **Opportunistic parasite** is a **parasite that normally does not infect or in which it does not normally cause disease**. However, it **takes advantage of particular circumstances to initiate an infection in a host.** For example, *Toxoplasma gondii* normally be held in check by a person with an intact immune system infection, but in an individual with a compromised immune system, such human immunodeficiency virus (HIV), it will produce infection.

Hosts: There are mainly two types of host namely definitive and intermediate hosts.

1. **Definitive host:** It is a host in which a parasite achieves sexual maturity, which is usually followed by sexual reproduction within that host.
2. **Intermediate host:** It is a host in which a parasite undergoes a required developmental step and may even reproduce asexually but does not reproduce sexually.

PROTOZOA

Protozoa are **single-celled** (unicellular) eukaryotic organisms. Protozoa usually range from 10 to 200 μm, in length. Most protozoa are motile and mainly belong to three general classes: **amebae, flagellates**, and **sporozoites**.

- **Amebae** move by projection of cytoplasmic extensions termed ***Pseudopoda.***
- **Flagellates** move through thread-like structures. Flagella extend out from the cell membrane of flagellates.
- **Sporozoites** do not have organelles of locomotion. They **differ from amebae and flagellates in their mode of replication.**

Mode of transmission: The protozoa are transmitted **by insects or by the fecal-oral route**.

Location: They are mainly located in the blood or intestine in humans **(Table 31)**.

Mechanism of disease by protozoa: Protozoa can cause human disease by different mechanisms.

- Some are extracellular parasites that **digest and invade human tissues** (e.g., *Entamoeba histolytica).*
- Some are **obligate** (obliged) **intracellular parasites that replicate in, and kill, human cells** (e.g., plasmodia).
- Some **damage human tissue largely by inflammatory and immunologic responses** (e.g., trypanosomes).
- Some protozoa (e.g., *T. gondii*) can **produce latent infections** and **cause reactivation disease in immunocompromised hosts.**

Diagnosis: Most protozoal infections are diagnosed by either microscopic examination of blood smears or lesions.

Malaria

Malaria is a mosquito-borne, hemolytic, febrile illness caused by the intracellular parasite *Plasmodium*. The name malaria (mal: bad, aria: air) was given in the 18th century in Italy, because it was thought to be caused by foul emissions from marshy soil.

Species of *Plasmodium*: *Plasmodium falciparum* (causes severe cerebral malaria) and the four other malaria parasites that infect humans (*P. vivax, P. ovale, P. knowlesi,* and *P. malariae*) are all **transmitted by female *Anopheles* mosquitoes**.

The relative prevalence of the four species of malaria parasites: It varies in different geographical regions. In India, malaria is a major public health threat.

1. ***P. vivax*:** Most widely distributed and most common in Asia, North Africa, and Central and South America.
2. ***P. falciparum:*** It is the predominant species in Africa, Papua New Guinea and Haiti. It is rapidly spreading in Southeast Asia and India.
3. ***P. malariae:*** It is present in most places but is rare, except in Africa.
4. ***P. ovale:*** It is almost confined to West Africa where it ranks second after *Falciparum*.
5. ***Plasmodium knowlesi:*** It is a monkey malaria and is distributed in Southeast Asia where the reservoir macaques (Old World monkeys) are prevalent.

Malaria may occur in endemic as well as epidemic patterns.

1. **Endemic**: It means that **occurs constantly in an area over a period of several successive years**.
2. **Epidemic**: It means when **periodic or occasional sharp rises occur in its incidence**.

Mode of transmission: Malaria is transmitted by the bite **of the female *Anopheles* mosquito**.

Incubation period: It varies with the type of species (**Table 32**).

Control measures: Mass spraying of DDT (dichloro-diphenyl-trichloroethane) was used to eliminate the mosquito vectors. After the initial success, now DDT has failed to eliminate and DDT was removed from the market due to environmental concerns. At present control of malaria is challenging because of insecticide-resistant mosquitoes and drug-resistant *Plasmodium* spp. Currently, to reduce the incidence of malaria a combination of mosquito control and antimalarial drugs is adopted.

Table 31: Location and disease caused in human by few protozoa.

Species	*Disease produced*
Location: Lumen or epithelium	
Entamoeba histolytica	Amebic dysentery; amebic liver abscess
Balantidium coli	Colitis
Giardia duodenalis	Diarrheal disease, malabsorption
Cystoisospora belli	Chronic enterocolitis or malabsorption or both
Trichomonas vaginalis	Urethritis, vaginitis
Location: Blood	
Plasmodium species	Malaria
Babesia species	Babesiosis
Trypanosoma species	African sleeping sickness
Location: Intracellular	
Trypanosoma cruzi	Chagas disease
Leishmania donovani	Kala-azar
Leishmania species	Cutaneous and mucocutaneous leishmaniasis
Toxoplasma gondii	Toxoplasmosis
Location: Central nervous system	
Naegleria fowleri	Meningoencephalitis
Acanthamoeba species	Meningoencephalitis or ophthalmitis

Life Cycle and Pathogenesis (Fig. 83)

Q. Write short essay on lifecycle of malaria.

The life cycles of the *Plasmodium* species are similar.

- ***P. vivax, P. ovale, P. knowlesi, and P. malariae:*** They produce **low levels of parasitemia**, mild anemia. Very rarely there may be splenic rupture and nephrotic syndrome.
- ***P. falciparum* infection:** It **produces high levels of parasitemia** and may lead to severe anemia, cerebral symptoms, renal failure, pulmonary edema, and death depending on the susceptibility of the host.

Two hosts: The life cycle of *Plasmodium* species is simple because it involves only two different hosts namely humans (intermediate host) and female mosquitoes (definitive host) and requires both these hosts. Distinguishing feature of the life cycle is the alternation of sexual and asexual phases in the two hosts.

1. **Human host** (intermediate host): The **asexual phase, called schizogony**, occurs in the human.

Table 32: Incubation period for various species of *Plasmodium*.

Species of Plasmodium	*Incubation period*	*Disease produced*
Plasmodium vivax	14 days (ranges 8–17 days)	Benign tertian malaria
Plasmodium falciparum	12 days (ranges 9–14 days)	Malignant tertian malaria
Plasmodium malariae	28 days (ranges 18–40 days)	Benign quartan malaria
Plasmodium ovale	17 days (ranges 16–18 days).	Benign tertian malaria

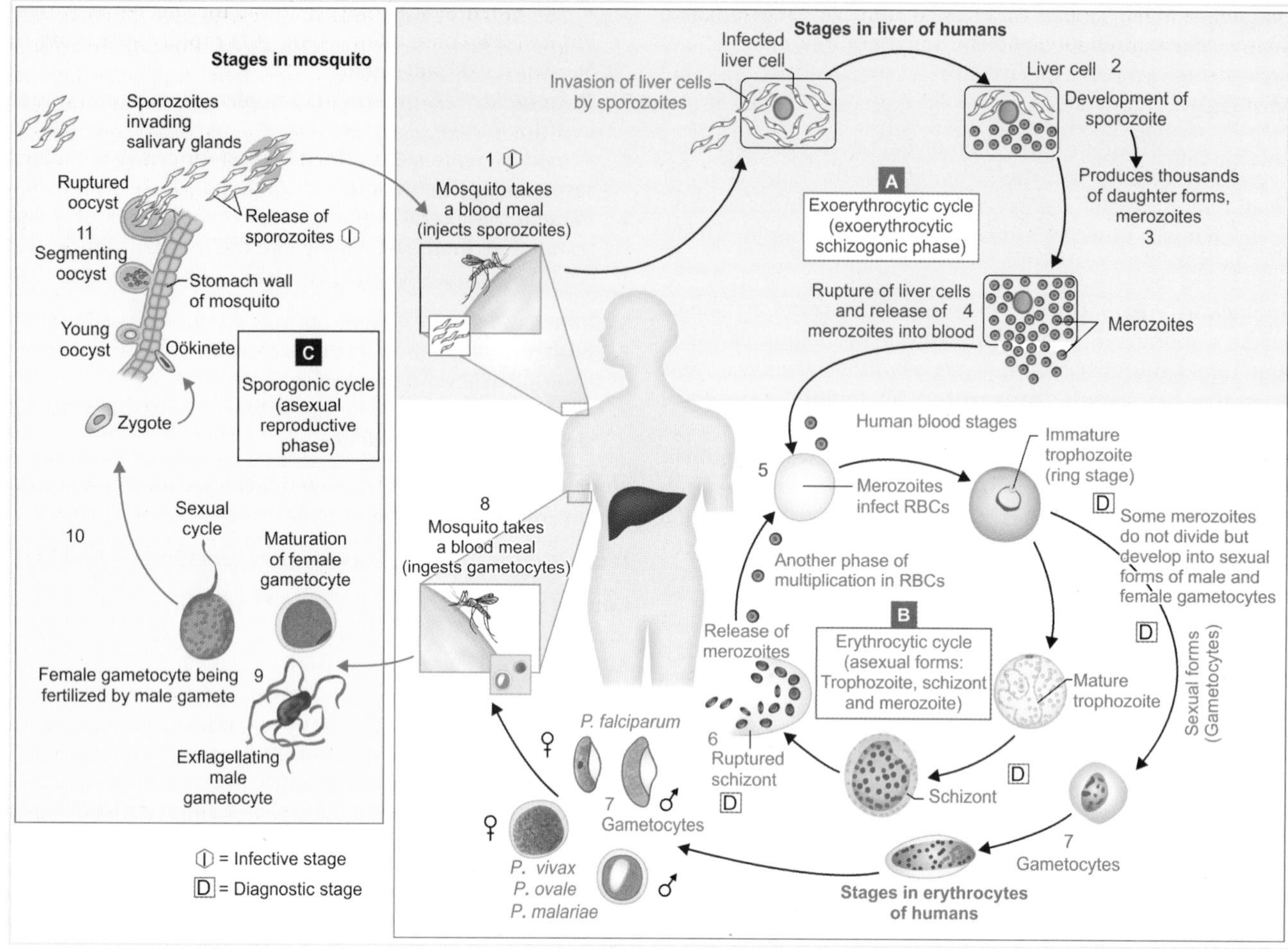

FIG. 83: Life cycle of malarial parasites (refer text for description).

2. **In the mosquito** (definitive host): First a **sexual phase** (gamogony) occurs; **followed by another asexual reproductive phase** (sporogony).

However, the development of the parasite is complex. The parasite passes through several morphologically distinct forms.

Human cycle

The asexual phase, called schizogony, occurs in the human. In this stage, the malaria parasite multiplies by division or splitting. Hence, this process is called as *schizogony* (from *schizo: to split,* and *gone: generation).*

Introduction of infectious *sporozoite* by mosquito bite: Human (intermediate host) cycle starts with the inoculation (introduction) of infectious stage of *Plasmodium*, the *sporozoite* into the human bloodstream by the bite of infected female *Anopheles* mosquito. This occurs when mosquito feeds on human blood after piercing the skin. The mouthparts of male *Anopheles* mosquito cannot penetrate human skin; hence, they feed solely on plant juices. Usually, 10–15 sporozoites are injected at a time, but occasionally it may be in hundreds. The sporozite is slender, curved, elongated, and minute measuring about 10–55 mm in length and about 1 mm in diameter. It has tapering at both ends, a central elongated nucleus and does not contain any pigment. The *sporozoite* is found in the salivary glands of mosquitoes. During mosquito bite, the mosquito takes a blood meal and sporozoites are released into the human's blood (1 in **Fig. 83**). In humans, schizogony occurs in two locations: (1) in the **liver cells** (**exoerythrocytic *schizogony*** or the tissue phase) and (2) in the **red blood cell** (RBC) (**erythrocytic *schizogony*).** The different stages of human cycle are:

Exoerythrocytic stage (pre-erythrocytic schizogony) (A in Fig. 81) Because schizogony in the liver is an essential step before the parasites can invade erythrocytes, it is called *pre-erythrocytic schizogony.* The **products of schizogony**, whether erythrocytic or exoerythrocytic, **are called *merozoites*** *(meros: a part, zoon: animal).*

The sporozoites function both in the vector (mosquito) and in the human hosts. They invade the cells of the salivary gland in the vector and the hepatocytes in the human.

In liver: Exoerythrocytic stage occurs in liver of humans. The spindle-shaped sporozoites pass into the bloodstream, where many are destroyed by the phagocytes. But some circulating sporozoites (infectious stage) within 30 minutes of entry rapidly attach to and invade liver cells (2 in **Fig. 83**) by binding to the hepatocyte receptor for the serum proteins thrombospondin (see **Fig. 85**) and properdin. Only few liver cells/ hepatocytes are infected by *Plasmodium*. Hence, liver damage does not occur in malaria. Within liver cells, the elongated spindle-shaped sporozoites become rounded. They enlarge in size and undergo repeated nuclear division to form several daughter nuclei; each of which is surrounded by cytoplasm. These **sporozoites yield numerous daughter *uninucleate* organisms**, termed **"merozoites"** (exoerythrocytic phase) (**3 in Fig. 83**). About 30,000 *merozoites* (asexual, haploid forms) are released when each infected liver cells ruptures (**4 in Fig. 83**). The infection of the liver and development of merozoites is referred to as the exoerythrocytic stage. This stage is asymptomatic. During this phase the parasites are not found in the peripheral blood and inoculation of such blood does not produce any infection (i.e., blood is sterile) inside the liver cells.

- In *P. falciparum* infection, rupture of liver cells usually occurs within 8–12 weeks.
- In *P. vivax* and *P. ovale,* sporozoites invade hepatocytes, where they **either enter a dormant (latent) hypnozoite stage or undergo merogony**. Some sporozoites of *P. vivax* and *P. ovale* do not develop further and may remain in liver as hypnozoites. The ability to form hypnozoites results in relapses that can occur in infected individuals' months or years postinfection. The release of "merozoites" occurs weeks to months after initial infection. This is responsible for relapses of malaria after many years.

Erythrocytic stage (B in Fig. 83) **Invasion of RBCs**–within 2–3 weeks of hepatic infection, the merozoites rupture the host hepatocytes and are released into the bloodstream. Merozoites are *pear-shaped* bodies, about 1.5 µm in length, possessing an ***apical complex*** *(rhoptery).* Once released from the liver, *Plasmodium* merozoites use a lectin-like molecule to bind to sialic acid residues on glycophorin molecules (major glycoprotein) on the surface of red cells and invade by RBC active penetration of the membrane (**5 in Fig. 83**).

Growth and reproduction in RBCs: Within the red cells (erythrocytic stage) merozoites grow in an intraerythrocytic membrane-bound digestive vacuole and feed on hemoglobin by hydrolyze hemoglobin through its enzymes. These **merozites (parasites) reproduce inside erythrocytes**.

Asexual forms (**6 in Fig. 83**): In the RBCs, parasite passes through three stages of asexual forms namely: **(1) trophozoite, (2) schizont, and (3) merozoite**. These asexual forms of parasite can be demonstrated in the thick blood smears 3 to 4 days after exposure. Each cycle of erythrocyte schizogony lasts 48–72 hours (in ***P. vivax, P. ovale, and P. falciparum*** it is 48 hours and in ***P. malariae*** it is 72 hours). The multiplication of parasites during this phase is responsible for clinical features of malaria. ***P. vivax*** has greater tendency to **invade younger RBCs**. ***P. falciparum*** has no special affinity and invade reticulocytes and young and old RBCs. ***P. malariae has a tendency to invade mature and older RBCs.***

1. **Trophozoite:** It is the first stage of the parasite in the red cell. In the erythrocyte, the merozoite loses its internal organelles and appears as a rounded body having a vacuole in the center with the cytoplasm pushed to the periphery and the nucleus (single chromatin mass) at one pole. These young parasites are, therefore, called the ***ring forms*** or early *trophozoites.* **First immature trophozoites (ring forms) are formed followed by mature trophozoites.**
   - **Ring (early trophozoite) form: Early trophozoite form** is called as ring form (**Fig. 83**). The **ring form,** as the name implies, refers to a ring-like appearance of the malarial parasite following invasion into a previously healthy RBC. When stained with Giemsa or Leishman's stain, the typical ring consists of a peripheral blue cytoplasmic circle (forming thin rim or ring) connected with or to, depending on the species, a red chromatin dot (mass), also referred as a nucleus (nucleal mass). The space inside the ring is known as central vacuole (unstained). **Ring forms are the first asexual form that can be demonstrated in the peripheral blood.** Ring form occupies one-third of RBC (ring form measures 2.5–3 µm in diameter; normal size of RBC is 7.2 µm), except in *P. falciparum* (ring form measures 1.25–1.5 µm in diameter*),* where it occupies one-sixth of RBC. *Plasmodium* feeds on hemoglobin of the erythrocyte. It does not metabolize hemoglobin completely. The undigested product of hemoglobin metabolism such as hematin, excess protein and iron porphyrin combine and leaves behind hematin-globin pigment. This is called as **malarial pigment (hemozoin pigment)**. The appearance of malarial pigment varies. Mostly it is brown black and numerous (except in *P. vivax* it is yellowish-brown and in *P. falciparum*, it is few in number). The malaria pigment released when the parasitized cells rupture. This is phagocytosed by the reticuloendothelial cells. Such pigment-laden cells in the internal organs provide histological evidence of previous malaria infection. Appearance of malaria pigments in different species of plasmodia is presented in **Table 33**.
   - **Late (growing/developing) trophozoite:** As the ring form develops, it **enlarges in size and become more irregular in shape and shows *ameboid motility*** (movement). This is called late trophozoite or ameboid form. Generally during this stage, the amount of RBC space invaded is significantly more than that of the ring form, because the active growth of the parasite.
2. **Schizont:** It is the next stage and **represents a full-grown trophozoite**. When late trophozoites reach a certain stage of development, it becomes compact, vacuoles disappear, pigments scatter throughout cytoplasm and nucleus becomes larger and lies at the periphery. Its nucleus starts dividing by mitosis (multiple nuclear divisions) followed by a division of cytoplasm. This form is called **schizont** and can be divided into immature and mature schizont. It shows multiple chromatin masses, each of which develops into a merozoite. Mature schizont (schizogony or merogony) contains 6–30 daughter merozoites arranged in the form of rosette. The mature schizont bursts releasing the merozoites into the circulation.
3. **Merozoites:** Lysis of the red cell containing merozoites occurs and the new merozoites infect additional naïve

Table 33: Appearance of malaria pigments in different species.

Plasmodia species	*Appearance of malarial pigment*
P. vivax	Numerous fine golden-brown dust-like particles
P. falciparum	Few 1–3 solid blocks of black pigment
P. malariae	Numerous coarse dark-brown particles
P. ovale	Numerous blackish-brown particles

(fresh) red cells. Merozoites attach to the erythrocytes by their apex. This initiates another cycle of erythrocytic parasitism and this cycle is repeated many times. This cycle of *erythrocytic schizogony* or ***merogony*** is repeated sequentially, leading to progressive increase in the parasitemia, till it is arrested by the development of host immune response. The characteristic clinical features of malaria such as paroxysmal fever, chills, and rigors develop during the release of these merozoites into the blood. The release of merozoites into the circulation of the host induces the host cells to produce cytokines such as tumor necrosis factor (TNF) that cause fever. The periodicity of such paroxysms (every 48–72 hours) of fever, chills and rigors varies with the species of the malarial parasite. Ruptured RBCs release the daughter merozoites, malarial pigments and toxins into the circulation. This is responsible for malarial paroxysm of fever at the end of each erythrocytic cycle. The interval between the entry of sporozoites into the human host and the earliest manifestation of clinical illness is the ***incubation period*** (refer **Table 32**).

Sexual forms (gametogony) (7 in Fig. 83): Female *Anopheles* mosquito represents definitive host, in which sexual forms takes place. It is to be noted that the sexual forms of the parasite ***(gametocytes)*** originate in human RBCs. Maturation and fertilization of sexual forms occur in the mosquito. This gives rise to a large number of **sporozoites** (from *sporos: seed).* Hence, this phase of sexual multiplication is called ***sporogony.*** Thus, there is an alternation of hosts as the asexual phase takes place in humans followed by sexual phase in mosquito.

Most malarial parasites within the red cells develop into merozoites. However, some parasites after entering into RBCs, under specific conditions instead of developing into trophozoites transform into sexual forms called gametocytes.

- **Site of gametocyte development:** The gametocytic development occurs in the blood vessels of organs such as spleen and bone marrow. Only the mature gametocytes appear in the peripheral blood.
- **Appearance:** The gametocytes are round in shape (except in *P. falciparum* in which they are crescent or banana shaped).
- **Types of gametocytes:** They are of two types namely: (1) **male gametocyte (or microgametocyte) and (2) female gametocyte (or macrogametocyte)**. Microgametocytes are smaller in size, lesser in number, their cytoplasm stains pale blue, and nucleus is larger, stains red and diffuse. In contrast, macrogametocytes are larger, numerous, their cytoplasm stains deep blue, nucleus is small, red and compact.
- **Significance:** Gametocytes neither cause any clinical illness nor they divide. Patient harboring gametocytes act as **carriers** or **reservoirs of infection**. They play an important role in the transmission of malarial disease. These gametocytes infect the mosquito when mosquito bites the infected human and takes its blood meal. Thus, completes the parasite's life cycle. It is to be noted that the parasitemia caused by ***P. vivax*** is suppressed if there is concurrent infection by ***P. falciparum.*** **Malaria** is **more severe when caused by *P. falciparum* than the other *Plasmodium* species.**

Latent stage (hepatic): After the blood infection is established, the initial tissue phase (pre-erythrocytic phase) disappears completely in *P. falciparum* whereas it persists in *P. vivax* and *P. ovale*. This resting phase of parasite is known as hypnozoite. This is capable of developing into merozoites. This is responsible for relapse in *P. vivax* and *P. ovale.*

Summary of phases of development of plasmodia in human (intermediate) host is presented in **Box 16.**

Mosquito cycle (C in Fig. 83)

The sexual cycle of malarial parasites first begins in the human host by forming gametocytes.

Ingestion of parasite by *Anopheles* mosquito: A female *Anopheles* mosquito (definitive host) during its blood meal from (**8 in Fig. 83**) an infected patient **ingests** parasitized erythrocytes containing both **sexual and asexual forms** of parasite. The asexual forms of malaria parasite get digested, and **only the mature sexual forms (gametocytes) that are capable of development** (hence considered as infective form of the parasite to mosquito). Probably in order to infect a mosquito, a human carrier must contain at least 12 gametocytes mm^3 of blood and also the number of female gametocytes should be more than the number of male gametocytes.

Development of gametocytes in the *Anopheles* mosquito: The gametocytes are set free in the midgut (stomach) of mosquito and undergo further development.

- **Maturation of male gametocyte:** Nucleus and cytoplasm of the male gametocytes divides to produce four to eight flagellated actively motile bodies called **microgametes**. Microgametes protrude out as long, actively motile, thread-like (whip-like) filaments, which move out for some time and then, break free. As this process of development can be observed outside in a moist preparation of blood, it is called **exflagellation** (**9 in Fig. 83; Fig. 84**). The exflagellation is complete in 15 minutes for *P. vivax* and P. *ovale* and 15–30 minutes for *P. falciparum.*

Box 16: Summary of phases of development of plasmodia in human (intermediate) host.

- **In the liver (tissue phase):** Pigment granules absent in this phase
    - **Pre-erythrocytic (primary exoerythrocytic) schizogony:** Neither any clinical features nor any pathological damage. Liberates merozoites into the circulation following rupture of infected liver cells
    - **Hypnozoite stage** (dormant *Plasmodium*-infected liver cells)**:** Responsible for relapse
- **Erythrocytic phase (inside the red blood cells):** Pigment granules present in this phase
    - **Erythrocytic schizogony:** Produces paroxysm symptoms of malaria
        - **Trophozoites:** Ring forms (early trophozoites) and late trophozoites
        - **Schizont**
        - **Merozoite**
    - **Gametogony:** If taken up by mosquito the life cycle gets completed
        - **Male gametocytes**
        - **Female gametocytes**

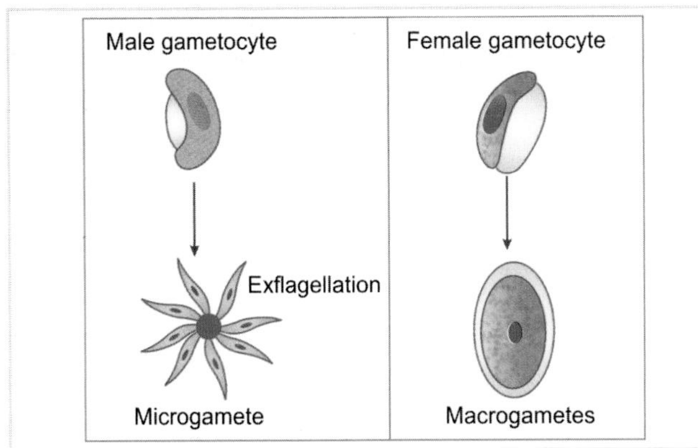

FIG. 84: Schematic diagram showing formation of microgamete and macrogamete.

- **Maturation of female gametocyte:** Female gametocytes do not divide and do not undergo exflagellation but it matures to form one **macrogamete or female gamete** (9 in **Fig. 83**).
- **Formation of zygote:** The **female gametocyte gets fertilized by one of the male microgametes by the process of chemotaxis**. This fusion forms nonmotile round **zygote** (**10 in Fig. 83**). Fertilization occurs in 0.5–2 hours after the blood meal by mosquito. Initially, the zygote is a motionless round body, gradually elongates and within 18–24 hours, transforms into vermicular motile elongated form with an apical complex anteriorly. This is called the ***ookinete (traveling vermicule)*** stage. Till this stage, the development takes place in the midgut of the mosquito.
- **Formation of oocyst in the stomach wall:** The ookinete penetrates the epithelial lining of the stomach wall of the mosquito and lies just beneath the basement membrane. It becomes rounded into a sphere with an elastic membrane. This stage is called the ***oocyst*** (**11 in Fig. 83**).
- **Production of sporozoites:** Oocyst is yet another multiplicatory phase. Oocysts undergo sporogony (meiosis) and produce thousands of spindle-shaped sporozoites. The mature oocyst measures about 500 µm in size bulges into body cavity of mosquito. When it ruptures, the sporozoites enter or released into the hemocele or body cavity.
- **Migration of sporozoites to salivary gland:** Sporozoites are distributed throughout the body but have a special affinity to salivary glands. Some **sporozoites** from body cavity **migrate or move to the salivary gland** (**12 in Fig. 83**). Mosquito is considered as infective when the sporozoites are present in salivary gland. Once infected, mosquito remains infective throughout its life. When these mosquitos feed on humans, the sporozoites are injected into skin capillaries to initiate human infection.

Extrinsic incubation period: The time taken for completion of sporogony in the mosquito is about **1–4 weeks** (extrinsic incubation period). This depends on the environmental temperature and the species.

Life Cycle of Plasmodium vivax

Plasmodium vivax has the widest geographical distribution and is found in the tropics, subtropics and temperate regions. It is responsible for about 80% of all malaria infections. It is the **most common species** of malaria parasite in Asia and America, but is much less common in Africa. It causes *benign tertian malaria* with frequent relapses. The sporozoites of *P. vivax* are narrow and slightly curved. The term vivax is derived from Latin (vivere = to live) and indicates the activity of movement.

Pre-erythrocytic schizogony

This phase occurs inside the liver cells (hepatocytes) and the parasite multiplies by asexual method (schizogony). The pre-erythrocytic schizogony consists of a single cycle and lasts for about 8 days. Fully developed pre-erythrocytic schizont is about 42 µm in diameter and the number of merozoites per schizont is 10,000–12,000. On entering the liver cells, the sporozoites initiate two types of infection. Some may enter into RBC in the circulation to begin the erythrocyte schizogony or re-enter into the liver cells to develop promptly into *exoerythrocytic schizonts.*

Erythrocytic schizogony

Asexual forms The **cycle of erythrocytic schizogony lasts for about 48 hours** and is mainly completed in the peripheral blood.

Type of RBC infected: After the release from liver cells, merozoites of *P. vivax* preferentially infect **reticulocytes and young erythrocytes** than mature erythrocytes.

Degree of parasitization: It is generally not heavy and not ***>2–5% of the red cells*** being affected. Each infected red cell usually has only one parasite.

Stages seen in peripheral blood: The parasite passes through three stages during erythrocytic schizogony namely: (1) trophozoite, (2) schizont, and (3) merozoite. **All stages of erythrocytic schizogony can be seen in peripheral smears.** The trophozoite is actively motile, as indicted by its name *vivax.*

Trophozoite: It consists of ring forms (early trophozoites) and late trophozoites.

- **Ring form (early trophozoite):** It is well-defined, with a prominent central nutrient vacuole. One side of the ring is thicker and the other side thin. Nucleus is situated on the thin side of the ring (signet ring appearance). The ring is about 2.5–3 µm in diameter, about a **one-third** of the size of an erythrocyte (normal size of RBC is 7.2 µm). The cytoplasm is blue and the nucleus red in stained films.
- **Late (growing) trophozoites:** The early trophozoite (ring form) shows very active ameboid movement and develops rapidly to the ameboid form and becomes late trophozoites. The trophozoites constantly put forth pseudopodia inside the infected RBC, giving rise to diverse forms of trophozoites. The infected erythrocytes are enlarged. The late trophozoites enlarge to become double its original size and become irregular in shape (distortion of the shape). These late trophozoites lose their red color, become pale and almost colorless and present a washed out appearance. After a period of growth, the portion of the cytoplasm of RBCs unoccupied by trophozoites shows dotted or stippled appearance known as ***Schuffner's*** (name of the discoverer) ***dots***. These are malarial pigments that appear as yellowish brown pigment or pinkish to red granules on in the cytoplasm of trophozoites.

Schizont: It appears after about 36–40 hours and represents the fully grown trophozoite.

- **Early (immature) schizont:** It has following characteristics.
    - **Shape:** As the late trophozoite grows, it becomes rounded in shape and loses all ameboid activities of trophozoite.
    - **Size:** Schizont becomes larger in size and occupies almost the whole of the infected enlarged RBC. It measures 9–10 µm in diameter.
    - **Nucleus:** The nucleus is larger and lies at the periphery.
    - **Vacuoles and granules:** The cytoplasmic vacuoles present in the trophozoite disappear and pigment granules are still scattered throughout the cytoplasm.
- **Intermediate schizont:** The schizont matures in the next 6–8 hours and becomes larger. Nuclear division takes place and gets completed. Depending on the stage of maturity, schizonts can be classified as immature schizont (nucleus is not divided) and mature schizont (in which nucleus is divided).
- **Mature schizont:** With further maturation 12–24 (average of 16) merozoites per schizont are produced. The red cell, which now measures about 10 µm in diameter is heavily stippled and often distorted. Each merozoite has a central nucleus and surrounding cytoplasm. The pigment granules aggregate into a few dark brown collections at the center. The merozoites area arranged around central pigment granules in the form of **rosette** (usually in two rows). This gives rise to mulberry-like (small purple berries) appearance to the schizont. Erythrocytic schizogony takes approximately 48 hours. When the maturation of **schizont** is completed, infected red cells are not able to hold the parasite and RBC bursts. This liberates the merozoites as well pigment present within the RBC. This produces the malaria paroxysm. The pigment is phagocytosed by reticuloendothelial cells.

Merozoites: Merozoites are oval in shape and consists of a central nucleus and surrounded by cytoplasm. It measures about 1.5–1.75 µm in length and 0.5 µm in breadth. It does not contain pigment. The free merozoites liberated from rupture of infected RBCs attack new RBCs and continue with erythrocytic schizogony. This cycle is repeated every 48 hours.

Sexual forms

Some schizonts instead of undergoing schizogony, they become modified biologically and differentiate into sexual forms. Merozoites present in a single schizont will differentiate either all males (microgametocytes) or all females (macrogametocytes). Changes in the infected red cells such as increase in size, pallor and the ***Schuffner's dots*** are also observed during the development of gametocyte. Both male and female gametocytes are large, nearly filling the enlarged red cell. The differences between male and female gametocytes of *P. vivax* are presented in **Table 34**. The gametocytes appear in the peripheral blood from the first day of fever (i.e., 16 days after inoculation of sporozoites by mosquito). This is equal to 4–5 days after initial appearance of asexual forms of the parasite (namely—trophozoite, schizont and merozoite). If these gametocytes are not taken up by the mosquito, they do not live for more than a week in the infected human host.

Table 34: Differences between male and female gametocytes of *Plasmodium vivax*.

Features	*Male gametocytes (microgametocyte)*	*Female gametocytes (macrogametocyte)*
Size	9–10 µm in length	10–12 µm in length
Shape	Round	Round
Color of the cytoplasm	Pale-staining cytoplasm staining light blue	Dense cytoplasm staining deep blue
Nucleus	Large, diffuse and lies laterally	Small, compact and lies peripherally

Various stages and morphological appearances of *P. vivax* infection are depicted in **Figure 85.**

Latent stage (hepatic): The latent hepatic stage is maintained throughout the course independent of erythrocytic schizogony. It may be there for several years and is responsible for relapses.

Life Cycle of Plasmodium falciparum

The name *falciparum* comes from the characteristic sickle shape of the gametocytes of this species *(falx: sickle, parere: to bring forth)*. *P. falciparum* is the highly pathogenic of all the plasmodia and hence, its infection is named as malignant tertian or pernicious malaria. It is associated with high rate of complications and unless treated, it is often fatal. This is responsible for almost all the deaths caused by malaria.

Pre-erythrocytic schizogony

The sporozoites are sickle-shaped. The tissue phase consists of only a single cycle of pre-erythrocytic schizogony and lasts for 6 days. **No hypnozoites occur.** The mature liver schizont releases about 30,000–400,000 merozoites into the blood on the 7th day of infection.

Erythrocytic schizogony

The parasite attack both **reticulocytes and erythrocytes (both young and mature)** and so the population of red cells affected is very large. Infected erythrocytes show a brassy coloration. The **cycle of erythrocytic schizogony is completed in 36–48 hours** and the periodicity of febrile paroxysms is 36–48 hours.

Trophozoite

- ***Ring form:*** The early ring form in the erythrocyte is very **delicate** and tiny and measures only a **one-sixth diameter of the red cell**. Rings are often seen attached along the margin or the edge of the red cell, the nucleus and a small part of the cytoplasm remains almost outside giving the characteristics so-called *form*, **"applique" or "accole"** (literally meaning joined or touching at the neck). Binucleate rings (double chromatin) are common resembling ***stereo headphones*** **(nucleus close together)** in appearance or nucleus situated at the opposite pole. Several rings may be seen within a single erythrocyte. In course of time, the rings become larger, about one-third of the size of the red cell and may have 1 or 2 grains of pigment in its cytoplasm.
- ***Late trophozoite, early and mature schizonts:*** Schizogony occurs only inside the capillaries of organs such spleen,

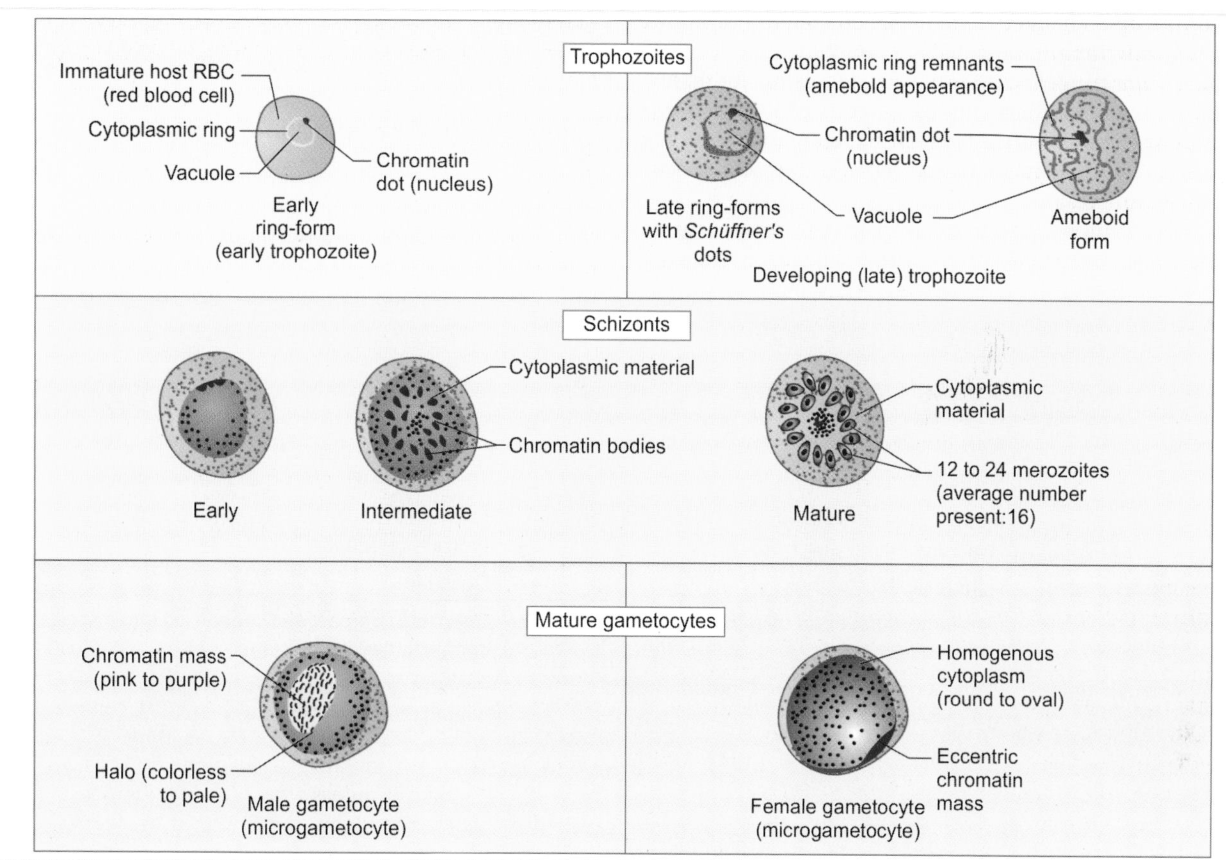

FIG. 85: Various stages and morphological appearances (diagrammatic) of *Plasmodium vivax* infection.

liver and bone marrow. Hence, in the peripheral blood only ring forms are seen. The subsequent **stages of the asexual cycle namely late trophozoite, early and mature schizonts are not ordinarily seen in peripheral blood, except in very severe or pernicious malaria**. The presence of *P. falciparum* schizonts in peripheral smears indicates a poor prognosis. In **very severe infections**, the rate of **parasitized cells may even be up to 50%**.

- As the late trophozoite grows, the nucleus divides into several masses ranging from 8 to 32 in number. The cytoplasm also divides into same numbers as nuclear division. They form many segments arranged around the central mass of pigment. The mature schizont is smaller than in any other measure about 4.5–5 µm in diameter and occupy about two-thirds of the diameter of infected RBC. In *P. falciparum,* erythrocytic schizogony always takes place inside the capillaries and vascular beds of internal organs. Therefore, in *P. falciparum* infections, schizonts and merozoites are usually not seen in the peripheral blood.
- The mature schizont species and has 8–24 (usually 16) merozoites. Very high intensity of parasitization is seen in *falciparum* malaria. The infected erythrocytes are of normal size. No Schüffner's dots seen. Instead they show a few (6–12) coarse brick-red dots which are called **maurer's clefts**. They stain brick red with Leishman stain. The pigment granules formed by the trophozoites are dark-brown or black in color and collect as a single mass. Some red cells show **basophilic stippling.**
- As soon as the pigment appears in the cytoplasm of trophozoites, the size of the ring increases to about 4 µm in diameter. These trophozoites come out of capillaries and enter the internal organs. In the organs, the vacuole of trophozoites disappears and trophozoites assume a compact solid appearance containing a single nucleus with pigment granules collected into a single dark brown or black mass.

Gametogony It begins after several generations of schizogony. The gametocytes appear in the peripheral blood about 10 days after the appearance of asexual ring forms of parasites. Gametogony occurs inside the capillaries of bone marrow and spleen. The early gametocytes seldom appear in peripheral circulation. If these gametocytes are not taken up by the mosquito, they persist in the peripheral blood of the infected host for a longer time (30–60 days or even more).

- The mature gametocytes, which are seen in peripheral smears appear as curved oblong structures, described as ***crescentic, sickle, sausage,*** **or** ***banana-shaped (Fig 83).*** They are usually referred to as *crescents*. As the gametocytes mature, the contents of infected RBC are gradually utilized by the mature gametocyte. The mature gametocyte is longer than the diameter of the red cell (about 1½ times that of RBC harboring it). Hence, RBC is stretched so much that its recognition is difficult and so produces gross distortion and sometimes even apparent disappearance of the infected red cell. The remaining RBC contents forms only a thin sheath (rim) on the concave side of the gametocyte projecting outward in the form of an arched rim. The differences between male and female gametocytes of *P. falciparum* are presented in **Table 35**.

- *Falciparum* crescents can survive in circulation for up to 60 days. This is much longer than in other species. Gametocytes are most numerous in the blood of young children (9 months to 2 years old). They, therefore, serve as the most effective source of infection to mosquitoes.

Various stages and morphological appearances (diagrammatic) of *P. falciparum* infection are depicted in **Figure 86**.

Latent stage (hepatic): Secondary exoerythrocytic (hepatic) stage is absent and there are usually no relapses. Recurrences may occur.

Pathogenesis of *Plasmodium falciparum*

Q. Write short essay on pathogenesis of falciparum malaria.

Plasmodium falciparum infestation produces **malignant malaria**. It is much more aggressive disease than the infestation by other plasmodia. Several features of *P.*

Table 35: Differences between male and female gametocytes of *Plasmodium falciparum*.

Features	*Male gametocytes (microgametocyte)*	*Female gametocytes (macrogametocyte)*
Size	8–10 µm in length and 2–3 µm in width	10–12 µm in length and 2–3 µm in width
Shape	Broader, shorter with blunt rounded ends (sausage-shaped or kidney-shaped)	Longer, narrower, (thinner) with pointed ends (more typically crescentic)
Color of the cytoplasm	Light (pale) blue or pink	Deep blue
Nucleus	Pink, large, diffuse and scattered in fine granules over a wide area	Deep red, compact and condensed into a small compact mass at the center
Distribution of pigment	Pigment granules scattered throughout the cytoplasm	Pigment granules are closely aggregated like a wreath around the nucleus

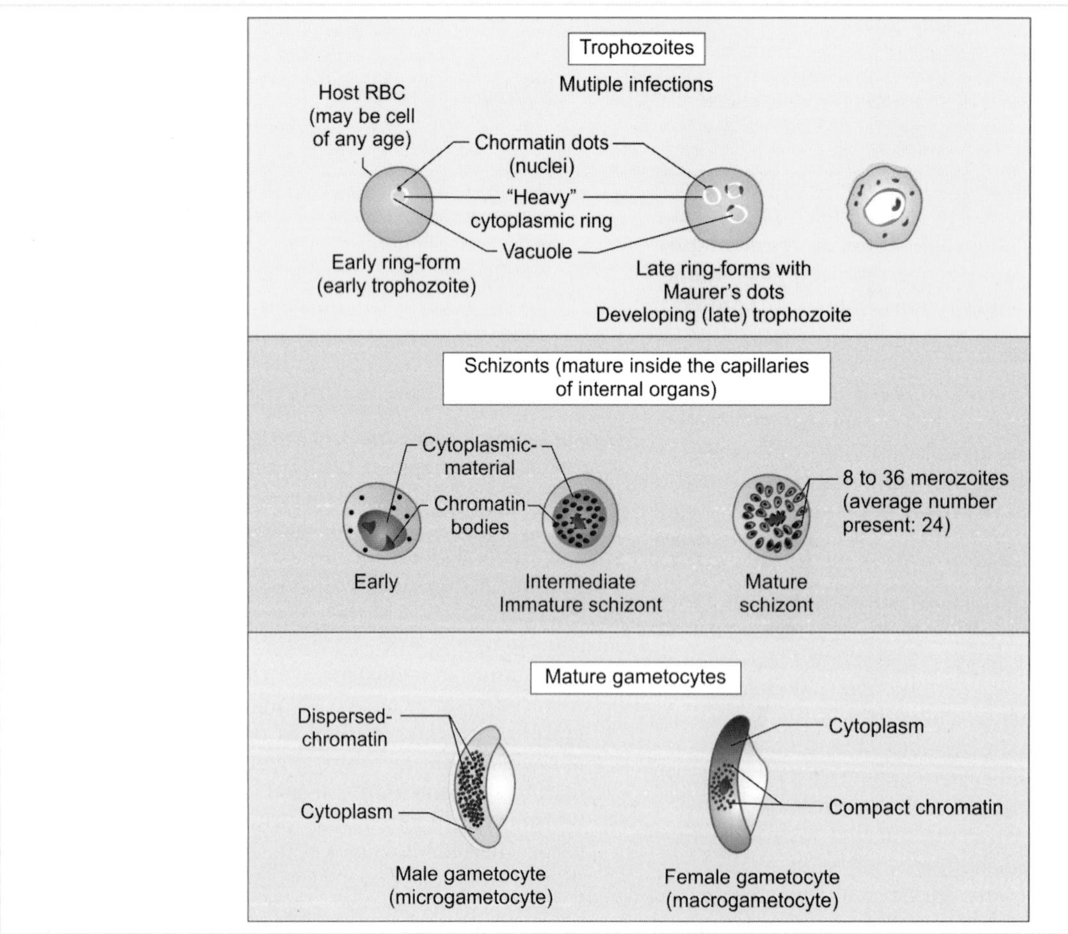

(RBC: red blood cell)

FIG. 86: Various stages and morphological appearances (diagrammatic) of *Plasmodium falciparum* infection.

falciparum are responsible for its greater pathogenicity. These are as follows:

- **Can infect red cells of any age:** *P. falciparum* is capable of infecting RBCs of any age causing marked parasitemia and anemia. In contrast other species of plasmodia infect only subpopulations of erythrocytes (e.g., only young or old red cells which constitute a smaller fraction of the red cell pool) leading to lower-level parasitemias and more modest anemias.
- **Causes sequestration of red cells:** The parasite-encoded proteins, found on the surface of infected erythrocytes, bind glycoproteins on the endothelium of capillaries. Thus, *P. falciparum* causes infected red cells to clump together (rosette) and to stick to endothelial cells lining small blood vessels. This process, called **sequestration (erythrocyte sequestration)**. Sequestration occurs in microvasculature ofvariousorgans.Thisblockstheblood flowandresultsinvery few circulating infected erythrocytes in which parasites are undergoing merogony. On the surface of infected red cells harboring late stage schizonts of *P. falciparum*, adhesive polypeptides, including *P. falciparum* erythrocyte membrane protein 1 (PfEMP1), associate and form knobs (**Fig. 87**) or **knob-like** deformities. The adhesive protein PfEMP1 (especially secreted by late stage schizonts of *P. falciparum*) on the surface of RBCs makes these infected RBCs to become sticky. **PfEMP-1** promotes aggregation of infected RBCs to other noninfected RBCs and also to the receptors of capillary endothelial cells. **PfEMP-1** causes adhesion of infected red cells to ligands on endothelial cells of small blood vessels. These ligands including CD36, thrombospondin, VCAM-1, ICAM-1, and E-selectin. By obstruction or blocking the blood flow in the small blood vessels, red cell sequestration decreases tissue perfusion and leads to severe tissue ischemia. This is probably the most important factor responsible for the manifestations of the organism's virulence especially in cerebral malaria.

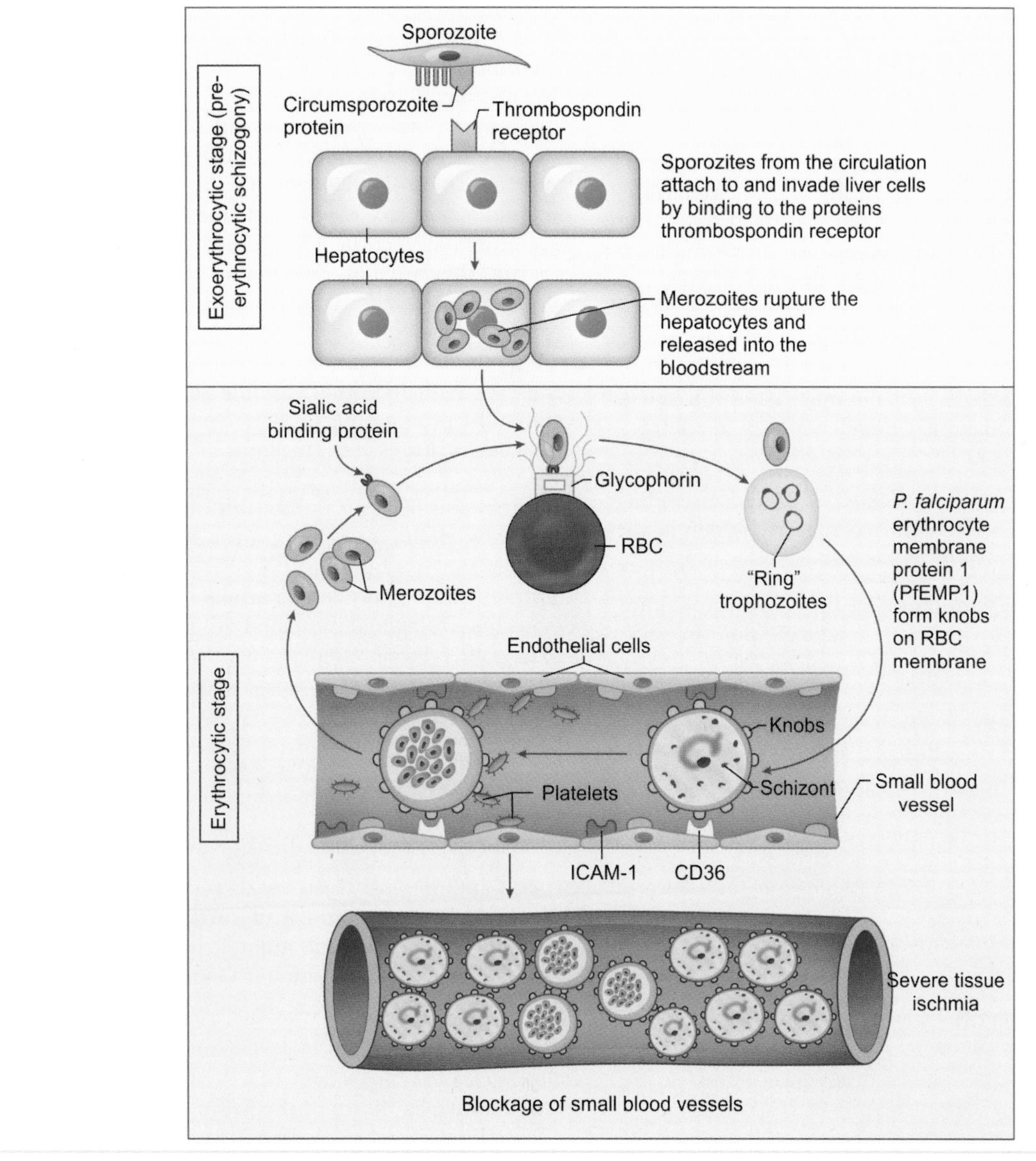

(ICAM-1: Intercellular adhesion molecule 1; RBC: red blood cell)

FIG. 87: Life cycle of *Plasmodium falciparum* shows both exoerythrocytic and erythrocytic stages in human intermediate host.

Cerebral malaria is the major cause of death in children with malaria. In cerebral malaria, these sequestrated RBCs cause **capillary plugging and obstruction** of cerebral microvasculature. This results in anoxia, ischemia, and hemorrhage in brain.

- **Induces cytokine production by host cells:** Other virulence factors of *P. falciparum* are histidine-rich protein II ***(HRP II)*** and glycosylphosphatidylinositol ***(GPI)***. In *P. falciparum* infection, GPI-linked proteins, (e.g., merozoite surface antigens) are released from infected red cells. They induce host cells to produce cytokines. These cytokines in turn increase fever, stimulate the production of reactive nitrogen species (causes tissue damage), and induce expression of endothelial receptors for PfEMP1 (thereby increasing sequestration).
- May be several parasites in a single infected red cell.
- No secondary exoerythrocytic (hepatic) stage.
- Unlike other plasmodia, *P. falciparum* is unable to form hypnozoites (dormant *Plasmodium*-infected liver cells) in the liver.

Cerebral malaria

Q. Write short essay on pathogenesis and pathology of cerebral malaria.

The most serious and fatal type of malaria is malignant tertian malaria caused by *P. falciparum.* If *falciparum* malaria is not treated timely or adequately, severe life-threatening complications may occur. In severe *falciparum* malaria, **parasitic load may be very high** and it **may affect >5% red cells.** The term pernicious malaria is also applied to cerebral malaria, blackwater fever, algid malaria, and septicemic malaria. The most serious complication of *P. falciparum* infection is cerebral malaria. It is the **most common cause of death** in malignant malaria. Complications of *falciparum* malaria are listed in **Box 17**.

Definition: Cerebral malaria is defined as **diffuse encephalopathy in a patient with falciparum malaria** which is not attributable to any other cause.

Symptoms of cerebral malaria The initial symptoms are nonspecific. It presents with fever, headache, pain in back, anorexia and nausea.

Box 17: Complications of *falciparum* malaria.

- Cerebral malaria
- Algid malaria
- Septicemic malaria
- Blackwater fever
- Pulmonary edema
- Acute renal failure
- Hypoglycemia (<40 mg/dL)
- Severe anemia (Hb <5 g/dL, PCV <1.5%)
- Hyperpyrexia
- Metabolic acidosis and shock
- Bleeding disturbances
- Hyperparasitemia

(Hb: hemoglobin; PCV: packed cell volume)

Anemia: The patient may be anemic and mildly jaundiced.

Hepatosplenomegaly: Liver and spleen are enlarged and non-tender.

Thrombocytopenia is common.

Neurological: After 4–5 days of high fever, cerebral malaria is manifested by features of **diffuse symmetric encephalopathy** such as headache, confusion, increased muscle tone, seizures, paralysis, slowly lapsing to coma.

- **Convulsions:** Usually generalized and often repeated. They occur in both children (50%) and adults (10%) but are more common in children.
- Most common neurological signs in adults are those of a symmetrical upper motor neuron lesion. The abdominal reflexes and cremasteric reflexes are absent.
- Mild neck stiffness may be seen, however, neck rigidity and photophobia and signs of raised intracranial tension are absent.
- Motor abnormalities such as decerebrate rigidity, decorticate rigidity and opisthotonus occur.
- Fixed jaw closure and tooth grinding (bruxism) are common.
- Neuropsychiatric manifestations, cerebellar signs, extrapyramidal syndromes and multiple cranial nerve involvement are common in Indian patients.
- **Residual neurological sequelae:** They develop in about 5% of adults and 10% of children. These include hemiplegia, cerebral palsy, cortical blindness, deafness aphasia, and ataxia. They are more frequent in patients with prolonged deep coma, repeated convulsions, those with hypoglycemia and severe anemia.

Hypoglycemia is common in patients following quinine therapy or with hyperparasitemia. In 10% of cases renal dysfunction progressing to acute renal failure may occur. Retinal hemorrhages occur in about 15% of cases, exudates are rare.

Other complications include **metabolic acidosis,** pulmonary edema and shock. Even with treatment, death occurs in 15% of children and 20% of adults who develop cerebral malaria. This occurs particularly when nonimmune persons have remained untreated or inadequately treated for 7–10 days after development of the primary fever.

For pathogenesis of cerebral malaria refer above pages 742–744 and **Fig. 87**.

MORPHOLOGY OF BRAIN

Q. Write short essay on Dürck granuloma.

Gross: Cerebral blood vessels and vessels in the pia matter show marked congestion. Cut surface shows slate-gray coloration of the cortex and multiple punctate hemorrhages in the subcortical white matter (**Fig. 88**). Areas of small infarcts may be seen in the brain substance.

Microscopy: In cerebral malaria caused by *P. falciparum*, following features are seen:

- The **entire capillary of the brain** (cerebral capillaries) are **dilatated and congested.** They are **plugged and filled with parasitized red cells**. They are more prominent in the white matter and evenly and uniformly distributed.

Continued

Continued

All the stages of erythrocytic cycle may occur in the capillaries of brain. Though trophozoites and schizonts are most common, gametocytes may also be seen (**Figs. 89A and B**).
- Around the vessels (**perivascular region**) show **hemorrhages having the appearance of "ring hemorrhages"**. They occur around the plugged vessels. RBCs of the hemorrhage are not parasitized.
- Scattered areas may show softening as a result of degeneration of nerve tissue.
- Later the softened areas may be invaded by glial cells and form so called local "malarial granulomas" of Dürck. This is due to reparative reaction to a local damage. A fully developed "granuloma" consists of a collection of proliferated glial cells radially arranged around the occluded blood vessel. When the lesion has advanced to the stage of "granuloma," some permanent damage may develop.

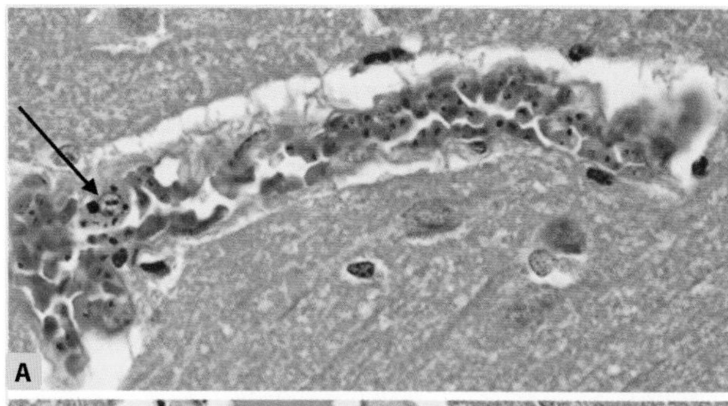

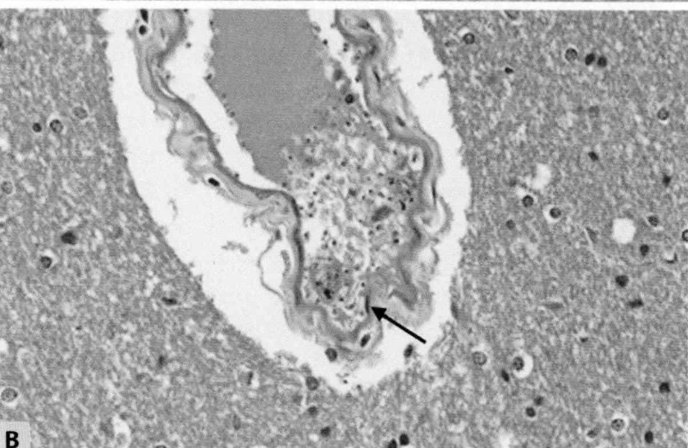

FIGS. 89A AND B: *Plasmodium falciparum*-infected red cells in the capillaries of brain in cerebral malaria marginating within a capillary in cerebral malaria. (A) The parasites appear as black dots in the red blood cells (arrow) when the tissue sections are stained with hematoxylin and eosin. (B) Cerebral blood vessel shows gametocyte also in the infected red blood cells (arrow)

Malarial hemoglobinuria (Blackwater fever)

- Malaria hemoglobinuria is uncommon, and is **usually associated with hyperparasitemia and/or severe disease**. It may or may not be accompanied by renal failure.
- Patients with glucose-6-phosphate dehydrogenase (G6PD) deficiency and other erythrocyte enzyme deficiencies may develop vascular hemolysis and hemoglobinuria when treated with oxidant drugs such as primaquine.
- **Blackwater fever** typically **occurs in nonimmune patients with chronic falciparum malaria, taking antimalarials** (especially quinine and primaquine) **irregularly**. It occurs **more commonly in patients with G6PD deficiency**. Patients with G6PD deficiency may develop this condition after taking oxidant drugs, even in the absence of malaria.
- The **hemolysis** can occur so rapidly that the hemoglobin may drop significantly within a few hours and it may recur periodically at intervals of hours or days.
- **Clinical manifestations**: Patient presents with headache, nausea, vomiting, and severe pain in the loins and prostration. Fever up to 39.4°C with a rigor is also seen. Urine is dark red to almost black due to hemoglobinuria **(black colored urine)**.
- **Pathogenesis**: It is probably due to massive intravascular hemolysis caused by antierythrocyte antibodies, leading to massive absorption of hemoglobin by the renal tubules **(hemoglobinuric nephrosis)**. Complications of blackwater fever include renal failure, acute liver failure, and circulatory collapse.

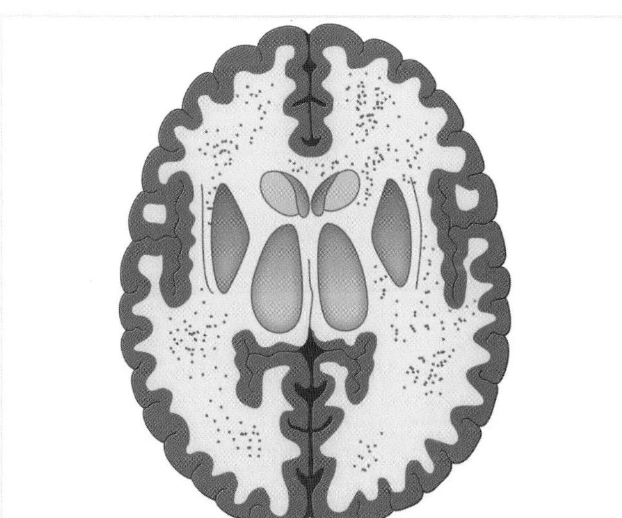

FIG. 88: Cut surface of brain in cerebral malaria shows slate-gray coloration of the cortex and multiple punctate hemorrhages in the subcortical white matter.

Circulatory collapse ("algid malaria")

Algid malaria or hypotension due to peripheral circulatory failure may develop suddenly in severe malaria or it may be the presenting feature in some cases of malaria, with low blood pressure, a cold, clammy, cyanotic skin, constricted peripheral veins, and rapid feeble pulse. There may be severe abdominal pain, vomiting, diarrhea and profound shock.

Septicemic malaria

It is characterized by high continuous fever with dissemination of the parasite to various organs, leading to multiorgan failure. Death occurs in 80% of the cases.

Life cycle of Plasmodium malariae

Plasmodium malariae was first discovered by Laveran in 1880 and he gave the name *malariae*. It causes ***quartan malaria,*** in which febrile paroxysms occur *every 4th day,* with *72 hours* interval between the bouts. The disease is generally mild, but is notorious for its long persistence in circulation in undetectable levels, for 50 years or more.

- **Slower development of parasite:** The development of *P. malariae* in man and mosquito is much slower than with other species. Chimpanzees may be naturally infected with *P. malariae* and may constitute a natural reservoir for quartan malaria.
- **Geographic distribution:** *P. malariae* occurs in tropical Africa, Sri Lanka, Myanmar and parts of India, but its distribution is patchy.
- The sporozoites are relatively *thick.*

Pre-erythrocytic schizogony

- Takes about *15 days,* much longer than in other species.
- Each schizont releases about 15,000 merozoites.
- *Hypnozoites do not occur.*
- The ***long latency*** of the infection is probably due to long time survival of few erythrocytic forms in some internal organs.

Erythrocytic schizogony

Plasmodium malariae preferentially infects **mature and older erythrocytes.** The degree of parasitization is *low.*

Trophozoites

- The ring forms resemble those of *P. vivax,* although thicker and more intensely stained. A characteristic feature is the late trophozoite often stretches right across the RBC and has a **broad band-like appearance**. These ***band forms*** are the **unique feature of *P. malariae*.** Coarse dark-brown to black granules appear in the cytoplasm when the trophozoites is 6–8 hours old. The infected RBC is not enlarged.
- Numerous large pigment granules are seen. The infected erythrocytes may be of the normal size or slightly smaller. Fine stippling, called ***Ziemann's stippling,*** *and* may be seen with special stains.

Schizonts

- The schizonts appear in about 50 hours and mature during the next 18 hours. The mature schizont has an average of eight merozoites, which usually present a *rosette* (daisey-head) appearance.
- The degree of parasitization is lowest in *P. malariae.*
- Erythrocytic schizogony takes *72 hours.*

Merozoite

- It measures 2–2.5 µm in diameter.

Gametogony

- The gametocytes develop in the internal organs and appear in the peripheral circulation when fully grown.
- Gametocytes are round and large nearly occupying the entire red cell.
- The male has pale blue cytoplasm with a large diffuse nucleus, while the female has deep blue cytoplasm and a small compact nucleus.

Various stages and morphological appearances (diagrammatic) of *P. malariae* infection are depicted in **Figure 90**.

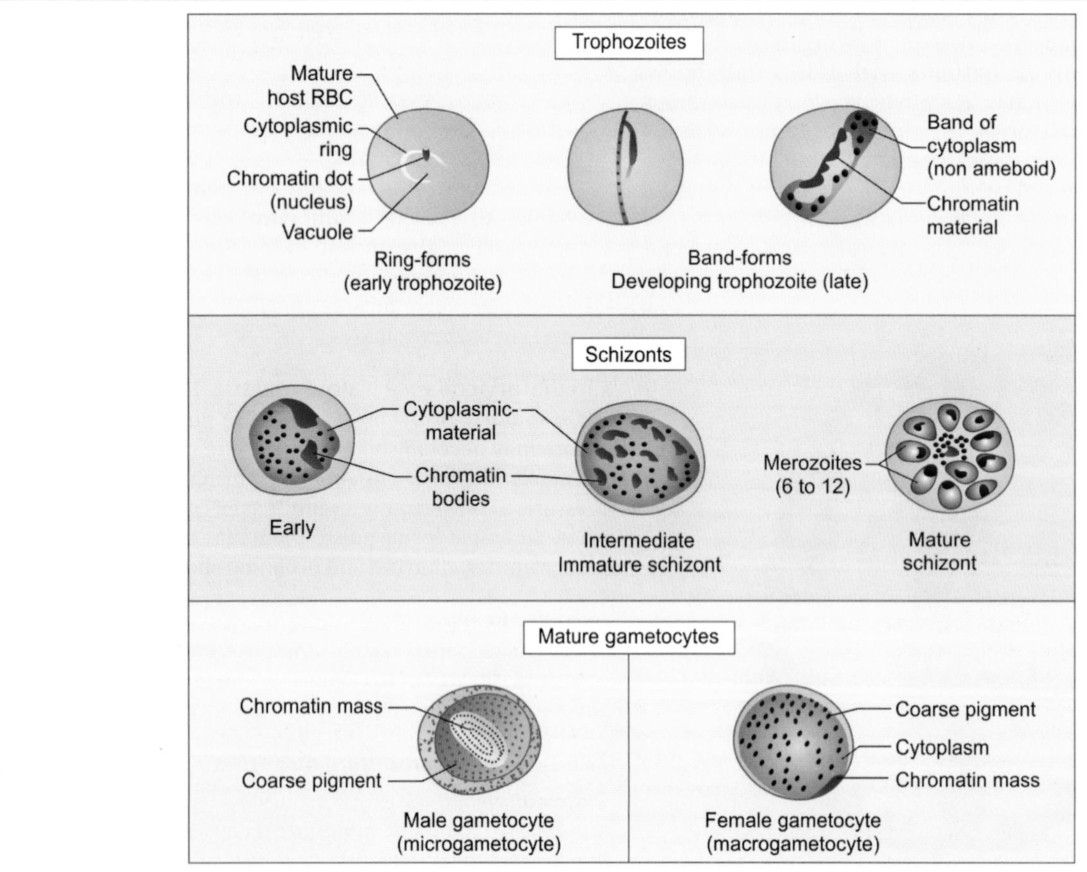

(RBC: red blood cell)

FIG. 90: Various stages and morphological appearances (diagrammatic) of *Plasmodium malariae* infection.

Plasmodium Ovale

The name of this parasite is derived from its shape and shape of the infected red cells, both appear oval. This parasite produces a tertian fever resembling *vivax* malaria, but with milder symptoms, prolonged latency and fewer relapses. It is the **rarest of all plasmodia** infecting humans and is seen mostly in tropical Africa, particularly along the West Coast.

Pre-erythrocytic schizogony

The pre-erythrocytic stage extends for 9 days. Hepatocytes containing schizonts usually have enlarged nuclei. The mature liver schizont releases about 15,000 merozoites. **Hypnozoites are present.**

Erythrocytic schizogony

Trophozoites

- Ring form resembles that of *P. malariae,* but there is no band-like appearance. The trophozoites resemble those in *vivax* malaria, but are usually more compact, with less ameboid appearance. Almost all infected RBCs show eosinophilic stippling. Infected RBC is slightly enlarged and oval with fimbriated edges (margins). This oval appearance of the infected erythrocyte is the reason for the name *ovale* given to this species.
- ***Schuffner's dots*** appear earlier and are more abundant and prominent than in *vivax* infection.

Schizonts

The schizonts resemble those of *P. malariae,* except that the pigment is *darker* and the erythrocyte is usually *oval,* with prominent Schuffner's dots.

Gametogony

Development of gametocytes is same as in other plasmodia.

Various stages and morphological appearances (diagrammatic) of *P. ovale* infection are depicted in **Figure 91**.

Plasmodium knowlesi (Quotidian Malaria)

- The infected RBC is not enlarged. The erythrocytic schizogony takes 24 hours.
- The ring stage of *P. knowlesi* resembles *P. falciparum.* Accole form, double chromatins and multiple infections are common in an infected RBC. The trophozoite stage resembles band form of *P. malariae.*
- The mature schizont has 10–16 merozoites. Pigment collects into 1 or more yellowish-black masses and eventually into a single mass in the mature schizont.
- Both male and female gametocytes occupy nearly the entire RBC.

Various stages and morphological appearances of *Plasmodium* (diagrammatic) are depicted in **Figure 92.**

Differences of erythrocytic phases of *P. vivax, P. falciparum, P. malariae,* and *P. ovale* are presented in **Table 36.**

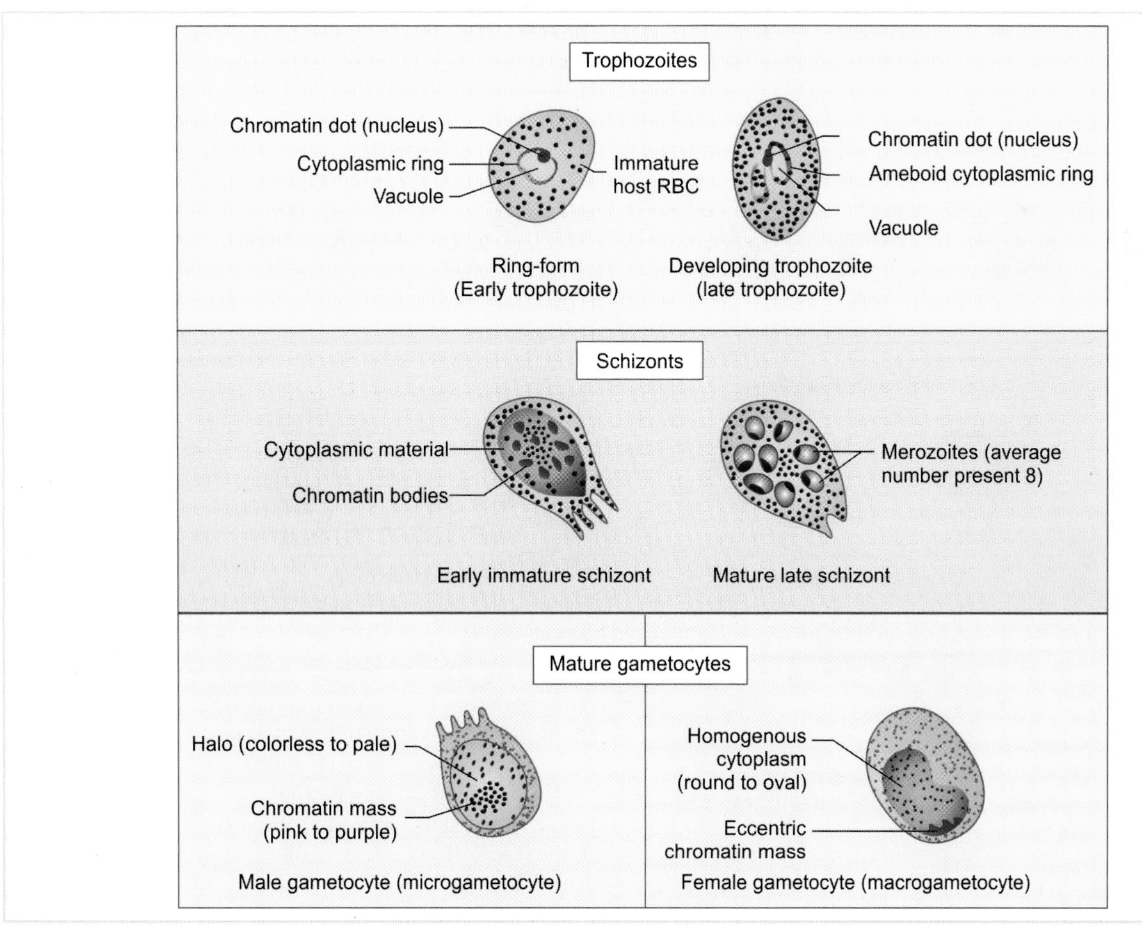

FIG. 91: Various stages and morphological appearances (diagrammatic) of *Plasmodium ovale* infection.

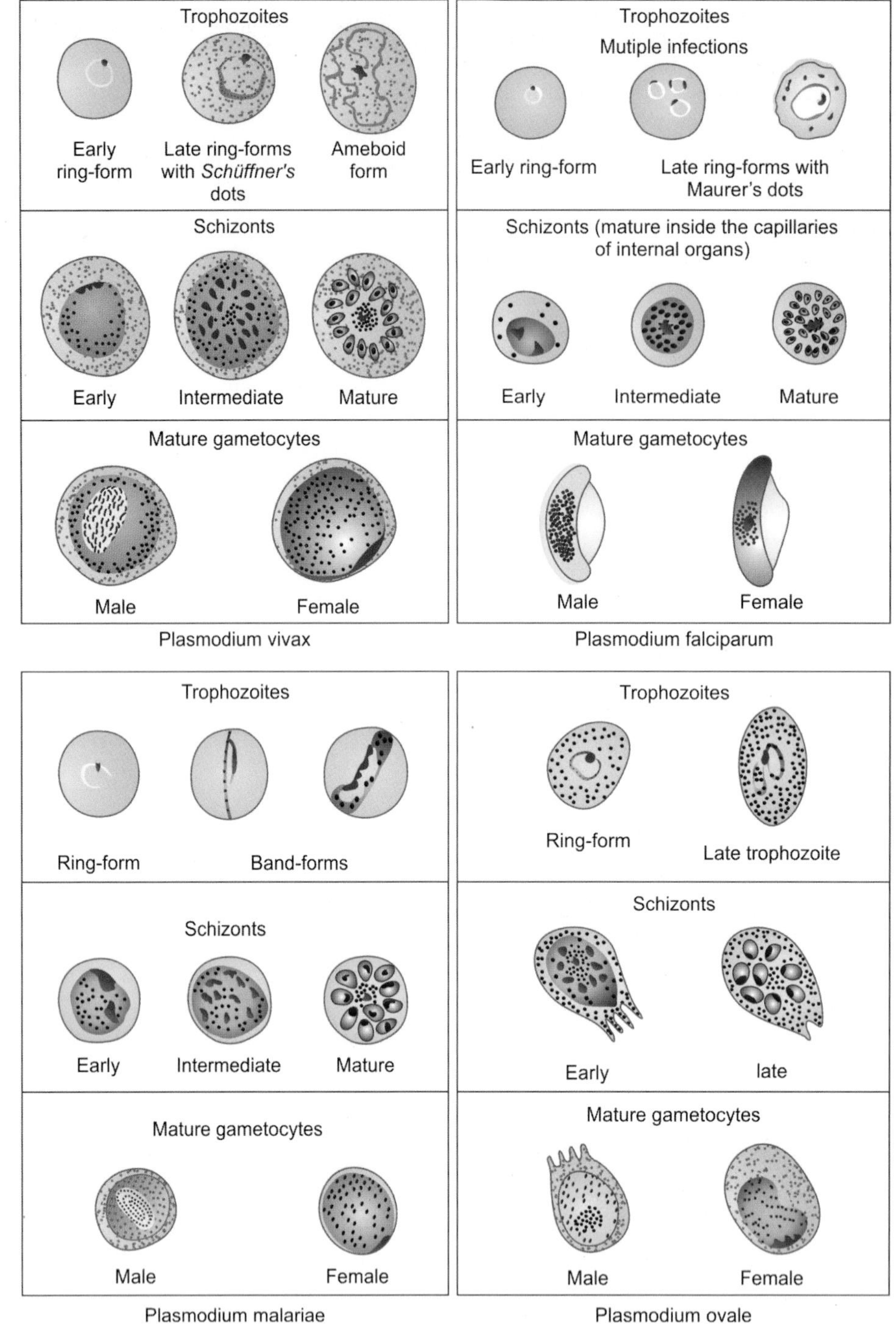

FIG. 92: Various stages and morphological appearances of *Plasmodium* (diagrammatic).

Mixed Infection

Different species of *Plasmodium* can infect the same mosquito. In endemic areas it is not uncommon to find mixed infections with ***two or more*** species of malaria parasites in the same individual.

- Mixed infection with *P. vivax* and *P. falciparum* is the most common combination with a tendency for one or the other to predominate.
- The clinical picture may be *atypical* with bouts of fever occurring ***daily.***
- Diagnosis may be made by demonstrating the characteristic parasitic forms in thin blood smears.

Clinical Features

In malaria the manifestation of the disease is due to local or systemic response of the host to parasite antigens. It is clinically present with periodic bouts of fever with chills and rigors. The febrile paroxysm follows the completion of erythrocytic schizogony when the mature schizont ruptures, releasing red cell fragments, merozoites, malaria pigments and other

Table 36: Differences of erythrocytic phases of *Plasmodium vivax, Plasmodium falciparum, Plasmodium malariae* and *Plasmodium ovale*.

Features	*P. vivax (tertian malaria)*	*P. falciparum (malignant tertian)*	*P. malariae (quartan malaria)*	*P. ovale (tertian malaria-rarest)*
Schizogony duration	48 hours	48 hours or less	72 hours	48 hours
Preference of type of red blood cells (RBCs)	Reticulocytes (young and immature RBCs)	Erythrocytes of any age	Older erythrocytes	Reticulocytes
Stages of parasites found in peripheral blood	Rings, trophozoites, schizonts, gametocytes	Only rings and gametocytes (crescents)	As in vivax	As in *vivax*
Ring (early trophozoite) forms				
Size (diameter)	2.5–3 µm. Delicate ring measuring one-third the size of RBC	Delicate and small, 1.25–1.5 µm	Resemble those of *P. vivax* but the cytoplasm is thicker	Resemble those in *P. vivax*, but are usually more compact
Appearance	One side of the cytoplasmic ring (opposite the nucleus) is thicker than the other	Fine and uniform cytoplasmic ring. Multiple rings may be seen within a single erythrocyte	Same as *P. vivax* although thicker and more intensely stained	Resembles that of *P. malariae*, but there is no band-like appearance
Nucleus	Nucleus is situated at the thinner part of the ring	Usually projects beyond the ring	Same as *P. vivax*	Same as *P. vivax*
Nature of nucleus	Single with no division	Nucleus is often divided into two parts which may be either remain close together or situated at opposite poles	Same as *P. vivax*	Same as *P. vivax*
Attachment of parasite to RBC and its position	No attachment to margin of RBC	Parasite usually attaches itself to the margin or edge of the infected RBC. Nucleus and a small portion of cytoplasm of parasite remains outside the infected RBC	Same as *P. vivax*	Same as *P. vivax*
Number of parasites infecting single RBC	Each red cell is invaded by single parasite and no more than 1 or 2 per red cell	Multiple infections of red cells. More than one parasite (from 2 to 6) invading single RBC	Same as *P. vivax*	Same as *P. vivax*
Late trophozoite				
Size of infected RBCs	Enlarged	Remains unaltered the infected erythrocytes are not enlarged	May be of the normal size or slightly smaller	Slightly enlarged, oval shape and fimbriated
Appearance	Large irregular, actively ameboid, prominent vacuole	Compact, seldom seen in blood smear	The trophozoites stretch across the diameter of the erythrocyte and seen as a band form	Many of them appear oval shape with fimbriated margins
Dots inside the cytoplasm of trophozoite	Schüffner's dots appear pink under Leishman stain	No Schüffner's dots but there are coarse dots which are Maurer's dots or clefts (6–12 in number). Stain brick red with Leishman stain	Fine stippling, called Ziemann's stippling may be seen with special stains	Schüffner's dots are present in the cytoplasm of the infected RBC
Schizont				
Size	9–10 µm	4.5–5 µm	6.5–7 µm	8.2 µm
Appearance	Regular, almost completely fills an enlarged red blood cell	Fills two-thirds of a red cell (red cell not enlarged)	Regular, almost fills an normal red blood cell	Fills ¾ of an slightly enlarged red blood cell
Number of merozoites inside mature schizont	12–24 (usually 18) merozoites per schizont in irregular grape-like cluster	About 8–24 (usually 16) merozoites in grape-like cluster	8–12 merozoites in daisy-head or rosette pattern	6–12 irregularly arranged
Duration of erythro-cytic schizogony	48 hours	36–48 hours	72 hours	48 hours

Continue

Continue

Features	***P. vivax (tertian malaria)***	***P. falciparum (malignant tertian)***	***P. malariae (quartan malaria)***	***P. ovale (tertian malaria-rarest)***
Malarial pigment	Yellowish-brown, fine granules	Dark-brown or blackish; one or two solid blocks	Dark-brown coarse granules	Dark yellowish-brown, coarser than *P. vivax*
Gametocyte				
Shape	Spherical or globular	Crescent or banana shaped	Round or oval	Oval
Size	Much larger than red cell filling almost the enlarged RBC	Larger than a red cell	Size of a red cell and occupy nearly the entire RBC	Size of a red cell and occupy nearly the entire RBC
RBC	Enlarged with Schüffner's dots	Hardly recognizable, Maurer's clefts sometimes basophilic stippling	Not enlarged, occasionally Ziemann's stippling	Slightly enlarged, oval fimbriated fimbriated, prominent with Schuffner's dots

parasitic debris. It is usually associated with severe headache, nausea, and vomiting.

Liver is enlarged and spleen is soft, moderately enlarged in acute infection. In chronic infection, the spleen undergoes fibrosis. Anemia is caused by rupture of infected RBCs and also due to complement-mediated, autoimmune hemolysis and hypersplenism. A decreased erythropoiesis in the bone marrow may also contribute to anemia.

Immunology of Malaria

Q. Write short essay on immunology of malaria.

Q. Write short essay on host resistance mechanism in malaria.

Immunity in malaria (host resistance to *Plasmodium*) can be two types: (1) **innate** (intrinsic) immunity and (2) **acquired** immunity.

Innate immunity

It is the inherent, non-immune, intrinsic mechanism of host resistance against malarial parasite. Innate immunity is due to inherited alterations that reduce the susceptibility of red cells to productive *Plasmodium* infections. **Several types of mutations involving red cells are highly prevalent in certain parts of the world where malaria is endemic and they are not observed in other parts of the world.** Most of these mutations are pathogenic in homozygous form. This suggests that they are maintained in populations due to a selective advantage for heterozygous carriers against malaria.

- **Duffy negative RBCs:** Mutations causing red cell membrane defects—absence of DARC (Duffy surface blood group), band 3, and spectrin protects against malaria. Attachment and invasion of red cells by merozoites to red blood cells requires the presence of specific glycoprotein receptors on the surface of erythrocyte. *P. vivax* enters red cells by binding to the Duffy blood group antigen (Fy^a or Fy^b). Individuals with Duffy negative blood group are protected from (refractory to infection by) *P. vivax infection.* This genetically determined blood group antigen is a specific receptor for *P. vivax* and *P. knowlesi.* Duffy antigen is absent in most of the West African population where *P. vivax* malaria is not prevalent.
- **Nature of hemoglobin:** RBCs containing hemoglobin F, C, or S impair growth of *P. falciparum* parasite.
  - **Hemoglobin E provides natural protection against *P. vivax.***
  - *P. falciparum* **cannot multiply properly within the sickled red cells containing HbS** (Point mutations in globin genes). Sickle cell anemia trait is very common in Africa, where *falciparum* malaria is hyperendemic and offers a survival advantage. Patients with hemoglobin S especially heterozygotes (sickle cell trait) are protected against the lethal complications of malaria.
  - **HbF** present in **neonates protects** them against all *Plasmodium* species.
  - Mutations leading to globin deficiencies such as α- and β-thalassemia and HbC disease (hemoglobinopathies) also provides protection against malaria.
- **Glucose-6-phosphate dehydrogenase deficiency:** Innate immunity to malaria has also been related to G6PD deficiency. G6PD deficiency is found in Mediterranean coast, Africa, Middle East and India. G6PD-deficient red cells are more resistant to infection by *P. falciparum.*
- **Human leukocyte antigen-B53:** Presence of human leukocyte antigen-B53 (HLA-B53) protects against cerebral malaria.
- **Nutritional status:** Patients with iron deficiency and severe malnutrition are relatively resistant to malaria.
- **Pregnancy:** *P. falciparum* infection is more severe in pregnancy, particularly in primigravida and may be enhanced by iron supplementation.
- **Splenectomy:** The spleen appears to play an important role in immunity against malaria. Splenectomy **increases the susceptibility of individual to malaria**.

Acquired immunity

Protective immunity and resistance against malaria may also be acquired following repeated or prolonged exposure to *Plasmodium* species This stimulates a partially protective immune response. Infection with malaria parasite induces specific immunity involving both humoral and cellular immunity.

Immunity in endemic regions: Individuals living in areas where *Plasmodium* is endemic often gain partial immune-mediated resistance to malaria. In highly endemic areas, it is likely that infected mosquitoes repeatedly bite almost everyone. The initial exposure to *Plasmodium* is likely to cause severe disease. In these regions, there is reduced clinical illness despite malarial infection but cannot eliminate parasites from the body. It can prevent superinfection, but is not powerful enough to defend against reinfection. Regular and repeated infection is required to prevent the onset of more serious and debilitating disease. This type of resistance in an infected host, which is associated with continued asymptomatic parasite infection despite parasitemia, is called ***premunition.*** This type of immunity disappears once the infection is eliminated. Most severe cases occur in young children, infected for the first time. Features of this immunity are: (1) it is not sterilizing, (2) it does not eradicate all parasites in an infected individual and (3) it is also of short duration. If an individual from a highly endemic area leaves that area for a year or two and then returns, that individual is once again vulnerable to serious disease. It is observed that the short-term and incomplete nature of immunity to malaria makes individuals living in highly endemic areas slightly protects against malarial infection better than those living in areas of sporadic transmission. The premunition in the individuals living in endemic area insures that if they survive infancy, they are unlikely to suffer from the worst complications of malaria.

Immune responses: The acquired immune responses are generated against each stage (including sporozoites, and intracellular liver and erythrocyte stages) in the *Plasmodium* life cycle. Immunity to malaria is limited partly because of its complex life cycle, during which each parasite stage expresses different antigens. Also these stage-specific antigens may change during successive waves of replication. It was found that the severity of disease is greatly reduced in individuals who are regularly exposed and this suggests that there is development of some protective immunity to *Plasmodium* infection. As in other immune responses, there are many humoral and cellular mechanisms involved. However, the precise role of these mechanisms is not yet completely resolved. Probably, the immunological memory is directed primarily at the merozoites infecting RBCs.

Major components and effector processes of the immune response to malaria: These are as follows:

- **Binding of pathogen-associated molecular patterns (PAMPs) in the malarial parasite with pattern recognition receptors (PRRs) on the surface of dendritic cells/antigen-presenting cells (APCs):** Immune response against *Plasmodium* is initiated by the engagement of PRRs on the surface of APCs by PAMPs in the malarial parasite. Glycosylphosphatidylinositol is known to bind TLR-2, whereas hemozoin binds TLR-9.
- **Activation of natural killer (NK) cells by IL-12 produced by APCs**: Upon activation APCs secrete interleukin (IL)-12 and this cytokine activates NK cells.
- **Production of IFN-γ by NK cells**: NK cells are important in the early response to intracellular pathogens, before the full activation of an adaptive response. Activated NK cells produce IFN-γ, which potentiate a Th1 response. IFN-γ also activates macrophages and increases their ability to produce toxic reactive oxygen and nitrogen species, with which they kill ingested parasites. Activated macrophages also secrete TNF-α to enhance inflammation. NK cells can lyse *Plasmodium*-infected erythrocytes directly and they secrete chemokines that recruit other cells during a malaria infection. Apart from NK cells other lymphocytes also appear to mediate an initial innate response to *Plasmodium.*
- **Activation of CD4+ T cells and differentiation into Th1 cells:** Meanwhile, APCs/dendritic cells migrate into secondary lymphatic structures. These dendritic cells present antigen and continue to release IL-12, activating naïve CD4+ T cells. The CD4+ T cells are induced to differentiate into effector T cells, primarily Th1 cells.
- **Functions of Th1 cells:** Th1 cells drive the primary adaptive response against liver-stage *Plasmodium* parasites.
  - Effector Th1 cells release IL-2, which activates CD8+ T cells. These active CD8+ T cells (cytotoxic T cells) are capable of recognizing and killing hepatocytes infected by *Plasmodium.*
  - Activated Th1 cells also produce IFN-γ, which promotes activation and enhanced killing by macrophages and also activate dendritic cells and CD8+ cytotoxic T cells.
  - Other effector CD4+ T cells activate B cells and cause antibody production, mainly to IgG.
  - Cytotoxic T cells can recognize and kill infected cells bearing their specific antigen. However, infected erythrocytes are not susceptible to cytotoxic T cell-mediated killing. This is because RBCs do not produce protein due to lose of their nuclei in erythrocytes during development.
  - This immune activation is counteracted by the suppressive actions of IL-10 and TGF-β, released by Treg (T-regulatory) cells. They in turn inhibit both inflammation and T-cell activation.

Humoral immunity: Humoral immunity is the primary adaptive effector mechanism once *Plasmodium* has left the liver. Most of the circulating antibody is of the IgM and IgG classes and rarely IgA. They are against asexual forms of plasmodia may give protection by inhibiting red cell invasion by parasite and antibodies against sexual forms reduce transmission of malaria parasite.

- **Functions of antibodies:** Antibodies produced against stages of *Plasmodium* in blood may help to reduce parasitemia in several ways.
  - May neutralize newly released merozoites before they can infect new erythrocytes, or
  - May bind to parasite antigens found on the membranes of infected erythrocytes, causing the agglutination of infected cells.
  - In *P. falciparum*, the antibodies may block sequestration of red cells in capillary beds by binding to the surface of infected red cells. Then these infected red cells which are unable to sequester themselves, may be transported and destroyed in the spleen.
- **Maternal transfer of antibodies:** Acquired antibody-mediated immunity is transferred from mother to fetus through the placenta. In endemic regions, the passive maternal antibodies protect infants below the age of 3 months from malarial infection.
- Young children are highly susceptible to malarial infection. As children grow up, they acquire immunity by subclinical or clinical infections. This is responsible for low incidence of malaria in older children and adults.

Cellular immunity: Sensitized T cells release cytokines that regulate macrophage activation and stimulate B cells to produce antibodies. The activated macrophages inside liver, spleen and bone marrow phagocytose both parasitized and nonparasitized RBCs.

- Antibodies and T lymphocytes specific for *Plasmodium* can reduce disease manifestations. However, the parasite has evolved strategies to evade the host immune response. *P. falciparum* escape from antibody responses to PfEMP1 and other surface proteins by antigenic variation. Each haploid *P. falciparum* genome contains many genes encoding variants of these parasite proteins. Some of the parasites switch genes during each generation, producing antigenically new surface proteins.
- Cytotoxic T cells may also be involved against resistance to *P. falciparum*.

Note: Protective immunity against malaria is species specific, stage specific and strain specific.

Major components and effector processes of the immune response to malaria is presented in **Figure 93.**

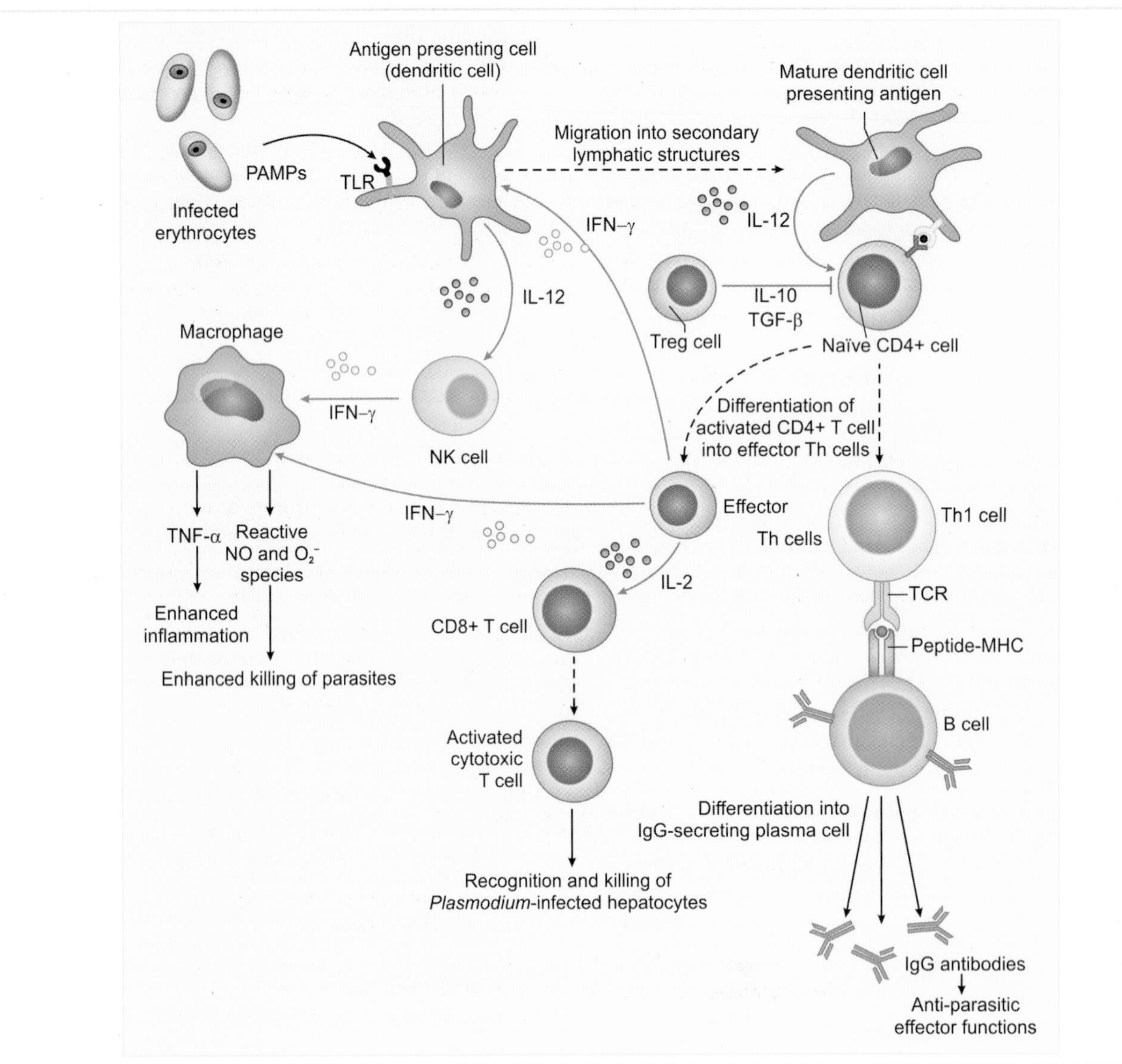

FIG. 93: Major components and effector processes of the immune response to malaria. The immune system is activated against *Plasmodium* when parasite pathogen-associated molecular patterns (PAMPs) bind toll-like receptors (TLRs) on antigen presenting cells [e.g. dendritic cell (DC)]. Dendritic cells secrete IL-12 and activate natural killer (NK) cells. NK cells in turn produce IFN-γ, which activates macrophages and increases their ability to produce toxic reactive oxygen and nitrogen species. This will help to kill ingested parasites. Activated macrophages also produce tumor necrosis factor alpha (TNF-α) and enhance inflammation. Meanwhile, dendritic cells migrate into secondary lymphatic structures and present antigen and continue to release IL-12. This cytokine IL-12 activates naïve CD4+ T cells and induces them to differentiate into effector T cells, primarily Th1 cell. Effector Th1 cells release IL-2, which in turn activates CD8+ T cells. These activated CD8+ T cells (cytotoxic T cells) are now capable of recognizing and killing hepatocytes infected by *Plasmodia*. Th1 cells also produce IFN-γ, which continues to activate macrophages and dendritic cells. Other effector CD4+T cells activate B cells and cause production of antibody mainly IgG type. This immune activation is counteracted by the suppressive effects of IL-10 and TGF-β, released by Treg (T regulatory cells) cells. This in turn inhibits both inflammation and T-cell activation.

Malaria Vaccine

Q. Write short essay on the development of malaria vaccine.

Malaria vaccine is an area of intensive research. Over past decades, there was a significant progress in the development of malaria vaccine. However, a completely effective vaccine is not yet available for malaria, though several vaccines are under development.

- **SPf66:** It is a cocktail of four antigens, three asexual blood stage antigens and circumsporozoite of *P. falciparum*. It was tested extensively in endemic areas in the 1990s, but found to be insufficiently effective.
- Other vaccine candidates targeting the blood stage of parasite's life cycle using merozoite surface protein 1 ***(MSP 1), MSP2, MSP 13*** and ring-infected erythrocyte surface antigens ***(RESAs)*** have also been in insufficient on their own.
- Several potential vaccines targeting the pre-erythrocytic stage are being developed, with ***RTS, S/ASOl*** showing the most promising results. The *RTS, S*/ASOl (commercial name, ***mosquirix***) was engineered using genes from the *outer protein of P. falciparum* and a portion *of hepatitis B virus,* plus a chemical adjuvant *(ASOL)* to boost immune response.

Pathological Changes in Organs in Malaria

All forms of malaria are associated with hepatosplenomegaly. The RBCs are sequestered by fixed mononuclear phagocytes present in organs such as liver, spleen, lymph nodes. These organs are darkened ("slate gray") by **macrophages filled with hemosiderin and malarial pigment, the end-product of parasitic digestion of hemoglobin**.

Spleen

In malaria, spleen acts as a filter for removing the parasite as well as the product of schizont from the blood. In all types of malaria, particularly *P. falciparum* infection, numerous parasites are found in the spleen in all the stages. The macrophages in the spleen actively phagocytosed malarial parasites as well as hematin pigments.

MORPHOLOGY

Gross (Fig. 94): Spleen is **moderately enlarged even in chronic malaria**. It will **never become massively enlarged** as in kala-azar or other conditions prevalent in the tropics. Spleen is **slate-gray or black in color** depending on the amount of pigmentation. The capsule is thin and stretched in acute *P. falciparum* infection and in chronic malaria it may be thickened due to perisplenitis. In acute cases, it is soft in consistency where as in chronic malaria it is fairly firm and is termed as "ague cake" (ague = malaria or another illness involving fever and shivering). On cut section. The parenchyma appears as a homogeneous dark brown or **slate gray** or even *black* due to dilated sinusoids, faintly birefringent hemozoin pigment accumulation and fibrosis. There are also scattered white fibrous trabeculae and gray white spot (Malpighian corpuscles).

Continued

Continued

Microscopy: It shows congestion of splenic sinusoids. **Abundant amount of both hematin and hemosiderin is found scattered all over the spleen**. Malarial parasites appear as black dots in the RBCs.

Liver

MORPHOLOGY

Gross

- Liver is uniformly enlarged due to congestion and proliferation of reticulo-endothelial cells. The color varies from dark chocolate-red to slate-gray or black. Cut surface shows dilated terminal hepatic venule and surrounded by yellow central zone of the lobule.

Microscopy

- Dilatation of terminal hepatic venules and sinusoids filled with parasitized RBCs.
- Kupffer cells are increased in number (hyperplasia) and their cytoplasm contains malarial pigment, parasitized RBCs, and cellular debris.
- Hepatocytes in the central zone of the lobule show fatty change (steatosis).

Laboratory Diagnosis

Q. Write short essay on laboratory diagnosis of malaria.

Demonstration of parasite by microscopy

A microscopic examination of a **peripheral blood film is one of the most important diagnostic methods in malaria**. Diagnosis of malaria can be made by examination and demonstration of a Giemsa/Leishman-stained peripheral blood smear for malarial parasite. It shows the **asexual stages of the parasite within infected red cells**. The timing of blood collection is important for the success in retrieving the malarial parasites. The various morphological forms of

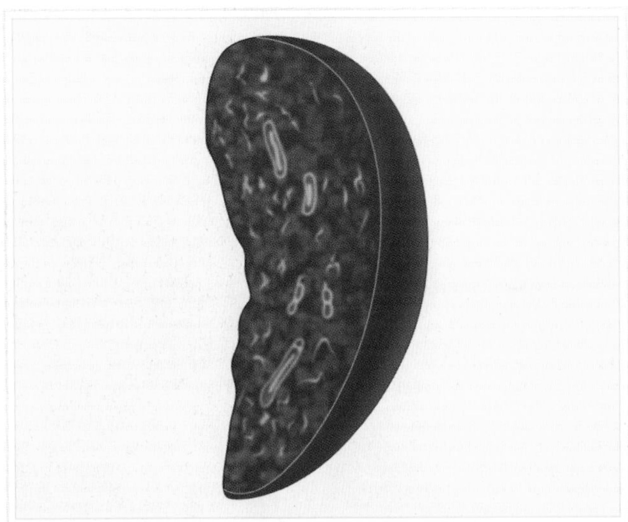

FIG. 94: Cut section of spleen in chronic malaria shows characteristic slate gray color (diagrammatic).

parasites seen at any given time in the smear depend on the stage of development of parasite at the time of specimen collection. The **greatest number of parasites is present in the blood in between characteristic bouts of fever and chills known as paroxysms.** During this period, there is release of merozoites and toxic waste products from infected RBCs. Thus, this is the optimal time to collect peripheral blood samples to determine the presence of *Plasmodium* species It is recommended that blood should be collected every 6–12 hours for up to 48 hours before considering a patient to be free of *Plasmodium* infection.

MORPHOLOGICAL FEATURE OF MALARIA PARASITES IN BLOOD SMEAR

Forms seen in peripheral smear
- In *P. vivax, P. ovale,* and *P. malariae* all asexual forms and gametocytes can be seen.
- In *P. falciparum* infection, only ring form alone or with gametocytes can be seen.

Appearance of ring forms: Ring forms of all species appear as streaks of blue cytoplasm with detached nuclear dots.
- They are large and compact in *P. vivax, P. ovale,* and *P. malariae.*
- In *P. falciparum,* they are delicate with binucleate rings (double chromatin) and resemble *stereo headphones* (nucleus close together) and multiple rings with "accole" forms are seen.

Gametocytes
- *Round* in *P. vivax, P. ovale, and P. malariae.*
- *Banana-shaped* (crescents) in *P. falciparum*

Continued

Continued

Infected red cell
- Enlarged RBCs with intracellular coarse brick-red stippling *(Schuffner's dots)* are characteristic in *P. vivax.*
- In *P. falciparum,* RBCs are normal in size with large red dots *(Maurer's dots)* and sometimes, with *basophilic stippling.* Careful search in blood should be made for *mixed infections.*

Types of smears Two types of smears are prepared from the peripheral blood namely: (1) *thin smear* and (2) *thick smear.* It is a good practice to prepare both thick and thin smears either on the same slide or on two different slides.

Thin smears: They are prepared from capillary blood of fingertip and spread over a good quality slide by a second slide held at an angle of 30–45° from the horizontal such that a tail is formed.
- A properly made thin film will consist of a **single layer of red cells**, ending in a tongue, which stops a little short of the edge of the slide.
- Thin smears are air dried rapidly, fixed in alcohol and stained by one of the Romanowsky stains such as Leishman, Giemsa, Field's, or JSB stain (named after Jaswant Singh and Bhattacharjee).
- Thin smears are used **for detecting the parasites** and ***determine the species.***
- In majority of patients with symptoms, a careful examination of thin film will almost always show the parasites.

Appearance of malarial parasite in thin smear is shown in **Figures 95A to D**.

Thick smears: They can be made either on the same slide of thin smear or separately.

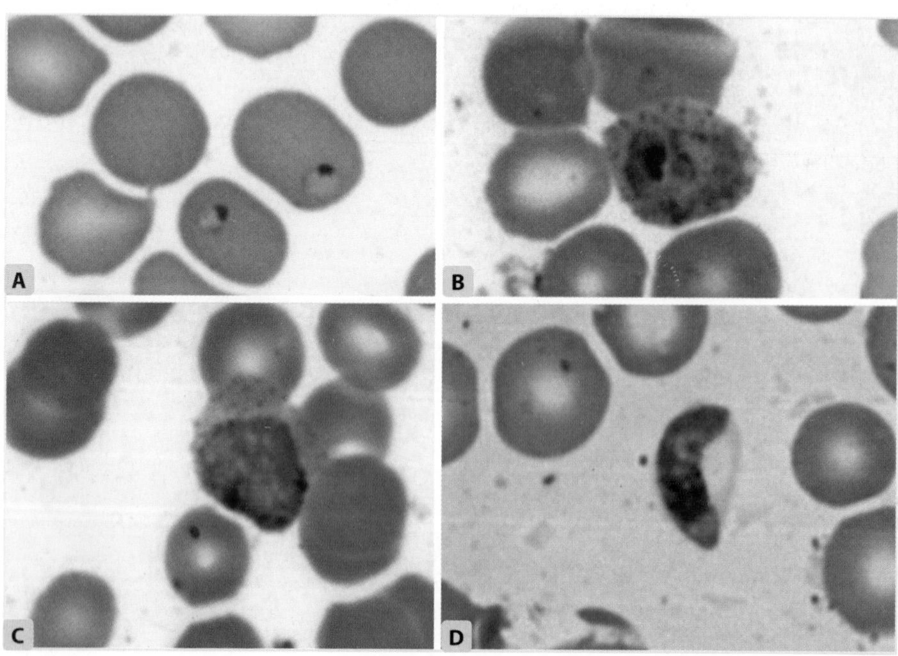

FIGS. 95A TO D: Appearance of malarial parasite *Plasmodium vivax* and *falciparum* in human. *Plasmodium vivax* ring forms (A) and schizont (B); *P. falciparum* schizont (C) and gametocyte (D).

- Thick film is usually prepared using **three drops** of blood that are **spread over a small area** (about 10 mm).
- The amount of blood in thin smear is about **1-1.5 μL,** whereas in a thick smear it is **3-4 μL.** The thickness of the film should be such that, it allow a newsprint to be read or the hands of a wrist-watch can be seen through after drying the smear.
- The thick film is dried in a horizontal position and covered by a petri dish. Drying during moist climate takes at least 30-60 minutes to dry at room temperature, Dry may be hastened by keeping the smear inside an incubator. Dehemoglobinization may be carried out by distilled water by keeping the smear in a vertical position in coplin jar with distilled water for 5-10 minutes. When the film appears white, it is taken out and allowed to dry in an upright position. After dehemoglobinization, the smear is stained with Leishman's or Giemsa stain in the same way as the thin smear. The smear is not fixed in methanol. The dehemoglobinized and stained thick film does not show any red cells, but only leukocytes, and, when present, the parasites. But the parasites are often distorted in form. The diagnostic changes in blood cells such as enlargement and stippling cannot be made out and identification of malarial species is difficult. Field's stain is a quick method of staining a thick film for malarial parasite (without fixation).
- Thick film is stained similar to thin film. The stained film is examined under the oil immersion objective of light microscope. It is recommended that 200 oil immersion fields should be examined before declaring a thick film as negative.
- First, thin film is examined at the tail end. If malarial parasites are found, there is no necessity to examine the thick film. If malarial parasites are not detected in thin film, then thick film should be examined.
- The thick film is more ***sensitive,*** when examined by an experienced individual, because it concentrates **20-30 layers** of blood cells in a small area.
- Thick film is more suitable for rapid detection of malarial parasite, particularly when the parasites are few in number (as low as **20 parasites/μL)** Quantification of parasites can be done by thick smear. The methods of counting of parasites are done to an approximate number as presented in **Table 37.**

Difficulties in detecting malarial parasites It may be encountered when blood smear is prepared under following situations:

1. After anti-malarial drugs.
2. During apyrexial interval of *P. falciparum* infection.
3. First 2-3 days of primary infection.

Table 37: Quantification of parasites by thick smear.

No. of parasite	*Expression of quantity*
1-10 parasite per 100 thick film fields	+
11-100 parasite per 100 thick film fields	++
1-10 parasite per thick film field	+++
More than 10 parasite per thick film field	++++

Quantitative buffy coat method

Principle: Staining of the centrifuged and compressed red cell layer with acridine orange and its examination under UV light source.

The quantitative buffy coat (**QBC**) test is a novel method for the diagnosis of malaria. In this method, a small quantity of blood (i.e., 50-110 μL) is spun in QBC centrifuge at 12,000 revolutions/minute (rpm) for 5 minutes.

- RBC containing malaria parasites are less dense than normal RBCs. When centrifuges they get concentrated just below the buffy coat of leukocytes at the top of the erythrocytic column.
- In this method, the hematocrit tube is precoated internally with acridine orange stain and potassium oxalate. Cylindrical float is inserted. The float occupies 90% of the internal lumen of the tube, the leukocyte and the platelet band widths and the top-most area of red cells are enlarged to 10 times normal. The QBC tube is placed on the tube holder and examined by fluorescent microscopy. Fluorescing parasites are then observed at the RBC/white blood cell (WBC) interface.
- Acridine orange induces a fluorescence on the parasites. The parasite contains deoxyribonucleic acid (DNA), but the mature RBCs do not contain DNA and ribonucleic acid (RNA). The acridine orange stains the DNA of the nucleus of the parasite and thus parasites can be readily seen under the oil immersion microscope. The parasites appear as fluorescent **greenish-yellow** against red background.
- **Advantage of QBC:** It is faster and more sensitive than thick blood smear.
- **Disadvantage:** Less sensitive than thick blood film and is expensive.
- A **careful smear examination is still remains as the "gold standard" in malaria diagnosis**.

Microconcentration technique

In microconcentration technique, blood sample is collected in micro hematocrit tube and centrifuged at high speed. The sediment obtained is mixed with normal serum and smear is prepared. Though it increases the positivity rate, it alters the morphology of the parasite.

Culture of malaria parasites

Culture is not needed for the diagnosis of malaria except in situations where it is difficult to differentiate trophozoites (ring-form) of *P. vivax* from *P. falciparum*. Culture provides a source of the parasites for study of their antigenic structure, in seroepidemiologic surveys, drug sensitivity tests and studies in monoprophylaxis.

Serodiagnosis

Serodiagnosis is not useful in clinical diagnosis. This is because they cannot differentiate between an active and past infection. It is used mainly for seroepidemiological survey and to identify the infected donors in transfusion malaria. The tests used include indirect hemagglutination (*IHA*), indirect fluorescent antibody (*IFA*) test and enzyme-linked immunosorbent assay (*ELISA*).

Tests used for demonstration of antibodies:

- *Indirect fluorescent antibody test*: Plasmodial schizonts are used as antigen in IFA.

- *ELISA*: Antigens-mixture of a total extract of cultured *P. falciparum* and recombinant *P. vivax* antigens (MSP1 and CSP) and so the test does not distinguish between IgG and IgM or between antibodies to *P. falciparum, P. vivax, P. ovale,* and *P. malariae.*

Newer methods of diagnosis

Fluorescence microscopy Fluorescent dyes such as acridine orange or benzothiocarboxy purine stain the parasites entering the RBCs but not WBCs. This is a method of differential staining. Acridine orange stains *DNA* as fluorescent green and cytoplasmic RNA as red. The stained slide is examined under fluorescent microscope. This method is mainly used for mass screening in field laboratory.

Rapid antigen detection tests

Immunochromatographic tests for malaria antigens: They are based on the detection of malarial antigens using immunochromatographic methods by using tagged monoclonal antibodies.

Principle: It is based on the capture of the parasite antigens from the peripheral blood using either monoclonal or polyclonal against the parasite antigen targets. These rapid antigen detection tests have been developed in different test formats such as the dipstick, card and cassette bearing monoclonal antibody, directed against the parasite antigens. Several kits are available in the market and they can detect *Plasmodium* in 15 minutes.

False positivity: These include persistent viable asexual-stage parasitemia, persistence of antigens due to sequestration and incomplete treatment, delayed clearance of circulating antigen (free or in antigen-antibody complexes) and cross reaction with nonfalciparum malaria or rheumatoid factor.

False negativity: These include genetic heterogeneity of PfHRP2 expression, deletion of *HRP-2* gene, presence of blocking antibodies of PfHPR2 antigen or immune complex formation and prozone phenomenon at high antigenemia.

Various tests are as follows:

- **ELISA malaria antigen test (Parasite-F test):** This test is based on detection of histidine rich protein-2 (HRP-2) antigen produced by the asexual stages of *P. falciparum* expressed on the surface of red cells. Monoclonal antibody produced against **HRP-2 antigen** (Pf band) is employed in the test strip.
  - **Advantages:** It is popular and has high sensitivity (98%) and specificity.
    - Test can detect low asexual parasitemia of >40 parasites/μL.
    - Test can be performed within 10 minutes.
    - Useful for screening blood donor, patient with a febrile illness with repeated blood smear negative, patient recently treated for malaria but in whom the diagnosis is questioned.
  - **Disadvantages:** These include:
    - It cannot detect the other three malaria species. Species-specific testing is available for the four human species: P. *falciparum, P. vivax, P. Malariae,* and *P. ovale.*
    - Remains positive up to 2 weeks after cure.
    - In *P. falciparum* infection, PfHRP-2 is not secreted in gametogony stage. Hence in "carriers", the Pf band may be absent.
    - Cross reactions often occur between *Plasmodium* species and *Babesia* species
- **Dual antigen test:** The test simultaneously detects parasite lactate dehydrogenase **(pfLDH)** produced by trophozoites and gametocytes of all *Plasmodium* species as well as **PfHRP-2 antigen** produced by *P. falciparum.* pfLDH is cleared rapidly within days of onset of treatment whereas from PfHRP-2 clears slowly from the blood and takes almost one month for it disappear after the acute disease.
  - One band (Pv band) produced is genus specific *(P. specific)* and other is *Plasmodium falciparum* specific (Pf band).
  - This is a rapid two-site sandwich immunoassay used for specific detection and differentiation of *P. falciparum* and *P. vivax* malaria in areas having high rates of mixed infection.
  - Provides good diagnostic sensitivity and helpful diagnostic method where microscopic examination of the smear for parasite is not possible. The **"Pv" band** can be used to monitor the success of antimalarial therapy in case of stained alone *P. vivax* infection. This is because the test will detect only live parasites and will be negative, if the parasite has been killed by the treatment.
  - Disadvantage of the test is that it is expensive and cannot differentiate between *P. vivax, P. ovale,* and *P. malariae.*

Flow cytometry On flow cytometric depolarized side scatter, the average relative frequency of pigment carrying monocyte was found to differ among semi-immune, nonimmune and malaria negative patients.

Automated hematology analyzers Diagnosis of malaria during routine blood counts: Abnormal cell clusters and small particles with DNA fluorescence, probably free malarial parasites, can be suspected based on the scatter plots produced on the analyzer. Automated detection of malaria pigment in WBCs may also suggest a possibility of malaria with a sensitivity of 95% and specificity of 88%.

Laser desorption mass spectrometry Detection of malaria parasites in blood can be done by using laser desorption mass spectrometry. Intact ferriprotoporphyin IX (heme) is sequestered by malaria parasites during their growth in human RBCs. They generate intense ion signals. The **laser desorption** mass spectrum of the heme is structure specific and the signal intensities. They correlate with the sample parasitemia. The sensitivity is 10 parasites/μL.

Molecular diagnosis

Deoxyribonucleic acid probe: DNA probe is a highly sensitive method for the diagnosis of malaria. It can detect <10 parasites/μL of blood. Polymerase chain reaction (**PCR**) is increasingly used now for species specification and for detection of drug resistance in malaria. PCR is ten times more sensitive than light microscopy. PCR are not yet accepted as the gold standard. Various PCR methods include real time PCR, nested PCR and multiplex real time PCR.

Ancillary tests

- Estimation of hemoglobin and packed cell volume (PCV) is needed in case of heavy parasitemia, particularly in children and pregnant woman.
- Total WBC and platelet count in severe *falciparum* malaria.
- Measurement of blood glucose to detect hypoglycemia, particularly in young children and pregnant women with *severe falciparum* malaria and patients receiving quinine.
- Coagulation tests such as measurement of antithrombin III level, plasma fibrinogen, fibrin degradation products (FDPs), partial thromboplastin time (PTT), if abnormal bleeding is suspected in *falciparum* malaria.
- Urine for free hemoglobin, if there is suspicion of blackwater fever.
- Blood urea and serum creatinine to monitor renal failure.
- G6PD screening before treatment with an antioxidant drug such as primaquine.

Salient laboratory investigations in malaria are summarized in **Box 18**.

Babesiosis

Babesiosis is a malaria-like infection (intraerythrocytic sporozoan parasites) caused by protozoa of the genus *Babesia.* The primary causes of babesiosis are *Babesia microti* and *Babesia divergens* with additional cases due to *B. duncani* and *B. venatorum.*

Mode of transmission: It is transmitted by hard-bodied ticks in a manner similar to Lyme disease and granulocytic ehrlichiosis. The ticks include *Ixodes scapularis* (deer tick) and *Ixodes ricinus* (sheep tick).

Reservoir of infection: *Babesia* infections are common in domestic and wild animals. The white-footed mouse is the reservoir for *B. microti.* In certain locations, nearly all mice have a persistent low-level parasitemia. *B. microti* survives well in refrigerated blood, and cases of transfusion-acquired babesiosis have been reported.

Pathogenesis: Human babesiosis is almost a medical curiosity. The parasites infect humans only when people intrude into the zoonotic cycle between the tick vector and its vertebrate host. *Babesia* species invade and parasitize red cells. They destroy erythrocytes, causing hemoglobinemia, hemoglobinuria and renal failure.

Clinical features: They cause fever and hemolytic anemia. Most infections are asymptomatic and self-limited. However, infection in debilitated or individuals who underwent splenectomy can cause severe, uncontrolled infections with fatal parasitemias. *Babesia* species are resistant to most antiprotozoal drugs.

MORPHOLOGY

Peripheral blood smear: *Babesia* species appear as intraerythrocytic round or pyriform, or ring form **superficially resembling ring stages of *P. falciparum*.** They **lack the central hemozoin pigment, show greater pleomorphism, and form characteristic tetrads (Maltese cross). If found,** tetrads are pathognomonic or **diagnostic of *B. microti* or *B. duncani* (Fig. 96).**

Severity of infection: Good indicator of the severity of infection of *B. microti* is the level of parasitemia. It is about 1–20% in mild cases (in immunocompetent patients) and up to 30% in splenectomized patients.

Fatal cases: It may produce shock and hypoxia. Findings related to shock and hypoxia include jaundice, hepatic necrosis, acute renal tubular necrosis, acute respiratory distress syndrome, erythrophagocytosis, and visceral hemorrhage.

Amebiasis

Amebiasis is an **infection caused by protozoan *E. histolytica*** (named so because of its lytic actions on involved tissue).

Principal site of involvement: Colon and occasionally, it spread beyond the colon to involve other organs. The most common site of extraintestinal disease is the liver, where *E. histolytica* causes slowly expanding, necrotizing abscesses the liver. Intestinal infection may range from asymptomatic colonization to severe invasive infection with bloody diarrhea.

Epidemiology: Amebiasis is found worldwide. But it is more common and more severe in tropical and subtropical areas, where there is poor sanitation.

Etiology

Entamoeba histolytica has three distinct stages:

1. **Trophozoite stage (Fig. 97A):** Amebic trophozoites are spherical or oval and measure 10–60 µm in diameter. They have a thin cell membrane, a single nucleus, condensed chromatin on the interior of the nuclear membrane and a central karyosome. The trophozoites may contain

Box 18: Laboratory investigations in malaria.

- Demonstration of malarial parasites in thick and thin blood smear stained by Leishman, Giemsa, or JSB stain
- Immunofluorescence staining and QBC smear
- Rapid immunochromatographic test (ICT) for detection of malaria antigen (PfHRP-2 and pLDH)
- Molecular diagnosis: DNA probe and PCR
- Routine blood examination for Hb, PCV and blood sugar

(DNA: deoxyribonucleic acid; Hb: hemoglobin; JSB: Jaswant Singh and Bhattacharjee; PCR: polymerase chain reaction; PCV: packed cell volume; PfHRP-2: Plasmodium falciparum histidine rich protein-2; pLDH: parasite lactate dehydrogenase; QBC: quantitative buffy coat)

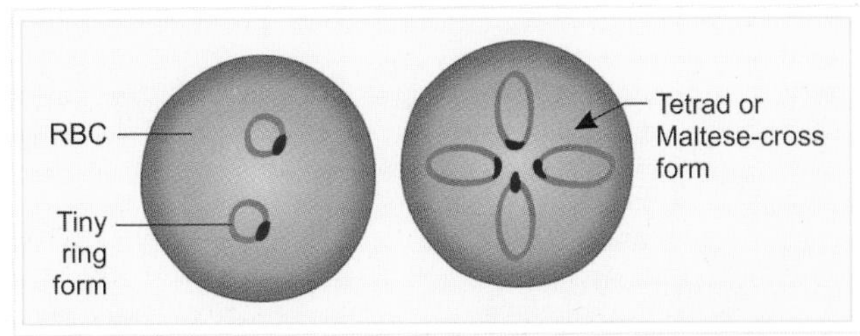

FIG. 96: Babesiosis showing ring-form and pathognomonic tetrads (Maltese cross).

phagocytosed erythrocytes (RBCs). They are seen in the stools of patients with acute symptoms. The cytoplasm of the trophozoites stain positively by periodic acid–Schiff (PAS) in tissue sections.

2. **Precyst stage (Fig. 97B):** In the colon, the trophozoite develops into a cyst through an intermediate form termed the precyst. Precyst is smaller in size than trophozoite. It is round or slightly oval with blunt pseudopodium projecting from the periphery. Nucleus is similar to trophozoite stage.
3. **Cyst stage (Figs. 97C to E):** During this process, trophozoites stop feeding. They become round and nonmotile, lose some digestive vacuoles and form glycogen masses and chromatoidal bodies (bars). They are spherical and have thick chitin walls. The cyst wall is a highly refractile membrane, which makes it highly resistant to gastric juice and unfavorable environmental conditions.
   - Early cyst contains a single nucleus and two other structures: (1) a **mass of glycogen** and (2) 1–4 ***chromatoid bodies*** *or chromidial bars,* which are cigar shaped refractile rods with rounded ends. The chromatoid bodies are so named because they stain with hematoxylin, like chromatin.
   - As the cyst matures, the glycogen mass and chromidial bars disappear and the nucleus undergoes two successive mitotic divisions to form two (**Fig. 95D**) and then four nuclei. The mature cyst is, thus **quadrinucleate** (**Fig. 97E**).

Amebic cysts are the infecting stage and are found only in stools since they do not invade tissue.

Source of infection: **Humans** are the only known reservoir for *E. histolytica.* It is reproduced in the colon of infected individual and passes in the feces.

Mode of infection: It is **acquired by fecal–oral route** through ingestion of materials contaminated with human feces containing *E. histolytica.*

Incubation period: About 8–10 days.

Pathogenesis

The amebic cysts are passed in the stool and the **cysts can contaminate water, food, or fingers**.

- On ingestion, *E. histolytica* cysts traverse the stomach. They are **resistant to the action of gastric acid.** They excyst in the lower ileum and pass to the colon.
- **Amebic cysts** then **colonize the epithelial surface of the colon and release trophozoites**. Each cyst containing four nuclei divides to form four small, immature trophozoites, which then mature to full size. In the colon, they feed on bacteria and human cells. They may colonize any part of the large intestine, but **most frequently in the cecum and ascending colon causing amebic colitis.** Patients with symptomatic amebic colitis pass both cysts and trophozoites in the stool.
- Trophozoite attaches the colonic epithelial cell and invades crypts, and burrow laterally into the lamina propria. The trophozoite kills the intestinal cell by producing a lytic protein that damages the cell membrane and creates a superficial ulcer. Recruitment of neutrophils causes tissue damage and creates a **flask shaped ulcer with a narrow neck and broad base.**
- **Trophozoite may penetrate blood vessels and reach the liver** to produce **abscesses** in about 40% of patients with amebic dysentery.

MORPHOLOGY

Entamoeba histolytica can produce intestinal or extraintestinal disease.

- **Intestinal disease:** It mainly involves the **colon** and ranges from **asymptomatic colonization to severe invasive infections** causing bloody dysentery.
- **Extraintestinal disease:** It can produce **amebic liver abscesses.**

Colon

- Amebic lesions start as small **foci of necrosis,** which progress to **ulcers**. The ulcer floor is **gray and necrotic**. The **chronic amebic ulcers** are described as **flask-shaped ulcer** with a narrow/bottle neck and broad base resembling a **flask** (**Figs. 98A and B**).
- Trophozoites can be detected on the surface of the ulcer and in the exudate. The ulcers show infiltration by acute and chronic inflammatory cells. PAS stain shows trophozoites of ameba in the exudate (**Fig. 98C**).
- **Ameboma:** It is a **rare complication** of amebiasis. The intestinal wall shows thickening due to inflammation (napkin-ring constriction) and may **resemble colon cancer**. Microscopically, **it consists of granulation tissue, inflammatory cells, fibrosis and clusters of trophozoites. Ameboma can also develop in brain (Fig. 99).**

Clinical Features

Intestinal amebiasis: It may be asymptomatic or produce dysentery of varying severity. The incubation period for acute amebic colitis is about 8–10 days. Amebic dysentery may present with **abdominal pain, bloody diarrhea, or weight loss. Liquid stools (up to 25/day) contain blood and mucus.**

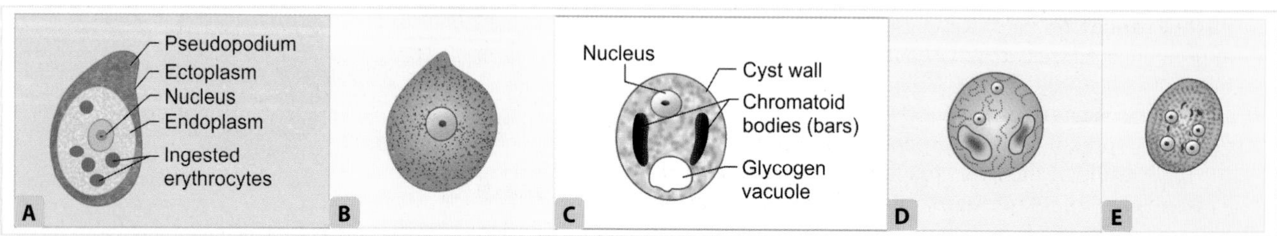

FIGS. 97A TO E: *Entamoeba histolytica.* (A) Trophozoite; (B) Precystic stage; (C) Uninucleate cyst; (D) Binucleate cyst; and (E) Mature quadrinucleate cyst.

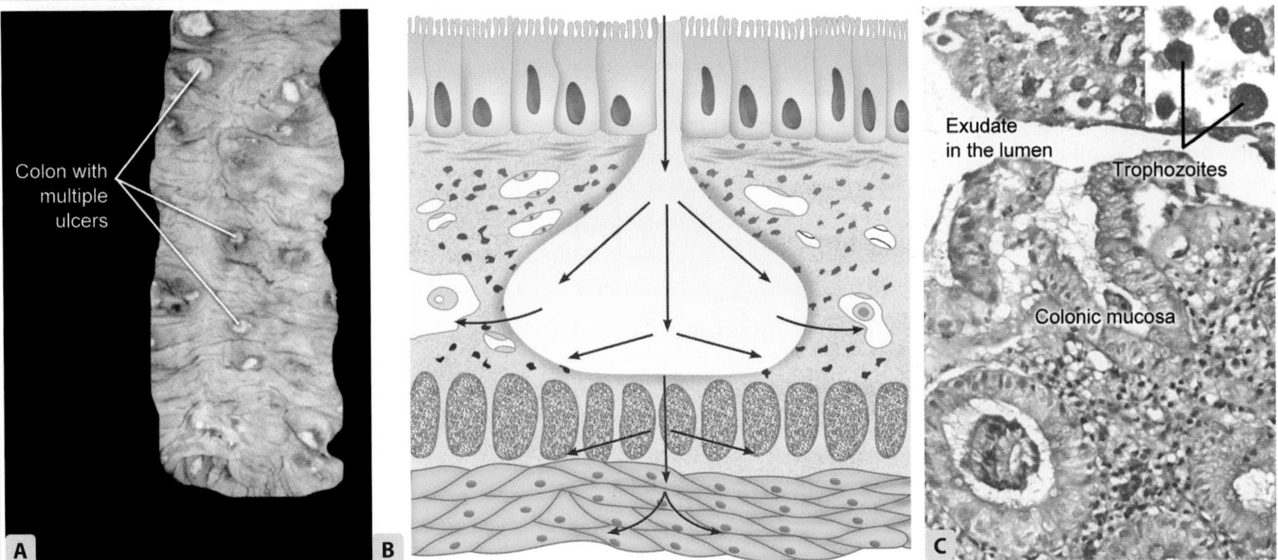

FIGS. 98A TO C: (A) Gross appearance of multiple amebic ulcers in the colon; (B) Microscopically appear as flask-shaped amebic ulcer (diagrammatic); (C) Microscopic appearance of amebic ulcer [periodic acid–Schiff (PAS) stain] shows PAS-stained trophozoites of ameba in the exudate (inset).

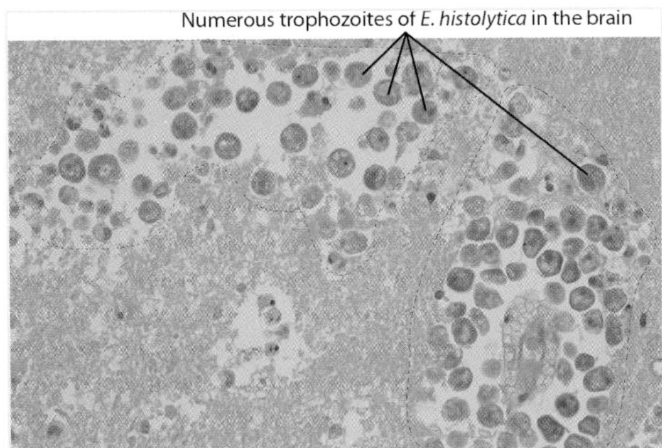

FIG. 99: Ameboma of brain showing clusters of trophozoites of *Entamoeba histolytica*.

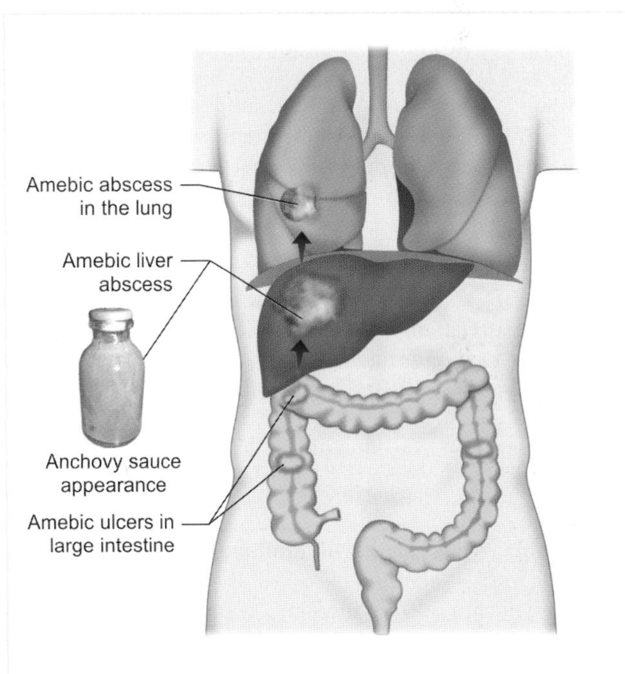

FIG. 100: Complications of amebiasis (diagrammatic).

Amebic Liver Abscess (Fig. 100)

- It is a **major complication of intestinal amebiasis**.
- *E. histolytica* **trophozoites from the colon may reach liver through the portal circulation.**
- **Trophozoites kill hepatocytes** and produce **abscess**.
- Abscess cavity is filled with a dark brown, odorless, semisolid necrotic material, which resembles **anchovy paste (sauce) in color and consistency**. The size of amebic liver abscess may vary and can exceed 10 cm in diameter.
- ***Spread of amebic liver abscess***:
  - **Local spread:** It may expand and rupture through the capsule of the liver® may directly **spread into the peritoneum, diaphragm, pleural cavity, lungs, or pericardium**.
  - **Hematogenous spread:** Rare and can spread to the **brain** and kidneys and produce necrotic lesions.

Clinical features of amebic liver abscess: It may present with severe right upper quadrant pain, low-grade fever and weight loss. The diagnosis is usually made by radiologic or ultrasound demonstration of the abscess, in conjunction with serologic testing for antibodies to *E. histolytica*.

Leishmaniasis

Introduction: Hemoflagellates are group of parasites located in blood and tissue that move by means of flagella. They belong to the genera *Leishmania* and *Trypanosoma*.

The genus *Leishmania* includes a numerous varieties and subspecies which differ in their natural habitats and the types of disease that they produce. There are about 21 species of *Leishmania* that infect humans. All members of the genus *Leishmania* are *obligate intracellular*, **kinetoplast-containing (kinetoplastid)** protozoan *parasites* that pass their life cycle in **two hosts:** (1) the mammalian host, and (2) the insect vector, female sandfly.

- **In humans and other mammalian hosts**, they multiply within macrophages. In the macrophages they occur exclusively in the **amastigote form** (described later).
- **In the sandfly**, they occur in the **promastigotes form** (described later).

Amastigote [Leishman–Donovan (LD) body]: They are round to oval and measures 5 × 3 µm in size (**Figs. 101A** and **103**). It contains a nucleus, a basal body structure (called a **blepharoplast**), and a small parabasal body. The large single nucleus is usually located off-center. Sometimes present more toward the edge of the organism. The dotlike blepharoplast gives rise to and is attached to an axoneme. The axoneme extends to the edge of the organism. The single parabasal body is located adjacent to the blepharoplast. **Kinetoplast** is a term usually used to refer to the blepharoplast and small parabasal body (**Kinetoplast** = blepharoplast + small parabasal body). It is typically intracellular, being found inside macrophages, monocytes, neutrophils, or endothelial cells. They are also known as ***LD bodies*** (see **Fig. 103**). Smears stained with Leishman, Giemsa, or Wright's stain show a pale blue cytoplasm enclosed by a limiting membrane. The large oval nucleus is stained red. Lying at the right angle to nucleus, is the red or purple-stained ***kinetoplast.*** Alongside the kinetoplast a clear unstained **vacuole** can be seen. Flagellum is absent.

Promastigotes: It is a flagellar stage and is present in insect vector, sandfly and in cultures. It usually measures 9–15 µm in length (**Fig. 101B**). The promastigotes, which are initially short, oval or pear-shaped forms, subsequently become long spindle-shaped cells, 15–25 µm in length and 1.5–3.5 µm in breadth. The large single nucleus is situated in or near the center of the long slender body. The kinetoplast lies transversely near the anterior end of the organism. A single, delicate free flagellum extends anteriorly from the axoneme and measures 15–28 µm.

Leishmaniasis is **a chronic inflammatory disease** caused by infection with *Leishmania* parasites. It causes a spectrum of clinical syndromes, from indolent, self-resolving cutaneous ulcers to fatal disseminated disease. **These spectrums include leishmaniasis of the skin, mucous membranes, or viscera.**

Mode of transmission: These parasites are **transmitted to humans through the bite of infected insect bites** (*Phlebotomus* sandflies). There are about 30 species of sandflies that serve as vectors.

Reservoirs of *Leishmania*: *Leishmanial* infection is **endemic in animal populations: dogs, ground squirrels, rodents, foxes, and jackals**. These are reservoirs of *Leishmania* species and potential sources for transmission to humans. *Phlebotomus* sandflies acquire the infection by feeding on these infected animals in many subtropical and tropical regions.

Epidemiology: Leishmaniasis is mainly a disease of less developed countries where humans live in close proximity to animal hosts and the fly vector. It is endemic throughout the Middle East, South Asia, Africa, and Latin America. It may also be epidemic, as it occurred in Sudan, India, Bangladesh, and Brazil.

Intracellular infection: **Leishmanial infection is an intracellular organism. Examples of other intracellular organisms include mycobacteria, *Histoplasma* species, *Toxoplasma* species, and trypanosomes.** All these infections by intracellular organisms are exacerbated by conditions that interfere with T-cell function, such as acquired immunodeficiency syndrome (AIDS).

Diagnosis: It is done by culture, PCR, or histologic examination of involved tissue.

Pathogenesis

The life cycle of Leishmania species ***(Fig. 102)*** involves two morphological forms: (1) the promastigote (develops and lives extracellularly in the sandfly vector), and (2) the amastigote (multiplies intracellularly in host macrophages).

- **Sandfly bite infected humans or animals:** When sandflies bite infected humans or animals, macrophages containing amastigotes are ingested. The amastigotes differentiate into flagellated promastigotes and multiply within the digestive tract of the sandfly. These infectious promastigotes migrate to the salivary gland and these are transmitted by the fly bite to the new host.
- **Infection of new host:** Infection begins when the infected sand fly bites a person. The slender, flagellated infectious promastigotes are inoculated into human skin by a sandfly bite. They are released into the host dermis along with the sandfly saliva, which potentiates parasite infectivity.
- **Transformation of promastigotes into amastigotes:** Shortly thereafter, the promastigotes are phagocytosed

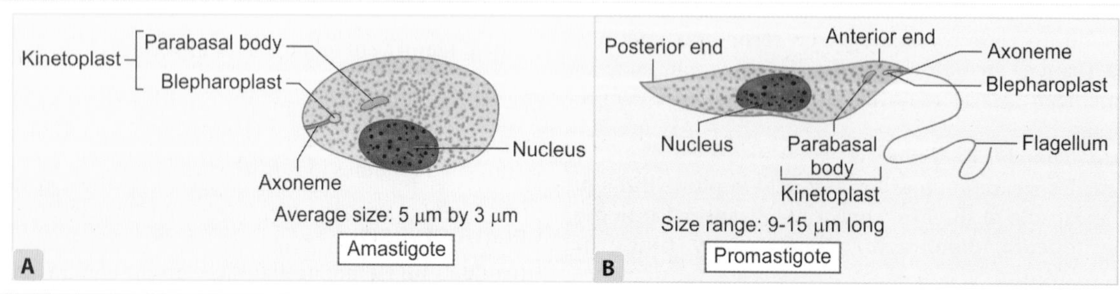

FIGS. 101A AND B: Two morphological forms (diagrammatic) of *Leishmania*. (A) Amastigote; and (B) Promastigotes.

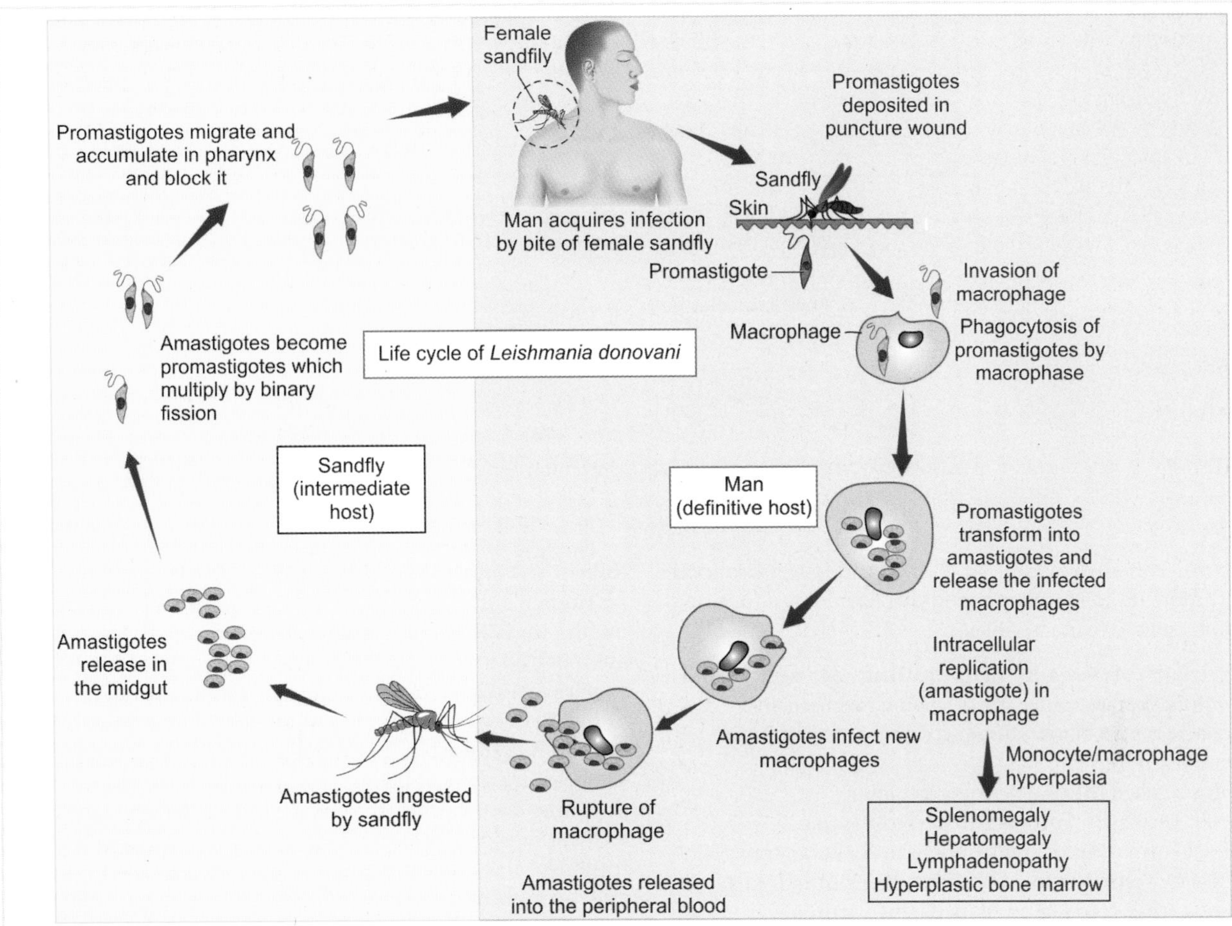

FIG. 102: Life cycle of leishmaniasis. Blood-sucking sandflies ingest amastigotes from an infected host. These amastigotes are transformed into promastigotes in the sandfly gut. They multiply in the sandfly. When the sandfly bite the new host, these are injected into the host. They invade macrophages, and revert to the amastigote form. They multiply in the macrophages and eventually rupture the infected macrophages. These released amastigotes then invade other macrophages, thus completing the cycle.

by macrophages (mononuclear phagocytes). The acidity within the phagolysosome induces promastigotes to transform into round amastigotes that lack flagella. The amastigote contains a single mitochondrion with its DNA massed into a unique suborganelle, the kinetoplast.

- **Proliferation and release of amastigotes:** The amastigotes are reproduced and they proliferate within the macrophage. When these macrophages containing daughter amastigotes die, they rupture and release progeny amastigotes. Released amastigotes infect additional macrophages and spread the infection. Reproduction continues in this way, and a cluster of infected macrophages forms at the site of inoculation. Extent of spread of the amastigotes and the extent of disease throughout the body depends on the specific *Leishmania* species and host.

Classification: *Leishmania* species can be classified on the basis of geographical distribution (**Flowchart 3**). Old World leishmaniasis include *L. major, L. tropica, L. donovani,* and *L. infantum* and refers to the Eastern Hemisphere [parts of Asia, the Middle East, Africa (particularly the tropical region and North Africa)], and southern Europe. New World leishmaniasis includes *L. mexicana, L. braziliensis,* and *L. chagasi* and refers to the Western Hemisphere (parts of Mexico, Central America, and South America).

Mechanism of escape from innate host defenses: *Leishmania* species handle innate host defenses to promote their entry and survival within the phagocytes. Promastigotes secrete two surface glycoconjugates that contribute to their virulence. These are lipophosphoglycan and Gp63.

- **Lipophosphoglycan:** It forms a dense glycocalyx that both activates and inhibits complement action. It activates complement and the C3b component gets deposited on the surface of the parasite. It also inhibits complement action and prevent the insertion of membrane attack complex (MAC = C5b-9) into the membrane of the parasite. Thus, though the parasite becomes coated with C3b, it avoids its destruction by the membrane attack complex. Instead, the C3b on the surface of the parasite binds to Mac-1 and CR1 on macrophages. This promotes phagocytosis of the promastigote by macrophages. This in turn helps in their proliferation inside macrophages.
- **Gp63:** It is a zinc-dependent proteinase. It is capable of cleaving the complement and some lysosomal

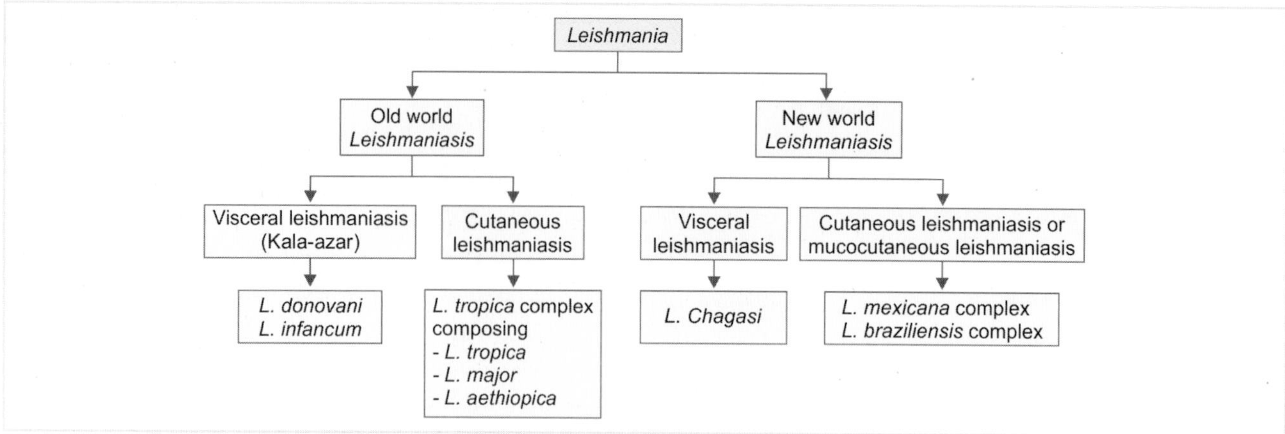

FLOWCHART 3: Classification of Leishmania based on geographical distribution and disease caused by *Leishmania* species.

antimicrobial enzymes. Gp63 also binds to fibronectin receptors on macrophages and this promotes adhesion of promastigote to macrophages.

Mechanism of escape from killing by neutrophils: *Leishmania* species utilize the following mechanisms:

- Prevent the formation of phagolysosomes and fusion with granules.
- Localize itself to nonlytic compartments.
- Resist destruction by reactive oxygen species.
- Resist formation of neutrophil extracellular trap (NET). This is achieved by producing endonucleases that digest the NETs and expressing protease-resistant molecules.

Mechanism to survive and replicate within macrophages: The amastigotes of *Leishmania* species also produce molecules that help for their survival and replication within macrophages.

- **Expressing a proton-transporting ATPase:** Normally phagolysosomes have a pH of 4.5 which is detrimental to the parasite. Amastigotes protect themselves from this adverse environment of low pH by expressing a proton-transporting ATPase. This maintains the phagolysosome pH at 6.5. Thus, amastigotes reproduce in macrophage phagolysosomes.
- **Stimulates iron entry into macrophage phagolysosomes:** *Leishmania* species need iron for survival. Normally macrophage phagolysosomes have low iron content. Amastigotes express an iron transporter from the ZRT-, IRT-like (ZIP) family of membrane proteins. This stimulates entry of iron into the macrophage phagolysosomes, thereby aid the survival of amastigotes.
    - **Mechanism by host to reduce iron in the macrophage phagolysosomes:** The host fights against increase of iron in the phagolysosome by using proinflammatory cytokines. These cytokines inhibit absorption of iron (partly by increasing production of hepcidin, the principal iron exporter), as well as activate synthesis of ferritin, which binds free iron. Also, macrophages downregulate the transferrin receptor and remove iron from the phagosome.

Role of Th1 and Th2 responses: The primary mechanisms of resistance and susceptibility to *Leishmania* species depend on Th1 and Th2 responses. Parasite-specific CD4+ Th1 cells are required for the control ***Leishmania* species. *Leishmania* species avoid host immunity by decreasing the development of the Th1 response**. In animal models, it was observed that mice that are resistant to *Leishmania* infection produce high levels of Th1-derived IFN-γ. This activates macrophages to kill the parasites. In contrast, mouse strains that are susceptible to leishmaniasis predominantly produce an effective Th2 response. Th2 cytokines (e.g., IL-4, IL-13, and IL-10) prevent effective killing of *Leishmania* species by suppressing the microbicidal activity of macrophages.

Disease Caused by Leishmania species

It depends on two factors: the immunologic status of the host and the infecting species of *Leishmania*. They produce four different types of lesions in humans: (1) visceral, (2) cutaneous (localized), (3) mucocutaneous, and (4) diffuse cutaneous.

Visceral leishmaniasis (Kala Azar)

Kala azar is produced by several subspecies of *L. donovani*. Reservoirs of the agent vary in different parts of the world. Humans are the reservoir in India.

Infection with *L. donovani begins* with localized collections of infected macrophages at the site of a sandfly bite. This is followed by spread the organisms throughout the body. This activates macrophages throughout the mononuclear phagocyte system. *L. donovani* are mostly destroyed by cell-mediated immune responses. In about 5% of patients, it produces visceral leishmaniasis. Especially it develops in children and malnourished individuals.

Manifestations: It causes a systemic inflammatory disease characterized by **hepatosplenomegaly, lymphadenopathy, pancytopenia, fever, and weight loss**. Often there is hyperpigmentation of the skin in individuals. Hence, the disease is called *kala-azar* (*black fever* in English). Advanced leishmaniasis may be associated with life-threatening secondary bacterial infections, such as pneumonia, sepsis, or tuberculosis. Hemorrhages due to thrombocytopenia may also be fatal.

MORPHOLOGY

The liver, spleen and lymph nodes become massively enlarged. Normal architecture of organ is gradually replaced by sheets of parasitized macrophages.

Spleen: It may weigh as much as 3 kg. Microscopically, it shows enlarged macrophages (phagocytic cells) filled with proliferating leishmanial amastigotes (LD bodies refer above on page 760 and **Fig. 103**). Many plasma cells are also present. Normal architecture of the spleen is obscured.

Liver: It is enlarged and in the late stages, it becomes increasingly fibrotic.

Phagocytic cells are seen in the **bone marrow (Figs. 103A and B)** and also may be found in the lungs, gastrointestinal tract, kidneys, pancreas, and testes.

Kidney: It may produce an immune complex-mediated mesangioproliferative glomerulonephritis. In advanced cases, there may be deposition of amyloid.

Laboratory diagnosis of Kala azar is presented in **Flowchart 4**.

Localized cutaneous leishmaniasis

Many species of *Leishmania* in Central and South America, Northern Africa, the Middle East, India and China cause a localized, ulcerating disorder skin disease. This also known as "oriental sore" or "tropical sore". It is a relatively mild, localized disease producing ulcers on exposed skin.

MORPHOLOGY

Localized cutaneous leishmaniasis begins as a papule surrounded by induration. It changes into a shallow and slowly expanding ulcer, usually with heaped-up borders. It usually heals by involution within 6–18 months without treatment.

Microscopically, the macrophages show amastigotes. These amastigotes are oval and measure 2 µm. They contain two internal structures, a nucleus and a kinetoplast. Amastigotes in macrophages appear as multiple regular cytoplasmic dots, **LD bodies (Fig. 103)**. As the cell-mediated immunity develops, the macrophages are activated and they kill the intracellular parasites. The lesion slowly shows granulomatous inflammation (epithelioid macrophages, Langhans giant cells, plasma cells and lymphocytes) usually with few parasites. Over the course of months, the cutaneous ulcer heals spontaneously.

Clinical features: Cutaneous leishmaniasis begins as an itching, solitary papule. This erodes to form a shallow ulcer with a sharp, raised border. The ulcer can grow to 6–8 cm in diameter. Satellite lesions develop along the course of draining

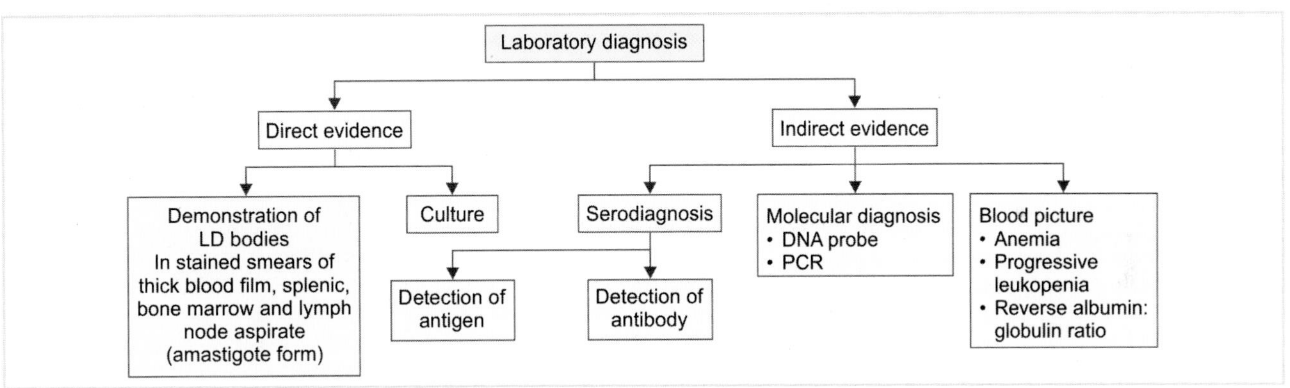

FLOWCHART 4: Laboratory diagnosis of kala-azar.

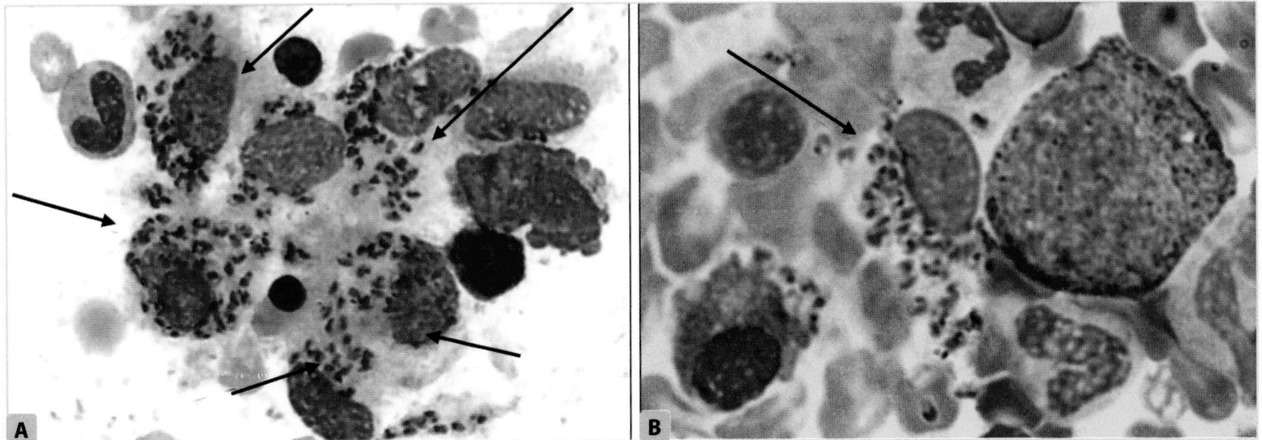

FIGS. 103A AND B: Leishman stain of a macrophage with *Leishmania donovani* (LD bodies) parasites (arrow) in the bone marrow aspiration.

lymphatics. The ulcers usually begin to resolve at 3–6 months. However, healing may take a year or longer.

Mucocutaneous leishmaniasis

Mucocutaneous leishmaniasis is found only in the New World and most cases occur in Central and South America, where rodents and sloths are reservoirs. It is caused by infection with *L. braziliensis* and is a late complication of cutaneous leishmaniasis.

MORPHOLOGY

The early course and pathological changes are like those of localized cutaneous leishmaniasis. A solitary ulcer occurs, expands and resolves. Years later, moist, ulcerating, or nonulcerating lesions develop at a mucocutaneous junction, such as the nasopharyngeal area, nasal septum, larynx, anus or vulva. The mucosal lesions may slowly progress to highly destructive and disfiguring lesions. They may erode mucosal surfaces and cartilage. Sometimes, destruction of the nasal septum can produce a "tapir nose" deformity. The patient may die if the ulcers obstruct the airways.

Microscopy: It shows a mixed inflammatory infiltrate composed of parasite-containing macrophages with lymphocytes and plasma cells. Later, the tissue inflammatory response becomes granulomatous, and the number of parasites in the macrophages decreases. The lesions heal and form scar. But, reactivation may occur after long intervals.

Diffuse cutaneous leishmaniasis

It is a rare form of dermal infection. It is found in Ethiopia and adjacent East Africa and in Central and South America. It can develop in few patients who lack specific cell-mediated immune responses to leishmaniae.

MORPHOLOGY

Diffuse cutaneous leishmaniasis begins as a single skin nodule, which slowly continues to spread by formation of adjacent satellite nodules. Ultimately the entire body is covered by nodular lesions. These lesions resemble lepromatous leprosy. Microscopically, they contain aggregates of foamy macrophages filled with *Leishmania* organisms.

African Trypanosomiasis

Q. Write short essay on trypanosomiasis.

African trypanosomes are kinetoplastid parasites, i.e., they contain a large mass of DNA called *kinetoplast* that proliferates as extracellular forms in the blood. They are curved flagellates, 15–30 µm in length. They can be demonstrated in blood or cerebrospinal fluid. However, they are difficult to find in infected tissues. They cause **African** trypanosomiasis, popularly termed as **sleeping sickness. They cause sustained or intermittent fevers, lymphadenopathy, splenomegaly, progressive brain dysfunction (sleeping sickness)** due to meningoencephalitis, **cachexia, and death.** It may be due to infection with hemoflagellate protozoa namely *Trypanosoma brucei gambiense* or *Trypanosoma brucei rhodesiense.*

Mode of transmission: It is transmitted by several species of blood-sucking tsetse flies of the genus *Glossina.*

Source/reservoir of infection: Tsetse flies transmit African *Trypanosoma* to humans either **from wild and domestic animals** *(T. brucei rhodesiense)* **or from other humans** *(T. brucei gambiense).* Natural reservoirs of *T. brucei rhodesiense* include antelope, other game animals and domestic cattle.

- *T. brucei rhodesiense* infection (Rhodesian trypanosomiasis) occurs in East Africa and is usually acute rapidly progressive, virulent that kills the patient in 3–6 months. It is a zoonotic infection and can be controlled by reducing infected fly (vector) populations.
- *T. brucei gambiense* infection (Gambian trypanosomiasis) occurs in West Africa spreads from human to human via fly bites. Gambian trypanosomiasis is a chronic infection usually lasts for more than a year. It needs active case detection and treatment.

Life Cycle (Fig. 104)

While the tsetse fly bites an infected animal or human, it ingests trypomastigotes with the blood. Within the fly, the trypomastigotes parasites lose their coat of surface antigen and multiply in the stomach of the fly. Then they migrate to the salivary glands before developing into nondividing trypomastigotes. During another bite (next blood meal), trypomastigotes are injected into the lymphatics and blood vessels of a new host (humans and animals). They disseminate

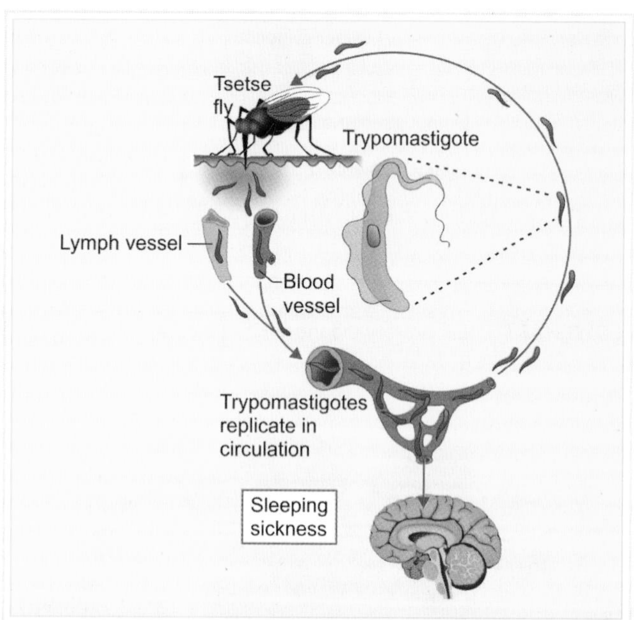

FIG. 104: African trypanosomiasis (sleeping sickness). When a tsetse fly bites an infected animal or human, it ingests trypomastigotes. In the fly, it multiplies into infective, trypomastigotes. When these flies bite a new host, these are injected into lymphatic and blood vessels. A primary chancre develops at the site of the bite. Trypomastigotes replicate further in the blood and lymph and produce a systemic infection. When another fly ingests trypomastigotes, the life cycle is completed. Invasion of the central nervous system by trypomastigotes leads to meningoencephalomyelitis.

to the bone marrow and tissue fluids. Some may invade the central nervous system (CNS). After replicating in blood, lymph and spinal fluid, trypomastigotes are ingested by another fly to complete the life cycle.

Pathogenesis

Normal mechanism of killing of parasite: African trypanosomes have a single, abundant, glycolipid-anchored protein covering called the **variant surface glycoprotein** (VSG). The parasites proliferate in the bloodstream and the host produces antibodies against VSG. These antibodies in association with phagocytes, destroy most of the parasites. This produces a spike of fever.

Escape of host immune response by parasites: A small number of trypanosome, however, evades immune attack by periodically undergoing a genetic rearrangement (genetically determined pattern and not by mutation). This produce a different glycoprotein antigen coat namely VSG on their surface, thereby escaping the host immune response. These successor trypanosomes multiply until the host produces a new anti-VSG response and kills most of them. Then another clone with a distinct VSG takes over. Thus, each wave of circulating trypomastigotes produces different antigenic variants. In this manner, African trypanosomes cause waves of fever before they finally invade the CNS. Trypanosomes have many *VSG* genes, only one of which is expressed at a time. The trypanosome uses an elegant mechanism to turn *VSG* genes on and off. *VSG* genes are found throughout the trypanosome genome. However, only *VSG* genes within bloodstream expression sites near the ends of chromosomes are transcribed. Periodically, new *VSG* genes move into these sites, chiefly by homologous recombination, generating a new VSG. A specialized RNA polymerase that transcribes *VSG* genes associates with only a single bloodstream expression site. Thus, it limits expression of one VSG at a time.

In African trypanosomiasis, immune complex formation may occur due to variable trypanosomal antigens and antibodies. Autoantibodies to antigens of erythrocytes, brain and heart may be involved in the pathogenesis.

MORPHOLOGY

Primary chancre: *T. brucei* multiplies at sites of inoculation and produce a localized, large, red, rubbery, nodular lesion at the site of the insect bite. This is termed "primary chancre." Microscopically, it shows numerous parasites surrounded by a dense, predominantly mononuclear, inflammatory infiltrate.

With chronicity, generalized involvement of lymph nodes and spleen becomes prominent. The lymph nodes and spleen enlarge due to infiltration by lymphocytes, plasma cells, and macrophages. The macrophages are filled with dead parasites.

Trypanosomes eventually localize to small blood vessels and concentrate in capillary loops (e.g., choroid plexus and glomeruli). When parasites breach the blood-brain barrier and invade the CNS, a leptomeningitis develops. This extends into the perivascular Virchow-Robin spaces, and produces a demyelinating panencephalitis. Plasma cells containing cytoplasmic globules filled with

Continued

Continued

termed as **Mott cells are frequently found**. Chronic disease leads to progressive cachexia.

Vasculitis: Lesions in the lymph nodes, brain, and various other sites (including the inoculation site) show vasculitis of small blood vessels. The vessels show endothelial cell hyperplasia and dense perivascular infiltrates of lymphocytes, macrophages and plasma cells. The vasculitis in CNS causes destruction of neurons, demyelination and gliosis.

Clinical features: Clinically, African trypanosomiasis is divided into three stages:

1. **Primary chancre:** It develops after 5–15 days of fly bite at the inoculation site. It appears as a papillary swelling topped by a central red spot and measures 3–4 cm in diameter. It usually subsides spontaneously within 3 weeks.
2. **Systemic infection:** Within 3 weeks of a fly bite, dissemination into the bloodstream is marked by intermittent fever, for up to a week. It is usually accompanied by splenomegaly and local and generalized lymphadenopathy. There is usually remitting irregular fevers, headache, joint pains, lethargy and muscle wasting.
3. **Brain invasion:** Invasion of CNS may occur early (weeks or months) in Rhodesian trypanosomiasis or late (months or years) in the Gambian trypanosomiasis. It is characterized by apathy, daytime somnolence and sometimes coma.

Diagnosis: Microscopic examination of blood smears (**Fig. 105**), lymph node, or chancre is used for the diagnosis. Cerebrospinal fluid should be examined to determine whether there is infection of the CNS.

Chagas Disease (American Trypanosomiasis)

***Trypanosoma cruzi* is a kinetoplastid, intracellular protozoan parasite. It causes American trypanosomiasis (Chagas disease).** Chagas disease is an insect-borne, zoonotic infection caused by *T. cruzi* and causes a systemic infection of humans. Acute manifestations and long-term sequelae are observed in the heart and gastrointestinal tract.

Mode of transmission: *T. cruzi* infection is endemic in wild and domesticated animals (e.g., rats, dogs, goats, cats, armadillos) in Central and South America (particularly Brazil).

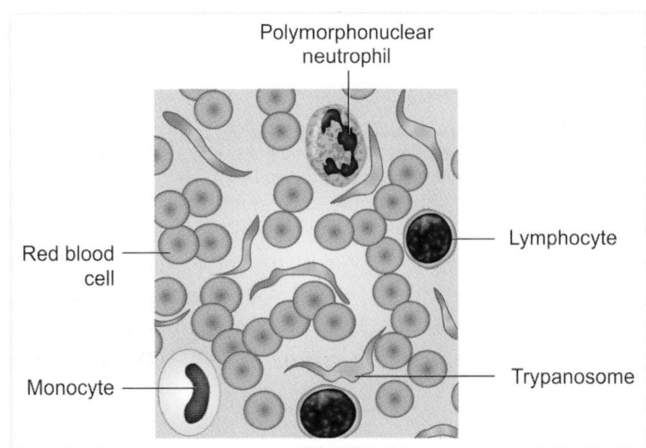

FIG. 105: *Trypanosoma rhodesiense* in blood smear (diagrammatic).

- **Through triatomine bugs:** The parasites are transmitted between animals and to humans by triatomine bugs (also known as kissing bugs or reduviids). These bugs hide in the cracks of loosely constructed houses. The bugs move out at night and feed on sleeping inhabitants (victims) and pass the parasites in feces. Infection is promoted by contact between humans and infected bugs. This usually occurs in mud or thatched dwellings of the rural and suburban poor. The infectious parasites enter the new host through damaged skin or through mucous membranes. At the site of skin entry of parasite, there may be formation of a transient, erythematous nodule.
- **Oral ingestion of the parasites:** This is another important route of infection is of the parasites. Ingestion occurs through contaminated food products with triatomine bugs and/or their feces.
- **Congenital infection:** It occurs with the passage of the parasite from mother to fetus.
- **Other modes of infection:** These include receipt of infected blood products and organ transplantation.

Habitat and morphological forms (Figs. 106A to C)

- *In humans, T. cruzi* exists in both *amastigote* and *trypomastigote* forms: Amastigotes are the intracellular parasites. They are found in muscular tissue (e.g., cardiac muscle), nervous tissue and reticuloendothelial system. Trypomastigotes are found in the peripheral blood.
- In *reduviid bugs,* epimastigote forms are found in the midgut and metacyclic trypomastigote forms are present in hindgut and feces.

Life cycle (Fig. 107): Infective forms of *T. cruzi* are passed in the feces of the reduviid bug as it takes its blood meal from the host. Contamination of the wound is promoted by itching and scratching at that site.

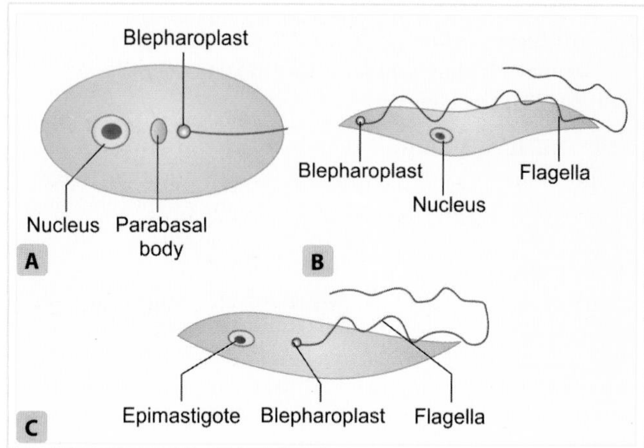

FIGS. 106A TO C: *Trypanosoma cruzi.* (A) Amastigote; (B) Trypomastigote; and (C) Epimastigote.

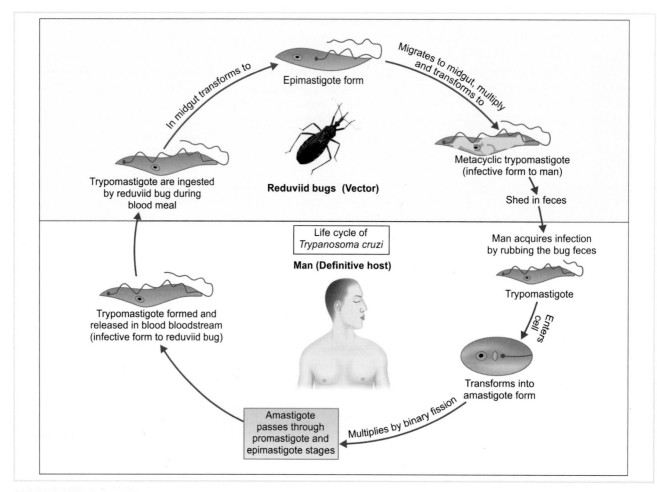

FIG. 107: Life cycle of *Trypanosoma cruzi.*

- The trypomastigotes penetrate at the site of the bite or at other abrasions, or enter the mucosa of the eyes or lips.
- Once they enter inside the body, the trypomastigotes (refer **Fig. 106**) lose their flagella and undulating membranes. They are round and become amastigotes (refer **Fig. 106A**) and enter macrophages.
- Inside the macrophages, the amastigote undergoes repeated divisions.
- Amastigotes also invade other sites such as cardiac myocytes and brain.
- Within host cells, amastigotes differentiate into trypomastigotes (refer **Fig. 106B**). They break out of the host cells and enter the bloodstream.
- These trypomastigotes are ingested in a subsequent bite of a reduviid bug.
- The trypomastigotes multiply in the alimentary tract of reduviid bug and are discharged in the feces.

Pathogenesis

- **Glycoprotein of parasite interacts with ligands of host involved in invasion:** *T. cruzi* has glycosylphosphatidylinositol anchored glycoprotein on their surface. They interact with multiple ligands (e.g., laminin, fibronectin, collagen, cytokeratin, and other extracellular proteins) in the host cells that are involved in cell adhesion and invasion.
- **Factors favoring survival in the phagolysosome:** After ingestion into macrophages, most intracellular pathogens avoid the toxic contents of lysosomes. However, for the intracellular development of amastigotes of *T. cruzi*, it actually needs a brief exposure to the acidic phagolysosome. To ensure exposure to lysosomes, *T. cruzi* trypomastigotes raise the concentration of calcium in the cytoplasm of the host cells. Increased intracytoplasmic calcium promotes fusion of the phagosome and lysosome. The low pH of the lysosome activates pore-forming proteins that destroy the lysosomal membrane and release the parasite into the cytoplasm of cell. This also enhances the development of amastigote.
- **Destruction of host cells and entry into the blood stream:** Parasites reproduce as rounded amastigotes in the cytoplasm of host cells. Then they develop flagella and destroy the host cells. These released parasites enter the bloodstream. They penetrate smooth, skeletal, and heart muscles. *T. cruzii* evades the complement system activation by expressing complement regulatory proteins.

Acute Chagas disease

Chagas disease mainly affects the heart. In endemic regions it is a major cause of sudden death due to cardiac arrhythmia. *T. cruzi* infects and reproduces in the host cells at sites of inoculation. There they form localized nodular inflammatory lesions called as **chagomas**. The parasite then disseminates throughout the body via the bloodstream. *T. cruzi* circulates in the blood as a 20 μm long, curved flagellate. They can be easily recognized on blood films. Within infected cells, it reproduces as a nonflagellated amastigote measuring 2–4 μm in diameter. Acute Chagas disease is mild in most patients. The cardiac damage is due to the direct invasion of myocardial cells by the parasite as well as the subsequent inflammation. Rarely, acute Chagas disease develops with high parasitemia, fever, or progressive cardiac enlargement, dilation and failure, usually with generalized lymphadenopathy or splenomegaly.

MORPHOLOGY

Acute myocarditis: In fatal cases**,** the changes are diffuse throughout the heart. The heart is pale and myocardium shows focal hemorrhage. Microscopically, many parasites are seen in the heart. Clusters of amastigotes cause swelling of individual myocardial fibers and create intracellular pseudocysts in myofibers. There is focal necrosis of myocardial cell. This is associated with extensive, dense, acute interstitial inflammatory infiltration throughout the myocardium. This is usually associated with dilation of the four-chamber heart.

Clinical features: Symptoms in acute Chagas disease develop 1–2 weeks after inoculation with *T. cruzi.* A chagoma develops at the site of infection. Parasitemia appears 2–3 weeks after inoculation. Acute Chagas disease is usually associated with a mild illness characterized by fever, malaise, lymphadenopathy, and hepatosplenomegaly. Systemic symptoms of acute Chagas disease are due to parasitemia and widespread cellular infection. Predominant target cells affected in acute Chagas disease depends on the strains of *T. cruzi*. Infections of cardiac myocytes, gastrointestinal ganglion cells and meninges are the causes of most significant disease. The disease can be fatal when there is extensive myocardial or involvement of meninges. With the onset of cell-mediated immunity, the acute manifestations subside, but chronic tissue damage may continue. Progressive destruction of cells at sites of infection especially those of the heart, esophagus and colon, leads to organ dysfunction and may manifest decades after the acute infection.

Chronic Chagas Disease

The most frequent and most serious consequences of *T. cruzi* infection develop in 20–40% of individual in 5–15 years after initial acute infection. In this phase of the disease, *T. cruzi* is no longer found in blood or tissue. However, the infected tissue become damaged due to chronic, progressive inflammation. It mainly affects the heart and gastrointestinal tract.

Chronic myocarditis

In endemic regions, chronic Chagas disease is a main cause of heart failure in young adults.

Mechanism of cardiac damage in chronic Chagas disease

- **Persistent inflammation:** The presence of persistent *T. cruzi* parasites leads to a continued immune response. Though there are usually only few parasites seen, there is chronic inflammatory infiltration of the myocardium.
- **Autoimmune response:** The parasite may also induce autoimmune responses. The antibodies and T cells recognize parasite proteins cross-react with host myocardial cells, nerve cells, and extracellular proteins (e.g., laminin). Thus, cross-reactive antibodies may induce electrophysiologic dysfunction of the heart.

MORPHOLOGY

Heart in chronic Chagas disease

It is characterized by: (1) a dilated, rounded heart with increased in size and weight, (2) prominent right ventricular outflow tract and (3) dilation of the valve rings. The interventricular septum is usually deviated to the right and this may cause immobilization of the adjacent tricuspid leaflet. Usually, mural thrombi are observed in about one-half of autopsy cases. These thrombi might lead to pulmonary or systemic emboli or infarctions. Chronic Chagas cardiomyopathy requires cardiac transplantation.

Microscopy: It shows interstitial and perivascular inflammatory infiltrates composed of lymphocytes, plasma cells, and monocytes. There are also foci of myocardial cell necrosis, extensive interstitial fibrosis hypertrophy of myofibers. This is especially found toward the apex of the left ventricle and may lead to and aneurysmal dilation and thinning. Fibrosis and inflammation also involves the cardiac conduction system. Damage to myocardial cells and to conductance pathways causes a dilated cardiomyopathy. Progressive cardiac fibrosis causes arrhythmias or congestive heart failure.

Gastrointestinal tract

Damage to the myenteric plexus causes dilation of the esophagus (megaesophagus) and colon (megacolon). Even with dilation of the esophagus and colon, parasites cannot be found within ganglia of the myenteric plexus. Gastrointestinal involvement is particularly common in endemic areas such as Brazil, where as many as 50% of the patients with lethal carditis have also colonic and esophageal disease.

Megaesophagus It is dilation of the esophagus and is common in chronic Chagas disease. It is caused by failure of the lower esophageal sphincter (achalasia) due to destruction of parasympathetic ganglia in the wall of the lower esophagus. It produces difficulty in swallowing and may be so severe that the patient can consume only liquids.

Megacolon It is characterized by massive dilation of the large bowel due to destruction of the myenteric plexus of the colon. Patient develops severe constipation due to progressive aganglionosis of the colon.

Congenital Chagas disease

It occurs in fetus or infants of pregnant women with parasitemia. Infection of the placenta and fetus may lead to spontaneous abortion. Even if there are live births, the infants die of encephalitis within a few days or weeks.

Diagnosis: It is done by examination of blood smear examination in the acute case and more commonly by serology.

Toxoplasmosis

Q. Write short essay on toxoplasmosis

Toxoplasmosis is a worldwide infectious disease caused by a **ubiquitous, parasitic protozoa *T. gondii*. Most infections are asymptomatic** (millions of individuals carry the *T. gondii* without symptoms due to control by their immune systems). But ***T. gondii*** **causes significant** devastating necrotizing **disease in the immunocompromised and in pregnant women and their offspring.**

Mode of infection: In the tropics, infection is generally acquired in childhood. Various modes of **acquiring infection in humans** are as follows:

- **Ingestion:** *T. gondii* infection can occur due to ingestion and include the following:
    - By eating uncooked or undercooked meat (particularly pork, lamb, venison) contaminated with the tissue cysts, or
    - By ingestion of mature oocysts through contaminated food, water or fingers contaminated with cat feces directly or indirectly or handling contaminated soil.
- **Vertical transmission:** Intrauterine infection from mother to fetus (*congenital toxoplasmosis*) during pregnancy.
- **Blood transfusion or organ transplantation**: From infected donors is very rare.

MORPHOLOGY

Trophozoites

Toxoplasma gondii has only two morphologic forms (stages) of trophozoites seen in human tissue, **tachyzoites and bradyzoites.** Both are crescent shaped and measure 2 × 6 μm.

- **Tachyzoites (Fig. 108A):** These are actively multiplying and crescent-shaped and range in size from 3 to 7 μm by 2 to 4 μm. One end of the organism usually appears more rounded than the other end. Each tachyzoite has a single centrally located nucleus, surrounded by a cell membrane.
- **Bradyzoites (Fig. 108B):** Basically, it has the same physical appearance as the tachyzoite but is smaller. These are slow-growing viable forms. They form clusters or groups inside a host cell, develop a surrounding membrane, and form a cyst in a variety of host tissues and muscles outside the intestinal tract. These cysts may contain fifty to several thousand bradyzoites. A typical cyst measures from 12 to 100 μm in diameter.

Oocyst (Fig. 108C)

The infective form of *T. gondii* for humans is the oocyst. The oocyst contains two sporocysts, each with four sporozoites. Oocyst is bordered by a clear, colorless, two-layered cell wall.

Life Cycle in Humans (Fig. 109)

Host: *T. gondii* completes its life cycle in two hosts.

1. **Definitive hosts:** Cats and other felines, in which both sexual and asexual cycles take place. The only final host is the cat. It becomes infected by ingesting toxoplasma cysts in tissues of an infected mouse or other intermediate host. In the intestinal epithelium of infected cat, five multiplicative stages take place and they excrete unsporulated oocysts. Oocysts sporulate in feces and soil (in the environment) and differentiate into sporocysts. These sporocysts contain sporozoites. The cat is the only definitive (final) host, and humans are a dead-end host.
2. **Intermediate hosts:** Man and other mammals, in which only the asexual cycle takes place. When these sporocysts containing sporozoites are ingested by intermediate

hosts (e.g., birds, mice/rodents or humans), they develop in the intermediate host to complete the life cycle of the parasite.

Life cycle of *Toxoplasma gondii* is presented in **Fig. 109**.

Pathogenesis

Toxoplasma gondii is an intracellular pathogen and can invade and infect any nucleated cell. This invasion is brought about by a unique form of actin-myosin moving junction and by forming a parasitophorous vacuole (PV) protected from lysosomal fusion. *T. gondii* also inhibits autophagy of the parasite-containing vacuole, thereby avoid clearance of the tachyzoites.

Types of infections

Acute phase of infection

- After ingestion of the oocysts, sporozoites are released from oocysts. These sporozoites invade the human intestinal epithelium, disseminating throughout the body.
- The sporozoites transform into tachyzoites that localize to tissues. The tachyzoite form is responsible for the tissue damage and initial infection.
- Tachyzoites multiply rapidly within intracellular vacuoles of parasitized cells and form "groups." Eventually these parasitized cells rupture. The released tachyzoites spread from the gut to a number of tissues and organs. Thus, it

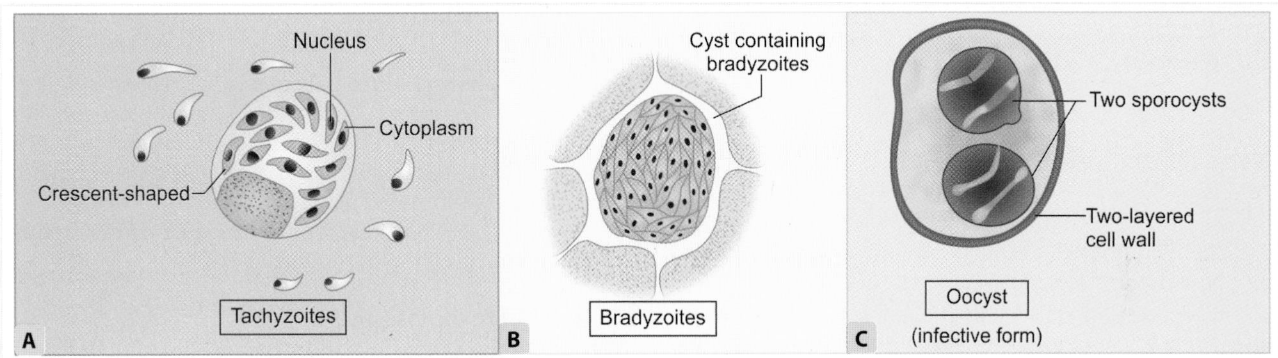

FIGS. 108A TO C: *Toxoplasma gondii.* (A) Crescentic tachyzoites-extracellular trophozoites and intracellular form within macrophage; (B) Thick-walled tissue cyst containing rounded forms bradyzoites; and (C) Oocyst containing two sporocysts with sporozoites inside.

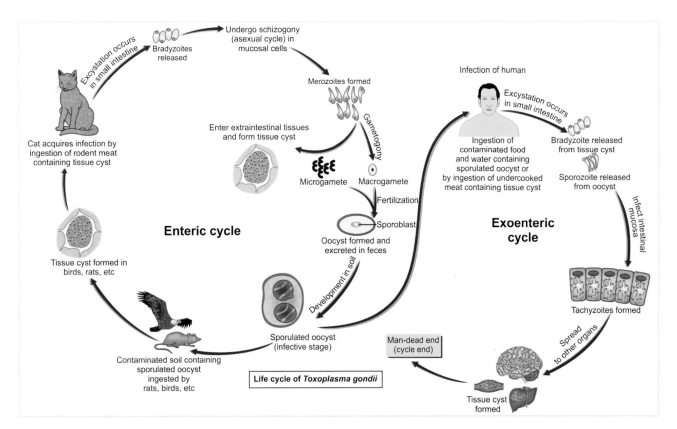

FIG. 109: Life cycle of *Toxoplasma gondii*.

migrates through lymphatics to regional lymph nodes, and through the blood to the liver, lungs, heart, brain and other organs. There they form tissue cysts filled with bradyzoites (**Fig. 108B**).

- Usually active infection is terminated by the development of cell-mediated immune responses. In most of the infections by *T. gondii,* there is no significant tissue destruction before the immune response develops. After the immune response, the active phase of the infection is brought under control, and those infected develop only few clinical effects.
- ***Toxoplasma* lymphadenopathy** occurs in immunocompetent persons. Lymphadenopathy is the most common (about 10–20% of patient) manifestation of *T. gondii* infection in immunocompetent hosts.

MORPHOLOGY

Patients usually present with nontender enlargement of regional lymph node. Any lymph node group may be involved, but usually enlarged cervical nodes are readily apparent. Sometimes, lymphadenopathy is accompanied by fever, sore throat, hepatosplenomegaly and circulating atypical lymphocytes. Rarely, hepatitis, myocarditis, and myositis may also accompany.

Microscopically, the affected lymph nodes have a distinctive appearance. They show numerous epithelioid macrophages surrounding and encroaching on reactive germinal centers. Lymphadenopathy usually resolves spontaneously in several weeks to several months, and treatment is seldom needed.

- Apart from swollen lymph nodes, these patients may present with muscle aches. They usually have a benign, self-limited course of weeks to months. This is followed by establishment of a latent infection by forming dormant tissue cysts in some infected cells. These tissue cysts survive for decades in host cells.
- The dormant bradyzoites inside the cyst may be reactivated following immunosuppression (if an infected individual loses cell-mediated immunity), such as after organ transplantation or in HIV infection. The bradyzoites can emerge from its encysted form. This causes renewal or re-establishment of a destructive infection in the host. Human infection is a dead end for the parasite.

Chronic infection

In chronic infection, the parasite is in the form of "bradyzoites," and it multiplies slowly. The bradyzoites store PAS positive material, and hundreds of parasites are tightly packed in "cysts". The cysts arise from intracellular vacuoles and when they enlarge beyond the usual size of the cell, they push the nucleus to the periphery. The **slowly** multiplying parasites within the cyst are called ***bradyzoites.***

***Toxoplasma* encephalitis:** It occurs due to reactivation of a latent infection. ***Toxoplasma* encephalitis** is the most common opportunistic pathogen of the CNS in in immunocompromised hosts especially in AIDS patients or those receiving immunosuppressive therapy.

Others: Myocarditis and pneumonitis are other common manifestations in AIDS patients.

MORPHOLOGY

***Toxoplasma* form cysts in skeletal muscle, myocardium, visceral organs, brain, and eyes.** Diagnosis is usually by serological tests. But cysts may be observed in biopsies (**Fig. 110**), or **tachyzoites** may be observed in stained fluid specimens (e.g., bronchoalveolar lavage fluid from an immunocompromised host). Tachyzoites may be detected by stains such as periodic acid-Schiff, Giemsa, or hematoxylin and eosin stains. Tissue cysts may vary in size from 5 to 100 µm. Intact cysts can remain for the life of the host without producing any inflammatory reaction. The wall of the cyst is thin and contains crescent-shaped bradyzoites of about 1.5 × 7 µm.

***Toxoplasma* encephalitis:** Infection with *T. gondii* produces a multifocal necrotizing encephalitis. Clinically, encephalitis may present with paresis, seizures, alterations in visual acuity and changes in mentation. *Toxoplasma* encephalitis in immunocompromised patients is fatal if not treated.

Polymerase chain reaction of blood or cerebrospinal fluid is a sensitive method for diagnosis.

Congenital toxoplasmosis

The symptoms of congenital toxoplasmosis may not be evident for months or many years after birth. *T. gondii* infection in a fetus is more destructive than postnatal infection. The fetus does not have the immunologic capacity to contain *T. gondii* infection. Prompt diagnosis and treatment at birth may reduce the sequelae.

MORPHOLOGY

Congenital toxoplasmosis can result in fetal death and abortion, or hydrocephalus, microcephaly, cerebral calcifications, neurocognitive deficits, and chorioretinitis. Congenital *toxoplasma* infections mainly affect the developing brain and eye.

Continued

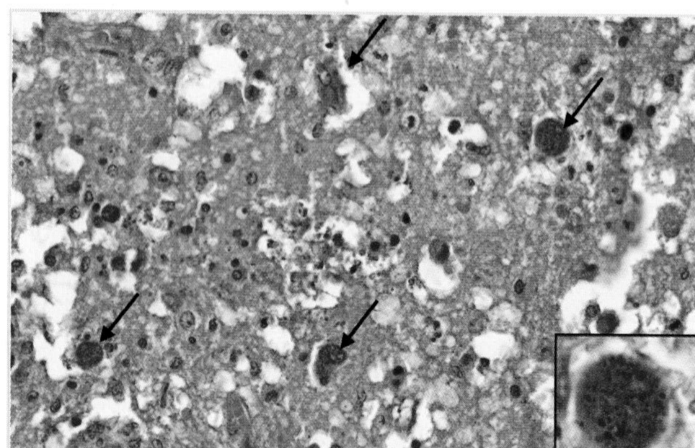

FIG. 110: A brain biopsy showing multiple cysts of bradyzoites of *Toxoplasma gondii (arrows)*. Right lower inset showing an enlarged cyst containing numerous bradyzoites.

Continued

Brain: In the congenital toxoplasmosis, brain involvement leads to a necrotizing meningoencephalitis. This if severe may cause loss of brain parenchyma, cerebral calcifications, and marked hydrocephalus.

Eye: In the eye, it can produce bilateral chorioretinitis (i.e., necrosis and inflammation of the choroid and retina). In contrast, in acquired ocular toxoplasmosis, chorioretinitis is usually unilateral.

Clinical features: If infection occurs early in pregnancy, it produces most severe fetal disease and usually leads to spontaneous abortion. In infants born with congenital toxoplasmosis, the brain involvement may produce severe mental retardation, seizures or psychomotor defects. Ocular involvement may cause congenital visual impairment. Latent ocular infection in utero may lead to visual loss later in life. Some newborns may develop *Toxoplasma* hepatitis characterized by large areas of necrosis associated with giant cells. Occasionally, adrenal necrosis may be seen.

Cryptosporidiosis

Cryptosporidia is protozoa of the genus *Cryptosporidium*. Humans can be infected by several different *Cryptosporidium* species, but two species of *Cryptosporidium* that usually cause human infections are C. *hominis* and *C. parvum*. Cryptosporidiosis was first discovered in the 1980s as an agent of chronic diarrhea in patients with AIDS patients. Now, it is recognized as a cause of acute, self-limited disease even in immunologically normal hosts. Cryptosporidiosis also causes persistent diarrhea in under-resourced countries. *Cryptosporidiosis* is an enteric infection due to Cryptosporidium. The infection ranges from a self-limited gastrointestinal infection to a potentially life-threatening illness. All can undergo entire life cycle (with asexual and sexual reproductive phases) in a single host.

Source of infection: *Cryptosporidium* oocysts are shed in feces of infected humans and animals. Many domesticated animals harbor the parasite and acts as a reservoir for human infection. The oocysts are killed by freezing. Oocysts are resistant to chlorine. Hence, they may persist in treated, but unfiltered, water. Contaminated drinking water continues to be the most common source of infection.

Mode of infection: It is acquired by ingestion of *Cryptosporidium* oocysts. Most infections probably result from person-to-person transmission. Contaminated drinking water is the most common mode of infection. Like giardiasis, cryptosporidiosis can spread to water sport participants. Food-borne infection is less frequent. *C. parvum* inhabits the small intestine. It may also be found in stomach, appendix, colon, rectum and pulmonary tree.

MORPHOLOGY

Oocyst (Figs. 111A and B): *Cryptosporidium* oocyst is the **infective form** of the parasite. The oocyst **is spherical** or oval and measures 4–6 μm in diameter. Oocysts are not always visible and do not stain with iodine. It is **acid-fast.** The mature oocyst consists of four small crescent-shaped sporozoites surrounded by a thick cell wall. But in 20% cases, wall may be thin. These thin-walled oocysts are responsible for autoinfection.

Schizonts and gametocytes: The other morphological forms needed to complete the life cycle of *Cryptosporidium* include schizonts containing four to eight merozoites, microgametocytes, and macrogametocytes. These morphological forms are not routinely seen in patient samples.

Organisms are typically most concentrated in the terminal ileum and proximal colon, but can be present throughout the gut, biliary tract, and even the respiratory tract of immunodeficient hosts. Diagnosis is based on finding oocysts in the stool.

Pathogenesis: Once ingested, as few as 10 encysted *Cryptosporidium* oocytes are enough to cause symptomatic infection. *Cryptosporidium* oocysts survive passage through the stomach and crescent-shaped sporozoites present are released following protease activation by gastric acid. The sporozoites are motile and have a specialized organelle that attaches to the brush border (microvillous surface) of the small bowel. This produces changes in the enterocyte cytoskeleton and induces the enterocyte to engulf the parasite and then it resides in an endocytic vacuole. They reproduce on the luminal surface of the gut, from stomach to rectum and form progeny that also attach to the epithelium of the gut. In immunocompetent individuals, immune responses terminate the infection. The parasite cannot be contained in patients with AIDS and in congenital immunodeficiencies. Hence, they develop chronic infections, which may spread from the bowel to involve the gallbladder and intrahepatic bile ducts. It may cause sodium malabsorption, chloride secretion, and increased tight junction permeability. These changes cause the nonbloody, watery diarrhea.

MORPHOLOGY

No grossly visible changes are observed in Cryptosporidiosis.

Microscopy: Mucosal changes are usually minimal. But persistent cryptosporidiosis in children and heavy infection in immunosuppressed patients can produce atrophy of intestinal villi, hyperplasia of crypts, and moderate or severe

Continued

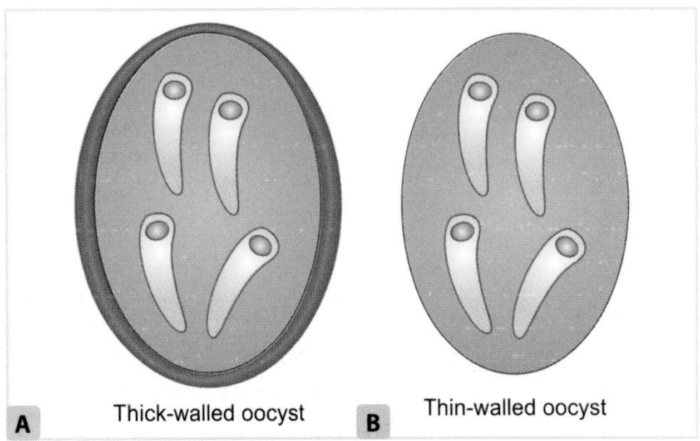

FIGS. 111A AND B: Oocysts of *Cryptosporidium parvum*. (A) Thick-walled oocyst; and (B) Thin-walled oocyst.

Continued

chronic inflammation in the lamina propria. These changes are directly related to the density of the parasites. The organisms are visible microscopically. Though the sporozoite is intracellular, it appears to sit on top of the epithelial apical membrane. The parasites appear as round, 2–4 μm blebs attached to the luminal surface of the epithelium. The colon shows chronic active colitis, with minimal disruption of architecture.

Clinical features: Clinically cryptosporidiosis presents as a profuse, watery diarrhea. Sometimes it may be accompanied by cramping abdominal pain or low-grade fever. Intensive fluid replacement is required when the volumes of fluid loss as diarrhea is heavy. In immunologically competent patients, diarrhea resolves spontaneously within 1–2 weeks. In immunocompromised individuals, diarrhea persists indefinitely and may lead to death.

Giardiasis

Giardia lamblia is a flagellated protozoan also referred to as *G. duodenalis* or *G. intestinalis.* It was initially described by Dutch scientist Antonie van Leeuwenhoek (the inventor of the microscope) in his own stool. *Giardia lamblia* causes infection of the small intestine known as giardiasis. It is characterized by abdominal cramping and diarrhea.

Epidemiology: *G. lamblia* has a worldwide distribution and it is the most common parasitic pathogen in humans. It is prevalent in warmer climates and crowded, unsanitary environments. Children are more susceptible than adults.

MORPHOLOGY

***Giardia lamblia* has two stages:** Trophozoites and cysts. The stools usually contain only cysts, but trophozoites may also be present in patients with diarrhea.

Trophozoites (Figs. 112A and B): They are flat, pear shaped (shape of a tennis racket/***heart shaped*/or *pyriform-shaped***), binucleate organisms with four pairs of flagella. They are rounded anteriorly and pointed posteriorly.

Continued

Continued

They are most numerous in the duodenum and proximal small intestine. A curved (concave), disk-like "sucker plate/disk" on their ventral surface which helps in its attachment to the intestinal mucosa.

Cysts (Fig. 112C): These are the infective forms of the parasite. The cysts are small and oval and they are surrounded by a hyaline cyst wall. Its internal structure includes two pairs of nuclei grouped at one end. A young cyst contains one pair of nuclei. The axostyle lies diagonally, forming a dividing line within cyst wall.

Source of infection: Infectious cysts are shed in the feces of infected humans and animals. These cysts are stable and resistant to chlorine. Thus, *Giardia* species are endemic in regions where there are unfiltered public water supplies. They are also common in rural streams (narrow rivers) during holiday camps who use these as a water source.

Mode of infection: Giardiasis is acquired by ingesting infectious cyst forms of the organism. Infection may occur after ingestion of as few as 10 cysts. Infection spreads directly from person to person and also in fecally contaminated water or food. *Giardia* can be acquired from wilderness water sources, where infected animals [e.g., beavers (large semiaquatic broad-tailed rodent native to North America), bears] act as the reservoir of infection. Infection may be epidemic, and outbreaks may occur in orphanages and institutions. Rarely, it may occur after accidental swallowing while swimming in contaminated water.

Pathogenesis: Ingested *Giardia* cysts contain 2 or 4 nuclei. These cysts survive gastric acidity and rupture in the duodenum and jejunum to release trophozoites. These trophozoites cause decreased expression of brush-border enzymes, produce microvillous damage, and apoptosis of small intestinal epithelial cells. They attach to small bowel epithelial microvilli and reproduce. For the clearance of *Giardia* infections, secretory IgA and mucosal IL-6 responses are important. Hence, it usually severely affects immunosuppressed, agammaglobulinemic, or malnourished individuals. *Giardia* can evade immune clearance through continuous modification of the major surface antigen, variant surface protein. It can persist for months or years, causing intermittent symptoms.

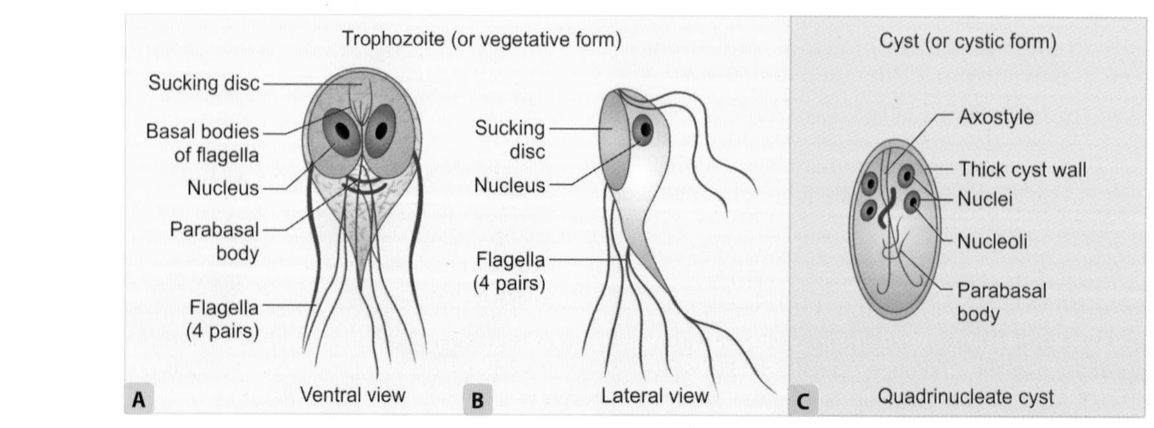

FIGS. 112A TO C: Stages of *Giardia lamblia*. Trophozoite—(A) Ventral view; (B) Lateral view: and (C) Quadrinucleate cyst.

MORPHOLOGY

Intestine

Gross: Giardiasis does not produce grossly visible changes.

Microscopy: It shows minimal mucosal changes. *Giardia* trophozoites can be found in duodenal biopsies on villous surfaces and within crypts. *Giardia* trophozoites can be identified based on their characteristic appearance. These include crescentic or pear or semilunar-shape and the presence of two equally sized nuclei. Though there may be large numbers of trophozoites, some of which are tightly bound to the brush border of villous enterocytes, there is no invasion, and small intestinal morphology may be normal. Heavy infections may be accompanied by villous blunting, increased numbers of intraepithelial lymphocytes and mixed lamina propria inflammatory infiltrates.

Clinical features: *G. lamblia* is usually a harmless commensal and giardiasis may be subclinical. But can cause acute or chronic diarrhea, malabsorption, and weight loss.

- **Acute giardiasis:** It presents with sudden onset of abdominal cramps frequently accompanied by foul smelling stools. The infection is highly variable. In some, symptoms resolve spontaneously within 1-4 weeks. Others may complain of persistent abdominal cramps and poorly formed stools for months.
- **Chronic giardiasis:** In children, chronic giardiasis may cause malabsorption, weight loss and growth retardation.

Diagnosis: Infection is usually diagnosed by examination of stool for cysts. The cysts in stool samples may also be detected by immunofluorescent technique.

Trichomonas Vaginalis

Trichomonas vaginalis is a pathogen that resides in the genital tract. It is the most common parasitic cause of sexually transmitted diseases (STDs). It was first detected by Donne in 1836 from the purulent genital discharge of a female. Though it is a eukaryote, its metabolism is similar to a primitive anaerobic bacterium. *Trichomonas vaginalis* commonly affects females than males.

MORPHOLOGY

It only exists in the trophozoite stage and there is no cystic stage.

Trophozoites (Fig. 113): It is pear (pyriform) shaped or ovoid, measures 10–30 μm in length and 5–10 μm in breadth. It has a short undulating membrane reaching up to the middle of the body. It has four anterior flagella and a fifth running along the outer margin of the undulating membrane and stops halfway down the side of the trophozoite. It doesn't come out free posteriorly. The undulating membrane is supported on to the surface of the parasite by a flexible rod like structure called as **costa**. A prominent ***axostyle*** runs throughout the length of the body and projects posteriorly like a tail. Trophozoite has a single nucleus. Trophozoites divide by *binary fission.* It is motile and shows characteristic rapid jerky or twitching type motility in saline mount preparation.

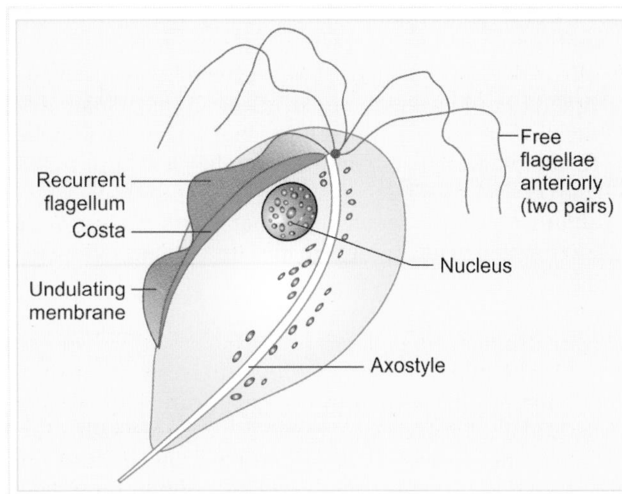

FIG.113: Diagrammatic representation of trophozoite of *Trichomonas vaginalis.*

Life cycle: Life cycle of *T. vaginalis* is completed in a *single* human *host* either male or female. There is no cystic stage and trophozoites represents both the infective and the diagnostic stage.

Mode of transmission: The trophozoite cannot survive outside and so infection is transmitted directly from person-to-person. **Sexual transmission** is the usual mode of infection. Trichomoniasis often coexists with other sexually transmitted diseases such as candidiasis, gonorrhea, syphilis, or human immunodeficiency virus (HIV). Neonates may get infected during the passage through vagina of infected mother during birth. Fomites such as towels have been implicated in transmission.

Incubation period: The incubation period is 4 days to 4 weeks and usually about 10 days.

Habitat: In females, it lives mainly in the vagina and cervix. It may also be found in Bartholin 's glands, urethra and urinary bladder. In males, it occurs mainly in the anterior urethra, but may also reside in seminal vesicle and prostate.

Pathogenesis: *Trichomonas vaginalis* particularly infects the squamous epithelium of vagina and secretes cysteine, proteases, adhesins, lactic acid and acetic acid. These secretions disrupt the glycogen levels and lower the pH of the vaginal fluid. Trophozoite are ***obligate parasites*** and cannot live without close association with the vaginal, urethral, or prostatic tissues. They do not invade the vaginal mucosa. Parasite produces petechial hemorrhage and mucosal capillary dilation ***(strawberry mucosa),*** metaplastic changes and desquamation of the vaginal epithelium. Intracellular edema and so-called *chicken-like epithelium* is the characteristic feature of trichomoniasis.

Clinical features: Infection by *Trichomonas vaginalis* can range from mild irritation to severe inflammation.

- **Males:** Infection is often asymptomatic, although some may develop urethritis, epididymitis and prostatitis.

- **Females:** It may produce severe itching in the genital area and presented as vulvovaginitis. This is characterized by offensive (foul smelling) yellowish green frothy discharge, dysuria, burning sensation with urination and dyspareunia. Rarely it is associated with complications such as pyosalpinx (pyosalpingitis), endometritis, infertility, low birth weight and cervical erosions.
- **Infants:** Rarely, neonatal pneumonia and conjunctivitis can develop in infants born to infected mothers.

Diagnosis

- Microscopic examination
  - **Wet (saline) mounting:** Fresh samples (within 10–20 minutes of collection) from vaginal or urethral discharge should be examined microscopically in saline wet mount preparation to demonstrate the characteristic jerky and twitching motility of the trophozoite and pus cells. In males, trophozoites may be found in urine or prostatic secretions.
  - **Permanent stain:** Fixed smears can be stained with acridine orange, Papanicolaou or Giemsa stains. Giemsa stain and Papanicolaou stain (**Fig. 114**) are routinely performed to demonstrate the morphology trophozoites.
  - **Direct fluorescent antibody:** Direct fluorescent antibody (DFA) is another method of detection of parasite and is more sensitive than the wet mount.
- **Culture:** Culture of clinical specimens in Johnson's and Trussel's medium is recommended when direct microscopy is negative. It is considered as a "gold standard" as well as the most sensitive (95%) method for the diagnosis of *T. vaginalis* infection.
- **Molecular diagnosis:** PCR on clinical specimens to detect *T. vaginalis* specific beta tubulin genes.

METAZOAL INFECTIONS

Metazoa are **multicellular, eukaryotic organisms having organ systems**. Metazoa live in many sites of the body, including the intestine, skin, lung, liver, muscle, blood vessels, and lymphatics. Parasitic metazoal infections are acquired by either consuming the parasite, usually in undercooked meat, or by direct invasion of the host through the skin or via insect bites. These infections are diagnosed by microscopic identification of larvae or ova in excretions or tissues, and by serological examination.

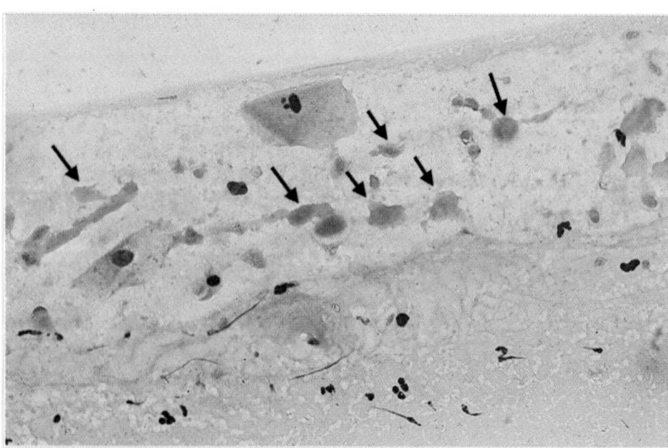

FIG. 114: Vaginal smear stained with Papanicolaou stain shows numerous trophozoites of Trichomonas *vaginalis* (arrows)

Helminthic infections: Helminths are among the **most common human pathogens**. Most of them that infect humans do little harm and are well adapted to human parasitism. They cause limited or no host tissue damage. However, some cause significant disease in humans. For example, schistosomiasis causes morbidity and mortality. Helminths are the largest and most complex organisms and are capable of living within the human body. Their adult forms of helminths range from 0.5 mm to over 1 m in length. Most can be seen by the naked eye. Helminths, or worms are ***multicellular*** (metazoa) ***bilaterally symmetrical*** parasites having three germ layers (*triploblastic metazoan*) and belong to the kingdom Metazoa.

- Helminths have differentiated tissues, including specialized nervous tissues, digestive tissues and reproductive systems. Their maturation from eggs or larvae to adult worms is complex process. It usually involves multiple morphologic transformations. Some helminths undergo metamorphoses in different hosts before becoming adult parasites. The human host supports this maturation process. Inside the human body, the helminths frequently migrate from the portal of entry into several organs and produce final infection.
- Helminths are acquired by ingestion, skin penetration or insect bites. Except two, they do not multiply in the human body, so a single parasite cannot cause an overwhelming infection. The two exceptions include: (1) *Strongyloides stercoralis* and (2) *Capillaria philippinensis*. These two can complete their life cycle and multiply within the human body.
- **Helminths cause disease in different ways**. These include:
  - Most parasites **cause dysfunction by producing destructive inflammatory and immunologic responses**. For example, morbidity in schistosomiasis is due to destructive helminthic infection that results from granulomatous responses to schistosome eggs deposited in tissue. **Basic proteins present in eosinophils** are **toxic to some helminths** and are a major component of inflammatory responses to these organisms.
  - Few compete with their human host for certain nutrients.
  - Some grow and block vital structures, thereby producing disease by mass effect.
- **Categories:** Parasitic helminths are classified depending on morphology and the structure of digestive tissues:
  - **Roundworms (nematodes):** These are elongate cylindrical parasites having tubular digestive tracts. Nematodes are said to be the most worm-like of all helminths.
  - **Flatworms (trematodes):** These parasites are dorsoventrally flattened with digestive tracts that end in blind loops.
  - **Tapeworms (cestodes):** These are segmented parasites with separate head and body parts. They do not have a digestive tract and absorb nutrients through their outer walls.

Cestodes: Intestinal Tapeworms

Taenia saginata, Taenia solium, Diphyllobothrium latum, and *Echinococcus granulosus* are cestode parasites (tapeworms) that infect humans. The source of human infection and diseases caused by these tapeworms in humans is presented in **Table 38**. Intestinal tapeworm infections are acquired by eating inadequately cooked beef (*T. saginata*), pork (*T. solium*) or fish (*D. latum*) containing larvae. These tapeworms have a complex life cycle. Tapeworm life cycles involve cystic larval stages in animals and worm stages in the human. Thus their life cycle requires two mammalian hosts: (1) a definitive host (in which the tapeworm reaches sexual maturity-humans), and (2) an intermediate host (in which the tapeworm does not reach sexual maturity—humans and animals). For the life cycles of beef and pork tapeworms, they require the animals to ingest material contaminated with infected human feces. The development of cystic larval forms occurs in the muscles of animals. In industrialized countries, modern cattle and pig farming practices have almost eliminated beef and pork tapeworms. However, in the underdeveloped countries, the infection is still common. Fish tapeworm infection is prevalent in region where raw, pickled or partly cooked freshwater fish are consumed. Presence of these adult tapeworms rarely damages the human host and is usually asymptomatic. The infected person passes portions of the tapeworm in the stool which may be frightening to the patient. The fish tapeworm (*D. latum*) consumes vitamin B_{12}, and few (<2%) may develop megaloblastic anemia.

General characteristics of adult tapeworms (Figs. 115A to C): The adult tapeworm consists of three parts: head (scolex), neck and trunk (strobila). The head (scolex) has suckers and hooklets that attach to the intestinal wall followed by a neck and trunk. The trunk consists of many flat segments that contain both male and female reproductive organs. The most distal segments are mature and contain many eggs, and they can detach and be shed in feces.

Cysticercosis—Taenia solium

- Cysticercosis is infection caused by larvae that develop after ingestion of eggs of tapeworm namely—***Taenia solium*** (pork tapeworm/armed tapeworm). **Cysticercus is the resting stage of larva in the intermediate host**.
- *Taenia solium* has a complex life cycle and requires two mammalian hosts: (1) a definitive host (in which the worm reaches sexual maturity—humans) and (2) an intermediate host (in which the worm does not reach sexual maturity-humans and pigs).

Mode of infection and pathogenesis (Fig. 116)

Taenia solium can be transmitted to humans in two ways with distinct outcomes.

Ingestion of larval cysts called cysticerci (present in uncooked pork infected with cysticerci) by humans. Pigs acquire cysticerci by ingesting eggs of *T. solium* in human feces. The *cysticerci* attach to the intestinal wall of human, where they develop into mature adult tapeworms. These adult tapeworms (**Fig. 117**) can grow to many meters in length and produce mild abdominal symptoms. The life cycle of the parasite is completed with this mode of infection. There is no development of disseminated cysticercosis. Adult tapeworms shed eggs in the feces of human beings. Adult tapeworm in the intestine can produce abdominal pain, diarrhea and loss of appetite. This cycle is essentially benign for both humans and pigs.

Ingestion of eggs present in contaminated food/water. This contamination is produced as follows:

- The intermediate hosts (pigs or humans) may ingest eggs in food or water contaminated with human feces.
- The embryo inside the egg is called the *oncosphere* (meaning *hooked ball)* because it is spherical and has hooklets. The ingested egg becomes an oncosphere in the lumen of the gut and hatches. It penetrates the gut wall, enter the blood stream.
- It disseminates hematogenously and lodges in tissue of many organs such as muscle, brain. In these tissues it can encyst and differentiate (undergo transition) to cysticercus. These **cystic larvae termed cysticercus cellulosae.** These cysticerci give rise to clinical symptoms of cysticercosis.

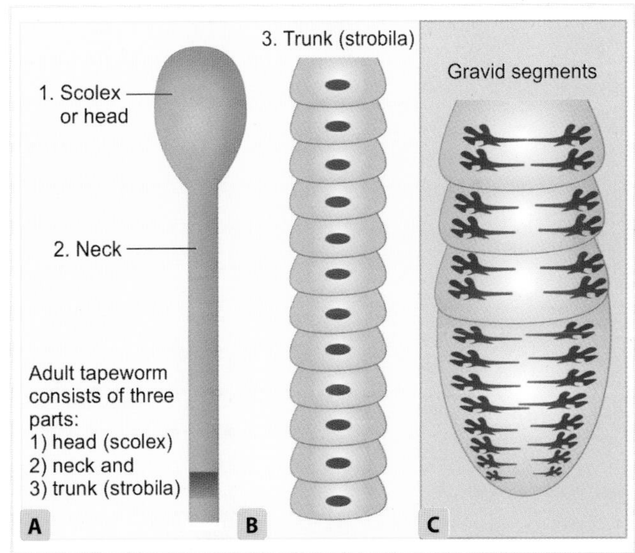

FIGS. 115A TO C: Parts of adult tapeworm (diagrammatic). (A) Scolex or head and neck that leads to the region of growth below, showing immature segments; (B) Mature segments; and (C) Gravid segments filled with eggs.

Table 38: Various infections in humans caused by tapeworm.

Species of tapeworm	*Source of human infection*	*Human disease*
Taenia saginata	Partly cooked beef	Adult tapeworm in intestine
Taenia solium	Partly/under cooked pork; human feces	Adult tapeworm in intestine; cysticercosis
Diphyllobothrium latum	Partly cooked freshwater fish	Adult tapeworm in intestine
Echinococcus granulosus	Dog feces	Hydatid cyst disease

- They spread to various sites.
- Most serious manifestations of cysticercosis is that when encyst occurs in the brain (neurocysticercosis). It can cause convulsions, increased intracranial pressure, and other neurologic disturbances.

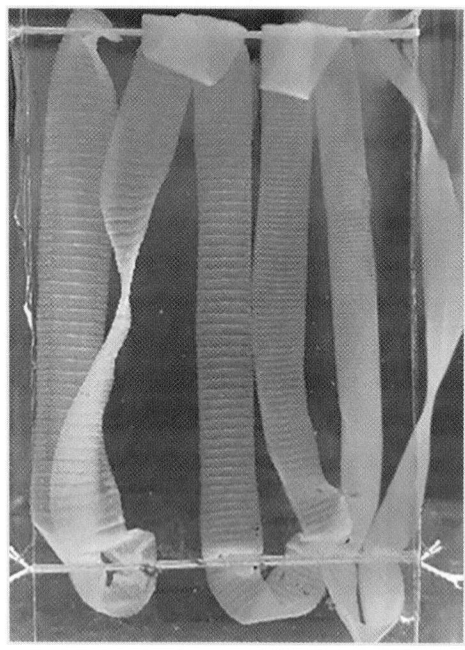

FIG. 117: Adult worm of *Taenia solium*.

- This mode of infection producing cysticerci cannot produce adult tapeworms. This is because larval cysts deposited in various tissues other than the intestine cannot develop into mature worms.
- Viable *T. solium* cysts usually do not produce symptoms. *T. solium* cysts can evade host immune defenses by producing taeniaestatin and paramyosin. These products probably inhibit complement activation. When the cysticerci degenerate and die, it produces an inflammatory response.

MORPHOLOGY

Organs affected: Cysticerci may be seen in any organ. More common locations include the **brain, skeletal muscles, skin, and heart**. When involves brain, cerebral symptoms depend on the precise location of the cysts. It may be intraparenchymal, attached to the arachnoid, or freely floating in the ventricular system.

Number: The cysticercus can be single or multiple.

Appearance of cysticercus cellulosae (Fig. 118): It is the larval form of *T. solium* and also the *infective form* of the parasite. It can develop in **various organs of pig as well as in man**. The **cysticercus cellulosae or "bladder worm"** is **round to oval opalescent milky-white, cyst** measuring 8–10 mm in breadth and 5 mm in length (often grape-sized). They contain little, clear cyst fluid. It **contains an invaginated scolex** (which has four suckers) **of the larva and circle of**

Continued

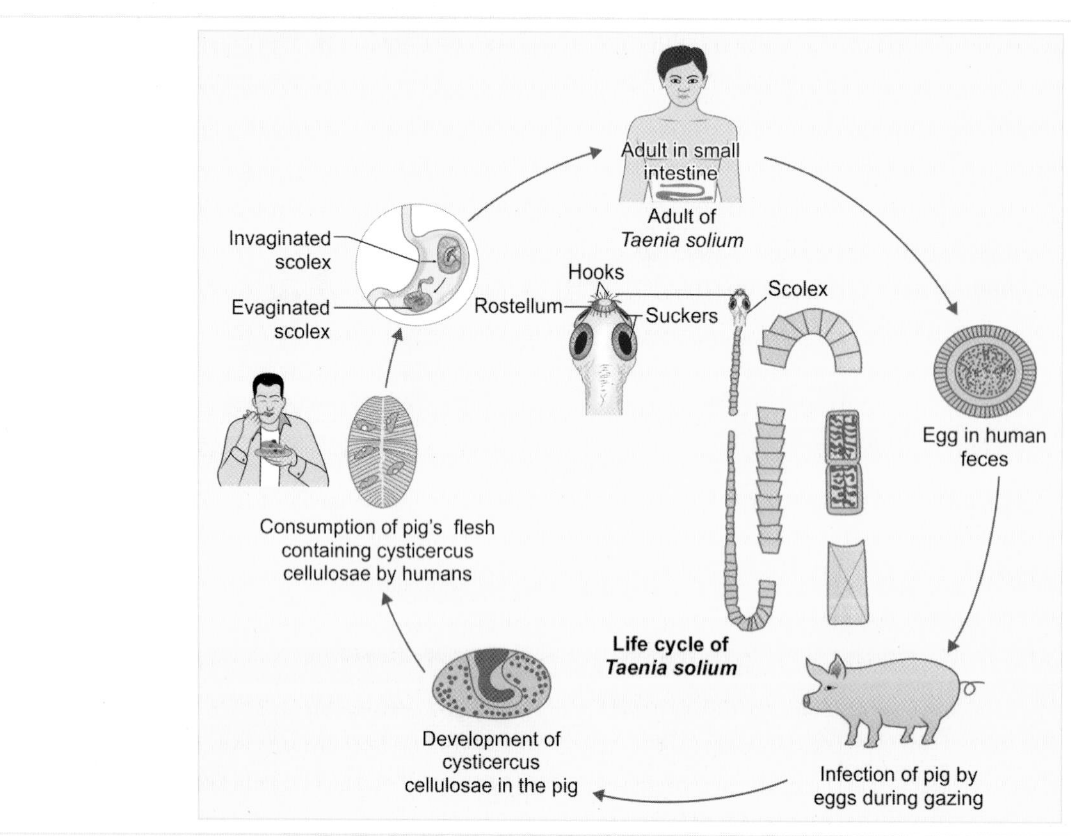

FIG. 116: Life cycle of *Taenia solium*.

Continued

birefringent hooks on its wall bathed in clear fluid in the cyst. This can be seen as a thick white spot. The cyst wall is usually >100 μm thickness and is rich in glycoproteins. There is seldom any host inflammatory response when cyst is intact. They remain viable for long time. Once the embryo dies, the cysts undergo degenerative changes. It induces granulomatous reaction with eosinophils and may later show scarring and calcification (may be visible by radiography).

Neurocysticercosis: The most serious manifestations of cysticercosis are due to involvement of the brain (neurocysticercosis). Cerebral symptoms depend on the location of the cysts. It can produce epilepsy (convulsions), headaches hydrocephalus, increased intracranial pressure, blurred vision and other neurologic disturbances. Multiple cysticerci in the brain may produce a "Swiss cheese" appearance to the tissue. Massive cerebral cysticercosis causes convulsions and death.

Cysticerci in the retina may cause blindness. In the heart, they may cause arrhythmias and sudden death.

Echinococcosis/Hydatid Disease

Q. Write short essay on hydatid disease.

Echinococcosis (hydatid disease) is a zoonotic, parasitic infestation caused by larval cestodes of the genus *Echinococcus*. Most commonly it **develops following ingestion of eggs of** cestode (tapeworms) namely ***Echinococcus granulosus*** which causes cystic hydatid disease. Rarely, human infestations are due to *Echinococcus multilocularis* and *Echinococcus vogeli*. **It is characterized by formation of cysts in organs where the parasite larvae are deposited.**

Echinococcus granulosus: The adult tapeworm *E. granulosus* measures 2–6 mm long (**Fig. 119**). It lives in the small intestines of carnivorous hosts (e.g., wolves, foxes, dogs). Adult *E. granulosus* has a scolex with suckers and numerous hooklets (arranged in two rows). These hooklets are used for its attachment to intestinal mucosa. A short neck is followed by three segments (proglottids). The terminal gravid proglottid breaks off and releases eggs. These eggs are excreted in feces and contaminate the grazing grass.

Life cycle (Fig. 120)

E. granulosus requires two mammalian hosts to complete its life cycle.

1. **Definitive host** (in which the worm reaches sexual maturity): These include dog, jackal, and fox.
2. **Intermediate host** (in which the worm does not reach sexual maturity): Usual intermediate hosts are sheep, pig, goat, cattle, man (accidental intermediate and is the dead end host).

For *E. multilocularis* the fox is the most important definitive host, and rodents are intermediate hosts.

- Infestation with *E. granulosus* is endemic in sheep, goats and cattle as well as their attendant dogs. Adult *E. granulosus* worm is found in small intestines of dogs and other canines. The dog is infected by eating the viscera of sheep containing hydatid cysts.
- The adult worm in small intestines of dogs, discharges eggs in feces. Dogs contaminate their habitats (and their human keepers) with infectious eggs. Eggs contaminate grass or other vegetable matters.
- Cestode eggs are ingested by herbivorous intermediate hosts, such as cattle, sheep, pigs, and other mammals during gazing in the field. The eggs hatch in the intestine and release larvae. These larvae penetrate the wall of the gut, enter the bloodstream, disseminate to various deep organs and grow to form hydatid cysts, containing brood capsules and scolices.
- When another dog ingests raw flesh from the cattle or sheep, the scolices are ingested and develop into mature worms in the dog's intestine to complete the cycle.

Infection of humans Humans are also become infected by inadvertently ingesting plant material contaminated by cestode (tapeworm) eggs.

Mode of infection: Humans are accidental intermediate hosts and humans acquire infection by:

- Handling dogs.
- Eating food/vegetables contaminated with eggs shed by dogs or foxes.

In the humans, the ingested eggs hatch release larvae in the duodenum. These larvae penetrate the gut wall are carried to the liver by portal venous system. They also enter

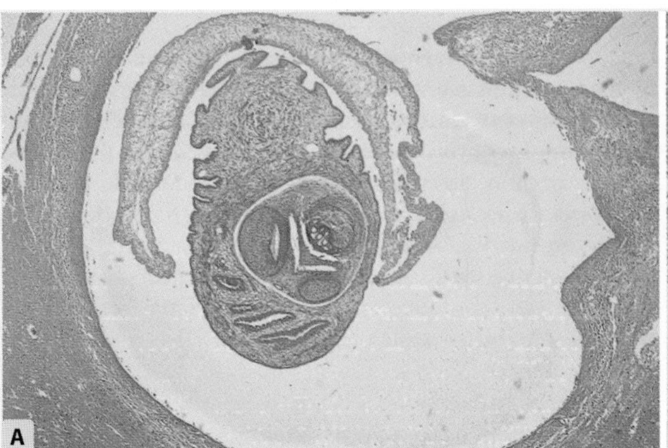

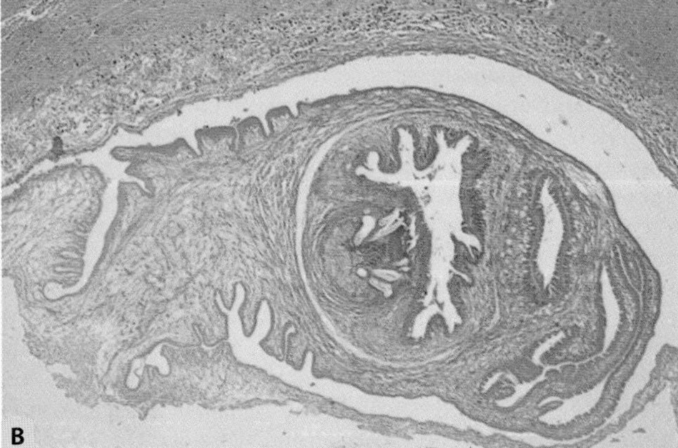

FIGS. 118A AND B: Cysticercus cyst in the brain.

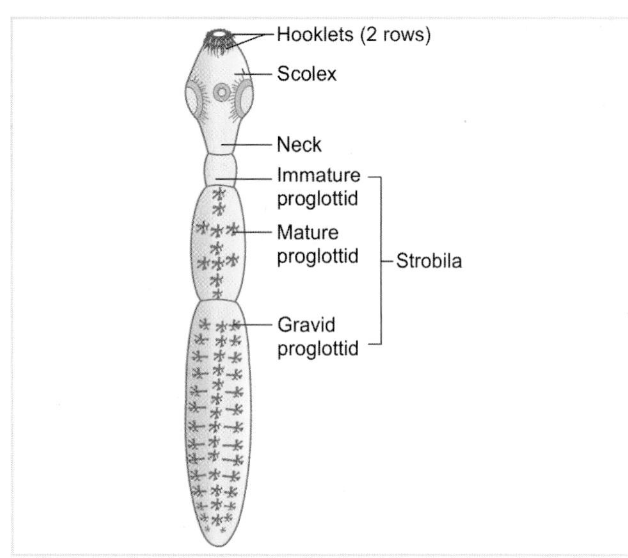

FIG. 119: *Echinococcus granulosus*. Schematic diagram of adult worm.

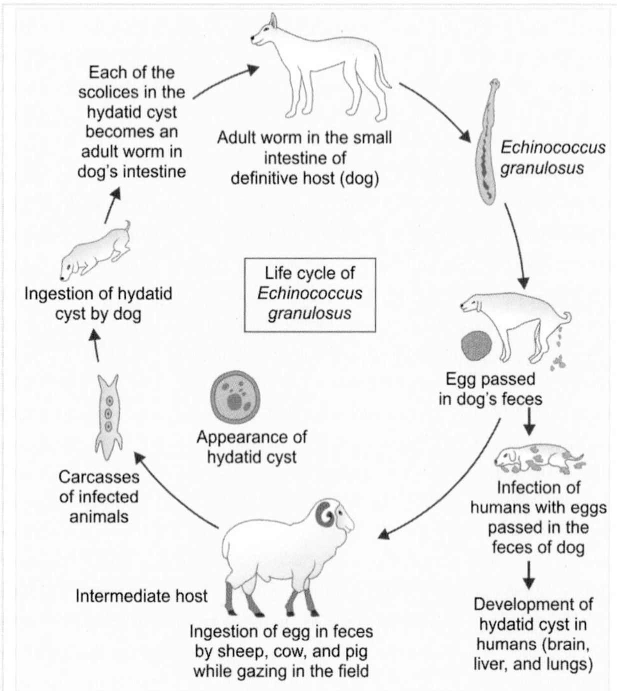

FIG. 120: Life cycle of *Echinococcus granulosus* and hydatid cystic disease. The adult tapeworm (cestode) lives in the small intestine of a dog (the definitive host). A terminal gravid proglottid of the cestode ruptures and releases cestode eggs into the dog's feces. Cestode eggs are ingested by cattle or sheep (the intermediate hosts) during gazing in the field. The eggs hatch in the intestine and release larvae. These larvae penetrate the wall of the gut and enter the bloodstream. They disseminate to various deep organs and grow to form hydatid cysts. These cysts contain brood capsules and scolices. When another dog eats raw flesh from the cattle or sheep containing the scolices of hydatid cysts, they develop into mature worms in the dog's intestine to complete the cycle. Humans are accidental intermediate hosts. Human can become accidently infected when cestode eggs in contaminated plant material are ingested. Ingested eggs hatch and release larvae that increase in size, but the parasite reaches a "dead end" without developing into an adult tapeworm. Hydatid cysts in humans occur mainly in the liver but may also involve lung, kidney, brain and other organs.

the bloodstream and disseminate to deep organs in other sites (e.g., lungs). Those which are trapped in the hepatic sinusoids develop into hydatid cyst. Large cysts contain brood capsules and scolices. In the liver it can produce abdominal pain or obstruction, and pulmonary cysts can cause pain, cough, and hemoptysis.

Echinococcus multilocularis: Dogs and cats are domestic definitive hosts and the domestic intermediate host is the house mouse. It causes alveolar hydatid disease in humans, but these infections are rare.

Echinococcus vogeli: Dogs are definitive hosts. Humans may become accidental intermediate hosts by ingesting eggs shed by domestic dogs. It causes polycystic hydatid disease.

MORPHOLOGY

Hydatid cysts slowly grow and they may be found by chance or become obvious when their size and position interfere with normal functions. Hydatid cyst in liver may manifest as a palpable right upper quadrant mass. Compression of intrahepatic bile ducts by the cyst can produce obstructive jaundice. Pulmonary cysts are usually asymptomatic and discovered incidentally on a chest radiograph.

Sites of hydatid cysts: About 65% human *E. granulosus* cysts are found in the **liver** and 5–15% in the **lung**, and the remaining 10–20% in **bones and brain** or other organs. In the involved organs, the larvae of *E. granulosus* lodge within the capillaries. They first provoke an inflammatory reaction consisting of mainly mononuclear leukocytes and eosinophils. Many of these larvae are destroyed, but few larvae become encysted.

Size: Hydatid cysts begin at microscopic cysts and progressively increase in size. The cysts may eventually attain a size over 10 cm in diameter in about 5 years.

Nature of cyst: *E. granulosus* usually produces unilocular hydatid cyst while *E. multilocularis* produces multilocular hydatid disease in the liver. They are white and opalescent (**Fig. 121**).

Microscopy (Figs. 122A to C): The cyst wall consists of three distinguishable zones enclosing an opalescent fluid:

1. **Pericyst (outer, capsular layer):** It shows inflammatory reaction and consists of fibroblasts, giant cells, and mononuclear cells and eosinophils. It forms a dense fibrous capsule.
2. **Ectocyst (intermediate opaque, non-nucleated layer):** It is distinctive and has innumerable delicate laminations.
3. **Endocyst (inner, nucleated, germinative layer with daughter cysts and scolices projecting into the lumen):** Daughter cysts usually develop within the large mother cyst. They appear initially as minute projections of the germinative layer. Then they develop central vesicles and form tiny brood capsules. Degenerating of the scolices of the worm produce a fine, grain-like (sand-like) sediment within the hydatid fluid (hydatid sand).

Clinical features

- Liver: Produces pressure effects due to cyst.
- Cerebral: Epilepsy
- Renal: Hematuria

- Rupture of cyst: The liberation of antigenic proteins in the hydatid fluid into the circulation produces eosinophilia and may even cause anaphylactic reactions.

Complications

Cyst rupture: If hydatid cyst ruptures, it seeds adjacent tissues with brood capsules and scolices. These "seeds" can germinate and produce many additional cysts and each has a capacity to grow as another new cyst. Parasites may disseminate from spillage of the cyst contents.

- **Hydatid cysts of liver or abdominal organ:** If the hydatid cyst of the liver or other abdominal organ undergoes traumatic rupture, it causes severe diffuse pain, resembling that of peritonitis.
- **Pulmonary cyst:** Rupture of a pulmonary cyst may cause pneumothorax and empyema.

Allergic reactions: Treatment of hydatid cysts requires careful surgical removal. It is very important to note that utmost caution is needed if surgical removal of the cyst is considered. Hydatid cysts must be sterilized with formalin before drainage or extirpation to prevent intraoperative anaphylactic shock. If a hydatid cyst ruptures into a body cavity or releases cyst contents fatal allergic reactions or anaphylaxis can occur.

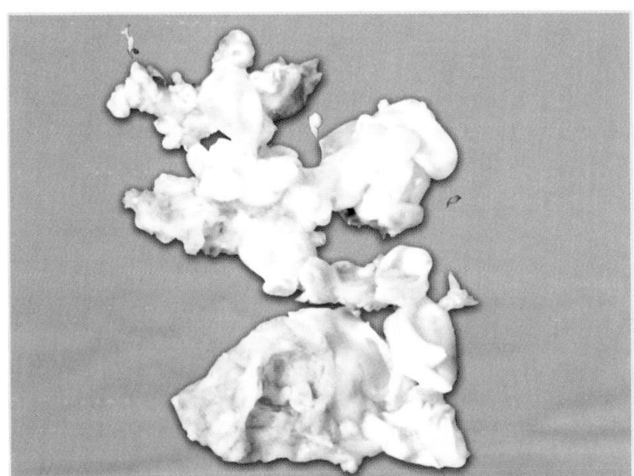

FIG. 121: Gross appearance of hydatid cysts consisting of multiple cysts.

Diagnosis

Radiological:

- **X-ray:** Routine chest radiographs are helpful in the diagnosis of hydatid cysts of lung. Lung lesions appear as round, irregular masses of uniform density. The "meniscus sign" or "crescent sign" is due to the presence of air between the pericyst and the laminated membrane. The "water lily sign" is due to an endocyst floating in a partially fluid-filled cyst.
- **CT scan (Fig. 123), ultrasonography and MRI** can identify the hydatid cysts by showing scolices and daughter cysts.

Casoni's skin test It is performed by intradermal injection of 0.2 mL of fresh sterile hydatid fluid. Positive test produces immediate hypersensitivity reaction (not routinely available).

Serological test:

- Precipitin reaction, complement fixation, immunofluorescent tests, and ELISA are positive in 70–90% of patients.
- Indirect hemagglutination test (IHAT), ELISA using specific echinococcal antigens.

Tissue Nematodes

Trichinosis

Trichinosis is produced by the infection with nematode parasite *Trichinella spiralis.*

Source and mode of infection: Humans acquire trichinosis **by eating** inadequately **or undercooked meat of infected animals (usually pigs, boars, or horses)** with encysted **larvae** of *T. spiralis.* The larvae are found in the skeletal muscles of various carnivorous or omnivorous wild and domesticated animals (e.g., pigs, rats, bears, and walruses). Pork (pig) is the most common source of human trichinosis. **The animals themselves** acquire trichinosis **by eating the flesh of other infected animals such as rats or meat products containing *T. spiralis.*** Infection is common among some wild animals and can be readily introduced into domesticated animals (e.g., pigs), when they feed on garbage or uncooked meat. Trichinosis occurs worldwide where undercooked meat, including noncommercial livestock and game (e.g., bear), is commonly eaten. Meat inspection programs and restriction of feeding practices in many developed countries have largely eliminated *T. spiralis* from domesticated pigs.

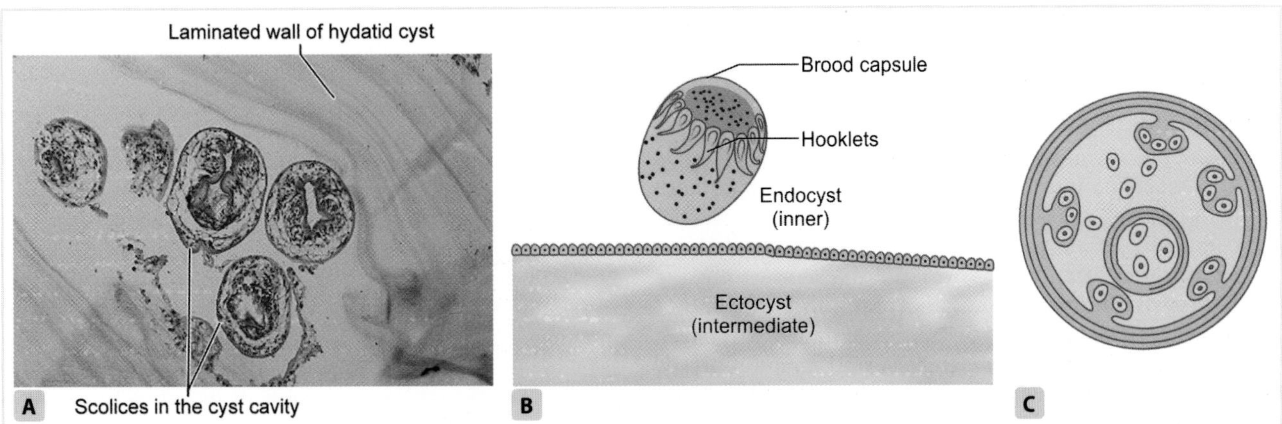

FIGS. 122A TO C: Hydatid cysts. (A and B) Wall of hydatid cyst showing a laminated, nonnuclear layer and a nucleated germinal layer with brood capsules attached and scolices in the cyst cavity. (C) Scolices inside the cyst (diagrammatic).

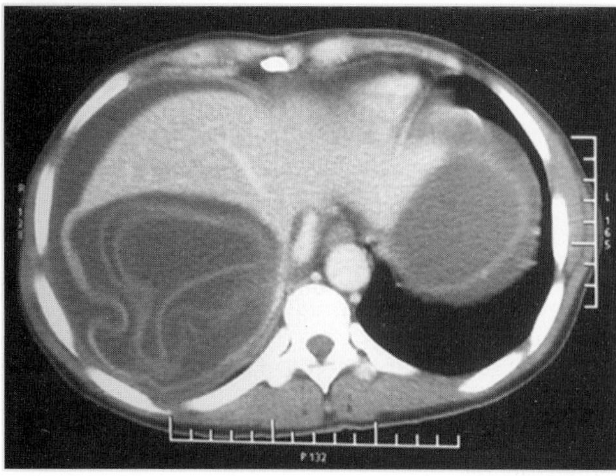

FIG. 123: Hydatid cyst on computed tomography (CT) abdomen.

Life cycle of *T. spiralis*

The life cycle of *T. spiralis* begins in the human intestine but ends within muscle of humans as humans are dead-end hosts.

- In the **small bowel of humans**, the **larvae** of *T. spiralis* **emerge from the ingested tissue cysts and burrow into the intestinal mucosa**. There **they develop into adult worms**. The adults mate, and the female **liberates larvae** that invade the intestinal wall.
- These larvae **enter the blood circulation** and disseminate hematogenously. These **larvae penetrate muscle cells** and cause fever, myalgias, marked eosinophilia, and periorbital edema. Less commonly, the larvae may lodge in the heart, lungs, and brain, and patients can present with dyspnea, encephalitis, and cardiac failure. Production of larvae in the intestine may continue for 1–4 months, until the worms are finally expelled from the intestine. The larvae can invade any tissue but they can survive only in striated skeletal muscle.
- **In striated skeletal muscle**, *T. spiralis* larvae become intracellular parasites. They encyst and remain viable in the skeletal muscles for years.

Molecular pathogenesis

- **Antibodies** may develop against larval antigens such as immunodominant carbohydrate epitope (called **tyvelose**). These antibodies may reduce reinfection and are also useful for serodiagnosis of the disease.
- **Th2 response:** *T. spiralis* (also other invasive nematodes) stimulate a Th2 response. Th2 cells produce cytokines such as IL-4, IL-5, IL-10, and IL-13. These cytokines activate eosinophils and mast cells. These inflammatory cells are associated with the inflammatory response to these parasites. Th2 response may be associated with increased contractility of the intestine. This may cause expulsion of adult worms from the gut. This in turn can subsequently reduce the number of larvae in the muscles. It is not known whether the intramuscular inflammatory response (consisting of mononuclear cells and eosinophils) is effective against the larvae.
- Sometimes the CNS or heart is also inflamed. This may cause meningoencephalitis or myocarditis.

MORPHOLOGY

During the invasive phase of trichinosis, heavy infections may cause widespread destruction of cells. This may be lethal.

Skeletal muscle: It is the major site of tissue damage in trichinosis. The larva of *T. spiralis* preferentially encysts in striated skeletal muscles with the richest blood supply. Thus, it is prominent in the **muscle of diaphragm, extrinsic ocular muscles, tongue, intercostal muscles, gastrocnemius, laryngeal, deltoid, and deltoids**.

- **Microscopy (Fig. 124):** The **larvae** infect a myocyte of the skeletal muscle and become **intracellular**. The intracellular parasites dramatically modify the myocyte. They **increase the size of the myocytes, produce basophilic degeneration, there is loss of its striations** and swelling. They also produce myositis. The larvae appear as coiled and measure about 1 mm in length. Larvae grow to 10 times their initial size, fold on themselves and develop a collagenous capsule. They are surrounded by intracellular membrane-bound vacuoles, which in turn are surrounded by plexus of new blood vessels. Early myocyte infection elicits an intense inflammatory infiltrate rich in eosinophils and macrophages. This infiltrate is abundant around dying parasites. With encapsulation, inflammation subsides. This cell-parasite complex is usually asymptomatic, and the **worm may persist for years and undergoes death followed by dystrophic calcification of cysts**. This may leave behind scars that are sufficiently characteristic to suggest the diagnosis of trichinosis.

Heart: It shows a patchy interstitial myocarditis characterized by many eosinophils and scattered giant cells. The myocarditis can lead to scarring. Larvae in the heart do not encyst. They are difficult to identify, because they die and disappear.

Lungs: The trapped larvae in the lung cause focal edema and hemorrhages. Sometimes it may show an allergic eosinophilic infiltrate.

CNS: The larvae cause a diffuse lymphocytic and eosinophilic infiltrate. There may be focal gliosis in and about small capillaries of the brain.

Small intestine: It is grossly unremarkable. In heavy infestations, adult worms may be found at the base of villi on microscopic examination. This may be accompanied by an inflammatory infiltrate.

Clinical features: Most human infections with small numbers of cysts of *T. spiralis* **are asymptomatic**. Symptomatic trichinosis is usually self-limited and they recover in a few months. If large numbers of cysts are ingested, patient may complain of abdominal pain and diarrhea due to invasion of small intestine by the worms. Fever, weakness and severe pain and tenderness of affected muscles may develop due to myositis. **Eosinophilia may be severe (>50% of all leukocytes).** Involvement of extraocular muscles can produce periorbital edema. Infection of the brain or myocardium can be fatal.

Cutaneous Larva Migrans (Creeping Eruption)

Definition: Cutaneous larva migrans (CLM) is a **creeping eruptions in the skin caused by the filariform larvae of nematodes** which **aimlessly wander/migrates through the skin for weeks or months producing a reddish itch papule along the path of travel of the larvae** (termed "larva migrans"). They provoke severe inflammation that appears as serpiginous urticarial trails.

Cause: CLM is particularly observed with nonhuman hookworms namely *Strongyloides stercoralis, Ancylostoma braziliense, Necator americanus,* and *A. caninum.* ***Strongyloides stercoralis*** may produce creeping eruptions and its filariform larvae moves rapidly in short line; hence it is termed **larva currens** (reflecting fast movement of strongyloides larva) (**Fig. 125**).

Sites affected: The main sites affected in CLM are the **dorsum and sole of the feet, buttocks, pelvic waist, legs and shoulders**. Infestation is usually self-limited. It can persist for a few days to months, but rarely for years.

Loeffler's syndrome (transient migratory pulmonary infiltrates, peripheral blood eosinophilia and sputum eosinophilia) is found in many cases of CLM.

Clinical features: There are usually no systemic symptoms and diagnosis is purely made on clinical grounds. Skin shows multiple, clearly defined, intensely pruritic, linear, and serpiginous tracts.

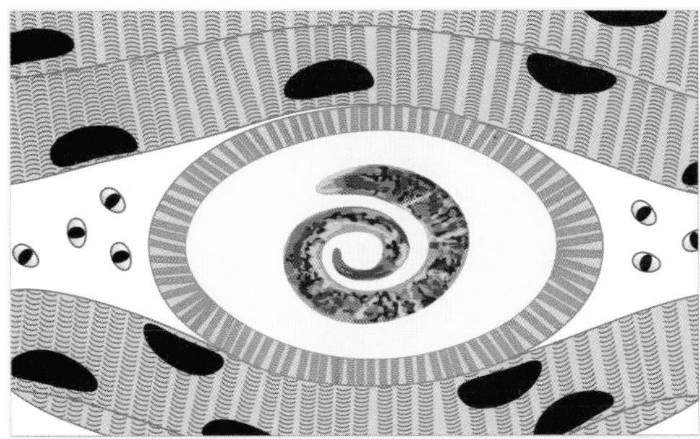

FIG. 124: Encysted larvae of *Trichinella spiralis* in skeletal muscle (diagrammatic).

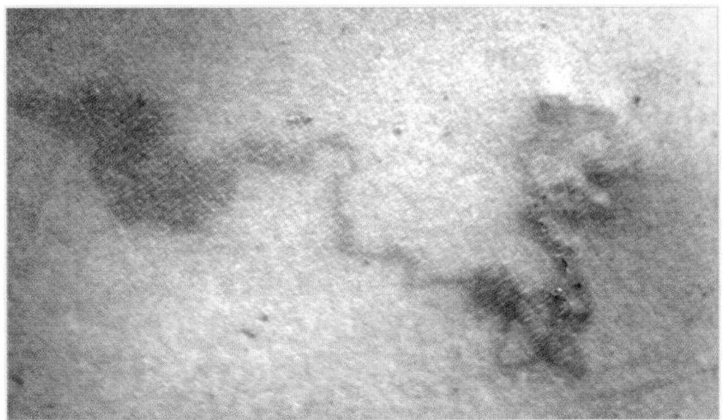

FIG. 125: Cutaneous larva migrans.

Trematodes (Flukes)

Trematodes are **leaf-shaped unsegmented, flat, and broad helminths** (hence the name *fluke,* from the *Anglo-Saxon* word *floe meaning flat fish).* The term *trematode* derived from their large prominent suckers with a hole in the middle (Greek *trema: hole, eidos: appearance).*

Schistosomiasis

Schistosomiasis **(bilharziasis)** is the **most important human helminthic disease** that **produces severe inflammatory and immune responses damage to the affected organ.** The affected organs and the site of major disease vary with the species. Three important species of schistosomes are: (1) *Schistosoma mansoni,* (2) *Schistosoma haematobium,* and (3) *Schistosoma japonicum. Schistosoma mansoni* (found in tropical Africa, parts of southwest Asia, South America and the Caribbean islands) and *S. japonicum* (found in parts of China, the Philippines, Southeast Asia and India) predominantly affect the liver (can lead to hepatic cirrhosis) or intestine. *S. haematobium* is found in Africa tropical Africa and parts of the Middle East and causes chronic granulomatous inflammation of the bladder that may lead to hematuria, obstructive uropathy, and carcinoma of urinary bladder. Diagrammatic appearance of eggs of *S. mansoni,* S. *haematobium,* and *S. japonicum* is presented in **Figures 126A to C. Schistosomiasis is responsible for greater morbidity and mortality than all other worm infections.**

Life cycle of schistosomes (Fig. 127)

Schistosomes have complicated life cycles. They alternate between asexual generations in their invertebrate host (snail) and sexual generations in the vertebrate host. The life cycle of *Schistosoma* species involves stepwise infection of several human tissues. Each step is associated with host inflammatory responses.

- The egg of s*chistosoma* requires passage through freshwater snails. These snails live in the slow-moving water of tropical rivers, lakes, and irrigation ditches (links agricultural development with spread of the s*chistosomiasis*). **Schistosome egg hatches in fresh water and releases a motile ciliated miracidium.**
- The ciliated **miracidium penetrates a snail**. In the snail, the miracidium larvae **mature into final infectious larval stage** called as **cercaria**.
- **Cercariae are released from snails** into the fresh water. They **swim through fresh water and penetrate human skin** with the help of powerful proteolytic enzymes that degrade the keratinized layer. There is minimal skin reaction at the site of penetration. During this process **cercariae lose their forked tails and become "schistosomula"**.
- The schistosomula migrate through the skin into the peripheral vasculature and lymphatics. Through blood vessels they migrate to the lungs and heart. From here they widely disseminate, including the mesenteric, splanchnic, and portal circulation **ultimately reaching the hepatic vessels, where they mature** (*S. mansoni* and *S. japonicum*).
- **In intestinal venules of the portal drainage, schistosomula mature** and form pairs of male and female worms. Mature male-female schistosoma worm pairs then migrate once again and settle in the venous system (commonly the portal or pelvic veins).

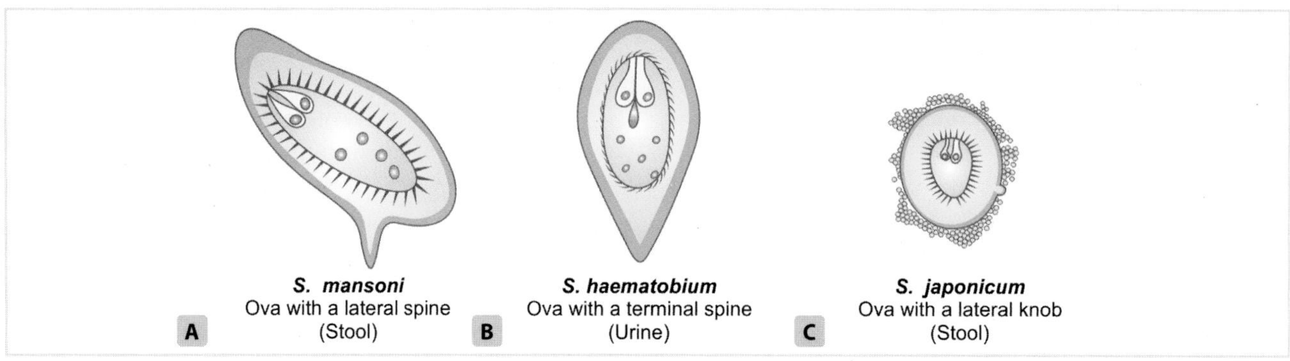

FIGS. 126 A TO C: Diagrammatic appearance of eggs of *Schistosoma mansoni* (A); Schistosoma *haematobium* (B); and *Schistosoma japonicum* (C).

Migrate to portal blood in liver
Circulation
Mature in intrahepatic portal veins into adults
Pairing of adult male and female worms
Adult worms in venous plexus
Egg in feces
Egg in urine
Schistosoma hematobium
Schistosoma mansoni
Schistosoma japonicum
Cercaria lose tails during penetration and become schistosomulae
Man (definitive host)
Life cycle of *Schistosoma* species
Eggs hatch releasing miracidia
Water
Penetrate skin of man (Definitive host)
Free-living ciliated miracidium hatches in water (16 hours)
Ingested by snail
Free-swimming cercaria released in water by snail (1–3 days)
1
2
3
Development within snail (Intermediate host) in 4–8 weeks
1. Primary sporocysts
2. Secondary sporocysts
3. Developing cercariae within secondary sporocysts

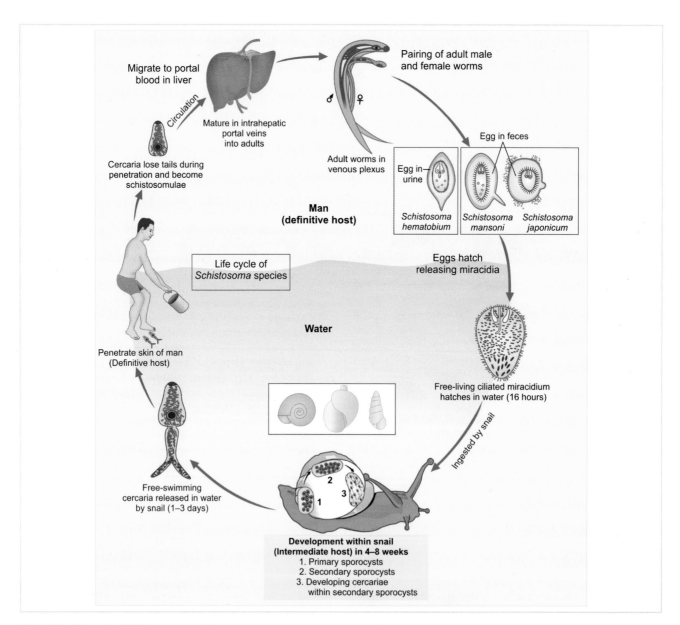

FIG. 127: Life cycle of *Schistosoma* species.

- **Females of schistosoma produce hundreds to thousands of eggs per day**. Theses eggs secrete proteases and produce localized inflammatory reactions. Female *S. mansoni* and *S. japonicum* deposit eggs in intestinal venules, whereas *S. haematobium* lays eggs in the urinary bladder.
- The local inflammatory response to egg helps in its migration and for passive transfer across the intestine and, in the case of *S. haematobium,* it is through bladder walls. This allows the eggs to be shed in stool in case of infection by *S. mansoni* and *S. japonicum* or urine in case of *S. haematobium.*
- **Embryos develop as the eggs pass through the respective tissues** (intestine or urinary bladder). The larvae are mature when eggs pass through the wall of the intestine or the bladder and are discharged in feces or urine.
- They hatch in fresh water and liberate miracidia. Infection of freshwater snails completes the life cycle.

Pathogenesis

Most of the pathological changes in schistosomiasis **are caused by host inflammatory reactions to different stages of the parasite.**

Liver Eggs carried by the portal circulation into the liver parenchyma can cause **severe chronic inflammation** in the liver. This immune response and inflammatory response to eggs of *S. mansoni* and *S. japonicum* in the liver produces **fibrosis**. This is responsible for the most serious complication of schistosomiasis. Adult schistosomes do not elicit inflammation while alive in the veins.

Helper T-cell response: Th1 and Th2 cells play a role depending on the phase of infection.

- **Th1 cell response during early phase**: In the early stage of **schistosomiasis,** helper T-cell response is dominated by Th1 cells. They produce IFN-γ, which stimulates macrophages to produce high levels of the cytokines TNF-α, IL-1, and IL-6 that cause fever.
- **Th2 response during chronic phase**: Chronic schistosomiasis is associated with a dominant Th2 response. This is associated with the presence of activated macrophages. Hepatic fibrosis is a serious manifestation of chronic schistosomiasis. Cells that play major role in portal ("pipestem") fibrosis and portal hypertension during chronic schistosomiasis in liver are Th2 cells and activated macrophages.

Female adult worms of schistosome deposit hundreds or thousands of eggs daily for 5–35 years. Most infected individuals harbor fewer than 10 adult females. Both types of helper T cells (i.e., Th1 and Th2) contribute to the formation of **circumscribed granulomas surrounding eggs in the liver**. If there is large burden of worms the granulomatous response against the large number of eggs laid by them produces significant problems. Granulomas formed around the eggs may also obstruct microvascular blood flow and produce ischemic damage to adjacent tissue. The result is progressive scarring and dysfunction in affected organs. There may be cellular infiltrate of eosinophils and neutrophils around an egg.

The site of involvement depends on the tropism of the particular schistosome species.

- *S. mansoni:* It lodges in the branches of the inferior mesenteric vein. Hence, they affect the distal colon and liver.
- *S. haematobium*: It has an affinity for the veins draining the rectum, bladder, and pelvic organs.
- *S. japonicum*: It lays eggs mainly in the branches of the superior mesenteric vein. Hence, they damage the small bowel, ascending colon, and liver.

MORPHOLOGY

***S. mansoni* or *S. japonicum* infections**

During early infections by *S. mansoni* or *S. japonicum,* white, pinhead-sized granulomas are seen scattered throughout the gut and liver. **Granulomas are formed around the schistosome egg**. Granuloma contains a miracidium and this degenerates over time and undergoes **dystrophic calcification**. The granulomas are composed of epithelioid macrophages, lymphocytes, neutrophils, and eosinophils (often predominate in early granulomas). These are characteristic for helminth infections. Giant cells may be prominent and the oldest granulomas are densely fibrotic. The eggs of the various schistosomal species are identified on the basis of their size and shape (see **Fig. 126**).

Liver disease: It is caused by *S. mansoni* or *S. japonicum.*

- **Gross:** The liver is darkened by regurgitated heme-derived pigments from the schistosome gut. They are like malaria pigments, which are iron-free and accumulate in Kupffer cells and macrophages in spleen. In late stages, the surface of the liver is bumpy. Cut surfaces show granulomas, widespread fibrosis and portal enlargement without intervening regenerative nodules of liver cells.
- **Microscopy:** It begins as periportal granulomatous inflammation and gradually progresses to dense periportal fibrosis. Because these fibrous tracts resemble the stem of a clay pipe, the lesion is named **pipe-stem fibrosis**. In severe hepatic schistosomiasis, fibrosis usually produces obstruction of portal venous blood flow. This leads to portal hypertension, severe congestive splenomegaly, esophageal varices, and ascites.

Colon: *S. mansoni* and *S. japonicum* also damage the intestine. In late stages of S. *mansoni* or *S. japonicum* infections, granulomatous responses may produce inflammatory patches or pseudopolyps and foci of mucosal and submucosal fibrosis.

Lung: Schistosome eggs, carried to the lung through portal collaterals, may produce granulomatous pulmonary arteritis. This is associated with intimal hyperplasia, progressive arterial obstruction, and progression to heart failure (cor pulmonale).

- **Microscopy:** The pulmonary arteries show disruption of the elastic layer by granulomas and scars. The lumen of the artery may show organizing thrombi, and angiomatoid lesions similar to those observed in idiopathic pulmonary hypertension.

Continued

Continued

Kidney: Patients with hepatosplenic schistosomiasis have an increased tendency to develop mesangioproliferative or membranous glomerulopathy. In such cases glomeruli show deposits of immunoglobulin and complement but rarely schistosome antigen.

***Schistosoma haematobium* infection**

Urogenital schistosomiasis: It is caused by *S. haematobium* infection. The eggs are most numerous in the bladder, ureter and seminal vesicles. They may also reach the lungs, colon and appendix. Inflammatory cystitis develops due to massive deposition of eggs in urinary bladder. Eggs in the bladder (**Figs. 128A** and **B**) and ureters provoke a granulomatous reaction during early phase. It may lead to mucosal erosions, inflammatory protuberances and patches of mucosal and mural fibrosis. This may cause hematuria. Later, the granulomas undergo dystrophic calcification and develop a sandy appearance. If calcification is severe, it may line the wall of the bladder and cause a dense concentric rim (calcified bladder) on radiographic films. The most frequent complication of *S. haematobium* infection is inflammation and fibrosis of the ureteral walls. These may obstruct urine flow, and may cause secondary inflammatory damage to the bladder, ureters and, kidneys. Obstruction may lead to obstructive uropathy, ureteral obstruction, chronic cystitis, hydronephrosis, and chronic pyelonephritis. Bladder disease produced by *S. haematobium* may lead to **squamous cell carcinoma of the urinary bladder**.

Clinical features: Sometimes the site of skin penetration by the schistosome larvae may be associated with a self-limited, intensely pruritic rash. Most of the cases of **schistosomiasis, the clinical manifestations are due to tissue damage produced by granuloma**. Hepatic involvement may be manifested by portal hypertension, splenomegaly, ascites and bleeding esophageal varices. Intestinal disease usually produces minimal symptoms, but some may complain of abdominal pain and bloody stools. Schistosomiasis of the bladder may be accompanied by hematuria, recurrent urinary tract infections and sometimes progressive urinary obstruction, leading to renal failure. Diagnosis is through identification of schistosome eggs in the urine or feces.

Intestinal Nematodes

Nematodes are the **most worm-like of all helminths**. They generally resemble the common earthworm in appearance, which is considered to be the prototype of "worms". However, taxonomically earthworms are not nematodes. Humans are the primary hosts for all of intestinal nematodes. The adult forms of several nematode species (**Table 39**) reside in the bowel of humans. Usually they do not cause symptomatic disease. Clinical symptoms develop almost always in patients having very large numbers of worms or who are immunocompromised. Infection spreads from person to person through eggs or larvae passed in the stool or deposited in the perianal region. Infection is most prevalent where there is lack of hand washing and hygienic disposal of feces (e.g., under developed countries). Many intestinal nematodes need warm, moist climates for their infectious forms to survive outside the body. Thus, these worms are endemic in tropical and subtropical regions.

Ascariasis

Ascaris lumbricoides is **commonly known as roundworm** and is the most common of human helminths. It is distributed worldwide. Its specific name *lumbricoides* is derived from its resemblance with earthworm (*Lumbricus*, meaning *earthworm* in Latin). **Infection by the *A. lumbricoides* is called ascariasis.** It usually does not produce any symptoms. Infection is most common in warm climates and with poor sanitation.

Life cycle (Fig. 129)

Life cycle of *Ascaris* involves only one host namely humans.

Mode of transmission: Infection occurs when the **egg containing the infective rhabditiform larva is swallowed**. A frequent mode of transmission is through fresh vegetables grown in fields manured with human feces (night soil). Infection may also be transmitted through contaminated drinking water.

Development in soil: The fertilized egg passed in stool/feces is not immediately infective. It has to undergo a period of incubation in soil before acquiring infectivity. The eggs are resistant to adverse conditions and can survive for several years. The development of the egg in soil depends on the

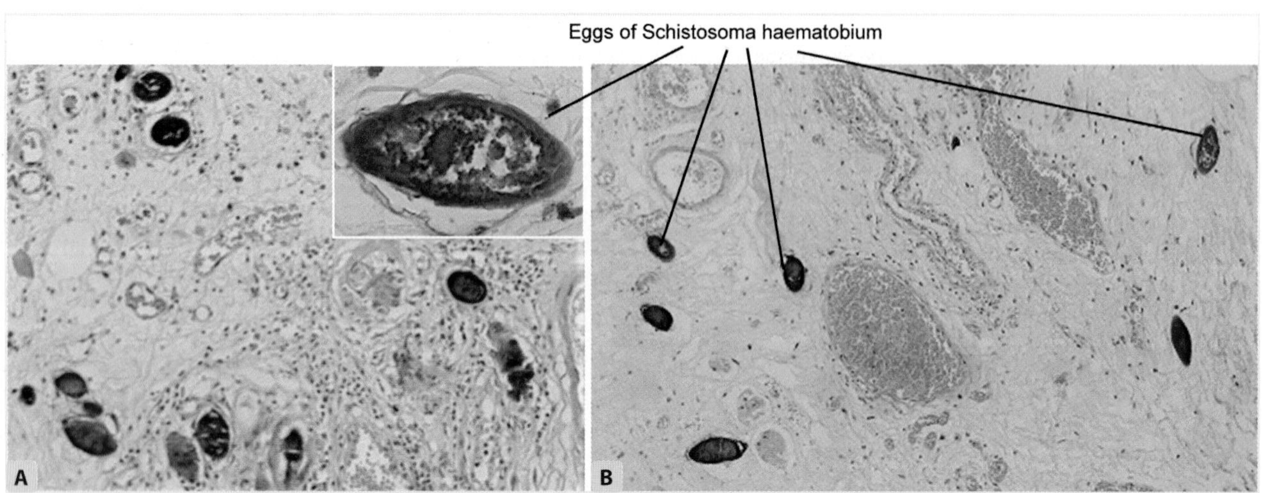

FIGS. 128A AND B: Eggs of *Schistosoma haematobium* in the urinary bladder. Inset in Figure 128A shows single ovum with calcification.

Table 39: Common intestinal nematodes and their usual clinical manifestations.

Species (common name)	*Clinical manifestations*
Site of adult worm: Small bowel	
Ascaris lumbricoides (roundworm)	• Allergic reactions to lung migration • Intestinal obstruction with heavy infestation
Ancylostoma duodenale (hookworm)	• Allergic reactions to cutaneous inoculation and lung migration • Blood loss in the intestine
Necator americanus (hookworm)	
Strongyloides stercoralis (threadworm)	• Abdominal pain and diarrhea • Dissemination to extraintestinal sites in immunocompromised persons
Site of adult worm: Large bowel	
Trichuris trichiura (whipworm)	• Abdominal pain and diarrhea • Rarely rectal prolapse
Enterobius vermicularis (pinworm) Mainly in cecum, appendix	Perianal and perineal itching

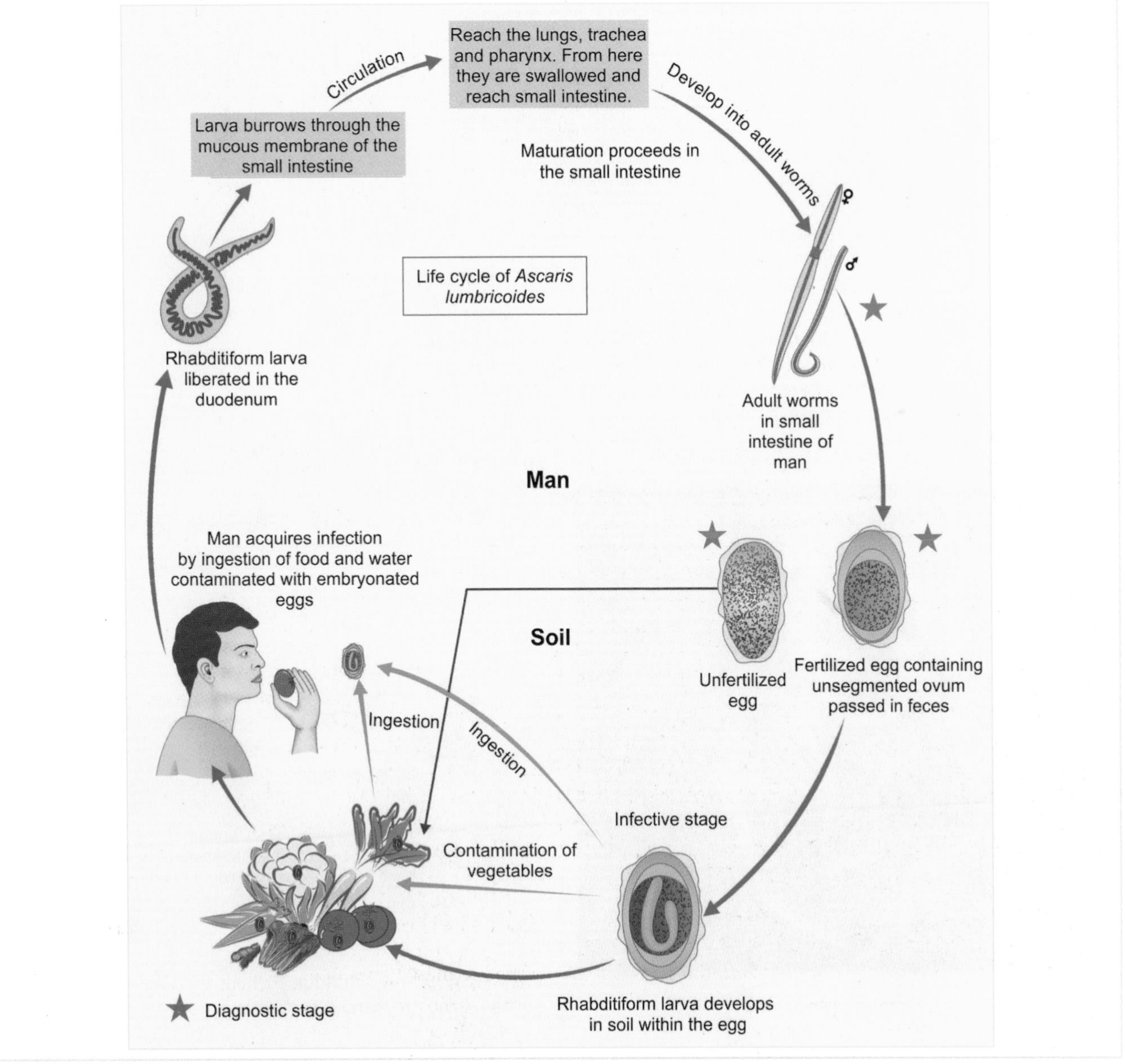

FIG. 129: Life cycle of *Ascaris lumbricoides*.

nature of the soil and various environmental factors. The development usually takes from 10 to 40 days, during which time the embryo becomes the infective rhabditiform larva, coiled up within the egg.

Development in humans: When the swallowed eggs reach the duodenum, the larvae hatch out. The **rhabditiform larvae** are actively motile. *Ascaris* larvae emerge in the small intestine, and penetrate the intestinal mucosa, enter the portal vessels and are carried to the *liver*. They then pass via the hepatic vein, inferior vena cava, and the right side of the heart. In about 4 days these reach the lungs through the venous circulation. In the lung they undergo growth and development. After development in the lungs, in about 10–15 days, the larvae pierce the lung capillaries and enter the alveoli. They crawl up and migrate up the trachea to the glottis and are swallowed. Thus, again they reach the small bowel. The larvae develop and mature into adult worms in the upper part of the *small intestine* and they live there. They become sexually mature in about 6–12 weeks. The gravid female worms start laying eggs. These eggs are discharged and are excreted in the feces to repeat the cycle. The adult worm has a lifespan of 12–20 months.

Clinical features: Adult round worms [15–35 cm long (**Fig. 130**)] usually do not cause any pathological changes. Heavy infections may be accompanied by vomiting, malnutrition and sometimes intestinal obstruction. Very rarely, adult worms enter the ampulla of Vater or pancreatic or biliary ducts. This may result in obstruction, acute pancreatitis, suppurative cholangitis, and liver abscesses. Eggs deposited in the liver or other tissues produce necrosis, granulomatous inflammation and fibrosis. When large numbers of larvae migrate within the air spaces of lungs, it may produce *Ascaris* pneumonia, which may be fatal. Diagnosis of ascariasis is by identifying eggs (**Fig. 131**) in the feces. Occasionally, adult worms may pass with the stools or even appear to come out through the nose or mouth.

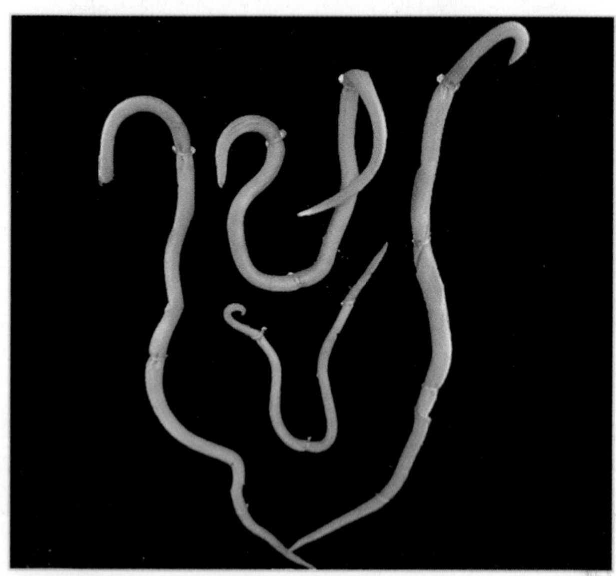

FIG. 130: Adult round worms (four in number).

Trichuriasis

Trichuriasis is caused by the intestinal nematode *Trichuris trichiura* ("**whipworm**"). Adult worm of *T. trichiura* measures about 3–5 cm in length. It has a long, slender anterior portion and a short, blunt posterior (**Fig. 132A**). Whipworm infection is most common in warm, moist places with poor sanitation. Children are more susceptible.

Life cycle: Humans acquire infection by ingestion of eggs in contaminated soil, food or drink. Larvae develop from ingested eggs in the small bowel. They migrate to the cecum and colon. Adult worms live in the cecum and upper colon of humans and they burrow their anterior portions into the superficial mucosa. This invasion produces small erosions and focal active inflammation of the mucosa. This may be accompanied by continuous loss of small quantities of blood. The adult female worms produce eggs and these eggs are passed in the feces. Excreted eggs embryonate in moist soil and become infective in 3 weeks.

Clinical features: Most infections of *T. trichiura* are asymptomatic. Heavy infestation may cause cramping abdominal pain, bloody diarrhea, weight loss and anemia. The diagnosis is by finding the characteristic eggs in the stool **(Fig. 132B).**

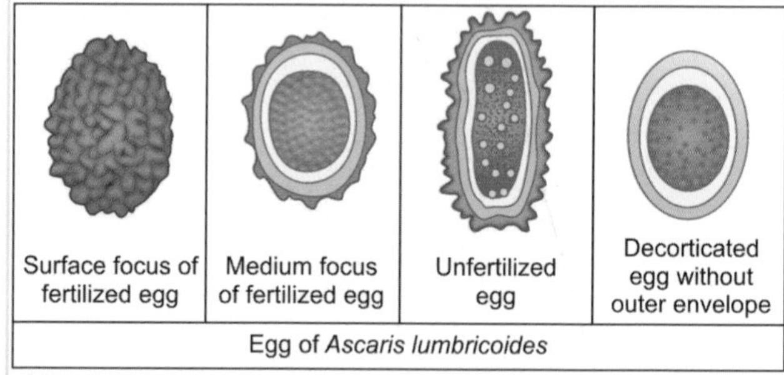

FIGS. 131: Diagrammatic appearance of eggs of *Ascaris lumbricoides.*

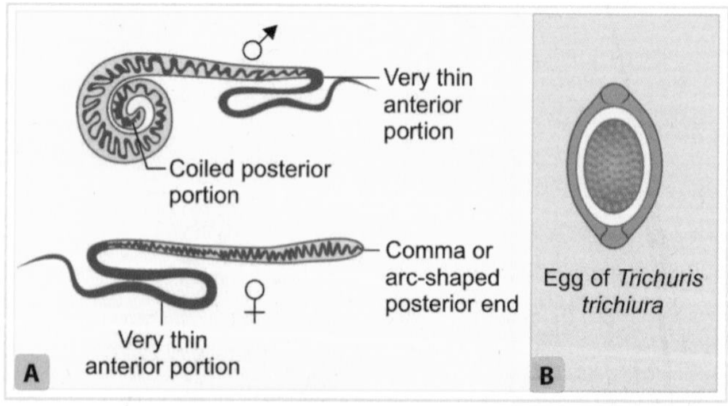

FIGS 132A AND B: (A) Adult Trichuris trichiura worms (male and female) (B) egg of Trichuris trichiura

Hookworms

Q. Write short essay on manifestations of hookworm infestation.

Ancylostomiasis is a symptomatic infection caused by parasitization with human hookworms *Ancylostoma duodenale* or *Necator americanus.* These hookworms are intestinal nematodes that infect the human small bowel. They produce laceration of the bowel mucosa thereby resulting in blood loss in the intestine. This can lead to anemia. Hookworm infection is one of the **major causes of anemia in the tropics and subtropics**. *A. duodenale* or old-world hookworm is found in East Asia, Africa, China, Japan, India and the Pacific Islands.

Necator americanus or new-world hookworm ("American" hookworm) is found in South and Central America and the Caribbean.

Mode of infection: It occurs through skin by filariform larvae when human walks bare-foot on the focally contaminated soil.

Life cycle (Fig. 133): Filariform larvae present in the contaminated soil directly penetrate the site of contact with human epidermis. Form skin they enter the venous circulation and travel to the lungs and lodge in alveolar capillaries. They rupture into the alveoli and larvae migrate up the trachea to the glottis and then are swallowed. In the duodenum, they attach to the mucosal wall with tooth-like buckle plates and clamp off a section of a villus and ingest it. When the infestations are extensive (especially with *A. duodenale*), they cause significant blood loss to cause anemia. Hookworms measure about 1 cm in length. Hence, these can be grossly seen attached to the small bowel mucosa alongside punctate areas of hemorrhages. There is usually no accompanying inflammation.

Clinical features: Most individual with light hookworm infection do not have any symptoms. Hookworm is the most important cause of chronic anemia.

Lesion in skin: Skin penetration is sometimes associated with **allergic dermatitis**/itching ("ground itch") dermatitis at the site of entry of the infective filariform larvae. The lesions are usually on the feet, particularly between the toes.

Pulmonary manifestations: The passage of larvae through the lungs in a heavy infection produces cough with bloodstained sputum and fever. There may be asthma-like

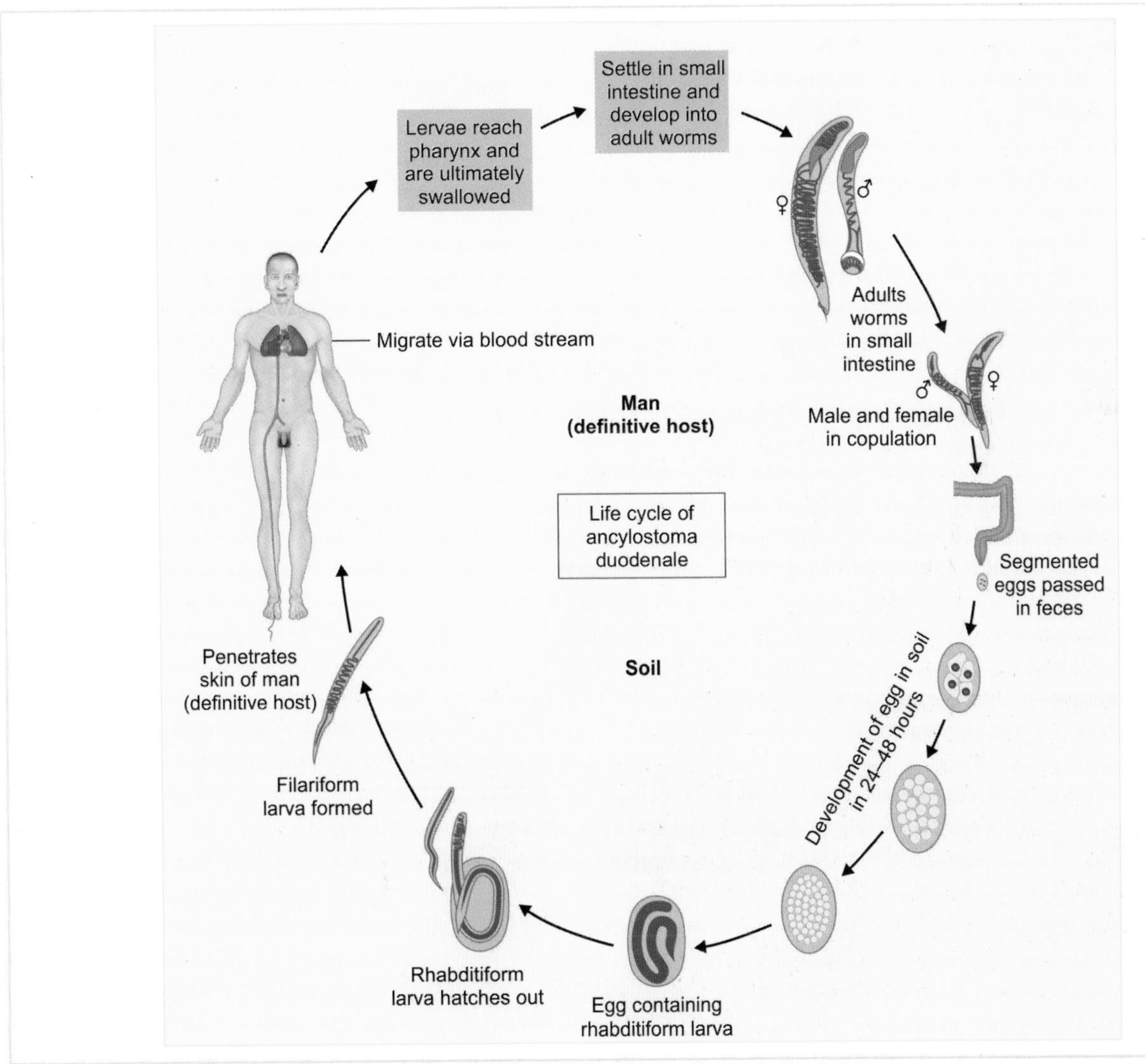

FIG. 133: Life cycle of Ancylostoma duodenale

symptoms, bronchitis, patchy pulmonary consolidation/ bronchopneumonia and eosinophilia.

Gastrointestinal manifestations: Light infections (especially in well-nourished individuals) are often asymptomatic. When the worms have reached the small intestine, heavier worm loads may be produce epigastric pain, nausea, and vomiting resembling peptic ulcer disease. Other symptoms include abdominal distension, pica, and small frequent loose stools.

Pathological effects: Chronic heavy infection, particularly on a background of malnourishment, may cause:

- **Iron deficiency anemia** due to chronic intestinal blood loss. In individuals with heavy burden of worm (particularly women who consume a diet low in iron) and in those who have inadequate iron intake, chronic intestinal blood loss can produce severe iron-deficiency anemia.
- **Hypoproteinemia/hypoalbuminemia** is a common in severe disease.
- **Retarded physical, mental and sexual development** may occur in older children with heavy infection in children.

Investigations and diagnoses

Stool examination

- **Microscopic examination** of **stool shows** the characteristic **eggs/ovum (Fig. 134A** and **B**). The eggs of both *A. duodenale* and *N. americanus* are 60–70 µm in length and bounded by an ovoid transparent hyaline membrane. Rarely rhabditiform larva may be seen in stool (**Fig. 134C**)
- **Occult blood:** The stools rarely show gross blood, but tests for occult blood are **usually positive**.

Blood

- **Peripheral blood smear:** It characteristically shows **microcytic hypochromic anemia.** There may be **eosinophilia** (as high as 70–80%) in some cases.
- **Hemoglobin** level is usually **low**.

Strongyloidiasis

Strongyloides stercoralis ("threadworm") is a nematode (elongated cylindrical worm) that causes infection of small intestinal infection and is called as Strongyloidiasis. *Strongyloides stercoralis (strongylus-round,* eidos-resembling, *stercoralis-fecal)* is the smallest of the intestinal nematodes and measure 0.2–0.3 cm in length (**Fig. 135A**). Infection is most frequent in areas with warm, moist climates, and poor sanitation. It is endemic in tropical and subtropical regions of South America, sub-Saharan Africa, and Southeast Asia. It occurs sporadically in other regions. In most cases, it is asymptomatic. But the infection can progress to lethal disseminated disease in immunocompromised individuals.

MORPHOLOGY

Eggs (Fig. 135B): Eggs are oval and are conspicuous within the uterus of gravid female. As soon as the eggs are laid, they hatch out to rhabditiform larva. Thus, it is the larva and not the egg, which is excreted in feces and detected on stool examination.

Larva

- **Rhabditiform larva (Fig. 135C)**: This is the first stage of larva. Eggs hatch to form rhabditiform larva in the small intestine. It is the most common form of the parasite found in the feces. The larva migrates into the lumen of the intestine and passes down the gut to be released in feces.
- **Filariform larva (Fig. 135D)**: It is long and slender. It has a long esophagus of uniform width and notched tail. It is the **infective stage** of the parasite to man.

Mode of infection: Through penetration of skin by the stage filariform larva, when an individual walks bare foot or by autoinfection.

Life cycle (Fig. 136): The worms live in the soil. They infect humans when larvae penetrate the skin. From skin they travel in the circulation to the lungs. Then travel up the trachea and are swallowed. Microscopically, the adult coiled female worm, along with eggs and developing larvae are embedded in the crypts of the duodenal mucosa and upper jejunum the human intestine (see **Fig. 137**). The female worms of parasite survive in the mucosa of the small intestine and produce eggs by asexual reproduction (parthenogenesis). There are no visible alterations and microscopically, there is no inflammation. The eggs laid in the mucosa hatch immediately and release ***rhabditiform*** **larva**. Most of the rhabditiform larva migrates into the lumen of the intestine and passes down the gut to be released in feces (stool). The rhabditiform larva may contaminate soil and in the soil become filariform the infective

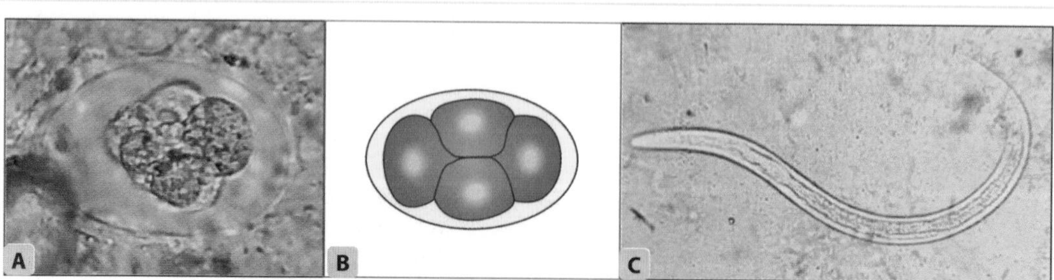

FIGS. 134A TO C: Hookworm (A) egg with blastomeres in stool sample; (B) diagrammatic appearance of egg with many blastomeres; (C) rhabditiform larva in stool.

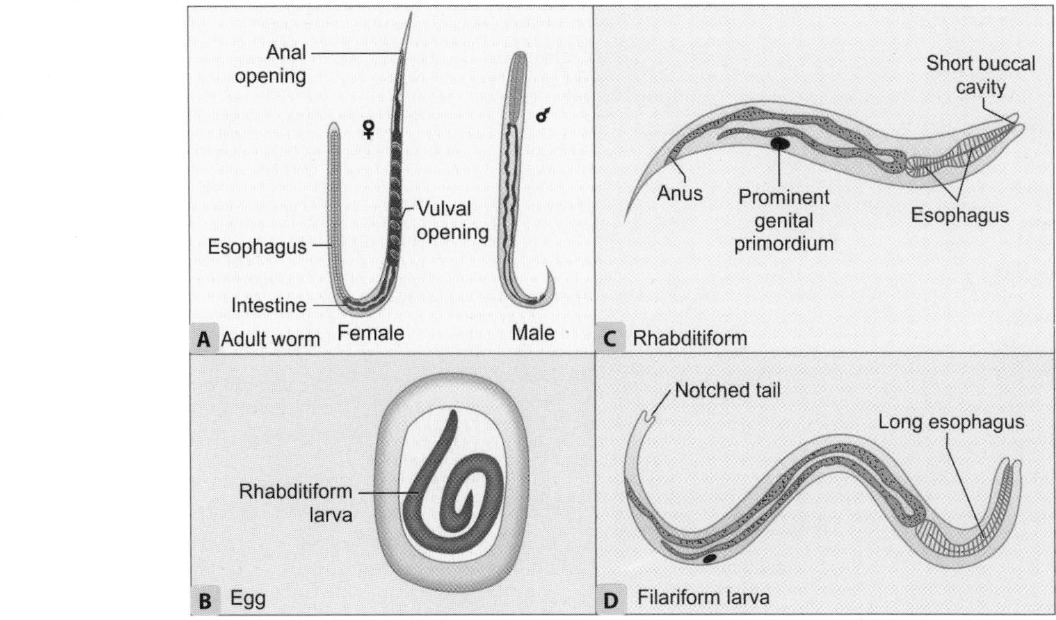

FIGS. 135A TO D: Diagrammatic appearance of adults worms, egg, and larvae of *Strongyloides stercoralis*. (A) Adult worms (male and female); (B) Egg; (C) Rhabditiform larva; (D) Filariform larva.

stage and thereby continue the cycle of infection. In some human hosts, unlike other intestinal nematodes, *S. stercoralis* may reproduce by a mechanism known as **autoinfection**. This autoinfection occurs when rhabditiform larvae become infective (filariform) larva during passage through the bowel of host's intestine. This filariform larva may repenetrate either the intestinal wall or the perianal skin without leaving the host and going to the soil. It provides a source of autoinfection. On entering the skin, *S. stercoralis* larvae again pass in the bloodstream to the lungs and then to the small bowel. The worms mature in the small bowel. This is similar to hookworms. Thus, parasite starts a new parasitic cycle within a single host. This ability to cause autoinfection explains the persistence of the infection in patients for long periods, even 30–40 years, after leaving the endemic areas.

Pathogenesis:

- **Infection in immunocompetent hosts:** *S. stercoralis* is usually asymptomatic, but may produce diarrhea, bloating, and occasionally malabsorption.
- **Infection in immunocompromised hosts:** Immunocompromise may be due to prolonged corticosteroid therapy. Corticosteroids inhibit the functions of eosinophils and other host immune cells that accumulate in tissues in response to infection. This stimulates female *Strongyloides* species to increase the production of infective larvae. This can result in very high worm burdens (hyperinfection or **disseminated strongyloidiasis**) due to uncontrolled autoinfection and produce fatal disease. Such patients have greatly increased internal autoinfection and extraordinary numbers of filariform larvae penetrate intestinal walls and disseminate to distant organs. Apart from prolonged corticosteroid therapy, other disease states that disturb immune control mechanisms (e.g., organ transplantation, lymphoma, HTLV-1) are also associated with increased risk. Hyperinfection can be complicated by sepsis due to gram-negative bacteria in the intestine. These bacteria enter the blood circulation through the damaged intestinal wall. The damage to the intestine is caused by the invading larvae. Disseminated strongyloidiasis is usually fatal.

MORPHOLOGY

Most infected individuals are asymptomatic, but moderate eosinophilia is common.

Mild strongyloidiasis: The worms, mainly larvae (**Figs. 137A and B**), are seen in the duodenal crypts. They are not seen in the underlying tissue. The lamina propria shows an eosinophil-rich infiltrate and mucosa shows edema.

Hyperinfection with *S. stercoralis*: It produces invasion of larvae into the colonic submucosa, lymphatics, and blood vessels. In disseminated strongyloidiasis, the gut may show ulceration, edema and severe mononuclear infiltrate. It may show adult worms, larvae, and eggs in the crypts of the duodenum and ileum (**Fig. 137**). Worms of all stages may be seen in other organs (e.g., skin and lungs), and also in sputum in large numbers.

Diagnosis

- **Stool examination**: Motile larvae (at least three samples) may be observed on microscopic examination of stool, especially after a period of incubation. Larvae may also be cultured from stool.
- **Blood:** Eosinophilia may be found in some patients.
- **Duodenal/jejunal aspirate** may show larvae.
- **Serological tests:** ELISA for antibody to *S. stercoralis*.
- **In patients with disseminated infection:** Stool examination, ELISA, and sputum and blood examination for larvae.

In the small intestine, larva mature into adult worms

Larva enters circulation and via heart, lungs, respiratory tree, and esophagus, reach small intestine

Adult female embedded in the mucosa of small intestine

Penetrates the perianal skin

Autoinfection

Filariform larva

Rhabditiform larva metamorphose in bowel

Egg containing the larva

Life cycle of strongyloides stercoralis

Filariform larva penetrates skin of man (Definitive host)

Man

Soil

Direct cycle
Rhabditiform larva directly metamorphose to infective filariform larva in soil

"Double bulb" esophagus

Indirect cycle

Filariform larva (infective stage)

♂

♀

Rhabditiform larva immediately released and passes out in feces

Free-living adult worms in soil

Rhabditiform larva in soil

Egg in soil

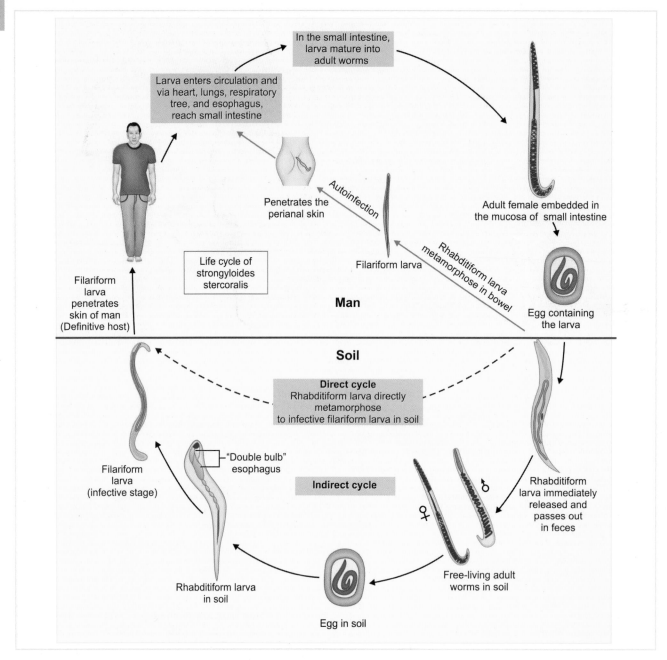

FIG. 136: Life cycle of *Strongyloides stercoralis*.

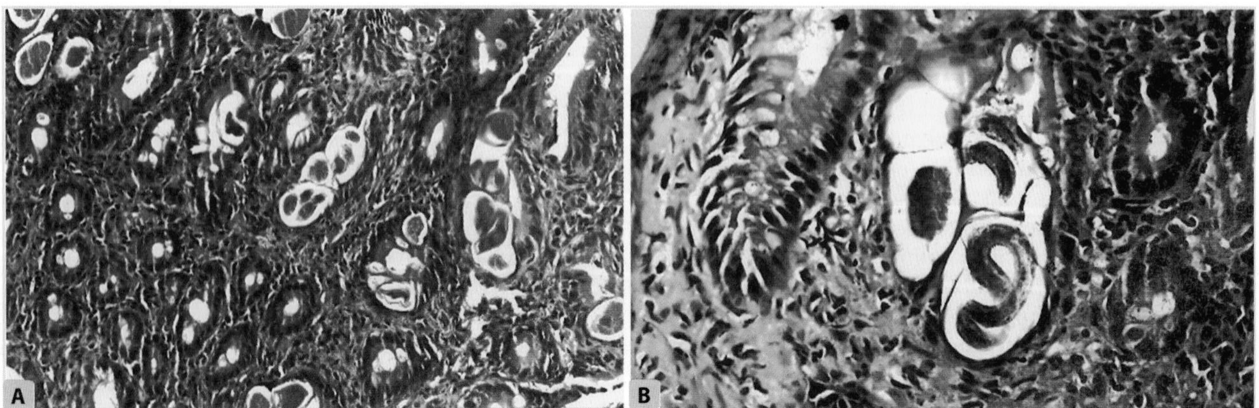

FIGS. 137A AND B: *Strongyloides stercoralis*. (A) Section of jejunum shows intestinal wall with mainly eggs and few larvae. (B) Larvae of *Strongyloides stercoralis* in the mucosal crypts.

Enterobiasis (Pinworm Infection)

Enterobiasis is an intestinal infection of humans caused by an intestinal nematode *Enterobius vermicularis* (threadworm). Though infection can develop at any age, parasitism is most common among young children.

Mode of infection: Humans are usually infected by the ingestion of eggs by direct transfer of eggs from the anus to the mouth by way of contaminated fingers or through contaminated food or water. The adult female worm resides in the cecum and appendix. But it migrates to the perianal and perineal skin to deposit eggs. The eggs stick to fingers, bed linens, towels, and clothing. These can be easily transmitted from person to person. Retroinfection occurs when the eggs hatch in the perianal region and the larvae migrate back into the bowel lumen.

Life cycle (Fig. 138): In the humans, the ingested eggs hatch in the small bowel and give rise to larvae. They mature into adult worms. Histopathological appearance of cut section of adult worm of *Enterobius vermicularis* in appendix is shown in **Figs. 139A** and **B**.

Clinical features: Some infected individuals are asymptomatic.

- **Perianal itching (pruritus ani):** It is the most common symptom, especially at night. This is due to the gravid female worm which migrates to anal region at night and lays ova around perianal region causing intense itching at night. The ova are carried to the mouth on the fingers and so reinfection or human-to-human infection is common (autoinfection). The adult worms may be seen moving on the buttocks or in the stool.
- **In females:** Migration of adult worm into the female genitalia may result in vaginal discharge, salpingitis, and endometritis.
- **Other symptoms** include irritability, insomnia, and enuresis.

Investigations and diagnoses

Direct visualizing the worms in the perineal and perianal region.

Stool examination for eggs (**Fig. 140**) may be positive in only 5–10% cases.

- **Cellophane tape test (preparation):** This test the specimen of choice for the detection of *Enterobius vermicularis* (pinworm) eggs. It may show adult female pinworms also. At night, typically in a child, when the body is at

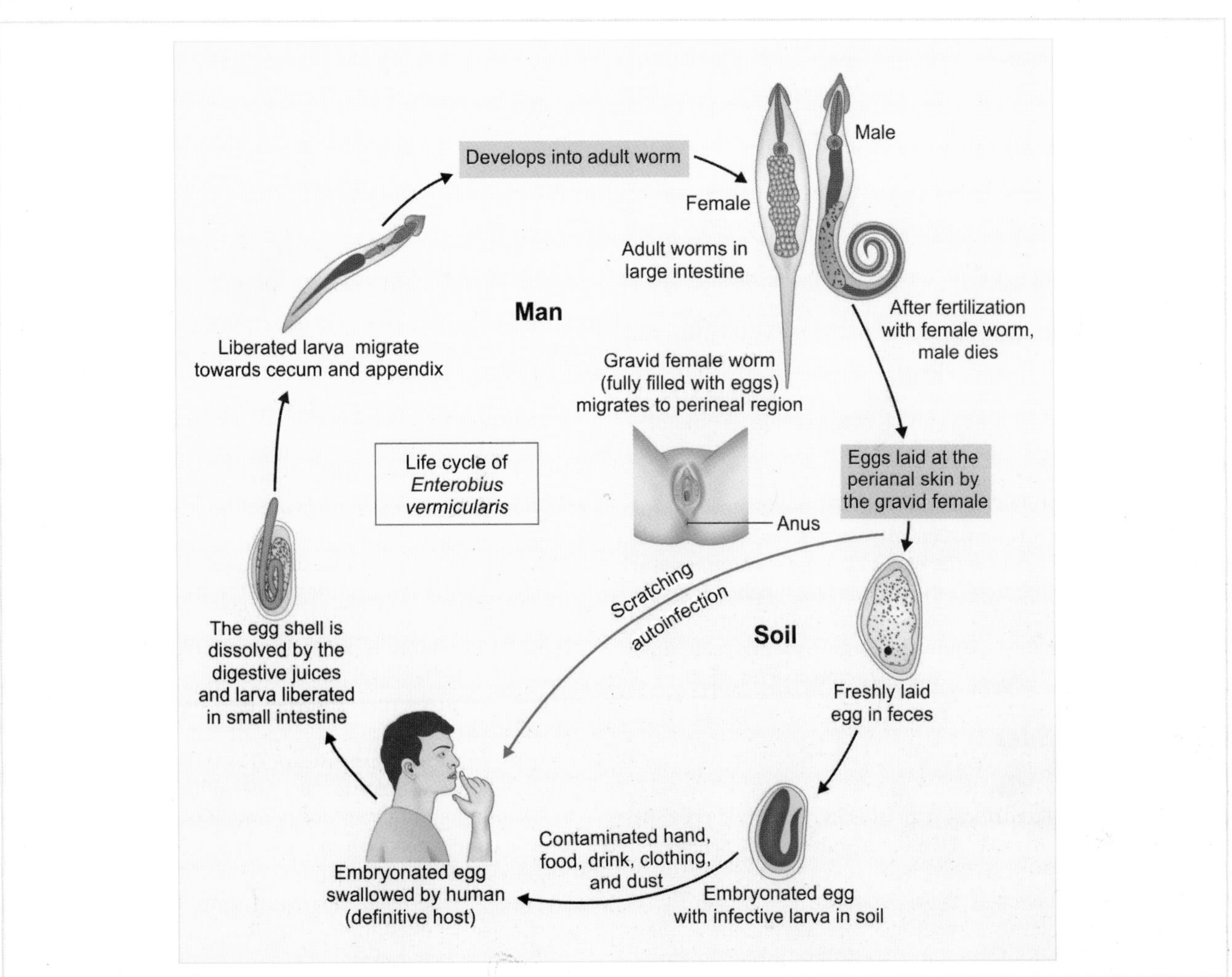

FIG. 138: Life cycle of *Enterobius vermicularis*.

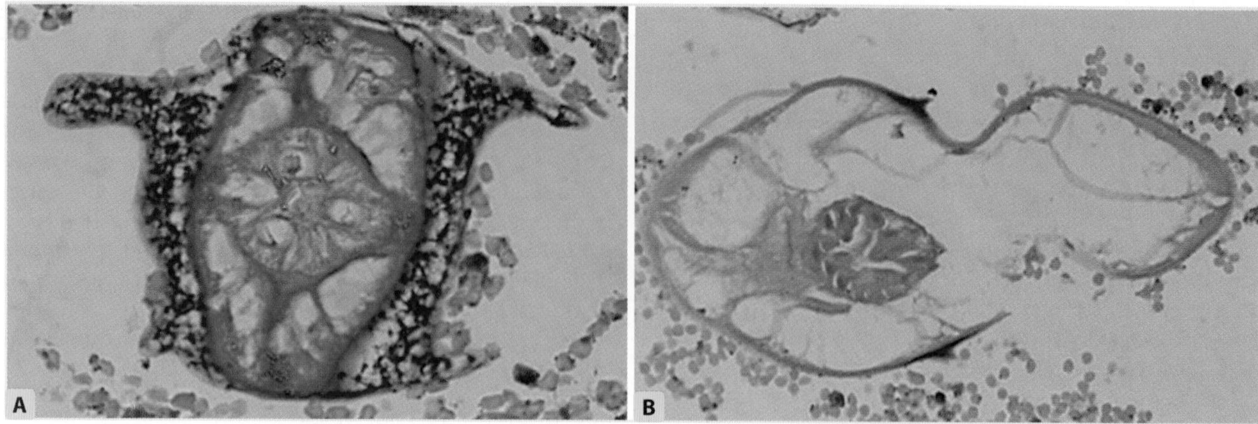

FIGS. 139A AND B: Adult worm of *Enterobius vermicularis* from the appendix. (A) Cross section; and (B) Longitudinal section.

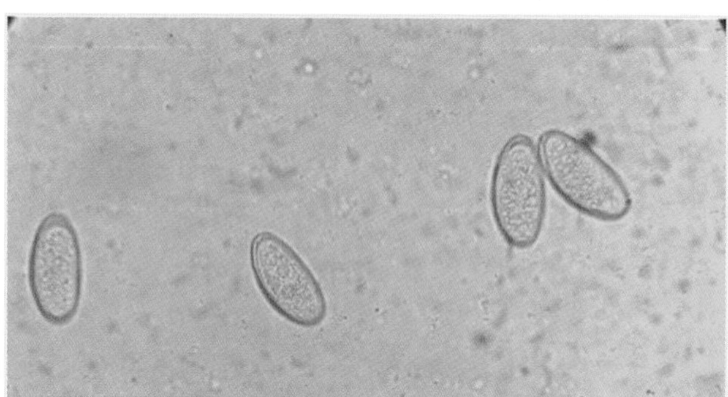

FIG. 140: Eggs of *Enterobius vermicularis* in the stool.

rest, pregnant adult female worms come out of the host through the rectum and lay numerous eggs in the perianal region. Therefore, it is important to collect the specimen in the morning before the patient washes or defecates. It is performed by firmly pressing (touching) the adhesive surface of cellophane tape to the skin of the perianal region of the patient several times in the morning. Using a rocking motion, cover as much of the region as possible. Remove and place the tape with adhesive side down, on a clean glass microscope slide. Avoid trapping of any air bubbles during this step. The slide is then examined for eggs under the low power of microscope. Reduced light is recommended because the eggs will appear colorless and make it difficult to detect them under high light intensity. Commercial collection kits are also available. Sensitivity of this test is about 90%. Apart from pinworm, this technique may be useful for the recovery of *Taenia* species eggs.

Filarial Nematodes

Filariasis

Q. Discuss the problem of filariasis/life cycle of *Wuchereria bancrofti*. Discuss about elephantiasis.

These nematodes belong to the *superfamily Filarioidea.* These are known as filarial worms because of their slender thread-like appearance (from the Latin *filum,* meaning "thread"). These are transmitted by the bite of blood-sucking insects. Various conditions included under filariasis are listed in **Box 19**.

Box 19: Conditions included under filariasis.

- Lymphatic filariasis: Caused by *Wuchereria bancrofti* and *Brugia malayi*
- Onchocerciasis (river blindness): Caused by *Onchocerca volvulus*
- Loiasis: Caused by *Loa loa*

Lymphatic filariasis

Lymphatic filariasis (bancroftian and Malayan filariasis) is an inflammatory parasitic infection of lymphatic vessels caused by closely related nematodes, *Wuchereria bancrofti* and *Brugia* species [*B. malayi* (90%) or *B. timori* (10%)]. It is transmitted by mosquitoes. Adult worms inhabit the lymphatics. Most frequent site being inguinal, epitrochlear and axillary lymph nodes, testis and epididymis.

Diseases: Lymphatic filariasis causes a spectrum of diseases. These are listed in **Box 20.**

Life cycle (Fig. 141): Humans, the only definitive host of these filarial nematodes and intermediate host is mosquito. Infection is acquired from the bites of at least 80 species of mosquitoes belonging to the genera *Culex, Aedes, Anopheles,* and *Mansonia.*

- During the mosquito bite to humans, the infective larvae are released by mosquitoes into the tissues. They migrate to lymphatics and lymph nodes. They develop within lymphatic channels and mature into adult males and females over several months. Adult worms mate and female releases microfilariae into lymphatics and the bloodstream.
- During the mosquito bite of the infected persons, the mosquitoes can take up the microfilariae. These micro-filariae undergo further development in the mosquito and they become infective and transmit the disease to humans.

Pathogenesis: Several filarial molecules of *W. bancrofti* and *B. malayi* may be responsible for invasiveness of the parasite and its mechanism of evasion or inhibition of immune defenses of host. These are as follows:

- **Elastases and trypsin-like proteases:** They *facilitate* invasion of host tissues by the parasite.

- **Surface glycoproteins with antioxidant function:** They may protect the parasite from the destructive effect of reactive oxygen species (ROS).
- **Homologs of cystatins (cysteine protease inhibitors):** These may impair the major histocompatibility complex (MHC) class II antigen-processing pathway.
- **Serpins (serine protease inhibitors):** These inhibit proteases released from neutrophils as well as inflammatory mediators
- **Homologs of host molecules:** Examples include TGF-β and macrophage migration inhibition factor, which could reduce the immune response.

Symbiotic *Wolbachia* bacteria: *Wolbachia* species bacteria infect filarial nematodes these are required for nematode development and reproduction. Thus, they contribute to pathogenesis of disease. It has been found that antibiotics that eradicate *Wolbachia* species impair survival and fertility of the parasite.

Immune responses by the host against the filarial worms cause damage to the human host. Similar to leprosy and leishmanial infections, the different manifestations (refer **Box 20**) of the lymphatic filariasis are probably related to variations in host T-cell responses to the parasites.

- **Chronic lymphatic filariasis:** In this, damage to the lymphatics is caused directly by the adult parasites and by a Th1-mediated immune response. Th1 response stimulates the formation of granulomas around the adult parasites.
- **Tropical pulmonary eosinophilia:** Hypersensitivity to microfilaria in the lungs is associated with tropical pulmonary eosinophilia. Filaria-specific Th2 helper T cells secrete IL-4 and IL-5 and these may stimulate IgE and eosinophils, respectively.

Box 20: Spectrum of diseases due to lymphatic filariasis.*

- Asymptomatic microfilaremia
- Recurrent lymphadenitis
- Chronic lymphadenitis with lymphatic obstruction. This may produce severe lymphedema (swelling) of the dependent limb or scrotum (elephantiasis)
- Acute lymphangitis
- Tropical pulmonary eosinophilia

*The elephantiasis characteristic of lymphatic filariasis was familiar in India even during 600 BC.

MORPHOLOGY

Adult parasite: The adult parasite is a white, thread-like worm. It is very convoluted within lymph nodes. Females are 80–100 mm in length and 0.2–0.3 mm in width and are twice the size of male parasites.

Microfilaria: The female parasite directly liberates sheathed microfilariae (embryo of the parasite) into lymph and they circulate in the blood. In blood films stained with Giemsa/Leishman, the microfilariae appear as curved **worms** (**Figs. 142 and 143B**). Microfilariae are also seen in blood vessels, lymphatics and body fluids.

Continued

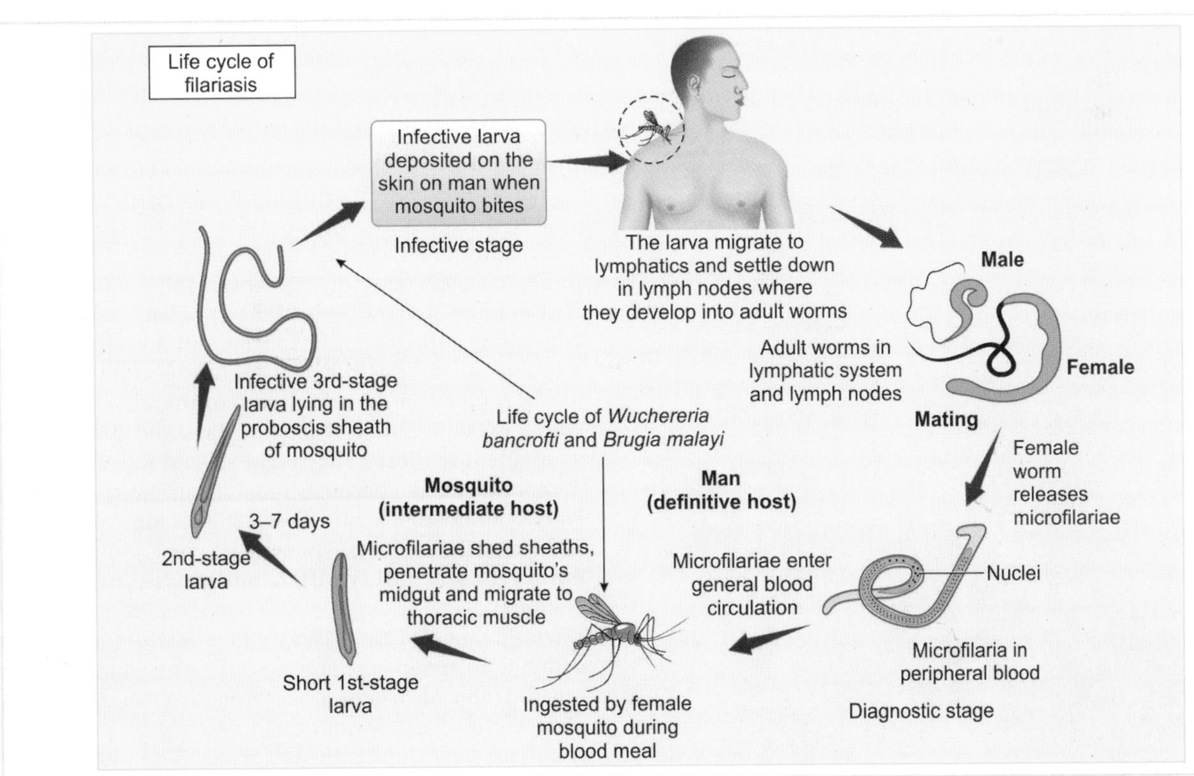

FIG. 141: Life cycle of filariasis.

Continued

Chronic filariasis: The adult parasites lodge in the lymphatics and cause dilatation of these lymphatics accompanied by thickening of the endothelial lining. In adjacent tissues, worms are surrounded by chronic inflammation, including eosinophils. Granuloma may be formed around the adult parasites and degenerating worms can provoke acute inflammation. After repeated attacks of lymphangitis, lymph nodes and lymphatics become densely fibrotic and usually contain calcified remnants of the worms. Chronic filariasis is characteristically show persistent lymphedema of the extremities (**Fig. 143A** and **C**), scrotum, penis, or vulva.

- **In severe and long-standing infections**, the swollen leg may develop tough subcutaneous fibrosis and epithelial hyperkeratosis, termed elephantiasis (**Fig. 143A and C**). Adult filarial worms (live, dead, or calcified) are observed in the draining lymphatics or nodes. The scrotum may also be markedly enlarged. Filariasis can also cause hydrocele and produce enlargement of involved lymph nodes. In longstanding cases, the dilated lymphatics develop polypoid infoldings.
- Microscopically, elephantoid skin shows thickening and hyperkeratosis of epidermis. The dermis shows dilation of the dermal lymphatics, infiltration of lymphocytes, and focal cholesterol deposits. Adult filarial worms (live, dead, or calcified) are present in the draining lymphatics or nodes. These are surrounded by (1) mild or no inflammation, (2) an intense eosinophilia with hemorrhage and fibrin (recurrent filarial funiculoepididymitis), or (3) granulomas. In the testis, hydrocele fluid may show cholesterol crystals, RBCs, and hemosiderin. It is associated with thickening and calcification of the tunica vaginalis.

Lung: Its involvement by microfilariae is characterized by either

- **Tropical eosinophilia:** Eosinophilia is due to Th2 responses and cytokine production, or
- **Meyers–Kouwenaar bodies:** In this, dead microfilariae are surrounded by stellate, hyaline, eosinophilic precipitates embedded in small epithelioid granulomas.

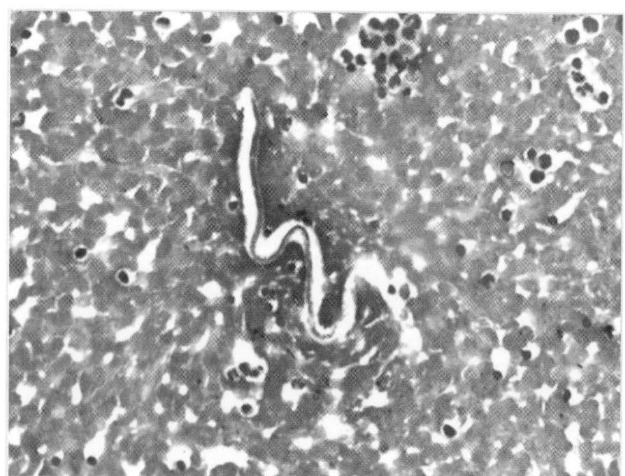

FIG. 142: Microfilaria in the peripheral blood.

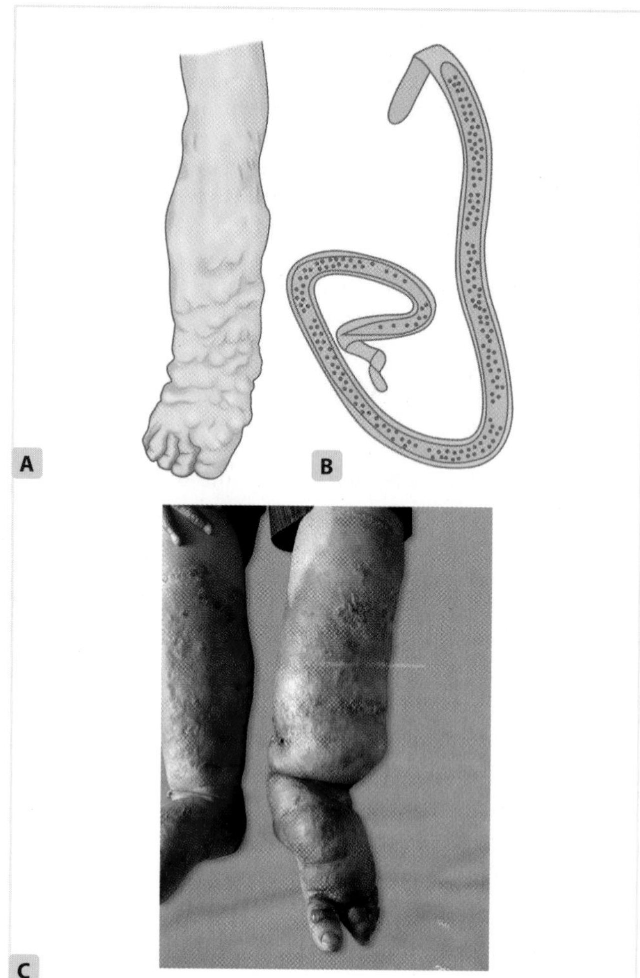

FIGS. 143A TO C: (A) Elephantiasis of leg (Diagrammatic); (B) Diagrammatic appearance of microfilaria (embryo of *Wuchereria bancrofti*) and (C) Elephantiasis of leg.

Clinical features: In endemic regions, most of the infected individuals have either antifilarial antibodies with no detectable infection or asymptomatic microfilaremia. The clinical manifestations of filariasis result from inflammatory responses to degenerating adult worms in the lymphatics.

- **Acute filarial lymphangitis:** It presents with fever, with chills and sweats, headache and muscle pain. On examination there will be **pain, tenderness and erythema along the course of inflamed lymphatic vessels**. The whole episode may last for few days and then resolve spontaneously. But it may recur several times in a year. Temporary edema becomes more persistent and regional lymph nodes (e.g., inguinal) enlarged painful and tender. Inflammation of the **spermatic cord (funiculitis), epididymis (epididymitis), and testis (orchitis)** is common.
- **Chronic stage of the disease:** Repeated infections are common in endemic regions which may lead to extensive scarring and obstruction of lymphatics over years. It is characterized by development of chronic permanent lymphedema ("**elephantiasis**") of legs (**Fig. 143 A and C**), scrotal edema, **chylous ascites, chylos pleural effusion, and chyluria**. Progressive enlargement of lymphedema

may produce coarsening, corrugation, fissuring and bacterial infection of the skin and subcutaneous tissue. This results in irreversible "elephantiasis". The scrotum may become very large in size because of hydrocele. Chyluria and chylous effusions appear as milky and opalescent which on standing shows fat globules on the top of chylous fluid.

- **Tropical pulmonary eosinophilia:** This is a manifestation of occult filariasis which presents with low-grade fever, loss of weight, and pulmonary symptoms such as dry nocturnal cough, dyspnea, asthmatic wheezing, and peripheral eosinophilia. **Occult filariasis** is characterized by indirect evidence of filarial infection (antifilarial antibodies). This condition is almost restricted to southern India and some Pacific Islands.

Investigations (laboratory findings) and diagnoses In the early stages of lymphangitis, diagnosis can be made on clinical grounds, and peripheral blood eosinophilia. Microfilariae are not seen in the peripheral blood during early infestation.

- **Peripheral blood:**
  - **Eosinophilia:** Host immune response to the parasite produces severe eosinophilia.
  - **Demonstration of microfilariaey**, in the peripheral blood at night.
- **Demonstration of microfilariae in other fluids:** Microfilariae can be demonstrated in the hydrocele fluid and may occasionally show an adult worm.
- **Diethylcarbamazine (DEC) provocation test:** In this test, administration of 100 mg DEC usually produces positive blood specimens within 30–60 minutes.
- **Radiology:** Calcified filariae may be demonstrable by radiography.
- **Serological tests: Antigen detection and antibody detection in the blood**—by ELISA or immunochromatic method.
- **PCR** for DNA detection.
- **Radionuclide lymphoscintigraphy:** It is used to detect widespread lymphatic abnormalities.

TECHNIQUES FOR DIAGNOSIS OF INFECTIOUS AGENTS

The gold standards for diagnosis of infections are: (1) identification of causative agent by culture, (2) serological methods, and (3) molecular techniques. Their selection depends on the suspected infectious agent.

Hematoxylin and eosin-stained tissue sections: Few infectious agents or their products can be directly seen in hematoxylin and eosin-stained sections. For example, inclusion bodies in cytomegalovirus (CMV) and herpes simplex virus (HSV) and bacterial clumps, which take up blue color.

Special stains: Many infectious agents can be best identified by special stains. The identification of the infectious agents is on the basis of characteristics of their cell wall or coat or by staining with specific antibodies (**Table 40**).

Serological examination: Acute infections can be diagnosed through serology by detecting pathogen-specific antibodies in the serum. The presence of specific IgM antibody shortly after the onset of symptoms is diagnostic of the disease. Also, specific antibody titers can be measured during the early infection and again 4–6 weeks later. A fourfold increase in the specific antibody titer is considered diagnostic.

Nucleic acid amplification tests: Examples include PCR and transcription-mediated amplification. These are used for rapid and early identification of microbes. Multiplex PCR panels for detection of several 20 pathogens are now available. In patients with viral infections such as HIV, HBV, or HCV, quantification of viral RNA is an important for the management of ART.

Next-generation sequencing can be used to detect bacteria, viruses, parasites, or fungi.

Table 40: Techniques for the diagnosis of infectious agents.

Techniques	*Infectious agents*
Routine stains	
• Hematoxylin and eosin	Cytomegalovirus (CMV) and herpes simplex virus (HSV)
Special stains	
• Gram stain	Most bacteria
• Acid-fast stain	*Mycobacteria* species, *Nocardia* species (modified)
• Fite-Faraco	*Mycobacteria leprae*
• Silver stains	Fungi, *Legionella* species, *Pneumocystis jirovecii*
• Periodic acid-Schiff	Fungi, amebae
• Mucicarmine	*Cryptococcus* species
• Giemsa	*Campylobacter* species, *Leishmania* species, malarial parasites
Other techniques	
• Antibody stains	All classes of infectious agents
• Culture	
• DNA probes	

11.7 Miscellaneous

CHAPTER OUTLINE

- Prion diseases
  - Pathogenesis
- Pyrexia (fever) of unknown origin
  - Causes
  - Investigation of classic FUO
- Laboratory diagnosis of urinary tract infections
  - Urine examination
- Emerging and re-emerging infections
  - General features
  - Factor influencing emergence of infections
- Agents of bioterrorism

PRION DISEASES

Q. Write short essay on prion diseases.

It has been noticed that infection can be transmitted and propagated solely by **proteins, without the participation of nucleic acids**. These causative infectious agents or particles called prions (**pro**teinaceous **in**fectious particles) and lack nucleic acids.

Definition: Prion diseases are a group of closely related rapidly progressive neurodegenerative conditions of humans and other mammals. They are caused by an accumulation, aggregated and intercellular spread of a misfolded prion protein (PrP) in the central nervous system (CNS). The hallmark of all PrP prion diseases is that they involve the aberrant metabolism of PrP.

Prion diseases: These are as follows: -

- **Diseases in humans (Box 21):** These include Creutzfeldt-Jakob disease (CJD), Gerstmann-Sträussler-Scheinker syndrome, fatal familial insomnia, and kuru.
- **Diseases in animals (Box 21):** These include scrapie in sheep and goats; mink-transmissible encephalopathy; chronic wasting disease of deer and elk; and bovine spongiform encephalopathy.

All prion diseases are morphologically characterized by "spongiform change" caused by intracellular vacuoles in neurons and glia, and clinically by a rapidly progressive dementia.

Transmission: Prion diseases may be sporadic, familial (dominantly inherited), or transmitted (acquired by infection). All prion diseases are transmissible, and inadvertent human iatrogenic transmission of CJD may follow administration of contaminated human pituitary growth hormone,

Tissue grafts such as corneal transplantation from a diseased donor, poorly sterilized neurosurgical instruments and surgical implantation of contaminated dura.

Pathogenesis

Prion diseases are degenerative disorders caused by "spreading" of misfolded proteins. These pathogenic proteins have some of the characteristics of an infectious organism. *PRNP* is the *PrP* gene located on human chromosome 20 and its product is prion protein (PrP). Normal prion protein (PrP) is a 30-kD cytoplasmic glycoprotein and is constitutively expressed cell surface glycoprotein. PrP is produced widely throughout the body by several tissues in mammals. But the highest levels of PrP messenger RNA (mRNA) are in CNS neurons. It binds

Box 21: Prion diseases in humans and animals.

Humans

- Creutzfeldt–Jakob disease (CJD)
  - Sporadic (85% of all CJD cases)
  - Inherited mutation of the prion gene, autosomal dominant transmission (15% of all CJD cases
  - Iatrogenic
    - Hormone injection: Human growth hormone, human pituitary gonadotropin
    - Tissue grafts: Dura mater, cornea, pericardium
    - Medical devices: Depth electrodes, surgical instruments (none definitely proven)
    - New variant CJD (vCJD)
- Gerstmann–Sträussler–Scheinker disease (GSS; inherited prion gene mutation, autosomal dominant transmission). Germline mutations in ***PRNP***
- Fatal familial insomnia (FFI; inherited prion gene mutation, autosomal dominant transmission)
- Kuru (confined to the Fore people of Papua New Guinea, formerly transmitted by cannibalistic funeral ritual)

Animals

- Scrapie in sheep and goats
- Bovine spongiform encephalopathy (BSE; "mad cow disease") in cattle
- Transmissible mink encephalopathy (TME)in mink
- Chronic wasting disease (CWD) of mule, deer and elk
- Feline spongiform encephalopathy (FSE) in cats
- Captive exotic ungulate spongiform encephalopathy in nyala, gemsbok, eland, Arabian oryx, greater kudu.
- Experimental transmission to many species, including primates and transgenic mice

neuronal plasmalemma via a glycolipid anchor. Its function is not known but it may play a role in copper metabolism. PrP prions reproduce by binding to the normal, cellular isoform of the prion protein (PrP^C). In prion diseases, there is stimulation of conversion of PrP^C into the disease-causing abnormal misfolded and aggregated isoform termed PrP^{SC} (for scrapie) and this PrP^{SC} accumulates. Normally, there are α-helical region in the PrP. Prion disease occurs when PrP is converted from its normal (native) α-helix-containing isoform (PrP^c) to an abnormal (pathogenic) β-pleated sheet-rich isoform, usually termed PrP^{sc}. This results in conformation change in PrP. The normal cellular prion protein, cellular PrP or PrP^C, and the pathogenic (infectious) prion protein, known as scrapie PrP or PrP^{SC}, have the same primary amino acid sequence. But they have different tertiary structures and patterns of glycosylation. Specifically, PrP^C is rich in α-helix configuration and has little β-structure, whereas PrP^{SC} has less α-helix and has high amount of β -pleated sheet configuration (**Fig. 144**). This α-to-β structural transition in PrP is the fundamental event underlying prion diseases. Pathogenic PrP^{SC} is able to recruit the normal form of PrP into the pathologic aggregate and the process is thus autocatalyzed. The pathogenic protein procures more pathogenic protein from the limitless supply of native protein. The pathogenic conformation is extremely stable so that PrP^{SC} strongly resists conventional microbial decontamination methods. If PrP^{SC} enters the brain either through infectious transmission or by spontaneous misfolding of native protein, it will change other PrP proteins into pathogenic PrP^{SC}. This leads to autocatalytic (self-propagating), exponentially expanding accretion of abnormal PrP^{SC}. PrP^{SC} formed tends to polymerize with subsequent fibril formation. These masses of PrP^{SC} formed compromise cell function and cause neurodegeneration. The exact mechanisms are not known but may be similar to those of other neurodegenerative diseases characterized by fibrillogenesis.

The pathogenic PrP^{SC} acquires resistance to digestion with proteases, such as proteinase K. Accumulation of PrP^{sc} in neural tissue is responsible for the pathologic changes in these diseases. Immunostaining for PrP after partial digestion with proteinase K can detect PrP^{SC} and this is diagnostic of prion diseases.

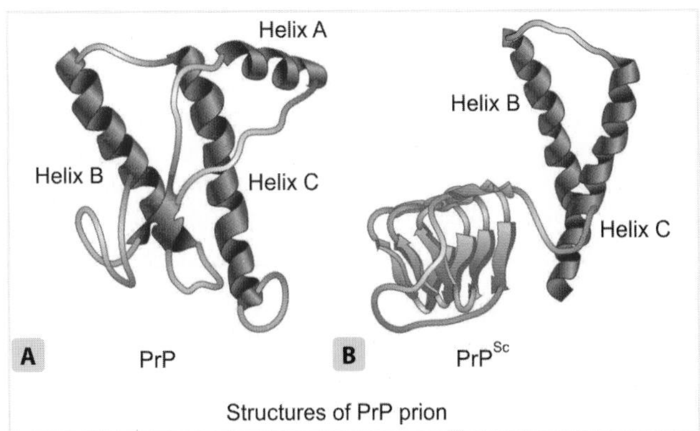

FIGS. 144A AND B: Structures of PrP prion proteins. (A). Diagrammatic structural model of PrP composed of the α-helical A (helix-A), B (helix-B) and C (helix-C) form. They resemble that of PrP^C. (B). Structural model of PrP^{SC} in which α-helical A region has been changes to a β-helical architecture whereas helices B and C are preserved as in PrP^C.(Copyrighted to be drawn)

The conformational change that result in PrP^{SC} may occur spontaneously. This may occur at an extremely low rate (resulting in sporadic cases of CJD) or at a higher rate if various mutations are present in PrP^C,as in familial forms of CJD, Gerstmann–Sträussler–Scheinker syndrome, and fatal familial insomnia. Whatever may be the means by which prions originates, PrP^{SC} then converts other PrP^C molecules to PrP^{SC} molecules and propagates PrP^{SC}. This accounts for the transmissible variants of prion diseases, which include iatrogenic CJD, variant CJD, and kuru.

Pathogenesis of prion disease is presented in **Fig. 145**. Characteristic features of prions are presented in **Box 22**.

Creutzfeldt–Jakob Disease (CJD)

CJD is a rare disorder and is the most common prion disease.

Clinical features: Symptoms begin insidiously. But usually within 6 months to 3 years, patients clinically manifest with progressive severe dementia leading to death.

- **Age:** CJD has a peak incidence in the seventh decade.
- **Signs and symptoms:** It presents with subtle changes in memory and behavior followed by a rapidly progressive dementia. It is often associated with pronounced involuntary jerking muscle contractions on sudden stimulation (startle myoclonus). Cerebellar involvement usually manifests in a minority of affected individuals as ataxia and this feature helps to distinguish CJD from Alzheimer disease.
- **Prognosis:** CJD is uniformly fatal and the average survival is only 7 months after the onset of symptoms. Few may live for several years, and these patients show extensive atrophy of involved gray matter.

Variants of Creutzfeldt–Jakob disease

CJD can be classified depend on etiology: sporadic, familial, iatrogenic and new variant.; Iatrogenic transmission can occur by corneal or dural transplantation, deep implantation of electrodes in the brain, and administration of contaminated preparations of cadaveric human growth hormone.

- **Sporadic (classical) CJD (sCJD):** The sporadic form accounts for 75% to 90% of CJD cases. The mode of acquisition is unknown. These patients neither show the mutations associated with inherited forms of CJD or other prion diseases nor have any history of iatrogenic exposure.
- **Inherited CJD (fCJD):** Familial CJD accounts for 15% of prion diseases and is caused by mutations in ***PRNP***, the gene that encodes PrP. Several different PRNP mutations in ***PRNP*** have been documented. In these patients, the PrP^C has a increased tendency to misfold into the pathogenic isoform. The mutated PRNP causes familial CJD, fatal familial insomnia and Gerstmann-Sträussler-Scheinker disease.
- **Iatrogenic CJD (iCJD):** Many iatrogenic causes of CJD are known and presently the most causes for iatrogenic CJD have been eliminated by precautionary measures. For example, recombinant human growth hormone has replaced human pituitary derived preparations for therapy. While performing brain biopsies or autopsies in prion disease cases, special protocols are used to limit exposure of staff and patients to prions. These infectious agents are characterized by the uncommon persistence of these agents. Normal methods of sterilization do not inactivate

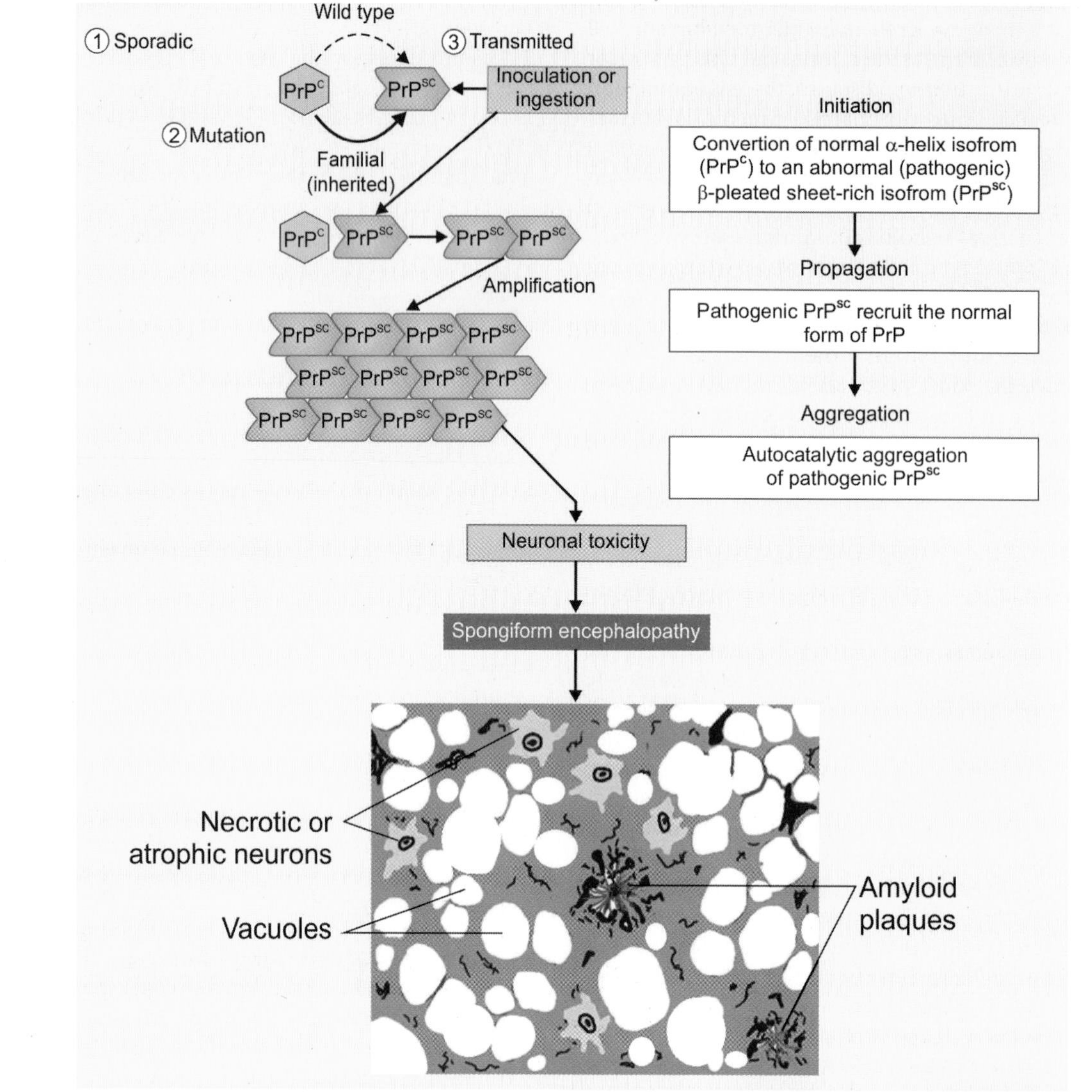

FIG. 145: Pathogenesis of prion disease. α-helical of PrP^{C} may undergo conversion to the β-sheet PrP^{SC} conformation spontaneously, mutations in *PRNP* or acquired. It occur spontaneously at a much higher rate in familial diseases associated with germline PrP mutations. PrP^{SC} may also be acquired from exogenous sources, such as contaminated food, medical instrumentation, or medicines. Once PrP^{SC} id formed, it converts additional molecules of PrP^{C} into PrP^{SC} through physical interaction. This will lead to the formation of pathogenic PrP^{SC} aggregates.Thus, prions are essentially misfolded proteins. They aggregate in the CNS and produce neuronal toxicity with progressive neurodegeneration.

Box 22: Characteristic features of prions.

- **Without nuclei acid:** Prions are the only known transmissible pathogens that does not have nucleic acid. All other infectious agents have genomes composed of either RNA or DNA that direct the synthesis of their progeny.
- **Wide spectrum of clinical manifestations:** Prion diseases may manifest as sporadic, genetic or infectious disorders. None of the other group of illnesses with a single etiology presents with such a wide spectrum of clinical manifestations.
- **Accumulation of PrP^{SC}:** Prion diseases are produced due to the accumulation of PrP^{SC}. The conformation of PrP^{SC} substantially differs from its precursor namely PrP^{C}.
- **Distinct strains of PrP prions exhibit different biologic properties:** Distinct strains of prions show different biologic properties, which are epigenetically heritable or inherited. PrP^{SC} can present in many different conformations.

them. They may be transmitted via surgical instruments or electrodes and hence use of disposable instruments can reduce its risk of transmission. Conventional autoclaving and most standard disinfectants do not eradicate this infectious agent. Hence, the surfaces and instruments are treated with 2 N NaOH.

- **New variant CJD (vCJD or nvCJD):** In 1995, a new CJD-like illness came to medical attention and was identified by a surveillance program in the United Kingdom after the BSE epidemic between 1980 and 1996. This group of patients were different in several important respects (key characteristics) from other patients with sporadic (classical) CJD. Most importantly is the age and this variant of CJD affected young adults (mean age is 26 years compared to about 65 years in sporadic CJD). Other features include prominent behavioral disorders (dysesthesias) or sensory disturbances in the early stages of the disease, the slower progression of neurologic syndrome than in individuals with other forms of CJD, a longer duration of illness (median, 12 months vs. 4 months) and none of the usual electroencephalographic (EEG) findings of sporadic CJD. At autopsy, vCJD showed prominent spongiform change in the basal ganglia and thalamus, and extensive PrP plaques in the cerebrum and cerebellum. The brain contained much more PrP than brains of sporadic CJD patients. The evidences indicated that the new variant of CJD (vCJD) was linked to exposure to bovine spongiform encephalopathy, either through consumption of contaminated foods or via transfusion of blood from patients in the asymptomatic/preclinical stage of vCJD. After this recognition, public health measures were taken to limit the spread of vCJD and it suddenly reduced the incidence in the United Kingdom that had peaked in 2000.

MORPHOLOGY

Characteristic features are seen in **brain**. The progression of the dementia in CJD is usually rapid. Hence, there is little time for any gross evidence of atrophy of brain.

Sites (Fig. 146): The pathognomonic finding in CJD is a **spongiform transformation of the cerebral cortex and deep gray matter structures** (caudate, putamen) and astrocytic gliosis.

Light microscopy: In CJD there is formation of multifocal foci of uneven small and apparently empty microscopic vacuoles of varying sizes within the neuropil and sometimes in the perikaryon of neurons. It is called as spongiform encephalopathy. Spongiform degeneration is characterized by many 1- to 5-μm vacuoles in the neuropil between nerve cell bodies. Advanced cases show severe loss of neurons, reactive gliosis, and sometimes expansion of the vacuolated areas into cystlike spaces ("status spongiosus"). **Absence of an inflammatory response** in CJD and other prion diseases is an important pathologic feature of these degenerative disorders. Astrocytic gliosis is a constant but nonspecific feature of prion diseases.

Electron microscopy: It shows the vacuoles to be membrane bound and located within the cytoplasm of neuronal processes.

Kuru plaques: They are extracellular deposits of aggregated abnormal PrP. They stain positively with Congo red- and PAS and usually occur in the cerebellum. But they are abundant in the cerebral cortex in cases of vCJD.

Immunohistochemistry: Immunohistochemical staining in all forms of prion disease, show the presence of proteinase K-resistant PrPsc in tissue.

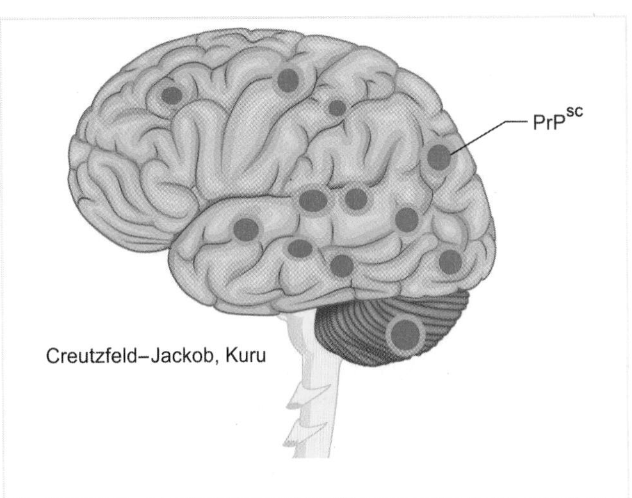

FIG. 146: Gross sites of involvement in Creutzfeldt–Jakob disease (CJD). The pathognomonic finding in CJD is a **spongiform transformation of the cerebral cortex and deep gray matter structures** (caudate, putamen).

Other Prion Diseases

Gerstmann-Sträussler-Scheinker syndrome: It is a rare transmissible spongiform encephalopathy and is usually familial. Rarely it may be sporadic. Patients may present with a variety of symptoms, but usually signs and symptoms of cerebellar degeneration are prominent. Later, patient develops dementia.

Fatal familial insomnia: It is also a rare inherited prion disorder. Hallmark of this disorder is progressive course of insomnia that worsens over time until the patient either barely or not at all sleeps. It is also characterized by autonomic instability, which manifests as increased sympathetic tone.

Kuru: Kuru is a progressive neurodegenerative disease. It is only found in the South Fore tribe/people in the remote highlands of Papua New Guinea. Kuru, the Foreword for "trembling," was transmitted by the consumption of brains from dead relatives during ritualistic cannibalism. After the cessation of ritualistic funerary cannibalism in the late 1950s, kuru nearly disappeared among the Fore and it disappeared within a generation.

PYREXIA (FEVER) OF UNKNOWN ORIGIN

Q. Discuss the laboratory diagnosis of PUO (FUO).

Normal body temperature: The homeostatic mechanisms of the body maintain a constant body temperature of 37°C (98.6°F). The daily fluctuation (circadian temperature rhythm) does not exceed ±1–1.5°C. Although 37°C (98.6°F) is considered as "normal", individuals vary in their body temperature; in some, it may be as low as 36°C, in others as high as 38°C.

Definition of fever: Fever is defined as an **abnormal increase in body temperature**. An oral temperature of >37.6°C (100.4°F) or a rectal temperature >38°C (101°F) is considered as fever. It is thought that fever may be a protective response by the host.

Continuous or intermittent: Fever may be continuous or intermittent.

- *Continuous fever*: In this, the body **temperature is elevated over the whole 24-hour period and swings <1°C**. For example, this type of fever is observed in typhoid and typhus fever.

- *Intermittent fever*: In this, the **temperature is above normal throughout the 24-hour period, but swings >1°C during that time**. A swinging fever is typical of pyogenic infections, abscesses, and tuberculosis.

Fever is a common complaint. The cause is usually immediately apparent or is discovered within a few days, or the temperature returns to normal spontaneously.

Pyrogens: These are substances that can produce a fever. Pyrogens may be exogenous or endogenous.
- **Exogenous pyrogen:** E.g., bacterial products, such as lipopolysaccharide (**LPS)** in gram-negative cell walls.
- **Endogenous pyrogen:** E.g., interleukin 1 (IL-1) and tumor necrosis factor (TNF) released from phagocytic cells.

Definition of fever of unknown origin (FUO): FUO is defined as **prolonged febrile illnesses without an established etiology in spite of intensive evaluation and diagnostic testing**.

According to new classification, pyrexia of unknown origin (PUO) is divided into four types:

1. **Classic PUO/FUO** is classically defined as:
   - **Temperature:** Daily temperature persistently elevated above 101°F (38.3°C) on at least two occasions.
   - **Duration:** Fever of at least 3 weeks' duration.
   - **No known immunocompromised state** (e.g., HIV or other immunosuppressing conditions).
   - **Remains undiagnosed** is spite of a thorough history-taking, physical examination, and the screening tests (or at least three outpatient visits or 3 days in hospital)
2. **Nosocomial PUO:**
   - **Temperature:** Daily temperature persistently elevated **above 101°F** (38.3°C) developing on several occasions.
   - In a **hospitalized patient (>24 hours) who is receiving acute care but no fever on admission.**
   - It is mandatory that the cause of fever is not found at least on 3 days of intelligent investigations, including at least 2 days' incubation of cultures.
3. **Neutropenic PUO:**
   - A temperature of >38.3°C (101°F) developing on several occasions.
   - **Neutrophil count is <500/mL** or is expected to fall to that level in 1 or 2 days.
   - It is mandatory that the cause of fever is not found at least on 3 days of intelligent investigations, including at least 2 days' incubation of cultures.
4. **HIV-associated PUO:**
   - A temperature of >38.3°C (101°F) developing on several occasions.
   - Duration of fever is >4 weeks for outpatients or >3 days for hospitalized patients.
   - **HIV infection confirmed.**
   - It is mandatory that the cause of fever is not found at least on 3 days of intelligent investigations, including at least 2 days' incubation of cultures.

Causes

Classic PUO is usually not due to a rare disease, but due to atypical presentation of common diseases. Common causes of prolonged fever are listed in **Box 23**.

Box 23: Causes of fever of unknown origin (FUO).

Infective causes (40% cases):
- **Bacterial infections:** Tuberculosis, enteric fevers, osteomyelitis, endocarditis, Brucellosis, abscesses (especially intra-abdominal), biliary system infections, urinary tract infections, Lyme disease, relapsing fever, leptospirosis, rat bite fever, typhus, spotted fever, psittacosis, and Q fever
- **Parasitic infections:** Malaria, trypanosomiasis, amoebic abscesses, and toxoplasmosis
- **Fungal infections:** Candidiasis, cryptococcosis, and histoplasmosis
- **Viral infections:** AIDS, infectious mononucleosis, and hepatitis

Noninfectious inflammatory diseases (20% cases):
- **Systemic rheumatic and autoimmune diseases:** E.g., ankylosing spondylitis, antiphospholipid syndrome, autoimmune hemolytic anemia, and autoimmune hepatitis
- **Vasculitis:** E.g., allergic vasculitis, eosinophilic granulomatosis with polyangiitis, giant cell vasculitis/polymyalgia rheumatica, granulomatosis with polyangiitis, and hypersensitivity vasculitis
- **Granulomatous diseases:** E.g., sarcoidosis
- **Autoinflammatory syndromes:** E.g., adult-onset Still's disease

Neoplasms (20% cases):
- **Hematologic malignancies:** Lymphoma and chronic leukemia
- **Solid tumors (nonhematological):** Renal cell carcinoma, hepatocellular carcinoma, pancreatic, breast, lung and colonic cancer, myelodysplastic syndrome, sarcomas, and atrial myxoma

Miscellaneous (10% cases): Drug fever, gout, postmyocardial infarction syndrome, adrenal insufficiency, and thermoregulatory disorders (e.g., brain tumor, hyperthyroidism, and pheochromocytoma)

Undiagnosed (10% cases)

Investigation of Classic FUO

Steps in the Investigative Procedure

FUO may be due to infectious and noninfectious causes of FUO, and it is not practical to perform specific investigations for each at the outset. Various steps in the investigation of classic FUO are discussed below.

Stage 1

Careful history taking, physical examination, and screening tests:

Careful history: It is essential. It should include about travel, occupation (e.g., Weil's disease), risk for venereal diseases, hobbies, contact with pet animals (e.g., cattle with brucellosis) and birds (e.g., psittacosis), exposure to animals (e.g., leptospirosis with cats and dogs and Q fever with cattle and sheep) and known infectious hazards, contact with patients with TB or other family members having infection, residence in endemic areas (vector-borne, e.g., malaria, kala-azar, and trypanosomiasis), antibiotic therapy within the previous 2 months, substance misuse, and other habits.

Physical examination: After history taking and the differential diagnosis, a complete physical examination of the patient with FUO is essential. This should, in particular, include the following:

- Examination of skin, eyes, lymph nodes, and abdomen.
- Auscultation of the heart.
- Others such as examination of temporal arteries, rectal digital examination, etc.
- Routine investigations (screening tests) such as blood tests and chest radiography should be performed at this stage. Guidelines for the minimum screening tests are presented in **Box 24**.

Stage 2

Review the history, repeating the physical examination, specific diagnostic tests, and noninvasive investigations:

Box 24: Stage-1 screening tests (routine investigations) done in patient with pyrexia.

Hematological tests:
- Full blood count with peripheral smear:
  - Leukocytosis: Increase in bands suggests an occult bacterial infection
  - Eosinophilia: Helminthiasis
  - Anemia
  - Leukemias
  - Lymphocytosis with atypical cells: Suspect herpesvirus infection
  - Atypical lymphocytes: Infectious mononucleosis
  - Thick and thin smear examination of the peripheral blood: Malaria, leishmaniasis, trypanosomiasis, and filariasis
- Erythrocyte sedimentation rate (ESR) and C-reactive protein (CRP) level
- Hemoglobin level
- Renal function tests
- Liver function tests
- Blood culture
- Serum virology for HIV, dengue, leptospira, and Widal test
- Urinalysis and culture
- Blood culture:
  - First specimen should be collected before antibiotics. Multiple blood samples (not <3 rarely >6 including samples for anaerobic cultures) should be cultured for at least 2 weeks to ensure that any HACEK group of organisms that may be present have ample time to grow
  - Typhoid, paratyphoid, subacute bacterial endocarditis, septicemia, and brucellosis
- Protein electrophoresis
- Sputum culture and sensitivity
- Stool routine and occult blood
- Mantoux test (tuberculin skin test—TST)
- Antinuclear antibodies and rheumatoid factor
- Malarial smear in endemic areas
- Investigations in pyrexia of unknown origin
- Serological tests directed by local epidemiological data

Radiological investigations:
- Chest X-ray
- Ultrasound abdomen, pelvis, and neck (if adenopathy, thyroid)

Review the history: A review of the patient's history, perhaps by a second physician, is valuable to check for omissions such as exposure to particular risk factors.

Repeating the physical examination: The physical examination should also be repeated.

Specific diagnostic tests: Clues to the diagnosis may be obtained by careful history taking and specific investigations can be carried out. Most common cause of FUO is infection. Hence, collection and careful examination of appropriate specimens are essential. The most important specimens include:

- Blood for culture.
- Blood for examination of antibodies. Serological tests help in the diagnosis of cytomegalovirus (CMV) and Epstein–Barr virus (EBV) infection, toxoplasmosis, psittacosis, and rickettsial infections.
- Direct examination of blood to diagnose malaria, trypanosomiasis, and relapsing fever.
- Review results of investigation and repeat investigation, if necessary. Laboratory investigations in stage 2 are presented in **Box 25**.

Stage 3

Comprises invasive tests: Biopsy of liver and bone marrow to be considered in classic cases of FUO and other tissues such as skin, lymph nodes, and kidney may also be biopsied.

LABORATORY DIAGNOSIS OF URINARY TRACT INFECTIONS

Q. Write short essay on laboratory diagnosis of urinary tract infections (UTI).

Box 25: Stage-2 laboratory investigations.

Hematological tests:
- Repeat blood counts, chemistry
- Protein electrophoresis
- Autoantibody screen (ANA, RF, ANCA, anti-dsDNA)
- Thyroid function tests
- Bone marrow examination with culture
- Lumbar puncture
- Coagulation workup
- Serum ferritin (adult onset Still's disease)
- Consider PSA, CEA, and LDH
- Paul–Bunnell test and Brucella agglutination test
- Weil–Felix reaction

Biopsy:
- Temporal artery biopsy
- Noninvasive investigative method
- Ultrasound, computed tomography (CT) scan, and magnetic resonance imaging (MRI)
- Gallium or technetium scans depending on the likely diagnosis
- Electrocardiogram (ECG)

(ANA: antinuclear antibodies; RF: rheumatoid factor; ANCA: anti-neutrophil cytoplasmic antibodies; anti-dsDNA: anti-double stranded DNA; CEA: carcinoembryonic antigen; LDH: lactate dehydrogenase; PSA: prostate-specific antigen)

Urinary tract infections are common, especially among women. The urinary tract is one of the most common sites of bacterial infection, particularly in females. UTIs in men are less common.

Various causative organisms causing UTI are presented in **Table 41**.

Viruses: Viruses usually do not cause UTI. But, they may be found in associations with hemorrhagic cystitis and other renal syndromes. Certain viruses may be recovered from the urine in the absence of urinary tract disease. These include the following:

- **Human polyomaviruses**: The human polyomaviruses, JC and BK, enter the body via the respiratory tract. They disseminate throughout the body and infect epithelial cells in the kidney tubules and ureter. In the epithelial cells of renal system, they establish latency with persistence of the viral genome. Thus, kidneys from healthy individuals may contain polyomavirus DNA sequences. Reactivation may occur in two situations.
  - Reactivation of the viruses may occur asymptomatically during normal pregnancy. This will result in appearance of large amounts of virus in the urine.
  - Reactivation also occurs in immunocompromised patients and may produce hemorrhagic cystitis.
- **Cytomegalovirus and rubella:** High titers of these viruses may be shed asymptomatically in the urine of congenitally infected infants.
- **Adenovirus**: Some of its serotypes may cause of hemorrhagic cystitis.
- **Rodent-borne hantavirus**: It is responsible for Korean hemorrhagic fever. It infects capillary blood vessels in the kidney and can cause a **renal syndrome** with proteinuria.
- **Other viruses infecting the kidneys**: These include mumps and HIV.

Urine samples are investigated by virus isolation, immunological and genomic detection methods.

Parasites: Only few can cause UTIs.

Others: These include—

- *Trichomonas vaginalis* is a protozoan, which can cause urethritis in both males and females, but usually cause vaginitis.
- Infections with *Schistosoma haematobium* result in inflammation of the bladder and commonly hematuria. The eggs penetrate the wall of the bladder and in severe infections, large granulomatous reactions can occur and the eggs may become calcified.

Urine Examination

Key feature in the diagnosis of UTI is the detection of significant bacteriuria.

Methods of Collection of Urine

- **Midstream specimen:** This is used for all types of urine examination. After voiding first half of urine into the toilet, a part of the next voided urine is collected as midstream urine (MSU) sample. An MSU sample should be collected into a sterile wide-mouthed container. First, carefully clean the labia or glans with soap (not antiseptic) and water. Then, allow the first part of the urine stream to be voided, as this helps to wash out contaminants in the lower urethra.
- **Clean catch specimen:** This is the method of collection for culture and sensitivity of urine. The external genitalia are cleaned with soap and water and specimen is collected as mentioned in the midstream sample.
- **Cather specimen:** It is used for culture and sensitivity in bed-ridden patients or patients with urinary tract obstruction.
- **Collection from infants:** It is usually collected by a clean plastic bag attached around the genitalia.

Urine specimens are usually collected by voiding into a sterile container. They may become contaminated with the periurethral flora during collection. However, infection is distinguished from contamination by quantitative culture methods. Bacteriuria is defined as "significant" when a properly collected MSU specimen contains $>10^5$ organisms/mL. Infected urine usually contains a single predominant bacterial species. Contaminated urine usually has $<10^4$ organisms/mL and usually contains >1 bacterial species. Ideally, urine samples should be collected before starting antimicrobial therapy. If the patient is receiving, or has received, therapy within the previous 48 hours, this should be mentioned on the request form.

Special urine samples: These are required to detect *Mycobacterium tuberculosis* and *Schistosoma haematobium*. These include—

- **For *M. tuberculosis:*** Three early morning urine samples on consecutive days for *M. tuberculosis*. These do not require the same precautions during collection as an MSU sample.

Table 41: Organisms causing urinary tract infection.

Bacteria:		
Gram-negative bacilli	***Gram-positive cocci***	***Miscellaneous***
Escherichia coli	*Enterococcus faecalis*	*Mycobacterium tuberculosis*
Klebsiella	*Staphylococcus saprophyticus*	*Citrobacter*
Proteus	*Staphylococcus aureus*	*Salmonella typhi*
Enterobacter	*Staphylococcus epidermidis*	*Streptococcus pyogenes*
Pseudomonas		*Streptococcus agalactiae*
Aeruginosa		*Gardnerella vaginalis*
Serratia		
***Fungus*:**		
Candida species and *Histoplasma capsulatum*		

This is because the culture technique prevents the growth of organisms other than mycobacteria. Molecular tests can also be used for the diagnosis of *M. tuberculosis*.

- **For *S. haematobium:*** Last few milliliters of a urine sample collected early afternoon after exercise are useful for detection of *S. haematobium*.

Preservation of Urine

Urine sample should be **examined within 2 hours** of collection. If delay is likely to occur, it should be preserved by one of the following methods:

- Refrigeration without any preservative.
- Use of preservatives such as toluene (add few drops to form a thin layer on the urine surface), concentrated Hcl (in the ratio of 1 mL for 125 mL of urine), thymol (one crystal/100 mL), chloroform (5 mL/100 mL), and formaldehyde (add 1 drop for 15 mL of urine—preserves cells and casts). Bacteriological examination urine is aspirated from bladder by needle.

Transport

Urine is a good culture medium for many bacteria, and multiplication of organisms in the specimen between collection and culture will give false results. Hence, it should be transported to laboratory as soon as possible (with minimum delay) or should be kept at 4°C.

Note: The criteria for "significant bacteriuria" do not apply to urine specimens collected from catheters or nephrostomy tubes or by suprapubic aspiration directly from the bladder. In these specimens, any number of organisms may be significant. This is because these specimens are not contaminated by periurethral flora.

Laboratory Investigations

Urine specimens should be examined macroscopically and microscopically and should be cultured by quantitative or semiquantitative methods.

Microscopic examination of urine

It is a very **useful method to provide a rapid preliminary report.** When bacteria are present in large numbers in the urine specimen, they may be seen on microscopy. However, they are not necessarily indicate the presence of infection. Because this may be due to poor collection of specimen or specimen must have been left at room temperature for a prolonged period of time. The presence of red and white blood cells (WBCs) in urine is abnormal, but may not necessarily indicative of UTI. Procedure for preparation of urine for microscopic examination by manual method:

- Centrifuge 10 mL of urine in a graduated conical centrifuge tube at a speed of 1,500–2,000 RPM for 5 minutes. The supernatant is poured off.
- Resuspend the sediment in 1 mL of urine.
- Take a small drop of the suspended urine on a glass slide.
- Mount with a coverslip and examine under the microscope.

Red blood cells (RBCs): Presence of RBCs [>2/hpf (hpf = high power field)] in the urine indicates bleeding at any point in the urinary system from the glomerulus to the urethra. Hematuria may be present in association with several conditions (**Box 26**).

White blood cells:

- White blood cells are present in the urine in very small numbers (e.g., <10/mL) in health. Increased number of WBCs (mainly neutrophils >5/hpf or a count of over 10/mL) in urine is considered abnormal and is termed as **pyuria (Box 27**). It is indicative of **UTI.** The causative organism of infection may be identified by bacteriological examination.
- Urinary casts indicate renal tubular damage. When pus cells are accompanied by **leukocyte casts** or mixed leukocyte-epithelial cell casts, increased urinary leukocytes are considered to be of **renal origin.**
- Pyuria need not always associated with bacteriuria. Sterile pyuria is an important finding and may be due to:
    - Concurrent antibiotic therapy.
    - Other diseases such as neoplasms or urinary calculi.
    - Infection with organisms not detected by routine urine culture methods.
- Renal tubular cells, seen in the urine of aspirin misusers, may be confused with WBCs.

Currently, for urine microscopy, instead of manual examination automated system is available. A machine aspirates a sample of the urine and then classifies the particles in the urine by size, shape, contrast, light scatter, volume, and other properties. In general, counts of bacteria are less accurate than are counts of red and WBCs.

Urine culture

A laboratory diagnosis of significant bacteriuria needs quantification of the bacteria. The detection of bacteria in a urine culture is the diagnostic gold standard for UTI. Conventional culture methods produce can give results within 18–24 hours. Rapid methods (e.g., based on bioluminescence, turbidimetry, leukocyte esterase/nitrate reductase test, etc.) are also commercially available. Usually, both culture and susceptibility (sensitivity) results are available within 24 hours.

Box 26: Few causes of hematuria.

Diseases of urinary tract:
- Infection of the urinary tract and elsewhere (e.g., bacterial endocarditis)
- Renal trauma
- Renal calculi
- Malignant tumors of urinary tract

Other causes:
- Infection elsewhere (e.g., bacterial endocarditis)
- Clotting disorders
- Thrombocytopenia

Note: Occasionally, red blood cells may contaminate urine specimens of menstruating women.

Box 27: Causes of pus cells in urine (pyuria).

- Pyelonephritis
- Urethritis
- Cystitis
- Urinary tract infection (UTI)

Urine specimens may become contaminated with the normal microbial flora present in the distal urethra, vagina, or skin. These contaminants can grow to high numbers, if the collected urine is allowed to stand at room temperature. In such situations, a culture that yields mixed bacterial species except in settings of long-term catheterization, chronic urinary retention, or the presence of a fistula between the urinary tract and the gastrointestinal or genital tract. **Interpretation of the significance of bacterial culture results depends upon a variety of factors such as**:

- **Collection:** Specimen collection must be carried out properly.
- **Storage:** Urine must be cultured within 1 hour of collection or held at 4°C for not >18 hours before culture.
- **Antibiotic treatment:** In a patient receiving antibiotics, smaller numbers of organisms may be significant and it may suggest an emerging resistant population.
- **Fluid intake:** If the patient is taking more or less fluid than usual, this will influence the quantitative result.

Interpretation of culture results: Criteria of active bacterial infection or urinary tract are presented in **Table 42**.

Indirect tests for UTI:

- Uncommonly significant UTIs may be present in high-risk individuals (e.g., elderly, pregnant, or diabetic, and those with a previous history of UTIs) without typical symptoms. If these patients are not treated, they may progress to severe renal damage.
- Rapid diagnosis of bacteriuria and leukocyturia can be done by indirect methods such as reagent strip nitrite and leukocyte esterase, respectively.
- Microscopic urinalysis is a rapid confirmatory test for identification of leukocytes and bacteria and bacteriological culture remains as the "gold standard" for detecting bacteriuria.

Nitrite test:

- Normally, nitrites are not found in the urine and ingested nitrites are converted to nitrates and excreted in the urine.
- Many bacteria causing UTIs (e.g., *Escherichia coli, Klebsiella, Enterobacter, Proteus, Staphylococcus,* and *Pseudomonas* species) can reduce nitrate to nitrite by their enzyme nitrate reductase, and this will cause a positive UTI.
- If the nitrite test is positive, a culture should be done. However, negative test does not indicate absence of urinary tract infection.

Leukocyte esterase test:

- Human neutrophil azurophilic (primary) granules contain proteins with esterolytic activity and presence of leukocyte esterase activity in the urine may be indicative of remnants of cells that are not visible microscopically.
- Positive leukocyte esterase results correlate with "significant" numbers of neutrophils (either intact or lysed).

Table 42: Criteria of active bacterial infection of urinary tract.

Criteria	*Interpretation*
Count >10^5 bacteria/mL	Significant bacteriuria
Count between 10^4 to 10^5 bacteria/mL	Doubtful bacteriuria
Count <10^4 bacteria/mL	No significant growth

EMERGING AND RE-EMERGING INFECTIONS

Q. Write short essay on emerging infections.

In the past several decades, there was antibiotic revolution, vaccinations, and modernization of public health measures. It was thought that the traditional global infectious diseases will be permanently disappeared. However, in the last few decades, there was emergence of microbial infections, including re-emergence of well-known agents (e.g., cholera, dengue fever, influenza, and anthrax), as well as previously unknown pathogens. Another new challenge was antibiotic resistance particularly against agents causing communicable diseases (e.g., multi-drug resistant tuberculosis).

Definition: Emerging infectious diseases are infections of following feature:

- Infections that have recently appeared in human population **(previously undetected or unknown infectious agents)**.
- Incidence or geographic range of infections is **rapidly increasing**.
- Infections that **threatens to increase in the near future**.
- **Re-emerging of infections** after a period of quiescence.

The rapidly expanding human population along with environmental lapse allows the emergence of new pathogens and the re-emergence of old infectious agents (previously thought to be under control). Examples of infections/diseases that have emerged over the past 50 years are presented in **Table 43.** This should serve as a reminder to us that the equilibrium between humans and the pathogens that confront them is a dynamic one. Hence, a continuous vigilance is necessary, and a sense of security invites disaster.

General Features

- Some infectious were not new, but were previously unrecognized because some of the infectious agents are difficult to culture. Examples include *Helicobacter pylori* gastritis, HBV and HCV, and *Legionella pneumophila*. The re-emergence of influenza virus as a pathogen caused the global influenza pandemics (e.g., H1N1 and H5N1).
- Some infectious agents are new to humans. New pathogens belonging to all classes are viruses, bacteria, parasites, and fungi. Examples include, HIV causing AIDS and *Borrelia burgdorferi* causing Lyme disease.
- Some infections have become much more common due to immunosuppression caused by AIDS or immunosuppressive therapy. Examples include CMV, Kaposi's sarcoma-associated herpesvirus (LSHV), *Mycobacterium avium intracellulare, P. jirovecii*, and *Cryptosporidium parvum*.
- Some infectious diseases that are common in one geographic area may be introduced into a new geographic region.

Table 43: List of emerging or re-emerging diseases.

Year of emergence/ re-emergence	*Causative agent*	*Human disease/association*
1973	*Rotavirus*	Severe watery diarrhea, vomiting, fever, and abdominal pain in infants and young children
1975	*Parvovirus B-19*	Asymptomatic cessation in erythropoiesis
1976	*Cryptosporidium parvum*	Acute watery and non-bloody diarrhea
1977	Ebola virus	Epidemic Ebola hemorrhagic fever
	Hantaan virus	Hemorrhagic fever with renal syndrome
	Legionella pneumophila	Legionnaire disease
	Campylobacter jejuni	Enteritis
1980	Human T-lymphotropic virus I (HTLV-I)	T-cell lymphoma or leukemia, HTLV associated myelopathy
1981	Toxin producing strains of *Staphylococcus aureus*	Toxic shock syndrome (TSS)
1982	*Escherichia coli* O157:H7	Hemorrhagic colitis and hemolytic–uremic syndrome (HUS)
	Borrelia burgdorferi	Lyme disease
1983	Human immunodeficiency virus-1 (HIV-1)	Acquired immunodeficiency syndrome (AIDS)
	Helicobacter pylori	*H. pylori*-induced gastric ulcers
1985	*Enterocytozoon bieneusi*	Intestinal and hepatobiliary microsporidiosis
1986	*Cyclospora cayetanensis*	Diarrhea
	Monkey pox	Similar to that of smallpox, but milder
	Human immunodeficiency virus-2 (HIV-2)	AIDS-like illness
	Human herpesvirus-6 (HHV6)	Roseola (exanthema subitum)
	Porogia virus	Hemorrhagic fever/renal syndrome (HFRS)
1988	Hepatitis E	Enterically transmitted hepatitis
1989	Hepatitis C	Hepatitis C
	Barmah Forest virus	Polyarthritis
	Chlamydia pneumoniae (TWAR)	Respiratory infection
	Ehrlichia chaffeensis	Ehrlichiosis
1990	Human herpesvirus-7 (HHV7)	Aseptic meningitis
	Anaplasma phagocytophilum	Human granulocytic anaplasmosis
	Haemophilus influenzae biotype *aegyptius*	Brazilian purpuric fever
1991	Guanarito virus	Venezuelan hemorrhagic fever (VHF)
	Encephalitozoon hellem	Disseminated microsporidiosis
	Ehrlichia chaffeensis	Human ehrlichiosis
	New species of Babesia	Babesiosis
1992	*Vibrio cholerae* O139	New epidemic cholera strain
	Bartonella henselae	Cat-scratch disease and bacillary angiomatosis
1993	*Sin Nombre virus*	Hantavirus cardiopulmonary syndrome (HCPS)
	Cyclospora cayetanensis	Coccidian diarrhea
	Balamuthia mandrillaris	Amebic meningoencephalitis
	Septata intestinalis (now *Encephalitozoon intestinalis*)	Intestinal and disseminated microsporidiosis
1994	*Ehrlichia phagocytophila*-like agent	Human granulocytic ehrlichiosis
	Sabia virus	Brazilian hemorrhagic fever
	Hendra virus	Acute respiratory syndrome
1995	Kaposi sarcoma-associated virus [human herpesvirus-8 (HHV8)]	Kaposi sarcoma in AIDS, body cavity lymphomas
	New variant Creutzfeldt–Jakob disease	Spongiform encephalopathy ("mad cow")

Continued

Continued

Year of emergence/ re-emergence	Causative agent	Human disease/association
1996	*Rickettsia africae*	African tick bite fever
1997	*Rickettsia slovaca* (tick-borne lymphadenopathy); TIBOLA	Lymph node enlargement
	Alkhurma hemorrhagic fever virus	Saudi Arabian hemorrhagic fever
1999	West Nile virus	West Nile fever, neuroinvasive disease, and West Nile encephalitis (WNV)
	Nipah virus	Acute respiratory syndrome
2000	Human metapneumovirus (hMPV)	Respiratory tract infection
	Rickettsia felis	Rickettsial spotted fever
2002	*Rickettsia aeschlimannii*	Rickettsial spotted fever
2003	Severe acute respiratory syndrome (SARS) coronavirus	Severe atypical pneumonia (SARS-CoV)
2004	*Rickettsia parkeri*	Rickettsial spotted fever
	Arcobacter species	Intestinal infection
	H5N1 "avian" influenza	Pneumonia
2005	Rickettsia *mongolotimonae*	Lymphangitis
	Coronavirus HCoV-HKU-1	Pneumonia
2006	*Mycobacterium tilburgii*	Multiorgan disease
	Rickettsia massiliae	Rickettsial spotted fever
2007	Zika virus	• Fever, rash, and Guillain–Barré syndrome • Fetal loss, microcephaly, and neurologic complications in newborns
	WU virus (WU PyV)	Respiratory
	KI virus (KI PyV)	Respiratory
	Saffold virus	Acute gastroenteritis
	Schineria larvae	Human myiasis
	Mycobacterium massiliense	Sepsis
	Segniliparus rugosus	Respiratory disease
2008	Human parvovirus-4 (PARV4)	Viremia
	Merkel cell polyomavirus (MC PyV)	Merkel cell carcinoma
2009	H1N1 "swine" influenza virus	Pneumonia
2010	*Listeria ivanovii*	Gastroenteritis and bacteremia
2011	*Candidatus Neoehrlichia mikurensis*	Sepsis
2012	*Exserohilum rostratum*	Fungal meningitis outbreak
	Heartland virus	Systemic disease
	Bas Congo virus	Hemorrhagic fever
	Novel coronavirus 2012	SARS-like respiratory infection
	GII.4 Sydney	Epidemic viral gastroenteritis
2013	H7N9 avian influenza virus	Pneumonia
2014	Ebola virus	Fever, rash, hemorrhage, and multisystem organ failure
	Middle east respiratory syndrome coronavirus (MERS CO-V)	SARS-like respiratory infection
2015	Bourbon virus	Tick-born febrile disease
2016	*Candida auris*	Candidemia, wound and ear infections resistant to antifungal agents

Continued

Continued

Year of emergence/ re-emergence	*Causative agent*	*Human disease/association*
2017	Zika virus	Congenital syndrome including microcephaly and fetal malformations
	Maguri virus	Febrile illness
2018	Human herpesvirus-1 (HHpgV-1) *Borrelia turicatae*	Tick-borne relapsing fever
2019	COVID-19	Fever, cough, dyspnea, and pneumonia

Factor Influencing Emergence of Infections

- **Human demographics** are important contributors for emergence of infectious diseases. High population density, global warming, large number of traveler, and increased hunger and malnutrition increase the possibility of spread of disease from person to person.
- **Behavior:** For example, outbreaks of Nipah virus infection in Bangladesh and India was due to consumption of date palm sap (fluid circulating in the plant). Infected bats shed the Nipah virus in their saliva and urine. They contaminate the palm sap by feeding on it. Nipah virus can also spread by person-to-person contact, and by transmission from pigs to people. Some of the recent outbreaks in India with high case fatality ratios were due to *Chandipura* virus.
- **International travel** facilitates movement of infections. For example, SARS was one of the fastest moving microorganisms passed on by international travel.
- **Environmental factors:** Changes in the environment may be one of the factors.
  - **Reforestation** of the eastern United States resulted in massive increase in the populations of deer and mice. They carry the ticks that transmit Lyme disease, babesiosis, and ehrlichiosis.
  - **Failure of DDT to control the mosquitoes** that transmit malaria and the **development of drug-resistant parasites** increased the morbidity and mortality of *Plasmodium falciparum* infection in Asia, Africa, and Latin America.
  - Microbial adaptation to antibiotics used leads to the emergence of **drug resistance** in many species of bacteria. Examples include *M. tuberculosis, Neisseria gonorrhoeae, Staphylococcus aureus,* and *Klebsiella pneumoniae.*
  - Human commercial use of domestic animals (e.g., pigs and chickens) and destruction of other disease reservoirs (e.g., bats and wild birds) have their consequences. This can lead to development of either unique trait in common pathogens (e.g., influenza) or evolution of unique viruses [e.g., severe acute respiratory syndrome (SARS) virus, West Nile virus, and Ebola virus]. Since, these pathogens are novel (new), humans lack immunity. Hence, they can quickly spread through the population as pandemics (e.g., influenza A H1N1 in 2009).
  - More recent emerging infectious diseases include Ebola virus, Zika virus, COVID-19, *Candida auris*, and some of the *Babesia* species.

AGENTS OF BIOTERRORISM

Q. Write short essay on Bioterrorism.

Bioterrorism is the use of biological or chemical agents as weapons.

History of bioterrorism (bio warfare): Biological agents have been used as weapons since ancient times.

- Earliest documentation was from 1,500 to 2,000 BC, in which victims of plague were driven into enemy lands.
- In 184 BC, Hannibal [the great Carthaginian (inhabitant of the ancient African city of Carthage) warrior] first used bioweapons. During a naval battle against King Eumenes of Pergamum, his army filled earthenware pots with serpents (large snakes) and hurled (thrown) them to the decks of the Pergamene ships.
- In 1346, the Tatars lay siege to the Genoese-controlled seaport of Caffa (modern-day Feodosiya, Ukraine). During the siege, the Tatars were affected by plague. The Tatar leader throwed his own dead soldiers affected by plague into the town to be seized so as to spread the epidemic. This forced the Genoese army to flee to Italy. Similar methods were used at Karlstein in Bohemia in 1422 and by Russian troops in fighting Swedish forces in Reval in 1710.
- In the 15th century, smallpox was used as a biological weapon by Francisco Pizarro for conquest of South America. He presented variola-contaminated clothing as gifts. In 1763, the English used a similar strategy in the French-Indian War. Sir Jeffrey Amherst presented smallpox laden blankets to the Delaware Indians loyal to the French.
- During the Revolutionary War, probably smallpox was used as weapon of terror from both sides. The British and their colonial allies planned to spread smallpox among the revolutionary American colonists.
- By 1777, General George Washington ordered smallpox inoculation as mandatory for all military recruits who had not had the disease.

Classification of biological agents used for bioterrorism (Table 44): They are classified into three categories based on an assessment of extent of danger that produce. The Centers for Disease Control and Prevention (CDC) classifies potential agents of bioterrorism into categories based on the risk and dissemination.

- **Category A agents**: They have the **highest risk** and can be **easily disseminated or transmitted** from person to

Table 44: Classification of biological agents of warfare and bioterror.

Bacteria	*Viruses*	*Biological toxins*
Category A • *Bacillus anthracis* • *Clostridium botulinum* and botulinum neurotoxin-producing species of *Clostridium* • *Yersinia pestis* • *Francisella tularensis*	***Category A*** • Filoviruses: Ebolavirus, Marburg virus • Arenaviruses: Lassa, Machupo, Sabia, Junin, Guanarito • Poxviruses: smallpox (variola) and monkeypox	***Category A*** Botulinum
Category B • Brucella abortus, Brucella suis, Brucella melitensis • Salmonella species¸ Escherichia coli O157:H7, Shigella • Burkholderia mallei, Burkholderia pseudomallei • Chlamydia psittaci • Coxiella burnetiid • Rickettsia prowazekii, Rickettsia rickettsii • Vibrio cholerae • Listeria monocytogenes	***Category B*** • Togaviruses: eastern equine encephalitis virus • Venezuelan equine encephalitis virus • Bunyaviruses: Rift Valley fever virus, Congo-Crimean hemorrhagic fever virus ***Category C*** • Nipah virus • Hantavirus	***Category B*** • *Clostridium perfringens* epsilon toxin • Staphylococcal enterotoxin B • Ricin
Parasite ***Category B*** *Cryptosporidium parvum*	***Other examples*** • Flaviviruses: Kyasanur Forest disease • Influenza, Kumlinge, Omsk hemorrhagic fever, Russian spring-summer encephalitis, tick-borne encephalitis	***Other examples*** Aflatoxins, shigatoxin, conotoxinsa abrin, tetrodotoxin, saxitoxin, T-2 toxin, diacetoxyscirpenol, microcystins, satratoxin H, palytoxin, anatoxin A

person. It can **produce high mortality**, might create panic in public, and might require public health preparedness. Smallpox is an example for category A agent. This is because, it has high transmissibility, its mortality rate of 30% or more, and it does not have an effective antiviral therapy. In the United States, vaccination against smallpox ended in 1972 and immunity has waned in citizens. Hence, the population is highly susceptible to smallpox. Other examples of category A agents include *Bacillus anthracis, Yersinia pestis,* and Ebola virus.

- **Category B agents:** They are relatively easy to disseminate and produce moderate morbidity but low mortality. They require specific diagnostic and disease surveillance. Many of these are food-borne or water-borne. Examples include *Brucella* species and *Vibrio cholerae.*
- **Category C agents:** These include emerging pathogens that could be engineered for mass dissemination. They are available, easy to produce, and disseminate. They can produce high morbidity and mortality, and great impact on health. Examples include Hantavirus and Nipah virus.

BIBLIOGRAPHY

1. Abel L, Fellay J, Haas DW, et al. Genetics of human susceptibility to active and latent tuberculosis: present knowledge and future perspectives. *Lancet Infect Dis.* 2018;18:e64.
2. Alanio A, Desnos-Ollivier M, Garcia-Hermoso D, et al. Investigating clinical issues by genotyping of medically important fungi: why and how?. *Clin Microbiol Rev.* 2017;30:671.
3. Awuh JA, Flo TH. Molecular basis of mycobacterial survival in macrophages. *Cell Mol Life Sci.* 2017;74:1625-48.
4. Barathi1 G, Thanka J, Shalini S. Diagnostic challenges of a spectrum of cases of Phaeohyphomycosis - A histopathological approach of rare dematiaceous (Melanized / pigmented) fungi. IP Archives of Cytology and Histopathology Research. https://doi.org/10.18231/j.achr.2020.025.
5. Baseler L, Chertow DS, Johnson KM, et al. The pathogenesis of Ebola virus disease. *Annu Rev Pathol.* 2017;12:387.
6. Brown JC. Herpes simplex virus latency: the DNA repair-centered pathway. *Adv Virol.* 7028194, 2017.
7. Buscher P, Cecchi G, Jamonneau V, et al. Human African trypanosomiasis. *Lancet.* 2017;390:2397
8. Centers for Disease Control and Prevention: https://www.cdc.gov/.
9. Chatterjee KD. Parasitology (Protozoology and Helminthology), 13th edition. New Delhi: CBS Publishersand distributors; 2011.
10. Coppens I. How Toxoplasma and malaria parasites defy first, then exploit host autophagic and endocytic pathways for growth. *Curr Opin Microbiol.* 2017;40:32.
11. Dal Peraro M, van der Goot FG. Pore-forming toxins: ancient, but never really out of fashion. *Nat Rev Microbiol.* 2016;14:77.
12. de Sousa JR, Sotto MN, Simoes Quaresma JA. Leprosy as a complex infection: breakdown of the Th1 and Th2 immune paradigm in the immunopathogenesis of the disease. *Front Immunol.* 2017;8:1635.
13. Duncan SM, Jones NG, Mottram JC. Recent advances in Leishmania reverse genetics. Manipulating a manipulative parasite. *Mol Biochem Parasitol.* 2017;216:30.
14. Dutta D, Clevers H. Organoid culture systems to study host-pathogen interactions. *Curr Opin Immunol.* 2017;48:15.
15. García-Elorriaga G, del Rey-Pineda G. Practical and Laboratory Diagnosis of Tuberculosis -From Sputum Smear to Molecular Biology. Switzerland: Springer International Publishing; 2015.
16. Ghosh S. Paniker's Textbook of Medical Parasitology, 9th edition. New Delhi: JP brothers; 2021.

17. Graham BS, Sullivan NJ. Emerging viral diseases from a vaccinology perspective: preparing for the next pandemic, *Nat Immunol.* 2018;19:20.
18. Grose C, Buckingham EM, Carpenter JE, et al. Varicella-zoster virus infectious cycle: ER stress, autophagic flux, and amphisome-mediated trafficking. *Pathogens.* 2016;5.
19. Grote A, Lustigman S, Ghedin E. Lessons from the genomes and transcriptomes of filarial nematodes. *Mol Biochem Parasitol.* 2017;215:23.
20. Hasnain SE, Ehtesham NZ, Grover S. Mycobacterium tuberculosis: Molecular Infection Biology, Pathogenesis, Diagnostics and New Interventions. Singapore: Springer; 2019.
21. Hinnebusch BJ, Jarrett CO, Bland DM. "Fleaing" the plague: adaptations of Yersinia pestis to its insect vector that lead to transmission. *Annu Rev Microbiol.* 2017;71:215.
22. Hoving JC, Kolls JK. New advances in understanding the host immune response to Pneumocystis. *Curr Opin Microbiol.* 2017;40:65.
23. Hryckowian AJ, Pruss KM, Sonnenburg JL. The emerging metabolic view of Clostridium difficile pathogenesis. *Curr Opin Microbiol.* 2017;35:42.
24. Jameson JL, Fausi AS, Kasper DL, et al. Harrison's principles of internal medicine (2 vols), 20th edition. New York: McGraw-Hill Medical Publishing. Division; 2018.
25. Jeffery-Smith A, Taori SK, Schelenz S, et al. Candida auris: a Review of the Literature. *Clin Microbiol Rev.* 2018;31.
26. Kilgore PE, Salim AM, Zervos MJ, et al. Pertussis: microbiology, disease, treatment, and prevention. *Clin Microbiol Rev.* 2016;29:449.
27. Koh WJ. Nontuberculous Mycobacteria-Overview, Microbiol Spectr 2017;5.
28. Kumar B, Kar HK. IAL Textbook of Leprosy, second edition. New-Delhi: JP Brothers; 2017.
29. Kumar V, Abbas AK, Aster JC. Robbins basic pathology, 10th edition. Philadelphia: Saunders Elsevier; 2018
30. Kumar V, Abbas AK, Fausto N, et al. Robbins and Cotran pathologic basis of disease, 10th edition. Philadelphia: WB Saunders; 2021.
31. Kumar V, Abbas AK, Aster JC, Deyrup AT. Robbins essential pathology, 1st edition. Philadelphia: Elsevier; 2021.
32. Lee PP, Lau YL. Cellular and molecular defects underlying invasive fungal infections-revelations from endemic mycoses. *Front Immunol.* 2017;8:735.
33. Mahmud R, Lim YAL, Amir A. Medical Parasitology-A Text Book. Malaysia: Springer International Publishing AG; 2017.
34. Marineli F, Tsoucalas G, Karamanou M, Androutsos G. Mary Mallon (1869-1938) and the history of typhoid fever. *Ann Gastroenterol.* 2013;26(2):132-4.
35. May RC, Stone NR, Wiesner DL, et al. Cryptococcus: from environmental saprophyte to global pathogen. *Nat Rev Microbiol.* 2016;14:106.
36. Mohan H. Textbook of pathology, 8th edition. New Delhi: Jaypee Brothers Medical Publishers (P) Ltd; 2018.
37. Musso D, Gubler DJ, Zika virus. *Clin Microbiol Rev.* 20216;29:487.
38. Nabarro L, Morris-Jones S, Moore DAJ. Peters' Atlas of Tropical Medicine and Parasitology. Seventh edition. United Kingdom: Elsevier; 2019.
39. Nash AA, Dalziel RG, Fitzgerald JR. Mims' Pathogenesis of Infectious Disease. 6th edition. London: Elsevier Ltd; 2015.
40. Noble SM, Gianetti BA, Witchley JN. Candida albicans cell-type switching and functional plasticity in the mammalian host. *Nat Rev Microbiol.* 2017;15:96.
41. Perlin DS, Rautemaa-Richardson R, Alastruey-Izquierdo A. The global problem of antifungal resistance: prevalence, mechanisms, and management. *Lancet Infect Dis.* 2017;17:e383.
42. Radolf JD, Deka RK, Anand A, et al. Treponema pallidum, the syphilis spirochete: making a living as a stealth pathogen. *Nat Rev Microbiol.* 2016;14:744.
43. Radoshevich L, Cossart P. Listeria monocytogenes: towards a complete picture of its physiology and pathogenesis. *Nat Rev Microbiol.* 2018;16:32.
44. Ralston SH, Penman ID, Strachan MWJ, et al. Davidson's principles and practice of medicine, 23rd edition. Edinburgh: Churchill Livingstone; 2018.
45. Ramirez-Toloza G, Ferreira A. Trypanosoma cruzi evades the complement system as an efficient strategy to survive in the mammalian host: the specific roles of host/parasite molecules and Trypanosoma cruzi calreticulin. *Front Microbiol.* 2017;8:1667.
46. Riedel S, Morse S, Mietzner T, Miller S. Jawetz, Melnick & Adelberg's Medical Microbiology-McGraw-Hill; 2019.
47. Santi-Rocca J, Blanchard N. Membrane trafficking and remodeling at the host-parasite interface. *Curr Opin Microbiol.* 2017;40:145.
48. Sardana K, Khurana A. Jopling's Handbook of Leprosy, 6th edition. New-Delhi: CBS Publishers and Distributors; 2020.
49. Sastry AS, Bhat SK. Essentials of Medical Parasitology, 2nd edition. New Delhi: JP Bros; 2019.
50. Strayer DS, Saffitz JE. Rubin's Pathology: Mechanism of Human Disease, 8th edition. Philadelphia: Wolters Kluwer; 2020.
51. Taylor GS, Long HM, Brooks JM, et al. The immunology of Epstein-Barr virus-induced disease. *Annu Rev Immunol.* 2015;33:787.
52. Thomer L, Schneewind O, Missiakas D. Pathogenesis of Staphylococcus aureus bloodstream infections. *Annu Rev Pathol.* 2016;11:343.
53. van de Veerdonk FL, Gresnigt MS, Romani L, et al. Aspergillus fumigatus morphology and dynamic host interactions. *Nat Rev Microbiol.* 2017;15:661.
54. Wahlgren M, Goel S, Akhouri RR. Variant surface antigens of Plasmodium falciparum and their roles in severe malaria. *Nat Rev Microbiol.* 2017;15:479.
55. Wheeler ML, Limon JJ, Underhill DM. Immunity to commensal fungi: detente and disease. *Annu Rev Pathol.* 2017;12:359.
56. Wing EJ, Schiffman FJ. Cecil Essentials of Medicine, tenth edition. Philadelphia: Elsevier; 2022.
57. Zeibig EA. Clinical Parasitology-A Clinical Approach, 2nd edition. Missouri: Saunders, an imprint of Elsevier; 2013.

CHAPTER 12

Genetic Disorders and Molecular Diagnosis

12.1 Genetic Disorders

CHAPTER OUTLINE

INTRODUCTION

Gene is defined as a **segment of deoxyribonucleic acid** (DNA) which **carries the genetic information**. Gene is the basic physical and functional unit that is regulated by transcription and encodes an ribonucleic acid (RNA) product, which is most commonly, but not always, translated into a protein that produces its activity within or outside the cell. Genetics is the study of heredity, or how the characteristics of living organisms are transmitted from one generation to the next via DNA (consists of genes that are the basic unit of heredity). Thus, **genetics is the study which deals with the science of genes, heredity, and its variation in living organisms. Human genetics** deals with the study of individual genes, their role and function in disease, and their mode of inheritance.

A **genome** is an **organism's complete set of genetic instructions. Genomics**, in contrast, is the **study of the entire genetic information of organism's genes**—called the genome. Each genome contains all of the information needed to build that organism and allow it to grow and develop. Thus, genomics includes the study of function and interaction of DNA within the genome, as well as with environmental or nongenetic factors, such as a person's lifestyle. With the characterization of the human genome, genomics not only complements traditional genetics in understanding the etiology and pathogenesis of disease, but also plays a prominent role in diagnostics, prevention, and therapy of disease.

Human genome project (HGP) was initiated in the mid-1980s as an effort to characterize the entire human genome and completed the DNA sequence for the last of the human chromosomes in 2006. HGP provided the first draft of the about 3 billion base pairs (bp)/nucleotides of DNA per haploid human genome. This has dramatically increased our understanding regarding the developmental and genetic disorders. The human genome contains about 20,000 protein-coding genes comprising 1.5% of the whole genome. Each gene varies in size. It is interesting to note that most of the protein-coding genes in the human genome are also found in genomes of other organisms including lower life forms (e.g., yeast). It is the remaining 98.5% of the human genome that is responsible for the remarkable complexity that ultimately determines the human species. This remaining 98.5% includes many non-protein-coding genes. These nonprotein-coding genes are transcribed into RNA molecules such as microRNAs and long noncoding RNAs. These are increasingly being recognized to play important regulatory functions. Recent advances in molecular genetics and cytogenetics technologies have greatly improved the understanding of the genetic basis of human disease including neoplasms.

Hereditary, familial, and congenital: Hereditary disorders are derived from one's parents and are transmitted in the germline through the generations. Hence, hereditary disorders are familial. Congenital means "born with" and some congenital diseases are not genetic (e.g., congenital syphilis). Not all genetic diseases are congenital. For example, Huntington disease is a genetic disease that begins to manifest only after 20s or 30s.

Genomic medicine, personalized medicine, or precision medicine is the study of our genes (DNA) and their interaction with our health. It aims at customizing medical decisions to an individual patient. The modern field of pharmacogenomics consists of study of how genes affect an individual's response to drugs. Now, it is possible to target drugs to specific genetic loci that are responsible for susceptibility to disease as well their prevention. This has created new classes of medicines targeting specific variants in gene and protein structure. This provides highly specific therapies with fewer side effects. Gene therapies also have great potential for treating genetic and many acquired diseases. Pharmacogenomics can be used to optimize drug therapy and predict efficacy, adverse events, and drug dosage of selected medications.

Diseases that manifest during the perinatal period may be caused due to factors in the fetal environment, genomic abnormalities or by combinations of genetic defects and environmental influences. For example, phenylketonuria (PKU) is disorder due to genetic deficiency of phenylalanine hydroxylase (refer pages 934 and 935). It produces mental retardation only if an infant with this disorder is exposed to dietary phenylalanine.

Genetic disorders are far more common than these are acknowledged. This is mainly because the genetic diseases diagnosed usually represent the tip of the iceberg and these remain hidden. Most of the time, genetic disorders with less extreme genotypic errors allow full development of embryonic and live birth.

Fetal death: About 50% of fetuses spontaneously aborted during the early months of gestation show a demonstrable chromosomal abnormality. The incidence of specific numerical chromosomal abnormalities in abortuses is several times more than in term infants. This indicates that most such chromosomal defects are lethal for survival of fetus and only a small number of fetuses with cytogenetic abnormalities are born alive. About 1% of all newborn infants reveal a gross chromosomal abnormality, and serious disease develops in about 5% of individuals younger than age of 25 years. Presently, advances in DNA sequencing have helped in detection of numerous smaller genetic errors. Probably the genomes contain at least 400 protein-damaging sequence variants and at least two bona fide disease mutations even in so-called healthy individuals. Thus, a potential disease-causing mutation need not produce disease. The expression of disease depends on complex interactions between genetic, epigenetic, and environmental factors.

Birth defects: A specific cause cannot be identified in more than two-thirds of all birth defects.

- **No known cause:** Presently in about 70% of birth defects, no known genetic or other cause is identifiable.
- **Genetic causes:** Genomic defects that cause birth defects include inherited traits or spontaneous mutations. Only small number due to chromosomal abnormalities.
- **Other causes:** Uterine factors, maternal disorders (e.g., metabolic imbalances or infections during pregnancy) or environmental exposures (e.g., drugs, chemicals, radiation) constitute not >6% of birth defects.

Reductions in the incidence of birth anomalies can be brought out by—(1) genetic counseling, (2) early prenatal diagnosis, (3) identifying high-risk pregnancies, (4) avoiding potential teratogens, and (5) implementation of preventive measures. For example, prenatal dietary supplement of folic acid can significantly reduce the incidence of congenital neural tube defects.

Infant mortality: In advanced countries, developmental and genetic birth defects are responsible for 50% of deaths during infancy and childhood. By contrast, in less developed countries, 95% of infant mortality is due to environmental causes (e.g., infectious diseases and malnutrition).

MUTATIONS

Q. Write short essay on principles and effects of gene mutations.

For synthesis of proteins, DNA is transcribed into RNA, which is processed into mRNA (messenger RNA). This, in turn, is translated into protein by ribosomes. Any changes in DNA can lead to corresponding changes in the amino acid sequence of its encoded protein or interfere with its synthesis.

The term mutation was coined by Müller in 1927. A **mutation is a permanent or stable change in the DNA** (genetic material) which can result in a disease. The term mutation is used to indicate the process to bring out genetic variations as well as the outcome of these alterations. It is to be noted that epigenetic events may also influence gene expression or facilitate genetic damage.

Definition: Mutation is defined as any permanent change in the primary nucleotide sequence of DNA regardless of its functional consequences though generally it has a negative significance.

Variation: This is a more neutral term and is now increasingly used to describe sequence changes in DNA and is recommended by many instead of mutation. Some variations may be lethal, others can be less injurious, and some may benefit as an evolutionary advantage.

Causes

Mutations drive evolution but can also be pathogenic.

- **Spontaneous mutation:** Majority of mutations occur spontaneously due to errors in DNA replication and repair.
- **Induced mutation:** Mutations can be caused due to exposure to mutagenic agents such as chemicals, viruses, and ultraviolet or ionizing radiation.
- **Polymorphism:** If the genetic material change/variant (sequence variations) does not cause obvious effect upon phenotype (i.e., it is not appreciable or perceptible), it is termed as polymorphism. A **polymorphism is defined as genetic variation that exists in population with a frequency of at least 1%** (or >1%). The allele frequency and functional consequences of polymorphism are usually not known, the term variation is now increasingly recommended to describe these sequence changes. Generally, polymorphism consists of single base-pair substitutions that do not alter the protein coding sequence because of the degenerate nature of the genetic code. In the human genome, about 1 in 1,000 base pairs is polymorphic. Evolution is based on the accumulation over time of such nonlethal variation/mutations that alter the ability of a species to adapt to its environment.

Consequences of mutations (or variations): These are highly variable.

- Some mutations have no functional consequences.
- Some are lethal. Hence, they are not transmitted to the next generation.
- Some may confer an evolutionary advantage (i.e., polymorphism). This is in between the above two extremes. This consists of a broad range of DNA changes that account for the genetic diversity of any species.

With the exception of triplet nucleotide repeats, which can expand, variations are usually stable.

Classification of Mutations

Depending on the cell affected, mutations can affect either somatic cells or germ cells.

- **Germ cell mutations:** Mutations that affect the germ cells or germline (sperm or oocytes) are transmitted to the progeny/descendants and can produce inherited/hereditary diseases.
- **Somatic cell mutations:** Mutations can occur during embryogenesis or in somatic tissues (i.e., somatic cells). They can produce some congenital malformations and cancers. The mutations that are not inherited and do not **cause hereditary diseases are known as de novo mutations.** Mutations that occur during development can lead to **mosaicism**. In this, tissues are composed of cells with different genetic constitutions. If the germline is mosaic, a mutation can be transmitted to some progeny but not others. Sometimes, somatic mutations that do not affect cell survival can be detected because of variable phenotypic effects in tissues. For example, café-au-lait skin pigmentations in McCune-Albright syndrome (characterized by mutation during early embryogenesis). Other somatic mutations are associated with neoplasia because they confer a growth advantage to cells.

Structural Chromosomal Mutations

The rearrangement of genetic material during mutation causes structural changes. Mutations structurally vary.

- Mutations can involve the entire genome. For example, triploidy characterized by one extra set of chromosomes.
- Gross numerical or structural alterations in chromosomes or individual genes.

Structural mutations may be—(1) visible during karyotyping or (2) submicroscopic (minute/subtle changes). The submicroscopic gene mutations can result in partial or complete deletion of a gene or more often, a single nucleotide base. Few examples of genetic mutations are discussed below.

Major Types of Mutations

Mutations cause rearrangement of genetic material. The changes in the genetic material can range from single base substitutions, through insertions and deletions of single or multiple bases to loss or gain of entire chromosomes. Thus, structural changes can be divided into—(1) visible during karyotyping or (2) submicroscopic (minute/subtle changes).

Submicroscopic (minute/subtle changes): The submicroscopic gene mutations can result in partial or complete deletion of a gene or more often, a single nucleotide base.

Point Mutation within Coding Sequences

Point mutation (single-base changes or base substitution or substitution mutation) is the replacement of one single **nucleotide base** (at a certain position in one strand of the DNA) **by another different nucleotide base within a gene.** Thus, one base pair in the DNA is altered. After DNA replication, a new base pair will appear in the daughter double helix. It may change the code in a triplet of bases and lead to the replacement of one amino acid by another in the gene product. These are the most common types of mutation and **point mutation is a common mechanism of oncogene activation.** Examples: Point mutations in one of the ***RAS*** genes (***HRAS, KRAS,*** or ***NRAS***) are observed in ~85% of pancreatic cancers and 45% of colon cancer, point mutations of ***RET*** in leukemia, and ***BRAF*** in melanoma. Point mutations (substitution) may be of two types—transition mutations and transversion mutations.

1. **Transition mutations (Figs. 1A and B):** It is a type of substitution in which the base of nucleotide is substituted by the same type of base in the nucleotide. Thus, a pyrimidine base [i.e., thymine (T) or cytosine (C)] is substituted by another pyrimidine (C for T or vice versa) or a purine base [i.e., adenine (A) or guanine (G)] is changed to another purine base (A for G or vice versa). Transition is more frequent than transversion (discussed below). Relatively high frequency of C to T transitions known as CpG dinucleotides (p represents the phosphate). This is because the methylated base in genomic DNA undergoes spontaneous deamination of methylcytosine converting them to thymine. CpG dinucleotides are termed as "hotspots" for mutation.
2. **Transversion mutations (Figs. 1A and C):** In this type, there is a substitution of a pyrimidine base by a purine base or vice versa. Thus, there are changes from a purine to either of the two pyrimidines or the change of a pyrimidine into either of the two purines. For example, TA or CG pair replaces the wild-type AT pair. It may occur in the coding region (the part of the gene that is translated into a protein) or noncoding region of the gene.

Functional groupings for point mutations: Majority of point mutations occur in the coding region of a gene. When the nucleotide sequence of a protein-coding gene containing the point mutation is transcribed into an mRNA molecule,

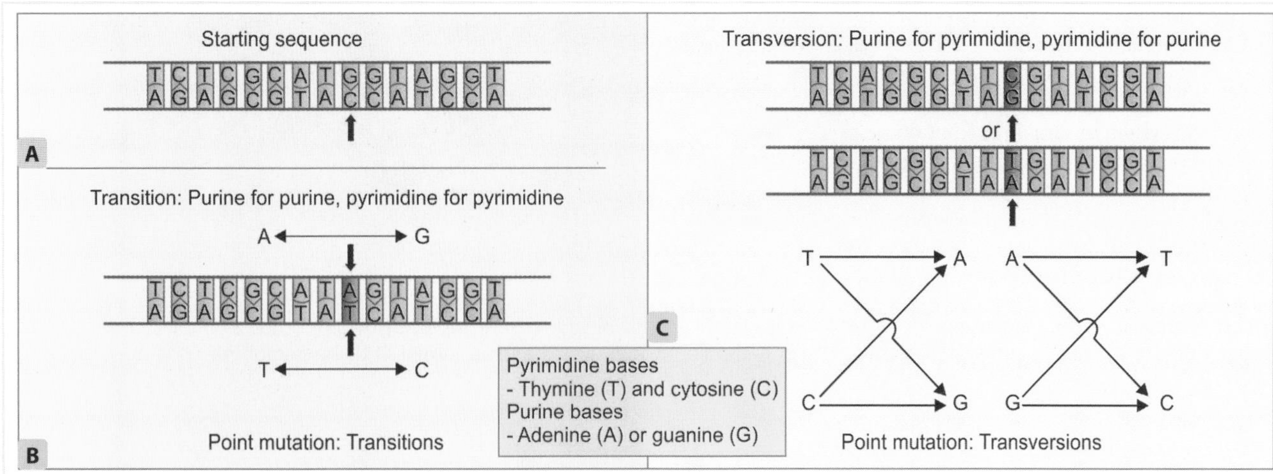

FIGS. 1A TO C: Schematic representation of transition and transversion mutations. (A) Starting sequence of DNA; (B) Transition is a type of substitution in which the base of nucleotide is substituted by the same type of base in the nucleotide, i.e., pyrimidine base by another pyrimidine or a purine base is changed to another purine base; (C) Transversion mutations.

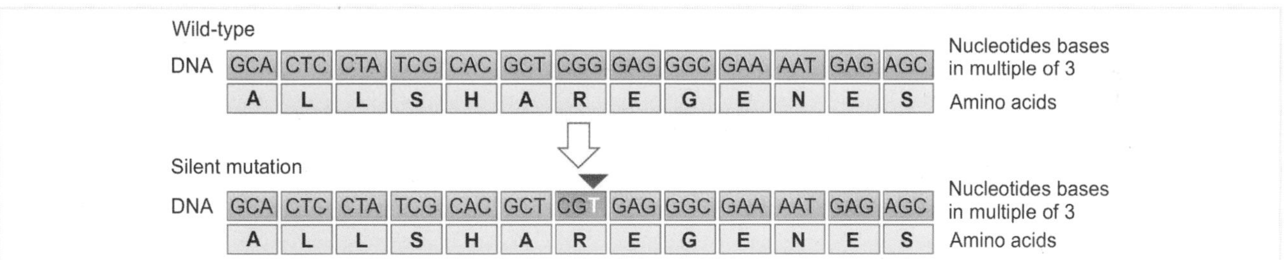

FIG. 2: Silent mutation. They do not change the primary structure of protein. In this example, CGG and CGT (point mutation where guanine is replaced by thymidine and vice versa) both encode amino acid arginine (one letter abbreviation for arginine is R).

then the RNA molecule will also show the base change at the corresponding location. Single-base changes in the mRNA are converted into a string of amino acids and may have one of the several effects when translated into protein. Thus, mutations often result as functional changes in the final protein product. Depending on the functional effect, point mutations can be divided into silent mutations, missense mutations, and nonsense mutations.

- **Silent (synonymous) mutations:** These occur when the point mutation causes altering of codon (produces a new genetic code) but still exactly encodes for the same amino acid as the original amino acid. For example, CGG and CGT (point mutation where guanine is replaced by thymidine and vice versa) both encoded amino acid arginine (one letter abbreviation for arginine is R) (**Fig. 2**). In some silent mutations, the new genetic code, codes for a different amino acid that has the same properties as the original amino acid. These point mutations do no show detectable effect.
- **Missense mutations:** It is a point mutation within coding sequences that changes the genetic code (change in the DNA sequence in a coding region) in a triplet of bases. If so, it alters an amino acid and leads to the replacement of one amino acid by another different amino acid in the gene product. Because these mutations alter the meaning of the sequence of the encoded protein, they are usually termed missense mutations (three-fourths of base changes in the coding region). In this type of point mutation change, the base substitution generates a genetic code that may code for a different amino acid. This results in incorporation of a different amino acid at the corresponding site in the protein molecule. This mistaken amino acid (or missense), depending on its location in the specific protein, may be acceptable, partially acceptable, or unacceptable to the function of that protein molecule.
    - **Conservative missense mutation:** In this type, the substituted amino acid has biochemical properties similar to the one it replaces (i.e., original). This change may have only little change or no effect on the function of the protein product.
    - **Nonconservative missense mutation:** In this type of missense mutations, new codon codes for a different amino acid and protein. The normal amino acid is replaced by biochemically a very different amino acid with very different properties. Thus, the result is change or loss of protein function. **Example, sickle cell anemia in which missense mutation affects the β-globin chain of hemoglobin** (**Fig. 3**). In this, the nucleotide triplet CTC (or GAG in mRNA), which encodes glutamic acid, is changed to CAC (or GUG in mRNA), which encodes valine. This single amino acid substitution (point mutation) changes the properties of hemoglobin and gives rise to sickle cell anemia.

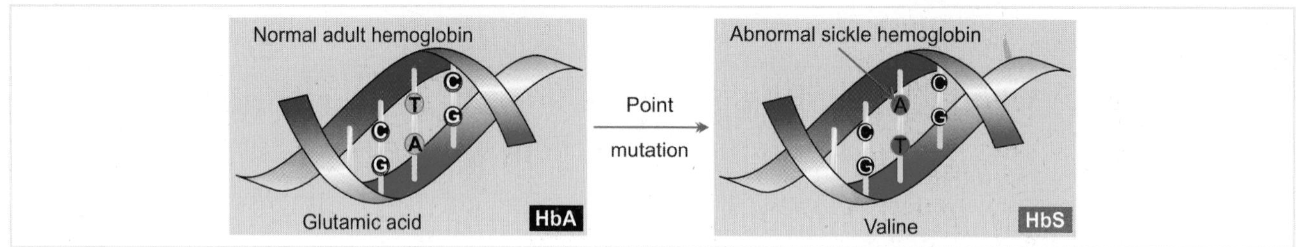

(HBA: hemoglobin A; HbS: hemoglobin S)

FIG. 3: Nonconservative missense point mutation in sickle cell anemia. When adenine replaces thymidine, the amino acid valine replaces glutamic acid in the sixth position of β-globin chain of hemoglobin and gives rise to abnormal sickle hemoglobin.

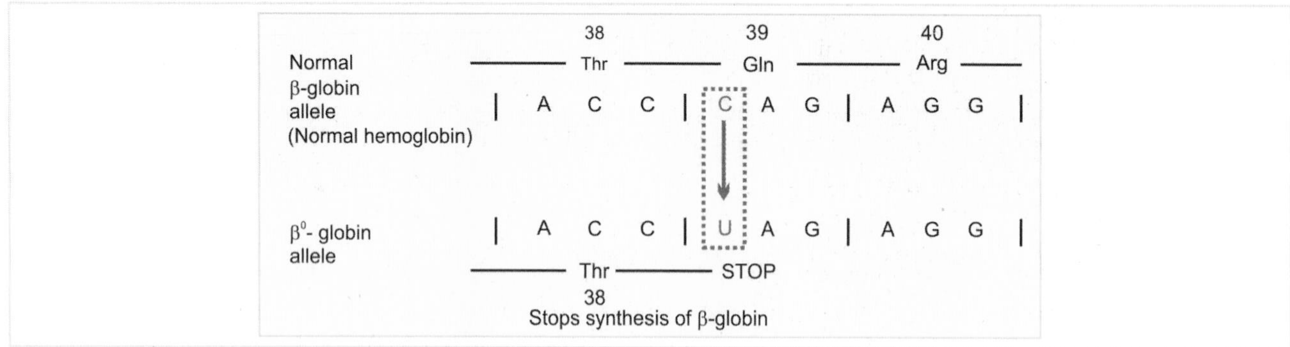

FIG. 4: Nonsense mutations shorten a polypeptide by replacing a codon with a stop signal leading to premature chain termination. In this example, a point mutation (C replaced by U) in codon 39 changes glutamine (Gln) codon to a stop codon. This stops the synthesis of protein at amino acid 38.

- **Nonsense mutation (stop codon):** It is a severe type of point mutation in which base substitution causes a stop (nonsense) codon resulting in the **premature termination**. There will be a premature termination codon (chain terminator or stop codon) of translation and the production of only a fragment of the intended protein molecule. The premature termination of protein synthesis leads to complete loss of function in the finished protein. Example, in β-globin chain, a point mutation affecting the codon for glutamine (CAG) creates a stop codon (UAG) if U replaces C (**Fig. 4**). This change leads to premature termination of β-globin gene translation. The short peptide produced due to this is rapidly degraded. It leads to deficiency of β-globin chains, thereby there is no synthesis of hemoglobin A. It produces a severe form of anemia called β_0-thalassemia.

Deletions and Insertions

Q. Write short essay on frameshift mutation.

In deletion, there is loss of one or more nucleotide pairs from a DNA molecule. In insertion, there is addition of one or more nucleotides into a gene. Deletions and insertions may be as small as a single base pair or as large as megabases (i.e., millions of base pairs).

Consequences of small deletions or insertions: If they involve the coding sequence, it can have three possible effects on the encoded protein.

1. **Intact reading frame:** If the number of base pairs involved is three or a multiple of three, the reading frame will remain intact. There will be synthesis of an abnormal protein lacking or gaining one or more amino acids.
2. **Frameshift mutation:** Amino acids are encoded by trinucleotide sequences. Frameshift mutation may occur due to small insertion or deletion of one or more nucleotides in the coding regions.
   i. If the number of nucleotide bases inserted or deleted is not a multiple of 3, the reading frame [is a way of dividing the sequence of nucleotides in a nucleic acid (DNA or RNA) molecule into a set of consecutive, nonoverlapping triplets] of the message is changed (**Fig. 5A**). This leads to alterations in the reading frame of the DNA strand; hence they are known as frameshift mutations. This changes the genetic the code (**Fig. 5A**). Frameshift mutations can also alter transcription, splicing or mRNA processing.
   ii. If the number of base pairs involved is three (**Fig. 5B**) or a multiple of three, frameshift does not occur. This may synthesize an abnormal protein lacking or gaining one or more amino acids followed by truncation resulting from a premature stop codon. Usually, the result is the incorporation of a variable number of incorrect amino acids.
3. **Large deletions:** Large deletions may affect a portion of a gene or an entire gene, or several genes. When deletions involve a large segment of DNA, the part or entire coding region of a gene may be entirely removed (**Fig. 5C**). There will be no protein product. Large deletions and insertions can reorganize genomes by changing either the order of genes along a chromosome, the number of genes in the genome, or even the number of chromosomes. A large deletion may also bring together coding regions of nearby

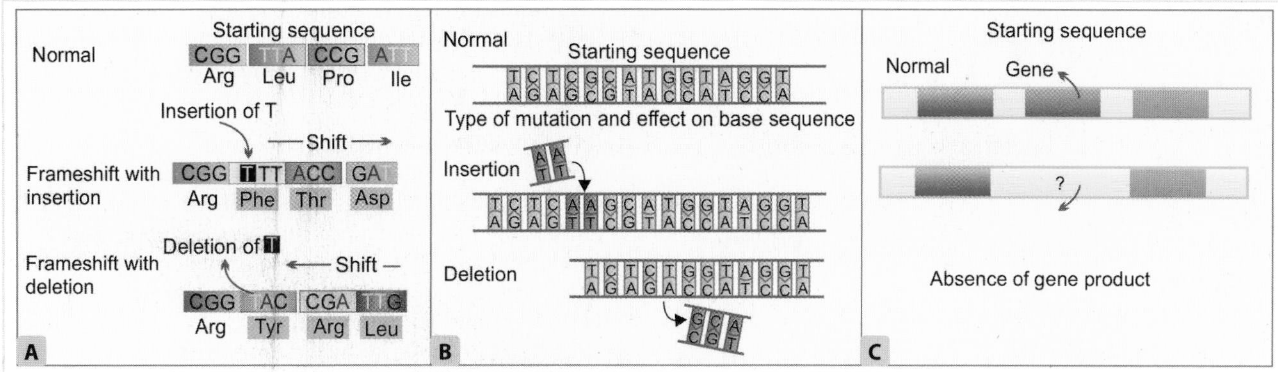

FIGS. 5A TO C: Frameshift mutations change the reading frame either by insertion or deletion. (A) Insertion or deletion of single nucleotide bases (not a multiple of 3), the code will be changed; (B) Insertion or deletion of more than one nucleotide bases; (C) Deletions involving a large segment of DNA in the coding region may entirely remove the gene.

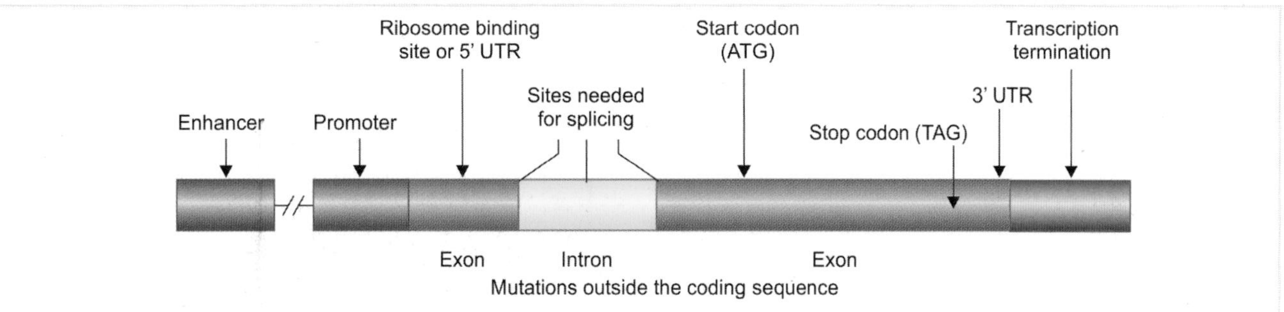

(ATG: translation initiation/start codon which codes for the aminoacid methionine; TAG: stop or termination codon; UTRs: untranslated regions)

FIG. 6: The exons (coding region) carry the code for the production of proteins. Mutations outside the coding region (includes promoter sequences, enhancers or other regulatory regions) can also disrupt gene expression.

genes. This can give rise to a fused gene that generates a hybrid protein in which part or all of one protein is followed by part or all of another.

Mutations within Noncoding Sequences

Mutations may also involve the noncoding regions (**Fig. 6**) of gene. Gene expression depends on several signals other than the actual coding sequence. Mutations in promoter sequences, enhancers or other regulatory regions can affect the level of gene expression. Hence, point mutations or deletions involving these regulatory regions may lead to either marked reduction in or total lack of transcription. Example, certain hereditary anemias. Mutations in miRNA or siRNA binding sites within untranslated regions (UTRs) can also result in disease.

Trinucleotide Repeat Mutation

The DNA contains several repeat sequences of three nucleotides (trinucleotide). Trinucleotide-repeat mutations belong to a special category of genetic anomaly. Many distinct trinucleotide repeats/expansions have been associated (and are identified) in human disease (**Table 1**). The number of copies of some such repeats varies among individuals. They represent allelic polymorphism of the genes in which they are found. When they are repeated directly adjacent to each other (one right after the other), they are known as tandem repeats (**Fig. 7**). As a rule, the number of repeats below a particular threshold does not change during mitosis or meiosis. When the repetitive trinucleotide sequences reach above this particular threshold, the number of repeats can expand or contract. Mutations characterized by amplification of a

Table 1: Examples of diseases associated with trinucleotide repeats.

Disease	*Normal length of sequence*	*Length of sequence in full mutation*	*Location of trinucleotide repeats sequence*
CAG sequence			
• Huntington disease	10–30	40–100	4p16.3
• Kennedy disease	15–25	40–55	Xq21
• Spinocerebellar ataxia	20–35	45–80	6p23
CGG sequence			
• Fragile X syndrome	5–44	200–1,000	Xq27.3
CTG sequence			
• Myotonic dystrophy	5–35	50–2,000	19q13
GAA sequence			
• Friedreich ataxia	7–30	120–1,700	9q13

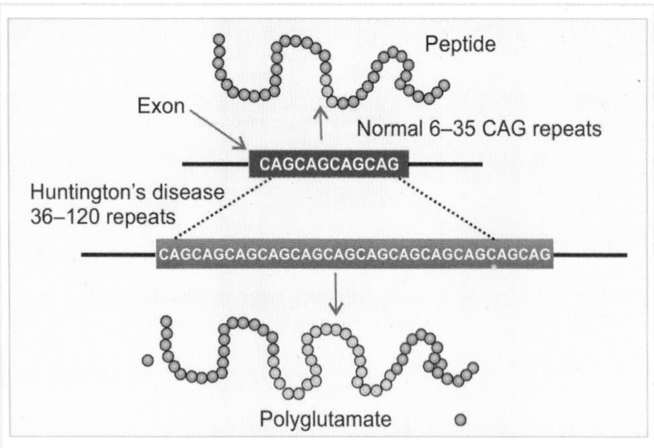

FIG. 7: Trinucleotide repeat disorder, e.g., Huntington's diseases. It results from expansion of a CAG (C is a pyrimidine base. A and G are purine bases) triplet repeat from a normal number of 6 to 35 repeats to greater than 36 repeats. This results in expansion of a polyglutamine sequence in the corresponding protein.

sequence of three nucleotides are more common. The specific nucleotide sequence that undergoes amplification differs in various disorders. However, almost all affected sequences share the nucleotides guanine (G) and cytosine (C) [G is a purine base and C is a pyrimidine base]. Fragile X syndrome (FXS) is a classic example of this category of disorders. In normal population, the number of tandem repeats of the sequence CGG within the regulatory region of a gene called familial mental retardation 1 *(FMR1)* is small with an average of 29. In FXS, there are 250–4,000 of these tandem repeats in *FMR1*. This expansion of the trinucleotide sequences prevents normal expression of the *FMR1* gene and gives rise to intellectual disability. One of the distinguishing features of these trinucleotide-repeat mutation is dynamic (i.e., the degree of amplification increases during gametogenesis). The number of these trinucleotide-repeat increases with each successive generation. This is also associated with increase in the severity of the disease and presents at younger age in successive generations. This mechanism is termed as genetic anticipation. Most trinucleotide repeat diseases are associated with expansions of a CAG (C is a pyrimidine base. A and G are purine bases) codon. This CAG encodes glutamine in the open reading frame of the gene. The tandem repeats of CAG result in polyglutamine tracts in the protein product. Hence, these disorders are associated with degeneration of neurons.

Functional Effects of Mutations on the Protein

Mutations in DNA can lead to either change in the amino acid sequence of a specific protein or may interfere with its synthesis. The consequences vary from those without any functional effect to those which have serious effects.

Loss-of-function (LOF) mutations: These mutations cause the reduction or complete loss of normal function of a protein (gene product). It is usually due to deletion of the whole gene but may also occur with a nonsense or frameshift mutation. LOF mutations involving enzymes are usually inherited in an autosomal or X-linked recessive manner. This is because the catalytic activity of the product of the normal allele is enough to carry out the reactions of most metabolic pathways.

- **Haploinsufficiency:** LOF mutations in the heterozygous state in which half normal levels of the gene product produce effect on phenotype, are called as haploinsufficiency mutations.

Gain-of-function mutations: These mutations result in either increased levels of gene expression or the development of a new function(s) of the gene product. These are usually due to missense mutations. In gain-of-function mutation, the protein function is altered in a manner that results in a change in the original function of the gene. The expanded triplet repeats mutations in the Huntington (*HTT*) gene cause qualitative changes in the gene product. These products aggregate in the central nervous system (CNS) causing its classic clinical features.

Lethal mutations: These lead to death of the fetus.

Alterations in Protein-coding Genes Other than Mutations

Apart from alterations in DNA sequence, coding genes also can undergo structural variations. These are copy number changes and include **amplifications or deletions—or translocations**. It may lead to aberrant gain or loss of protein function. Similar to mutations, structural changes may occur in the germline, or be acquired in somatic tissues. Many pathogenic germline changes involve a contiguous portion of a chromosome rather than a single gene (e.g., 22q microdeletion syndrome). Next-generation sequencing (NGS) technology is used for assessing genome-wide DNA copy number variation (CNV) at very high resolution Somatically acquired structural alterations (e.g., amplifications, deletions, and translocations) are often seen in cancers. For example, "Philadelphia chromosome"—translocation t (9;22) between the *BCR* and *ABL* genes in chronic myeloid leukemia (refer Fig. 25 of Chapter 10).

Alterations in Noncoding RNAs

There are very large number of genes that do not encode proteins but produce transcripts. The nonencoded products of these genes, so-called "noncoding RNAs (ncRNAs)", play important regulatory functions [e.g., small RNA molecules called microRNAs (miRNAs) and long noncoding RNAs (lncRNAs)].

Mutations can interfere with gene expression at various levels. Deletions and point mutations involving promoter sequences in a gene may suppress transcription. Mutations involving introns or splice junctions or both, may lead to abnormal mRNA processing. Translation can be affected if a nonsense mutation produces a stop codon (chain termination mutation) within an exon. Mutations may lead to expression of normal amounts of a dysfunctional protein (e.g., amyloidosis).

GENETIC DISORDERS

There are many types of genetic abnormalities that affect the structure and function of proteins. This may disrupt the cellular homeostasis and produce disease. The mode of inheritance for a given phenotypic trait or disease is determined by pedigree analysis using standard symbols. Definition of symbols in a standard pedigree is presented in **Figure 8**.

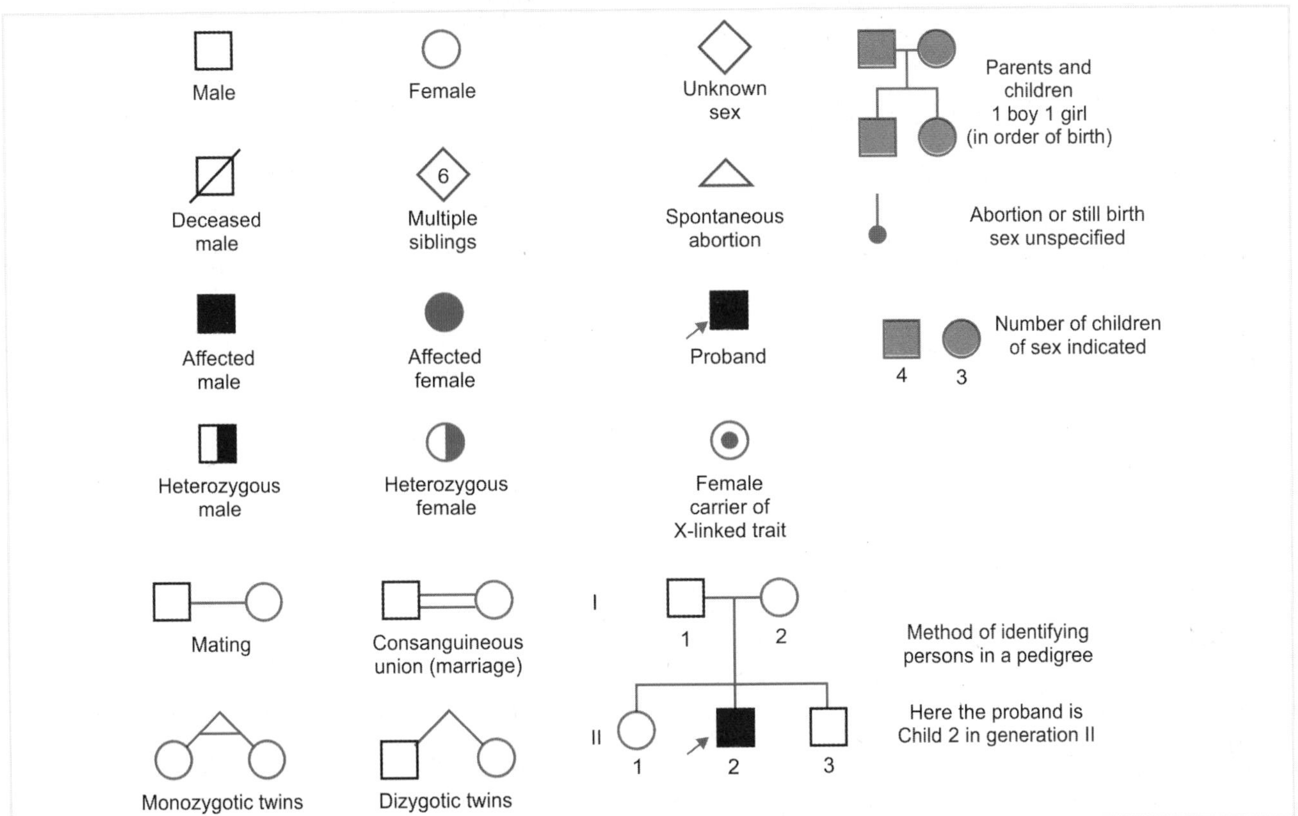

FIG. 8: Definition of symbols in a standard pedigree. Males = squares; females = circles. A line drawn between a square and a circle indicates a mating of that male and female. Two lines drawn between a square and a circle indicate a consanguineous mating in which the two individuals are related (usually as second cousins). Children of a mating are connected to a horizontal line, called the sibship line represented by short vertical lines. The children of a sibship are always listed in order of birth (the oldest on the left). Others are indicated in the figure.

Classification of genetic disorders: Genetic disorders are classified into different categories (**Box 1**).

Mendelian Disorders/Single-gene or Monogenic Disorders

Q. Write short essay on molecular and biochemical basis of Mendelian disorders/single gene disorders.

Disorders related to mutations in single genes with large effects: Single gene disorders result from mutations in single gene and are called as **monogenic human diseases**. They usually follow the principles of classic Mendelian pattern of inheritance (genetic transmission) originally put forth by Gregor Mendel. Hence, they are frequently termed as **Mendelian disorders**. The classic laws of mendelian inheritance are:

- **Mendelian trait:** It is determined by **two copies of the same gene called as alleles**. These alleles are present at the same locus on two homologous chromosomes. In the case of the X and Y chromosomes in males, a mendelian trait is determined by one allele only.
- **Location of defective gene**
  - In autosomal disorders (both dominant and recessive), the defective gene is on autosomes (autosomal inheritance) and is present on one of the 22 autosomes.
  - **Sex-linked traits:** These are encoded by loci on the X chromosome. In sex-linked disorders, it is on the sex chromosomes (sex-linked inheritance).
- **Dominant phenotypic trait:** Genes are inherited in pairs—one gene from each parent. However, the inheritance may not be equal, and one gene may overpower the other in their coded characteristic. The **gene that overshadows the other is called the dominant gene;** the **overshadowed gene is the recessive one. Dominant phenotype needs only one allele of a homologous gene pair**. The phenotype is expressed irrespective whether the allelic genes are homozygous or heterozygous.
- **Recessive phenotypic trait:** It **needs both alleles to be identical** (i.e., homozygous) for the expression of the phenotype.
- **Codominant inheritance:** Though mendelian traits are usually described as dominant or recessive, sometimes **both of the alleles in a heterozygous gene pair are fully expressed and contribute to the expression of phenotype**. It is called codominance. One of the classical examples for codominance is the AB blood group genes.
- **Homozygous versus heterozygous:** Most of the mutations occurring in autosomal genes produce partial expression in the heterozygote and full expression in the homozygote. For example, in sickle cell anemia, the normal hemoglobin A (HbA) is replaced by abnormal hemoglobin S (HbS). If an individual is homozygous for the mutant gene (i.e., sickle cell anemia), all the hemoglobin will be abnormal, HbS, type. Even with normal saturation of oxygen, this disorder is fully

Box 1: Classification of genetic disorders.

Disorders related to mutations in single genes with large effects (monogenic Mendelian disorders)
- Autosomal dominant
- Autosomal recessive
- X-linked dominant
- X-linked recessive

Cytogenetic disorders—chromosomal disorders (aberrations/abnormalities)
- Numerical aberrations aneuploidy (trisomy, monosomy), polyploidy, and mosaicism
- Structural aberrations
  - Translocations
  - Balanced reciprocal translocations
  - Robertsonian translocations
  - Inversion
  - Isochromosome
  - Ring chromosome
  - Deletions
  - Insertions

Complex/multifactorial multigenic/polygenic disorders
- Diabetes mellitus
- Hypertension

Single-gene disorders with nonclassical patterns of inheritance
- Disorders caused by trinucleotide repeat mutations
- Disorders due to mutations in mitochondrial DNA (mtDNA)
- Disorders influenced by genomic imprinting or gonadal mosaicism

expressed (i.e., sickling deformity occurs in all red blood cells (RBCs) leading to hemolytic anemia). In the heterozygote, only a proportion of the hemoglobin is HbS and the remainder being normal HbA. Hence, sickling of RBCs develops only under unusual circumstances such as exposure to lowered oxygen tension. This heterozygous state is known as the sickle cell trait to differentiate it from homozygous full-blown sickle cell anemia.

One dominant (A) allele and one recessive (a) allele can display three Mendelian modes of inheritance. These are—(1) autosomal dominant (~65%), (2) autosomal recessive (~25%), and (3) X-linked (~5%). Presently, these disorders can be identified by genetic testing.

Almost all Mendelian disorders are due to mutations in single genes that have large effects. Every individual carries several deleterious genes and most of them are recessive. Hence, they do not have any serious phenotypic effects. About 80–85% of mutations in single genes are familial and the remaining are due to new mutations that occur de novo.

Pleiotropism and genetic heterogeneity: A single mutant gene may produce many end effects. These are termed as pleiotropism. Mutations at several genetic loci may produce the same trait (genetic heterogeneity).

- Example for pleiotropism**:** Sickle cell anemia is a classic example of pleiotropism. This is a hereditary disorder in which the point mutation in the β-globin gene gives rise to HbS, that predisposes hemolysis of RBCs, but also the abnormal RBCs with HbS tend to cause a blockage of small vessels resulting in several end effects such as splenic fibrosis/infarct, infarcts in organs, and changes in the bone. All these different derangements in end organs are related to the primary defect in hemoglobin synthesis.
- Example for genetic heterogeneity**:** Childhood deafness is an example of genetic heterogeneity. It is an apparently homogeneous clinical condition. It can be produced by many different types of autosomal recessive mutations. Recognition of genetic heterogeneity is important in genetic counseling as well as in the understanding of the pathogenesis of some common disorders, such as diabetes mellitus.

Study of these single genes and mutations with large effects has been extremely informative in medicine. Several physiologic pathways (e.g., cholesterol transport, chloride secretion) that are presently known to us have been learned from analysis of single-gene disorders. However, these disorders are usually rare.

Transmission patterns of single-gene disorders: Mutations involving single genes generally belong to one of the three patterns of inheritance—(1) autosomal dominant, (2) autosomal recessive, and (3) X-linked.

Autosomal Dominant Disorders

In autosomal dominant disorders, **mutations in a single allele** (only one mutated allele) are **sufficient to cause the disease** and at least one parent of an index case is usually affected. The mutant trait is considered to be dominant. Autosomal dominant disorders are manifested in the heterozygous state (expressed in heterozygotes). When an affected individual marries an unaffected one, every child has one chance in two of having the disease. The general features of autosomal dominant disorders traits are as follows:

- **Location of mutant gene:** It is on autosomes.
- **Required number of defective genes:** Only one copy.
- **Both sexes equally affected:** Both males and females are affected equally because the defective (mutant) gene is on one of the 22 autosomes. Both sexes can transmit the condition. Thus, father-to-son transmission (which is absent in X-linked disorders) may occur.
- **Transmission to successive generation (Fig. 9):** In autosomal dominant disorders, individuals are affected in successive generations (unless reproductive capacity is compromised). Since most affected individuals are heterozygous, and their normal mates do not carry the defective gene, normal unaffected members of a family do not transmit the disorder to their offspring or children.
- **Risks of transmission and offspring affected:** Autosomal dominant mutations alter one of the two alleles at a given locus. Because the alleles segregate randomly at meiosis, the probability of proportions of normal and diseased offspring of patients with this disorder is about equal (i.e., offspring affected is 50% and unaffected is also 50%). Affected males and females have an equal risk of passing on the disorder to children.
- **One affected parent:** Unless there is a new germline mutation, every affected individual has an affected parent. Unaffected members of a family (with a normal genotype) do not transmit the trait to their offspring/siblings.

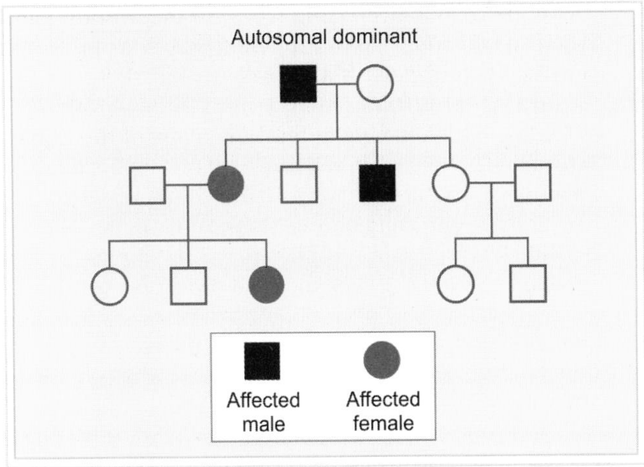

FIG. 9: Pedigree analysis of autosomal dominant mode of transmission (Refer Fig. 8 for definition of symbols in a standard pedigree).

- **New mutations:** It should be recognized; however, some individuals do not have affected parents. They acquire a mutated gene from an unaffected parent. Such disease represents a new mutation involving either the egg or the sperm from which they were derived. De novo germline mutations occur more frequently during later cell divisions in gametogenesis, which explains why siblings are rarely affected. Siblings of patients with new mutations are neither affected nor at increased risk for development of disease. The proportion of patients who develop the disease due to a new mutation depends on the effect of the disease on reproductive capability. If a disease markedly reduces reproductive capability, most cases occur due to new mutations. Many new germline mutations occur more frequently in fathers of advanced (older fathers). For example, the average age of fathers with new germline mutations that cause Marfan syndrome (MFS) is ~37 years compared to fathers who transmit the disease by inheritance have an average age of ~30 years.
- **Clinical features** of autosomal dominant disorders may be variable due to differences in penetrance or expressivity. The mechanisms of incomplete penetrance and variable expressivity are not clearly known. Probably, they are likely to be due to the effects of other genes or environmental factors that modify the phenotypic expression of the mutant allele.
    - **Penetrance:** It is the percentage of individuals (with mutant gene) having clinical symptoms. Penetrance is expressed in mathematical terms. Thus 50% penetrance means that 50% of those who carry the mutant gene express the disease. With complete penetrance (100% penetrance), all individuals show clinical symptoms. With incomplete penetrance, only some individuals inherit the mutant gene but are phenotypically normal. In non-penetrance, individuals may not show any symptoms.
    - **Variable expressivity** (qualitatively or quantitatively) of disorder: If a trait is seen in all individuals (even within the same family). carrying the mutant gene but is expressed differently among individuals. This phenomenon is called variable expressivity. Examples are as follows:
        - **Neurofibromatosis type 1:** Its manifestations range from brownish spots on the skin to multiple skin tumors and skeletal deformities.
        - **Sickle cell anemia:** It is due to mutation at the β-globin locus. The phenotype of a patient with sickle cell anemia is influenced by the genotype at the α-globin locus. This is because the genotype at the α-globin influences the total amount of hemoglobin.
        - **Familial hypercholesterolemia (FH):** In these patients, the expression of the disease in the form of atherosclerosis is influenced by environmental factors namely, the dietary intake of lipids.
    - **Delayed onset:** Symptoms and signs may be delayed and may not appear until adulthood in many autosomal dominant disorders. For example, Huntington's disease manifests after adulthood.

Molecular (biochemical) mechanisms of autosomal dominant disorders: Molecular mechanisms depend on the nature of the mutation and the type of protein affected due to this mutation. Most mutations are associated with reduced production of a gene product or produce a dysfunctional or inactive protein. Whether any mutation causes a dominant or recessive disease depends on the remaining copy of the gene. Thus, if remaining copy of the gene is capable of compensating for the loss, it produces recessive disease and if not, a dominant disease (LOF mutations give rise to dominant). Many autosomal dominant diseases arising from detrimental mutations fall into one of the following familiar patterns:

- **Metabolic pathways with feedback inhibition:** Diseases may be associated with abnormalities in the regulation of complex metabolic pathways with feedback inhibition. If the product of a gene is rate limiting in a complex metabolic network (e.g., a receptor or an enzyme), and mutant gene produces <50% of the normal product and this may be insufficient for a normal phenotype. This is known as haploinsufficiency. For example, membrane receptors for low-density lipoprotein (LDL). In FH, if there is a 50% loss of LDL receptors (LDLRs) on hepatocytes, it leads to secondary elevation of serum cholesterol. This, in turn, predisposes to atherosclerosis in affected heterozygotes.
- **Involvement of key structural proteins:** Mutations in genes for structural proteins (e.g., collagens, cytoskeletal constituents) can cause abnormal molecular interactions. This disrupts the normal morphologic patterns. Examples of key structural proteins include collagen and cytoskeletal elements of the red cell membrane (e.g., spectrin) and osteogenesis imperfecta (OI).
- **Mutant allele disturbs normal proteins:** In some cases, when the gene encodes one subunit of a multimeric protein, the protein product of the mutant allele can interfere with the assembly of a functionally normal multimer. For example, the collagen molecule is a trimer and consists of three collagen chains arranged in a helical configuration. For the assembly and stability of the collagen molecule, each of the three collagen chains in the helix must be normal. Even if there is a single mutant collagen chain, it cannot form normal collagen trimers and this leads to a marked deficiency of collagen. This mutant allele (LOF mutations) impairs the function of a normal allele and is called dominant negative. For example, in OI (osteogenesis

imperfecta), there is marked deficiency of collagen and severe skeletal abnormalities.

- **Gain-of-function mutations:** It may be in two forms.
  i. **Increase in normal function of a protein:** Mutations may increase in normal function of a protein (e.g., excessive enzymatic activity).
  ii. **New activity of the protein:** Some mutations may grant a new activity to the affected protein, that is completely unrelated to its normal function. For example, in Huntington disease, the trinucleotide-repeat mutation affects the HTT (Huntingtin). It produces an abnormal protein, called huntingtin, which is toxic to neurons. Hence, even heterozygotes develop a neurologic deficit.
- **Mutant protein insensitive to normal regulation:** For example, mutations in the RET proto-oncogene in families with multiple endocrine neoplasia type 2 increase the activity of a tyrosine kinase. This stimulates cell proliferation.

There are more than 1,000 human diseases that are inherited as autosomal dominant traits and most of them are rare. Examples of few common human autosomal dominant disorders are presented in **Table 2**.

Autosomal Recessive Disorders

Q. Write short essay on autosomal recessive disorders.

Autosomal recessive disorders constitute the largest group of Mendelian disorders.

General features of autosomal recessive disorders are as follows:

- **Location of mutant gene:** It is on autosomes.
- **Required number of defective gene:** Symptoms of the disease **appear only when an individual has two copies** (both alleles at a given gene locus) **of the mutant gene**. When an individual has one mutated gene and one normal gene, this heterozygous state is called as a carrier.
- **Pattern of inheritance:** For a child to be at risk, both parents must be having at least one copy of the mutant gene. For example, all inborn errors of metabolism.
- **Parents:** Both parents are usually heterozygous for the trait and are clinically normal. In most cases, an affected individual is the offspring of heterozygous parents. In such situation, there is a 25% chance that the offspring will have a normal genotype, 50% probably of a heterozygous state, and 25% have risk of homozygosity for the recessive alleles (**Fig. 10**). The trait does not usually affect the parents of the affected individual, but siblings may show the disease. If one parent is unaffected heterozygous and other one is affected homozygous, the probability of disease increases to 50% for each child. In such cases, the pedigree analysis (**Fig. 11**) appears similar to an autosomal dominant mode of inheritance (pseudodominance). However, in contrast to autosomal dominant disorders, new mutations in recessive alleles are rarely manifested because they usually result in an asymptomatic carrier state.
- **Sex affected:** Females and males are equally affected.
- **Consanguineous marriage:** If the mutant gene occurs with a low frequency in the population, most probably the affected individual (proband) is the product of a consanguineous marriage. Thus, parental consanguinity is a common predisposing factor.
- **Risks of transmission (Fig. 10):** Symptoms appear in about 25% of their children (i.e., the recurrence risk is 25% for each birth). Half of all offsprings are heterozygous for the trait and are asymptomatic. Thus, two-thirds of unaffected offsprings are heterozygous carriers.
- **Expression of disease:** It is more uniform than in autosomal dominant disorders.
- **Penetrance:** Complete penetrance is common.

Table 2: Examples of common autosomal dominant disorders.

System affected	*Examples*
Nervous system	• Huntington disease • Neurofibromatosis • Tuberous sclerosis • Myotonic dystrophy
Musculoskeletal system	• Marfan syndrome • Osteogenesis imperfecta (types I–IV) • Achondroplasia • Ehlers–Danlos syndrome (some variants)
Hematopoietic system	• Hereditary spherocytosis (major forms) • von Willebrand disease • Hereditary elliptocytosis (all forms)
Renal system	• Polycystic kidney disease • Wilms tumor
Gastrointestinal system	• Familial polyposis coli
Metabolic disorders	• Familial hypercholesterolemia • Acute intermittent porphyria
Others	• Retinoblastoma • Hereditary amyloidosis

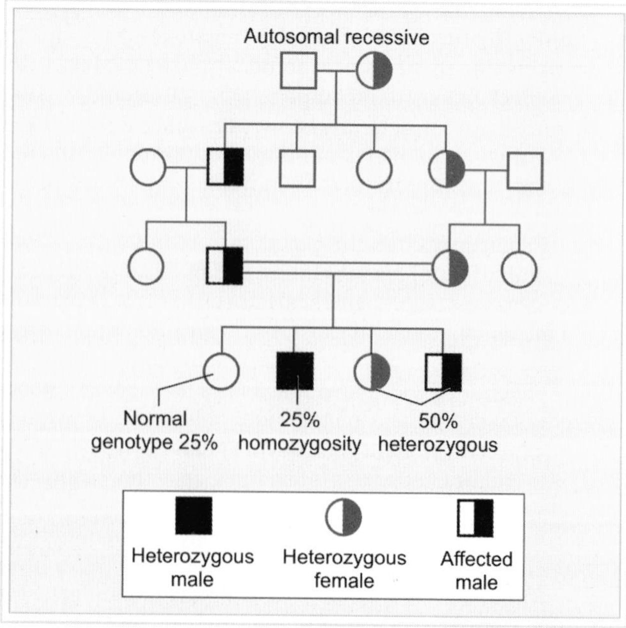

FIG. 10: Pedigree analysis of autosomal recessive mode of transmission (Refer Fig. 8 for definition of symbols in a standard pedigree).

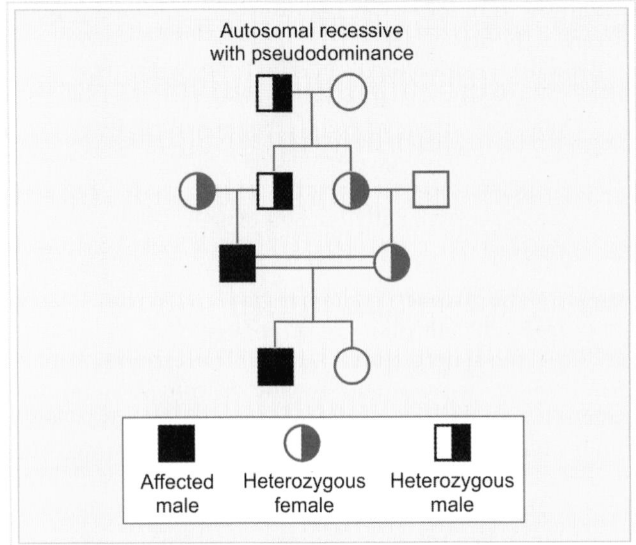

FIG. 11: Pedigree analysis of autosomal recessive with pseudodominance mode of transmission (Refer Fig. 8 for definition of symbols in a standard pedigree).

- **Onset:** It frequently manifests early in life.
- **New mutations:** Though new mutations can occur with recessive disorders, they are difficult to identify clinically. This is because heterozygotes are asymptomatic.
- **Clinical features of autosomal recessive disorders:** They tend to be more consistent than in autosomal dominant diseases. Hence, they present more commonly in childhood, while dominant disorders may initially appear in adults.
- Some autosomal recessive diseases show variability in clinical expression. This may be due to residual functionality of the affected protein. Such variability manifests in—(1) different degrees of clinical severity, (2) age at onset, or (3) as acute and chronic forms of the specific disease.

Most mutant genes causing autosomal recessive disorders are rare in the general population. This is because the homozygotes for the trait usually die before reproductive age. However, a few autosomal recessive diseases, such as sickle cell anemia and cystic fibrosis (CF), are common.

Biochemical (molecular) basis of autosomal recessive disorders

In **autosomal recessive disorders, many of the mutated genes encode enzymes and usually produce deficiencies in enzymes rather than structural proteins.** The enzymes are involved in metabolic pathways, receptors, or proteins in signaling cascades. The mutated alleles result in a complete or partial loss of enzyme function.

- Autosomal recessive diseases, due to mutation that inactivates an enzyme, rarely cause an abnormal phenotype in heterozygotes. This is because in heterozygotes, equal amounts of normal and defective enzyme are synthesized. There is usually natural "margin of safety" and the enzyme functions normally.
- In autosomal recessive diseases caused by impaired catabolism of dietary substances [e.g., PKU (phenylketonuria), galactosemia] or cellular constituents (e.g., Tay–Sachs, Hurler), the partial lack of enzymes is compensated by an increase in the concentration of substrate in heterozygotes. This is because most cellular enzymes operate at substrate concentrations well below saturation and an enzyme deficiency can be easily corrected simply by increasing the amount of substrate.
- By contrast, in a homozygote, there is loss of both alleles and it results in complete loss of enzyme activity. This cannot be corrected by such mechanisms mentioned earlier.

Autosomal recessive disorders include almost all inborn errors of metabolism. Examples of autosomal recessive disorders are shown in **Table 3**.

Table 3: Examples of autosomal recessive disorders.

System affected	Examples
Inborn errors of metabolism	• Phenylketonuria (PKU) • Galactosemia • Cystic fibrosis (CF) • Homocystinuria • Hemochromatosis • Lysosomal storage diseases • Glycogen storage diseases • Wilson disease • α_1-antitrypsin deficiency • Myeloperoxidase deficiency
Hematopoietic system	• Sickle cell anemia • Thalassemias (α and β)
Skeletal system	• Alkaptonuria • Ehlers–Danlos syndrome (some variants)
Nervous system	• Neurogenic muscular atrophies • Friedreich ataxia • Spinal muscular atrophy
Endocrine system	Congenital adrenal hyperplasia

X-linked Pattern of Inheritance

Q. Write short essay on X-linked inheritance.

Males have only one X chromosome. Linked traits are not transmitted from father to son. A son inherits the Y normal chromosome from his symptomatic father and one X chromosome from mother. A daughter always inherits her father's X chromosome and one of her mother's two X chromosomes. Thus, the characteristic features of X-linked pattern of inheritance are—(1) no transmission from father-to-son and (2) all the daughters of an affected male are obligate carriers of the mutant allele **(Fig. 12)**. Thus, the X-linked disease skips a generation in males, as female carriers transmit it to grandsons of a symptomatic male. Almost all sex-linked Mendelian disorders are X-linked and almost all are recessive. Several genes are located in the male-specific region of Y. All of these genes are related to spermatogenesis. Males with mutations involving the Y-linked genes are generally infertile, and hence there is no Y-linked inheritance.

Expression of an X-linked disorder: Risk of developing disease due to a mutant X-chromosomal gene is different in male and females.

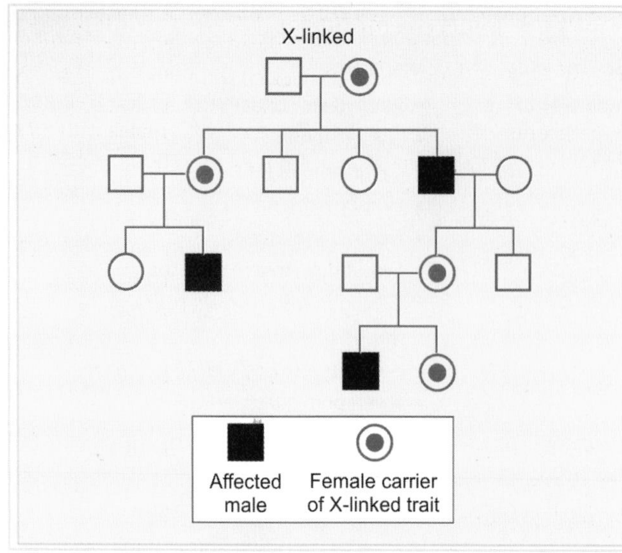

FIG. 12: Pedigree analysis of X-linked mode of transmission (Refer Fig. 8 for definition of symbols in a standard pedigree).

- **Males:** Males have only one X chromosome and they are hemizygous for the mutant allele. Mutation affecting X-chromosome is likely to be fully expressed even with one copy, regardless of whether the mutation is dominant or recessive.
- **Females:** Females have two X chromosome. Thus, they may be either heterozygous or homozygous for the mutant allele. The clinical expression of the X-linked disease is variable, depending on whether it is dominant or recessive. Females are rarely affected by X-linked recessive diseases; however, they are affected by X-linked dominant disease. Therefore, the terms X-linked dominant or X-linked recessive are only applicable to expression of the mutant phenotype in females.

X-linked recessive inheritance

Most X-linked traits are recessive, and they constitute a small number of well-defined clinical conditions. For the most part, the Y chromosome is not homologous to the X chromosome. So mutant genes on the X chromosome do not have corresponding alleles on the Y chromosome. Hence, males are hemizygous for X-linked mutant genes. So, X-linked disorders are expressed in males.

General features

- **Location of mutant gene:** It is on the X chromosome and there is no male-to-male transmission.
- **Required number of defective gene:** One copy for the manifestation of disease in males, but two copies are needed in females.
- **Sex affected:** Males are more frequently affected than females; daughters of affected male are all asymptomatic carriers. Affected male does not transmit the disorder to his sons. Heterozygous females do not manifest clinical disease. Symptomatic homozygous females can rarely occur due to mating of an affected male with an asymptomatic, heterozygous female, or, lyonization may preferentially inactivate the normal X chromosome and very rarely may lead to an affected heterozygous female.
- **Pattern of inheritance:** Transmission is through female carrier (heterozygous).
- **Risks of transmission to children (offspring):**
    - An affected male does not transmit the disorder to his sons. But all daughters are asymptomatic carriers.
    - Sons of heterozygous female have 50% (one chance in two) chance of receiving the mutant gene. Daughters are not symptomatic, but 50% of daughters will also be carriers.

Expression of disease: A heterozygous female usually does not express the full phenotypic change. This is because they have the paired normal allele. The expression of X chromosomal genes in the female is influenced by the random inactivation of one of the X chromosomes. Hence, females have a variable proportion of cells in which the mutant X chromosome is active. Very rarely, it is possible for the normal allele to be inactivated in most cells and allow full expression of heterozygous X-linked conditions in females. More commonly, the normal allele is inactivated in only some of the cells, and thus a heterozygous female partially expresses the disorder. **One of the classical examples is glucose-6-phosphate dehydrogenase (G6PD) deficiency**. It is X-linked disorder in which G6PD enzyme deficiency predisposes to hemolysis of red cell when the patients are receiving certain types of drugs; it is mainly expressed in males. In females, a proportion of the RBCs may be derived from precursors with inactivation of the normal allele of G6PD. Such RBCs are at the same risk for undergoing hemolysis as the RBCs in hemizygous males. Thus, these females are not only carriers of this disorder but also are susceptible to drug-induced hemolytic reactions. In heterozygous females, the proportion of defective RBCs depends on the random inactivation of one of the X chromosomes. The hemolytic reactions are less severe in heterozygous females than in hemizygous males.

Localization of various inherited diseases on the X chromosome is depicted on **Figure 13**. Examples of X-linked recessive disorders are shown in **Table 4**.

X-linked dominant inheritance

General features

- They are very rare. Examples for X-linked dominant inheritance: Vitamin D-resistant rickets and Alport syndrome.
- **Location of mutant gene:** It is on the X chromosome and there is no transmission from affected male to son. They are caused by dominant disease-associated alleles on the X chromosome.
- **Required number of defective gene:** One copy of mutant gene is required for its effect.
- Often lethal in males and so may be transmitted only in the female line.
- Often lethal in affected males and they have affected mothers.
- No carrier states.
- More frequent in females than in males.
- **Risks of transmission to children (offspring):**
    - Transmitted by an affected heterozygous female to 50% (half) of her sons and 50% (half) of her daughters.
    - Transmitted by an affected male parent to all his daughters but none of his sons, if the female parent is unaffected.

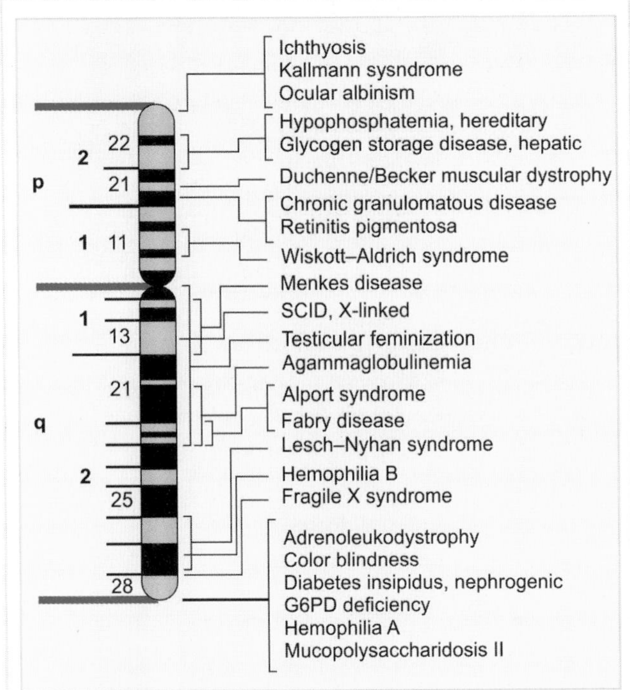

[G6PD: glucose-6-phosphate dehydrogenase; SCID: severe combined immunodeficiency (syndrome)].

FIG. 13: Diagrammatic representation of localization of various inherited diseases on the X chromosome.

Table 4: Examples of X-linked recessive disorders.

System affected	*Examples*
Blood	• Hemophilia A (factor VIII deficiency) and B (factor IX deficiency) • Glucose-6-phosphate dehydrogenase deficiency • Chronic granulomatous disease
Musculoskeletal system	Duchenne muscular dystrophy
Nervous system	Fragile X syndrome
Metabolic disorders	• Diabetes insipidus • Lesch–Nyhan syndrome [hypoxanthine-guanine phosphoribosyltransferase (HPRT) deficiency]
Immune systems	• X-linked agammaglobulinemia • Wiskott–Aldrich syndrome • X-linked severe combined immunodeficiency

Y-linked Disorders

The Y chromosome contains relatively small number of genes. One gene, namely, the sex-region determining Y factor (SRY), encodes the testis-determining factor (TDF). It is important for normal development of male. Infrequently exchange of sequences on the Y chromosome can occur with the X chromosome. The SRY region is situated adjacent to the pseudoautosomal region (PAR) of Y chromosome. This PAR of Y chromosomes has a high degree of homology with that of X chromosome. Occasionally, during meiosis in the male, a crossing-over event may involve the SRY region of Y-chromosome with the distal tip of the X chromosome. This translocation can result in XY females with the Y chromosome without the *SRY* gene or XX males with *SRY* gene on one of the X chromosomes. Point mutations in the *SRY* gene can also result in individuals with an XY genotype and an incomplete female phenotype. Majority of these mutations occur de novo. Males with oligospermia/azoospermia may have microdeletions on the long arm of the Y chromosome involving one or more of the azoospermia factor (*AZF*) genes.

Biochemical and Molecular Basis of Single Gene (Mendelian) Disorders

Mendelian disorders result from alterations in single genes. The genetic defect may lead to the formation of an abnormal protein or a reduced production of the gene product. In single-gene disorders, almost any type of protein may be affected and by a different mechanism **(Table 5)**. The mechanisms involved in single-gene disorders can be classified into four categories **(Box 2)**. The pattern of inheritance of the disease is, to some extent, related to the type of protein affected by the mutation.

Mendelian disorders can be studied under the broad categories as listed in **Box 3.**

Defects in Enzyme and their Consequences

Q. Write short essay on diseases associated with enzyme deficiencies.

Mutations may result in the synthesis of either reduced amount of a normal enzyme or an enzyme with reduced activity. Both lead to block in the concerned metabolism. An example of normal metabolic pathway showing different steps in the conversion of a substrate into an end product is depicted in **Figure 14**. This involves a series of intracellular enzymes (depicted as enzyme 1, 2, and 3) and reactions. Intermediate substrates A and B are produced during the process. M1 and M2 represent the products of a minor pathway. The biochemical consequences of an enzyme defect in such a reaction may have three major consequences as discussed below.

Accumulation of the substrate

Mutation in single gene may produce reduced amount of a normal enzyme or an enzyme with reduced activity. The site of block varies depending on the enzyme involved in the metabolic pathway.

- **Accumulation of substrate:** It may be due to the deficiency or reduced activity of the initial enzyme (enzyme 1).
- **Accumulation of intermediates:** It may produce accumulation of one or both intermediates (intermediate A and B).
- **Excess of products of a minor pathway:** An increased accumulation of intermediate B may stimulate the minor pathway. This can produce an excess of products of a minor pathway namely, M1 and M2.

Tissue injury: The high concentrations of accumulated substrate (precursor) or the intermediates, or the products of alternative minor pathways may be toxic to tissues. Examples are as follows:

Table 5: Examples of biochemical and molecular basis of some Mendelian disorders.

Protein type/Function	*Example*	*Disease*
Defects in enzyme		
• Enzyme deficiency	Phenylalanine hydroxylase	Phenylketonuria (PKU)
	Hexosaminidase	Tay–Sachs disease
	Galactose-1-phosphate uridylyltransferase (GALT)	Galactosemia
	Various lysosomal enzymes	Lysosomal storage diseases
	Adenosine deaminase	Severe combined immunodeficiency
	Tyrosinase	Albinism
	Hypoxanthine guanine phosphoribosyl transferase (HGPRT)	Lesch–Nyhan syndrome
• Enzyme inhibitor	α_1-antitrypsin	Emphysema and liver disease
Defects in membrane receptor	Low-density lipoprotein receptor	Familial hypercholesterolemia
	Vitamin D receptor	Vitamin D-resistant rickets
Defects in transport		
• Oxygen	Defective hemoglobin structure	Sickle cell anemia
	Reduced amount of α-globin chain	α-thalassemia
	Reduced amount of β-globin chain	β-thalassemia
• Ion channels	Cystic fibrosis transmembrane conductance regulator	Cystic fibrosis
Defects in structure		
• Extracellular	Fibrillin	Marfan syndrome
	Collagen	Ehlers–Danlos syndrome, Osteogenesis imperfecta
• Cell membrane	Dystrophin	Duchenne/Becker muscular dystrophy
	Spectrin, ankyrin, or protein 4.1	Hereditary spherocytosis
Defects in function, or quantity of nonenzyme proteins		
• Hemostasis	Factor VIII	Hemophilia A
• Growth regulation	Rb protein	Hereditary retinoblastoma
	Neurofibromin	Neurofibromatosis type 1
Genetically determined adverse reactions to drugs		
G6PD enzyme deficiency	G6PD enzyme	G6PD enzyme deficiency

Box 2: Classification of mechanisms involved in single gene disorders.

- Defects in enzyme or enzyme inhibitors
- Defects in membrane receptors
- Defects in transport systems
- Alterations in the structure, function, or quantity of nonenzyme proteins
- Mutations resulting in unusual reactions to drugs

Box 3: Broad categories of Mendelian disorders.

- Disorders associated with defects in structural proteins:
  - Marfan syndrome
  - Ehlers–Danlos syndromes (EDSs)
- Disorders associated with defects in receptor proteins:
  - Familial hypercholesterolemia
- Disorders associated with enzyme defects:
  - Lysosomal storage diseases
  - Glycogen storage diseases (glycogenoses)
- Disorders associated with defects in proteins that regulate cell growth

- **Galactosemia:** This is due to the deficiency of galactose-1-phosphate uridylyltransferase and causes accumulation of galactose. These metabolic intermediates produce damage to tissue.
- **Lysosomal storage diseases:** Deficiency of degradative enzymes in the lysosomes produces excessive accumulation of complex substrates within the lysosomes in lysosomal storage diseases. These complex substrates produce tissue damage.

Decreased amount of end product

- **Decreased end product with loss of its normal function:** An enzyme defect can block the metabolic pathway with resultant decrease in the amount of end product that may be necessary for normal function. For example, in albinism there is deficiency of melanin. This is due to the absence of an enzyme called tyrosinase, which is necessary for the biosynthesis of melanin from its precursor, tyrosine.
- **Lack of feedback inhibition due to lack of end product:** If the end product is a feedback inhibitor of the enzymes involved in the early reactions of the metabolism, the deficiency of the end product may allow excessive

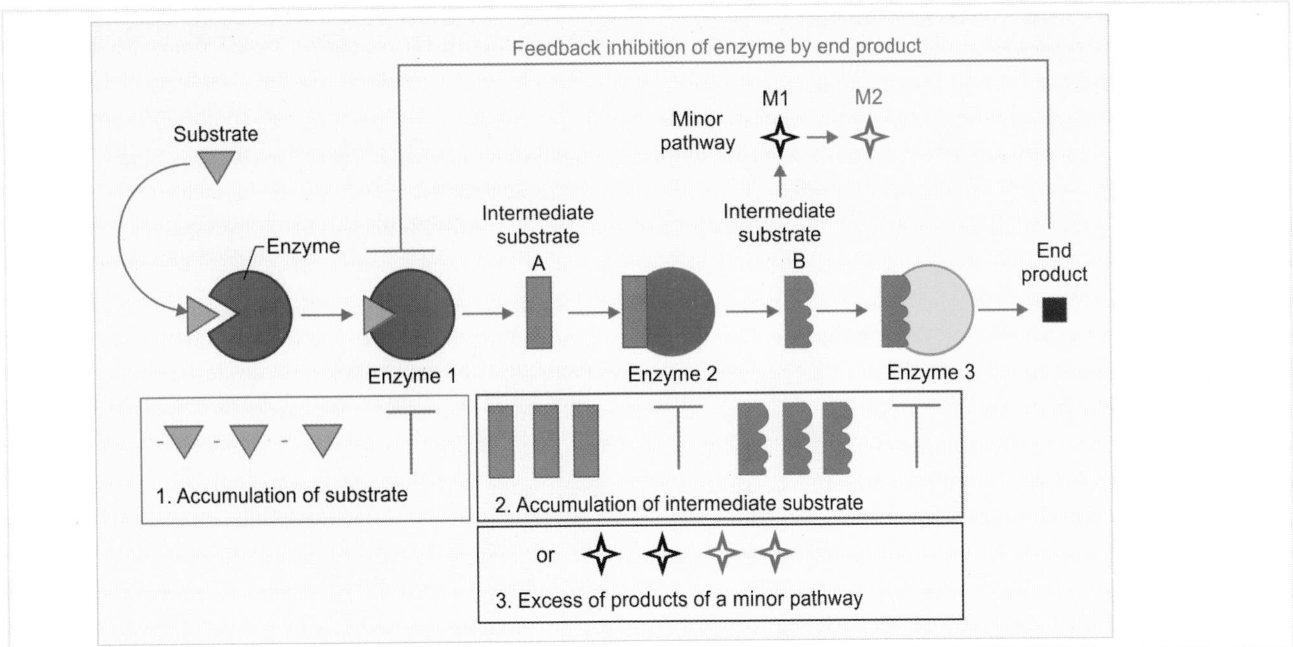

FIG. 14: Metabolic pathway showing possible steps in the conversion of a substrate into an end product. This involves a series of intracellular enzymes (depicted as 1 2, and 3) and reactions. M1, M2 represents the products of a minor pathway. End product in certain metabolism may inhibit the enzymes.

production of intermediates and their catabolic products. High concentrations of some of these intermediates and the catabolic products may injure tissue. For example, Lesch–Nyhan syndrome is a condition characterized by neurological and behavioral abnormalities due to overproduction of uric acid (hyperuricemia) in the body. It is due to complete absence of enzyme hypoxanthine guanine phosphoribosyl transferase (HGPRT) that results in hyperuricemia.

Failure to inactivate a tissue-damaging substrate

There are certain enzymes which are capable of inactivating a tissue-damaging substrate (enzyme inhibitors). Deficiency of such enzymes (e.g., α_1-antitrypsin) will allow the damage by the substrate. For example, individuals with inherited deficiency of serum α_1-antitrypsin cannot inactivate protease called as neutrophil elastase in their lungs. Unchecked activity of neutrophil elastase causes destruction of elastin in the walls of lung alveoli. This leads to emphysema in the lung.

Defects in receptors and transport systems

Biologically active substances need active transport across the cell membrane. In some, transport is through receptor-mediated endocytosis. A genetic defect can occur due to defect in receptor-mediated transport system. Examples are as follows:

- **Familial hypercholesterolemia:** It is characterized by reduced synthesis or function of LDLRs (low density lipoprotein receptors). This causes defect in the transport of LDL into the cells and secondarily to excessive cholesterol synthesis by complex intermediary mechanisms (refer **Fig. 18**).
- **Cystic fibrosis:** In this condition, there is a defect in transport system for chloride and bicarbonate ions in exocrine glands, sweat ducts, lungs, and pancreas. This impaired anion transport produces serious damage to the lungs and pancreas (refer Figs. 17 and 18 of chapter 13).

Alterations in Structure, Function, or Quantity of Nonenzyme Proteins

Genetic defects that alter nonenzyme proteins usually produce widespread secondary effects. Examples include:

- **Sickle cell disease:** It is a hemoglobinopathy, characterized by structural defect (qualitative defect) in the globin molecule of hemoglobin.
- **Thalassemias:** In contrast to hemoglobinopathy, these are due to mutations in globin genes that affect the amount (quantitative defect) of globin chains synthesized. Thalassemias are associated with reduced amounts of structurally normal α-globin or β-globin chains.
- **Genetic disorders with defective structural proteins:** Examples include osteogenesis imperfecta (defect in collagen), hereditary spherocytosis (defect in spectrin), and muscular dystrophies (defect in dystrophin).

Genetically Determined Adverse Reactions to Drugs

Some single gene disorders may produce enzyme deficiencies that are unmasked only after exposure of the affected individual to certain drugs. This special area of genetics is called as pharmacogenetics and has gained considerable clinical importance. Examples include:

- **Deficiency of the enzyme G6PD:** It is one of the classic examples of drug-induced injury in the genetically susceptible individuals. Under normal conditions, the individual with G6PD deficiency does not have any disease. But on administration of certain drugs (e.g., antimalarial drug primaquine), a severe hemolytic anemia develops.

Disorders Associated with Defects in Structural Proteins

Several diseases can be produced due to mutations in genes that encode structural proteins (**Table 5**). Three of the most common and best-studied diseases namely, MFS, Ehlers-Danlos syndromes (EDSs) and osteogenesis imperfecta (OI) affect connective tissue and hence involve multiple organ systems.

Marfan Syndrome

Q. Write short essay on Marfan syndrome.

Marfan syndrome (MFS) is a disorder of connective tissues affecting many organs. It primarily affects skeleton, cardiovascular system (CVS) (heart and aorta), eyes, and skin. About 70–85% of cases are familial and transmitted by autosomal dominant inheritance. The remainder are sporadic and arise from new mutations.

Pathogenesis

MFS results from an **inherited defect due to missense mutations in the gene for extracellular glycoprotein called fibrillin-1** (FBN1) on the long arm of chromosome 15 (15q21.1).

Fibrillins These are a family of collagen-like connective tissue proteins. There are many genetically distinct fibrillins. Fibrillin is the major component of microfibrils present in the extracellular matrix in many tissues. Microfibrils are threadlike filaments that form larger fibers. These large fibers are organized into rods, sheets, and interlaced networks. During embryonic development, these fibrils form scaffolds on which tropoelastin is deposited to form elastic fibers. After birth, they remain as a component of elastic tissues (e.g., elastin is deposited on lamellae of microfibrillar fibers in the concentric rings of elastin in the aortic wall). Though microfibrils are widely distributed in the body, they are abundant in the aorta, ligaments, and the ciliary zonules that support the lens. These tissues are mainly affected in MFS. In MFS, abnormal microfibrillar fibers can be seen in all affected tissues by immunofluorescent microscopy. Fibrillin occurs in two homologous forms, FBN1, and FBN2. They are encoded by two separate genes, *FBN1* and *FBN2*, mapped on chromosomes 15q21.1 and 5q23.31, respectively. FBN1 is a large, cysteine-rich glycoprotein and forms 10-nm microfibrils in the extracellular matrix of many tissues. The ciliary zonules that suspend the lens of the eye consist almost exclusively of fibrillin but does not contain elastin. Dislocation of the lens is one of the characteristics of MFS. Mutations in the *FBN2* gene, which is structurally similar to the *FBN1* gene, are less common. They are found in patients with MFS-like syndrome of congenital contractual arachnodactyly (an autosomal dominant disorder characterized by skeletal abnormalities).

Molecular pathogenesis There are two fundamental mechanisms by which loss of fibrillin produces clinical features of MFS namely—(1) loss of structural support in microfibril-rich connective tissue and (2) increased activation of transforming growth factor (TGF)-β signaling.

1. **Loss of structural support in microfibril-rich connective tissue:** MFS is due to mutations of *FBN1*. It has been revealed that about 1,000 distinct mutations involving *FBN1* gene have been identified in individuals with MFS. Most of these mutations are missense mutations and give rise to abnormal FBN1. These abnormal FBN1 can inhibit polymerization of fibrillin fibers (dominant negative effect). Also, the reduction of fibrillin content below a certain threshold weakens the connective tissue (haploinsufficiency).
2. **TGF-β bioavailability:** Many clinical features of MFS can be explained by changes in the mechanical properties of the extracellular matrix resulting from abnormalities of fibrillin. However, several features such as bone overgrowth and myxoid changes in mitral valves cannot be explained due to changes in tissue elasticity. It is observed that FBN1 also binds to TGF-β. TGF-β multifunctional protein regulates cell proliferation and is upregulated in a variety of inflammatory diseases. Normal microfibrils sequester TGF-β in the extracellular matrix and thus, FBN1 controls the bioavailability of TGF-β. Reduced or altered forms of FBN1 give rise to abnormal and excessive activation of TGF-β. Patients with MFS have increased TGF-β in their aortas, cardiac valves, and lungs, probably due to decreased FBN1, which normally sequesters this cytokine. Excessive TGF-β signaling, in turn, produces different effects. These include—(1) upregulates to inflammation, (2) deleterious effects on vascular smooth muscle development, and (3) increases the activity of metalloproteases, causing loss of extracellular matrix. The evidence are supported by following observations:
   - **Gain-of-function mutations in the TGF-β type II receptor:** This produces a related syndrome, called Marfan syndrome type 2 (MFS2). Also, patients with germline mutations in one isoform of TGF-β, called TGF-β3, are predisposed to aortic aneurysm and other cardiovascular manifestations similar to those in classic MFS. Treating FBN1-deficient mice with a TGF-β antagonist decreases the severity of their "Marfan phenotype." This suggests the potential therapeutic approach in this disease that does not directly target the genetic mutation.
   - **Angiotensin receptor II blockers:** They inhibit TGF-β activity. In mouse models of MFS, they markedly reduce the aortic root diameter.

MORPHOLOGY

Skeletal System

Skeletal changes are the most characteristic of MFS.

- **General features:** Usually (but not always) the patient is unusually tall with greater lower body length (pubis to sole) than upper body length. They have exceptionally long thin extremities and long, tapering fingers (arachnodactyly/spider fingers) and toes.
- **Ligaments:** The joint ligaments, joint capsules, and tendons in the hands and feet are lax and weak. This leads to hyperextensibility of the joints suggesting that the patient is double-jointed; typically, the thumb can be hyperextended back to the wrist.
- **Head:** The head (skull) is commonly long (dolichocephalic) with prominent of the frontal eminences and prominent supraorbital ridges.

Continued

- **Spinal deformities:** Various deformities such as kyphosis, scoliosis, or rotation or slipping of the dorsal or lumbar vertebrae may be seen.
- **Chest:** It is classically deformed. Disorders of the ribs may cause either pectus excavatum (deeply depressed or concave sternum) or a pectus carinatum (pigeon breast deformity).

Cardiovascular System

CVS lesions are the most life-threatening features of MFS. The two most common lesions are as follows:

Mitral valve prolapse: It is seen in 40–50% of cases. The mitral valve typically has redundant leaflets and chordae tendineae-leading to mitral valve prolapse syndrome.

Dilation of the ascending aorta due to cystic medionecrosis: The most important defect is in the aorta, where the tunica media is weak and is of greater importance. Loss of medial support due to cystic medionecrosis results in progressive dilation of the aortic valve ring and the root of the aorta, weakening of the media predisposes to an intimal tear. This may initiate an intramural hematoma that cleaves the layers of the media to produce aortic dissection. There is high incidence of development of aortic dissection usually of the ascending aorta in MFS. After cleaving the aortic layers for considerable distances, sometimes these dissections may rupture back to the root of the aorta or into the pericardial cavity, extend down the aorta, iliac arteries, and rupture into the retroperitoneal space. Dilation of the aortic ring may produce dilation of the ascending aorta and severe aortic incompetence or regurgitation. This may be severe enough to produce angina pectoris and congestive heart failure. Patients most often die of cardiovascular disorders.

- **Microscopy:** The aorta shows marked fragmentation and loss of elastic fibers, with increased metachromatic mucopolysaccharide. This mucopolysaccharide may accumulate in discrete pools. These features are sometimes called cystic medial necrosis of the aorta. These changes in the media are almost similar to those found in cystic medionecrosis not related to MFS. Smooth muscle cells are enlarged and lose their orderly circumferential arrangement.

Eyes

Ocular changes are common in MFS and may take many forms. Most characteristic is bilateral subluxation or dislocation (usually outward and upward) of the lens. This is termed as ectopia lentis. This is due to the weakening of ciliary zonules. Finding of bilateral ectopia lentis should raise the suspicion of MFS even in individuals who do not have this disease. Other eye changes may be severe myopia due to elongation of the eye and retinal detachment.

Clinical features

This genetic disorder shows great variation in the clinical expression of the disease. Variability in clinical expression may be seen within a family. But interfamilial variability is much more common and extensive. Major involvement of two of the four organ systems (skeletal, cardiovascular, ocular, and skin) and minor involvement of another organ is needed for diagnosis of MFS.

Cardiovascular system

- **Valvular lesions:** Mitral valve lesions are more common but are clinically less important than aortic lesions. In the mitral valve, the loss of connective tissue support in leaflets makes them soft and billowy. This is responsible for so-called floppy valve. Valvular lesions in association with lengthening of the chordae tendineae, can result in mitral regurgitation. Similar changes may affect the tricuspid and, rarely, the aortic valves.
- **Aortic lesions:** Majority of deaths in MFS are caused by rupture of aortic dissections, followed by cardiac failure.
- **Echocardiography:** It helps to detect the cardiovascular abnormalities and is therefore, extremely valuable in the diagnosis of MFS.

Eyes Patients with prominent eye or cardiovascular changes may show only few skeletal abnormalities. Patients with striking changes in body habitus may not have any eye changes.

Prognosis: Untreated men with MFS usually die in their 30s and untreated women often die in their 40s.

Ehlers–Danlos Syndromes

Q. Discuss in detail about EDS.

Ehlers–Danlos syndromes (EDS) comprise a clinically and genetically heterogeneous group of inherited disorders of connective tissue. They result from some mutations in genes that encode collagen, enzymes that modify collagen, and less commonly other proteins present in the extracellular matrix. Other disorders caused due to mutations affecting collagen synthesis include OI, Alport syndrome, and epidermolysis bullosa.

Collagen: Biosynthesis of collagen is a complex process and involves many genes. Collagen synthesis can be disturbed by many genetic errors. These genetic errors may involve mutations in any one of the structural genes involved in the formation of collagen or genes involved in enzymatic post-transcriptional modifications of collagen.

Mode of inheritance: Mode of inheritance of EDSs may be any of the three Mendelian patterns. Thus, different forms of EDSs may be inherited as autosomal dominant or recessive (autosomal or X-linked) traits depending on the specific mutation.

Classification: Depending on the clinical and molecular characteristics, 11 molecular types/variants of EDSs have been recognized (**Table 6**).

Tissues involved and their consequences

In most variants of EDS, whatever may be the underlying biochemical defect, there is deficient or defective collagen.

- **Ligaments and joints:** It frequently involves tissues rich in collagen. These include skin, ligaments, and joints. The abnormal collagen fibers formed due to mutations lack adequate tensile strength. This produces hyperextensible skin and hypermobile joints with laxity. These features allow strange flexibility such as bending the thumb backward to touch the forearm and bending the knee forward to create almost a right angle. Probably most gymnast with unbelievable flexibility have one of the EDSs. However, one of the prices to be paid for this profession is predisposition to dislocation of joint. In more severe forms, surgical repair may be needed.

Table 6: Different forms of Ehlers–Danlos syndromes (EDSs).

EDS type (previous numerical equivalents)*	*Inheritance*	*Gene defects*	*Protein defect*
Classic (EDS I—severe and EDS II—mild)	AD (autosomal dominant)	*COL5A1, COL5A2*	Collagen V
Hypermobile (EDS III)	AD	*TNXB*	Tenascin X
Vascular (EDS IV)	AD	*COL3A1*	Collagen III
Ocular-scoliotic (Kyphoscoliosis) EDS VI (EDS VIA and EDS VIB)	AR (autosomal recessive)	*PLOD1 (Lysyl hydroxylase)*	Deficiency of procollagen-lysine 5-dioxygenase activity (EDS VIA)
Arthrochalasic EDS VII (EDS VIIA and EDS VIIB)	AD	*COL1A1, COL1A2*	Mutations that prevent cleavage of the N propeptides
Dermatosparactic EDS VII C	AR	*ADAMTS2 (Procollagen N-peptidase)*	Deficiency of procollagen I N-terminal proteinase
Periodontal EDS VIII	AD	*C1R, C1S*	Components of the complement pathway
EDS due to tenascin X deficiency	AR	*TNXB*	Tenascin X
EDS, cardiac valvular form	AR	*COL1A2*	Type I collagen deficiency
EDS, progeroid form	AR	*B4GALT7*	Deficiency of galactosyltransferase 7 [defective synthesis of dermatan sulfate (DS) proteoglycans]
EDS, musculocontractural form	AR	*CHST14* *DSE*	Dermatan 4-O-sulfotransferase 1 (CHST14) and DS epimerase 1 (DSE) leading to defective synthesis of DS proteoglycans

*EDS types were previously classified by Roman numerals.

- **Skin:** All types of EDSs show soft, extremely fragile, and hyperextensible (extraordinarily stretchable) skin. The skin is easily bruised. Minor injuries produce gaping defects and serious wounds. The surgical repair by sutures do not hold well and surgical incisions often dehisce (burst open). Surgical intervention may be difficult because of the lack of normal tensile strength.
- **Other organs:** The basic defect in connective tissue may cause serious internal complications. These include rupture of the colon, large arteries (vascular EDS), gravid uterus, ocular fragility with rupture of cornea and retinal detachment (kyphoscoliosis EDS), and diaphragmatic hernia (classic EDS).

Biochemical and molecular basis

Only few types of EDSs are discussed below.

Kyphoscoliosis (ocular-scoliotic) type of EDS: It is the most common autosomal recessive form of EDS. It results from mutations in the *PLOD1* gene encoding enzyme lysyl hydroxylase. Lysyl hydroxylase is an enzyme necessary for hydroxylation of lysine residues during collagen synthesis. This produces hydroxylysine which is required for intermolecular and intramolecular cross-linking of collagen fibers. These patients have markedly reduced levels of lysyl hydroxylase, and this results in the synthesis of collagen without normal structural stability.

Vascular type of EDS: It results from mutations affecting the *COL3A1* gene encoding collagen type III. There is abnormal type III collagen. It is genetically heterogeneous and at least three distinct types of mutations can affect the *COL3A1* gene giving rise to different variants. These mutations may—(1) affect the rate of synthesis of pro-α1 (III) chains, or (2) affect the secretion of type III procollagen, or (3) lead to the synthesis of structurally abnormal type III collagen. Vascular-type EDS results from mutations involving a structural protein (rather than an enzyme protein). The blood vessels and intestines are rich in collagen type III. Hence, it produces severe structural defects (e.g., vulnerability to spontaneous rupture) in these organs. The skin is not usually hyperextensible in this type.

EDS—arthrochalasia type and dermatosparaxis type: The defect in these two types of EDS is in the conversion of type I procollagen to collagen. In this step of collagen synthesis (**Fig. 15**), there is cleavage of noncollagen peptides at the N terminus and C terminus of the procollagen molecule. This is brought out by N-terminal-specific and C-terminal-specific proteases (peptidases).

- **Arthrochalasia type of EDS:** In this type of EDS, the defect is in the conversion of procollagen to collagen. It is due to mutations that affect one of the two type I collagen genes, *COL1A1* and *COL1A2*. It results in production of structurally abnormal pro-α1 (I) or pro-α2 (I) chains. These products resist cleavage of N-terminal peptides. If the patient has a single mutant allele, only 50% of the type I collagen chains are abnormal. But these abnormal chains interfere with the formation of normal collagen helices. Hence, heterozygotes manifest the disease.
- **Dermatosparaxis type of EDS:** It is caused due to mutations in the *ADAMTS2* gene that encodes procollagen-N-peptidase. This enzyme is needed for the cleavage of procollagens. Because this is due to an enzyme deficiency, it is transmitted as an autosomal recessive disorder.

Classic type of EDS: It is found that genes other than those that encode collagen may also be involved in EDS. In about 90% of cases of classic type of EDS, there are mutations involving the genes for type V collagen (*COL5A1* and *COL5A2*). Surprisingly, in the remaining cases, though they are clinically

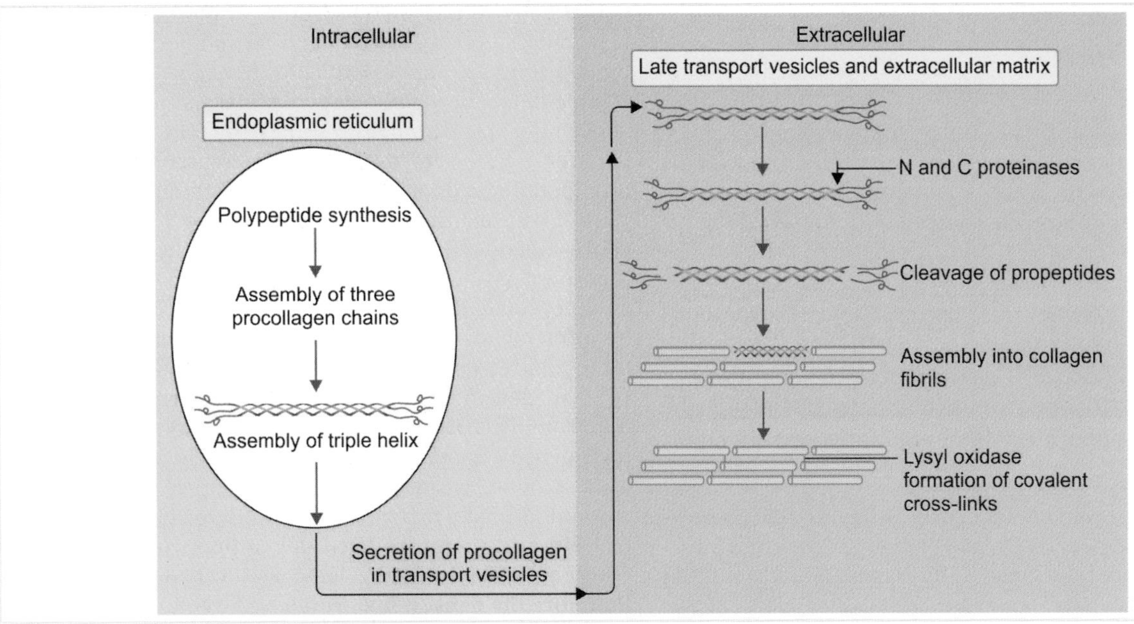

FIG. 15: Major steps in involved in the biosynthesis of fibrillar collagens (Schematic). The process of collagen synthesis occurs mainly in the fibroblasts. Collagen synthesis occurs both intracellularly and extracellularly. (A) Various intracellular events in collagen formation. First, transcription of mRNA in the nucleus followed by translation. Post-translational modification in the endoplasmic reticulum (ER) produces polypeptide chains. Assembly of three procollagen chains occurs followed by assembly of triple helix. This produces pro-collagen in transport vesicle (B) Events in late transport vesicles and extracellular matrix. Enzymes known as collagen peptidases preform propeptide cleavage and remove the ends of the procollagen molecule and the molecule becomes tropocollagen. Lysyl oxidase a copper-dependent enzyme acts on lysine and hydroxylysines, and covalent bonding between tropocollagen molecules form a collagen fibril .

similar to the classic type EDS, there are no abnormalities in collagen gene. Probably, in some cases, genetic defects that affect the biosynthesis of other extracellular matrix molecules that influence collagen synthesis may be indirectly involved. One example is a classic EDS-like condition due to mutation in the *TNXB* gene encoding tenascin-X. Tenascin-X is a large multimeric protein that interacts with fibrillar types I, III, and V collagens.

Diagnosis: It is based on clinical criteria and on DNA sequencing.

Osteogenesis Imperfecta

Osteogenesis imperfecta (OI), or brittle bone disease (type 1 collagen disease), is the most common inherited disorder of connective tissue. It is a phenotypically heterogenous group in which a generalized abnormality of connective tissue is caused by deficiencies in type I collagen synthesis. OI mainly affects bone (expressed mainly as fragility of bone), but it also involves other tissues rich in type I collagen (joints, eyes, ears, skin, and teeth). OI is inherited as an autosomal dominant trait, although rarely it may be transmitted as autosomal recessive.

Pathogenesis

It is caused by mutations in genes *COL1A1* and *COL1A2* that encode α1 and α2 chains of type I collagen. More than 800 mutations have been identified. There is a point mutation with replacement of a glycine residue within the α-helical structure of type I collagen with another bulkier amino acid. This disrupts the triple-helical formation. Collagen synthesis and extracellular transport need triple-helix formation. Thus, these mutations result in misfolding of collagen polypeptides and defective assembly of higher order collagen chains. Mutant collagens also interfere with assembly of normal wild-type collagen chains (i.e., they exert a dominant negative effect). These are inherited in autosomal dominant pattern. Rarely, it may involve other structural proteins in bone.

Clinical subtypes: The fundamental abnormality is too little bone. This leads to extreme skeletal fragility. OI is divided into four major clinical subtypes of varying severity.

- **Type I:** It is characterized by a normal appearance at birth. Fractures of many bones occur during infancy and at the time the child starts walking. Such patients have been described as being as "fragile as a china doll." They have blue sclerae caused by decreased collagen fibers. This makes the sclera translucent and allows partial visualization of the underlying choroidal veins. Patient may develop hearing loss due to both a sensorineural deficit and impaired conduction due to fractures and fusion of the bones of the middle ear restrict their mobility. Type I collagen is normal, but the quantity is reduced by half (haploinsufficiency).
- **Type II:** It is usually fatal in utero or shortly after birth. Those who are born alive usually die of respiratory failure within their first month.
- **Type III:** It produces progressive deformities. It is usually detected at birth due to the baby's short stature and misshapenness caused by fractures in utero. There may be dental defects (small, misshapen, and blue-yellow teeth) secondary to dentin deficiency. Hearing loss is common. It is often inherited as an autosomal recessive trait.
- **Type IV:** It resembles type I, but sclerae are normal and the phenotype is more variable.

Disorders Associated with Defects in Receptor Proteins

Familial Hypercholesterolemia

Q. Write short essay on FH and its mechanism.

Q. Write short essay on hypercholesterolemia and its consequences.

Q. Write short essay on lipoprotein metabolism in disease.

Familial hypercholesterolemia (FH), also known as autosomal dominant hypercholesterolemia (ADH), is an autosomal codominant disorder. It is characterized by high levels of plasma low-density lipoprotein cholesterol (LDL-C) in the absence of hypertriglyceridemia.

Basics of lipids

Lipids are mainly found in three compartments in the body—(1) plasma, (2) adipose tissue, and (3) biological membranes.

Fatty acids are the simplest form of lipids, found mainly in plasma.

Triglycerides [TGs, triacylglycerols (TAG)] are the storage form of lipids and are stored in solid form mainly in adipose tissue. Fatty acids in tissues are commonly esterified to glycerol, forming a TAG (TGs). The source of TGs is food and it is also produced by liver. TAG produced in the liver on the smooth endoplasmic reticulum can only be stored transiently. The liver has the unique capacity to offload stored TAG by producing lipoprotein complexes. These lipoprotein complexes also contain cholesterol, phospholipids, and apolipoproteins (also synthesized on the endoplasmic reticulum) and are exported in the form of very low-density lipoprotein (VLDL). The VLDL is then assembled in the endoplasmic reticulum and transferred to the Golgi apparatus. From here, VLDL is released into the bloodstream.

Phospholipids are the major class of lipids in biological membranes of all cells.

Cholesterol is an essential component of cell membranes and also essential for cell function. Cholesterol is also a precursor of the steroid hormones, vitamin D, and the bile acids.

Lipoproteins are large macromolecular complexes consisting of lipids and specialized proteins. Lipoproteins play a main role in the absorption of poorly soluble lipids [e.g., cholesterol, TGs (TGs), and fat-soluble vitamins] from the intestine They are essential for transport of these poorly soluble lipids through body fluids (plasma, interstitial fluid, and lymph) to and from tissues. They also transport lipids from the liver to peripheral tissues and the transport of cholesterol from peripheral tissues to the liver. Structurally, lipoproteins consist of a central core of hydrophobic lipids (TGs and cholesteryl esters) surrounded by a shell of hydrophilic lipids (phospholipids, unesterified cholesterol) and proteins (called apolipoproteins) that interact with body fluids. The plasma lipoproteins are classified into five major classes based on their relative density and size (**Fig. 16A**)—chylomicrons, very low-density lipoproteins (VLDLs), intermediate-density lipoproteins (IDLs), low-density lipoproteins (LDLs), and high-density lipoproteins (HDLs). Lipid is less dense than water and the density of a lipoprotein particle depends on the amount of lipid per particle. **Chylomicrons are the richest in lipid and therefore least dense lipoprotein particles, whereas HDLs have the least amount of lipid and are therefore the densest lipoproteins**. The composition of each type of lipoprotein class varies in percentage of proteins, TGs, and cholesterol and cholesterol esters (**Fig. 16B**). The proteins associated with lipoproteins are called as apolipoproteins. They are required for the assembly, structure, function, and metabolism of lipoproteins. ApoB is a very large protein and is the major structural protein present in chylomicrons, VLDLs, IDLs, and LDLs. HDLs have most abundant ApoA-I which is synthesized in both the liver and intestine and also ApoA-II.

Normal cholesterol metabolism and transport

Exogenous pathway of lipoproteins: Cholesterol may be derived from the diet or from endogenous synthesis and plasma cholesterol level depends on endogenous cholesterol synthesis in liver and dietary intake of cholesterol. Cholesterol is circulated via special carriers called lipoproteins (refer below). One of the main roles of lipoproteins is the transport of lipids in the diet from the intestine to tissues that require fatty acids for energy or store and metabolize lipids and of intestinal cholesterol to the liver.

- Dietary TGs and cholesterol are incorporated into chylomicrons in the intestinal mucosa. These chylomicrons (**Fig. 17**) are the primary form of circulating lipids with

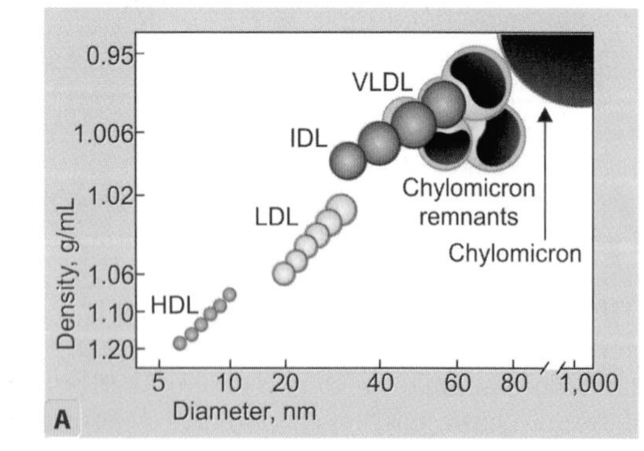

Lipoprotein	% protein	% triacylglycerol	% cholesterol and cholesteryl ester
Chylomicrons	1–2	85–90	4–8
VLDL	5–10	50–65	15–25
IDL	10–20	20–30	40–45
LDL	20–25	7–15	45–50
HDL	40–55	3–10	15–20

B

(HDL: high-density lipoprotein; IDL: intermediate-density lipoprotein; LDL: low-density lipoprotein; VLDL: very low-density lipoprotein)

FIGS. 16A AND B: Lipoproteins classifications. (A) Lipoproteins are classified depending on the size and density of lipoprotein particles. These are inversely related; (B) Various components of lipoproteins.

a protein content of only 1–2%. The primary function of chylomicrons is to transport dietary lipids to adipose tissue as free fatty acids and cholesterol to the liver. After intestinal absorption, dietary cholesterol is transported from the intestine by gut lymphatics to the blood.

- In the capillaries of muscle and fat, these chylomicrons are hydrolyzed by an endothelial lipoprotein lipase (LPL) and form chylomicron remnants. These chylomicron remnants are rich in cholesterol and are rapidly removed from the circulation by the liver.
- From liver, some of the cholesterol enters the metabolic pool, and some is excreted as free cholesterol or as bile acids into the biliary tract.

Endogenous pathway of lipoproteins: The endogenous synthesis of cholesterol and LDL begins in the liver (**Fig. 17**).

- The first step consists of the secretion of VLDL from the liver into the blood. VLDL particles are rich in TGs and contain lesser amounts of cholesteryl esters (**Fig. 17**). VLDLs on their surface also carry apolipoproteins ApoB, ApoC, and ApoE.
- In the capillaries of adipose tissue and muscle, VLDL undergoes lipolysis and it is converted to VLDL remnant (also called IDL). These IDL particles have reduced content of TGs and an increase in cholesteryl esters in comparison with VLDL. Apolipoprotein ApoC present on the surface of VLDL is lost during its conversion to IDL (VLDL remnant), but ApoB and ApoE are retained.
- The IDL (VLDL remnant) particles, after their release from the capillary endothelium, can have one of the two fates:
    - About 50% of newly formed IDL is quickly taken up by the liver by receptor-mediated transport. The receptor for the IDL present on the liver cell membrane recognizes both ApoB and ApoE. This receptor is called as ApoB/E and is commonly known as the LDLR, because of its involvement in the hepatic clearance of LDL. IDL is recycled to the liver cells to produce VLDL.
    - The IDL particles that are not taken up by the liver are subjected to further metabolic processing. In this process, most of the remaining TGs and ApoE are removed and form ApoB carrying cholesterol-rich LDL particles.

LDLR pathway: Many cell types have high-affinity LDLRs (low-density lipoprotein receptors). These include fibroblasts, lymphocytes, smooth muscle cells, hepatocytes, and adrenocortical cells. But about 70% of the plasma LDL (low-density lipoprotein) is cleared by the liver, using a quite sophisticated transport process (**Fig. 17**).

- **Binding of LDL to cell-surface receptors:** The cell-surface receptors for LDL are clustered in specialized regions of the plasma membrane called coated pits. The first step in LDL pathway is binding of LDL to these cell-surface receptors.

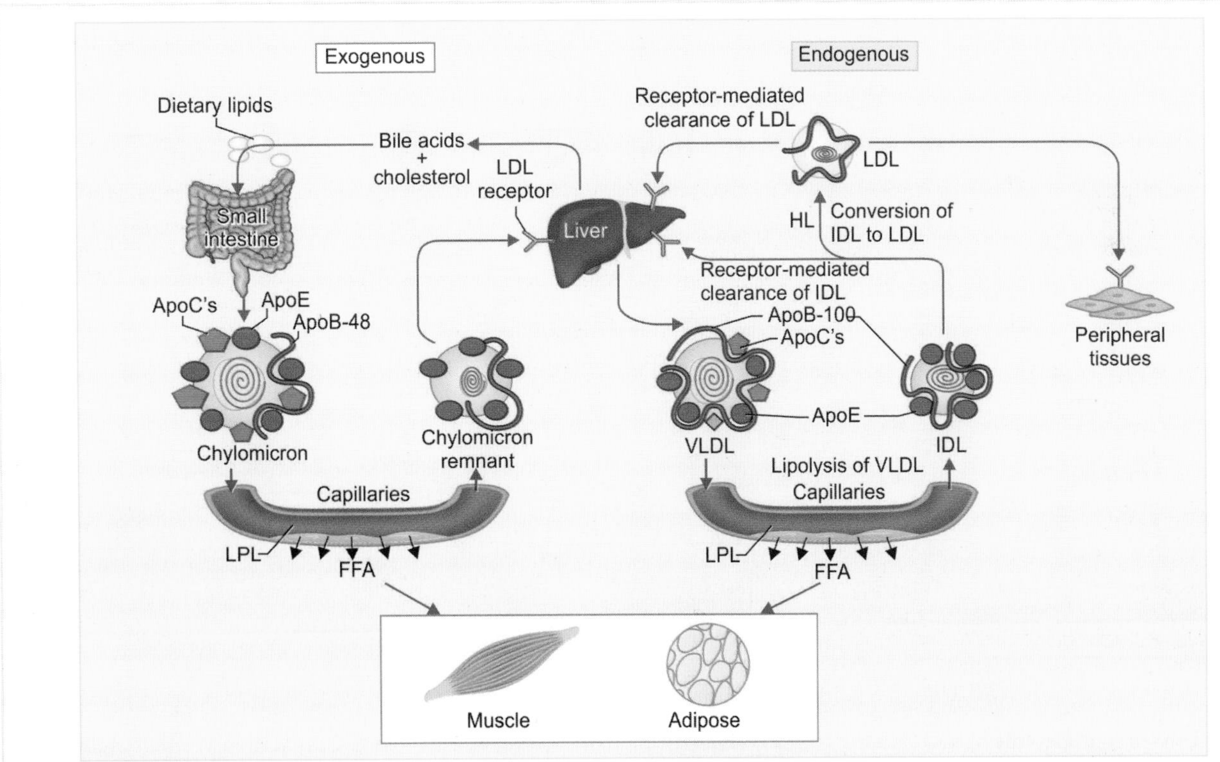

(ApoC: apolipoprotein C; ApoE: apolipoprotein E; ApoB-100: apolipoprotein B-100; FFA: free fatty acid; HL: hepatic lipase; IDL: intermediate-density lipoprotein; LDL: low-density lipoprotein; LDLR: low-density lipoprotein receptor)

FIG. 17: The exogenous and endogenous metabolic pathways of lipoprotein and the role of liver in its synthesis and clearance. In the exogenous pathway, dietary lipids are transported to the periphery and the liver. In the endogenous pathway, hepatic lipids are transported to the periphery. Lipolysis of very low-density lipoprotein (VLDL) by lipoprotein lipase (LPL) in the capillaries releases triglycerides and free fatty acids, which are then stored in adipose tissue and used as a source of energy in skeletal muscles.

- **Internalization of LDL:** After binding to the receptors, the coated pits containing the receptor-bound LDL are internalized by invagination and form coated vesicles. The coated vesicles migrate and form endosomes within the hepatocytes. These endosomes fuse with the lysosomes.
- **Dissociates of the receptor and recycling:** The LDL dissociates from the receptor and is recycled to the surface of the cell. The recycling of LDLRs is regulated by proprotein convertase subtilisin/kexin type 9 (PCSK9). This PCSK9 binds to LDLRs on the surface of hepatocytes and degrades them after endocytosis.
- **Degradation of LDL in the lysosome:** Inside the lysosomes of the hepatocyte, the LDL molecule is enzymatically degraded. The apoprotein part of LDL is hydrolyzed to amino acids, whereas the cholesteryl esters are split into free cholesterol. The free cholesterol in the lysosome crosses the membrane of lysosomes and enters the cytoplasm. In the cytoplasm, free cholesterol is utilized for synthesis of membrane and also acts as a regulator of cholesterol homeostasis. The exit of cholesterol from the lysosomes needs the action of two proteins, called NPC1 and NPC2 (NPC is Niemann–Pick disease type C). The release of intracellular cholesterol can follow four separate processes **(Fig. 18):**
  - **i. Suppression of cholesterol synthesis within the cells:** Cholesterol can suppress synthesis of further cholesterol within the cell. This is achieved by inhibiting the activity of the enzyme 3-hydroxy-3-methylglutaryl coenzyme A (HMG CoA) reductase. HMG CoA reductase is the rate-limiting enzyme in the synthetic pathway of cholesterol.
  - **ii. Activation of acyl-coenzyme A: cholesterol acyltransferase:** Cholesterol activates the enzyme called acyl-coenzyme A: cholesterol acyltransferase. This **favors esterification and causes storage of excess cholesterol**.
  - **iii. Cholesterol suppresses the synthesis of LDLRs:** This protects the cells from excessive accumulation of cholesterol.
  - **iv. Cholesterol upregulates the expression of PCSK9:** This **reduces recycling of LDLRs and causes degradation of endocytosed LDLRs**. This protects the cells from excessive accumulation of cholesterol.

Synthesis of LDL receptors (Fig. 18): The LDLRs are made in the endoplasmic reticulum, transferred to the Golgi apparatus, and transported to the cell surface. In the cell surface, it is present in clathrin-coated pits.

Causes of familial hypercholesterolemia (Box 4)

Familial hypercholesterolemia results from various mutations in the gene encoding the receptor for LDL (i.e., *LDLR*) or the two genes that compromise its function. The impact of these gene mutations in FH is as follows:

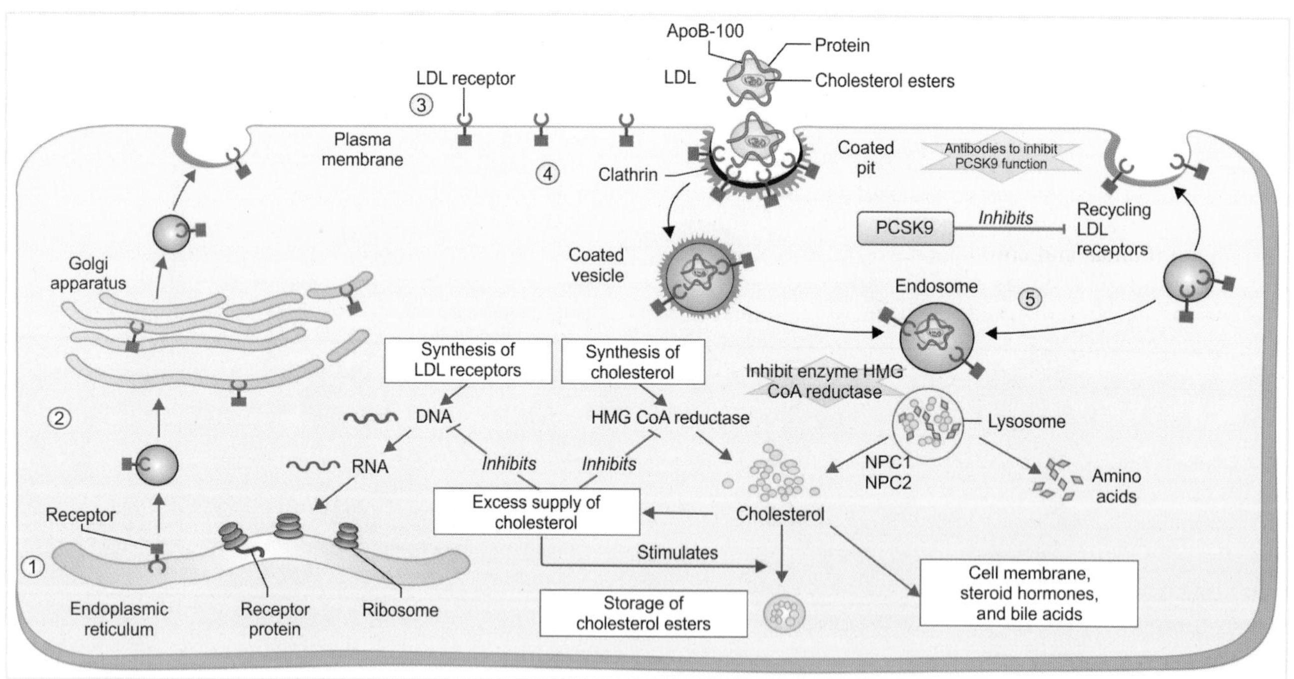

(ApoB-100: apolipoprotein B-100; HMG CoA: 3-hydroxy-3-methylglutaryl coenzyme A; PCSK9: proprotein convertase subtilisin/kexin type 9; NCP: Niemann–Pick disease type C)

FIG. 18: Low-density lipoprotein (LDL) receptor pathway and regulation of cholesterol metabolism. Classification of LDL receptor (LDLR) mutations depends on abnormal function of the mutant protein. Various mutations include the—(1) class I mutation (abnormality of LDL receptor synthesis): may reduce LDLR synthesis in the endoplasmic reticulum; (2) class II mutation (abnormality of transport to Golgi complex): may reduce transport of LDLR to the Golgi complex; (3) class III mutation (abnormality of LDL binding by receptor): may reduce binding of apoprotein ligands, (4) class IV mutation (abnormality of receptor clustering in coated pit): may reduce clustering in coated pits, and (5) class V mutation (abnormality in recycling in endosomes): may reduce recycling in endosomes. In class VI mutation (not depicted in Figure), initial targeting of the receptor to basolateral membrane does not occur. Drugs can be used to lower plasma cholesterol by increasing the number of LDLRs. Two classes of drugs that are used include drugs to inhibit the enzyme HMG CoA reductase (statins) and antibodies to inhibit PCSK9 function. Both of them lower cholesterol by different mechanisms.

Box 4: Mutations in familial hypercholesterolemia.

- Mutation in the LDL receptor gene (LDLR) is seen in about 80–85% of cases
- Mutation in the gene that encodes apolipoprotein B-100 (ApoB), the ligand for LDLR on the LDL particle, is observed in 5–10% of cases
- Mutation in the gene that encodes proprotein convertase subtilisin/kexin type 9 (commonly known by its abbreviation PCSK9) is seen in 1–2% of cases

(LDL: low-density lipoprotein; LDLR: low-density lipoprotein receptor)

Mutations in the LDL receptor gene (LDLR gene) FH is most commonly caused by mutations in the gene encoding the receptor for LDL (*LDLR*). This leads to reduced function or activity of the LDLR and results in inadequate/reduced rate of removal (clearance) of circulating plasma LDL by the liver. Most (80–85%) of the cases of FH are due to mutations in the *LDLR* gene on the short arm of chromosome 19. FH caused by LDLR mutations is one of the most frequent Mendelian disorders.

- Heterozygous individuals of FH have one mutant *LDLR* gene and one normal *LDLR* gene. They possess only 50% of the normal number of high-affinity LDL receptors (due to normal *LDLR* gene). This results in defect in transport and impairs the catabolism of LDL by the receptor-dependent pathways. These patients have twofold to threefold rise in circulating plasma LDL and cholesterol levels from birth and cholesterol deposition in arteries, tendons, and skin. This leads to premature atherosclerosis and tendinous xanthomas in adult life.
- Homozygous individuals have two mutant *LDLR* genes and do not have any normal LDLRs in their cells. They have fivefold to sixfold rise in circulating plasma LDL and cholesterol levels and are much more severely affected. Skin xanthomas and coronary, cerebral, and peripheral vascular atherosclerosis may develop at an early age. Myocardial infarction may develop before age 20 years.

Both the homozygotes and the heterozygotes have defective LDL clearance and increased synthesis of LDL. The increased synthesis leading to hypercholesterolemia is also due to lack of LDLRs. IDL (the immediate precursor of plasma LDL) also uses hepatic LDLRs (ApoB/E receptors) for its transport into the liver cells. Hence, in FH, impaired IDL transport into the liver secondarily diverts more amount of plasma IDL into the precursor pool for plasma LDL.

Other mutations Much less commonly, FH is due to mutations in two other genes involved in removal or clearance of plasma LDL. These are as follows:

- Mutations in gene encoding apolipoprotein B-100 (ApoB): ApoB on the surface of LDL particles is the ligand for LDL receptors. Mutation of gene encoding ApoB reduces the binding of LDL molecules with LDLRs. This in turn increases serum LDL cholesterol. This is responsible for 5-10% cases of FH.
- Activating mutation in the *PCSK9* gene: The proprotein convertase subtilisin/kexin type 9 is an enzyme, commonly known by its abbreviation PCSK9. This enzyme reduces expression of LDLRs by downregulating their recycling and consequent increased degradation in lysosomes during the recycling process. Activating mutation in the PCSK9 greatly reduces the number of LDLRs on the cell. This is responsible for 1-2% cases of FH.

All these three types of mutations impair hepatic clearance of LDL and this in turn increases the plasma level of LDL such that the rate of production of LDL equals the rate of clearance of LDL by residual LDLR as well as non-LDLR mechanisms. This increases the serum levels of cholesterol and predisposes to premature development of atherosclerosis and a markedly increased risk of myocardial infarction.

Scavenger receptor pathways for LDL: Apart from LDLRs in the hepatocytes, the transport of LDL partly can also occur through the scavenger receptor. These are found in the cells of the mononuclear phagocyte system. Thus, monocytes and macrophages of the mononuclear phagocyte system have receptors for chemically altered (e.g., acetylated or oxidized) LDL. Normally, the amount of LDL transported through these scavenger receptor pathways is less than that mediated by the LDL receptor-dependent mechanisms. But in patients with hypercholesterolemia, there is a marked increase in the scavenger receptor-mediated transport of LDL cholesterol into the cells of the mononuclear phagocyte system and probably the vascular walls. This increase in scavenger receptor pathways is responsible for the development of xanthomas and involved in the pathogenesis of premature atherosclerosis.

Molecular genetics of familial hypercholesterolemia

Molecular genetics of FH is very complex. More than 2,000 mutations involving the LDL receptor gene have been detected. These include DNA CNVs, insertions, deletions, and missense and nonsense mutations. LDL receptors mutations can be classified into six groups (**Figs. 18** and **19**):

1. **Class I mutations:** These are characterized by complete failure of synthesis of the nascent LDL receptor protein (LDLR protein) in the endoplasmic reticulum. This is mostly due to large deletions in the gene (null alleles). This

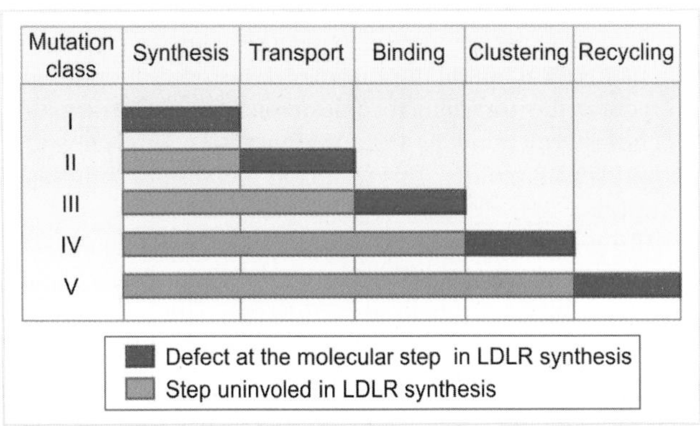

FIG. 19: Classification of low-density lipoprotein receptor (LDLR) mutations depends on abnormal function of the mutant protein. Mutation can involve any steps involved in the synthesis of LDLR. Various mutations include—(1) class I mutation: may reduce LDLR synthesis in the endoplasmic reticulum; (2) class II mutation: may reduce transport of LDLR to the Golgi complex; (3) class III mutation: may reduce binding of apoprotein ligands; (4) class IV mutation: may reduce clustering in coated pits, and (5) class V mutation: may reduce recycling in endosomes. In class VI mutation (not depicted in Figure), there is failure of initial targeting of the LDLR to the basolateral membrane.

leads to absence of the LDL receptor in the cell membrane. These are relatively uncommon.

2. **Class II mutations:** These mutations block transfer of nascent LDL receptors from the endoplasmic reticulum to the Golgi (transport-defective alleles). They cause folding defects in LDLR and make it impossible for LDLR to be transported from endoplasmic reticulum to the Golgi complex. Thus, LDLR does not reach the cell surface and LDLR proteins accumulate in the endoplasmic reticulum. These are the fairly common defects.
3. **Class III mutations:** They affect the ApoB binding site of the LDL receptor. The mutant LDL receptors reach the cell surface but are defective in the ligand-binding domain (binding-defective alleles). So, there is either failure or poor binding of LDL to LDLR.
4. **Class IV mutations:** In this, LDLRs are efficiently synthesized and transported to the cell surface. LDL binds normally to LDLR, but the receptor does not localize (not cluster) in coated pits. Thus, the internalization of bound LDL by endocytosis is blocked (internalization-defective alleles) and there is no internalization. These are rare mutations.
5. **Class V mutations:** In this, LDLRs expressed on the cell surface can bind LDL as well as they can be internalized. However, internalized LDLR complexes remain in endosomes and there is failure of pH-dependent dissociation of the receptor and the bound LDL. Such LDLRs are trapped in the endosome and are degraded there. Hence, receptors do not recycle to the plasma membrane or the cell surface (recycling-defective alleles).
6. **Class VI mutations:** It is characterized by failure of initial targeting of the LDLR to the basolateral membrane.

Cholesterol lowering drugs

The understanding of the critical role of LDLRs in cholesterol homeostasis has helped to design drugs that lower plasma cholesterol by increasing the number of LDLRs (**Fig. 18**).

- Drugs to inhibit the enzyme HMG CoA reductase: Normally, the enzyme HMG CoA reductase promotes the synthesis of intracellular cholesterol. One of strategy is to use drugs (statins) that inhibit the enzyme HMG CoA reductase. This reduces the intracellular cholesterol. Lowered intracellular cholesterol removes the braking action of cholesterol on LDLR synthesis. This results in increased synthesis of LDLRs.
- Antibodies to inhibit PCSK9 function: Normally, PCSK9 inhibits recycling of LDLRs. In another strategy, antibodies are used to inhibit PCSK9 function. This reduces the degradation of LDLRs, thereby increasing the LDLRs on the cell membrane and consequent increased clearance of LDL cholesterol from the blood.

Disorders Associated with Enzyme Defects

Lysosomal Storage Diseases

Q. Write short essay on lysosomal storage disorders (LSD).

Introduction

Lysosomes are heterogeneous subcellular organelles and form the key components of the intracellular digestive system. Lysosomes are membrane-bound intracellular structures containing numerous hydrolytic enzymes. These enzymes degrade (digest) virtually all types of biological macromolecules including proteins, glycoproteins, mucopolysaccharides, nucleic acids, carbohydrates, and lipids.

Special properties of lysosomal enzymes: The hydrolytic enzymes in lysosomes have two special properties namely—(1) they **function in the acidic milieu of the lysosomes** and (2) these enzymes constitute a special category of secretory proteins. These lysosomal enzymes are **destined for intracellular organelles and not for the extracellular fluids.** Lysosomal digestive enzymes are sometimes called "acid hydrolases" because their optimal activities occur at acidic pHs (pH 3.5–5.5). The action of these enzymes on intracellular organelles requires special processing within the Golgi apparatus.

Types of lysosomal enzymes: There are several types of degradative enzymes. These include nucleases, proteases, glycosidases, lipases, phosphatases, sulfatases, and phospholipases.

Biosynthesis and intracellular transport of lysosomal enzymes (Fig. 20): Most of the lysosomal enzymes are N-linked glycoproteins. Similar to all other secretory proteins, lysosomal enzymes are also synthesized and glycosylated in the endoplasmic reticulum and transported to the Golgi apparatus. Within the Golgi complex, they undergo a variety of post-translational modifications. Such post-translational modifications are important for the functioning of the enzyme and defects can result in multiple enzyme/protein deficiencies. These include phosphorylation, sulfation, and additional proteolytic processing, etc. One of these post-translational modifications is the attachment of terminal mannose-6-phosphate groups to some of the oligosaccharide side chains. The phosphorylated mannose residues serve as an "address label." This is recognized by specific receptors present on the inner surface of the Golgi membrane. Lysosomal enzymes bind these receptors present on the inner surface of the Golgi membrane. This allows segregation of lysosomal enzymes from the numerous other secretory proteins within the Golgi apparatus. Subsequently, small transport vesicles containing these receptor-bound enzymes are pinched off from the Golgi apparatus. These vesicles fuse with the lysosomes. Thus, the enzymes are transferred to the lysosomes. The empty vesicles are returned back to the Golgi apparatus (**Fig. 20**).

Catalyzation of macromolecules by lysosomal enzymes (Fig. 20): The lysosomal enzymes catalyze the breakdown of almost all variety of complex macromolecules. These large molecules (macromolecules) may be derived from either extracellular or intracellular source. Extracellular macromolecules may be acquired from outside the cells that are internalized by endocytosis or phagocytosis (heterophagy) and are digested in lysosomes to their basic components. The intracellular constituents are derived from metabolic turnover of intracellular organelles (autophagy). End-products may be transported across lysosomal membranes into the cytosol. In the cytoplasm (cytosol), they are reused in the synthesis of new macromolecules.

Pathogenesis of lysosomal storage disorders (Fig. 21)

Abnormalities at any step involved in the biosynthesis of lysosomal enzymes can impair activation of enzymes and lead to a LSDs (lysosomal storage disorders). Majority of lysosomal

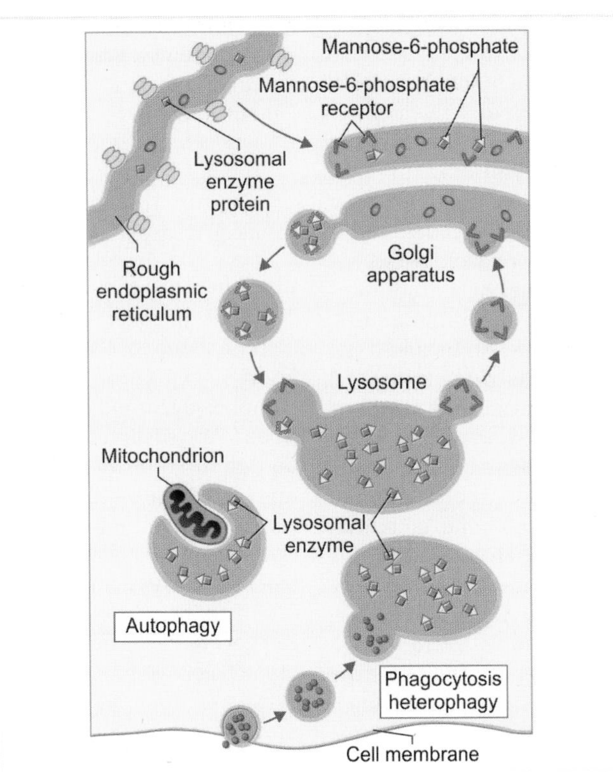

FIG. 20: Various steps in synthesis and intracellular transport of lysosomal enzymes. Lysosomal enzymes are synthesized and glycosylated in the rough endoplasmic reticulum and transported to the Golgi apparatus. Within the Golgi complex, they undergo a variety of post-translational modifications. One of these post-translational modifications is the attachment of terminal mannose-6-phosphate groups to some of the oligosaccharide side chains. The phosphorylated mannose residue is recognized by specific receptors present on the inner surface of the Golgi membrane. Lysosomal enzymes bind these receptors present on the inner surface of the Golgi membrane. Subsequently, small transport vesicles containing these receptor-bound enzymes are pinched off from the Golgi apparatus. These vesicles fuse with the lysosomes. Thus, the enzymes are transferred to the lysosomes. The empty vesicles are returned back to the Golgi apparatus. The lysosomal enzymes catalyze the breakdown of almost all variety of complex macromolecules. These molecules may be derived from either extracellular or intracellular source. Extracellular macromolecules are internalized by endocytosis or phagocytosis (heterophagy) and are digested in lysosomes to their basic components. The intracellular constituents are derived from metabolic turnover of intracellular organelles (autophagy).

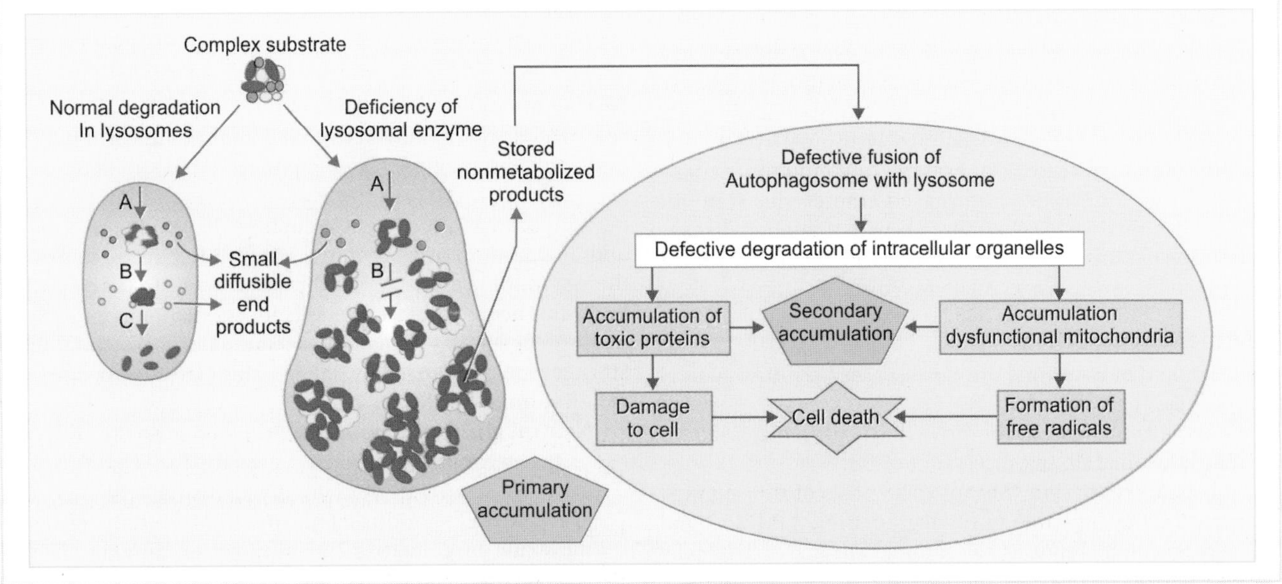

FIG. 21: Pathogenesis of lysosomal storage diseases. Normally a complex substrate is degraded by a series of lysosomal enzymes (e.g., A, B, and C) into soluble end products. Deficiency or defect in one of the enzymes (e.g., B) leads to incomplete catabolism of complex substrate. There will be accumulation of insoluble intermediates in the lysosomes and it is called primary accumulation. The toxic effects also result from defective autophagy and lead to secondary accumulation.

enzyme deficiencies are due to point mutations or genetic rearrangements at a locus that encodes a single lysosomal hydrolase. An inherited deficiency of a functional lysosomal enzyme can have two pathologic consequences:

1. **Incomplete catabolism of the substrate of the missing enzyme:** Deficient or missing enzyme can prevent catabolism of the normal macromolecular substrate of that enzyme. This leads to the accumulation of the undigested or partially degraded insoluble substrate (metabolite) within the lysosomes. This is called as "**primary accumulation**." Loaded with incompletely digested macromolecules, lysosomes become large and numerous and expand the lysosomal compartment of the cell. Resulting lysosomal distention impairs or interferes with normal cell functions and critical cellular activities. Particularly in the brain and heart, this can lead to poor cellular function or cell death. Common final pathway for LSDs is the accumulation of specific macromolecules within tissues and cells that normally have a high flux of these substrates.
2. **Defective degradation of organelles by autophagy by lysosomes:** There is a tight link between autophagy, mitochondrial functions, and lysosomes. A wide range of cellular organelles and molecules are degraded by autophagy. These include complex lipids, polyubiquitinated proteins, mitochondria, and fragments of the endoplasmic reticulum. Autophagy is needed particularly for turnover of mitochondria by a process called **mitophagy**. This process acts as a quality control system in which dysfunctional mitochondria are degraded. In lysosomal disorders, the accumulated undigested macromolecules in the lysosomes markedly reduce the rate of processing of organelles (especially mitochondria) delivered by autophagocytic vacuoles to the lysosomes. This causes persistence of dysfunctional and leaky mitochondria with poor capacity to buffer calcium and altered membrane potentials in the lysosomes. Damaged mitochondria also produce free radicals and release molecules that stimulate the intrinsic pathway of apoptosis. Impaired autophagy results in secondary accumulation of autophagic substrates. These include ubiquitinated and aggregate-prone polypeptides (e.g., α-synuclein, Huntingtin protein). This is the basis of a close link at the molecular level between neurodegenerative disorders and lysosomal storage diseases such as Gaucher disease. There may be association of lysosomal dysfunction with common diseases. For example, an important genetic risk factor for Parkinson disease is the carrier state for Gaucher disease, and almost all with Gaucher disease develop Parkinson disease. NPC disease (LSD) is associated with an increased risk of Alzheimer disease.

Treatment approach

The treatment of lysosomal storage diseases has three general approaches. These include:

1. **Enzyme replacement therapy:** This is presently used for may lysosomal storage diseases.
2. **Substrate reduction therapy:** The basis of this therapy is that if the substrate to be degraded by the lysosomal enzyme can be reduced, the residual enzyme activity may be enough to catabolize it and prevent its accumulation.
3. **Molecular chaperone therapy:** It is based on the molecular basis of enzyme deficiency. In many LSDs (e.g., Gaucher disease), the enzyme activity is low. This is because the mutant proteins are unstable and undergo misfolding and are degraded in the endoplasmic reticulum. In such disorders, an exogenous competitive inhibitor of the enzyme can be given. This binds to the mutant enzyme and acts as the folding template. This in turn assists proper folding of the enzyme and prevents its degradation.

Apart from the above, other therapies include hematopoietic stem cell transplants and gene therapy in specific cases.

Classification of lysosomal storage diseases (Table 7)

The lysosomal storage diseases are a heterogeneous group of disorders due to LOF (loss of function) mutations in various lysosomal enzymes. This results in an inability to break down complex glycolipids or other intracellular macromolecules. About 70 lysosomal storage diseases are known. These may be due to abnormalities of lysosomal enzymes or proteins involved in substrate degradation, endosomal sorting, or lysosomal membrane integrity. Lysosomal storage diseases are classified into categories based on the enzyme involved and the biochemical nature of the retained or accumulated metabolite or substrates (material) in the lysosomes (**Table 7**). Within each category of LSDs, there are many subgroups. Each result from the deficiency of a specific enzyme. Thus, when accumulated substrates are sphingolipids, they are termed sphingolipidoses. Storage of mucopolysaccharides [glycosaminoglycans (GAGs)] leads to the mucopolysaccharidoses (MPSs). They are categorized as lipidoses/sphingolipidoses, MPSs, mucolipidoses (MLs), glycoproteinoses, glycogenoses, and others.

Sphingolipidoses **Phospholipids** are the predominant lipids of cell membranes. There are two classes of phospholipids; those that have glycerol (from glucose) as a backbone and those that have sphingosine (from serine and palmitate).

- **Glycerophospholipids (or phosphoglycerides):** These are phospholipids that contain glycerol.
- **Sphingophospholipids (sphingomyelin):** The backbone of sphingomyelin is the amino alcohol sphingosine, rather than glycerol. Sphingomyelin is degraded by sphingomyelinase (a lysosomal enzyme that removes phosphorylcholine) to produce a ceramide. Ceramides are the precursors of both phosphorylated and glycosylated sphingolipids.

Glycosphingolipids: Glycolipids, more precisely called glycosphingolipids, are molecules that contain both carbohydrate and lipid components. Like the phospholipid sphingomyelin, glycosphingolipids are derivatives of ceramides to which carbohydrates have been attached. Normally, synthesis and degradation of glycosphingolipids are balanced, so that their amount present in membranes is constant. If a specific lysosomal acid hydrolase needed for degradation is partially or totally deficient, a sphingolipid accumulates. **Lysosomal lipid storage diseases caused by deficiencies of these enzymes are called sphingolipidoses.**

- **Neutral glycosphingolipids:** Adding one sugar molecule to the ceramide produces a cerebroside. Cerebrosides are the simplest neutral glycosphingolipids These are ceramide monosaccharides that contain either a molecule of galactose (forming ceramide-galactose or galactocerebroside, the most common cerebroside found in myelin) or glucose (forming ceramide-glucose or glucocerebroside, an intermediate in the synthesis and degradation of the more complex glycosphingolipids).

Table 7: Classification of lysosomal storage diseases.

Disease (mode of inheritance)	*Enzyme deficiency*	*Major accumulating metabolites*
Sphingolipidoses (including sphingolipid activator defects)		
G_{M1} gangliosidosis		
• Type 1—infantile, generalized (AR) • Type 2—juvenile (AR)	G_{M1} ganglioside β-galactosidase	G_{M1} ganglioside, galactose-containing oligosaccharides
G_{M2} gangliosidosis		
• Tay–Sachs disease (AR)	β-Hexosaminidase A	G_{M2} ganglioside
• Sandhoff disease (AR)	β-Hexosaminidase A and B	G_{M2} ganglioside, globoside
• G_{M2} gangliosidosis variant (activator defect) AB (AR)	Ganglioside activator protein	G_{M2} ganglioside
Neutral glycosphingolipidoses		
• Fabry disease (X-linked)	α-Galactosidase A	Ceramide trihexoside
• Niemann–Pick disease: types A and B (AR)	Sphingomyelinase	Sphingomyelin
• Gaucher disease (AR)	Glucocerebrosidase (acid β-glucosidase)	Glucocerebroside
Leukodystrophies (sulfatidoses)		
• Metachromatic leukodystrophy (MLD) (AR)	Arylsulfatase A	Cerebroside sulfate (sulfatide)
• Multiple sulfatase deficiency (AR)	Arylsulfatase A, B, C; steroid sulfatase; iduronate sulfatase; heparin N-sulfatase	Sulfatide, steroid sulfate, mucopolysaccharides (heparan sulfate, dermatan sulfate)
• Krabbe disease (AR)	Galactosylceramidase	Galactocerebroside
Mucopolysaccharidoses (MPSs)		
• MPS I-H (Hurler)(AR)	α-L-Iduronidase	Dermatan sulfate, heparan sulfate
• MPS II (Hunter) (X-linked)	Iduronate 2-sulfatase	–
Mucolipidoses (MLs)		
• I-cell disease (ML II) and pseudo-Hurler Polydystrophy (AR)	UDP-N-acetylglucosamine-1-phosphotransferase	Mucopolysaccharide, glycolipid
Glycoproteinoses (oligosaccharidoses)		
• Fucosidosis (AR)	α-fucosidase	Fucose-containing sphingolipids and glycoprotein fragments
• α-mannosidosis (AR)	α-mannosidase	Mannose-containing oligosaccharides
• Aspartylglycosaminuria (AR)	Aspartylglucosaminidase (aspartylglycosamine amide hydrolase)	Aspartyl-2-deoxy-2-acetamido-glycosylamine
• Sialidosis (AR)	Neuraminidase	Sialyloligosaccharides
Disorders of neutral lipids		
• Infantile-onset LALD (AR)	Acid lysosomal lipase	Cholesteryl esters; triglycerides
• Childhood/adult-onset LALD (AR)	Acid lysosomal lipase	Cholesteryl esters
• Farber disease (AR)	Acid ceramidase	Ceramide
Glycogenosis (disorders of glycogen)		
• Type 2—Pompe disease (AR)	α-1,4-glucosidase (lysosomal glucosidase)	Glycogen
Lysosomal membrane and transport defects		
• Cystinosis (AR)	Cystinosin (cysteine transporter)	Cystine
Other lysosomal storage diseases		
• Wolman disease	Acid lipase	Cholesterol esters, triglycerides

(AD: autosomal dominant; AR: autosomal recessive; LALD: lysosomal acid lipase deficiency)

In **neutral glycosphingolipidoses [e.g.,** Niemann–Pick disease (types A and B) Gaucher disease**], there is an accumulation of neutral glycosphingolipids in the cells.**

- **Acidic glycosphingolipids:** These are negatively charged at physiologic pH.
  - **Gangliosides:** These are the most complex glycosphingolipids and are found mainly in the ganglion cells of the CNS, particularly at the nerve endings. They are derivatives of ceramide oligosaccharides. The notation for these gangliosides is G (for ganglioside) plus a subscript M, D, T, or Q to indicate whether there is one (mono), two (di), three (tri), or four (quatro) molecules of NANA (N-acetylneuraminic acid) in the ganglioside, respectively. **Gangliosidoses (e.g., G_{M1} and G_{M2} gangliosidosis)** are lipid storage disorders with accumulation of glycosphingolipids in cells.
  - **Sulfatides:** These sulfoglycosphingolipids are sulfated galactocerebrosides that are negatively charged at physiologic pH. Sulfatides are found predominantly in the brain and kidneys. Sulfatidoses (leukodystrophies) are disorders characterized by the intralysosomal accumulation of sulfur-containing lipids (sulfatides). Examples include Krabbe disease, metachromatic leukodystrophy, and multiple sulfatase deficiency.

Degradation of sphingolipid with the various lysosomal enzymes involved is depicted in **Figure 22**. An overview of sphingolipid synthesis is presented in **Figure 23**.

Organ and tissue involvement in LSDs: Usually, the organs involved and the distribution of the stored substrate depend on tissues and location that are normally involved in degradation of most of the substrate. Examples are as follows:

- **Brain is rich in gangliosides**, and defective hydrolysis of gangliosides (e.g., in G_{M1} and G_{M2} gangliosidoses) causes accumulation of metabolites within neurons and produces neurologic symptoms.
- **Mucopolysaccharides are widely distributed** in the body. Hence, any defects in degradation of mucopolysaccharides involves almost every organ in the body.
- Cells of the **mononuclear phagocyte system** such as the spleen and liver are rich in lysosomes. Hence, liver and spleen are involved in the degradation of many substrates and are frequently enlarged in several forms of LSDs.

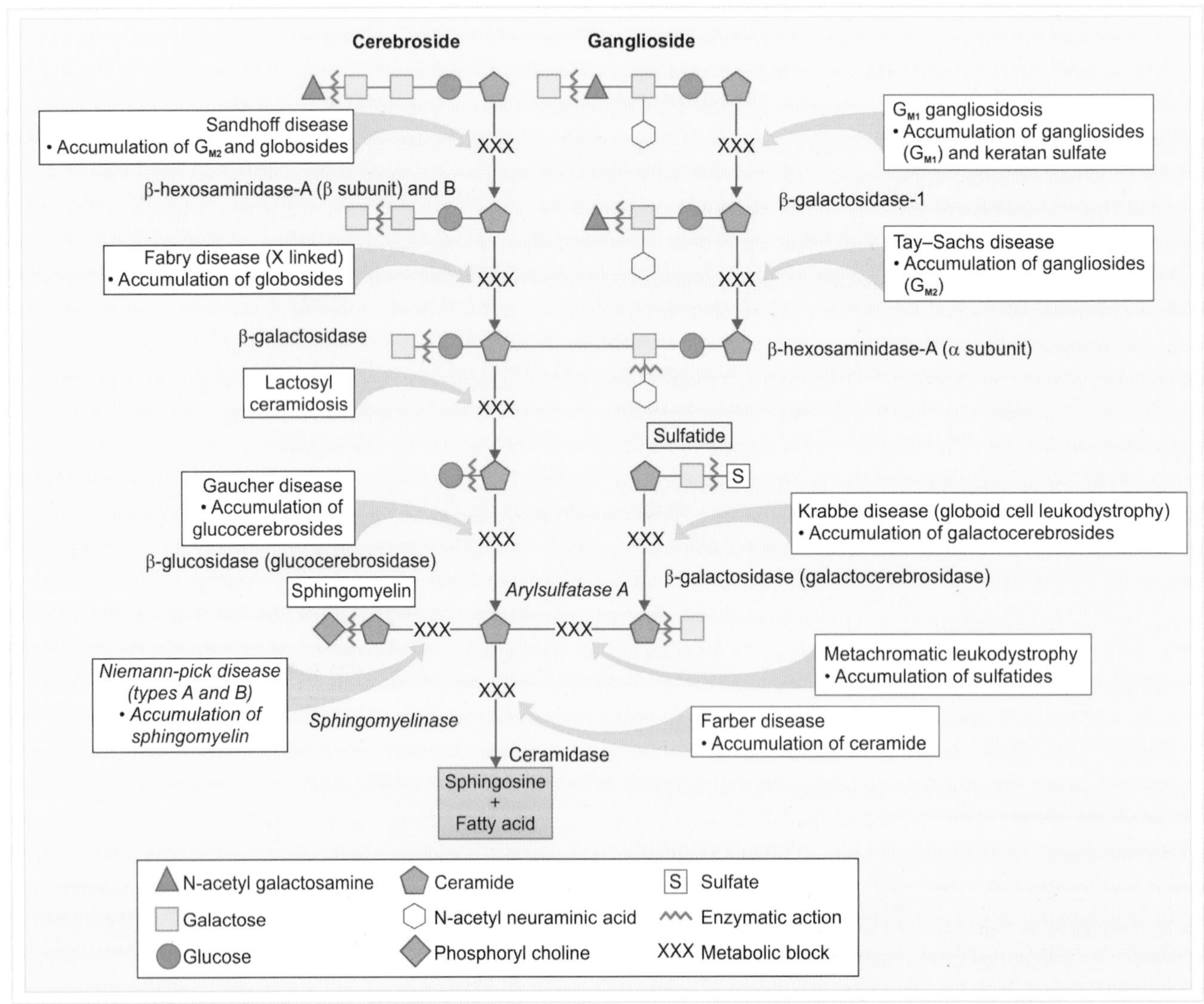

FIG. 22: Lysosomal degradation/catabolism of some sphingolipids with the various lysosomal enzymes involved. Disturbances of lipid metabolism in various sphingolipidoses, related genetic diseases, and lysosomal enzymes involved are also shown.

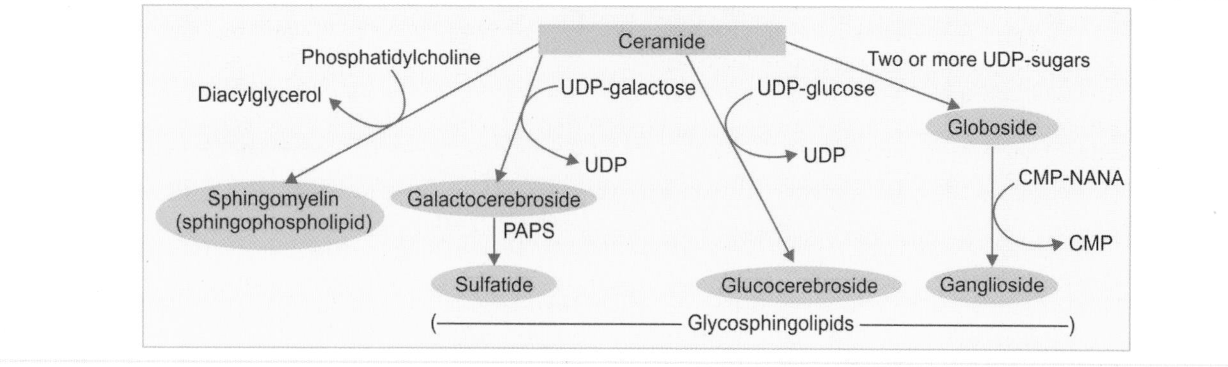

(CMP: cytidine monophosphate; NANA: N-acetylneuraminic acid; PAPS: 3′-phosphoadenosine-5′-phosphosulfate; UDP: uridine diphosphate)

FIG. 23: An overview of sphingolipid synthesis.

Tay–Sachs disease (G_{M2} gangliosidosis: Hexosaminidase α-subunit deficiency)

Q. Write short essay on Tay–Sachs disease.

The gangliosidoses are a clinically heterogeneous group of disorders that are due to hereditary defects of the metabolism of sialic acid-containing glycoconjugates caused by primary deficiencies of the lysosomal hydrolases, β-galactosidase or β-N-acetylgalactosaminidase (β-hexosaminidase). They are neurodegenerative disorders and non-neurological manifestations are usually clinically minimal.

Tay–Sachs disease is a catastrophic infantile form of lysosomal storage diseases also known as the G_{M2} gangliosidoses or hexosaminidase α-subunit deficiency. G_{M2} gangliosidoses consist of a group of three lysosomal storage diseases caused due to deficiency of the enzyme β-hexosaminidase. Tay–Sachs disease is inherited as an autosomal recessive trait.

β-hexosaminidase enzyme and its isoenzymes: It has two isoenzymes namely—(1) Hex A, consisting of two subunits, α and β, and (2) Hex B, a homodimer of β-subunits. These enzymes are involved in the catabolism of G_{M2} gangliosides. Degradation or catabolism of G_{M2} gangliosides needs three polypeptides. These polypeptides are encoded by three distinct genes namely—

1. *HEXA* (on chromosome 15): It encodes the α-subunit of Hex A.
2. *HEXB* (on chromosome 5): It encodes the β-subunit of Hex A and Hex B.
3. *GM2A* (on chromosome 5): It encodes the activator of hexosaminidase.

Genetics: The genetic basis of the different variants of G_{M2} gangliosidosis is depicted in **Figure 24**.

Deficiency of the enzyme β-hexosaminidase: It results in an inability to catabolize G_{M2} gangliosides. This ganglioside is deposited in CNS neurons due to a failure of lysosomal degradation. The phenotypic effects of mutations affecting all these genes mentioned above are similar. This is because all of them result in accumulation of G_{M2} gangliosides. However, the underlying enzyme defect is different for each of these mutations.

- **Mutations in the α-subunit locus on chromosome 15:** This is the most common form of G_{M2} gangliosidosis. It is associated with severe deficiency of hexosaminidase A and hexosaminidase A enzyme is absent in almost all the tissues. It is more prevalent among Jews, particularly among those of Eastern European (Ashkenazic) origin.

Molecular pathogenesis: Gangliosides are glycosphingolipids with a ceramide and an oligosaccharide chain that contains N-acetylneuraminic acid. They are present in the outer leaflet of the plasma membrane, particularly in brain neurons.

- **Misfolding of mutant protein:** More than 100 mutations have been identified in the HEXA α-subunit gene and most of them affect protein folding. Because the mutant protein is misfolded (refer pages 181 and 182), it induces the unfolded protein response.
- **Proteasomal degradation of misfolded proteins:** Usually misfolded proteins are stabilized by chaperones. If they are not stabilized by chaperones, they undergo proteasomal degradation. This leads to accumulation of toxic substrates and intermediates within neurons.
- **Molecular chaperone therapy:** The above findings indicate that molecular chaperone therapy for some variants of late-onset Tay–Sachs and other selected lysosomal storage diseases may be useful. In this therapy, synthetic chaperones that can cross the blood-brain barrier are used. They bind to the mutated protein and produce proper folding. Sufficient functional enzyme can then be rescued to relieve the effects of the inborn error.

MORPHOLOGY

Hexosaminidase A is absent in almost all the tissues. So G_{M2} ganglioside accumulates in many tissues such as CNS, retina, heart, liver, and spleen. But the involvement of neurons in the central and autonomic nervous systems and retina produces the characteristic clinical features. The size of the brain varies with the length of survival of affected infants. In early stages, there may be marked atrophy of brain.

Continued

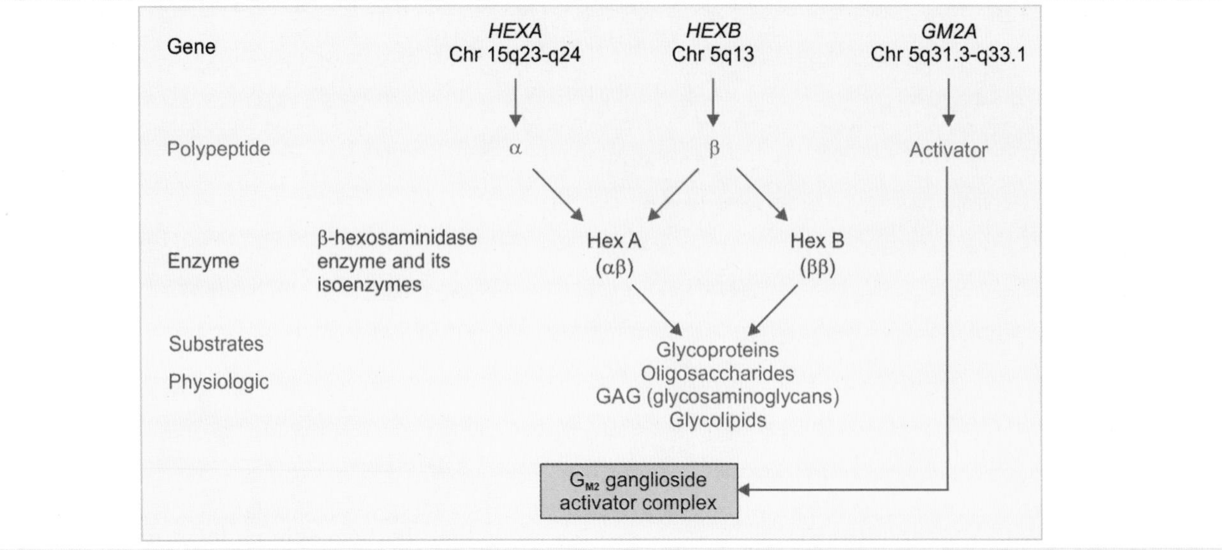

FIG. 24: Genetics of G_{M2} gangliosidosis.

Continued

Light microscopy

- **Neurons:** They are **ballooned and markedly distended due to many vacuoles in the cytoplasm.** Each **vacuole represents a markedly distended lysosome filled with gangliosides.** The progressive accumulation is followed by destruction of neurons, proliferation of microglia, and accumulation of lipids in phagocytes within the brain substance.
- **Retina: Ganglion cells in the retina are also distended with G_{M2} ganglioside.** They are more prominent at the margins of the macula. It gives rise to characteristic **cherry-red spot** in the macula. Cherry-red spot is due to accentuation of the normal color of the macular choroid contrasted with the pallor produced by the swollen ganglion cells in the remainder of the retina. Cherry-red spot is also seen in other storage disorders (**Box 5**) affecting the neurons.

Electron microscopy: Several types of cytoplasmic inclusions can be seen. Most prominent is **lysosomes with whorled configurations due to onion-skin layers of membranes.** This is characteristic of Tay-Sachs disease as well as other storage disorders affecting the neurons.

Special stains: Special stains for fat such as oil red O and Sudan black B stain positive with gangliosides.

Box 5: Storage disorders with cherry-red spot.

- G_{M1} gangliosidosis
- G_{M2} gangliosidosis
  - Tay–Sachs/B1 variant
  - Sandhoff
- Krabbe leukodystrophy
- Niemann–Pick A
- Sialidosis
- Galactosialidosis

Clinical features

Infantile form: It is a fatal neurodegenerative disease. Affected infants appear normal at birth, but begin to show signs and symptoms between 6 and 10 months of age. Clinical features are mainly due to neuronal involvement in the central and autonomic nervous systems and retina. Symptoms include progressive motor and mental deterioration, loss of motor skills, blindness, and increasing dementia. Sometime during the early course of the disease, ophthalmoscopy shows characteristic, but not pathognomonic, cherry-red spot in the macula of the eye in almost all patients. Over the span of 1 or 2 years, a complete vegetative state is reached. Most children die before 3 years of age.

Juvenile-onset form: It presents with ataxia and dementia. Death occurs by age of 10–15 years.

Adult-onset disorder: It is characterized by clumsiness in childhood; progressive motor weakness in adolescence. Additional spinocerebellar and lower motor neuron signs and dysarthria develop in adulthood. Antenatal diagnosis and carrier detection: It can be done by enzyme assays and DNA-based analysis.

Niemann–Pick disease types A and B

Q. Write short essay on Niemann–Pick's disease A, B, and C.

Niemann–Pick disease types A and B are two related **autosomal recessive** LSDs. It is characterized by accumulation of sphingomyelin in lysosomes due to an inherited deficiency of acid sphingomyelinase. Similar to Tay–Sachs disease, Niemann–Pick disease (both types A and B) is common in Ashkenazi Jews.

Type A disease: It is a severe infantile form. It shows severe neurologic involvement, marked accumulations of sphingomyelin in viscera, and progressive wasting. Usually, early death occurs within the first 3 years of life.

Type B disease: They have organomegaly and usually without involvement of CNS. These patients usually survive into adulthood.

Genetics: The gene for the lysosomal enzyme acid sphingomyelinase is located on chromosome 11p15.4. It is one of the imprinted genes that is preferentially expressed from the maternal chromosome as a result of epigenetic silencing of the paternal gene. About 180 mutations have been identified in the acid sphingomyelinase gene. In the classic infantile type, A variant, a missense mutation is associated with almost complete deficiency of sphingomyelinase. There is correlation between the type of mutation, the severity of enzyme deficiency, and the phenotype. Usually, it is inherited as an autosomal recessive. However, heterozygotes who inherit the mutant allele from the mother can develop Niemann–Pick disease.

MORPHOLOGY

Classic infantile type A variant is associated with almost complete deficiency of sphingomyelinase. Sphingomyelin is a ubiquitous component of cellular (including organellar) membranes. The deficiency of enzyme sphingomyelinase blocks degradation of the lipid and the lipid progressively accumulates within lysosomes. They are particularly observed within cells of the mononuclear phagocyte system. The involvement of the **spleen** usually causes **massive enlargement** and sometimes it may be 10 times of its normal weight. Hepatomegaly is usually not prominent. The lymph nodes usually show moderate to marked enlarged throughout the body. Brain shows shrunken gyri and widened sulci.

Microscopy: Affected cells become enlarged due to the distention of lysosomes with sphingomyelin and cholesterol. Sometimes these cells **may be 90 µm in diameter**. The cells contain **numerous small vacuoles (foam cells)** of relatively uniform size that gives a foamy appearance to the cytoplasm. The lipid-laden phagocytic foam cells are distributed in several organs such as the spleen, liver, lymph nodes, lymphatic vessels, bone marrow, tonsils, gastrointestinal (GI) tract, and in alveoli of lungs and pulmonary arteries. In frozen sections, vacuoles take up fat stains.

Electron microscopy: The vacuoles represent engorged secondary lysosomes. These lysosomes usually contain membranous cytoplasmic bodies resembling concentric lamellated myelin figures, sometimes called as **zebra bodies.**

Neuronal involvement: This disorder diffusely affects all parts of the nervous system. The dominant microscopic feature is **vacuolation and ballooning of neurons**. As the time progresses, it leads to cell death and loss of brain substance.

Retina: A **cherry-red spot,** similar to that of Tay-Sachs disease, is observed in about 30–50% of patients.

Clinical features: Type A disease may be present at birth or is evident by age of 6 months. Infants usually present with a protuberant abdomen due to hepatosplenomegaly. The clinical manifestations are followed by progressive failure to thrive, vomiting, fever, generalized lymphadenopathy, and progressive deterioration of psychomotor function. Death occurs generally within the first or second year of life.

Diagnosis: It is by biochemical assays for sphingomyelinase activity in nucleated cells such as leukocytes or bone marrow biopsy. They show markedly decreased (1–10% of normal) sphingomyelinase activity. Patients affected by both types A and B as well as carriers can be detected by DNA analysis.

Niemann–Pick disease type C

Previously Niemann–Pick disease type C was considered to be related to types A and B of Niemann–Pick disease, however, it is distinct from them both at the biochemical and genetic levels. It is also more common than types A and B combined.

Genetics: It is due to mutations in two related genes namely—*NPC1* (Niemann–Pick disease, type C1) and *NPC2* (Niemann–Pick disease, type C2). Mutation in *NPC1* is responsible for 95% of cases. Unlike most other storage diseases where the defect is an enzyme, primary defect in Niemann–Pick disease type C is nonenzymatic lipid transport. NPC1 is membrane bound, whereas NPC2 is soluble. Both NPC1 and NPC2 are lysosomal proteins involved in the transport of free cholesterol from the lysosomes to the cytoplasm.

Clinical features: Niemann–Pick disease type C is a progressive CNS disease and clinically heterogeneous. It can present as hydrops fetalis and stillbirth, or liver (neonatal hepatitis) or splenic disease. Most commonly and major manifestations as a chronic form characterized by progressive CNS disease with neurologic damage. The clinical course is marked by childhood with ataxia, vertical supranuclear gaze palsy, dystonia, dysarthria, and psychomotor regression.

Gaucher disease

Q. Write short essay on Gaucher disease and its molecular biology and a note on Gaucher cell.

Gaucher disease is the **most common LSD**. It constitutes a group of **autosomal recessive** disorders resulting from **mutations in the gene encoding glucocerebrosidase**. Normally, glucocerebrosidase cleaves the glucose residue from ceramide. The enzyme defect causes **accumulation of glucocerebrosides** (also called glucosylceramide) **mainly in lysosomes of phagocytes** (e.g., macrophage). But in some subtypes, it also accumulates in the CNS. Glucocerebrosides are basic glycolipid component of the cell membrane. It is continually formed from the catabolism of glycolipids derived mainly from the cell membranes of senescent leukocytes and red cells.

Genetics: Gaucher disease is due to mutations in the gene encoding glucocerebrosidase. The affected gene encodes an enzyme glucocerebrosidase (a lysosomal acid β-glucosidase). The enzyme deficiency occurs due to a variety of single base mutations in the β-glucosidase gene, on the long arm of chromosome 1 (1q21). Each of the clinical types shows heterogeneous mutations in this gene.

- **Risk factor for Parkinson disease:** Mutation of the glucocerebrosidase gene is the most common genetic risk factor for Parkinson disease. Patients with Gaucher disease have a 20 times higher risk of Parkinson disease than controls, and 5–10% of patients with Parkinson disease have mutations in the gene encoding glucocerebrosidase. α-synuclein is the protein involved in the pathogenesis of Parkinson disease. There is a reciprocal relation between the level of enzyme glucocerebrosidase and aggregation of α-synuclein. In patients with lysosomal diseases, there is impaired autophagy. This is responsible for aggregation and persistence of proteins such as α-synuclein.

Causes of pathologic changes in Gaucher disease: These are due to two factors namely—(1) accumulation of glucocerebrosides (storage material) and (2) activation of macrophages that secrete cytokines such as interleukin (IL)-1, IL-6, and tumor necrosis factor (TNF).

Clinical subtypes of Gaucher disease Disease variants are classified depending on the absence or presence and progression of neuronopathic involvement into **three subtypes:**

- **Type 1 (chronic non-neuronopathic):** It is the **most common type** and accounts for 99% of cases. In this type, **accumulation of glucocerebrosides is limited to the mononuclear phagocytes throughout the body**. Involvements of **spleen and skeleton** dominate this type of the disease. In this type, there is either no involvement of the brain or if involved it does not manifest early. It is found principally in Jews of European stock. These individuals have reduced but detectable levels of glucocerebrosidase activity. Longevity is shortened, but not markedly.
- **Type 2 (acute neuronopathic):** It is the infantile acute cerebral pattern. In these patients, there is almost no detectable glucocerebrosidase activity in the tissues. The clinical picture is dominated by **progressive involvement of CNS and leads to death at an early age**. Hepatosplenomegaly is also seen.
- **Type 3 (subacute neuronopathic):** It is intermediate between types I and II. These patients have the **systemic involvement similar to type I but have progressive disease of CNS**. It usually begins in adolescence or early adulthood.

MORPHOLOGY

In all types of Gaucher disease, **glucocerebrosides accumulate in massive** amounts within phagocytic cells throughout the body.

Gaucher cells: The **hallmark of Gaucher disease** is the presence of Gaucher cells. These are **lipid-laden distended, phagocytic cells** (i.e., macrophages). Gaucher cells are **found in the spleen** (seen in the red pulp), **liver** (Kupffer cells in sinusoids), **bone marrow, lymph nodes, tonsils, thymus, and Peyer patches.** Similar cells may also be seen in both the alveolar septa and the air spaces in the lung. **In other lipid storage disorders, cells appear vacuolated.** The Gaucher cells rarely appear vacuolated, but they have a **fibrillary type of cytoplasm likened to crumpled/wrinkled tissue paper** (**Figs. 25A** and **B**). Gaucher cells are usually enlarged and measure sometimes up to 100 µm in diameter. They have one or more dark, eccentrically placed nuclei.

- **Periodic acid–Schiff stain:** The cytoplasm of Gaucher cells stains **intensely positive** with Periodic acid–Schiff stain.
- **Electron microscope:** The fibrillary cytoplasm represents elongated, distended lysosomes, containing the stored lipid arranged in parallel layers of tubular structures (stacks of bilayers).

Continued

Continued

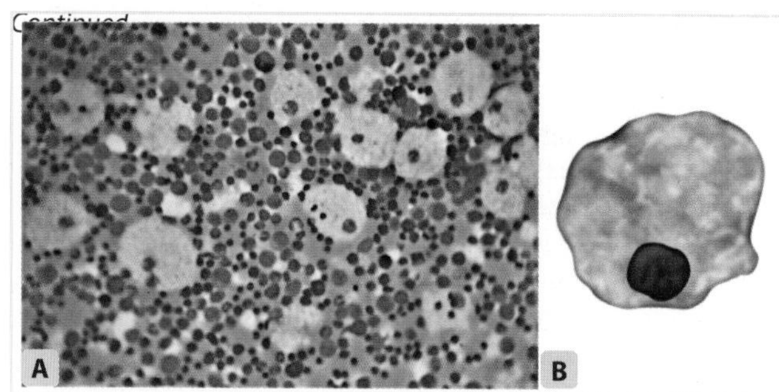

FIGS. 25A AND B: (A) Bone marrow aspiration showing Gaucher cells. The Gaucher cells have a fibrillary type of cytoplasm likened to crumpled/wrinkled tissue paper; (B) Appearance of Gaucher cells (diagrammatic).

Continued

Splenomegaly: It is **universal** in Gaucher disease. In type I disease, the spleen is enlarged, sometimes up to 10 kg. The cut surface of the enlarged spleen is firm and pale. It may show sharply demarcated infarcts. The **red pulp shows nodular and diffuse infiltrates of Gaucher cells** and moderate fibrosis.

Lymph node: Lymphadenopathy is mild to moderate and is generalized.

Liver: It is usually enlarged by Gaucher cells within sinusoids. There is no involvement of hepatocytes. In severe cases, hepatic fibrosis and even cirrhosis may develop.

Skeletal changes: It may involve bone marrow and bone.

- **Bone marrow:** Accumulation of **Gaucher cells in the bone marrow** (**Fig. 25**) is found in 70–100% of cases of type I Gaucher disease. Bone marrow involvement spreads from proximal to distal in the limbs.
- **Bone:** There is defective bone remodeling with loss of total bone calcium leading to osteopenia, osteonecrosis, avascular infarction. It produces areas of **bone erosion.** These erosions may be small or may be sufficiently large to produce **pathologic fractures.** The cytokines secreted by activated macrophages are responsible for destruction of bone.

CNS: In the patients in which there is cerebral involvement, **Gaucher cells** are seen **in the Virchow–Robin spaces, and arterioles are surrounded by swollen adventitial cells.**

Lipids are not stored in the neurons and **neurons appear shriveled** and undergo progressive destruction. Probably the damage to neurons is due to cytokine secreted by lipids that accumulate in the phagocytic cells around blood vessels.

Clinical features: The course of Gaucher disease depends on the clinical subtype.

- **Type 1:** Symptoms and signs first appear in adult life. They present as slowly to rapidly progressive visceral disease and symptoms related to splenomegaly or bone involvement. Most commonly pancytopenia (anemia, leukopenia, and thrombocytopenia) or thrombocytopenia develop secondary to hypersplenism. Splenic infarctions can resemble an acute abdomen. Bone pain and pathologic fractures may occur due to extensive expansion of the marrow space. Though it is a progressive disease in adults, the life expectancy of most patients is normal and is compatible with long life.

- **Type 2:** It is rare and usually presents by the age of 3 months with hepatosplenomegaly. Within a few months, infants show progressive CNS disease and present with neurologic signs. These include classic triad of trismus, strabismus, and backward flexion of the neck. Further neurologic deterioration rapidly develops and leads to death by the age of 3 years in most patients.
- **Type 3:** This type is also rare and shows combined features of types 1 and 2. In this type, neurologic deterioration starts later. They present with CNS dysfunction, convulsions, and progressive mental deterioration. The organs such as the liver, spleen, and lymph nodes are also affected. It progresses more slowly and most live until about age of 30 years.

Diagnosis: It can be made as described below:
- **In homozygotes:** Diagnosis can be made by measuring glucocerebrosidase activity in peripheral blood leukocytes or in extracts of cultured skin fibroblasts.
- **In heterozygotes:** The enzyme assay is not useful in heterozygotes because the levels of glucocerebrosidase are difficult to distinguish from those in normal cells. Though heterozygotes can be identified by detection of mutations, since there are more than 150 mutations in the glucocerebrosidase gene causing Gaucher disease, presently there is no single genetic test available. If the causative mutation in a patient is known, a heterozygote can be identified with molecular tests such as NGS.

Treatment: Replacement therapy with recombinant enzymes is effective, and patients with type I disease can expect normal life expectancy. However, it is extremely expensive. The fundamental defect is in mononuclear phagocytic cells arising from marrow stem cells. Hence, allogeneic hematopoietic stem cell transplantation can be curative. Other treatment modalities include correction of the enzyme defect by transfer of the normal glucocerebrosidase gene into the patient's hematopoietic stem cells.

Mucopolysaccharidoses (glycosaminoglycan storage disorders)

Mucopolysaccharidoses are lysosomal diseases in which there is accumulation of GAGs (glycosaminoglycan and formerly called as mucopolysaccharides) in many organs. They constitute a group of closely related syndromes that occur due to genetic deficiencies of enzymes involved in the degradation of mucopolysaccharides (GAGs). GAGs refer pages 88 and 89.

Mucopolysaccharides: Mucopolysaccharides are GAGs and chemically consist of long polymers (chain complex carbohydrates) of repeating disaccharide units containing N-acetylhexosamine and a hexose or hexuronic acid. Either disaccharide may be sulfated. GAGs may be attached to a protein molecule to form proteoglycans. Proteoglycans are abundant in extracellular matrix, joint fluid, and connective tissue. The proteoglycans provide the ground or packing substance of connective tissue. In MPSs, GAGs that accumulate in lysosomes are dermatan sulfate, heparan sulfate, keratan sulfate, and chondroitin sulfate.

Enzyme deficiency: There are 11 enzymes involved in the degradation of long-chain complex carbohydrates of mucopolysaccharides (GAGs) molecules. They cleave terminal sugars from the polysaccharide chains disposed along a polypeptide or core protein. In the absence of enzymes, these chains accumulate within lysosomes in various tissues and organs of the body. All the GAGs accumulated (i.e., dermatan sulfate, heparan sulfate, keratan sulfate, and chondroitin sulfate) in MPSs are derived from cleavage of proteoglycans (important extracellular matrix constituents). GAGs are degraded in a stepwise manner by removing sulfates (by sulfatases) or sugar (by glycosidases) residues (**Fig. 26**). MPSs are rare diseases caused by deficiencies in any of the lysosomal enzymes that catabolize GAGs. Thus, a deficiency in any one of the glycosidases or sulfatases causes undegraded GAGs to accumulate. Deficiency of an N-acetyltransferase leads to deposition of heparan sulfate in Sanfilippo C disease.

Clinical variants of MPSs: These are rare diseases and there are 11 clinical variants of MPS, and each is due to the deficiency of one specific enzyme. Some variants have subvariants. All the MPSs are inherited as autosomal recessive traits, except for Hunter syndrome, which is inherited as an X-linked recessive trait. Within a given group (e.g., MPS I, characterized by a deficiency of α-L-iduronidase), there are subgroups. These subgroups result from different mutant alleles at the same genetic locus. Thus, the severity of enzyme deficiency and the clinical features even within subgroups are generally different.

MORPHOLOGY

Sites of accumulation: The mucopolysaccharides are accumulated usually in **mononuclear phagocytic cells, endothelial cells, intimal smooth muscle cells, and fibroblasts throughout the body**. Common sites involved are spleen, liver, bone marrow, lymph nodes, blood vessels, and heart.

Microscopy: The affected cells are distended with mucopolysaccharides and show apparent **clearing of the cytoplasm. This creates so-called balloon cells.** Metachromasia confirms the presence of GAGs.

Periodic acid–Schiff: The vacuoles give **positive** reaction with periodic acid–Schiff stain.

Electron microscope: The clear cytoplasm consists of numerous minute vacuoles. These vacuoles represent swollen lysosomes containing a finely granular periodic acid–Schiff-positive material.

Biochemical evaluation: The vacuoles contain mucopolysaccharide.

Central nervous system: Lysosomal changes described above can also be found in the neurons of those MPSs with CNS involvement. Some of the lysosomes in neurons may be replaced by lamellated zebra bodies similar to those seen in Niemann–Pick disease.

Other organs: These include **hepatosplenomegaly, skeletal deformities, valvular lesions, and subendothelial arterial deposits**, particularly in the coronary arteries, and lesions in the brain are common in all the MPSs. In severe cases, coronary subendothelial lesions can produce myocardial ischemia. Thus, myocardial infarction and cardiac decompensation are important causes of death in MPSs.

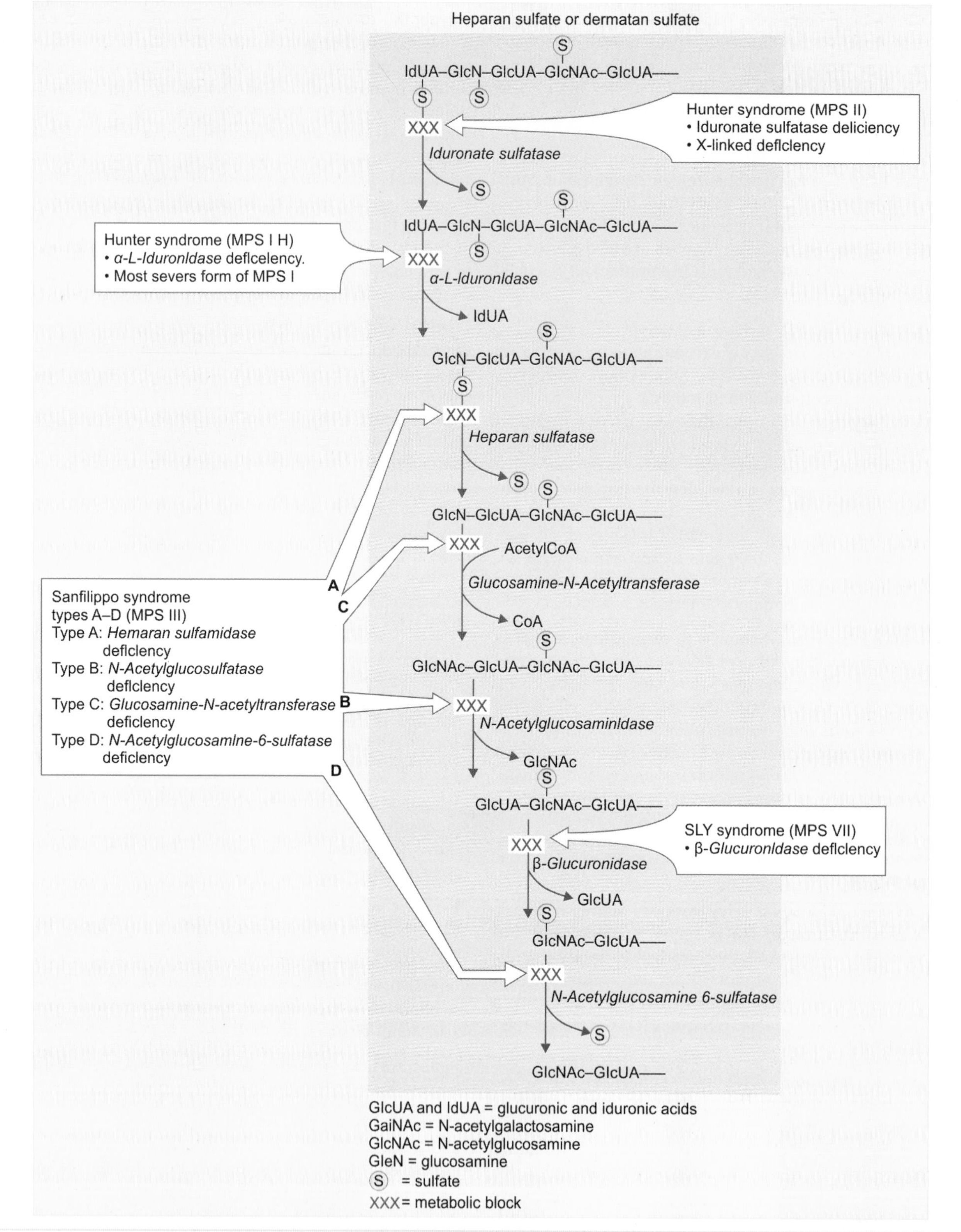

FIG. 26: Degradation of the glycosaminoglycan (mucopolysaccharides namely, heparan sulfate and dermatan sulfate) by lysosomal enzymes. Shows metabolic blocks indicating various sites of enzyme deficiencies that affect the degradation of heparan sulfate and some representative resulting in mucopolysaccharidoses (MPS).

Clinical features: There are 11 recognized variants of MPSs and only two well-characterized syndromes.

- **General features of MPSs:** Generally, MPSs are progressive disorders. They are characterized by coarse facial features, clouding of the cornea, joint stiffness, and intellectual disability. The accumulated mucopolysaccharides are usually excreted in increased quantity in urine and are used as a diagnostic tool.
- **Hurler syndrome:** It is also called as MPS I-H and is one of the most severe forms of MPS. It is due to deficiency of α-L-iduronidase and there is accumulation of heparan sulfate and dermatan sulfate in various tissues (**Fig. 25**). It is the prototype for MPSs. Affected children appear normal at birth but symptoms appear at 6 months to 2 years of age. They develop hepatosplenomegaly, retardation of growth, and, as in other forms of MPS, they develop characteristic coarse facial features and skeletal deformities (e.g., joint stiffness). The combination of coarse facial features and dwarfism is reminiscent of gargoyles on Gothic cathedrals and the old term used for this syndrome was gargoylism. Death occurs usually by age of 6–10 years and is usually due to cardiovascular complications.
- **Hunter syndrome:** It is also called as MPS II and is due to deficiency in iduronate sulfate sulfatase. It is similar to but differs from Hurler syndrome in mode of inheritance (X-linked), absence of corneal clouding (or other eye disease), and milder clinical course.

Glycoproteinoses

The glycoproteinoses **(see Table 7)** constitute a group of lysosomal disorders that result from deficiency of glycoprotein catabolism. It includes α-mannosidosis, β-mannosidosis, aspartylglucosaminuria (AGU), sialidosis, α-N-acetylgalactosaminidase deficiency (Schindler disease, Kanzaki disease), and fucosidosis.

Glycogen Storage Diseases (Glycogenoses)

Q. Write short essay on glycogen storage disorders.

Introduction

Carbohydrate metabolism plays an important role in cellular function by providing the energy needed for most of the metabolic processes. Glucose is the main substrate of energy metabolism. Metabolism of glucose generates adenosine triphosphate (ATP) through glycolysis and mitochondrial oxidative phosphorylation (OXPHOS). Glycogen is the storage form of glucose.

Glycogenoses [glycogen storage diseases (GSDs)] are a group of inherited disorders characterized by glycogen accumulation. The GSDs develop due to hereditary deficiency of one of the enzymes involved in the synthesis or sequential degradation of glycogen **(Fig. 27)**. With the exception of type 0 disease, defects in glycogen metabolism usually produce accumulation of glycogen in the tissues—hence the designation GSDs. Depending on the normal tissue or organ distribution of the specific enzyme, glycogen storage disorders may be restricted to a few tissues, may be more widespread (not involving all tissues), or may be systemic. Glycogen is mainly accumulated in the liver, skeletal muscle, and heart. The structure of stored glycogen can be normal or abnormal in the various disorders.

Normal metabolism of glycogen

To understand the significance of a specific enzyme deficiency in glycogen storage disorders, it is essential to know the normal metabolism of glycogen (**Fig. 27**). Glycogen is a storage form of glucose and is a complex carbohydrate/large glucose polymer (20,000–30,000 glucose units per molecule). Glycogen is composed of glucose residues joined in straight chains by α1–4 linkages and branched at intervals of 4–10 residues by α1–6 linkages. Glycogen is stored in most cells as a ready source of energy during fasting. However, its function is different in each organ. Liver and muscle are rich in glycogen. The liver stores glycogen not for its own use but to supply glucose to the blood quickly, particularly to supply glucose to the brain. By contrast, glycogen in skeletal muscle is used as a local fuel when there is fall in the supply of oxygen or glucose.

Glycogen synthesis Glycogen is synthesized and degraded by several enzymes.

Various steps involved in synthesis of glycogen from glucose are as follows:

- First glucose is converted to glucose-6-phosphate by the action of an enzyme hexokinase (glucokinase).
- Glucose-6-phosphate is converted to glucose-1-phosphate by the action of an enzyme phosphoglucomutase.
- Glucose-1-phosphate is then converted to uridine diphosphoglucose.
- It is followed by building of a highly branched, large polymer (molecular weight as high as 100 million), containing many (as many as 10,000) glucose molecules. These glucose molecules are linked together by α-1,4-glucoside bonds.
- The elongation of glycogen chain and branches continues by the addition of glucose molecules by the action of enzyme glycogen synthetases.

Degradation of glycogen

Major pathway of degradation: During degradation, distinct phosphorylases present in the cytoplasm of liver and muscle split glucose-1-phosphate from the glycogen until about four glucose residues remain on each branch. This leaves a branched oligosaccharide containing four glucose residues, called limit dextrin. This dextrin can be further degraded only by the debranching enzyme.

Minor pathway of degradation: Apart from the major pathways, glycogen can also be degraded in the lysosomes by the enzyme acid alpha-glucosidase. If these enzymes are deficient in lysosomes, the glycogen present in lysosomes is not accessible to degradation by cytoplasmic enzymes such as phosphorylases.

Subgroups of glycogen storage diseases

Glycogen is synthesized (formed) and degraded (broken down) by many/several enzymes, and deficiency of any of these enzymes leads to accumulation of glycogen. Significant organ involvement depends on the specific enzyme defect. Some enzyme defect mainly affects the liver, whereas others mainly cause dysfunction of cardiac or skeletal muscle. Symptoms of glycogenosis may be due to accumulation of glycogen itself (Pompe disease, Andersen disease) or due to absence of the glucose normally derived from degradation of glycogen (von Gierke disease, McArdle disease). Clinical manifestations differ markedly and the symptoms range from

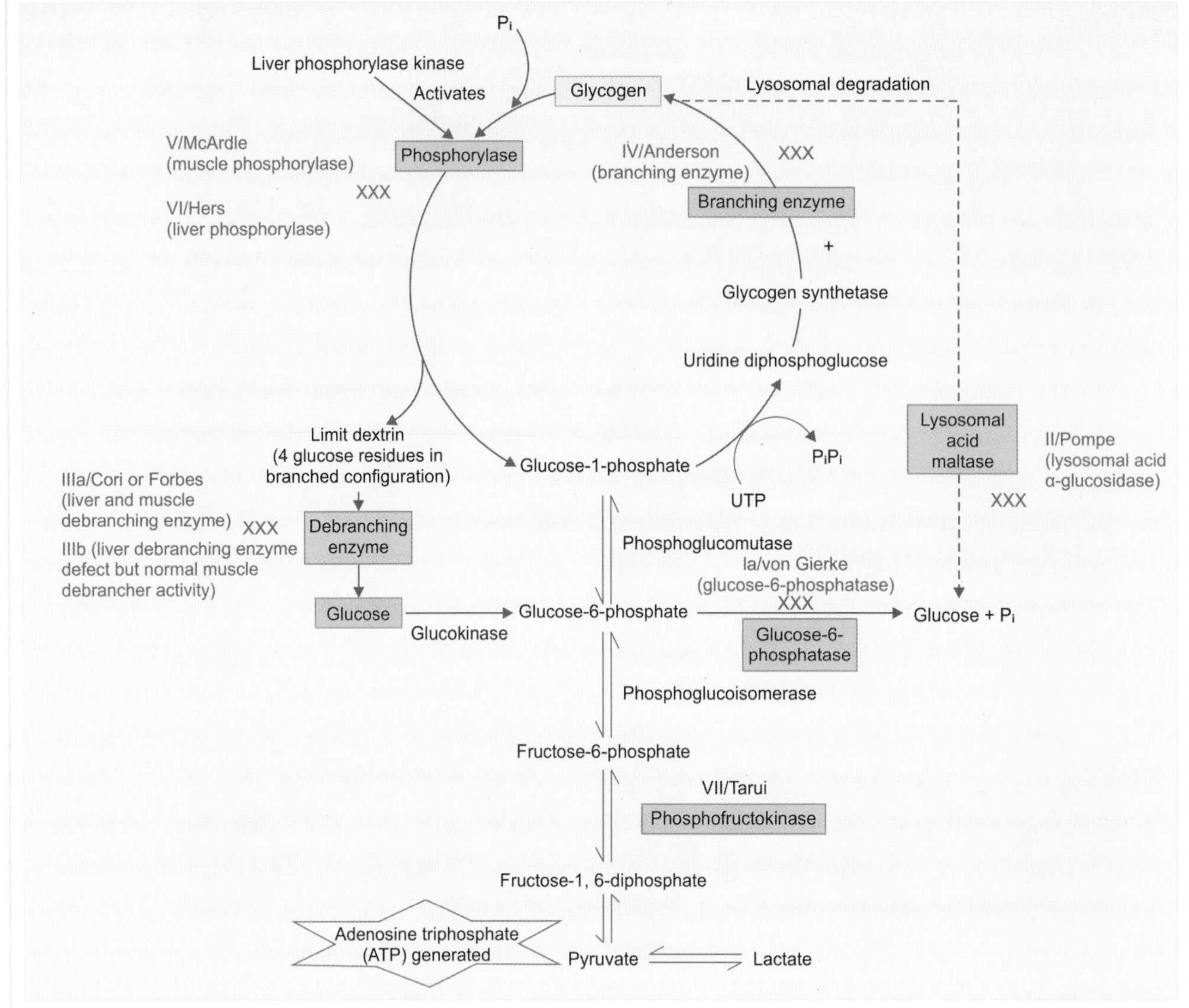

FIG. 27: Steps involved in glycogen metabolism. Enzyme deficiencies associated with glycogen storage diseases (in Roman numerals) are mentioned in red colored font.

minimally harmful to lethal. There are several major types of GSDs. Depending on the specific enzyme deficiencies and the clinical pictures, glycogenoses are traditionally divided into at least 14 syndromes designated by Roman numerals, by the name of the defective enzyme or eponymously after the physician who first described the condition. Diagnosis of GSD is usually made on the basis of the symptoms, physical examination, and results of biochemical tests. Occasionally, a muscle or liver biopsy is needed to confirm the enzyme defect.

Depending on the pathophysiology of glycogenosis, they are divided into three major subgroups (**Table 8**).

Liver glycogenoses (disorders with hepatomegaly and hypoglycemia) The liver is a main organ involved in the metabolism of glycogen. Liver contains enzymes that are involved in the synthesis of glycogen for storage and also degradation or breakdown of glycogen into free glucose. The glucose is then released from liver into the blood. An inherited deficiency of hepatic enzymes that are involved in degradation of glycogen causes not only accumulation of glycogen in the liver but also reduces the glucose levels in the blood (hypoglycemia) (**Fig. 28**). In these disorders, glycogen is stored in many organs, but hepatic enlargement and hypoglycemia are the dominant features.

Q. Write short essay on Von Gierke disease.

Type I GSD (glucose-6-phosphatase or translocase deficiency, Von Gierke disease): Type I GSD is an **autosomal recessive** disorder due to the **deficiency of the enzyme glucose-6-phosphatase in liver, kidney, and intestinal mucosa.** There are two subtypes of GSD I:

1. **Von Gierke disease (type Ia glycogenosis):** It is a classical main example for the hepatic hypoglycemic form of GSD. There is a deficiency of glucose-6-phosphatase enzyme.
2. **Type Ib glycogenosis:** There is a deficiency of the translocase that transports glucose-6-phosphate across the microsomal membrane.

In both subtypes, there is **inadequate conversion of glucose-6-phosphate to glucose in the liver and glycogen**

Table 8: Main subgroups and examples of glycogenoses (glycogen storage disorders).

Clinicopathologic category	*Specific type/common name*	*Basic enzyme deficiency*
Liver glycogenoses (disorders with hepatomegaly and hypoglycemia)	Hepatorenal—von Gierke disease (type Ia)	Glucose-6-phosphatase
	Type Ib	Glucose-6-phosphate translocase
	IIIa/Cori or Forbes	Liver and muscle debranching enzyme
	IV/Andersen	Branching enzyme
	0/liver glycogen synthase deficiency	Glycogen synthase
Muscle glycogenosis (disorders with muscle energy impairment)	V/McArdle	Muscle phosphorylase
	VII/Tarui	Phosphofructokinase M subunit
	Phosphoglycerate kinase deficiency	Phosphoglycerate kinase
Disorders with progressive skeletal muscle myopathy and/or cardiomyopathy	Generalized glycogenosis—Pompe disease (type II)	Lysosomal acid alpha-glucosidase

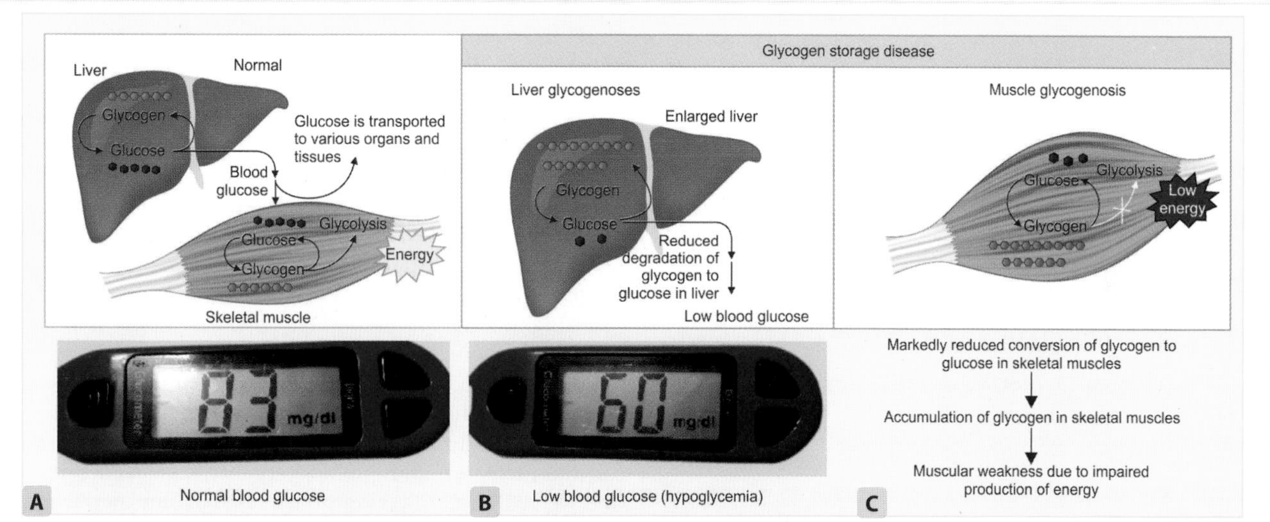

FIG. 28: Glycogen storage disorder. (A) Normal metabolism of glycogen in the liver and skeletal muscles; (B) Effects of a genetic deficiency of hepatic enzymes involved in glycogen metabolism; (C) Effects of a genetic deficiency of the enzymes involved in glycogen metabolism in skeletal muscles.

accumulates in the liver. The symptoms are due to the inability of the liver to convert glycogen to glucose. This leads to hepatomegaly and reduced glucose level in the blood (hypoglycemia). It usually presents in infancy or early childhood. These individuals are susceptible to fasting hypoglycemia and lactic acidosis during the neonatal period. Generally, these **children have doll-like facies with fat cheeks, relatively thin extremities, retarded growth** (short stature), and a **protuberant abdomen that is due to massive hepatomegaly**. The kidneys are enlarged. Spleen and heart are normal in size. The cytoplasm of hepatocytes is distended due to accumulated glycogen and fat (large and prominent lipid vacuoles). The liver enzyme levels are usually normal or near normal. Type Ib patients also develop neutropenia and impaired neutrophil function. This results in recurrent bacterial infections and ulceration of oral and intestinal mucosa. With treatment, the prognosis for normal mental development and longevity is usually good.

Type III GSD (debrancher deficiency, limit dextrinosis): Type III GSD is an autosomal recessive disorder caused by a deficiency of glycogen debranching enzymes. Debranching and phosphorylase enzymes are required for the complete degradation of glycogen into glucose. Deficiency of glycogen debranching enzymes leads to incomplete breakdown of glycogen, resulting in abnormal glycogen accumulation with short outer chains, resembling limit dextrin (**Fig. 27**).

Andersen disease (type IV glycogenosis): It is a very rare condition characterized by deficiency of the branching enzyme (amyloglucantransferase; at 3p12). Normally this enzyme creates the branch points in normal glycogen molecules. Due to the absence of the branching enzyme, there is formation and accumulation of an abnormal, toxic form of glycogen called amylopectin. This is a starch-like material that is deposited mostly in the liver, but also in the heart, skeletal muscles, and nervous system. Typically, children with this disease die between 2 and 4 years of age from cirrhosis of the liver. Liver transplantation is curative for this disorder. It is observed that after a liver transplant, cardiac and other extrahepatic deposits of amylopectin are markedly reduced by an unknown mechanism.

Muscle glycogenosis (disorders with muscle-energy impairment) In this type of glycogenosis, glycogen in skeletal muscles is predominantly used as a source of energy during physical activity and not the glycogen in liver. ATP is the source of energy. It is produced by glycolysis, which leads to the formation of lactate **(Fig. 27)**. If there is deficiency of enzyme involved in glycolytic pathway, glycogen accumulates in the muscles **(Fig. 28B)**. This is associated with muscular weakness due to impaired production of energy. Generally, patients present with muscle cramps after exercise. The lactate levels in the blood fail to rise after exercise due to a block in glycolysis. Examples include deficiencies of muscle phosphorylase (McArdle disease or type V glycogenosis), muscle phosphofructokinase (type VII GSD), etc.

Q. Write short essay on McArdle's disease.

McArdle disease (type V glycogenosis, muscle phosphorylase deficiency): McArdle disease is an autosomal recessive disorder caused by deficiency of muscle phosphorylase. This enzyme releases glucose-1-phosphate from glycogen. McArdle disease is a typical muscle energy disorder as the enzyme deficiency limits generation of ATP by glycogenolysis (breakdown of the molecule glycogen into glucose). This results in glycogen accumulation in skeletal muscles. There are two forms namely, childhood onset and adult onset. The gene for myophosphorylase, *PYGM* (the muscle type of the glycogen phosphorylase gene), is situated on chromosome 11q13. About 100 different mutations have been associated with this disorder. Symptoms generally manifest in adolescence or early adulthood. They complain of myalgia, muscle cramps, and spasms during exercise, which may lead to myocytolysis and myoglobinuria (dark-colored urine). Lack of an increase in blood lactate and exaggerated elevations of blood ammonia after an ischemic exercise test indicates muscle glycogenosis. It indicates a defect in the conversion of glycogen or glucose to lactate. Aerobic exercise and high-protein diets may be effective in some patients.

Disorders with progressive skeletal muscle myopathy and/or cardiomyopathy GSDs associated with—(1) deficiency of acid alpha-glucosidase (acid maltase) and (2) lack of branching enzyme, do not fit into the above two categories (i.e., liver or muscle glycogenosis). These are associated with accumulation or storage of glycogen in many organs and death occurs early in life.

Pompe disease, type II glycogenosis (acid α-1,4 glucosidase deficiency): Pompe disease is a **lysosomal storage disease** transmitted as an autosomal recessive disorder. It is caused due to a deficiency of lysosomal acid α-1,4 glucosidase (acid alpha-glucosidase), a lysosomal enzyme necessary for the degradation of glycogen in the lysosomes. The mutation occurs in the gene for the lysosomal enzyme acid maltase/acid α-glucosidase (GAA) located on the long arm of chromosome 17 at 17q25.2-q25.3. It leads to excessive accumulation of undegraded glycogen in lysosomes of many different cells. Since this disease is due the lysosomal enzyme deficiency, accumulation of glycogen is in the lysosomes. This is in contrast to accumulation in cytoplasm in the other glycogenoses. Glycogen accumulates in almost all organs, but cardiomegaly is the most prominent feature. Patients do not develop hypoglycemia, because there is no involvement of cytoplasmic metabolic pathways of glycogen synthesis and degradation. Normally, a small proportion of cytoplasmic glycogen is degraded within lysosomes after an autophagic sequence. This disorder has a range of phenotypes. Each phenotype has myopathy but differs in the age of onset, extent of organ involvement, and clinical severity. The most severe is the infantile form, with cardiomegaly and hypotonia. Without enzyme replacement therapy, the hearts of babies with infantile form of Pompe disease progressively thicken and enlarge. These babies die before 2 years of age due to heart failure, cardiorespiratory failure or respiratory infection. Juvenile and adult form of this disorder are less common and have a better prognosis. For patients with late-onset Pompe disease, prognosis depends on the age of onset. Usually, the later the age of onset, the slower is the disease progression. Prognosis depends on the extent of involvement of respiratory muscle.

Lysosomal Membrane and Transport Defects

Cystinosis

Cystinosis is a lysosomal storage disease transmitted as an autosomal recessive disorder. It is caused by mutations in the *CTNS* gene at chromosome 17p13. This gene encodes the lysosomal cystine/proton transmembrane transporter (cystinosin). Deficiency of cystinosin leads to accumulation of crystalline cystine inside lysosomes due to its poor solubility. The cysteine is derived from protein degradation. Three clinical forms are recognized that depend on the degree of impairment of transporter function. The most severe form is classic nephropathic cystinosis and it causes renal Fanconi syndrome starting at 6–12 months of age (i.e., during the first year of life). It presents with polydipsia, excretion of large amounts of dilute urine, dehydration, electrolyte imbalances, growth retardation, and rickets. Without treatment, it progresses to renal failure during childhood usually by the age of 10 years. In intermediate nephropathic cystinosis, renal failure develops between 15 and 25 years of age. Ocular non-nephropathic cystinosis is caused by deposition of cystine crystals in the cornea producing photophobia. Impaired lung and brain functions are usually observed in older patients. Almost all cells and organs show cystine crystals. Renal transplantation may be useful in patients with renal involvement. Administration of cysteamine decreases lysosomal cysteine. The cysteamine enters lysosomes and forms a mixed disulfide with cysteine. This is exported from the lysosome using a cationic amino acid transporter. This therapy greatly slows disease progression and improves survival.

Disorders Associated with Defects in Proteins that Regulate Cell Growth

Two main classes of genes regulate normal growth and differentiation of cells. These are proto-oncogenes and tumor suppressor genes. The products of these genes either promote or restrain growth of cells. It is discussed in detail on pages 441–453. Mutations in these two classes of genes are important in the pathogenesis of neoplasms. Majority of the cancer-causing mutations involve somatic cells and not the germ cells. Hence, these are not inherited in 95% of malignant tumors. In about remaining 5% cancers, these genetic mutations are transmitted through the germline as familial cancers. Most familial cancers are inherited in an autosomal dominant fashion and only few are transmitted as autosomal recessive disorders.

COMPLEX MULTIGENIC DISORDERS

Q. Write short essay on polygenic inheritance.

Multifactorial inheritance: Most human disorders are not inherited as simple dominant or recessive Mendelian disorders. Many disorders caused due to **interactions between multiple genes and environment, epigenetic, and other factors**. These reflect multifactorial inheritance and constitute complex multigenic disorders. Such inheritance leads to familial aggregation and they do not obey simple Mendelian rules. In monogenic inheritance, there is a specific risk of disease (e.g., 25%, 50%), whereas in polygenic disease, it is usually only about 5–10%. Several normal phenotypic characteristics are determined by multifactorial inheritance. Examples for such phenotypes include height, hair color, eye color, skin color, height, body habitus, and intelligence. Similarly, many chronic disorders of adults such as diabetes, atherosclerosis, many types of cancer, arthritis, and hypertension "run in families" but they do not follow simple patterns of inheritance. Examples of complex multigenic disorders are listed in **Table 9**.

Common disease/common variant hypothesis: A gene has at least two alleles. Each allele occurs at a frequency of at least 1% in the population and is called polymorphic. In polymorphic, each variant allele is termed as polymorphism. According to the common disease/common variant hypothesis, complex genetic disorders develop when many polymorphisms, each with a modest effect and low penetrance, are coinherited. Two additional features of common complex disorders, such as type 1 diabetes mellitus (T1DM) are:

1. **Variable significance of different polymorphisms:** When complex disorders occur from the collective inheritance of many polymorphisms, different polymorphisms have variable significance. For example, there are about 20–30 genes involved in T1DM. Out of these, only 6 or 7 are most important, and a few HLA alleles form >50% of the risk for T1DM.
2. **Polymorphisms and disease:** Some polymorphisms are common to many diseases of the same type, while other polymorphisms are disease specific. This is true with regards to autoimmune diseases.

Environmental influences: These also significantly modify the phenotypic expression of complex multigenic disorders. For example, type 2 diabetes mellitus (T2DM) has many features of a multifactorial disorder. It usually first manifests after gain of weight. Thus, obesity and other environmental factors unmask the diabetic genetic trait. More than one-fourth of all genes in normal humans have polymorphic alleles. Such heterogeneity is responsible for wide variability in susceptibility to many diseases. It is made more complex by interactions with the environment.

Table 9: Examples of complex multigenic disorders.

Adults	*Children*
Hypertension	Pyloric stenosis
Atherosclerosis	Cleft lip and palate
Type 2 diabetes mellitus	Congenital heart disease
Ankylosing spondylitis	Meningomyelocele and anencephaly
Schizophrenia	Hypospadias
Psoriasis	Hirschsprung disease
Gout	Congenital hip dislocation

General features: Complex multigenic disorders have following common features—

- Expression of symptoms of diseases due to multifactorial inheritance is proportional to the number of mutant genes. Close relatives of an affected individual have more mutant genes than the general population and are also more likely to express the disease. The probability is highest in identical twins.
- Environmental factors influence expression of the diseases due to multifactorial inheritance. Thus, concordance for the disease may be observed in only one-third of monozygotic twins.
- Risk of developing disease in first-degree relatives (parents, siblings, children) is the same (5–10%). The probability is much lower in second-degree relatives.
- The more severe the disorder, the greater the risk of transmitting it to the offspring. Probably, patients with more severe polygenic defects have more mutant genes. Hence, their children will more likely inherit more abnormal genes than children of less severely affected parents.
- Some diseases with multifactorial inheritance also have gender predilection. For example, pyloric stenosis is more common in males, whereas congenital hip dislocation is more common in females.

CHROMOSOMAL DISORDERS

Q. Discuss about cytogenetics and its applications.

Q. Write short essay on techniques employed for diagnosis of chromosomal disorders.

Normal Karyotype

Cytogenetics is defined as the science that combines the methods and findings of cytology and genetics. This allows the investigation of heredity at the cellular level. Cytogenetics is a branch of genetics that deals with the study of the chromosomes. Karyotype (study of chromosomes) is one of the basic tools of cytogenetics. The **chromosomal constitution of a cell or individual is known as the karyotype.** The normal somatic cells in humans contain 46 chromosomes. These include 22 homologous pairs of autosomal chromosomes and one pair of sex chromosomes (i.e., XX in the female and XY in the male). Normal karyotype for females is denoted as 46, XX and for males as 46, XY.

Techniques of cytogenetics: These can be broadly divided into—

- **Conventional (traditional) cytogenetics:** It is the routine chromosome analysis.
- **Molecular cytogenetics:** Molecular genetics (often called as "DNA technology") is the study of the genetic material at the level of the individual nucleotide bases of DNA.

Box 6: Common uses of conventional cytogenetic analysis.

Evaluation of congenital disorders
- To diagnose syndromes associated with abnormalities of chromosomal number or structure
- To establish the chromosomal sex in cases of sexual ambiguity
- To screen for karyotypic abnormalities in patients with multiple birth defects

Prenatal diagnosis

Surgical pathology
- Evaluation of neoplastic disorders (e.g., lymphoma and leukemia, soft tissue neoplasms)
- Aids targeted therapy and prognosis

Conventional (Traditional) Cytogenetics

Common uses of conventional cytogenetic analysis are presented in **Box 6**.

Limitations of conventional cytogenetic analysis: It can be performed only on viable tissue specimens that contain proliferating cells and only suitable for detecting numerical abnormalities and gross structural rearrangements. Hence, it is not sensitive to detect mutations such as small deletions, duplications, and amplifications, or single base pair substitutions.

Karyotyping

Study of structural patterns of the chromosomes in a sample of cells is known as karyotyping. This includes both the number and appearance (photomicrograph) of complete set of chromosomes.

Source of chromosome: To produce karyotype, it is necessary to obtain cells capable of growth and division. Cells for chromosomal study may be obtained from either by culture or directly.

- **Culture:** The source may be fibroblast or cells obtained by amniocentesis (amniotic fluid) or peripheral blood. The more commonly used cell for chromosomal study is circulating lymphocyte obtained from the blood sample cultured in a media.
- **Direct:** Lymphocytes are generally used as they are easily stimulated to divide. Cells obtained from bone marrow and chorion villous biopsy samples may be used without culture.

Arrest of cells in metaphase: Karyotyping requires cells to be in a state of division and arresting this cell division at the metaphase of cell cycle. The arrest of dividing cells in metaphase is by using mitotic spindle inhibitors [e.g., N-diacetyl-N-methylcolchicine (colcemid)] and then to stain the chromosomes. In a metaphase spread, the individual chromosomes appear as two chromatids connected at the centromere. A karyotype is obtained by arranging each pair of autosomes according to length, followed by sex chromosomes.

The different techniques used for staining metaphase chromosomes can be divided into two major categories (**Table 10**)—(1) methods that produce specific alternating light and dark regions (bands) along the length of each chromosome and (2) methods that stain only a defined region of specific chromosomes.

Table 10: Major chromosome staining and banding techniques.

Method	*Staining pattern*
Methods that produce alternating light and dark bands	
Giemsa banding (G banding)	Dark bands (AT rich) and light bands (CG rich)
Quinacrine banding (Q-banding)	Bright regions (AT rich)
Reverse banding (R-banding)	AT rich regions stain lightly (dull fluorescence), CG rich regions stain darkly (bright fluorescence)
4,6-diamidino-2-phenylindole staining (DAPI staining)	Binds AT rich regions and produces a pattern similar to Q-banding
Methods that stain defined region of specific chromosome	
Constitutive heterochromatin banding (C-banding)	Stains heterochromatin around the centromeres. Also used to demonstrate some inherited polymorphisms
Telomere banding (T-banding)	Technical variation of R-banding used to stain telomeres
Silver staining for nucleolar organizer regions (AgNOR staining)	Stains the NORs (which contain rRNA genes) on the satellite stalks of acrocentric chromosomes
Fluorescence in-situ hybridization (FISH)	Staining pattern depends on the probe

Staining: There are many staining methods using specific dyes to identify individual chromosomes. Different stains produce different banding patterns of the chromosomes. The stain used depends on what the karyotyping is trying to identify. Identification is done on the basis of distinctive and reliable patterns of alternating light and dark bands. Currently, the most commonly used stain is Giemsa stain, hence the banding technique is called G-banding. In this, the chromosomes are digested by trypsin before staining with a Giemsa stain, creating lightly (GC rich regions) and darkly (AT rich regions) stained bands on the chromosomes. Each individual chromosome has a characteristic banding pattern. So, cytogenetic changes can be identified based on changes in the banding pattern.

Classification of chromosomes in karyotyping

There are various systems used for studying the morphology of the chromosomes.

Denver system of classification: In this system, the chromosomes are grouped from A to G according to the length and position of the centromere of the chromosomes.

Paris system of classification: This is a universally accepted classification. According to this, the chromosomes are identified based on the various banding patterns.

Common indications for chromosome analysis are listed in **Box 7**.

Chromosomal banding

Banding is a method to study the structure of a chromosome. In this method, chromosomes are stained by a special stain (e.g., Giemsa) which binds to specific bands of chromosome. Each

Box 7: Common indications for chromosome analysis.

- Multiple congenital abnormalities
- Presence of dysmorphic features
- Unexplained mental retardation and neurodevelopmental disorders
- Sexual ambiguity or disorder of sexual development
- Infertility
- Recurrent miscarriage
- Unexplained stillbirth
- Malignancy and chromosome breakage syndromes

chromosome shows a characteristic banding pattern (light and dark bands) which will help to identify them. The chromosomes in metaphase are arranged in order of decreasing length.

Techniques: Different banding techniques are:

- **G-banding (G for Giemsa):** It is most commonly used and shows a series of light and dark stained bands (**Fig. 29A**). Giemsa stain (hence "G") is specific for the phosphate groups of DNA. In G-banding, AT-rich (A=adenine, T=thymine) regions stains darkly and GC-rich (G=gaunine, C=cytosine) regions stain lightly.
- **Q-banding (stains with quinacrine fluorescent stain):** Stained with quinacrine that causes a fluorescent pattern similar to G-banding (thus, "Q").
- **R-banding (Fig. 29B):** It is the reverse images of G and Q bands (the R stands for "reverse") such that dark G bands are light R bands and vice versa. In reverse of G-banding, AT-rich regions stains lightly and GC-rich regions stain darkly.
- **C-banding (centromeric) (Fig. 29C):** This method stains centromeres (hence "C") and other portions of chromosomes containing constitutive heterochromatin, highly condensed, repetitive DNA sequences. These are transcriptionally silent. In contrast, facultative heterochromatin, which forms the inactive X chromosome (Barr body), is not repetitive but it shares the condensed structure of constitutive heterochromatin.
- **Nucleolar organizing region (NOR) staining:** It demonstrates secondary constrictions (stalks) of chromosomes with satellites.
- **T-banding:** It preferentially stains telomere (terminal/telomeric) regions/ends of chromosomes (hence "T").
- **High resolution banding:** It provides greater sensitivity.

With standard G-banding, about 400–800 bands per haploid set are usually detected. By obtaining the cells in prophase, the resolution by banding can be markedly improved. With this, the individual chromosomes appear markedly elongated, and about 1,500 bands per karyotype can be recognized. The banding techniques allow to identify each chromosome and roughly delineate breakpoints and other gross alterations in chromosome.

Karyotype analysis The final step in cytogenetic analysis is the production of a karyotype. It consists of the chromosomal complement of the cell displayed in a standard sequence on the basis of size, centromere location, and banding pattern. International System for Human Cytogenetic Nomenclature is used for structural and numerical chromosomal abnormalities.

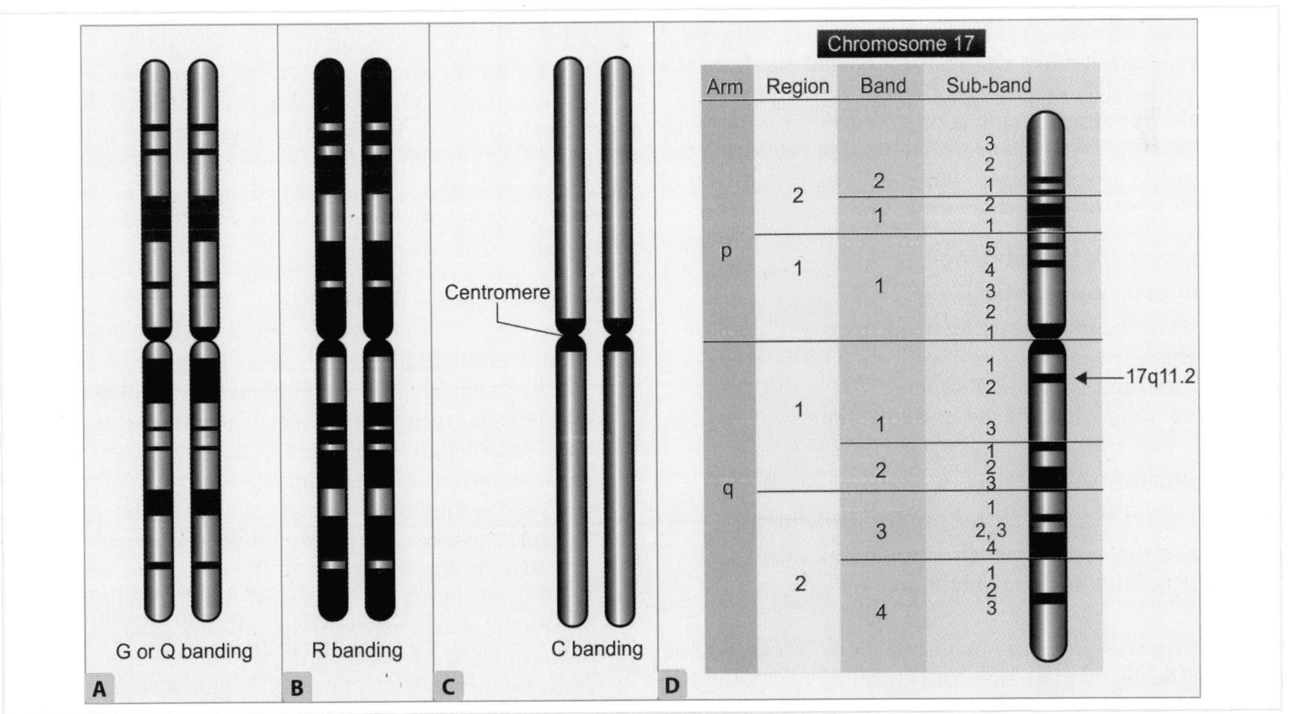

FISG. 29A TO D: Staining patterns on chromosomes are used for identification and site location. (A) Heterochromatin stains darkly by G or Q banding; (B) Euchromatin stains darkly by R banding; (C) C banding stains centromeres and (D) Identification of chromosomal location by G-band patterns. Locations are designated by the chromosome number, the arm, the region, the band, and the sub-band. In Figure (D), the location is depicted as 17q21.2 on the right side. The 17q21.2 represents that the chromosome number is 17, the arm is q (long arm), the region is 2, the band is 1, and the sub-band is 2.

Commonly used terminology in cytogenetics: Karyotypes are generally described using a standard shorthand format in the following order:

- **Total number of chromosomes.**
- **Designation (number) of affected chromosomes:** Sex chromosome constitution or component.
- **Nature and location of the defect on the chromosome:** Description of abnormalities in ascending numerical order
  - **Short arm or long arm:** The short arm of chromosome is designated "p" (petit) and the long arm "q" (queue). Each chromosome arm ends in a terminus, designated pter and qter for the short and long arms, respectively.
  - **Region:** In a banded karyotype (**Fig. 29D**), each arm of the chromosome (i.e., short and long arm) is divided into two or more regions bordered by prominent bands. The regions are numbered (e.g., 1, 2, 3) from the centromere outward.
    - **Bands and sub-bands:** Each region is further subdivided into bands and sub-bands, and these are ordered numerically as well. This will help for precise localization of the gene.
- **Structural changes in chromosomes and their corresponding abnormalities.**

Examples for Human Cytogenetic Nomenclature are as follows:

- Male with trisomy 21 is designated 47, XY + 21.
- The notation Xp21.2 (read as "X P two one point two") refers to a chromosomal segment located on the short arm of the X chromosome, in region 2, band 1, and sub-band 2.
- The notation 3p22.1 is read as "three P two two point one."

Uses of karyotyping

- **For diagnosis:** Diagnosis of genetic disorders including prenatal diagnosis.
- **To detect the cause of repeated abortions:** Many chromosomal aberrations can cause repeated spontaneous abortions and they can be identified by karyotyping.
- **Prognostic value:** Identification of specific chromosomal anomalies in certain cancers will help in predicting the course and prognosis (e.g., Philadelphia chromosome in chronic myeloid leukemia).

Disadvantages of karyotyping (conventional cytogenetics)

- Cannot detect minor (subtle/submicroscopic) deletions/mutations.
- Cannot identify gene amplifications.
- Metaphasic arrest is difficult in solid tumors.

Chromosomal Aberrations

Q. Write short essay on chromosomal disorders.

Q. Write short essay on chromosomal quantitative abnormalities and translocations.

Different types of chromosomal aberrations in cytogenetic disorders (**Box 8**) may be numerical (i.e., an abnormal number of chromosomes), structural chromosomal aberrations (i.e., alterations in the structure of one or more chromosomes) or different cell lines (i.e., different chromosome constitutions in two or more cell lines).

Box 8: Different types of chromosomal aberrations in cytogenetic disorders.

Numerical chromosomal aberrations:
- Aneuploidy
- Monosomy
- Trisomy
- Tetrasomy
- Polyploidy
  - Triploidy
  - Tetraploidy

Structural chromosomal aberrations:
- Translocations
  - Reciprocal
  - Robertsonian (centric fusion)
- Deletions
- Inversions
  - Paracentric
  - Pericentric
- Isochromosomes
- Ring chromosome (rings)
- Insertions

Different cell lines (mixoploidy):
- Mosaicism
- Chimerism

Numerical Chromosomal Aberrations

The normal chromosome is expressed as 46, XX for females and 46, XY for males. **Haploid is a single set of each chromosome** (23 in humans). Normally, only germ cells have a haploid number (n) of chromosomes. **Diploid is a double set of each of the chromosomes (46 in humans)**. Somatic cells have a diploid number (2n) of chromosomes. Any exact multiple (from n to 8n) of the haploid number of chromosomes (23) is called euploid. Total number of chromosomes may be either increased or decreased. The **deviation from the normal number of chromosomes is called as numerical chromosomal aberration**.

Types of numerical aberrations

- **Aneuploidy:** It is defined as a **chromosome number** that is **not a multiple of 23** (the normal haploid number-n). It may be due to an error either in meiosis or mitosis. **Many cancer cells are aneuploid, which usually corresponds to aggressive cell division**. Usually, aneuploidies are caused due to nondisjunction and anaphase lag.
  - **Nondisjunction:** Nondisjunction is **failure of paired chromosomes or chromatids to separate and move to opposite poles of the spindle at anaphase**, during mitosis or meiosis. If nondisjunction occurs during gametogenesis (**Fig. 30**), the gametes formed have either an extra chromosome (n + 1) or one less chromosome (n – 1). Fertilization of such gametes by normal gametes produces two types of zygotes—trisomic (2n + 1) or monosomic (2n – 1) (**Fig. 30**).
  - **Anaphase lag:** Anaphase lag is a consequence of an event occurring during cell division where sister

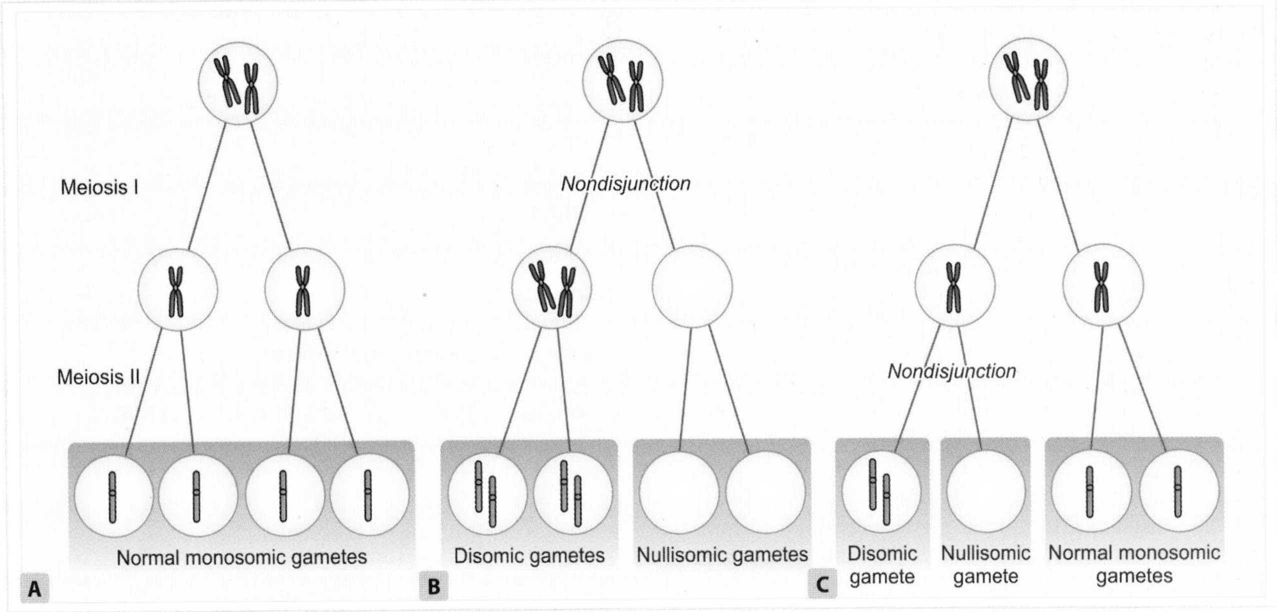

FIG. 30: Nondisjunction. Segregation at meiosis of a single pair of chromosomes in—(A) normal meiosis; (B) nondisjunction in meiosis I; and (C) nondisjunction in meiosis II.

chromatids do not properly separate from each other because of improper spindle formation. The chromosome or chromatid does not properly migrate during anaphase and the daughter cells will lose some genetic information. In this, one homologous chromosome in meiosis or one chromatid in mitosis lags behind and is left out of the cell nucleus. The result is one normal cell and one cell with monosomy.

- **Trisomy:** It is numerical abnormality with the **presence of one extra chromosome** (2n + 1). It may involve either autosomes or sex chromosomes.
  - **Trisomy of autosomes:** Several autosomal trisomies permit survivals but all (except trisomy 21) have severe malformations and almost invariably die at an early age. Most cases of Down's syndrome (trisomy 21) are due to the presence of an additional number 21 chromosome. Thus, they have total three copies of chromosome 21 (47, XX, +21) instead of normal two copies (refer **Fig. 37**). Other examples of autosomal trisomies compatible with survival to term are Patau syndrome (trisomy 13) and Edwards syndrome (trisomy 18). Most other autosomal trisomies such as trisomy 16 lead to early pregnancy loss (spontaneous miscarriages). Trisomy can result from nondisjunction in meiosis (**Fig. 31**).
  - **Trisomy of sex chromosomes:** The presence of an additional sex chromosome (X or Y) produces only mild phenotypic effects.
- **Monosomy:** It is the numerical abnormality with the absence or loss of one (single) chromosome (2n – 1) in a somatic cell of a homologous pair. It may involve autosomes or sex chromosomes. As with trisomy, monosomy can result from nondisjunction in meiosis (**Fig. 31**),. If one gamete receives two copies of a homologous chromosome (disomy), the other corresponding daughter gamete will have no copy of the same chromosome (nullisomy). Monosomy can also be caused by loss of a chromosome as

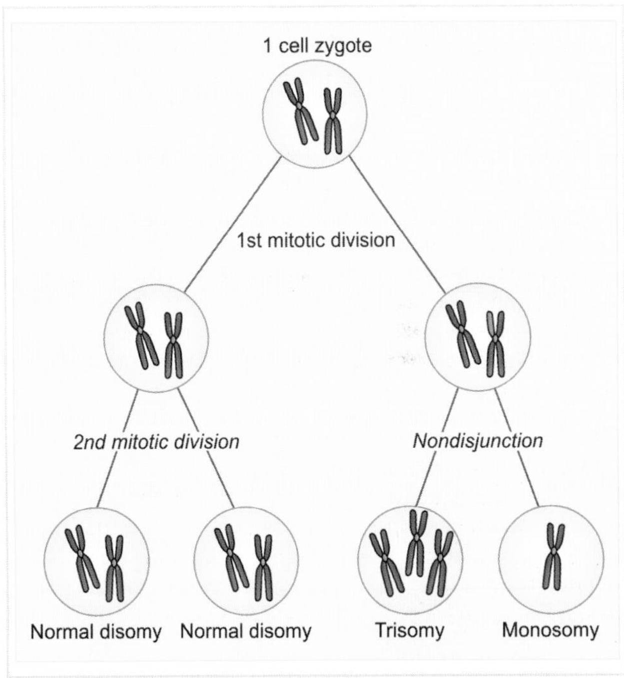

FIG. 31: Somatic mosaicism caused by mitotic nondisjunction.

it moves to the pole of the cell during anaphase, an event called as anaphase lag.
  - **Monosomy of sex chromosomes:** Lack of contribution of an X or a Y chromosome results in a 45, X karyotype. For example, Turner syndrome 45 XO instead of normal 46, XX.
  - **Monosomy of autosomes:** Monosomy involving an autosome usually causes loss of too much genetic information. Hence, it does not permit live birth or even embryogenesis.

- **Polyploidy:** This term is used when the chromosome number is a multiple greater than two of the haploid number (multiples of haploid number 23). Polyploid cells contain multiples of the haploid number of chromosomes such as 69, triploidy, or 92, tetraploidy.
  - **Triploidy:** It is found in material grown from spontaneous miscarriages, but they do not survive beyond mid-pregnancy. Even if triploid live births occur, they die soon after birth. Triploidy can be due to failure of a maturation meiotic division in an ovum or sperm. Alternatively, it can occur due to fertilization of an ovum by two sperms; this is known as dispermy.

Genesis of numerical aberrations: Exact causes of chromosomal aberrations are not fully known. Exogenous factors, such as radiation, viruses, and chemicals, can affect mitotic spindles or DNA synthesis. They can disturb mitosis and meiosis and produce breakage in human chromosomes. They have increased risk of chromosome alteration. Changes in chromosome numbers arise mainly due to nondisjunction in maternal and paternal gametes (usually of older people).

Structural Abnormalities of Chromosomes

Structural chromosomal aberration: The frequency of structural abnormalities varies. Spontaneous abortions show the highest frequency, whereas newborns show the lowest frequency. Aberration of structure (changes in the structure) of one or more chromosomes may occur **during either mitosis or meiosis.** Somatic cells undergo mitosis, while gametes undergo meiosis.

Cell division: Mitotic cell division (refer pages 72 and 73) in somatic cells gives rise to two daughter cells. These daughter cells are identical to the original parent cell in chromosome number and genetic content. Mitosis results in a diploid (2n) number of chromosomes in the daughter cells. Meiosis only occurs in male and female germline cells (refer page 73). It results in gametes with half the diploid chromosome content (23 chromosomes, plus either an X or a Y sex chromosome). This is the haploid number (n) of chromosomes.

Detection of structural chromosomal abnormalities: To be visible under routine banding techniques, there must be involvement of structural abnormalities in a fairly large amount of DNA [about 2–4 million base pair (bp)], containing many genes. The resolution is much higher with fluorescence in-situ hybridization (FISH) and it can detect chromosomal changes as small as kilobases.

Consequences of chromosome breakage: Structural abnormalities or changes in chromosomes usually result from chromosome breakage with subsequent reunion in a different configuration. There may be **loss or rearrangement of chromosomal material**.

- **Chromosomal rearrangement:** It can be balanced or unbalanced.
  - **Balanced rearrangements:** In these, there is no loss or gain of genetic material, and these are generally harmless with the exception of rare cases in which one of the breakpoints damages an important functional gene. However, carriers of balanced rearrangements have risk of producing children with an unbalanced chromosomal complement.
  - **Unbalanced rearrangements:** In unbalanced chromosome rearrangement, the chromosomal complement contains an incorrect amount of chromosome material. Its clinical effects are usually serious. This gives rise to early fetal loss, particularly when there are significant unbalanced rearrangements.
- **Chromosomal loss: It causes loss of genetic material.**

The various structural chromosomal aberrations (**Box 8**) are discussed below.

Translocations

A chromosome translocation is an abnormal **structural alteration between two nonhomologous chromosomes** (e.g., chromosomes 11 and 22) in which **segment of one chromosome gets detached and is transferred to another chromosome**. Thus, in translocation there is transfer of genetic material (cross over and exchange genetic material) from one chromosome to another. This exchange of chromosome material can be balanced or unbalanced.

Nomenclature: Chromosomal translocations are classified as per the International System for Human Cytogenetic Nomenclature. Examples are as follows:

- Balanced reciprocal translocation involving the chromosomes 11 and 22 is relatively common. Nomenclature for this translocation between chromosomes "11" and "22" is written as t (11;22).
- Nomenclature for sites of the translocation is further defined by Giemsa bands. Thus, the nomenclature t (11;22) (q23;q11) means that the region of the chromosome 11 long arm (symbol "q") broken at band q23 translocated to the long arm (symbol "q") of chromosome 22 at band q11. After translocation, the region from 22q11 forms part of the long arm at 11q23.

Major types of translocations: There are two major types of translocations namely—(1) reciprocal and (2) Robertsonian.

- **Reciprocal translocations (Fig. 32A):** It is characterized by single breaks in each of the two chromosomes (at least two chromosomes) with exchange of genetic material (segments) distal to the break. There is exchange of chromosomal segments between different (nonhomologous) chromosomes. This forms two new derivative chromosomes. Usually, the chromosome number remains at 46.
  - **Nomenclature:** For example, a balanced reciprocal translocation between the long arm (symbol "q") of chromosome 2 and the short arm (symbol "p") of chromosome 5 would be written 46, XX, t (2;5) (q31;p14). This individual has 46 chromosomes with altered morphology of one of the chromosomes 2 and one of the chromosomes 5.
  - **Significance:** Reciprocal translocations are balanced if there is no net loss of genetic material. In this, each chromosomal segment is translocated in its entirety. It is not usually associated with loss of genetic material (or little loss) and most carriers of balanced translocations are phenotypically normal. However, a balanced translocation carrier is likely to have an increased risk of producing abnormal gametes (sperm or ova). In balanced translocation in gametes (sperm or ova), all somatic cells in the progeny inherit the abnormal chromosomal structure. Balanced

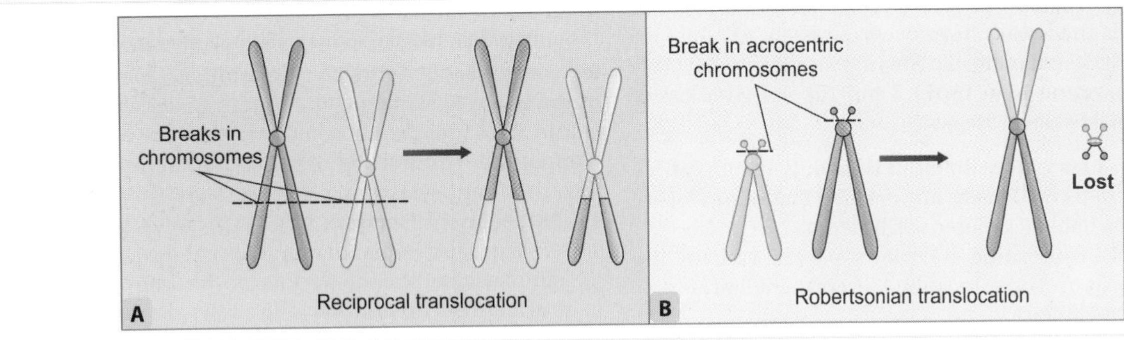

FIGS. 32A AND B: Chromosomal translocation. (A) Balanced reciprocal translocation; (B) Robertsonian translocation (centric fusion).

reciprocal translocations can be inherited for many generations. For example, in the case mentioned above, there may be formation of a gamete containing one normal chromosome 2 and another gamete containing translocated chromosome 5. Such a gamete would be unbalanced because it may not contain the normal complement of genetic material. Subsequent fertilization by a normal gamete can lead to the formation of an abnormal (unbalanced) zygote. This leads to spontaneous abortion or birth of a malformed child.

- ○ **Detection:** If the exchanged fragments (segments or genetic material) are of roughly equal size, a reciprocal translocation can be identified only by **detailed chromosomal banding studies or FISH**.

- **Robertsonian translocation (centric fusion) (Fig. 32B):** It is a particular type of reciprocal translocation between two nonhomologous acrocentric chromosomes (numbers 13, 14, 15, 21, and 22). Robertsonian translocations of chromosomes 13 and 14 are most common. The breaks are usually located at, or close to the centromeres of each chromosome. When chromosomes break near the centromere, transfer of the segments leads to combination of two long arms that fuse to form one large chromosome and one extremely small one. The small one (product) is because of fusion of short arms of both chromosomes which lack a centromere. This small acentric chromosomal fragment lacks a centromere and is usually lost in subsequent divisions. This loss is not clinically important and compatible with life because it carries only highly redundant genes (e.g., ribosomal *RNA* genes). This is because there are multiple copies of genes for ribosomal RNA on the various other acrocentric chromosomes. However, its significance lies in that it may produce abnormal progeny. The total chromosome number is reduced to 45. Similar to reciprocal translocations, a Robertsonian translocation is balanced if there is no loss of genetic material. The carrier is also usually phenotypically normal. But they may be infertile because a Robertsonian translocation can reduce the number of chromosomes. These are then asymmetrically segregated during meiosis. However, if a carrier is fertile, their gametes may produce unbalanced translocations and the offspring may have congenital malformations.
  - ○ **Significance of Robertsonian translocations:** The major practical importance is that a Robertsonian translocation of chromosome 21 has greater risk of having a child with Down/trisomy 21 syndrome. This is as a result of the embryo inheriting two normal number 21 chromosomes (one from each parent) plus a translocation chromosome involving a number 21 chromosome. In such situation, maternal transmission is more common than paternal.

Deletion

It is the **loss of any portion or part of a chromosome**. By definition, such chromosome alterations are **unbalanced with the loss of one or multiple genes present in the deleted chromosome segment**.

Causes of deletion: Chromatid breaks during mitosis in somatic cells may produce chromosomal fragments that do not recombine with any other chromosome. These chromosomal fragments are lost in subsequent cell divisions. Deletions may also result from **unequal crossover during meiosis**.

Types: It is of two types namely—interstitial (middle) and terminal (rare). Most deletions are interstitial and terminal deletions are rare.

- **Interstitial deletions (Fig. 33A)** are produced when there are two breaks within a chromosome arm. These are followed by loss of the chromosomal material between the breaks and fusion of the broken ends of chromosome.
- **Terminal deletions (Fig. 33B)** result from a single break in a chromosome arm. This produces a fragment without centromere. This deleted fragment is then lost at the next cell division. The deleted end of the retained chromosome is protected by acquiring telomeric sequences.

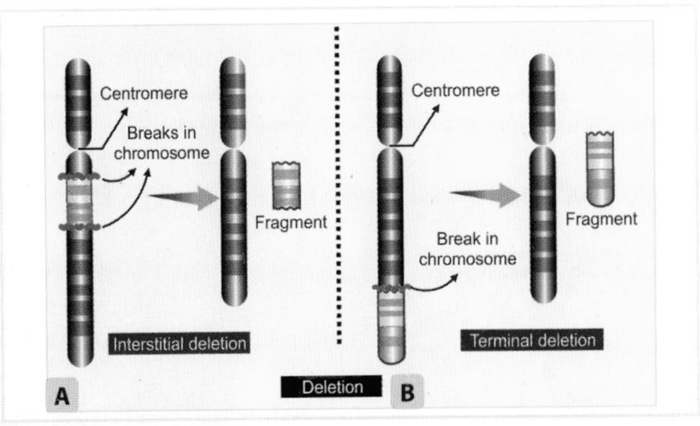

FIGS. 33A AND B: Chromosomal deletion. (A) Interstitial; and (B) Terminal deletion.

Nomenclature: Example for the specification of the regions, and the bands the breaks have occurred is 46, XY, del (16) (p11.2p13.1). It describes breakpoints in the short arm (symbol "p") of chromosome 16 at 16p11.2 and 16p13.1 with loss of genetic material between breaks.

Significance: A very large deletion is usually incompatible with survival to term. Usually, any deletion that causes loss of >2% of the total haploid genome will be lethal.

- **Cancer:** Chromosome deletions play a role in the pathogenesis of cancer, including several hereditary forms. Examples include:
  - **Familial retinoblastomas** are associated with **deletions in the long arm of chromosome 13** containing the *RB1* gene locus at 13q14.1-q14.2.
  - Individuals with **chromosome 11 deletions** may develop **WAGR syndrome.** The components of this syndrome include **Wilms tumor, aniridia, genitourinary malformations, and mental retardation**. The gene involved in WAGR syndrome is WT1 (a tumor suppressor gene in region 11p13).

Recognition: Deletions can be recognized at two levels.

1. **Large chromosomal deletion:** It can be detected under the light microscope by **routine chromosome analysis**. Examples of such large deletion syndromes include Wolf–Hirschhorn and cri du chat. These are characterized by loss of material from the short arms of chromosomes 4 and 5, respectively.
2. **Minute deletions:** Deletions of specific genes or chromosomal regions can be detected by **FISH and higher resolution techniques**. The high-resolution techniques such as array comparative genomic hybridization (aCGH) detect gene CNVs related to ploidy. aCGH can be used to profile whole genomes and to detect very small or cryptic (obscure) deletions in unidentified regions of the chromosome. These minute cryptic (obscure) deletions, or submicroscopic microdeletions, involve definitive genes in specific chromosomes. Many microdeletion syndromes are characterized by using unique sequence DNA probes for the specific gene involved, such as the *ELN* gene (elastin). Deletion of this gene in chromosome region 7q11.2 leads to Williams syndrome. *ELN* gene (elastin) is too small to be detected by routine chromosome analysis. It is readily detected by FISH and aCGH. Prader–Willi (PWS) and Angelman syndromes (AS) have microdeletions of the long arm of chromosome 15.

Inversion

It involves two **breaks within a single chromosome, the affected segment inverts with reattachment (reincorporation) of the inverted segment**. The genetic material is transferred within the same chromosome. Inversions are **usually fully compatible with normal development** because no genetic material is lost. Two types of inversions are:

1. **Paracentric inversions (Fig. 34A)** result from breaks on the same arm (either the short arm or the long arm) of the chromosome. They do not involve the centromere region.
2. **Pericentric inversions (Fig. 34B)** result from breaks on the opposite sides of the centromere (and include the centromere) where both the short and long arms are involved. A pericentric inversion involving chromosome number 9 [inv (9) (p11q12)] occurs as a common structural variant or polymorphism that is observed in up to 1% of all people. It is also known as a heteromorphism and is not thought to be of any functional importance.

Isochromosome

It is formed due to faulty centromere division. Normally, centromeres divide in a plane parallel to long axis of the chromosome and give rise to two identical hemichromosomes. If a centromere divides in a plane transverse to the long axis, it results in pair of isochromosomes (**Fig. 35A**). One pair consists of two short arms only and the other has two long arms with the lower part of the centromere. Thus, an isochromosome shows loss of one arm with duplication of the remaining arm. An isochromosome has morphologically identical genetic information in both arms.

Significance: The most common isochromosome encountered in live births is that which consists of two long arms of the X chromosome and is designated i(X)(q10). The Xq isochromosome is associated with monosomy for genes on the short arm of X and with trisomy for genes on the long arm of X. This accounts for up to 15% of all cases of Turner syndrome.

Ring chromosome

Ring chromosome is a **rare and a special form of deletion**. Ring chromosomes are **formed by a break at both the telomeric ends of a chromosome**, deletion of the acentric (without a centromere) fragments, and end-to-end fusion of the remaining centric portion (damaged ends) of the chromosome (**Fig. 35B**). The consequences depend on the amount of genetic material lost due to the break. If the ring contains a centromere, it is usually somewhat stable. However, due to abnormal

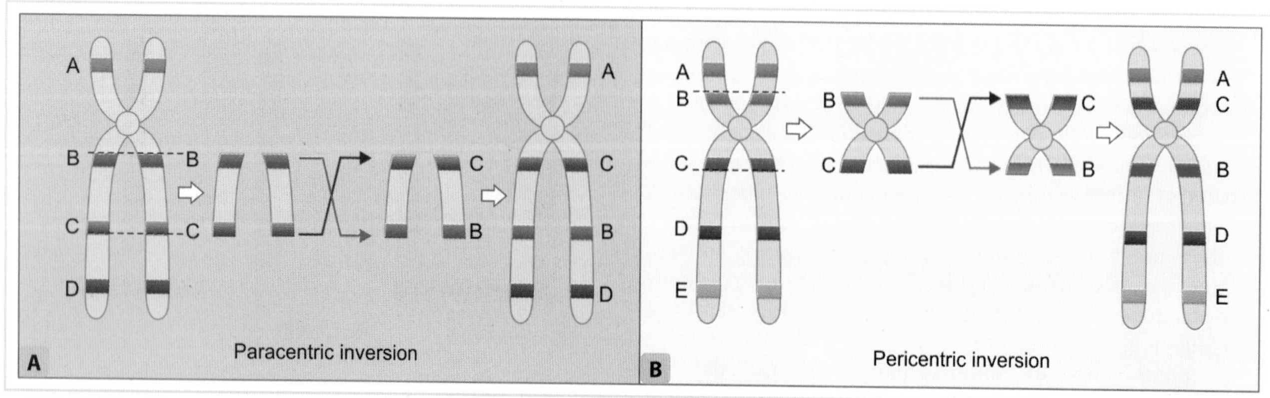

FIGS. 34A AND B: Types of inversions. (A) Paracentric; (B) Pericentric inversion.

anomalies, and limited hip abduction. Fetuses with trisomy with severe anomalies abort spontaneously. Fetuses with trisomy 18 occur in women older than 35 years.

Trisomy of chromosome 13

Trisomy 13, or Patau syndrome, is rare. It is associated with severe mental and growth retardation. Significant malformations include cleft lip and cleft palate, persistent fetal hemoglobin, severe malformations nervous system and heart, polycystic kidneys, polydactyly, umbilical hernia, and simian crease. Increased maternal age is risk factor.

Trisomy 21, trisomy 18, and trisomy 13 are the only known trisomies in liveborn infants. Their chromosomal changes and clinical features are briefly summarized in **Table 13**. **Figures 38A** and **B** show features of trisomy 18 and trisomy 13.

Chromosomal Deletion Syndromes

Chromosomal deletion syndromes are almost always characterized by deletion of parts of one or more chromosomes. Deletion of an entire autosomal chromosome (i.e., monosomy) is usually incompatible with life. However, several syndromes arise from deletions of parts of several chromosomes (**Tables 12** and **14**). Most of these congenital syndromes are sporadic, but in a few cases, reciprocal translocations occur in the parents. Almost all of these deletion syndromes have phenotypes such as low birth weight, mental retardation, microcephaly and craniofacial and skeletal abnormalities, and cardiac and urogenital malformations.

5p– syndrome (cri du chat)

This deletion syndrome calls for attention because of the high-pitched cat-like cry of the affected infant. The clinical features in infant include intellectual disability and delayed development, microcephaly, low birth weight, and hypotonia. They have distinctive facial features, with widely set eyes (hypertelorism), low-set ears, a small jaw, and a rounded face. Some may have congenital heart diseases. Most are sporadic and reciprocal translocations may be found in 10–15% of the parents. The size of the 5p deletions varies. Larger deletions cause more severe intellectual disability and developmental delay. Loss of a specific gene, *CTNND2*, present on the short arm of chromosome 5 is associated with severe intellectual disability.

Table 13: Examples of trisomic syndromes with clinical features.

Trisomic syndromes	*Clinical features*
Chromosome 21 (Down syndrome 47, XX or XY, +21)	Epicanthic folds, speckled irides, flat nasal bridge, congenital heart disease, simian crease of palms, Hirschsprung disease, increased risk of leukemia (AML/ALL)
Chromosome 18 (Edwards syndrome 47, XX or XY, +18)	Female preponderance, micrognathia, micro-ophthalmia, congenital heart disease, horseshoe kidney, deformed fingers, limited hip abduction, rocket-bottom feet
Chromosome 13 (Patau syndrome 47, XX or XY, +13)	Cleft lip and cleft palate, persistent fetal hemoglobin, microcephaly, congenital heart disease, polycystic kidneys, polydactyly, umbilical hernia, simian crease, rocket-bottom feet

(ALL: acute lymphocytic leukemia; AML: acute myeloid leukemia)

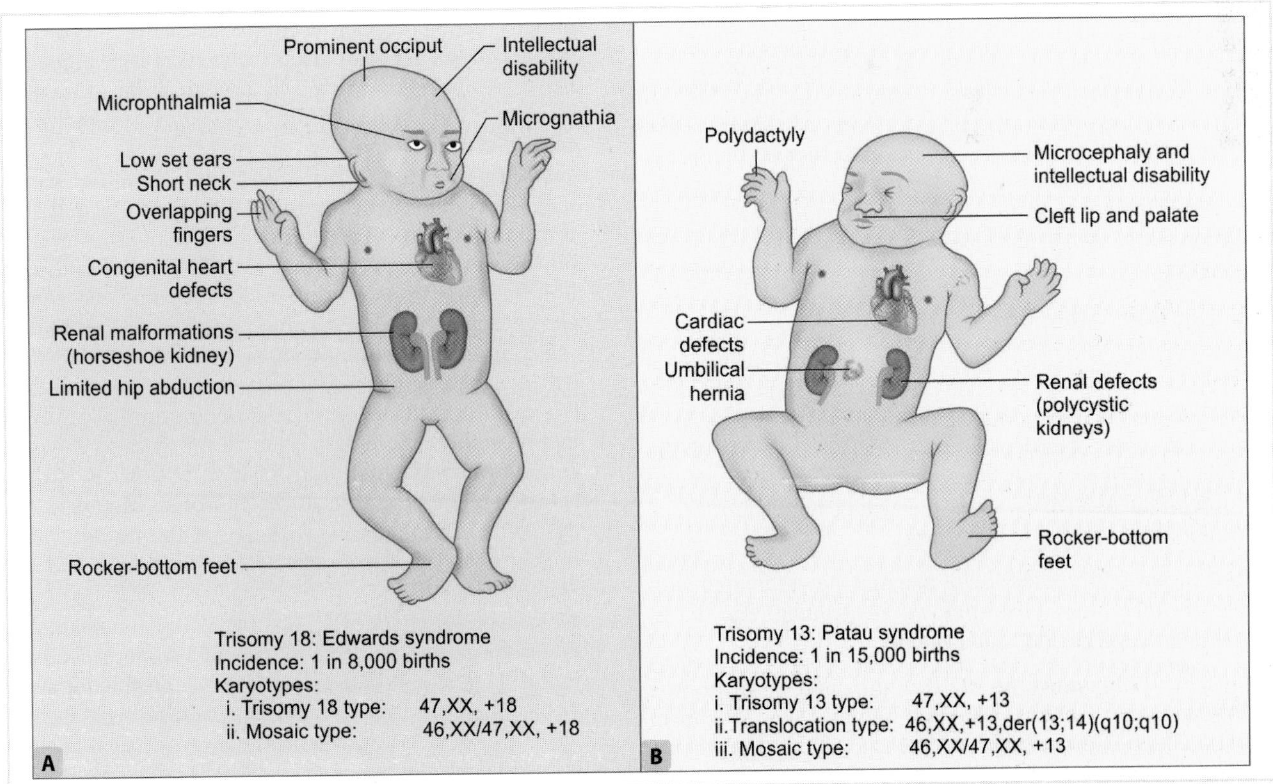

FIGS. 38A AND B: Clinical features and karyotypes of—(A) Trisomy 18 and (B) Trisomy 13.

Chimerism

Chimerism is defined as the presence, in an individual, of two or more genetically distinct cell lines derived from more than one zygote (i.e., they have a different genetic origin). The term chimera is derived from the mythological Greek monster that had the head of a lion, the body of a goat, and the tail of a dragon. In humans, there are two kinds of chimeras namely—dispermic chimeras and blood chimeras.

Dispermic chimeras These are produced as a result of double fertilization in which two genetically different sperms fertilize two ova and the resulting two zygotes fuse to form one embryo. If the two zygotes are of different sex, the chimeric embryo can develop into an individual with true hermaphroditism and an XX/XY karyotype.

Blood chimeras Blood chimeras are produced due to exchange of cells between nonidentical twins in utero via the placenta. For example, 90% of one twin's cells can have an XY karyotype with RBCs of blood group B, whereas 90% of the cells of the other twin can have an XX karyotype with RBC of blood group A.

Cytogenetic Disorders Involving Autosomes

Trisomy 21 (Down Syndrome)

Q. Write short essay on Down syndrome and its mechanism.

Q. Write short essay on underlying maternal age causing fetal trisomy.

Down syndrome was first described by Dr John Langdon Down. It is a **cytogenetic disorder involving autosomes.** It is the **most common chromosomal disorder** and the **most common (leading) cause of mental retardation and intellectual disability**. Liveborn infants constitute only a fraction of all conceptuses with this defect and about two-thirds abort spontaneously or die in utero. About **95% of individuals have trisomy 21 (extra copy of chromosome 21)**, resulting in chromosome count of 47 instead of normal 46. FISH with chromosome 21-specific probes shows an extra copy of chromosome 21 in such individuals. Parents of children with Down syndrome are normal and have a normal karyotype.

Etiology and pathogenesis

Maternal age: Maternal age has a strong influence on the incidence of trisomy 21 and rises dramatically with increasing maternal age. Older mothers (above 45 years of age) have much greater risk of having children with Down syndrome. The correlation of Down syndrome with maternal age suggests that in most (about 95%) of the cases, the meiotic nondisjunction of chromosome 21 occurs in the ovum.

Other factors: Increased incidence may be associated with exposure of mother to pesticides, electromagnetic fields, anesthetic drugs, alcohol, and caffeine.

Features of chromosome 21: It is the smallest autosome in humans and contains <2% of all human DNA. All known functional genes (except ribosomal RNA genes) of chromosome 21 are present on the long arm (21q). Chromosome 21 is a "gene-poor" acrocentric chromosome and contains only 200–250 genes. The region responsible for the full Down syndrome phenotype (usually have typical Down syndrome facial features) is in band 21q22.2, a 4-Mb region of DNA. It is called as the **Down syndrome critical region (DSCR)**. Genes in DSCR involved in Down syndrome are designated as *DSCR1, DSCR2,* and so forth. It has a high ratio of AT to GC sequences. Down syndrome probably results from gene dosage imbalance rather than the action of a few genes. This is supported by the following observations:

- **Gene dosage:** Majority of the protein coding genes mapped to chromosome 21 are overexpressed. One of them is gene for amyloid-beta precursor protein (APP). Aggregation of amyloid-beta proteins is the important initiating event in the development of Alzheimer disease. This may be responsible for the early onset of Alzheimer disease in individuals with Down syndrome.
- **Mitochondrial dysfunction:** About 10% of the genes overexpressed in Down syndrome are directly or indirectly involved in regulation of mitochondrial functions. Mitochondria are abnormal both morphologically and functionally in several tissues of patients with Down syndrome. Morphologically, the cristae of mitochondria are broken or swollen and functionally there is production of reactive oxygen species and activation of apoptosis.
- **Noncoding RNAs:** Chromosome 21 has the highest density of lncRNAs (long non-coding RNAs).

Mechanism of trisomy 21: The three copies of chromosome 21 in somatic cells cause Down syndrome. Trisomy 21 may be due to:

- **Nondisjunction in the first meiotic division of gametogenesis** is responsible for trisomy 21 in most (95%) of the patients. The extra chromosome 21 is maternal in origin in about 95% of such individuals. Almost all maternal nondisjunction probably occurs in meiosis I.
- **Robertsonian translocation** (refer page 855, **Fig. 32B**): Down syndrome is caused by translocation of an extra portion of long arm of chromosome 21 to another acrocentric chromosome (e.g., 22 or 14) in about 4–5% of cases. This occurs in two situations—(1) either parent may be a phenotypically normal carrier of a balanced translocation, or (2) a translocation may arise de novo during gametogenesis. These translocations are usually Robertsonian translocation and affect only acrocentric chromosomes, with short arms consisting of a satellite and stalk (chromosomes 13, 14, 15, 21, and 22). Translocations between these acrocentric chromosomes are common. This is because they cluster during meiosis and are likely to break and recombine more than other chromosomes. The most common Robertsonian translocation in Down syndrome is fusion of the long arms of chromosomes 21 and 14. It is designated as rob (14;21) (q10;q10). Other Robertsonian translocation is fusion involving two chromosomes 21, rob (21;21) (q10;q10).
- **Mosaicism for trisomy 21:** It is caused by nondisjunction of chromosome 21 during mitosis of a somatic cell early in the stage of embryogenesis. It is responsible for about 1–2% of cases of Down syndrome. These individuals have a mixture of cells with 46 or 47 chromosomes. In these individuals, symptoms are variable and milder, depending on the proportion of abnormal cells.

Table 12: Chromosome abnormalities in Down syndrome.

Abnormality	*Frequency (%)*
Trisomy 21	95
Translocation (14, 21)	4
Mosaicism	1

Down syndrome due to translocation or mosaicism is not related to maternal age. Chromosome abnormalities in Down syndrome are presented in **Table 12**.

Clinical features

Diagnosis of Down syndrome is usually apparent even at the time of birth by the infant's significant hypotonia (flaccid state) and characteristic craniofacial appearance. These include flat facial profile, upward sloping of (oblique) palpebral fissures, epicanthic folds, small ears, and protruding tongue (**Fig. 36**). The diagnosis is confirmed by cytogenetic analysis (**Fig. 37**). or FISH analyses. Down syndrome is a major cause of severe intellectual disability. But some mosaics with Down syndrome have mild phenotypic changes and may even have normal or near-normal intelligence. Characteristic features appear as the child grows.

Mental status: Children are invariably mentally retarded with low IQ (25–50). They are at higher risk for Alzheimer disease.

Craniofacial features: Diagnostic craniofacial clinical features are—

- Flat face and occiput, with a low-bridged nose, reduced interpupillary distance, and oblique palpebral fissures.
- Epicanthal folds of the eyes impart an Asian/oriental appearance (obsolete term mongolism).
- Speckled appearance of the iris (Brushfield spots).
- Enlarged low set and malformed ears.
- A prominent tongue (macroglossia), which characteristically lacks a central fissure. It protrudes through an open mouth.

Cardiac anomalies: Cardiac malformations are found in about 40% of children with Down syndrome. The incidence is even higher in aborted fetuses. Congenital cardiac anomalies are responsible for majority of the deaths in infancy and early childhood. The cardiac defects are:

- Septal and atrioventricular (AV) defect: These defects may involve atrial septum (atrial septal defect), ventricular septum (ventricular septal defect), one or more AV valves, and common atrioventricular canal.
- Other cardiac anomalies: Tetralogy of Fallot and patent ductus arteriosus.

Skeletal abnormalities: These children are small because of shorter bones of the ribs, pelvis, and extremities. The hands are broad and short and show a "Simian crease" (a single transverse crease across the palm). The middle phalanx of fifth finger is hypoplastic and curves inward. There is a wide gap between first and second toes.

GI tract: It may show esophageal/duodenal stenosis or atresia, imperforate anus, and Hirschsprung disease (megacolon). This may be observed in 2–3% of children with Down syndrome.

Reproductive system: Men are usually sterile because of spermatogenesis arrest. Few women with Down syndrome may give birth to children, 40% of which have trisomy 21.

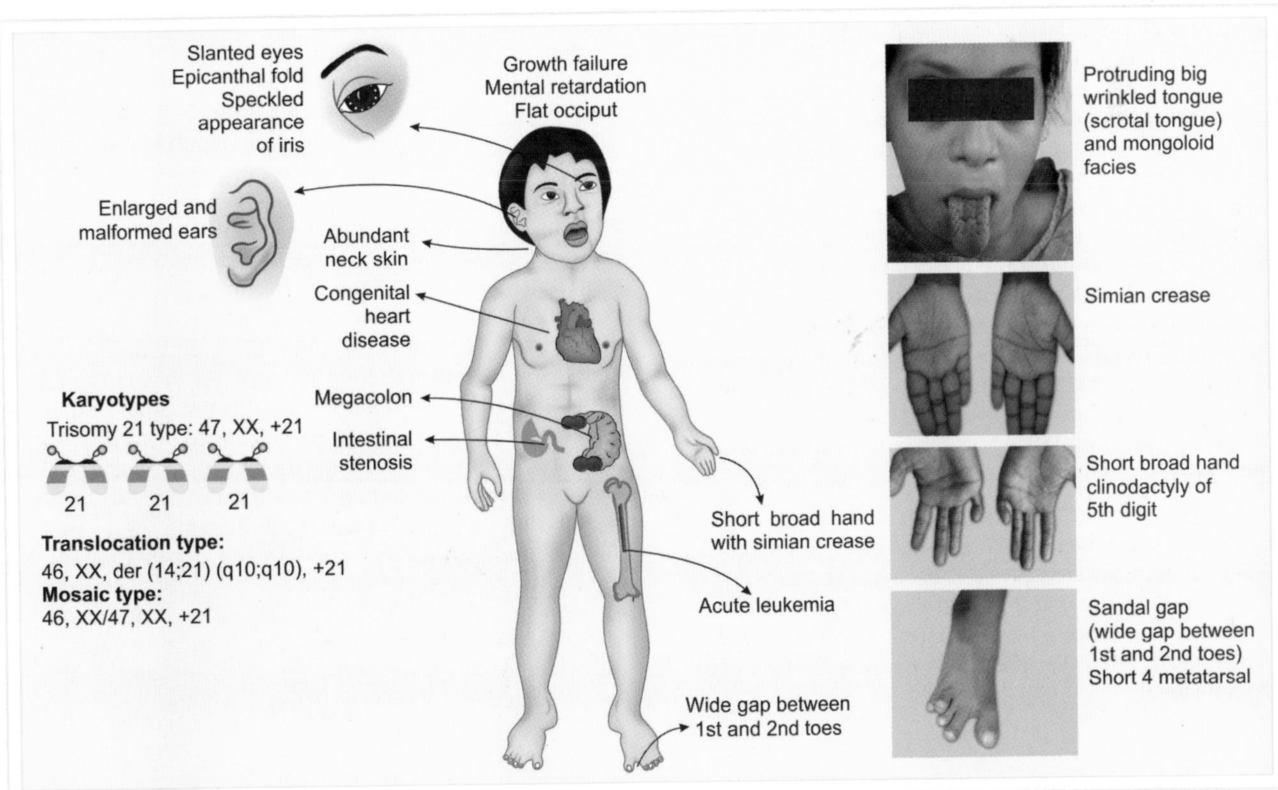

FIG. 36: Major clinical features of Down syndrome.

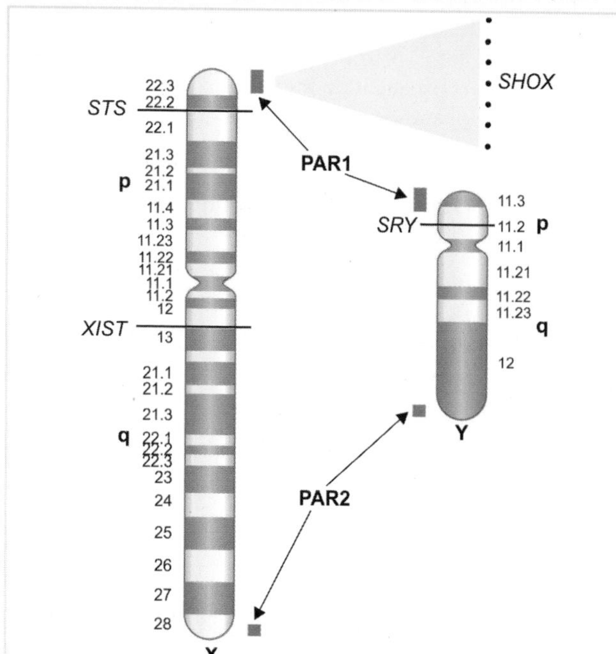

FIG. 40: The X and Y chromosomes showing the pseudoautosomal regions (PARs), PAR1 and PAR2, at the tips of Xp-Yp and Xq-Yq, respectively, and the relative positions of the *XIST*, *SHOX*, and *STS* genes in X chromosome and *SRY* gene in Y chromosome.

seeming disparity is explained by the Lyon effect or **Lyon hypothesis**.

Lyon hypothesis

Q. Write short essay on Lyon hypothesis.

In 1961, Mary Lyon defined the concept of X-inactivation. It is now commonly known as the Lyon hypothesis (**Box 10**). Lyonization is a normal process in which each cell only has one active X chromosome. Thus, the great preponderance of (almost all) normal females (XX) is in reality mosaics for paternal and maternal X chromosomes. Thus, they have two population of cells, one with an inactivated maternal X chromosome and the other with an inactivated paternal X chromosome (**Fig. 41**). Mosaicism in females for G6PD was main factor in demonstrating the monoclonal origin of neoplasms. In females, one X chromosome is irreversibly inactivated early in embryogenesis. The **inactive X chromosome remains in a condensed form and is detectable in interphase** (during interphase) **nuclei**. It appears in the interphase nuclei as a darkly staining small mass (as a clump of heterochromatin) attached to the inner nuclear membrane (in contact with the nuclear membrane) as **"sex chromatin", Barr body or X chromatin**.

Molecular basis of X inactivation: A unique gene, called *XIST*, and its product, a lncRNA, are retained (switched on) in the nucleus of active X chromosome. The lncRNA "coats" the X chromosome that it is transcribed from and initiates a gene-silencing process by chromatin modification and DNA methylation. The XIST allele is switched off in the active X chromosome.

Box 10: Features of Lyon hypothesis.

- Only one of the X chromosomes is genetically active
- X-chromosome inactivation (lyonization): Other X chromosome of either maternal or paternal origin undergoes heteropyknosis and is rendered inactive
- Inactivation of either the maternal or the paternal X chromosome occurs at random among all the cells of the blastocyst on or about day 5.5 of embryonic life. X-chromosome inactivation (XCI) is often referred to as lyonization
- X-chromosome inactivation is permanent. Inactivation of the same X chromosome persists in all the daughter (progeny) cells derived from each precursor cell. It may be paternally or maternally derived
- Inactivation of the X chromosome is virtually complete*
- X chromosomes are propagated clonally

*The inactive X chromosome is extensively methylated at gene control regions and transcriptionally repressed. But not all of the X chromosome is inactivated. However, minority of X-linked genes escape inactivation and continue to be expressed by both X chromosomes. Genes that escape inactivation and remain active are in the pseudoautosomal region (PAR) at the tip of the short arm (**Fig. 40**). Other loci elsewhere on both long and short arms include XIST. XIST is an X-linked nonprotein-coding *RNA* gene expressed only by the inactive X chromosome. The probability that an X chromosome is inactive correlates with levels of XIST.

Q. Write short essay on *SHOX* gene.

Genes remaining active in inactivated X chromosome: It was thought that all the genes on the inactive X chromosome are inactivated or "switched off". This is not so simple and not all genes on the inactive X chromosome are inactivated and many genes escape X inactivation. If all loci on one X chromosome were inactivated and entirely nonfunctional, then all women would have Turner syndrome and individuals with XO (Turner) karyotypes should have been phenotypically normal. And also, more than one X in a male [e.g., 47, XXY (Klinefelter)], or two in a female (e.g., 47, XXX), would have no phenotypic effects. But these individuals are not phenotypically normal. This indicates that inactivated X chromosomes still function, at least in part. Molecular studies revealed that about 30% of genes on Xp (short arm of X chromosome) and a smaller number (3%) on Xq (long arm of X chromosome) escape X inactivation. The tips of short and long arms of X and Y chromosomes have regions of homology that recombine during meiosis and are therefore inherited as autosomal loci. For this reason, they are called **PARs** (see **Fig. 40**). There are two PARs in X chromosome namely, Xp (PAR1) and Xq (PAR2). This PAR shares homology with the Yp (short arm) and Yq (long arm) of Y chromosome (which escapes X-inactivation). During meiosis, pairing occurs between the homologous Xp and Yp chromosomal regions and undergo meiotic recombination. As a result of a meiotic cross-over, a gene could be transferred from the X to the Y chromosome, or vice versa. This allows the possibility of male-to-male transmission. Genes for PAR are present in two functional copies in both males and females. Thus, individuals with Turner syndrome (45, X) are haploinsufficient for these genes, whereas individuals with more than two X

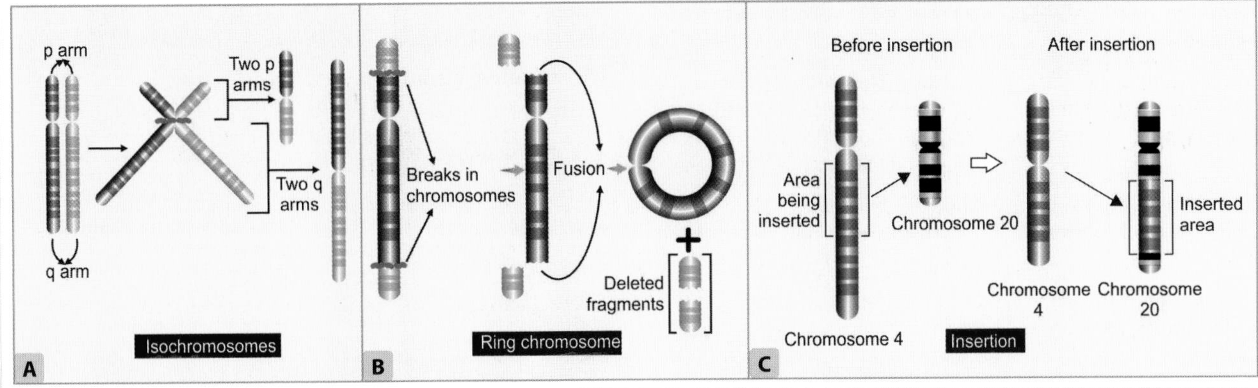

FIGS. 35A AND B: (A) Isochromosome; (B) Ring chromosome.

shape of ring chromosome, it may be lost during meiotic cell division. Loss of significant amount of genetic material will result in phenotypic abnormalities. It is expressed as 46, XY, r (14). Ring chromosomes do not behave normally in meiosis or mitosis. Ring chromosomes have been found in some patients with epilepsy (chromosome 20); mental retardation and dysmorphic facies (chromosomes 13 and 14); mental retardation, dwarfism, and microcephaly (chromosome 15); and Turner syndrome (chromosome X).

Insertion

It is a form of nonreciprocal translocation in which a fragment of chromosome is transferred and inserted into a nonhomologous chromosome. Two breaks occur in one chromosome, which releases a chromosomal fragment (**Fig. 35C**). This fragment is inserted into another chromosome following one break in the receiving chromosome to insert this fragment.

Chromosomal nomenclature for chromosomal aberrations is presented in **Table 11**.

Different Cell Lines (Mixoploidy)

Mosaicism

Mosaicism can be defined as the presence of two or more population of cells lines with different chromosomal complement in the same individual or in a tissue, but are derived from a single zygote (i.e., they have the same genetic origin). It can result from mitotic errors (e.g., nondisjunction) during the cleavage of the fertilized ovum or in somatic cells.

- **Mosaicism affecting the sex chromosomes:** It is relatively common. During the division of the fertilized ovum, an error may lead to one of the daughter cells receiving three sex chromosomes, whereas the other receives only one. For example, this may give rise to 45, X/47, XXX mosaic. All descendant cells derived from each of these precursors thus have either a 47, XXX complement or a 45, X complement.
- **Mosaicism affecting the autosomes:** Autosomal mosaicism is much less common than that involving the sex chromosomes. An error during an early mitotic division involving the autosomes usually leads to a nonviable mosaic due to autosomal monosomy. Rarely, the nonviable cell population may be lost during embryogenesis. This may yield a viable mosaic (e.g., 46, XY/47, XY, +21).

Table 11: Chromosomal nomenclature for chromosomal aberrations.

Terminology	*Nomenclature/ abbreviation/symbol*
Numerical designation of autosomes	1–22
Sex chromosomes	X, Y
Addition of a whole or part of a chromosome	Plus sign (+)
Loss of a whole or part of a chromosome	Minus sign (–)
Numerical mosaicism (e.g., 46/47) (i.e., separates cell lines or clones)	Slash (/)
Short arm of chromosome	(petite) p
Long arm of chromosome	q
Translocation	t
Deletion	del
Isochromosome	i
Ring chromosome	r
Insertion	ins
Derivative chromosome (carrying translocation)	der
Terminal	ter
Additional material of unknown origin	add
Centromere	cen
Break	single colon (:)
Break and reunion	double colon (: :)
Separates chromosome number, sex chromosomes, and abnormalities	comma (,)
Double minute(s)	dmin
Duplication	dup
Identical abnormalities as in prior clone	idem
Inversion	inv
Marker chromosome	mar
Uncertainty of chromosome identification or abnormality	question mark (?)
Reciprocal	rcp
Separates chromosomes and breakpoints in rearrangements involving more than one chromosome	semicolon (;)

Table 14: Examples of deletion syndromes and their clinical features.

Syndromes	*Clinical features*
Chromosome 5p– syndrome (cri du chat 46, XX or XY, 5p–)	Cat-like cry, low birth weight, microcephaly, epicanthic folds, congenital heart disease, short hands and feet, and simian crease
Chromosome 11p– syndrome (46, XX or XY, 11p–)	Aniridia, Wilms tumor, gonadoblastoma, and male genital ambiguity
Chromosome 13q– syndrome (46, XX or XY, 13q–)	Low birth weight, microcephaly, retinoblastoma, congenital heart disease

Microdeletion syndromes

These syndromes are characterized by small deletions (≈5 Mb) of a chromosomal segment. High-resolution karyotyping (2–5 Mb) usually cannot detect such microdeletions. FISH using probes for the critical deleted interval can be used for their diagnosis. Various microdeletion syndromes are discussed in **Table 15**.

Table 15: Examples of microdeletion syndromes.

Microdeletion syndrome	*Abnormality detected*
Microdeletion in autosomes	
• 1p36 microdeletion	1p36 deletion
• Wolf Hirschhorn	4p16.3 deletion
• Cri du chat	5p15.2 deletion
• Williams	7q11.23 deletion
• Prader–Willi	15q11.2 deletion
• Angelman	15q11.2 deletion
• Miller–Dieker	17p13.3 deletion
• Smith–Magenis	17p11.2 deletion
• Chromosome 22q11.2 deletion (DiGeorge/velocardiofacial)	22q11.2 deletion
Microdeletion in sex chromosomes	
• Kallmann	Xp22.3 deletion
• X-linked ichthyosis	Xp22.3 deletion
• Sex reversal/ambiguous genitalia	Yp11.3 deletion

Chromosome 22q11.2 deletion syndrome Chromosome 22q11.2 deletion syndrome consists of a group of disorders characterized by a small deletion (3-Mb microdeletion) of band q11.2 on the long arm of chromosome 22. The syndrome is reasonably common, but usually missed because of its variable clinical features. The variable clinical presentation includes congenital heart disorders, abnormalities of the palate, facial dysmorphism, developmental delay, and variable degrees of T-cell immunodeficiency and hypocalcemia. These spectra of clinical features were previously considered to represent two different disorders namely, DiGeorge syndrome and velocardiofacial syndrome. In a very small number of patients, there is a deletion of 10p13-14.

- **DiGeorge syndrome:** These patients have thymic hypoplasia associated with T-cell immunodeficiency, parathyroid hypoplasia producing hypocalcemia, various cardiac malformations affecting the outflow tract, and mild facial anomalies. Also, there may be associated atopic disorders (e.g., allergic rhinitis) and autoimmune disorders (e.g., thrombocytopenia).
- **Velocardiofacial syndrome:** Its clinical features include facial dysmorphism (prominent nose, retrognathia), cleft palate, cardiovascular anomalies, and learning disabilities. Immunodeficiency is less frequent.

The above two different apparently unrelated syndromes have overlapping clinical features (e.g., cardiac malformations, facial dysmorphology) and were found to be associated with a similar cytogenetic abnormality. By FISH test, about 90% of individuals having DiGeorge syndrome and 80% with the velocardiofacial syndrome have a deletion of 22q11.2. Apart from numerous structural malformations, individuals with the 22q11.2 deletion syndrome have a high risk for psychotic illnesses, such as schizophrenia (seen in about 25% with this syndrome) and bipolar disorders. Conversely, 22q11.2 deletion can be seen in 2–3% of individuals with childhood-onset schizophrenia.

Molecular basis: It is not completely understood. The deleted region is large (approximately 1.5 Mb) and contains 30–40 genes. The clinical heterogeneity, with predominant immunodeficiency in some individuals (DiGeorge syndrome) and predominant dysmorphology and cardiac malformations in other individuals, is probably due to the variable position and size of the deleted segment from this genetic region. Of the 30 genes, *TBX1*, a T-box transcription factor, is most closely related with the phenotypic features of chromosome 22q11.2 deletion syndrome. *TBX1* gene is expressed in the pharyngeal mesenchyme and endodermal pouch. The facial structures, thymus, and parathyroid are derived from this pharyngeal mesenchyme and endodermal pouch. The targets of *TBX1* include *PAX9* (gene that controls the development of the palate, parathyroid, and thymus).

Diagnosis of 22q11.2 deletion: It can be established only by detection of the deletion by FISH.

Deletions and rearrangements of telomeric/subtelomeric sequences

Telomeres are specialized protein-DNA complexes present at the ends of chromosomes (refer page 212 of Chapter 7). Telomeres prevent chromosomal degradation and end-to-end fusion. Telomeric DNA has 3–20 kb of TTAGGG repeats. Subtelomeres are segments of DNA adjacent to telomeric caps. They are rich in genes. Deletions and rearrangements of telomeric/subtelomeric regions are major causes of mild-to-severe mental retardation and dysmorphic features. These deletions and rearrangements can be demonstrated by FISH.

Chromosomal Breakage Syndromes

Q. Write short essay on chromosomal breakage syndrome.

A small number of hereditary disorders are characterized by an excess of chromosome breaks and gaps. These disorders have defects in DNA repair or genomic instability and there is an increased susceptibility to neoplasia. The chromosome breakages are acquired, i.e., occur as somatic events and predispose to malignancy. These include xeroderma pigmentosum, Bloom syndrome, ataxia telangiectasia, and Fanconi anemia (constitutional aplastic pancytopenia). They are discussed in pages 525 and 526.

Cytogenetic Disorders Involving Sex Chromosomes

Q. Discuss the cytogenetic disorders involving sex chromosomes.

Genetic diseases associated with changes involving the sex chromosomes are **more common** than those involving autosomal chromosomes. Also, numerical aberrations of sex chromosomes (excess or loss) usually cause **less severe** clinical syndromes and are much better tolerated than are similar aberrations in autosomes. This may be due to two factors that are peculiar to the sex chromosomes—(1) lyonization or inactivation of all but one X chromosome and (2) the Y chromosome carries only the moderate amount of genetic material. Various numerical aberrations of sex chromosomes are depicted in **Figure 39**.

Sex Chromosomes

X and Y are sex chromosomes. There is a striking contrast between the X and Y chromosomes. X chromosome is one of the larger chromosomes and contains about 2,000 genes. Y chromosome is much smaller and has only 78 genes, and one of this is gene is called as the testis-determining gene (SRY). About 95% portion of the human Y chromosome is unable to recombine. Only the tip of the Y chromosome, called the PAR, is capable of recombining with the X chromosome. The rest of the Y chromosome is passed on to the next generation relatively intact. Thus, the Y chromosome can be used for investigating male human evolution.

Y chromosome (Fig. 40)

Genes on the Y chromosome are main determinants of gender phenotype and regardless of the number of X chromosomes, the presence of a single Y chromosome determines the male sex. Y chromosome is both necessary and sufficient for male development. Thus, individuals who are XXY (Klinefelter syndrome) have a male phenotype, and those who are XO (Turner syndrome) have a female phenotype.

***SRY* (sex-determining region Y gene):** The short arm of the Y chromosome at Yp11.3, near the distal end of its short arm, has an intron-less *SRY* gene. This gene dictates testicular development. It encodes a transcription factor belonging to the *SOX* (SRY-like box) gene family of DNA-binding proteins. It is the therian TDF, also termed as the sex-determining region Y protein or SRY protein. This SRY protein initiates male sex determination. Mutations in SRY in Y chromosome lead to XY females, whereas translocations that add SRY from Y chromosome to an X chromosome produce XX males. A small proportion of infertile males having azoospermia or severe oligospermia show small deletions in parts of the Y chromosome. The sizes and locations of these deletions vary. But they do not correlate with the severity of spermatogenic failure.

Male-specific Y region, or MSY region: It was considered that only *SRY* gene is of significance on the Y chromosome. However, it was found that there are several gene families in the so-called **male-specific Y region, or MSY region**. They harbor 75 protein-coding genes. All of these are believed to be testis-specific and are involved in spermatogenesis. Y chromosome deletions are associated with azoospermia.

X chromosome

Males have only one X chromosome. But males have the same amount of X chromosome gene products as do females. This

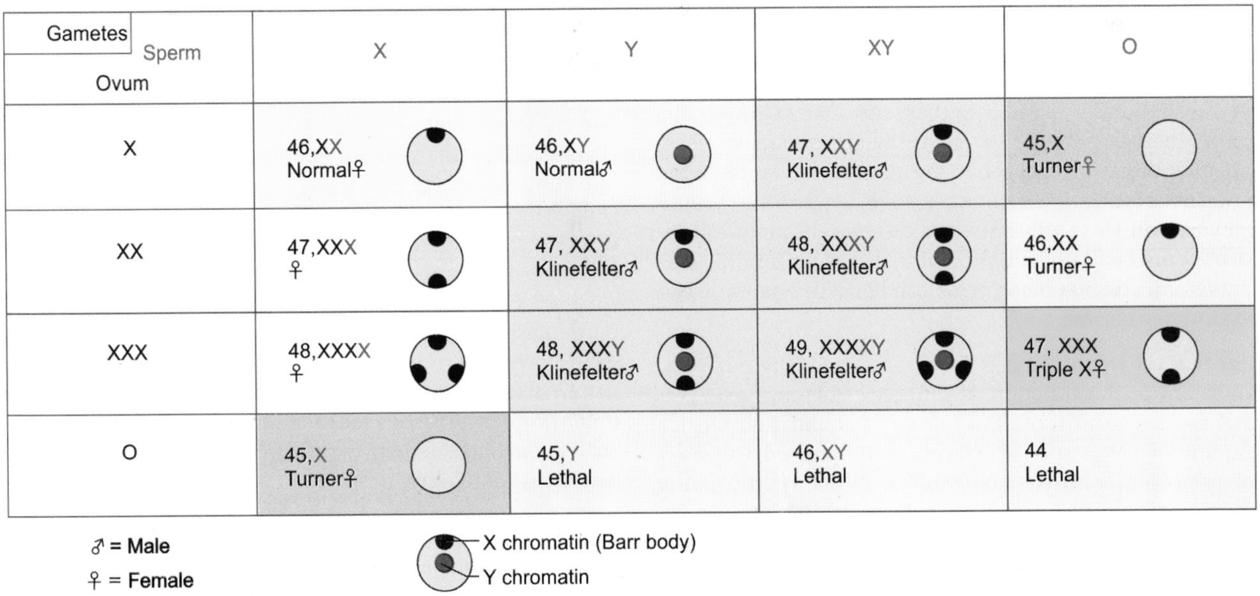

Gametes / Sperm / Ovum	X	Y	XY	O
X	46,XX Normal♀	46,XY Normal♂	47, XXY Klinefelter♂	45,X Turner♀
XX	47,XXX ♀	47, XXY Klinefelter♂	48, XXXY Klinefelter♂	46,XX Turner♀
XXX	48,XXXX ♀	48, XXXY Klinefelter♂	49, XXXXY Klinefelter♂	47, XXX Triple X♀
O	45,X Turner♀	45,Y Lethal	46,XY Lethal	44 Lethal

♂ = Male
♀ = Female
X chromatin (Barr body)
Y chromatin

FIG. 39: Various numerical aberrations of sex chromosomes. Main cause of these abnormalities is nondisjunction in either the male or female gamete.

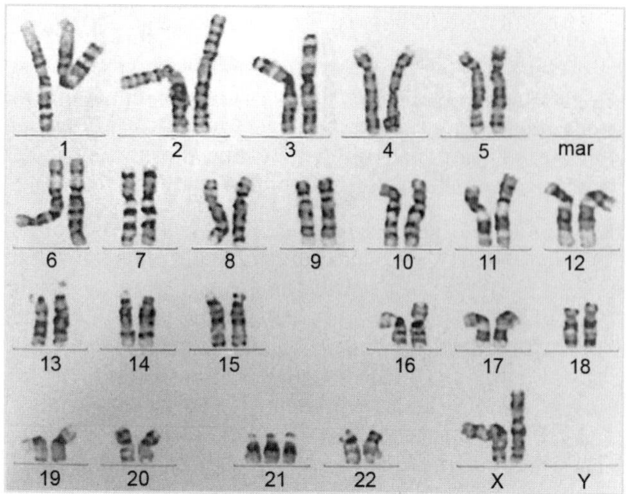

FIG. 37: G-banded karyotype from an individual with Down syndrome showing trisomy 21.

Box 9:	**Summary of common clinical findings in Down syndrome.**

Newborn period: Hypotonia, sleepy, excess nuchal skin

Craniofacial features: Brachycephaly (flat facial profile), oblique palpebral fissures, epicanthic folds, protruding tongue, small ears, and upward sloping palpebral fissures

Cardiac anomalies: Atrial and ventricular septal defects, common atrioventricular canal, tetralogy of Fallot, and patent ductus arteriosus

Skeletal abnormalities: Short stature, single palmar crease ("Simian crease"), small middle phalanx of fifth finger, and wide gap between first and second toes

Gastrointestinal tract: Esophageal/duodenal stenosis or atresia, anal atresia, imperforate anus, and Hirschsprung disease (megacolon)

Immune system: Children with Down syndrome have abnormal immune responses. They are susceptible to infections particularly of the lungs, and to autoimmune diseases of thyroid.

Endocrine system: Antithyroid antibodies may cause hypothyroidism.

Hematologic disorders: They have increased risk of both acute myeloid (under 4 years of age and 500-fold increased risk) and acute B lymphoblastic (in older individuals and 20-fold increased risk) leukemia. The acute myeloid is most commonly acute megakaryoblastic leukemia type. Leukemoid reactions (transient pronounced neutrophilia) are common in newborns with Down syndrome.

Neurologic disorders: There is neither clear pattern of neuropathology nor are there characteristic changes on the electroencephalogram in Down syndrome. Almost all patients with trisomy 21 older than age of 40 years develop neuropathologic changes characteristic of Alzheimer disease. Alzheimer disease is a degenerative disorder of the brain and shows neuropathologic changes such as granulovacuolar degeneration, neurofibrillary tangles, senile plaques, and loss of neurons. β-amyloid protein is always present in senile plaques and cerebral blood vessels in both Alzheimer disease and Down syndrome.

Atlantoaxial instability: It is characterized by excessive movement at the junction of the atlas (C1) and axis (C2) vertebrae, due to laxity of either bone or ligament. Neurological symptoms develop when spinal cord is compressed. Clinically, it may present with easy fatigability, difficulty in walking, abnormal gait, restricted neck mobility, torticollis, etc.

Major clinical features of Down syndrome and common clinical findings are presented in **Figure 35** and **Box 9**, respectively.

Life expectancy: It depends on the age and associated abnormalities.

- **First decade of life:** It depends on the presence or absence of congenital heart disease. Only 5% with normal hearts die before age 10, whereas 25% with heart disease die by first decade.
- **Patients above 10 years of age:** Life expectancy is about 55 years, which is 20 years or more lower than that of the general population.
- Only 10% reach age 70.

Diagnosis

Prenatal diagnosis: In the maternal blood, about 5–10% of the total cell free DNA is derived from the fetus. This can be identified by polymorphic genetic markers. It is possible to determine, with great precision, the gene dosage of chromosome 21 linked genes in fetal DNA by using NGS.

Next-generation sequencing is a noninvasive screening test for prenatal diagnosis of trisomy 21 and other trisomies. Most laboratories confirm a positive screening test by performing conventional karyotyping (see **Fig. 37**).

Other Trisomies

Many other trisomies may involve chromosomes 8, 9, 13, 18, and 22. Only trisomy 18 (Edwards syndrome) and trisomy 13 (Patau syndrome) are common and they share several karyotypic and clinical features with trisomy 21. Most cases of trisomy 18 (Edwards syndrome) and trisomy 13 (Patau syndrome) are due to meiotic nondisjunction and therefore, carry a complete extra copy of chromosome 18 or 13, respectively. About 10% of cases are caused by mosaicism or unbalanced rearrangements, particularly Robertsonian translocations in Patau syndrome. As in Down syndrome, these are also associated with increased maternal age. In contrast to trisomy 21, the malformations are much more severe and wide ranging. Hence, only rarely infants survive beyond the first year of life and most die within a few weeks to months after birth.

Trisomy of chromosome 18

Trisomy 18 or Edwards syndrome is the second most common autosomal trisomy syndrome. It causes mental retardation and females to male ratio is 3:1. Almost all infants with trisomy 18, born with severe cardiac malformations, die within 1 week and rarely survive for few months. Other anomalies include clenched hands with overlap of fingers, intrauterine growth retardation (IUGR), rocker bottom feet, micrognathia, prominent occiput, micro-ophthalmia, low-set ears, renal

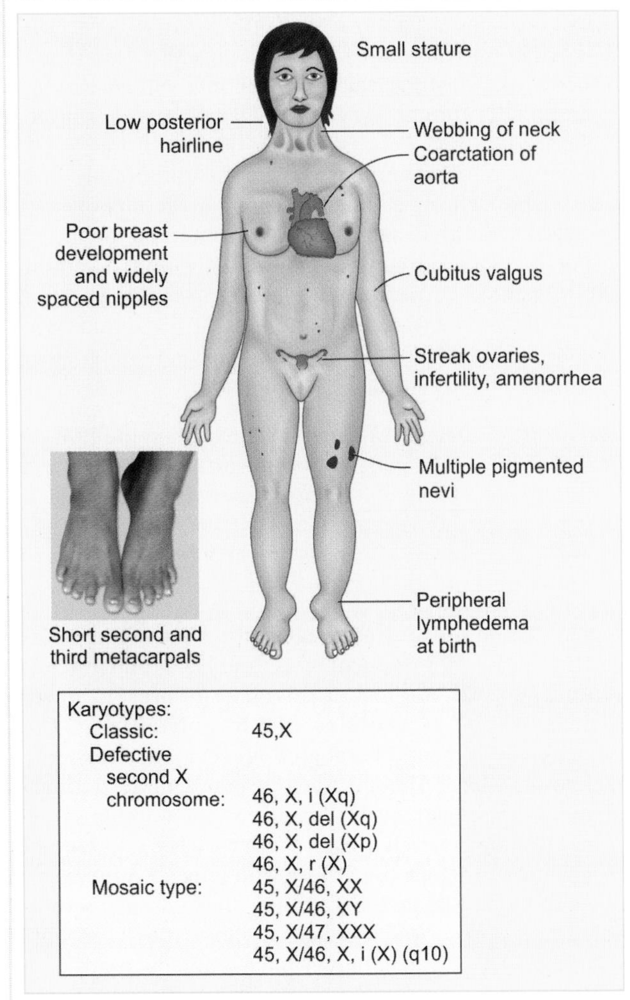

FIG. 46: Clinical features of Turner syndrome.

True hermaphrodite: It indicates the presence of both ovarian and testicular tissues.

Pseudohermaphrodite: It indicates a disagreement between the phenotypic and gonadal sex. Thus, a female pseudohermaphrodite has microscopically ovaries but male external genitalia and a male pseudohermaphrodite has microscopically testicular tissue but female-type genitalia.

SINGLE-GENE DISORDERS WITH NONCLASSIC INHERITANCE

Transmission of some single-gene disorders does not follow classic Mendelian principles of Mendelian disorders. They can be classified into four categories (**Box 11**).

Box 11: Single-gene disorders with nonclassic inheritance.

- Diseases due to trinucleotide repeat mutations
- Disorders due to mutations in mitochondrial genes
- Disorders associated with genomic imprinting
- Disorders associated with gonadal mosaicism

Diseases due to Trinucleotide Repeat Mutations

The DNA contains several repeat sequences of three **nucleotides** (trinucleotide). **Expansion of trinucleotide repeats is an important genetic cause of human disease**. This is particularly observed in neurodegenerative disorders (**Tables 1** and **16**). Trinucleotide repeat mutations belong to a special category of genetic anomaly. Many distinct trinucleotide repeats/expansions have been associated (and are identified) in human disease. In 1991, it was discovered that expanding trinucleotide repeats cause FXS (Fragile X syndrome). It was a landmark in human genetics. From then onward, several (about 40) human diseases were traced to be due to unstable nucleotide repeats (**Tables 1** and **13**). All these disorders are associated with neurodegenerative changes.

General Principles

- **Nucleotides shared are guanine (G) and cytosine (C):** Mutations associated with the expansion of trinucleotides usually share the nucleotides G and C (e.g., CGG, CAG, GAA, CTG triplet). Trinucleotide repeats may be unstable and their expansion beyond a critical number (threshold) impairs gene function in various ways. Recently, diseases associated with unstable tetranucleotides, pentanucleotides (5 nucleotides), and hexanucleotides (6 nucleotides) have also been discovered. Thus, unstable nucleotides act as a fundamental mechanism of neuromuscular diseases.
- **Sex of the transmitting parent:** The tendency to expand these nucleotides strongly depends on the sex of the transmitting parent. For example, in Huntington disease, nucleotide expansions occur during spermatogenesis and in FXS, they occur during oogenesis.
- **Mechanism causing disease (Fig. 47):** Mutations may affect coding regions or noncoding regions and their pathogenetic mechanisms are different. Main mechanisms by which unstable repeats cause diseases are:
    - **Loss of function of the affected gene:** It is usually by **silencing of transcription** (e.g., in FXS). In such cases, usually the trinucleotide repeats are in the noncoding region of the gene. There is loss of function of proteins produced by gene.
    - **Toxic gain of function:** It is by changing the protein structure of the gene product (e.g., Huntington disease and spinocerebellar ataxias). In these cases, the trinucleotide expansions occur in the coding regions of the genes. They usually involve CAG repeats coding for polyglutamine tracts in the corresponding proteins. These polyglutamine diseases are characterized by progressive neurodegeneration and usually occur in midlife. Polyglutamine expansions lead to toxic gain of function. They produce abnormal protein which may interfere with the function of the normal protein (a dominant negative activity) or acquire a new pathophysiologic toxic activity. In most cases, the abnormal proteins are misfolded and tend to aggregate. These aggregates may suppress transcription of other genes. This in turn causes dysfunction of mitochondria or stimulates the unfolded protein stress response and apoptosis.

- **Intellectual disability and X chromosome:** Usually, greater the number of X chromosomes (both in males and females), the greater the likelihood of intellectual disability.

The two most clinically important disorders due to aberrations of sex chromosomes are discussed below.

Klinefelter Syndrome (47, XXY)

Q. Write short essay on Klinefelter syndrome and its mechanism.

It is one of the most frequent forms of cytogenetic disorders involving sex chromosomes and also one of the most common causes of male hypogonadism and male infertility (associated with reduced spermatogenesis). In Klinefelter syndrome, phenotype is male, and they have a Y chromosome plus two more X chromosomes. It is the most important genetic disease involving trisomy of sex chromosomes.

Definition: Klinefelter syndrome (testicular dysgenesis) is male hypogonadism characterized by two or more X chromosomes and one or more Y chromosomes.

Molecular pathogenesis

- **Classic Klinefelter syndrome (47, XXY karyotype) (Fig. 43):** Most (80–90%) of the male patients with Klinefelter syndrome have one extra X chromosome (47, XXY karyotype instead of normal 46, XY). This complement of chromosomes results from nondisjunction during the meiotic divisions (meiotic nondisjunction during gametogenesis) in one of the parents. Roughly there is equal involvement of both maternal and paternal nondisjunction at the first meiotic division. There is no phenotypic difference observed between those individuals who receive the extra X chromosome from their father and those who receive it from their mother. In 50% of cases, nondisjunction in paternal meiosis I leads to formation of sperm with both X and Y chromosomes (XY). Fertilization of a normal egg (X) by such a sperm produces a 47, XXY karyotype. Advanced maternal age (>40 years) is a risk factor.

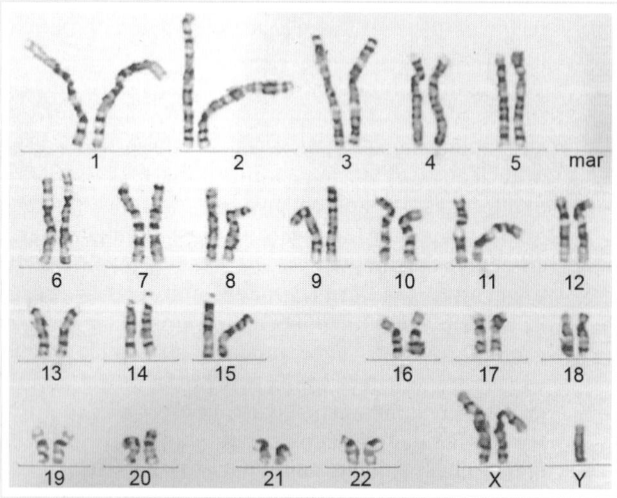

FIG. 43: G-banded karyotype from an individual with Klinefelter syndrome showing 47, XXY karyotype.

- **Minority of Klinefelter syndrome:** A minority (about 10–15%) of individuals with Klinefelter syndrome have variety of mosaic patterns. Most of them are 46, XY/47, XXY or have more than two X chromosomes (e.g., 47, XXY/48, XXXY) and in some, there is a cell line with structurally abnormal X chromosome (e.g., 47,iXq,Y) or one or more Y chromosomes.

Regardless of the number of extra X chromosomes (even up to 4), the Y chromosome results in a male phenotype. In Klinefelter syndrome, as is the case with normal females, all but one X chromosome undergoes inactivation. Additional X chromosomes correlate with more abnormal phenotypes, in spite of the inactivation of these extra X chromosomes. Probably in Klinefelter syndrome, the same genes that escape inactivation in normal females are functional.

***Short-stature HomeobOX* gene:** It is present on the PAR (see **Fig. 40**) of Xp. *SHOX* gene is growth-related and associated with expression of height. PAR (see **Fig. 40**) is one of the genes that is not inactivated during X-inactivation. An extra copy of this growth-related *SHOX* gene is probably responsible for the tall stature and long legs typical of Klinefelter syndrome.

Gene encoding the androgen receptor: A second important gene in Klinefelter syndrome is the gene that encodes the androgen receptor, and this gene is present on the X chromosome. It contains highly polymorphic CAG (trinucleotide) repeats. Through this receptor, testosterone mediates its effects. The functional response of the androgen receptor to androgen partly depends on the number of CAG repeats. Androgen receptors with shorter CAG repeats are more sensitive to androgens than those with long CAG repeats. In individuals with Klinefelter syndrome, the androgen receptor allele (on X chromosome) with the shortest CAG repeat is preferentially inactivated. In XXY males with low testosterone levels, there is expression of less sensitive androgen receptors with long CAG repeats. This exacerbates the hypogonadism and probably responsible for certain aspects of the phenotype, such as small penis size.

Clinical features

The clinical features of Klinefelter syndrome are mainly due to two major factors—(1) aneuploidy and the influence of increased gene dosage by the extra X and (2) the presence of hypogonadism.

Klinefelter syndrome (**Fig. 44**) is usually diagnosed after puberty because manifestations of hypogonadism are not observed before early puberty.

Body built: Most of these individuals have a distinctive body figure. They are tall and thin with relatively long legs. Increase in length between the soles and the pubic bone creates the appearance of an elongated body. Other characteristics are eunuchoid body habitus (i.e., a sexually deficient individual especially one lacking in sexual differentiation) with abnormally long legs and small atrophic testes usually with a small penis. There is also absence of secondary male characteristics such as deep voice, beard, and male distribution of pubic hair. Female characteristics include a high-pitched/deep voice, gynecomastia (breast enlargement), and a female pattern of pubic hair.

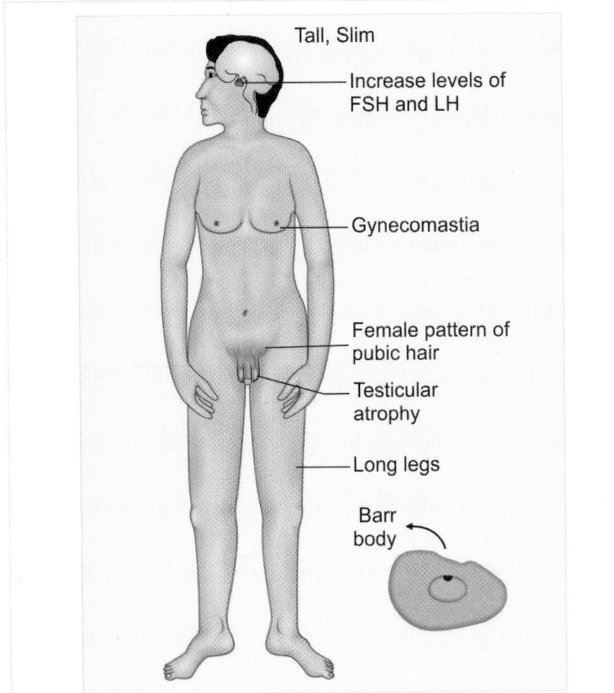

FIG. 44: Features of Klinefelter's syndrome.

Mental status: Gross mental retardation is uncommon, although average IQ is reduced. Klinefelter syndrome should be suspected in all boys with some mental deficiency and/ or severe behavioral problems. There may be moderate deficit in verbal skills particularly in reading and language comprehension.

Development of comorbid conditions: These include increased incidence of T2DM and the metabolic syndrome with insulin resistance, increased risk for congenital heart disease (e.g., mitral valve prolapse), higher prevalence of atrial and ventricular septal defects, and an increased incidence of osteoporosis and fractures due to sex hormonal imbalance.

Risk of other diseases: There is a 20- to 30-fold higher risk of developing extragonadal germ cell tumors (mostly mediastinal teratomas). Also, there is an increased frequency of breast cancer and autoimmune diseases (e.g., systemic lupus erythematosus).

Reduced spermatogenesis and male infertility: Klinefelter syndrome is an important genetic cause that is associated with reduced spermatogenesis and male infertility. Hypogonadism, reduced levels of testosterone, and remarkably high levels of follicle-stimulating hormone (FSH) and luteinizing hormone (LH) are seen in Klinefelter syndrome. Mean plasma estradiol levels are elevated. The ratio of estrogens and testosterone determines the degree of feminization.

Testis: The findings vary. In some, the seminiferous tubules show total atrophy and are replaced by pink, hyaline, collagenous ghosts. In others, there are apparently normal tubules interspersed with atrophic tubules. In some, all seminiferous tubules are primitive and appear embryonic. They consist of cords of cells without a lumen or that have not progressed to mature spermatogenesis. Leydig cells are prominent due to the atrophy and crowding of the tubules and raised gonadotropin levels. Reduced spermatogenesis causes azoospermia and leads to infertility.

Turner Syndrome

Q. Write short essay on Turner syndrome and its mechanism.

It is a cytogenetic disorder involving sex chromosomes. It is characterized by hypogonadism and is the most common sex chromosome abnormality in females.

Definition: Turner syndrome is a spectrum of abnormalities that results from complete or partial monosomy of the X chromosome in a phenotypic female.

Karyotypic abnormalities

Three types of karyotypic abnormalities are found with routine cytogenetic methods in Turner syndrome.

1. **Missing of an entire X-chromosome** (about 57%): It results in a 45, X karyotype (**Fig. 45**); sometimes erroneously, it is referred to as 45, XO. In 75% of these cases, the single X chromosome is of maternal origin, suggesting that the meiotic error tends to be paternal. The incidence of Turner syndrome is not related with maternal age.
2. **Structural abnormalities of the X chromosomes** (about 14%): The common feature of these abnormalities is production of partial monosomy of the X chromosome. The structural abnormalities of the X chromosome according to the order of frequency are—(1) isochromosome of the long arm, 46,X,i(X)(q10), resulting in the loss of the short arm; (2) deletion of portions of both long and short arms, resulting in the formation of a ring chromosome, 46,X,r(X); and (3) deletion of portions of the short or long arm, 46X,del(Xq) or 46X,del(Xp).
3. **Mosaics** (about 29%): These patients have a 45, X cell population along with one or more karyotypically normal or abnormal cell types. Examples—(1) 45, X/46, XX; (2) 45, X/46, XY; (3) 45, X/47, XXX; or (4) 45, X/46, X,i(X)(q10). Mosaics with a 45, X/46, XX karyotype tend to have a milder phenotype and may even be fertile and are

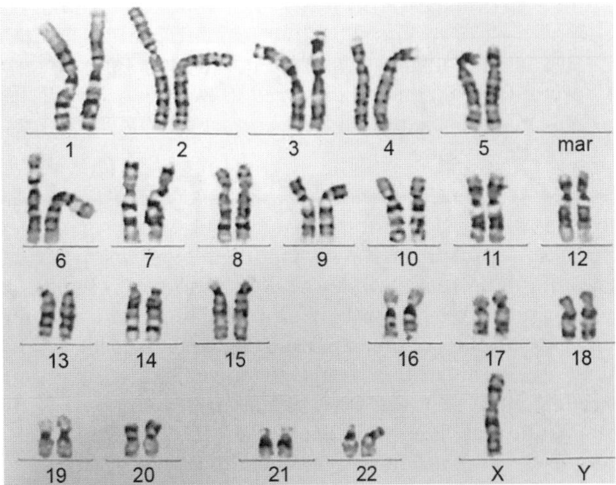

FIG. 45: G-banded karyotype from an individual with Turner syndrome showing 45, X karyotype.

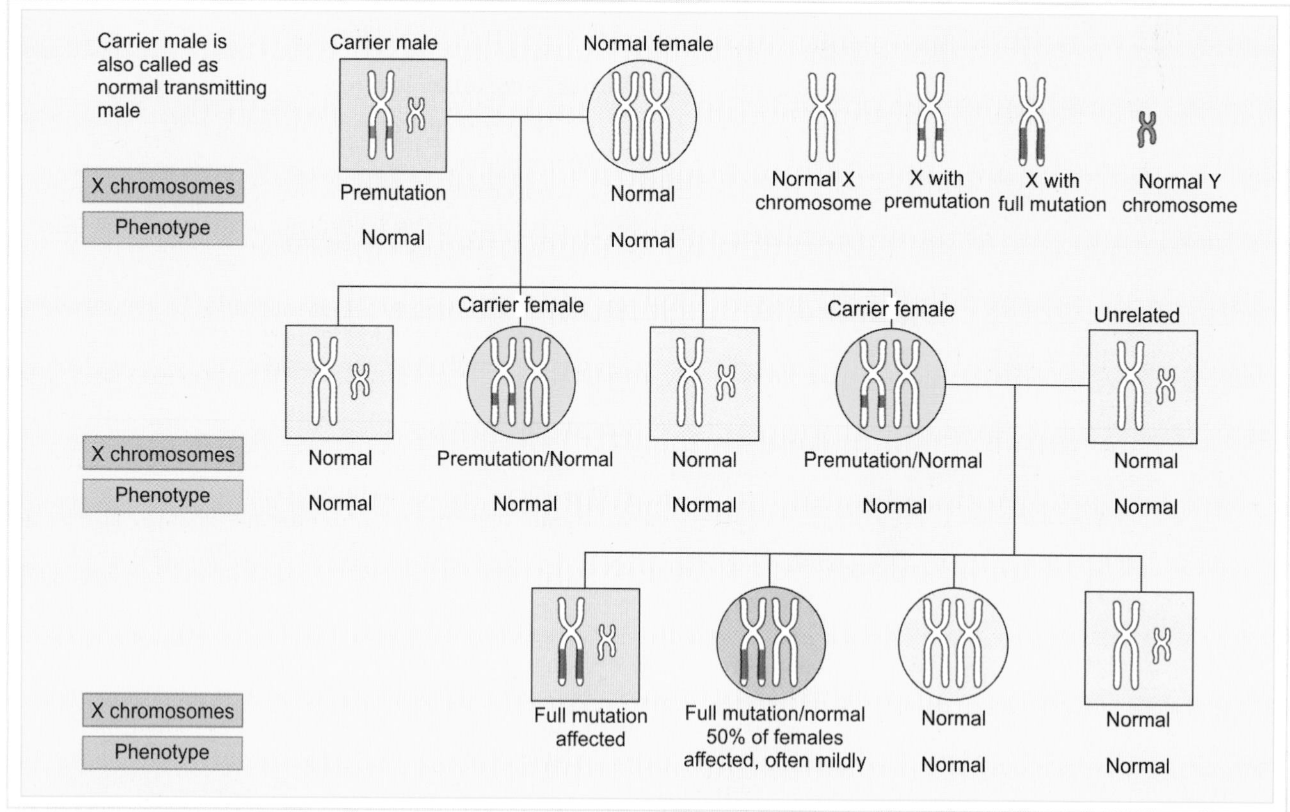

FIG. 49: Fragile X pedigree. In first generation, all sons are normal and all females are carriers. In the carrier female, premutation expands to full mutation during oogenesis. So, in the next generation, all males who inherit the X with full mutation are affected. However, only 50% of females who inherit the full mutation are only mildly affected.

of transmitting males. This is because grandsons are subjected to the risk of inheriting a **premutation from their grandfather** that is **amplified to a full mutation in their mothers' ova**. By comparison, brothers of transmitting (carrier) males, being higher up in the pedigree, are less likely to have a full mutation.

- **Transmission from carrier females with premutation:** When the premutation is passed on by a carrier female, there is a high probability of a dramatic amplification of the CGG repeats. This leads to intellectual disability in most male offsprings and 50% of female offsprings. In these 50% female offsprings, during the process of oogenesis, premutations can be converted to mutations by triplet-repeat amplification. This is the reason behind the unusual inheritance pattern.

Fragile X mental retardation protein (FMRP) It is the product of *FMR1* gene and FMRP is a widely expressed cytoplasmic protein. LOF of the FMRP underlies the molecular basis of intellectual disability and other somatic changes in FXS. As mentioned earlier, the normal *FMR1* gene contains range from 6 to 55 (average 29) CGG repeats in its 5′ UTR. When the number of trinucleotide repeats in the *FMR1* gene exceeds about 230, the DNA of the entire 5′ region of the gene undergoes abnormal methylation. Methylation also extends into the promoter region of the gene. This results in transcriptional suppression of *FMR1*. Absence of FMRP causes the phenotypic changes. FMRP is most abundant in the brain and testis. Hence, these are the two organs most affected in FXS. Functions of FMRP in the brain are as follows:

- **Regulates intracellular transport of mRNAs to dendrites (Fig. 50):** FMRP selectively binds mRNAs associated with polysomes. FMRP regulates the intracellular transport of mRNAs to dendrites. Unlike other cells, in neurons, protein is synthesized both in the perinuclear cytoplasm and in dendritic spines. Newly produced FMRP translocates to the nucleus. In the nucleus, FMRP assembles into a complex containing mRNA transcripts that encode presynaptic and postsynaptic proteins. The FMRP-mRNA complexes are then exported to the cytoplasm. From the cytoplasm they are trafficked to dendrites near neuronal synapses.
- **FMRP acts as a translation regulator**. FMRP helps to regulate production of other proteins and plays a role in synapse development. At synaptic junctions, FMRP suppresses protein synthesis from the bound mRNAs and acts as a translation regulator. This is a response to signaling through group I metabotropic glutamate receptors (mGlu-R). The reduction of FMRP in FXS results in increased translation of the bound mRNAs at synapses. This in turn leads to an imbalance in the production of proteins at the synapses. The imbalances result in loss of synaptic plasticity—the ability of synapses to change and adapt in response to specific signals. Synaptic plasticity is required for learning and memory. This is the molecular basis of intellectual disability in FXS.

Demonstration of an abnormal karyotype can identify FXS. Molecular DNA diagnostic testing (DNA-based analysis of triplet repeat) is available to identify fragile X premutation carriers as well as full FXS mutation. Polymerase chain reaction

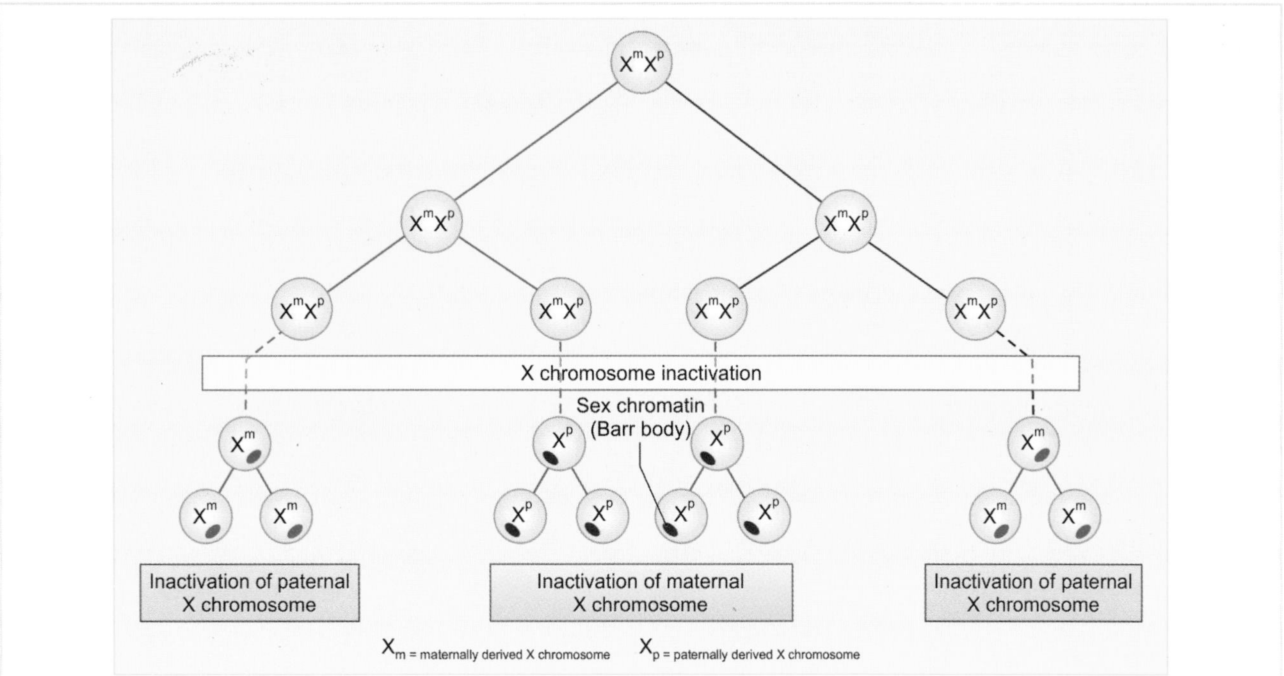

FIG. 41: Diagrammatic representation of X-chromosome inactivation during development (lyonization).

chromosomes (e.g., Klinefelter patients) have more than two functional copies. Several other genes outside the PAR also escape X inactivation and remain active in inactivated X chromosome. They are present in other loci on both long and short arms and one of the examples is *XIST* gene. At least some of the genes that are expressed from both X chromosomes are important for normal growth and development. A gene located in the PAR namely, ***short-stature HomeobOX (SHOX)* gene** (see **Fig. 40**), is associated with height. This notion is supported by the fact that patients with monosomy of the X chromosome (Turner syndrome: 45, X) have short stature and gonadal abnormalities. If a single dose of X-linked genes were sufficient, no detrimental effect would be expected in such individuals. This is due to haploinsufficiency of *SHOX* gene in Turner syndrome. Haploinsufficiency is as a condition in which the normal phenotype requires the protein product of both alleles, and reduction of 50% of gene function results in an abnormal phenotype. Extra copies of *SHOX* may be responsible for the increased stature in other sex chromosome aneuploidy conditions such as 47, XXX; 47, XYY; 47, XXY; 48, XXYY; and so forth. Mental retardation in phenotypic males and females with extra X chromosomes correlates roughly with the number of X chromosomes.

Demonstration of sex chromatin: There are two simple methods—

1. **Buccal smear for Barr body (sex chromatin) (Fig. 42A):** Barr and Bertram in 1949 identified the presence of tiny dark granule adjacent to the nuclear membrane. This granule is known as the Barr body, or X chromatin or sex chromatin. It represents one inactive and condensed X-chromosome in a female. The inactive X can be seen in the interphase nucleus as a darkly staining small mass in contact with the nuclear membrane.

   The number of Barr bodies in a cell depends upon the number of X chromosomes. It is always one less than the number of X chromosomes. Thus, normal cells in female (XX) have one Barr body and presence of Barr bodies indicates female genotype. Normal cells in male (XY) have no Barr bodies, because they have only one active X chromosome. The XXXY cells have two Barr bodies.

   Demonstration: Buccal smears used for demonstration of Barr body are prepared with a thin wooden spatula, by scraping the buccal mucosa. Smears are stained by Papanicolaou stain.

2. **Leukocytes—nuclear sexing (Fig. 42B):** Neutrophils in the peripheral smear may also be examined for nuclear sexing. Abnormalities of sex chromosomes can be diagnosed by nuclear sexing. In a normal female (XX), the neutrophils in a peripheral smear show a drumstick which is counterpart of Barr body in buccal smear.

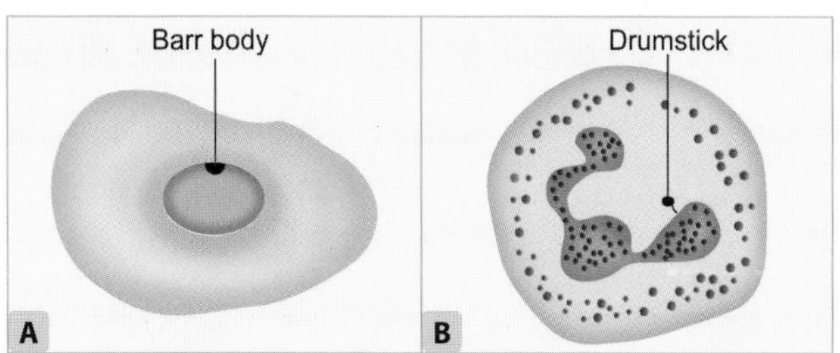

FIGS. 42A AND B: (A) Nuclei of intermediate squamous cell with Barr body; (B) Neutrophil with drumstick.

General features of disorders of sex chromosome

- **Subtle disorder:** Disorders of sex chromosome generally cause subtle, chronic problems relating to sexual development and fertility.
- **Diagnosis:** Disorders of sex chromosome are usually difficult to diagnose at birth, and many are first diagnosed at the time of puberty.

Table 16: Examples of trinucleotide repeat disorders.

Disease (trinucleotide repeat)	*Gene*	*Locus*	*Protein involved*
Expansions affecting noncoding regions			
Fragile X syndrome (CGG)	*FMRI (FRAXA)*	Xq27.3	FMR-1 protein (FMRP)
Friedreich ataxia (GAA)	*FXN*	9q21.1	Frataxin
Myotonic dystrophy (CTG)	*DMPK*	19q13.3	Myotonic dystrophy protein kinase (DMPK)
Expansions affecting coding regions (all have CAG trinucleotide repeat)			
Spinobulbar muscular atrophy (Kennedy disease)	*AR*	Xq12	Androgen receptor (AR)
Huntington disease	*HTT*	4p16.3	Huntingtin
Dentatorubral-pallidoluysian atrophy (Haw River syndrome)	*ATNL*	12p13.31	Atrophin-1
Spinocerebellar ataxia type 1	*ATXN1*	6p23	Ataxin-1
Spinocerebellar ataxia type 2	*ATXN2*	12q24.1	Ataxin-2
Spinocerebellar ataxia type 3 (Machado–Joseph disease)	*ATXN3*	14q21	Ataxin-3
Spinocerebellar ataxia type 6	*Ataxin-6*	19p13.3	α1A-voltage-dependent calcium channel subunit
Spinocerebellar ataxia type 7	*Ataxin-7*	3p14.1	Ataxin-7

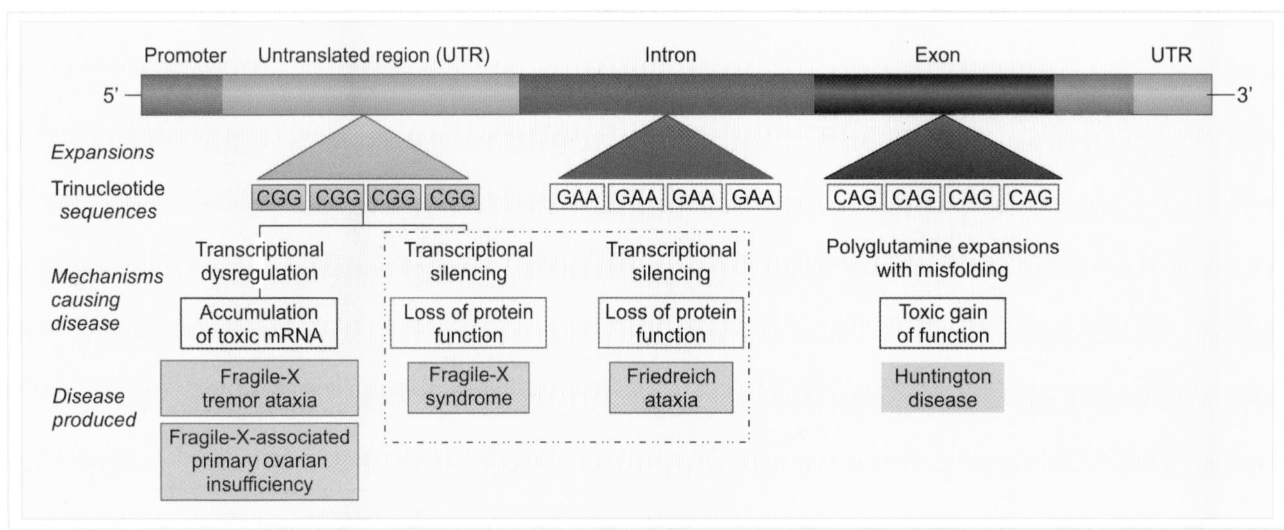

FIG. 47: Trinucleotide repeat mutations. Various sites of expansion, trinucleotide sequences involved, and mechanism of causing disease in few diseases.

- **Toxic gain of function mediated by RNA:** It is seen in fragile X-associated tremor/ataxia syndrome. The trinucleotide expansions involve the noncoding region of the gene.

- **Morphologic hallmark:** The diseases due to trinucleotide repeats are morphologically characterized by the **accumulation of aggregated mutant proteins** and form large **intranuclear inclusions**. Formation of aggregates is common to many polyglutamine diseases. But direct toxic role of aggregates is not common. According to some, these aggregations sequestrate the misfolded protein and thus may be protective.

Fragile X Syndrome

Q. Write short essay on FXS and *FMR* gene.

Fragile X syndrome (FXS) is the most common genetic cause of intellectual disability in males. It is second only to Down syndrome as a genetic cause of mental retardation. It results from a **trinucleotide expansion mutation in the *familial mental retardation 1*** *(FMR1)* gene. It was initially discovered as the cause of FXS. However, it is now known that expansion mutations affecting the *FMR1* gene are also present in two other well-defined disorders—fragile X-associated tremor/ataxia syndrome and fragile X-associated primary ovarian insufficiency.

Fragile X chromosome: The FXS derived its name from an inducible cytogenetic abnormal alteration (appearance) in the X chromosome within which the *FMR1* **gene** maps. When cells are cultured in a folate-deficient medium (impair DNA synthesis by methotrexate, floxuridine), the cytogenetic alteration was discovered as a **discontinuity of staining or as a constriction in the long arm of the X chromosome. Because it appears that the chromosome is "broken" at this site (Fig. 48), it was named as a fragile site.** This fragile site is close

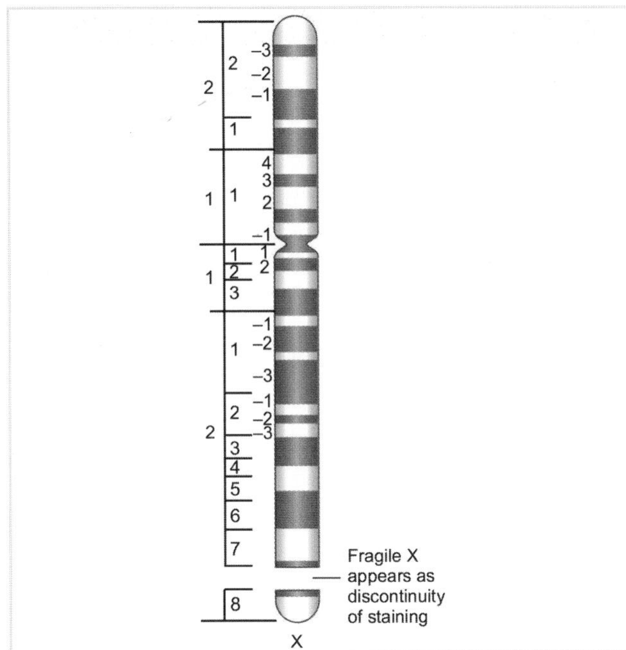

FIG. 48: X chromosome shows fragile X that appears as discontinuity of staining in the end of the long arm at Xq27.3.

to the telomere at the end of the long arm at Xq27.3. A fragile site is a nonstaining gap or constriction, represents a specific locus, or band usually involving both chromatids. This fragile site at the chromosome easily breaks (liable to break) under certain conditions.

Clinical features

Males with FXS

Physical features: It is an X-linked disease and affects mainly males. These patients have marked intellectual disability. They have a characteristic physical phenotype that includes increased head circumference, an elongated face with a large mandible, large protruding/everted ears, and large testicles (macroorchidism). In some patients, presence of hyperextensible joints, a high arched palate, and mitral valve prolapse mimics FXS to connective tissue disorder. However, these abnormalities are not always present, and in some, they are subtle. The most distinctive feature is macroorchidism, which is seen in about 90% of affected postpubertal males. A significant proportion of autistic boys has a fragile X chromosome.

Neurological features: Apart from intellectual disability, these patients have several neurologic and neuropsychiatric manifestations. These include epilepsy (in 30%), aggressive behavior (in 90%), autism spectrum disorder (includes several conditions such as autism and Asperger syndrome), and anxiety disorder/hyperactivity disorder.

Mode of transmission: Similar to other X-linked diseases, FXS affects mainly males. However, it shows some patterns of transmission that are not typically seen with other X-linked recessive disorders (**Fig. 49**).

- **Carrier males:** About 20% of males (as revealed by pedigree analysis and by molecular tests) are known to carry a fragile X mutation and they appear clinically normal. These carrier males transmit the trait through all their phenotypically normal daughters to affected grandchildren. Hence, they are called **normal transmitting males**. All of the daughters of a normal transmitting male will carry the premutation (refer below on page 871). Their sons are at risk of inheriting either the premutation or a full mutation.
- **Affected females:** About 30–50% of carrier females are affected (i.e., have intellectual disability and other features). Thus, the number of females affected are much higher than that observed in other X-linked recessive disorders.
- **Genetic anticipation (Sherman paradox) and risk of phenotypic effects:** Within fragile X families, the risk (probability of being affected) depends on the position of the individual in the pedigree. Later generations are more likely than earlier ones to be affected. The clinical features worsen with each successive generation, as if the mutation becomes increasingly deleterious as it is transmitted from a man to his grandsons and great grandsons (through daughters).

Molecular pathogenesis

The first breakthrough came to light when linkage studies localized the mutation responsible for FXS to Xq27.3, within the cytogenetically abnormal region. *FMR1* gene is located in this region of X chromosome. Mutation was characterized by multiple tandem repeats of the nucleotide sequence CGG in its 5′ UTR (see **Fig. 47**).

Normal CGG repeats: In the normal population, the number of CGG repeats in the DNA of a normal person is small and it range from 6 to 55 (average 29). These repeats are inherited in a stable fashion.

Premutations: Normal average of CGG repeat is about 29. Expansions of size of these CGG repeat region in males and females with 50–200 repeats of the CGG segment are said to have premutation. Normal transmitting males and carrier females carry 50–200 CGG repeats, thereby have premutations. During the process of oogenesis, but not during spermatogenesis, premutations can be converted to mutations. This convertion of premutations to mutations is by triplet-repeat amplification. Most individuals with premutation are intellectually normal. A male who carries a premutation is known as a "normal transmitting male". All of the daughters of a normal transmitting male will carry the premutation.

Full mutations: Patients with FXS have an **extremely large expansion of the CGG repeat region** (200–4,000 repeats) and this is termed as full mutation. Full mutations are the result of further amplification of the CGG repeats seen in premutations. Expansion of a premutation to a full mutation during gametogenesis occurs only in females (process of oogenesis). The presence and severity of clinical symptoms of FXS depend on the amplification (number) of the CGG repeats. In a female who carries a full mutation, there is a 50% risk that each of her sons will be affected with the full syndrome and that each of her daughters will inherit the full mutation (not depicted in **Fig. 49**).

The peculiar pattern of inheritance can be explained as follows:

- **Transmission from carrier (transmitting) males:** Carrier males transmit the CGG repeats to their progeny with **small changes in repeat number.** The probability of intellectual disability is much higher in grandsons than in brothers

able to conceive. About 5–10% of patients with Turner syndrome have Y chromosome sequences either as a complete Y chromosome (e.g., 45, X/46, XY karyotype) or as fragments of Y chromosomes translocated on other chromosomes. These mosaic karyotypes (i.e., 45, X/46, XY) have a 20% higher risk for development of a gonadal tumor (gonadoblastoma) and therefore prophylactic removal of the abnormal gonads is advisable.

The karyotypic heterogeneity in Turner syndrome is responsible for significant variations in phenotype. In individuals with high proportion of 45, X cells, the phenotypic changes are more severe than in those who have readily detectable mosaicism. The latter may appear almost normal and may have only primary amenorrhea.

Molecular pathogenesis

It is not completely understood. It is observed that in about 80% of cases, the X chromosome is maternal in origin. This point toward an abnormality in paternal gametogenesis.

Normal changes in ovary: Normally, both X chromosomes are active during oogenesis and are needed for normal development of the ovaries. During normal fetal development, ovaries have about 7 million oocytes. The oocytes gradually disappear and by menarche their numbers are reduced to almost 400,000, and when menopause occurs, <10,000 remain.

Ovary in Tuner syndrome: Ovaries of women with Turner syndrome show an acceleration of normal aging. In Turner syndrome, fetal ovaries develop normally early during the first 18 weeks of gestation. But due to the absence of the second X chromosome, there is an accelerated loss of oocytes. None of these oocytes remain by 2 years of age. Thus, in children with Turner syndrome, menopause may be considered to occur long before menarche ("menopause occurs before menarche"). The ovaries undergo atrophy forming fibrous strands/ streaks, without ova and Graafian follicles (streak ovaries). But the uterus, fallopian tubes and vagina develop normally.

Somatic features and *SHOX* gene in Turner syndrome: Many of the somatic features in Turner syndrome are determined by genes on the short arm of chromosome X, whereas genes on the long arm of chromosome X affect fertility and menstruation. Most important gene involved in the Turner phenotype is the critical regulator of growth *SHOX* gene at Xp22.33 (refer page 864). *SHOX* maps at the PAR of the X and Y chromosomes and escapes X inactivation (**Fig. 40**). Thus, both normal males and normal females have two copies of *SHOX* gene. Haploinsufficiency of SHOX in Turner syndrome is responsible for short stature. Deletions of the *SHOX* gene are observed in 2–5% of otherwise normal children with short stature. During fetal life, *SHOX* is expressed in the growth plates of many long bones such as the radius, ulna, tibia, and fibula as well as in the first and second pharyngeal arches. Loss of *SHOX* is associated with short stature, whereas excess copies of *SHOX* gene (in Klinefelter syndrome) are associated with tall stature. Though haploinsufficiency of *SHOX* can be responsible for growth retardation in Turner syndrome, it cannot explain other clinical features (e.g., cardiac malformations and metabolic abnormalities). Hence, several other genes on the short arm of X chromosome may be involved.

Clinical features (Fig. 46)

Infancy: Most severely affected infants usually present with edema of the dorsum of the hand and foot due to lymph stasis. They may also have swelling of the nape of the neck due to markedly distended lymphatic channels, producing cystic hygroma (cystic or nuchal lymphangioma). As these infants develop, the swellings subside but usually bilateral neck webbing and looseness of skin on the back of the neck persists.

Adults: Turner syndrome is usually not discovered before puberty. It is usually discovered when absence of menarche at puberty brings the child to medical attention. Important diagnostic features are:

- Adult women with short stature (<5 ft tall), primary amenorrhea and sterility. At puberty, normal secondary sex characteristics fail to develop. Turner syndrome is the most important cause of primary amenorrhea and is responsible for about one-third of the cases.
- Webbed neck (pterygium coli), low posterior hairline, wide carrying angle of the arms (cubitus valgus), broad chest with widely spaced nipples, and hyperconvex fingernails
- Failure to develop normal secondary sex characteristics such as infantile genitalia, inadequate breast development, and little pubic hair. The ovaries are converted to fibrous streaks.
- Pigmented nevi become prominent as the age advances.
- CVS anomalies such as congenital heart disease, particularly coarctation of the aorta and bicuspid aortic valve. About 5% of young women initially diagnosed with coarctation of aorta have Turner syndrome. Dilatation of aortic root is observed in 30% of cases, and there is a 100-fold higher risk of dissecting hematoma (aortic dissection). CVS abnormalities are the most important cause of increased mortality in children.
- Development of autoantibodies: About 50% show autoantibodies that react with the thyroid gland and about 50% of them may develop hypothyroidism.
- Mental status is usually normal.
- Others: Glucose intolerance, metabolic syndrome, obesity, nonalcoholic fatty liver disease, and insulin resistance in some patients. Renal anomalies such as horseshoe kidney and malrotation in 50% of patients.

Hermaphroditism and Pseudohermaphroditism

Sex of an individual can be defined on several levels. There are various criteria for determining sex.

- **Genetic sex:** It is determined by the presence or absence of a Y chromosome. Irrespective of number of X chromosomes, a single Y chromosome directs the testicular development and the genetic male sex. In the embryos, the initially indifferent gonads of both male and female have an inherent tendency to feminize, unless they are influenced by Y chromosome-dependent masculinizing factors.
- **Gonadal sex:** It is based on the microscopic features of the gonads.
- **Ductal sex:** It depends on the presence of derivatives of the Müllerian or wolffian ducts.
- **Phenotypic, or genital, sex:** It is based on the appearance of the external genitalia.

Sexual ambiguity is considered to be present if there is disagreement among the various criteria for determining sex.

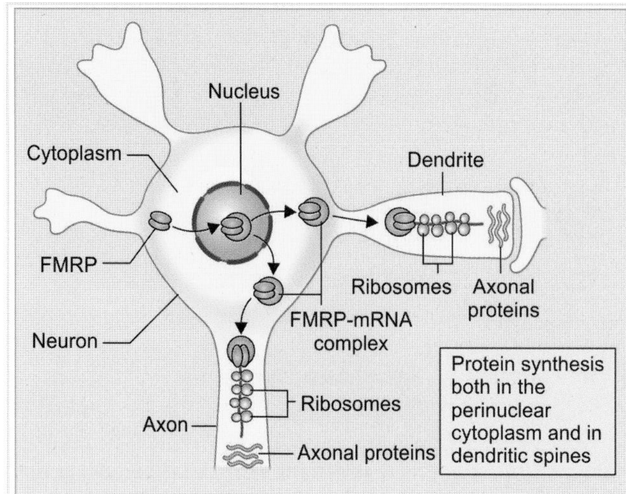

FIG. 50: Action of familial mental retardation protein (FMRP) in neurons. FMRP regulates intracellular transport of mRNAs to dendrites In neurons, FMRPs synthesized both in the perinuclear cytoplasm and in dendritic spines. Newly produced FMRP translocates to the nucleus and forms FMRP-mRNA complex These complexes are exported to the cytoplasm and trafficked to dendrites near neuronal synapses.

(PCR)-based detection of the repeats is presently the method of choice for diagnosis.

Fragile X-associated Tremor/Ataxia Syndrome and Fragile X-associated Primary Ovarian Failure

The CGG premutations in the *FMR1* gene can cause two other disorders that are phenotypically different from FXS and occur through a different involving a toxic gain-of-function.

Fragile X-associated primary ovarian failure

It was found that about 20% of females carrying the premutation (carrier females) have premature ovarian failure (before the age of 40 years). This condition is termed as fragile X-associated primary ovarian failure. Affected females have menstrual irregularities and decreased fertility. There are increased levels of FSH and decreased levels of anti-Müllerian hormone. Both the markers indicate declining function of the ovary. These patients develop menopause 5 years earlier than normal individuals. Aggregates containing FMR1 mRNA are seen in granulosa cells and ovarian stromal cells. Perhaps these aggregates are responsible for premature death of ovarian follicles.

Fragile X-associated tremor/ataxia

About 50% of premutation-carrying males (transmitting males) show a progressive neurodegenerative syndrome beginning in the sixth decade. This syndrome is termed as fragile X-associated tremor/ataxia. It is characterized by intention tremors and cerebellar ataxia and may progress to parkinsonism.

Pathogenesis: In this condition, the *FMR1* gene instead of being methylated and silenced, continues to be transcribed and CGG-containing FMR1 mRNAs, so formed, are "toxic." These toxic CGG-containing FMR1 mRNAs recruit RNA-binding proteins. They impair the function of RNA-binding by sequestration from their normal locales. The expanded FMR1 mRNA and the sequestered RNA-binding proteins aggregate in the nucleus. They form intranuclear inclusions both in the central and the peripheral nervous systems. Similar to FXS, males are affected much more frequently and more severely than female permutation carriers.

Mutations in Mitochondrial Genes

Mitochondria are cytoplasmic organelles. Their major function in all tissues and cells is to generate ATP by the process of OXPHOS (oxidative phosphorylation) under aerobic conditions. Other functions are free radical production, calcium homeostasis, and apoptosis (programmed cell death).

Mitochondrial Genes

Majority of genes (1,400+) are located on chromosomes in the nucleus of cell (nuclear genes or nDNA). These genes follow the rules and patterns of classic nuclear genomic Mendelian inheritance. There are also several genes (total 37) in mitochondria (mtDNA). Proteins in mitochondria are encoded by both nuclear (nDNA) and mitochondrial (*mtDNA*) genes. Most mitochondrial respiratory chain proteins are encoded by nuclear genes, but 13 such proteins are products of the mitochondrial genome.

- **Maternal inheritance:** Mitochondrial DNA is inherited in quite a different manner than nuclear genes or nDNA. A unique feature of these mtDNA is maternal inheritance, i.e., **only the maternal DNA is transmitted to the offspring**. This is because ova contain abundant cytoplasm with numerous mitochondria, whereas spermatozoa contain few, if any. The fertilized oocyte degrades mtDNA carried from the sperm in a complex process on the inner membrane of the oocyte. Hence, the mtDNA complement of the zygote is entirely derived from the ovum. Thus, although mothers transmit their mtDNA to all their offsprings, sons and daughters, only the daughters, but not her sons, are able to transmit the inherited mtDNA to future generations (**Fig. 51**).
- **Variability of mtDNA copies:** The number of mitochondria and the number of copies of mtDNA per mitochondrion vary in different tissues. Each aerobic cell in the body contains many (multiple) mitochondria generally numbering hundreds or more in cells with extensive energy production requirements. The number of copies of mtDNA within each mitochondrion varies from several to hundreds. This is true of both somatic as well as germ cells, including oocytes in females.

Mutations in Mitochondrial Genes

- **High mutation rate:** Most inherited defects in mitochondrial function are due to mutations in the mitochondrial genome itself. The rate of mtDNA mutation is much higher than that of nuclear DNA. This may be partly due to their lesser capacity to repair DNA.
- **Heteroplasmy (Fig. 52):** Each mitochondrion contains thousands of copies of mtDNAs within each cell, including the maternal germ cells. Generally, harmful mutations of mtDNA affect some but not all of these copies. Thus, tissues and, indeed, individuals may contain both normal (wild-type) and mutant mtDNA. Mutations in mtDNA lead to mixed populations of mutant and normal (wild-type) mitochondrial genomes. This phenomenon or situation

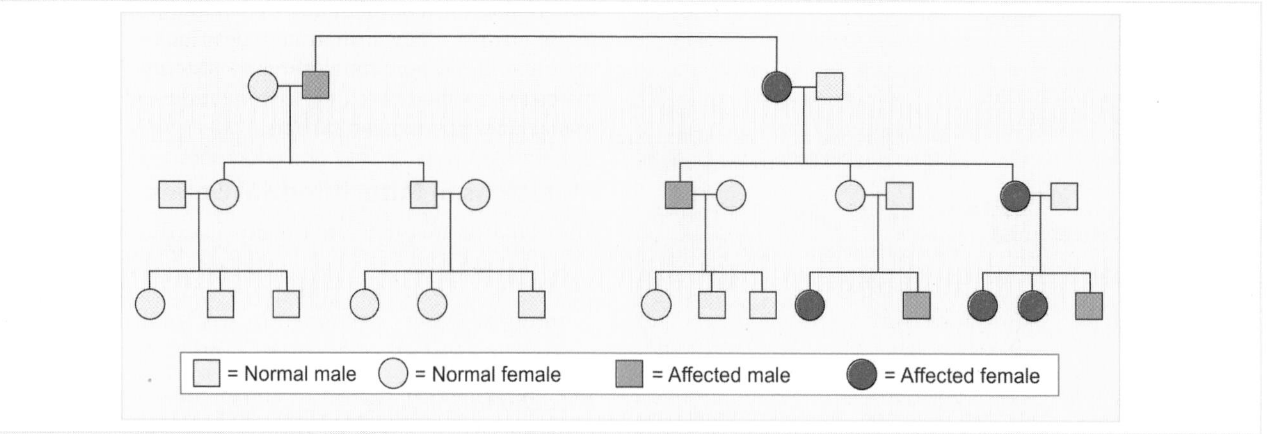

FIG. 51: Pedigree of maternal inheritance of mitochondrial DNA (mtDNA) disorders and heritable traits [e.g., Leber hereditary optic neuropathy (LHON), a disorder caused by mutation in mitochondrial DNA]. Affected males (green squares) do not transmit the trait to any of their offspring. Affected females (red circles) transmit the trait to all their children, male and female.

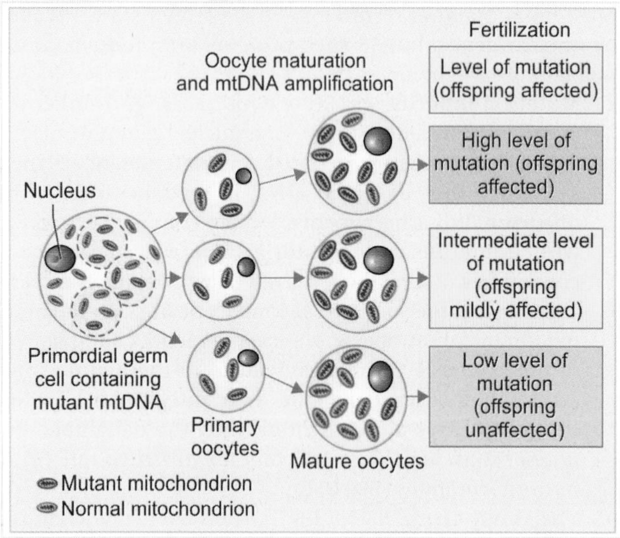

FIG. 52: Heteroplasmy. Mutations in mtDNA of primordial cells lead to mixed populations of mutant and normal mitochondrial genomes. This situation is called heteroplasmy and these primordial cells contain both normal and mutant mitochondria. During the production of primary oocytes from primordial germ cell, only a selected number of mitochondrial DNA (mtDNA) molecules (both normal and mutant) are transferred into each oocyte. During oocyte maturation, there is rapid replication of this mtDNA population. There is a random shift of mtDNA mutational load between generations. This is responsible for the variable levels of mutated mtDNA in affected offspring from mothers with pathogenic mtDNA mutations. Depending on the level of mutations, the offspring may be unaffected, mildly affected, or fully affected.

is called heteroplasmy. Heteroplasmy for a given mtDNA sequence variant or mutation arises as a result of the coexistence within a cell, tissue, or individual of mtDNA molecules bearing more than one version of the sequence variant. This is in contrast to much greater uniformity (homoplasy) of somatic nuclear DNA sequence.

- **Effects of mutations depend on ATP demand by tissue:** The phenotype of mtDNA mutations depends on the severity of the mutation, the proportion of mutant genomes, and the tissue's demand for ATP. Human mtDNA contains 37 genes. Of these 37, 22 are transcribed into transfer RNAs and 2 into ribosomal RNAs. The remaining 13 genes encode respiratory chain enzymes involved in OXPHOS. Different tissues require different amounts of ATP to sustain their metabolism. Thus, mutations affecting *mtDNA* genes exert their harmful effects mainly on the organs most dependent on OXPHOS. These particularly include the **CNS (brain), skeletal muscle, cardiac muscle (heart),** liver, and kidneys, that have high energy demands.
- **Threshold effect:** There should be minimum number of mutant mtDNAs in a cell or tissue before oxidative dysfunction produces a disease. This is called the "threshold effect." This threshold is most easily reached in the metabolically active tissues such as CNS (brain), skeletal muscle, cardiac muscle (heart), liver, and kidneys.
- **Variable expression of disease:** During cell division, mitochondria and their DNA are randomly distributed to the daughter cells. Similarly, when a cell containing normal and mutant mtDNA divides, the proportion of the normal and mutant mtDNA in daughter cells is extremely variable. This is responsible for the quite variable expression of disorders resulting from mutations in mtDNA.

Leber Hereditary Optic Neuropathy

Diseases associated with mitochondrial inheritance are rare. Many of the diseases caused by mutations in the mitochondrial genome mainly affect the nervous system, heart, and skeletal muscle. Functional deficits in all of these disorders are due to impaired OXPHOS.

Leber hereditary optic neuropathy is the first human mtDNA disease described. It is a model of disorder due to mitochondrial inheritance. It is a neurodegenerative disease characterized by progressive bilateral loss of central vision. Visual impairment is first brought to notice between 15 and 35 years of age. This finally progresses to blindness (loss of vision). Males in affected pedigrees are much more likely to develop visual loss than females. In some families, defects in cardiac conduction and minor neurologic manifestations have been observed.

Disorders Associated with Genomic Imprinting

Q. Write short essay on implications of genomic imprinting in human disease.
Q. Write short essay on gene silencing/imprinting.
Q. Write short essay on genetic disorders associated with maternal imprinting.

All individuals inherit two copies of each autosomal gene, carried on homologous maternal and paternal chromosomes. It was earlier thought that there is no functional difference between the alleles derived from the mother or the father. Now definite evidence has been found that, at least with respect to some genes, important **functional differences exist between the paternal allele and the maternal allele**. These **differences are due to an epigenetic process, called imprinting** (genomic/genetic imprinting). Epigenetics is the mechanisms and phenotypic changes that are not due to variation in the primary DNA nucleotide sequence, but are caused by secondary modifications of DNA or histones. Epigenetic gene inactivation on selected chromosomal regions is a phenomenon referred to as genomic imprinting. Mostly, **imprinting selectively inactivates either the maternal or paternal allele**. In **maternal imprinting**, there is transcriptional **silencing** (inactivation) **of the maternal allele**, whereas **in paternal imprinting**, there is **inactivation of paternal allele**. Imprinted genes, either the maternal or paternal allele, are maintained in an inactive state. Probable number of imprinted genes is the range from 200 to 600.

Mechanism of imprinting: Genomic imprinting is a normal physiologic process.

- **CpG methylation:** Similar to other epigenetic regulations, imprinting is associated with differential patterns of DNA methylation at CG nucleotides [i.e., predominantly on cytosines followed by guanine residues (**CpG methylation**) and "p" refers to the phosphodiester bond between cytosines and guanine]. CpG dinucleotides are abundant throughout the genome. The genomic imprinting by **CpG methylation occurs in regulatory regions of imprinted allele**, so that the **nonimprinted allele provides the sole biological function for that locus**. If the nonimprinted allele is damaged by mutation, the imprinted allele remains inactive and cannot compensate for the missing function.
- **Other mechanisms of genomic imprinting:** These include histone H4 deacetylation (deacetylation by histone deacetylases) and methylation (involves the addition of a methyl group to lysine residues in histone proteins).

Time and site of imprinting: Regardless of the mechanism, the imprinting of paternal and maternal chromosomes **occurs in meiosis during gametogenesis**. Thus, it occurs in the ovum or the sperm, before fertilization. From the moment of conception, some chromosomes remember whether they are paternal and maternal in origin. This pattern of imprinting is maintained to variable degrees in different tissues. This is stably transmitted to all somatic cells through mitosis. Imprinting is reset during meiosis in the next generation, so the selection of a given allele for imprinting can vary from one generation to the next. Though imprinted genes may occur in isolation, commonly they are found in groups. These groups are regulated by common cis-acting elements called imprinting control regions.

Genomic imprinting is best illustrated by certain hereditary diseases whose phenotype is determined by the parental source of the mutant allele. Two uncommon genetic disorders of genomic imprinting provide excellent examples of the effect of imprinting on genetic diseases. These are—(1) Prader-Willi syndrome (PWS) and (2) Angelman syndrome (AS). Both disorders are associated with (heterozygous) deletion in the region of 15(q11-13), but have remarkably different phenotypes.

Prader–Willi Syndrome and Angelman Syndrome

Prader–Willi syndrome: It is characterized by short stature, intellectual disability (learning difficulty), hypotonia, obesity, profound hyperphagia, small hands and feet, hypogonadism, and characteristic facies. In 65–70% of cases, there is an approximate 5 Mb **interstitial deletion of band q12 in the long arm of chromosome 15**, del (15) (q11.2q13) visible by conventional cytogenetics. In most cases, the breakpoints are the same. In 15% of patients, a submicroscopic deletion can be demonstrated by FISH or molecular methods. This deletion is striking that in all cases the deletion involves the **paternally derived chromosome 15**.

Angelman syndrome: Patients with AS also have intellectual disability, but also, they present with microcephaly, unsteady or ataxic gait, seizures (epilepsy), hyperactivity, and inappropriate laughter. Because of their hyperactivity, inappropriate laughter (happy affect), and unsteady or ataxic gait, these patients have been referred to as "happy puppets." In contrast to PWS, patients with the phenotypically distinct AS have a deletion of the same chromosomal region i.e., deletion involves the chromosome 15. But it is maternally derived (derived from their mothers) chromosome 15 and not from the father (not paternal). These two syndromes demonstrate the parent-of-origin effects on gene function.

Molecular basis: The molecular basis of PWS and AS depends on whether the genomic imprinting involves paternal or maternal chromosome (**Fig. 53**). Three molecular mechanisms are involved:

- **Deletions:** Deletions are responsible for about 70% cases. It may involve paternal gene or maternal gene.
    - **Deletion of paternal gene on chromosome 15:** Normally, genes or set of genes present on maternal chromosome 15q12 are imprinted (and hence silenced). The functional alleles of this chromosome are provided by the paternal chromosome. PWS develops because critical genes in the maternal locus are normally silenced by imprinting and the same region on the paternal chromosome is deleted. Because the functional alleles of paternal origin are lost due to deletion, there is a lack in its expression and the individual develops PWS.
    - **Deletion of maternal gene on chromosome 15:** The converse applies in AS. Normally, a distinct gene that maps to the same region of chromosome 15 is imprinted (and hence silenced) on the paternal chromosome.

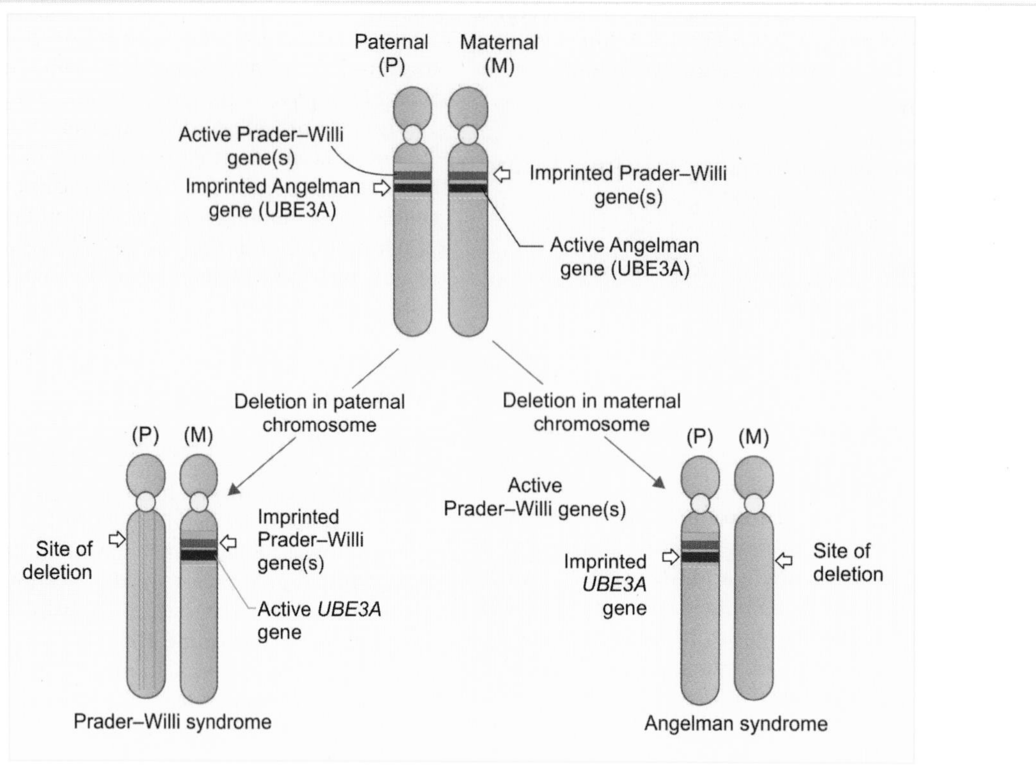

FIG. 53: Molecular basis of Prader–Willi syndrome and Angelman syndrome. It depends on whether the genomic imprinting involves paternal or maternal chromosome (for details refer text).

Only the maternally derived allele of this gene is normally active. Deletion or mutation of this maternal gene on chromosome 15 inactivates it and gives rise to the AS.

- **Uniparental disomy (UPD):** Normally, an individual inherits one of a pair of homologous chromosomes from each parent. Occasionally, however, **individuals may inherit both homologs of a chromosome pair** (both chromosomes of a pair) **from only one parent**. This is called as UPD. PWS without the deletion was found to have two maternal copies of chromosome 15. This UPD produces the same net effect. There is no functional set of genes from the (nonimprinted) paternal chromosomes. AS can also result from UPD of paternal chromosome 15. This is the second most common mechanism, accounting for 20–25% cases.
- **Defective imprinting:** In minority of patients (1–4%), there is a defect in genomic imprinting. Thus, in few patients with PWS, the paternal chromosome carries the maternal imprint, whereas in AS, the maternal chromosome carries the paternal imprint, this leads to absence of functional alleles.

Genetic basis: The genetic basis of PWS and AS is as follows:

- **Angelman syndrome:** In AS, the affected gene is a ubiquitin ligase. This catalyzes the transfer of activated ubiquitin to target protein substrates. The active Angelman gene is called *UBE3A* and maps within the 15q12 region. Normally, it is imprinted on the paternal chromosome, and is expressed from the maternal allele mainly in specific regions of the brain. Absence of this *UBE3A* gene inhibits synapse formation and synaptic plasticity. *UBE3A* is expressed from both alleles in most tissues. Thus, its imprinting is tissue specific.
- **Prader–Willi syndrome:** In this syndrome, there is no single gene implicated, but a series of genes located in the 15q11.2-q13 interval is probably involved. These series of genes is imprinted on the maternal chromosome and expressed from the paternal chromosome. These genes include the SNORP family of genes (encode small nucleolar RNAs) and cluster of small nucleolar RNAs (snoRNAs). The small nucleolar RNAs are noncoding molecules and they are involved in post-transcriptional modifications of ribosomal RNAs and other small nuclear RNAs. Probably loss of SNORP functions leads to PWS.

Molecular diagnosis: It depends on assessment of methylation status of marker genes, FISH, and array CGH.

It is to be kept in mind that genomic (genetic) imprinting is not restricted to only rare chromosomal disorders. Parent-of-origin effects are involved in a variety of inherited diseases such as Huntington disease and myotonic dystrophy and in tumorigenesis. In some tumors of childhood such as Wilms tumor, osteosarcoma, bilateral retinoblastoma, and embryonal rhabdomyosarcoma, the maternal allele of a putative tumor suppressor gene is lost. In these tumors, the remaining allele is on a chromosome of paternal origin.

Disorders Associated with Gonadal Mosaicism

Q. Write short essay on mosaicism.

New mutation during gametogenesis: In every autosomal dominant disorder, few patients may not have affected parents. In such patients, the autosomal dominant disorder is due to a new mutation occurring in the egg or the sperm of their parents. Hence, the siblings of such patients are neither affected nor have an increased risk for development of the disease.

Gonadal mosaicism: In few autosomal dominant disorders (e.g., OI), phenotypically normal parents have more than one affected child. This is clear violation of the laws of Mendelian inheritance. Such unusual pedigrees may be due to gonadal mosaicism. This mosaicism results from a mutation occurring postzygotically during early (embryonic) development. Postzygotic mutation may occur in cells destined to form germ cells or somatic cells. If the mutation occurs in only cells destined to form the gonads, then only the gametes carry the mutation. The somatic cells of this individual are completely normal. A phenotypically normal parent with gonadal mosaicism can transmit the disease-causing mutation to the offspring. This is through their mutated gametes. Since the progenitor cells of the gametes carry the mutation, it is possible that such a parent can transmit the disease to more than one child. Of course, such an occurrence depends on the proportion of germ cells carrying the mutation.

12.2 Molecular Diagnosis

CHAPTER OUTLINE

INTRODUCTION

A disease constitutes any abnormality in the living system. Causative agents for disease can be bacteria, virus, fungus, and parasites. Apart from this, mutation in genes can also cause many types of disorders and/or disease. Sequencing of human genome has made it easier to identify sequences that are altered or linked to a particular disease. It is not enough to identify such sequences but also necessary to develop a therapy or cure. Molecular biology tools are of great use for all these purposes.

Various uses of molecular diagnostic testing for genetic alterations are that they—(1) facilitate detection of disease detection, (2) aid in disease classification (diagnosis), (3) predict disease outcomes (prognostication), and/or (4) guide therapy. Apart from genetic alterations, nongenetic alterations can affect the expression of key genes. This is termed as epimutations. They contribute to the genesis of disease at many tissue sites. Epigenetic alterations can lead to gene silencing that are equivalent to inactivating mutations or gene deletions. Major types of genetic and epigenetic alterations causing disease are presented in **Box 12**.

During the initial half of the 20th century, the diagnosis of genetic diseases was by labor-intensive and low throughput methods. These included conventional karyotyping for diagnosis of cytogenetic disorders (e.g., Down syndrome) and DNA-based assays such as Southern blotting (e.g., for the diagnosis of Huntington disease). In the latter half of the 20th century, molecular genetic diagnostics came to use for diagnosis of genetic diseases. Molecular diagnostics needs techniques to detect sequence variations that are minute changes in complex genomes. In general, molecular diagnostics usually requires—(1) selection and amplification to the nucleic acid of interest, (2) visualization of the amplified nucleic acids, and (3) specific identification and often quantification of individual nucleic acid species.

Box 12: Major types of genetic and epigenetic alterations causing disease.

Genetic alterations

Nucleotide sequence abnormalities:

- Changes in individual genes
  - Involving single nucleotide changes (missense and nonsense)
    - Point mutations
  - Small insertions or deletions
    - Frameshift mutations
  - Trinucleotide repeat mutations

Chromosomal abnormalities:

- Gain or loss of one or more chromosomes (aneuploidy)
- Chromosomal rearrangements resulting from DNA strand breakage (translocations, inversions, and other rearrangements)
- Gain or loss of portions of chromosomes (amplification, large-scale deletion)

Epigenetic Alterations

- DNA methylation
- Modifications of histone proteins (by methylation and acetylation) and chromatin structure

Presently, many technologic breakthroughs and advances have led to improvement in terms of speed and cost. Various advances include the development of Sanger DNA sequencing (1977) and PCR (1983) and high throughput, massively parallel sequencing strategies (late 1990s). The high throughput, massively parallel sequencing strategies usually together come under the term next-generation sequencing (NGS). NGS has increased the speed of diagnosis. Nucleic acid-based testing is now taking a central role in the diagnosis and management of many diseases, and "old" technologies are being slowly supplanted by more comprehensive NGS-based approaches.

Nature of the sample: Following considerations will determine the nature of the sample used for the genetic test—

- **Constitutional versus somatic cell:** The genetic markers can be either constitutional (i.e., present in every cell of the affected individual; for example, CFTR mutation in a patient with cystic fibrosis) or somatic (i.e., found only in specific tissue types or lesions, for example, RAS mutations in human cancers).
- **Infections restriction to particular cells or tissues:** In case of suspected infections, nucleic acids that are specific to the infectious agent may be restricted to particular cells or body sites.

The nature of the sample used for the assay includes peripheral blood cells, tumor tissue, nasopharyngeal swab, etc.

DIAGNOSTIC METHODS AND INDICATIONS FOR TESTING

There are many techniques and indications for the molecular genetic diagnostic tests. Their choice is often problematic to both for molecular pathologists and for clinicians (who advise the optimal test for their patients).

Laboratory Considerations

Pathologists focus on the sensitivity, specificity, accuracy, and reproducibility of different methods. Apart from these, other factors such as cost, labor, reliability, and turnaround time also to be kept in mind. To select the most appropriate diagnostic technique, it is necessary to have a thorough knowledge of the spectrum of genetic anomalies that are responsible for the disease. Disease causing genetic diseases may be single base substitutions in the chromosome to gains or losses of entire chromosomes. It is necessary to have a close communication between clinicians, medical genetics specialists, and diagnosticians to select the optimal test strategy in difficult cases.

Indications for Analysis of Inherited Genetic Alterations

Mendelian disorders: Most genetic testing is performed during the prenatal or postnatal/childhood periods. However, it is not unusual for inherited genetic disorders to present in adulthood. There are thousands of Mendelian disorders caused by mutations in specific genes and definitive diagnosis is possible by DNA sequencing tests in most of these disorders.

Chromosomal aberrations: Other inherited disorders are due to chromosomal aberrations that usually present prenatally or at birth.

Timing of Genetic Tests

Depending on the timing of performing, these genetic tests can be divided into four types.

Preimplantation testing These test are done before conception (i.e., when one or two of the parents are carriers of a certain trait) on embryos created in vitro prior to uterine implantation to detect genetic changes in embryos. This is performed when parents are known to be at risk of having a child with a genetic disorder. It eliminates the chance of generational transmission of a familial disease.

Prenatal testing

Q. Write short essay on prenatal diagnosis methods and its utility.

Prenatal testing should be performed in all fetuses having a risk of a cytogenetic abnormality. Indications for prenatal testing are presented in **Box 13**. These are done after conception. Prenatal testing may also be needed for fetuses at known risk for Mendelian disorders (e.g., CF, spinal muscular atrophy) depending on family history. At present, these genetic tests are usually performed on cells obtained by amniocentesis, chorionic villus biopsy, or umbilical cord blood. About 10% of the free DNA in a pregnant mother's blood is of fetal origin. The new noninvasive **sequencing technologies** are performed by using this source of **DNA**.

Methods of prenatal diagnosis: There are various techniques available to determine the health and genetic disorders of fetus. These are discussed below.

Amniocentesis: Amniotic sac surrounds the fetus and contains amniotic fluid. Amniotic fluid consists of fetal urine and cells from fetal skin. The method of obtaining a small sample of amniotic fluid from the amniotic sac is known as amniocentesis. It is a well-established, reliable, safe, and widely available method for prenatal diagnosis of congenital disorders. It is usually performed between the 13 and 18 weeks of pregnancy. Amniocentesis is performed under ultrasound guidance to avoid damage to placenta and the fetus.

- **Procedure of amniocentesis (Fig. 54):** First the placenta, fetus, and amniotic fluid are located with the help of the ultrasound. With or without local anesthesia, a thin, hollow needle (22 gauge with a stylet) is inserted into the uterus through the abdomen. When the needle enters the amniotic sac, patient may feel a sharp pain for few seconds. About 10–20 mL of the amniotic fluid is aspirated. The fluid is normally clear and yellow. Remove the needle and apply bandage at the skin puncture site. Monitor the fetal activity

Box 13: Indications for prenatal testing.

- A mother of advanced age (>35 years) who has increased risk of trisomies
- A parent known to carry a balanced chromosomal rearrangement which increases the frequency of abnormal chromosome segregation during meiosis and the risk of aneuploidy in the fertilized ovum
- A fetus with abnormalities detected by ultrasound
- Routine maternal blood screening, indicating an increased risk of Down syndrome (trisomy 21) or another trisomy

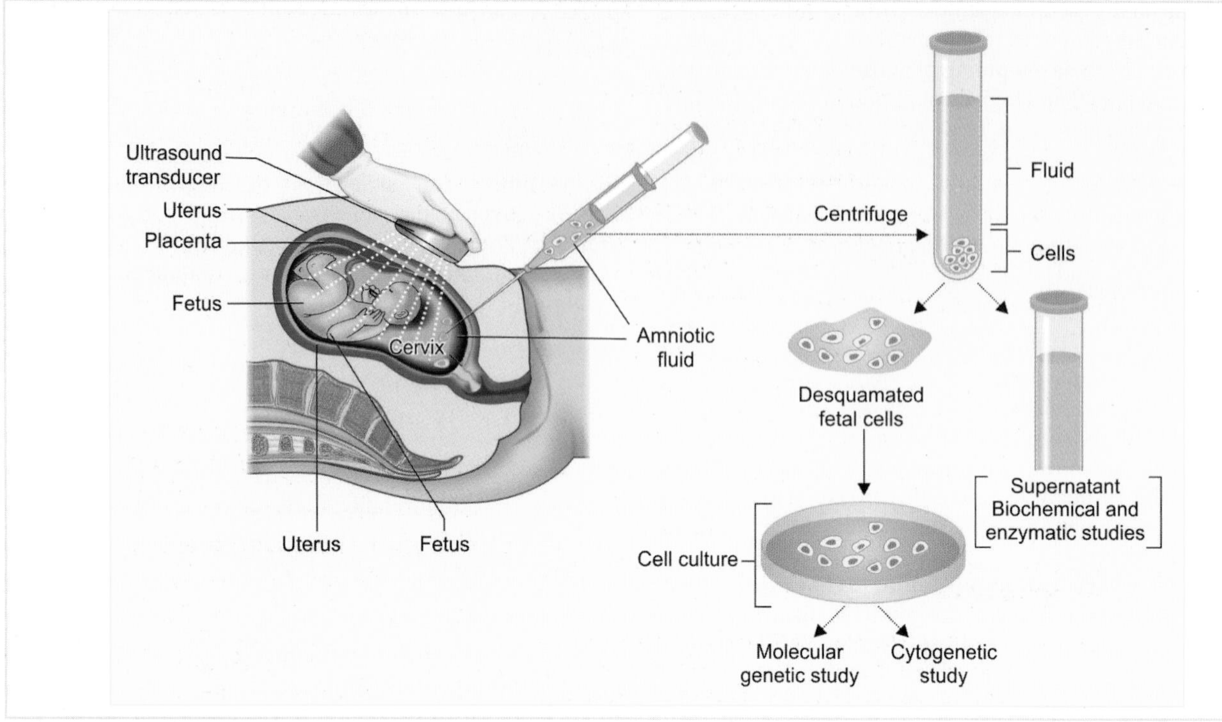

FIG. 54: Amniocentesis and its use for prenatal diagnosis.

by ultrasound. The amniotic fluid is centrifuged to separate the cells. The cells are then cultured for further karyotyping studies and DNA studies. The fluid is subjected to various biochemical tests for the detection of substances such as the α-fetoprotein, carcinoembryonic antigen, and others.

- **Indications for amniocentesis:** (1) For cytogenetic and chromosomal analysis of pregnancies at increased risk of Down syndrome or other chromosomal abnormalities; (2) In specific cases, biochemical analysis of amniotic fluid or cultured cells may be required for diagnosing inborn errors of metabolism; (3) It is performed in high-risk women (including those in whom the quadruple serum test is abnormal); (4) Sex determination for an X-linked disorder; and (5) For estimating α-fetoprotein concentration and acetylcholinesterase activity in amniotic fluid in pregnancies at increased risk of neural tube defects.

Q. Write short essay on chorionic villous sampling.

Chorionic villus biopsy/sampling: It is an invasive technique in which a piece of chorionic villus material of placenta is obtained. It is generally performed between 10 and 12 weeks of pregnancy. It is done either transcervically with a flexible catheter passing through the vagina and cervix into the uterus (**Fig. 55**) or by a needle inserted through the abdomen (transabdominal puncture). Both the methods are performed under ultrasound guidance, and piece of developing placenta is obtained. The viability of fetus is checked before and after the procedure.

- **Indications:** It is indicated for the diagnosis of chromosomal disorders or various genetic conditions by DNA analysis.
- **Advantages:** It can be performed during much earlier weeks of gestation than the amniocentesis. Results are usually ready within 1–2 weeks which permit earlier termination of pregnancy, if required. Earlier termination of pregnancy is safer than late pregnancy. More cells for study are obtained than amniocentesis.
- **Disadvantage:** Chorionic villus sampling (CVS) is not routinely done because it carries a risk of miscarriage and other complications.

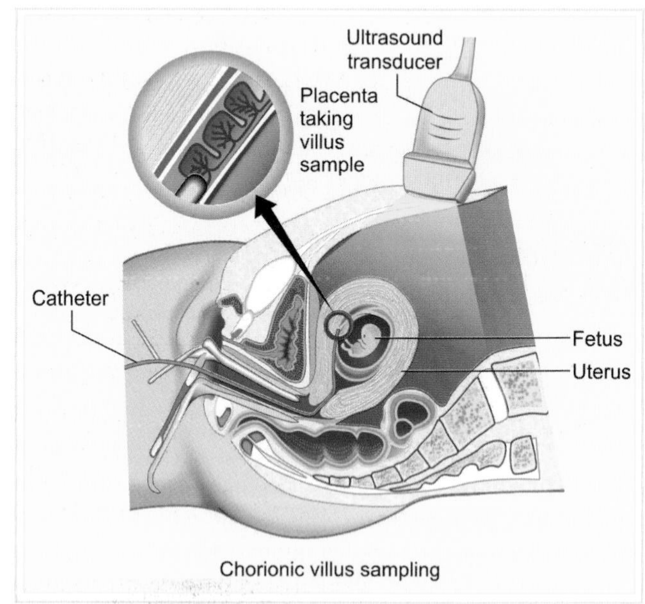

FIG. 55: Method of transcervical chorionic villus sampling.

Newborn and children genetic testing They are used to identify genetic disorders just after birth. It is done as soon as

Box 14: Indications for newborn and children genetic analysis.

- Major/multiple congenital anomalies
- Suspicion of a metabolic syndrome (e.g., phenylketonuria)
- Unexplained mental retardation (intellectual disability) and/or developmental delay
- Suspected aneuploidy (e.g., features of Down syndrome) or other syndromes associated with chromosomal abnormality (e.g., deletions, inversions)
- Suspected monogenic disease (previously described in the family or new)

Box 15: Indications for genetic test in adolescence and adulthood.

- Inherited cancer syndromes (family history of cancer with a known or suspected inherited predisposition or an unusual cancer presentation such as multiple cancer types or unusually young age at diagnosis)
- Atypically mild monogenic disease (e.g., attenuated cystic fibrosis)
- Family history of an adult-onset of neurodegenerative disorders (e.g., familial Alzheimer disease, Huntington disease)

the possibility of constitutional genetic disease arises so that it can be treated early in life. Indications for newborn and child genetic analysis are shown in **Box 14**. It is **usually performed on peripheral blood DNA**.

Genetic test in adults and older individuals In this age group, testing is more focused toward genetic diseases that manifest at later stages of life. More common indications are listed in **Box 15**.

Indications for Analysis of Acquired Genetic Alterations

In the present era, molecular targeted therapies are being increasingly used. So, it is important to identify nucleic acid sequences or aberrations that are specific for acquired diseases. It is especially useful in diagnosis and management of cancer and infectious disease. Common indications are listed in **Box 16**.

Box 16: Common indications for analysis of acquired genetic alterations.

Diagnosis and management of cancer

- To detect tumor-specific acquired mutations and cytogenetic alterations that are characteristic of specific tumors; for example, *BCR-ABL* fusion genes in chronic myelogenous leukemia or CML
- To identify specific genetic alterations which help in choosing therapy; for example, *HER2* (official gene name *ERBB2*) amplification in breast cancer and *EGFR* (official gene name *ERBB1*) mutations in lung cancer
- To determine the efficacy of treatment; for example, to detect minimal residual disease in patients with CML by quantitative PCR for BCR-ABL
- To determine clonality as an indicator of a neoplastic condition
- To detect drug-resistant secondary mutations in malignant tumors treated with target therapies to specific proteins (e.g., mutated EGFR)

Diagnosis and management of infectious disease

- To detect microorganism-specific genetic material for definitive diagnosis; examples include human immunodeficiency virus (HIV), mycobacteria, human papillomavirus, and herpes virus in central nervous system
- To identify specific genetic alterations in the genomes of microbes in case of drug resistance
- To determine efficacy of treatment, e.g., to assess viral loads in HIV, hepatitis C virus infection, and Epstein–Barr virus

(EGFR: epidermal growth factor receptor; PCR: polymerase chain reaction)

TOOLS OF MOLECULAR DIAGNOSTICS

Q. Write short essay on laboratory diagnosis of genetic diseases.

Q. Write short essay on techniques employed for diagnosis of chromosomal disorders.

Q. Write short essay on diagnostic applications of molecular techniques related to genetic disorders.

Molecule is the smallest physical unit of an element or compound, consisting of one or more like atoms in an element and two or more difficult atoms in a compound. Moleculardiagnostics is a term used for a family of techniques used to analyze biological markers in an individual's genetic code (genome) and to analyze how their cells express their genes as proteins (proteome). In simple terms, it is the analysis of molecules namely, nucleic acids and proteins. Recent advances in molecular knowledge have revolutionized the field of diagnostic medicine.

Nucleotide is the smallest basic unit of genetic information. It consists of a deoxyribose (five carbon sugar) with an attached nitrogenous base and a phosphate group. The nitrogenous base can either be a purine (A or G) or a pyrimidine (C or T). Nucleotides attach to each other linearly and form long strands (polynucleotides). These strands serve as the basic genetic code and are referred to as DNA. DNA isolation is an essential technique in molecular biology. Molecular diagnostics is one of the fastest growing segments of laboratory medicine.

At present, it is possible to clone disease-causing genes and the proteins that they encode. It is possible to detect the presence of these genes and proteins in the serum and other body fluids and tissues of patients, even though they may be present in small amount. This detection is possible because of development of new, highly sensitive methods/techniques by which gene or protein molecules may be amplified. These methods include PCR, branched-DNA (BDNA), FISH, and MS (mass spectrometry). MS is very useful for the identification of proteins that are involved in causing disease. All these diagnostic approaches constitute diagnostic or clinical molecular biology or molecular diagnostics. Many of these techniques are capable of analyzing single patient samples for multiple genes or proteins. The expression of multiple genes and also whole genomes can be assayed on microarrays. Some of these processes are completely automated.

Uses of Molecular/Diagnostics (Box 17)

For the diagnosis of disease: There is a growing demand for molecular diagnostics in many different clinical indications. These include infectious disease, medical genetics, and molecular oncology. They are useful in diagnosis and treatment of the patient. In many, such diseases are associated with well-defined, reproducible chromosomal abnormalities. It is possible to identify increasing numbers of genes on chromosomes that are strongly responsible in causing disease by the FISH technique. FISH is major advancement in the diagnosis of disease, and it can detect gene rearrangements and gene deletions in a number of diseases (e.g., cancer).

Infectious organisms: Molecular diagnostic tests are used for rapid detection of certain infectious agents and are especially useful for agents that are difficult to culture or take a long time to grow on culture media. Molecular pathology techniques are used to genotype infectious agents such as HIV.

Forensic purposes: It is possible to identify single gene mutations in patients' DNA that may either be resulting disease or may simply be polymorphisms. Identification of polymorphisms can be used in establishing the parentage of children and the investigation of crime. Thus, molecular diagnostics laboratory can also be used for forensic purposes.

Personalized medicine: The patients can be genetically tested for the most appropriate drug therapy. This is most successfully used for anticoagulant and antiplatelet therapies.

Applications of molecular diagnostics are depicted in **Figure 56.**

Steps in Molecular Pathology

The various steps for many molecular pathological tests follow a similar scheme (**Fig. 57**).

Nucleic Acid Extraction

Starting step in almost all molecular diagnostic applications is efficient extraction of high-quality nucleic acids, DNA and RNA (including mRNA, miRNA), from biological samples.

Box 17: Uses of molecular diagnostics.

- For the diagnosis and monitor of disease
- To detect risk or predict the occurrence of disease
- To predict the prognosis of diagnosed disease
- To guide therapy: Personalize therapies by determining which treatments will work best for an individual patient

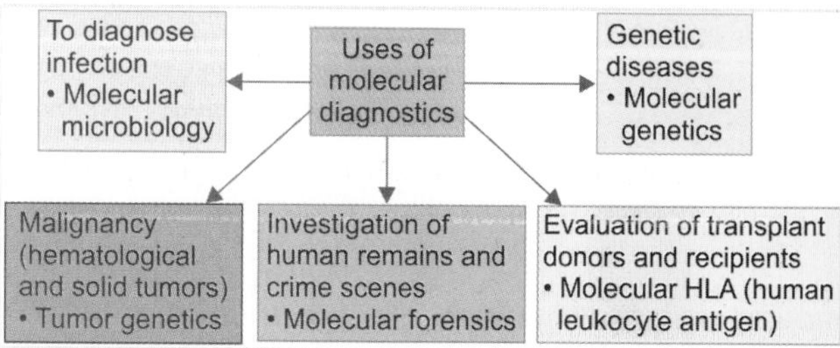

FIG. 56: Application of molecular diagnostics.

- **Manual extraction methods:** They range from chemical-based extractions depending on manual phenol-chloroform purification, to the use of manufactured extraction kits. These kits utilize silica-based spin column or magnetic bead nucleic acid purifications. In this method, in silica-based spin column method, a digested sample is loaded onto a column to which nucleic acids bind in the presence of chaotropic salts. Microcentrifugation of the column followed by washing removes proteins and other macromolecules. Then, nucleic acids are eluted with buffer or water. The biological samples used in the molecular diagnostics laboratory are of wide variety (**Box 18**). Hence, the manual extraction methods vary with the sample used and require highly trained technologist with significant expertise in specific extraction method.
- **Automated techniques** for nucleic acid extraction: Advantages are—(1) it increases extraction efficiency, and quality; (2) it reduces turnaround time; and (3) it reduces inter- and intra-operator variability and results. Commonly used automated nucleic acid extraction is performed using magnetized glass beads techniques. After the cell

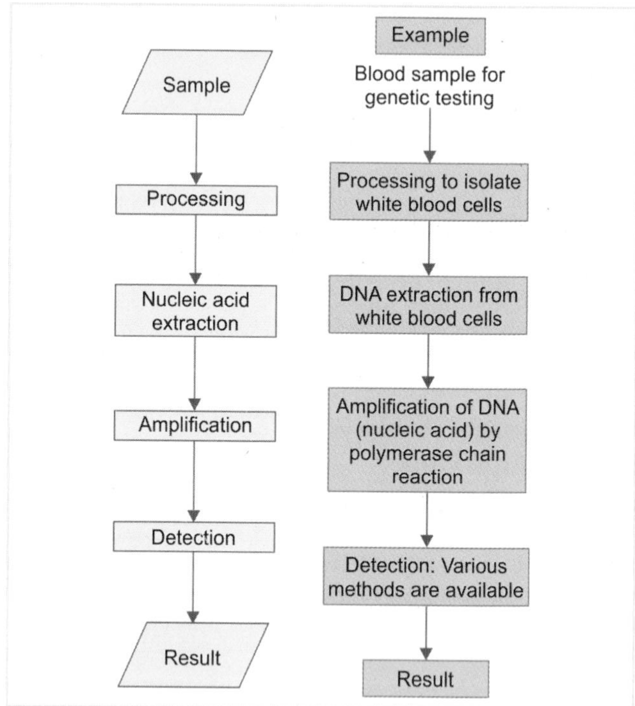

FIG. 57: The general steps in molecular diagnostic protocols.

Box 18: Various biological samples used in the molecular diagnostics laboratory.

- Whole blood
- Urine
- Saliva
- Feces
- Buccal and nasopharyngeal swabs
- Bone marrow biopsies
- Fresh and frozen tissues
- Formalin-fixed paraffin-embedded tissue

lysis, nucleic acids bind to the glass beads, which can be robotically manipulated with a magnet. The beads are washed, and then nucleic acids are eluted with water or a buffer. These machines are capable of processing various sample types (e.g., plasma, whole blood, fresh tissue, and formalin-fixed tissue). They are used for isolation of total nucleic acid, DNA, and RNA.

Basic Techniques used in Molecular Diagnostics

One of the main purposes in molecular diagnostics is to identify aberrations in the genetic code. It can be done by using many methods. A molecular technique is selected depending on the genetic aberration that is to be detected.

- **Techniques that provide an overview of the entire DNA genome:** In general, an overview of the entire DNA genome is provided by a cytogenetic technique such as **conventional karyotyping, virtual karyotyping, or FISH**. It is comparable (analogous) to having an aerial overview of a forest.
- **Techniques that provide information on specific parts of the DNA genome: PCR techniques** provide information on specific parts of the DNA genome. It is comparable (analogous) to looking at individual trees in a forest.
- **Techniques that provide detailed view of the DNA genome: Sequencing techniques** give a detailed view of the DNA genome. It is comparable (analogous) to data on how many leaves or branches are on an individual tree.

TECHNIQUES THAT PROVIDE AN OVERVIEW OF THE ENTIRE DNA GENOME

These include conventional karyotyping, virtual karyotyping, special karyotyping or FISH.

Cytogenetic Karyotyping

Cytogenetic karyotyping is a cytogenetic technique used for an overview of cytogenetic abnormalities of the patient's chromosomes. Examples of these abnormalities include aneuploidy (changes in chromosome numbers), translocations, inversions, and deletions. In classic karyotyping, cells from various sources (e.g., blood, bone marrow, tumor, or amniotic fluid) are cultured to grow on cell plates. This is followed by addition of a mitotic inhibitor such as colchicine to the cell culture to stop the mitosis at metaphase. Then the inhibitor is removed and the cells are placed in a hypotonic solution. Hypotonic solution lyses the RBCs and more importantly produces swelling of the white blood cells. This allows for the individual chromosomes from the white blood cells to spread out for analysis. Next the cells are fixed and stained with different types of stains. Then they are arranged by a cytogenetic specialist. The chromosomes are arranged in pairs from chromosome 1 (largest) to chromosome 22 (smallest) with the sex chromosomes at the end. The short arm of the chromosome is oriented toward the top and the long arm is oriented toward the bottom. It is analyzed by a cytogenetic specialist (It is discussed on pages 849–851).

Virtual Karyotyping

Virtual karyotyping is a relatively newer technology in the cytogenetics. In virtual karyotyping, **copy number changes** (e.g., gains, deletions, and amplification) **can be identified at a higher resolution** (10–20 kb) than in conventional karyotyping (5–10 Mb). However, it **cannot identify balanced translocations, inversions, and ringed chromosomes** because there are no copy number changes. Therefore, it serves as an adjunct to traditional cytogenetic techniques and not as a replacement. Virtual karyotyping is performed by hundreds to millions of probes. These probes are attached to an array hybridizing to fragmented DNA. These fragments of DNA are both from normal DNA and DNA from tissue of interest. The ratio of the hybridization signal between DNA of interest and normal DNA is captured by the virtual karyotyping hardware. Since the location of the probes on the chromosomes is known; the software is capable to reconstruct in silico the chromosomes visually on a computer. Since it is possible to see the ratio between the normal and the tissue in question, the pathologist interpreting the virtual karyotype is able to determine whether copy number changes are present. Two main types of virtual karyotype used are—(1) aCGH (see page 77 and 78) and (2) SNP array (see page 78 and 79). SNP arrays are popular due to the added advantage of being able to detect copy number neutral loss of heterozygosity.

Spectral Karyotyping

Q. Write short essay on SKY.

Special karyotyping (SKY) is a novel multicolor probe hybridization-based cytogenetic technique. It unambiguously (not open to more than one interpretation) displays and identifies all 24 human chromosomes at one time without any prior knowledge of any abnormalities involved. SKY **can recognize the aberrations that cannot be detected by conventional banding technique and FISH**. Hence it is very accurate and sensitive. It can analyze chromosome rearrangements involving the whole or a portion of a chromosome(s), translocations involving two or more chromosomes, and to identify marker chromosomes not resolvable by banding technique (e.g., G-band karyotype analysis).

Spectral karyotyping and multicolor FISH (refer page 897) are both advanced molecular cytogenetic techniques for chromosome analysis. They are based on the principle of FISH. Both these techniques visualize all the chromosomes simultaneously by labeling them with a combination of different colors that are spectrally distinguishable fluorochromes. But different methods are used to detect and discriminate the different combinations of fluorescence after ISH (in situ hybridization).

- **SKY:** The images are captured by charge-coupled device (CCD) imaging and analyzed by using optical microscopy. Image processing software then assigns a pseudo color to each spectrally different combination. This allows the visualization of the individually colored chromosomes.
- **Multicolor FISH:** In this, each homologous pair of chromosomes is uniquely labeled with five fluorochromes set which are spectrally distinct in different combinations. The images are captured by band-pass filter sets. The defined emission spectra are measured by M-FISH software.

Components: SKY combines spectroscopy, CCD imaging, and optical microscopy, to measure simultaneously at all

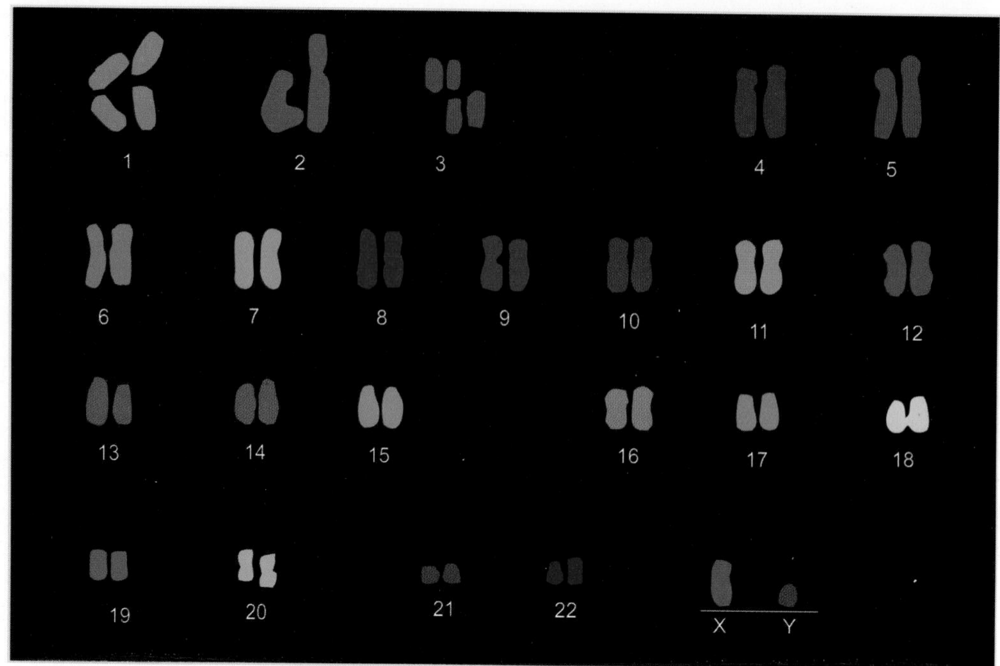

FIG. 58: Spectral karyotyping in a normal male (diagrammatic).

points in the sample emission spectra in the visible and near-infrared range. Thus, it allows the use of multiple spectrally overlapping probes. Hybridization signals are captured using a fluorescent microscope equipped with special devices and image processing software.

Major steps in SKY: These include—(1) hybridization, (2) image acquirement, and (3) analysis of results. Metaphase chromosomes from a specimen of interest are required for this analysis.

Characteristics of SKY: These are FISH-based methods that allow the simultaneous display of all chromosomes in different colors (**Fig. 58**) using five fluorochromes, alone and in combination in a single experiment. This employs a different approach to acquire image. The advantage of SKY is that it can immediately identify interchromosomal aberrations (e.g., translocations cause two color differences on the derivative chromosome), as well as the identification of complex rearrangements. However, small deletions, duplications, and intrachromosomal inversions do not produce recognizable color change. The resolution of SKY for the detection of interchromosomal rearrangements is between 500 and 2,000 kb (FISH is discussed in detail on pages 897–900).

TECHNIQUES THAT PROVIDE INFORMATION ON SPECIFIC PARTS OF THE DNA GENOME

PCR and Detection of DNA Sequence Alterations

Q. Write short essay/note on PCR.

Kary Mullis in 1983 discovered PCR and has revolutionized molecular diagnostics. PCR is an in vitro technique in molecular biology. The basic goal of PCR is to selectively amplify minute amount (single or a few copies to several orders of magnitudes) of specific target nucleic acid sequences (i.e., target DNA) within a few hours. The amplification is achieved by using primers specific for the target region to be amplified. It produces many copies of a target DNA in order to examine that particular focus of DNA more closely. It is a very simple technique for characterizing, analyzing, and synthesizing DNA from virtually any living organism (plant, animal, virus, bacteria).

For the last few decades, PCR analysis has been a mainstay of molecular diagnostics. It is a widely used powerful tool in the molecular diagnosis of human disease.

Principle: PCR involves synthesis of relatively short DNA fragments from a DNA template. It is achieved by using and thermal cycling. DNA sequence information is used to design two oligonucleotide primers (amplimers) of approximately 20 bp in length. These primers are complementary to the DNA sequences flanking the target DNA fragment. The first step in PCR is to denature the double-stranded DNA of interest and separate it into two individual strands by heating. Each strand is then allowed to hybridize with a primer. The primers then bind to the complementary DNA (cDNA) sequences of the single-stranded DNA templates of target DNA. Appropriate heat-stable DNA polymerases extend the primer DNA in the presence of the deoxynucleotide triphosphates (dATP, dCTP, dGTP, and dTTP) to synthesize the cDNA sequence. Subsequent heat denaturation of the double-stranded DNA, followed by annealing of the same primer sequences to the resulting single-stranded DNA, will result in the synthesis of further copies of the target DNA. About 30–35 successive repeated cycles result in more than 1 million copies (amplicons) of the DNA target. The specific fragment of DNA (target DNA) is amplified to generate large quantities (thousands to millions of copies usually <1,000 bp) of particular DNA fragments of interest. PCR is mostly used to amplify DNA fragments up to 1 kb. Long-range PCR allows the amplification of larger DNA fragments of up to 20–30 kb.

Source of material: PCR can analyze DNA from any cellular source containing nuclei. Thus, it includes blood as well less invasive samples, such as saliva, buccal scrapings, or pathological archival material.

Quantity of DNA required: It is possible to start with quantities of DNA as small as that from a single cell (e.g., in preimplantation genetic diagnosis). Great care is needed with PCR because DNA from a contaminating extraneous source (e.g., desquamated skin from a laboratory worker) will also be amplified. This can give false-positive results.

Components required for a basic PCR are listed in **Box 19**.

Basic steps (Fig. 59) Synthesis and amplification of DNA are done through multiple thermal cycles. This cycle consists of three steps—denaturing, annealing, and extension. This is followed by a final elongation and hold step.

- **Denaturation:** In this step, the double-stranded template DNA is denatured by heat (temperature of around 92–96°C) into single-stranded DNA.
- **Annealing:** DNA primers of interest are added along with the four basic deoxynucleotides and the solution is cooled. It causes binding of DNA probes to their specific target regions of the single-stranded DNA at a temperature of around 50–65°C.
- **Extension/elongation:** The primers are extended at a temperature of around 68–78°C in the presence of DNA polymerase, dNTPs, and Mg^{2+} ions. The newly synthesized DNA strand acts as a template for the next cycle. This cycle is repeated several times (around 25–30 times) and produces millions of copies of the original specific target DNA. To retain the activity of DNA polymerase enzyme at such high denaturation temperature, Taq DNA polymerase, extracted from a microorganism (*Thermus aquaticus*), is used in the PCR reaction.

Various steps involved in amplification of a DNA segment by the polymerase chain reaction are presented in **Fig. 60**.

Final elongation: This single step is occasionally performed at a temperature of 70–74°C for 5–15 minutes after the last PCR cycle. This is done to ensure that any remaining single-stranded DNA is fully extended. Denaturation, annealing, and extension steps are repeated 20–30 times in an automated thermal cycler that can heat and cool the reaction mixture in tubes within a very short time. This results in exponential accumulation of specific DNA fragments, ends of which are defined by 5′ ends of the primers. The doubling of the number

Box 19: Components required for a basic polymerase chain reaction (PCR).

- **Target DNA** (to be examined)
- **DNA template** or cDNA that contains the region to be amplified
- **Two primers** complementary to the 3′ ends of each of the sense and antisense strand of the DNA which sets up the boundaries to the DNA to be amplified.
- Thermostable **DNA polymerase** such as Taq, Vent, and Pfu
- **Deoxynucleoside triphosphates** (dNTP): These include mixtures of deoxyadenosine triphosphate (dATP), deoxycytidine triphosphate (dCTP), deoxyguanosine triphosphate (dGTP), and deoxythymidine triphosphate (dTTP). These are the building blocks from which the DNA polymerase synthesizes a new DNA strand by adding nucleotides (A, G, T, C)
- **Buffer solution** which provides a suitable chemical environment for optimal activity and stability of DNA polymerase
- **Bivalent cations** such as magnesium or manganese (Mg^{2+} or Mn^{2+}) are necessary for maximum Taq polymerase activity and influence the efficiency of primer to template annealing
- **Monovalent cation** such as K^+ to facilitate correct primer annealing

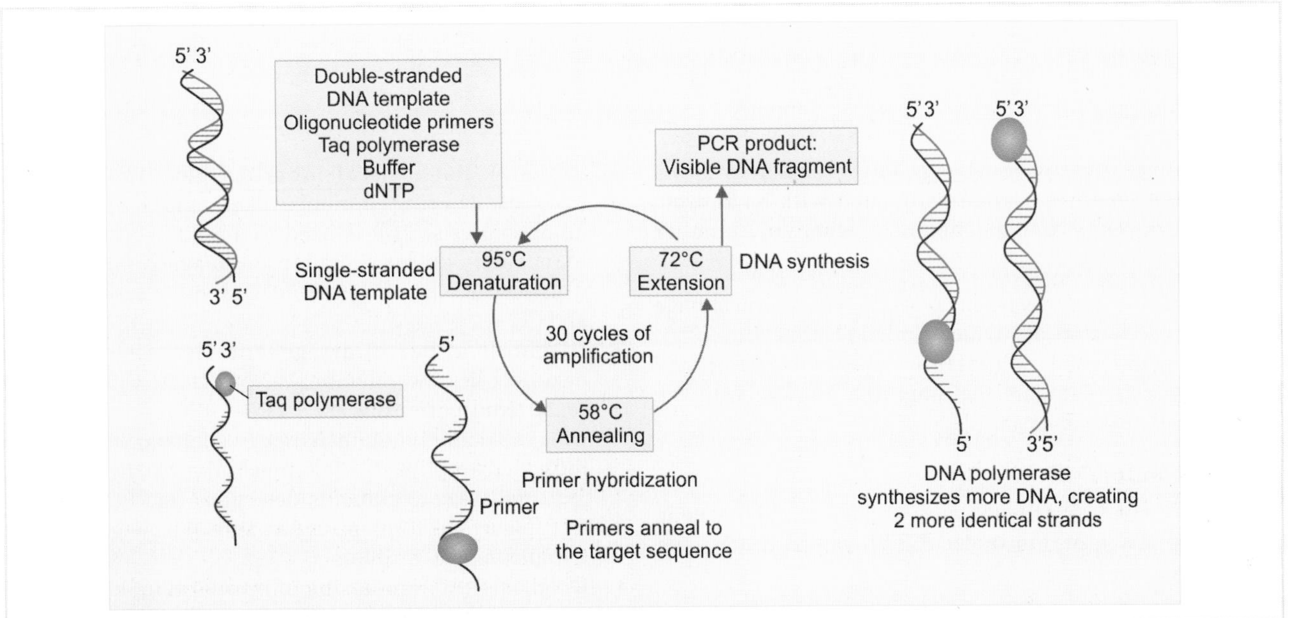

FIG. 59: Three steps and typical temperatures for each step in a single polymerase chain reaction (PCR) cycle. One cycle of PCR amplification is shown. Each cycle consists of three steps—(1) template denaturation, (2) primer annealing, and (3) primer extension. Each step usually occurs over 15–30 seconds and can vary depending on the instrument.

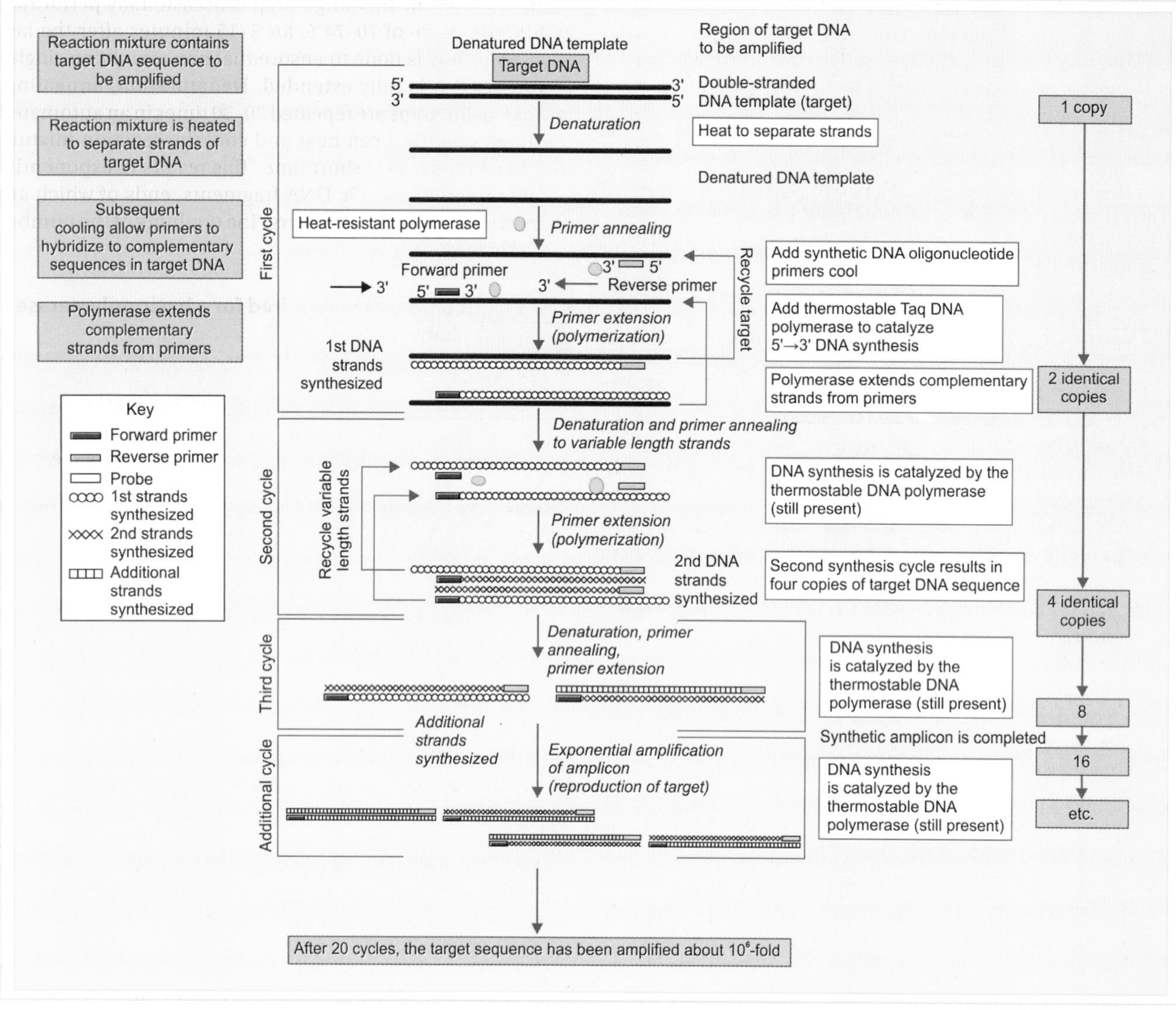

FIG. 60: Amplification of a DNA segment by the polymerase chain reaction (PCR). The PCR procedure has three steps. DNA strands are separated by heating, followed by annealing to an excess of short synthetic DNA primers. These primers flank the region to be amplified and a new DNA strand is synthesized by polymerization catalyzed by DNA polymerase. The three steps are repeated for 25 or 30 cycles in an automated process carried out in a thermocycler.

of DNA strands corresponding to the target sequences allows to estimate the amplification associated with each cycle using the formula—Amplification = 2n, where n = number of cycles.

Final hold: This step may be employed for short-term storage of the reaction mixture at 4°C for an indefinite time.

After completion of the PCR, perform agarose gel electrophoresis. Compare the amplified product with the ladder and determine its size.

Applications of PCR

PCR is the starting test used in most of the molecular genetic tests. It is very useful in molecular biology and has wide applications.

PCR in clinical diagnosis: It is useful in the diagnosis of various diseases such as inherited disorders (genetic diseases), viral diseases, and bacterial diseases.

- **Prenatal diagnosis of inherited/genetic disorders/diseases:** By using chorionic villus samples or cells from amniocentesis. PCR is used to amplify gene segments that contain known mutations for diagnosis of inherited diseases such as sickle cell anemia, β-thalassemia, PKU, and CF.
- **Diagnosis of hereditary/genetic diseases:** In genetic disorders, genetic mutations can be detected by PCR alone (e.g., Huntington disease), PCR followed by digestion with restriction endonucleases (e.g., diagnosis of spinal muscular atrophy), PCR followed by dot-blot hybridization (e.g., thalassemia mutation detection), and PCR followed by capillary electrophoresis for genotyping (e.g., detection of triplet repeat disorders).
- **Diagnosis and monitoring of retroviral infections:** PCR from cDNA is a valuable tool for diagnosis and monitoring of retroviral infections, including use of reverse transcriptase enzyme for RNA viruses (e.g., HIV infection).

- **Diagnosis/detection of bacterial infections:** For example, tuberculosis by *Mycobacterium tuberculosis*.
- **Diagnosis of cancers:** Several virally induced cancers (e.g., cervical cancer caused by human papilloma virus) and some cancers which occur due to chromosomal translocation (e.g., chromosome 14 and 18 in follicular lymphoma, chronic myeloid leukemia).
- **PCR in sex determination of embryos:** Sex of human and livestock embryos fertilized in vitro can be determined by PCR. It is also useful to detect sex-linked disorders in fertilized embryos.

PCR in DNA sequencing: PCR technique is simple and quick for amplification of the DNA. Hence, it is used for sequencing. For this purpose, single strands of DNA are required.

In transplantation: PCR has been used to establish precise tissue types for transplants.

PCR in comparative studies of genomes: These include the following:

- **PCR in forensic medicine:** DNA sequences that are unique to each individual. A single molecule of DNA from any source (e.g., blood strains, hair, and semen) can be amplified by PCR. Thus, PCR is very important for identification of criminals as well as genetic fingerprinting and paternity test.
- **To study evolution:** PCR is useful in archeology and in paleontology. By this technique, even minute quantities of DNA from any source such as fossils, mummified tissues, and hair/bones can be studied.
- **To determine viral load:** By real-time quantitative PCR (qPCR), the "viral load" can be quantitated. This is useful for diagnosis and monitoring the progress of an infection (e.g., hepatitis B and C, HIV).

Advantages and disadvantages of PCR are presented in **Boxes 20** and **21**, respectively.

Modifications and developments of PCR

The procedure described above is that of a basic standard PCR amplification. The basic technique of PCR can be modified depending on the specific demands of the situation. Some of the variants of PCR are listed in **Box 22**.

Nested polymerase chain reaction Nested PCR is used because of its increased sensitivity and specificity than PCR. In this method, **two pairs of amplification primers are used along with two successive rounds of PCR.**

- **First round with first pair of primers:** Usually one pair of primer is used in the first round of PCR of 15–30 cycles.
- **Second round with second pair of primers:** The PCR products obtained after the first round of amplification are then subjected to a second round of amplification using the second set of primers. These second set of primers anneal to a sequence internal to the sequence amplified by the first primer set (i.e., first-round products). It allows products to be generated from as little as a single cell.

Disadvantage: The major disadvantage is the high rate of contamination. This may occur during the transfer of first-round products to the second tube for the second round of amplification. This can be prevented either by physically separating the first- and second-round amplification mixtures using a layer of wax or oil, or by designing single-tube amplification protocols.

Inverse polymerase chain reaction In this technique, DNA sequence flanking the target region is determined. Its determination depends on the presence of one restriction site inside the target region and a different restriction site in the flanking regions. A segment of DNA containing the target sequence and flanking regions is obtained by one restriction enzyme or by reverse transcriptase. A second strand of DNA is obtained to yield a double-stranded DNA. This DNA is

Box 20: Advantages of polymerase chain reaction (PCR).

- Wide range of samples: PCR allows analysis of DNA from any cellular source containing nuclei
- Small quantity required: PCR needs very small quantity of genetic material and can amplify DNA from even single cell
- High sensitivity and specificity
- Simple, quick, and inexpensive: Rapid turnaround time of samples for analysis. It produces DNA fragments in a matter of hours. Real-time PCR machines have reduced this time to <1 hour. Fluorescence technology is used to monitor the generation of PCR products during each cycle. This eliminates the need for gel electrophoresis
- PCR products are easily labeled for detection
- Phenotype–genotype correlations are possible

Box 21: Disadvantages and limitations of polymerase chain reaction (PCR).

- It requires knowledge of the nucleotide sequence of the target DNA fragment
- It can amplify DNA fragments usually up to 1 kb
- Analyzes only the target region
- Amplifies intact target regions
- Amplification bias: Some DNA templates are preferentially amplified versus other templates within the same reaction
- Technical factors: Several technical factors can lower the sensitivity and specificity of PCR. These include presence of nonspecific inhibitors of PCR such as heparin in patient samples and uncharacterized components of CSF, urine, and sputum

Box 22: Variations of polymerase chain reaction (PCR).

- Nested PCR*
- Inverse PCR*
- Anchored PCR
- Asymmetric PCR*
- Allele specific PCR
- Reverse transcription PCR (RT-PCR)*
- Multiplex PCR*
- Real-time quantitative PCR (qPCR)*
- Rapid-cycle PCR*
- Digital PCR*
- Random amplified polymorphic DNA (RAPD)
- Amplified fragment length polymorphism (AFLP)
- Rapid amplification of cDNA ends (RACE)

* only these are briefly discussed below.

then circularized by DNA ligase. A linear DNA is obtained by restriction enzyme cleavage in the target region and a PCR product is obtained by primers directed "out" from opposing ends of the target region. Inverse PCR is used for chromosome walking. Chromosome walking is a method of positional cloning used to find, isolate, and clone a particular allele in a gene library.

Asymmetrical polymerase chain reaction It is used preferentially to amplify one strand of the original DNA more than the other. Used in some types of sequencing and hybridization probing where having only one of the two complementary stands is required.

Reverse-transcriptase polymerase chain reaction Original PCR is a technique used for amplification of DNA. Reverse-transcriptase PCR (RT-PCR) was developed if **the template of interest is a RNA**. This technique uses an enzyme namely, reverse transcriptase that works like DNA polymerase but uses RNA as a template and makes RNA/DNA complex, then replaces the RNA with DNA. The resulting strand is referred to as cDNA or complementary DNA. After the cDNA strand is made from the RNA template, the remaining cycles can be carried out with DNA polymerases, using standard PCR protocols. RT-PCR basically consists of four steps: (1) RNA isolation, (2) Reverse transcription, (3) PCR amplification, and (4) PCR product analysis.

Multiplex polymerase chain reaction Multiplex PCR is a widespread molecular biology technique for amplification of multiple targets in a single PCR experiment. In multiplex PCR, two or more primer pairs designed for amplification of different targets (i.e., more than one target sequence/fragment) are used in one reaction tube. It can determine more than one target sequence in a single specimen in a single tube by adding further primer pairs. It is necessary to carefully select the primers having similar annealing temperatures and they must be noncomplementary to each other to avoid primer dimers and inefficient reactions. Multiplex PCR is used for diagnosis of genomic rearrangements and identification of pathogens. As an extension to the practical use of PCR, this technique has the potential to produce considerable savings in time and effort within the laboratory without compromising on the utility of the experiment.

Real-time (homogeneous, kinetic) quantitative polymerase chain reaction (qPCR) PCR protocols can also be used to estimate the relative copy numbers of particular DNA sequences in a sample. This is called quantitative PCR (qPCR) or real-time PCR. For example, if certain genes are amplified in tumor cells, qPCR can reveal the increased representation of that DNA sequence. Real-time PCR monitors the amplification of a targeted DNA molecule during the PCR, i.e., quantifies the PCR product in real-time (immediate), and not at its end, as in conventional PCR. In real-time PCR, both the target amplification and detection steps occur simultaneously in the same tube (homogeneous). It uses specific labeling probes with fluorescence emission (intercalating fluorophores) as well as equipment with the ability to detect this fluorescence during the reaction. It is used to quantify the amount/number of copies of input DNA/RNA. The abbreviation qPCR is used for quantitative real-time PCR and that RT-qPCR be used for reverse transcription–qPCR.

Real-time PCR is carried out in a special thermal cycler with precision optics. These thermal cyclers have the capacity to illuminate each sample with a beam of light and detect the fluorescence emitted by the excited fluorophore. The thermal cycler is also able to rapidly heat and chill sample. The optics monitor the fluorescence emission from the sample wells. The computer software supporting the thermocycler monitors the data throughout the PCR at every cycle (kinetic) and generates an amplification plot for each reaction. Advantages of real-time PCR are presented in **Box 23**.

Box 23: Advantages of real-time polymerase chain reaction (qPCR).

- Very sensitive
- Reproducible
- Rapid procedure
- Less risk of carryover contamination (sealed reactions)
- High sample throughput (~200 samples/day)
- Easy to perform
- The detection and visualization of amplicon as the amplification progresses
- Can quantify the results
- Software-driven operation

Methylation-specific PCR Methylation of CpG sites in DNA causes transcriptional inactivation of imprinted genes and is important in the inactivation of X chromosome. Methylation of CpG is also an important mechanism for developmentally regulated and tissue-specific gene regulation. Altered pattern of methylation is characteristic of many human diseases. For example, changes in the CpG methylation pattern in some malignancies are associated with differences in response to specific chemotherapeutic agents and overall survival.

Rapid-cycle polymerase chain reaction Reducing the assay time is the advantage of rapid-cycle PCR. The polymerases used in usual PCR can incorporate 35–100 nucleotides per second. More time is utilized for performing PCR in temperature equilibration for the solution so that efficient annealing and extension occur, and also for changing the temperature. The time needed can be significantly reduced by reducing the thermal profile of the solution using thin-walled tubes or capillaries. They force the reaction solution into thin columns or sheets of fluid.

Digital polymerase chain reaction (dPCR) PCR exponentially amplifies nucleic acids. By computing the number of amplification cycles, and the amount of amplicon, it is possible to quantify the starting targeted nucleic acid. However, many factors can complicate this calculation. These include the quality and source materials of the standard curve and choice for signal threshold. These factors can cause uncertainties and inaccuracies, especially when the starting concentration is low. This can be overcome by using digital PCR which transforms the exponential data from conventional PCR to digital signals. These digital signals indicate whether amplification occurred or not. A count of the individual nucleic acid molecules in PCR product is a direct measure of the absolute quantity of nucleic acid in the sample. The capture or isolation of individual nucleic acid molecules may be done in capillaries, microemulsions, arrays of miniaturized chambers, or on surfaces that bind nucleic acids. Its applications are:

- For the detection and absolute quantification of low levels of pathogens or viral load, rare genetic variants, gene

expression (in single cells or circulating nucleic acids), and clonal amplification of nucleic acids for sequencing mixed nucleic acid samples.
- Target amplification as part of NGS methods.

Other PCRs

Allele-specific PCR: It is used to determine the genotype of SNPs (single base differences in DNA) by using primers whose ends overlap the SNP and differ by that single base.

Assembly PCR: It is the completely artificial synthesis of long gene products by performing PCR on a pool of long oligonucleotides with short overlapping segments.

Immuno-PCR: It conjugates the antibody detection system to fragment of DNA and subsequent amplification by PCR.

Single-cell PCR: Used for analysis of CF gene in a single cell removed from human eight-celled embryo, sperm analysis, and evaluation of gene expression in a single Reed–Sternberg cell.

Hot-start PCR: This can be performed manually by simply heating the reaction components briefly at the melting temperature (e.g., 95°C) before adding the polymerase. Hot-start PCR is achieved with new hybrid polymerases that are inactive at ambient temperature and are instantly activated at elongation temperature.

Colony PCR: By this, bacterial clones (*E. coli*) can be rapidly screened for correct DNA vector constructs.

Long-range amplification: Fragments above 10 kb can now be generated by PCR using modified polymerases.

Automation: High-throughput PCR amplification can be achieved through the use of robots and 96-well plate technology.

Automated fragment analysis: The method of gel electrophoresis is modified for the detection of fluorescently labeled PCR products on DNA fragment analyzers.

Emulsion PCR: It is an extension of digital PCR in which the components of a PCR are separated into oil droplets. Solid-phase reaction technology with beads is used in emulsion PCR. Emulsion PCR is used for amplification of single DNA molecules.

Troubleshooting guide for PCR is presented in **Table 17**.

Table 17: Troubleshooting guide for polymerase chain reaction (PCR).

Observation/ problem	*Possible cause*	*Solution/comments*
Nonspecific/ spurious bands observed	Template DNA or deoxynucleotide triphosphates (dNTPs) concentration, inappropriate, high load	Take the same amount of template DNA and dNTPs as specified in the procedure
	Prolonged waiting after adding Taq	Start reaction immediately after adding Taq
	Template DNA is degraded	Minimize damage to template DNA by avoiding vigorous mixing
No or poor amplification yield	Template or dNTPs may be degraded, enzymes may have been inactive	Store the kit at -20°C and avoid repeated freeze and thaw. Also, keep all the materials in ice while performing the experiment
	Thermocycler operation or program improper	Ensure proper functioning of Thermocycler. Run positive control with every reaction
	Inadequate mixing of the reaction tube	Mix the reaction mixture using a micro pipette, avoid air bubble
Smearing of the product	DNA degraded	Work in sterile conditions to avoid contamination. Avoid vigorous mixing of the DNA samples
Primer-dimer observed	Concentration of primers and dNTPs may be inappropriate	Use recommended concentration of primers and dNTPs

Subsequent Analysis of DNA Fragments

DNA fragments are only amplified by PCR and their detection usually requires indirect different detection techniques. PCR product may be analyzed for the presence of a pathogenic mutation, gene rearrangement, or infectious agent. The indirect different detection techniques include—(1) sequencing-based methods (e.g., Sanger sequencing, pyrosequencing, NGS), (2) single-base primer extension, (3) restriction fragment length analysis, (4) amplicon length analysis, and (5) real-time PCR. However, these DNA fragments can be directly visualized by ultraviolet fluorescence after ethidium bromide staining, without the need to use indirect detection techniques.

Sequencing-based Methods

Deoxyribonucleic acid sequence is the order or sequence of nucleotides in the DNA molecule. Sequencing is any method that determines the exact order of bases in a DNA fragment. DNA sequence is used for many purposes including detecting mutations, typing microorganisms, identifying human haplotypes, and designating polymorphisms.

Sequencing (literally means arrange in a particular order) is the general term for any technique designed to determine the order of nucleotides in a nucleic acid molecule. Sequencing methods are the most commonly used techniques for mutation "screening" where a patient is suspected of having a mutation within a specific gene or genes. These include Sanger sequencing, pyrosequencing, and next-generation sequencing (NGS).

Sanger (first-generation) sequencing (Fig. 61)

The "gold standard" method of mutation screening is DNA sequencing using the di-deoxy chain termination method. It was developed in the 1970s by Fred Sanger. Sanger sequencing is also known as dideoxy or capillary electrophoresis sequencing. In this, a single-stranded DNA template (a template strand is the strand used by DNA polymerase or RNA polymerase to attach complementary bases during DNA replication or RNA transcription, respectively) of PCR product is used to synthesize new complementary strands. The single-stranded DNA template is mixed with a DNA polymerase, an appropriate specific oligonucleotide primer, and nucleotides.

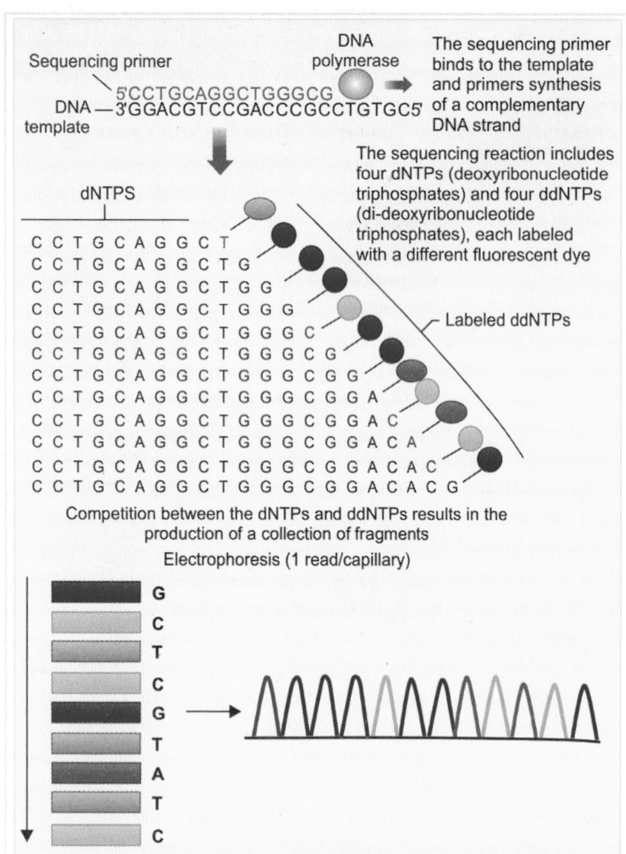

FIG. 61: Sanger sequencing. It generates a ladder of ddNTP-terminated, dye-labeled products. These products are subjected to high-resolution electrophoretic separation within capillaries of a sequencing instrument. As fluorescently labeled fragments of discrete sizes pass a detector, the four-channel emission spectrum is used to generate a sequencing trace.

In addition, four dead-end (di-deoxy terminator) normal nucleotides (A, T, G, and C) labeled with different fluorescent dye (tags) are also used. There is no hydroxyl group at the 3′ carbon position of di-deoxynucleotides (di-deoxy terminator). This prevents phosphodiester bonding and results in each reaction container consisting of a mixture of DNA fragments of different lengths. They terminate in their respective dideoxynucleotide due to di-deoxy chain termination. This occurs at random in each reaction mixture at the respective nucleotide. When the reaction products are separated by capillary electrophoresis, the reaction produces a ladder of DNA molecules of all possible lengths (i.e., DNA sequences of differing length). Each labeled with a fluorescent tag corresponding to the base at which the reaction stopped due to incorporation of a terminator nucleotide. The size separation is done by electrophoresis. The DNA sequence complementary to the single-stranded DNA template is generated by the computer software. The DNA sequence is then read and compared with the normal sequence to detect mutations. The position of a mutation may be highlighted with an appropriate software package.

Disadvantages: Sanger sequencing can only be performed on one target per reaction. The target has a maximum size of a few hundred nucleotides. The sensitivity of Sanger sequencing is less.

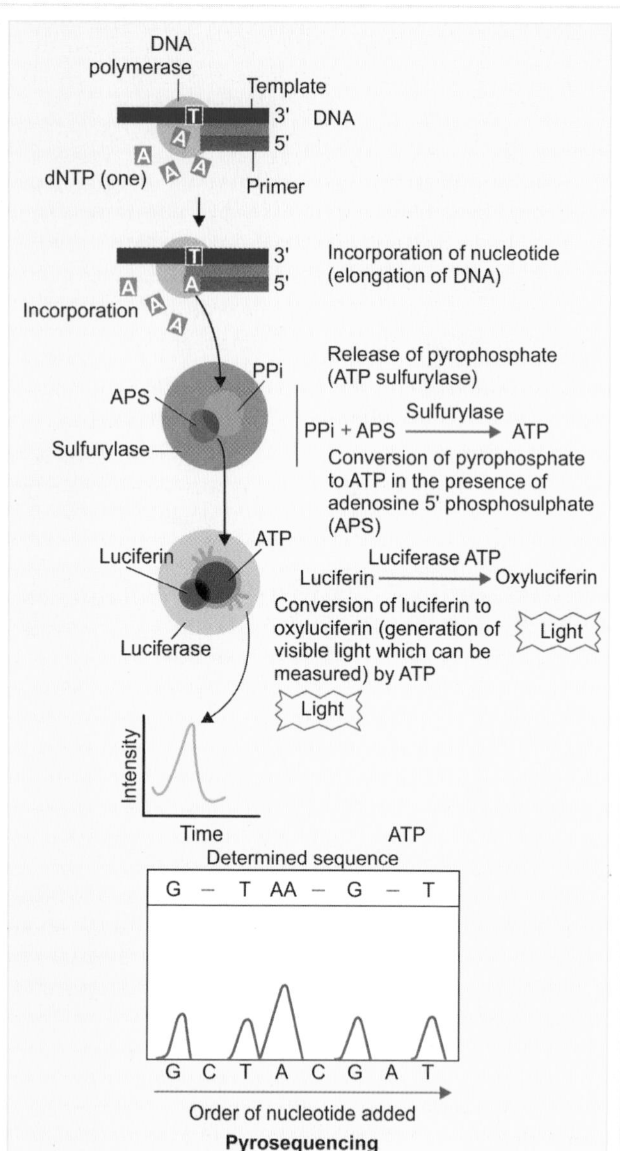

FIG. 62: Different steps in pyrosequencing. First individual deoxynucleotide triphosphates (dNTPs) are added one by one to the single-stranded template along with a primer, and a polymerase. Pyrophosphate (PPi) is generated if the dNTP is complementary to the next base on the template. Any PPi produced reacts with adenosine-5′-phosphosulfate (APS) to produce adenosine triphosphate (ATP). This ATP in turn generates light in the presence of luciferase. The sequence can be determined from the order of dNTP addition and the intensity of light produced.

Pyrosequencing

Pyrosequencing uses sequencing by synthesis approach. In this method, modified nucleotides are added and removed one at a time, with chemiluminescent signals produced after the addition of each nucleotide. It determines the nucleic acid sequence of short segments without electrophoresis. This technology produces quantitative sequence data rapidly. For example, it is used in the identification of *KRAS* mutations in patients with colorectal cancer.

Technique (Fig. 62): In this technique, first a sequencing primer is hybridized to a single-stranded template previously generated by PCR. Next, a single nucleotide [one of the four deoxynucleotide triphosphates (dNTPs)] is added to the sequencing chip. If the nucleotide base is complementary to the template strand, DNA polymerase catalyzes nucleotide incorporation in a template-dependent manner. The sequencing reaction is monitored through the release of the pyrophosphate (PPi) during nucleotide. The incorporation of nucleotide to the template strand releases pyrophosphate. After enzyme-linked chemical reactions, PPi release generates visible light. Light emission is detected by a camera which records the appropriate sequence of the cluster. Any unincorporated bases are degraded by apyrase before the addition of the next nucleotide. This cycle is repeated by adding one dNTP at a time to determine the nucleotide sequence. It is continued till the sequencing reaction is complete. This is an automated technique and is useful when the sequences of a large number of short segments need to be determined.

Next-generation sequencing

The demand for low-cost sequencing has led to the development of high-throughput sequencing technologies. Next-generation sequencing (NGS) is designed to sequence large numbers of templates simultaneously, which yields not just one, but hundreds of thousands of sequences in a run within few hours. It is a "massively parallel sequencing" because of its ability to sequence multiple nucleic acid molecules at the same time. Next (or second) generation sequencing produces millions of sequences at once. In NGS technique, PCR using primers for many different genomic regions is performed simultaneously. The resulting mixture of PCR products enriched for regions of interest is subjected to NGS (refer page 904). NGS is more sensitive than Sanger sequencing, because it can accurately identify the presence of mutations in only a small percentage of the individual sequencing reads. This is observed frequently in cancers, either because the mutation is only present in a small fraction of tumor cells or because the tumor cells are heavily contaminated with usually normal stromal cells. In the clinical diagnostic setting, NGS is particularly useful for the genetic diagnosis of rare diseases that show genetic heterogeneity. In a single test, NGS can simultaneously analyze all the genes in which mutations have been reported to cause the disease. NGS is useful for detecting genetic anomalies of essentially any size scale ranging from SNPs (single nucleotide polymorphisms—SNPs is pronounced "snips") to very large rearrangements including aneuploidy.

Single-base Primer Extension

This is useful for identification of mutations at a specific nucleotide position. For example, an oncogenic mutation in codon 600 of the *BRAF* gene. A primer is added to the PCR product. This primer hybridizes one base upstream of the target. Differently colored terminator fluorescent nucleotides are added (corresponding to normal and variant bases). This is followed by performance of a single base polymerase extension. The relative amounts of normal/variant fluorescence are then detected (**Fig. 63**). This technique is very sensitive. Disadvantage is that it only produces 1 bp of sequence data.

Restriction Fragment Length Analysis

This is simple approach in which the digestion of DNA is performed with endonucleases known as restriction enzymes.

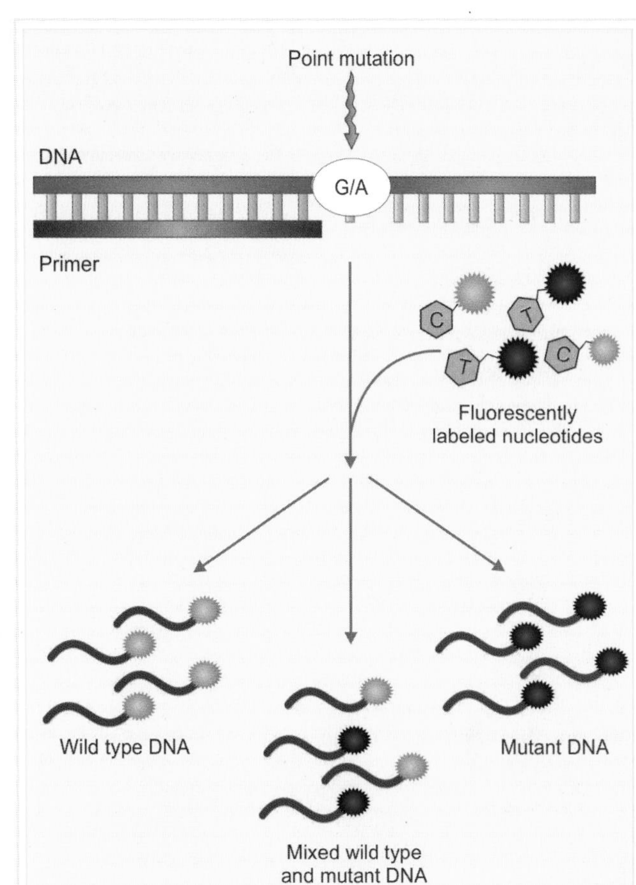

FIG. 63: Single-base extension analysis of a product of polymerase chain reaction. A primer to interrogate a single base position is used. Nucleotides complementary to the mutant (in this figure mutant nucleotide is G/A) and wild-type bases at the site of point mutation are labeled with different fluorophores. In this figure, C and T nucleotides are fluorescently labeled. They produce fluorescent signals of varying intensity depending on the ratio of mutant to wild-type (normal) DNA present.

These enzymes recognize and cut DNA at specific sequences. If the specific mutation is known to affect a restriction site, the amplified PCR product may be digested. The normal and mutant PCR products will yield fragments of different sizes. It is possible to test for the mutation by digesting a PCR product with the appropriate enzyme and separating the products by electrophoresis. They can be easily distinguished. It is useful for molecular diagnosis when the causal mutation always occurs at an unchanged nucleotide position.

Amplicon Length Analysis

Mutations that involve the length of DNA (e.g., deletions or expansions) can be easily detected by PCR. For example, in FXS, there are alterations in trinucleotide repeats and PCR analysis can be used to detect this mutation. In **Figure 64**, for the diagnosis of FXS, two primers that flank the region containing the trinucleotide repeats at the 5′ end of the *FMR1* gene are used to amplify the intervening sequences. Because there are large differences in the number of repeats, the size of the PCR products obtained from the DNA of normal individuals, or those with a premutation, is different and can

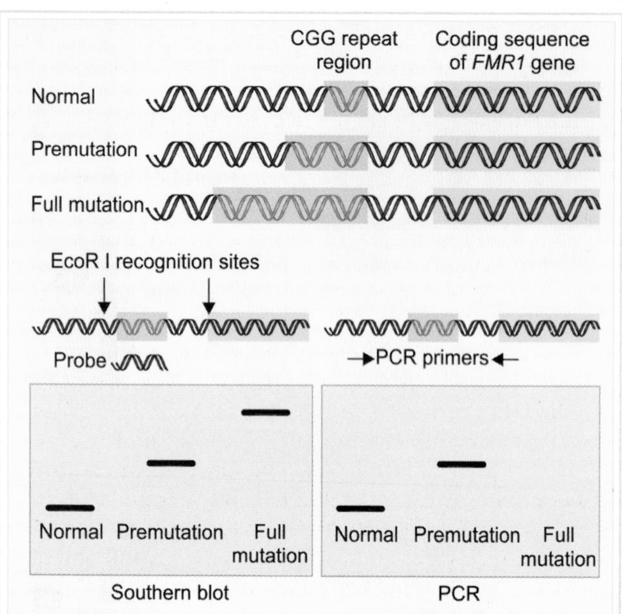

[EcoR I (pronounced "eco R one"): A restriction endonuclease enzyme isolated from species *Escherichia coli*].

FIG. 64: Diagnostic use of polymerase chain reaction (PCR) and Southern blot analysis in fragile X syndrome. With PCR, the differences in the size of CGG repeats between normal and premutation produce products of different sizes and mobility. However, with a full mutation, the region between the primers is too large to be amplified by conventional PCR. In Southern blot analysis, the DNA is cut by enzymes that flank the CGG repeat region. This is then probed with cDNA that binds to the affected part of the gene. In Southern blot, a single small band is observed in normal males, a band of higher molecular weight is observed in males with premutation, and a very large (usually diffuse) band is observed in males with the full mutation.

be distinguished by gel electrophoresis. If the trinucleotide expansion is very large, it cannot be amplified by convention PCR. Hence, Southern blot analysis of genomic DNA may have to be performed.

Real-time PCR

Real-time PCR combines the amplification steps of traditional PCR with simultaneous detection steps. It does not need post-PCR manipulation or interrogation of amplified products. Many PCR-based technologies that use fluorophore indicators can detect and quantify the presence of particular nucleic acid sequences in real time (i.e., during the exponential phase of DNA amplification rather than post-PCR). It is usually used to monitor the frequency of cancer cells bearing characteristic genetic lesions in the blood or in tissues [e.g., the level of *BCR-ABL* fusion gene sequences in chronic myelogenous leukemia (CML)], or the infectious load of certain viruses (e.g., HIV, Epstein–Barr virus).

TECHNIQUES THAT PROVIDE DETAILED VIEW OF THE DNA GENOME

Various techniques that can be used to detect and analyze products of PCR are depicted in **Figure 65**.

Mass spectrometry is discussed on page 911.

Hybridization array technologies

Q. Write short essay on DNA microarray/cytogenomic array.

DNA microarray (gene/DNA chip) is a technique used to analyze the differential expression of multiple genes.

Principle: In hybridization array technology, known DNA probes (molecules) are immobilized on a small area of a

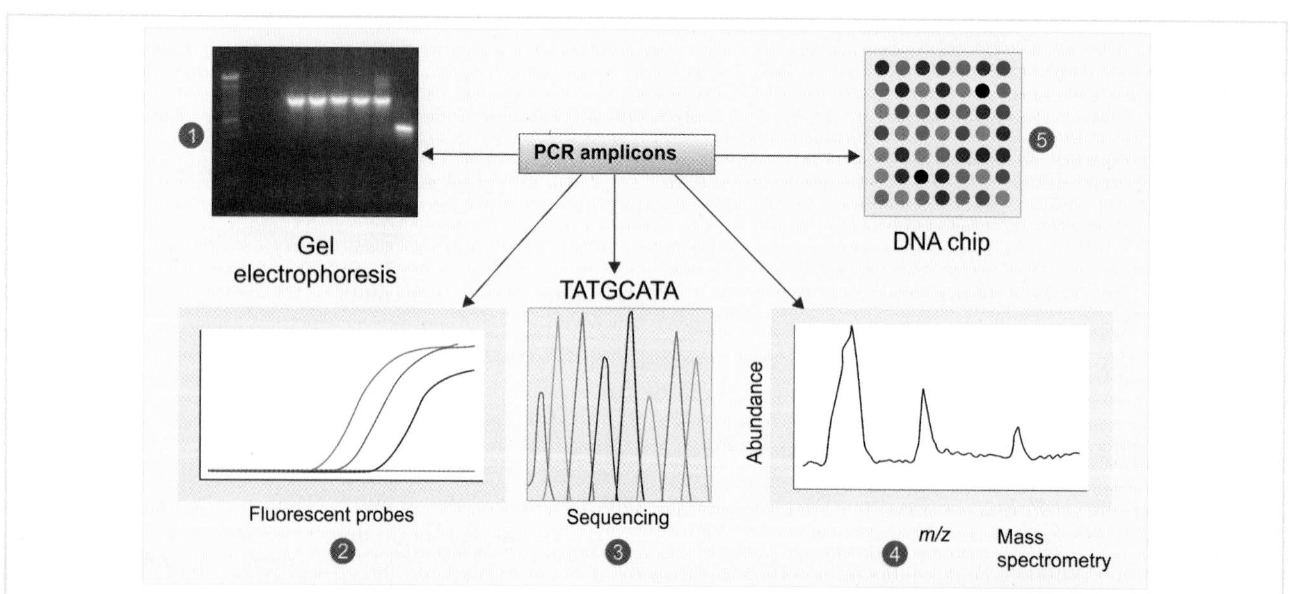

FIG. 65: Various techniques that can be used to detect and analyze products of polymerase chain reaction (PCR) called as amplicons. Amplicons can be (1) sized by gel electrophoresis, (2) detected in real time with fluorescent probes, and (3) sequenced with a variety of methods. (4) Mass spectrometry is useful for precise sizing of fragment or for determination of base composition. (5) DNA "chips" allow parallel hybridization of amplicon and thousands of probes.

solid support on planar surface of silicon, polymer or glass material (usually a glass slide). The length of the DNA probe varies according to the nature or role of the array. DNA, usually generated by PCR, is then incubated on the slide with fluorescent markers. DNA is only incorporated if an exact match occurs between test DNA and known DNA on the chip. The result is a picture of gene expression on the microarray. For example, microarrays can be used for genotyping for blood group antigens.

Advantages: It can be used to perform thousands of simultaneous hybridization reactions on a solid substrate within a single analytical procedure. This is useful for diagnostic purpose ranging from gene sequencing and detection of genetic polymorphisms to measurement of gene expression profiles in cancer cells. Microarray-based systems can quantify the expression of thousands of genes at the same time. Thus, it is useful for analysis of whole cassettes of genes, or patterns of gene expression, instead of just analysis of one, two, or three genes at a time.

General steps in microarray processing (Fig. 66)

- Generation of nucleic acid (i.e., DNA) complementary to genes of interest. This single-stranded DNA (probe) is laid in microscopic quantities on solid surfaces at defined positions. This attachment of the "probe" to the surface involves coupling reagents, spacer molecules, and customized surface chemistry.
- The nucleic acid (genomic DNA or cDNA) from samples is added over the surface.
- The cDNA in the sample binds to the probe.
- A fluorescent tag is added to the sample to facilitate the detection of successful hybridization. Detection of the hybridization is affected with the array reader which detects the level of fluorescence and identifies the location of the spot.

Hybridization array technology has revolutionized the approach to the study of disease. The one gene–one protein–one function approach is no longer used. In array technology, multiple functions, multiple proteins, and multiple genes approach is used. This technology has the ability to determine changes in the patterns of genes, identifying multiple genes acting in concert. The patterns obtained are grouped into functional categories (e.g., respiratory genes, inflammatory genes), and are used to derive signatures diagnostic of disease or to generate novel hypotheses about pathogenesis and cell function. The relationship of these genes to one another (increased vs. decreased expression) is determined.

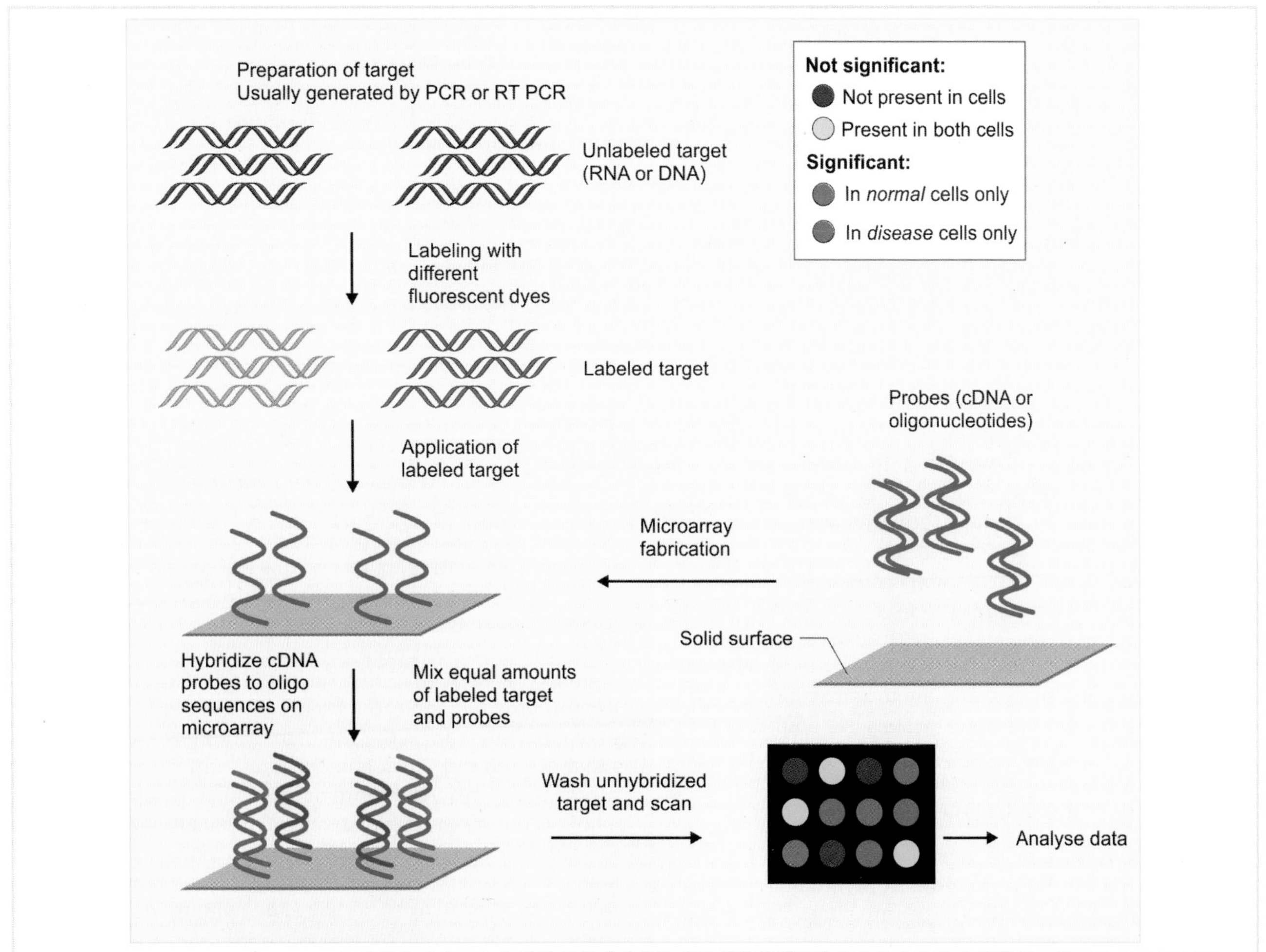

FIG. 66: Various steps of microarray technique. DNA or mRNA from more than one sources are obtained by PCR or RT PCR. They are tagged with fluorescent tags and are mixed in equimolar concentration. This mixture is hybridized to a slide which has been pre-spotted with specific cDNA. After hybridization scanning and data analysis is performed. The pattern of hybridization can be calculated for determination of gene expression.

Array technologies: A hybridization array is the molecular equivalent of a spreadsheet. In this, each cell or address reveals a specific piece of data, usually inferred from the binding of a ligand to its specific target. The first array-based methods were used in immunoassays. Similar to antigen-antibody interactions on immunoarrays, the nucleic acid arrays detect specific hybridization between complementary strands. The solid-support hybridization formats use nitrocellulose membranes for dot blots, line probes, and Southern blots. Changing the labeled entity from the probe to the sample was first called as reverse line-blot (or dot blot) hybridization.

Macroarray: It is the formats in which areas of probe localization (usually called features) are large and can be visualized without magnification. These are manufactured on nylon or nitrocellulose membranes or as plastic strips with linear arrays of bound target. Because of the large size of the features, the density of macroarrays is much lower than microarrays. They range from a few dozen to hundreds or even thousands of probes. They are usually deposited onto the membrane by printing or dot blotting. Then they are dried and stored for future use. Standard supports used to make macroarrays include nylon, plastic, and glass (silicon wafer). Silicon is a preferred matrix for hybridization arrays. Since nylon is porous and displays high autofluorescence, it limits the sensitivity of fluorescence-based detection because of high background values. Presently, macroarrays are used for targeted applications. For example, for cytokine genes or those within specific signal transduction pathways that are activated during infectious and inflammatory processes. Other applications (usually in kit format) are used to detect and type specific PCR products, such as in the CF mutation screen, human leukocyte antigen typing, or human papilloma virus typing. Advantages of macroarrays are that they have ability to use standard hybridization equipment, simplified reading or scanning, and affordability.

Microarrays: Miniaturization of assay saves time and reduces costs in biomedical diagnostic applications and research. In microarray, smaller volumes are used which reduces reagent consumption, increases sample concentration, and improves reaction kinetics. It allows to determine hundreds or thousands of results in the time formerly required for a single experiment.

In contrast to macroarray, nonporous solid (plastic, glass, or silicon substrates) support is used in microarrays. This prevents diffusion of the target nucleic acids and allows faster hybridization kinetics and easier washing steps. In order to allow spatial discrimination of numerous reactions performed simultaneously, the molecular probes are bound to a solid surface in defined arrays. Deposition of probes on a solid substrate is also more amenable to automation and enables higher array densities with optimal image definition.

Clinical applications of array technology The use of microarray technology ranging from molecular staging of tumors to the identification and characterization of microbial agents. Next to PCR, microarray technology is assuming as a core technology in the clinical molecular diagnostics laboratory.

Array technology in the clinical laboratory

- It can be used to detect common respiratory pathogens and when compared with conventional culture, the sensitivities of the array assay are higher.
- Tissue microarrays (TMAs) can be used as a tool for internal quality control to improve the interpretation of immunohistochemical staining.
- Drug detection assays: To optimize drug dosing and minimize side effects on the basis of individual genotype. The cytochrome genes coding for liver enzymes are important in drug metabolism. Hence, it can be used for drug dosage and minimize side effects of drug.
- For pre-, peri-, and postnatal screening and pediatrics diagnosis.
- Nucleic acid sequencing.

Array technology in clinical disease To screen genes that are differentially regulated: Microarray technology has the ability to screen genes that are differentially regulated and help in correlation of selected genes with their function.

To evolve therapeutic targets, diagnostic or prognostic indicators: Examples in melanoma, leukemias, lymphomas, myelodysplastic syndromes, and carcinomas of prostate, bladder, kidney, colon/rectum, breast, ovary, and endometrium.

Others:

- To study of the effect of ionizing radiation.
- Detection of microbial, viral, and other pathogens.
- Karyotyping of cell-free DNA in amniotic fluid.
- Provide molecular markers for allergic, urologic, cardiac, and inflammatory disorders; Alzheimer's disease; multiple sclerosis; dystonia; diabetes; transplant rejection; and pulmonary hypertension.
- To predict adverse drug reactions, response to therapy, drug sensitivity, and toxicity profiles.

Tissue Microarrays

Q. Write short essay on tissue microarray (TMA).

Tissue microarray is a method used to evaluate numerous samples of tissue in a short period. By this mechanism, multiple tissue samples can be arranged in a single paraffin block using precision tools to prepare the recipient block.

Tissue microarrays are paraffin blocks produced by extracting cylindrical tissue cores from different paraffin donor blocks and re-embedding these tissues cores into a single recipient (microarray) block. By this technique, up to 1,000 or more tissue samples can be arrayed (ordered arrangement) into a single paraffin block. In TMAs, tissue from many paraffin-embedded conventional histologic blocks from different patients can be seen on the same slide. TMAs are commonly used in research and can be routinely used in histopathology practice. TMA reduces the size of the sampled tissue, simplifies the mechanics of block construction, and allows the donor blocks to be preserved more or less intact. In this technique, a hollow punch/needle is used to take 100 or more tissue core samples from specific areas of pre-existing blocked tissue. They are placed in a single array block. Sections are then taken from this block. It produces a single slide containing hundreds of tissue cores for the pathologist to review.

Purpose of TMA: Conventional fresh frozen or paraffin wax embedded tissue sections are too expensive and time consuming to be applied to the characterization of 100s or

1,000s of genes or gene clusters. These genes may be associated with distinct tumor entitles or other diseases. By TMA, hundreds of samples to be analyzed simultaneously for in situ analysis of DNA, RNA, and protein targets. TMA should not be confused with DNA microarrays (discussed above on page 892). In DNA microarrays, each tiny spot represents a unique cloned cDNA or oligonucleotide. TMA is useful to study and evaluate many diseases at an early stage.

- Due to the development of molecular biology, TMA has become a powerful diagnostic tool. It helps in conserving tissue samples and also saves time for both research (including cancer) and clinical work.
- In clinical pathology, it serves as a quality control for new antibodies. The production of antibodies is an expensive and lengthy process.
- TMA can help in the streamlining of the cumbersome validation and quality control of archival tissue as well as daily immunohistochemistry (IHC) controls.

Types of Tissue Microarrays

- **Prevalence TMAs:** These are used to determine the prevalence of a given alteration in a specific area of interest in a tumor. Thus, TMAs are assembled from tumor samples of one or several types.
- **Progression TMAs:** They are used to discover associations between tumor genotype and phenotype. In this, samples of different stages of one tumor type are assembled. For example, a breast cancer progression TMA contain samples of—(1) normal breast from patients with and without a history of breast cancer, (2) various non-neoplastic breast diseases, (3) ductal and lobular carcinoma in situ, (4) invasive cancer of all stages, grades, and histological subtypes, and (5) breast cancer with metastases and recurrences after initially successful treatment.
- **Prognosis TMAs:** They represent a fast and reliable method for the evaluation of clinical importance of new detected disease-related genes. In this, samples from tumors available with clinical follow-up data are used. This can establish the associations between molecular findings and clinical outcomes.
- **Experimental TMAs:** They are assembled from cell lines or samples from TMA archives for testing new antibodies and looking for gene targets.

Steps of TMA Construction

Preparing the tissue microarray is a multistep project.

Tissue selection

Donor paraffin block: Carefully identify, select the blocks to be arrayed (donor block) by reviewing the file slides and appropriate paraffin wax blocks that contains donor tissue. Examine representative H&E stained sections of the donor tissue to select the suitable donor blocks and also to select the region of interest. The area of interest (e.g., biopsy, tumor tissue) to be included in the TMA is marked by circling with a pilot pen or permanent fine point marker on the H&E slides. The blocks are marked in the corresponding area after matched to the corresponding glass slide. It is important that the block is marked in the same area of interest as the marked slide. The punching is aided by using an H & E stained slide placed on the donor block surface and is used for the orientation. Precisely record their localization details. After initial review and selection of the region, all selected tissue blocks are arranged and kept in the same order to be represented in the TMA. Transfer the marked slide and paraffin block to the person who will build the TMA. The cores of tissue in microarray can be of any diameter.

Limitations to tissue selection: The donor blocks should contain a 2–3 mm thickness of the target tissue. This will permit the greatest number of serial tissue section to be cut from the TMA block. Hence, control of core placement depth in the recipient block is important. All cores should contain tissue of the same depth and should be positioned in such a way that the tissues begin and end in two planes parallel to the block face. If this is not followed, TMA sections cut from the beginning and end of a block will contain variable numbers of "empty" core positions. These reflect the variable core lengths. One way to avoid rectify this is to use tissue arrayer punches fitted with depth stop. A single, well-prepared TMA can routinely yield 100–300 sections before the number of exhausted cores makes the array unusable.

Type of tissue: It is important that the sample of tissue present in a TMA core must be adequate for diagnostic purposes. Some tissues are easier to sample than others. Relatively uniform solid tissues usually do not pose problems. For example, if the entire block consists of only tumor, the cores punching from the predefined region of the donor paraffin blocks do not have much challenges. However, tissues with large-scale architectural variations (e.g., lymph nodes, GI tract) or tissues with microscopically fine diagnostic features (e.g., epithelial, mucosal, and serosal surfaces) present challenges for selection. The diagnostic utility of any TMA core depends on sampling representative donor tissue sites.

Punch/needle sizes: A hollow needle/punch is used to remove small tissue cores (size depending on the punch size) from marked regions of interest in paraffin-embedded tissues. The size of the punch is important in planning the TMA. There are four different sizes of punches namely, 0.6, 1.0, 1.5, and 2.0 mm; and 1.0 or 1.5 mm needles are recommended for general use. Punch used for skin biopsy may also be used. The process of punching tissue cores from a donor block usually does not produce any significant distortion either in the tissue core or in the donor block. Multiple cores can be removed from donor blocks without compromising the remaining tissue.

Array design and preparation

Arrays are divided into sub-arrays of smaller dimensions (e.g., 5 rows, 5 columns) with "empty" spaces between successive sub-arrays. Donor tissue core of varying diameter can be used but 0.6 mm diameter allows a large number of samples to be arranged. The 0.6 mm tissue cores are arranged at a 0.8–1.0 mm intercore space in a regular grid and require precise control. Marker core of various types can be placed to help to orientate the array unambiguously which consists of characteristic tissue type, or colored crayons or marker inks. Cores designed as positive and negative controls for specific assays can also be incorporated into arrays. A single well-made TMA can routinely yield 100–300 sections.

TMA core placement and size

Recipient paraffin array block: The commercially available tissue arrayers are preferred. A blank/empty paraffin block (using soft paraffin) is prepared and used as the recipient for the tissue samples. There should not be any holes in the block due to air bubbles. The number of specimens per array depends on the size of the punches and the desired array density. Tissue cores are transferred and inserted into a recipient paraffin wax block. They are placed in array pattern in the readymade holes, guided by defined X-Y position (X-Y axis block position). Usually, donor blocks should contain 2–3 mm thickness of the target tissue. This will help to procure many serial histological sections from the TMA block. An array uses a series of 50 or more samples, set into one or several blocks. Assembling a TMA needs patience and skill. TMA cores are slip-fit into recipient block holes without added bonding material. After placing all the cores in the array, the block is incubated at 37°C for 10–15 minutes which adheres the core to the wall of the block. TMA can also be performed on frozen tissue. But its preparation and using them is more challenging.

Smoothing and sectioning: The array block should be smooth and level before sectioning. Smoothing can be done by heating a clean microscopic slide to around 70–80°C and touching it to the surface of array block. The surface of the block will begin to melt. Move the slide in a circular motion and place the slide and block in the refrigerator or freezer. Section yield is maximized by cutting the entire TMA block in one sitting. Store all slides obtained for future use. One important drawback of this is that while antigenicity of tissue stored in paraffin wax blocks can be retained for up to 70 years, some epitopes degrade on storage of unstained histological sections. For example, decreased staining intensity or percent tissue reactivity or both are observed for p53, estrogen receptor, androgen receptor, Factor VIII, bcl-2, chromogranin, CD3, Ki67, EGFR, and PSA immunoreactivity. One method that can reduce this possibility is by storing cut TMA sections under nitrogen or after recoating the glass-mounted section in paraffin wax. The surface of the block is pressed with a glass slide after incubation for even sectioning.

Sectioning array

Microtomy: The sectioning of TMA slides is performed on microtomes used for the conventional paraffin sections. Gently face off the array block on a dedicated microtome. Sections of 4–5 µm are cut from this block, mounted on a microscope slide, and then analyzed by any method of standard histological analysis. Tests commonly performed in TMA include IHC and FISH. Sectioned TMA blocks should be dipped in paraffin to seal the surface. This will help in avoiding loss of antigens.

Method of preparation of tissue microarray is summarized in **Figure 67**.

Staining of TMA

Uses: TMA technique can be used for a wide range of staining procedures. These include **IHC, ISH, FISH, RNA-ISH, special stain control samples, and quality control sections for H&E stains**.

All slides are incubated in one jar so as to make sure of identical reagent concentrations and temperatures.

TMA Informatics—Source Tissue Data Management

A large tissue array can contain up to 1,000 cores. Each core has source data and it must be recorded, along with pathological diagnosis. Additional information such as patient-specific (e.g., stage of the disease, treatment history), tissue-specific (tissue type and pathological diagnosis), and core-specific (e.g., location within the donor tissue-tumor center, tumor margin, normal tissue adjacent to tumor) also must be recorded. These can be managed using sophisticated data management tools on computer-based spread sheets.

TMA Applications

Use of many tissue samples on a single TMA slide allows high volume, well-controlled parallel histological assays to be performed with a minimum of reagent and effort. The whole range of routine tissue-based analyses such as IHC, mRNA ISH, and chromosomal FISH can be successfully performed on TMAs. TMA facilitates standardization of IHC staining procedures and interpretation by introduction of external and internal quality assurances (QAs). TMA along with other

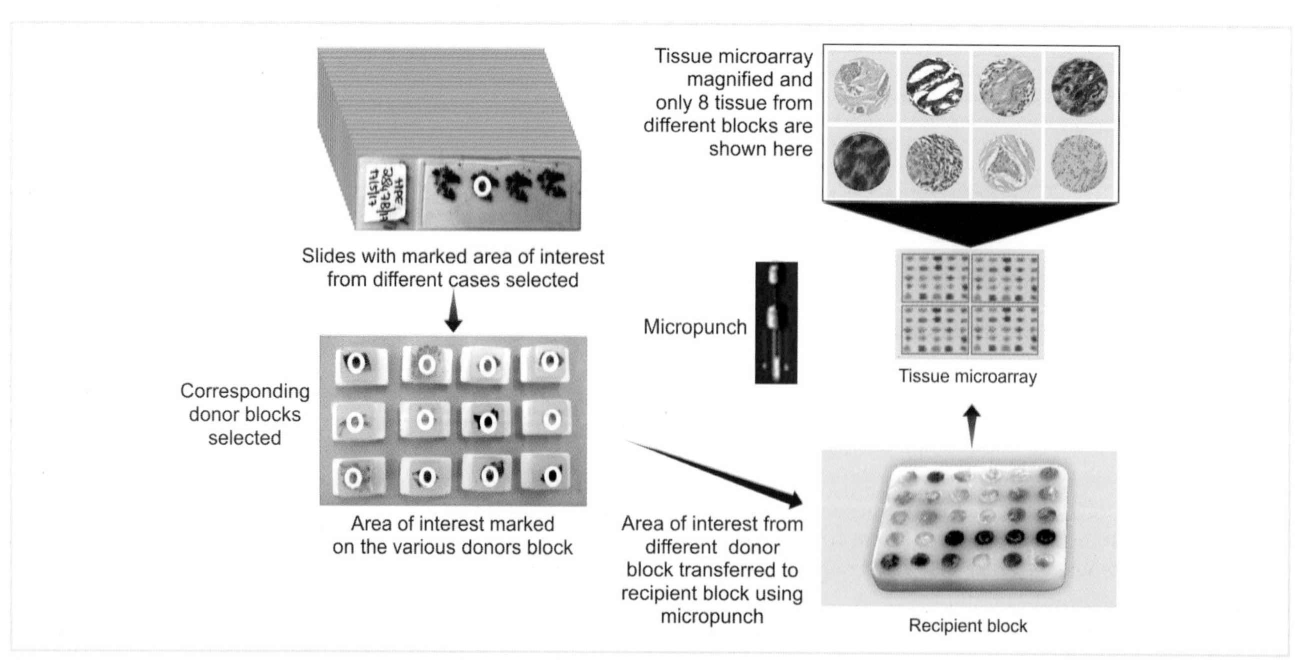

FIG. 67: Method of preparation of tissue microarray.

high-throughput techniques (e.g., gene chip) have contributed to our present understanding in carcinogenesis. TMA is an ideal tool for tissue anonymization.

Advantages

- Only a small amount of reagent is used to analyze each slide. Thus, TMA is a cost-effective technique particularly with IHC and ISH techniques.
- TMA method has become integral to pathology research and for experimental purposes.
- TMA is used in IHC for quality control and assurance.
- Useful for amplification of scarce resource.
- Experimental uniformity.
- Decreased assay volume.
- Does not destroy original donor block.

Molecular Analysis of Genomic Alterations

Genetic lesions with large deletions, duplications, or more complex rearrangements form a significant number of genetic lesions. These **cannot easily be assayed by standard PCR or DNA sequencing approaches**. Such genomic-scale changes can be studied by many hybridization-based techniques.

Nucleic Acid Hybridization Techniques

Principle: Nucleic acid hybridization assay is a technique based on the ability of single-stranded nucleic acids (DNA or RNA) allowed to form specific double-stranded hybrids. These hybrids are formed by molecules with similar, complementary sequences. The hybridization process requires that—(1) probe and target nucleic acids are mixed under conditions that allow complementary base pairing and (2) there is a method to detect the newly produced double-stranded nucleic acids.

Nucleic acid hybridization involves mixing DNA from two sources (one of them is DNA probe). These DNAs are denatured by heat or alkali to make them single stranded. Then they are allowed for complementary base pairing of homologous sequences. If one of the DNA sources is labeled (i.e., is a DNA probe), this allows identification of specific DNA sequences in the other source. Many methods of DNA analysis involve the use of nucleic acid probes and the process of nucleic acid hybridization.

Nucleic acid probes: Nucleic acid probes are usually single-stranded DNA sequences and are radioactively or nonradioactively labeled. These can be used to detect DNA or RNA fragments with sequence homology.

- **Source of DNA probes:** It may be from variety of sources and includes random genomic DNA sequences, specific genes, cDNA sequences or oligonucleotide DNA sequences. These are produced synthetically based on knowledge of the protein amino acid sequence.
- **Labeling of DNA probes:** A DNA probe can be labeled by a variety of processes. These include isotopic labeling with ^{32}P and nonisotopic methods using modified nucleotides containing fluorophores (e.g., fluorescein or rhodamine).
- **Detection:** Hybridization of a radioactively labeled DNA probe with cDNA sequences on a nitrocellulose filter can be detected by autoradiography. DNA fragments that are fluorescently labeled can be detected by exposure to the appropriate wavelength of light (e.g., fluorescent in-situ hybridization). **Various methods of detecting nucleic acid hybridization are Southern blotting, Northern blotting, DNA microarrays, aCGH, and FISH.**

Fluorescence In-situ Hybridization

Q. Write short essay on FISH.

Fluorescence in-situ hybridization is a **combination of molecular and cytogenetic technologies**. It has expanded the ability to investigate chromosome anomalies. FISH is a method widely used to detect protein and RNA as well as DNA structures in place in the cell, or in situ. FISH is a more rapid assay with higher resolution and flexibility than karyotyping. FISH is a cytogenetic technique developed by Christoph Lengauer. In this, fluorescent-labeled DNA probes (molecules) are used to detect the absence or presence and localize the specific (particular) regions/sequences on chromosomes. FISH offers higher resolution than karyotyping for specific targets. But it is limited to the regions complementary to the FISH probes. Probes are designed to hybridize to critical areas that are amplified, deleted, translocated, or otherwise rearranged in disease states. Karyotyping is performed under a light microscope. But FISH analysis requires a fluorescence microscope that will excite fluorescent emission for the probes and special filters for detection of fluors emitting at different wavelengths.

***Types of FISH*:** FISH can be performed on interphase nuclei or nuclei in metaphase.

- ***Interphase FISH*:** In contrast to karyotyping, **interphase FISH** does not require culturing of cells. Because growing cells in culture is not required, interphase FISH methods are used commonly to study prenatal samples, tumors, and hematological malignancies, that are not conveniently brought into metaphase in culture.
- ***Metaphase FISH*: In this, the** fluorescent probes bind to metaphase chromosomal regions or to whole chromosomes. **Metaphase FISH** allows analysis of small regions not visible by regular chromosome banding. Probes that cover the entire chromosome, or **whole chromosome paints,** are useful for detecting these small or complex rearrangements.

Principle: Large fragments of cloned genomic DNA (probes) that extend up to 200 kb are labeled with fluorescent dyes. These probes with fluorescent dyes are applied to **metaphase chromosome preparations or interphase nuclei** that are pretreated so as to "melt" the genomic DNA. The probe hybridizes to its homologous genomic sequence. Thus, probe labels a specific chromosomal region. This can be visualized under a fluorescent microscope.

Sample required: FISH can be performed on a cytogenetic slide preparation on prenatal samples, peripheral blood cells (blood smear), or other types of slide preparation (e.g., bone marrow smear, formalin fixed paraffin embedded tissue sections, cytology spin preparations, touch preparations from cancer biopsies).

Requirements

Q. Write short essay on DNA probes.

Fluorescent-labeled probes Almost all in-situ hybridization (ISH) analyses are performed using probes. Probes are predetermined sequence of DNA or RNA complementary to gene that is required to be seen. These probes are either directly or indirectly labeled with variety of fluorophores. The choice of labels largely depends on practical issues, such as the excitation and emission filters on the microscope that will be used to view the chromosome spreads. In FISH, fluorescent labeled probes are designed to be complementary to specific regions/locus/sequences of interest on the chromosome. Hence, they bind to only those parts of the chromosome with which they show a high degree of sequence similarity. To create a probe, first a target DNA of interest is chosen, and the relevant DNA is isolated. A single stranded copy of that DNA is labeled with a fluorescent dye. FISH probes are classified in different groups, i.e., according to their chemical properties, labeling, or target size. The FISH probes may also be classified into four main groups **(Fig. 68)** namely—(1) repetitive probes; (2) locus-specific probes; (3) whole chromosome probes/paints, and (4) partial chromosome probes/paints.

Commercial probes are available for single, dual, and multicolor applications.

- **Repetitive (repeat) sequence probes:** Most commonly used are repetitive sequence probes. They bind to α-satellite sequences of centromeres and produce strong signals. This is because α-satellite sequences are present in hundreds of thousands of copies. Based on differences in α-satellite sequences, chromosome-specific centromere-specific probes are available for most of the human chromosomes. These probes are particularly useful for chromosome enumeration (i.e., to detect the gain or loss of specific chromosomes such as aneuploidy). For this purpose, usually chromosome-specific pericentromeric and subtelomeric probes are used. They can be used on both metaphase and interphase preparations. Simultaneous analysis of more than one locus is possible by using a cocktail of differentially labeled probes in the same hybridization. Other repetitive sequence probes include probes that recognize β-satellite sequences (located on the short arms of acrocentric chromosomes), and probes that recognize the telomeric repeat sequence TTAGGG.

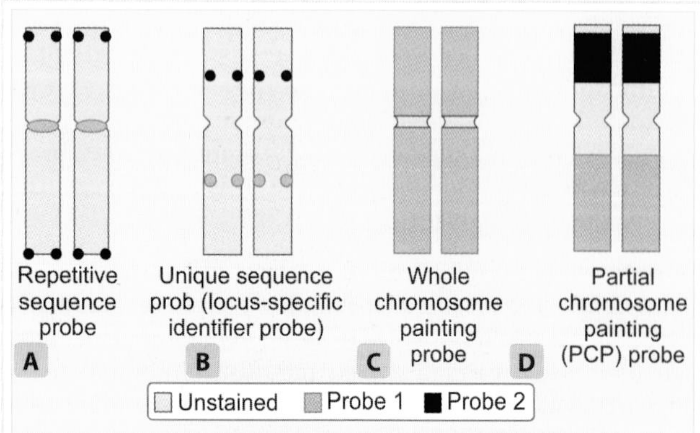

FIGS. 68A TO D: Four different kinds of fluorescence in-situ hybridization probes according to their target size. (A) Two probes specific for repetitive sequences like telomeric (probe 1) and centromeric regions (probe 2); (B) Two locus-specific (unique sequence probes) single-copy probes; (C) Whole chromosome painting probe; and (D) Two partial chromosome painting probes.

- **Unique sequence probes (locus-specific identifier probes, or LSI probes):** This type of probes is used to detect sequences that are present only once in the genome. They are usually isolated (derived) from cloned DNA of a disease-causing gene or a fragment of DNA of known location associated with a particular gene. But they can also be produced from cDNA or by PCR. These probes are mainly used to identify the presence or absence of a gene, gene region, or chromosomal rearrangement of interest that cannot be identified by examination of chromosomes stained by routine banding methods. Subtelomere probes are a subset of this category, and chromosome-specific subtelomere probes are used to characterize cryptic (mysterious or obscure) subtelomeric deletions or rearrangements that have been associated with unexplained mental retardation.
- **Whole chromosome probes (WCPs):** They are also known **as chromosome painting probes or chromosome libraries**. They consist of cocktail of many unique DNA fragments (i.e., thousands of overlapping probes) that recognize unique and moderately repetitive sequences along the entire length of individual chromosomes. Thus, following hybridization, the entire chromosome fluoresces. WCPs are used to identify rearrangements that are not detected by routine banding methods, to confirm the interpretation of aberrations identified by routine banding methods, or to establish the chromosomal origin of rearrangements that are difficult to evaluate by other techniques. These probes are designed for use only with metaphase chromosome preparations. For example, a probe to any unique region on chromosome 22 should produce an image of two signals per nucleus. This reflects the two copies of chromosome 22 in the somatic cell nucleus (**Fig. 69**). If the cell has a deletion or duplication of the DNA, the hybridized probe will result in a nucleus with only one signal in case of deletion or more than two signals in case of duplication.
- **Partial chromosome painting** (PCP) probes can also be useful for the characterization of chromosomes.

Many different types of probes are also available to detect different alterations on chromosomes. These alterations may be in the centromeres, telomeres, chromosome bands, genes, translocation break points, etc.

- **Basic FISH probe:** In this, a single probe is used to detect presence or absence of a specific sequence (e.g., mutation, deletion).

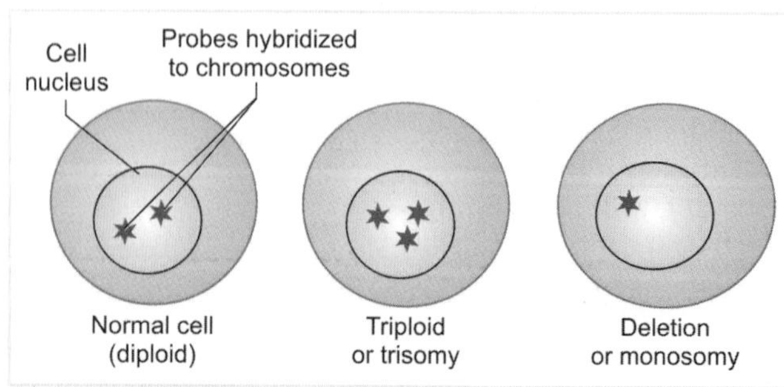

FIG. 69: FISH analysis using centromeric probes for a normal diploid cell (A), triploidy or trisomy (B), and deletion or monosomy (C).

- **Break-apart probe:** It is another type of FISH probe. If there is no translocation present involving the area where the probe is attached (annealed) to, it produces one signal. This will be considered a negative result. However, when there is a translocation present in the area the probe anneals to, the translocation causes a break in the middle of the probe. This produces two separate signals, and this will be considered a positive result. This is useful for examining genes, such as *EWSR1,* that have many fusion partners. When the *EWSR1* probe breaks apart into two signals, it means that a fusion has occurred. However, by this test alone, the fusion partner is not known.
- **Fusion probe:** This is another type and commonly used probe. In this, two probes with different fluorescent colors sit on two different chromosomes. When there is fusion of the two chromosomes, the two probes will come together and result in just one signal instead of two. This signifies a fusion. For example, a common fusion probe is for the BCR-ABL1 transcript. In this, one probe of one fluorescent color sits on the ABL1 on chromosome 9 and another probe of another fluorescent color sits on BCR on chromosome 22. In cells with a BCR-ABL1 transcript, these two probes will come together. This allows to identify the fusion transcript in the cells.

Fluorophore It is a component of a molecule that causes a molecule to be fluorescent. They absorb energy of a specific wavelength and re-emit energy at a different wavelength. Fluorescein isothiocyanate (FITC) is a reactive derivative of fluorescein. It is one of the most common fluorophores chemically attached to other, nonfluorescent molecules to create new fluorescent molecules for a variety of applications.

In this method, the slide is aged in a salt solution, dehydrated with ethanol, and then fluorescent probes are added. The DNA on the slide preparation and the probes are heated. This allows both DNA and probes to denature. Then the preparation is cooled so that both DNA and probes are allowed to anneal to each other. The remaining unbound probes are removed by washing. It is counterstained with 4′6-diamidino-2-phenylindole (DAPI). The slides are analyzed by examining 200–1,000 cells.

Fluorescent microscope The presence or absence of the signal can be seen using a fluorescence microscope. Fluorescence microscope is used at find out where the fluorescent probe is bound to the chromosomes. It exposes a specimen to ultraviolet, violet or blue light and forms an image of the object with the resulting fluorescent light.

Technique

The FISH can be performed on either metaphase (metaphase FISH) or interphase (interphase FISH) cells. For metaphase FISH, cells are cultured and harvested as for a routine karyotype analysis. But for interphase FISH, no culture is needed. Fixed cells are collected, and slides are prepared as described for karyotyping (refer pages 849–851). FISH has following basic steps (**Figs. 69** and **70F**):

- Probe and metaphase or interphase target DNA on the slide are denatured by a high temperature and formamide.
- Fluorescently labeled single-stranded molecular probe is allowed to hybridize to the chromosomal DNA. This is achieved by using an annealing temperature that favors hybridization of homologous regions of DNA in the chromosome.

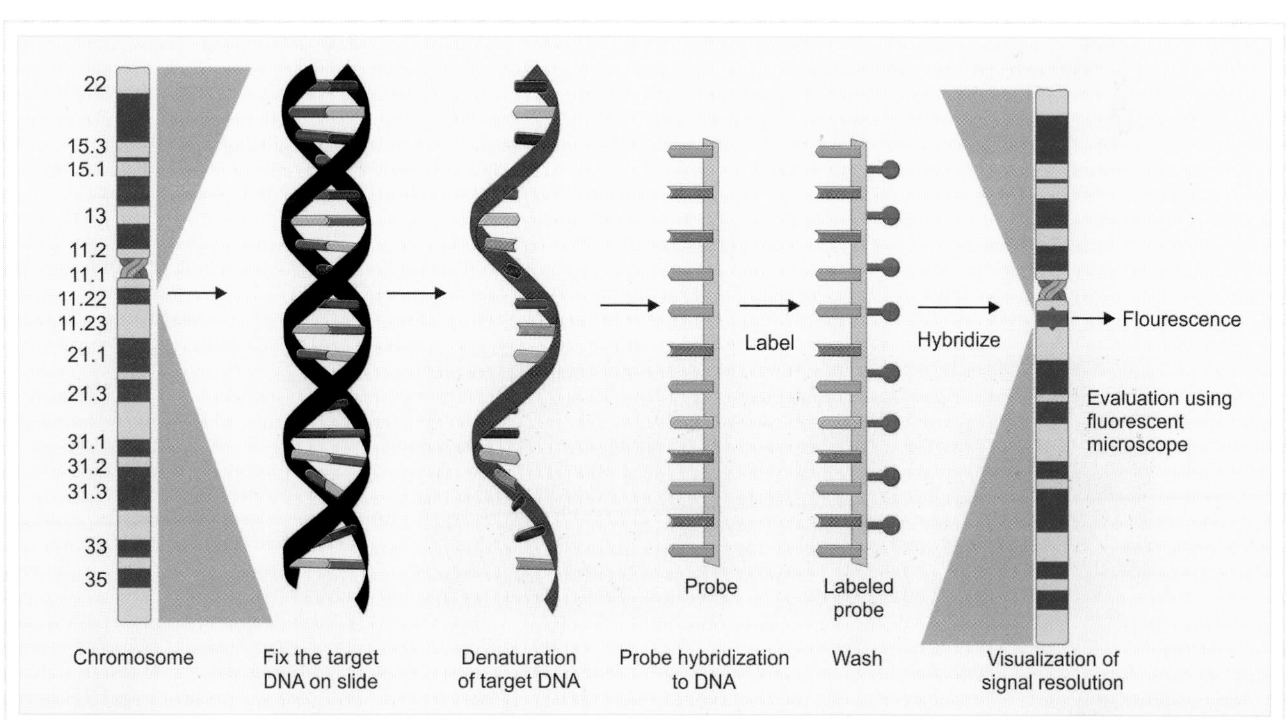

FIG. 70: Various steps in fluorescence in-situ hybridization (FISH). The target DNA derived from a known gene is fixed onto the slide surface and rendered single stranded. It is denatured. Same time, the probe DNA labeled with a fluorescent tag is also denatured. Probe DNA is then hybridized back to the chromosomes of a metaphase cell. Washing is done to remove unbound single-stranded DNA as well as nonspecifically bound DNA. FISH is ready for inspection under the fluorescence microscope.

- After an appropriate period of hybridization, excess unbound probe is removed by post-hybridization washes. The nonhybridized DNA is counterstained with another fluorochrome-based counterstain to allow visualization of the entire chromosome.
- A fluorescent microscope with appropriate sets of exciter filters allows evaluation of the cells. Bound probe is viewed in regard to its distribution and location by fluorescence microscopy. For documentation, images are captured using a computer-assisted system.

Interpretation (Fig. 70)

Selection of a specific probe or probes is one of the most critical elements in FISH. For example, one of the most useful clinical applications of FISH is the detection of microdeletions too small to be identified under classical cytogenetics. For its detection by FISH, the gene must be known, and the probe used must be homologous to the critical region of the deleted gene. Hybridization with the probe produces a fluorescent signal only at the target locus. If a signal is present, it indicates that DNA complementary to the probe is present. This means there is no deletion (**Fig. 71A**). If the particular signal is absent, it indicates the presence of deletion. This is because there is no DNA sequence present on the chromosome that is complementary to the probe. Hence, there is no hybridization (**Fig. 71C**). A control probe to a different region of the chromosome is usually used as a hybridization control (**Fig. 71B**). Hence, when interpreting a disease-related probe in FISH, an unaffected individual should have two signals per cell for each autosomal gene (i.e., one signal for each chromosome of the pair). An affected individual with a deletion will show only one single signal per cell, showing one normal and one deleted chromosome. The control probe should show two signals per cell in all cells that are scored, both in affected and unaffected individuals. Absence of a signal may also be due to technical failure of hybridization. Hence, to avoid this, a minimum of 20 cells must be evaluated. FISH is a targeted assay, and the probes will only provide information about the locus from which they are derived. Hence, it is important to know the probe while interpreting the results (**Figs. 71D** and **E**).

Multicolor fluorescence in-situ hybridization (multiplex metaphase FISH)

One of the features of FISH is its ability to hybridize multiple probes to a single slide. This will provide a better understanding of chromosome rearrangements. In most of the fluorescent microscopes, the maximum number of FISH probe colors that can be used and viewed by naked eye is three. One for target sequence, one for control sequence, and one for counterstain. If more than three colors are required, it needs a computer-assisted imaging system, by which multiple colors become possible. It is not that the computer actually "sees" more colors, but it can detect subtle differences in shades better than the human eye. So, two fluorochromes are used and mixed in varying proportions to give a range of colors.

Multiplex FISH and spectral karyotyping (SKY) are related techniques in which metaphase chromosome spreads are hybridized with a combination of probes labeled with different fluorophores. In this, each chromosome is painted with different fluorophores and it helps to visualize genetic abnormalities. Since N (number of color probes) different fluorophores can produce (2^N-1) different color combinations; in this, use of five different fluorophores yields sufficient

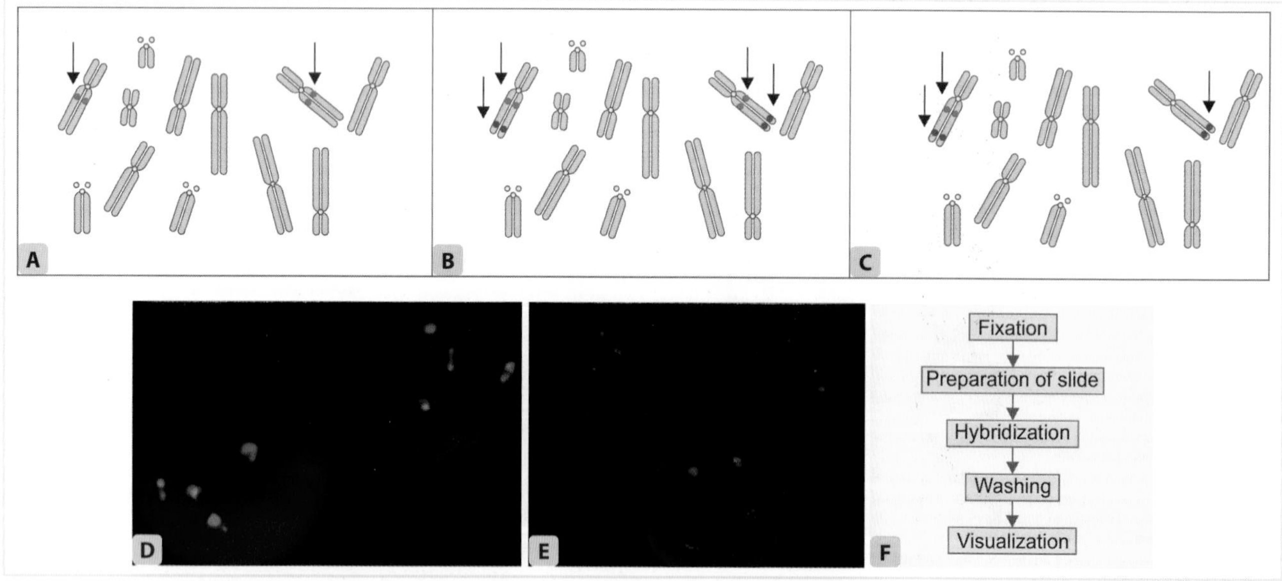

FIGS. 71A TO E: Interpretation of fluorescence in-situ hybridization (FISH). Metaphase cell with chromosomes (only few shown in this figure) processed using FISH technology. The labeled probes hybridized to targets (arrows). (A) Dual signals (both red) indicating hybridization to both alleles of target gene; (B) A control probe to a different region of the chromosome is usually tested as a hybridization control. It shows target gene (red signal) and a control probe (green signal) with complete hybridization to all alleles; (C) Hybridization of both controls (green) but presence of only a single target gene indicates deletion of one allele; (D) Positive for BCR/ABL1 fusion: 2F1R1G. Fusion signals on translocated (derivative) chromosomes 9 and 22. Green and red signals on normal chromosomes [t (9;22): Dual color, dual fusion probe used]; (E) Positive for c-myc/IgH fusion: 2F1R1G. Fusion signals on translocated (derivative) chromosomes 8 and 14. Green and red signals [t (8;14): Dual color, dual fusion probe used]. (F) Basic steps in FISH.

different color combinations to uniquely label WCPs so that all 24 different human chromosomes can be identified in one hybridization. In both multiplex FISH and SKY, a cocktail of labeled probes for each of the 24 chromosomes is hybridized to metaphase chromosome spreads. The fluorescent emitted are measured by computerized imaging systems.

- **Uses:** Both multiplex FISH and SKY are used to detect aneuploidy, detect interchromosomal rearrangements, and identify marker chromosomes (chromosomal material of unknown origin). By using a multicolor FISH, it is possible to detect common abnormalities such as aneuploidies for chromosomes 13, 18, 21, and the sex chromosomes in a single hybridization.
- **Disadvantages**. The minimum size of individual DNA chromosomal fragments that can be visualized by either FISH or SKY technique is in the range of 1–2 Mb. They will reveal intrachromosomal deletions and duplications that are large enough to produce a change in size of the affected chromosome. Thus, these techniques cannot be used to detect intrachromosomal rearrangements such as inversions. The probe sets are expensive.

Quantitative FISH (Q-FISH): This uses labeled (Cy3 or FITC) synthetic DNA mimics called peptide nucleic acid (PNA) oligonucleotides to quantify target sequences in chromosomal DNA using fluorescent microscopy and analysis software. Most commonly used to study telomere length located at the distal end of chromosomes that prevents DNA damage responses as well as genome instability.

Uses of FISH

Most common goal of FISH is **to determine whether a gene, a specific mutation, or a particular chromosomal rearrangement is present**. FISH is **used to detect numeric abnormalities of chromosomes (e.g., aneuploidy), subtle microdeletions, and complex translocations that cannot be detected by routine karyotyping and gene amplification** (e.g., *NMYC* amplification in neuroblastomas, *HER2* in breast cancer). It is also used when rapid diagnosis is needed. For example, before deciding to treat a patient with suspected acute promyelocytic leukemia with retinoic acid. This is because retinoic acid is effective only when there is presence of a particular chromosomal translocation involving the retinoic acid receptor gene in the tumor cells. Examples of diseases that are diagnosed using FISH include Down syndrome, PWS and AS, 22q13 deletion syndrome, CML, and acute lymphoblastic leukemia. Common applications of FISH are presented in **Box 24**. Features of FISH are presented in **Box 25**.

Box 24: Common applications of fluorescence in-situ hybridization (FISH).

Genetics
- Prenatal diagnosis of inherited chromosomal aberrations
- Application in cytogenetics: It can detect submicroscopic deletions and cryptic translocations of genes associated with unexplained mental retardation and miscarriages
- Postnatal diagnosis of carriers of genetic disease
- Evaluation of structural or numeric chromosomal abnormalities, including translocations, gene deletion/ amplification, and aneusomy
- Gene mapping, detection of aberrant gene expression, and microdeletions
- Tumor cytogenetic diagnosis and to study tumor biology
- For mapping chromosomal genes

Diagnosis of infectious disease: Viral and bacterial disease

Box 25: Features of fluorescent in-situ hybridization.
- Identify known deletions irrespective of size
- Identify translocation by different probes
- Identify gene amplification
- No need of metaphasic arrest
- Cannot detect unknown chromosomal changes

Cytogenomic Array Technology

Fluorescent in-situ hybridization needs prior knowledge of the one or few specific chromosomal regions suspected of being altered in the test sample. However, genomic abnormalities without prior knowledge of chromosomal changes can be detected by using microarray technology to perform a global genomic survey. First generation technology was designed for CGH, whereas newer platform technology uses SNP genotyping approaches and has multiple benefits.

Array-based comparative genomic hybridization (Fig. 72)

This technique was described in the early 1990s. It is now used for the identification and characterization of chromosomal abnormalities in different cell types.

Principle: Chromosomal deletions and duplications are detected by comparison of equal amounts of genomic DNA from a patient and a normal control.

In aCGH (array comparative genomic hybridization), both the test DNA (patient DNA) and a reference (normal) DNA are labeled with two different fluorescent dyes. The samples are then mixed and hybridized to a microarray (array means display of ordered series or arrangement). Microarray consists of large numbers of DNA target sequences representing the entire set of genes. These DNA target sequences are oligonucleotides (up to 1 million). They are bound (spotted) to glass microscope slides using robotics to create a microarray in which each DNA target has a unique location. Following hybridization, washing is done to remove unbound DNA. At each chromosomal probe location, the binding of the labeled DNA from the two samples (i.e., patient and control DNA) is compared.

Interpretation: Following are the different types of fluorescence—

- **Equal hybridization:** If the two samples (test/patient and control DNA) are equal (i.e., the test sample is diploid), all spots on the microarray will fluoresce yellow. This is due to equal admixture of green and red dyes.
- **DNA dosage loss:** If the test/patient sample has a deletion, the probe spots corresponding to it will show skewing toward red (on gain of material).
- **DNA dosage gain:** If the test/patient sample has duplication, the probe spots corresponding to it will show skewing toward green (on loss of material).

The microarray scanner measures the fluorescent signals. The relative levels of fluorescence are measured using computer software. Computer software analyzes the data and produces a plot.

Advantages: aCGH is **faster and more sensitive** than conventional metaphase analysis for the identification of

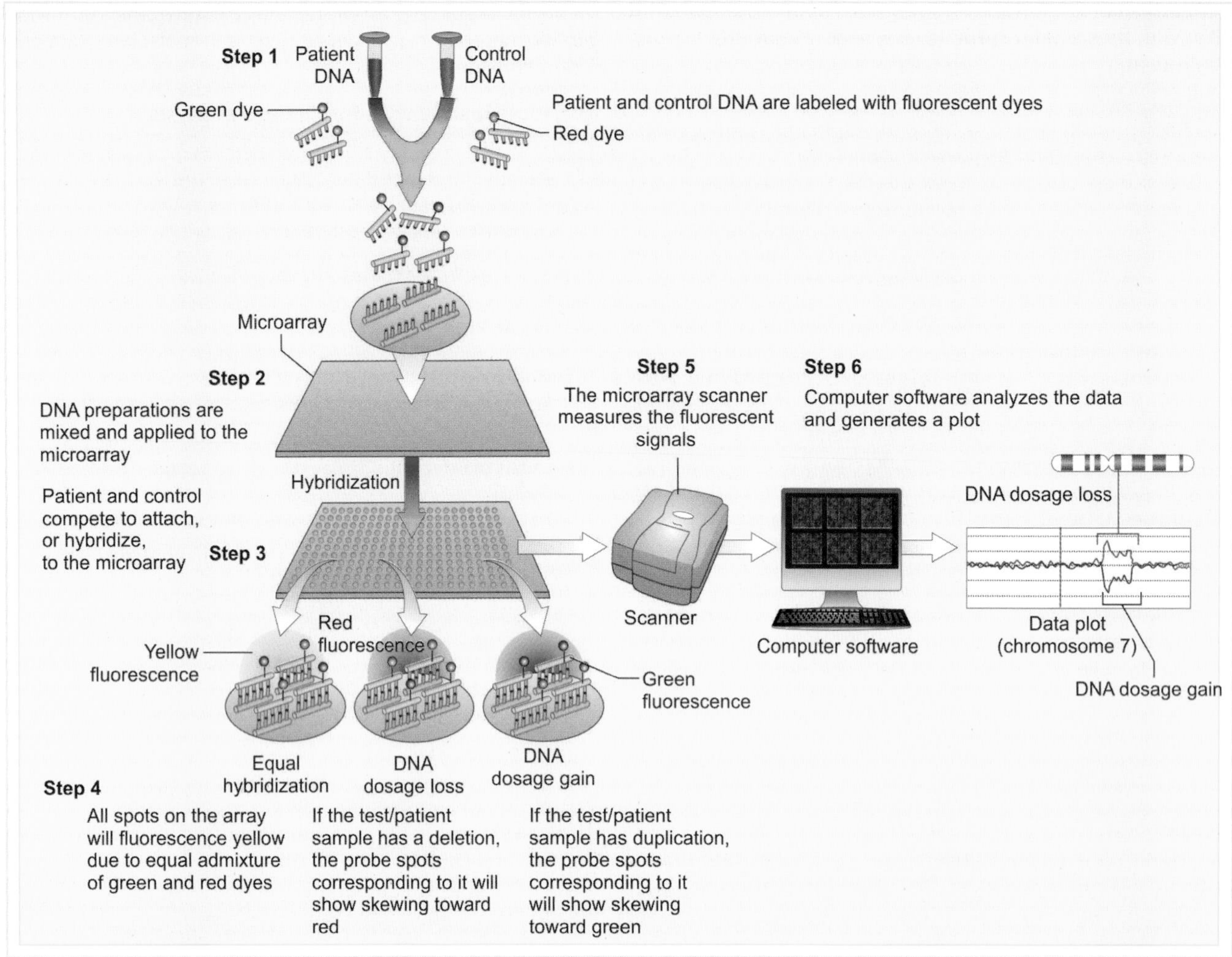

FIG. 72: Various steps involved in array comparative genomic hybridization methodology. Step 1: Patient's DNA is labeled with a green dye and a control genomic DNA preparation is labeled with red dye. Step 2: The DNA preparations are mixed and applied to the microarray. Step 3: These are cohybridized to an array of oligonucleotides on a glass slide. Step 4: The DNA bound to each spot (known as a feature) of the array is analyzed. Step 5: The fluorescence signals are measured and quantified using a laser scanner. In the patient's DNA, normal regions will be indicated by a yellow balanced color. The regions of duplication will be identified as red, and regions of deletion will be identified as green. Step 6: Computer software analyzes the data and produces a plot.

constitutional gene rearrangements. It is capable of detecting copy number changes in the genome to a resolution of 5–10 kb DNA. It allows highly accurate determination of even focal copy number gain or loss anywhere in the genome. aCGH is the first-line investigation in patients with severe developmental delay/learning difficulties and/or congenital abnormalities. It is also used in the prenatal setting when abnormalities are detected by ultrasound scanning.

Disadvantage: It cannot **detect balanced translocations or inversions**.

Single nucleotide polymorphism genotyping arrays

There is an enormous number variation of DNA sequence in the human genome. Two main types are SNPs (single nucleotide polymorphisms) and hypervariable tandem repeat DNA length polymorphisms. These are predominantly used in genetic analysis. SNPs are the most common type of DNA polymorphism. Approximately 1 in 1,000 nucleotide bases throughout the genome shows variation. SNPs are most frequently biallelic and occur in both coding and noncoding regions. SNPs are characterized by a change in the individual base and are the most common polymorphism. For example, the alteration of a DNA fragment ACGT to ACTT by replacement of the third base from a guanine to a thymine. Two unrelated individuals will have about 3 million SNPs that differ between them. Comprehensive mapping of an individual's SNP pattern is termed genotyping. In genotyping, one form of the known gene sequence (allele) can be compared with an alternative form at a specific predetermined site.

There are several different methodologies to analyze SNPs. The current generation of SNP genotyping array is quite comprehensive. The largest contains greater than 4 million SNP probes. In the clinical laboratory, SNP arrays are routinely used to detect copy number abnormalities in pediatric patients. This is performed when the karyotype is normal but there is still a suspicion of a structural chromosomal abnormality.

Indications: Common indications include **congenital abnormalities, dysmorphic features, developmental delay, and autism**.

Advantages: Unlike CGH arrays, SNP arrays can identify loss of heterozygosity. This is important in the diagnosis of disorders caused by UPD (e.g., in PWS and AS). In these conditions, despite diploid genomic copy number, the SNP in the affected chromosomal regions shows reduction to homozygosity. SNP data can also help to reveal other anomalies, such as mosaicism, which produce complex but distinctive skewing of zygosity plots.

Third-generation (or single molecule) sequencing

New instruments that utilize a revolutionary new technology, referred to as third-generation (or single molecule) sequencing, are presently available. Unlike all the previous sequencing strategies, third-generation sequencers neither need amplified DNA, nor do they involve enzymatic activities. Third-generation (or single molecule) sequencing is able to determine the nucleotide sequence of individual DNA molecules which are isolated directly from a genome. They achieve sequencing by pulling each DNA molecule through a tiny hole, or "nanopore". Then each nucleotide is identified one at a time, as it passes through the opening.

Applications: The knowledge of genetic and genomic sequence alterations is useful in clinical pathology.

- To find out the causes of inherited diseases, or to use genome-wide mutation profiles for individualized medicine, care, and treatment.
- Direct sequencing is used to determine viral types (e.g., human papillomavirus), bacteria, and other pathogens.
- Oncology: To identify key mutations in oncology (e.g., BRCA1 and BRCA2)

Markers and Molecular Diagnosis

It is possible to detect disease-specific mutations only if we know the gene responsible for the disorder and its sequence has been identified. If the exact nature of the genetic aberration is not known, diagnostic laboratories can make use of the phenomenon called linkage.

Genetic Linkage Analysis

Genetic linkage analysis is a powerful tool to detect the chromosomal location of genes producing disease. In humans, even if two DNA loci are 100,000 bp apart on the same chromosome, they are almost certain to co-segregate during meiosis. This is due to the extremely low chance of the crossover event happening between them. Thus, the **genes that are physically closer in two loci remain linked during meiosis**. There is a high probability that they will move together in family pedigrees. Positional cloning is the identification of a disease gene through its location in the human genome, without prior knowledge of its function. It is also termed as reverse genetics because it involves an approach opposite to that of functional cloning, in which the protein is the starting point.

If the pathogenic allele is not known, a diagnostic laboratory can choose this genetic linkage property of alleles. Thus, if the exact nature of the genetic aberration is not known, examination of nearby marker loci of the family pedigree will be useful in the diagnosis. Linkage analysis, also known as genetic mapping, can be performed for a single, large family or for multiple families.

Polymorphism useful for linkage analysis

The two types of genetic polymorphisms are most useful for linkage analysis. These are SNPs (refer above on page 902) and repeat length polymorphisms. Repeat length polymorphisms are known as minisatellite and microsatellite repeats.

Repeat length polymorphisms Human DNA contains short repetitive sequences of DNA called repeat length polymorphisms.

Types: Repeat length polymorphisms are usually subdivided on the basis of their length into two types namely, microsatellite repeats and minisatellite repeats.

- **Microsatellites repeats:** These are usually **<1 kb** and are characterized by a repeat size of 2–6 bp.
- **Minisatellite repeats**; These are **larger (1–3 kb),** and the repeat motif is usually 15–70 bp.

In both microsatellites and minisatellites, the number of repeats is extremely variable within a given population. Hence, both these stretches of DNA can be utilized for establishing genetic identity for linkage analysis. Different microsatellites and minisatellites can be distinguished based on size. The size can be measured by performing PCR amplification using primers that flank this repeat region.

Other uses of assays to detect genetic polymorphisms: Detection of genetic polymorphisms is also important in many other areas of medicine. These include determination of **relatedness and identity in transplantation, cancer genetics, paternity testing, and forensic medicine**. Microsatellite markers are scattered throughout the human genome and they have a high level of polymorphism. Hence, they are useful for differentiating between two individuals and to follow transmission of the marker from parent to child. They are routinely used for determining paternity and for criminal investigations. They play a central role in forensic identifications. They are used in patients following allogeneic hematopoietic stem cell transplant to detect and quantify chimerism.

Epigenetic Alterations

Definition of epigenetics: It is defined as the study of heritable chemical changes (modification) of DNA or chromatin that does not alter the protein-encoding DNA sequence itself. Thus, these are heritable changes to gene expression that are not due to differences in the genetic code. Important epigenetic modifications (see pages 433–436) include methylation of DNA and methylation and acetylation of histones. The epigenetic modifications are important for normal human development. They are involved in the regulation of tissue-specific gene expression, X chromosome inactivation, imprinting, aging, and cancer expression, and frequently correlate negatively with the level of methylation of DNA. Methylation particularly involves cytosine residues in CG dinucleotide-rich promoter regions known as CpG islands. Increased methylation of CpG islands is associated with decreased gene expression and is accompanied by changes in methylation and acetylation of histone.

Technique of identifying DNA methylation: This requires special techniques. One method is to treat genomic DNA with sodium bisulfite (chemical that converts unmethylated cytosine to uracil). Methylated cytosines remain unchanged. After this, the unmethylated (modified) DNA from the methylated (unmodified) DNA is identified by DNA sequencing.

RNA Analysis

Deoxyribonucleic acid exerts its effects on the cell through RNA expression. The mature mRNA contains the coding sequences of all expressed genes. RNA can be used as a main substitute for DNA in several diagnostic applications. DNA is much more stable than RNA. So, DNA-based diagnosis is usually preferred. However, RNA analysis is important in several areas of molecular diagnostics.

Applications of RNA analysis: It is useful for the detection and quantification of RNA viruses such as HIV and hepatitis C virus. It is also used **to evaluate cancer**. mRNA expression profiling is an important tool for molecular stratification of certain tumors (e.g., breast cancer). In some malignant tumors, cancer cells with particular chromosomal translocations are detected with greater sensitivity by analyzing mRNA (e.g., the BCR-ABL fusion transcript in CML). This is mainly because most translocations occur in scattered locations within particular introns, which can be very large. This may complicate its detection by PCR amplification of DNA. During the formation of mRNA, introns are removed by splicing. By using reverse transcriptase, RNA is first converted to cDNA and it is then analyzed by PCR. Real-time PCR performed on cDNA is the method of choice for monitoring residual disease in CML and certain other hematologic malignancies.

Next-generation Sequencing

Q. Write short essay on NGS.

Next-generation sequencing (NGS) is a term used to describe several newer DNA sequencing technologies. They produce very large amounts of sequence data in a massively parallel manner. NGS technologies have revolutionized biomedical research and have a great impact on molecular diagnostics. NGS allows to perform previously impossible analyses at relatively low cost. In principle, the concepts behind Sanger and NGS technologies are similar. In both NGS and Sanger sequencing, DNA polymerase adds fluorescent nucleotides one by one onto a growing DNA template strand. Each incorporated nucleotide is identified by its fluorescent tag. Comparison of Sanger sequencing with NGS is presented in **Table 18**.

Advantage: Any DNA from almost any source can be used and is well suited to heterogeneous DNA samples. It not only allows the simultaneous sequencing of many genes, but also allows the simultaneous detection of CNVs and even low-level single nucleotide variants (SNVs).

Sequencing by synthesis (Fig. 73): Sequencing by synthesis (SBS) is a widely adopted NGS technology. This method for DNA sequencing utilizes the step-by-step incorporation of reversibly fluorescent and terminated nucleotides. In this method, the nucleotides have been modified in two ways—(1) each nucleotide is reversibly attached to a single fluorescent molecule with unique emission wavelengths and (2) each nucleotide is also reversibly terminated ensuring that only a single nucleotide will be incorporated per cycle. There are four nucleotides in DNA and all four nucleotides are added to the sequencing chip.

Method

- First the genomic DNA strand is fragmented into short strands/fragments of 100–500 bp in length. Adaptors are added to ends of the DNA fragments (**Fig. 73A**). These short fragments are immobilized on a solid-phase platform (e.g., glass slide) by using universal capture primers. These primers are complementary to adaptors that have previously been added to ends of the template fragments.
- The addition of fluorescently labeled complementary nucleotides, one per template DNA per cycle, occurs in a "massively parallel" fashion, at millions of templates immobilized on the solid phase at the same time (**Fig. 73B**). A four-color imaging camera is used to capture the fluorescence originating from each template location (corresponding to the specific incorporated nucleotide). After nucleotide incorporation, the remaining DNA bases are washed away. Following this, the fluorescent signal is read at each cluster and recorded. This is followed by cleaving and washing away of both the fluorescent molecule and the terminator group. The entire cycle is repeated until the sequencing reaction is complete. Powerful computational programs can convert the images to generate sequences complementary to the template DNA at the end of one run. These sequences are then mapped back to the reference genomic sequence to identify alterations in the DNA fragment. This method overcomes the disadvantages of the pyrosequencing system in which only a single nucleotide is incorporated at a time.

Analysis of heterogeneous DNA samples can be performed in NGS due to its three common basic principles:

1. **Spatial separation:** In NGS, individual DNA molecules are physically isolated from each other in space. This occurs at the beginning of the procedure. The specification of this process is platform-dependent.
2. **Local amplification:** After the individual DNA molecules are physically separated, these individual molecules are amplified in place using a limited number of PCR cycles. Amplification is needed so that sufficient signal can be produced. This helps in easy detection and increases accuracy.
3. **Parallel sequencing:** Then the amplified DNA molecules are simultaneously sequenced by the addition of polymerases and other reagents. With each spatial separation and amplification, original molecule yields a "read" corresponding to its sequence. Sequence reads from NGS instruments are usually short, <500 bp.

Bioinformatics

Bioinformatics is the application of computational technology to handle the rapidly growing repository of information related to molecular biology. Bioinformatics is the merger of biology with information technology (IT). Bioinformatics uses computers and statistics to perform extensive omics-related research by searching biological databases and comparing gene sequences and protein. Thus, bioinformatics used to identify vast scale of sequences or proteins that differ between

Table 18: Comparison of Sanger sequencing with next-generation sequencing.

Sanger sequencing	*Next-generation sequencing*
Needs a single homogeneous template DNA (usually a specific polymerase chain reaction product)	No such requirement; any DNA from almost any source can be used
Volume: One sequence read/sample (only sequences a single DNA fragment at a time)	Volume: Massively parallel sequencing (massively parallel, sequencing millions of fragments simultaneously per run)
500–1,000 bases/read	100–400 bases/read
Approximately 1 million bases/day/machine	Approximately 2 billion bases/day/machine
Low-throughput process	High-throughput process translates into sequencing hundreds to thousands of genes at one time; Can detect novel or rare variants

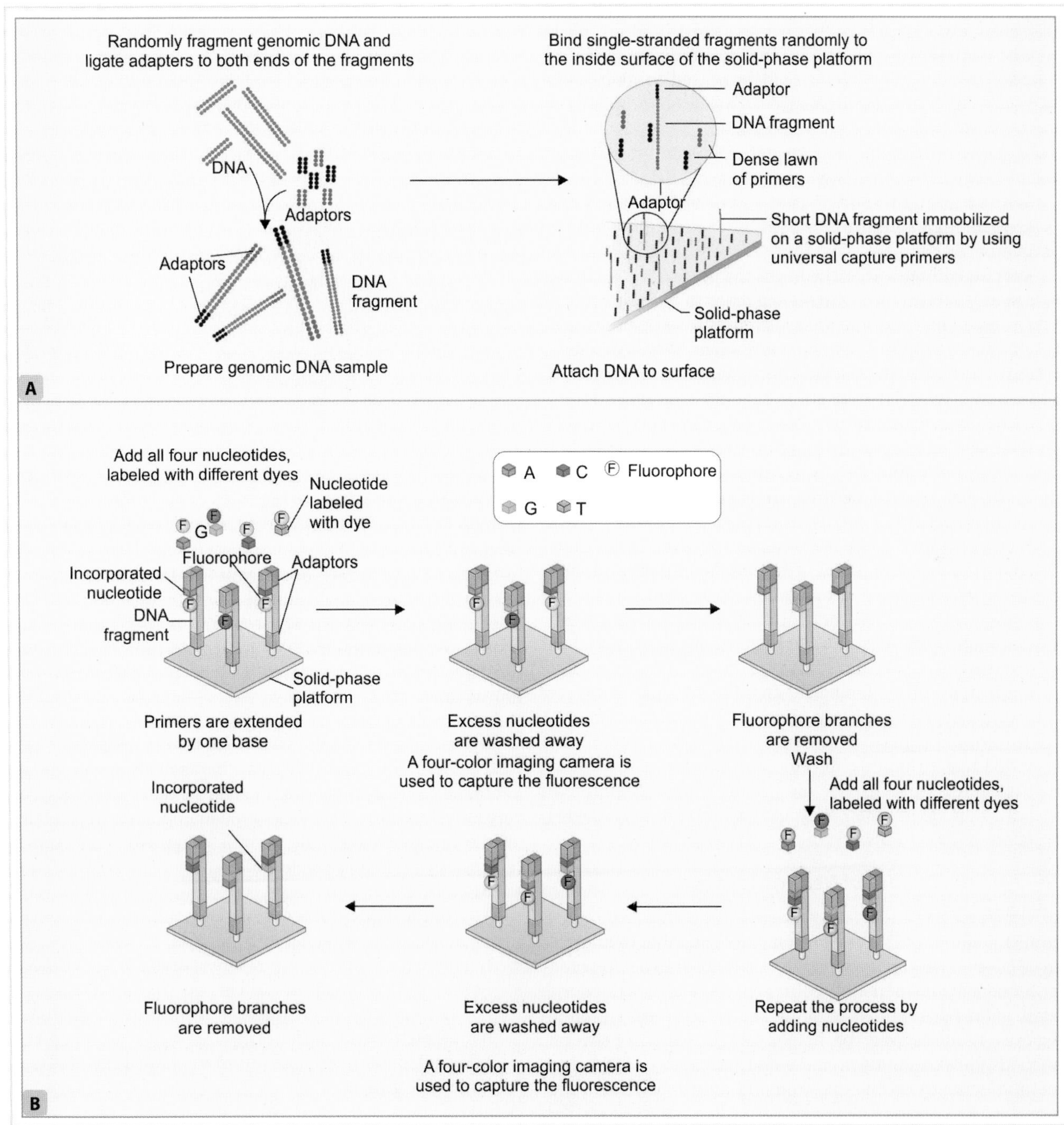

FIGS. 73A AND B: Basic steps in next-generation sequencing [sequencing by synthesis (SBS)] (read the text for description).

diseased and healthy tissues, or between different phenotypes of the same disease. Following the sequencing reaction, each NGS analysis produces an astonishing amount of sequence raw data (i.e., it generates millions of individual molecules, each with a specific sequence). For a high-throughput sequencing instrument, this may amount to 400 billion bp or more of sequence per day. It is enough to produce a high-quality sequence extending an entire human genome. The next integral step in creating a massively parallel sequencing report is bioinformatic processing. The data obtained is far too much for an individual or group of people to analyze and interpret by hand. Fortunately, there are powerful computational tools designed to compile the most salient sequencing data into a format that is understandable to a molecular pathologist. The **raw data obtained from the instrument is first translated into individual sequences** known as "**reads**." Then, **each read is "mapped" by identifying its targeted region in the genome**. Finally, the aligned reads are used to determine differences in nucleotide sequence between the sample DNA and a standardized reference sequence. These basic steps are sequence alignment, and variant calling and mutational signature calling. They are explained in further detail below.

- **Sequence alignment:** It is the process by which the sequencing reads from a sample are mapped onto a reference genome.
- **Variant calling:** Variant calling is the process by which we identify variants from sequence data. In variant calling, all the sequence data from a sample are systematically compared with the reference sequence. The more reads that cover a particular location (sequencing depth), it is more likely that a variant will be detected if present. If a locus shows sufficient evidence of a difference from the reference sequence, a variant call is made.
- **Variant annotation and interpretation:** Variant annotation is the process of assigning functional information to DNA variants. Called variants can be annotated with various features. These features include name of the gene, coding change and protein effect predictions, information from databases listing benign and pathogenic variants, clinical information, etc. After completion of variant annotation by the clinical laboratory, the annotated data are ready for reporting. It is essential to provide a brief description of the biological and clinical significance of each pathogenic variant as a part of this report.
- **Mutational signature calling:** In addition to totaling up individual mutations, develop an informatics algorithm that detects patterns of mutations. This may point to particular environmental exposures (e.g., ultraviolet light) or any defects in DNA repair.

Clinical Applications of Next-generation DNA Sequencing

In next-generation DNA sequencing, it is possible to analyze any DNA sample. However, first the DNA needs to be prepared for sequencing by preparing a library of short DNA sequences. These short DNA sequences should be enriched for genomic regions of interest (e.g., particular exons). There are several methods for NGS library preparation from genomic DNA. The method depends on the question and desired result. In the clinical laboratories, most applications of NGS are for detection of constitutional genetic disease and cancer diagnostics. Few different basic techniques are discussed below.

Targeted sequencing

It captures multiple genes and loci with hybridization techniques followed by deep sequencing. For targeted sequencing, a careful selection of panel of genes is done. This maximizes sequencing depth and minimizes costs and the time and expense required for interpretation and clinical reporting. Sample is prepared for targeted sequencing either by enriching for sequences of interest through hybrid capture via custom complementary probes or by multiplex PCR. NGS assays are also used for inherited disorders, genetic diseases such as cardiomyopathy and congenital deafness. In cancer, gene panels are widely used to perform detailed tumor profiling. Each tumor has a unique set of somatic mutations. Hence, these assays can detect as many treatable or prognostic mutations as possible. This helps in individually tailored patient care. Repeat testing at the time of disease recurrence helps providing information regarding the mechanisms of drug resistance. This in turn can guide the selection of second-line therapies.

Whole-exome sequencing

Whole-exome sequencing (WES) is an unbiased approach and analysis can be performed without reference sequences from parents or siblings. It is a more expansive type of targeted sequencing. In this, hundreds of thousands of custom probes are used to enrich for the roughly 1.5% of the genome that consists of protein encoding exons prior to NGS. It is not commonly used in the evaluation of suspected germline disorders. WES is also used in oncology mostly in the research setting.

Whole-genome sequencing

It is the most comprehensive type of DNA analysis that can be performed on an individual. Presently, its use is mostly limited to cases where exome sequencing has failed to provide an answer, but there is high clinical suspicion of genetic disease. In cancer, it can detect novel structural rearrangements (e.g., insertions, deletions, translocations) that may be clinically relevant. However, its cost is relatively high, and the turnaround time is slow.

Future Applications of Next-generation Sequencing

Next-generation sequencing can be used to detect genetic anomalies of essentially any size. It can detect from SNPs to very large rearrangements and even aneuploidy. Thus, almost all the presently available genetic diagnostic tests can be replaced by NGS. These include:

- RNA analysis.
- Microbiome (combined genetic material of the microorganisms in a particular environment) analysis.
- Blood screening for early markers of diseases (e.g., cancer).
- Assess the response of cancers to therapy (i.e., using circulating "free" DNA released from tumor cells that is harvested from the blood).

Few molecular techniques used in clinical diagnosis are presented in **Table 19**

Table 19: Techniques used in clinical diagnosis.

Techniques to detect		
Known mutation	***Unknown mutation***	***Gene copy number change***
Southern/restriction fragment length polymorphism (RFLP)	Gradient gel electrophoresis (GGE)/denaturing	Southern blot
Pyrosequencing	Denaturing high-performance liquid chromatography (DHPLC)	Multiplex ligation-dependent probe amplification (MLPA)
Real-time , polymerase chain reaction (PCR)	Protein truncation test (PTT)	Array comparative genomic hybridization (aCGH)
Sanger sequence analysis in case of known mutation	Sanger sequence analysis	Single-nucleotide polymorphism (SNP) arrays

GENE THERAPY

Q. Write short essay on gene therapy.

Genes are the units of heredity and code for protein synthesis. Many disease have been shown to have molecular basis. One of the recent advances in molecular biology is the development of successful gene therapy. In the gene therapy, functioning gene is introduced into cells in order to produce a protein product that is missing or defective, or to supply a gene that has a novel function. Gene therapy uses genes to treat or prevent disease.

Definition: Gene therapy is defined as the insertion of genes (replacement of a deficient gene product or repair of an abnormal gene) into an individual's cells and tissues to treat a disease, such as a hereditary disease in which a deleterious mutant allele is replaced with a functional one.

To be effective, the gene therapy requires methods that ensure the safe, efficient, and stable introduction of genes into human cells. Gene therapy uses genes to treat or prevent disease. First done on September 14, 1990 for Ashanthi DeSilva suffering from SCID where the missing gene was introduced through processed WBC.

Approaches for Correcting Faulty Genes

- A normal gene may be inserted into a nonspecific location to replace a nonfunctional gene.
- An abnormal gene could be swapped through homologous recombination.
- Repair through selective reverse mutation.
- The regulation of a particular gene could be altered.

Applications of Gene Therapy

Gene therapy should only be used to treat serious diseases that are thought to be incurable. It has certain side effects. The various applications are:

- **Introduction of normally functioning gene** (gene augmentation/gene addition) into the genome: When there is a defective (mutated or abnormal) gene in the cells, it cannot produce the respective protein, which normal gene produces. In order to produce a protein product, the defective gene causing the disease is replaced by a healthy copy of the gene. This will compensate for underproduction of an important gene product (e.g., CF).
- **Introduction of toxic gene:** Genes whose products are toxic may be introduced to cause direct death of malignant cells or infective organisms in the cells.
- **Introduction of prodrug gene:** The products of introduced genes may act as prodrugs and kill the cells by conventionally administered cytotoxic agents.
- **Introduction of antigen or cytokine gene:** This may stimulate immune response against neoplastic cells or infective diseases and result in immune-mediated destruction.
- **Inactivating or "knocking out" a gene:** The nonfunctional defective gene may be removed by this approach.

Types of Gene Therapy

The cells in the body can be divided into two main categories—somatic cells and germ cells.

1. **Somatic cell therapy:** It involves delivering a corrective gene to somatic cells in the affected tissues. Somatic cells are the nonreproductive cells and its therapeutic effect ends with the individual receiving it and is not passed on to the future generations. Hence, somatic cell therapy is considered as a safer approach. The effects of therapy are short-lived and repeated gene therapies are required to maintain the therapeutic effect. This type of gene therapy is used for disorders such as CF, muscular dystrophy, cancers, and certain infectious diseases. There are three basic forms of somatic gene therapy—(1) ex vivo and (2) in vivo and (3) antisense therapy.
   i. **Ex vivo gene therapy:** In this, somatic cells from an affected individual are collected. The isolated cells are grown in culture outside the body. These cells are then transfected by retroviral cloning vectors containing the remedial gene construct. The cells are further grown and those cells which contain the gene of interest are selected. They are subsequently transplanted or transfused back into the patient (**Fig. 74**). These transplanted transfected cells will synthesize the gene product (i.e., the protein). For example, sickle cell anemia, thalassemia, etc., can be cured by this type of treatment.
   ii. **In vivo gene therapy:** In this type of treatment, there is the direct delivery of the remedial gene into the cells of a particular tissue of the patient. The gene may be transferred by a viral (retroviral) vector or by a nonviral method (**Fig. 74**). This type of treatment may be used to cure patients with neuronal degeneration, muscular dystrophy, and tumors of brain.
   iii. **Antisense therapy:** This is aimed to prevent or lower the expression of a specific gene (**Fig. 75**). Few genetic diseases and cancers are associated with dysregulation or over expression of the genes. This results in either production of excessive amount of gene product or its continuous presence in the cell leading to disruption of the normal functioning of the cell. In such conditions, addition of a normal gene will not be sufficient. It

would be more useful to block the synthesis of the gene product (protein). Thus, in antisense therapy a nucleic acid sequence complementary to complete or a part of that specific mRNA is introduced into the target cell. The mRNA produced by the normal transcription of the gene will hybridize with the antisense oligonucleotide by base pairing. This in turn prevents the translation of this mRNA and results in reduced amount of target protein. The antisense therapy can be used in treatment of sickle cell anemia, various cancers, atherosclerosis, AIDS, and leukemia.

2. **Germ cell therapy:** In germ cell therapy, germ cells (egg or sperms) are used, and it results in permanent changes that are passed on to the future generations. Thus, it offers the possibility of permanently eliminating some diseases from a particular family and ultimately from the population. It is not accepted at present due to ethical reasons.

Arguments for Germline Gene Therapy

- Medical utility: The potential of a true "cure".
- Medical necessity: May be only way to cure some diseases.
- Prophylactic efficacy: Better to prevent a disease rather than to treat pathology.
- Parental autonomy: Parents can make choices about what is best for their children.
- Easier, more effective than somatic gene therapy.
- Eradication of disease in future generations.
- Part of being human: Supporting human improvement.

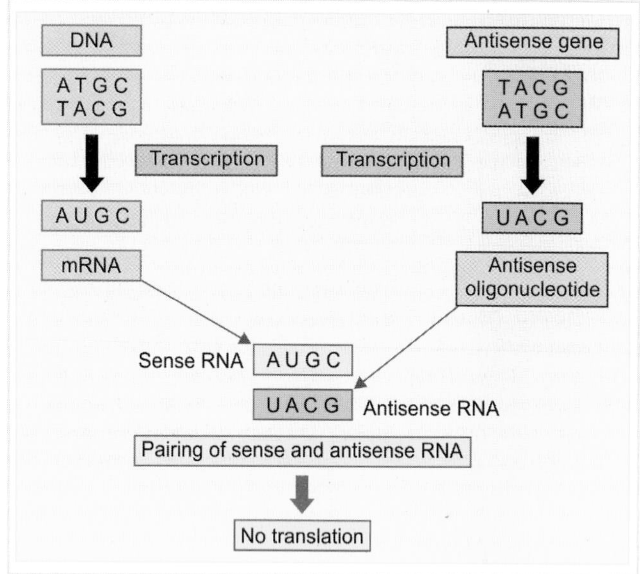

FIG. 75: Basic principle of antisense gene therapy.

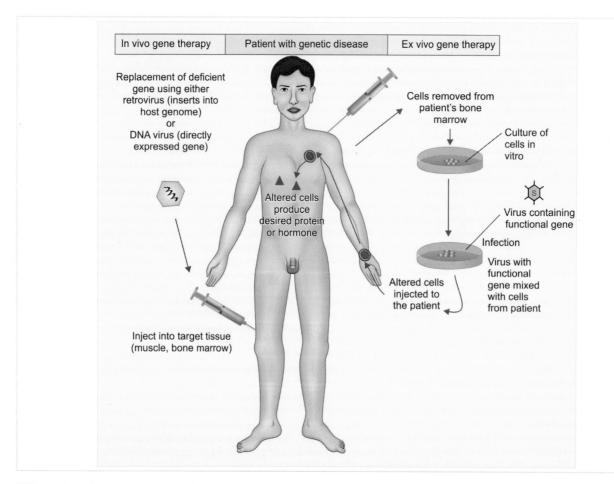

FIG. 74: Gene therapy. In vivo gene therapy delivers genetically modified cells directly to the patient. Ex vivo gene therapy removes cells from the patient which are modified in vitro and then returned to the patient.

Methods of Gene Therapy (Fig. 73)

Vectors in Gene Therapy

The most common form of gene therapy involves insertion of normal gene into the genome with the help of certain carriers called vectors. These vectors can be divided into two main types—viral and nonviral vectors.

1. **Viral vectors:** They are the most commonly used vectors. These viruses are genetically modified such that they do not cause disease in patients who receive gene therapy. The viral vectors deliver the therapeutic human gene into the target cells (such as the patient's liver or lung cells) by infecting these target cells. The therapeutic gene produces the functional protein product and restores the target cell to a normal state. Various viruses that can be used as vectors for gene therapy include retroviruses, adenoviruses, adeno-associated viruses, and herpes simplex viruses.
2. **Nonviral methods:** Gene delivery can also be carried by nonviral methods. These have some advantages. They do not elicit an immune response, are safer and simpler to use, and allow large-scale production. The nonviral methods include:
   i. Direct introduction/naked DNA.
   ii. Liposome-mediated DNA transfer: Liposomes are lipid bilayers surrounding an aqueous vesicle/core. This liposome is capable of transferring the foreign DNA into a target cell by linking with target cell's membrane.
   iii. Gene gun method
   iv. Dendrimers
   v. Oligonucleotides

Problems/Limitations of Gene Therapy

- **Short-lived nature of gene therapy:** Hence, patients will have to undergo multiple rounds of gene therapy.
- **Immune response:** Gene therapy may stimulate the immune response against introduced gene and reduce the effectiveness of gene therapy.
- **Problems with viral vectors:** Viral vectors may sometimes cause potential problems to the patient such as toxicity and inflammatory responses. In addition, the viral vector, once inside the patient, may recover its ability to cause disease.
- **Multifactorial disorders:** Genetic disorders due to single gene mutations usually show best response to gene therapy. Unfortunately, some of the most commonly occurring disorders (e.g., atherosclerosis, hypertension, diabetes, Alzheimer's disease, and rheumatoid arthritis) are multifactorial and are difficult to treat effectively using gene therapy.
- **Risk of inducing a tumor** (insertional mutagenesis): If the gene is integrated in the wrong place in the genome (e.g., in a tumor suppressor gene), it could induce a tumor.
- **Risk of death:** Deaths have occurred due to gene therapy.

Therapeutic Applications (Box 26)

- It has not been approved for clinical use.
- Trials are being conducted on using gene therapy in the treatment of various genetic disorders, cancers, infectious diseases, and other diseases such as Alzheimer's disease and atherosclerosis.

Box 26: Gene therapy in medicine.

- Cancers
- Parkinson disease
- Vascular diseases
- Metastatic melanoma
- Thalassemia
- Hemophilia
- Cystic fibrosis
- Infectious diseases
- Severe combined immunodeficiency (SCID)
- Muscular dystrophy
- Sickle cell anemia
- Leber's congenital amaurosis

HUMAN GENOME PROJECT

Q. Write short essay on HGP/genomic library.

Genome: A genome is the entire DNA in an organism, including its genes. The human genome is estimated to contain ~21,500 genes that are divided among the 23 chromosomes. Of the 23 different chromosomes, 22 are autosomes (numbered 1–22) and one pair of sex chromosomes (X and Y). The function of over 50% of discovered genes is not known. In the genome, about 3 billion bases are arranged along the chromosomes in a particular order for each individual. Storing all this information is a challenge to bioinformatics.

Gene mapping: It is the process of identifying and sequencing each and every human gene of the human genome. The map of the human genome provides a picture of locations, and structures of genes. There are two different types of mappings—physical mapping and genetic mapping. These maps are interdependent and complementary.

Genetic mapping (linkage analysis): A genetic map describes the order of genes and defines the position of a gene relative to other loci on the same chromosome.

Physical mapping: Physical mapping indicates the position of genes in a chromosome, which is determined by physical distances (measured in base pairs) between genes.

Organisms and their genomic sizes are presented in **Table 20**.

Table 20: Organisms and their genomic size.

Organism	*Genomic size in base pairs*
Epstein–Barr virus	0.172×10^6
Bacteria (*Escherichia coli*)	4.6×10^6
Yeast	12.1×10^6
Nematode worm (*Caenorhabditis elegans*)	95.5×10^6
Fruit fly	180×10^6
Human	$3{,}200 \times 10^6$

The **HGP** is an international scientific research project to understand the genomes of humans and other organisms. It was started in 1990 under Dr James D Watson at the United States National Institute of Health. In addition to the United States, the international consortium comprised geneticists in the United Kingdom, France, Germany, Japan, China, and India.

Goals of Human Genome Project

- Understand and identify all genes of the human genome.
- Determine the human DNA sequence: For the entire human genome; also to map human inherited diseases.
- Develop software for large-scale DNA analysis, store all found information in databases, and improve tools for data analysis.
- Transfer related technologies to the private sector.
- Collect and distribute data.
- Study the ethical, legal, and social issues (ELSI) of genetic research that may arise from the project.

Components involved in human genome are diagrammatically shown in **Figure 76.**

All human beings have unique gene sequences. The HGP is a scaffold for future work in identifying differences among individuals.

Uses of Human Genome Project

The understanding of the genome provides clues for:

- Etiology of cancers, Alzheimer's disease, etc.
- Defining the pathogenesis of a disease and to study the disease processes at molecular level.
- Susceptibility of an individual to a variety of illnesses, e.g., carcinoma breast, disorders of hemostasis, liver diseases, CF, etc.
- Precise new ways to prevent a number of diseases that affect human beings.
- To diagnose and treat disease. Target genes for treatment and management of diseases.
- Human development and anthropology: Analysis of similarities between DNA sequences from different organisms helps to study evolution.
- Researcher: By visiting the human genome database on the World Wide Web, a researcher can examine what other scientists have written about the gene.

Ethical Issues (Box 27)

Human genome project helps to identify disease-causing genes, thereby can lead to improvements in diagnosis, treatment, and prevention. It is estimated that most of the individuals harbor several serious recessive genes. However, completion of the human genome sequence and determination of the association of genetic defects with disease have raised many new issues with implications for the individual and mankind.

PROTEOME AND PROTEOMICS

Q. Write short essay on proteomics.

The term proteome is derived from proteins expressed by a genome. It refers to all the proteins produced by an organism and proteins are the functional units. Thus, proteome represents full sets of proteins produced by the body and is similar to the term genome for the entire set of genes. Human body contains more than 2 million different proteins, each having different functions.

Proteomics: It is the study of the proteome (full set/entire library of proteins in a cell type or tissue) and its variation/relationship to disease. It includes the identification, characterization, and quantitation of the entire complement of proteins in cells, tissues or whole individual with a view to understand their function in relation to the life of the cell.

Amino acids are the basic units of proteins and are very small. Each amino acid consists of atoms ranging from 7 to 24 and cannot be identified under even the powerful microscopes.

Box 27: Ethical issues in human genome project.

- Fairness in the use of genetic information
- Privacy and confidentiality
- Psychological impact and stigmatization
- Genetic testing
- Reproductive issues
- Education, standards, and quality control
- Commercialization
- Conceptual and philosophical implications

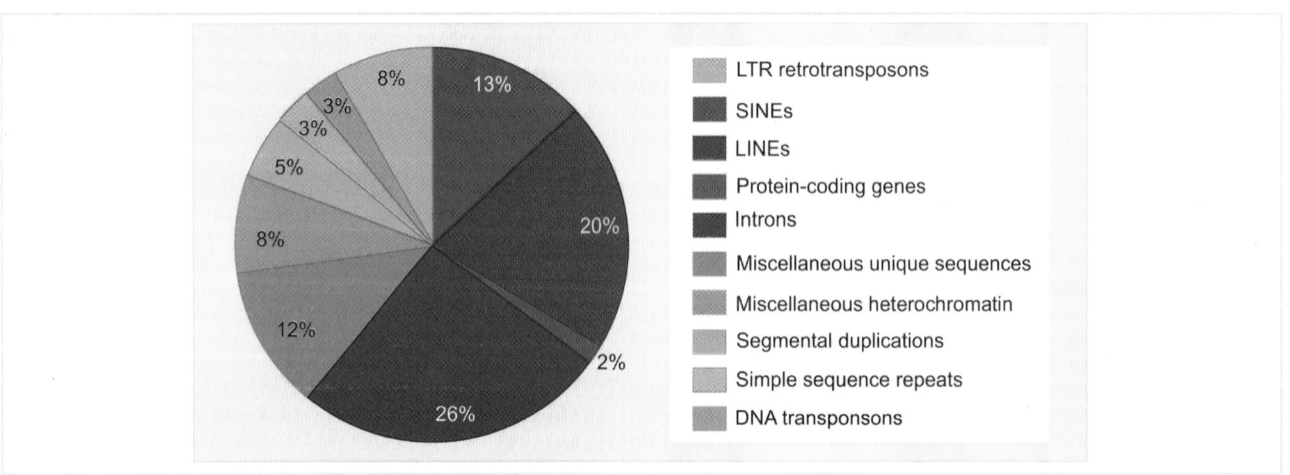

(LTR: long terminal repeat; LINEs: long interspersed nuclear elements; SINEs: short interspersed nuclear elements)

FIG. 76: Components of human genome.

Box 28: Applications of proteomics.

- Medicine, biotechnology, environmental surveillance
- Protein changes during normal processes (e.g., differentiation, development, and aging)
- Abnormal protein expression in disease (e.g., diseases of multigenic origin)
- Identification of novel drug targets and mechanism of drug action
- Surrogate markers
- Targets for gene therapy
- Toxicology
- To detect tumors at an early stage

Uses: Proteomic technologies play an important role in drug discovery, diagnostics, and molecular medicine. When a defective protein causing particular diseases is found, new drugs can be developed to either alter the shape of a defective protein or mimic a missing one. Applications of proteomics arelisted in **Box 28**. The presence or absence of particular proteins in the circulation or in cells is useful for diagnostic and disease-screening purposes.

Mass Spectrometry

Spectrometry is the measurement of the interactions between light and matter, and the reactions and measurements of radiation intensity and wavelength. Mass spectrometry (MS) is an analytical technique that measures the mass-to-charge ratio of ions. MS is based on fragmentation and ionization of molecules using a suitable source of energy. The resulting fragment masses and their relative abundance produce a characteristic mass spectrum of the parent molecule. The results are usually presented as a mass spectrum, a plot of intensity as a function of the mass-to-charge ratio. MS is the major tool used in proteomics and is a powerful method of protein identification (**Fig. 77**). Before a compound can be detected and quantified by MS, the compound must be isolated by another method. This may be either by gas chromatography (GC) or high-performance liquid chromatography (HPLC). Proteins to be analyzed are first digested with a protease (commonly used protease is trypsin). This cleaves proteins into small fragments (peptides) in the range of about 20 amino acid residues long. The peptides are then ionized by irradiation with a laser or by passage through a field of high electrical potential. These are introduced into a mass spectrometer, which measures the mass-to-charge ratio of each peptide. This produces a mass spectrum in which individual tryptic peptides are indicated by a peak corresponding to their mass-to-charge ratio. The results are compared (by using computer algorithms) to a database of theoretical mass spectra of all known proteins for protein identification. This allows identification of the unknown protein.

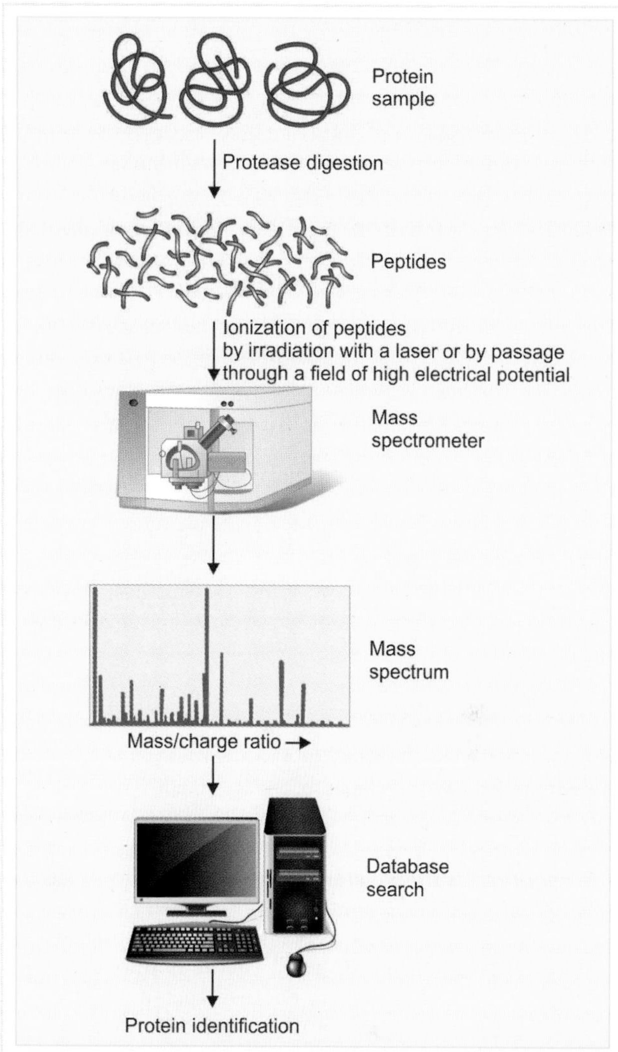

FIG. 77: Mass spectrometry for identification of proteins. First protein is digested with a protease that cleaves it into small peptides. The peptides are then ionized and analyzed in a mass spectrometer. This determines the mass-to-charge ratio of each peptide. The results are displayed as a mass spectrum. It is then compared to a database of theoretical mass spectra of all known proteins for protein identification.

DNA RECOMBINANT TECHNOLOGY

Q. Write short essay on DNA recombinant technology.

Genetic recombination: It is a common phenomenon that occurs during normal sexual reproduction. It mainly **consists of the breakage and re-joining of DNA fragments of the chromosome**. This is essential and useful in reassortment of genetic material.

Gene Cloning

Q. Write short essay on merits (advantages) and demerits (disadvantages) of cloning.

Gene cloning (molecular cloning) is the process of isolating a DNA sequence (genetic material) of interest and creating identical copies of it by growing it artificially.

Basic Steps in Gene Cloning (Fig. 78)

1. **Selection and isolation of DNA:** First a DNA fragment coding for the gene of interest (that has to be cloned) is selected and cut. Usually, isolation of gene is done by PCR. Then this DNA segment is isolated enzymatically. This **DNA segment of interest is termed as DNA insert** (foreign/target/cloned DNA).

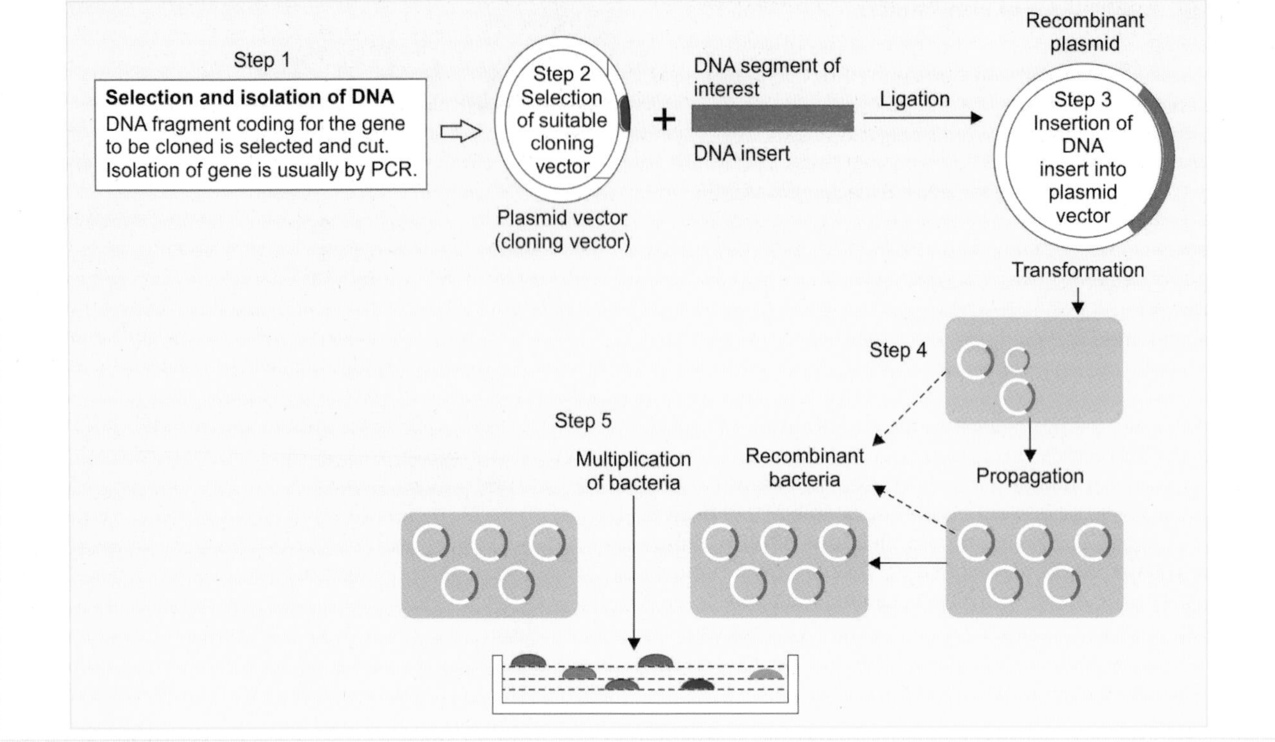

FIG. 78: Steps in gene cloning.

2. **Selection of suitable cloning vector:** A cloning vector is a self-replicating DNA molecule into which DNA insert is to be integrated. Next step is selection of suitable cloning vector. **Most commonly used vector is plasmid DNA.** Plasmid is known as a vector because it acts as a vehicle for the transport of the gene into the host cell. The host cell can be bacterium, yeast or animal cells.
3. **Introduction of DNA insert into vector:** The DNA insert that has been extracted and cleaved enzymatically by the selective restriction endonuclease enzymes (in step 1) is inserted into the vector. It is ligated (joined) by the enzyme ligase to vector DNA. The resultant product is known as recombinant DNA molecule. This is often called as cloning vector–insert DNA construct.
4. **Recombinant DNA molecules are introduced into suitable host:** Suitable hosts are selected and the recombinant DNA molecules are introduced into the host cells. Usually selected host cells are bacterial cells such as *Escherichia coli*. However, yeast and fungi can also be used. This process of entry of recombinant DNA molecule is termed as transformation. After introduction into the host cell, the carrier is known as recombinant host. The plasmid through the process of replication gets amplified and produces large number of copies.
5. After multiple divisions of bacterium, a clone of identical colonies is produced. Each cell in the colony contains a single clone to multiple copies of the recombinant plasmid.

The gene cloning is the process of making recombinant molecules to create recombinant organisms which can produce any drug or protein of interest in bulk amounts.

Recombinant DNA Techniques

It comprises of all the cloning steps and is another way of mimicking natural genetic recombination.

Recombinant DNA technology is defined as "the joining together of DNA molecules from different organisms and inserting it into a host organism to produce new genetic combinations."

It is produced in the laboratory by genetic combination. The genetic material from different sources is brought together to create a genetic sequence that would not otherwise be found in the genome.

Applications

- **Production of hormones:** Different hormones such as insulin, somatostatin, and p-endorphin.
- **Production of vaccines:** For example, polio, hepatitis, rabies, smallpox, cholera, and malaria.
- **Biosynthesis of interferon and antibiotics.**
- Prevention and diagnosis of diseases by using monoclonal antibodies.
- **Gene therapy.**
- **Production of transgenic plant and animals.**

GENE SILENCING

Q. Write short essay on gene silencing/imprinting.

Gene silencing is the **process of regulation of gene expression in a cell to prevent the expression of a particular gene.** Gene silencing is a modern gene-editing technique used for genetic engineering experiments. It is often used in research.

Difference between gene silencing and gene knockdown: When a gene is silenced, its expression is reduced to some extent and not completely. In contrast, when a gene is knocked out, it is completely removed from the genome. Thus, it has no expression and there is no production of protein usually produced by that particular gene.

Methods used to silence genes include RNAi, CRISPR, or siRNA. They usually reduce the expression of a gene by about 70% and do not completely eliminate it.

Types of Gene Silencing

The mechanism of gene silencing may be genetic or epigenetic ways. Gene silencing can occur during either transcription or translation.

Gene Silencing Pathway by Epigenetic Factors

Epigenetic factors such as methylation, acetylation, histone modifications, and chromatin remodeling also cause gene silencing.

Transcriptional Gene Silencing

- **Transposons in gene silencing:** The transposons are the mobile natural genetic elements involved in gene silencing. They can move from one place to another in a genome. There are two types of transposon systems namely—DNA transposons and retrotransposons. Transposable element jumps from one location to the active gene and inserts in it. After its insertion, the active gene has some extra gene sequence that is not a part of it actually. Hence, it cannot perform translation.
- **Antisense oligonucleotides:** By designing some short-nucleotide sequences specific to the mRNA, it is possible to silence the gene and make it inactive. This method is known as antisense oligonucleotides. The complementary antisense nucleotides hybridize to its complementary region on mRNA. Antisense oligonucleotides may either cleave mRNA by using the RNase H or block the translation by some other means. In both the cases, the mRNA cannot form a protein. This method is known as antisense RNA technology.
- ***CRISPR-CAS9* gene silencing:** CRISPR-CAS9 is used for gene editing (refer pages 114 and 115). In normal CAS9 activity, the single-stranded guided RNA recognizes the nuclease CAS9 and guides it to cleave the nucleic acid sequence. The gene cannot form protein. A special type of nuclease, namely CAS9 nuclease, can bind to the target nucleic acid or gene but cannot cut it. Consequently, the polymerase and other transcriptional factors cannot identify the sequence. Thereby there is no protein formation from it.
- **Genomic imprinting:** Somatic cells have two copies of the gene in the genome, one inherited from the father and one from the mother. Genomic imprinting is discussed on page 875.
- **Transgene silencing:** In this, transgene is delivered as DNA or by a virus vector, thereby silencing the gene.
- **Position effect:** It is the effect on the expression of a gene when its location is changed in a chromosome. Position effect is usually by translocation.
- **Paramutation:** Paramutation is an interaction between two alleles at a single locus. In this, one allele induces a heritable change in the other allele and may silence the gene.

Post-transcriptional Gene Silencing

Post-transcriptional gene silencing is due to destruction or blocking of mRNA of a particular gene. The destruction of the mRNA prevents translation to form an active gene product (in most cases, a protein).

- **RNA interference-mediated gene silencing:** It is the common mechanism of post-transcriptional gene silencing. RNA interference (RNAi) is a process in which RNA molecules inhibit gene expression or translation by neutralizing targeted mRNA molecules. In the RNAi mechanism, the process of gene silencing is governed by either siRNA (small interfering RNA) or miRNA (microRNA). Both are noncoding RNAs that regulate gene expression by different mechanisms. Both types of RNA consist of 20–30 nucleotides in length. They bind to the mRNA (messenger) for performing a specific action. They are discussed in detail on page 110–112 (refer **Figs. 22 A and B** of **chapter 5**)
  - siRNA: It binds to the mRNA and cleaves it, thereby making it unavailable to form protein.
  - miRNA: It binds to the target mRNA transcript, and blocks binding of translational factors. Thus, **it blocks translation**.
- **Nonsense-mediated decay:** Nonsense-mediated mRNA decay (NMD) is a surveillance pathway. Its main function is to reduce errors in gene expression by eliminating mRNA transcripts that contain premature stop codons.

Meiotic Gene Silencing

- **Transection:** It is an epigenetic phenomenon that results from an interaction between an allele on one chromosome with the corresponding allele on the homologous chromosome. Transection can either activate or silence gene.
- **Meiotic silencing of unpaired DNA:** If a gene is not paired with a homolog in prophase I of meiosis, it generates a signal that transiently silences all sequences homologous to it.

Applications of Gene Silencing

- **AIDS:** The siRNA-mediated gene silencing is used for treating infectious diseases such as HIV. siRNAs bind to viral *RNA* gene and inactive it transcriptionally thereby effectively inhibiting replication of HIV replication. HIV infection can also be inhibited by targeting either viral genes (for example, gag, rev, tat, and env) or human genes (for example, CD4, the principal receptor for HIV) that are involved in the life cycle of HIV.
- **Viral hepatitis:** Hepatitis B and hepatitis C may also be targeted by gene silencing.
- **Cancer:** RNAi may be a promising way to treat cancer by silencing genes that are differentially upregulated in tumor cells or genes involved in cell division.
- **Others:** It may be useful for the treatment of macular degeneration, respiratory syncytial virus, asthma, CF, chronic obstructive pulmonary disease, chronic myeloid leukemia, and neurodegenerative disorders.

DIGITAL PATHOLOGY AND TELEPATHOLOGY

Conventional Light Microscopy

It is the core tool in diagnostic surgical pathology. Presently, electronic modes of image presentation are used in routine practice in addition to conventional light microscopy. In conventional light microscopy, the magnification, focus, and condenser setting can be adjusted at any time.

Digital Pathology

It is the acquisition, management, sharing, and interpretation of pathology information, including slides and data, in a digital environment. Digital slides are created when glass slides are captured with a scanning device, to provide a high-resolution digital image that can be viewed on a computer screen or mobile device. These digital images can be integrated with the respective pathology reports.

Digital pathology is advantageous in surgical pathology. There are various devices to capture digital images of gross and microscopic specimens. Virtual microscopy is the technique in which entire glass slides or selected areas of slides are scanned and converted to digital data files (also termed as virtual slides). These can then be viewed on a computer screen. The characteristics of the displayed image, in terms of resolution and range of magnification, mainly depend on the optical features of the scanning system. Overall, these are comparable with those of glass slide microscopy. In conventional light microscopy, in digital scanning, the so-called "scanning depth" must be determined before the acquisition of the image. The "scanning depth" includes the region of interest, the scanning power [scanning power includes the physical magnification (e.g., 20×) and resolution (e.g., 2,048 × 4,800 pixels)], and the number of horizontal levels to be obtained in the plane of the tissue section. The number of horizontal levels (so-called z-stacking) is dependent on the thickness of section.

Whole Slide Imaging

Whole slide imaging (WSI) is the scanning of entire glass slides to produce electronic images. The average time required to digitize a 15 × 15 region of tissue on glass slide at 40 × of a single horizontal level of a slide (non-z stacked) may range from 2 to 4 minutes. This produces a large data file (may range from about 200 MB to 2.5 GB).

Parts: Each virtual file consists of multiple parts and are termed as file segments. These include an identification tag, a barcode [generated by the laboratory information system (LIS)], a low-power overview, and the images at the selected power. The methods of image acquisition vary and are usually of three types namely—(1) linear, (2) meander, or (3) array. Most systems produce tiled images. These tiled images are small images that are retrieved and stitched together to form the final image on the computer screen at the selected power. Most interfaces permit electronic zooming (i.e., additional magnification) beyond the original scanned magnification.

Image acquisition and resolution: Currently, resolution and functionality of virtual slides are comparable to those of conventional light microscopes. Though scanning time has improved over time, it still consumes time. The scanning time is mainly dependent on computational speed and optical physics. The optical physics in turn depends on the magnification of the scanning objective. The actual image acquisition step occurs through a CCD. CCD consists of several hundred thousand individual picture elements (pixels) that transform the optical image into a virtual image. Thus, the whole slide images are acquired by the movement of an optical lens over the slide. Some instruments reduce scanning time to acquire images by using a meander (follow a winding course) rather than a linear scanning pattern. However, both the meander and linear methods have inherent physical limitations. The third type of technology for image acquisition is known as "lens array microscopy." It uses arrays of detectors (miniaturized lenses) to simultaneously capture information from larger areas of the tissue section. This can reduce the scanning time.

Image Stitching

It is the technology by which several smaller images that have overlapping areas are combined to produce a larger image. The computational process employed by smartphones can produce panoramic photographs from a single lens moved slowly across a field of view. Image stitching for virtual microscopy is a simple process and it offers several advantages over conventional WSI.

Implementation of Virtual Microscopy

For virtual microscopy in the cytopathology or surgical pathology laboratory, it needs an electronic and organizational infrastructure and a slide scanning instrument. The infrastructure needs an efficient interaction between IT and LIS personnel. Dedicated and trained technical personnel (e.g., image technologists) are needed to load and maintain the scanning instrument, perform screening (and rescanning if required), monitor quality of scan, and to distribute the virtual files in a manner that can be conveniently viewed by the pathologist.

Diagnostic and Clinical Applications

These include diagnostic consultations, archiving, primary diagnosis, and QA.

Diagnostic consultation: It is also called e-consultation. This is one of the most useful applications. Apart from its convenience (no need to pack or mail the slides), other advantages include instantaneous electronic distribution permits consulting pathologists to review the scanned slides at any time and location. Also, online, real-time conferencing and simultaneous viewing by two or more pathologists can be easily achieved. There are no risks of losing the primary data (i.e., tissue blocks or glass slides).

Scanning of selected cases for archiving: Virtual slide prepared by scanning of selected cases that are sent in consultation makes it permanent record of the diagnostic slides for the consulting institution. These archives enhance patient care and guide frozen section diagnosis, or final diagnosis at the time of definitive excision. These archives also can be utilized for subsequent clinicopathologic conferences.

Primary diagnosis: Primary diagnosis based on review of virtual slides has the same accuracy as primary diagnosis based on routine conventional light microscopy.

Quality assurance: QA programs may be enhanced by reviewing the virtual slides of cases that had discrepancies in diagnosis.

Education

Virtual microscopy is an important tool for medical education in pathology. This includes teaching medical students (includes histology), pathology residents, postgraduates and fellows, and continuing medical education for practicing pathologists. Presently, many national/regional pathology conferences and slide seminars post virtual slides on websites before the conferences/meeting.

Research Applications

In surgical pathology, research applications include consensus review of slides, quantitative image analysis, and imaging of tissue microarrays. These are used to study patterns of gene and protein expression. In diagnostic pathology, it is easy to share virtual slides of specimens among investigators at different sites, anytime. Virtual slides also allow for the electronic publication of whole slides rather than selected fields of slides, that provides new useful information to practicing pathologists.

Telepathology

Q. Write short essay on telepathology.

Captured digital images can be transferred electronically to any part of the globe.

Definition: Telepathology is the practice in which pathologists provide diagnoses from a distance. Pathologists view electronically transmitted images from a distance rather than by examining the glass slides themselves by conventional light microscopy. Thus, telepathology means practice of pathology and viewing at a distance.

Histological, cytological or macro images can be transmitted along telecommunication pathways on a video monitor rather than directly through a microscope. Thus, telepathology is the practice of medical diagnosis facilitated by digital transmission of pathological data.

Mode of transmission of digital images: Transmission can be done at various levels, from the e-mail attachment of a few static photographs by ordinary telephone lines, high-speed digital lines, or satellites. Presently, via the Internet, sophisticated systems that duplicate almost to perfection the examination of slides under the microscope are available.

Advantages/Benefits

- Telepathology makes it faster and easier to share medical images. Biopsies can be cut, stained, scanned, magnified, and sent digitally. A pathologist can read the slides remotely in real-time and provide with an immediate diagnosis.
- Pathologists in different locations can view images simultaneously and discuss diagnoses through teleconferencing. It brings expert services closer to the patient. Thus, eliminates the unnecessary shifting of patients to referral hospital.
- Pathologist can consult pathologists who are specialized in area of concern, such as liver pathology or lung pathology.
- It allows pathologists, surgeons, and radiologists to communicate with each other over diagnostic dilemmas and overcoming the barrier of distance.
- It is easier to get second opinions on the particular case when needed.
- Provides higher quality of education. The acquisition of images may be useful for diagnosis, consultation or continuing medical education.

Components

The various components of telepathology network include:

- A conventional microscope.
- Device to capture the image, i.e., a camera mounted on a microscope.
- Telecommunication link between the sending and receiving sites.
- A workstation at the receiving site with a high-quality video monitor.

Main Categories of Telepathology

Currently three main types/systems (with some overlap) of telepathology are available namely—dynamic, static, and virtual.

Dynamic telepathology (real-time) systems

This is also termed robotic interactive telepathology and real-time telepathology. In this, the recipient pathologist view images in real time by electronic control of a distant robotic microscope that has motorized optics and a motorized stage. These are real time images that are viewed on a high-resolution monitor. The section can be viewed entirely and this eliminates the inadequate or inappropriate selection of fields. These instruments allow the remote user (pathologist) to remotely control the movement of the slide on the microscope in any direction, to change magnifications, and even to change the focus (particularly useful for cytological preparations). The resolution of the images is practically the same as that obtained with the actual slide under the microscope. Reported diagnostic accuracy is comparable to that of conventional light microscopy. Dynamic-robotic telepathology is mainly useful to provide intraoperative frozen section diagnoses to hospitals without on-site pathologists. This technique is suitable for routine histological preparations, immunostains, cytology preparations, and electron micrographs. Usually, in less than a minute, a digital overview of the slide is created.

A variation of the dynamic method is the submission of a live ("streaming") image from the remotely located microscope. In this, the slide and magnification are controlled through instructions to the person using the microscope.

Advantages: Selection of field of interest by expert is fast and resolution of image is high.

Disadvantages: It is a complex technology and is expensive. It needs extra time to review the virtual slides compared with standard slides. Implementation requires substantial planning, communication, and training of both pathologists and support personnel.

Static telepathology systems

Static image-based systems: In static telepathology, static images (e.g., .jpeg or .tiff files) are captured from a digital camera connected to a microscope. These selected images are stored and transmitted (forwarded) to the pathologist. A limited number of images (1–40) are captured and stored in the hard drive of the computer or compact disc-read only memory (CD-ROM) for transmission. Static systems are mainly used to obtain second opinions on difficult cases. The diagnostic accuracy almost approaches conventional glass slide optical microscopy.

Advantages: It is economical, simple, and requires only a standard telephone and internet connection. There is no need for any special software and transfer size is small.

Disadvantages: Selection of field for images should be done by expert and if done by a nonexpert, may miss the important areas. The number of images is limited and sampling error due to inability to view the entire slide. Selection of images may be biased by a pathologist who may take images of field to support his/her diagnosis. The image quality depends on the camera and interpretation at the receiving end depends on the skill and pathologist in viewing static images. To a pathologist who is trained to see slide in continuity may feel it as suboptimal approach.

Differences between static and real-time telepathology are listed in **Table 21**.

Table 21: Differences between static and real-time telepathology.

Features	*Static*	*Real-time*
Image system	Still	Live
Microscope	Conventional good microscope	Motorized bidirectional microscope
Robotic remote control	No	Present
Images per case	5 or more	Unlimited
Specimen sampling	Limited	Comprehensive
Image selection	By referring pathologist	Pathologist at receiving end
Transmission time per image	45 seconds	1/15 second
Average duration for diagnosis	15 minutes	3–10 minutes
Video conferencing facility	Not available	Available
Network capacity	Low (28.8 kbps)	High (1.54 Mbps)

Virtual slide telepathology

Virtual slide systems: Pathology specimen slides are scanned and high-resolution digital images created for transmission. The virtual microscopy in telepathology has clinical utility, even in intraoperative frozen section diagnosis.

Disadvantages: The scanning time needed to produce a WSI, the required infrastructure, and the large file sizes may limit the usefulness of virtual slide telepathology.

Box 29: Applications of telepathology.

- Validation: Intraoperative frozen section, surgical pathology consultation, expert-to-expert consultation, distance education teaching, and quality control programs
- Provisional: Cytogenetics, cytometry imaging, cytopathology, fine needle aspirates, autopsy pathology, hematopathology, and immunohistochemistry
- Future: Point-of-care pathology services, proficiency testing, ultra-rapid turnaround time (TAT) in surgical pathology especially for difficult cases and research tool

Uses of Telepathology (Box 29)

Whether telepathology will ever replace the time-honored practice of mailing the slides for consultation remains to be seen. Most pathologists prefer to look at a section on a glass slide than an image. This is because this is what they have been doing since the beginning of recorded pathology history.

BIBLIOGRAPHY

1. Aflaki E, Westbroek W, Sidransky E. The complicated relationship between Gaucher disease and Parkinsonism: insights from a rare disease. *Neuron*. 2017;93:737.
2. Alberts B, Johnson A, Lewis J et al. Molecular Biology of the Cell, second edition. New York: Garland Science, Taylor & Francis Group; 2015.
3. Almal, S., Padh, H. Implications of gene copy-number variation in health and diseases. J Hum Genet 57, 6–13 (2012). https://doi.org/10.1038/jhg.2011.108. [Last accessed on 2021 January 19].
4. Anastasiadou E, Jacob LS, Slack FJ. Non-coding RNA networks in cancer. *Nat Rev Genet*. 2018;18:5-18.
5. Angulo MA, Butler MG. Cataletto ME: Prader-Willi syndrome: a review of clinical, genetic, and endocrine findings. *J Endocrinol Invest*. 2015;38:1249.
6. Antonarakis SE. Down syndrome and the complexity of genome dosage imbalance, Nat Rev Genet 18:147, 2017. Benito-Vicente A, Uribe KB, Jebari S et al: Familial hypercholesterolemia: the most frequent cholesterol metabolism disorder caused disease. *Int J Mol Sci*. 2018;19(11):3426.
7. Bagni C, Zukin RS. A synaptic perspective of fragile X syndrome and autism spectrum disorders. *Neuron*. 2019;101:1070.
8. Berberich AJ, Hegele RA. The complex molecular genetics of familial hypercholesterolaemia. *Nat Rev Cardiol*. 2019;16:9.
9. Breiden B, Sandhoff K: Ganglioside metabolism and its inherited diseases. *Methods Mol Biol*. 2018;1804:97.
10. Buckingham L. Molecular Diagnostics Fundamentals, Methods, and Clinical Applications, third edition. Philadelphia: F.A. Davis Company; 2019.
11. Buiting K, Williams C, Horsthemke B: Angelman syndrome—insights into a rare neurogenetic disorder. *Nat Rev Neurol*. 2016;12:584.
12. Cagle PT, Allen TC. Basic Concepts of Molecular Pathology. London: Springer Science; 2009.
13. Coleman WB, Tsongalis GJ. Diagnostic Molecular Pathology: A Guide to Applied Molecular Testing. London: Elsevier Inc; 2017.
14. Coleman WB, Tsongalis GJ. Essential Concepts in Molecular Pathology. London: Elsevier Inc; 20107.
15. Cooper GM. The Cell: A Molecular Approach, eight editions. United States of America: Oxford University Press; 2019.
16. Cortini F, Villa C, Marinelli B et al. Understanding the basis of Ehlers-Danlos syndrome in the era of the next-generation sequencing. *Arch Dermatol Res*. 2019;311:265.

17. Defesche JC, Gidding SS, Harada-Shiba M et al. Familial hypercholesterolaemia. *Nat Rev Dis Primers*. 2017;3(17093):1.
18. Dietz HC: New therapeutic approaches to mendelian disorders. *N Engl J Med*. 2010;363:852.
19. Elles R, Mountford R. Molecular Diagnosis of Genetic Diseases, second edition. New York: Human Press; 2010.
20. Elliott D, Ladomery M. Molecular Biology of RNA, Second edition. United Kingdom: Oxford University Press; 2016.
21. Ferreiraa CR, Gahlc WA. Lysosomal storage diseases. *Transl Sci Rare Dis*. 2(1):2017.
22. Filocamo M, Tomanin R, Bertola F et al. Biochemical and molecular analysis in mucopolysaccharidoses: what a paediatrician must know. *Ital J Pediatr*. 2018;44(2):129.
23. Guest PC. Multiplex Biomarker Techniques- Methods and Applications. Brazil: Springer Science; 2017.
24. Hall DA, Berry-Kravis E. Fragile X syndrome and fragile X-associated tremor ataxia syndrome. *Handb Clin Neurol*. 2018;147:377.
25. Hartwell LH, Goldberg ML, Fischer JA, Hood L. Genetics. From Genes to Genomes, 6th edition. New York: McGraw-Hill Education; 2018.
26. Horst H. Molecular Pathology. London: CRC Press, Inc; 2018.
27. Iwarsson E, Jacobsson B, Dagerhamn J et al. Analysis of cell-free fetal DNA in maternal blood for detection of trisomy 21, 18 and 13 in a general pregnant population and in a high-risk population—a systematic review and meta-analysis. *Acta Obstet Gynecol Scand*. 2017;96:7.
28. Iwasa J, Marshall W. Karp's cell and Molecular Biology: Concepts and Experiments, 8th edition. USA: John Wiley & Sons, Inc; 2016.
29. Jameson JL, Fausi AS, Kasper DL, et al. Harrison's principles of internal medicine (2 vols), 20th edition. New York: McGraw-Hill Medical Publishing. Division; 2018.
30. Kanakis GA, Nieschlag E. Klinefelter syndrome: more than hypogonadism. *Metab Clin Exp*. 2018;86:135.
31. Karp G. Cell and Molecular Biology: Concepts and Experiments. 6th edition. USA: John Wiley & Sons; 2010.
32. Keller A, Meese E. Nucleic Acids as Molecular Diagnostics. Germany: Wi;ey-VCH; 2015.
33. Kohler L, Puertollano R, Raben N. Pompe disease: from basic science to therapy. *Neurother*. 2018;15:928.
34. Korf BR, Irons MB. Human Genetics and Genomics, 4th edition. West Sussex: Wiley-Blackwell; 2013.
35. Kumar V, Abbas AK, Aster JC. Robbins basic pathology, 10th edition. Philadelphia: Saunders Elsevier; 2018.
36. Kumar V, Abbas AK, Fausto N, et al. Robbins and Cotran pathologic basis of disease, 10th edition. Philadelphia: WB Saunders; 2021.
37. Levitsky LL, O'Donnell Luria AH, Hayes FJ et al: Turner syndrome: update on biology and management across the life span. *Curr Opin Endocrinol Diabetes Obes*. 2015;22(1):65.
38. Lewis R. Human Genetics: Concepts and Applications,11th edition. Penn Plaza: McGraw-Hill Education; 2015.
39. Lodish H, Berk A, Kaiser CA et al. Molecular Cell Biology, eight edition. New York: W. H. Freeman and Company; 2016.
40. Man L, Lekovich J, Rosenwaks Z et al. Fragile X-associated diminished ovarian reserve and primary ovarian insufficiency from molecular mechanisms to clinical manifestations. *Front Mol Neurosci*. 2017;12:1.
41. Mila M, Alvarez-Mora MI, Madrigal I et al. Fragile X syndrome: an overview and update of the FMR1 gene, Clin Genet 93:197, 2018.
42. Morsheimer M, Whitehorn TFB, Heimall J et al: The immune deficiency of chromosome 22q11.2 deletion syndrome. *Am J Med Genet*. 2017;173A:2366.
43. Ohashi T. Gene therapy for lysosomal storage diseases and peroxisomal diseases. *J Hum Genet*. 2019;64:139.
44. Plotegher N, Duchen MR. Mitochondrial dysfunction and neurodegeneration in lysosomal storage disorders. *Trends Mol Med*. 2017;23(2):116.
45. Priyadarshini A, Pandey P. Molecular Biology: Different Facets. Canada: Apple Academic Press; 2018.
46. Pyeritz RE. Etiology and pathogenesis of the Marfan syndrome: current understanding. *Ann Cardiothorac Surg*. 2017:6(6):595.
47. Ralston H, Penman ID, Strachan MWJ, Hobson RP. Davidson's Principles and Practice of Medicine, 23rd edition. Edinburgh: Elsevier; 2018.
48. Rapley R, Harbron S. Molecular Analysis and Genome Discovery, Second edition.UK: John Wiley & Sons; 2012.
49. Sabatine MS. PCSK9 inhibitors: clinical evidence and implementation. *Nat Rev Cardiol*. 2019;16:155.
50. Salcedo-Arellano MJ, Dufour B, McLennan Y et al. Fragile X syndrome and associated disorders: clinical aspects and pathology. *Neurobiol Dis*. 2020;136:1.
51. Salik I, Rawla P: Marfan syndrome. [Updated 2019 Feb 28]. In StatPearls [internet], Treasure Island, FL, 2019, StatPearls Publishing.
52. Schuchman EH, Desnick RJ. Types A and B Niemann-Pick disease. *Mol Genet Metab*. 2017;120(1–2):27.
53. Seranova E, Connolly KJ, Zatyka M et al. Dysregulation of autophagy as a common mechanism in lysosomal storage diseases. *Essays Biochem*. 2017;61:733.
54. Skuse D, Printzlau F, Wolstencroft J. Sex chromosomal aneuploidies. In Geschwind DH, Paulson HL, Klein C, editors: Handbook of clinical neurology, 2018, p 147. (3rd series) Neurogenetics, Part 1 355.
55. Stirnemann J, Belmatoug N, Camou F et al. A review of Gaucher disease pathophysiology, clinical presentation and treatments. *Int J Mol Sci*. 2017;18(441):1.
56. Strayer DS, Saffitz JE. Rubin's Pathology: Mechanism of Human Disease, 8th edition. Philadelphia: Wolters Kluwer; 2020.
57. Tinkle B, Castori M, Berglund B et al. Hypermobile Ehlers-Danlos syndrome (a.k.a. Ehlers-Danlos syndrome Type III and Ehlers-Danlos syndrome hypermobility type): clinical description and natural history. *Am J Med Genet Part C Semin Med Genet*. 2017;175C:48.
58. Turnpenny PD, Ellard S. Emery's Elements of Medical Genetics.15th edition. Philadelphia: Saunders Elsevier; 2017.
59. Weinstein DA, Steuerwald U, De Souza CFM et al. Inborn errors of metabolism with hypoglycemia: glycogen storage diseases and inherited disorders of gluconeogenesis. *Pediatr Clin North Am*. 2018;65(2):247.
60. Wong LJC. Next Generation Sequencing Based Clinical Molecular Diagnosis of Human Genetic Disorders, Texas: Springer International Publishing; 2017
61. Zamponi Z, Helguera PR. The shape of mitochondrial dysfunction in Down syndrome. Dev Neurobiol Epub 2019.

CHAPTER 13

Diseases of Infancy and Childhood

CHAPTER OUTLINE

- Introduction
- Congenital anomalies
  - Definitions and terminologies
  - Causes of anomalies
- Prematurity and fetal growth restriction
  - Major risk factors for prematurity
  - Fetal growth restriction
  - Neonatal respiratory distress syndrome
  - Necrotizing enterocolitis
- Perinatal infections
  - Transcervical (ascending) infections
  - Transplacental (hematologic) infections
  - Sepsis
- Fetal hydrops
  - Immune hydrops
  - Nonimmune hydrops
  - Clinical features
- Inborn errors of metabolism and other genetic disorders
  - Inborn errors of amino acid metabolism
  - Galactose and fructose disorders
  - Cystic fibrosis (mucoviscidosis)
- Sudden infant death syndrome
  - Epidemiology
  - Risk factors
  - Pathogenesis
  - Diagnosis
- Tumors and tumor-like lesions of infancy and childhood
  - Tumor-like conditions
  - Benign neoplasms (tumors)
  - Malignant neoplasms
  - Neuroblastic tumors
  - Wilms tumor (nephroblastoma)

INTRODUCTION

Development from birth to puberty (i.e., infant to child) can be divided into different groups or stages (**Table 1**).

Each of these groups has its own anatomic, physiologic, and immunologic characteristics. Each group is susceptible to different types of disorders. Many conditions occurring in childhood are unique. Causes and mechanisms of morbidity and mortality in the neonatal period differ from those in infancy and childhood.

- **Perinatal period:** Diseases during the perinatal period (the period immediately before and after birth) account for significant morbidity and mortality. Diseases that manifest during the perinatal period may be caused due to factors in the fetal environment, due to genomic abnormalities or by interactions between genetic defects and environmental influences. For example, phenylketonuria (PKU) is due to genetic deficiency of phenylalanine hydroxylase (PAH). It causes mental retardation only if an affected infant is exposed to phenylalanine in the diet.
- **First 12 months of life:** Leading causes of death in the first 12 months of life include congenital anomalies, prematurity and low birth weight, sudden infant death syndrome (SIDS), and maternal complications and injuries. The chances for survival of infants improve as the week passes. Once the infant survives the first year of life, the outlook significantly improves.

Table 1: Traditional different stages from birth to puberty.

Stages/groups	*Range of age*
Neonatal age/period	First 4 weeks of life
Infancy	First year of life
Early childhood	1–4 years of age
Late childhood	5–14 years of age

- **From 1 to 9-year age group:** In the two age groups namely 1 to 4 years and 5 to 9 years, accidental injuries are the leading cause of death. In this group major important natural diseases are congenital anomalies and malignant neoplasms.
- **From 10 to 14-year age group:** Leading causes of death are accidents, malignancies, suicide, homicide, and congenital malformations.

CONGENITAL ANOMALIES

Congenital anomaly (birth defect/congenital defect/congenital disorder): The term congenital means "born with". All types of the structural abnormalities or defects that are present at birth are termed as congenital anomalies. However, few (e.g., cardiac defects, renal anomalies) may not evident at birth but become clinically apparent years later.

Actually, congenital anomalies found in live-born infants represent the less serious developmental failures in embryogenesis. This is because they have resulted in live birth. Less severe anomalies allow more prolonged intrauterine survival. Some of them may terminate in stillbirth (intrauterine death of fetus). The serious congenital anomalies cause spontaneous abortion.

Definitions and Terminologies

Definitions

The process of organ and tissue development is known as morphogenesis. It can be impaired by different errors.

Malformations: Malformations are morphologic defects or abnormalities of an organ, part of an organ or anatomic region. It is due to disturbed or error in morphogenesis (i.e., an intrinsically abnormal developmental process).

- **Cause:** Malformations can be result of a single gene or chromosomal defect, but more commonly it is multi-factorial in origin.
- **Patterns:** Developmental anomalies due to interference with morphogenesis may present in several patterns. Some involve single body systems [e.g., congenital heart defects (e.g., ventricular or atrial septal defects), anencephaly (absence of part or all of the brain) **Fig. 1**], cleft lip and/or palate and neural tube defects. Others involve many organs together.

Disruptions: They result from secondary destruction of an organ or body region in which there was normal development. Thus, in contrast to malformations, disruptions occur due to an extrinsic disturbance in morphogenesis. The classic example of a disruption includes amniotic bands. These bands develop following rupture of amnion and formation of "bands". They encircle, compress, or attach to parts of the developing fetus. Many environmental agents may cause disruptions. Disruptions are not heritable. Hence, they are not associated with increased risk of recurrence in subsequent pregnancies.

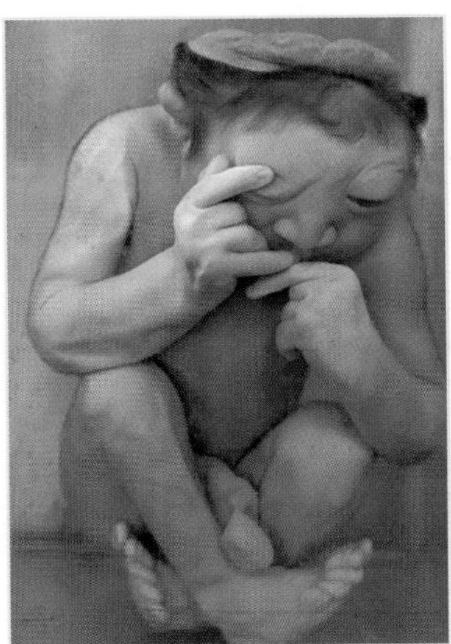

FIG. 1: Anencephaly.

Deformations: These are abnormalities of form, shape or position of a part of the body due to an extrinsic disturbance (mechanical forces) of development rather than an intrinsic error of morphogenesis. Most anatomic defects that occur in the last two trimesters of pregnancy fall into this category. It is common and is similar to disruptions.

- **Pathogenesis:** It is due to localized or generalized compression of the growing fetus. Responsible forces may be external (e.g., amniotic bands in the uterus) or intrinsic (e.g., fetal hypomobility caused by CNS injury). The most common underlying factor is uterine limitations or restrictions. For example, equinovarus foot may be caused by uterine wall compression in oligohydramnios or by spinal cord abnormalities that lead to defective innervation and movement of the foot. Between 35 and 38 weeks of gestation, the size of the fetus grows faster the growth of the uterus, and the relative amount of amniotic fluid (which normally acts as a cushion) decreases. Thus, even the normal fetus is subjected to some degree of uterine limitations or restrictions.
- **Predisposing factors:** Several factors may increase excessive compression of the fetus leading to deformations.
  - **Maternal factors:** These include first pregnancy, small uterus, malformed (e.g., bicornuate) uterus, and uterus with leiomyomas.
  - **Fetal or placental factors:** These include oligohydramnios, multiple fetuses, and abnormal fetal presentation. For example, clubfeet can occur as a component of Potter sequence (**Fig. 2**).

Developmental sequence anomaly (anomalad or complex anomaly): It is a cascade (pattern) of anomalies (defects) arising from a single anomaly or pathogenetic mechanism. These patterns are activated by one initiating aberration (departure from normal). Almost 50% of the time, congenital anomalies occur singly and in the remaining 50% of cases, they are multiple. In some cases, the sequence of anomalies may be explained by a single localized aberration in organogenesis (malformation, disruption, or deformation). This begins to produce secondary effects in other organs. Oligohydramnios (severely reduced amount of amniotic fluid) sequence (or Potter complex) is an example for sequence (**Fig. 2**). Potter sequence is the atypical physical appearance of a baby due to oligohydramnios and occurs within the uterus. It includes clubbed feet, pulmonary hypoplasia and cranial anomalies related to the oligohydramnios. The sequences are as follows:

- **Oligohydramnios** (decreased amniotic fluid) may be caused by different unrelated maternal, placental, or fetal abnormalities.
  - Maternal causes: The most common cause of oligohydramnios is chronic leakage of amniotic fluid due to rupture of fetal membranes.
  - Fetal causes: Fetal urine is a major component of amniotic fluid. Fetal causes include renal agenesis and urinary tract obstruction in the fetus.
  - Placental causes: Uteroplacental insufficiency due to maternal hypertension or severe pre-eclampsia.
- The features of Potter complex occur regardless of the cause of oligohydramnios. Significant oligohydramnios produces intrauterine fetal compression and morphologic changes of the amnion are all related to oligohydramnios. The compression produces a classic phenotype in the

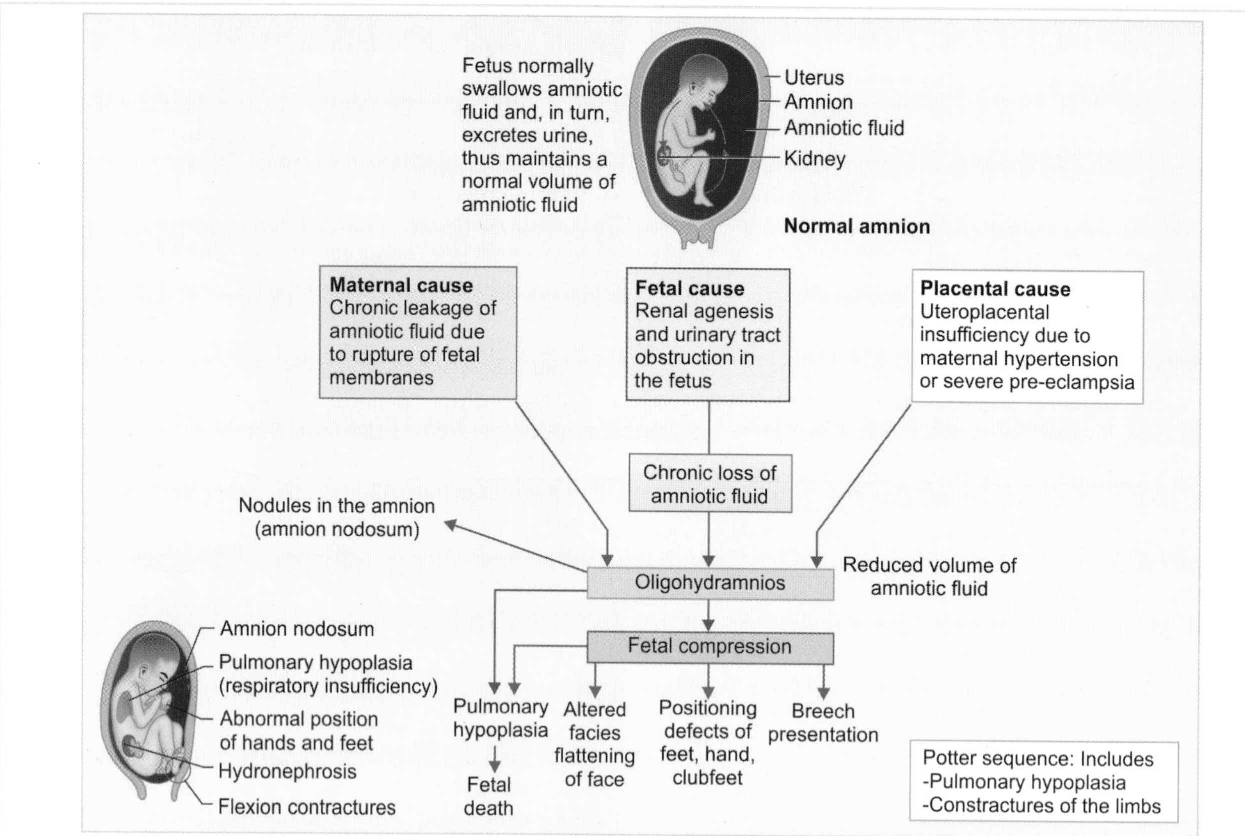

FIG. 2: Steps involved in the pathogenesis of oligohydramnios sequence. Oligohydramnios results in a spectrum of congenital abnormalities called Potter sequence. This includes pulmonary hypoplasia and contractures of the limbs. The amnion has a nodular appearance.

newborn infant. These phenotypic changes include flattening of face, positional abnormalities of the hands, clubfeet and may be accompanied by dislocation of hip. Compression reduces the growth of the chest wall and accompanied by **hypoplastic lungs**. This may result in fetal death. Frequently nodules in the amnion termed as amnion nodosum, are present.

Malformation (developmental) syndrome: It refers to multiple congenital anomalies arising from a common pathogenic mechanism. It is pathologically related to a sequence, but in contrast to a sequence, malformation cannot be explained on the basis of a single, localized, initiating defect. Syndromes are usually caused by a single etiologic agent (e.g., viral infection or specific chromosomal abnormality) and it simultaneously affects several tissues.

Developmental association or syntropy: It describes multiple anomalies that arise concurrently but have different pathogeneses.

Terminologies

Agenesis: It is the complete absence of an organ and its associated primordium (organ in the earliest stage of development). Agenesis may manifest as (1) total absence of an organ (e.g., unilateral or bilateral renal agenesis); (2) absence of part of an organ (e.g., agenesis of the corpus callosum of the brain); or (3) absence of specific cell types in an organ (e.g., absence of testicular germ cells in congenital Sertoli cell-only syndrome). Congenital Sertoli cell-only syndrome is unusual syndrome. It is characterized by severely reduced or absent spermatogenesis even with the presence of both Sertoli and Leydig cells. It is due to microdeletions in the Yq11 region of the Y chromosome, known as the AZF (azoospermia factor) region.

Aplasia: It is closely related to agenesis. Aplasia refers to the absence of a mature organ but there is persistence of an organ anlage or rudiment (undeveloped or immature part), without the mature organ. It is due to failure of growth of the existing primordium (earliest stage of development). For example, in pulmonary aplasia, the main bronchus ends blindly in a nondescript mass of rudimentary ducts and connective tissue.

Atresia: It describes the absence or incomplete formation of a normal body orifice (opening) or tubular passage of a hollow visceral organ (e.g., trachea, esophagus, intestine). Many hollow organs/viscera originate as cell strands and cords whose centers undergo apoptosis to produce a central cavity or lumen. For example, esophageal atresia is characterized by localized absence of the lumen, which was not fully developed during embryogenesis.

Hypoplasia: It refers to incomplete development of all or part of an organ or decreased (reduced) size of an organ with decreased numbers of cells. For example, micrognathia (small jaw) and microcephaly (small brain and head).

Dysraphic anomalies: These are defects due to failure of apposed structures to fuse. For example, in spina bifida, the spinal canal does not close completely, and there is no fusion of overlying bone and skin. This leaves a defect in the midline.

Involution failures: It is the persistence of embryonic or fetal structures that normally involute or disappear during development. For example, persistent thyroglossal duct is due to incomplete involution of the tract that connects the base of the tongue with the developing thyroid.

Division failures: These are caused by incomplete apoptosis in embryonic tissues. For example, fingers and toes are formed at the distal ends of limb buds by loss of cells between cartilage-containing primordia. If these cells do not undergo apoptosis, fingers are conjoined or incompletely separated (syndactyly).

Dystopia: It is an inadequate migration of an organ from its site of development to its normal location. For example, kidneys originate in the pelvis and then move in a cephalad direction. Dystopic kidneys remain in the pelvis. Another example is dystopic (undescended) testes remain in the inguinal canal and do not enter the scrotum (cryptorchidism).

Hyperplasia is defined as the enlargement of an organ due to increased numbers of cells. It is discussed under cellular adaptation on page 195.

Hypertrophy or hypotrophy: An abnormality in an organ or a tissue due to an increase or a decrease in the size (rather than the number) of individual cells is termed as hypertrophy or hypotrophy, respectively.

Dysplasia: Dysplasia may be seen as precancerous condition also. But in the context of malformations, dysplasia (versus precancerous epithelial lesions in neoplasia—refer page 412) describes an abnormal organization of cells. It is caused by abnormal histogenesis. For example, in tuberous sclerosis, aggregates of normally developed cells are arranged into grossly visible "tubers."

Box 1: Causes of congenital anomalies in live-born infants.

Cause (frequency in %)
- Genetic factors
  - Chromosomal aberrations (10–15)
  - Mendelian inheritance (2–10)
- Environmental factors
- Maternal/placental infections (2–3)
  - Rubella
  - Toxoplasmosis
  - Syphilis
  - Cytomegalovirus
  - Human immunodeficiency virus
- Maternal disease (6–8)
  - Diabetes
  - Phenylketonuria
  - Endocrinopathies, including severe obesity
- Drugs and chemicals (1)
  - Alcohol
  - Smoking
  - Cytotoxic drugs, folic acid antagonists
  - Anticonvulsants, e.g., phenytoin
  - Thalidomide
  - Androgens
  - Warfarin (oral anticoagulant)
  - 13-*cis*-retinoic acid (used in the treatment of severe acne)
  - Heavy metals
  - Others
- Irradiation (1)
- Multifactorial (20–25)
- Unknown (40–60)

Causes of Anomalies

The exact cause of congenital anomalies is unknown in 40–60% of cases. The commonly known causes of congenital anomalies can be divided into three major categories: (1) Genetic, (2) Environmental, and (3) Multifactorial (**Box 1**).

Genetic Causes

Chromosomal aberrations: Almost all chromosomal syndromes are associated with congenital malformations. Examples of chromosomal syndromes include Down syndrome and other trisomies, Turner syndrome, and Klinefelter syndrome. Most of these chromosomal disorders develop during gametogenesis and hence are not familial.

Mendelian inheritance: Some major malformations may be due to single-gene mutations with Mendelian inheritance. For example, Hedgehog signaling pathway plays a critical role in the morphogenesis of forebrain and midface in humans. Loss-of-function mutations of individual components within Hedgehog signaling pathway is responsible for holoprosencephaly (HPE). This HPE is a cephalic disorder in which the prosencephalon (the forebrain of the embryo) fails to develop into two hemispheres. It is the most common developmental defect of the forebrain and midface.

Environmental Factors

The environmental factors that may cause fetal anomalies include viral infections, drugs, and maternal irradiation.

Viral infections

In 19th and early 20th centuries, rubella was a major cause of congenital anomalies. Maternal rubella vaccination has almost eliminated maternal rubella and the resultant rubella embryopathy.

Drugs and chemical

Teratology is the study of developmental anomalies (Greek teraton, "monster"). Teratogens (**Table 1**) are drugs, chemical, physical and biological agents that cause developmental anomalies.

Relatively few teratogens have been proven in humans. Many drugs and chemicals are teratogenic in animals and should thus be considered potentially dangerous for humans. However, only less than 1% of congenital malformations are caused by teratogenic agents. Exposure to a teratogen may result in a malformation, but not invariably.

General principles of teratology

Variable susceptibility to teratogens: Main factors that decide the susceptibility are the genotypes of the fetus and mother, but other factors also play a role. For example, the fetal alcohol syndrome (FAS) affects some children of alcoholic mothers but not others. Diagnosis of FAS can be made in an infant of an alcoholic mother born with characteristic facial features, small size and central nervous system (CNS) damage. But alcoholic mothers often abuse other substances. Thus, the teratogenic effects of prenatal alcohol exposure may be confounded by many variables.

Susceptibility to teratogens is specific for each embryologic stage. Most agents are teratogenic only at particular times in development of fetus. For example, maternal rubella infection can cause congenital rubella syndrome (CRS) only when the mother is infected within the first 20 weeks of pregnancy.

Mechanisms of teratogenesis: They are specific for each agent. Teratogenic drugs may inhibit crucial enzymes or receptors. This interferes with formation of mitotic spindles or impairs energy production. Thus, it may inhibit metabolic steps important for normal morphogenesis. Many drugs and viruses affect specific tissues and damage some developing organs more than others.

Teratogenesis is dose dependent and may be idiosyncratic. Thus, an absolutely safe dose cannot be predicted for each woman.

Outcome of teratogens: Teratogens may produce death, growth retardation, malformation or functional impairment. The outcome depends on complex interactions between a teratogen, the maternal factors and the fetal-placental unit.

- **Thalidomide:** Thalidomide is not teratogenic in mice and rats, but it caused complex malformations in humans. It was once used as an antiemetic or as a tranquilizer during the first trimester of pregnancy. It produced high incidence (50–80%) of limb malformations.
- **Alcohol:** Alcohol is an important environmental teratogen, even if it is consumed in modest amounts during pregnancy can cause FAS. Affected infants with FAS show prenatal and postnatal growth retardation, facial anomalies (microcephaly, short palpebral fissures, maxillary hypoplasia) in the newborn and reduction in mental functions (psychomotor disturbances) as the child grows older. It is difficult to establish the minimal amount of alcohol consumption that can produce FAS. But consumption of alcohol during the first trimester of pregnancy is particularly harmful.
- **Smoking:** Nicotine present in cigarette smoke has not been proved to be a teratogen. However, it is associated with a high incidence of spontaneous abortion, premature labor, and placental abnormalities in pregnant women who smoke. Babies born to mothers who smoke usually have a low birth weight and are susceptible to SIDS. Hence, it is advised to avoid nicotine exposure altogether during pregnancy.

Maternal disease states

Diabetes mellitus: In spite of advances in antenatal obstetric monitoring and glucose control, the incidence of major malformations in infants of diabetic mothers constitutes about 6–10% of malformations. Maternal hyperglycemia induces hyperinsulinemia in fetus. This results in fetal macrosomia (organomegaly and increased body fat and muscle mass); cardiac anomalies, neural tube defects, and other CNS malformations in diabetic embryopathy.

Multifactorial Inheritance

Interaction of environmental influences with two or more genes of small effect is the most common genetic etiology of congenital malformations. Examples of multifactorial inheritance include relatively common malformations such as cleft lip, cleft palate, and neural tube defects. The incidence of neural tube defects has been dramatically reduced due to intake of folic acid during periconceptional period even though contributing genes have not been eliminated.

Pathogenesis

The pathogenesis of congenital anomalies is complex and not completely known. Two general principles of developmental pathology irrespective of the etiologic agent are discussed here.

1. **The timing of the teratogenic exposure:** It is an important factor that has a role on the occurrence and the type of anomaly produced (**Fig. 3**). The intrauterine development can be divided into two phases: (1) the early embryonic period (include the first 9 weeks of pregnancy); and (2) the fetal period (from 9 weeks till birth).
    - **Early embryonic period:** This is the period consisting of first 3 weeks after fertilization. Exposure to an injurious agent during this period damages either: (1) sufficient cells to cause death and abortion or (2) only a few cells and allow the embryo to recover without developing defects.
    - **Between the 3rd and the 9th weeks:** During this period, the embryo is extremely susceptible to teratogenesis. Peak sensitivity is between the 4th and the 5th weeks of gestation. During this period, organs are being shifted out of the germ cell layers.
    - **Fetal period:** It follows organogenesis and this period is marked mainly by further growth and maturation of the organs. There is great reduction in the susceptibility to teratogenic agents. However, the fetus is susceptible to growth restriction or injury to already formed organs. Thus, any given agent may produce different anomalies if exposure occurs at different times of gestation.
2. **Interaction between environmental teratogens and intrinsic genetic defects:** There is interaction between environmental insults and intrinsic genetic defects. Examples for these interactions are as follows:
    - **Cyclopamine:** It is a plant teratogen present in the corn lily. If a pregnant sheep feed this plant, it gives birth to lambs with severe craniofacial abnormalities such as HPE and "cyclopia" (single fused eye, hence the origin of the moniker cyclopamine). Cyclopamine is an inhibitor of Hedgehog signaling in the embryo, and

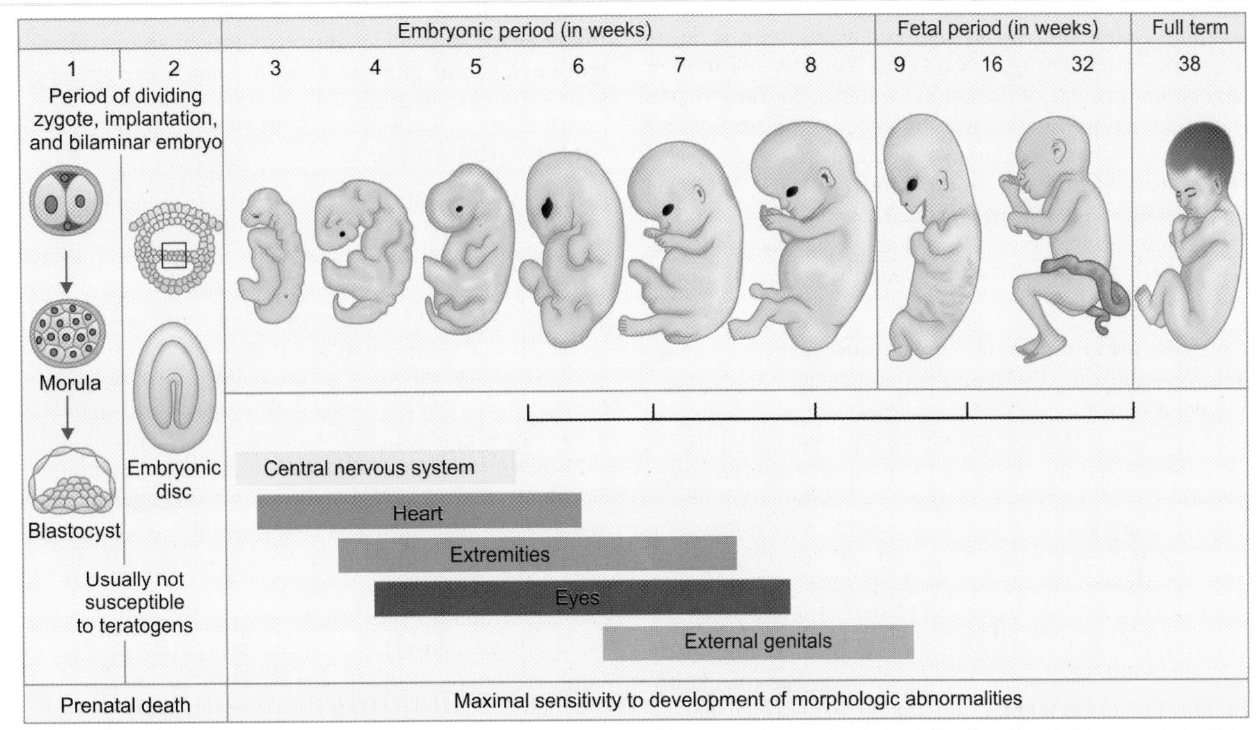

FIG. 3: Sensitivity of specific organs to teratogenic agents at critical periods of human embryogenesis and the resultant malformations. Exposure to adverse influences during preimplantation and early postimplantation stages of development (far left) leads to prenatal death. Periods of maximal sensitivity to teratogens (horizontal bars) vary for different organ systems. Most are limited to the first 8 weeks of pregnancy.

mutations of Hedgehog genes are present in subsets of patients with HPE.

- **Valproic acid:** It is an antiepileptic drug and is teratogen if taken during pregnancy. Valproic acid suppresses the expression of a family of highly conserved developmentally critical transcription factors known as homeobox (HOX) proteins. HOX proteins are necessary in the patterning of limbs, vertebrae, and craniofacial structures. Hence, mutations in the *HOX* family of genes are responsible for congenital anomalies in valproic acid embryopathy.
- **All-trans-retinoic acid:** Vitamin A (retinol) derivative all-trans-retinoic acid is essential for normal development and differentiation of cells. If it is absent during embryogenesis, it can produce constellation of malformations affecting multiple organ systems. These include the eyes, genitourinary system, cardiovascular system, diaphragm, and lungs. On the contrary, excessive exposure to retinoic acid is teratogenic. Infants born to mothers treated with retinoic acid for severe acne can develop a predictable phenotype called retinoic acid embryopathy. These malformations include CNS, cardiac, and craniofacial defects, such as cleft lip and cleft palate. The components of the transforming growth factor-β (TGF-β) signaling pathway are involved in palatogenesis. The retinoic acid deregulation the components of the TGF-β signaling pathway and is responsible for cleft palate. Mice with knockout of the *Tgfb3* gene develop cleft palate.

PREMATURITY AND FETAL GROWTH RESTRICTION

Human pregnancy normally lasts for 40 ± 2 weeks, and most newborns weigh 3,300 ± 600 g. The World Health Organization **defines prematurity as a gestational age less than 37 weeks** (timed from the first day of the last menstrual period). Traditionally, in prematurity birth weight is below 2,500 g, regardless of gestational age. However, since full-term infants may also weigh below 2,500 g because of intrauterine growth retardation rather than prematurity. Hence, the term low-birth-weight infants (<2,500 g) should be used. This low-birth-weight infants may be either appropriate for gestational age (AGA) or small for gestational age (SGA).

Prematurity is the second most common cause of neonatal mortality, first being congenital anomalies.

Major Risk Factors for Prematurity

Preterm premature rupture of membranes (PPROM): PPROM develops as complicates about 3% of all pregnancies and is responsible for about one-third of all preterm deliveries. Rupture of membranes (ROM) before the onset of labor can be spontaneous or induced.

- **Preterm premature rupture of membranes (PPROM):** PPROM is the spontaneous ROM occurring before 37 weeks of gestation. Hence termed as "preterm." Clinical risk factors for PPROM, include prior history of preterm delivery, preterm labor and/or vaginal bleeding during the current pregnancy, maternal smoking, low socioeconomic status, and poor maternal nutrition. Both fetal and maternal outcomes after PPROM depend on the gestational age of the fetus (second-trimester PPROM has a dismal prognosis) and the effective prophylaxis of infections that occurs due to exposure of amniotic cavity.

- **Premature rupture of membranes (PROM):** PROM is spontaneous ROM occurring after 37 weeks of gestation.

This distinction between PPROM and PROM is important because after 37 weeks, there is considerably decrease in the associated risk to the fetus.

Intrauterine infection: This is a major cause of preterm labor and may be associated with and without intact membranes. Intrauterine infection is present in about 25% of all preterm births. Earlier the gestational age at delivery, there will be higher the frequency of intra-amniotic infection. Microscopically, intrauterine infection is characterized by inflammation of the placental membranes (chorioamnionitis) and inflammation of the fetal umbilical cord (funisitis). The most common microorganisms involved in intrauterine infections that lead to preterm labor are *Ureaplasma urealyticum, Mycoplasma hominis, Gardnerella vaginalis* (the dominant organism observed in "bacterial vaginosis," a polymicrobial infection), *Trichomonas,* Gonorrhea, and *Chlamydia.* In underdeveloped and low-income countries, malaria and HIV are responsible for preterm labor and prematurity.

- **Molecular mechanisms of inflammation-induced preterm labor:** Endogenous Toll-like receptors (TLRs), bind bacterial components as natural ligands. They are the key players in molecular mechanisms of inflammation-induced preterm labor. The signals produced by TLR engagement deregulate prostaglandin expression. This induces contractions of uterine smooth muscle and preterm labor.

Structural abnormalities of uterus, cervix, and placenta: They are associated with an increased risk of prematurity. Examples include uterine distortion by uterine fibroids, compromised structural support of the cervix due to "cervical incompetence", placenta previa, and abruptio placentae.

Multiple gestations (twin pregnancy): It is also one of the risk factors for prematurity.

Hazards of prematurity are listed in **Box 2**.

Fetal Growth Restriction

Birth weights of preterm infants are low. However, it is adjusted for their gestational age, it is usually appropriate. In contrast, almost one-third of infants who weigh <2,500 g are born at term. These infants are therefore considered as undergrown rather than immature. These SGA infants suffer from fetal growth restriction (FGR). This FGR may be due to maternal, fetal, or placental abnormalities. In many cases the specific cause cannot be identified.

Box 2: Hazards of prematurity.

- Neonatal respiratory distress syndrome (hyaline membrane disease)
- Necrotizing enterocolitis (NEC)
- Sepsis
- Intraventricular and germinal matrix hemorrhage

Maternal Abnormalities

Most common factors associated with SGA infants are maternal conditions that cause decreased blood flow to placental. Usually, maternal conditions include vascular diseases such as pre-eclampsia (toxemia of pregnancy) and chronic hypertension. There are several other maternal conditions associated with SGA infants. Some of these conditions are avoidable such as maternal narcotic abuse, alcohol intake, and heavy cigarette smoking. Drugs that can cause FGR include both classic teratogens (e.g., chemotherapeutic agents), and some commonly administered therapeutic agents (e.g., antiepileptic drug phenytoin). Maternal malnutrition (especially prolonged hypoglycemia) may also affect fetal growth.

Fetal Abnormalities

Fetal abnormalities intrinsically reduce growth of the fetus despite an adequate supply of nutrients from the mother. Most prominent fetal conditions are (1) Chromosomal disorders, (2) Congenital anomalies, and (3) Congenital infections.

- **Chromosomal abnormalities:** It may be seen in about 17% of fetuses with FGR and in about 66% of fetuses with documented ultrasonographic malformations. The chromosomal abnormalities include triploidy (7%), trisomy 18 (6%), trisomy 21 (1%), trisomy 13 (1%), and deletions and translocations (2%).
- **Congenital fetal infection:** It should be considered as a cause in all infants with FGR. Most common infections for FGR are the **TORCH group of infections** (***t***oxoplasmosis, ***o***ther viruses and bacteria such as syphilis, ***r***ubella, ***c***ytomegalovirus, and ***h***erpes virus).

Infants who are SGA because of fetal factors usually have symmetric growth restriction (also termed as proportionate FGR). Thus, all organ systems are similarly affected.

Placental Abnormalities

During the third trimester of pregnancy, fetus grows vigorously and needs heavy supply of the uteroplacental blood. Therefore, in the preceding midtrimester, the adequacy of placental growth is very important, and uteroplacental insufficiency is an important cause of restriction of fetal growth. The uteroplacental insufficiency may be due to umbilical-placental vascular anomalies (such as single umbilical artery and abnormal cord insertion), placental abruption, placenta previa, placental thrombosis and infarction, chronic villitis of unknown etiology, placental infection, or multiple gestations. In some cases, the placenta (and the baby) may be small without any identifiable cause. Placental causes of FGR usually produce asymmetric (or disproportionate) growth restriction of the fetus with relative sparing of the brain. The SGA infant struggles for survival even during the perinatal period, in childhood and adult life. Depending on the underlying cause of FGR and the degree of prematurity, there is a significant risk of morbidity in the form of cerebral dysfunction, learning disability, or hearing and visual impairment.

Neonatal Respiratory Distress Syndrome

Respiratory distress syndrome (RDS) is also known as **hyaline membrane disease**. It is characterized by **deposition of a layer of hyaline proteinaceous material in the peripheral airspaces of infants who die to this condition.**

Causes: Respiratory distress in the newborn has many causes. The most common cause is neonatal RDS. Others causes include excessive sedation of the mother, fetal head injury during delivery, aspiration of blood or amniotic fluid by fetus, and intrauterine hypoxia due to coiling of the umbilical cord about the neck of fetus (**Fig. 4**). The incidence of RDS increases with decreasing gestational age. Neonatal RDS is the leading cause of morbidity and mortality among premature infants. Other risk factors that predispose to RDS include: (1) neonatal asphyxia, (2) maternal diabetes, (3) delivery by cesarean section, (4) precipitous delivery, and (5) twin pregnancy.

Pathogenesis

The fundamental defect in the pathogenesis of RDS is **pulmonary immaturity and deficiency of surfactant**.

Surfactant: It predominantly **consists of dipalmitoyl phosphatidylcholine (lecithin), small amounts of phosphatidylglycerol, and two groups of surfactant-associated proteins.**

- **First group of surfactant-associated protein:** It is composed of hydrophilic glycoproteins SP-A (surfactant protein-A) and SP-D. They play a role in pulmonary host defense (innate immunity).
- **Second group of surfactant-associated protein:** It consists of hydrophobic surfactant proteins SP-B and SP-C. Along with the surfactant lipids, these are involved in the reduction of surface tension at the air-liquid barrier in the alveoli of the lung. With reduced surface tension in the alveoli, less pressure is needed to keep them patent and hence lung gets aerated. Thus, these surfactant proteins are important for normal lung function. So, a severe respiratory failure in neonates develops when there is congenital deficiency of surfactant caused by mutations in the *SFTPB (surfactant protein B)* or *SFTPC (surfactant protein C)* genes.

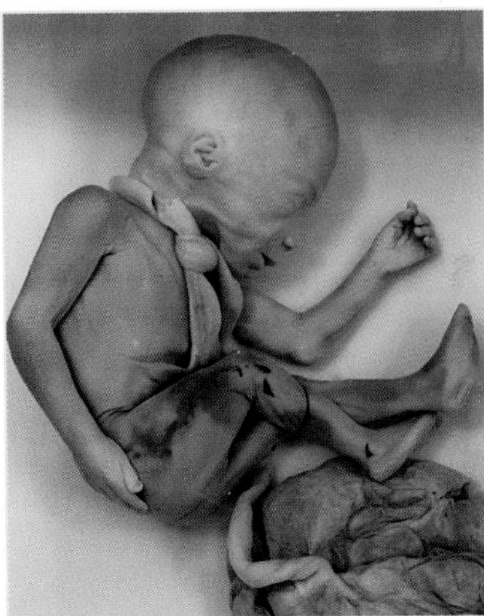

FIG. 4: Umbilical cord around neck of a fetus.

Sequence of events when a newborn starts breathing: Surfactant is produced by type II alveolar cells and its production is accelerated after the 35th week of gestation in the fetus. At birth, the first breath of life by newborn needs high inspiratory pressures to expand the lungs. When a newborn starts breathing, type II cells release their surfactant stores. Surfactant reduces surface tension by decreasing the affinity of alveolar surfaces for each other. Normal levels of surfactant allow alveoli to remain open when the baby exhales and reduces resistance to reinflating the lungs. The lungs retain up to 40% of the residual air volume after the first breath; thus, subsequent breaths need far lower inspiratory pressures.

Consequences of deficiency of surfactant (Fig. 5): Surfactant function is inadequate in many premature infants with immature lungs. If surfactant function is inadequate, the alveoli of the lungs collapse when the baby exhales and resists expansion with the next breath. Lungs collapse with each successive breath. Hence, infants must work as hard with each successive breath as it did with the first breath. The energy needed for the second breath must overcome the stickiness within alveoli. Inspiration, therefore, needs considerable effort. The problem of stiff atelectatic lungs is compounded by the soft thoracic wall that is pulled in as the diaphragm descends.

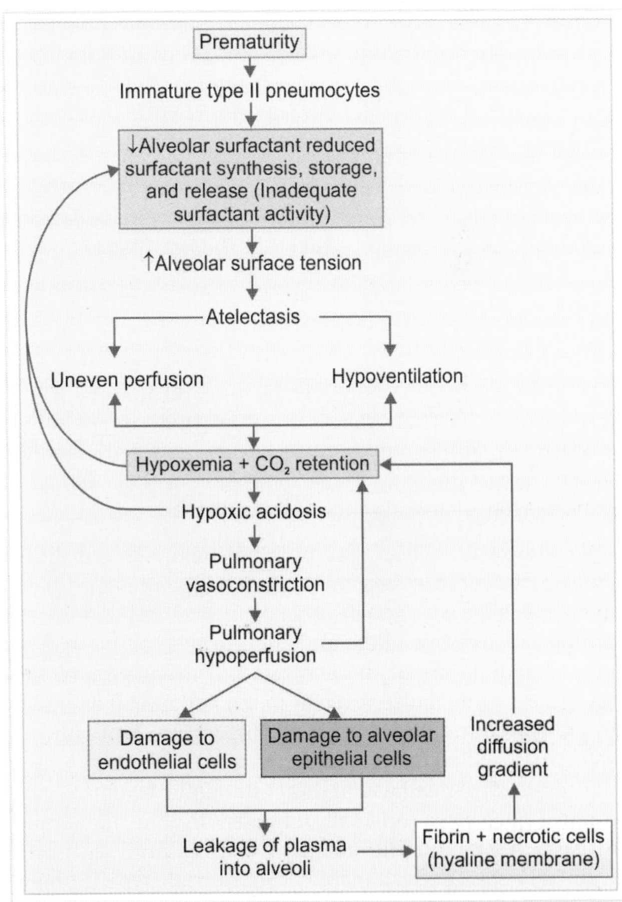

FIG. 5: Pathogenesis of respiratory distress syndrome in the neonate. The sequence of events that leads to the formation of hyaline membranes.

There is progressive atelectasis and reduced lung compliance. The alveolar lining becomes damaged when adherent alveolar walls pull apart. The injured alveoli leak protein-rich (including albumin), fibrin-rich exudate into the alveolar airspaces and form hyaline membranes. The proteins bind surfactant and further impair function of lung, thus exacerbating respiratory insufficiency. Many alveoli are perfused with blood but not ventilated by air. The fibrin-hyaline membranes are barriers to gas exchange, leading to carbon dioxide retention, hypoxemia and acidosis. The hypoxemia itself further impairs surfactant synthesis by type II pneumocytes. Intra-alveolar hypoxia induces pulmonary arterial vasoconstriction. This increases right-to-left shunting through the ductus arteriosus, through the foramen ovale and within the lung itself. This results in further pulmonary ischemia and aggravates alveolar epithelial damage and injures alveolar capillary endothelium. Thus, a vicious cycle develops.

Factors modifying synthesis of surfactant: Surfactant synthesis is modulated by many different hormones and growth factors. These include cortisol (glucocorticoids), insulin, prolactin, thyroxine, and TGF-β.

- **Corticosteroid:** Any conditions associated with intrauterine stress and FGR (fetal growth restriction) increase the release of corticosteroid. The corticosteroid **reduces the risk of developing RDS** (respiratory distress syndrome).
- **Insulin:** Synthesis of surfactant can be suppressed by insulin levels in infants and thereby **increases the risk of developing RDS**. Compensatory high blood levels of insulin are observed in infants of diabetic mothers. This insulin counteracts the effects of steroids. Thus, this is one of the factors for higher risk of developing RDS in infants of diabetic mothers.

Labor versus cesarean delivery: It is found that normal labor increases the synthesis of surfactant whereas **cesarean delivery** before the onset of labor may **increase the risk of RDS.**

MORPHOLOGY

Gross: The lungs in neonatal RDS have distinctive gross appearance. Though size is normal, they are solid in consistency, airless, and reddish purple (dark red), similar to the color of the liver. They usually sink in water and this indicates the relative absence of entrapped air.

Microscopy: The alveoli are poorly developed, and those that are present in the sections appear collapsed. If the infant dies early in the course of the disease, necrotic cellular debris proteinaceous edema fluid and erythrocytes can be seen in the terminal respiratory bronchioles and alveolar ducts. The respiratory bronchioles, alveolar ducts, and alveoli are lined by **conspicuous, eosinophilic, fibrin-rich, amorphous structures, called hyaline membranes.** The necrotic material gets incorporated within this eosinophilic hyaline membrane. Hence, it was originally termed as hyaline membrane disease. The membranes mainly consist of fibrin admixed with cell debris derived mainly from necrotic type II pneumocytes. Collapsed alveoli have thick walls, capillaries are congested, and lymphatics contai proteinaceous material.

Continued

Continued

There is usually no neutrophilic inflammatory reaction associated with these membranes. It is to be noted that hyaline membrane disease is never found in stillborn infants (intrauterine death). If the infant survives more than 48 hours, progressive reparative changes develop in the lungs. The alveolar epithelium proliferates under the surface of the membrane. This epithelium may detach into the airspace and undergoes partial digestion or phagocytosis by macrophages. If epithelium does not detach, fibroblasts grow into the membrane, and it becomes incorporated into the alveolar wall.

Clinical Features

The newborn infant with RDS is almost always preterm. Their weight may be appropriate for gestational age, and appear normal at birth. It is strongly but not invariably associated with male gender, maternal diabetes, and cesarean delivery. The first symptom usually appears within 30 minutes to an hour of birth and it is in the form of increased respiratory effort (difficulty in breathing) with forceful intercostal retraction and the use of accessory neck muscles. Respiratory rate may increase to more than 100 breaths per minute. Within a few hours cyanosis develops in the untreated infant. On auscultation, fine rales can be heard over both lung fields. At this time, a chest radiograph usually shows uniform minute reticulogranular densities, producing a so-called characteristic "ground-glass" picture/ granularity. In terminal stages, the fluid-filled alveoli appear as complete "white-out" of the lungs. In the full-blown severe cases, the respiratory distress persists, cyanosis increases, and infant becomes progressively obtunded (lessened interest in the environment) and flaccid. Even the administration of 80% oxygen by ventilatory methods fails to improve the situation. Long periods of apnea ensue and infants eventually die of asphyxia. However, if the therapy can save the infant from death for the first 3 or 4 days, the infant has an excellent chance of recovery.

Course and prognosis: It varies depending on the maturity and birth weight of the infant and the promptness of therapy. Recent therapeutic advances have improved survival in infants with RDS and reduced the incidence of many complications of RDS.

Prevention: Major importance is given to prevention of RDS, either by **delaying labor until the fetal lung reaches maturity** or by **inducing maturation of the lung by use of antenatal steroids**. If labor threatens a preterm pregnancy, administration of corticosteroids to mothers accelerated the maturation of fetal lung and reduces the incidence of RDS in preterm babies. To achieve these preventive objectives, it is necessary to accurately assess fetal lung maturity. Pulmonary secretions of fetus are discharged into the amniotic fluid. Hence, analysis of amniotic fluid phospholipids is valuable guide to the level of surfactant in the alveolar lining. Prophylactic administration of exogenous animal-derived surfactant (porcine or bovine), at birth to very small premature infants (gestational age <28 weeks) has been found to be very beneficial. Together with newer improved assisted ventilation techniques has dramatically improved pulmonary function, resolution of symptoms and shortened the course, and markedly reduced mortality. Currently, even extremely premature infants have an 85–90% chance of survival. In uncomplicated cases, recovery starts within 3 or 4 days. Complications of RDS such as retrolental fibroplasia (retinopathy of prematurity) in the eyes, and bronchopulmonary dysplasia (BPD) are now less frequent and less severe.

Complications of RDS

Major complications of RDS are as follows:

- **Retinopathy of prematurity (retrolental fibroplasia):** Its pathogenesis has two phases.
    - Phase I (hyperoxic phase of RDS therapy): During this phase, there is markedly decreased expression of the proangiogenic vascular endothelial growth factor (VEGF). This causes apoptosis of the endothelial cells.
    - Phase II (relatively hypoxic room air ventilation): VEGF levels rebound after return to relatively hypoxic room air ventilation. This induces proliferation of retinal vessels (neovascularization) in the retina.
- **Bronchopulmonary dysplasia:** It is a late complication of RDS usually in infants who weigh less than 1,500 g. It is characterized by marked reduction in alveolar septation (seen as large, simplified alveolar structures) and a dysmorphic capillary configuration. The BPD is caused by a potentially reversible impairment in the development of alveolar septation at the so-called "saccular" stage. Chest radiographs show a change from almost complete opacification to a sponge-like appearance, with small lucent areas alternating with denser foci. Many factors such as hyperoxemia, hyperventilation, prematurity, inflammatory cytokines, and vascular maldevelopment contribute to BPD. Increased levels of many proinflammatory cytokines [TNF, interleukin-1β (IL-1β), IL-6, and IL-8] are found in the alveoli of infants who develop BPD. Probably these cytokines have a role in arresting pulmonary development. Treatment with mesenchymal stem cells may cause secretion of soluble factors that suppress inflammation and favors repair of the air spaces.
- **Intraventricular cerebral hemorrhage:** The periventricular region in the newborn brain contains dilated, thin walled veins. These periventricular capillaries can rupture easily probably due to anoxic injury, venous sludging and thrombosis and impaired vascular autoregulation. This produces hemorrhage.
- **Persistent patent ductus arteriosus:** The ductus arteriosus remains patent in about one-third of newborns who survive RDS. With recovery from the pulmonary disease, pulmonary arterial pressure declines. The higher pressure in the aorta reverses the direction of blood flow in the ductus arteriosus. This leads to a persistent left-to-right shunt. Congestive heart failure may develop and correction of the patent ductus may be needed.
- **Necrotizing enterocolitis**

Necrotizing Enterocolitis

It is the most common acquired gastrointestinal emergency in newborns. Necrotizing enterocolitis (NEC) is most common in premature infants and occurs in approximately 1 in 10 very-low-birth-weight infants (<1,500 g). The incidence of the disease is inversely proportional to the gestational age. It is an intestinal complication of RDS.

Pathogenesis: The exact pathogenesis is not known and it is multifactorial.

- **Infection:** Apart from prematurity, most cases of NEC are associated with enteral feeding. This suggests that some postnatal insult such as introduction of bacteria, sets in a cascade of events leading to destruction of tissue. Though infectious agents may be responsible in the pathogenesis of NEC, no single bacterial pathogen has been correlated with the disease. Probably alteration in the microbiome occurs due to enteral feeding. It is probably due to ischemia of the intestinal mucosa that leads to bacterial colonization, usually with *Clostridium difficile*.
- **Inflammatory mediators:** Many inflammatory mediators are associated with NEC. One important mediator is platelet activating factor (PAF). PAF promotes apoptosis of enterocytes and damages the intercellular tight junctions. Thus, PAF increases the mucosal permeability and adds "fuel to the fire". Stool and serum samples of infants with NEC show higher PAF levels than control. Breakdown of mucosal barrier functions by PAF allows transluminal migration of gut bacteria. This leads to a vicious cycle of inflammation, mucosal necrosis, and further bacterial entry. This may finally lead to sepsis and shock.

Clinical Course

It begins with the onset of bloody stools, abdominal distention, and may lead to circulatory collapse. Abdominal radiographs may show gas within the intestinal wall (pneumatosis intestinalis). When detected early, NEC usually managed conservatively. However, about 20–60% of cases need resection of the necrotic segments of bowel. NEC is associated with high perinatal mortality. Those infants who survive usually develop post-NEC strictures due to fibrosis caused by the healing process.

MORPHOLOGY

Site of involvement: NEC usually involves the terminal ileum, cecum, and right colon. However, any part of the small or large intestine may be involved.

Gross: The involved intestinal segment is distended, friable, and congested, or it may be frankly gangrenous (**Figs. 6A** and **B**). Complications such as intestinal perforation may be accompanied by peritonitis.

Microscopy: It shows mucosal or transmural coagulative necrosis, ulceration, bacterial colonization, and submucosal gas bubbles. Shortly after the acute episode, reparative changes may develop. These include the formation of granulation tissue and fibrosis.

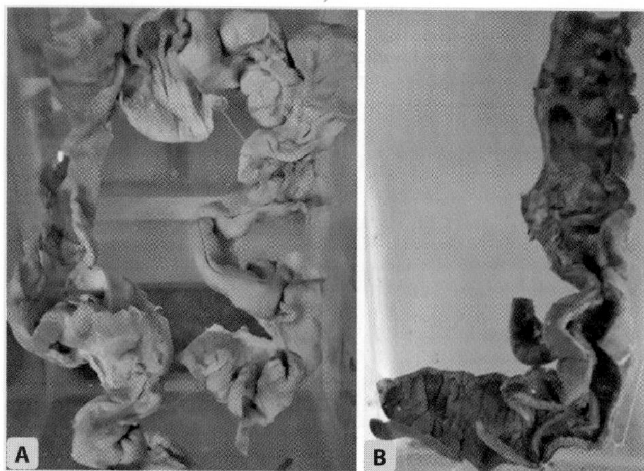

FIGS. 6A AND B: Necrotizing enterocolitis (NEC). (A) NEC shows markedly distended small bowel; (B) The congested ileum with areas of hemorrhagic infarction and transmural necrosis.

PERINATAL INFECTIONS

Usually fetal and perinatal infections are acquired through one of two primary routes namely—transcervically (also called as ascending) or transplacentally (hematologic). Rarely, infections can occur by a combination of these two routes, i.e., an ascending microorganism (transcervically) infects the endometrium and then these organisms invade the fetal bloodstream through the chorionic villi (transplacentally).

Transcervical (Ascending) Infections

Many bacterial and a few viral (e.g., herpes simplex II) infections are acquired transcervically (by cervicovaginal route). These infections may be acquired in utero or during delivery via infected birth canal.

Rote of entry of infection: Usually, the infection enters the fetus either by inhalation of infected amniotic fluid into the lungs shortly before birth or during the passage through an infected birth canal during delivery.

- **Infected amniotic sac:** Usually preterm birth is a common consequence of infection. Preterm birth due to infection may be either due to damage and rupture of the amniotic sac by direct inflammation, or to the induction of labor by prostaglandins released from infiltrating neutrophils. The most common sequelae in fetus infected by inhalation of amniotic fluid are pneumonia, sepsis, and meningitis.
- **Inflammation of the placental membranes and cord:** They are usually seen. However, there need not be correlated with the severity of the fetal infection and the presence or absence and severity of chorioamnionitis (inflammation of chorion and amnion).

Transplacental (Hematologic) Infections

Most parasitic (e.g., *Toxoplasma*, malaria) and viral infections and a few bacterial infections (i.e., *Listeria, Treponema*) enter the fetal bloodstream transplacentally (hematogenous transmission) through the chorionic villi of placenta. This transmission of infection may occur at any time during gestation. Occasionally (e.g., hepatitis B and HIV), the infection may be acquired at the time of delivery via maternal-to-fetal transfusion.

Clinical manifestations: These are highly variable and depend on the gestational timing and microorganism involved.

Parvovirus B19

It causes erythema infectiosum or "fifth disease of childhood" in immunocompetent older children. Parvovirus B19 can infect 1–5% of seronegative (nonimmune) pregnant women, and majority of these women have a normal pregnancy outcome. In a minority of intrauterine infections, it can result in spontaneous abortion (especially in the second trimester), stillbirth, hydrops fetalis, and congenital anemia. Parvovirus B19 has a particular affinity for erythroid cells. Diagnostic viral inclusions can be detected in early erythroid progenitors in infected infants.

TORCH Complex

Q. Write short essay on TORCH complex.

TORCH refers to a complex of signs and symptoms produced by fetal or neonatal infection with different infection. These include toxoplasma (T), rubella (R), cytomegalovirus (C) or herpes simplex virus (H). The "O" in TORCH represents "others" and includes syphilis, varicella-zoster virus (chicken pox), fifth disease (parvovirus B19) and HIV. The TORCH infections are grouped together because they may produce similar clinical and pathologic manifestations. These include fever, encephalitis, chorioretinitis, hepatosplenomegaly, pneumonitis, myocarditis, hemolytic anemia, and vesicular or hemorrhagic skin lesions. This reminds that these fetal and newborn infections may be indistinguishable from one another. Hence, testing should be done for all TORCH agents in suspected cases.

TORCH infections are major causes of neonatal morbidity and mortality. If they occur early in gestation, they may cause chronic sequelae in the child, including growth retardation and intellectual disability, cataracts, congenital cardiac anomalies, and bone defects. These organisms produce severe damage and are largely irreparable. Hence, they should be prevented. Suspicion of congenital infection and awareness of its prominent features helps for its early diagnosis. The specific organisms of the TORCH complex are discussed in detail on page 928 and 929.

MORPHOLOGY

Both clinical and pathologic features in symptomatic newborns vary. Only a minority of newborn show the entire spectrum of abnormalities (**Box 3**).

Common findings include growth retardation and abnormalities of the brain, eyes, liver, hematopoietic system and heart.

CNS lesions: They are the most serious changes in TORCH infected children.

- Acute encephalitis: Foci of necrosis are seen in the brain and are surrounded by inflammatory cells.
- Later lesions: The lesions in brain calcify and are most prominent in congenital toxoplasmosis.

Continued

Continued

Other common lesions: Microcephaly, hydrocephalus and abnormally shaped gyri and sulci (microgyria). Severe CNS injury may lead to psychomotor retardation, neurologic defects, and seizures.

Radiological findings: It may show abnormal cerebral cavities (porencephaly), missing olfactory bulbs, and other major brain defects.

Ocular defects: It may also be prominent, especially with rubella infection. In rubella infections, majority of patients develop cataracts and microphthalmia. Other defects include glaucoma and retinal malformations (coloboma). Choroidoretinitis (usually bilateral), is common with rubella, Toxoplasma and CMV. In neonatal herpes infection, keratoconjunctivitis is the most common eye lesion.

Cardiac anomalies: They are seen in many children with the TORCH complex, mostly with congenital rubella. These anomalies include patent ductus arteriosus and septal defects. Occasionally, pulmonary artery stenosis and complex cardiac anomalies may be found.

Sepsis

Perinatal sepsis can be divided into early onset (within the first 7 days of life) and late onset (from 7 days to 3 months) sepsis.

- **Early onset sepsis:** Most infections are acquired at or shortly before birth. They produce clinical signs and symptoms of pneumonia, sepsis, and occasionally meningitis within 4 or 5 days of life. Group B *Streptococcus* is the most common cause of early-onset sepsis and also early-onset bacterial meningitis.
- **Late onset sepsis:** Infections with Listeria and Candida have longer latent periods between the time of inoculation of these microorganisms and the development of clinical symptoms. Hence, they produce late-onset sepsis.

Box 3: Common pathologic findings in the fetus and newborn with TORCH infections.

- General features
  - Prematurity
  - Intrauterine growth retardation
- Central nervous system
  - Encephalitis
  - Microcephaly
  - Hydrocephaly
  - Intracranial calcifications
  - Psychomotor retardation
- Ear
  - Damage to inner ear and hearing loss
- Eye
  - Microphthalmia (R)
  - Glaucoma (R)
  - Pigmented retina (R)
  - Keratoconjunctivitis (H)
  - Cataracts (RH)
  - Chorioretinitis (TCH)
  - Visual impairment (TRCH)
- Liver
  - Hepatomegaly
  - Liver calcifications (R)
  - Jaundice
- Hematopoietic system
  - Hemolytic and other anemias
  - Thrombocytopenia
  - Splenomegaly
- Skin and mucosae
  - Vesicular or ulcerative lesions (H)
  - Petechiae and ecchymoses
- Respiratory system
  - Pneumonitis
- Cardiovascular system
  - Myocarditis
  - Congenital heart disease
- Skeletal system

(R: rubella virus; C: cytomegalovirus; H: herpesvirus; T: Toxoplasma)

FETAL HYDROPS

Q. Write short essay on hydrops fetalis. What are its causes and laboratory diagnosis?

Fetal hydrops is characterized by the **accumulation of edema fluid in the fetus during intrauterine growth.**

Types and causes: It can be divided into immune and nonimmune hydrops.

- **Immune hydrops:** In the past, immune hydrops due to hemolytic anemia resulting from Rh blood group incompatibility between mother and fetus was the most common cause. Presently the successful prophylaxis available for this disorder during pregnancy. Hence it is not the common cause.
- **Nonimmune hydrops:** Currently, it is more common.

Severity of fluid accumulation: The intrauterine fluid accumulation can be quite variable. It may range from focal to generalized edema. The generalized edema of the fetus (hydrops fetalis) may be progressive and is usually lethal condition. Localized edema may present as isolated pleural and peritoneal effusions, or postnuchal fluid accumulation (cystic hygroma) that are compatible with life.

Immune Hydrops

Immune hydrops is the result of hemolytic disease caused by incompatibility of blood group antigen between mother and fetus. If the fetus inherits red cell antigenic determinants from the father that are foreign to the mother red cell antigens, a maternal immune reaction may occur.

Etiology and Pathogenesis

The major antigens that can produce clinically significant immunologic reactions are certain **Rh antigens** and the **ABO blood groups**. The reaction usually occurs in second and subsequent pregnancies in a Rh-negative mother with a Rh-positive father. In immune hydrops there is immunization of the mother by blood group antigens on fetal red cells. The red cells may reach the maternal circulation either during the last trimester of pregnancy (when the cytotrophoblast is no longer present as a barrier), or during childbirth (there is placental separation and opening of uterine vessels). The initial exposure to Rh antigen causes the production of IgM antibodies. These antibodies, unlike IgG antibodies, do not cross the placenta.

Immune hydrops due to Rh incompatibility (Fig. 7)

The Rh blood group system consists of numerous antigen (about 25 components), of these only the alleles cde/CDE are very important. Of these antigens in the Rh system, only the D is of major importance. Antibodies against D antigen is the major (about 90%) cause of Rh incompatibility. In Rh incompatibility, mother is Rh (D antigen) negative and fetus is Rh positive. The anti-D antibodies are responsible for the fetal hydrops. Sequence of events is as follows:

Sensitization of mother: It occurs when fetal Rh positive RBCs (in >1 mL fetal blood) enter into Rh negative mothers' circulation. Rh positive red cells enter maternal circulation only at the time of delivery or during miscarriage. Fetal hydrops due to Rh incompatibility does not manifest in the first pregnancy.

Production of anti-Rh antibodies in the mother The fetal Rh antigens cause sensitization of mother to the foreign antigen (i.e., fetal red cell Rh antigens). The antibodies are produced in the Rh-negative mother against the Rh antigen. Thus, Rh disease is uncommon during the first pregnancy. Exposure during a subsequent pregnancy generally leads to a brisk

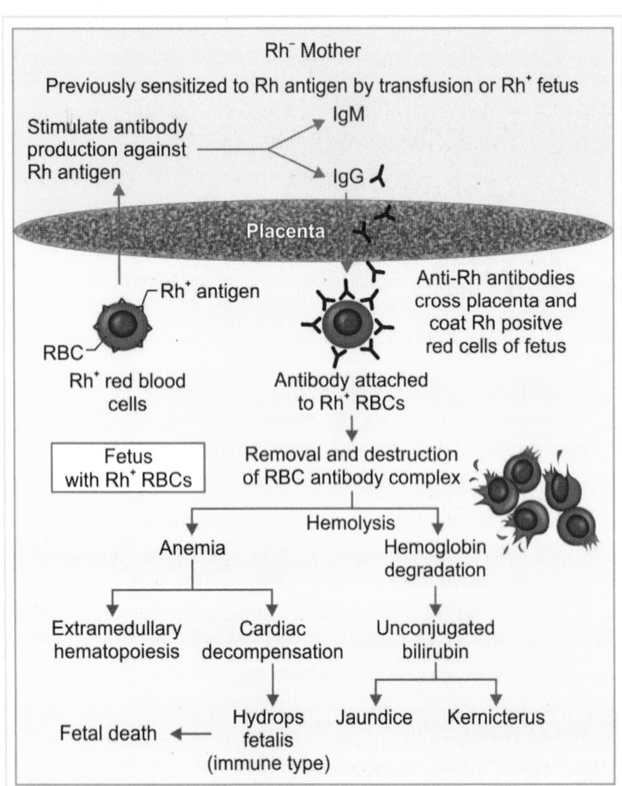

FIG. 7: Pathogenesis of immune hydrops fetalis due to Rh incompatibility between mother and fetus.

IgG antibody response and the risk of immune hydrops. Two important factors that influence the immune response to RhD positive fetal RBCs that reach the maternal circulation are as follows:

- **Concurrent ABO incompatibility:** If there is associated ABO incompatibility between mother and fetus, it protects the mother against Rh immunization. This is because the fetal RBCs are quickly coated and removed from the maternal circulation by anti-A or anti-B IgM antibodies that do not cross the placenta.
- **Dose of immunizing antigen:** The antibody response depends on the dose of immunizing antigen. Hence, hemolytic disease of new-born develops only when the mother has a significant transplacental bleed (>1 mL of Rh-positive fetal red cells).

Passage of anti-Rh antibodies from mother to fetus during second pregnancy In subsequent pregnancy, anti-Rh antibodies from mother freely pass through (cross) placenta to the fetus. In the fetus, these anti-Rh antibodies coat the Rh positive fetal red cells. These antibodies cause immune destruction of fetal red cells and results in severe hemolytic anemia leading to jaundice of the new-born.

Rhesus immune globulin (RhIg): The incidence of maternal Rh isoimmunization has markedly reduced with the use of RhIg containing anti-D antibodies. Time of administration of RhIg is as follows:

- **During pregnancy and delivery:** RhIg is administered to Rh-negative mothers at 28 weeks of gestation and within 72 hours of delivery. This significantly reduces the risk for hemolytic disease in Rh-positive neonates and in subsequent pregnancies.
- **Following abortions:** RhIg is also administered following abortions. This is because abortions are associated with uteroplacental bleeding and can lead to immunization.

Antenatal identification of fetus at risk: Antenatal identification of the fetus at-risk can be done by amniocentesis and chorionic villus and fetal blood sampling. Also cloning of the *RHD* gene using fetal DNA in maternal serum to determine fetal Rh status.

Antenatal management of severe intrauterine hemolysis in fetus: If severe intrauterine hemolysis is identified, it may be treated by fetal intravascular transfusions via the umbilical cord and early delivery of fetus.

Immune hydrops due to ABO Incompatibility

The pathogenesis of fetal hemolysis due to maternofetal ABO incompatibility is slightly different from that caused by Rh incompatibility. Though ABO incompatibility occurs in about 20–25% of pregnancies, laboratory evidence of hemolytic disease is found in only 1 in 10 of such infants. ABO incompatibility is less severe and severe hemolytic disease that needs treatment is only 1 in 200 cases. Several factors account for these features of ABO incompatibility.

- Most anti-A and anti-B antibodies are of IgM type. The IgM antibodies do not cross the placenta.
- Neonatal red cells poorly express blood group antigens A and B.
    - Many cells other than red cells such as fetal fluids and tissues express A and B antigens. This results in consumption (adsorption) of major portion of the

transferred maternal antibodies by these cells other than RBCs. The small portion which is left combines with fetal red cells causing only mild hemolysis.

Mother O group and fetus A or B group: ABO hemolytic disease occurs almost exclusively in fetus/infants either of group A or B who are born of mother's with blood group is O. Either anti-A or anti-B antibodies cause hemolysis. For unknown reasons, certain mother with blood group O have IgG antibodies directed against group A or B antigens (or both) even without prior sensitization. The IgG antibodies against blood group A or B from maternal blood cross placenta and enter the fetal circulation. Therefore, the firstborn (new born of first pregnancy) may be affected. Fortunately, even with transplacentally acquired antibodies, hemolysis of the infant's RBCs is minimal. In contrast to Rh, there is no effective protection against ABO reactions.

Consequences of excessive destruction of RBCs in the neonate

There are two main consequences of excessive destruction of RBCs in the neonate (**Fig. 7**). The severity of these consequences markedly varies. It depends on the degree of hemolysis and the maturity of the infant.

Anemia It is due to destruction accompanied by direct loss of red blood cells. If there is only mild hemolysis, compensatory mechanism causes increased production of red cell and may maintain near-normal levels of red cells.

Hypoxic injury: If hemolysis is more severe, progressive anemia develops and produces hypoxia in fetus/infant. Hypoxia may cause hypoxic injury to the fetal heart and liver.

- **Hypoxic injury to liver:** It causes reduced synthesis of plasma protein resulting in decreased levels of these proteins. It may be as low as 2–2.5 mg/dL and leads to reduced plasma oncotic pressure.
- **Hypoxic injury to heart:** Cardiac hypoxia may lead to cardiac decompensation and cardiac failure in fetus/infant. Cardiac failure produces increased hydrostatic pressure in the circulation.

The combination of decreased plasma oncotic pressure and increased hydrostatic pressure in the circulation results in generalized edema and anasarca. This finally leads to hydrops fetalis (immune type).

Jaundice Hemolysis produces raised unconjugated bilirubin in fetus/infant. The infant's blood-brain barrier is poorly developed. Hence, water-insoluble unconjugated bilirubin passes through blood brain barrier. Unconjugated bilirubin blinds to lipids in the brain and can damage the CNS. This bilirubin induced brain damage is termed as kernicterus.

Nonimmune Hydrops

Various causes of nonimmune hydrops are listed in **Box 4**. Three major causes of nonimmune hydrops are cardiovascular defects, chromosomal anomalies, and fetal anemia.

Cardiovascular Defects

Both structural (congenital malformations of CVS) and functional cardiovascular defects (e.g., arrhythmias) may produce intrauterine cardiac failure and hydrops.

Box 4: Causes of hydrops fetalis.

- **Immune hydrops**
  - Rh incompatibility
  - ABO incompatibility
- **Nonimmune hydrops**
  - Cardiovascular defects*
    - Structural defects such as congenital malformations
    - Functional defects such as arrhythmias
  - Chromosomal anomalies accompanied by structural cardiac anomalies*
    - Turner syndrome
    - Trisomies 21 and 18
  - Fetal anemia*
    - Severe anemia due to homozygous α-thalassemia (deletion of all four α-globin genes)
  - Transplacental infection by parvovirus B19
  - Monozygous twin pregnancies and twin-to-twin transfusion
  - Unknown

*Major causes of nonimmune hydrops

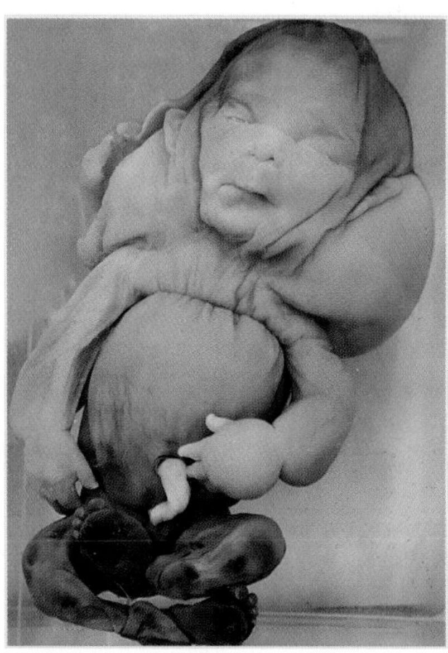

FIG. 8: Hydrops fetalis with cystic hygroma.

Chromosomal Anomalies

Chromosomal anomalies such as 45, X karyotype (Turner syndrome) and trisomies 21 and 18 are associated with fetal hydrops. It is due to the accompanying structural cardiac anomalies in these chromosomal anomalies. In Turner syndrome, abnormalities of lymphatic drainage from the neck may also produce accumulation of fluid in the postnuchal region (cystic hygromas) (**Fig. 8**).

Fetal Anemia

Fetal anemia due to Rh- or ABO-associated antibodies produces immune hydrops. Hydrops may develop due to anemia which is nonimmune type. The most common cause of nonimmune hydrops is severe fetal anemia due to homozygous α-thalassemia. This anemia is due to **deletion of all four α-globin genes.**

Other Causes

- **Transplacental infection by parvovirus B19** can also cause hydrops. The virus preferential infects the erythroid precursors (normoblasts) and replicates within them. It leads to apoptosis of red cell progenitors and results in red cell aplasia. Parvoviral intranuclear inclusions can be found within circulating and marrow erythroid precursors.
- About 10% of nonimmune hydrops are related to monozygous twin pregnancies and twin-to-twin transfusion occurring through anastomoses between the two circulations. In about 20% of cases of nonimmune hydrops, the cause is not known.

MORPHOLOGY

Morphological features in fetuses with intrauterine fluid accumulation vary depending on the severity of the disease and the underlying cause. **Hydrops fetalis is the most severe and generalized manifestation**. Lesser degrees of edema may manifest as isolated pleural, peritoneal, or postnuchal fluid collections (**Fig. 8**). Accordingly, fetus may be stillborn (intrauterine death), infant may die within the first few days, or recover completely.

- **Chromosomal abnormality:** It may show the presence of dysmorphic features and postmortem examination may reveal an underlying cardiac anomaly.
- **Fetal anemia:** In hydrops associated with fetal anemia, both the fetus and placenta are characteristically pale. In most of the cases both the liver and spleen are enlarged due to cardiac failure and resulting congestion. The bone marrow shows compensatory hyperplasia of erythroid precursors (except that due to parvovirus-associated red cell aplasia). Extramedullary hematopoiesis is found in the liver, spleen, lymph nodes, and in other tissues also (e.g., kidneys, lungs, heart). The increased hematopoietic activity is accompanied by large numbers of immature red cells including reticulocytes and erythroblasts **(erythroblastosis fetalis)** in the peripheral blood,

Kernicterus or bilirubin encephalopathy: The term kernicterus is derived from the German kern, "nucleus" and icterus "jaundice". The most serious condition in fetal hydrops is damage to the CNS and is known as kernicterus. In kernicterus, brain is enlarged and edematous. On cut section it has a bright yellow color due to bile staining, particularly the basal ganglia, pontine nuclei, thalamus, cerebellum, cerebral gray matter (cerebellar dentate nuclei), and spinal cord. The exact level of bilirubin that produces kernicterus is unpredictable. Usually in full term infants, neural damage develops when the bilirubin level in the blood is >20 mg/dL. In premature infants this level needed may be considerably lower (as low as 12 mg/dL). Probably bilirubin injures the cells of the brain by interfering with mitochondrial function.

Clinical Features

The clinical features of fetal hydrops vary depending on severity of the disease. Minimally affected infants have pallor and hepatosplenomegaly. Most severely affected neonates present with rapidly develop progressive jaundice (hyperbilirubinemia), generalized edema, and signs of neurologic damage. Severe kernicterus initially produces loss of the startle reflex and athetoid movements and progresses to lethargy and death in 75% of cases. Those who survive, most have severe choreoathetosis and mental retardation.

INBORN ERRORS OF METABOLISM AND OTHER GENETIC DISORDERS

Inborn errors of metabolism are genetic disorders producing defects in metabolism. This term was coined by Sir Archibald Garrod in 1908. Most inborn errors of metabolism are rare diseases and are usually inherited as autosomal recessive or X-linked traits (Chapter 12). Mitochondrial disorders form a distinct group with mutations in mitochondrial genes (refer page 873). The clinical features are usually due to either abnormal accumulation of metabolite or deficiency of the desired product. Some of the common clinical features suggest a metabolic disorder in a neonate (**Box 5**). Most important inborn errors of metabolism are phenylketonuria (PKU), galactosemia, and cystic fibrosis. Early diagnosis (through neonatal screening) of PKU and galactosemia are particularly important. Because early death or intellectual disability can be prevented with proper dietary treatment. Cystic fibrosis is one of the most common, potentially lethal diseases.

Box 5: Common clinical features that suggest a metabolic disorder in a neonate.

- **General features**
  - Dysmorphic features
  - Deafness
  - Abnormal body or urine odor, e.g., "sweaty feet"; "mousy or musty"; "maple syrup"
  - Self-mutilation
  - Abnormal hair
  - Hepatosplenomegaly
  - Cardiomegaly
  - Hydrops
- **Neurologic features**
  - Hypotonia/hypertonia
  - Persistent lethargy
  - Seizures
  - Coma
- **Gastrointestinal features**
  - Poor feeding
  - Recurrent vomiting
  - Jaundice
- **Eyes**
  - Cataracts
  - Cherry red macula
  - Glaucoma
  - Dislocated lens
- **Muscle and Joints**
  - Myopathy
  - Abnormal mobility

Inborn Errors of Amino Acid Metabolism

Metabolism is the term used to describe the all chemical reactions involved (interconversion of chemical compounds) in the body. The basic pattern of metabolism depends on the nature of the diet. There is a need to process the products of digestion of dietary carbohydrate (glucose), lipid (fatty acids and glycerol), and protein (amino acids). Basic outline of the pathways for the catabolism of carbohydrate, protein, and fat is presented in **Figure 9**. Metabolic disorders of carbohydrate and lipid are discussed in Chapter 12.

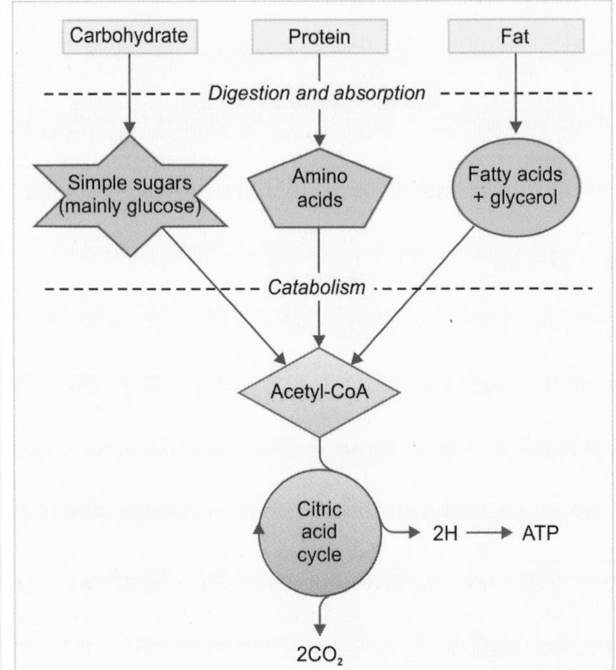

FIG. 9: Basic outline of the pathways for the catabolism of carbohydrate, protein, and fat.

Amino acids: The terms "essential" and "nonessential" with regard to amino acids are misleading since all 20 common amino acids are essential for health. There are 20 amino acids, of which eight must be present in the human diet, and thus are best termed "nutritionally essential". The other 12 amino acids are "nutritionally nonessential" since they need not be present in the diet

Inherited disorders of the metabolism of many amino acids have been identified (**Box 6**). They vary greatly in severity. Some of them are lethal in early childhood and others are clinically insignificant. Only examples of defects in the metabolism of phenylalanine and tyrosine (**Fig. 10**) are discussed here.

Box 6: Examples of inherited disorders of amino acid metabolism.

- Phenylketonuria (hyperphenylalaninemia)
- Tyrosinemia, alkaptonuria, albinism
- Histidinemia
- Hypermethioninemia
- Maple syrup urine disease (branched-chain ketoaciduria)
- Ornithine transcarbamylase deficiency (ammonia intoxication)
- Carbamyl phosphate synthetase deficiency (ammonia intoxication)
- Argininosuccinic acid synthetase deficiency (citrulline accumulation)
- Arginase deficiency
- Homocystinuria
- Cystinosis

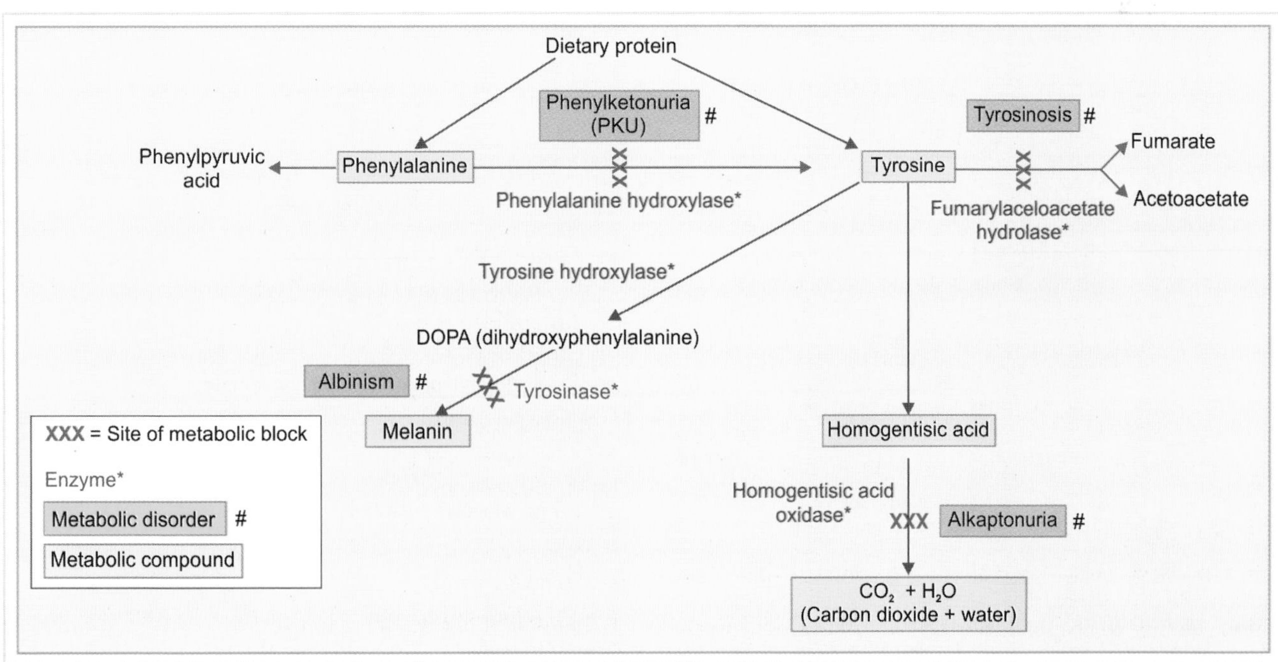

FIG. 10: Diseases caused by disturbances of phenylalanine and tyrosine metabolism include phenylketonuria, tyrosinosis, albinism, and alkaptonuria.

Phenylketonuria (PKU)

Phenylketonuria (hyperphenylalaninemia) is an autosomal recessive disorder due to the severe deficiency of the hepatic enzyme namely phenylalanine hydroxylase (PAH) leading to hyperphenylalaninemia. There are several variants of this inborn error of metabolism and the most common form, referred to as classic PKU.

Infants with PKU are normal at birth but within a few weeks develop high circulating levels of plasma phenylalanine level. This impairs brain development leads to progressive severe mental deterioration [intellectual disability with low IQ (intelligence quotient)] in the first few years of life (usually by 6 months of life). About two-thirds children with PKU cannot talk and one-third of them are never able to walk. In untreated children, the intellectual disability is usually accompanied by seizures, other neurologic abnormalities, decreased pigmentation of hair and skin, a characteristic musty odor, and eczema.

Dietary restriction of phenylalanine in children with PKU: To prevent hyperphenylalaninemia and the resultant intellectual disability, diagnosis and initiation of dietary treatment of should occur before the child is 2 weeks of age. Dietary treatment is usually started if blood phenylalanine levels are >360 µmol/L (6 mg/dL). Dietary treatment consists of restricting intake of phenylalanine. Thus, a special diet low in phenylalanine and supplementation with tyrosine is given. Tyrosine becomes an essential amino acid in PAH deficiency. The plasma phenylalanine concentrations should be maintained between 120 and 360 µmol/L (2 and 6 mg/dL). Dietary restriction should be continued and monitored indefinitely.

Maternal phenylketonuria: A number of females with PKU, if treated with dietary restriction since infancy, will reach childbearing adulthood and become pregnant. It is necessary to strictly control phenylalanine levels in these pregnant females both before and during pregnancy. Most of them discontinue dietary treatment after they reach adulthood and have marked hyperphenylalaninemia. If phenylalanine levels are not strictly controlled, 75–90% of their children are develop severe intellectual disability, growth retardation and are microcephalic. About 15% the children have congenital heart disease, even though the infants themselves are heterozygotes. This syndrome is termed as maternal PKU. These defects are due to the teratogenic effects of phenylalanine or its metabolites. These metabolites cross the placenta and affect specific fetal organs during development. The presence and severity of the fetal anomalies directly correlate with the level of phenylalanine in the mother. Pregnancy risks can be minimized by continuing lifelong phenylalanine-restricted diets and strict maternal dietary restriction of phenylalanine 2 months before the conception and continued throughout pregnancy.

Molecular pathogenesis

Phenylalanine is an essential amino acid exclusively derived from the diet. In normal children, less than 50% of the dietary intake of phenylalanine is needed for protein synthesis. The remainder phenylalanine is converted in the liver to tyrosine by PAH system (**Fig. 11A**). If the diet contains adequate quantities of the phenylalanine, tyrosine is nutritionally nonessential. However, since the PAH reaction is irreversible, dietary tyrosine cannot replace phenylalanine (essential amino acid).

Deficiency of PAH: In PKU there is deficiency of functional PAH. Thus, there is a biochemical defect of inability to convert phenylalanine into tyrosine and causes hyperphenylalaninemia. Blocking of the phenylalanine metabolism activates the minor alternative (shunt) pathways, producing several off-pathway metabolites (**Fig. 11B**). There is formation of phenylketones by the transamination of phenylalanine. These phenylketones metabolites include phenylacetate and phenylpyruvate and its derivatives. These are excreted in large

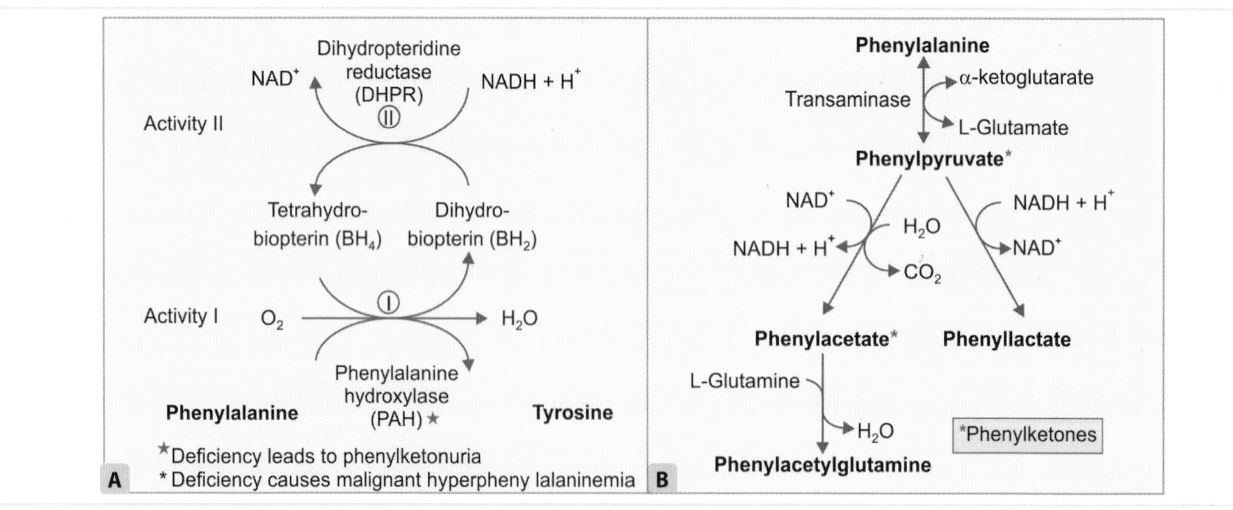

[NAD: nicotinamide adenine dinucleotide (oxidized); NADH: nicotinamide adenine dinucleotide (reduced)].

FIGS. 11A AND B: (A) The phenylalanine hydroxylase (PAH) system. Conversion of phenylalanine to tyrosine is by PAH. Two distinct enzymatic activities are involved. Activity I—the reduction of O_2 to H_2O and of phenylalanine to tyrosine. Activity II catalyzes reduction of dihydrobiopterin to tetrahydrobiopterin by NADH. Phenylketonuria may develop due to deficiency of either PAH or dihydropteridine reductase (DHPR). Deficiency of DHPR leads to malignant hyperphenylalaninemia. (B) Alternative pathways of phenylalanine catabolism in phenylketonuria. The reactions also occur in normal liver tissue but are of minor significance.

amounts in the urine and sweat. These metabolites impart a strong musty or mousy odor to affected infants. Excess of phenylalanine or its metabolites causes the brain damage in PKU. PKU is accompanied by lack of tyrosine (see **Fig. 10**) which is a precursor of melanin. Hence, the hair and skin of these children have a light color.

Milder forms: PAH activity is not always totally lacking. These are few milder forms of disease than classic PKU. In such patients, phenylpyruvic acid is not excreted in the urine.

Genetic basis: More than 500 mutant alleles of the *PAH* gene causing deficiency in PAH have been identified.

- **Mutations in PAH:** Classic PKU is caused by mutations in the *PAH* gene on the long arm of chromosome 12 (12q22–24.1). Mutations in both PAH alleles are needed for the development of the disease. Mutations that cause markedly reduced PAH activity, infants present with markedly raised blood phenylalanine levels, and the classic features of PKU. Infants with up to 6% residual PAH activities usually have milder disease. Patients with less than 1% of the normal PAH activity usually have a PKU.
    - **Benign hyperphenylalaninemia:** Some PAH mutations are associated with only moderately raised levels of phenylalanine levels in blood without any neurologic damage. This condition is called benign hyperphenylalaninemia. It is important to recognize this, because these patients may have positive screening tests but do not have the stigmata of classic PKU. Measurement of serum phenylalanine levels is required to differentiate benign hyperphenylalaninemia from PKU. In PKU, the levels are usually five times or more than normal.
- **Non-PKU hyperphenylalaninemia:** About 98% of PKU is due to mutations in PAH. In about 2% of cases, there are mutations different from those in classic PKU. These are termed as malignant hyperphenylalaninemia. In these patients, dietary restriction of phenylalanine does not arrest neurologic deterioration. It may be caused due to abnormalities in synthesis (deficiency) or recycling of the cofactor tetrahydrobiopterin (BH_4). Tetrahydrobiopterin is a cofactor required for hydroxylation of phenylalanine by PAH (see **Fig. 11A**). Sometimes there may be failure to regenerate BH_4, due to an absence of dihydropteridine reductase (DHPR). DHPR is the enzyme that reduces dihydrobiopterin (BH_2) to the tetrahydro form BH_4. The mutant *DHPR* gene is present on the short arm of chromosome 4, and it is so distinct from the *PAH* gene on chromosome 12. Phenotypically, infants with malignant hyperphenylalaninemia are indistinguishable from those with classic PKU. But, BH_4 deficiency also interferes with synthesis of the neurotransmitters dopamine (tyrosine hydroxylase dependent) and serotonin (tryptophan hydroxylase dependent). Thus, brain damage in malignant hyperphenylalaninemia is probably due to other factors apart from a simple elevation in phenylalanine levels.

Clinical features

Phenylketonuria is a classic example to illustrate the interaction between genetic and environmental factors in the pathogenesis of disease. It is caused by a genetic defect, but its expression needs a dietary constituent (an environmental factor). Infants with PKU appear normal at birth, but mental retardation is observed within a few months. In untreated infants, by 1 year of age, there is loss of about 50 IQ points due to severe mental retardation. These infants usually have fair skin, blond hair and blue eyes. These are due to the reduced melanin synthesis due to inability to convert phenylalanine to tyrosine (see **Fig. 10**). These are excreted in large amounts of phenylacetic acid (phenylacetate) in the urine and sweat. These metabolites impart a strong "musty" or "mousy" odor to affected infants. Hyperphenylalaninemia can be diagnosed by a simple blood test (Guthrie test).

Tyrosinemia

Tyrosinemia is inborn error of tyrosine catabolism. There are three types of tyrosinemia. The most severe and rare is type I (hepatorenal). It is transmitted as an autosomal recessive disorder due to the deficiency of the enzyme fumarylacetoacetate hydrolase (FAH) (see **Fig.10** and **Fig. 12**). In early infancy, it manifests as acute liver disease or in children it may present as a more chronic disease of the liver, kidneys, and brain. Other types are tyrosinemia type II (oculocutaneous) and tyrosinemia type III.

Molecular pathogenesis

Tyrosinemia is characterized by elevated levels of tyrosine and its metabolites in blood.

Fumarylacetoacetate hydrolase (15q23–25) is the last enzyme in the catabolic pathway that converts tyrosine to fumarate and acetoacetate (**Fig. 12**). FAH is deficient in both acute and chronic forms of type I tyrosinemia. In the acute form, there is complete absence of enzyme activity, whereas children with chronic disease have variable residual enzyme activity. In hereditary tyrosinemia, cell injury is caused by abnormal toxic metabolites (succinylacetone and succinylacetoacetate).

Clinical features

Acute tyrosinemia: It manifests in the first few months of infancy. It is characterized by hepatomegaly, edema, failure to thrive and a cabbage-like odor. Within a few months, infants develop hepatic failure and die.

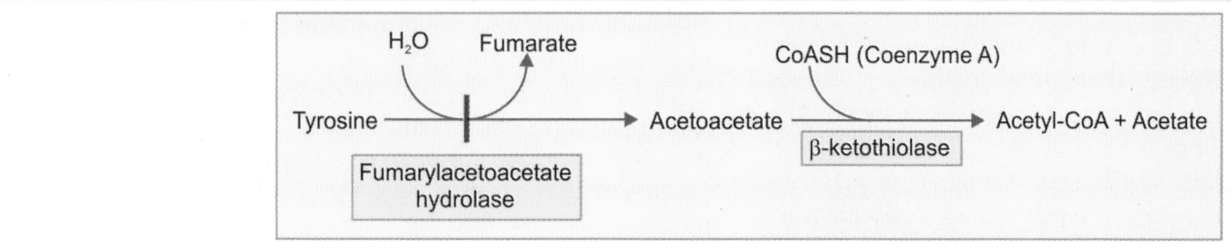

FIG. 12: Intermediates in tyrosine catabolism. Fumarylacetoacetate hydrolase is deficient in both acute and chronic forms of type I tyrosinemia.

Chronic tyrosinemia: It is characterized by cirrhosis of the liver, renal tubular dysfunction (Fanconi syndrome) and neurologic abnormalities. Hepatocellular carcinoma develops in more than one-third of patients. Most children die before the age of 10.

Prenatal diagnosis: It is done by analysis of amniotic fluid for succinylacetone or of fetal cells for FAH (fumarylacetoacetate hydrolase).

Alkaptonuria (Ochronosis)

This is a rare autosomal recessive metabolic disease.

Pathophysiology

Alkaptonuria is due to a deficiency of the enzyme homogentisate oxidase (i.e., homogentisate 1,2-dioxygenase/HGD). This enzyme is involved in the degradation of tyrosine. Homogentisic acid is an intermediate gene product in phenylalanine and tyrosine metabolism. Deficiency of enzyme HGD (homogentisate 1,2-dioxygenase) prevents catabolism of homogentisic acid. This result in accumulation of homogentisic acid (see **Fig. 10**) and its oxide, alkapton in the blood and are excreted in urine in large amounts. Excessive accumulation of homogentisic acid causes damage to cartilage (ochronosis, leading to osteoarthritis), heart valves and precipitates as kidney stones.

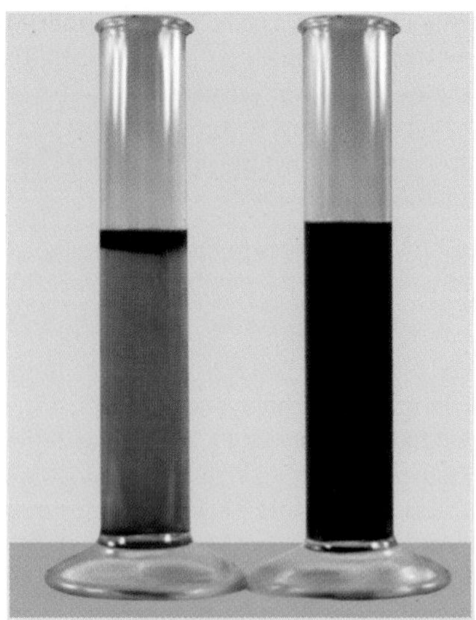

FIG. 13: Urine in alkaptonuria. (A) (left), Urine that has been standing for 15 minutes shows darkening at the surface due to the oxidation of homogentisic acid. (B) (right), After 2 hours the urine has become entirely black in color.

MORPHOLOGY

Patients with alkaptonuria excrete urine that darkens rapidly on standing. This is due to formation of a pigment on the nonenzymatic oxidation of homogentisic acid (**Fig. 13**). In long-standing alkaptonuria, a similar pigment namely benzoquinone acetate is formed from homogentisic acid. The benzoquinone acetate polymerizes and binds to connective tissue (**Fig. 14**). It is deposited in many tissues, particularly the sclerae, cartilage in many areas (ribs, larynx, trachea), tendons and synovial membranes. The pigment is bluish black on gross examination. However, it is brown under the microscope, hence the term ochronosis (color of ocher = earthy pigment containing ferric oxide with clay). The term ochronosis was coined by Rudolf Virchow. A degenerative and disabling arthropathy ("ochronotic arthritis") usually develops after years of alkaptonuria. Though alkaptonuria affects many organs, it does not reduce longevity of the patient.

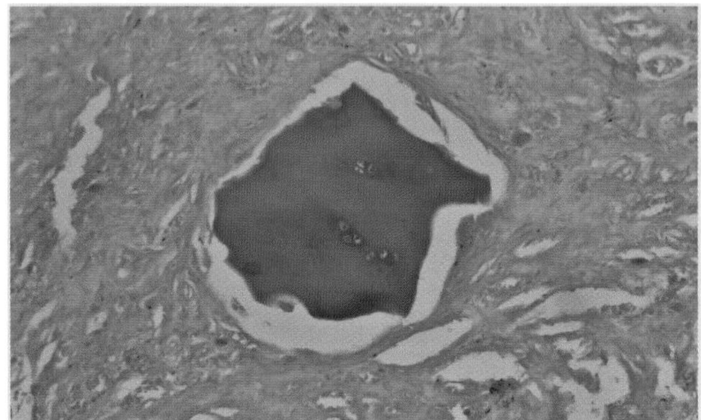

FIG. 14: Ochronosis characterized by accumulation of homogentisic acid in cartilage. The affected cartilage appears brown in color.

Albinism

Albinism is a heterogeneous group of inherited disorders due to absent or reduced biosynthesis of melanin and it causes hypopigmentation.

- **Type 1 albinism:** It is caused by defects in production of melanin pigment.
- **Type 2 albinism:** It is due to a defect in the *"P"* gene, which interferes with metabolism of tyrosine. Tyrosine is a precursor of melanin (see **Fig. 10**). Individuals with type 2 albinism have slight coloring at birth.
- **Hermansky-Pudlak syndrome (HPS):** It is a form of oculocutaneous albinism. It is caused by recessive mutations in various genes. Depending on the affected gene, it can be associated with a bleeding disorder, immunodeficiency and/or lung and bowel diseases.
- **Localized albinism:** Certain complex diseases may be associated with loss of coloring in only a certain area (localized albinism). Examples include Chédiak-Higashi syndrome (lack of coloring all over the skin, but not complete); tuberous sclerosis (small areas of loss of skin coloring); Waardenburg syndrome (no coloring in one or both irises).

The most common type of albinism is oculocutaneous albinism (OCA). OCA is a family of closely related diseases with autosomal recessive mode of inheritance (except one). In OCA, there is absent or reduced melanin pigment in the skin, hair follicles and eyes (optic fundus with visual loss and photophobia). Ocular albinism is another type of albinism due to deficiency of different enzymes or transporters and is characterized by hypopigmentation of optic fundus and visual loss.

Forms of oculocutaneous albinism: Tyrosinase is the first enzyme involved the biosynthesis that converts tyrosine to melanin (**Fig. 10**). There are two major forms of OCA. They are distinguished by the presence or absence of tyrosinase.

- **Tyrosinase-positive OCA:** It is the most common type of albinism. Patients usually have complete albinism, but with age, a small amount of clinically detectable pigment accumulates. It is due to defect in the *P* gene (15q11.2-13) that encodes a tyrosine transport protein and prevents synthesis of melanin.
- **Tyrosinase-negative OCA:** It is the second most common type of albinism. There is complete absence of tyrosinase (11q14-21) and melanin. Melanocytes are present but contain unpigmented melanosomes. These individuals have snow-white hair, pale pink skin, blue irides and prominent red pupils (due to the absence of retinal pigment). They have severe eye problems such as photophobia, strabismus, nystagmus and poor visual acuity.

Skin of all patients with albinism have marked sensitivity to sunlight. They have increased risk for development of squamous cell carcinomas of sun-exposed skin.

Galactose and Fructose Disorders

Galactose and fructose disorders and their basic defects are given in **Table 2**.

Galactosemia

Galactosemia is an autosomal recessive disorder of galactose metabolism. It is due to lack of enzyme namely galactose-1-phosphate uridyl transferase. This enzyme is involved in the conversion of galactose-1-phosphate to glucose-1-phosphate. It leads to accumulation of galactose-1-phosphate and its metabolites in the liver and other organs and tissues.

Lactose is the major carbohydrate present in mammalian milk. Normally, lactose is split into glucose and galactose by lactase in the intestinal microvilli. Galactose is then converted to glucose (**Fig. 15**) in several steps involving distinct enzymes.

Variants of galactosemia: There are two variants of galactosemia.

1. More common variant: In this there is total absence of galactose-1-phosphate uridyl transferase (GALT). It is discussed in detail here.
2. Rare variant: It is characterized by deficiency of galactokinase. Deficiency of galactokinase leads to a milder form of the disease and is not associated with intellectual disability.

Table 2: Galactose and fructose disorders.

Type/common name	*Basic defect*
Galactose disorders	
Galactosemia with uridyltransferase deficiency	Galactose 1-phosphate uridyl transferase
Galactokinase deficiency	Galactokinase
Uridine diphosphate galactose 4-epimerase deficiency	Uridine diphosphate galactose 4-epimerase
Fructose disorders	
Essential fructosuria	Fructokinase
Hereditary fructose intolerance	Fructose 1,6-bisphosphate aldolase B
Fructose 1,6-diphosphatase deficiency	Fructose 1,6-diphosphatase

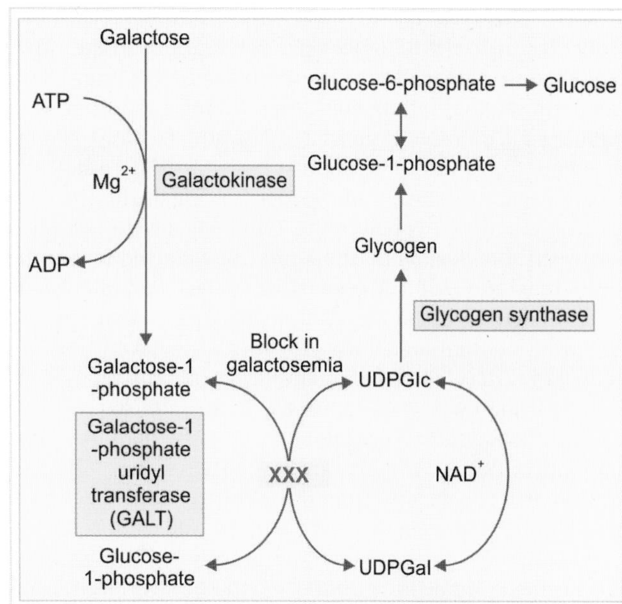

(UDPGal: uridine diphosphate galactose; UDPGlc: uridine diphosphate glucose)

FIG. 15: Pathway of conversion of galactose to glucose in the liver.

Galactosemia due to GALT deficiency

Deficiency of GALT leads to **accumulation of galactose-1-phosphate in many organs and tissues. These include the liver, spleen, lens of the eye, kidneys, heart muscle, cerebral cortex, and erythrocytes**. Blocking of the galactose metabolism causes activation of alternative metabolic pathways. This leads to the production of galactitol (a polyol metabolite of galactose) and galactonate, an oxidized byproduct of excess galactose. Both these products also accumulate in the tissues. These metabolic intermediates are responsible for long-term toxicity observed in galactosemia. Heterozygotes may have a mild enzyme deficiency and the clinical and pathologic consequences are less than in the homozygous state.

MORPHOLOGY

Liver: Within 2 weeks of birth, the liver shows extensive and uniform accumulation of fat (**fatty change/steatosis**) and is responsible for hepatomegaly. Fatty change is accompanied by marked **proliferation of bile ductule** in and around portal tracts. Cholestasis is usually observed in canaliculi and bile ductules. Bile plugs fill many of these pseudoacini. By about 6 weeks of age, **fibrosis** begins. Fibrosis extends from portal tracts into the lobules and may progresses to widespread scarring to produce cirrhosis by 6 months. This closely resembles the cirrhosis of alcohol abuse. Institution of a galactose-free diet improves the disease and reverses many of the morphologic changes.

Eyes: Lens develops opacity (cataract). This is probably galactitol, produced by alternative metabolic pathways, it accumulates and increases osmotic pressure. Hence, the lens absorbs water and swells.

CNS: Nonspecific changes appear in the CNS. These include loss of nerve cells, gliosis, and edema. These changes are mainly observed in the dentate nuclei of the cerebellum and the olivary nuclei of the medulla. Similar changes may also develop in the cerebral cortex and white matter.

Clinical features The clinical presentation is variable, probably due to the heterogeneity of mutations in the *GALT* gene. Mainly damaged organs are the liver, eyes (cataracts), and brain (mental retardation). Affected infants present with vomiting and diarrhea within a few days after feeding the milk. These infants fail to thrive almost from birth. Jaundice and hepatomegaly usually become evident during the first week of life. There may be hypoglycemia. Cataracts develop within a few weeks. Intellectual disability may be detected within the first 6–12 months of life. Galactose and galactose-1-phosphate accumulation in the kidney impairs transport of amino acid and produces aminoaciduria. These infants have increased frequency of developing fulminant *Escherichia coli* septicemia. This is probably due to depressed neutrophil bactericidal activity. Hemolysis and coagulopathy may also manifest in the new born period.

Removal of galactose from the diet early during newborn period and for at least the first 2 years of life can prevent or alleviate many of the clinical and morphologic changes of galactosemia. If this is instituted soon after birth, it prevents the cataracts and liver damage and allows almost normal development. However, even with dietary restrictions, older patients may be frequently affected by a speech disorder and gonadal failure (especially premature ovarian failure) and, less commonly, ataxia. However, even in untreated infants the disability is usually not as severe as that observed in PKU.

Diagnosis: Screening test based on fluorometric assay of GALT enzyme activity can be performed on a dried blood spot. A positive screening test must be confirmed by assay of GALT levels in red blood cells. **Antenatal diagnosis** is possible by **assay of GALT activity in cultured amniotic fluid cells** or by **determination of galactitol level in amniotic fluid** supernatant.

Essential fructosuria

Q. Write short essay on fructosuria.

Essential fructosuria is a benign and asymptomatic condition characterized by the incomplete metabolism of fructose in the liver, leading to its excretion in urine. It is caused due to deficiency of the enzyme hepatic fructokinase. Fructose is either excreted unchanged in the urine or metabolized to fructose-6-phosphate by alternate pathways (most commonly by hexokinase in adipose tissue and muscle). This defective degradation does not cause any clinical symptoms.

It is an autosomal recessive disorder caused by mutation in *KHK* gene located to chromosome 2p.

Diagnosis: Fructose is a reducing substance and can be detected in the urine.

Cystic Fibrosis (Mucoviscidosis)

Q. Write short essay on mucoviscidosis/cystic fibrosis.

Cystic fibrosis (CF) is an inherited autosomal recessive disorder of ion transport. It affects fluid secretion in exocrine glands (exocrinopathy) and in the epithelial lining of the respiratory, gastrointestinal, and reproductive tracts. In many patients, the abnormal viscous inspissated/thickened mucus secretions obstruct organ passages and produce most of the clinical features. These features include chronic lung disease secondary to recurrent infections, pancreatic insufficiency, steatorrhea, malnutrition, hepatic cirrhosis, intestinal obstruction, and male infertility. These clinical features may develop at any time from before birth, childhood or adolescence. The **primary defect in cystic fibrosis is abnormal transport of chloride and bicarbonate ions mediated by an anion channel** (i.e., ion transporter) **(Fig. 16)**.

Cystic fibrosis is the **lethal genetic disease**. Though it is an autosomal recessive disorder, even heterozygote carriers have an increased incidence of respiratory and pancreatic disease. It shows a wide degree of phenotypic variation. This results from three additional factors namely: (1) diverse mutations in the gene associated with cystic fibrosis, (2) the tissue-specific effects of the encoded gene product, and (3) the influence of modifier genes.

Cystic Fibrosis Gene: Normal Structure and Function

The **cystic fibrosis transmembrane conductance regulator *(CFTR)* gene** is present on the long arm of chromosome 7 (7q31.2). It encodes a CFTR protein of 1,480 amino acids. **CFTR is an integral membrane protein** that is **involved in passive conduit for chloride and bicarbonate transport** (as an ion transporter) across plasma membranes of most epithelial tissues. The direction of ion flow dependent on the electrochemical driving force.

Structure of CFTR: CFTR (cystic fibrosis transmembrane conductance regulator) is situated in the apical plasma membranes of acinar and other epithelial cells. In these cells, it regulates the amount and composition of secretion by exocrine glands. **CFTR has two transmembrane domains** (each containing six α-helices), **two cytoplasmic nucleotide-binding domains** (NBDs), and a **regulatory domain (R domain) that contains protein kinase A and C phosphorylation sites (Fig. 16)**. The two transmembrane domains form a channel and chloride passes through this channel.

Steps in CFTR activation: Activation of CFTR channel involves cyclical structural change with opening and closing of channel pore.

- Activation of the CFTR channel is mediated agonists (e.g., acetylcholine) which bind to epithelial cells. These agonists increase levels of cyclic adenosine monophosphate (cAMP).
- In normal mucus-secreting epithelia, the cAMP activates a protein kinase A (PKA) that phosphorylates the R domain of CFTR and permits channel opening.
- Adenosine triphosphate (ATP) binding and hydrolysis occurs at the NBD. Hydrolysis of ATP further enhances activation CFTR. CFTR has two adenosine triphosphate (ATP)-hydrolyzing domains and they drive ion transporter function. Utilization of the energy provided from ATP hydrolysis is a central feature of ion channel mechanochemistry.
- The binding of ATP to NBD is essential for opening and closing of the channel pore. This opening of channel pore is enhanced by the presence of phosphorylated R domain.

Regulation of CFTR activity: CFTR activity is regulated by the balance between kinase (i.e., phosphorylation) and phosphatase activities (i.e., dephosphorylation). Phosphorylation of the R domains, mainly by PKA (protein kinase A), stimulates activity of chloride channel. Secretion of chloride anions by mucus-secreting epithelial cells controls the parallel secretion

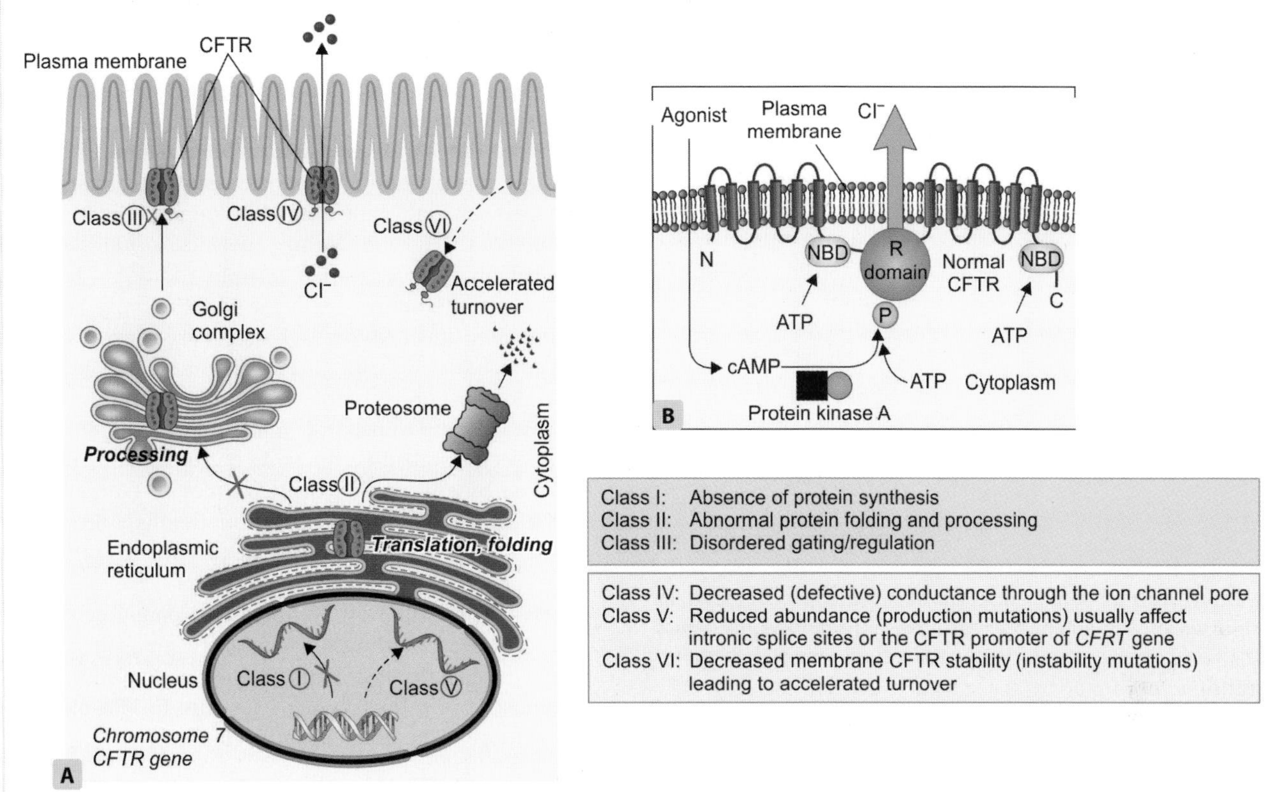

(ATP: adenosine triphosphate; Cl^-: chloride ion)

FIGS. 16A AND B: (A) Steps involved in formation of CFTR from gene to protein and categories of CFTR mutations. (B) Normal structure and activation of cystic fibrosis transmembrane conductance regulator (CFTR). CFTR consists of two transmembrane domains, two nucleotide binding domains (NBDs), and a regulatory R domain. Agonists (e.g., acetylcholine) bind to epithelial cells and increase levels of cyclic adenosine monophosphate (cAMP). This in turn activates protein kinase A and phosphorylates the CFTR R domain using ATP. This opens the chloride ion channel.

of fluid. This in turn controls the viscosity of the mucus. In normal mucus-secreting epithelia, cAMP activates PKA, which phosphorylates the regulatory domains of CFTR. This allows opening of the ion channel.

Recent advances of CFTR function and its role in cystic fibrosis: These are as follows:

CFTR regulates multiple ion channels and cellular processes: Initially CFTR was considered as only chloride-conductance channel, but it is now recognized that it can regulate additional multiple ion channels and cellular processes (**Box 7**).

Of these, the most important with regard to with cystic fibrosis is ENaC (epithelial sodium channel). The ENaC is present on the apical surface of epithelial cells. It is responsible for uptake of sodium from the luminal fluid and makes the luminal fluid hypotonic. Normally functioning CFTR inhibits ENaC whereas in cystic fibrosis, there is increased activity of ENaC. This causes marked increase in the uptake of sodium across the apical membrane and makes the luminal fluid hypotonic. However, human sweat gland duct is one exception for this, where ENaC activity decreases as a result of *CFTR* mutations. This leads to formation of hypertonic fluid with high sodium chloride (the *sine qua non* of classic cystic fibrosis). This is the basis for the "salty" sweat in cystic fibrosis and usually the mothers of affected infants detect this.

Box 7: Multiple channels and cellular processes regulated by CFTR.

- Outwardly rectifying chloride channels
- Inwardly rectifying potassium channels (Kir6.1)
- Epithelial sodium channel (ENaC)
- Gap junction channels
- Cellular processes involved in ATP transport and mucus secretion

Functions of both CFTR and mutated CFTR are tissue-specific: These are discussed as follows:

- **In sweat gland ducts:** The major function of CFTR in the sweat gland ducts is to reabsorb chloride ions from luminal fluid and increase sodium reabsorption via the ENaC (see above). Loss of CFTR function in cystic fibrosis leads to decreased reabsorption of sodium chloride in the sweat ducts and the produces hypertonic sweat (**Fig. 17**).
- **In the respiratory and intestinal epithelium:** CFTR is one of the most important ways for active luminal secretion of chloride in the respiratory and intestinal epithelium. At these sites, CFTR mutations result in loss or reduction of chloride secretion into the lumen from epithelium

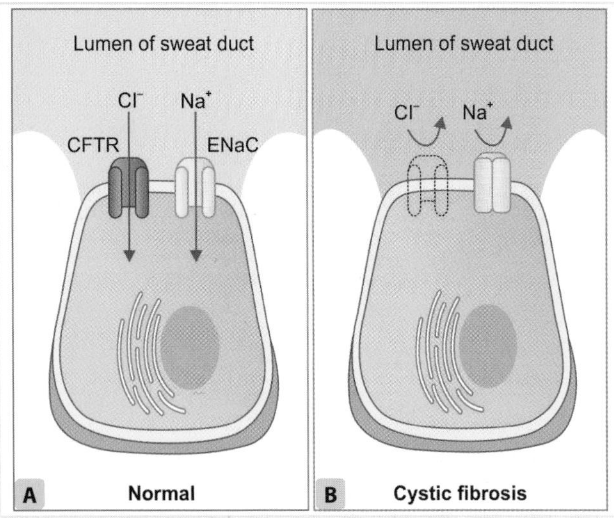

(CFTR: cystic fibrosis transmembrane conductance regulator; Cl⁻: chloride ion; ENaC: epithelial sodium channel)

FIGS. 17A AND B: (A) Role of CFTR chloride channel and ENaC in normal sweat ducts and epithelium. (B) In cystic disease, the defect in the sweat ducts causes increased sodium chloride concentration in sweat.

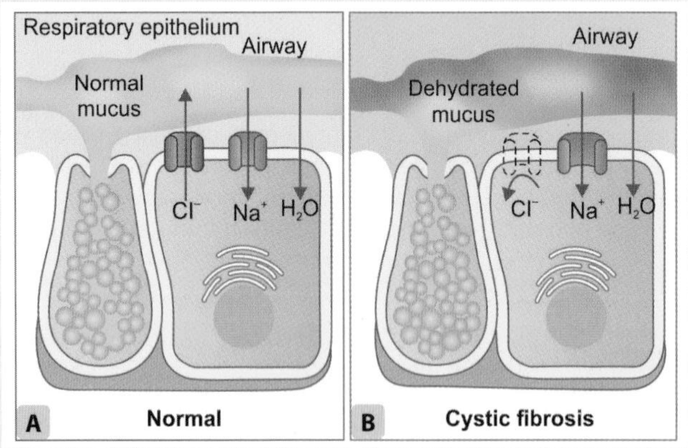

(CFTR: cystic fibrosis transmembrane conductance regulator; Cl–: chloride ion; ENaC: epithelial sodium channel)

FIG. 18A AND B: Role of CFTR chloride channel and ENaC in respiratory epithelium. (A) Normal airway and the mechanism of maintenance of normal mucus. (B) Airway in patients with cystic fibrosis have decreased chloride secretion and increased sodium and water reabsorption. This leads to dehydration of the mucus layer coating epithelial cells, defect in the mucociliary function, and mucus plugging of airways.

(**Fig. 18**), and there is increased active luminal absorption of sodium due to loss of inhibition of ENaC activity. These changes in ion distribution causes increased passive water reabsorption from the lumen and reduced the water content of the surface fluid layer coating mucosal cells. Thus, unlike in the sweat ducts, there is no difference in the salt concentration of the surface fluid layer coating respiratory and intestinal mucosal cells in patients with cystic fibrosis when compared with normal individuals. The pathogenesis of respiratory and intestinal complications in cystic fibrosis is due to an isotonic but low-volume surface fluid layer. In the lungs, this dehydration causes defective mucociliary action and the accumulation of hyperconcentrated, viscid secretions. These secretions obstruct the air passages and predispose to recurrent pulmonary infections.

- **CFTR regulates transport of bicarbonate ions:** CFTR also involved directly and indirectly in regulating bicarbonate transport across the apical epithelial membrane. The anion channel of CFTR is not entirely specific for chloride and it is permeable to bicarbonate also. In addition, CFTR has reciprocal interactions with the SLC26 family of anion exchangers. These anion exchangers are coexpressed on the apical surface with CFTR. In some CFTR mutants, chloride transport is completely or substantially preserved, and bicarbonate transport is markedly abnormal. Normal tissue secretes alkaline fluids. In contrast, fluids that are secreted by epithelia in these mutant CFTR alleles are acidic (due to absence of bicarbonate ions). The acidity of secretions causes decrease in the pH of lumen and can lead to a variety of adverse effects. These include increased precipitation of mucin and plugging of ducts and increased binding of bacteria to plugged mucins. Pancreatic insufficiency is a feature of classic cystic fibrosis, is almost always found when there are CFTR mutations with abnormal bicarbonate conductance.

Categories of CFTR Mutations

CFTR gene was cloned in 1989. About more than 2,000 disease-associated mutations have been identified in cystic fibrosis of which only five mutations are important for disease-causing genotypes. Most of the mutations are missense mutations but frameshift, splicing, and nonsense mutations are also seen. The mutations can be divided into six classes depending on their effect on the CFTR protein (**Fig. 16**). The relationship between genotypes and the clinical severity of CF is complicated and not always consistent. These mutations may be "severe" or "mild." Class I to III mutations are associated with less than 10% residual CFTR activity and are termed "severe" mutations. Class IV to VI mutations are associated with less than 20% residual CFTR activity and are termed "mild" mutations.

Class I: Defective (absence of) protein synthesis (null mutations) (I in Fig.16A): These mutations result in complete absence or failure of CFTR synthesis. There are no CFTR at the apical surface of epithelial cells. These mutations result in premature termination of protein translation that interferes with synthesis of the full-length CFTR protein. There is no CFTR-mediated chloride secretion occurs in involved epithelia.

Class II: Abnormal protein folding, processing, and trafficking (processing mutations) (II in Fig.16A): It is characterized by defective protein maturation and premature degradation. These mutations result in defective processing of the protein from the endoplasmic reticulum to the Golgi apparatus. These mutations prevent proper folding of the nascent protein. These protein does not become fully folded and glycosylated. So, it is then targeted for proteasomal degradation before it is transported to the plasma membrane (surface of the cell). Most common

CFTR mutation is a class II. It is caused by deletion of three nucleotides coding for phenylalanine at amino acid position 508 (ΔF508/DeltaF508 = deletion of three nucleotides spanning positions 507 and 508 of the *CFTR* gene. The symbol Δ, means "change" and ΔF508 = deletion of phenylalanine 508. In class II mutations, there is near-complete lack of CFTR protein at the apical surface of epithelial cells.

Class III: Defective regulation (gating mutations) (III in Fig.16A): Class III mutations allow CFTR proteins to reach the plasma membrane but affect ATP-binding domains. These mutations prevent activation of CFTR by diminished (defective) ATP binding to CFTR and hydrolysis of ATP. This is an essential prerequisite for ion transport. Thus, there is a normal amount of CFTR on the apical surface, but it is non-functional. Defective ATP binding to CFTR interferes with channel regulation and limiting, but not abolishing, secretion of chloride.

Class IV: Decreased (defective) conductance (conduction mutations) through the ion channel pore (IV in Fig.16A): These mutations occur in the transmembrane domain of CFTR, which forms the ionic pore for chloride transport. These mutations are associated with normal amount of CFTR at the apical membrane, but with reduced conduction of chloride. There is defective chloride secretion by mutant CFTR. Thus, in the channel pore there is inhibition of chloride secretion.

Class V: reduced abundance (production mutations) (V in Fig. 16A): These mutations usually affect intronic splice sites or the *CFTR* promoter of *CFRT* gene. This causes reduced number of CFTR transcripts and there is a reduced amount of normal protein.

Class VI: Decreased membrane CFTR stability (instability mutations) (VI in Fig. 16A): These mutations give rise to fully processed and functional proteins but there is accelerated turnover from the cell surface and markedly reduced membrane stability. **Cystic fibrosis** being an **autosomal recessive disease, affected patients have mutations on both alleles**. However, the nature of mutations on each of the two alleles can produce remarkable effect on the phenotype and organ-specific manifestations.

Genetic and Environmental Modifiers

Modifier genes

Cystic fibrosis is one of the well-known examples of the "one gene, one disease". However, genes other than CFTR can modify the frequency and severity of certain organ-specific manifestations. This is especially true with regard to pulmonary manifestations and neonatal meconium ileus. Products of certain genes modulate neutrophil function in response to bacterial infections. In cystic fibrosis, polymorphisms in such genes act as modifier loci for the severity of pulmonary disease. Examples of such modifier genes include mannose binding lectin 2 (*MBL2*), transforming growth factor β1 (*TGF-β1*), and interferon-related developmental regulator 1 (*IFRD1*). Polymorphisms in these modifier genes regulate the resistance of the lungs to exogenous infections with virulent microbes. Thus, they modify the natural history of cystic fibrosis.

Environmental modifiers

Some of the significant phenotypic differences between individuals who share the same CFTR genotype may be due to environmental modifiers. For example, in pulmonary disease, CFTR genotype-phenotype correlations can be very puzzling. Deficient hydration of the mucus causes defective mucociliary action and thereby results in an inability to clear bacteria from the airways. *Pseudomonas aeruginosa* species, in particular, colonize the lower respiratory tract, first intermittently and then chronically. Such colonization is favored by concurrent viral infections. The static mucus produces a hypoxic microenvironment in the surface fluid in airway. This favors the production of alginate, a mucoid polysaccharide capsule, by the colonizing bacteria. Alginate production in turn allows the formation of a biofilm that protects the bacteria from antibodies and antibiotics. Thus, organisms evade host defenses and produce a chronic destructive lung disease. Organisms induce antibody- and cell-mediated immune reactions but they are ineffective against the organism and they produce further destruction of lung tissue. About 80% of patients with cystic fibrosis have colonization by *Pseudomonas aeruginosa* by 20 years of age. Chronic colonization by these bacteria is a significantly responsible for the morbidity and mortality of cystic fibrosis. Thus, apart from genetic factors (e.g., class of mutation), many environmental modifiers (e.g., intercurrent and concurrent infections by microorganisms) can influence the severity and progression of lung disease in cystic fibrosis.

MORPHOLOGY

Morphological changes are highly variable both in distribution and severity. It affects many organs that produce exocrine secretions.

- In individuals with nonclassic cystic fibrosis, the disease is usually mild and does not disturb the growth and development.
- In others, the involvement of pancreas is severe and impairs intestinal absorption because of pancreatic insufficiency. Thus, malabsorption disturbs the development and postnatal growth.
- In others, the defect in mucus secretion leads to defective mucociliary action, obstruction of bronchi and bronchioles, and crippling fatal pulmonary infections.
- In all variants of cystic fibrosis, the sweat glands are morphologically not affected.

Pancreatic abnormalities: They are found in about 85–90% of patients with cystic fibrosis.

- **Milder cases:** There may be only accumulation of mucus in the small ducts with **mild dilation of the exocrine glands.**
- **More severe cases:** It is usually seen in older children or adolescents. The ducts are completely plugged and may become simply cystic. It produces **atrophy of the exocrine glands and progressive fibrosis**. It may leave only islets of Langerhans within a fibrofatty stroma. The finding of pancreatic cysts and fibrosis led to the original

Continued

Continued

name of cystic fibrosis. The loss of pancreatic exocrine secretion impairs absorption of fat, and fat-soluble vitamin mainly vitamin A. Avitaminosis A may produce squamous metaplasia of the epithelium lining the pancreatic duct, which is already damaged by the inspissated mucus secretions. The tenacious exocrine secretions (sometimes called as concretions) obstruct pancreatic ducts. This impairs production and flow of digestive enzymes from pancreas to the duodenum.

The complete name of the disease, cystic fibrosis of the pancreas, refers to severe tissue destruction of the exocrine pancreas (loss of pancreatic acinar tissue), with fibrotic scarring and/or replacement by fat, cyst formation, and loss of normal architecture of pancreas Cystic fibrosis of the pancreas was also known as mucoviscidosis of pancreas.

Intestine: A normal new born, shortly after birth, passes the intestinal contents that have accumulated in utero (meconium). Thick viscid plugs of mucus may be observed in the small intestine of infants with cystic fibrosis. Sometimes these may lead to obstruction of small-bowel, known as meconium ileus. **Figures 19A** and **B** shows intestinal gland distended with mucus secretion.

Liver involvement: It shows plugging of the bile canaliculi by mucus material, accompanied by ductular proliferation and portal inflammation. Hepatic steatosis is not an uncommon finding. Later, focal biliary cirrhosis may develop in about one-third of patients. Eventually this involves the entire liver, resulting in diffuse hepatic nodularity. Such severe hepatic involvement is observed in less than 10% of patients.

Salivary glands: They show changes similar to those in the pancreas namely: (1) progressive dilation of ducts, (2) squamous metaplasia of the lining epithelium, and (3) glandular atrophy followed by fibrosis.

Pulmonary changes: They are the **most serious complications of cystic disease** and cause most morbidity and mortality. These changes are due to the **viscous mucus secretions** of the submucosal glands of the respiratory tree. This viscous mucus **produces secondary obstruction and infection of the air passages mainly bronchioles**. CF airway secretions are exceedingly difficult to clear. The bronchioles are usually distended with thick mucus accompanied by marked hyperplasia and hypertrophy of the mucus-secreting cells. Recurrent cycles of obstruction and infection result in chronic bronchiolitis and bronchitis and may lead to secondary pulmonary hypertension. Secondary infections lead to severe chronic bronchitis and bronchiectasis. In many patients it may be complicated by forming lung abscesses. Three most common organisms responsible for lung infections are: (1) *Staphylococcus aureus*, (2) *Haemophilus influenzae*, and (3) *Pseudomonas aeruginosa*. A mucoid form (phenotype) of *P. aeruginosa* (due to release of alginate exoproduct, i.e., alginate-producing) is particularly frequent and produces chronic inflammation This confers selective advantage for the pathogen (i.e., *P. aeruginosa*) and poor prognosis for the host. Even more dangerous is the infection with another group of pseudomonads, the *Burkholderia cepacia* complex. This includes at least nine different species;

Continued

Continued

of these, infections with *B. cenocepacia* are the most common in patients with cystic fibrosis. Infection with *B. cenocepacia* is associated with severe illness ("cepacia syndrome") and it is highly resistant to antibiotics and is commonly fatal. Other opportunistic bacterial pathogens in cystic fibrosis include *Stenotrophomonas maltophilia* and nontuberculous mycobacteria. Allergic bronchopulmonary aspergillosis also observed.

Azoospermia and infertility: They are seen in 95% of males with cystic fibrosis who survive to adulthood. It may show atrophy or fibrosis of the reproductive duct system, including the vas deferens, epididymis and seminal vesicles. A frequent finding is the congenital bilateral absence of the vas deferens and in some this may be the only feature suggesting an underlying *CFTR* mutation (bi-allelic *CFTR* mutations in 80% of cases).

Clinical Features

Cystic fibrosis is one of the classical examples of childhood diseases that produce protean clinical manifestations. It produces extremely variable symptoms that may appear at birth to years later, and can involve one organ system or many systems. Only 5–10% of cases come to clinical attention at birth or soon after because of meconium ileus. Distal intestinal obstruction can also develop in older individuals. This may manifest as recurrent episodes of right lower quadrant pain sometimes accompanied by a palpable mass of meconium. This may or may not be associated intussusception, in the right iliac fossa.

In cystic fibrosis, decreased chloride conductance in CFTR results in failure of chloride reabsorption by cells of sweat gland ducts. This leads to accumulation of sodium chloride in the sweat. The skin in children is salty and may even show salt crystals after severe sweating.

Pancreatic manifestations

Exocrine pancreatic insufficiency: It is observed in the majority (85–90%) of patients with cystic fibrosis and is associated with "severe" CFTR mutations on both alleles (e.g., ΔF508/ΔF508). In 10–15% of patients there is one "severe" and one "mild" CFTR mutation (e.g., ΔF508/R117H) or two "mild" CFTR mutations. In these patients, pancreatic exocrine function is retained enough so that there is no need for enzyme supplementation (pancreas-sufficient phenotype).

Consequences of pancreatic insufficiency: Failure of pancreatic exocrine secretion leads to fat and protein malabsorption and their increased loss in feces. Malabsorption manifest as bulky (large) foul-smelling stools (steatorrhea), abdominal distention, and poor weight gain. They may appear during the first year of life. Persistent diarrhea may result in rectal prolapse in about 10% of children.

- **Defective fat absorption:** The faulty fat absorption may lead to nutritional deficiency of the fat-soluble vitamins. These manifests as avitaminosis A, D, E, or K.
- **Defective protein absorption:** It produces hypoproteinemia which may be severe enough to cause generalized edema.

Pancreas-sufficient phenotype: It is usually not associated with other gastrointestinal complications. Usually, these

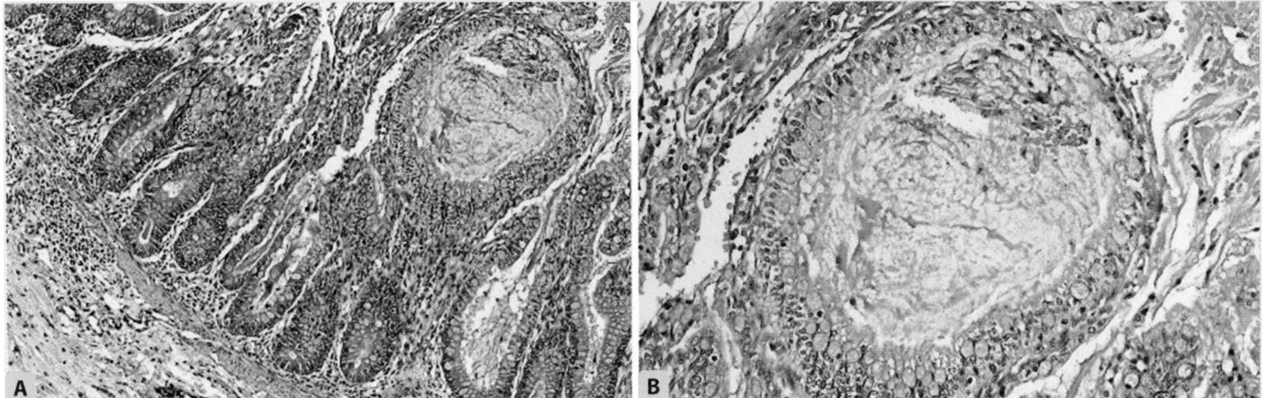

FIGS. 19A AND B: Low (A) and high (B) magnifications showing intestinal gland distended with mucus secretion in cystic fibrosis.

individuals have normal growth and development. Few patients may present with recurrent episodes of pancreatitis associated with acute abdominal pain and occasionally, life-threatening complications. These patients have other features of classic cystic fibrosis (e.g., pulmonary disease).

Idiopathic chronic pancreatitis: It can develop as an isolated late-onset finding without other features of cystic fibrosis. Majority of these individuals show biallelic CFTR mutations (usually one "mild," one "severe").

Endocrine pancreatic insufficiency It can produce diabetes mellitus and may develop in up to 50% of adults with cystic fibrosis. It is likely to be multifactorial in nature due to severe progressive destruction of endocrine pancreas (islets of Langerhans), insulin resistance due to stress hormones, and additional factors.

Respiratory manifestations

It begins with productive cough with large amounts of tenacious, hyperviscous and purulent sputum. The hyperviscous and adherent pulmonary secretions obstruct small and medium-sized airways. CF airway secretions are exceedingly difficult to clear and predispose to recurrent or persistent infection of lung. Persistent lung infections, obstructive pulmonary disease, and cor pulmonale, are the major morbidity and mortality in cystic fibrosis. Repeated bouts of infectious bronchitis and bronchopneumonia become progressively more frequent. This will eventually produce dyspnea. Respiratory failure and cardiac complications of pulmonary hypertension (cor pulmonale) occur late. Patients with one "severe" and one "mild" *CFTR* mutation may develop late-onset mild pulmonary disease (i.e., nonclassic or atypical cystic fibrosis). There is usually little or no pancreatic disease in patients with mild pulmonary disease.

Organisms: In CF, there is a complex bacterial flora and the organisms routinely cultured from CF sputum include *Staphylococcus aureus, Haemophilus influenzae,* and *Pseudomonas aeruginosa.* About 80% of patients with classic cystic fibrosis harbor *P. aeruginosa*, and 3.5% harbor *B. cepacia.* With the indiscriminate use of antibiotic prophylaxis against *Staphylococcus*, infections by resistant strains of *Pseudomonas* are found in many patients.

Recurrent sinonasal polyps can be observed in 10–25% of individuals with cystic fibrosis.

Hepatic manifestations

Significant liver disease develops late in the natural history of cystic fibrosis. It is becoming clinical important as life expectancies increase. Asymptomatic hepatomegaly may be observed in up to one-third of individuals. Symptomatic or biochemical liver diseases are usually detected at or around puberty. Obstruction of the common bile duct may occur due to stones or sludge. It presents with pain abdomen and the acute onset of jaundice. Diffuse biliary cirrhosis develops in less than 10% of case.

Diagnosis

In most cases of cystic fibrosis, the diagnosis is based on:

- **Persistently elevated sweat electrolyte concentrations:** Usually mother recognizes infant's abnormally salty sweat. An increased sweat chloride concentration is observed. Minority of individuals, especially those with at least one "mild" CFTR mutation, may have a normal or near-normal sweat test (<60 mm). In such circumstances, measurement of nasal transepithelial potential difference in vivo can be a useful adjunct. Individuals with cystic fibrosis show abnormal epithelial nasal ion transport (nasal potential difference). There is significantly more negative baseline nasal potential difference than controls.
- **Characteristic clinical findings:** Sinopulmonary disease and gastrointestinal manifestations
- **Abnormal new born screening test:** The most common newborn screening test is based on measurement of the blood level of immunoreactive trypsinogen. This is produced by the pancreas, and its levels are elevated due to injury to pancreas.
- **Family history**.
- **Molecular diagnosis:** In individuals with a positive screening test, suggestive clinical findings, or family history (or more than one of these), genetic analysis should be performed. Sequencing the *CFTR* gene is the gold standard for diagnosis of cystic fibrosis. Molecular prenatal diagnosis of CF is accurate in 95% of cases

Recent advances in the management

A massive effort has identified novel and promising approaches to CF therapy. This includes the management of both acute and chronic complications with more potent antimicrobial therapies, pancreatic enzyme replacement, and bilateral lung transplantation.

Potentiation of mutant CFTR gating: Depending on the molecular defect, three classes of therapeutic agents are being developed.

Potentiators: These agents keep the "gate" of the CFTR channel open and stimulate ion transport. Hence, these agents are most useful in mutations that involve gating (class III) and conduction (class IV). They are also helpful in production mutations (class V), in which they improve the function of reduced amounts of CFTR.

Correctors: These agents help in proper folding and maturation of the CFTR protein. This in turn increases its CFTR transport to the surface of cell. Hence, they are useful in patients with mutations in processing (class II) of CFTR. These include patients with ΔF508 which is the most common CFTR mutation.

Amplifiers: These agents increase the amount of production of CFTR protein by the cell. Thus, these can be useful for patients with mutations in production (class V) of CFTR.

The mentioned, the most common CFTR mutation involve two copies (alleles) of ΔF508. These patients can be treated with a combination therapy consisting of a "potentiator" agent and a small molecule that is a CFTR "corrector." With overall improvements in the management of cystic fibrosis, presently the median life expectancy has extended to 50 years.

SUDDEN INFANT DEATH SYNDROME

Definition: SIDS is defined as "the sudden death of an infant under 1 year of age is unexpected by history (remains unexplained after a thorough case investigation), including thorough postmortem examination (i.e., complete autopsy), examination of the death scene, and review of the clinical history fails to demonstrate an adequate cause of death."

Diagnosis by exclusion: A diagnosis of SIDS should be made only after excluding other specific causes of sudden death (e.g., infection, hemorrhage, aspiration). Its diagnosis requires careful examination of the death scene and a complete postmortem examination. Autopsy may reveal congenital anomalies, diseases of prematurity and low birth weight, and maternal complications. Homicide must be excluded as a potential cause of SIDS, especially when more than one sibling has died of apparent SIDS. It many cases of sudden death in infancy may have an unexpected anatomic or biochemical basis detected at autopsy (**Box 8**). These should not be termed as SIDS, but rather called sudden unexpected infant death (SUID). Infant usually dies while asleep, mostly in the prone or side position. Hence, it is falsely (the pseudonyms) known as "crib death" or "cot death."

Box 8: Major postmortem abnormalities in sudden infant death syndrome (SIDS).

- Infections
- Viral myocarditis
- Bronchopneumonia
- Congenital anomaly: Unsuspected congenital anomalies such as aortic stenosis, anomalous origin of the left coronary artery from the pulmonary artery
- Traumatic child abuse
- Genetic and metabolic defects

Epidemiology

Typically, victims of SIDS are apparently healthy young infants. They went to sleep without any hint of the impending death but did not wake up. Infant deaths due to nutritional factors and infections have been markedly reduced. As more predisposing factors and environmental, biochemical, structural and genetic contributors are identified, the number of deaths without any identifiable pathogenesis has markedly reduced.

Age and time: About 90% of all SIDS deaths occur during the first 6 months of life, mostly between 2 and 4 months of age. Most infants die at home, usually during the night after a period of sleep.

MORPHOLOGY

Postmortem findings in SIDS

In infants who have died of suspected SIDS, a variety of findings have been observed at postmortem examination. They are usually minimal, of uncertain significance and are not seen in all cases. It is important to perform a postmortem examination to identify other causes of SUID. These include presence of unsuspected infection, congenital anomaly, or a genetic disorder, the presence of any findings that excludes a diagnosis of SIDS; and in ruling out the unfortunate possibility of traumatic child abuse.

Multiple petechiae: These are the most common finding in more than 80% of cases. They are usually present on the thymus, visceral and parietal pleura, and epicardium.

Lungs

- **Gross:** Lungs are usually congested
- **Microscopy:** It may show vascular engorgement with or without pulmonary edema in the majority of cases.

Upper respiratory system: Larynx and trachea may be some microscopic evidence of recent infection.

Central nervous system

- There may be astrogliosis of the brainstem and cerebellum.
- Sophisticated morphometric studies: There may be quantitative brainstem abnormalities (e.g., hypoplasia of the arcuate nucleus) or a decrease in brainstem neuronal populations in several cases.

Other nonspecific findings: These include persistence of hepatic extramedullary hematopoiesis and periadrenal brown fat.

Risk Factors (Box 9)

Sudden infant death syndrome is generally accepted as a multifactorial condition. Risk factors for SIDS are difficult to find out. Infant is vulnerable to sudden death during the critical developmental period (i.e., the first 6 months of life). A "triple-risk" model of SIDS has been proposed for this vulnerability. It consists of: (1) parental, (2) infant and environmental (exogenous stressor) risk (vulnerable) factors (**Box 9**). There is intersection of these three overlapping factors.

Channelopathies: Inherited abnormalities in cell membrane ion channels (see pages 14–5 of chapter 1) may be responsible for 10–12% of cases of SIDS.

- **Inherited arrhythmia syndromes:** Most common of these is long QT syndrome. It is probably due to loss-of-function mutations in cardiac potassium channels (KCNQ1, KCNH2) or in some cases it may be sodium channel (SCN5A) and L-type calcium channel (CACNA1C). Long QT syndrome is characterized by prolonged QT intervals on electrocardiogram.
- **Other channelopathies:** Include catecholaminergic polymorphic ventricular tachycardia (CPVT due to mutations in ryanodine receptor 2), Brugada syndrome (mutations in the SCN5A sodium channel, and n calcium channels) and short QT syndrome (gain-of-function mutations in cardiac potassium channels, causing accelerated repolarization of cardiac muscle).

Box 9: Risk factors associated with sudden infant death syndrome (SIDS).

Parental
- Young maternal age (younger than 20 years of age at first pregnancy)
- Maternal cigarette smoking and/or alcohol consumption during and after pregnancy
- Use of illicit drugs during pregnancy: Drug abuse in either parent, specifically paternal marijuana and maternal opiate, cocaine use
- Short intergestational intervals
- Late or no prenatal care
- Low socioeconomic group/status (poor education, unmarried mother, poor prenatal care)
- Increased parity

Infant
- Prematurity (born before term) and/or low birth weight
- Decreased gestational age
- SIDS in a prior sibling (indicates genetic predisposition)
- Antecedent (immediate prior history of) respiratory infections within the last 4 weeks before death
- Brainstem abnormalities, associated with delayed development of arousal and cardiorespiratory control
- Male sex
- Product of a multiple birth
- Germline polymorphisms in autonomic nervous system genes

Environment stressors
- Prone or side sleep position
- Sleeping on a soft surface
- Hyperthermia (thermal stress)
- Cosleeping in first 3 months of life
- Sleeping with parents in the first 3 months

Pathogenesis

Abnormalities in serotonin-dependent signaling: Most accepted hypothesis is that SIDS reflects a delayed development of "arousal" and cardiorespiratory control. The brainstem (particular the medulla oblongata) plays a critical role in the body's "arousal" response to noxious stimuli (e.g., episodic hypercarbia, hypoxia, and thermal stress) exposed during sleep. The serotonergic (5-HT) system of the medulla is involved in these "arousal" responses and also in the regulation of other critical homeostatic functions (e.g., respiratory drive, blood pressure, and upper airway reflexes). Abnormalities in serotonin-dependent signaling in the brainstem may be the responsible for SIDS in some infants.

Laryngeal chemoreceptors: Probably, laryngeal chemoreceptors may form a link between upper respiratory tract infections, the prone position, and SIDS. Antecedent (immediate prior history of) respiratory infections may predispose to impairment of cardiorespiratory control and delayed arousal. When laryngeal chemoreceptors are stimulated, they produce an inhibitory cardiorespiratory reflex. Stimulation of the chemoreceptors is increased by respiratory tract infections. This increases the volume of secretions, and by the prone position, impairs swallowing and clearing of the airways, even in healthy infants. In a vulnerable infant with impaired arousal, the resulting inhibitory cardiorespiratory reflex may be fatal.

Genetic vulnerability: These include polymorphisms of genes related to serotonergic signaling and autonomic innervation. This points to the importance of these processes in the pathophysiology of SIDS.

Diagnosis

Diagnosis of SIDS is by exclusion. It needs careful examination of the death scene and a complete postmortem examination. Autopsy can reveal an unsuspected cause of sudden death.

TUMORS AND TUMOR-LIKE LESIONS OF INFANCY AND CHILDHOOD

Q. Write essay on tumors of infancy and childhood.

Malignancies in children 1–14 years old are uncommon and only 2% of all malignant tumors occur in infancy and childhood. But cancer (including leukemia) remains the leading cause of death from disease in this age group. Only accidental trauma cause significantly more deaths than cancers. In adults most cancers are of epithelial origin (e.g., carcinomas of the lung, breast and GI tract). In contrast, most malignant tumors in children arise from hematopoietic, nervous and soft tissues. Many childhood cancers are part of developmental complexes.

Tumor-like Conditions

Two tumor-like lesions in infancy and childhood are hamartoma and choristoma.

Hamartomas

Definition: It is a disorganized (jumbled) mass of benign-appearing cells, indigenous to the particular site.

These lesions are focal, benign overgrowths of one or more mature cellular elements of a normal tissue native/indigenous to the organ in which it occurs. Though the cellular elements are mature and identical to those found in the remainder of the organ, they do not reproduce the normal architecture of the surrounding tissue. They are often arranged irregularly. Example: Pulmonary chondroid hamartoma (see Fig 8 of chapter 10) consists of islands of disorganized, but histologically normal cartilage, bronchi and vessels. Many hamartomas are clonal and have defined DNA rearrangements. Hence, they may be classified as true neoplasms. Because both hamartomas and benign tumors can be clonal, there is no clear line of demarcation between them. Benign tumors such as hemangiomas, lymphangiomas, rhabdomyomas of the heart, adenomas of the liver, and developmental cysts within the kidneys, lungs, or pancreas are considered as hamartomas by some.

Choristomas

Definition: It is tiny microscopic aggregates (island) of normal tissue components in aberrant (ectopic/abnormal) locations (i.e., normal tissue in an abnormal site). It is a congenital anomaly and not a true tumor. Example: Presence of small nodular mass of normally organized pancreatic tissue in the submucosa of the stomach, duodenum, or small intestine, a small mass adrenal tissue in the renal cortex (kidney), lungs, or ovaries, heterotopic parathyroid glands within the thymus in the anterior mediastinum.

It also called **heterotopias** or **ectopia**. They are usually of little significance, but they can be confused clinically with neoplasms. Rarely, they are sites of origin of true neoplasms, producing paradoxes (e.g., an adrenal carcinoma arising from choristoma contains adrenal cells in the ovary).

Benign Neoplasms (Tumors)

Benign tumors are more common than cancers in children. Most benign tumors are of little concern. Almost any benign neoplasm may develop in the pediatric age group. In adults, most common tumors, benign or malignant, are of epithelial origin. In contrast, most common neoplasms in childhood are soft-tissue tumors derived from mesenchyme. Only hemangiomas, lymphangiomas, and teratomas are discussed here.

Hemangiomas

They are the most common neoplasms of infancy. Architecturally, they are same as those occurring in adults. It is not clear whether they are true neoplasms or hamartomas, but 50% of them are present at birth. Hemangiomas may enlarge along with the growth of the child, but in most cases, they spontaneously regress with age.

Sites: It has diverse locations. Most hemangiomas in children are found in the skin, particularly on the face and scalp.

Appearance: They vary in size and appear as flat to elevated, irregular, red-blue masses. Hemangiomas especially on the head or neck, may produce large masses and may rapidly grow causing serious problems. Hemangiomas may enlarge as the child grows, but many a times they may spontaneously regress. Majority of superficial hemangiomas have only a cosmetic significance.

Some of the flat, larger lesions congenital capillary hemangiomas (some consider it as vascular ectasias) of the skin of the face and scalp are called as port-wine stains. They are often disfiguring and produce dark purple coloration of the affected area. Unlike many small hemangiomas, they persist for life.

Rarely, hemangiomas may be the manifestation of a hereditary disorder associated with disease within internal organs (e.g., von Hippel-Lindau syndrome). Few cavernous hemangiomas of CNS can occur in the familial setting and the affected families show mutations in one of three cerebral cavernous malformation (CCM) genes (*KRIT1, CCM2, or PDCD10*).

Histological types: It may be cavernous or capillary hemangiomas. Capillary hemangiomas are often more cellular in children than in adults.

Capillary hemangioma

It is most common type of hemangioma.

Sites: Most commonly in the skin, subcutaneous tissues, and mucous membranes of the oral cavities and lips. It may also develop in internal organs (e.g., liver, spleen and kidneys).

MORPHOLOGY

Gross: Bright red to blue in color. Size varies from few millimeters to several centimeters in diameter. It may be in level with the surface of the skin or slightly raised. The skin overlying it is usually intact.

Microscopy (Figs. 20A and B)

- Unencapsulated lesion.
- Composed of aggregates of closely packed, thin-walled vascular channels. The size and structure of these vascular channels resemble normal capillaries.
- Capillaries are lined by flattened endothelium and their lumen is usually filled with blood. The lumens may contain partially or completely organized thrombus.
- The vessels are separated by scant connective tissue stroma.

Cavernous hemangioma

It consists of large, dilated vascular channels; compared with small vascular spaces in capillary hemangiomas.

MORPHOLOGY

Gross: Red-blue, soft, spongy masses and measure 1–2 cm in diameter. More frequently involve deep structures. They are found in the skin, on the mucosal surfaces and visceral organs, such as the spleen, liver and pancreas.

Microscopy (Figs. 21A and B)

- Consist of sharply defined unencapsulated mass.
- Composed of large, cavernous blood-filled vascular spaces, separated by a moderate amount of connective tissue stroma. Intravascular thrombosis and dystrophic calcification are common.

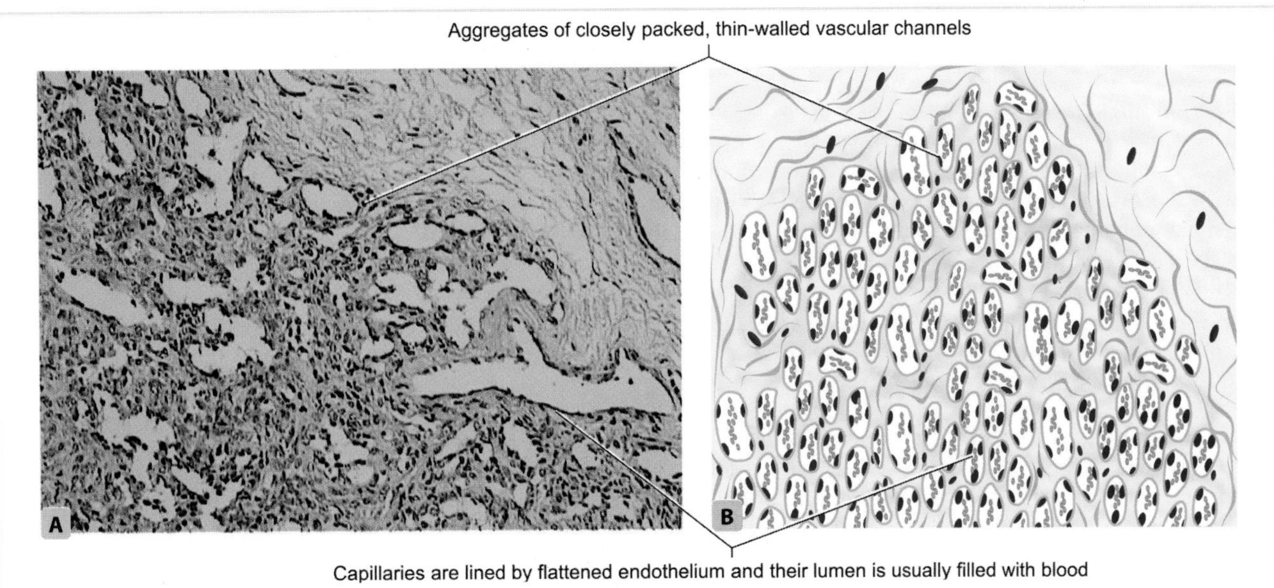

FIGS. 20A AND B: Microscopic appearance of capillary hemangioma: (A) Photomicrograph; (B) Diagrammatic.

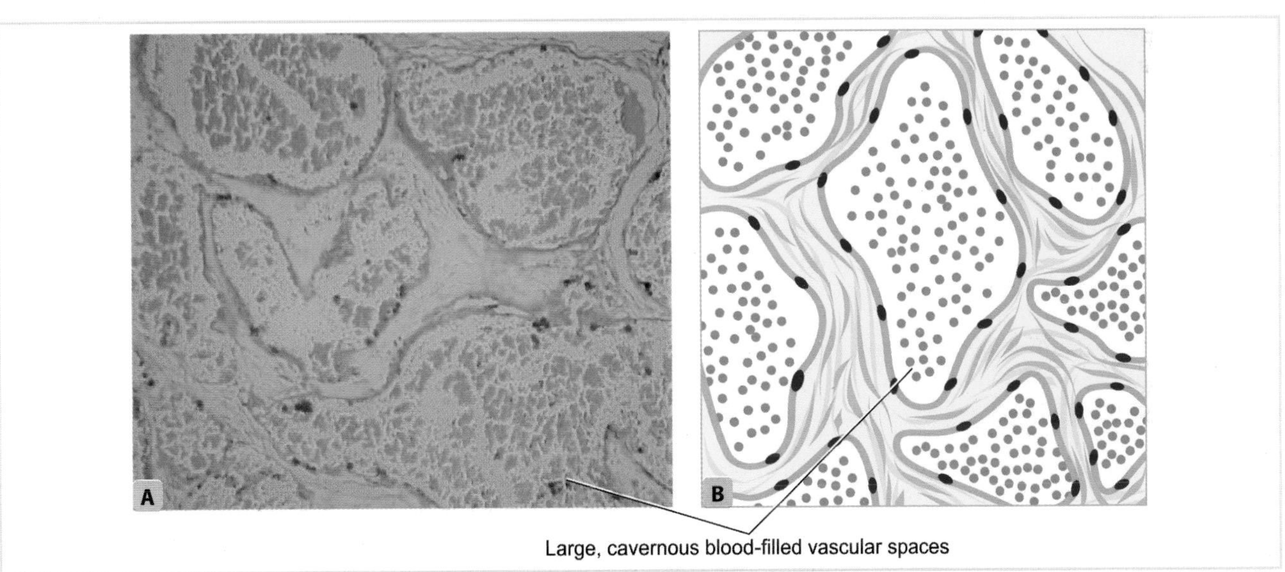

FIGS. 21A AND B: Microscopic appearance of cavernous hemangioma: (A) Photomicrograph; (B) Diagrammatic

Lymphangiomas

They represent the lymphatic counterpart of hemangiomas and also called as cystic hygromas (see **Fig. 8**). Unlike hemangiomas, these lesions do not regress spontaneously and should be resected.

Site: They are poorly circumscribed swellings that are usually present at birth. They may be found on the skin but, more commonly, they are seen in the deeper regions of the head and neck, axilla, mediastinum, floor of the mouth, and retroperitoneum. They may increase in size after birth and may compress the mediastinal structures or nerve trunks in axilla.

Microscopy: They may be unilocular or multilocular. They show cystic and cavernous spaces lined by endothelial cells and surrounded by lymphoid aggregates. The lumen/spaces usually contain pale straw-colored fluid.

Fibrous Tumors

Fibrous tumors that occur in infants and children include sparsely cellular proliferations of spindle-shaped cells (termed as fibromatosis) and richly cellular lesions indistinguishable from fibrosarcomas occurring in adults (termed as congenital-infantile fibrosarcomas). Biological behavior of these tumors cannot be predicted based on microscopy alone. However, is spite of microscopic similarities of congenital-infantile fibrosarcomas with adult fibrosarcomas, it has an excellent prognosis. Congenital infantile fibrosarcomas is characteristically shows chromosomal translocation, t (12;15) (p13; q25), that produces an ETV6-NTRK3 fusion transcript. The normal *ETV6* gene product is a transcription factor, and the *NTRK3* gene product (also known as TRKC) is a tyrosine kinase. Similar to other tyrosine kinase fusion proteins found in neoplasms, ETV6-NTRK3 is constitutively active. It stimulates signaling through the oncogenic RAS-MAPK and PI3K/AKT pathways. ETV6-NTRK3 fusion transcript is a useful diagnostic marker for congenital infantile fibrosarcomas.

Teratomas

In teratomas, there is a relationship between histologic maturity of tissue components and biologic behavior.

Types

- Mature teratomas: These are benign, well-differentiated cystic lesions.
- Immature teratomas: Lesions of indeterminate potential or
- Malignant teratomas: They are unequivocally malignant. Usually admixed with another germ cell tumor such as an endodermal sinus tumor (yolk sac tumor).

Age group: Teratomas have two peaks in its presentation: the first at about 2 years of age and the second in late adolescence or early adulthood. The first peak is congenital neoplasms and the second peak lesions may also be of prenatal origin but are more slowly growing.

Sacrococcygeal teratomas: These rare germ cell tumors. They present as masses near the sacrum and buttocks. They are the most common (about 40%) teratomas of childhood. About 10% of sacrococcygeal teratomas may be associated with congenital anomalies such as primarily defects of the hindgut and cloacal region and other midline defects (e.g., meningocele, spina bifida). They are four times more common in girls than in boys. They present as masses near the sacrum and buttocks. They may be large, lobulated tumors, sometimes they may be as big as the infant's head. About 75% of these tumors are mature teratomas with a benign course. About 12% may be malignant and lethal. The remaining 13% of tumors are immature teratomas, and their malignant potential depends on the amount of immature tissue elements present usually immature neuroepithelial elements. Most benign teratomas occur in younger infants (<4 months), whereas malignant lesions tend to occur in older children. Microscopically, the teratomas contain multiple tissues derived from more than one germ cell layer.

Other sites for teratomas in childhood: These include the testis, ovary, and various midline locations, such as the mediastinum, retroperitoneum, and head and neck.

Malignant Neoplasms

Malignant neoplasms developing during infancy and childhood are biologically and microscopically different from their counterparts occurring later in life. These differences are:

- Incidence and type of tumor
- Presence of genetic abnormalities or familial syndromes that predispose to cancer. For example, short arm deletions of chromosome 11, causing Wilms tumor associated with aniridia, genitourinary malformations and mental retardation (WAGR complex); Loss of the long arm of chromosome 13 is associated with retinoblastoma due to the loss of the Rb tumor suppressor gene.
- Frequently a close relationship between abnormal development (teratogenesis) and tumor production (oncogenesis).
- Tendency of malignancies to regress spontaneously or to undergo "differentiation" into mature elements. For example, neuroblastoma, which may show differentiation to ganglioneuroblastoma and ganglioneuroma.
- Improved survival or cure rate in many childhood tumors. Hence, in survivors more attention is needed to minimize the delayed adverse effects of chemotherapy and radiation therapy. This includes even the development of second malignancies following therapy.

Incidence and Types

Malignant neoplasms in infancy and childhood are uncommon and their distribution according to their age is presented in **Figure 22**. Most common of these include neoplasms of the hematopoietic system, neural tissue, and soft tissues. This distribution is unlike in that in adults, in whom most cancers are of epithelial origin such as carcinomas of the lung, breast, prostate, and GI tract. The most frequent malignant tumors in childhood arise in the hematopoietic system, nervous tissue (including the central and sympathetic nervous system, adrenal medulla, and retina), soft tissue, bone, and kidney. In contrast, most common tumors in adults arise in skin, lung, breast, prostate, and colon. Leukemia alone is responsible for more deaths in children under 15 years of age than all of the other tumors combined.

Origin: Most malignant tumors in childhood are of mesodermal origin.

Microscopy

Primitive appearing tumor cells: Many of the malignant nonhematopoietic pediatric neoplasms have unique microscopic features. Usually, they consist of primitive (embryonal) undifferentiated appearing cells rather than pleomorphic-anaplastic microscopic appearance characteristic of malignant tumors in adult.

Small, round, blue-cell tumors: Because of their primitive appearance of cells, many childhood tumors have been collectively called as small, round, blue-cell tumors. These cells have small, round nuclei and are arranged in sheets. The differential diagnoses of such tumors are listed in **Box 10**. These primitive cells frequently show features of organogenesis specific to the site of tumor origin. Hence, these tumors are frequently designated by adding the suffix—blastoma. These include nephroblastoma (Wilms tumor), hepatoblastoma, neuroblastoma, retinoblastoma and medulloblastoma.

Diagnosis: These tumors usually show distinctive microscopic features by which a definitive diagnosis is possible. Diagnosis is usually possible on microscopic examination alone, if the site of origin of tumor is known. However, occasionally a combination of molecular studies (e.g., chromosome analysis), immunoperoxidase stains, or electron microscopy is required. They are becoming increasingly useful, both for diagnosis and prognosis.

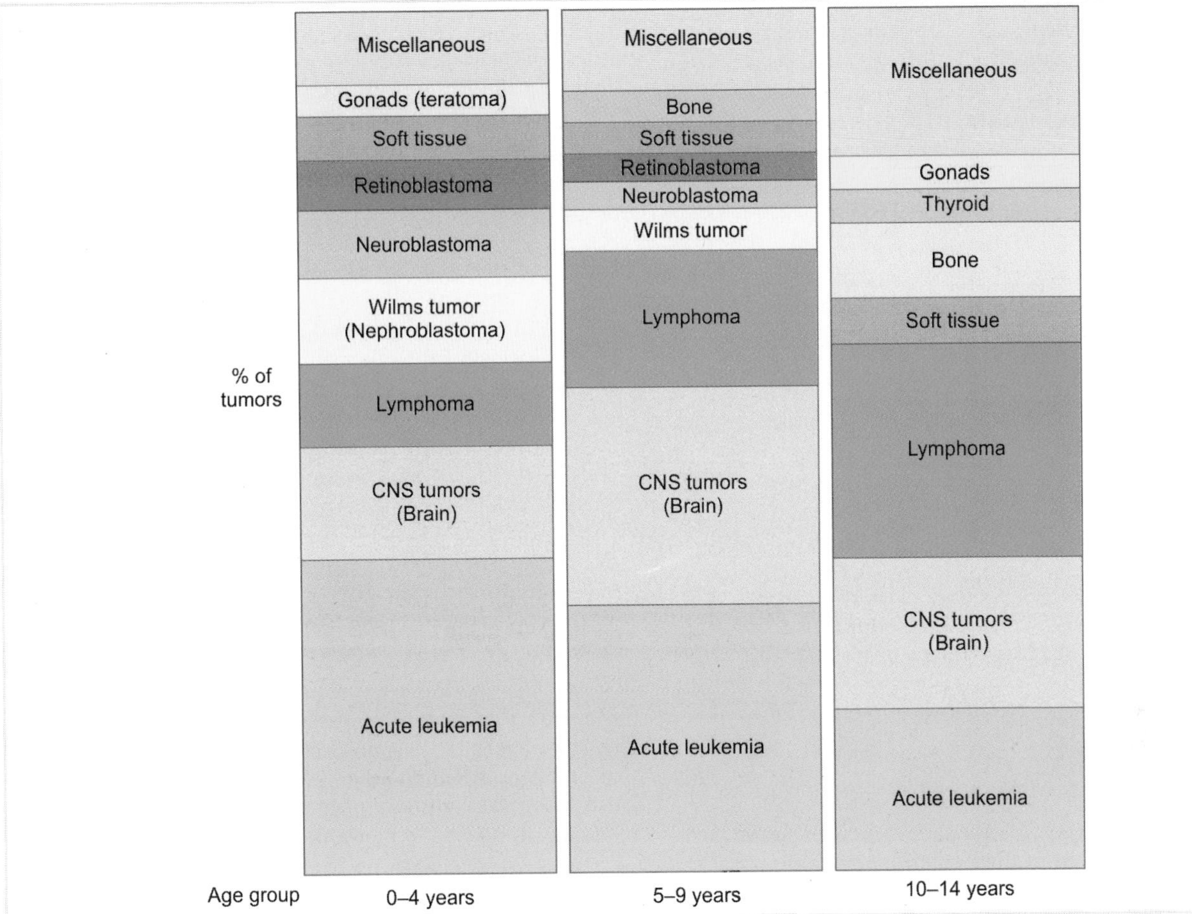

FIG. 22: Distribution of common malignant neoplasms of infancy and childhood according to age group.

Box 10: List of small, round, blue-cell tumors.

- Neuroblastoma
- Lymphoma
- Rhabdomyosarcoma
- Ewing sarcoma (primitive neuroectodermal tumor)
- Some cases of Wilms tumor
- Medulloblastoma
- Retinoblastoma

Neuroblastic Tumors

Neuroblastic tumor is a tumor group (**Fig. 21**) that includes tumors of the sympathetic ganglia and adrenal medulla that are derived from primordial neural crest cells present in these sites.

Neuroblastoma

Q. Write short essay on neuroblastoma.

Neuroblastoma is the most important embryonal malignant neuroblastic tumor of neural crest origin. They are composed of neoplastic neuroblasts. Neuroblasts are derived from primitive sympathogonia and represent an intermediate stage in the development of sympathetic ganglion neurons (**Fig. 23**). The term neuroblastoma includes a spectrum of tumors showing variable degrees of differentiation, including neuroblastoma, ganglioneuroblastoma, and ganglioneuroma.

Age: It is the most common extracranial childhood solid tumor. It is most frequently diagnosed malignancy during infancy (median age at diagnosis is 18 months). It is the second most common solid malignancy of childhood after brain tumors.

Sporadic and familial types: Most of them occur sporadically, but 1–2% is familial. In familial cases, it may involve both of the adrenals or multiple primary autonomic sites. Germline mutations in the anaplastic lymphoma kinase (*ALK*) gene are observed in majority having familial predisposition to neuroblastoma. Germline mutations in *PHOX2A* or *KIF1B* genes may also be responsible for familial cases. Somatic gain of function (ALK) mutations are also found in a few (10%) sporadic neuroblastomas. Tumors having ALK mutations respond to drugs that target their activity. Amplification of *N-MYC* (MYC family of proto-oncogenes) is found in about 30% of neuroblastomas.

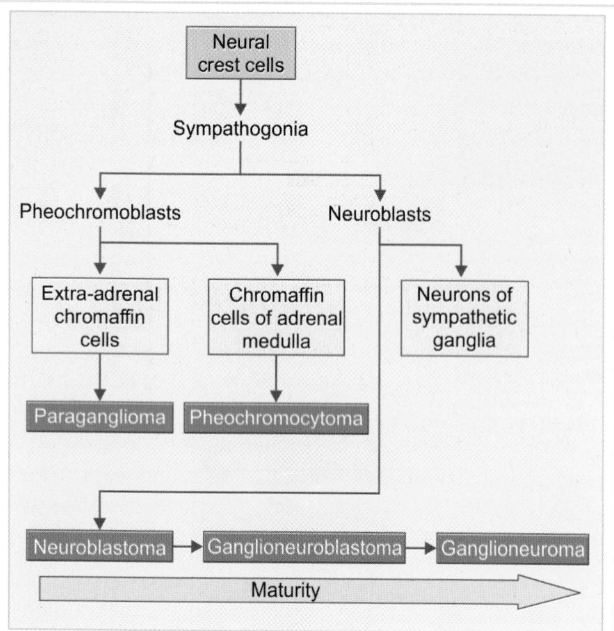

FIG. 23: Histogenesis of tumors derived from neural crest.

MORPHOLOGY

Gross

Site: Neuroblastomas can arise at any site with neural crest-derived cells (i.e., from the posterior cranial fossa to the coccyx). About 40% of childhood neuroblastomas occur in the adrenal medulla. Remaining can arise anywhere along the sympathetic chain (paravertebral sympathetic ganglia and sympathetic paraganglia). These sites include:

- Paravertebral region of the abdomen (25%).
- Posterior mediastinum (15%).
- Pelvis, the neck, and brain (cerebral neuroblastomas)

Size: Vary from minute, barely noticeable nodules (as in situ lesions) to large tumors weighing 1 kg that are readily palpable through the abdominal wall (in case of tumors of adrenal).

Nature: Majority of these are silent and regress spontaneously.

Gross: They are round, irregularly lobulated masses and weigh 50–150 g or more. They may be sharply demarcated with a fibrous pseudocapsule or infiltrate the surrounding structures (kidneys, renal vein, and vena cava, and can envelop the aorta).

Cut section: Soft, friable, brain-like tissue and gray-tan or variegated maroon in color. Large tumors may show areas of necrosis, hemorrhage, cystic change, and calcification.

Microscopy

The microscopic features of classic neuroblastomas are as follows:

- **Tumor cells:** The tumor cells are arranged in solid sheets. The pattern of growth is vaguely nodular or nested due to the presence of delicate, incomplete fibrovascular septa. The tumor cells appear as:

Continued

Continued

  - Typical neuroblasts are small, regular, round, primitive-appearing cells having dark/deeply staining (hyperchromatic) nuclei resembling lymphocytes. They are slightly larger than lymphocytes
  - Scant pink cytoplasm is present and cell borders are poorly defined.
  - Others: Mitotic activity, karyorrhexis (breakdown of nuclear material), and pleomorphism may be prominent.
  - These tumors may be difficult to differentiate morphologically from other small round blue cell tumors.
- **Stroma/background:** The tumor cells are continuous with the intermixed neuropil. Neuropil appears as a faintly/lightly eosinophilic fibrillary material. It represents tangled mass of the neuritic processes of the primitive neuroblasts as revealed by silver stains, immunohistochemistry, or electron microscopy.
- **Homer–Wright pseudorosettes:** They may be seen in about one-fourth to one-third of the cases. These consist of rim of dark tumor cells concentrically arranged (circumferential arrangement) around a central pale fibrillar core (area or space) filled with neuropil (**Figs. 24A** and **B**). Because of the absence of an actual central lumen they are called pseudorosettes.
- **Immunohistochemistry:** Cells show positive immunohistochemical reactions for neuron-specific enolase, chromogranin, synaptophysin, microtubule-associated proteins, and NB-84 (antineuroblastoma antibody). Recently, it is found that immunohistochemistry for PHOXB2 (transcription factor PHOX2B) represents the most sensitive and specific marker for neuroblastoma.
- **Electron microscopy:** The malignant neuroblasts show small, peripheral, membrane-bound, dendritic processes with longitudinally oriented microtubules and catecholamine-containing neurosecretory granules and filaments in the cytoplasm.`
- Some neoplasms show signs of maturation that can be spontaneous or therapy-induced. Larger cells having more abundant cytoplasm, large vesicular nuclei, and a prominent nucleolus, representing ganglion cells in various stages of maturation, may be found in tumors admixed with primitive neuroblasts (ganglioneuroblastoma).

International Neuroblastoma Pathology Classification (INPC)

Neuroblastomas have several unique features in their natural history. Some neoplasms may show spontaneous or induced (by therapy) maturation.

Based on INPC, the tumor cells show a spectrum of differentiation from primitive neuroblasts to ganglion cells. Thus, the classification of neuroblastoma depends on the relative amounts of these components (**Table 3**). It is to be noted that this classification is used only for untreated neuroblastomas. Chemotherapy usually induces maturation and/or nuclear anaplasia. Hence, postchemotherapy neuroblastoma should be interpreted as "neuroblastoma with chemotherapy effect."

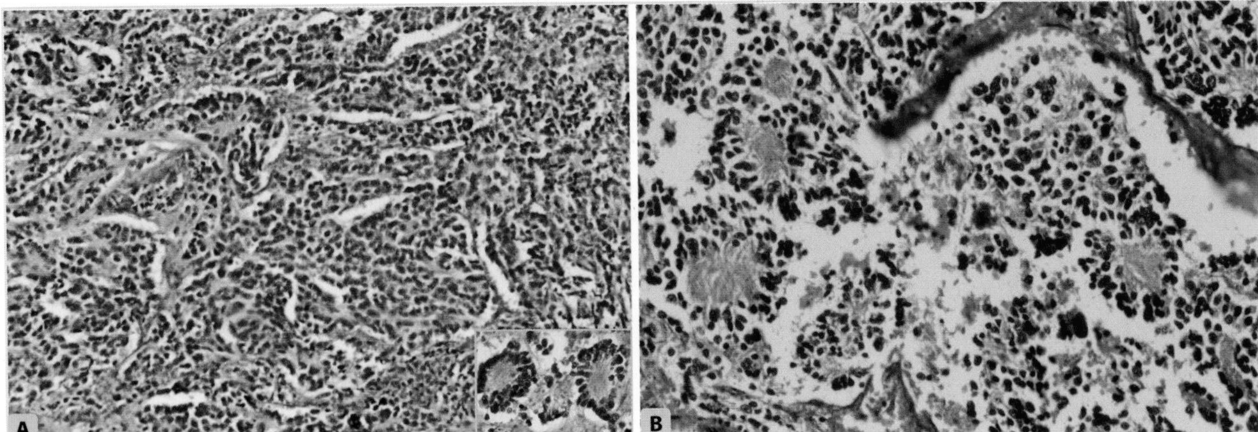

FIGS. 24A AND B: Microscopic appearance of neuroblastoma. (A) Poorly differentiated neuroblastoma consisting of small primitive appearing cells with scant cytoplasm embedded in a finely fibrillar matrix. Inset of A shows two Homer–Wright rosettes. (B) Higher magnification showing Homer–Wright rosettes consisting of rim of dark tumor cells concentrically arranged (circumferential arrangement) around a central pale fibrillar core (area or space) filled with neuropil.

Table 3: The International Neuroblastoma Pathology Classification (INPC).

Nature of stroma	*Microscopic features/comments*	*Diagnosis*
Schwannian stroma poor	• No Schwannian stroma/no neuropil • Needs adjunctive diagnostic tests	Neuroblastoma, undifferentiated
	• Presence of neuropil allows for H&E diagnosis • <5% differentiating neuroblasts	Neuroblastoma, poorly differentiated
	• More abundant neuropil • >5% differentiating neuroblasts	Neuroblastoma, differentiating
Schwannian stroma rich (>50%)	• Schwannian stroma comprises >50% of the tumor • Microscopic foci of neuropil contain neuroblastic cells at varying stages of maturation • No macroscopic nodules present	Ganglioneuroblastoma, intermixed
Schwannian stroma dominant	• Schwannian stroma is the predominant element of the tumor • Scattered ganglion cells are mature or maturing • No neuropil is present	Ganglioneuroma, maturing
	• Schwannian stroma is the predominant element of the tumor • Scattered ganglion cells are mature with surrounding satellite cells • No neuropil is present	Ganglioneuroma, mature
Composite stroma rich/dominant and stroma poor	• Grossly visible nodule consists of any type of stroma poor neuroblastoma • Background of ganglioneuroblastoma or ganglioneuroma • Nodular component should also be classified	Ganglioneuroblastoma, nodular

Undifferentiated neuroblastoma: The most primitive neuroblast does not show visible cytoplasm. Tumors consisting entirely of these primitive cells without any associated neuropil are classified as "undifferentiated neuroblastoma". These have significant morphological overlap with lymphoma or other small round blue cell tumors. The process of neuroblast differentiation and development of Schwannian stroma go hand in hand.

Poorly differentiated neuroblastoma (Fig. 24): When less than 5% of neuroblasts in a tumor show ganglion cell differentiation (equal volumes of nucleus and cytoplasm) the tumor is termed as "poorly differentiated neuroblastoma". These tumors show a definite component of neuropil. Hence, its diagnosis is more straightforward than the undifferentiated form.

Differentiating neuroblastoma: When a tumor has more than 5% ganglion cell differentiation, but consists of less than 50% Schwannian stroma, it is called "differentiating neuroblastoma."

Ganglioneuroblastoma, intermixed: When the Schwannian stroma is more than 50% of the tumor (always associated with more than 5% ganglion cell differentiation), it is classified as "ganglioneuroblastoma, intermixed."

Ganglioneuroma: When the tumor is composed completely of Schwannian stroma and ganglion cells, it is diagnosed as ganglioneuroma. In children, caution should be exercised in diagnosing ganglioneuromas. Before diagnosing, it is necessary to thoroughly sample the specimen. By definition, it should not show any persistent nests of neuroblastic cells and no recognizable neuropil. Ganglioneuroma is further classified in children as follows:

- **Ganglioneuroma, maturing:** When the tumor shows clusters of maturing ganglion cells (without associated neuropil), it is called "ganglioneuroma, maturing."
- **Ganglioneuroma, mature (Fig. 25):** When ganglion cells are scattered throughout the Schwannian stroma individually (in association with surrounding sustentacular cells), the tumor is termed "ganglioneuroma, mature". In adults, ganglioneuromas are almost always mature.
- **Ganglioneuroblastoma, nodular type:** Few neuroblastic tumors may show any type of Schwannian "stromal-rich" neuroblastic tumor (otherwise typical ganglioneuroma or ganglioneuroblastoma, intermixed). This is seen with a distinct grossly identifiable nodule composed of more primitive "stromal-poor" microscopic features, which is most commonly poorly differentiated neuroblastoma or differentiating neuroblastoma. Such tumors are termed as "ganglioneuroblastoma, nodular type." It is very important to carefully examine all gross specimens with thin sectioning to assess for such macroscopic nodules.

Spread and metastases

Local infiltration: Adrenal neuroblastomas locally infiltrate the surrounding tissues. They may show intraspinal (dumbbell) extension or spread into the kidney.

Lymph node spread: It spreads to lymph nodes.

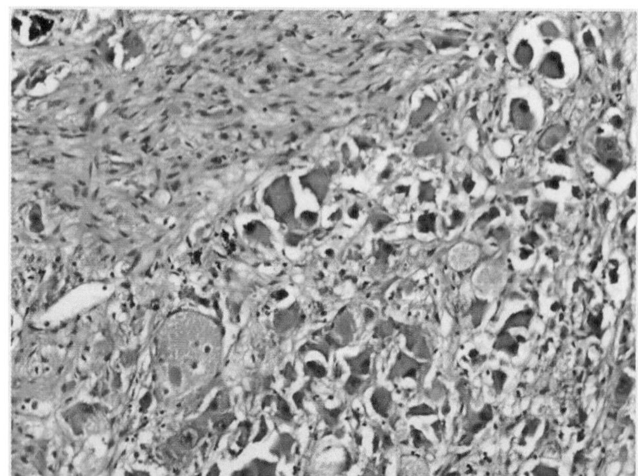

FIG. 25: Ganglioneuroma maturing with numerous large cells with vesicular nuclei and abundant eosinophilic cytoplasm, representing neoplastic ganglion cells. Spindle-shaped Schwann cells are present in the background stroma.

Blood spread: The most common sites of distant metastases are liver, lungs, bone marrow, bones, liver, orbit, and dura. Intracranial and pulmonary metastases are rare. Bone metastases are usually multiple and sometimes symmetrical. This point has to be remembered while in the differential diagnosis with Ewing sarcoma. Morphologic evaluation of bone marrow for neuroblastoma cells is a routinely used for clinical staging.

Staging

Staging systems directly related to surgical pathology for neuroblastoma is the International Neuroblastoma Staging System (INSS) and is presented in **Box 11**. At the time of gross evaluation and sectioning, for correct staging it is necessary that lymph nodes attached to and removed with the primary tumor should be evaluated separately from other submitted lymph nodes. The staging system is important to determine prognosis.

Clinical course

- **Children below 2 years of age:** Usually present as large abdominal masses, fever, and weight loss.

Box 11: International Neuroblastoma Staging System (INSS).

Stage I
- Localized tumor completely excised, with or without microscopic residual disease
- Representative ipsilateral "non-adherent" lymph nodes microscopically negative for tumor
- Nodes adherent to the primary tumor may be positive for tumor

Stage IIA
- Localized tumor incompletely gross resected
- Representative ipsilateral "non-adherent" lymph nodes negative for tumor microscopically

Stage IIB
- Localized tumor with or without complete gross excision
- Ipsilateral "non-adherent" lymph nodes positive microscopically for tumor
- Any enlarged contralateral lymph nodes, which are negative for tumor microscopically

Stage III
- Unresectable unilateral tumor infiltrating across the midline with or without regional lymph node involvement
- Localized unilateral tumor with contralateral regional lymph node involvement

Stage IV
- Any primary tumor with dissemination to distant lymph nodes, bone, bone marrow, liver, skin, and/or other organs (except as defined for stage IVS)

Stage IVS (S, Special)
- Localized primary tumor (as defined for stage I, IIA, or IIB) with dissemination limited to skin, liver, and/or bone marrow (<10% of nucleated cells are constituted by neoplastic cells; >10% involvement of bone marrow is considered as stage 4)
- Stage 4S limited to infants younger than 1 year (12 months) of age

- **Older children:** Symptoms develop due to metastases such as bone pain, respiratory symptoms, or gastrointestinal complaints. Spread to the periorbital region may produce proptosis and ecchymosis. In neonates, disseminated neuroblastomas may produce multiple cutaneous metastases. This can cause deep blue discoloration of the skin which is unfortunately designated as "blueberry muffin baby."
- Ganglioneuromas may present either as asymptomatic mass or symptoms related to compression.

Laboratory finding

- Majority (~90%) of neuroblastomas, irrespective of their location, secrete catecholamines (similar to pheochromocytomas). This is an important diagnostic feature.
- The elevated levels of catecholamines in blood leads to elevated urine levels of their metabolites vanillylmandelic acid (VMA) and homovanillic acid (HVA), norepinephrine, and dopamine. However, hypertension is less frequent.

Course: It is extremely variable.

Prognosis factors

Many clinical, histopathologic, molecular, and biochemical factors influence the prognosis. The tumors are classified as "low," "intermediate," or "high" risk. The most important prognostic factors are as follows:

Tumor stage and patient age at time of diagnosis Neuroblastomas at stage I, IIA, or IIB (see **Box 11**) tend to have an excellent prognosis, irrespective of age ("low" or "intermediate" risk). However; exception are tumors with amplification of the *MYCN* oncogene. Infants with localized primary tumors and metastases to the liver, bone marrow, and skin (stage 4S) form a special subtype. In these tumors, spontaneous regression is not uncommon. Children below 18 months of age, and especially those in the first year of life, have an excellent prognosis regardless of the stage of the neoplasm. Children above 18 months of age usually fall into at least the "intermediate" risk category. Patients with higher-stage tumors or with unfavorable prognostic features such as MYCN amplification in the neoplastic cells are considered "high" risk.

Tumor morphology It is an independent prognostic factor. Accordingly, tumors are divided into "favorable" or "unfavorable" histologic subtypes in combination with patient age and MKI (**Table 4**).

MYCN amplification status *MYCN* amplification occurs in 20–25% of primary tumors. Presence of amplification of the *MYCN* proto-oncogene in neuroblastomas shifts the tumor to the "high"-risk category, irrespective of age, stage, or histology. *MYCN* is located on the distal short arm of chromosome 2 (2p23-p24). Amplification of *MYCN* does not occur at the 2p23-p24 site. But it occurs as extrachromosomal multiple, small, structures called "**double minutes"/dmins** or **homogeneous staining regions (HSR),** if increased copies of gene are integrated within other chromosomes (refer Fig. 27 of Chapter 10). Increased copies of gene may be inserted into new location in the chromosome, which may be distant from the normal location of the involved genes. The HSRs represent amplification *of N-myc* (*MYCN*). Most *MYCN* amplification is seen as the disease advances and the degree of amplification correlates with poorer prognosis. Presently, *MYCN* amplification is the most important genetic abnormality used for risk stratification of neuroblastic tumors. HSR regions containing amplified genes lack a normal banding pattern and appear as homogeneous in G-banded karyotype This amplification can be detected by FISH or PCR techniques. Rare cases with genotype-phenotype discordance have been reported (i.e., *MYCN* amplification with favorable histology). In these, there are two prognostic subgroups, i.e., neuroblastomas with the poor prognostic group is characterized by prominent nucleoli (i.e., "bull's eye" tumor).

Chromosomal abnormalities Tumors with *MYCN* amplification may show chromosome 1p deletions (especially del 1p36.3). In patients without MYCN amplification, allelic gain of 17q and 11q deletion indicates more aggressiveness.

Ploidy of the tumor cells Ploidy is the number of complete sets of of chromosomes and all humans are diploid organism. Ploidy of the tumor cells correlates with outcome in children below 2 years of age and an independent prognostic importance. In DNA ploidy analyses, the DNA content per nucleus is calculated for all the nuclei from a tumor specimen. This gives a histogram of the distribution of DNA content in the measured sample. DNA ploidy is a measure of large-scale genomic instability and discriminates between specimen

Table 4: International Neuroblastoma Pathology Classification: Favorable and unfavorable histology groups.

Age at the time of diagnosis	*Favorable histology*	*Unfavorable histology*
Any age	• Ganglioneuroblastoma, intermixed • Ganglioneuroma, mature or maturing	• Neuroblastoma, undifferentiated • Neuroblastoma of any subtype, with high MKI
<18 months	• Neuroblastoma, poorly differentiated, with low or intermediate MKI • Neuroblastoma, differentiating, with low or intermediate MKI	
18–60 months	• Neuroblastoma, differentiating, with low MKI (Mitosis–karyorrhexis index)	• Neuroblastoma, poorly differentiated • Neuroblastoma, differentiating, with intermediate MKI
>60 months	• None	• Neuroblastoma of any subtype

Note: For Ganglioneuroblastoma, nodular subtype favorable versus unfavorable histology is based on the subtype of the Schwannian stroma poor neuroblastoma component using the same age and MKI-based criteria.

with a normal DNA content and nuclei with an abnormal and often unstable DNA content. DNA ploidy has less prognostic value in patients older than 2 years. Neuroblastomas can be broadly divided into two categories: (1) near-diploid and (2) hyperdiploid (whole-chromosome gains).

- A DNA index near the diploid/tetraploid range is unfavorable. These near-diploid tumors harbor generalized genomic instability, with multiple segmental chromosomal
- *Aberrations*: This result in a complex karyotype. Hyperdiploid or near-triploid is associated with a more favorable prognosis. Neuroblastomas with hyperdiploidy have an underlying defect in the mitotic machinery. This leads to nondisjunction and whole-chromosome gains, but otherwise relatively bland karyotypes. One peculiar form of segmental aberration in aggressive neuroblastomas is termed as chromothripsis (refer page 432). It is characterized by localized fragmentation of a chromosome segment followed by random assembly of the fragments. In some patients of neuroblastomas, chromothripsis can lead to amplification of MYCN or other oncogenes, or losses in tumor suppressor loci.

Clinical outcome is favorable in association with an aneuploid stem line and a low percentage of tumor cells in the S, G_2, and M phases of the cell cycle.

Mitosis-karyorrhexis index (MKI) The MKI is a count of all mitotic and karyorrhectic figures found per 5,000 neuroblasts. The number of mitotic and karyorrhectic figures can vary in different fields in a large pretreatment resected specimen. But the reported MKI should be representative of all tumors on the slides. Once at least 5,000 neuroblasts are exceeded in the denominator, one calculates the percentage for the MKI (mitotic + karyorrhectic figures/neuroblasts). This index is divided into low (<100/5000; 2%), intermediate (100–200/5,000; 2%–4%), or high (>200/5,000; >4%). The following features may help in determining the appropriate MKI:

- **Karyorrhectic figures:** They are recognized by small pyknotic nuclei. These nuclei may appear crescentic, angulated, or round, and should have recognizable eosinophilic cytoplasm. Should avoid counting lymphocytes.
- **MKI averaging method:** Unlike other mitotic count methods, MKI should be weighted. It should not determine by areas of highest count. First identify whether the tumor is homogeneous or heterogeneous with respect to mitotic-karyorrhectic figures. If heterogeneous, then determine regions that may be high, intermediate, or low.
- **Counting and magnification:** The MKI should not be estimated visually. Use a manual differential counter and count 40X fields, Record the number of mitotic-karyorrhectic figures over the denominator of neuroblasts present. Most poorly differentiated neuroblastomas have average 600–800 neuroblasts per 40X field. In differentiating neuroblastoma there may be as low as 100–200. For the average poorly differentiated neuroblastoma, a count of ten 40X fields will give more than 5,000 neuroblasts.
- **Necrosis:** Areas of necrosis should be avoided when counting MKI.

Alterations in gene Whole-genome sequencing has discovered alterations in a variety of genes. Some of these genetic alterations may have prognostic value. The products of some genes are involved in neural crest development (neurogenesis). Neurogenesis is a process in neuronal differentiation and includes the sprouting of neurites, which later forms dendrites and axons. Examples of mutated genes involved in neurogenesis include alpha-thalassemia/mental retardation, X linked (*ATRX*); genes involved in chromatin remodeling, such as AT-rich interaction domains 1A and 1B (*ARID1A and ARID1B*); and neurotrophin receptors (*NTRK1, NTRK2*, and *NTRK3*). Several genes such as *ALK*, and paired-like homeobox 2B (*PHBX2B*) genes may also become oncogene.

Tyrosine kinase neurotropin receptors Neuroblastomas can express several tyrosine kinase neurotropin receptors (TRKs). These include TrkA, TrkB and TrkC. High levels of TrkA is found with younger age, lower stage, absence of MYCN amplification and has favorable prognosis. Conversely, TrkB expression is associated with an invasive phenotype, high-risk disease and chemoresistance. TrkC occurs in lower-stage tumors. Higher expression of EPHB6, CD44, EFNB2 and EFNB3 correlates with good prognosis.

Prognostic factors in neuroblastomas are summarized in **Table 5**.

Wilms Tumor (Nephroblastoma)

Q. Write short essay on Wilms tumor.

Wilms tumor is also known as nephroblastoma (currently the preferred term) is the most common primary renal tumor of childhood. It is highly malignant primary embryonal tumor of kidney.

Age group: Most common between 2 and 5 years of age, and more than 95% occur below 10 years of age.

Location: Wilms tumor is classically located in the kidney. Both kidneys are equally affected. In most (90%) cases, the Wilms tumor is sporadic and unilateral. About 5–10% of Wilms tumors involve both kidneys, either simultaneously (synchronous) or one after the other (metachronous). However, Wilms tumor as a congenital neoplasm is exceptional.

It is one of the classical examples of a neoplastic process that faithfully recapitulates embryogenesis at the morphologic and molecular levels. The biology of Wilms tumor highlights several important aspects of childhood neoplasms. These are as follows:

- Relationship between malformations and neoplasia
- Histologic similarities between organogenesis and oncogenesis
- Two-hit theory of recessive tumor suppressor genes
- Role of premalignant lesions
- Potential for treatment to affect prognosis and outcome.

Pathogenesis and Genetics

Two genetic loci predisposing to Wilms tumor have been identified namely *WT1* and *WT2*. Alterations of these genes have been implicated in congenital malformations with Wilms tumor but they may also be identified in sporadic tumors. There is a relationship between the level of expression of these genes and the microscopic features of the tumor.

- *WT1* is located in 11p13 and encodes a zinc finger transcription factor (DNA-binding transcription factor) that is expressed within several tissues, early development of the urogenital system (kidney) and gonads, during

Table 5: Prognostic factors in neuroblastomas.

Variable feature	*Favorable*	*Unfavorable*
Stage of disease	Stage I, IIA, IIB, IVS	Stage III, IV
Age of patient	<18 months (1½ years)	>18 months (1½ years)
Microscopy: Evidence of Schwannian stroma and gangliocytic differentiation	Present	Absent
MYCN amplification	Not present	Present
Chromosomal abnormalities		
• Chromosome 1p loss	Absent	Present
• Chromosome 11q loss	Absent	Present
DNA ploidy of tumor cells	Hyperdiploid (whole chromosome gains)	Near-diploid (segmental chromosome losses; chromothripsis)
Mitosis-karyorrhexis index (MKI)	<200/5,000 cells	>200/5,000 cells
Tyrosine kinase neurotrophin receptor (TRK/Trk)		
• TRKA expression	Present	Absent
• TRKB expression	Absent	Present
Mutations of neuritogenesis genes	Absent	Present

embryogenesis. The product of *WT1* gene is WT1 protein which is critical for normal development of renal system and gonads. Germline point mutation and deletion of *WT1* is the underlying genetic alteration found in Denys–Drash syndrome and WAGR syndrome, respectively. WT1 has multiple binding partners. The choice of this partner can affect whether WT1 functions as a transcriptional activator or repressor in a given cellular context. There are numerous transcriptional targets of WT1, including genes encoding glomerular podocyte-specific proteins and proteins involved in induction of renal differentiation. Even though WT1 is important in nephrogenesis and also acts as a tumor suppressor gene, only about 10% of patients with sporadic (nonsyndromic) Wilms tumors have WT1 mutations. This suggests that the majority (90%) of these tumors are caused by mutations in other genes. WT1 is a tumor-suppressor protein that regulates transcription of several other genes. These include insulin-like growth factor-II (*IGF-II*), Snail, E-cadherin (*Cdh1*) and platelet-derived growth factor (*PDGF*).

- *WT2* is located in 11p15.5, which contains the gene for insulin growth factor II. It is implicated in Wilms tumors associated with Beckwith–Wiedemann syndrome.

Congenital syndromes with Wilms tumor

Increased risk of Wilms tumor is observed in three groups of congenital malformations associated with distinct chromosomal loci. Though Wilms tumors arising in these congenital syndromes are responsible for not more than 10% of Wilms tumor, they have provided important insight into the biology of this tumor.

- **WAGR syndrome:** This syndrome is characterized by **W**ilms tumor, **a**niridia, **g**enitourinary anomalies, and intellectual disability (formerly called mental **r**etardation). The lifetime risk of developing Wilms tumor in this syndrome is about 33%. WAGR syndrome is caused by constitutional (germline) deletions in the short arm of chromosome 11 (11p13). Affected genes include the aniridia gene (*PAX6*) and Wilms tumor gene 1 (*WT1*) and both are located on chromosome 11p13. *WT1* was first identified Wilms tumor-associated gene and detected in this syndrome. WT1 protein is expressed in kidneys, thymus, spleen and gonads. Loss or mutation of one *WT1* allele leads to genitourinary anomalies. *PAX6* is an autosomal dominant gene for aniridia and defect in *PAX6* causes aniridia. Patients with deletions restricted to *PAX6*, with normal *WT1* function, develop aniridia, but they are not at increased risk for Wilms tumors. The germline *WT1* deletion mutation in one *WT1* allele in WAGR syndrome represents the "first hit" in the development of Wilms tumor in these patients. This produces loss of heterozygosity (LOH) at this locus. The second mutation in remaining *WT1* allele ("second hit") is needed for Wilms tumor to occur (as in retinoblastomas.) This second hit frequently develops as an acquired somatic mutation in the *WT1* allele with a nonsense or frameshift mutation.
- **Denys–Drash syndrome:** This is a second congenital syndromes associated with higher risk for Wilms tumor (~90%). This is characterized by gonadal dysgenesis (male pseudohermaphroditism) and early-onset nephropathy leading to renal failure. The characteristic glomerular lesion is diffuse mesangial sclerosis. As in WAGR, these patients also have germline abnormalities in WT1. Unlike germline deletions of *WT1* in WAGR syndrome), the genetic abnormality in patients with Denys-Drash syndrome is a dominant-negative missense mutation in the zinc-finger region of the WT1 protein. This affects its DNA-binding properties. This mutation interferes with the function of the remaining wild-type (normal *WT1*) allele. Surprising though it interferes with wild-type, it is sufficient only to produce genitourinary abnormalities but not tumorigenesis. Thus, Wilms tumors arising in Denys–Drash syndrome reveal biallelic inactivation of *WT1*. In addition to Wilms tumors, individuals with Denys–Drash

syndrome have also increased risk for developing germ cell tumors called gonadoblastomas. This is as a consequence of disruption in normal gonadal development.

- **Beckwith–Wiedemann syndrome (BWS):** It is third type of congenital syndromes with an increased risk of developing Wilms tumor. BWS is characterized by gigantism to hemihypertrophy, enlargement of body organs (organomegaly/visceromegaly) and macroglossia, omphalocele, and abnormal large cells in the adrenal cortex (adrenal cytomegaly). Beckwith–Wiedemann syndrome is a model for tumorigenesis associated with genomic imprinting (refer page 875). The chromosomal region involved in BWS is located in band 11p15.5 (so-called WT2 locus), distal to the WT1 locus. This region contains multiple genes that are normally expressed from only one of the two parental alleles. Other parental homolog allele is transcriptionally silenced (i.e., imprinting) by methylation of the promoter region. Compared to WAGR and Denys–Drash syndromes, the genetic basis for BWS is considerably more heterogeneous in that no single 11p15.5 gene is involved in all cases. Also, the phenotype of BWS, including the predisposition to tumorigenesis, depends on the presence of specific *WT2* gene imprinting abnormalities. Normally, one of the genes in the *11p15.5* region-insulin-like growth factor-2 (IGF2)-is expressed only from the paternal allele, and the maternal allele is silenced by imprinting. In some Wilms tumors, there is loss of imprinting (i.e., re-expression of the maternal IGF2 allele) leading to overexpression of the IGF2 protein. In some case, there is selective deletion of the imprinted maternal allele combined with duplication (i.e., germline duplications of the paternal locus) of the transcriptionally active paternal allele in the tumor (uniparental paternal disomy). This has the similar functional effect of IGF2 overexpression. IGF2 protein is an embryonal growth factor. Hence, it can explain both the features of overgrowth (enlargement of body organs which is a feature) and increased risk for Wilms tumors BWS.

Sporadic Wilms tumors

Sporadic (i.e., nonsyndromic) Wilms tumors account for 90% of cases in children. In contrast with syndromic Wilms tumors, the knowledge about molecular abnormalities underlying sporadic (i.e., nonsyndromic) tumors are recently beginning to understand. Examples are as follows:

- **Mutations in β-catenin gene (*CTNNB1*):** Gain-of-function (activating) mutations of the gene encoding **β-catenin** (refer Chapter 10) seen in about 10% of sporadic Wilms tumors. It results in disturbance of the Wnt signaling pathway. It may be found in tumors with *WT1* mutation, but not with *WT1* wild-type.
- **Inactivation of the *WTX* gene:** The *WTX* gene is located on the X chromosome. It is mutated and inactivated in 6–30% of cases of sporadic Wilms tumor. There may be either somatic deletion (in two-thirds of cases) or, less commonly, inactivating mutation of the gene on the single X chromosome in tumors of males or the active X chromosome in tumors of females. WTX may act as a tumor suppressor. The downregulation of WTX may cause degradation of β-catenin. This may downregulate WNT/β-catenin signaling. It leads to increased signaling in the Wnt pathway. Thus, activation of WNT/β-catenin signaling may be important in Wilms tumorigenesis. About 3/4 of Wilms tumors with mutant *WT1* also have *CTNNB1* mutations. This suggests that WT1 loss does not fully activate WNT/β -catenin signaling.
- **Mutations in micro-RNA (miRNA):** Other recurrent mutations occur in genes encoding proteins involved in micro-RNA (miRNA) processing (DROSHA, DGCR8, and DICER1). These are found in 15–20% of Wilms tumors with predominantly blastemal component on microscopy (see later). Probably aberrations in miRNA processing lead to reduced levels of many mature miRNAs, in particular in the miR-200 family. This miR-200 family is involved in "mesenchymal to epithelial transformation" during renal morphogenesis. Absence of mesenchymal to epithelial transformation probably leads to persistent blastemal "rests" in the kidney, which later evolve into Wilms tumors.
- ***TP53* mutations:** Tumors with *TP53* mutations (in 5%) are associated with poor (unfavorable) prognosis and often have a distinctive anaplastic histologic appearance (see below).
- Abnormalities in other chromosomes—1, 7q, 8, 12, and 16 are also been found. Rarely, MYCN amplification is found in association with aggressive behavior, most commonly with diffuse anaplasia. Other includes mutations in the SIX/2 pathway.

MORPHOLOGY

Gross (Fig. 26)

- Wilms tumor is usually large, single, round, well-circumscribed mass and of soft consistency. Usually unilateral but 10% is either bilateral or multicentric. Size is extremely variable, and their median weight is 550 g. It may be enclosed by a thin rim of renal cortex and capsule.
- Cut section:
  - Tumor is predominantly solid, soft, bulging, homogeneous, and pale gray or tan.
  - Foci of hemorrhage, cyst formation, and necrosis may be seen.

Microscopy (Figs. 27A and B)

Wilms tumors are microscopically characterized by recognizable attempts to recapitulate different stages of nephrogenesis.

1. **Blastemal component:** These areas are very cellular and composed of small, round to oval primitive, blue cells with very scanty cytoplasm. Adjacent nuclei commonly appear to overlap. The pattern of growth may be diffuse, nodular, trabecular, cordlike (serpentine), or basaloid (with peripheral palisading).
2. **Immature stromal (mesenchymal) component:** It consists of undifferentiated fibroblast-like spindle cells or myxoid tissue. They may show smooth muscle, skeletal muscle or fibroblast differentiation.
3. **Immature epithelial component:** Epithelial cells show differentiation in the form of small abortive (embryonic) tubules or immature glomeruli. The structures closely recapitulate the appearance of normal developing metanephric tubules (and glomeruli) at the light microscopic, ultrastructural, and by lectin histochemistry. The tubular structures can be small and round, thus simulating the rosettes of neuroblastoma. Features that favor tubules of Wilms tumor over rosettes of

Continued

Continued

neuroblastoma are: (1) presence of a lumen, (2) single cell layer, (3) distinct basal lamina, and (4) surrounding fibromyxoid stroma.

Rarely, other heterologous elements can be found. These include squamous, mucinous ciliated, mucinous, or transitional epithelium; smooth muscle; adipose tissue; cartilage; and osteoid and neurogenic tissue.

Classically, tumor shows triphasic combination of (all three major components) namely undifferentiated blastema, mesenchymal (stromal) tissue, and epithelial cell types in the majority of tumors. The percentage of each component varies. They resemble normal fetal tissue. Most Wilms tumors show a representation of all three components, but percentage of each component is widely variable from case to case and sometimes from region to region in the same tumor. Some tumors contain only two elements (biphasic) or even only one (monophasic).

Anaplasia: About 5% of Wilms tumors have anaplasia. It is defined as the presence of cells with large, hyperchromatic, pleomorphic nuclei and atypical mitotic figures. Anaplasia is associated with acquired *TP53* mutations and such tumors do not respond to chemotherapy. Normally, whenever there is DNA damage, p53 elicits proapoptotic signals. The loss of p53 function is responsible for unresponsiveness of anaplastic cells to cytotoxic chemotherapy.

Nephrogenic rests: These are supposed to be precursor lesions of Wilms tumors. They are seen in the renal parenchyma adjacent to about 25–40% of unilateral tumors. In bilateral Wilms tumors, they may be observed in nearly 100% of cases. In many cases these nephrogenic rests share genetic alterations observed in the adjacent Wilms tumor. This points them to be preneoplastic lesions. The microscopic appearance of nephrogenic rests varies. It may appear as expansile masses that resemble Wilms tumors (hyperplastic rests resembling small foci of persistent primitive blastemal cells) to sclerotic rests consisting predominantly of fibrous tissue and occasional admixed immature tubules or glomeruli. It is important to mention the presence of nephrogenic rests in the resected specimen of Wilms tumor. This is because these patients are at an increased risk of developing Wilms tumors in the contralateral kidney and need frequent and regular check-up for many years.

Clinical Features

- Most children present with a large abdominal mass that may be unilateral or when large it may extend across the midline and down into the pelvis.
- Others: Hematuria, pain in the abdomen after a traumatic incident, intestinal obstruction, hypertension and pulmonary metastases are other patterns of presentation.

Spread

- **Local Spread:** It spreads to perirenal soft tissues. The tumor may directly involve the adrenal glands, bowel, liver, vertebrae, and paraspinal region. In the paraspinal region it may produce compression of spinal cord.
- **Lymphatic spread:** It spreads to regional lymph nodes.
- **Hematogenous spread:** Invasion of the renal vein is common. Hematogenously it can spread to lungs, liver and peritoneum. In a child with a retroperitoneal neoplasm, the presence of lung metastases strongly favors a diagnosis of Wilms tumor over that of neuroblastoma. The presence of bone metastases suggests a diagnosis other than Wilms tumor, because bone metastasis occurs in only 1% of the Wilms tumor.

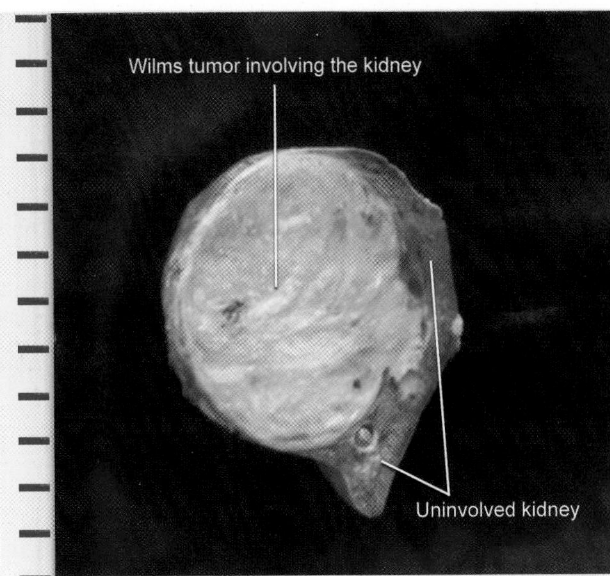

FIG. 26: Wilms tumor of the kidney with well-circumscribed margins.

Prognosis

Most patients with Wilms tumor can be almost cured and the overall cure rate for unilateral Wilms tumor is 80–90%. Few long-term survivors of Wilms tumor develop a second malignant neoplasm, either due to a genetic predisposition to neoplasia or secondary to therapy. The prognostic factors are as follows:

1. **Age:** Patients under 2 years of age usually have fewer metastases. Hence, they have better 5-year survival rate than those over 2 years.
2. **Stage:** Clinicopathological staging of Wilms tumor is the most important prognostic factor. Staging based on the COG (Children's Oncology Group) systems is presented in **Table 6**. Staging is mainly based on capsular invasion, rupture at surgery, extrarenal vein invasion, tumor implants, lymph node metastases, distant metastases, and bilaterality. During grossing, it is important to take sections from the renal sinus, the junction between tumor and normal kidney, the tumor capsule, and the uninvolved renal parenchyma.
3. **Size:** Tumor mass is measured by the weight of the excised specimen and is an important prognostic factor.

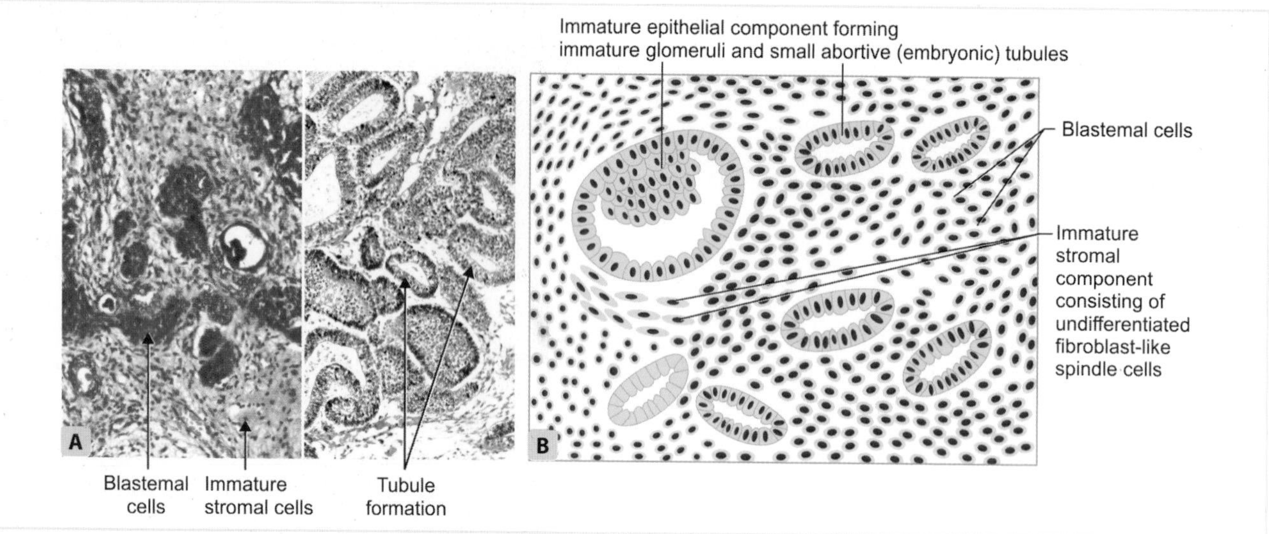

FIGS. 27A AND B: (A) Hematoxylin and eosin (H&E); (B) Diagrammatic—Wilms tumor shows highly cellular areas composed of tightly packed blue cells (undifferentiated blastema) separated by loose stroma containing undifferentiated mesenchymal cells, and immature (primitive) tubules.

Table 6: Staging of nephroblastoma of the kidney (Children's Oncology Group).

Stage	*Description*
Stage I	Completely resected tumor limited to the kidney. No intraoperative rupture or biopsy of the tumor prior to removal. No involvement of the vessels of the renal sinus. No evidence of tumor beyond the margins of resection. Microscopically, regional lymph nodes confirmed negative
Stage II	Completely resected tumor with no evidence of tumor at or beyond margins of resection. Tumor extends beyond the kidney as evidenced by regional extension of the tumor (through renal capsule, extensive invasion of the soft tissue of the renal sinus) or tumor in blood vessels within the nephrectomy specimen, but outside renal parenchyma. This includes blood vessels of the renal sinus
Stage III	Residual tumor present after surgery, confined to abdomen. This includes the following: • Lymph nodes within the abdomen/pelvis are involved by tumor • Tumor has penetrated through the peritoneal surface • Tumor implants are on the peritoneal surface • Gross or microscopic tumor remains postoperatively (positive surgical margins on microscopic examination) • Involvement of vital structures precludes complete resection • Tumor spillage before or during surgery • Tumor is treated with preoperative chemotherapy (with or without any prior biopsy, including fine-needle aspiration) • Tumor is removed in more than one piece (e.g., tumor is found in tissues separate from nephrectomy specimen, such as separately excised adrenal, or separately removed thrombus from renal vein) • Extension of primary tumor into thoracic vena cava and/or heart
Stage IV	Hematogenous metastases or lymph node metastases outside the abdominopelvic region
Stage V	Bilateral renal involvement present at diagnosis. Each kidney should be substaged separately by above criteria

4. **Anaplasia:** To place a Wilms tumor into the anaplastic category, the tumor should meet three criteria (**Box 12**). Anaplastic histology is perhaps the most important factor of adverse prognosis. Even anaplasia restricted to the kidney (i.e., without extrarenal spread) is associated with an increased risk of recurrence and death. Hence, it is necessary to accurately identify anaplasia on microscopic examination. It is very uncommon in tumors from patients under 2 years of age and is one of the reasons for the better prognosis in this age group. Sometimes anaplasia is found in the metastases and not in the primary tumor. The term focal anaplasia is used when anaplasia is restricted to one or a few discrete loci within the primary tumor, with no anaplasia or marked nuclear atypia elsewhere. If a tumor with localized anaplasia, the background tumor shows a degree of "marked" atypia (i.e., nuclear pleomorphism without other features), it is termed as showing "nuclear unrest" and are classified as diffuse anaplasia. Wilms tumors with anaplasia are referred to as having "unfavorable histology". Thus, these tumors have a lesser

Box 12: Three criteria for anaplastic category of Wilms tumor.

1. Marked enlargement of nuclei in the blastemal, epithelial, or stromal cell lines (except skeletal muscle cells) to at least three times the diameter of adjacent nuclei of the same cell type
2. Hyperchromasia of the enlarged nuclei
3. Multipolar mitotic figures

response to chemotherapy. This terminology is greater value when the anaplasia is diffuse rather than focal, and since anaplasia predicts response to therapy.

5. **Extensive tubular differentiation:** This is considered as a good prognostic sign.
6. **Skeletal muscle differentiation:** This does not have a significant effect on prognosis, except when present in massive amounts. Massive skeletal muscle differentiation is associated with a better prognosis.
7. **Post-chemotherapy morphology:** Based on response to chemotherapy, tumor is categorized into three types: (1) completely necrotic (low risk), (2) blastemal predominant (high risk), and (3) "others" (intermediate risk).
8. ***TP53* mutation.** Mutations of the *TP53* gene are evaluated indirectly through the immunohistochemistry for detection of P53 protein overexpression. *TP53* mutation correlates with the presence of anaplasia at the histologic level and has an unfavorable outcome.
9. **LOH at 1p and 16q:** Molecular parameters that indicate adverse prognostic factor in favorable histology of Wilms tumors include loss of heterozygosity of chromosomes 1p and 16q, and gain of chromosome 1q in tumor cells.

Improvements in cure rates for Wilms tumor (from previous 30% to current 90%) represent one of the greatest successes of pediatric oncology. Increased survival of patients with Wilms tumor may have an increased risk of developing second primary tumors. These include bone and soft tissue sarcomas, leukemia and lymphomas, and breast cancers. Some of these second primary neoplasms may be the result from the presence of a germline mutation in a cancer predisposition gene, whereas others are as a consequence of therapy.

BIBLIOGRAPHY

1. Ahn SY, Chang YS, Kim JH, et al. Two-year follow-up outcomes of premature infants enrolled in the phase I trial of mesenchymal stem cell transplantation for bronchopulmonary dysplasia. *J Pediatr*. 2017;185:49-54.e2.
2. Bellini C, Hennekam RC. Non-immune hydrops fetalis: a short review of etiology and pathophysiology. *Am J Med Genet A*. 2012;158A(3):597-605.
3. Coelho AI, Rubio-Gozalbo ME, Vicente JB, et al. Sweet and sour: an update on classic galactosemia. *J Inherit Metab Dis*. 2017;40(3): 325-42.
4. Cohn SL, Pearson ADJ, London WB, et al. The International Neuroblastoma Risk Group (INRG) classification system: an INRG Task Force report. *J Clin Oncol*. 2009;27(2):289-97.
5. Cutting GR. Cystic fibrosis genetics: from molecular understanding to clinical application. *Nat Rev Genet*. 2015;16(1):45-56.
6. Dome JS, Perlman EJ, Graf N. Risk stratification for Wilms tumor: current approach and future directions. *Am Soc Clin Oncol Educ Book*. 2014;215-23.
7. Donlon J, Sarkissian C, Levy H, et al. Hyperphenylalaninemia: phenylalanine hydroxylase deficiency. In Valle D, Beaudet AL, et al, editors: The online metabolic and molecular bases of inherited disease. New York, NY: McGraw-Hill.
8. Elborn JS. Cystic fibrosis, *Lancet*. 2016;388(10059):2519-31.
9. Farrell PM, White TB, Ren CL, et al. Diagnosis of cystic fibrosis: consensus guidelines from the Cystic Fibrosis Foundation. *J Pediatr*. 2017;181S:S4-S15.e1.
10. Gadd S, Huff V, Walz AL, Ooms AHAG, Armstrong AE, Gerhard DS, et al. A Children's Oncology Group and TARGET initiative exploring the genetic landscape of Wilms tumor, *Nat Genet*. 2017;49(10):1487-94.
11. Goldblum JR, Lamps LW, McKenney JK, et al. Rosai and Ackerman's surgical pathology (2 vols), 11th edition. Philadelphia: Elsevier; 2018.
12. Jameson JL, Fausi AS, Kasper DL, et al. Harrison's principles of internal medicine (2 vols), 20th edition. New York: McGraw-Hill Medical Publishing. Division; 2018.
13. Kumar V, Abbas AK, Aster JC. Robbins basic pathology, 10th edition. Philadelphia: Saunders Elsevier; 2018.
14. Kumar V, Abbas AK, Fausto N, et al. Robbins and Cotran pathologic basis of disease, 10th edition. Philadelphia: WB Saunders; 2021.
15. Matthay KK, Maris JM, Schleiermacher G, Nakagawara A, Mackall CL, Diller L, et al. Neuroblastoma. *Nat Rev Dis Primers*. 2016;2:16078.
16. McCloskey B, Endericks T. The rise of Zika infection and micro-cephaly: what can we learn from a public health emergency? *Public Health*. 2017;150:87-92.
17. Mone F, Quinlan-Jones E, Ewer AK, et al. Exome sequencing in the assessment of congenital malformations in the fetus and neonate. *Arch Dis Child Fetal Neonatal Ed*. 2019;104:F452-F456.
18. Murphy SL, Mathews TJ, Martin JA et al: *Annual summary of vital statistics*. 2013-2014, Pediatrics. 139(6):2017.
19. Moon RY, AAP Task Force on Sudden Infant Death Syndrome. SIDS and other sleep-related infant deaths: evidence base for 2016 updated recommendations for a safe infant sleeping environment. Pediatrics. 2016;138(5):e20162940.
20. Pierro M, Ciarmoli E, Thébaud B. Bronchopulmonary dysplasia and chronic lung disease: stem cell therapy. *Clin Perinatol*. 2015;42(4):889-910.
21. Ralston SH, Penman ID, Strachan MWJ, et al. Davidson's principles and practice of medicine, 23rd edition. Edinburgh: Churchill Livingstone; 2018.
22. Solebo AL, Teoh L, Rahi J. Epidemiology of blindness in children. *Arch Dis Child*. 2017;102(9):853-7.
23. Strayer DS, Saffitz JE, Rubin E. Rubin's Pathology: Mechanism of Human Disease, 8th edition. Philadelphia: Wolters Kluwer; 2020.
24. Thakkar HS, Lakhoo K. The surgical management of necrotising enterocolitis (NEC). *Early Hum Dev*. 2016;97:25-8.

CHAPTER 14

Environmental and Nutritional Diseases

CHAPTER OUTLINE

- Environmental diseases
- Effects of climate change on health
  - Heath effects due to climate change
- Toxicity of chemical and physical agents
  - Basic principles of the effects of toxic chemicals and drugs
- Environmental pollution
  - Air pollution
  - Metals as environmental pollutants
- Occupational health risks: industrial and agricultural exposures
  - Volatile organic solvents and vapors
  - Agricultural chemicals
  - Aromatic halogenated hydrocarbons
  - Bisphenol A
  - Mineral dusts
  - Cyanide
- Smoking
  - Types of tobacco
  - Constituents of tobacco smoke
  - Effects of tobacco
- Alcoholism
  - Metabolism of ethanol
- Injury by therapeutic drugs and drugs of abuse
  - Injury by therapeutic drugs (adverse drug reactions)
  - Injury by nontherapeutic agents (drug abuse)
- Injury by physical agents
  - Mechanical trauma
  - Thermal injury
  - Electrical injury
- Radiation
  - Types of radiation
  - Quantitation of radiation
  - Ionizing radiation
  - Ultraviolet rays
  - Nonionizing radiation
- Nutritional diseases
  - Dietary insufficiency
  - Severe acute malnutrition
  - Anorexia nervosa and bulimia nervosa
- Vitamin deficiencies
  - Fat-soluble vitamins
  - Water-soluble vitamins
  - Water-soluble vitamins—vitamin B complex
- Trace elements
- Obesity
  - Types of obesity
  - Physiologic regulation of energy balance
  - Etiology and pathogenesis
  - Pathologic consequences of obesity (complications of obesity)
  - Diet and cancer
  - Diet and systemic diseases
- Starvation
  - Metabolic changes in starvation

ENVIRONMENTAL DISEASES

Environment includes the various indoor, outdoor, and occupational atmospheres in which we live and work. Environmental diseases are conditions or diseases caused by exposure to harmful external agents and deficiencies of vital substances. The external agents include chemical or physical agents in the ambient, workplace, and personal environment. Deficiency of vital substances is diseases of nutritional origin. Many diseases are either caused or influenced by environmental factors. Humans breathe air, consume food and water, and are exposed to many toxic agents. These are environmental agents that are major determinants of health. The environmental factors that influence our health also depend on the behavior of individual ("personal environment"). This personal environment includes use of tobacco, ingestion of alcohol, consumption of recreational drug, diet, etc., or the external (ambient and workplace) environment. The environmental diseases are major causes of disability and suffering.

EFFECTS OF CLIMATE CHANGE ON HEALTH

Climate is the average weather in a given area over a longer period of time. Climate includes the usual temperature, humidity, atmospheric pressure, wind, rainfall, and other meteorological elements in an area of the Earth's surface for a long time. Climate change will become the preeminent universal cause of environmental disease in the 21st century and beyond. During the early 20th century, global atmospheric and oceanic temperatures have warmed significantly. The rising temperatures have led to a large number of effects that include changes in storm frequency, drought, and flood. The climate change is mainly man-made. These causes include rising atmospheric level of greenhouse gases (i.e., gases in Earth's atmosphere that trap heat), particularly carbon dioxide (CO_2) released through the burning of fossil fuels, ozone (O_3) (an important air pollutant), and methane. These gases, along with water vapor absorbing energy radiated from Earth's surface that otherwise would be lost into space. This produces the so-called greenhouse effect. This increase is not only due to increased production CO_2 but also from deforestation and the attendant decrease in conversion of carbon dioxide to oxygen by plants.

Heath Effects due to Climate Change

Climate change increases the incidence of a number of diseases. These are as follows:

- **Cardiovascular, cerebrovascular, and respiratory diseases:** These are exacerbated by heat waves and air
- **Gastrointestinal diseases:** These include **gastroenteritis, cholera**, and **other foodborne and waterborne infectious diseases**. These are caused due to contamination following disruption of clean water supplies and sewage treatment. This may be the consequence of floods after heavy rains or other environmental disasters.
- **Vector-borne infectious diseases:** These include **malaria** and **dengue fever**. They result from changes in vector number and geographic distribution as it occurs due to increased temperatures, crop failures, and more extreme weather variation.
- **Malnutrition:** The changes in local climate can disrupt crop production especially most severe in tropical locations. In these regions, the average temperatures may be already near or above crop tolerance levels. Reduction in crops can lead to malnutrition.

Apart from these disease-specific effects, a rise in sea level can submerge the land mass. This in-turn results in displacement of people and can disrupt lives and commerce. It may create political unrest, war, malnutrition, sickness, and death.

TOXICITY OF CHEMICAL AND PHYSICAL AGENTS

We are surrounded by, breathe in and consume many chemicals that are added to, or appear as contaminants in, foods, water, and air. **Toxicology** is traditionally defined as the science of poisons. More descriptive definition toxicology is **"the study of the adverse effects of chemical, physical** (e.g., radiation and heat), **or biological agents on living organisms and the ecosystem, including the prevention and amelioration of such adverse effects**." Thus, the study involved the distribution, effects, and mechanisms of action of toxic agents. There are wide variations in individual sensitivity to toxic agents. It depends on the complex interaction between toxic agent, age, genetic predisposition, and different tissue sensitivities of exposed individual. This is the drawback of establishing "safe levels" of an agent for entire populations. However, such cut-offs are useful for comparative studies of the effects of agents between different populations and for estimating risk of disease in individuals exposed heavily.

Basic Principles of the Effects of Toxic Chemicals and Drugs

Many important mechanisms govern the effect of toxic agents. These include the toxin's absorption, distribution, metabolism, and excretion.

Definition of a poison: It is defined as a **substance that is capable of causing the illness or death of a living organism when introduced or absorbed**. It is a quantitative concept and it depends on dosage. In the 16th century, Swiss physician and chemist Paracelsus expressed the basic principle of toxicology: "All substances are poisons and nothing is without poison; only the right dosage differentiates a poison from a remedy." This is often condensed to: "The dose makes the poison." It is still valid today and many pharmaceutical drugs have potentially harmful effects.

Q. Write short essay on xenobiotic metabolism.

Xenobiotics: These are defined as **exogenous chemicals** in the environment in air, water, food, and soil. These are **not used by organism as a nutrient chemical** and is **not essential to the organism for normal homeostasis**. Xenobiotics include **pesticides and industrial-process residues** (e.g., pharmaceutically active compounds, organochlorides, dyes etc.). They **may be absorbed into the body through inhalation, ingestion, and skin contact** (**Fig. 1**).

Absorption: Chemical may be absorbed through lung, gastrointestinal or skin and depends largely on the chemical. For example, insecticides chlordane and heptachlor are lipid soluble and rapidly absorbed and stored in body fat. In contrast, the water-soluble herbicide paraquat is easily eliminated.

Transport: Most solvents and drugs are lipophilic (dissolve in fats, oils, lipids). This helps their transport in the blood by lipoproteins and also their penetration through the plasma membrane into cells.

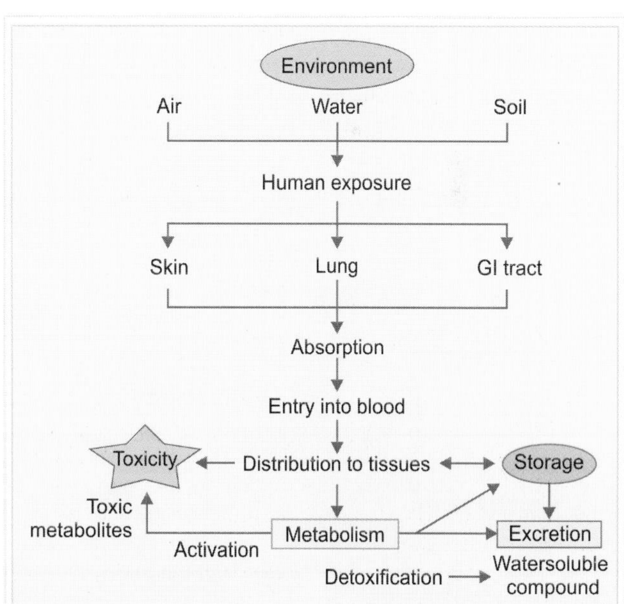

FIG. 1: Human exposure to pollutants in environment. Xenobiotics are exogenous chemicals in the environment. These pollutants may be in the air, water, and soil. They are absorbed through the lungs, gastrointestinal (GI) tract, and skin. In the body they may act at the site of absorption, but are usually enter the blood stream. Through blood they are distributed to various organs. In the organs, they may be stored or metabolized. These xenobiotics may be metabolized to water-soluble compounds that are excreted or converted to toxic metabolites. This process of conversion into toxic metabolites is termed as activation (Copyrighted).

Site of action: The chemicals may act at the site of entry or at other sites following transport through the blood.

Fate of xenobiotic: They may have one or more of the following fates:

- Water-soluble compounds are readily excreted in urine or feces
- Disposed of in expired air
- Accumulate in bone, fat, brain, or other tissues.

Metabolism of Xenobiotic (Fig. 2A and B)

Most solvents, drugs, and xenobiotics are metabolized to inactive water-soluble products (detoxification) or are activated to form toxic metabolites.

Detoxification of xenobiotic (Fig. 2A)

The reactions that metabolize xenobiotics into nontoxic products or that activate xenobiotics to produce toxic compounds (**Figs. 1 and 2**) occur in **two phases**.

- **Phase I reactions:** During this phase, chemicals undergo hydrolysis, oxidation, or reduction.
- **Phase II reactions:** Usually the products of phase I reactions are metabolized into water-soluble compounds during phase II reactions. The phase II reactions include glucuronidation, sulfation, methylation, and conjugation with glutathione (GSH).

Cytochrome P-450 enzyme system (P-450 system): The cytochrome P-450 enzyme system is the most important catalyst of phase I reactions. Cytochrome P-450 enzymes (CYPs) are a large family of heme-containing enzymes, each with preferred substrate specificities. These enzymes are mainly present in hepatocytes and are localized to the endoplasmic reticulum. But CYPs can also be present in skin, lungs, gastrointestinal mucosa, and other organs.

Activation of xenobiotic (Fig. 2B)

The P-450 system reactions either detoxify xenobiotics or, less commonly, convert xenobiotics into active compounds that cause cellular injury. Both types of reactions may generate reactive oxygen species (ROS) as a by-product. ROS can produce cellular damage. CYPs are involved in the metabolism of alcohol and many common therapeutic drugs (e.g., acetaminophen, barbiturates, warfarin, anticonvulsants). Examples of metabolic activation of chemicals into active compounds through CYPs are as follows:

- Production of the toxic trichloromethyl free radical from carbon tetrachloride in the liver
- Production of a DNA binding metabolite from benzo[a] pyrene. Benzo[a]pyrene is a carcinogen present in cigarette smoke in the lung.

Polymorphisms in CYPs: Activity of CYPs shows great variation among individuals. Though these variations may be due to genetic polymorphisms in specific CYPs, more commonly it is due to exposure to drugs or chemicals that induce or diminish CYP activity.

- **CYP inducers:** These increase the CYP activity. Examples include environmental chemicals, drugs, smoking, alcohol, and hormones. These inducers act by binding to specific nuclear receptors. After binding to these receptors, they heterodimerize with the retinoic X receptor (RXR) to form a transcriptional activation complex. This associates with promoter region located in the 5'-flanking regions of CYP genes. Nuclear receptors participating in CYP induction include the aryl hydrocarbon receptor, the peroxisome proliferator-activated receptors (PPARs) and two orphan nuclear receptors, constitutive androstane receptor (CAR), and pregnane X receptor (PXR).
- **Diminish CYP:** Examples include fasting or starvation. They can decrease CYP activity.

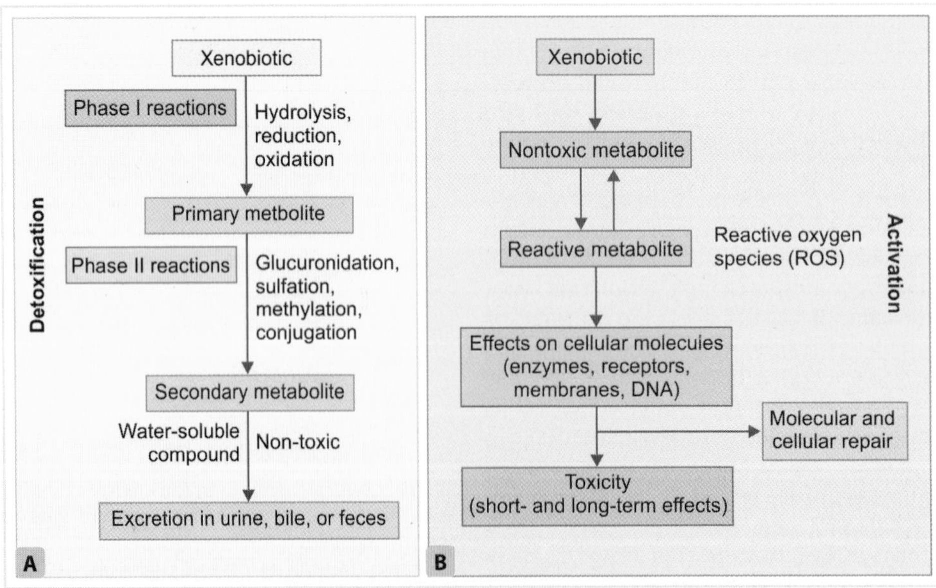

FIG. 2A and B: Metabolism of xenobiotic. (A) Xenobiotics can be metabolized to nontoxic metabolites (detoxification) and excreted from the body in urine or feces. (B) Xenobiotic metabolism may also form a reactive metabolite that is toxic to cellular components. If repair is not effective, it may produce short-term and long-term toxic effects.

ENVIRONMENTAL POLLUTION

Pollution is the introduction of harmful materials into the environment. These harmful materials are called pollutants.

Air Pollution

Q. Write short essay on air pollution.

It is essential to have a clean air to breathe and to maintain good health. Air pollution is responsible for a significant cause of morbidity and mortality, especially among individuals with pre-existing lung or heart disease. Air pollution is usually invisible, except on days when the pollution is particularly bad. Air is precious to life, but air that we breathe also contains many potential substances that can cause disease. Microorganisms present in air are responsible for major morbidity and death. Air pollutants also include chemical and particulate pollutants. Air pollutants may be found in both outdoor and indoor air.

Sources of air pollution: There are many sources of air pollution. These can be classified in different ways. Depending on the source they can be classified as follows:

- **Mobile sources:** These include motor vehicles such as cars, trucks, buses, trains, and airplanes.
- **Stationary sources:** These include a variety of commercial and industrial operations/activities (e.g., oil refineries, iron, and steel plants). It can be further broken down as point sources and area source.
    - **Point sources:** Pollution is emitted from a specific point like a smokestack.
    - **Area sources:** In this, pollution emerges from a large number of smaller sources. For example, smaller everyday activities (e.g., dry cleaning, auto body shop painting). Air pollutants can be from indoors, e.g., from gas appliances, cleaning agents, pesticides, and personal-care products.

Classification of air pollution according to the type of pollutant is presented in **Box 1**.

Outdoor Air Pollution

The outdoor air is contaminated with an unpleasant mixture of gaseous and particulate (matter in the form of minute separate particles) pollutants. They are heavier in cities and in near the industries. Collectively, six pollutants namely sulfur dioxide, carbon monoxide (CO), ozone (O_3), nitrogen dioxide (NO_2), lead, and particulate matter produce the well-known smog (smoke and fog). Sometimes they suffocate large cities such as New Delhi. Major effects of outdoor air pollutants on health are summarized in **Table 1**.

Organs affected: The lungs are the most common organ affected by air pollution, but air pollutants can affect many organ systems.

Box 1: Classification of air pollution according to the type of pollutant.

- **Criteria pollutants:** For example, carbon monoxide, nitrogen dioxide, lead, ozone, particulate matter, and sulfur dioxide. They are widespread and are usually associated with respiratory discomfort and distress.
- **Hazardous (toxic) air pollutants (air toxics):** For example, asbestos, benzene, cadmium, chromium, dioxin, mercury, methylene chloride, and toluene. They are more localized and can cause serious, sometimes can cause cancer. (Hazardous air pollutants are also known as air pollutants.

Table 1: Major effects of outdoor air pollutants on health.

Individuals at risk	*Major effects*
Ozone	
• Healthy adults and children	Reduces lung function, increases airway reactivity, inflammation of lung
• Athletes, outdoor workers	Decreases exercise capacity
• Asthmatics	Increases hospitalizations
Nitrogen dioxide	
• Healthy adults	Increases airway reactivity
• Asthmatics	Reduces lung function
• Children	Increases respiratory tract infections
Sulfur dioxide	
• Healthy adults	Increases respiratory symptoms
• Individuals with chronic lung disease	Increases mortality
• Asthmatics	Increases hospitalization, reduces lung function
Acid aerosols	
• Healthy adults	Alters mucociliary clearance
• Children	Increases respiratory tract infections
• Asthmatics	Increases hospitalization, decreases lung function
Particulates	
• Children	Increases respiratory tract infections
• Individuals with chronic lung or heart disease	Reduces lung function
• Asthmatics	Increases mortality, increases frequency of attacks

The most important air pollutants are generated by combustion of fossil fuels, industrial, and agricultural processes. In this section, major effects of outdoor pollutants on health and five outdoor pollutants namely (i) ozone (O_3), (ii) nitrogen dioxide, (iii) sulfur dioxide, (iv) particulates, and (v) carbon monoxide (CO) are discussed.

Ozone (O_3)

Earth's atmosphere can be divided into three layers namely (i) troposphere, (ii) stratosphere, and (iii) mesosphere. The troposphere is the lowest layer near the ground of earth. Stratosphere is the second layer of the atmosphere above the troposphere. The next higher layer above the stratosphere is the mesosphere.

Stratospheric ozone: Ozone is a highly reactive gas composed of three oxygen atoms. It has a distinctive odor of the air after a thunderstorm or around electrical equipment. Ozone is produced by interaction of ultraviolet (UV) radiation and oxygen (O_2) in the stratosphere (second layer in the atmosphere). Ozone naturally accumulates in the so-called O_3 layer 10 to 30 miles (15 to 45 km) above the Earth's surface. This O_3 layer absorbs the most dangerous UV radiation emitted by the sun and protects life on earth. It was discovered in 1985 that O_3 was nearly completely depleted over Antarctica (Earth's southernmost continent) and also was thinned elsewhere. This depletion of O_3 is the result of the widespread use of chlorofluorocarbon gases in air conditioners and refrigerators and as aerosol propellants. When released into the atmosphere, these gases flow up into the stratosphere. There they participate in chemical reactions that destroy O_3. Due to current stratospheric air currents, the depletion is most severe in polar regions, particularly over Antarctica during the winter months. These observations resulted in international agreements to complete phase-out the use of chlorofluorocarbon by 2040. Over the past 30 years, decreased use of chlorofluorocarbons has reduced the size of the yearly O_3 "hole" over Antarctica.

Mediators of ozone toxicity: It is mainly mediated **by the production of free radicals**. These free radicals injure or damage epithelial cells lining of the respiratory tract and type I alveolar cells in the alveoli. They stimulate the release of inflammatory mediators.

Effects: Low levels of O_3 can be tolerated by healthy individuals. Normal individuals they experience upper respiratory tract inflammation and mild symptoms due to reduced lung function and chest discomfort. But exposure is more dangerous especially in patients suffering from asthma or emphysema.

Nitrogen dioxide

Tropospheric (ground-level) ozone: The O_3 in the stratosphere is "good" O_3. In contrast O_3 that accumulates in the lower atmosphere (ground-level/tropospheric O_3) is one of the most dangerous air pollutants. Tropospheric O_3 is O_3 near the ground of earth as opposed to in the upper atmosphere O_3 in stratosphere. **Ground-level O_3 is a gas mainly formed by the reaction of sunlight on nitrogen oxides (NO_2) and volatile organic compounds**, especially on warm, sunny days. These chemicals are released from emissions by industries and exhaust of motor vehicles.

Sulfur dioxide

Ozone often combines with other agents such as sulfur dioxide and particulates to create more damage than O_3 alone.

Source: Sulfur dioxide (SO_2) is produced by burning coal and oil (derived from burning fossil fuels) in power plants, from copper smelting, and as a by-product of paper mills. After release of sulfur dioxide into the air, it may be converted into sulfuric acid and sulfuric trioxide.

Effects: These substances produce a burning sensation in the nose and throat, difficulty in breathing, and asthma attacks in susceptible individuals.

Particulate matter

Particulate matter is present in the form of minute separate particles in the air and is known as "soot." It is associated with morbidity and mortality due to pulmonary inflammation and secondary cardiovascular effects.

Source: Particulates are produced by coal- and oil-fired power plants, by industrial processes burning these fuels, and by diesel exhaust.

Effects: Fine or ultrafine particles <10 µm in diameter are the most harmful. They are inhaled into the alveoli. In the alveoli, they are phagocytosed by macrophages and neutrophils. These inflammatory cells release many inflammatory mediators. Particles larger than 10 µm in diameter are of lesser important because usually they are either removed in the nose or trapped by the mucociliary epithelium of the airways.

Carbon monoxide

Carbon monoxide is a nonirritating, colorless, tasteless, and odorless gas.

Source: It is produced by the incomplete combustion (oxidation) of hydrocarbons (hydrogen and carbon materials). The most important environmental source of CO is the burning of carbonaceous materials, as in automotive engines (exhaust), furnaces, and cigarette smoke. CO is short-lived in the atmosphere. It is rapidly oxidized to CO_2. Hence, raised levels in ambient air are transient and occur only in close proximity to sources of CO.

Pathogenesis: Carbon monoxide is a systemic asphyxiant with its affinity for hemoglobin that is 200 times more than that of oxygen. CO binds to hemoglobin and forms carboxyhemoglobin. Carboxyhemoglobin cannot carry oxygen. The oxygen from carboxyhemoglobin does not dissociate as readily as in oxyhemoglobin. Carboxyhemoglobin concentrations below 10% are common in smokers and usually do not produce symptoms. When the hemoglobin is 20 to 30% saturated with CO, it produces systemic hypoxia. With 60 to 70% saturation, it can produce unconsciousness and death.CO kills partly by inducing depression of central nervous system (CNS).

Effects: Carbon monoxide is a **systemic asphyxiant**. It is an important cause of accidental and suicidal death.

- **Chronic toxicity:** The low levels of CO usually found in air may produce impaired respiratory function but are not usually life-threatening. However, certain individuals may develop chronic poisoning. Examples include individuals working in confined environments with high exposure to fumes (e.g., tunnel and underground garage workers) and highway toll booths with high exposures to automobile fumes. Carboxyhemoglobin, once formed is remarkably stable. This is responsible for chronic poisoning by CO. Even with low-level, but persistent exposure to CO, the level of carboxyhemoglobin may rise to life-threatening levels in the blood. The diagnosis is made by estimating carboxyhemoglobin levels in the blood.

- **Acute toxicity:** It may develop in a small and closed garage. The average running car can produce sufficient CO to induce coma or death within 5 minutes. Rapid rise of CO concentrations to toxic levels can also occur during improper use of gasoline-powered generators (e.g., during power outages) or following mine fires. CO can cause of accidental and suicidal death. Treatment of acute CO poisoning (e.g., who attempt suicide or are trapped in fires) consists mainly of the administration of 100% oxygen.

MORPHOLOGY

Chronic poisoning: It slowly produces hypoxia. Hypoxia can insidiously cause widespread ischemic changes in the CNS. These changes are more marked in the basal ganglia and lenticular nuclei. Though cessation of exposure to CO, the patient usually recovers; there may be permanent neurologic sequelae. These include impairment of memory, vision, hearing, and speech.

Acute poisoning: Acute poisoning in light-skinned individuals shows a characteristic generalized **cherry-red color of the skin and mucous membranes**. It is due to high levels of carboxyhemoglobin in the superficial capillaries. If death occurs rapidly, there may not be morphologic changes. With longer survival, the brain may be slightly edematous, with punctate hemorrhages and hypoxia-induced neuronal changes. The morphologic changes are due to systemic hypoxia and not specific.

Bhopal: On December 3, 1984, a pesticide plant in Bhopal, India, released about 40 tons (36 metric tons) of methyl isocyanate into the atmosphere. Methyl isocyanate is a highly toxic gas. It quickly spread to the nearby villages and killed 8,000 in the following days. It also led to >20,000 mortalities. More than half-million survivors who were exposed to the gas developed serious side effects such as respiratory problems, blindness, skin burns, anxiety, and depression.

Indoor Air Pollution

In the modern world, we try to exclude the environment in our homes. This increases the likely pollution of the indoor air. The most common pollutant is tobacco smoke (discussed later), others include CO, NO_2, and asbestos. In low income parts of the world, volatile substances containing polycyclic aromatic hydrocarbons produced by cooking oils and coal burning are important indoor pollutants.

Smoke from burning of organic materials: They contain various oxides of nitrogen and carbon particulates. These are irritants and predispose to lung infections and may also contain carcinogenic polycyclic aromatic hydrocarbons. It is generated by burning carbon-containing material (e.g., wood, dung, or charcoal) in homes for cooking, heating, and light.

Bioaerosols: Bioaerosols (biological aerosols) are particles released from terrestrial (earth) and marine (aquatic) ecosystems into the atmosphere. They consist of both living and non-living components, such as fungi, pollen, bacteria, and viruses. They may contain pathogenic microbiologic agents and can cause infectious diseases such as Legionnaires' disease, viral pneumonia, and the common cold. They may also contain allergens derived from pet dander, dust mites, and fungi and molds that can cause rhinitis, eye irritation, and asthma.

Radon: It a radioactive gas derived from uranium. It is present in soil and in homes. Radon exposure in uranium miners (especially in smokers) can cause lung cancer. In smokers, low-level chronic exposures in the home likely to increases the risk of lung cancer. Radon is the main cause of lung cancer in nonsmokers.

Formaldehyde: It is used in the manufacture of building materials such as cabinetry (cabinets collectively), furniture, adhesives, resins, leathers, rubber, metals, and woods. Exposure also occurs in laboratory workers (especially pathology and anatomy); embalmers and it is emitted from urethane foam insulation. In poorly ventilated house, it may accumulate in the air. At concentrations of 0.1 ppm (parts per million) or higher, it produced difficulties in breathing and burning sensation in the eyes and throat. It can also trigger attacks of asthma. Formaldehyde is a carcinogenic (nasopharyngeal carcinoma).

Sick building syndrome (SBS) describes the discomfort building occupants sometimes experience while inside the building. SBS is most common in office buildings. But it can also occur in apartments, schools, and other buildings with multiple occupants. Common symptoms include headache, cough, dry and itchy skin, dizziness, nausea, loss of concentration, fatigue, odor sensitivity, and irritation of the eye, nose, or throat. It may be due to exposure to one or more indoor pollutants due to poor ventilation.

Metals as Environmental Pollutants

Metals are group of environmental chemicals that can cause disease in humans. The various heavy metals that can produce harmful effects in humans include lead, mercury, arsenic, and cadmium.

Lead

Q. Write short essay on lead poisoning.

Lead is a universal heavy metal commonly present in the environment of industrialized countries.

Source: Exposure to lead occurs through contaminated air, food, and water.

- During 20th century, the major sources of lead in the environment were house paints and gasoline (gasoline or petrol is a derivative of crude oil/petroleum). The use of lead-based paints and leaded gas has been greatly decreased in 21st century. In children, lead poisoning was related to pica—the habit of chewing on cribs, toys, furniture and woodwork—and eating painted plaster and fallen paint flakes.
- Presently, the level of exposure to lead is markedly reduced due to the several measures taken to prevent exposure to lead (e.g., removal of lead from gasoline, use of titanium instead of lead in paints, and control of industrial point

sources). Currently, the main sources of lead in the environment include mines, foundries, manufacturing of auto batteries, lead crystal, ceramics, fishing weights; batteries, and spray paints, all of which are occupational hazards. Occupational exposure occurs in individuals engaged in lead smelting (releases metal fumes and deposits lead oxide dust). Lead oxide is a constituent of battery grids and an occupational exposure occurs in individuals working in the manufacture and recycling of automobile batteries. Other sources of lead are demolition or sanding of lead-based paint in older houses in which the flaking (separate or fall away from the surface as flakes), plumbing, lead pipes, soldering, contaminated herbal remedies, and soil contamination.

- In children living in older homes with lead-contaminated dust, blood levels of lead are usually >5 µg/dL. Ingested lead is harmful mainly to children because they absorb >50% of lead present in the food, whereas adults absorb about 15%. The blood–brain barrier in children is more permeable and produces a high concentration in the brain and produce brain damage. Main clinical features of lead poisoning in children and adults are shown in **Figures 3 and 4**.

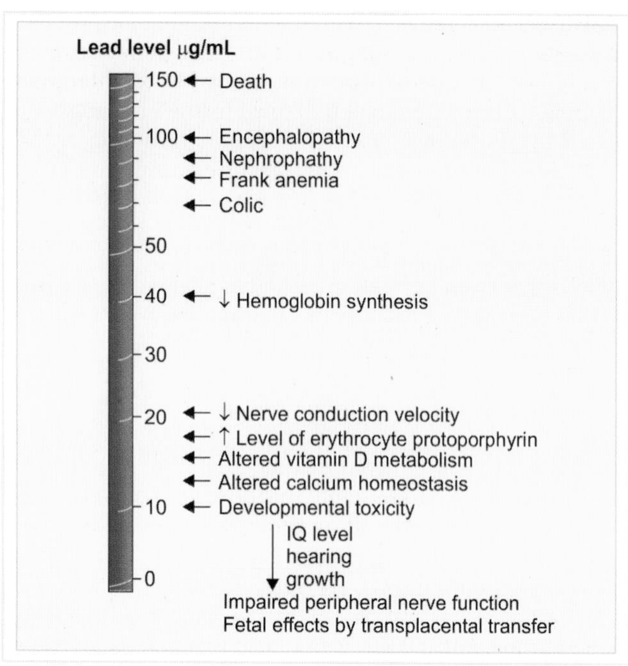

FIG. 3: Various effects of lead poisoning in children according to blood levels.

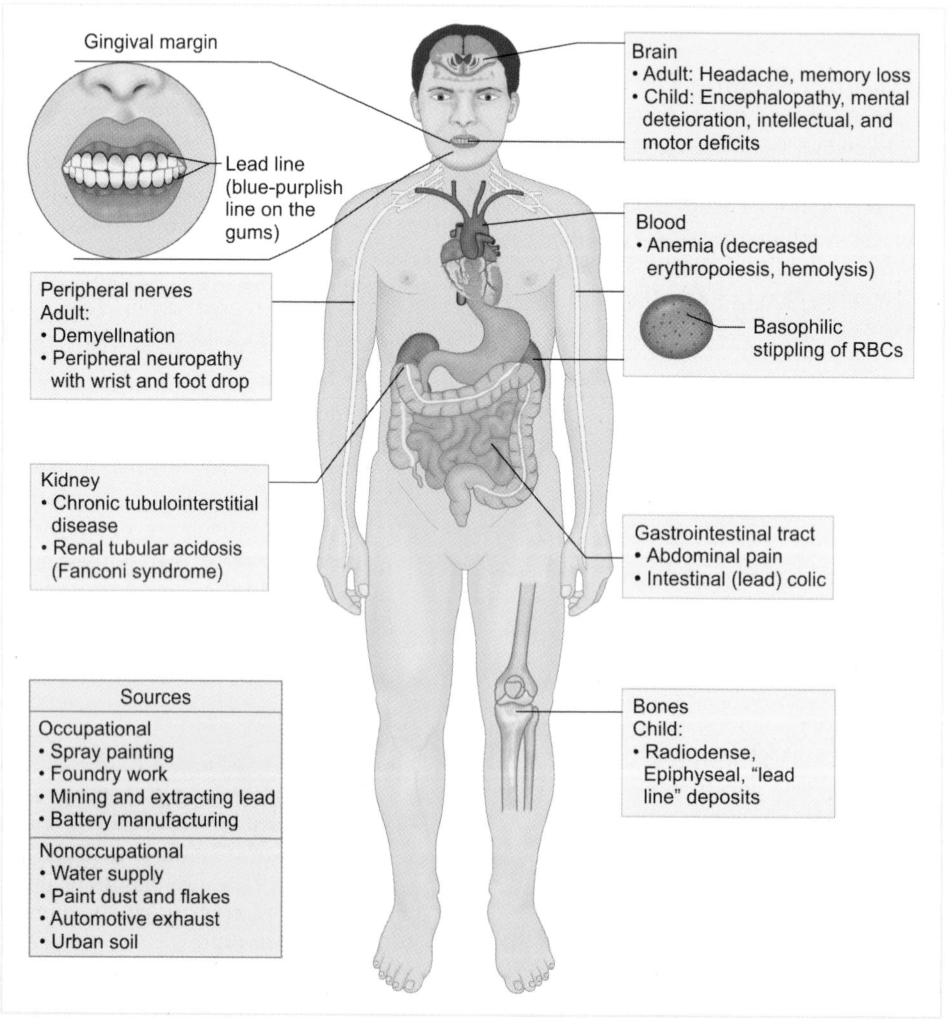

FIG. 4: Pathologic features and complications of lead intoxication.

Pathophysiology

Absorption: Lead is easily absorbed through inhalation into the lungs or through ingestion into the gastrointestinal tract or absorbed dermally [organic lead (e.g., tetraethyl lead)].

Distribution: Most absorbed lead (80–85%) is taken up by the developing teeth and bone (15% of dose sequestered in bone). In these sites, lead competes with calcium, binds phosphates, and this phosphate bound lead has a half-life of 20 to 30 years. Once in the blood, it freely circulates in the blood, and 95–99% is sequestered in RBCs, hence, must measure lead in whole blood (not serum). The remaining lead is distributed widely in soft tissue, with half-life ~30 days. It is excreted mostly by the kidneys into urine but also appears in other fluids including breast milk. Lead can easily cross the blood–brain barrier. Lead is concentrated in the brain, liver, kidneys, and bone marrow.

Mode of toxicity: Lead interferes with mitochondrial oxidative phosphorylation, ATPases, calcium-dependent messengers; enhances oxidation and cell apoptosis. Lead binds to sulfhydryl groups in proteins and interferes activities of zinc (Zn)-dependent enzymes and also calcium metabolism (lead competes with calcium). This leads to hematologic, skeletal, neurologic, gastrointestinal, and renal toxicities. In bones, teeth, nails and hair, it forms a tightly bound pool of lead which is harmful. It also interferes with enzymes involved in the synthesis of steroids and cell membranes.

Toxicity: Lead affects many tissues and produces various manifestations.

- **Acute exposure:** When blood lead levels are >60–80 μg/dL, it causes impaired neurotransmission and neuronal cell death (with central and peripheral nervous system effects); impaired hematopoiesis and renal tubular dysfunction. With blood levels of lead are higher [e.g., BPb (blood lead) >80–120 μg/dL], it can produce acute encephalopathy with convulsions, coma, and death. Children with lead encephalopathy are irritable and ataxic. They may develop convulsions or display altered states of consciousness (drowsiness to frank coma). Children with low blood lead levels may present with mild CNS symptoms, such as clumsiness, irritability, and hyperactivity.
- **Subclinical exposures in children:** When blood lead levels are between 25 and 60 μg/dL, it can cause anemia, mental retardation motor function, impaired hearing, and behavior. Impairment of IQ can occur even at lower levels of exposure.
- **Chronic subclinical exposures in adults:** When lead levels are >40 μg/dL, it is associated with anemia, demyelinating peripheral neuropathy (mainly motor), impaired hearing, hypertension, ECG higher risk of cardiovascular disease (CVD) and death, interstitial nephritis and chronic renal failure, diminished sperm counts, and spontaneous abortions.

MORPHOLOGY

Lead toxicity mainly affects the blood and bone marrow, bone, nervous system, gastrointestinal tract, and kidneys.

Blood and bone marrow changes

Lead produces rapid and characteristic changes in blood and bone marrow. Lead has a high affinity for sulfhydryl groups and interferes with two enzymes involved in heme synthesis

Continued

Continued

in bone marrow erythroblasts. These enzymes are (i) delta-aminolevulinic acid dehydratase and (ii) ferrochelatase.

Bone marrow: Inhibition of ferrochelatase by lead may result in the appearance of a few ring sideroblasts. These ring sideroblasts are red cell precursors containing iron-laden mitochondria. They are detected by using Prussian blue stain.

Peripheral blood: Lead impairs incorporation of iron into heme and produces defect in hemoglobin synthesis. It leads to microcytic (small red cells) and hypochromic anemia. Anemia is a cardinal and one of the earliest signs of lead intoxication. Lead also inhibits sodium- and potassium-dependent adenosine triphosphatases (ATPases) in cell membranes. This may increase the fragility of red cells, causing mild hemolysis. RBC in lead intoxication shows prominent punctate basophilic stippling of the red cells. This reflects clustering of ribosomes. Lead also inhibits sodium- and potassium-dependent ATPases in cell membranes. This may increase the fragility of red cells causing hemolysis (reduced life span). Thus, anemia in lead intoxication is due to ineffective hematopoiesis and accelerated RBC turnover. There is formation of zinc-protoporphyrin instead of heme.

Bone

Excess lead in bone interferes with the normal remodeling of calcified cartilage and primary bone trabeculae in the epiphyses in children. It causes increased bone density and is detected as radiodense lead lines. Lead lines of a different category also may be seen in the gums. In the gums, excess lead stimulates hyperpigmentation to produce lead line. This is called as Burton's line. It is a blue-purplish line on the gums seen in lead poisoning. It is caused by a reaction between circulating lead with sulphur ions released by oral bacterial activity. The lead sulphide is formed at the junction of the teeth and gums. Lead also inhibits the healing of fractures by increasing chondrogenesis and delaying mineralization of cartilage.

Nervous system

Excess lead is toxic to nervous tissues in both adults and children. In adults it predominantly produces peripheral neuropathies, whereas in children effects on CNS are more common.

- **Children:** Lead toxicity in a pregnant woman may impair development of brain in the fetus. Children are prone to brain damage due to lead. The effects of chronic low-dose lead exposure in children may be slight. This includes sensory, motor, intellectual, psychological disturbances and mild dysfunction such as reduced IQ, learning disabilities, and delayed psychomotor development. The microscopic changes with subtle functional deficits are not well defined. At higher doses, lead produces destructive results and produce lead encephalopathy. It may produce blindness, psychoses, seizures, coma, and even death. Microscopically, higher doses of lead produce marked brain edema, demyelination of the cerebral and cerebellar white matter, and necrosis of cortical neurons. These may be accompanied by of cortical neurons. These may be accompanied by diffuse astrocytic proliferation. Both peripheral nervous

Continued

Continued

system and CNS abnormalities in children usually are irreversible (permanent).

- **Adults:** In adults CNS is less often affected. But it frequently produces a peripheral demyelinating neuropathy. Neuropathy involves the motor nerves of the most commonly used muscles. Thus, it first affects the extensor muscles of the wrist and fingers and causes wrist drop. This is followed by paralysis of the peroneal muscles and causes foot drop. Lead-induced peripheral neuropathies in adults usually diminish with the elimination of lead exposure.

Gastrointestinal tract: Lead-induced neuropathy may produce paroxysms of extremely severe, poorly localized abdominal pain known as lead colic.

Kidney: Lead is mainly excreted through the kidneys in the urine. Acute lead exposures may cause damage to proximal tubules. Lead nephropathy is due to the toxic effect of the lead on the proximal tubular cells of the kidney. It is characterized by aminoaciduria, glycosuria, and hyperphosphaturia (Fanconi syndrome). Microscopically, characteristic intranuclear inclusions consisting of protein aggregates are seen in the nuclei of the proximal tubular cells in lead nephropathy.

These inclusions are composed of a lead-protein complex containing >100 times the concentration of lead in the whole kidney. Chronic renal damage produces interstitial fibrosis and renal failure. It may decrease excretion of uric acid can lead to gout (saturnine gout).

Laboratory diagnosis: The diagnosis of lead poisoning needs constant vigilance. Lead poisoning may be suspected on the basis of neurologic changes in children or unexplained microcytic anemia with basophilic stippling in RBCs in adults and children. In milder cases of lead exposure, anemia may be the only abnormality. Definitive diagnosis of lead poisoning and intoxication requires demonstration of elevated lead in blood and red cell free protoporphyrin levels (greater than 50 μg/dL). Alternatively, raised blood levels of zinc-protoporphyrin levels or its product are required for definitive diagnosis. In milder cases of lead exposure, anemia may be the only obvious abnormality. The chronic and cumulative exposure to lead is best measured in bone, rather than blood. The level of lead in blood reflects more ongoing exposure.

Treatment: Lead poisoning is treated with chelating agents namely ethylenediaminetetraacetic acid (EDTA), either alone or in combination with dimercaprol (BAL). Usually, hematologic and renal manifestations of lead intoxication are reversible whereas the alterations in the CNS are usually irreversible.

Mercury

It is one of the heavy metals that has had many uses throughout history. Humans have used inorganic mercury since prehistoric times and it has been known to be an occupation-related hazard. It was used as a pigment in cave paintings, a cosmetic, for treating syphilis, and a component of diuretics.

Source: There are three forms of mercury are: (i) metallic mercury (also called as elemental mercury), (ii) inorganic mercury compounds (mostly mercuric chloride), and (iii) organic mercury (mostly methyl mercury).

Currently, the main sources of exposure are organic mercury derived from living matter that has contaminated fish. Other source is mercury vapors released from metallic mercury in dental amalgams dental amalgams and it may be and occupational hazard for dental workers. Mercury is also used in thermometers and batteries. It is still used as a medicine in homeopathy though in dilutions. Mercury is also released into the environment by power plants, gold mining, fertilizer and plastics factory and other industrial sources. This is discharged into and contaminate the rivers.

Inorganic mercury may be released during the natural degassing (removal of unwanted or excess gas) of the earth's crust or from industrial wastes. Exposures may occur in some chemical, metal-processing, electrical-equipment, and automotive industries. Mercury is dispersed by waste incineration. The inorganic mercury is converted to highly neurotoxic organic compounds such as methyl mercury by environmental bacteria. The organic mercury then may be bioconcentrated. Bioconcentration refers to substances that are taken up strictly from water. Fish are said to bioconcentrate contaminants from their environment through uptake over the gills. Consequently, their body concentrations of many contaminants can be much greater than they are in the environment. Thus, mercury enters the aquatic food chain. Bacteria in bays and oceans also can convert inorganic mercury compounds from industrial wastes into highly neurotoxic organomercurials. These compounds are then transferred up the food chain. Methyl mercury is then taken by the large predatory (preying naturally on others) carnivorous fish (e.g., swordfish, shark, tuna, pike, and bluefish). The mercury levels in these fishes may be 1 million times higher than in the surrounding water. These form a substantial part of the diet in many countries. Consumption of such fish contaminated with mercury can produce mercury poisoning. Children exposed in utero showed delayed developmental milestones and abnormal reflexes. To protect potential fetal brain damage, the CDC (Centers for Disease Control and Prevention) has recommended that pregnant women avoid consumption of fish known to contain high levels of mercury.

Pathophysiology

Absorption: Elemental (metallic) mercury (Hg) is not well absorbed but it will volatilize into highly absorbable vapor. Inorganic mercury is absorbed through the gastrointestinal tract and skin. Organic mercury is well absorbed through inhalation and ingestion. Ingested mercury can damage the GI tract and cause ulcerations and bloody diarrhea.

Distribution: Elemental (metallic) and organic mercury are soluble in lipid. So, they can cross the blood-brain barrier and placenta. This allows their accumulation in the brain, disturbing neuromotor, cognitive, and behavioral functions.

Excretion: Mercury is excreted in urine and feces. It has a half-life in blood of ~60 days. However, mercury deposits will remain in the kidney and brain for years. Exposure to mercury stimulates the kidney to produce metallothionein. This provides some detoxification benefit.

Mechanism of action: Mercury binds to sulfhydryl groups (like lead) in certain proteins with high affinity. It interferes with a wide variety of critical enzymatic processes. The kidney is the main target of the toxicity of inorganic mercury and the CNS (brain) is damaged by organic mercury. It can also damage the GI tract. Intracellular GSH (reduced glutathione) acts as a sulfhydryl donor and this is the main protective mechanism against mercury-induced CNS and kidney damage.

Minamata disease: Exposure of the fetus to high levels of mercury in utero may lead to Minamata disease, characterized by cerebral palsy, deafness, and blindness. Contamination of many ecosystems was followed by many well-known outbreaks of methyl mercury poisoning. These episodes occurred in Japan, first in Minamata Bay in the 1950s and then in Niigata. In both cases, local inhabitants developed severe, chronic organic mercury intoxication. This poisoning was following the consumption of fish contaminated with mercury. The mercury had been discharged into the environment from a fertilizer and a plastics factory.

Toxicity

In the olden days, mercuric chloride was widely used as an antiseptic and acute mercuric chloride poisoning was much more common. It was ingested by accident or for suicidal purposes.

Acute inhalation of mercury (Hg) vapor: It causes pneumonitis and noncardiogenic pulmonary edema and can cause death. It also produces CNS symptoms, and polyneuropathy.

Chronic high exposure: It causes CNS toxicity. Lower exposure to mercury impairs renal function, memory, and coordination.

Acute ingestion of inorganic mercury: It causes gastroenteritis, nephritic syndrome acute renal failure, and hypertension.

Ingestion of organic mercury: It causes gastroenteritis, arrhythmias.

High exposure during pregnancy; It causes severe mental retardation.

Mild exposures during pregnancy (from fish consumption): Reduced neurobehavioral performance in offspring.

Dimethyl mercury: It is a compound only found in research labs. It is "supertoxic" and a few drops of exposure through skin absorption or inhaled vapor can cause severe cerebellar degeneration and death.

MORPHOLOGY

Neurotoxicity: Children exposed in utero showed delayed developmental milestones and abnormal reflexes, cerebral palsy, deafness, blindness, and major CNS defects. The developing brain is very sensitive to methyl mercury. Pathologically, there will be cerebral and cerebellar atrophy. Microscopically, the cerebellum shows atrophy of the granular layer, without loss of Purkinje cells and spongy softening in the visual cortex and other cortical regions.

Nephrotoxicity: Mercury can produce acute tubular necrosis (proximal tubular necrosis) and accompanied by oliguric renal failure. Chronic exposure can cause nephrotic syndrome. Microscopically, it shows membranous glomerulonephritis with subepithelial electron-dense deposits, suggesting immune complex deposition.

Arsenic

The toxic properties of arsenic are well known. Arsenic was used as poison of choice by skilled practitioners in Renaissance Italy. It was used as an instrument of assassination among royal families; arsenic has been called "the poison of kings and the king of poisons."

Sources: Unintentional exposure to arsenic is an important health problem in many areas of the world. Arsenic compounds have been used as insecticides, herbicides, pesticides, fungicides, weed killers, other agricultural products, and wood preservatives. Arsenic is present in Chinese, Indian herbal, and homeopathic medicine, and folk remedies. Arsenicals may also be found naturally in soil and deep-water wells (in countries, such as Bangladesh, Chile, and China) as a result of naturally occurring arsenic-rich rock formations, from coal burning or from use of arsenical pesticides. It may contaminate the environment by the mining smelting (process of applying heat to ore in order to extract a base metal) microelectronics industry.

Metabolism: Organic arsenic (arsenobetaine, arsenocholine) is ingested in seafood and fish and is nontoxic. Inorganic arsenic is readily absorbed through lung and GI tract. Arsenic is stored in liver, spleen, kidneys, lungs, and GI tract. It persists in skin, hair, and nails and detoxified by biomethylation.

Toxic effects

Most toxic forms of arsenic are the trivalent compounds arsenic trioxide, sodium arsenite, and arsenic trichloride. Arsenic interferes with many aspects of cellular metabolism; its interference with mitochondrial oxidative phosphorylation by replacing the phosphates in ATP by the trivalent arsenic. However, arsenic also has pleiotropic effects on the activity of a many other enzymes and ion channels. These may also be responsible for certain toxicities of arsenic. Arsenic produces its toxic effects mainly in the gastrointestinal tract, nervous system, skin, and heart.

Acute arsenic poisoning: Present days, acute arsenic poisoning is almost always due to accidental or homicidal ingestion. Ingestion of large quantities of arsenic causes acute gastrointestinal, cardiovascular, and CNS toxicities that usually leads to death. In the GIT, it produces severe abdominal pain, diarrhea and is accompanied by necrosis of intestinal mucosa with hemorrhagic gastroenteritis, fluid loss, hypotension. It may also produce cardiac arrhythmias, shock, respiratory distress syndrome, and acute encephalopathy. GI, cardiovascular, and CNS toxicity may be severe and cause death.

Chronic arsenic exposure: Chronic arsenic intoxication affects many organ systems. It produces nonspecific symptoms such as malaise and fatigue.

- **Neurologic effects:** It usually occurs 2 to 8 weeks after exposure. It consists of a sensorimotor peripheral neuropathy and produce paresthesias, numbness, and pain.
- **Cardiovascular effects:** These include hypertension and prolonged Q-Tc interval with ventricular arrhythmias.
- **Skin changes:** With chronic exposure, hyperpigmentation and hyperkeratosis occur.

- **Increased risk for the development of cancers:** It is the most serious consequence of chronic exposure. It can produce cancer of skin, lung, liver (angiosarcoma), bladder, and kidney. Skin tumors produced by arsenic differ from those induced by sunlight. Arsenic-induced skin cancers are generally multiple and usually appear on the palms and soles. Probable mechanisms of arsenic carcinogenesis in skin and lung are defects in nucleotide excision repair mechanisms that protect against DNA damage.
- **Others:** It can produce diabetes, vasospasm, peripheral vascular insufficiency, and gangrene.

Lethal dose: 120–200 mg (adults); 2 mg/kg (children).

Cadmium

Cadmium is a plasticizer and a pigment and is relatively a modern toxic agent. It is one of the heavy metals.

Sources: It is an occupational and environmental pollutant. It is produced by mining, electroplating other metals (e.g., automobile parts and musical instruments), production of rechargeable nickel-cadmium batteries, manufacturing alloys, smelting, and plastics industries. These are usually disposed of as household waste. Cadmium may contaminate the soil and plants directly or through fertilizers and irrigation water. Ingestion of food that concentrates cadmium (grains, cereals) is the most important source of cadmium exposure for the general population. Both plant- and animal-derived foodstuffs may contain significant amount of cadmium.

Metabolism: The main routes of exposure of cadmium are ingestion and inhalation. It is bound by metallothionein, filtered at the glomerulus, but reabsorbed by proximal tubules. This causes its poor excretion. It binds cellular sulfhydryl groups, competes with zinc, calcium for binding sites. Toxic effects of cadmium require its uptake into cells via transporters such as ZIP8. Normally, ZIP8 acts as a transporter for zinc. Cadmium is mainly concentrated in liver and kidneys. It is toxic to the kidneys and the lungs. It is probably through increased production of ROS (reactive oxygen species).

Biologic half-life: It accumulates in the human body with a half-life 10–30 years. It is rarely recycled.

Toxic effects

- **Acute cadmium toxicity:** Acute inhalation of cadmium irritates the respiratory tract. It causes pneumonitis and pulmonary edema after 4–24 hours. Acute ingestion causes gastroenteritis.
- **Chronic exposure:** It is mainly toxic to the lungs and kidneys. It can lead to obstructive lung disease (emphysema) by necrosis of alveolar epithelial cells. In the kidney, initially it produces proteinuria due to renal tubular damage (rather than glomerular damage). It may progress to end-stage renal disease. Cadmium can also cause skeletal abnormalities due to calcium loss. Cadmium-containing water used to irrigate rice fields in Japan caused a disease in postmenopausal women known as itai-itai ("ouch-ouch"). This is characterized by a combination of osteoporosis and osteomalacia associated with renal disease. Cadmium exposure increases the risk of lung cancer. Though cadmium is not directly genotoxic, it may produce DNA damage through the production of ROS. Other manifestations include anosmia, yellowing of teeth, minor LFT (liver function test) elevations, microcytic hypochromic anemia unresponsive to iron therapy, increased urinary β_2-microglobulin, and calciuria.

Chromium

Chromium (Cr) is used in several industries, such as metal plating and some types of manufacturing. Chronic exposure is highly genotoxic and increases the risk of lung cancer and other tumors.

Nickel

Nickel is used in electronics, coins, steel alloys, batteries, and food processing.

The most frequent effect of exposure to nickel is contact dermatitis ("nickel itch") and can develop due to contact with metals containing nickel, such as coins and costume jewellery.

Exposure to nickel increases the risk of lung cancer and cancer of the nasal cavities.

OCCUPATIONAL HEALTH RISKS: INDUSTRIAL AND AGRICULTURAL EXPOSURES

Q. Discuss common disease due to environmental and occupational exposures.

Present day industrial revolution is associated with a rise in the number of chemicals manufactured and a corresponding increase in the risk of human exposure to these chemicals. The risks include acute poisoning and chronic toxicity. Occupational injuries and illnesses are one of the important health risks. Toxic agents causing diseases vary depending on the industry. Industrial exposures may produce diseases that range from irritations of respiratory airways (e.g., formaldehyde or ammonia fumes) to lung cancers (arising from exposure to asbestos, arsenic, or uranium). Various diseases associated with occupational exposures are presented in **Table 2**.

Toxic metals produce environmental diseases and are discussed above. Apart from these other important agents that produce to environmental diseases are briefly discussed below:

Volatile Organic Solvents and Vapors

Volatile organic solvents and vapors are widely used in industry in large quantities throughout the world. Exposures to these compounds (with few exceptions) are industrial or accidental. They usually produce short-term dangers rather than long-term toxicity. Most of these organic solvents exposure is by inhalation rather than by ingestion.

Chloroform ($CHCl_3$) and carbon tetrachloride (CCl4): Chloroform and carbon tetrachloride are solvents used in degreasing and dry-cleaning agents and paint removers. These solvents are CNS depressants (anesthetics), but are known hepatotoxins.

- **Acute exposure** to high levels of both these agents, but classically with carbon tetrachloride, lead to **acute hepatic necrosis, fatty liver, and liver failure**. Clinically they cause dizziness and confusion, CNS depression, and even coma. At lower levels, they are toxic to liver and kidney. Usually, long-term exposure to carbon tetrachloride would not be permitted, because each exposure to it causes recognizable clinical liver injury.

Table 2: Various diseases associated with occupational exposures to toxic substances.

Diseases caused	*Toxic substances/occupation causing diseases*
Respiratory system	
Nasal cancer	Isopropyl alcohol, wood dust, furniture, and shoe manufacturing
Paranasal sinus cancer	Nickel
Lung cancer	Radon, asbestos, silica, nickel, arsenic, chromium, mustard gas, uranium, bis(chloromethyl) ether, tars, and oils. Hematite mining
Mesothelioma (pleura and peritoneum), lung cancer (in smokers)	Asbestos
Chronic obstructive pulmonary disease	Grain dust, coal dust, cadmium
Hypersensitivity	Beryllium, isocyanates
Irritation	Ammonia, formaldehyde, sulfur oxides
Fibrosis	Silica, asbestos, cobalt
Gastrointestinal tract	
Cancers of gastrointestinal tract	Tars and oils
Liver angiosarcoma	Vinyl chloride
Hematopoietic system	
Leukemia, multiple myeloma	Benzene
Cardiovascular system	
Heart disease	Carbon monoxide, lead, cadmium, solvents, cobalt
Urinary system	
Renal toxicity	Mercury, lead, glycol ethers, solvents
Bladder cancer	Naphthylamines, 4-aminobiphenyl, benzidine, rubber products
Reproductive system	
Male infertility	Lead, cadmium, phthalate plasticizers
Female infertility and stillbirths	Lead, mercury
Teratogenesis	Mercury, polychlorinated biphenyls
Nervous system	
Peripheral neuropathies	Solvents, acrylamide, methyl chloride, mercury, lead, arsenic, dichlorodiphenyltrichloroethane (DDT)
Diseases caused	*Toxic substances/occupation causing diseases*
Ataxic gait	Mercury, chlordane, toluene, acrylamide
Central nervous system (CNS) depression	Alcohols, ketones, aldehydes, solvents
Eye	
Cataracts	Ultraviolet radiation
Skin	
Folliculitis and acneiform dermatosis	Polychlorinated biphenyls, dioxins, herbicides
Cancer	Ultraviolet radiation

Benzene (C_6H_6): Benzene is the classical aromatic hydrocarbon. It must be distinguished from benzine, which is a mixture of aliphatic hydrocarbons. Benzene is one of the most extensively used chemicals in industrial processes. It is a starting point for innumerable syntheses and a solvent. It is also a part of fuels and accounts for about 3% of gasoline; tobacco smoke also contains benzene. Both (gasoline and tobacco smoke) contribute to increased benzene levels in the urban atmosphere. Almost all cases of acute and chronic benzene toxicity occur due to industrial exposures, e.g., in shoemakers and workers in shoe manufacturing. These occupations were heavily exposed to benzene-based glues.

- **Acute benzene poisoning:** It mainly affects the CNS and death occurs due to respiratory failure.
- **Long-term exposure:** The long-term effects of benzene and 1,3-butadiene exposure are mainly on the bone marrow. Individuals exposed develop characteristic hematologic abnormalities namely **hypoplasia or aplasia of the bone marrow and pancytopenia**. Aplastic anemia develops while the workers are still exposed to high concentrations of benzene. In a significant proportion of patients of benzene-induced anemia, myelodysplastic syndromes, acute myeloid leukemia, erythroleukemia, or multiple myeloma develop. These may occur either during continuing exposure to benzene or after a variable latent period after the worker is removed from the hazardous environment. Some individuals develop acute leukemia without a prior history of aplastic anemia. Though chronic myeloid and chronic lymphocytic leukemia have been reported, causal role of benzene exposure is less convincing than that of acute leukemia. There is 60-fold increase in the risk of leukemia in workers exposed to the highest atmospheric concentrations of benzene.
- **Mechanism:** The toxic effects of benzene are related to its metabolites. **Benzene is oxidized to an epoxide** (an organic compound molecule containing a three-membered ring involving an oxygen atom and two carbon atoms) through hepatic CYP2E1, a component of the P-450 enzyme system. The epoxide and other metabolites **disrupt progenitor cell differentiation in the bone marrow**. This may lead to marrow aplasia and acute myeloid leukemia. Two closely related compounds namely toluene and xylenes are also widely used as solvents. They do not cause of hematologic abnormalities, probably because they are metabolized through different pathways.

Polycyclic hydrocarbons: These are released during the combustion of coal and gas. They are mainly released at the high temperatures used in steel foundries. They are also present in tar and soot. Polycyclic hydrocarbons are the most potent carcinogens. Its industrial exposures can cause cancer of lung and bladder. Polycyclic hydrocarbons are discussed in detail on pages 530 and 531.

Methanol (CH_3OH): Methanol, unlike ethanol, is not taxed and is cheaper. It is used by some alcoholics who are poor as a substitute for ethanol. It may also be illegally used for adulterating alcoholic beverages, especially in regions where there is poverty. In methanol poisoning, intoxications are similar to that produced by ethanol. It also produces gastrointestinal symptoms, visual dysfunction, seizures, coma, and death. The major toxicity of methanol is due to its metabolism; it first converted to formaldehyde and then to formic acid. Metabolic acidosis is common following ingestion of methanol. The most characteristic features of methanol toxicity are that it produces **necrosis of retinal ganglion cells and subsequent degeneration of the optic nerve, leading to blindness**. Severe poisoning may produce lesions in the putamen and globus pallidus.

Ethylene glycol ($HOCH_2CH_2OH$): Ethylene glycol has low vapor pressure and is commonly used in antifreeze. It produces toxicity following ingestion. Chronic alcoholics use this as a substitute for ethanol. Owing to its sweet taste and solubility it was used to adulterate wines. The toxicity of ethylene glycol is mainly due to its metabolites. Main metabolite is oxalic acid and produces toxicity within minutes of ingestion. It produces metabolic acidosis, CNS depression, nausea and vomiting, and hypocalcemia-related cardiotoxicity. Oxalate crystals in renal tubules and oxaluria may be observed and may cause renal failure.

Gasoline and kerosene: These are used as fuels. They consist of mixtures of aliphatic hydrocarbons and branched, unsaturated, and aromatic hydrocarbons. Chronic exposure is by inhalation. Prolonged exposure to gasoline is seen in gas station attendants and auto mechanics. There is no evidence that inhalation of gasoline over the long term is particularly injurious. Gasoline is an irritant, but causes systemic problems only if inhaled in very high concentrations. Kerosene is used for domestic purposes and accidental poisoning can occur in children.

Trichloroethylene (C_2HCl_3): It is also used as an industrial solvent. In high concentrations, it depresses the CNS, but has minimal hepatotoxicity. There is no evidence that it produces disease, even after ordinary long-term industrial exposure.

Agricultural Chemicals

For modern agriculture, to increase productivity, it is necessary to use pesticides, fungicides, herbicides, fumigants, and organic fertilizers. However, many of these chemicals persist in soil and water and may constitute a potential long-term hazard. Exposure to these chemicals at industrial concentrations or accidentally contaminated food can cause severe acute illness. Children are particularly susceptible. They may ingest home gardening preparations.

Organochlorines

Organochlorines and halogenated organic compounds are synthetic products that resist degradation and are lipophilic. Organochlorine may be pesticides or nonpesticides.

Organochlorine pesticides

Organochlorines that are used as pesticides include dichlorodiphenyltrichloroethane (DDT) and its metabolites and agents (e.g., lindane, aldrin, and dieldrin), chlordane, and others. They accumulate in soils and in human tissues and break down very slowly. High levels of such pesticide can be harmful to humans in acute exposures. Acute DDT poisoning causes neurologic toxicity. Acute toxicity of most organochlorine insecticides is due to inhibition of CNS GABA responses. Symptoms of acute toxicity are usually depends on the mode of action of the toxin. For example, organophosphate insecticides, which have largely replaced organochlorine compounds, are acetylcholinesterase inhibitors. These are absorbed through the skin. Thus, acute toxicity is due to neuromuscular disorders such as visual disturbances, dyspnea, mucous hypersecretion, and bronchoconstriction. Death may occur due to respiratory failure. Most organochlorines are endocrine disruptors and in laboratory animals they have antiestrogenic or antiandrogenic activity. However, long-term health effects in humans have not been well established. Some of these compounds (e.g., aldrin and dieldrin) are associated with tumor development. Long-term exposure to substantial concentrations of these chemical produces symptoms similar to those of acute exposure.

Paraquat

Human exposure to herbicides namely paraquat (chemical herbicide, or weed killer) is common. Occupational exposure to paraquat is usually through the skin. It is very corrosive and causes burns or ulcers of whatever it comes into contact. It is actively transported to the lung and it can damage the pulmonary epithelium. This can cause edema and even respiratory failure. High-level exposures may lead to death from cardiovascular collapse. Lower doses may produce pulmonary fibrosis and ultimately death.

Aromatic Halogenated Hydrocarbons

Nonpesticide organochlorines: Organochlorines can be nonpesticide such as polychlorinated biphenyls (PCBs) and dioxin [2,3,7,8-tetrachlorodibenzo-p-dioxin (TCDD)]. These are halogenated aromatic hydrocarbons. Dioxins and PCBs can cause skin disorders such as folliculitis and acneiform dermatosis known as chloracne. Chloracne consists of acne, cyst formation, hyperpigmentation, and hyperkeratosis. They usually develop around the face and behind the ears. It can be associated with abnormalities in the liver and CNS. PCBs induce the P-450 enzyme system. Hence, workers exposed to PCBs may show altered drug metabolism. In the late 1960s, environmental disasters in Japan and China were caused by the consumption of rice oil contaminated by PCBs. It poisoned around 2000 individuals in each episode. The main presenting features of the disease (yusho in Japan, yu-cheng in China) were chloracne and hyperpigmentation of the skin and nails.

Bisphenol A

Bisphenol A (BPA) is a chemical compound that is used in the production of hard plastics used for baby bottles and food storage containers. They are also used for synthesis of epoxy resins that coats the insides line almost all food bottles and cans. When heated in microwaves, the plastic breaks down, allowing BPA to leach into food. Hence, exposure to BPA is almost always is universal in humans. In animal studies, BPA has been shown to cause mammary and prostate cancer. BPA is known as a potential endocrine disruptor. Elevated urinary BPA levels may predispose to heart disease in adult populations. In addition, infants who drink from BPA-containing containers may be particularly susceptible to the endocrine effects of BPA. In 2010, Canada listed BPA as a toxic substance. This led to stoppage of using BPA in the manufacturing of baby bottles and "sippy" cups by the largest manufacturers.

Vinyl chloride: It is used in the synthesis of polyvinyl resins. It can cause a rare type of liver tumor known as **angiosarcoma of the liver**.

Mineral Dusts

Inhalation of mineral dusts causes chronic, nonneoplastic lung diseases called pneumoconioses. Pneumoconioses include diseases caused by organic and inorganic particulates, and chemical fume- and vapor-induced non-neoplastic lung diseases. Most common pneumoconiosis includes those due to coal dust, silica, asbestos, and beryllium. Pneumoconioses usually occur in the workplace. There is increased risk of cancer due to asbestos exposure.

Cyanide

Cyanide blocks cellular respiration. This is achieved by reversible binding of cyanide to mitochondrial cytochrome oxidase that is the terminal acceptor in the electron transport chain. This reduces the molecular oxygen to water. The pathologic consequences of cyanide are similar to those produced by any acute generalized anoxia.

SMOKING

Q. Describe the role of tobacco in human diseases.

Smoking tobacco is the single largest, exogenous, most readily preventable cause of death. It is responsible for about 90% of lung cancers. The main offender is cigarette smoking. However, smokeless tobacco (e.g., snuff, chewing tobacco) is an important cause of oral cancer. Apart from death due to various types of cancers, tobacco can cause deaths from cardiovascular and metabolic diseases, deaths from nonmalignant lung diseases and perinatal deaths. The use of tobacco products not only produces risk to the smoker, but can cause lung cancer in these nonsmokers who passively inhales tobacco from the environment (second hand smoke).

Dose-dependency and cumulative effect: Tobacco reduces overall life expectancy. Overall mortality is dose-dependent and proportional to the amount and duration of cigarette smoking. It is commonly quantitated and expressed as "pack-years" (i.e., the average number of cigarette packs smoked each day multiplied by the number of years of smoking). Smoking has a cumulative effect. However, cessation of smoking reduces the risk of overall mortality and the risk of death from CVD (cardiovascular disease) within 5 years.

Types of Tobacco

Tobacco may be used either for smoking or as smokeless tobacco.

Smoking: It is the main culprit and may be used in the form of cigarette, *beedi*, cigar, or pipe smoking, or reverse smoking (smoking a cheroot with the burning end inside the mouth is practiced in certain regions of India). Regular marijuana use has also been associated with oropharyngeal cancer. Life expectancy is reduced by cigarette smoking and overall mortality is proportional to the amount (dose dependent) and duration of smoking. Tobacco smoking not only produces personal risk, but passive tobacco inhalation from the environment ("second-hand smoke") can also cause lung cancer in nonsmokers. Cessation of smoking greatly decreases the risk of death from lung cancer.

Smokeless tobacco: It is also harmful to health and is an important cause of oral cancer. It may be used in its various forms such as chewing tobacco or snuff. Betel quid/pan is a type of tobacco chewing that contains several ingredients, such as areca nut, slaked lime, and tobacco which are wrapped in a betel leaf. It is commonly used in India and Southeast Asia, and is associated with marked increase in oral cancer. Betel quid appears to be the major carcinogen. However, it may also be related to slaked lime and the areca nut. Other methods of tobacco consumption include snuff dipping and tobacco chewing. Oral cancers are found on the buccal and gingival surfaces in the sites where tobacco products are held in contact with the mucosa for long periods.

Constituents of Tobacco Smoke

Tobacco contains >2,000 substances (potentially noxious) and >60 have been identified as carcinogens. Many mucosal toxins and ciliotoxic agents have also been found. Few of these substances along with the type of injury produced by these agents are listed in **Table 3**.

Nicotine and its effects: Tobacco leaves contain an alkaloid called nicotine. It does not directly cause tobacco-related diseases, but is strongly addictive and is responsible for tobacco addiction. Nicotine in the tobacco binds to nicotinic acetylcholine receptors in the brain. This binding stimulates the release catecholamines from sympathetic neurons. The catecholamines are responsible for the acute ill effects of smoking. These ill effects are increase in (i) heart rate, (ii) blood pressure, (iii) cardiac contractility, and output. Apart from being an addictive, nicotine has other untoward effects especially fetus of pregnant women. Nicotine affects the development of fetal brain and can lead to preterm birth and still birth.

Effects of Tobacco

The major diseases responsible for increased mortality in cigarette smokers are, in order of frequency: **(i) cancers,**

Table 3: Effects of selected tobacco smoke constituents.

Constituent of tobacco smoke	*Effect(s)*
Cigarette, tar	Carcinogenesis
Polycyclic aromatic hydrocarbons	
Benzo[a]pyrene	
Nitrosamine	
Nicotine	Release catecholamine, cause ganglionic stimulation and depression. Promotes tumor
Phenol	Promotes tumor and causes irritation of mucosa
Carbon monoxide (CO)	Impaired oxygen transport and use
Formaldehyde	Toxic to cilia and causes irritation of mucosa
Oxides of nitrogen	

(ii) CVD (iii) metabolic diseases, and (iv) chronic pulmonary diseases. Any irritating smoked product increases the risk for tumors of the oral cavity. Nicotine and other tobacco components cause cancer. Carcinogens in tobacco can act as initiators, as well as promoters. Risk increases with amount and duration of tobacco use. **Various cancers** that are more common in smokers than in nonsmokers include those of the **oral cavity, larynx, esophagus, pancreas, bladder, kidney, colon, liver, and cervix**. Increased mortality in smokers is also from tuberculosis, atherosclerotic aortic aneurysms, and peptic ulcers. The effects of cigarette smoking on the various organs in smokers are shown in **Fig. 5**.

Respiratory System

The most common diseases caused by cigarette smoking involve the respiratory system mainly lung.

Smoking and lung cancer

Components particularly polycyclic hydrocarbons and nitrosamines present in cigarette smoke, (**Table 4**), are potent carcinogens. They are directly involved in the development of lung cancer in humans.

CYPs (cytochrome P-450 enzymes) and phase II enzymes (refer page 962) increase the water solubility of the carcinogens present in tobacco smoke. This helps in their excretion through urine. However, few intermediates produced by CYPs during phase II that are electrophilic. These electrophilic intermediates combine with DNA and form DNA adducts. These adducts may be repaired DNA repairing machinery. If DNA adducts persist, they can cause oncogenic **mutations in oncogenes and tumor suppressors**. The risk of developing lung cancer in smokers depends on the intensity of exposure to cigarettes smoke. It is usually expressed in terms of number of "pack years" (e.g., one pack daily for 20 years is equal to 20 pack years) or cigarettes smoked per day and duration of smoking habit.

Smoking is also an important factor in the production of lung cancer that is associated with certain occupational exposures. Thus, smoking increases the risk of other carcinogens (e.g., asbestos, uranium). For example, there is a 10-fold higher incidence of lung carcinomas in asbestos workers and uranium miners who smoke over those who do not smoke. There is also interaction between tobacco and alcohol in the development of oral and laryngeal cancers. In nonsmokers, passive environmental smoke inhalation is also associated with risk of lung cancer than those who are not exposed to passive smoke. The risk of lung cancer declines after one quits smoking.

Nonneoplastic diseases

Chronic bronchitis, emphysema, and chronic obstructive pulmonary disease (COPD): Mucosal toxins and ciliotoxic agents present in smoke have a direct irritant effect on the tracheobronchial mucosa. They produce inflammation and increased production of mucus (bronchitis). Cigarette smoke also recruits leukocytes to the lung, and increases the local production of elastase. This injures lung tissue leading to emphysema. Smoking also exacerbates asthma and increases the risk for pulmonary tuberculosis. Children living along with adult smokers are susceptible to increase respiratory illnesses and asthma.

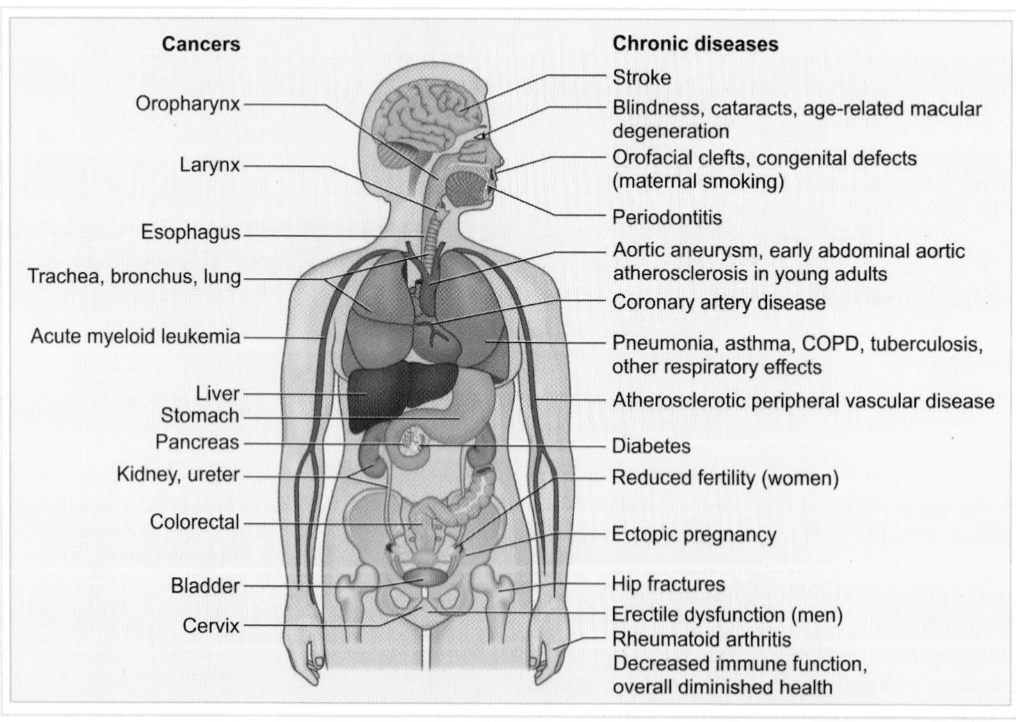

(COPD: chronic obstructive pulmonary disease)

FIG. 5: Organs affected by active cigarette smoking in smokers.

Table 4: Organ-specific suspected carcinogens in tobacco smoke.

Organ involved	*Carcinogen responsible for cancer*
Lung, larynx	Polycyclic aromatic hydrocarbons, 4-(Methylnitrosoamino)-1-(3-pyridyl)-1-butanone (NNK), Polonium 210
Esophagus	N′-Nitrosonornicotine (NNN)
Oral cavity (smoking)	Polycyclic aromatic hydrocarbons, NNK, NNN
Oral cavity (smokeless tobacco: Snuff, tobacco chewing)	NNK, NNN, polonium 210
Pancreas	NNK
Bladder	4-Aminobiphenyl, 2-naphthylamine

Other Cancers

Apart from lung cancer, tobacco smoking is a risk factor for many other malignant and non-malignant disorders of many organ systems. Tobacco consumption interacts with alcohol in multiplying the risk of oral, laryngeal, and esophageal cancer.

- **Oral cancers:** Smokeless tobacco along with alcohol consumption is important (>90%) cause of oral cancer. These include cancers of the **lip, tongue, and buccal mucosa**. All forms of tobacco use-cigarette, cigar and pipe smoking, and tobacco chewing are associated with oral cancer.
- **Cancer of the larynx:** It is also associated with smoking.
- **Cancer of the esophagus**
- **Cancer of the pancreas**
- **Carcinoma of the kidney**
- **Cancer of the bladder:** There is a clear relationship between incidence of bladder cancer, numbers of cigarettes smoked per day, and duration of cigarette smoking.
- **Cancer of the uterine cervix** is significantly more in women smokers.
- **Colon and rectum cancers:** They are more common in active smokers, especially heavy smokers, than in nonsmokers. Smokers also have an increased risk for colonic adenomatous polyps. These are considered as premalignant precursors of adenocarcinomas.
- **Breast cancer:** There is a relationship between risk for tobacco-related breast cancer and rapid acetylator phenotypes for the enzyme N-acetyltransferase-2.
- **Ovarian tumors:** There is a slightly increased incidence of borderline mucinous tumors of the ovary with cigarette smoking.
- **Liver cancers**
- **Acute myeloid leukemia (AML)**

Cardiovascular System

Atherosclerosis and myocardial infarction: Cigarette smoking is one of the major risk factors and strongly linked to the development of atherosclerosis and its major complication is myocardial infarction. Smoking also increases the incidence of sudden cardiac death. Atherosclerosis of the coronary arteries and aorta is more severe and extensive in cigarette smokers than among nonsmokers. As a consequence, cigarette smoking is a strong risk factor for atherosclerotic aortic aneurysms. If smoking is combined other risk factors, such as hypertension (elevated blood pressure) and hyper-cholesterolemia (raised blood cholesterol levels), this multiplies the risk of atherosclerosis and myocardial infarction. The cigarette smoking is a strong risk factor for atherosclerotic aortic aneurysms.

Cerebrovascular disease and peripheral vascular disease: Smoking is a risk factor for atherosclerotic peripheral vascular disease and cerebrovascular disease. Cigarette smoking is an independent risk factor for cerebrovascular diseases such as ischemic stroke and certain forms of intracranial hemorrhage.

Buerger's disease: It is an inflammatory and occlusive disease of the lower leg vasculature. It occurs almost only in heavy smokers.

Other Nonneoplastic Diseases

Peptic ulcer disease: These are more common in male cigarette smokers than in nonsmokers.

Type 2 diabetes mellitus (T2DM): It may develop in smokers. It may be due to nicotine-related insulin resistance and beta cell apoptosis, increased central obesity and altered metabolism of estrogens and androgens in smokers.

Severe course of tuberculosis: The course of tuberculosis is more severe in smokers and tuberculosis-related death is more in smokers.

Asthma: Its incidence and exacerbations are more in smokers than in nonsmokers.

Impaired immune function: Smoking affects both innate and adaptive immune system.

Seropositive rheumatoid arthritis: It can result from cigarette smoking and smokers are more prone to develop rheumatoid arthritis.

Osteoporosis in women: It is exacerbated by tobacco use.

Thyroid diseases: Cigarette smoking is associated with Grave's disease, and particularly when hyperthyroidism is complicated by exophthalmos.

Ocular diseases: These include macular degeneration and cataracts.

Brain development may be impaired by nicotine in adolescent smokers.

Reproductive Function

Men: Those who smoke are more susceptible to erectile dysfunction.

Women: Menopause occurs early in smoking women than do nonsmokers, probably because of the effects of tobacco on estrogen metabolism.

Maternal Smoking

Smoking increases the risk of spontaneous abortions and preterm births and results in intrauterine growth retardation. Ectopic pregnancy is more common in smokers.

Fetal tobacco syndrome (FTS): FTS is group of adverse fetal and infant health effects associated with maternal smoking during pregnancy. Maternal cigarette smoking impairs the fetal development and retards fetal growth (fetal tobacco syndrome). Infants born to women who smoke during pregnancy are smaller and on average, weigh 200 g less than infants born to comparable non-smoking women. These infants are small for gestational age at every stage of pregnancy.

Perinatal mortality is higher among offspring of smokers and due to effect of smoking on the uteroplacental system. There are increased incidences of abruptio placentae, placenta previa, uterine bleeding, and premature rupture of membranes in smokers. These complications usually develop when the fetus is not viable or is at great risk (i.e., 20–32 weeks of gestation).

Children born of smoking mothers are more susceptible to several respiratory diseases, including respiratory infections and otitis media. Maternal cigarette smoking impairs physical, cognitive, and emotional development of children. Thus, these children have measurable deficits in physical growth, intellectual maturation, and emotional development. There is also increased risk of certain types of attention deficit hyperactivity disorder (ADHD) in these children. Deficits in cognitive and auditory function may persist for years and are detectable well into adolescence. Generally, boys are more vulnerable to many of the psychosocial problems than girls. Maternal smoking greatly increases (about 4 times) the risk of sudden infant death syndrome (SIDS).

Environmental Tobacco Smoke

Involuntary exposure to tobacco smoke in the environment is called environmental tobacco smoke (ETS). It is also called second-hand smoke, passive smoking and is harmful to nonsmokers. It is associated with some of the same harmful effects that result from active smoking. It is a risk factor for some diseases in nonsmokers (**Table 5**). Nonsmoking spouses of smokers have 20–30% increased risk of developing cancer of lung. The World Health Organization (WHO) classifies ETS as a carcinogen and recognizes that it is responsible for some lung cancers in nonsmokers. ETS is also associated with an increased risk of cancer of breast in premenopausal nonsmoker women. An increased incidence of respiratory illnesses (such as asthma) and hospitalizations is observed among infants living in a household with an adult/parents who smokes. Also, mild impairment of pulmonary function was found in children of smokers and exacerbation of preexisting asthma. ETS is associated with an increased risk for sudden infant death syndrome (SIDS). A metabolite of nicotine is called cotinine. By measuring the blood levels of cotinine passive smoke inhalation in nonsmokers can be estimated.

Electronic Cigarettes (e-Cigarettes)

These devices simulate cigarette smoking by delivering vaporized nicotine and flavorings. They are becoming more popular. The use of flavored e-cigarettes is called "vaping." It is being increasingly used in recent times, mainly by among young adults. Though the e-cigarettes had no significant recorded untoward effects, in the summer of 2019 an outbreak of vaping-associated acute lung injury occurred in the United States. By the end of 2019 about 2000 cases had been reported with 42 fatalities. The pathogenesis of this outbreak is not known.

ALCOHOLISM

Q. Describe the role of alcohol in human diseases.

Usually consumption of alcohol (ethanol) in moderate amount is not injurious to health and may even protect against some disorders. Unmoderated alcohol consumption can lead to addiction and also known as alcoholism. Excessive amounts of alcohol can cause marked physical and psychological damage.

Types of alcohol: Human uses three types of alcohol: **ethanol, methanol, and isopropanol**. Ethanol is used for drinks. Other two types of alcohol namely methanol and isopropanol are used for cleaning and manufacturing and not suitable for drinks. This is because, methanol and isopropanol are metabolized as toxic substances and can cause liver failure. Hence, consuming even a small amount of methanol or isopropanol can be fatal. Methanol (or methyl alcohol) is a component in fuel for cars and boats. It is also used to manufacture antifreeze, paint remover, windshield wiper fluid, etc. Isopropanol (or isopropyl alcohol) is used for cleaning and disinfecting (including the alcoholic rub on hand disinfectant advised during covid-19 epidemic!). Henceforth, in this section the term alcohol is used for ethanol.

Different types of alcoholic drinks by alcohol content: There are many different kinds of alcohol drinks. Some of them contain more alcohol than others. Alcoholic beverages can be mainly categorized into two: (i) Undistilled and (ii) distilled (liquors and spirits) drinks.

- **Undistilled (fermented) drinks:** Fermentation is the process by which bacteria or yeast chemically converts sugar into ethanol. Examples of undistilled drinks are wine (ferment grapes) and beer (ferment barley, wheat, and other grains).
- **Distilled (liquors and spirits) drinks:** Distillation is a process that follows fermentation. Distillation concentrates

Table 5: Consequences of environmental tobacco smoke.

During childhood	*Respiratory and others*	*Cardiac and vascular*	*During pregnancy*
• Development of asthma • Acute otitis media • Pulmonary infections • Lower respiratory illness • Respiratory symptoms • Impaired lung function	• Development of asthma • Pulmonary infections • COPD • Nasal irritation • Lung cancer • Breast cancer • Stroke	• Acute myocardial infarction • Coronary atherosclerosis • Ischemic stroke • Sudden cardiac death (SCD) • Angina	• Stillbirth • IUGR • SIDS • Neurologic and behavioral disorders • Preterm delivery

(COPD: chronic obstructive pulmonary disease; IUGR: intrauterine growth retardation; SIDS: sudden infant death syndrome)

a fermented substance into a higher concentration of alcohol by separating the water and other components of a fermented substance. Liquors and spirits are distilled alcoholic beverages. They contain more alcohol by volume (ABV) than undistilled drinks. Examples include gin (made from juniper berries and have 35–55% ABV), brandy (distilled wine and have 35–60% ABV), whiskey (made from fermented grain and have 40–50% ABV), and vodka (made from fermented grains and potatoes and has 40% ABV).

Measures of alcohol content: There are two measures of alcohol content, or the concentration of alcohol in a drink. These are ABV (alcohol by volume) and alcohol proof. ABV is the number of milliliters of ethanol per 100 mL (or 3.4 fl oz) in a solution. Alcohol proof is twice the percentage of ABV. For example, a drink which has 50% ABV will be 100 proof.

Calculation of pure alcohol mass: Pure alcohol mass in a serving can be calculated if **concentration, density and volume of alcohol** are known. For example, a 350 mL beer with an ABV of 5.5% contains 19.25 mL of pure alcohol, which has a density of 789.24 g/L (at 20°C). Therefore, has a pure alcohol mass of 15.19 grams (concentration × density × volume = 5.5 × 789.24 × 350 = 15.19). **Average alcohol density is 800g/L.**

One "standard" drink (or one alcoholic drink equivalent) contains roughly 10–14 g of pure alcohol [10 g alcohol = 1 oz, or 30 mL, of 86 proof (43%) spirits]. Using the above formula, various volumes of alcohol (in round figures) containing 14 g (in a standard drink) of pure alcohol are as follows: 340 mL (12 oz) of regular beer (usually contains 5% alcohol; calculation 5 × 340 × 800 = 13.6 g), 115 mL (4 oz) of nonfortified (not strengthened or enriched) wine (about 12% alcohol; calculation 12 × 115 × 800 = 11.04 g), and 43 mL (1.5 oz) of 80-proof liquor (distilled spirits, e.g., whisky contains about 40% alcohol; calculation 40 × 43 × 800 = 13.76 g). Other examples include 0.5 L (1 pint) of 80-proof beverage (contains about 40% alcohol; calculation 40 × 500 × 800 = 160 g) contains ~160 g of ethanol (about 16 standard drinks), and 750 mL of wine (contains about 12% alcohol; calculation 12 × 750 × 800 = 11.04 g contains ~72 g of ethanol (about 6 standard drinks).

Metabolism of Ethanol

Absorption of ethanol: After consumption, alcohol is absorbed unaltered in small amounts from mucous membranes of the mouth and esophagus, in moderate amounts from the stomach and large bowel. The major site of absorption is from the proximal portion of the small intestine. The rate of absorption is increased by rapid gastric emptying (as seen with carbonation = process of dissolving CO_2 in a liquid such as carbonated soft drink; commonly used as soda along with drinks) and by the absence of proteins, fats, or carbohydrates (which interfere with absorption). The rate of absorption is increased by dilution to a moderate percentage of ethanol (maximum at ~20% by volume).

Distribution: After absorption, ethanol is distributed to all the tissues and fluids of the body which is directly proportional to its level in the blood. Less than 10% of the alcohol is excreted directly without any change in the urine, sweat, and breath.

Blood levels of ethanol: They are expressed as milligrams or grams of ethanol per deciliter (e.g., 100 mg/dL = 0.10 g/dL). Usually level of ~0.02 g/dL (20 mg/dL) results from the ingestion of one typical drink. The amount of alcohol exhaled in the breath is proportional to the blood level of ethanol. This is the basis for the breath test used by traffic police for drunken driving. Usual legal definition of drunk driving is an alcohol concentration of 80 mg/dL in the blood. In most individual, this alcohol concentration may be observed after consumption of three standard drinks, e.g., three (12 oz) bottles of beer, 15 oz of wine, or 4–5 oz of 80-proof distilled spirits (e.g., whisky, gin). When the alcohol level reaches 200 mg/dL, drowsiness develops, at 300 mg/dL level stupor, and with more than this level, coma with respiratory arrest may develop.

Though there are no firm rules, for most individuals, daily consumption of >45 g (e.g., ~135 mL whisky) alcohol should be discouraged. Consumption of 100 g (e.g., ~300 mL of whisky) or more ethanol per day may be injurious or dangerous.

Factors affecting alcohol levels in blood: Apart from amount of alcohol consumed other factors also affect the alcohol levels in blood. The rate of metabolism affects the alcohol level in blood. Chronic alcoholics develop tolerance to alcohol and alcohol is metabolizes at a higher rate in them than in normal individual. Hence, in chronic alcoholics, the blood levels of alcohol are lower than that is observed in others for the same amount of alcohol consumed.

Metabolism in Liver (Fig. 6)

The liver is the main organ involved in the ethanol metabolism. Only 2% (at low blood alcohol concentrations) and 10% (at high blood alcohol concentrations) of ethanol is excreted directly through the lungs, urine, or sweat. But most is metabolized primarily in the liver.

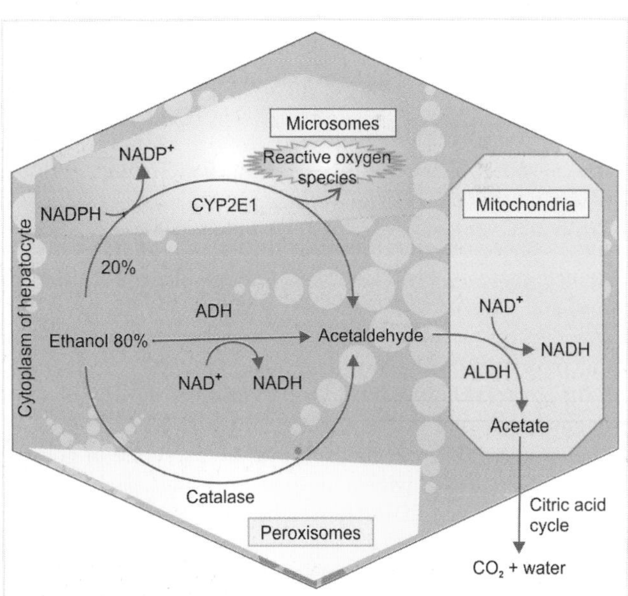

(NADP+: nicotinamide-adenine dinucleotide phosphate; NADPH: reduced form of nicotinamide-adenine dinucleotide phosphate; NAD+: nicotinamide adenine dinucleotide; NADH: reduced form of nicotinamide adenine dinucleotide)

FIG. 6: Ethanol metabolism in hepatocyte. Ethanol is converted to acetaldehyde by three different routes: (1) Most important route is in the cytosol by alcohol dehydrogenase (ADH) (2) in the microsomes (by CYP2E1), and (3) in the peroxisomes (by catalase). Acetaldehyde is oxidized by aldehyde dehydrogenase (ALDH) to acetic acid in mitochondria. Oxidation through CYPs (cytochrome P-450 enzymes) in the microsomes may also generate reactive oxygen species.

Formation of acetaldehyde

Most of the **ethanol** in the blood is metabolized in the liver. It is **converted into acetaldehyde by three enzyme systems** present in the liver, namely:(i) alcohol dehydrogenases (ADHs), (ii) CYPs (cytochrome P-450 enzymes), and (iii) catalase (least important).

- **ADH:** ADH (alcohol dehydrogenase) is present in the cytoplasm of the liver cells and is the **main enzyme system involved in alcohol metabolism at low concentrations**. It is the most important pathway in the cytosol where ADH **produces acetaldehyde**.
- **CYPs (cytochrome P-450 enzymes):** When blood alcohol levels are high, the microsomal (present in microsomes) ethanol-oxidizing system (MEOS) participates in ethanol metabolism. It is responsible for ≥10% of ethanol oxidation high blood alcohol concentrations. The system involves CYPs particularly the CYP2E1 isoform, present in the smooth ER. It can also generate ROS (reactive oxygen species). Alcohol induces P-450 enzymes. Hence, alcoholics have increased susceptibility to other compounds metabolized by the same enzyme system. These include drugs (acetaminophen, cocaine), anesthetics, carcinogens, and industrial solvents. However, when alcohol level in the blood is at high concentrations, alcohol competes with other CYP2E1 substrates and may delay the catabolism of other drugs. This may potentiate the effects of these drugs.
- **Catalase:** It is present in peroxisomes and is of minor importance. It metabolizes only about 5% of alcohol.

Formation of acetate

Acetaldehyde (produced by the three systems mentioned above) is **converted to acetate** by acetaldehyde dehydrogenase (ALDH) present in the mitochondria. The acetate is then used in the mitochondrial respiratory chain or in lipid synthesis.

Toxic Effects of Alcohol

Ethanol metabolism produces several toxic effects and the most important of are as follows:

Low expression of aldehyde dehydrogenase (ALDH): Acetaldehyde is the direct product of alcohol oxidation produced in liver and has many toxic effects. Some of the acute effects of alcohol are due to acetaldehyde. The efficiency of alcohol metabolism varies among populations. It depends on the expression levels of two enzymes involved in alcohol metabolism namely ADH (alcohol dehydrogenase) and ALDH (acetaldehyde dehydrogenase) and the presence of genetic variants that alter activity of these two enzymes. Normal allele of ALDH is termed ALDH2*1. In some populations, there is very low ALDH activity due to the substitution of lysine for glutamine at residue 487. This produces an inactive variant of ALDH designated as ALDH2*2. The ALDH2*2 protein has dominant-negative activity. Thus, even one copy of the ALDH2*2 allele significantly reduces ALDH enzyme activity. **Individuals homozygous for the ALDH2*2 allele is completely unable to oxidize acetaldehyde and cannot tolerate alcohol**. They develop nausea, flushing, tachycardia, and hyperventilation after the alcohol ingestion.

Decreased NAD and increased NADH: Alcohol is oxidized to acetaldehyde by ADH (alcohol dehydrogenase). During this process of alcohol oxidation, there is reduction of nicotinamide adenine dinucleotide (NAD) to NADH (reduced form of nicotinamide adenine dinucleotide). This results in decrease in NAD and increase in NADH. In the liver, NAD is required for oxidation of fatty acid as well for the conversion of lactate into pyruvate. Deficiency of NAD due to alcohol is a main cause of the fat accumulation in the liver of alcoholics. The increase in the NADH/NAD ratio in alcoholics also causes lactic acidosis.

Generation of ROS and cytokines: Metabolism of ethanol in the liver by CYP particularly by CYP2E1 isoform produces ROS (reactive oxygen species). ROS cause lipid peroxidation of cell membranes of hepatocyte and damages the cells. Also, alcohol also stimulates the release of endotoxin (lipopolysaccharide) from gram negative bacteria in the intestinal flora. This in turn stimulates the generation of tumor necrosis factor (TNF) and other cytokines from macrophages and Kupffer cells. All these produce damage to liver cells.

Adverse Effects of Ethanol

Alcohol abuse (improper/bad use) is a widespread hazard and claims many more lives hazardous than illicit drugs (e.g., cocaine and opiates). Worrisome feature is that many present young generations suffer from alcohol abuse disorder (AUD). AUD is a chronic relapsing brain disease. It is characterized by an impaired ability to stop or control alcohol use in spite of adverse social, occupational, or health consequences. Alcohol abuse may lead to death either directly or due to accidents caused by drunken driving and alcohol-related homicides and suicides, and due to cirrhosis of the liver. The adverse effects of ethanol can be classified as acute or chronic.

Acute alcoholism

Alcohol produces its effects mainly on the CNS. Alcohol acutely reduces neuronal activity and has similar behavioral effects as in other depressants, (e.g., benzodiazepines and barbiturates). It may also produce reversible hepatic and gastric damage, if alcohol consumption is discontinued. Acute alcohol intoxication may cause fatalities from motor vehicle accidents.

- **Liver:** Even moderate intake of alcohol produces fatty change or hepatic steatosis. It is characterized by accumulation of multiple fat droplets in the cytoplasm of hepatocytes.
- **Gastric damage:** It may induce acute gastritis and ulceration.
- **Central nervous system:** In the CNS, alcohol acts as a depressant. It first affects subcortical structures (probably the high brain stem reticular formation) that modulate cerebral cortical activity. As a result, there is stimulation and produces disordered cortical, motor, and intellectual behavior. In a normal individual, intellectual behavioral changes can be observed at low alcohol concentrations (below 50 mg/dL). Levels above 80 mg/dL are usually associated with slower reaction times and gross incoordination. The cortical neurons and then lower medullary centers become depressed, including those that regulate respiration. Most individuals become comatose at levels above 300 mg/dL, and at concentrations above 400 mg/dL, death from respiratory arrest/failure is common.

Chronic alcoholism

Q. Write a short note on diseases and cancers associated with chronic alcoholism.

Chronic alcoholism: It is defined as regular intake of sufficient amount of alcohol (ethanol) to injure an individual socially, psychologically, or physically. Alcoholism is addiction to ethanol in which there are features of dependence and withdrawal symptoms. It can cause acute and chronic toxic effects on the body. Alcoholism is more common in men, but the number of female alcoholics is gradually increasing.

Chronic alcoholics usually develop CNS tolerance to alcohol and may easily tolerate blood alcohol levels of 100–200 mg/dL. Most alcohol-related disorders are due to the toxic effects of alcohol itself. Chronic alcoholism can affect any organs and tissues, but main effects are found in the liver and stomach. Chronic alcoholics have significant morbidity and shortened life span. This is mainly due to damage to the liver, GI tract, CNS, cardiovascular system, and pancreas.

Liver: It is the main organ affected by chronic alcoholism. It can produce alcoholic liver disease which includes (i) fatty change (steatosis), (ii) alcoholic hepatitis, and (iii) cirrhosis. Cirrhosis is associated with portal hypertension and also is a risk factor for hepatocellular carcinoma. Any alcoholic beverage (beer, wine, whiskey, hard cider, etc.) consumed in excess produces cirrhosis which in turn depends on the total dose of alcohol.

Gastrointestinal tract: Esophagus and stomach are directly affected by alcohol. Chronic alcoholism can cause reflux esophagitis, massive bleeding from gastritis, peptic/gastric ulcer, or esophageal varices (complication of cirrhosis). Violent retching may cause tears at the esophageal-gastric junction (Mallory-Weiss syndrome). Small intestine mucosal cells may show variety of absorptive abnormalities and ultrastructural changes. Alcohol inhibits active transport of amino acids, thiamine, and vitamin B_{12}.

Nervous system: General cortical atrophy, cerebellar degeneration of the brain, and optic neuropathy are common in chronic alcoholics. Most of the characteristics of brain diseases in alcoholics are probably due to nutritional deficiency.

- **Wernicke encephalopathy:** It is due to nutritional thiamine (vitamin B1) deficiency which is common in chronic alcoholics. It is characterized by mental confusion, ataxia, abnormal ocular motility, and polyneuropathy.
- **Korsakoff psychosis:** It is due to thiamine deficiency. Thiamine deficiency may be associated with chronic alcoholism. Korsakoff psychosis is a late complication of persistent Wernicke encephalopathy. It is characterized by memory deficits (amnesia), confusion, and behavioral changes.
- **Alcoholic cerebellar degeneration:** It produces progressive unsteadiness of gait, ataxia, incoordination, and reduced deep tendon reflex activity.
- **Central pontine myelinolysis:** It is caused by electrolyte imbalance, usually after electrolyte therapy following an alcoholic binge or during withdrawal. In this condition, patient presents with a progressive weakness of bulbar muscles that terminates in respiratory paralysis.
- **Polyneuropathy:** Peripheral neuropathy is common in chronic alcoholics. It is usually due to deficiencies of thiamine and other B vitamins. The most common complaints include numbness, paresthesias, pain, weakness, and ataxia.
- **Amblyopia (impaired vision):** It may be due to alcohol-related decreases in tissue vitamin A.

Cardiovascular system: Chronic alcoholism produces various effects on the cardiovascular system.

- **Alcoholic (congestive) cardiomyopathy:** Chronic alcoholism can cause myocardial injury and produce dilated congestive cardiomyopathy called as alcoholic cardiomyopathy.
- **Arrhythmias:** Alcoholics are more susceptible to arrhythmias and sudden, fatal arrhythmias may cause sudden death.
- **Coronary heart disease:** Heavy alcohol consumption and the liver injury associated with it may be associated with decreased levels of high-density lipoprotein (HDL). This increases the risk of coronary heart disease. On the contrary moderate amounts of alcohol consumption, or "social drinking" (one to two drinks a day) may increase serum levels of HDLs and inhibit platelet aggregation. This may provide significant.
- **Hypertension:** There may be increased incidence of hypertension in chronic alcoholics.

Pancreatitis: Excess alcohol intake increases the risk of both acute and chronic pancreatitis. Chronic calcifying pancreatitis in alcoholism produces severe pain, pancreatic insufficiency, and pancreatic stones.

Effects on fetus: Infants born to mothers who consume alcohol (even in low amounts) during pregnancy (especially during the first trimester) can show a group of abnormalities that together constitute the **fetal alcohol syndrome** (FAS). These abnormalities in the new-born consists of microcephaly, growth retardation and facial abnormalities (dysmorphology, neurologic dysfunction), and other congenital anomalies. However, about 6% of the infants of alcoholic mothers develop the full syndrome. More commonly it is associated with less severe abnormalities, such as mental retardation (reduction of mental functions in older children), intrauterine growth retardation, and minor dysmorphic features.

Carcinogenesis: Chronic alcohol consumption is associated with an increased incidence of cancers of the oral cavity, esophagus, larynx, liver (increased in patients with alcoholic cirrhosis), and probably, breast in females than in the general population. The mechanisms of the carcinogenic effect are not known. The risk is markedly more if there is concurrent smoking or the use of smokeless tobacco.

Malnutrition: Alcohol provides substantial energy, but is often consumed at the expense of food (empty calories). Thus, chronic alcoholism may be associated with malnutrition and deficiencies, particularly of the B vitamins (such as thiamine deficiency).

Hematopoietic system: Megaloblastic anemia is not uncommon in alcoholics. It may be due to dietary deficiency of folic acid and decreased absorption of folate by the small intestine in alcoholics. Chronic ethanol intoxication may directly increase the mean corpuscular volume (MCV) of RBCs. In patients with alcoholic cirrhosis, the spleen is often enlarged by portal hypertension. In these patients, hypersplenism may cause hemolytic anemia. Transient thrombocytopenia may develop after acute alcohol intoxication and may produce bleeding. Platelet aggregation is impaired by alcohol and may also contribute to bleeding.

Endocrine system: Male alcoholics may develop feminization and loss of libido and potency. They may also develop gynecomastia (enlargement of breasts), loss of body hair, and a female distribution of pubic hair (female escutcheon). Some of these are due to impaired estrogen metabolism in chronic liver disease. But many of the changes (especially testicular atrophy) may occur even without any liver disease. Chronic alcoholics have lower levels of circulating testosterone. Alcohol has a direct toxic effect on the testes and causes male sexual impairment.

Bone: Chronic alcoholism, especially in postmenopausal women predisposes to osteoporosis. Interestingly, it may be noted that moderate consumption of alcohol may be protective against osteoporosis. Male alcoholics are likely to have high incidence of aseptic necrosis of the head of the femur.

Immune system: Chronic alcoholics may be prone to many infections (particularly pneumonias) with microorganisms that are unusual in the general population (e.g., *Haemophilus influenzae*).

Chronic alcoholism and associated diseases (main effects) are summarized in **Box 2**.

INJURY BY THERAPEUTIC DRUGS AND DRUGS OF ABUSE

Drug injury may be due to use of therapeutic drugs (adverse drug reactions) or nontherapeutic agents (drug abuse).

Box 2: Chronic alcoholism and associated diseases (main effects).

Liver: Fatty liver, alcoholic hepatitis, cirrhosis, and an increased risk of hepatocellular carcinoma

GI tract: Massive bleeding from gastritis, gastric ulcer, or esophageal varices (associated with cirrhosis). Impaired small intestinal absorption

CNS: Thiamine deficiency resulting in peripheral neuropathies and the Wernicke–Korsakoff syndrome, cerebral atrophy, cerebellar degeneration, and optic neuropathy

CVS: Dilated congestive cardiomyopathy (alcoholic cardiomyopathy), arrhythmias, and increased incidence of hypertension

Pancreas: Increased risk of acute and chronic pancreatitis

Effects on fetus: Consumption during pregnancy can cause fetal alcohol syndrome

Carcinogenesis: Increased incidence of cancers of the oral cavity, esophagus, liver, and, possibly, breast in females

Malnutrition and deficiencies of B vitamins

Hematopoietic system: Megaloblastic anemia, hemolytic anemia

Endocrine system: Feminization, loss of libido and potency, gynecomastia, and testicular atrophy in male alcoholics

Bone: Osteoporosis and aseptic necrosis of bone

Injury by Therapeutic Drugs (Adverse Drug Reactions)

The beneficial effects of drugs are also associated with the inescapable risk of untoward effects. Iatrogenic drug injury refers to the unintended side effects and risks associated with therapeutic or diagnostic drugs prescribed by physicians. These side effects are also called adverse drug reactions (ADRs). Thus, ADRs are untoward effects of drugs that develop following conventional therapeutic settings. ADRs to pharmaceuticals drugs are extremely common in the practice of medicine. It is observed in almost 5–7% of patients admitted to the hospitals and of these reactions, 2–12% are fatal. Untoward effects of drugs may result from (i) overdose, (ii) exaggerated physiologic responses, (iii) a genetic predisposition, (iv) hypersensitivity reactions, (v) interactions with other drugs, and (vi) other unknown mechanism. Commonly ADRs are due to direct actions of the drug (due to exaggerated physiologic responses or a genetic predisposition), or to immunologically based hypersensitivity reactions. Drug-induced hypersensitivity reactions most commonly present as skin rashes. Sometimes adverse reactions may mimic autoimmune disorders such as systemic lupus erythematosus (SLE) or produce immunohemolytic anemia or immune thrombocytopenia. ADRs much more likely to develop in older individuals (above 65 years).

Adverse reactions can also be classified in two broad groups. **Type A reactions** develop due to exaggeration of an intended pharmacologic action of the drug (e.g., increased bleeding with anticoagulants or bone marrow suppression with antineoplastic agents). **Type B reactions** develop due to toxic effects unrelated to the intended pharmacologic actions. Common ADRs and the drugs or agents causing reactions are presented in **Table 6**.

Anticoagulants

The two oral anticoagulants drugs that most frequently cause adverse reactions are the **warfarin and dabigatran**. Warfarin is an antagonist of vitamin K, and dabigatran is a direct inhibitor of thrombin. Two main complications with both of these anticoagulant drugs are (i) **bleeding**, which can be fatal, and (ii) **thrombotic complications** such as embolic stroke following undertreatment. Warfarin is inexpensive drug and its effects are easy to monitor. However, many drugs and foods rich in vitamin K either interfere with its metabolism or nullify its function. So, it is difficult to maintain anticoagulation in a relatively safe therapeutic range. Though there are no pharmacologic interactions of drugs with dabigatran metabolism, many bleeding complications can occur. This drug is mainly used to prevent thromboembolism in patients with at high risk for thrombotic stroke (e.g., atrial fibrillation).

Menopausal Hormone Therapy

Menopausal hormone therapy (MHT) previously known as hormone replacement therapy (HRT).

MHT preparations are of different types such as oral estrogen only and oral combined estrogen plus progestogen combinations. The most common type of MHT consists of the estrogens together with a progestogen. It was found that the risk of uterine cancer with estrogen alone therapy was more. Hence, presently it is used only in hysterectomized women. MHT is given to women for diverse reasons. These include to

Table 6: Common adverse drug reactions and the drugs or agents causing reactions.

Common adverse drug reaction	*Major drugs/agents causing reactions*
Bone marrow and blood cells	
• Granulocytopenia, aplastic anemia, pancytopenia	Antineoplastic agents, immunosuppressive drugs, chloramphenicol
• Hemolytic anemia, thrombocytopenia	Penicillin, quinidine, methyldopa, heparin
Cutaneous manifestations	
• Urticaria, macules, papules, vesicles, exfoliative dermatitis, petechiae, fixed drug eruptions, abnormal pigmentation	Antineoplastic agents, sulfonamides, hydantoins, few antibiotics, and many other agents
Systemic manifestations	
• Anaphylaxis	Penicillin
• Lupus erythematosus syndrome (drug-induced lupus)	Hydralazine, procainamide
• Bleeding	Warfarin, dabigatran
Cardiac manifestations	
• Arrhythmias	Theophylline, hydantoins, digoxin
• Cardiomyopathy	Doxorubicin, daunorubicin
Pulmonary manifestations	
• Asthma	Salicylates
• Acute pneumonitis	Nitrofurantoin
• Interstitial fibrosis	Busulfan, nitrofurantoin, bleomycin
Hepatic manifestations	
• Fatty change	Tetracycline
• Diffuse liver damage	Halothane, isoniazid, acetaminophen
• Cholestasis	Chlorpromazine, estrogens, contraceptive agents
Renal manifestations	
• Glomerulonephritis	Penicillamine
• Acute tubular necrosis	Aminoglycoside antibiotics, amphotericin B, cyclosporin
• Tubulointerstitial disease with papillary necrosis	Phenacetin, salicylates
Central nervous system manifestations	
• Tinnitus and dizziness	Salicylates
• Acute dystonic reactions and parkinsonian syndrome	Phenothiazine antipsychotics
• Respiratory depression	Sedatives

reduce the severity of distressing symptoms of menopause, protect from osteoporosis and, more recently, to protect from cardiovascular, cerebrovascular and CNS diseases that occur in older women. Initially MHT was given to reduce hot flashes and other symptoms of menopause, and was thought to prevent or slow the progression of osteoporosis and reduce the likelihood of myocardial infarction. However, subsequent studies failed to support some of the presumed beneficial effects of the MHT. Recently it was found that combination MHT treatment increased the risk of breast cancer, stroke, and venous thromboembolism (VTE) and had no effect on the incidence of coronary heart disease. Newer analyses showed that effects of MHT depend on several factors. These include (i) the type of hormone therapy regimen used (combination estrogen-progestin versus estrogen alone), (ii) the age and risk factor status of the woman at the beginning of treatment, (iii) the duration of the treatment, and (iv) probably the dose of hormone, formulation, and route of administration. The current risk/benefit can be summarized as follows:

- **Increased risk of carcinoma of breast:** Use of combination of estrogen-progestin therapy, increases the risk of breast cancer after a median time of 5 to 6 years. When estrogen alone was used in women with hysterectomy there was a borderline reduction in risk of breast cancer. There is no increased risk for ovarian cancer.
- **Protective effect on the development of atherosclerosis:** In women younger than 60 years, MHT may have a protective role on the development of atherosclerosis and coronary disease. There is no protection in women who started MHT at an older age. This protective effects in younger women partly depend on the response of estrogen receptors in healthy vascular endothelium. However, MHT should not be advised for prevention of CVD (cardiovascular disease) or other chronic diseases.
- **Increases the risk of stroke and venous thromboembolism:** MHT increases the risk of stroke and VTE. Thus, there is more risk of developing deep vein thrombosis and pulmonary embolism. The increase in VTE is more during the first 2 years of treatment. It is more in women who have other risk factors. These risk factors for thrombosis include immobilization and hypercoagulable states (e.g., due to prothrombin or factor V Leiden mutations) (refer page 371 and 372). The risks of VTE and stroke are lower when estrogen is given transdermally than by oral route.

Oral Contraceptives

Orally administered hormonal contraceptives (OCs) are the most commonly used method of birth control. Current formulations of OCs contain a synthetic estradiol and a variable amount of a progestin, but some OCs contain only progestins. They act either by preventing ovulation or preventing implantation. Currently used OCs contain a much smaller amount of estrogens (as little as 20 μg of ethinyl estradiol) than the earliest formulations. Transdermal and implantable formulations are also available.

Complications (Fig. 7)

Currently used OCs are associated with fewer side effects. Nevertheless, OCs carry a small risk of complications. These are as follows:

Vascular complications OCs including the newer low-dose (<50 μg of estrogen) preparations are associated with a 2- to 4-fold increased risk of **venous thrombosis (deep vein thrombosis) and pulmonary thromboembolism**. The risk may be even higher with newer third-generation OCs that contain synthetic progestins. Risk of thromboembolism is due to a hypercoagulable state produced by increased synthesis of

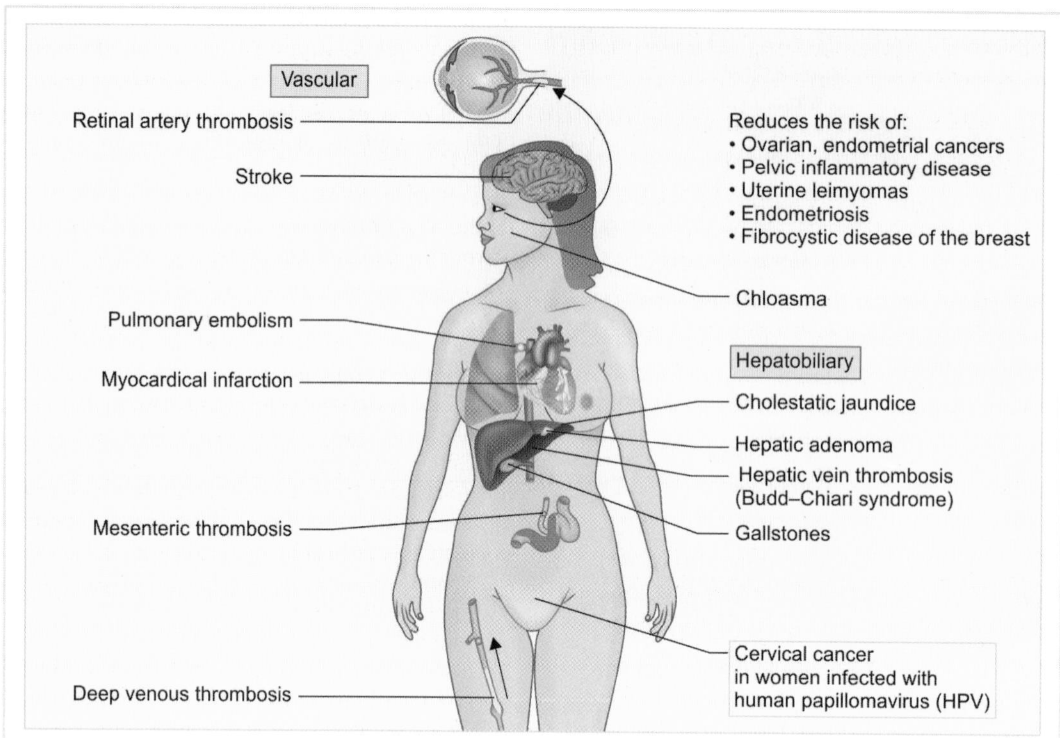

FIG. 7: Complications of oral contraceptives.

coagulation factors by liver. The risk is particularly higher in women who have factor V Leiden mutation.

Neoplastic complications Tumors of female reproductive organs: Several female reproductive organs, especially ovary, endometrium, and breast, are strongly influenced by female hormones.

- **Breast carcinoma:** OCs **do not increase breast cancer** risk.
- **Endometrial cancer and ovarian cancers:** OC use **decreases risk of ovarian and endometrial cancers** by about half, probably by suppressing the production of pituitary gonadotropins. Thus, OCs have a protective effect against these tumors. This effect may last for decades following cessation of OC use.
- **Cervical cancer:** OCs may increase risk of squamous carcinoma of the cervix in women infected with human papillomavirus (HPV).
- **Hepatic adenoma:** It is a rare benign hepatic neoplasm. There is a significant increase in incidence of benign hepatic tumor with use of OCs. This is especially in older women who have used OCs for prolonged periods. The risk increases conspicuously with the duration of use, particularly after 5 years.

Cardiovascular disease Probably OCs do not increase the risk of coronary artery disease in women younger than 30 years or in older women who are nonsmokers. However, the risk is double in women older than 35 years who smoke.

Other complications

- **Chloasma:** OCs may produce increased pigmentation of the malar eminences, called chloasma. This pigmentation is increased by sunlight and persists for a long time even after the discontinuation of contraceptives.
- **Cholelithiasis:** It is more frequent (2-fold increase) with the use of OCs for 4 years or less. OCs accelerate gallstone formation but do not increase its incidence.

Benefits of oral contraceptives

There are certain benefits of OCs. Apart from a significant **reduction in the risk of ovarian and endometrial cancers,** OCs **decrease the risk of pelvic inflammatory disease, uterine leiomyomas, endometriosis, and fibrocystic disease of the breast**.

Acetaminophen

Acetaminophen is the **most commonly used analgesic** and may be used alone or in combination with other therapeutic drugs. It can cause acute liver failure. It may be either due to intentional overdose (attempted suicide) or unintentional therapeutic overdose.

Metabolism (Fig. 8): Normally, after ingestion of acetaminophen, about 95% of its reactive metabolites are detoxified in the liver by phase II enzymes. Detoxification occurs by combining with hepatic GSH (glutathione). It is excreted in the urine as glucuronate or sulfate conjugates. About 5% or less of acetaminophen is metabolized through the activity of CYPs (mainly CYP2E) to N-acetyl-p-benzoquinoneimine (NAPQI). NAPQI is a highly reactive metabolite and normally it conjugates with GSH. But when acetaminophen is taken in large doses, unconjugated NAPQI accumulates and hepatocellular damage or injury occurs. It produces centrilobular necrosis that may progress to liver failure. There are two mechanisms of producing injury by NAPQI namely:

1. Covalent binding of NAPQI to hepatic proteins and forming protein adducts, which causes damage to cellular membranes and mitochondrial dysfunction, and

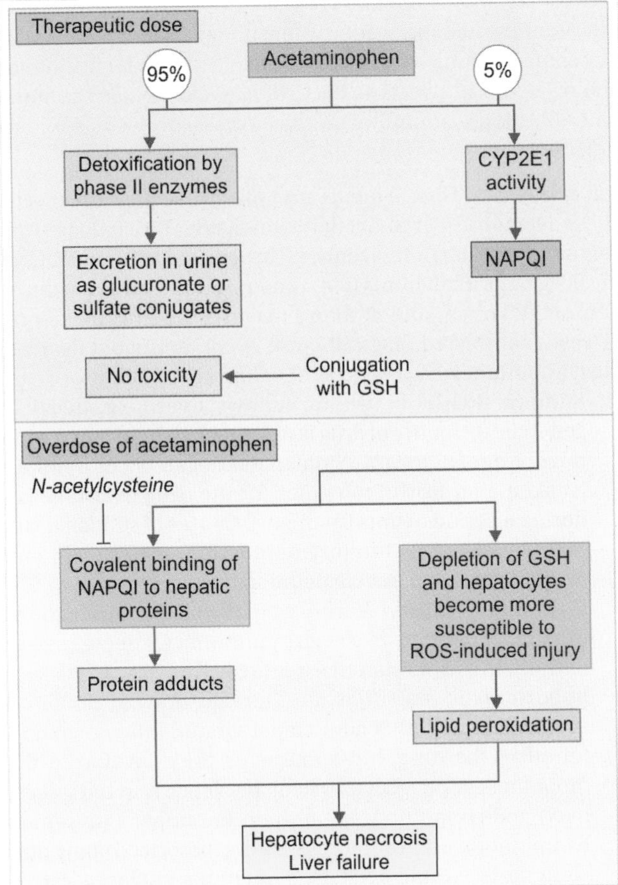

(CYP: cytochrome P-450 enzyme; GSH: glutathione; NAPQI: N-acetyl-p-benzoquinoneimine; ROS: reactive oxygen species)

FIG. 8: Acetaminophen metabolism and toxicity.

2. Depletion of GSH and hepatocytes become more susceptible to ROS-induced injury.

The risk of acetaminophen-related hepatic necrosis is increased in patients receiving drugs such as phenobarbital or phenytoin, which increase the rate of drug metabolism. Both acetaminophen and alcohol use CYP2E in the liver exhausting GSH stores. Hence, acetaminophen toxicity can occur at lower therapeutic doses in chronic alcoholics.

The difference between the usual therapeutic dose (0.5 g) and the toxic dose (15–25 g) of acetaminophen is large. So, acetaminophen is ordinarily very safe drug. Toxicity presents with nausea, vomiting, diarrhea, and sometimes shock. It may be followed, in a few days, by jaundice.

Treatment of overdose of acetaminophen: Early stages (within 12 hours) acetaminophen toxicity is treated by administration of *N*-acetylcysteine. *N*-acetylcysteine reduces the binding of electrophilic metabolites to hepatic proteins and restores GSH levels. However, when there is a serious overdose, liver failure develops. Microscopically, it begins with centrilobular necrosis which may extend to entire lobules of liver. In such cases, only liver transplantation can save life. Some patients may also show concurrent damage to the kidney.

Aspirin (Acetylsalicylic Acid)

Aspirin overdose may occur as an accidental ingestion of a large number of tablets by young children. In adults, overdose is usually suicidal. Rarely, salicylate poisoning may occur due to the excessive use of ointments containing oil of wintergreen (methyl salicylate).

Acute toxicity

Aspirin is usually given in the doses of 75–325 mg/day. Fatal oral dose for children is 2–4 g and for adults, it is about 10–30 g. However, there are reports of survival even after the ingestion of doses five times larger. Acute salicylate overdose causes alkalosis due to stimulation of the respiratory center in the medulla. This is followed by metabolic acidosis. There will be accumulation of pyruvate and lactate caused by uncoupling of oxidative phosphorylation and inhibition of the Krebs cycle. Metabolic acidosis increases the formation of nonionized forms of salicylates. These nonionized forms diffuse into the brain and produce effects ranging from nausea to coma.

Chronic aspirin toxicity (salicylism)

It may develop in individuals who take 3 g or more daily for long periods. They are usually taken for the treatment of chronic pain or inflammatory conditions. Chronic salicylism clinically presents with headaches, dizziness, ringing in the ears (tinnitus), hearing impairment, mental confusion, drowsiness, nausea, vomiting, and diarrhea. Later, individual may develop convulsions and coma.

Morphological features of chronic salicylism Morphological features vary. Usually, it produces an acute erosive gastritis which may manifest as gastrointestinal bleeding and can lead to gastric ulceration. Aspirin acetylates platelet cyclooxygenase and irreversibly blocks the production of thromboxane A_2. Thromboxane A_2 is an activator of platelet aggregation. Hence, chronic toxicity may produce bleeding tendency. This may manifest as petechial hemorrhages in the skin and internal viscera. It may also exacerbate bleeding from gastric ulcerations. Previously analgesic mixtures of aspirin, phenacetin or its active metabolite, and caffeine were used, commonly known as APC. These can cause tubulointerstitial nephritis with renal papillary necrosis, termed as analgesic nephropathy. Currently, these mixtures are taken over by acetaminophen.

Injury by Nontherapeutic Agents (Drug Abuse)

Q. Write short essay on pathological changes in organs in narcotic drug abuse.

Drug abuse is defined as "the use of any substance in a manner that deviates from the accepted medical, social or legal patterns within a given society." In drug abuse, individual repeatedly or chronically uses mind-altering substances (that alter mood and perception) beyond therapeutic or social norms. This may lead to drug addiction and overdose, both serious public health problems. Common drugs of abuse with examples of each class are listed in **Table 7**.

Opioid Narcotics and Its Derivatives

Opioids may be natural and synthetic and opiates include morphine and codeine, derived from poppy plants.

Table 7: Common class of drugs of abuse with examples.
Class (molecular target) with examples
Opioid narcotics and its derivatives [μ **(Mu)** and δ (delta) opioid receptor (agonist)]
• Heroin, hydromorphone
• Oxycodone
• Methadone
• Tramadol
• Meperidine
• Morphine
• Fentanyl
• Codeine
Sedative-hypnotics [GABAA receptor (agonist)]
• Barbiturates
• Ethanol
• Tranquilizers
• Methaqualone
• Glutethimide
• Ethchlorvynol
Psychomotor stimulants [Dopamine transporter (antagonist)]
• Cocaine
Psychomotor stimulants [Serotonin receptors (toxicity)]
• Amphetamines
• 3,4-Methylenedioxymethamphetamine
Phencyclidine-like drugs [NMDA glutamate receptor channel (antagonist)]
• Phencyclidine [PCP (phencyclidine), angel dust]
• Ketamine
Cannabinoids [Endocannabinoids, CB1 cannabinoid, 2-arachidonoylglycerol receptors (agonist)]
• Marijuana
• Hashish
Hallucinogens [Serotonin 5-HT2 receptors (agonist)]
• Lysergic acid diethylamide (LSD)
• Mescaline
• Psilocybin
Inhalants
• Amyl nitrite
• Organic solvents such as those in glue

(GABA: gamma-amino-butyric acid; 5-HT: 5-hydroxytryptamine; NMDA: N-methyl-D-aspartate)

Opioid drugs of abuse include prescription drugs such as oxycodone, hydrocodone, fentanyl, tramadol, and methadone. These oral opioids are prescribed for treatment of pain and may lead to abuse of opoid narcotics.

Heroin

Heroin is a common illicit (forbidden by law) opiate (street drug) used to induce euphoria. Heroin is derived from the poppy plant that is closely related to morphine. Heroin use is more harmful than the use of cocaine. It is a street drug sold on the street. It is cut (diluted) with an agent (usually talc or quinine). This creates not only variable size of the dose and usually the dose is not known to the buyer. Heroin is usually self-administered intravenously or subcutaneously along with any contaminating substances. The usual dosage is effective for about 5 hours. Its effects on the CNS vary and include euphoria, hallucinations, somnolence (sleepiness/drowsiness), and sedation.

Adverse effects Heroin has a range of adverse physical effects. These depend on—(1) the action of the agent, (2) reactions to the contaminants or cutting agents, (3) hypersensitivity reactions to the drug or its adulterants (e.g., quinine adulteration produces neurologic, renal, and auditory toxicity), and (4) incidental diseases contracted due to the use of contaminated needles. Most important adverse effects of heroin are as follows:

- **Sudden death:** It usually follows overdose, because generally the purity of drug is unknown. It may show a wide range from 2% to 90%. Sudden death can occur if heroin is taken after loss of tolerance for the drug over time (as during a period of imprisonment). Causes of sudden death include severe respiratory depression, arrhythmia and cardiac arrest, and severe pulmonary edema.
- **Pulmonary injury:** Various pulmonary complications include moderate to severe pulmonary edema, septic embolism from infective endocarditis, lung abscess, opportunistic infections, and foreign body granulomas against talc and other adulterants. Granulomas are mainly found in the lung, but sometimes they develop in the mononuclear phagocyte system, particularly in the spleen, liver, and lymph nodes that drain the upper extremities. Examination of granulomas under polarized light may show trapped talc crystals, sometimes enclosed within foreign body giant cells.
- **Infections:** Infectious complications are common and usually involve four sites. These sites are—(1) the skin and subcutaneous tissue, (2) heart valves, (3) liver, and (4) lungs. In the endocarditis, vegetations involve right-sided heart valves, particularly the tricuspid valve. Most cases are due to *Staphylococcus aureus*, but fungi and other organisms may also be responsible for infective endocarditis. Sharing of dirty needles may produce viral hepatitis, high incidence of human immunodeficiency virus (HIV) infection in intravenous drug addicts.
- **Skin:** Lesions in the skin are probably the most frequent tell-tale sign of heroin addiction. It may produce acute changes such as abscesses, cellulitis, and ulcerations at the site of subcutaneous injections. Repeated intravenous inoculations produce sequelae at injection sites such as scarring, hyperpigmentation over commonly used veins, and thrombosed veins.
- **Kidneys:** Two kidney diseases frequently observed are—(1) amyloidosis (generally secondary to skin infections) and (2) focal and segmental glomerulosclerosis. Both conditions produce proteinuria and nephrotic syndrome.

Psychomotor Stimulants

Cocaine

Cocaine is an alkaloid extracted from the leaves of the coca plant. It is usually prepared as a water-soluble powder, cocaine hydrochloride. Cocaine is diluted with talcum powder, lactose, or other look-alikes. It can be snorted/sniffing (inhalation through nose), smoking, or dissolved in water and injected subcutaneously or intravenously or orally. Crystallization of the pure alkaloid produces hard nuggets (small lump) of crack. This is called so because when heated to produce smaller pieces and vapors for inhalation, it makes cracking or popping sound. The pharmacologic actions of cocaine and crack are identical, but crack is far more potent. The half-life of cocaine in the blood is about 1 hour.

Cocaine users report extreme euphoria (intense feelings of well-being and happiness) and neurologic stimulation. There is heightened sensitivity to a variety of stimuli. These features make it as one of the most addictive drugs.

Mode of action: Cocaine facilitates neurotransmission both in the CNS and at adrenergic nerve endings. Neurotransmitters are chemical messengers that transmit a message from a nerve cell across the synapse to a target cell. Main neurotransmitters involved are dopamine and norepinephrine. These neurotransmitters are first released from the axon and then bind to the receptor site on the dendrite.

- **Central nervous system:** In the CNS, cocaine blocks/inhibits the reuptake of neurotransmitter dopamine. The euphoria effect of cocaine is due to increased dopamine activity in the brain, especially in the so-called mesolimbic dopamine reward pathway.
- **Adrenergic nerve terminals**: Adrenergic nerve terminals are found in the secondary neurons of the sympathetic nervous system (sympathetic nervous system is one of the two divisions of the autonomic nervous system). At adrenergic nerve endings, cocaine blocks/inhibits the reuptake of both epinephrine and norepinephrine but stimulates the presynaptic release of norepinephrine.

Presenting features These include euphoria, paranoia, and hyperthermia due to dopamine activity. With addiction, paranoid states and conspicuous emotional lability occurs. Cocaine overdose produces anxiety and delirium and occasionally produces seizures. The acute and chronic effects of cocaine on various organ systems are as follows:

Cardiovascular effects: These are due to sympathomimetic activity of cocaine which blocks the reuptake of both epinephrine and norepinephrine at adrenergic nerve endings (**Fig. 9**). This leads to the accumulation of these two neurotransmitters (i.e., epinephrine and norepinephrine) in synapses and results in excess stimulation. Clinically it is manifested by tachycardia, hypertension, and peripheral vasoconstriction.

- **Myocardial ischemia:** Cocaine may also produce ischemia of the myocardium by causing coronary artery vasoconstriction and by increasing platelet aggregation and formation of thrombus. These two effects of cocaine increase myocardial oxygen demand and decrease coronary blood flow. Thus, it may lead to myocardial ischemia and myocardial infarction.
- **Arrhythmias:** Cocaine increases sympathetic activity and also disturbs normal ion (K^+, Ca^{2+}, Na^+) transport in the myocardium. This can precipitate lethal arrhythmias.
- **Dilated cardiomyopathy:** Chronic abuse of cocaine may also be associated with the occasional development of a characteristic dilated cardiomyopathy, which may be fatal.

The toxic effects of cocaine on CVS need not be related to dose, and a fatal event can occur in a first-time user with a typical mood-altering dose. Cigarette smoking may aggravate the cocaine-induced coronary vasospasm. Sudden death in otherwise apparently healthy individual due to cardiac arrhythmias and other effects on the heart may occur.

CNS: The most common acute effects of cocaine on the CNS are hyperpyrexia and seizures. Hyperpyrexia is probably due to aberrations of the dopaminergic pathways that control body temperature.

Effects on pregnancy: In pregnant women, cocaine may cause acute reduction in the flow of blood to the placenta. This may produce fetal hypoxia and spontaneous abortion. The fetus of a pregnant woman who is a chronic drug user may show impaired neurologic development.

Other effects in chronic cocaine uses include—(1) perforation of the nasal septum in snorters (who inhales cocaine) and (2) decreased lung diffusing capacity in individuals who inhale the smoke.

Amphetamines and related drugs

Amphetamine is a synthetic, addictive, mood-altering drug.

Methamphetamine: It is an addictive drug, commonly known as "speed" or "meth." Methamphetamines are most commonly

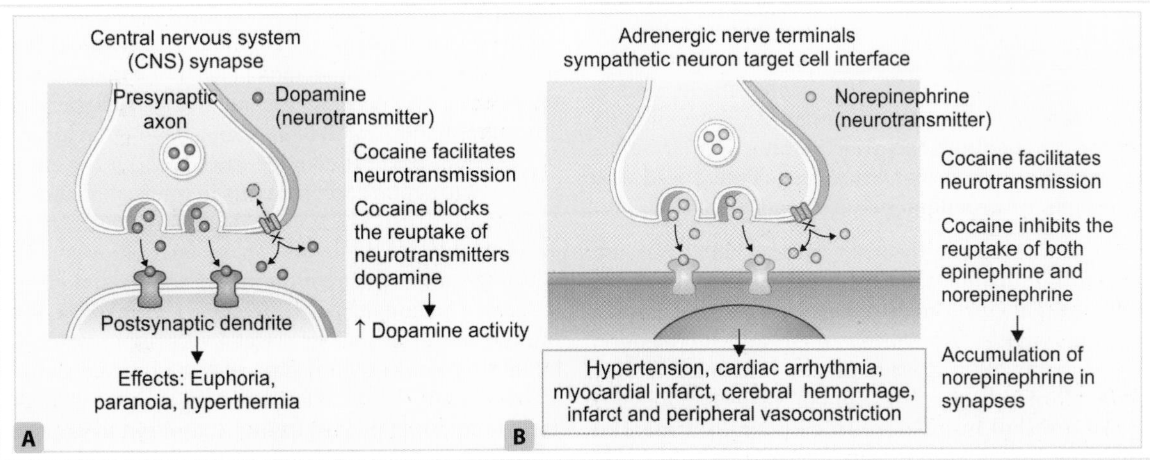

FIGS. 9A AND B: Effect of cocaine on neurotransmission. Cocaine facilitates neurotransmission both in the CNS and at adrenergic nerve endings. (A) In the CNS, cocaine blocks the reuptake of neurotransmitter dopamine. (B) At adrenergic nerve endings, cocaine blocks the reuptake of both epinephrine and norepinephrine but stimulates the presynaptic release of norepinephrine.

used as "crystal meth," which is produced by hydrogenation of ephedrine or pseudoephedrine. Methamphetamine is closely related to amphetamine but has stronger effects in the CNS. In the brain, they are sympathomimetic and act by releasing dopamine. The dopamine inhibits presynaptic neurotransmission at corticostriatal synapses and slows the release of glutamate. Methamphetamine induces euphoria followed by a "crash." The features resemble cocaine in their effects, but have a longer duration of action. Chronic use leads to violent behaviors, confusion, and psychosis marked by paranoia and hallucinations. Amphetamine use may lead to vasculitis of the CNS, and can produce both subarachnoid and intracerebral hemorrhages. Most serious complications of the abuse of amphetamines are seizures, cardiac arrhythmias, and hyperthermia.

Phencyclidine-like Drugs

These include 1-(1-phenylcyclohexyl) piperidine (PCP), or phencyclidine, and ketamine (related anesthetic agents).

Phencyclidine: It is an anesthetic agent having psychedelic or hallucinogenic effects. As a recreational drug, it is known as "angel dust." It may be taken orally, intranasally or by smoking. The anesthetic properties of PCP effect cause reduced capacity to perceive pain. Hence, in addicts it may lead to self-injury and trauma. Apart from the behavioral effects, PCP produces tachycardia and hypertension. High doses may lead to deep coma, seizures, and decerebrate posturing.

Ketamine derivatives: They are taken in low doses approved for treatment of severe depression.

Cannabinoids

Marijuana

Marijuana (or "pot") is one of the illicit drugs and most commonly used. Marijuana is prepared from the leaves of the *Cannabis sativa* plant. It contains the psychoactive substance Δ^9-tetrahydrocannabinol (THC). It is smoked in a hand-rolled cigarette ("joint") and about 5–10% of THC is absorbed during smoking. Marijuana produces euphoria and a sense of relaxation. Many individuals experience a heightened sensory perception (e.g., brighter colors), laughter, altered perception of time, and increased appetite. Marijuana can be used to treat nausea secondary to cancer chemotherapy and to decrease pain in some chronic conditions that are otherwise difficult to treat. During its use, it distorts sensory perception and impairs motor coordination. These acute effects usually disappear within 4–5 hours. With continued use, these changes may progress to cognitive and psychomotor impairments. These impairments include inability to judge time, speed, and distance and may cause automobile accidents.

Effects: Marijuana increases the heart rate and blood pressure (sometimes). In individuals with coronary artery disease, it may produce angina. Chronic smoking of marijuana causes laryngitis, pharyngitis, bronchitis, cough and hoarseness, and may cause asthma-like symptoms with mild airway obstruction. Marijuana cigarettes contain many carcinogens that are also present in tobacco. In contrast to a tobacco cigarette, a marijuana cigarette increases three times the amount of tar inhaled and retained in the lungs. This may be because in marijuana smoking, there is a larger puff volume, deeper inhalation, and longer breath holding. Few heavy users develop cannabis hyperemesis syndrome, characterized by intractable nausea and vomiting that subside with cessation of use. Chronic use of marijuana, especially if the exposure started during adolescence, may give rise to marijuana use disorder.

Hallucinogens

Hallucinogens are a group of chemically unrelated drugs. They alter perception and sensory experience.

Lysergic acid diethylamide (LSD): It is a most potent hallucinogen that is currently not used. It causes perceptual distortion of the senses, interferes with logical thought, alters time perception, and a sense of depersonalization. Acutely, LSD has unpredictable effects on mood, affect, and thought, sometimes leading to bizarre and dangerous behaviors. It produces sympathomimetic effects such as tachycardia, hypertension, and hyperthermia. Large overdoses cause coma, convulsions, and respiratory arrest.

Organic Solvents

Various commercial preparations that contain organic solvents include fingernail polish, glues, plastic cements, and lighter fluid. Recreational inhalation of these organic solvents may be observed among adolescents. All these organic solvents are sniffed. The active ingredients of these organic solvents include benzene, carbon tetrachloride, acetone, xylene, and toluene. Many of these organic solvents are also industrial solvents and reagents. Hence, chronic low level occupational exposure occurs. They are all CNS depressants, though initial effects (e.g., with xylene) may be excitatory. Acute intoxication with organic solvents resembles intoxication with alcohol. Large doses may produce nausea and vomiting, hallucinations, and eventually coma. Respiratory depression and death may occur. Either chronic exposure or abuse of organic solvents may damage the brain, kidneys, liver, lungs, and hematopoietic system. For example, benzene is a bone marrow toxin and associated with the acute myelogenous leukemia.

Complications of Intravenous Drug Abuse (Fig. 10)

Similar to oral drug abuse, intravenous drug abuse may develop reactions related to pharmacologic or physiologic effects of substance abuse. Apart from these, the most common complications are caused due to introduction of infectious organisms by a parenteral route. Most infections occur at the site of injection and include cutaneous abscesses, cellulitis, and ulcers. When these infections heal, "track marks" will persist. These areas may become hypopigmented or hyperpigmented. Thrombophlebitis of the veins may develop at draining sites of injection. Bacteria may be introduced intravenously and may lead to septic complications in internal organs. Bacterial endocarditis, usually due to *Staphylococcus aureus*, occurs on both sides of the heart. These infected vegetations may embolize and cause pulmonary, renal, and intracranial abscesses; meningitis; osteomyelitis; and mycotic aneurysms. Intravenous drug abusers are at a very high risk for AIDS and hepatitis B and C. Viral hepatitis may progress to chronic active hepatitis. They may also develop necrotizing angiitis, and glomerulonephritis. Immune reaction to impurities that contaminate illicit drugs may produce immune complexes. This may give rise to a focal glomerulosclerosis ("heroin nephropathy"). Intravenous injection of talc (used to dilute pure drug) may produce foreign body granulomas in the

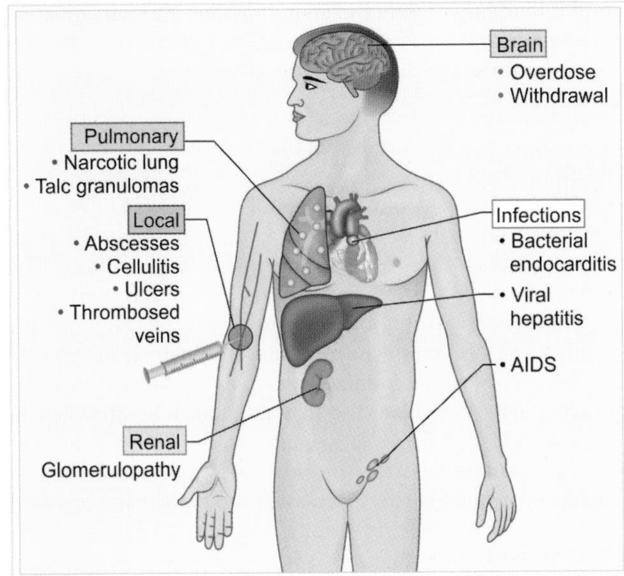

FIG. 10: Complications of intravenous drug abuse.

lung. These may be severe and produce interstitial pulmonary fibrosis.

Drug Addiction in Pregnant Women

Use of drugs by pregnant women may cause addiction of newborn infants. These infants often show a full-blown withdrawal syndrome. Development of the drug withdrawal syndrome in the fetus during labor may result in excessive fetal movements and increased oxygen demand. This increases the risk of intrapartum hypoxia and meconium aspiration. If labor occurs when maternal drug levels are high, the born infants usually have respiratory depression. Higher incidence of toxemia of pregnancy and premature labor is common in mothers who are addicted to drugs. There are other ways by which illicit drugs used during pregnancy injure the developing fetus. For example, pregnant women using cocaine more commonly develop abruptio placenta and premature labor. Infants of such mothers are usually of low birth weight and develop CNS and other anomalies and show impaired brain function after birth.

INJURY BY PHYSICAL AGENTS

Injury induced by physical agents can be divided into the four different categories—(1) Mechanical trauma, (2) Thermal injury, (3) Electrical injury, and (4) Injury produced by ionizing radiation.

Mechanical Trauma

Mechanical trauma may cause a variety of forms of physical injuries/damage. The effect of mechanical trauma is related to the—(1) shape of the object causing mechanical trauma, (2) the amount of force transmitted (energy exerted) to the tissue, (3) the rate at which the transfer occurs, and (4) the area of the body (tissue or organs) involved. The damage produced by bone and head injuries is unique. All soft tissues react similarly to mechanical trauma. Destruction of cells and tissues resulting from mechanical trauma ranges from mild abrasion to severe lacerating trauma. These **patterns of injury can be divided into abrasions, contusions, lacerations, incised wounds, and puncture wounds**. Other wounds include those produced by shooting, stabbing, blunt force, traffic accidents, and other causes. Direct trauma to cell causes cell death, blood loss or obstruction of blood flow, and hypoxia. Nonpenetrating trauma usually results from physical impact with a blunt object (e.g., fist, a car steering wheel, or the pavement). Surgery is a common cause of tissue trauma. Trauma-induced inflammatory swelling may further compromise injured tissues.

Contusion: Contusion is a localized mechanical injury with focal hemorrhage. A mechanical force with sufficient energy may disrupt capillaries and venules within an organ or tissue. It may result in hemorrhage in tissue spaces outside the vascular compartment. It forms a discrete extravascular blood pool within the tissue and is called as hematoma. Initially, the deoxygenated blood produces blue to blue-black discoloration of the area (classical example is "black eye"). Macrophages ingest the RBCs in the hematoma and convert their hemoglobin to bilirubin. This changes the color of area from blue to yellow. Both mobilization of the pigment by macrophages and further metabolism of bilirubin cause the yellow color to fade to yellowish green. Then it gradually disappears.

Abrasion: It is a skin defect caused by crushes or scrapes. The disruptive mechanical force may be a site for portal of entry for microorganisms.

Laceration: It is a split or tear of the skin. Lacerations result from mechanical force that has an impact stronger than that causing an abrasion. Usually it is the result of unidirectional displacement. When lacerations have crushed margins, they are called abraded lacerations.

Wounds: These are mechanical disruptions of tissue integrity. An incision is an intentional opening in the skin by a sharp cutting instrument (e.g., a surgeon's scalpel). Incisions have sharp edges and, there is no or only minimal loss of tissue. Deep penetrating wounds occur due to high-velocity projectiles (e.g., bullets) and are often misleading. This is because the energy of the missile (object which is forcibly propelled at a target) as it passes through the body may be released at sites distant from the entrance itself. For example, bullets rotate and produce a well-defined and usually round entrance wound. Once they enter the flesh, they may fragment, tumble, or actually explode. This may produce considerable tissue damage and the exit wound is large and ragged.

Thermal Injury

Both excessive heat and excessive cold cause injury. Burns are the most common cause of thermal injury.

Thermal Burns

Majority burns are caused by fire or by scalding. Scalding is burn that develops with hot liquid or steam and is the major cause of injury in children. Following factors determine the clinical significance of a burn injury:

- Depth of the burns
- Percentage of body surface involved
- Internal injuries due to inhalation of hot and toxic fumes
- Promptness and efficacy of therapy: This includes fluid and electrolyte management and prevention or control of infections of burn wounds.

Classification of burns (Fig. 11)

Burns were formerly classified according to the depth of the injury as first degree to fourth degree burns. First-degree burns are the most superficial. Currently, burns are classified as superficial, partial-thickness, and full-thickness.

- **Superficial burns:** These were formerly known as first-degree burns. In this type, the wounds are confined to the epidermis.
- **Partial-thickness burns:** These were formerly known as second-degree burns. They involve injury to the dermis.
- **Full-thickness burns:** These were formerly known as third-degree burns. In this, injury extends to the subcutaneous tissue. Full-thickness burns may also involve and damage to underlying muscle tissue underneath the subcutaneous tissue. These types of full-thickness burns were formerly known as fourth-degree burns.

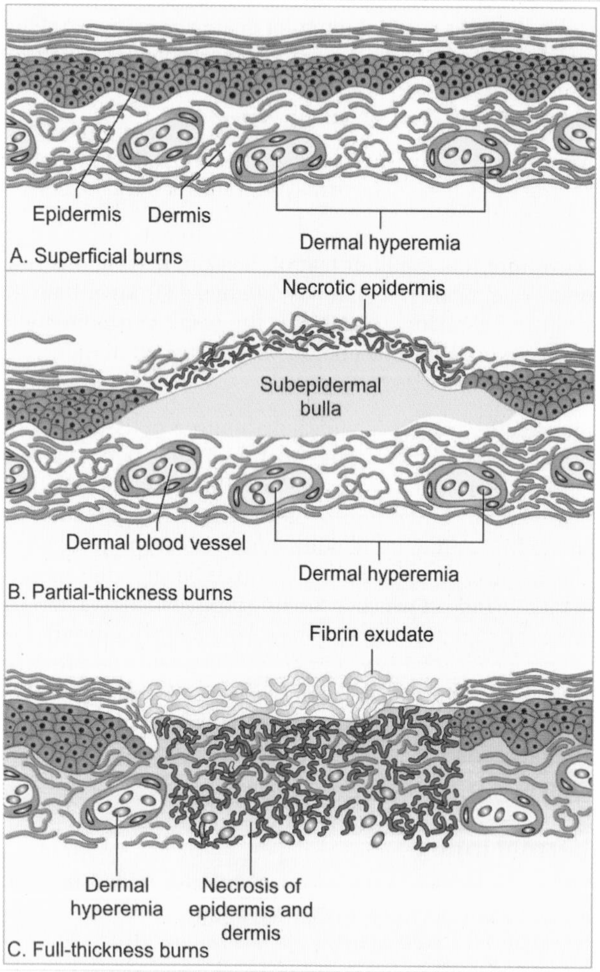

FIGS. 11A TO C: Classification of cutaneous burns. (A) Superficial skin burn shows only dilation of the dermal blood vessels. (B) In partial-thickness burn, there is necrosis of the epidermis and fluid collects below the necrotic epidermis to form a bulla. (C) In full-thickness burn, both the epidermis and dermis show necrosis.

Complications: Sepsis, shock, and respiratory insufficiency are the main complications that may be greatest threats to life in burn patients.

- **Widespread vascular leakage:** When burns involve >20% of the body surface, there is a rapid (within hours) shift of body fluids from the circulating blood into the interstitial compartments due to widespread vascular leakiness. This occurs throughout the body due to the systemic inflammatory response syndrome (refer page 323) and may lead to shock. Generalized vascular leakiness produces generalized edema, including pulmonary edema and it can be severe.
- **Hypermetabolic state:** In burns, a hypermetabolic state develops due to excess loss of heat and there is an increased requirement for nutritional support. When the burn involves >40% of the body surface, the resting metabolic rate doubles.
- **Infections:** The burn area is an ideal site for the growth of microorganisms. Almost all burns become colonized with bacteria. The factors favoring infections are—(1) the serum and debris provide nutrients, (2) the burn injury reduces blood flow to the site of wound and prevent the effective inflammatory responses. Infections are defined by the presence of>10^5 bacteria per gram of tissue, and invasive local infection is defined by the presence of >10^5 bacteria per gram in unburned adjacent tissue. The most common opportunist bacteria producing infections is *Pseudomonas aeruginosa*. However, antibiotic-resistant strains of other common hospital-acquired bacteria may also cause infections. These include methicillin-resistant *S. aureus*, and fungi (e.g., *Candida* species). There may also be impairment of both innate and adaptive immune responses due to systemic inflammatory response syndrome (SIRS). The organism from local site may seed the bloodstream to produce bacteremia and also release toxic substances such as endotoxin. Septic shock with renal failure and/or acute respiratory distress syndrome may develop.
- **Injury to the airways and lungs:** Within 24–48 hours after the burn, injury to the airways and lungs may develop. This may be due to the direct effect of heat on the mouth, nose, and upper airways or the inhalation of heated air and noxious gases in the smoke.
  - **Inflammation of the upper airways by water-soluble gases:** Especially in the upper airways, water-soluble gases (e.g., chlorine, sulfur oxides, ammonia) may react with water to form acids or alkalis. They produce inflammation and swelling thereby causing partial or complete airway obstruction.
  - **Inflammation of lower airways by lipid-soluble gases:** For example, lipid soluble gases such as nitrous oxide and products of burning plastics, may reach deeper airways, producing pneumonitis.
- **Hypertrophic scars:** They may develop at the site of the original burn and is a common complication of burn injury. It is characterized by excessive deposition of collagen in the healing wound bed. There may be also development of contractures (Fig. 64 of Chapter 8).

MORPHOLOGY

Gross: Full-thickness burns appear white or charred, dry, and painless. This painless is due to destruction of nerve endings. Partial-thickness burns, depending on the depth of burns, are pink or mottled with blisters. These are painful.

Microscopy: The devitalized tissue in the burn site shows coagulative necrosis, adjacent to vital tissue. It is accompanied by quick accumulation of inflammatory cells and marked exudation of fluid.

Hyperthermia

Q. Write short essay on hyperthermia.

Definition: Hyperthermia or fever is defined as an elevation of the core body temperature above the normal diurnal range of 36–37.5°C due to failure of thermoregulation.

Hyperthermia occurs due to the following mechanisms namely—(1) increased production of heat, (2) reduced elimination of heat from the body (due to an abnormal response of the thermal regulatory center) **or (3) a disturbance of the thermal regulatory center itself. Hyperthermia can also develop due to conduction of heat into the body faster than the system can clear it.** Prolonged exposure to elevated ambient (immediate surroundings) temperatures can cause heat cramps, heat exhaustion, and heat stroke.

Heat cramps: This is produced due to the loss of electrolytes through sweating. Cramping is sudden, involuntary, spasmodic contraction of a muscle or group of voluntary muscles. It is the hallmark of heat cramps. It is usually in association with vigorous exercise. Heat-dissipating (heat drive off) mechanisms are able to maintain normal core body temperature during heat cramps.

Heat exhaustion: It develops suddenly, with prostration and collapse. It is associated with hypovolemia due to dehydration. Heat exhaustion occurs due to failure of the cardiovascular system to compensate for hypovolemia. Collapse is brief usually if the individual victim is rehydrated. Usually after rehydration, equilibrium is spontaneously re-established.

Heat stroke: It develops in association with high ambient temperatures, high humidity, and exertion. It is not mediated by endogenous pyrogens. Individuals who are at a high risk for heat stroke are older adults, persons undergoing intense physical activities (e.g., young athletes and military exercises), and individuals with CVD (cardiovascular disease). In the heat stroke, there is failure of thermoregulatory mechanisms, sweating stops, and the core body temperature rises to >40°C. These lead to multiorgan dysfunction and can be rapidly fatal. Heat stroke is accompanied by marked generalized vasodilation, with peripheral pooling of blood. This reduces the effective volume of circulating blood. Other systemic effects include hyperkalemia, tachycardia, and arrhythmias. Sustained contractions of skeletal muscle in heat stroke can exacerbate the hyperthermia and lead to muscle necrosis (rhabdomyolysis). These are due to nitrosylation of ryanodine receptor 1 (RYR1), present in the sarcoplasmic reticulum of skeletal muscle. The release of calcium from the sarcoplasm is regulated by RYR1. Heat stroke deranges RYR1 function and permits calcium to leak into the cytoplasm. In the cytoplasm, calcium stimulates muscle contraction and heat production.

Malignant hyperthermia: Though the term hyperthermia is used, it is not caused by exposure to high temperatures. It is a genetic disorder due to mutations in genes such as *RYR1* that control calcium levels in skeletal muscle cells. In these individuals, exposure to certain anesthetics during surgery stimulates a rapid increase in levels of calcium in skeletal muscle. This leads to rigidity of muscle and increases production of heat. If untreated, it has a mortality rate of approximately 80%. If this condition is promptly recognized and muscle relaxants are administered, mortality rate falls below 5%.

Hypothermia

Definition: Hypothermia is defined as a core temperature below 35°C (95°F). Prolonged exposure to low ambient temperature causes hypothermia. Hypothermia can result in systemic or focal injury. Examples of focal injury include trench foot or immersion foot. In localized hypothermia of these types, actual tissue freezing does not occur. In frostbite, there is crystallization of tissue water.

Mechanisms of injury by hypothermia:

- **Direct effects:** Hypothermia causes crystallization of intracellular and extracellular water (frostbite). Direct effects are probably due to physical disruptions within cells by high salt concentrations due to crystallization of water.
- **Indirect effects:** They are due to circulatory changes. These effects vary depending on the rate and duration of the reduction of temperature.
    - **Slow chilling:** It may cause vasoconstriction and increase vascular permeability. This in turn produces edema and hypoxia. Such changes are typical of trench foot. Trench foot, or immersion foot syndrome, is a serious condition in which feet being wet for too long. It developed in soldiers during World War I (1914–1918), who spent long time in waterlogged trenches. It causes gangrene and needs amputation.
    - **Sudden and persistent chilling:** It produces vasoconstriction and increases the viscosity of the blood in the local area. This may cause ischemic injury and degenerative changes in peripheral nerves. The vascular injury and edema in this situation, become obvious, only after the temperature begins to return to normal. If the period of ischemia is prolonged, it will produce hypoxic changes and infarction of the affected region (e.g., gangrene of toes or feet).

Generalized hypothermia

Hypothermia may occur in a number of settings. It happens because of overwhelming exposure to cold air temperatures and is frequent in homeless persons. High humidity and wet clothing, sometimes exacerbated by dilation of superficial blood vessels especially after taking agents that impair thermoregulation (e.g., alcohol and some drugs and pharmacologic agents), speeds up the lowering of body temperature. When the body temperature reaches about 90°F, there will be loss of consciousness, bradycardia, and atrial fibrillation.

Cold water immersion: It is acute immersion in water at 4–10°C (39.2–50°F). It reduces central blood flow. Along with reduced core body temperature, there is cooling of the blood perfusing the brain and this results in mental confusion. Tetany makes swimming impossible. This is accompanied by increased vagal discharge and leads to premature ventricular contractions, ventricular arrhythmias, and even fibrillation. The most important factor in causing death is cardiac arrhythmia or sudden cardiac arrest.

Electrical Injury

Electrical injuries develop from contact with low-voltage currents (i.e., in the home and workplace) or high-voltage currents carried by high-power lines or produced by lightning. It is usually fatal. Electrical injury may occur when the cells of the body act as conductors of electricity.

Types: Injuries produced by electrical injury are of two types—(1) burns (by hyperthermic destruction of tissues) and (2) ventricular fibrillation or cardiac and respiratory center failure (result from disruption of nerve impulse conduction such as neural and cardiac impulses). The electric current follows the path of least resistance—through neurons and body fluids. It causes violent muscle contractions, thermal injury, and coagulation in blood vessels.

Extent of damage: Resistance to the flow of electrons results in heat production, which damages the tissues. The type of injury, its severity, and extent of burns depend on the strength (amperage), duration, and path of the electric current within the body.

- **Low voltage current:** Voltage in the household and workplace is usually 220V. Low resistance at the site of contact may occur when the skin at the area of contact is wet. The voltage of 220V is high enough when applied to a low-resistance area (e.g., wet skin) at the site of contact. With this, sufficient current can pass through the body to cause serious injury, including ventricular fibrillation. If the current flow is sustained, the heat generated at the site is sufficient to produce burns at the site of entry and exit as well as in internal organs. Alternating current is usually supplied to most homes. Its peculiarity is that it induces tetanic muscle spasm. So, when a live wire or switch is grasped, irreversible clutching occurs and thereby prolongs the period of current flow. This results in more extensive electrical burns. In some cases, it may induce spasm of the muscles of chest wall producing death from asphyxia.
- **High-voltage current:** Currents generated from high-voltage sources cause similar damage. In these, there is generation of large current flows. Hence, they are more likely to produce paralysis of medullary centers and extensive burns. One of the classic examples of cause of high-voltage electrical injury is lightening.

RADIATION

Q. Write short essay on biological effects of radiation.

Q. Write short essay on delayed complications of ionizing radiations.

Definition: Radiation is emission energy [energy given off by matter (anything that has mass and volume)] that travels in the form of waves (rays) or high-speed particles through space or through a material medium. It can also be simply defined as emission of energy by one body, its transmission or through an intervening medium, and its absorption by another body.

By above definition, radiation consists of the entire electromagnetic spectrum and certain charged particles emitted by radioactive elements. All matter is composed of atoms. An **atom is defined as the smallest particle of a substance that can exist by itself or be combined with other atoms to form a molecule**. Atoms are made up of various parts (**Fig. 12**). Atom has a nucleus that contains minute particles called protons and neutrons. The outer shell of atom contains other particles called electrons. The nucleus of the atom carries a positive electrical charge, whereas the electrons carry a negative electrical charge. These forces within the atom work toward a strong, stable balance by getting rid of excess atomic energy (radioactivity). In that process, unstable nuclei may emit a quantity of energy, and this spontaneous emission is called as radiation.

Physical forms of radiation: Matter gives off energy (radiation) in two basic physical forms.

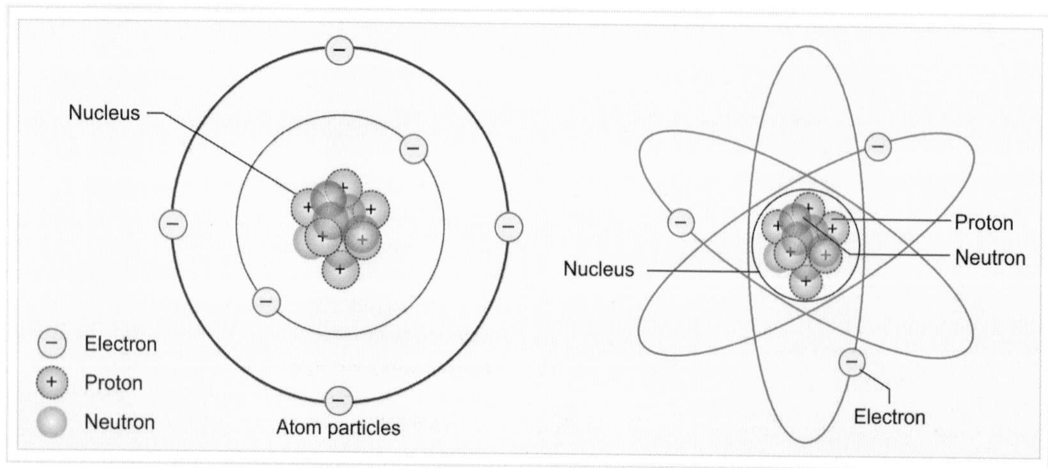

FIG. 12: Various parts of atom has a nucleus that contains minute particles called protons (+) and neutrons. The outer shell of atom contains other particles called electrons. The nucleus of the atom carries a positive electrical charge, whereas the electrons carry a negative electrical charge.

- **Electromagnetic radiation:** This form of radiation is pure energy with no weight and is known as electromagnetic radiation. It is like vibrating or pulsating rays or "waves" of electrical and magnetic energy. Examples of electromagnetic radiation include **sunlight (cosmic radiation), X-rays, radar, and radio waves**.
- **Particle radiation:** It is tiny fast-moving particles that have both energy and mass (weight). Examples includes **alpha (α) particles, beta (β) particles, and neutrons**.

Radioactive decay: Large unstable atoms become more stable by emitting radiation to get rid of excess atomic energy (radioactivity). This radiation can be emitted in the form of positively charged alpha particles, negatively charged beta particles, gamma (γ) rays, or X-rays. Radioisotopes are radioactive isotopes of an element. These are atoms that contain an unstable combination of neutrons and protons, or excess energy in their nucleus. **Radioisotopes lose their radioactivity over time and this process is called radioactive decay**. This gradual loss of radioactivity is measured in half lives. A half-life of a radioactive material is the time it takes one-half of the atoms of a radioisotope to decay by emitting radiation. This time can range from fractions of a second (e.g., radon-220) to millions of years (e.g., thorium-232).

Types of Radiation

Radiation consists of a wide range of energies. Radiation can be divided into two types—(1) Ionizing radiation, and (2) Nonionizing radiations depending on how they affect matter.

Ionizing Radiation

Ionization is the ability of the radiant energy to split water molecules by knocking off orbital electrons (radiolysis). Radiolysis creates activated free radicals. They remove (steal) electrons from other molecules and disrupt chemical bonds. Ionizing radiation (e.g., X-rays, cosmic rays) has sufficient energy and is more energetic than nonionizing radiation. Ionizing radiation passes through material and interacts with atoms. Consequently, it deposits enough energy to break molecular bonds and release (displace or remove) electrons from atoms in a reaction cascade. This electron displacement creates two electrically charged particles (ions). This electron release reaction cascade is termed ionization. They can cause molecular damage and remove tightly bound electrons. Ionizing radiation is a double-edged sword. It is used in medical practice in the treatment of cancer, in diagnostic imaging, and in therapeutic or diagnostic radioisotopes. Electromagnetic (X-rays, γ rays) and particulate (α particles, β particles, protons, neutrons) radiations are all carcinogenic. Radiation is teratogens and can cause developmental anomalies.

Sources and uses: The main sources of ionizing radiation are—(1) High-energy electromagnetic radiations such as X-rays and γ rays (i.e., electromagnetic waves of very high frequencies), (2) High energy neutrons, alpha particles (composed of two protons and two neutrons), and (3) Beta particles, which are essentially electrons.

- **X-rays and γ rays:** They consist of high-energy waves that can travel great distances at the speed of light and usually have a longer and deeper course. They have great ability to penetrate other materials. They produce considerably less damage per unit of tissue. X-rays are used to provide static images of body parts (e.g., teeth, bones), and are also used in industry to find defects in welds (joining together metal parts by heating). Gamma rays (e.g., from cobalt-60) are used to treat cancer and sterilize medical instruments. Though these are able to penetrate other materials, in general, neither γ rays nor X-rays have the ability to make anything radioactive. Several feet of concrete or a few inches of dense material (e.g., lead) are able to block these types of radiations.
- **Alpha particles:** These are charged particles and produce heavy damage in a restricted area. Alpha particles are emitted from naturally occurring materials (e.g., uranium, thorium, and radium) and man-made elements (e.g., plutonium and americium). These alpha emitters are mainly used in very small amounts (e.g., as smoke detectors).
- **Beta particles:** These are similar to electrons and are emitted from naturally occurring materials (e.g., strontium-90). Beta particles are lighter than alpha particles, and usually have a greater ability to penetrate other materials. Thus, beta particles can travel a few feet in the air, and can penetrate skin. However, a thin sheet of metal or plastic or a block of wood can stop beta particles.

Alpha particles and the beta particles of elements such as tritium (^{3}H) and carbon 14 (^{14}C) are of great use scientifically and have few hazards for humans.

Neutrons: These are high-speed nuclear particles that have an ability to penetrate other materials. Neutrons can make objects radioactive.

Major types of ionizing radiations are presented in **Figure 13**.

Ionizing radiation is human-made and mostly originating from medical devices and radioisotopes. These include computed tomography (CT) scans, radionucleotide scans, and radiotherapy. It can produce short- and long-term effects such as fibrosis, mutagenesis, carcinogenesis, and teratogenesis. Ionizing radiation is also used in smoke detectors and to sterilize medical equipment.

Penetrating radiation

It includes uncharged neutrons or high-energy electromagnetic radiations such as X-rays and γ rays.

X-rays and γ rays dissipate energy over a longer, deeper course, and produce considerably less damage per unit of tissue. They affect the skin and deeper tissues.

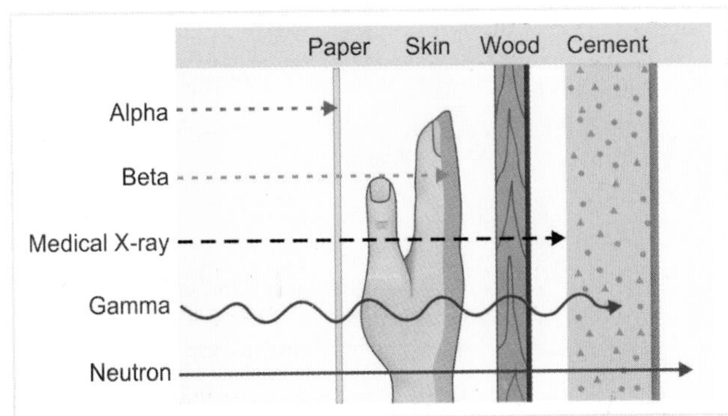

FIG. 13: Major types of ionizing radiations.

Nonpenetrating radiation

It includes charged subatomic alpha and beta particles. Alpha (composed of two protons and two neutrons) and the beta (essentially electrons) particles of elements such as tritium (^3H) and carbon 14 (^{14}C) are of immense use scientifically and have few hazards for humans. Alpha particles induce heavy damage in a restricted area.

Nonionizing Radiations

The energy of nonionizing radiation includes UV rays of sunlight, visible light, laser, infrared, microwave radio waves, and sound waves. Nonionizing radiation can move atoms in a molecule or cause them to rotate and vibrate, but their energy is not enough to displace (or remove) bound electrons from atoms or to break molecular bonds. The rotational and vibrational energy is then converted to heat. The localized hyperthermia may result in cellular injury It affects only skin. Nonionizing UV is used for therapy in skin diseases and laser therapy for diabetic retinopathy.

There are many forms of electromagnetic radiation. They range from low-energy radio waves to high-energy γ rays or photons (**Fig. 14**).

Quantitation of Radiation

Several terms are used to describe radiation dose. Radiation can be quantified according to—(1) the amount of radiation emitted by a source, (2) the amount of radiation that is absorbed by a person, and (3) the biologic effect of the radiation. Various radiation units are described below.

- **Roentgen:** It is a measure of the emission of radiant energy from a source. This unit refers to the amount of ionization produced in air.
- **Rad (radiation absorbed dose):** It is abbreviated as R. It measures absorption of radiant energy and is biologically the most important parameter. A rad defines the energy, expressed as ergs, absorbed by a tissue. One rad is equal to 100 ergs per gram of tissue. One rad is equivalent to 0.01 Gray (Gy) = 0.01 sievert (Sv).
- **Gray:** It is a unit that expresses the energy absorbed by the target tissue per unit mass. One Gray corresponds to absorption of 10^4 erg/g of tissue. A Centigray (cGy), which is the absorption of 100 erg/g of tissue, is equivalent to 100 Rad (1 joule/kg of tissue). In medical practice. the cGy terminology has replaced the Rad.
- **Curie (Ci):** It represents the disintegrations/second of a radionuclide (radioisotope). One Ci is equal to 3.7×10^{10} disintegrations/second. This is an expression of the amount of radiation emitted by a source.
- **Rem:** It is used to describe the biological effect caused by a rad of high-energy radiation, since low energy particles produce more biological damage than gamma or X-rays. One rem is equivalent to 0.01 Sv (sievert).
- **Sievert:** It is the dose in Gray multiplied by an appropriate quality factor Q, so that 1 Sv of radiation is roughly equivalent in biological effectiveness to 1 Gy of γ rays. Thus, it depends on the biologic rather than the physical effects of radiation. The relative biologic effectiveness depends on the type of radiation, the type and volume of the exposed tissue, the duration of the exposure, and some other biologic factors. The effective dose of X-rays in radiographs and CT is usually expressed in milliSieverts (mSv). For X-radiation, 1 mSv = 1 mGy.

Following discussion is restricted to ionizing radiation.

Ionizing Radiation

Factors Determining the Biologic Effects of Ionizing Radiation

Apart from the physical properties of radiation, the biologic effects of ionizing radiation depend mainly on the following factors:

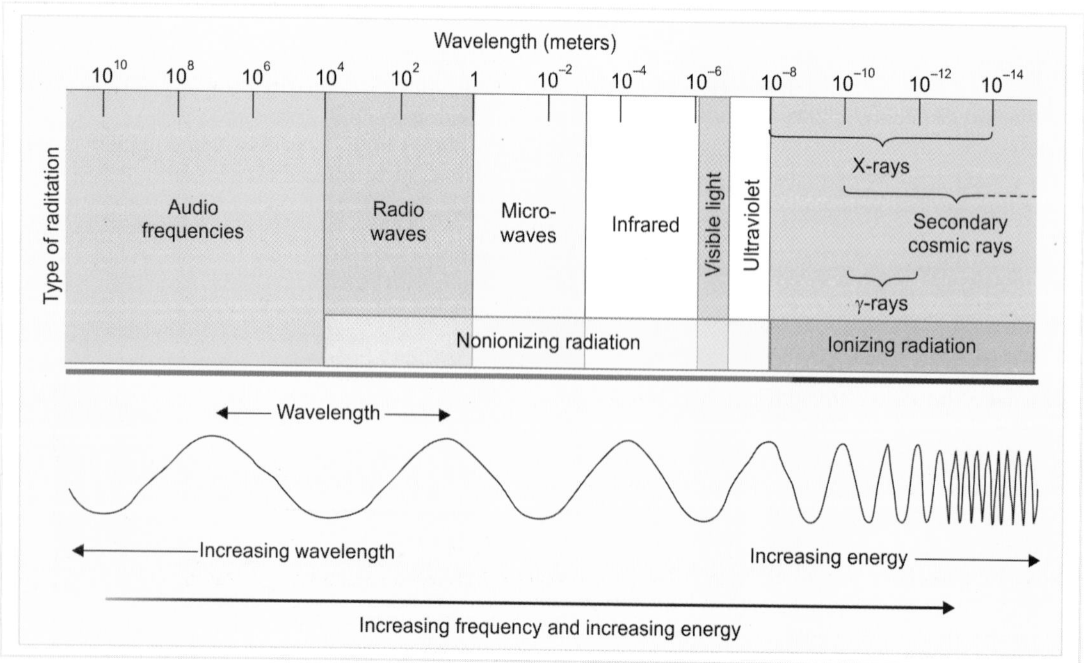

FIG. 14: Types of electromagnetic radiation and their wavelength.

- **Rate of delivery of radiation:** It has significant role in the biologic effect. The effect of radiant energy is cumulative. But in divided doses (called fractionated doses), the time between exposures gives time for cells to repair some of the damage. With radiation therapy of tumors, normal cells have more and rapid capability to repair and recover than tumor cells. The normal cells do not have much cumulative radiation damage.
- **Field size:** It has a major influence on the consequences of irradiation. The body can withstand relatively high doses of radiation when delivered to small, carefully shielded fields. But if smaller doses are delivered to larger fields, it may be lethal. Thus, doses of radiation delivered to shielded smaller fields are safer than smaller doses delivered to larger fields, which may be lethal.
- **Cell proliferation:** The vulnerability of a tissue to radiation-induced damage depends on its proliferative rate of the constituent cells. Ionizing radiation damages DNA and thus rapidly dividing cells are more susceptible to radiation injury than are quiescent cells. Examples of tissues with a high rate of cell division, such as gonads, hematopoietic bone marrow, lymphoid tissue, and the mucosa of the gastrointestinal tract. Injury to these cells is manifested early after exposure. Examples of nondividing cells include neurons (brain) and muscle cells. Except at extremely high doses that impair DNA transcription, irradiation does not kill nondividing cells. In dividing cells, DNA damage is detected by sensors that produce signals leading to the upregulation of p53 (the "guardian of the genome"). p53 upregulates the expression of genes that initially lead to cell cycle arrest. If the damage to DNA is severe to be repaired, there is upregulation of genes that cause cell death through apoptosis.
- **Oxygen effects and hypoxia:** The major mechanism of DNA damage by ionizing radiation is by the production of ROS (reactive oxygen species). Free radicals such as ROS are generated by radiolysis of water by ionizing radiation. Tissues with poor vascularization and low oxygen, such as the central region of rapidly growing tumors, are usually less sensitive to radiation therapy than nonhypoxic tissues.
- **Vascular damage:** The endothelial cells are moderately sensitive to radiation. Damage to endothelial cells may cause narrowing or occlusion of blood vessels. This may lead to impaired healing, fibrosis, and chronic ischemic atrophy of the area exposed to radiation. These changes may be seen months or years after exposure to radiation. The late effects in tissues with a low cell proliferation, such as the brain, kidney, liver, muscle, and subcutaneous tissue, may include cell death, atrophy, and fibrosis.

Pathophysiology

Ionizing radiation may injure cells directly or indirectly. Indirectly, it generates free radicals from hydrolysis of water or molecular oxygen. At the cellular level, radiation has two main effects namely:

1. **Somatic effect:** Radiation causes acute death of cells. Radiation-induced cell death is caused by the acute effects of the radiolysis of water. It produces activated oxygen species which causes lipid peroxidation, injury to cell membrane injury, and interact with macromolecules of the cell. Rapid somatic cell death occurs only with very high doses of radiation (excess of 10 Gy). Morphologically, it is coagulative type of necrosis.
2. **Genetic damage:** It is caused indirectly by a reaction of DNA with oxygen radicals. DNA damage may be repaired by DNA repair genes. If DNA is not adequately repaired, the cells may undergo apoptosis. If cells with DNA damage are neither repaired nor undergo apoptosis, they may undergo neoplastic transformation. These cells with genetic damage may be either as mutation or as reproductive failure. Both may lead to delayed cell death, and mutation is responsible for the development of radiation-induced neoplasia. Effects and consequences ionizing radiation on DNA are presented in **Figure 15**.

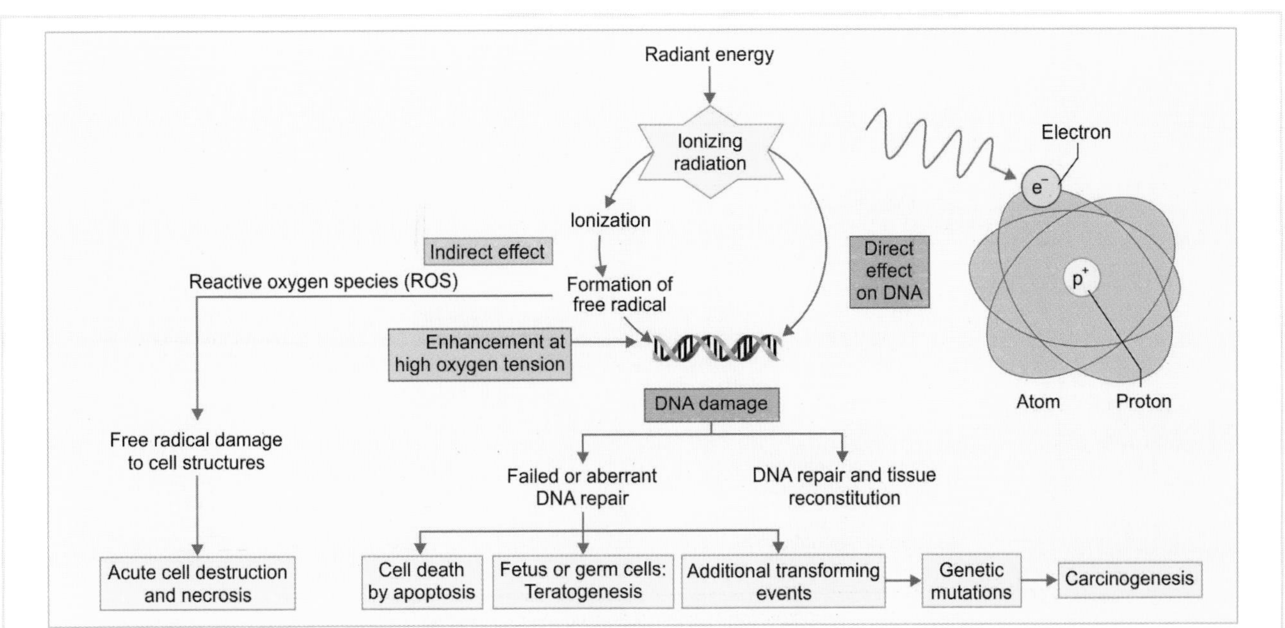

FIG. 15: Effects and consequences of ionizing radiation on DNA. Radiation can produce direct effects on DNA or more indirectly through generation of free radicals such as reactive oxygen species (ROS).

Localized Complications of Radiation Therapy

Q. Write short essay on morphology of radiation injury.

Radiation therapy is one of the methods of treating malignant neoplasms. In the course of radiotherapy for cancer, some normal tissue also is inevitably irradiated (expose to radiation). Almost any organ or tissue can be damaged by radiation. However, the skin, lungs, heart, kidney, bladder, and intestine are susceptible and difficult to shield. Localized damage to the bone marrow is of little functional significance. This is because of the great reserve capacity of the hematopoietic system.

MORPHOLOGY

Chromosomal changes: Cells which survive radiant energy damage show many structural changes in chromosomes.

- **Beak in the double-stranded DNA (dsDNA):** These include deletions, translocations, and fragmentation. The mitotic spindle often becomes disorderly and may show polyploidy and aneuploidy.
- **Nuclear changes:** These include nuclear swelling and condensation, clumping of chromatin, and disruption of the nuclear membrane. Cells may undergo apoptosis.
- **Abnormal nuclear morphology:** There may be giant cells with pleomorphic nuclei or more than one nucleus. These cells may persist for years after exposure. At very high doses of radiant energy, nuclear pyknosis and lysis may appear quickly.

Cytoplasmic changes: Radiant energy may produce variety of cytoplasmic changes. These include cytoplasmic swelling, distortion of mitochondria, degeneration of the endoplasmic reticulum, and focal breaks and defects in plasma membrane.

Changes in cells mimic cancer cells: The above microscopic changes in the radiation-injured cells such as cellular pleomorphism, formation of giant-cell, changes in nuclei, and abnormal mitotic figures produce an appearance similar to cancer cells. Hence, pathologist should be careful when

Continued

Continued

evaluating irradiated tissues while assessing for the possible persistence of tumor cells.

Persistent damage to radiation exposed tissue can be due to—(1) reduction of the vascular supply and (2) a fibrotic repair reaction to acute necrosis and chronic ischemia.

Vascular changes: Radiation-induced tissue injury mainly affects small arteries and arterioles. The endothelial cells are the most sensitive elements in the blood vessels. During the immediate post-irradiation period, the vessels in the irradiated tissues may show only dilation. With time or with higher doses, many degenerative changes develop. These include swelling and vacuolation of endothelial cells or necrosis and ruptures of the walls of small vessels (e.g., capillaries and venules). The involved vessels may show thrombus. With time, vascular walls become thickened due to endothelial cell proliferation and there may be collagenous hyalinization and thickening of the intima of vessels in the irradiated region. These morphological changes can produce marked narrowing or obliteration of the vessel lumens. During this period, there is evidence of increase in interstitial collagen in the irradiated region.

Collagen deposition leads to scarring and contractions of the irradiated area. Striking vacuolization of intimal cells (called foam cells) is typical of radiation damage.

Interstitial fibrosis: May be prominent in irradiated tissues.

Effects of Ionizing Radiation

Q. What is ionizing radiation? Add a note on effects of ionizing radiation injury and their consequences.

Effects of ionizing radiation are presented in **Figure 16**. Major morphologic consequences of ionizing radiation injury are presented in **Figure 17**. Acute radiation effects on specific organs and corresponding threshold doses of radiation are presented in **Table 8**.

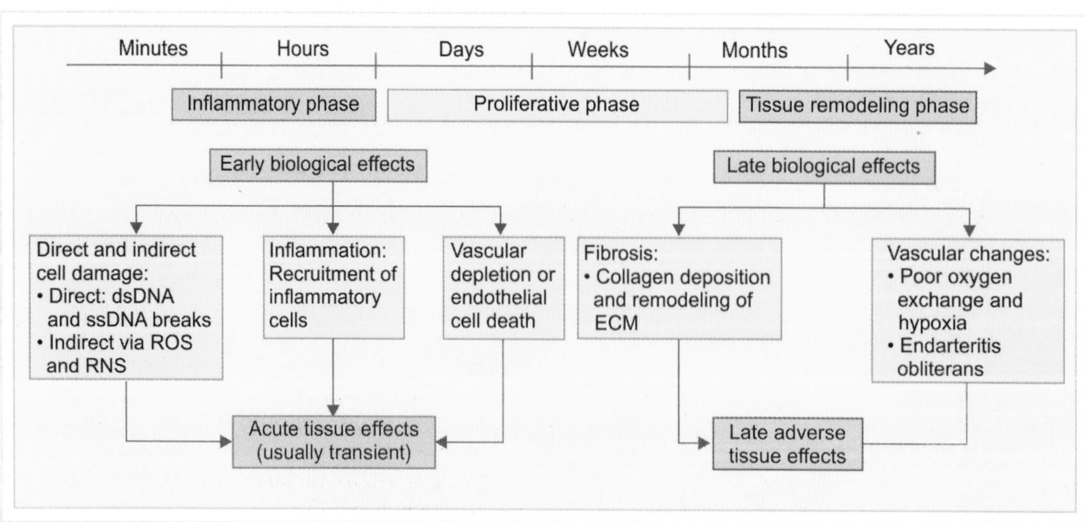

(dsDNA: double-stranded DNA; ROS: reactive oxygen species; RNS: reactive nitrogen species; ssDNA, single-stranded DNA)

FIG. 16: Effects of ionizing radiation. Early biologic events cause acute effects that are normally transient and resolve within 3 months of completing therapy. Late biologic events can lead to late adverse tissue effects such as fibrosis and vascular changes. Severity of these effects is increased with higher radiation dose per fraction.

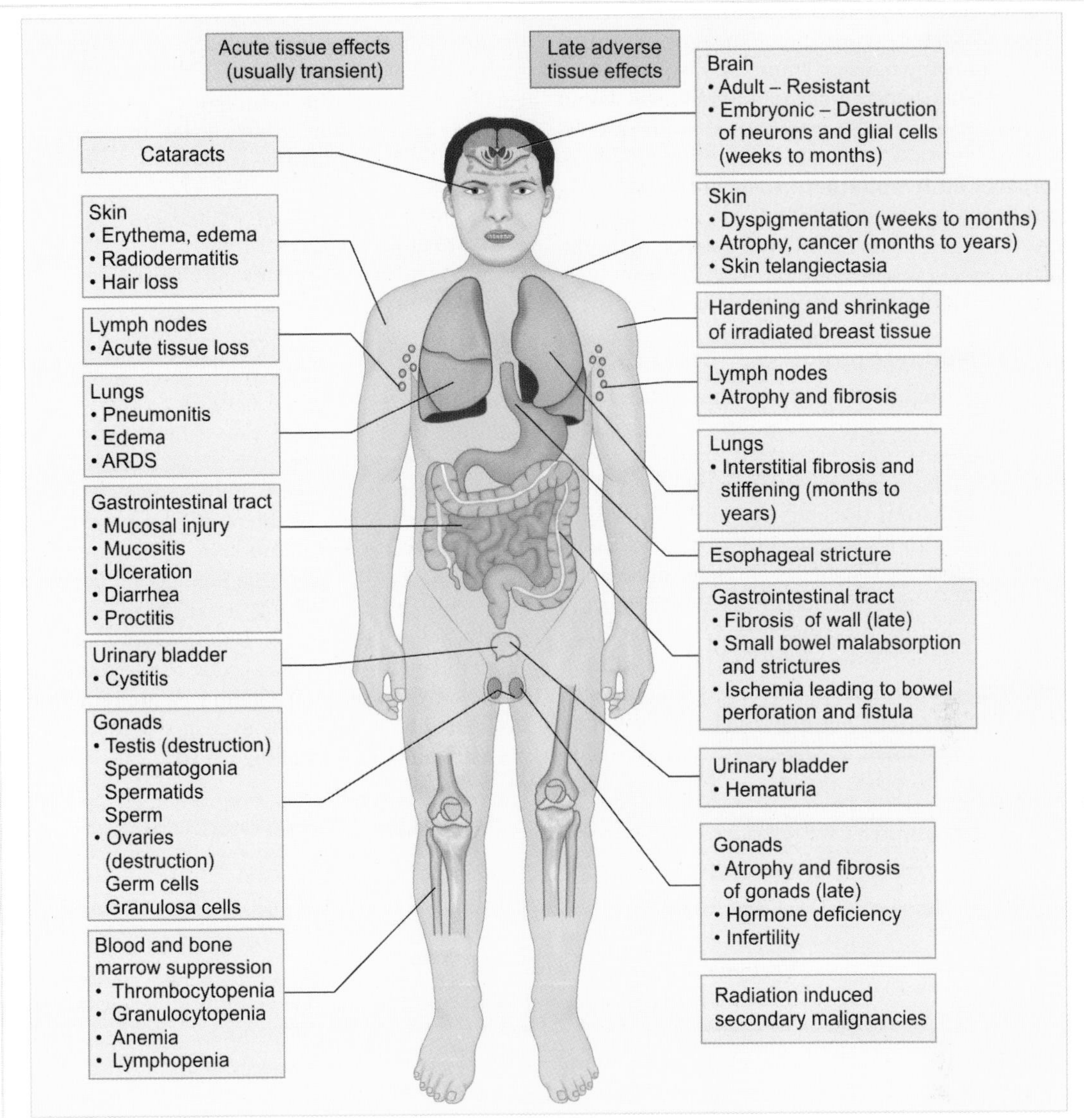

(ARDS: acute respiratory distress syndrome)

FIG. 17: Major morphologic consequences of ionizing radiation injury. Early tissue effects occur within hours to weeks and late adverse tissue effects occur in months to years.

Table 8: Acute radiation effects on specific organs and corresponding threshold doses of radiation.

Organ and acute radiation effect	*Radiation dose in sievert (Sv)*
Testes: Temporary sterility	0.15
Bone marrow: Suppression of hematopoiesis	0.50
Skin: Reversible skin effects (e.g., erythema)	1–2
Ovaries: Permanent sterility	2.5–6
Skin: Temporary loss of hair	3–5
Testis: Permanent sterility	3.5
Lens of eye: Cataract	5

Tissue vulnerability

- **Tissue with labile cells:** Tissues with actively dividing cells (labile cells), such as bone marrow and gastrointestinal mucosa, are more sensitive to ionising radiation.
- **Hemopoietic system:** Lymphocyte depletion is the most sensitive indicator of bone marrow injury and after exposure to a fatal dose, marrow aplasia is the most common cause of death.
- **Gastrointestinal mucosal toxicity:** May cause death due to severe diarrhea, vomiting, dehydration, and sepsis
- **Gonads:** Highly radiosensitive and may cause temporary or permanent sterility
- **Eye:** Cataracts
- **Skin:** Radiation dermatitis (radiation burns) characterized by skin erythema, purpura, blistering, and secondary infection may occur. Complete loss of body hair after an exposure >5 Gy.

- **Lung:** Acute inflammatory reactions, pulmonary fibrosis
- **Central nervous system syndrome:** Exposures of >30 Gy are followed rapidly by nausea, vomiting, disorientation, and coma. Death due to cerebral edema can follow within 36 hours. It may also cause permanent neurological deficit.
- **Bone necrosis and lymphatic fibrosis** occur following regional irradiation, particularly for breast cancer.
- **Thyroid gland** due to its capacity to concentrate iodine is responsible for its susceptibility to damage even after exposure to relatively low doses of radioactive.

Whole-Body (Total-Body) Irradiation

It is important to distinguish between whole-body (total-body) irradiation and localized irradiation. Though high-dose irradiation precedes bone marrow transplantation, a significant level of whole-body irradiation results only from industrial accidents or from nuclear weapons explosions, or nuclear power plants and hospitals. It may be also due to deliberate nuclear explosions designed to eliminate population and rarely by poisoning, e.g., with polonium. Hence, most of information regarding human diseases caused by whole-body irradiation has been derived from studies of Japanese atom bomb survivors and small sample of individuals who survived when accidently exposed at the Chernobyl nuclear power plant in Ukraine in 1986. By contrast, localized irradiation is used for many diagnostic radiologic procedures and for radiation therapy. Rapid somatic cell death occurs only with extremely high doses of radiation, well in excess of 0.1 Sv. Morphologically, this cell death is indistinguishable from coagulative necrosis produced by other causes. In contrast, irreversible damage to the replicative capacity of cells needs far lower doses as few as 0.05 Sv.

Acute radiation syndromes

Q. Write short essay on acute radiation sickness/acute radiation syndrome.

Damaging effects can be observed with exposure of large areas of the body to even very small doses of radiation. Minimal symptoms are produced with doses below 1 Sv. However, exposure to higher doses causes health effects termed **acute radiation syndromes**. Acute radiation sickness involves several systems and the extent of damage depends on the dose of radiation. Commonly involved systems are hematopoietic, gastrointestinal, CNS, and skin. With progressively higher doses, radiation involves the hematopoietic, gastrointestinal, and CNS. In whole-body irradiation, radiant energy is transmitted to all organs. The development of the different acute radiation syndromes is due to variation in vulnerability of the target tissues to radiation. Acute radiation syndromes associated with total-body exposure to ionizing radiation are presented in **Table 9** and **Figure 18**.

Table 9: Major effects, time of presentation, and lethality of total-body ionizing radiation.

Features	*0–1 sievert (Sv)*	*1–2 Sv*	*2–10 Sv*	*10–20 Sv*	*>50 Sv*
Major organ/cells injured	None	Lymphocytes	Bone marrow	Small bowel	Brain
Signs and symptoms	Nil	Moderate granulocytopenia, lymphopenia	Leukopenia, hemorrhage, hair loss, vomiting	Diarrhea, vomiting, fever, electrolyte imbalance	Ataxia, vomiting, coma, convulsions,
Time of presentation (latency)	–	1 day to 1 week	2–6 weeks	5–14 days	1–4 hours
Extent of lethality	Nil	Nil	Variable (0–80%)	100%	100%

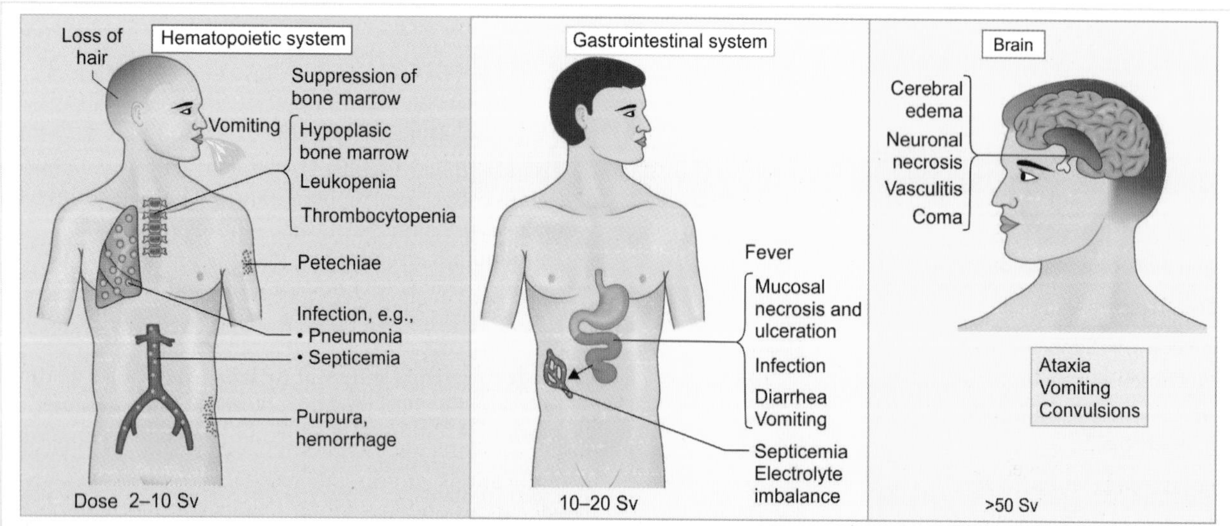

FIG. 18: Acute radiation syndromes. At a dose of approximately 2–10 sievert (Sv) of whole-body radiation, a syndrome characterized by hematopoietic failure develops within 2 weeks. With 10–20 Sv, a gastrointestinal syndrome with a latency of only 5–14 days develops. With doses of 50 Sv or more, disease of the central nervous system appears within 1–4 hours and death occurs rapidly.

- **Mild acute radiation sickness:** It is characterized by nausea, vomiting, and malaise which follow doses of about 1 Gy. Individual develops lymphopenia within several days, followed 2–3 weeks later by a fall in all WBCs and platelets.
- **2–10 Sv:** At this dose of whole-body radiation, a syndrome of hematopoietic failure develops within 2 weeks.
- **10–20 Sv:** At this dose, the main cause of death is related to the gastrointestinal system. The entire epithelium of the gastrointestinal tract is destroyed within 5 days. It may cause severe diarrhea leading to dehydration. Because of loss of epithelial barrier in the intestine, the organisms in intestinal lumen invade and disseminate throughout the body. This can lead to septicemia and shock resulting in death.
- **50 Sv or more:** Doses of 50 Sv and above may cause damage to CNS and death within hours. With very high doses, necrosis of neurons can develop leading to convulsions, coma, and death.

Acute effects on hematopoietic and lymphoid systems Hematopoietic and lymphoid systems are extremely susceptible to radiation injury.

High dose levels (0.3 Sv) of radiation and large exposure fields kill lymphocytes directly, both in the circulation and in tissues (lymph nodes, spleen, thymus, gut). It first produces severe lymphopenia (decrease of circulating lymphocytes) within hours of irradiation, along with shrinkage of the lymph nodes and spleen. This is followed by a progressive decrease in all formed elements of the blood. This leads to bleeding (due to decreased platelets), anemia (due to decreased RBCs), and infection (due to decreased WBCs). Infection is often the cause of death.

With sublethal doses of radiation, prompt regeneration of lymphocytes from precursors occurs. This leads to restoration of a normal blood lymphocyte count within weeks to months.

Very high doses kill hematopoietic precursors (i.e., marrow stem cells) in the bone marrow. This can produce a dose-dependent marrow aplasia and permanent aplasia (aplastic anemia). The acute effects of marrow irradiation on peripheral blood counts depend on the normal turnover and half-lives of the formed elements namely, the granulocytes, platelets, and red cells. Half-life is the length of time required for the concentration of a particular cell to decrease to half of its level in the body. The granulocytes have a half-life of less than a day, platelets have 10 days, and red cells have 120 days.

- **Granulocytes:** After a brief increase in the circulating neutrophil count, neutropenia develops within several days. During the second week, neutrophil counts reach their lowest level, often it may be near zero. If the patient survives, it may need 2–3 months for recovery and have a normal granulocyte count.
- **Platelets:** Thrombocytopenia is observed by the end of the first week. Platelet counts reach their lowest level somewhat later than that of granulocytes and recovery is also similarly delayed.
- **RBCs:** Anemia develops after 2–3 weeks and it may persist for months.

Higher doses of radiation produce more severe cytopenias and need more prolonged periods for recovery. Very high doses destroy hematopoietic stem cells and produce permanent aplasia (aplastic anemia). The permanent aplasia is characterized by a failure of blood count recovery. With lower doses of radiation, the aplasia is transient.

Fibrosis

- Fibrosis in the tissues included in the irradiated field is a common consequence of radiation therapy for cancer. Fibrosis may be observed within weeks or months after irradiation. Fibrosis is due to replacement of dead parenchymal cells by connective tissue. Fibrosis leads to scar formation and adhesions.
- **Mechanism of radiation-induced fibrosis:** Radiation produces damage to vessels and the death of tissue stem cells. This is accompanied by release of cytokines and chemokines. These promote inflammation and fibroblast activation leading to the development of fibrosis.
- **Common sites of fibrosis:** After radiation treatment for head and neck cancers, fibrosis develops in lungs and the salivary glands. Fibrosis involves colorectal and pelvic areas after treatment for cancer of the prostate, rectum, or cervix.

Fetal effects The effects of whole-body irradiation on the human fetus were documented in studies of Hiroshima nuclear bomb survivors. Pregnant women who were exposed to 0.025 Sv or more whole-body irradiation gave birth to infants with decreased size of head, decreased overall growth, and mental retardation. If pregnant women were exposed to therapeutic doses of radiation between the 3rd and 20th weeks of gestation, the fetus showed growth retardation and microcephaly. Other effects of irradiation in utero include hydrocephaly, microphthalmia, spina bifida, chorioretinitis, blindness, cleft palate, clubfeet, and genital abnormalities.

Major congenital malformations are unlikely at doses below 0.025 Sv after 14th day of pregnancy. However, lower doses may produce more subtle effects (e.g., decrease in mental capacity).

Genetic effects The risk of genetic damage to future generations from radiation appears to be small. After long-term follow-up, in survivors of the atomic bomb explosion at Hiroshima and Nagasaki, there was no evidence of genetic damage (both congenital abnormalities or heritable diseases in subsequent offspring).

Aging There is no evidence to show that whole-body irradiation leads to premature aging.

DNA damage and carcinogenesis Ionizing radiation can produce multiple types of DNA damage. These include single-base damage, single- and double-stranded breaks (DSBs), and DNA–protein cross-links. In surviving cells, simple defects may be repaired by various enzyme and DNA repair systems present in most of the cells. The most serious DNA damage is DSBs. Two types of repair mechanisms are involved in the repair of DSBs in cells. These are homologous recombination and nonhomologous end joining (NHEJ), with NHEJ being the most common repair pathway. These are discussed in detail on pages 514–527. DNA repair through NHEJ often produces mutations. These mutations may be short deletions or duplications or gross chromosomal aberrations such as translocations and inversions. Replication of cells with DSBs can be prevented by cell cycle checkpoint controls. If not, these cells with chromosomal damage persist and may initiate carcinogenesis many years later.

Cancer risks from exposures to radiation Any cell capable of cell division, if undergoes mutation, can become cancerous. Exposure to ionizing radiation can cause mutation. Hence, there is an increased incidence of neoplasms in any organ exposed to ionizing radiation. Radiation is a well-known carcinogen. Extremely long latent period is common and it has a cumulative effect. Radiation has also additive or synergistic effects with other potential carcinogenic agents.

Medical or occupational exposure and cancer: Increased risk of cancer is associated with occupational exposures.

- **X-ray instruments:** During early part of the 20th century, scientists and radiologists used to test their X-ray equipment by placing their hands in the path of the beam. They developed basal and squamous cell carcinomas of the exposed skin. Radiologists of that era suffered an unusually high incidence of leukemia. This is rectified with the use of modern shielding and protective equipment.
- **Radium used for watch dials:** Olden days watches with luminous radium-containing dials were used. An unusual occupational exposure to radiation occurred among these workers. They were painting radium-containing material onto watches to create luminous dials. These workers were in the habit of licking their paint brushes to produce a point. During this, they unknowingly ingest the radium in the brush. Body handles radium similar to calcium. Hence, radium subsequently localized in the bones of these workers. They were exposed to a long-lived isotope and it persisted in their bones indefinitely. These workers had high incidence of cancer of the bone and of the paranasal sinuses.
- **Radon:** Radon radioactive noble gas is a ubiquitous product of the spontaneous decay of uranium 238 (^{238}U). Radon is itself inert. Environmental hazards and carcinogenic effects of radon are due to its two radioactive decay products, which are called "radon daughters". These radon daughters are polonium 214 and polonium 218. They emit alpha particles. Polonium 214 and polonium 218 (half-life is 103 years) produced from inhaled radon get deposited in the lung. High rate of lung cancer was found in uranium miners who are chronically exposed to inhalation of radioactive dust and radon gas. Most of these workers were also smokers. Both have a synergistic effect in lung carcinogenesis. Radon may also be formed from the decay of uranium which is found in soil and rock formations. If the levels of radon in homes are very high comparable to those found in mines, it also is a risk factor for lung cancer.
- **Therapeutic radiation and cancer:** Iatrogenic cancer resulted in Great Britain from widespread use of low-dose spinal irradiation to treat ankylosing spondylitis. These patients later developed aplastic anemia, acute myeloid leukemia, and other tumors. Papillary carcinoma of the thyroid followed irradiation of head and neck region. An increase in brain tumors was found in patients who had received cranial irradiation for tinea capitis infection of the scalp during childhood. Radioactive thorium dioxide (Thorotrast) was used a few decades ago for radionuclide imaging to visualize the arterial tree. The persistence of this long-lived radioisotope in the liver resulted in development of hepatic angiosarcomas.
- **Development of second malignancy:** The risk of secondary cancers following irradiation is greatest in children. The risk of solid tumors (especially breast cancer) was high among adult women who were treated with radiation to thoracic region for Hodgkin disease as children. Long-term survivors of childhood Hodgkin disease, who were treated with radiation therapy, also had almost a 20-fold increased risk of developing a second neoplasm.

It is difficult to determine the level of radiation needed to increase the risk of cancer development. Acute or prolonged exposures in doses of >100 mSv are found to produce serious consequences, including cancer. Evidence that radiation can lead to cancer comes from many sources (**Fig. 19**). These are as follows:

- Increased incidence of leukemias and solid tumors in several organs (e.g., thyroid, breast, and lungs) in survivors of the atomic bomb explosion in Hiroshima and Nagasaki. Survivors of the atomic bomb explosion (dropped on Hiroshima and Nagasaki) had increased incidence of number of cancers. They had more than 10-fold increase in the incidence of leukemia, which peaked 5–10 years after exposure, then declined to background rates. Two-thirds were acute leukemia; the remainder were of chronic myelogenous leukemia. There was no increase in incidence of chronic lymphocytic leukemia. The risk of multiple myeloma increased 5-fold and there was a small increase in the incidence of lymphoma. Subsequently, the frequency of solid tumors, although not as great as that for leukemia, was also increased. These solid tumors include that of the

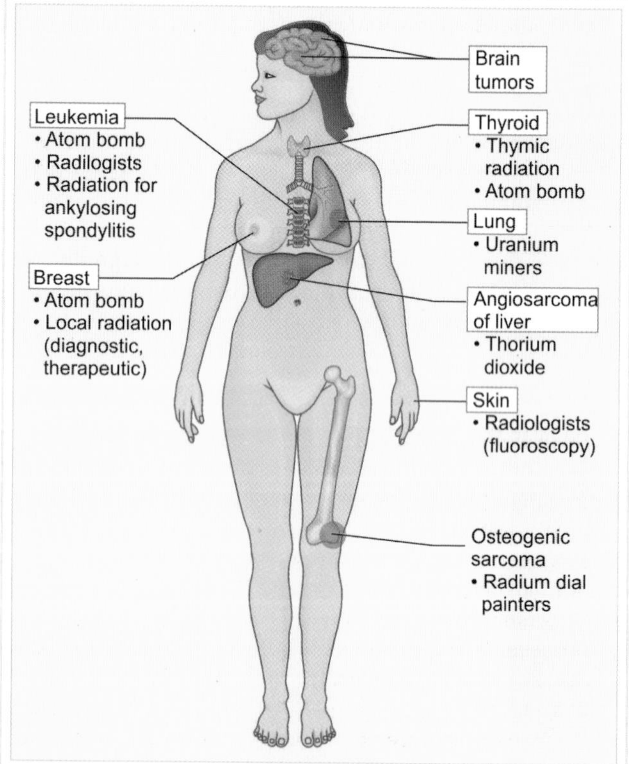

FIG. 19: Various radiation-induced cancers.

breast, lung, thyroid, gastrointestinal tract (e.g., colon), and urinary tract. The development of malignant tumors, including leukemia, showed a dose-response relationship.

- Increased number of carcinomas of thyroid in survivors of the Chernobyl accident. Iodine is concentrated by the thyroid. Inhalation or ingestion of radioactive iodine isotopes causes high concentration of radioactive iodine. Marked increase in the incidence of thyroid cancer was found among children in geographical areas contaminated by the nuclear catastrophe at Chernobyl in Ukraine in 1986. It was due to release of radioactive iodine isotopes in that incident.
- High incidence of tumors of thyroid, leukemias, and birth defects in inhabitants of the Marshall Islands exposed to nuclear fallout.
- Nuclear plant accidents: Risk of lung cancers

Cancer risks caused by radiation exposures in the range of 5–100 mSv are not well established. However, for X-rays and γ rays, there is a statistically significant increase in the risk of cancer at acute doses >50 mSv and acute doses >5 mSv. A single posteroanterior chest radiograph, a lateral chest radiograph, and a CT scan of the chest deliver effective doses to the lungs of 0.01 mSv, 0.15 mSv, and 10 mSv, respectively. Tissues which are relatively resistant to radiation-induced neoplasia—skin, bone, and the gastrointestinal tract.

Ultraviolet Rays

They are derived from the sunlight. Sun emits large spectrum of electromagnetic radiation and exposure to UV light (100–400 nm) derived from sunlight has different effects on the human body.

- **DNA damage and cancer:** UV light can damage DNA and lead to skin cancer. These are—(1) squamous cell carcinoma, (2) basal cell carcinoma, and (3) malignant melanoma. They are more common on parts of the body regularly exposed to sunlight and UV light.
- **Modulation of immune functions:** UV radiation is absorbed by photoreceptors in the skin and it may release many substances that suppress cell-mediated immunity. Thus, UV can modulate both local and systemic immune functions.
- **Effect on autoimmune diseases:** UV light may have beneficial effect on the severity of some autoimmune diseases (e.g., multiple sclerosis).
- **Endogenous production of vitamin D:** Exposure to UV radiation stimulates endogenous production of vitamin D in the skin. UV wavelength between 270 nm and 300 nm is called UVB. It results in production of a precursor for vitamin D from a cholesterol derivative.

Risk factors: The amount of damage caused by UV light depends on:

- Type of UV rays
- Intensity of exposure
- Protective mantle of melanin:
  - Melanin absorbs UV radiation and has a protective effect.
  - Skin cancers are more common in fair-skinned people and those living in geographic location receiving a greater amount of sunlight (e.g., Queensland, Australia, close to the equator).

Pathogenesis

- UV radiation leads to formation of pyrimidine dimers in DNA, which is a type of DNA damage which is responsible for carcinogenicity.
- DNA damage is repaired by the nucleotide excision repair pathway.
- With excessive sun exposure, the DNA damage exceeds the capacity of the nucleotide excision repair pathway and genomic injury becomes mutagenic and carcinogenic.
- **Xeroderma pigmentosum:** It is a rare hereditary autosomal recessive disorder characterized by congenital deficiency of nucleotide excision repair DNA. These individuals develop skin cancers (basal cell carcinoma, squamous cell carcinoma, and melanoma) due to impairment in the excision of UV-damaged DNA.

It is discussed on pages 525 and 526.

Nonionizing Radiation

Microwaves: Nonionizing radiation does not produce ionization. Microwaves are produced by ovens, radar and diathermy are electromagnetic waves that penetrate tissue but are nonionizing. In contrast to X- and gamma radiation, absorption of microwave energy produces only heat. The energy of microwave radiation is too low to modify chemical bonds or change DNA. Under ordinary circumstances, exposure to microwave radiation is not likely to produce any injury or any increased incidence of cancer.

Ultrasound: In ultrasound, the vibrational waves in air are above the audible range. They produce mechanical compression and there is no ionization. They are commonly used for diagnostic ultrasound and are unlikely to produce any tissue damage.

NUTRITIONAL DISEASES

Q. Write short essay on malnutrition.

Malnutrition includes the full continuum of undernutrition and over-nutrition (obesity). It refers to deficiencies, excesses or imbalances in an individual's intake of energy and/or nutrients. Malnutrition is usually a consequence of inadequate intake of proteins and calories or deficiencies in the digestion or absorption of proteins. It results in the loss of fat and muscle mass, weight loss, and generalized weakness. In lower income nations, malnutrition is due to starvation. In the higher income nations and in some lower income countries, obesity is a major public health problem and is associated with diseases such as diabetes, atherosclerosis, and cancer.

Malnutrition can be primary or secondary. Primary malnutrition is caused by inadequate energy intake. In secondary malnutrition, individual's dietary intake is sufficient, but energy is not adequately absorbed by the body. This may occur due to infectious conditions such as diarrhoea, measles or parasitic infections, or medical or surgical disorders affecting the digestive system.

In 2010, an International Consensus Guideline Committee incorporated a new appreciation for the role of inflammatory response. Hence, they suggested the following categories of malnutrition:

- **Starvation-associated malnutrition:** In this category, there is chronic starvation without inflammation (anorexia nervosa or major depression with lack of interest in eating).
- **Chronic disease-associated malnutrition:** In this type, inflammation is chronic and of mild to moderate degree (e.g., organ failure, pancreatic cancer, or sarcopenic obesity).
- **Acute disease or injury-associated malnutrition:** In this category, inflammation is acute and of severe degree (e.g., major infection, burns, trauma, or closed head injury).

Dietary Insufficiency

Diet: An appropriate diet should provide the following:

- **Sufficient energy:** It should be in the form of carbohydrates, fats, and proteins required for the body's daily metabolic requirements.
- **Amino acids and fatty acids:** These are used as building blocks for synthesis of proteins and lipids.
- **Vitamins and minerals:** They function as coenzymes or hormones in important metabolic pathways or as an important structural component (e.g., calcium, phosphate).

In primary malnutrition, one or all of these components are not present in the diet whereas in secondary malnutrition there may be malabsorption, impaired utilization or storage, excess loss, or increased need for nutrients.

Predisposing Factors for Malnutrition

Many conditions may produce primary or secondary malnutrition.

- **Poverty:** In lower income nations, poverty, crop failures, famine and drought, especially during war and political disturbances, create the setting for the malnourishment in both children and adults. Poorly, elderly individuals, and children of the poor family develop severe malnutrition and deficiencies of trace nutrients.
- **Acute and chronic illnesses:** In many acute and chronic illnesses, the basal metabolic rate rises. This leads to increased daily demand for all nutrients. Malnutrition is common in patients with wasting diseases (e.g., advanced cancers and AIDS) and are complicated by cachexia.
- **Chronic alcoholism:** Chronic alcoholics may suffer from malnutrition. More commonly, they have deficiencies of vitamins (e.g., thiamine, pyridoxine, folate, and vitamin A). This may be due to poor diet, defect in absorption from gastrointestinal tract, abnormal utilization nutrient and storage, increased metabolic needs, and excessive loss. For example, thiamine deficiency in chronic alcoholics may result in irreversible brain damage (e.g., Wernicke encephalopathy and Korsakoff psychosis).
- **Ignorance:** Infants, adolescents, and pregnant women require increased nutritional needs. Ignorance about the nutritional content of foods and failure of diet supplementation may also produce malnutrition. Examples are—(1) iron deficiency in infants fed only on artificial milk diets, (2) thiamine deficiency due to use of polished rice as staple/predominant diet, and (3) lack of iodine from food and water.
- **Self-imposed dietary restriction:** In anorexia nervosa, bulimia, and other eating disorders, individuals are concerned about body image and are obsessed with body weight. They themselves impose dietary restriction
- **Other causes:** These include diseases of gastrointestinal tract and malabsorption syndromes, genetic diseases, certain drugs that block uptake or utilization of particular nutrients, and inadequate **total parenteral nutrition.**

Severe Acute Malnutrition

Definition: According to WHO, severe acute malnutrition (SAM) is defined as a state characterized by a weight for height ratio that is 3 standard deviations below the normal range.

Severe acute malnutrition was previously termed as protein energy malnutrition (PEM) or protein–calorie malnutrition. SAM manifests as a spectrum of clinical syndromes, all resulting from an inadequate dietary intake of protein and calories, that is inadequate to meet the body's requirement. At two ends of spectrum of SAM are marasmus and kwashiorkor with intermediate states of marasmus–kwashiorkor.

Protein compartments: Functionally, there are two protein compartments in the body—(1) the **somatic compartment** and (2) **visceral compartment**. Somatic compartment consists of proteins in skeletal muscles, and the visceral compartment is composed of protein stores in the visceral organs, mainly liver. Both these two compartments are differently regulated. In marasmus, the somatic compartment is more severely affected whereas in kwashiorkor the visceral compartment is more severely depleted.

Diagnosis of SAM: In most severe forms of SAM, diagnosis is easy. Usual approach for diagnosis in mild to moderate forms of SAM is to compare the body weight for a given height against standard tables. Other parameters that help in diagnosis include fat stores, muscle mass, and levels of certain serum proteins [e.g., albumin, prealbumin, transferrin, retinol-binding protein, C-reactive protein (CRP)]. Loss of fat is measured by assessing the skinfold thickness. Skin thickness includes skin and subcutaneous tissue and is reduced in SAM.

- If the somatic protein compartment is catabolized, it reduces muscle mass and thereby reduces circumference of the midarm.
- Adequacy of the visceral protein compartment can be assessed by measuring serum proteins (albumin, transferrin, and others).
- **Gut microbiome:** Substantial difference was found between the gut microbial flora of children with SAM and normal children. Microbiome is involved in the pathogenesis of SAM. Evidence for this came from fecal transplants from children with SAM into germ-free mice. Malnutrition was induced in host mice by fecal transplants from affected but not well-nourished children.

Marasmus

Marasmus is a type of SAM that develops when there is severe lack of calories in the diet. In marasmus, the weight of the affected child falls to 60% of normal for sex, height, and age. In a marasmic child, catabolism and depletion of the somatic protein compartment causes retardation of growth and loss of muscle mass. This is an adaptive response that provides the body with amino acids as a source of energy. There is only marginal depletion of the visceral protein compartment. Visceral protein is more important for survival and in marasmus, serum albumin levels are either normal or only mildly reduced. Apart from muscle proteins, there is also mobilization of subcutaneous fat and this is used as fuel. Leptin production is low. This may stimulate the hypothalamic-pituitary adrenal axis to produce high levels of cortisol. This leads to lipolysis. Due to losses of muscle and subcutaneous fat, the extremities in marasmus are emaciated. The head comparatively appears too large for the body. There is anemia, multivitamin deficiencies, and immune deficiency, particularly of T-cell-mediated immunity. This leads to concurrent infections and causes additional stress on a weakened body. There is no edema. The hair is thin and dry.

The marasmic child does not appear as apathetic or anorexic as with kwashiorkor. Diarrhea occurs frequently.

Kwashiorkor

Kwashiorkor develops when protein deprivation is relatively greater than the reduction in total intake of calories. This is the most common SAM (severe acute malnutrition) observed in African children. These children have been weaned too early and subsequently fed, almost exclusively, a carbohydrate diet. The name kwashiorkor is derived from the Ga language in Ghana. It describes the illness in a young child that appears after the arrival of another baby. Kwashiorkor is found commonly in lower income nations of Southeast Asia. Less severe forms occur in children with chronic diarrheal disorders (protein is not absorbed), or in individuals with chronic protein loss (e.g., protein-losing enteropathies, the nephrotic syndrome, or following extensive burns). Rarely, it may result from craze diets or replacement of milk by rice-based beverages.

Features (Fig. 20): In contrast to marasmus, in kwashiorkor, there is marked lack of protein. It is associated with severe loss of the visceral protein compartment. This produces hypoalbuminemia and gives rise to generalized or dependent edema. Children with severe kwashiorkor have typically 60–80% of normal weight. The true loss of weight is masked because of the increased fluid retention (edema). Also, there is relative sparing of subcutaneous fat and muscle mass which is unlike that of marasmus.

- **Skin lesions:** Children with kwashiorkor have characteristic skin lesions. This consists of alternating zones of hyperpigmentation and hypopigmentation, producing "**flaky paint**" appearance.
- **Hair changes:** These include loss of color or alternating bands of pale and darker hair. There is also straightening, fine texture, and loss of firm attachment of hair to the scalp.
- **Other features:** The other features that differentiate kwashiorkor from marasmus are as follows:
  - Presence of enlarged **fatty liver**. It is due to reduced synthesis of the carrier protein component of lipoproteins.
  - Development of apathy, listlessness, and loss of appetite
  - Presence of vitamin deficiencies
  - Defects in immunity and secondary infections. This produces inflammation and a catabolic state and aggravates the malnutrition.

Marasmus and kwashiorkor are two ends of a spectrum, and there may be considerable overlap between the two.

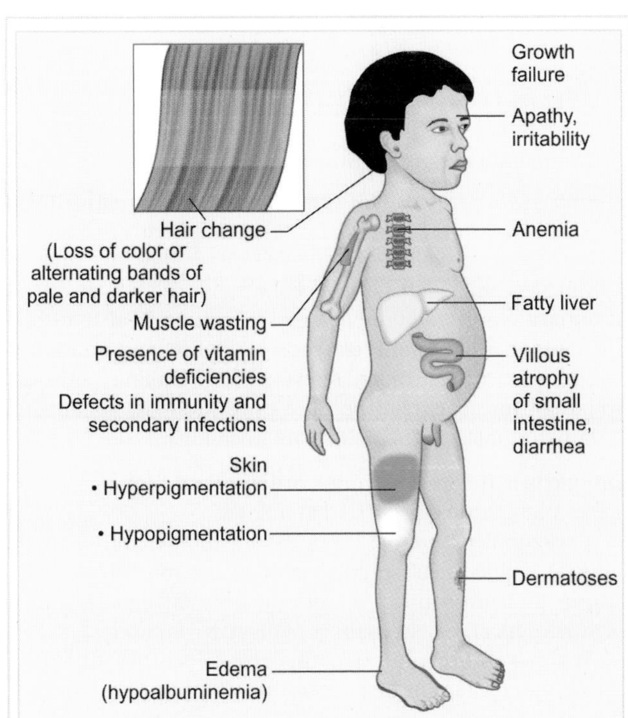

FIG. 20: Features and complications of kwashiorkor.

Secondary Malnutrition

It develops in chronically ill, aged, and bedridden patients. The signs of secondarymalnutrition include—(1) depletion of subcutaneous fat (e.g., arms, chest wall, shoulders, or metacarpal regions), (2) wasting of the muscles (e.g., quadriceps and deltoid); and (3) edema in the ankle or sacral region. Bedridden or malnourished individuals are prone to infection, sepsis, impaired wound healing, and death after surgery.

MORPHOLOGY

Main morphological changes in SAM are—(1) failure of growth; (2) peripheral edema in kwashiorkor; and (3) loss of body fat and atrophy of muscle, more marked in marasmus.

Liver: In kwashiorkor, but not in marasmus, liver is enlarged and fatty (steatosis). Superimposed cirrhosis is rare.

Small intestine: In marasmus, there is reduction in mitotic cells in the crypts of the glands. There is also atrophy of mucosa and loss of villi and microvilli. These changes are associated with loss of small intestinal enzymes and manifest as disaccharidase deficiency. Hence, initially these infants with kwashiorkor may not respond well to full-strength, milk-based diets. Mucosal changes are reversible with treatment.

Bone marrow: Both in both kwashiorkor and marasmus, bone marrow may be hypoplastic mainly due to decreased numbers of red cell precursors.

Peripheral blood smear: Shows mild to moderate anemia. Anemia is often multifactorial in origin. It may be due to nutritional deficiencies of iron, folate, and protein, and suppression due to infection (anemia of chronic inflammation). Depending on the predominant factor, the RBCs may be microcytic, normocytic, or macrocytic.

Brain: Infants born to malnourished mothers and who have SAM during the first 1 or 2 years of life show cerebral atrophy, a reduced number of neurons, and impaired myelinization of white matter.

Continued

Continued

Other changes: These include—(1) thymic and lymphoid atrophy (more in kwashiorkor than in marasmus), (2) changes produced by intercurrent infections, particularly with endemic worms and other parasites, and (3) deficiencies of other nutrients (e.g., iodine and vitamins).

Cachexia: Secondary malnutrition is a common complication in acquired immunodeficiency syndrome
(AIDS) or advanced cancers. In these settings, it is called as cachexia. It is discussed on page 547.

Differences between kwashiorkor and marasmus are listed in **Table 10**.

Anorexia Nervosa and Bulimia Nervosa

Anorexia nervosa and bulimia nervosa are eating disorders that occur mainly in previously healthy young women who have developed an obsession with body image and thinness. Anorexia nervosa is self-induced starvation. It results in marked weight loss. Bulimia nervosa is a condition in which the patient binges on food (excessive satisfaction in eating) and then induces vomiting. Probably altered serotonin metabolism may be an important component of these disorders.

Anorexia nervosa: In anorexia nervosa, they restrict their caloric intake to a degree that their body weight deviates significantly from age, gender, health, and developmental norms. Patients with anorexia nervosa have the highest death rate similar to any psychiatric disorder. The clinical findings of anorexia nervosa are usually similar to those of SAM (severe acute malnutrition). Also, they have prominent effects on the endocrine system.

- **Amenorrhea:** This is due to decreased secretion of gonadotropin-releasing hormone. This in turn results in reduced secretion of luteinizing hormone and follicle-stimulating hormone. Amenorrhea is common and its presence is diagnostic feature of anorexia nervosa.
- **Decreased thyroid hormone release:** This causes cold intolerance, bradycardia, constipation, changes in the skin and hair, dehydration, and electrolyte abnormalities. The skin appears dry and scaly.

Table 10: Main differences between kwashiorkor and marasmus.

Feature	*Kwashiorkor*	*Marasmus*
Definition	Inadequate protein intake with reasonable caloric (energy) intake	Inadequate intake of both protein and calories
Age	Children aged between 6 months and 3 years	Infants under 1 year
Growth failure	Present	Present
Edema	Localized or generalized	Absent
Liver	Enlarged fatty	Not enlarged

- **Gelatinous transformation of bone marrow:** Though fat is reduced elsewhere, fat is paradoxically increased in the marrow. This is associated with a peculiar deposition of mucinous matrix material in the marrow. This is termed as gelatinous transformation and almost **pathognomonic for anorexia nervosa**.
- **Reduced bone density:** It is probably due to low levels of estrogen and mimics the postmenopausal acceleration of osteoporosis.
- **Other features:** Anemia, lymphopenia, and hypoalbuminemia may be seen.
- **Complication of anorexia nervosa (and bulimia):** Increased susceptibility to cardiac arrhythmia and sudden death, resulting from hypokalemia.

Bulimia nervosa: It is more common than anorexia nervosa and usually has a better prognosis.

In bulimia, binge eating is normally present. Individuals engage in recurrent and frequent (at least once a week for 3 months) periods of binge eating. Binge eating is defined as excessive food intake in a prescribed period of time, usually <2 hours. During this, large amounts of food, mainly carbohydrates, are ingested, followed by induced self-induced vomiting, purging, enemas, use of laxatives, or excessive exercise to avoid weight gain.

- **Menstrual irregularities:** They are common, but amenorrhea is observed in <50% of bulimic patients. This is because both weight and gonadotropin levels remain near normal.
- **Complications:** They are due to frequent vomiting and the chronic use of laxatives and diuretics. These complications include—(1) electrolyte imbalances (hypokalemia), which predispose to cardiac arrhythmias, (2) aspiration of gastric contents into lung, and (3) esophageal and gastric rupture.
- **Diagnosis:** There are no specific signs or symptoms of bulimia. Hence, its diagnosis depends on a comprehensive psychologic assessment.

VITAMIN DEFICIENCIES

Q. Write short essay on micronutrients.

Vitamins are vital organic micronutrients or substances required in limited amounts. Most of them are used as necessary precursors of coenzymes and play key roles in certain metabolic pathways. Micronutrients are a diverse array of dietary components necessary to sustain health. Micronutrients include vitamins, trace elements, and additional compounds with nutritional relevance [e.g., choline (necessary precursor for acetylcholine) and phospholipids (needed to sustain normal levels of biologic methylation)].

Categories: Thirteen vitamins are necessary for health and these vitamins are categorized as follows:

- **Fat-soluble vitamins:** These include four vitamins namely, A, D, E, and K. Fat-soluble vitamins are stored in the body, but their absorption may be poor in fat malabsorption disorders or in disturbances of digestive functions.
- **Water-soluble vitamins:** This group includes all other 9 vitamins (vitamins of the B complex group and vitamin C).

It is important to distinguish fat-soluble from water-soluble vitamins. Fat-soluble vitamins may be poorly absorbed in fat malabsorption disorders due to disturbances of digestive functions. Some vitamins can be synthesized endogenously. For example, vitamin D is synthesized from precursor steroids; vitamin K and biotin by the intestinal microflora; and niacin from tryptophan (an essential amino acid). However, dietary supply of all vitamins is necessary for health.

Deficiency of vitamins: It may be primary (deficiency in diet) or secondary to defect in intestinal absorption, transport in the blood, tissue storage, or metabolic conversion. Deficiency of a single vitamin is uncommon. Single or multiple vitamin deficiencies may be found in SAM.

Fat-soluble Vitamins

Q. Write short essay on fat soluble vitamins.

Vitamin A (Retinol)

Vitamin A (retinol) is a fat-soluble vitamin. It is a part of the family of retinoids which is present in food and the body as esters combined with long chain fatty acids. The family of retinoids consists of vitamin A in its various forms. This group includes both natural and synthetic chemicals that are structurally related to vitamin A. However, all retinoids may not have vitamin A-like biologic activity. Vitamin A group of related compounds includes retinol, retinal, and retinoic acid, that have similar biologic activities.

- **Retinoids/retinol (vitamin A alcohol):** Vitamin A occurs naturally as retinoids or as a precursor, β-carotene. Retinoid is the generic term used for vitamin A in its various forms. It includes both natural and synthetic chemicals that are structurally related to vitamin A. Its oxidized metabolites, namely retinaldehyde and retinoic acid (vitamin A acid), are biologically active compounds. It is the chemical name of vitamin A. Retinol and retinoic acid is the transport form and retinol ester is also the storage form.
- **Carotenoids:** The most common carotenoid in the food having provitamin A activity is β-carotene. Major portions of carotenoids are absorbed as such and are stored in liver and fat.

Sources of vitamin A: Various sources are as follows:

- **Animal-derived foods:** Main dietary sources of preformed vitamin A. Vitamin A is found only in animal derived foods. These include liver, fish, eggs, milk, butter, and cheese. Fish livers are a particularly rich source of vitamin A itself (retinoids).
- **Yellow and green leafy vegetables:** The source of the precursor-carotene is mainly leafy and green vegetables. Dark green and deeply colored fruits and vegetables are the vegetable sources of provitamins A carotenoids. Vegetable sources include yellow and leafy green vegetables such as carrots, squash, and spinach. These vegetable sources provide large amounts of carotenoids and provitamins. Moderate cooking of vegetables increases the release of carotenoid, thereby improves absorption in the gut. Carotenoids constitute about 30% of the vitamin A in human diets and most important being β-carotene. In the body, carotenoids (including β-carotene) can be metabolized to active vitamin A.

Metabolism of vitamin A (Fig. 21)

Absorption: Vitamin A is a fat-soluble vitamin. For its absorption, it requires bile, pancreatic enzymes, and some

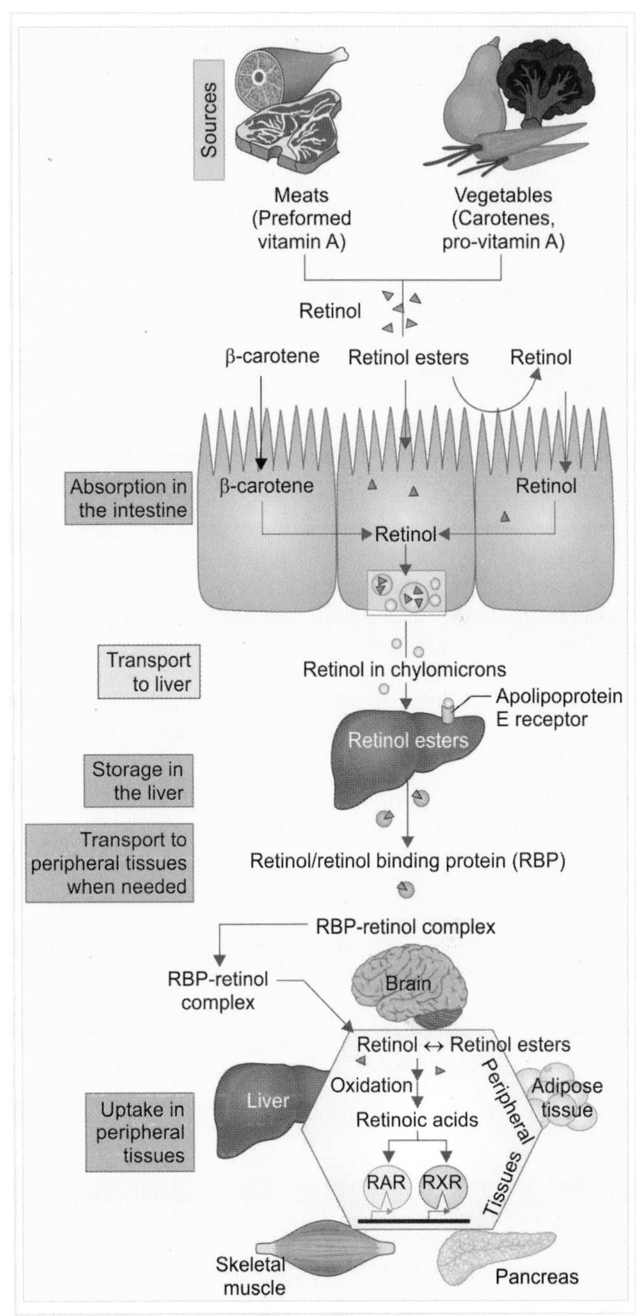

(RAR: retinoic acid receptors; RXR: retinoid X receptor)

FIG. 21: Metabolism of vitamin A. Retinol (usually ingested as retinol ester) and β-carotene are absorbed in the intestine. In the intestine, the β-carotene in the diet is also converted to retinol. These are absorbed with chylomicrons. From intestine, retinol is transported in chylomicrons to the liver. The liver cells uptake retinol through the apolipoprotein E receptor. Retinol esters are stored in the liver and can be transported to peripheral tissues when needed. Before retinol esters are released from liver, retinol binds to a specific retinol-binding protein (RBP) and forms RBP-retinol complex. The uptake of RBP-retinol in peripheral tissues depends on cell surface receptors specific for RBP.

level of antioxidant activity in the food. Fatty meal facilitates the absorption of carotenoids. Retinol (usually ingested as retinol ester) and β-carotene are absorbed in the intestine. In the intestine, the β-carotene in the diet is also converted to retinol. These are absorbed with chylomicrons.

Transport to liver: From intestine, retinol is transported in chylomicrons to the liver.

Storage in liver: In the liver, the liver cells uptake retinol through the apolipoprotein E receptor. Then retinol is esterified and stored in the liver. More than 90% of the body's vitamin A reserves are stored in the liver, mainly in the perisinusoidal stellate (Ito) cells. In healthy individual who takes an adequate diet, these vitamin A reserves are enough to meet the body's requirement for at least 6 months.

Transport to peripheral tissues: Retinol esters are stored in the liver. It can be transported to peripheral tissues when needed. Before retinol esters are released from liver, retinol binds to a specific retinol-binding protein (RBP) and forms RBP-retinol complex. RBP is synthesized in the liver.

Uptake in peripheral tissues: The uptake of RBP-retinol in peripheral tissues depends on cell surface receptors specific for RBP. After retinol is taken up into peripheral tissues, the retinol may also be stored as retinol ester or may be oxidized to form retinoic acid. This retinoic acid has important effects on epithelial differentiation and growth.

Functions of vitamin A

Vitamin A has several metabolic roles. The main functions of vitamin A in humans are as follows:

Maintenance of normal vision: It is one of the major functions of vitamin A. The visual process involves four forms of vitamin A containing pigments. These are rhodopsin in the rods and three iodopsins in cone cells. Rods are the most light-sensitive pigment and therefore important in reduced light. Each iodopsins in cone cells is responsive to specific colors in bright light.

- The synthesis of rhodopsin from retinol involves mainly three steps (**Fig. 22**) namely—(1) oxidation of retinol to all-trans-retinal, (2) isomerization to 11-*cis*-retinal, and (3) covalent association with the 7-transmembrane rod protein opsin to form rhodopsin.
- A photon (a particle representing a quantum of light) of light causes the isomerization of 11-*cis*-retinal to all-*trans*-retinal, which dissociates from rhodopsin. This produces a conformational change in rhodopsin and generates a series of downstream events. This in turn generates a nerve impulse. Through neurons, the nerve impulse is transmitted from the retina to the brain.
- Vitamin A is essential for dark adaptation During dark adaptation, some (but not all) of the all-*trans*-retinal is reconverted to 11-*cis*-retinal. But most of the *all*-trans-retinal is reduced to retinol and lost to the retina. That is the reason for the need of continuous supply of vitamin A. Deficiency of vitamin A causes nyctalopia (a condition characterized by an abnormal inability to see in dim light or at night known as night blindness).

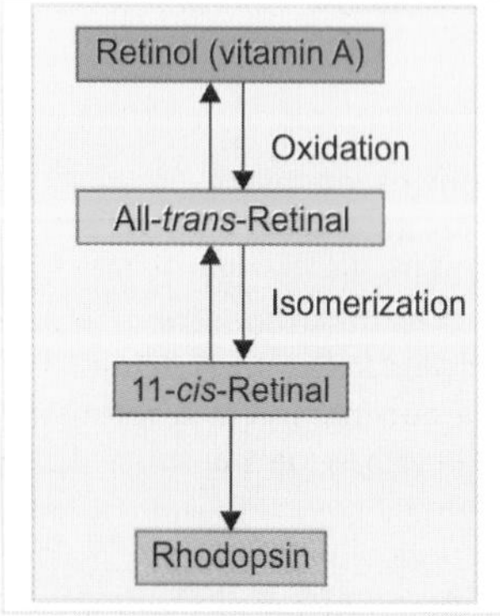

FIG. 22: Steps in the synthesis of rhodopsin.

Regulation of cell growth and differentiation: It is another major function of vitamin A. Retinol and retinoic acid are involved in the control of proliferation (growth), differentiation, and repair of epithelial cells and integrity of the epithelial cells of the respiratory, urinary, and intestinal tracts. Vitamin A and retinoids play an important role in the orderly differentiation of mucus-secreting epithelium. In vitamin A deficiency, mucus-secreting cells are replaced by keratin-producing cells and this process is known as squamous metaplasia. Vitamin A is needed for the maintenance of the surface linings of the eyes. Activation of retinoic acid receptors (RARs) occurs by binding of these receptors by their ligands. The ligand namely vitamin A derivative all-*trans*-retinoic acid has the highest affinity for RARs compared with other retinoids. This binding causes the release of corepressors and the obligatory formation of heterodimers with another retinoid receptor, RXR. Both RAR and RXR are nuclear receptor and have three isoforms namely, α, β, and γ. The RAR/RXR heterodimers bind to retinoic acid response elements present in the regulatory regions of genes. These regulatory regions encode receptors for growth factors, tumor suppressor genes, and secreted proteins. By these mechanisms, retinoids (vitamin A) regulate cell growth and differentiation, cell cycle control, and other biologic responses.

Metabolic effects of retinoids: The RXR can be activated by 9-cis-retinoic acid and can form heterodimers with other nuclear receptors. These nuclear receptors include those involved in drug metabolism, peroxisome proliferator-activated receptors (PPARs), and vitamin D receptors. PPARs are key regulators of lipid metabolism including fatty acid oxidation in fat cells and muscle, adipogenesis, and lipoprotein metabolism. This association of RXR and PPARγ is responsible for the metabolic effects of retinoids on adipogenesis.

Enhancing immunity to infections: Morbidity and mortality rates from diarrhea may be reduced by giving vitamin A supplementation. Vitamin A is able to stimulate the immune system. Retinol binding protein (RBP) is a negative "acute phase protein". Probably, infections reduce the bioavailability of vitamin A by inducing the acute phase response. This in turn can inhibit synthesis of RBP in the liver. The reduced levels of RBP in liver lead to decreased levels of circulating retinol. So, there is reduced availability of vitamin A to tissue. Also, retinoids, β-carotene, and some related carotenoids act as photoprotective and antioxidant agents. Retinoids are required for normal growth, fetal development, fertility, hematopoiesis, and immune function.

Antioxidant: Retinoids, β-carotene, and some related carotenoids act as photoprotective and antioxidant agents.

Other functions: Vitamin A is involved in growth of bone, reproduction, embryonic development, and the regulation of adult genes.

Clinical uses: Retinoids are used in the treatment of skin disorders such as severe acne (13-*cis*-retinoic acid) and certain forms of psoriasis (isotretinoin). Tretinoin, i.e., all-*trans* retinoic acid, is also used in the treatment of acute promyelocytic leukemia (APL). All-*trans*-retinoic acid induces the differentiation and subsequent apoptosis of APL cells. This is achieved by binding of retinoids to a PML-RARα fusion protein present in promyelocytic leukemia (refer page 512 and 513). A different isomer, called 13-cis-retinoic acid, has been used in the treatment of childhood neuroblastoma.

Vitamin A deficiency

Causes of deficiency (Table 11): Vitamin A deficiency may be primary (due to malnutrition or undernutrition with deficiency in the diet) or secondary to conditions which cause malabsorption of fats. In newborn infants, the absorption of the vitamin is poor. In children, infections cause depletion of vitamin A stores. In adults, malabsorption syndromes such as celiac disease, Crohn disease, and colitis can produce deficiency of vitamin A as well other fat-soluble vitamins. Bariatric surgery and continuous use of mineral oil as a laxative in older individual may lead to deficiency.

Pathologic effects (clinical features) of vitamin A deficiency

Effects in the eye: Vitamin A is a component of rhodopsin and other visual pigments. Its various effects are as follows:

- **Night blindness:** Vitamin A is a component of rhodopsin and other visual pigments. Hence, impaired vision particularly impaired adaptation to the dark (night blindness) is one of the earliest manifestations of vitamin A deficiency.
- **Xerophthalmia:** Vitamin A is needed for maintaining the differentiation of epithelial cells. Persistent deficiency of vitamin A produces epithelial metaplasia and keratinization. In the eyes, it produces keratinization of the cornea termed as xerophthalmia (dry eye). Initially, there is dryness of the conjunctiva (xerosis conjunctivae) because of the replacement of the normal lacrimal and mucus-secreting epithelium by keratinized epithelium. Subsequently, there is a gradual accumulation of keratin debris in small opaque plaques which gives rise to characteristic Bitot spots (**Fig. 23**). They may progress to erosion of the roughened corneal surface, softening and destruction of the cornea (keratomalacia), scarring, and irreversible blindness.

Table 11: Causes of vitamin A deficiency.	
Primary causes	***Secondary causes***
Prolonged dietary deprivation	Sprue
Vegetarians	Cystic fibrosis
Refugees	Pancreatic insufficiency
Chronic alcoholics	Duodenal bypass
Toddlers	Chronic diarrhea
Preschool children	Bile duct obstruction
	Giardiasis, and cirrhosis

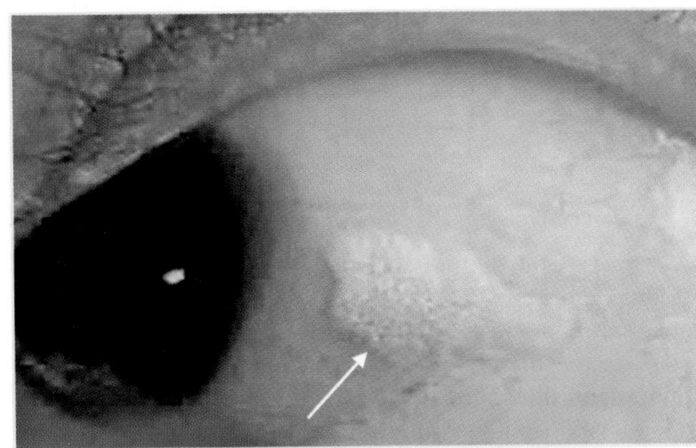

FIG. 23: Bitot's spot.

Effects on other epithelia: Deficiency of vitamin A also causes squamous metaplasia of the epithelium lining the upper respiratory passage and urinary tract. Loss of the mucociliary epithelium lining the upper airways predisposes to secondary infections of lung. Desquamation of keratin debris in the urinary tract predisposes to renal and urinary bladder stones. In the skin, it produces hyperplasia and hyperkeratinization of the epidermis. This leads to plugging of the ducts of the adnexal glands and may produce follicular or papular dermatosis. Advanced metaplasia may increase the risk of squamous cell carcinoma.

Immune deficiency: It is responsible for higher mortality rates from common infections, such as measles, pneumonia, and infectious diarrhea. In individuals with vitamin A deficiency, dietary supplements reduce mortality by 20–30%.

Pathological effects of vitamin A deficiency are depicted in **Figure 24**.

Vitamin A toxicity

Q. Write short essay on vitamin A toxicity.

Types of toxicity: Vitamin A may be due to short-term or long-term excesses and both may produce toxic manifestations.

Vitamin A toxicity can be acute (usually due to accidental ingestion by children) or chronic. Both types of toxicity cause headache and increased intracranial pressure (pseudotumor cerebri).

- **Acute toxicity** also produces headache, dizziness, nausea, vomiting, stupor, and blurred vision. Single doses of 300 mg in adults or 100 mg in children can be harmful.
- **Chronic toxicity** also causes changes in skin, hair (loss), and nails; liver and bone damage; double vision, ataxia, hyperlipidemia, weight loss, anorexia, nausea, vomiting and bone and joint pain. It stimulates osteoclast production and activity. Thus, there is increased resorption of bone predisposing to the risk of fractures. Retinol (retinoic acid) is teratogenic and incidence of birth defects in infants is high with vitamin A intakes of >3 mg a day during pregnancy. The synthetic retinoids used for the treatment of acne are not associated with chronic toxic symptoms. However, their use in pregnancy should be avoided because of teratogenic effects of retinoids.

Carotenemia is common among infants and toddlers who eat large amounts of carrots and green leafy vegetables. It is benign and the skin appears yellow. It can be confused with jaundice, but discoloration of skin spontaneously resolves once the intake of carotenoid rich food is reduced.

Recommended dietary allowances (RDAs)/adequate intake of fat-soluble vitamins for individuals are shown in **Table 12**.

Vitamin D

Q. Write short essay on vitamin D and rickets.

Vitamin D is a fat-soluble vitamin. Vitamin D is responsible for enhancing intestinal absorption of calcium, iron, magnesium, phosphate, and zinc. It is required for the maintenance of adequate plasma levels of calcium and phosphorus. These calcium and phosphorus support metabolic functions, bone mineralization, and neuromuscular transmission.

Physiology: Vitamin D is a fat-soluble steroid hormone **found in two forms—vitamin D_3 (cholecalciferol) and vitamin D_2 (ergocalciferol)**. Both have equal biological potency in humans.

- **Vitamin D_3 (Cholecalciferol):** It is produced in skin with direct sunlight.
- **Vitamin D_2 (Ergocalciferol):** It is derived from plant ergosterol. It is less effective as precursor to 1,25$(OH)_2$-vitamin D.

Vitamin D prevents rickets (in children whose epiphyses have not already closed), osteomalacia (in adults) and hypocalcemic tetany. Vitamin D maintains the correct concentration of ionized calcium in the extracellular fluid compartment and thereby prevents tetany. When there is deficiency of vitamin D, there is reduced ionized calcium in the extracellular fluid. This results in continuous excitation of muscle (tetany). However, if there is any reduction in the level of serum calcium, it causes increased secretion of parathyroid hormone (PTH). It leads to bone resorption and serum calcium levels are usually corrected. Hence, tetany is quite uncommon with reduced serum calcium level.

Metabolism of vitamin D (Fig. 25)

The main steps of vitamin D metabolism are as follows:

Sources of vitamin D: Photochemical synthesis of vitamin D from 7-dehydrocholesterol in the skin (endogenous synthesis) and absorption of vitamin D from foods (exogenous sources) in the gut.

- **Endogenous synthesis:** The major source of vitamin D is by endogenous synthesis from a precursor called 7-dehydrocholesterol. Vitamin D is formed in a photochemical reaction that needs solar or artificial UV

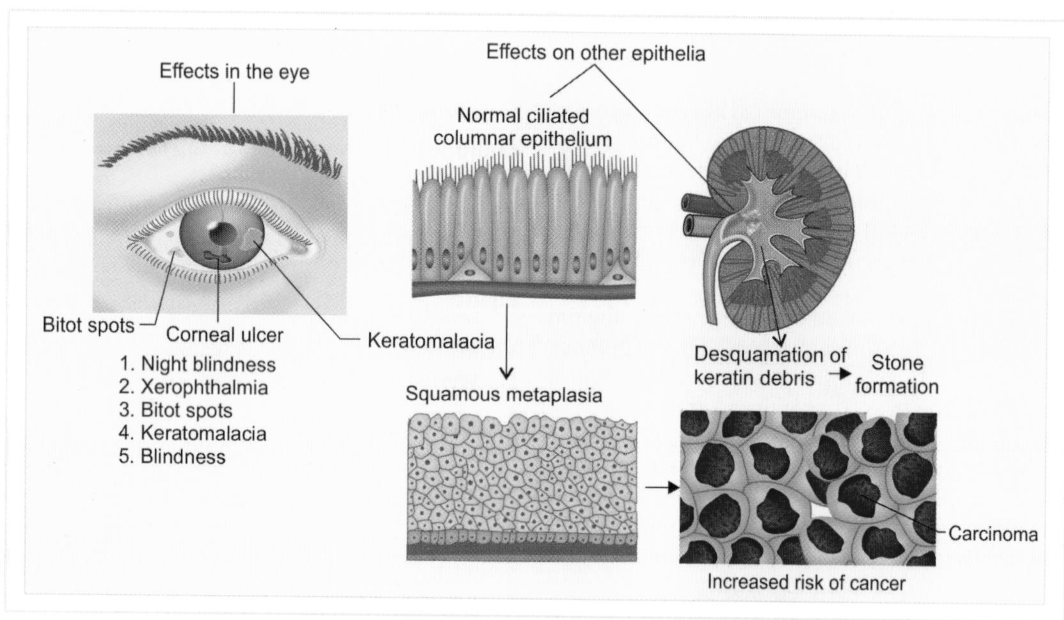

FIG. 24: Pathological effects of vitamin A deficiency. It produces various changes in the eye and epithelial metaplasia.

Table 12: Recommended dietary allowances (RDAs)/adequate intake of fat-soluble vitamins for different age group.

Age group	*Vitamin A(RAE*)*	*Vitamin D (µg/day)*	*Vitamin E (µg/day)*	*Vitamin K (µg/day)*
Infants	400–500	5	4–5	2–2.5
Children (1–13 years) >14 years	300–600	5	6–11	30–60
• Males	900	5–15	15	75–120
• Females	600–700	5–15	11–15	75–90
Pregnancy	750–770	5	15	75–90
Lactation	1,200–1,300	5	19	75–90

*1 RAE (retinol activity equivalents) = 1 µg retinol, 12 µg β-carotene; 1 µg calciferol = 40 IU vitamin D

Note: The Recommended Dietary Allowance for vitamin A is expressed in retinol equivalents. It takes into account both preformed vitamin A and β-carotene.

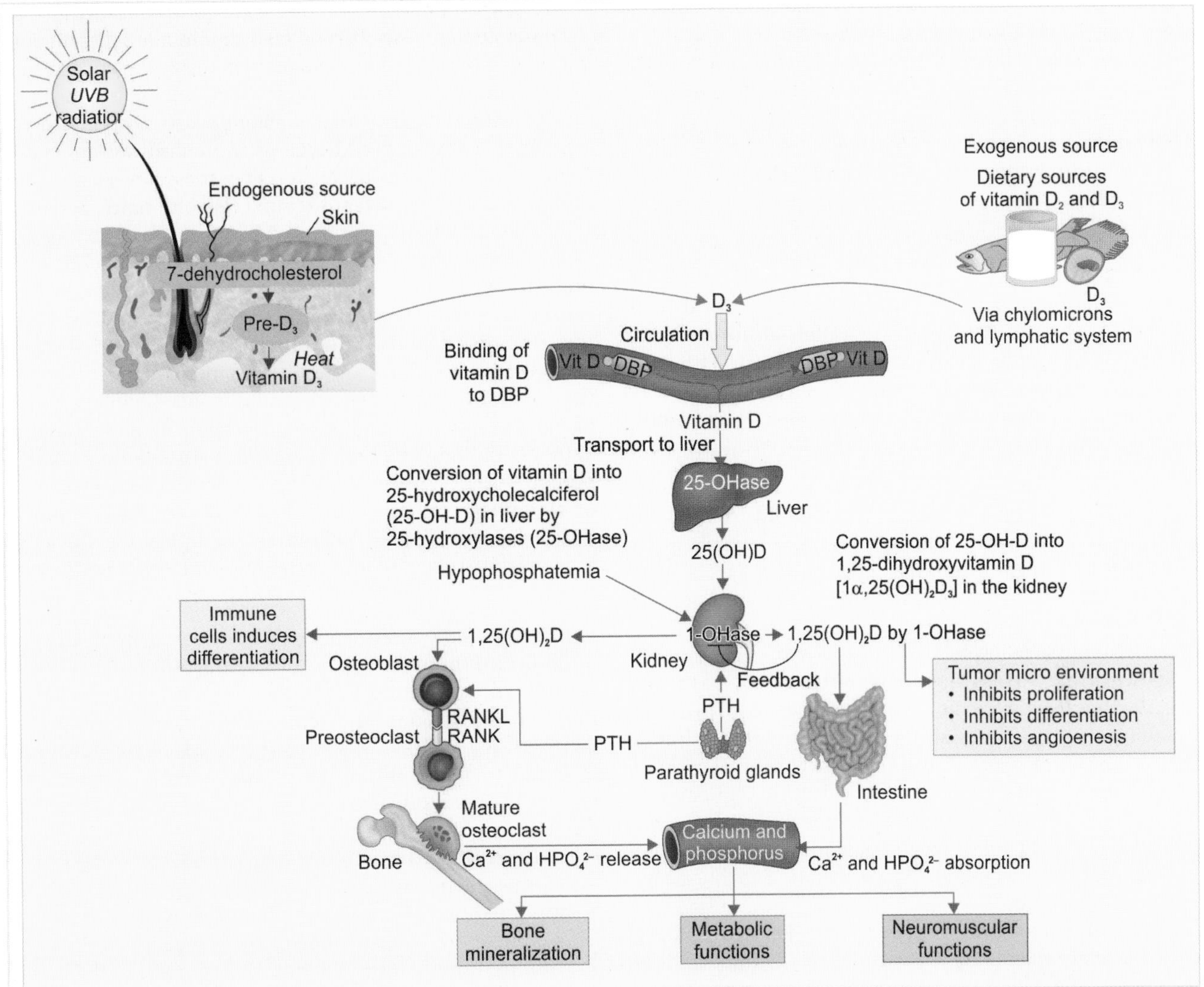

(DBP: vitamin D-binding protein).

FIG. 25: Metabolism of vitamin D. Vitamin D is endogenously produced from 7-dehydrocholesterol in the skin or is ingested in the diet. Vitamin D (D_3) is converted in the liver into 25(OH)D and in the kidney into 1,25-dihydroxyvitamin D [1,25(OH)$_2$D$_3$]. 1,25(OH)$_2$D$_3$ is the most active form of the vitamin. 1,25(OH)$_2$D$_3$ stimulates the expression of RANKL. RANKL is an important regulator of osteoclast maturation and function on osteoblasts. 1,25(OH)$_2$D$_3$ also increases the intestinal absorption of calcium and phosphorus, induces immune differentiation, and involved in tumor microenvironment.

light in the range of 290–315 nm (UVB radiation). This reaction produces cholecalciferol, known as vitamin D_3. The term vitamin D is used for vitamin D_3. Normally, the skin endogenously synthesizes about 90% of the required vitamin D by sun exposure. Generally, vitamin D production in individuals with dark skin is low because of melanin pigmentation.

- **Exogenous sources:** Dietary sources of vitamin D include deep-sea fish, plants, and grains. They contribute to the remaining vitamin D required. The vitamin is absorbed in the jejunum and its absorption depends on adequate fat absorption by the intestine. In plants, vitamin D is present in a precursor form (ergosterol), Ergosterol is a biological precursor of vitamin D_2 (ergocalciferol). Ergosterol is converted to vitamin D in the body.

- **Binding of vitamin D to vitamin D-binding protein (DBP) and transport to liver:** Vitamin D from both the sources binds to plasma α_1-globulin (DBP) and is transported to the liver.
- **Conversion of vitamin D into 25-hydroxycholecalciferol (25-OH-D) in the liver:** It is by the action of 25-hydroxylases, including CYP27A1 and other CYPs.
- **Conversion of 25-OH-D into 1,25-dihydroxyvitamin D [1α,25(OH)$_2$D$_3$] in the kidney:** It is carried out by the enzyme 1α-hydroxylase in the kidney and the product formed 1,25-dihydroxyvitamin D [1α,25(OH)$_2$D$_3$] is the most active form of vitamin D.

Regulation of production of 1,25-dihydroxyvitamin D in the kidney (Fig. 25): It is regulated by three main mechanisms—

1. **Parathyroid hormone:** Hypocalcemia stimulates secretion of PTH from parathyroid. PTH increases the conversion of

25-OH-D into 1,25-dihydroxyvitamin D by upregulating the expression of 1α-hydroxylase in the kidney.
2. **Hypophosphatemia:** It also upregulates 1α-hydroxylase expression in the kidney thereby increasing the production of 1,25-dihydroxyvitamin.
3. **Through a feedback mechanism:** Increased levels of 1,25-dihydroxyvitamin D downregulate its own synthesis by feedback mechanism by inhibiting the activity of 1α-hydroxylase in the kidney.

Functions

Similar to retinoids and steroid hormones, 1,25-dihydroxyvitamin D also acts by binding to a **high-affinity nuclear receptor (vitamin D receptor)** namely, RXR. This RXR heterodimeric complex binds to vitamin D response elements present in the regulatory sequences of vitamin D target genes.

Skeletal homeostasis

Regulation of plasma levels of calcium and phosphorus: Most cells of the body have receptors for 1,25-dihydroxyvitamin D. In the small intestine, bones, and kidneys, signals transduced through these receptors regulate levels of calcium and phosphorus in the plasma. The main functions of 1,25-dihydroxyvitamin D on calcium and phosphorus homeostasis are as follows:

- **Stimulates intestinal absorption of calcium:** 1,25-dihydroxyvitamin D stimulates absorption of calcium in the duodenum. It is via interaction of 1,25-dihydroxyvitamin D with nuclear vitamin D receptor and the formation of a complex with RXR. The complex binds to vitamin D response elements and activates the transcription of TRPV6 (a member of the transient receptor potential vanilloid family). TRPV6 encodes a main calcium transport channel.
- **Stimulates calcium reabsorption in the kidney:** 1,25-dihydroxyvitamin D increases calcium influx in distal tubules of the kidney. It is via the increased expression of TRPV5, another member of the transient receptor potential vanilloid family. TRPV5 expression is also regulated by PTH in response to hypocalcemia.
- **Interaction with PTH in the regulation of blood calcium:** The levels of calcium and phosphorus in the plasma are maintained by Vitamin D. The parathyroid glands play a main role in the regulation of extracellular concentrations of calcium. Parathyroid glands sense even small changes in blood calcium concentrations though a calcium receptor. Both 1,25-dihydroxyvitamin D and PTH increase the absorption of calcium in the intestine and also increase the expression of RANKL (receptor activator of NF-κB ligand) on osteoblasts. RANKL binds to its receptor (RANK) present in preosteoclasts. This binding induces the differentiation of preosteoclasts into mature osteoclasts. These osteoclasts dissolve bone by secreting hydrochloric acid and activation of proteases such as cathepsin K. Thus, they release calcium and phosphorus from the bone into the circulation.
- **Mineralization of bone:** Vitamin D plays a role in the mineralization of osteoid matrix and epiphyseal cartilage in both flat and long bones. Vitamin D stimulates osteoblasts to secrete the calcium-binding protein osteocalcin. Osteocalcin is involved in the deposition of calcium during development of bone. Flat bones develop by intramembranous bone formation. During this process, the mesenchymal cells differentiate directly into osteoblasts. These osteoblasts synthesize the collagenous osteoid matrix and on this matrix calcium gets deposited. Long bones develop by endochondral ossification. During this, the growing cartilage at the epiphyseal plates is provisionally mineralized. It is then progressively resorbed and replaced by osteoid matrix. Osteoid matrix becomes mineralized by deposition of calcium and forms bone.

When hypocalcemia develops due to vitamin D deficiency (**Fig. 26**), production of PTH by parathyroid is increased. This causes—(1) activation of renal 1α-hydroxylase and increases the amount of active vitamin D and thereby increases absorption calcium from intestine, (2) increased resorption of calcium from bone by osteoclasts, (3) reduced renal excretion of calcium, and (4) increased excretion of phosphate by kidneys. Though these mechanisms restore and maintain a normal level of calcium in the serum, there will be persistence of hypophosphatemia. This impairs the mineralization of bone. Tumor-induced osteomalacia and some forms of hypophosphatemic rickets may be due to increased production of FGF-23.

Other functions Apart from skeletal homeostasis, vitamin D has immunomodulatory and antiproliferative effects. 1,25-dihydroxyvitamin D can also act through alternative mechanisms without the need of the transcription of target genes. In these alternative mechanisms, 1,25-dihydroxyvitamin D binds to a membrane-associated vitamin D receptor (mVDR). This activates protein kinase C and opening of calcium channels.

- **Antiproliferative effects:** The vitamin D receptor is expressed in the parathyroid gland, and $1,25(OH)_2D_3$ has an antiproliferative effect on parathyroid cells and it suppresses the transcription of the *PTH* gene.
- **Immunomodulatory:** Vitamin D is involved in the innate and adaptive immune system.

Vitamin D deficiency

The normal reference range for circulating 25-(OH)-D is 20–100 ng/mL. In vitamin D deficiency, its concentrations are <20 ng/mL. Milder forms of vitamin D deficiency, also called as vitamin D insufficiency, lead to an increased risk of bone loss and hip fractures in older adults.

Causes of vitamin D deficiency: (1) Impaired cutaneous production due to limited exposure to sunlight; (2) Diets deficient in calcium and vitamin D; and (3) Malabsorption. Impaired production occurs in heavily veiled women and in children born to mothers who have frequent pregnancies followed by lactation. Less commonly, renal disorders can cause decreased synthesis of 1,25-dihydroxyvitamin D or some rare inherited disorders. Some genetically determined variants of the vitamin D receptors may be associated with increased loss of bone minerals during aging and some familial forms of osteoporosis. Vitamin D deficiency can be prevented by providing a diet high in fish oils.

Skeletal effects of vitamin D deficiency Vitamin D deficiency produces **rickets in growing children and osteomalacia in adults.** Both **rickets and osteomalacia** result in an **excess of unmineralized matrix**.

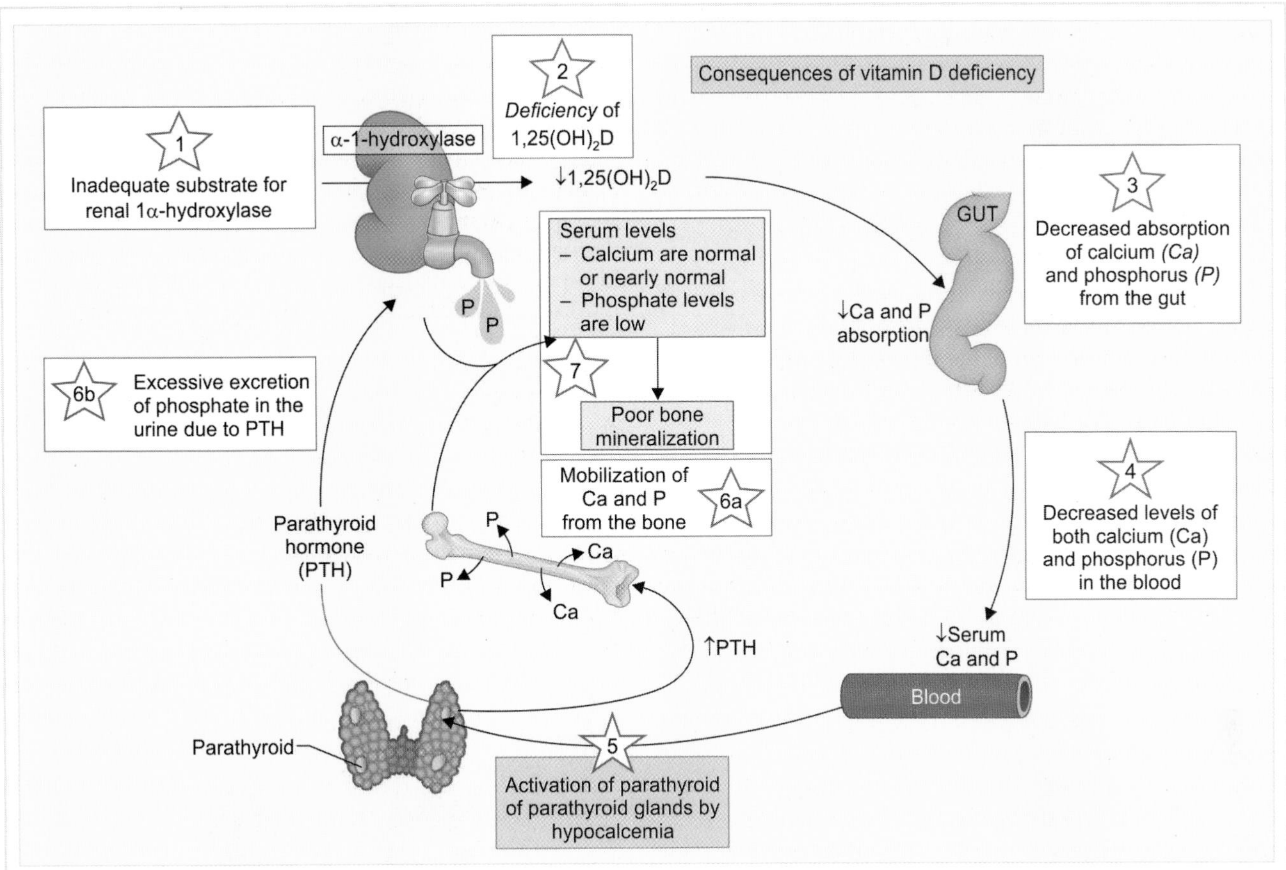

FIG. 26: Consequences of vitamin D deficiency. (1) Vitamin D deficiency is associated with inadequate substrate for renal 1α-hydroxylase. (2) This will produce a deficiency of 1,25(OH)2D, and (3) deficient absorption of calcium (Ca) and phosphorus (P) from the gut; (4) There will be reduced serum levels of calcium and phosphorus. (5) The hypocalcemia activates the parathyroid glands to secrete parathyroid hormone (PTH). (6a) PTH causes mobilization of calcium and phosphorus from bone. (6b) The parathyroid hormone (PTH) also induces excessive excretion of phosphate in the urine and calcium retention. (7) Due to this the serum levels of calcium are normal or nearly normal, but phosphate levels are low. This in turn causes poor mineralization of bone.

Rickets in children In children, before the closure of epiphyses, vitamin D deficiency causes retardation of growth associated with an expansion of the growth plate known as rickets.

MORPHOLOGY

Rickets in Children

In the normal growth plate, there are three layers of chondrocytes namely—(1) the reserve zone, (2) the proliferating zone, and (3) the hypertrophic zone. The following are the sequence in rickets:

- Overgrowth of epiphyseal cartilage: It is due to inadequate provisional calcification and defect of the cartilage cells to mature and disintegrate.
- Persistence of distorted, irregular masses of cartilage: These masses project into the bone marrow cavity.
- On inadequately mineralized cartilaginous remnants, there will be deposition of osteoid matrix.
- Disruption of the orderly replacement of cartilage by osteoid matrix: There will be enlargement and lateral expansion of the osteochondral junction.

Continued

Continued

- Abnormal overgrowth of capillaries and fibroblasts in the disorganized zone: This results from microfractures and stresses on the inadequately mineralized, weak, poorly formed bone
- Deformation of the skeleton: This is due to the loss of structural rigidity of the developing bones.
- Rickets due to impaired vitamin D action is characterized by expansion of the hypertrophic chondrocyte layer. In vitamin D deficiency, the hypophosphatemia due to secondary hyperparathyroidism is responsible for the development of the rachitic growth plate.

Gross skeletal changes in rickets (Fig. 27A): It depends on the severity and duration of the vitamin D deficiency and also the on the stresses on individual bones.

- **During the nonambulatory stage of infancy:** During this stage, there is greatest stress on head and chest.
  - **Craniotabes:** The occipital bones are softened and become flattened. The parietal bones fold inward by pressure and with the release of the pressure, elastic recoil brings the bones back into their original

Continued

Continued

original positions (craniotabes). The skull appears square and box-like and there is delayed closure of anterior fontanelle.
  - **Frontal bossing:** Excess of osteoid produces frontal bossing and the head develops a squared appearance.
  - **Rachitic rosary:** Overgrowth of cartilage or osteoid tissue at the costochondral junction causes deformation of the chest. This produced the "rachitic rosary." Rosary means string of knots or beads.
  - **Pigeon breast/chest deformity:** The weakened metaphyseal areas of the ribs are subject to the pull of the respiratory muscles. Thus, chest bends inward and produces anterior protrusion of the sternum. This results in pigeon breast deformity (pectus carinatum).
  - **Harrison's sulcus/groove:** It is due to indrawing of ribs on inspiration.
- **During the ambulatory stage:**
  - **Lumbar lordosis:** This occurs when an ambulating child develops rickets. It is characterized by deformities affecting the spine, pelvis, and tibia.
  - **Bowing of the legs (Fig. 27B):** Due to effect on tibia

Continued

Continued

Osteomalacia in Adults

Vitamin D deficiency in adults is accompanied by hypocalcemia and hypophosphatemia. This results in impaired (hypo/under/inadequately) mineralization of bone matrix proteins, a condition known as osteomalacia. Lack of vitamin D deranges the normal bone remodeling that occurs throughout life. The newly formed osteoid matrix produced by osteoblasts is inadequately mineralized. Thus, it produces the excess of persistent osteoid that is characteristic of osteomalacia.

This hypomineralized bone matrix is biomechanically inferior (weak) to normal bone. Though the contours of the bone are not affected, the bone is weak. These bones are prone to bowing of weight-bearing extremities and gross skeletal fractures or microfractures. These fractures mostly affect vertebral bodies and femoral necks.

Microscopically, the unmineralized osteoid appears as a thickened layer of matrix. It stains pink in hematoxylin and eosin stain. Theis unmineralized osteoid is arranged about the more basophilic, normally mineralized bone trabeculae.

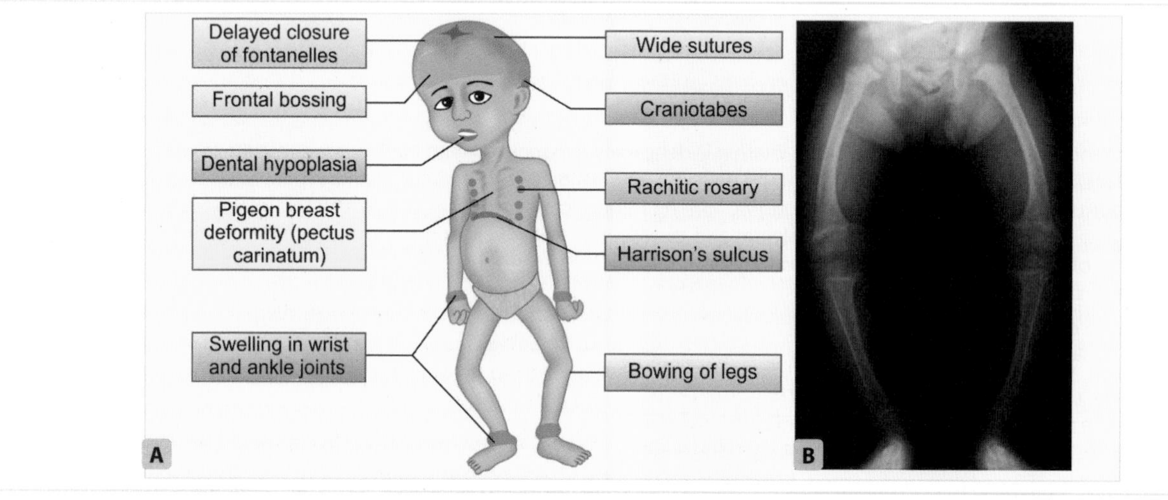

FIGS. 27A AND B: (A) Features of rickets; (B) X-ray of rickets showing splaying of epiphyses and bow legs.

Nonskeletal effects of vitamin D

Proximal myopathy: It is observed both in children and in adults with severe vitamin D deficiency. It rapidly resolves by vitamin D treatment.

Hypocalcemic tetany: Calcium is required for normal neural excitation and the relaxation of muscles. Hypocalcemic tetany is a convulsive state caused by an insufficient extracellular concentration of ionized calcium.

Vitamin D receptor is present in many cells and tissues that are not involved in calcium and phosphorus homeostasis. Many cells can produce 1,25-dihydroxyvitamin D. Examples include macrophages, keratinocytes, and tissues, such as breast, prostate, and colon. In the macrophages, synthesis of 1,25-dihydroxyvitamin D occurs through the activity of CYP27B. This CYP27B is in the mitochondria. Probably pathogen-induced activation of Toll-like receptors in macrophages causes increased expression of vitamin D receptor and CYP27B. This causes local synthesis of 1,25-dihydroxyvitamin D. It also activates vitamin D-dependent gene expression in macrophages and other neighboring immune cells. Low levels of 1,25-dihydroxyvitamin D (<20 ng/mL) may increase in the incidence of cancers of colon, prostate, and breast cancers, but whether vitamin D supplement can reduce cancer risk has not known.

Vitamin D toxicity

Prolonged exposure to normal sunlight does not produce an excess of vitamin D. The most common cause of excess vitamin D is administration of megadoses orally. This leads to hypervitaminosis D. The initial response to excess vitamin D is hypercalcemia. This leads to nonspecific symptoms such as weakness and headaches. Increased renal calcium excretion results in nephrolithiasis or nephrocalcinosis. Metastatic calcification can occur in blood vessels, heart, and lungs. In children, hypervitaminosis D may cause metastatic calcifications of soft tissues such as the kidney. In adults, it causes bone pain and hypercalcemia. The large doses of vitamin D is a potent rodenticide.

Vitamin E

Vitamin E is a collective name for eight stereoisomers of tocopherols and tocotrienols. The most important dietary form is α-tocopherol.

Functions

- Antioxidant: It prevents oxidation of low-density lipoproteins (LDLs) and polyunsaturated fatty acids in cell membranes by free radicals. Other antioxidants (e.g., vitamin C, glutathione) and enzymes maintain vitamin E in a reduced state. Acts in conjunction with other antioxidants, such as selenium.
- It helps to maintain cell membrane structure.
- It affects DNA synthesis and cell signaling.
- Anti-inflammatory: Vitamin E also inhibits prostaglandin synthesis and the activities of protein kinase C and phospholipase A_2.
- Immune systems

Deficiency

- Dietary deficiency of vitamin E is very rare.
- Vitamin E deficiency is seen only in premature infants and in severe and prolonged malabsorption diseases, such as celiac disease, or after small intestinal resection.
- It can cause mild hemolytic anemias, ataxia, and visual scotomas.

Vitamin K

Forms of vitamin K: There are two natural forms—Vitamin K1 (phylloquinone) derived from vegetable (green leafy vegetables, such as kale and spinach) and animal sources (liver), and vitamin K2 (menaquinone) which is synthesized by bacterial flora in the colon and in hepatic tissue. Phylloquinone can be converted to menaquinone in some organs.

Functions

- **Coagulation:** Vitamin K is a cofactor for carboxylation of glutamic acid which is necessary for the production of carboxyglutamate (gla). Gla residues are found in four of the coagulation factor proteins (II, VII, IX and X). Thus, it is involved in coagulation process.
- **Others:** Other important gla proteins include osteocalcin (in bone) and matrix gla protein (vascular smooth muscle) that are important in mineralization of bone. However, the importance of vitamin K for mineralization of bone and prevention of vascular calcification is unknown.

Deficiency

Various cause are as follows:

- Chronic small intestinal disease (e.g., celiac disease, Crohn's disease).
- Obstruction of biliary tracts: In obstructive jaundice, dietary vitamin K is not absorbed and it is necessary to administer the vitamin in parenteral form before surgery.
- After small bowel resection
- Broad-spectrum antibiotics: They can precipitate vitamin K deficiency by reducing gut bacteria which synthesize menaquinones, and by inhibiting the metabolism of vitamin K.
- Warfarin and related anticoagulants: Warfarin type drugs prevent the conversion of vitamin K to its active hydroquinone form.
- **Deficiency in newborn:** It is because of—(1) low-fat stores, (2) low breast milk levels of vitamin K, (3) sterility of the infantile intestinal tract, (4) liver immaturity, and (5) poor placental transport.

Effects of deficiency

- Vitamin K deficiency leads to delayed coagulation and bleeding. Hence, the symptoms of vitamin K deficiency are due to hemorrhage.
- **Newborn:** In breastfed newborns, it may cause hemorrhagic disease of the newborn. Intracranial, gastrointestinal, and skin bleeding can occur in vitamin K-deficient infants 1–7 days after birth. Thus, vitamin K (1 mg IM) is given routinely to newborn babies to prevent hemorrhagic disease.

Water-soluble Vitamins

Vitamin C (Ascorbic Acid)

Q. Write short essay on pathology of vitamin C deficiency.

It is a water-soluble vitamin. The effects of vitamin C deficiency (scurvy) were described 5,000 years ago in Egyptian hieroglyphs. It was mentioned by Hippocrates in 500 BC. Sailors of the British Royal Navy were nicknamed scurvy as "limeys" for the seamen. This term is called so because at the end of the 18th century, the Navy started providing lime and lemon juice (rich sources of vitamin C) to sailors. This was given to prevent scurvy during their long temporary stay at sea. It was only in 1932, ascorbic acid was identified and synthesized.

Functions

Ascorbic acid has many functions and affects a variety of processes.

Synthesis of collagen: Vitamin C is necessary for the formation of collagen from procollagen. Vitamin C is involved in the hydroxylation of proline and lysine in procollagen to hydroxyproline and hydroxylysine in mature collagen. This is achieved by activation of prolyl and lysyl hydroxylases from its inactive precursors and causes hydroxylation of procollagen by vitamin C. Inadequately hydroxylated procollagen cannot have a stable helical configuration. This procollagen is poorly secreted from the fibroblast. Those molecules of procollagen that are secreted by fibroblast are inadequately cross-linked. These molecules do not have tensile strength, and are more soluble and prone to enzymatic degradation. Normally, collagen has the highest content of hydroxyproline and is most affected in vitamin C deficiency. Collagen particularly in blood vessels is usually affected and this is responsible for the predisposition to hemorrhages in scurvy. Vitamin C is important for chondroitin sulfate synthesis.

Synthesis of neurotransmitter: Neurotransmitters (e.g., norepinephrine, dopamine) are chemical messengers that transmit a message from a nerve cell across the synapse to a target cell. Synthesis of norepinephrine needs hydroxylation of dopamine. Vitamin C is needed for this step.

Antioxidant properties: Ascorbic acid is the most active powerful reducing agent controlling the redox potential within cells. Vitamin C can scavenge free radicals directly and can act indirectly by regenerating the antioxidant form of vitamin E.

Other functions include modulating the immune response, intracellular electron transfer, and promotion of nonheme iron absorption. The effect of vitamin C as antioxidant and modulation of immune response has formed the basis of clinical trials based on supplementation of vitamin C in sepsis.

Causes of vitamin C deficiency

Ascorbic acid is not synthesized endogenously in humans. Hence, humans are entirely dependent on the diet for this nutrient. Vitamin C is present in milk and some animal products (liver, fish) and is abundant in many fruits and vegetables. The best dietary sources of vitamin C are citrus fruits, green vegetables, and tomatoes. All but the most restricted diets provide adequate amounts of vitamin C. Causes of vitamin C deficiency include:

- Infants fed only on boiled cow's milk during the first year of life are at risk. Infants who are maintained on formulas of evaporated milk without supplementation of vitamin C may also develop deficiency.
- Individuals who do not eat vegetables such as elderly people who live alone (singly) and chronic alcoholics.
- Pregnant and lactating women and those with thyrotoxicosis require more vitamin C because of increased utilization.
- Individuals at risk of deficiency:
  - Anorexia nervosa or anorexia from other diseases such as AIDS or cancer
  - Type 1 diabetics require increased vitamin C
  - Patients undergoing peritoneal dialysis and hemodialysis
  - Diseases of small intestine such as Crohn's, Whipple, and celiac disease
  - Food faddists

Effects of vitamin C deficiency

Deficiency of vitamin C leads to the development of **scurvy**. It is mainly characterized by bone disease in growing children and by hemorrhages and healing defects in both children and adults.

- **Bone disease:** More **common in growing children** and manifests after 1–3 months. It is characterized by deranged formation of osteoid matrix and bone pain. Fractures, dislocations, and tenderness of bones are common in children.
- **Hemorrhages:** Hemorrhage is a hallmark feature of scurvy and can occur in any organ. Hair follicles are one of the common sites of cutaneous bleeding. Marked tendency to bleed into the skin (easy bruising, petechiae, ecchymosis, perifollicular hemorrhages), bleeding into muscles, joints, and underneath peritoneum are observed. Bruising and hemorrhage may be spontaneous. They are most common on the legs and buttocks where hydrostatic pressure is the greatest.
- **Delayed/poor wound healing** and breakdown of old scars
- **Anemia:** It may cause high-output heart failure.
- **Gums:** Inflamed spongy gums (gum swelling) friability, bleeding, and infection with loosening of teeth; mucosal petichiae are common.
- **Skin changes:** Roughness, keratosis of hair follicles with "corkscrew" hair, perifollicular hemorrhages
- **Nails:** Splinter hemorrhages
- **Other features:** Emotional changes, shortness of breath

Major consequences and complications of vitamin C deficiency (scurvy) caused by impaired formation of collagen are presented in **Figure 28**.

Vitamin C excess

Whether megadoses of vitamin C protect against the common cold or relieve the symptoms, is not clearly known. Mild relief as may be probably due to the mild antihistamine action of ascorbic acid. Similarly, there is no evidence that large doses of vitamin C protect against development of cancer. The availability of excess vitamin C is limited because—(1) it has inherent instability, (2) poor absorption in the intestine, and (3) rapid urinary excretion. Fortunately, toxicities due to high doses of vitamin C are rare. It may be developed with iron overload (due to increased absorption), hemolytic anemia in individuals with glucose-6-phosphate dehydrogenase (G6PD) deficiency, and calcium oxalate kidney stones.

Water-soluble Vitamins—Vitamin B Complex

Vitamins in the B group are water-soluble vitamins and consist of eight distinct vitamins.

Thiamine (Vitamin B_1)

Thiamine was the first B complex vitamin identified and is referred to as vitamin B_1.

Functions

Thiamine is an important water-soluble vitamin. It is involved in carbohydrate, fat, amino acid, glucose, and alcohol metabolism. Thiamine functions as a coenzyme in many α-ketoacid decarboxylation and transketolation reactions. Vitamin B_1 is essential for the coenzyme, thiamine pyrophosphate (TPP). It is required for the following reactions:

- Decarboxylation of pyruvate (glycolytic pathway) to acetyl CoA (Krebs cycle)
- Transketolase in the hexose monophosphate (HMP/pentose) shunt pathway
- Decarboxylation of α-ketoglutarate to succinate (Krebs cycle)
- It has an additional role in neuronal conduction.

Inadequate thiamine results in inadequate adenosine triphosphate (ATP) synthesis and abnormal carbohydrate metabolism.

Sources

Thiamine can be produced by plants and some microorganisms. However, animals cannot synthesize them.

- Source of thiamine for humans is diet, though small amounts may be synthesized by intestinal bacteria.

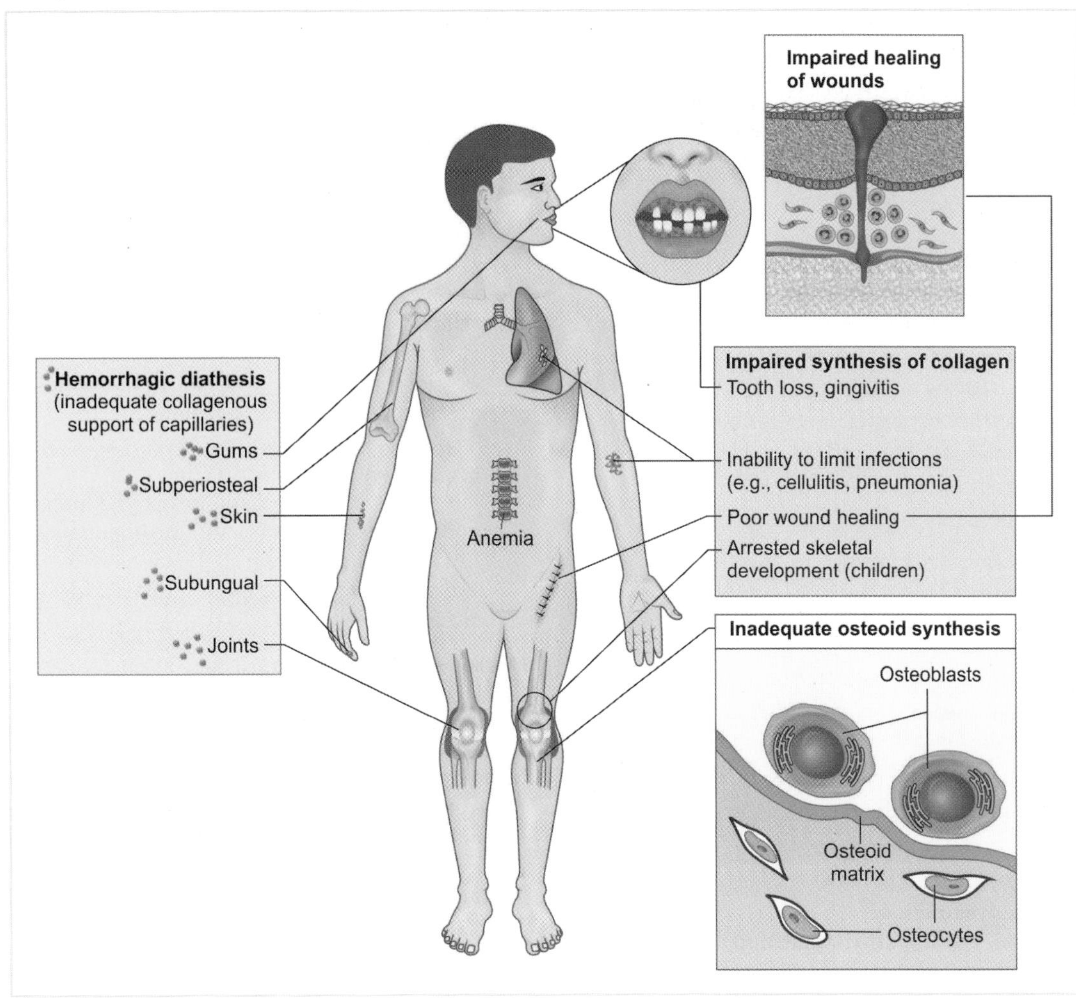

FIG. 28: Major consequences and complications of vitamin C deficiency (scurvy) caused by impaired formation of collagen.

- Dietary sources: Good dietary sources of thiamine are whole wheat flour, unpolished rice, cereals, grains, beans, nuts, and yeast. There is little or no thiamine in milled rice and grains. Thus, thiamine deficiency is more common in individuals who consume mainly a rice-based diet.
- It is also present in liver, meat, and eggs.

Requirement: Up to 30 mg of thiamine can be stored in body tissues. Required daily allowance (RDA) is 1–1.5 mg/day. Requirement increases with increased carbohydrate intake, pregnancy and lactation, smoking, alcoholism, prolonged antibiotic intake, and serious or prolonged illness.

Causes of deficiency (Box 3)

Most dietary deficiency of thiamine is due to poor dietary intake. Alcoholism, chronic renal dialysis, and chronic illnesses, such as cancer, are common precipitant factors. High carbohydrate intake increases need for vitamin B_1. Alcohol interferes with the absorption of thiamine and also with the synthesis of thiamine pyrophosphate.

Women with prolonged hyperemesis gravidarum can develop thiamine deficiency. Maternal thiamine deficiency can lead to infantile beriberi in breastfed children.

Consequences of thiamine deficiency

Consequence of thiamine deficiency is impaired glucose oxidation.

- Cells cannot metabolize glucose aerobically to generate energy as ATP. Neuronal cells are most susceptible, because they depend almost exclusively on glucose for energy requirements.
- Causes an accumulation of pyruvic and lactic acids. This in turn produces vasodilatation and increased cardiac output.

Effects of deficiency

Mild deficiency Thiamine deficiency in its early stage is characterized by irritability, decrease in short-term memory, anorexia, fatigue, and headaches.

More severe deficiency—beriberi Prolonged thiamine deficiency causes beriberi. It is classically categorized as wet or dry or a combination of two. It is the classic deficiency syndrome observed in individuals consuming polished rice diet. It shows **combinations of peripheral neuropathy, cardiovascular dysfunction, and cerebral dysfunction**.

Peripheral neuropathy: Complaints of pain and paresthesia associated with diminished reflexes. The neuropathy affects the legs most markedly, and these patients have difficulty rising from a squatting position.

Cardiovascular dysfunction ("wet beriberi"): Congestive heart failure and low peripheral vascular resistance.

Box 3: Causes of thiamine deficiency.

Lack of thiamine intake:
- Food items like milled rice, raw freshwater fish, raw shellfish, and ferns that have a high level of thiaminase
- Food high in antithiamine factor, such as tea, coffee, and betel nuts
- Alcoholic state
- Starvation state, anorexia
- With overall poor nutritional status on parenteral glucose

Increased consumption states:
- Diets high in carbohydrate or saturated fat intake
- Pregnancy and lactation
- Hyperthyroidism
- Fever—severe infection
- Increased physical exercise

Increased depletion:
- Diarrhea
- Peritoneal dialysis, hemodialysis, chronic diuretic therapy due to increased urinary thiamine losses
- Hyperemesis gravidarum

Decreased absorption:
- Chronic intestinal disease
- Alcoholism
- Malnutrition
- Gastric bypass surgery (bariatric bypass surgery)
- Malabsorption syndrome—celiac and tropical sprue

Cerebrovascular dysfunction:
- **Wernicke's encephalopathy:** Acute appearance of nystagmus, ophthalmoplegia, ataxia, and psychotic symptoms. The acute symptoms are reversible when treated with thiamine. However, if untreated, they may be followed by a prolonged and largely irreversible condition, called Korsakoff syndrome.
- **Korsakoff syndrome:** Characterized clinically by hallucinations, disturbances of short-term memory, and confabulation. The syndrome is common in chronic alcoholics but may also be seen with thiamine deficiency resulting from gastric disorders including carcinoma, chronic gastritis, or persistent vomiting.

Wet beriberi presents primarily with cardiovascular symptoms.

Dry beriberi presents with a symmetric peripheral neuropathy of the motor and sensory systems with diminished reflexes.

Clinical syndromes of thiamine deficiency are listed in **Box 4**.

Diagnosis: Immediate and dramatic response to parenteral administration of thiamine is the most reliable diagnostic test for thiamine deficiency. Biochemical tests useful for diagnosis include measurement of thiamine, pyruvate and lactate levels in blood or urine, and erythrocyte thiamine transketolase activity.

Riboflavin (Vitamin B_2)

It is a water-soluble vitamin.

Source: Riboflavin is derived from many plant and animal sources.

Box 4: Clinical syndromes of thiamine deficiency.

- Wet beriberi—high cardiac output failure
- Dry beriberi—peripheral neuropathy
- Wernicke's encephalopathy
- Korsakoff's psychosis
- Leigh syndrome (progressive subacute necrotizing encephalomyopathy

Functions

- It is important for the metabolism of fat, carbohydrate, and protein. It also plays a role in drug and steroid metabolism including detoxification reactions.
- Serves as a coenzyme for a diverse array of biochemical reactions and as an electron donor.
- The primary coenzymatic forms of riboflavin are flavin mononucleotide (FMN) and flavin adenine dinucleotide (FAD) and are known as flavoenzymes (e.g., succinic acid dehydrogenase, monoamine oxidase, glutathione reductase).

Causes of deficiency: Almost always is due to dietary deficiency and is usually seen in conjunction with deficiencies of other B vitamins.

Effects of deficiency (Fig. 29)

Nonspecific and mainly manifests as lesions of the mucocutaneous surfaces of the mouth and skin. These include hyperemia and edema of nasopharyngeal mucosa, **cheilosis, angular stomatitis, glossitis** and **seborrheic dermatitis**. Other lesions include **corneal vascularization** (**corneal interstitial keratitis)**, normochromic-normocytic anemia and personality changes.

Niacin (Vitamin B_3)

The term niacin refers to nicotinic acid and the corresponding amide, nicotinamide, and their biologically active derivatives. Niacin is a water-soluble vitamin.

Source: Nicotinic acid is derived from dietary sources or biosynthesized from tryptophan. Niacin is available in many

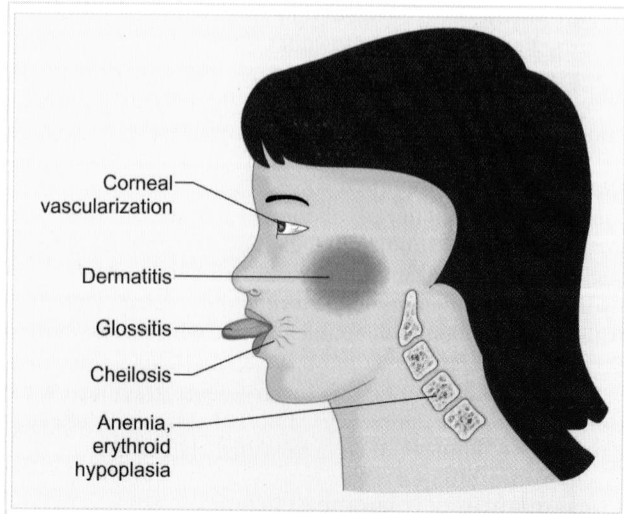

FIG. 29: Features of riboflavin deficiency.

types of grain. Animal protein (e.g., meat, eggs, and milk) is high in tryptophan and is therefore a good source of endogenously synthesized niacin. In the body, nicotinic acid is converted to nicotinamide.

Functions

- Nicotinic acid and nicotinamide serve as precursors of two coenzymes, NAD and NADP, which are important in numerous oxidation and reduction reactions.
- NAD (nicotinamide adenine dinucleotide) and NADP (nicotinamide adenine dinucleotide phosphate) are active in adenine diphosphate–ribose transfer reactions involved in DNA repair and calcium mobilization.

Causes of deficiency

- **Inadequate intake:** Maize or jowar (sorghum) diet, malnutrition, chronic alcoholism (who eat little), anorexia nervosa
- **Generalized malabsorption** (rare)
- **Drug-induced:** Prolonged isoniazid therapy, pyrazinamide, 6-mercaptopurine, 5-fluorouracil, azathioprine, ethionamide, carbamazepine, phenytoin, and phenobarbitone
- **Other disorders:**
  - **Hartnup's disease:** It is a rare genetic disorder in which there is reduced absorption of basic amino acids including tryptophan by the gut.
  - **Carcinoid syndrome and pheochromocytoma:** In these conditions, tryptophan metabolism is diverted away from the formation of nicotinamide to form amines producing pellagra-like symptoms.

Deficiency states (Fig. 30)

Pellagra: Niacin deficiency causes pellagra ("rough skin"). It is found mostly in population in which corn is the major source of energy in parts of China, Africa, and India.

- **Early symptoms:** Loss of appetite, generalized weakness and irritability, abdominal pain, and vomiting
- **Early signs:** Bright red glossitis, stomatitis, vaginitis, esophagitis, vertigo, and burning dysesthesias
- **Advanced stages:** Characteristic skin rash develops that is pigmented and scaling that develops in skin areas exposed to sunlight. This rash is known as **Casal's necklace (Fig. 31)** because it forms a ring around the neck.
- **Six Ds:** Diarrhea (in part due to proctitis and in part due to malabsorption), **d**epression, seizures and **d**ementia (or associated symptoms of anxiety or insomnia), and **d**ermatitis are part of the pellagra syndrome. Myelin degeneration of tracts in the spinal cord resembles the subacute combined **d**egeneration of vitamin B_{12} deficiency. Severe longstanding pellagra adds another "**D**," namely, death.

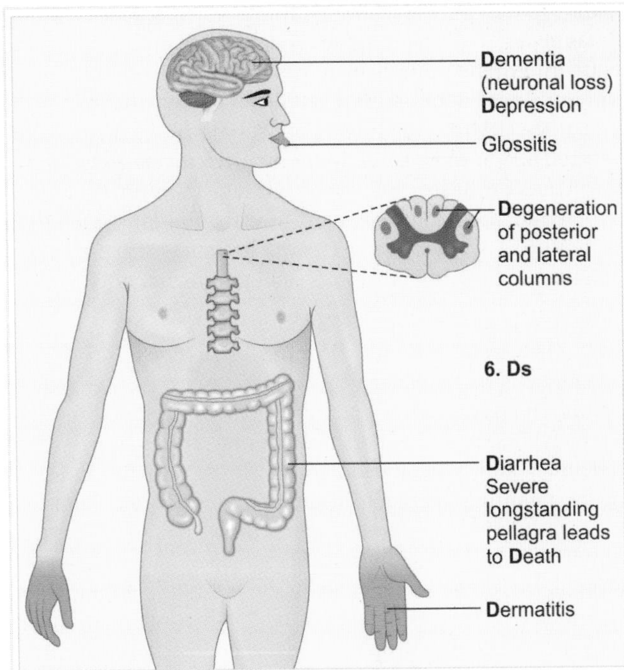

FIG. 30: Features and complications of niacin deficiency (pellagra).

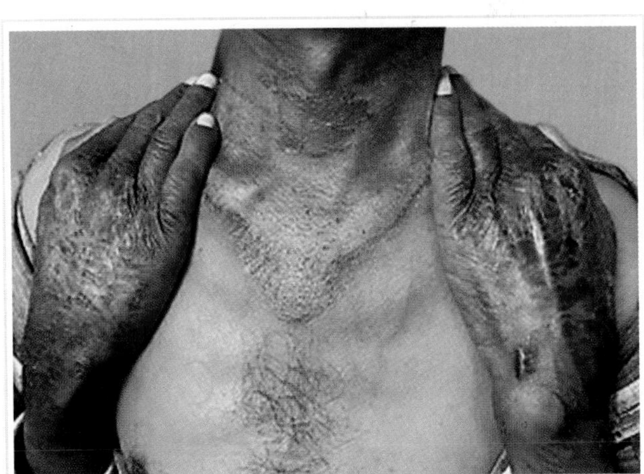

FIG. 31: Casal's necklace (ring around the neck) and dermatitis.

Pantothenic Acid (Vitamin B_5)

It is one of the water-soluble vitamins.

Source: Major sources of pantothenic acid include beef, chicken, liver, eggs, grains, and many vegetables.

Function: Pantothenic acid acts as a component of coenzyme A (CoA) and is an essential cofactor in the biosynthesis of fatty acids and certain peptides.

Deficiency of pantothenic acid: It is uncommon, except in severe malnutrition. Deficiency produces a syndrome characterized by behavioral, neurologic, and gastrointestinal disturbances. No adverse effects were found with overconsumption of pantothenic acid.

Pyridoxine (Vitamin B_6)

Vitamin B_6 (pyridoxine) refers to several (mainly three) naturally occurring derivatives of pyridine that include pyridoxine (PN), pyridoxal (PL), and pyridoxamine (PM), which are interconvertible in the body.

Sources: Pyridoxine compounds are widely distributed in vegetable and animal foods.

Functions: Vitamin B_6 functions as a coenzyme in numerous metabolic pathways. These include those related to amino acids, lipids, steroids, methylation and decarboxylation, metabolism of glycogen (gluconeogenesis), and synthesis of heme and many neurotransmitters. The coenzymatic forms are pyridoxal-5-phosphate (PSP) and pyridoxamine-5-phosphate (PMP). 5′-pyridoxal phosphate (PLP) is a cofactor for >100 enzymes involved in amino acid metabolism including transaminases and carboxylases. Vitamin B_6 is also involved in sphingoid bases and several vitamins, including the synthesis of niacin from tryptophan. It may also play a role in maintaining normal B- and T-cell immune function.

Deficiency: Deficiency is usually seen in conjunction with other water-soluble vitamin deficiencies. Pyridoxine deficiency is rarely caused by an inadequate diet. However, infants who have been fed poorly prepared powdered formula in which pyridoxine was destroyed during preparation develop deficiency and may develop convulsions. A higher demand for the vitamin may occur in pregnancy. This may lead to a secondary deficiency state. Certain prolonged medications can inhibit vitamin B_6 metabolism. These include many drugs such as isoniazid, cycloserine, penicillamine, l-dopa, ethanol, and theophylline. Pyridoxine should be given concurrently with isoniazid to avoid neuropathy. Because vitamin B_6 interferes with the action of l-dopa, it should not be given with this drug. Occasionally, deficiency state can occur in alcoholics.

Effects of deficiency pyridoxine: These include—

- Stomatitis, angular cheilosis, glossitis, irritability, depression, and confusion occur in moderate to severe depletion.
- Microcytic hypochromic anemia is due to diminished hemoglobin synthesis, since it is the first enzyme involved in heme biosynthesis. It may also produce normochromic-normocytic anemia.
- In infants: In the CNS, it has a role in the formation of pyridoxal-dependent decarboxylase of the neurotransmitter GABA. In infants and children, diarrhea, seizures/convulsions, and anemia can occur.
- Severe vitamin B_6 deficiency: Peripheral neuropathy and abnormal electroencephalograms
- Increased risk of atherosclerosis
- Low blood levels of vitamin B_6 have also been correlated with a number of conditions such as aging, impaired renal function, and inflammatory conditions.
- Low blood levels of the active form of vitamin B_6, namely, PLP, correlated with increased risk of developing colorectal cancer.

Biotin (Vitamin B_7)

Sources: Most biotin is found in meats and cereals. In these, it is largely bound to protein.

Functions: Biotin is an obligatory cofactor for five carboxylases that participate in intermediary metabolism, including the Krebs cycle.

Deficiency: It can develop in individuals who consume large amounts of raw eggs, in those with prolonged malabsorption syndrome and in children with severe protein-calorie malnutrition. Chronic administration of anticonvulsant drugs can also produce depletion of biotin.

Effects of deficiency: These include seborrheic and eczematous skin rash. In adults, it can produce neurologic symptoms such as lethargy, hallucinations, and paresthesias. In infants, it can produce hypotonia and developmental delay. Administration of high dose of biotin does not produce adverse consequences.

Folic Acid (Vitamin B_9)

Folic acid is also known as pteroylmonoglutamic acid and is a heterocyclic derivative of glutamic acid. It is yellow, crystalline, and one of the water-soluble vitamins. Folates are a group of related pterin compounds. Folic (pteroylglutamic) acid is the parent compound of a large family of natural folate compounds. Thus, folate is the naturally occurring form of vitamin B_9. The fully oxidized form is called folic acid which is not found in nature but is the pharmacologic (synthetic) form of vitamin B_9. Folate differs from folic acid in three respects—(1) they are partly or completely reduced to dihydrofolate (DHF) or tetrahydrofolate (THF/FH_4/tetrahydrofolic acid) derivatives; (2) they usually contain a single carbon unit; and (3) 70–90% of natural folates are folate-polyglutamates.

Sources: Humans are entirely dependent on dietary sources for their folic acid requirement. The daily requirement is 50–200 mg. Folates are produced by plants and bacteria. Folates are present in almost all foods. Green vegetables (spinach, broccoli, lettuce, legumes), fruits (bananas, melons), nuts (>100 µg/100 g), dairy products, yeast, cereals, and animal proteins (liver, kidney, seafood) are the richest sources and most normal diets contain sufficient amounts of folic acid.

Requirements: Total body folate in the adult is small and ~10 mg and the liver contains the highest store. Daily adult requirements are ~100 µg and so stores are sufficient for only 3–4 months in normal adults. Hence, severe folate deficiency may develop rapidly within a matter of weeks.

Folic acid metabolism: The folic acid in the foods is mostly in the form of polyglutamates. Polyglutamates are sensitive to heat, particularly in large volumes of water (thermolabile); boiling, steaming or frying, and cooking destroy most of the folate.

- **Absorption:** Intestinal conjugases split (hydrolyze) the polyglutamates in the food into monoglutamates. These monoglutamates are easily absorbed in the proximal jejunum. The monoglutamates are actively transported across the enterocyte by a proton-coupled folate transporter (PCFT, SCL46A1). This transporter is present at the apical brush border and is most active at pH 5.5 (it is the pH of the duodenal and jejunal surface). Genetic mutations of this transporter protein can cause hereditary malabsorption of folate.
    - **At lower doses:** All dietary folic (pteroylglutamic) acid/folates are converted to 5-methyltetrahydrofolate (5-MTHF/5-methyl THF) within the small intestinal mucosa before entering portal plasma. The 5-methyl THF is the normal transport form of folic acid.
    - **At higher doses:** Folic (pteroylglutamic) acid at doses >400 µg is absorbed largely unchanged and converted to natural folates in the liver.
- **Transport:** From the intestine, folate is transported to plasma. In plasma, about one-third is loosely bound to plasma proteins such as albumin and two-thirds is unbound. There is an enterohepatic circulation of folate. In all body fluids (plasma, cerebrospinal fluid, milk, bile), folate is mainly (if not entirely) 5-MTHF in the monoglutamate form.

- **Delivery to cells:** Three types of folate-binding proteins are involved in delivery of folate to cells.
  i. **Reduced folate transporter (RFC, SLC19A1):** It is the major route of delivery of plasma folate (5-MTHF) to cells.
  ii. **Folate receptors (FRs):** There are two folate receptors (FRs) namely, FR2 and FR3, embedded in the cell membrane by a glycosyl phosphatidylinositol anchor. Folate binds to FR2 and FR3. Folate is and transported into the cell through receptor-mediated endocytosis.
  iii. **Proton-coupled folate transporter (PCFT):** It is the third folate-binding protein, namely PCFT; transports folate at low pH from the vesicle to the cell cytoplasm. The reduced folate transporter also mediates uptake of methotrexate by cells.
- **Excretion:** Everyday about 60–90 μg of folate passes through the bile and is excreted into the small intestine. This loss of folate, along with the loss of folate present in sloughed intestinal cells, increases the speed of development of folate deficiency in malabsorption conditions.

Causes of deficiency: Deficiency is usually a consequence of a generally poor diet (e.g., in some alcoholics), rather than a diet deficient in any single constituent. Isolated folate deficiency is rare. Various causes of folic acid deficiency are listed in **Box 5.**

Role of folic acid

Metabolism of vitamin B_{12} and folic acid is closely related and both are essential for normal DNA synthesis and nuclear maturation. The active form of folic acid is tetrahydrofolate (THF/FT_4). All folate functions relate to its ability to transfer one carbon groups. Synonyms and abbreviations used for folic acid and its derivatives are presented in **Table 13**.

Table 13: Synonyms used for folic acid, vitamin B_{12}, and their derivatives.

Term	*Synonyms and abbreviations*
Tetrahydrofolate	Tetrahydrofolic acid, THF, FH_4
Methyl-THF	N^5-methyl FH_4, 5-methyltetrahydrofolate (5-MTHF)
$N^{5,10}$-Methylene FH_4	5,10-methylenetetrahydrofolic (5,10-methylene-THF) and 5,10-Methylene THF
Dihydrofolate	DHF, FH_2
Vitamin B_{12}	Cyanocobalamin

Box 5: Causes of folic acid deficiency.

Decreased intake: Inadequate diet—alcoholism, malnutrition

Impaired absorption
- **Malabsorption states:** Nontropical and tropical sprue
- Diffuse infiltrative diseases of the small intestine (e.g., lymphoma)
- Drugs—anticonvulsant phenytoin and oral contraceptives

Increased loss: Hemodialysis

Increased demand: Pregnancy, infancy, disseminated cancer, markedly increased hematopoiesis

Impaired utilization: Folic acid antagonists, such as methotrexate

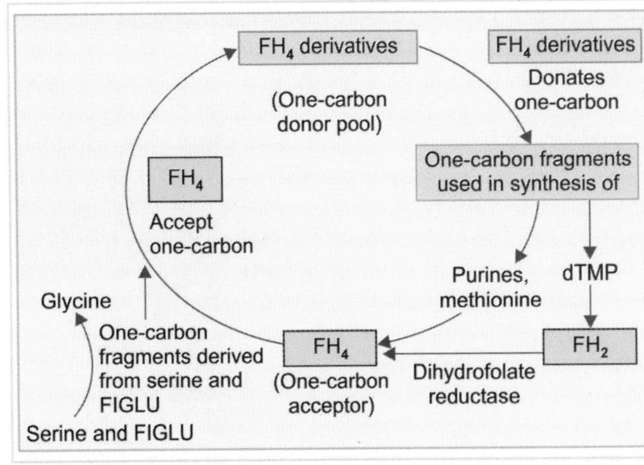

(dTMP: deoxythymidine monophosphate; FH_4: tetrahydrofolic acid; FH_2: dihydrofolic acid; FIGLU: formiminoglutamate)

FIG. 32: Various roles of folate derivatives in the transfer of one-carbon fragments for synthesis of biologic macromolecules. Tetrahydrofolic acid (FH_4) accepts one-carbon from serine and FIGLU and forms FH_4 derivative. This FH_4 derivative donates one carbon for the synthesis of purine, and methionine as well deoxythymidine monophosphate (dTMP).

Transfer of single-carbon units (Fig. 32): FH_4 (tetrahydrofolic acid/tetrahydrofolate/THF) is the active form of folates and its derivatives act as coenzymes (intermediates) in the transfer of single-carbon (one-carbon) units such as formyl and methyl groups to various compounds (**Fig. 32**). FH_4 serves as an acceptor of one-carbon unit from compounds such as serine and formiminoglutamic acid (FIGLU). Conversion of serine to glycine reaction yields one-carbon units, which enter the THF cycle. Also, conversion of forminoglutamic acid to glutamic acid in histidine catabolism donates one-carbon. THF (FH_4) is the acceptor of single carbon units. After accepting one-carbon fragment, THF (FH_4) generates FH_4 derivatives. This derivative in turn donates the acquired one-carbon fragments in reactions synthesizing various metabolites. Thus, FH_4 is a biologic "middleman" involved in accepting and donating one-carbon moieties. The most important metabolic processes that depend on such transfers are as follows:

1. **Synthesis of purine (Fig. 33):** Folate is critical in the generation of purine nucleotides and the conversion of uracil to thymidine. Purine derivatives, particularly adenine and guanine, are building blocks of DNA and RNA. In folate deficiency causing megaloblastic anemia, this reaction is blocked.
2. **Conversion of homocysteine to methionine (Figs. 33 and 34):** Homocysteine is a sulfur-containing amino acid and is a metabolite of the essential amino acid methionine. Folate is also a coenzyme for methionine synthesis. Thus, conversion of homocysteine to methionine requires folic acid as well as methylcobalamin (vitamin B_{12}). During this process, THF is regenerated. Folate together with vitamin B_{12} is a key cofactor in methylation reactions and serves as a methyl group donor. Methionine produced during conversion of homocysteine to methionine is also a precursor for S-adenosylmethionine (SAM). SAM is a universal key methyl donor involved in >100

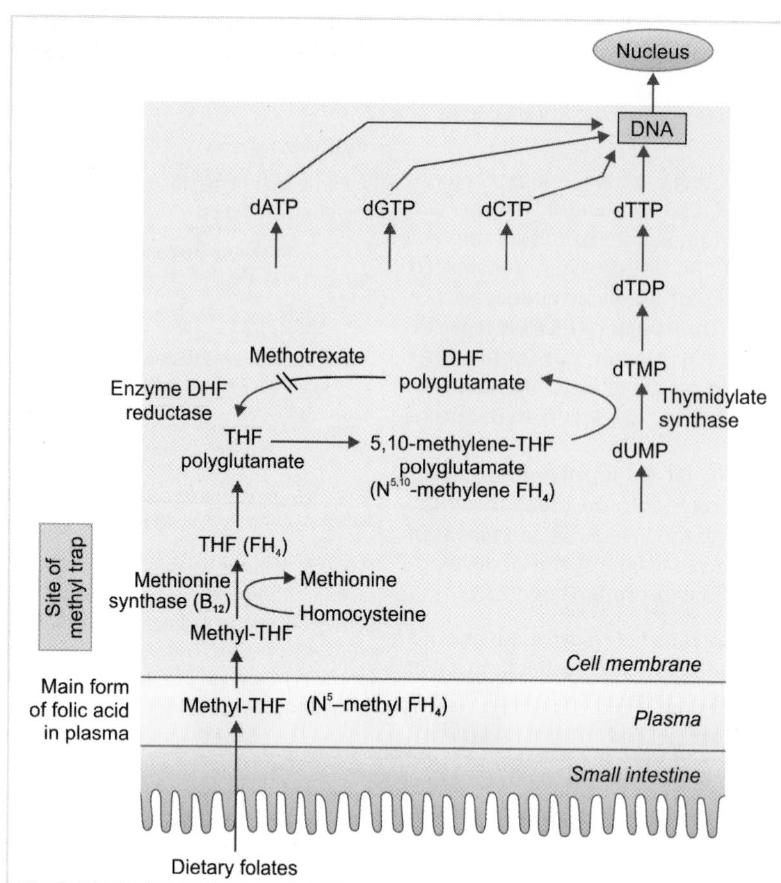

(A: adenine; B_{12}: vitamin B_{12}, cobalamin; C: cytosine; d: deoxyribose; DHF: dihydrofolate; dTMP: deoxythymidine monophosphate; dUMP: deoxyuridine monophosphate; FH_4: tetrahydrofolic acid/tetrahydrofolate; G: guanine; MP: monophosphate; T: thymine; THF/FH_4: tetrahydrofolate; TP: triphosphate)

FIG. 33: Interrelation and role of vitamin B_{12} and folate (folic acid) and its derivative 5,10-methylene-THF polyglutamate in the synthesis of DNA. In vitamin B_{12} deficiency, folate is sequestered as N^5-Methyl FH_4 (Methyl-THF/5-methyl tetrahydrofolate). This ultimately reduces the availability of thymidylate synthetase of its folate coenzyme ($N^{5,10}$-methylene FH_4) and leads to impaired synthesis of DNA.

methyltransferase reactions. These reactions include the synthesis of neurotransmitters (DOPA, epinephrine), phospholipids (phosphatidylethanolamine to phosphatidylcholine), myelin basic protein, methylated nucleotides, and histones.

3. **Synthesis of dTMP (Figs. 33 and 34):** Thymidylate is a component of DNA. **Conversion of deoxyuridine monophosphate (dUMP) to deoxythymidine monophosphate (dTMP)** is needed during the synthesis of DNA. For conversion of dUMP to dTMP, 5,10 methylene THF polyglutamate is required. This is a rate-limiting step in pyrimidine synthesis. During this process, 5,10-methylene-THF is oxidized to DHF (**Fig. 33**). The enzyme DHF reductase converts DHF to THF. The drugs methotrexate, pyrimethamine, and trimethoprim inhibit DHF reductase. Thus, these drugs prevent formation of active THF coenzymes from DHF. Pyrimidine is one of the two classes of heterocyclic nitrogenous bases found in the nucleic acids namely, DNA and RNA. In DNA, the pyrimidines are cytosine and thymine, in RNA uracil replaces thymine.
4. **Metabolism of histidine (Fig. 35):** Histidine is a semi-essential amino acid. Histidine is metabolized to FIGLU which combines with THF to form glutamic acid (**Fig. 33**). In folic acid deficiency, this reaction cannot take place and therefore FIGLU accumulates and is excreted as such in urine. This was used as a test to measure folic acid deficiency.

In the above, in first two reactions namely, (1) and (2), FH_4 is regenerated from its one-carbon carrier derivatives. It is available to accept another one carbon moiety and re-enter the donor pool. In the synthesis of dTMP [i.e., reaction (3)] dihydrofolic acid (FH_2) is produced. This must be reduced by dihydrofolate reductase for re-entry into the FH_4 pool. The reductase step is important because various drugs can inhibit this enzyme. Among all the molecules that are dependent on folates for their synthesis, dTMP is biologically most important. This is because it is needed for DNA synthesis. Suppressed synthesis of DNA occurs in both folic acid and vitamin B_{12} deficiency and they cause megaloblastic anemia.

Biochemical reactions of folate coenzymes are presented in **Table 14**.

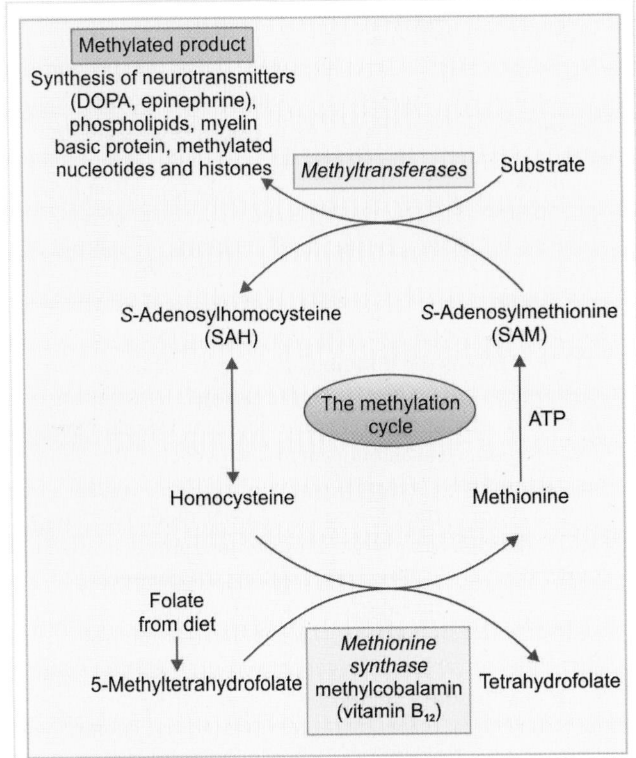

(ATP: adenosine triphosphate; DOPA: dihydroxyphenylalanine)

FIG. 34: The role of folates is in the formation of S-adenosylmethionine (SAM). SAM is involved in many methylation reactions.

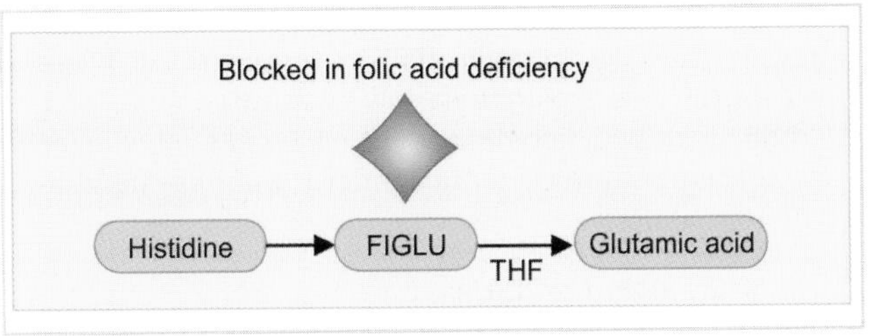

(FIGLU: formiminoglutamate; THF: tetrahydrofolate)

FIG. 35: Role of folic acid in metabolism of histidine.

Effects of folic acid deficiency: Megaloblastic anemia and diarrhea. Folate supplements given during early pregnancy reduce the incidence of fetal neural tube defects.

Cobalamin (Vitamin B_{12})

Vitamin B_{12} is also known as cobalamin. Vitamin B_{12} is a group of closely related compound known as cobalamin and belongs to water-soluble vitamins. Cobalamin (vitamin B_{12}) exists in many different chemical forms and all have a cobalt atom at the center of a corrin ring. In nature, the vitamin is mainly in the 2-deoxyadenosyl (ado) form and is present in mitochondria. It is the cofactor for the enzyme L-methylmalonyl coenzyme A mutase. The other major natural cobalamin is methylcobalamin. Methylcobalamin is present in plasma and in cell cytoplasm. It is the cofactor for methionine synthase. There are also small amounts of hydroxocobalamin

Table 14: Biochemical reactions of folate coenzymes.

Reaction	*Coenzyme form of folate involved*
Purine synthesis	
• Formation of glycinamide ribonucleotide	5,10-Methylene-THF
• Formylation of aminoimidazole carboxamide ribonucleotide (AICAR)	10-Formyl (CHO)-THF
Pyrimidine synthesis	
• Methylation of deoxyuridine monophosphate (dUMP) to thymidine monophosphate (dTMP)	5,10-Methylene-THF
Amino acid interconversion	
• Serine–glycine interconversion	THF
• Homocysteine to methionine	5-Methyl(M)THF
• Forminoglutamic acid to glutamic acid in histidine catabolism	THF

(DHF: dihydrofolate; THF: tetrahydrofolate)

to which methyl- and adocobalamin are converted rapidly by exposure to light.

Source: Cobalamin is synthesized solely by microorganisms and humans are totally dependent on food of animal origin (e.g., meat, fish, eggs, and dairy products) for vitamin B_{12} requirement. Vegetable sources such as vegetables, fruits, and other foods of nonanimal origin are free from vitamin B_{12} (cobalamin) unless they are contaminated by bacteria. Therefore, strict vegetarians do not get an adequate quantity of vitamin B_{12}.

Requirements: A balanced diet (not rigid vegetarian!) contains significantly large amounts (5–30 µg of cobalamin daily) of vitamin B_{12}, which accumulates in the body (liver).

Daily requirement of vitamin B_{12} is about 2–3 µg. Body stores are of the order of 2–3 mg, sufficient for several (3–4) years if supplies are completely cut off. Due to this adequate storage, if there is any dietary deficiency or malabsorption of vitamin B_{12}, its clinical manifestations appear only after about 2–4 years.

Metabolism of vitamin B_{12} (Fig. 36)

There are two mechanisms for absorption of cobalamin. The normal physiologic major mechanism is active and occurs through the ileum. Various steps involved in active absorption are as follows:

- Vitamin B_{12} in food is usually in coenzyme form (as deoxyadenosyl cobalamin and methylcobalamin) and bound to binding proteins in the diet.
- In the stomach, peptic digestion at low pH is required for release of vitamin B_{12} from binding protein in the food.
- The released vitamin B_{12} binds with salivary protein called haptocorrin (HC), which is secreted in salivary juices.
- These haptocorrin B_{12} complexes leave the stomach along with unbound special protein called intrinsic factor (IF), which is produced by gastric (fundus and cardia) parietal (oxyntic) cells (intrinsic factor is also called as Castle intrinsic factor). Normally, vast excess of IF is produced.

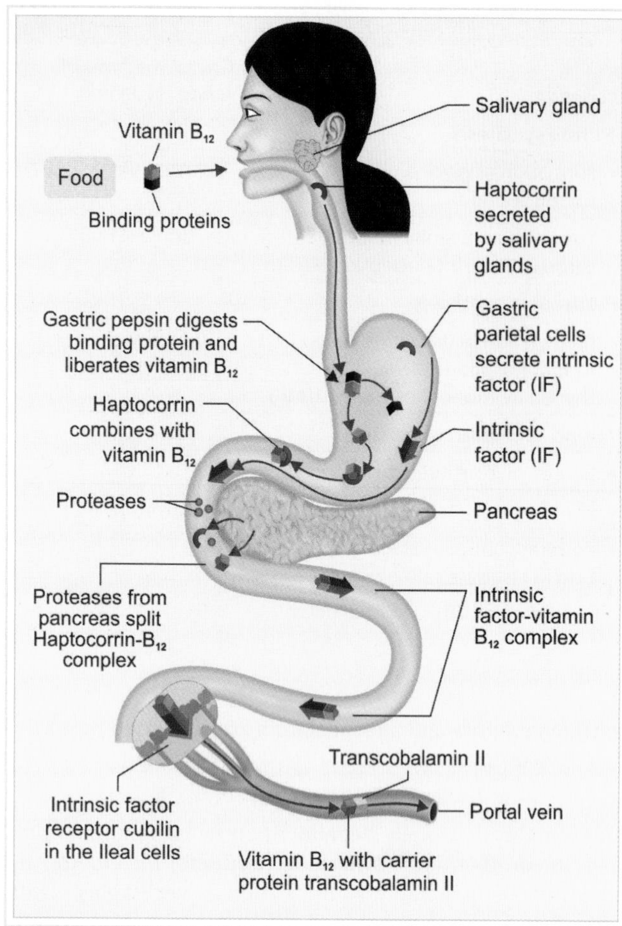

FIG. 36: Mechanism of vitamin B_{12} absorption.

- As the haptocorrin B_{12} complexes pass into the second part of the duodenum, pancreatic proteases release vitamin B_{12} from haptocorrin. Vitamin B_{12} then associates with the intrinsic factor and forms IF-B_{12} complex.
- This stable IF-vitamin B_{12} complex is transported to the ileum, where it is endocytosed by ileal enterocytes. These ileal enterocytes express a receptor on their surfaces for the intrinsic factor. These receptors are called cubilin. IF is destroyed in the ileal cell.
- In the ileal epithelium, vitamin B_{12} combines with a major carrier protein, transcobalamin II, and is actively transported into the mucosal cells and then into the blood.
- Transcobalamin IIvitamin B_{12} complex delivers vitamin B_{12} to the liver and other cells of the body, particularly rapidly proliferating cells in the bone marrow and mucosal lining of the gastrointestinal tract.

Other mechanism of vitamin B_{12} absorption is passive diffusion. This occurs inefficiently and equally through buccal, duodenal, and ileal mucosa. It is rapid but extremely inefficient, with <1% of an oral dose being absorbed by this process.

Functions (role) of vitamin B_{12}

Vitamin B_{12} is indirectly required for DNA synthesis (**Fig. 37**) and its deficiency impairs DNA synthesis. Only two reactions in humans require vitamin B_{12}. The two active coenzyme forms of vitamin B_{12} are deoxyadenosylcobalamin and methylcobalamin.

- **Conversion of homocysteine to methionine (Figs. 33 and 37):** Methylcobalamin is the main form of vitamin B_{12} in plasma. Methylcobalamin serves as an essential cofactor in the conversion of homocysteine to methionine by methionine synthase. During the process, methylcobalamin (vitamin B_{12}) loses (yields) a methyl group that is recovered (replaced) from N^5-methyltetrahydrofolic acid (N^5-methyl FH_4/methyl THF), the main form of folic acid present in plasma. In the same reaction, N^5-methyl FH_4 is converted to tetrahydrofolic acid (FH_4/THF) (**Fig. 33**). FH_4 is crucial because it is needed (through its derivative N5,10-methylene FH_4) for the conversion of dUMP to dTMP. dTMP is the building block for DNA. In vitamin B_{12} deficiency, the main cause of impaired DNA synthesis is that N^5-methyl FH_4 is not converted into THF and thereby there is reduced availability of FH_4. Most of FH_4 is "trapped" as N^5-methyl FH_4 and methyl THF (N^5-methyl FH_4) accumulates in the cell and is known as methyl THF trap.
- **Isomerization of methylmalonyl coenzyme A to succinyl coenzyme A (Fig. 38):** Isomerization, the chemical process by which a compound is transformed into any of its isomeric forms, *i.e.,* forms with the same chemical composition but with different structure or configuration. The isomerization of methylmalonyl coenzyme A to succinyl coenzyme A is achieved by the enzyme methylmalonyl coenzyme A mutase, which requires adenosylcobalamin. This is other reaction that depends on vitamin B_{12}. Deficiency of vitamin B_{12} blocks this isomerization and leads to increased levels of methylmalonic acid in plasma and urine. This can lead to the formation and incorporation of abnormal fatty acids into neuronal lipids. This biochemical abnormality predisposes to myelin breakdown and is probably responsible for producing subacute combined degeneration of the spinal cord (neurologic complications of vitamin B_{12} deficiency). However, this explanation may be not true, because rare individuals with hereditary deficiencies of methylmalonyl-coenzyme A mutase do not suffer from these neurologic abnormalities.

Cobalamin-folate relations

- Folate is required for many reactions (refer pages 1017–1019) whereas only two reactions require cobalamin (vitamin B_{12}). Methylmalonyl- coenzyme A (CoA) isomerization to CoA requires cobalamin (**Figs. 37** and **38**), and the methylation of homocysteine to methionine requires both methylcobalamin and 5-methlyl tetrahydrofolate (N^5-methyl FH_4 /MTHF). This reaction is the first step in the pathway by which 5-methlyl tetrahydrofolate, enters bone marrow and other cells from plasma. The 5-methlyl tetrahydrofolate is converted into all the intracellular folate coenzymes. The folate coenzymes are all polyglutamated (the larger size aiding retention in the cell). But, the enzyme folate polyglutamate synthase (**Fig. 37**) can use only THF, not 5-methlyl tetrahydrofolate, as substrate.
- In cobalamin deficiency: Methylcobalamin serves as an essential cofactor in the conversion of homocysteine to methionine by methionine synthase. In the same reaction, 5-methyl FH_4 is converted to tetrahydrofolic acid (FH_4/THF) (**Fig. 33**). In cobalamin deficiency, 5-methlyl tetrahydrofolate (MTHF) is not converted to THF in the cell and MTHF accumulates in plasma. Due to failure of

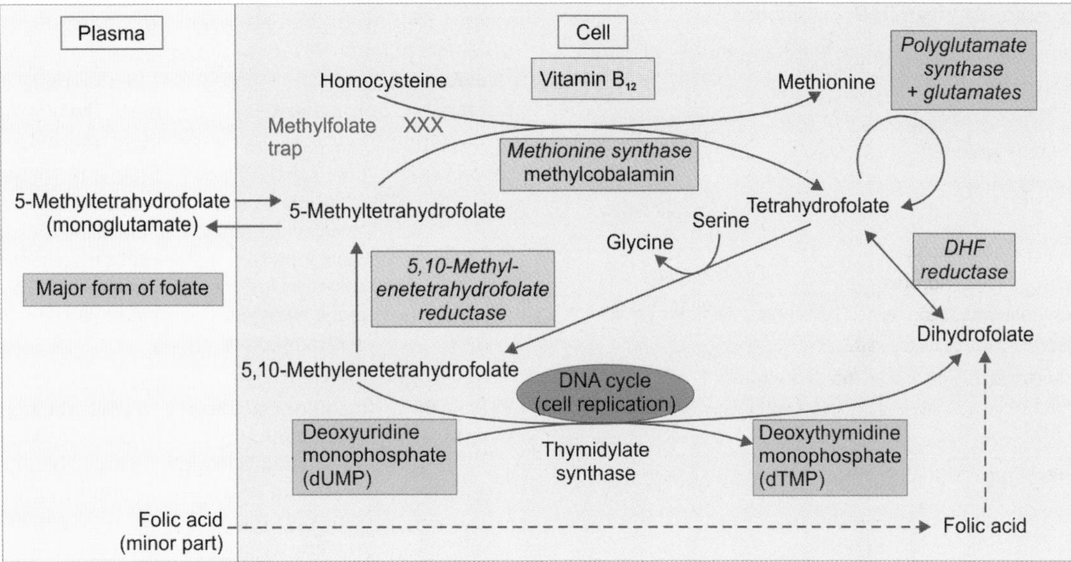

(DHF: dihydrofolate)

FIG. 37: The role of folates and vitamin B_{12} in the synthesis of DNA synthesis.

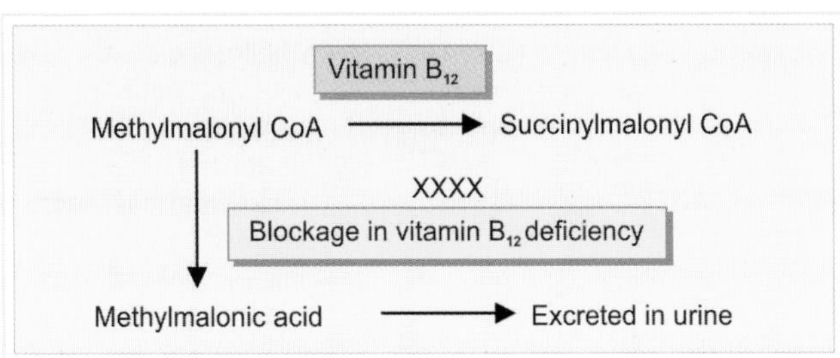

FIG. 38: Role of vitamin B_{12} in methylmalonyl CoA metabolism.

formation of THF, the intracellular concentrations of folate fall. THF is the substrate on which folate polyglutamates are built (**Fig. 37**). This has been termed THF starvation, or the methylfolate trap (**Fig. 37**). This is the abnormality of folate metabolism that occurs in cobalamin deficiency. This is characterized by high serum folate, low cell folate, positive purine precursor aminoimidazole carboxamide ribonucleotide (AICAR) excretion. This is also the reason why the anemia due to cobalamin deficiency responds to large doses folic acid. However, the neurologic complications associated with vitamin B_{12} deficiency are not improved (and may actually be worsened) by folate administration.

Causes of vitamin B_{12} deficiency

Dietary inadequacy is a rare cause of deficiency except in strict vegetarians. Mostly due to loss of intestinal absorption. These include pernicious anemia, pancreatic insufficiency, atrophic gastritis, small bowel bacterial overgrowth, or ileal disease. **Box 6** shows the causes of megaloblastic anemia.

Effects of deficiency

Hematological changes: Megaloblastic anemia and megaloblastic changes in other epithelia.

Neurologic complications: Demyelination of peripheral nerves, posterior and lateral columns of spinal cord, and nerves within the brain. Altered mentation, depression, and psychoses occur.

Vitamins, major functions and their principal clinical manifestations/deficiency syndromes are summarized in **Table 15**.

TRACE ELEMENTS

Q. Write a short essay on role of trace elements in health and disease.

- The term "trace" is used for concentrations of elements not exceeding 250 μg/g of extracellular matrix. Trace elements are naturally occurring, homogeneous, inorganic substances required in humans in amounts <100 mg/day.
- Classification of trace elements is presented in **Box 7**.
- There are about 15 trace elements of which only 10 are essential nutrients in humans. These include: Iron, zinc, copper, chromium, selenium, iodine, fluorine, manganese, tin, molybdenum, nickel, cobalt vanadium, silicon and fluorine.
- Essential trace minerals are mostly components of enzymes and cofactors. Dietary deficiencies of these trace elements are clinically important in the case of iron and iodine.

Selected trace elements, function, causes of deficiency and deficiency syndromes are presented in **Table 16**.

OBESITY

Q. Discuss obesity and its recent advance.

Q. Write a short essay on obesity.

Introduction: Food supplies may be intermittent in certain region at certain times. The ability to store energy in excess than that is needed for immediate use is essential for survival.

Box 6: Causes of vitamin B_{12} deficiency.

Decreased intake: Inadequate diet, "pure vegetarians" (vegans)

Impaired absorption

- Gastric: Deficiency of gastric acid or pepsin or intrinsic factor
  - Pernicious anemia
  - Post-gastrectomy
- Intestinal
  - Loss of absorptive surface
    - Malabsorption syndromes
    - Diffuse intestinal disease, e.g., lymphoma, systemic sclerosis
    - Ileal resection, Crohn disease
  - Bacterial or parasitic competition for vitamin B_{12}
    - Bacterial overgrowth in blind loops and diverticula of bowel
    - Fish tapeworm infestation (*Diphyllobothrium latum*)

Increased demand: Pregnancy, hyperthyroidism, disseminated cancer

Table 15: Summary of vitamins, major functions and their principal clinical manifestations/deficiency syndromes.

Vitamin (biochemical name)	*Functions*	*Clinical manifestation/ deficiency syndromes*
Fat-soluble		
Vitamin A	Component of visual pigment	Xerophthalmia, night blindness, Bitot's spots
	Maintenance of specialized epithelia	Squamous metaplasia, follicular hyperkeratosis
	Maintenance of resistance to infection	Vulnerability to infection, particularly measles, immune dysfunction
Vitamin D	Facilitates absorption of calcium and phosphorus in the intestine and mineralization of bone	• Rickets in children: Skeletal deformation, rachitic rosary, bowed legs • Osteomalacia in adults
Vitamin E	Antioxidant and scavenges free radicals	Peripheral neuropathy, spinocerebellar ataxia, skeletal muscle atrophy, retinopathy, hemolytic anemia
Vitamin K	Cofactor in hepatic carboxylation of pro-coagulants: Factors II (prothrombin), VII, IX, and X and protein C and protein S	Elevated prothrombin time, bleeding diathesis
Water-soluble		
Vitamin B_1 (thiamine)	Pyrophosphate is coenzyme in decarboxylation reactions	Beriberi (dry or wet): Neuropathy, muscle weakness and wasting, cardiomegaly, edema, ophthalmoplegia, confabulation, Wernicke syndrome, Korsakoff syndrome
Vitamin B_2 (riboflavin)	Converted to coenzymes flavin mononucleotide and flavin adenine dinucleotide, cofactors for many enzymes in intermediary metabolism	Magenta tongue (glossitis), angular stomatitis, seborrhea, cheilosis, glossitis, seborrheic dermatitis, ariboflavinosis, corneal vascularization
Vitamin B_3 (niacin)	Incorporated into nicotinamide adenine dinucleotide (NAD) and NAD P (nicotinamide adenine dinucleotide phosphate), involved in a variety of redox reactions	• Pellagra: Pigmented rash of sun-exposed areas, bright-red tongue, diarrhea, apathy, memory loss, disorientation • Six Ds: Dementia, dermatitis, diarrhea, depression, degeneration of myelin and death
Vitamin B_6 (pyridoxine)	Derivatives serve as coenzymes in many intermediary reactions	• Cheilosis, glossitis, seborrhic dermatitis, convulsions, peripheral neuropathy, depression, confusion, anemia • Maintenance of myelinization of spinal cord tracts
Vitamin B_9 (folate, folic acid)	Essential for transfer and use of one-carbon units in DNA synthesis	Megaloblastic anemia, atrophic glossitis, neural tube defects ion fetus
Vitamin B_{12} (cobalamin)	Required for normal folate metabolism and DNA synthesis	Megaloblastic anemia, degeneration of posterolateral spinal cord tracts, loss of vibratory and position sense, abnormal gait, dementia
Vitamin C (ascorbic acid)	Involved in many oxidation-reduction (redox) reactions and hydroxylation of collagen	Scurvy: Petechiae, ecchymosis, inflamed and bleeding gums, joint effusion, poor wound healing, fatigue
Vitamin B_5 (pantothenic acid)	Incorporated in coenzyme A	No syndrome recognized
Vitamin B_7 (biotin)	Cofactor in carboxylation reactions	No defined clinical syndrome

Fat cells are widely distributed in deposits of adipose tissue are capable of storing excess energy as triglyceride (TG). When needed, they release stored energy as free fatty acids for use at other sites. This physiologic system is controlled through endocrine and neural pathways. This allows us to survive starvation for as long as several months.

Food supplies may be in abundance in certain nations. This along with a sedentary lifestyle and genetic factors may increase stores of adipose energy to such an extent that may produce adverse health effects.

Definition: Obesity is defined as a state of excess adipose tissue mass. It is characterized by an accumulation of excess body fat (adipose tissue) that is of sufficient degree to weaken health.

Prevalence of obesity: Obesity is a major health problem in developed countries and an emerging health problem in developing countries, including India.

Measurement of fat accumulation: Body mass index (BMI) is not a direct measure of adiposity. But it is most commonly used for measurement of fat accumulation and to determine obesity. It is calculated by using the formula mentioned here:

$$\text{BMI (kg/m}^2) = \frac{\text{Weight (in kilograms)}}{\text{Height squared (in meters)}}$$

The normal range of BMI range differs for different countries due to differences in ethnicity and genetic backgrounds. Classification of overweight and obesity by BMI is presented in **Table 17**. In both men and women, BMI of 30 is most commonly used as a threshold for obesity. Other methods of quantifying obesity include anthropometry (skinfold thickness), densitometry (underwater weighing), computed tomography (CT) or magnetic resonance imaging (MRI), and electrical impedance.

Box 7: Classification of trace elements.

Essential trace elements: Iodine, zinc, selenium, copper, molybdenum, chromium, cobalt, iron

Trace elements that are probably essential: Manganese, nickel, silicon, boron, vanadium

Potentially toxic elements with possible essential functions in low doses: Fluoride, lead, cadmium, mercury, arsenic, lithium, tin, aluminum

Types of Obesity

The distribution of the stored fat is important in obesity and according to body fat distribution obesity is divided into:

- **Central (abdominal/visceral/android/apple shaped) obesity:** This type of obesity shows increased accumulation of fat preferentially in the trunk and in the abdominal cavity/intra-abdominal (in the mesentery and around viscera). It is associated with a greater risk for several

Table 16: Selected trace elements, function, causes of deficiency and deficiency syndromes.

Trace element and their function	*Causes of Deficiency*	*Clinical Features*
Iron: Essential component of hemoglobin and many iron-containing metalloenzymes	• Inadequate diet • Chronic blood loss • Increased demand	Microcytic hypochromic anemia
Iodine: Component of thyroid hormone	Inadequate supply in food and water	Goiter and hypothyroidism
Zinc: Component of enzymes, mainly oxidases	• Inadequate supplementation in artificial diets • Interference with absorption by other dietary constituents • Inborn error of metabolism	• Acrodermatitis enteropathica (inherited disorder of zinc metabolism): Rash around eyes, mouth, nose, and anus • Anorexia and diarrhea • Growth retardation in children • Hypogonadal dwarfism in boys • Depressed mental function • Delayed wound healing and impaired immune response and night vision • Infertility
Copper: Component of cytochrome c oxidase, dopamine β-hydroxylase, tyrosinase, lysyl oxidase, and involved in cross-linking collagen	• Inadequate supplementation in artificial diet • Impaired absorption	• Weakness of muscle • Neurologic defects • Abnormal cross-linking of collagen • Microcytic anemia
Fluoride: Unknown mechanism	Inadequate supply in soil and water	Dental caries
Trace element and their function	*Causes of Deficiency*	*Clinical Features*
Selenium: Component of glutathione peroxidase Antioxidant with vitamin E	Inadequate amounts in soil and water	• Myopathy • Cardiomyopathy (Keshan disease)
Manganese: Component of several metalloenzymes. Most of it is in mitochondria as a component of manganese superoxide dismutase	Not demonstrated	Hypocholesterolemia, weight loss, hair and nail changes, dermatitis, and impaired synthesis of vitamin K–dependent proteins
Molybdenum: A cofactor in several enzymes, most prominently xanthine oxidase and sulfite oxidase	Secondary to parenteral administration of sulfite	Hyperoxypurinemia, hypouricemia, and low sulfate excretion

diseases (e.g., T2DM, the metabolic syndrome and CVD) than generalized obesity (with subcutaneous fat).
- **Generalized' (gynoid/pear-shaped) obesity:** This type is characterized by excess accumulation of fat diffusely in the subcutaneous tissue.

Distinction between two is made clinically by determining the waist-to hip ratio, with a ratio >0.9 in women and >1.0 in men is considered as abnormal.

Diseases associated with obesity: Most important diseases associated with obesity are: Insulin resistance, T2DM, hypertension, hyperlipidemia, CVD, and cancer and hyperandrogenism in women. This association depends on both the quantity and distribution of excess fat.

Physiologic Regulation of Energy Balance

Q. Write a short essay on pathophysiology of obesity.

The two sides of the energy equation are **energy intake and energy expenditure**. They are **regulated by both endocrine and neural components** (mechanisms). Most adults regulate the average energy balance with greater than 1% precision. They maintain body weight within a narrow range for many years. This complex regulatory system is required because even small imbalances between energy intake and expenditure will have effects on body weight. Regulation of both energy intake and energy expenditure occurs through conscious and unconscious processes. Regulation or dysregulation of body weight depends on a complex interplay of hormonal and neural signals. The fine balance between energy intake and energy expenditure is controlled by an internal set-point, or "lipostat". Lipostat senses the quantity of energy stores (adipose tissue) and accordingly regulates intake of food as well as energy expenditure. The **master regulator of energy homeostasis is the hypothalamus**. It receives inputs from the periphery about the state of energy stores. If energy stores are inadequate, it triggers anabolic circuits, whereas energy stores are adequate, catabolic circuits are activated.
- **Effect of the anabolic circuits:** It increases the food intake and reduces energy expenditure.
- **Effects of catabolic circuits:** It reduces intake of food and increases energy expenditure.

Neurohumoral Mechanisms That Regulate Energy Balance (Fig. 39)

Neurohumoral mechanisms that regulate energy balance can be subdivided into three components namely **peripheral or afferent system, central processing system and afferent system** (**Figs. 39** and **40**).

Table 17: Classification of overweight and obesity by body mass index.

Category	*BMI Kg/m²*
Underweight	<18.5
Normal	18.5–24.9
Overweight	25.0–29.9
Obesity—Class I	30.0–34.9
Obesity—Class II	35.0–39.9
Extreme obesity—Class III	≥40

Peripheral or Afferent System

Peripheral or afferent system generates signals from various sites. These signals may be divided into appetite stimulating and suppressing signals (**Fig. 39**). Appetite is influenced by many factors. The afferent signals are transmitted to the central processing system and are integrated by the brain mainly within the hypothalamus. These signals include neural afferents, hormones, and metabolites.

Appetite suppressing signals: Its main components are:
- **Adiponectin** (discussed on pages 1029 and 1030)
- **Gut peptides:** These are as follows:
    - Peptide YY (PYY): It is secreted by the endocrine cells (L cells) in the ileum and colon. It reduces appetite.
    - Glucagon-like peptide 1 (GLP-1): It is secreted from the ileum and colon. It produces peripheral appetite suppressing signals
    - Insulin: It is secreted by cells of the pancreas and acts centrally to activate the appetite suppressing pathway.
    - Cholecystokinin (CCK): It is produced in duodenal and jejunal mucosa. It is released after fat and protein intake. It acts on two distinct receptors. CCK stimulates release of enzymes from the pancreas and gallbladder. These enzymes help in digestion, slow gastric emptying and reduce intake of food. Regulation of intake food intake is mediated through vagal afferent signals to the brain.
    - Amylin: It is a peptide secreted with insulin from pancreatic β-cells. It is also found in gut endocrine cells, visceral sensory neurons and the hypothalamus. It is a potent inhibitor of gastric emptying and decreases food intake.

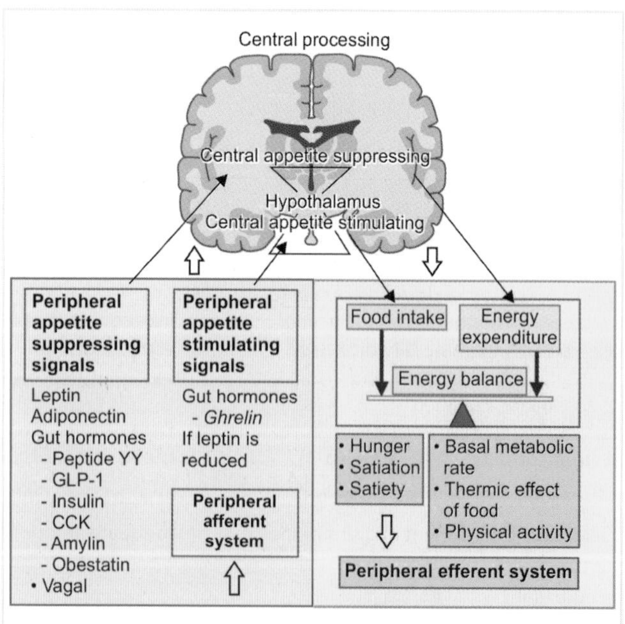

(CCK: cholecystokinin; GLP-1: glucagon-like peptide 1)

FIG. 39: Regulation of energy balance. Peripheral afferent system (appetite suppressing and stimulating signals) influences the activity of the hypothalamus, which is the central regulator of appetite and satiety. Signals from hypothalamus in turn act on peripheral efferent system (food intake and energy expenditure).

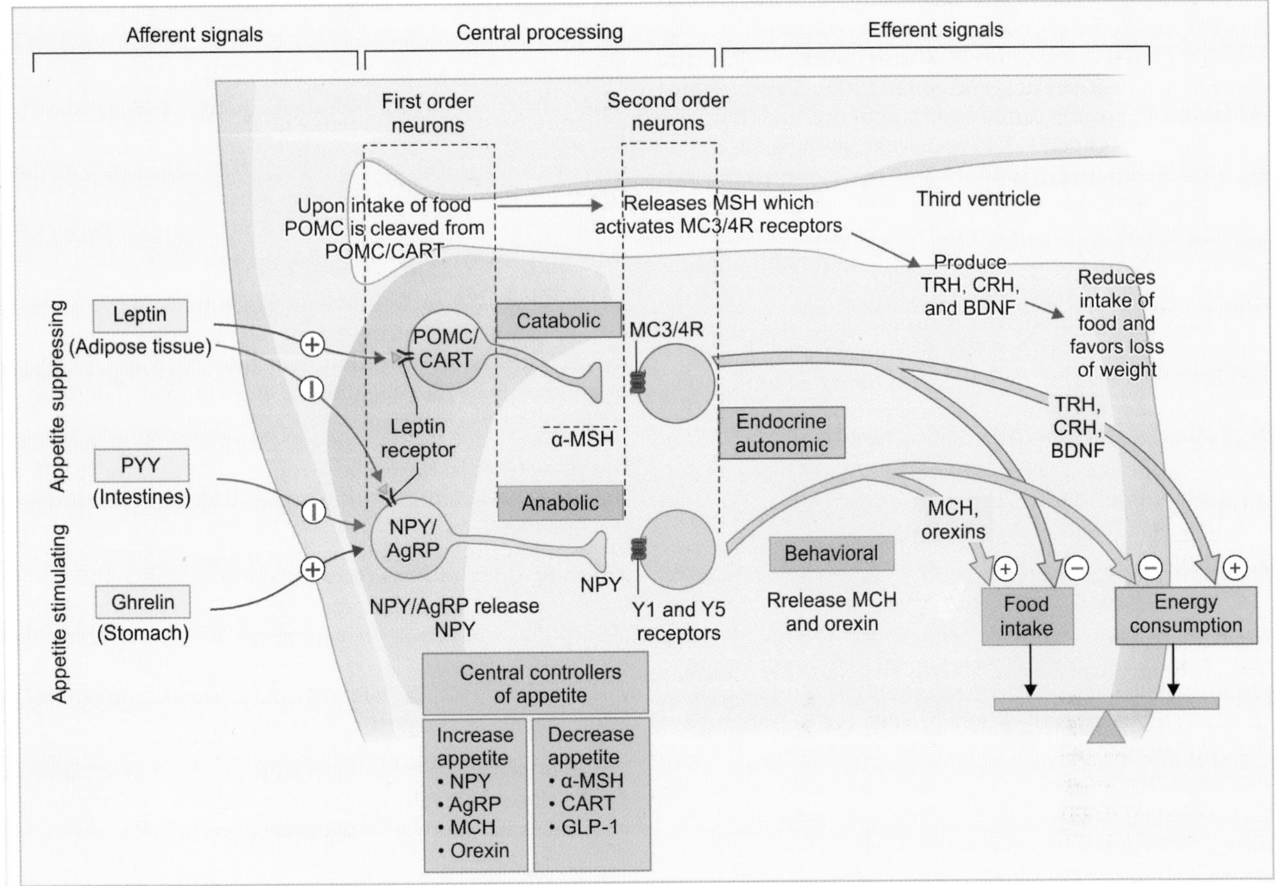

(α-MSH: α-melanocyte–stimulating hormone; AgRP: agouti-related peptide; BDNF: brain-derived neurotrophic factor; CART: cocaine and amphetamine-regulated transcript; CRH: corticotropin-releasing hormone; GLP-1: glucagon-like peptide 1; MC3/4R: melanocortin-3 and -4 receptor; MCH: melanin-concentrating hormone; NPY: neuropeptide Y; PYY: peptide YY; TRH: thyroid-releasing hormone)

FIG. 40: Neurohumoral mechanisms that regulate energy balance in the hypothalamus. Pathways of POMC/CART anorexigenic neurons and NPY/AgRP orexigenic neurons in the hypothalamus.

  - Obestatin: It is a peptide produced by the same gene that encodes ghrelin. It counteracts the increase in food intake induced by ghrelin.
  - Other peripheral appetite suppressing signals are derived from oxyntomodulin.
- **Vagal inputs:** They bring out information from viscera, such as gut distention.
- Resistin (resistance to insulin): It is primarily produced by macrophages and not fat cells. It causes insulin resistance and inhibit appetie.
- **Metabolites:** Glucose, ketones. Decreased appetite during a ketogenic diet may be due to elevated plasma ketone levels

***Appetite stimulating signals:* Its main components are:**
Reduced leptin: It stimuletes appetite.
- Ghrelin from the stomach stimulates appetite (discussed on page 1030).
- Leptin is a **hormone** produced by fat cells (discussed on page 1028).

Central processing system

It is present in the arcuate nucleus of the hypothalamus. In the hypothalamus neurohumoral peripheral signals are integrated to generate efferent signals. Two sets of neurons participate in central processing of peripheral systems (**Fig. 40**).

- **A pair of first-order neurons:** These are: (1) pro-opiomelanocortin (POMC) and cocaine and amphetamine-regulated transcript (CART) neurons; and (2) neurons containing neuropeptide Y (NPY) and agouti-related peptide (AgRP). These first-order neurons communicate with second-order neurons.
- **A pair of second-order neurons:** These include: (1) neurons that bear melanocortin receptors 3 and 4 (MC3/4R) and receive signals from first-order POMC/CART neurons; and (2) neurons that bear Y1 and Y5 receptors and receive signals from first-order NPY/AgRP neurons.

Functioning of hypothalamic centers that regulate energy balance

- **Central appetite suppressing (anorexigenic pathway or leptin melanocortin pathway):** This pathway enhances energy expenditure and weight loss. Upon intake of nutrient or food, POMC is cleaved from POMC/CART by proenzyme convertase 1 (PC-1) in first order neurons. This gives rise to α-melanocyte–stimulating hormone (MSH), MSH in turn activates MC3/4R receptors (melanocortin-3 and -4 receptor) in second-order neurons. These second-order neurons produce brain-derived neurotrophic factor (BDNF), thyroid-releasing hormone (TSH), and corticotropin-releasing hormone (CRH). These reduce intake of food by suppressing appetite and increase expenditure of energy. This favors loss of weight.

- **Central appetite stimulating (orexigenic pathway):** Orexigenic means appetite stimulant. In this pathway, fasting activates the NPY/AgRP in first order neurons and release neuropeptide Y (NPY). Released NPY activates neuropeptide Y receptor type 1 and type 5 (Y1 and Y5 receptors) in second-order neurons. These second-order neurons in turn release melanin-concentrating hormone (MCH) and orexin. They increase intake of food intake and reduce expenditure of energy by downregulation of sympathetic output (characterized by the release of large quantities of epinephrine). NPY/AgRP neurons also directly inhibit POMC/CART neurons. This weaken the anorexigenic effect of POMC/CART neurons.

The orderly functioning of the above two pathways maintains energy homeostasis.

Efferent system

This consists of signals generated by second order neurons. These signals are organized along two pathways and both of these pathways control food intake and energy expenditure

- **Catabolic** (downstream of MC3/4R) pathways: The products of this pathway cause decreased food intake with or without increased energy expenditure.
- **Anabolic** (downstream of Y1 and Y5 receptors) pathways: The products of this pathway cause increased food intake with or without decreased energy expenditure.

Apart from these circuits within the hypothalamus, the hypothalamic nuclei also communicate with forebrain and midbrain centers. This in turn control the autonomic nervous system.

Energy intake (food intake) Biologic regulation of food intake depends on peripheral or afferent signals. These signals may affect different aspects of eating behavior. They can affect three main components of energy intake: **(1) hunger, (2) satiation or (3) satiety**. Hunger is the compelling need or desire for food. Satiation is the state of being satisfactorily full and unable to take on more. Satiety is the sense of no longer being hungry and includes a complex set of postprandial events that affect the interval to the next meal or the amount consumed at the next meal.

Control of appetite: Signals may affect different aspects of eating behavior. Some signals may alter one aspect of eating behavior whereas others may affect multiple aspects. For example, ghrelin (a peptide produced by the stomach), increases hunger but does not affect satiation or satiety. Cholecystokinin causes satiation, but has no effect on satiety. Leptin acts on multiple pathways. Leptin deficiency is associated with increased hunger and reduced satiation and satiety.

Peripheral satiety signals inhibit further intake food at some point during consumption of meal. The route of afferent signals reaching the brain may be through the vagus nerve and through the systemic circulation. Examples of the factors modulating appetite are presented in **Figure 39**. These signals are triggered both by mechanical stimuli (e.g., the fullness of the stomach) and the presence of nutrients in the jejunum and ileum.

Food: The increase in obesity can be related to the type of food consumed (i.e., food containing sugar and fat) and also psychological factors.

Following a meal, substances, such as CCK, bombesin and GLP-1 are released from the small intestine and glucagon and insulin from the pancreas. These hormones are involved in the control of satiety. The control of appetite is extremely complex.

Energy expenditure Daily energy expenditure in adults varies depending on physical activity of the individuals and energy needs. Daily energy expenditure can be divided into resting (or basal) metabolic rate, the thermic effect of food, and physical activity energy expenditure.

Basal metabolic rate: The basal metabolic rate (BMR) is the energy expenditure during rest, awake, in the overnight postabsorptive state.

Thermic effect of food (thermogenesis): About 10% of the energy content of food is spent in the process of digestion, absorption, and metabolism of nutrients. This is irrespective of physical activity. There is a significant interindividual variability. This is called dietary induced thermogenesis which is lower in obese and post-obese individuals.

Physical activity energy expenditure (discussed on page 1028). Obese individuals tend to spend more energy during physical activity as they have a larger mass to move.

Etiology and Pathogenesis

Q. Describe the etiology and pathogenesis of obesity. Write its role in carcinogenesis.

Q. Describe the pathogenesis of obesity and its consequences.

The etiology of obesity is complex and not completely understood. There are significant genetic, constitutional influences and environmental factors involved in obesity. Obesity can be simply considered as a disorder of energy homeostasis.

Role of Genes

Obesity is commonly seen in families and genetic influences play a strong role toward the regulation of body weight. It is known that height is heritable and similar to that body weight is also heritable. Currently, both common and rare genetic variants, account for <5% of the variance of body weight. Usually, inheritance of obesity is not Mendelian pattern.

Extremely rare monogenic forms of human obesity may be due to mutations in the leptin gene and leptin receptor gene. This results in actual or functional deficiency of leptin and is much like that seen in *ob/ob* or *db/db* mice animal models (ob/ob = obese mice and db/db = diabetic mice). Inherited forms of human obesity may also develop due to mutations of genes that regulate appetite neuropeptide synthesis. Genome wide association studies have shown that several genes (about 100) linked to obesity and are associated with higher BMI. These include obesity-associated (*FTO*) gene (which is of unknown function), melanocortin-4 receptor (*MC4R*) gene, *TMEM18, KCTD15, GNPDA2, SH2B1, MTCH2, and NEGR1*.

Specific genetic syndromes: Obesity in rodents has been known to be caused by a number of distinct mutations distributed through the genome. Mutations of the *ob* gene mutation in genetically obese (*ob*/*ob*) mice were the major breakthrough. The *ob*/*ob* mouse develops severe obesity and insulin resistance. The product of the *ob* gene is the peptide leptin. Another mouse mutant *db*/*db*, which is resistant to leptin. It has a mutation in the leptin receptor and develops a similar syndrome. The *ob* gene is present in humans and it is also expressed in fat. Mutations in several genes that cause severe obesity in humans and mice are presented in **Table 18**. These genetic defects mainly involve a pathway through which leptin (by stimulating POMC and increasing α-MSH) restricts food intake and limits weight (See **Fig. 41**). These syndromes are rare.

- **Inactive mutations in leptin or the leptin receptor:** Several families have been described with early-onset obesity caused by inactivating mutations in either leptin or the leptin receptor. However, mutations in the leptin or leptin receptor genes do not play a prominent role in common forms of obesity.
- **Mutations in the gene encoding proopiomelanocortin:** It causes severe obesity through failure to synthesize key neuropeptides that inhibit appetite in the hypothalamus. These neuropeptides are α-MSH, and β-MSH. The absence of POMC also causes secondary adrenal insufficiency due to absence of adrenocorticotropic hormone (ACTH), as well as pale skin and red hair due to absence of α-MSH.
- **Mutations in proenzyme convertase 1:** Mutations in PC-1 cause obesity by preventing synthesis of α-MSH from its precursor peptide, POMC.
- **Mutations in type 4 melanocortin receptor:** α-MSH binds to a key hypothalamic receptor namely the type MC4R. This inhibits eating. Heterozygous loss-of-function mutations of this receptor are responsible for about 5% of severe obesity. Rarely, loss of function of MRAP2 (a protein required for normal MC4R signaling) has been found to produce severe obesity.

Table 18: Examples of obesity genes involved in humans and mice.

Gene	*Gene product*	*Mechanism of obesity*
Both in humans and mice		
Lep (ob)	Leptin (hormone derived from adipocyte)	Mutation prevents leptin from delivering satiety signal; brain recognizes starvation
LepR (db)	Leptin receptor	
POMC	Proopiomelanocortin (a precursor of many hormones and neuropeptides)	• Mutation prevents synthesis of melanocyte-stimulating hormone (MSH) • MSH is a satiety signal
MC4R	Type 4 receptor for MSH	Mutation prevents reception of satiety signal from MSH
TrkB	TrkB (neurotrophin receptor)	Hyperphagia due to hypothalamic defect
Fat (recently identified in human)	Carboxypeptidase E (a processing enzyme)	Mutation prevents synthesis of neuropeptide (probably MSH)
Tub (recently identified in human)	Tub (hypothalamic protein function of which is not known)	Hypothalamic dysfunction
Only in humans		
PC-1	Prohormone convertase 1 (a processing enzyme)	Mutation prevents synthesis of neuropeptide (probably MSH)
Only in mice		
AgRP	Agouti-related peptide (a neuropeptide expressed in the hypothalamus)	Overexpression inhibits signal through MC4R

Other genes: Mutations in TUB and carboxypeptidase-E (CPE) have recently been identified in humans.

- **Mutation of tub gene:** Tub gene encodes a hypothalamic peptide of unknown function. Mutation of this gene causes late-onset obesity.
- **Mutations in fat gene:** The fat gene encodes a peptide-processing enzyme called CPE. Probably, mutation of this gene cause obesity by disrupting production of one or more neuropeptides.
- **Overexpression of AgRP:** AgRP is coexpressed with NPY in arcuate nucleus neurons. AgRP antagonizes α-MSH action at MC4 receptors. Overexpression of AgRP induces obesity.

Few complex human syndromes with defined inheritance are associated with obesity. Examples of single gene defects resulting in obesity are syndromes such as Prader–Willi and Laurence–Moon–Biedl.

- **Prader–Willi syndrome:** It is a multigenic neurodevelopmental disorder in which obesity coexists with other features. These include short stature, mental retardation, hypogonadotropic hypogonadism, hypotonia, small hands and feet, fish-shaped mouth, and hyperphagia. Most patients have reduced expression of imprinted paternally inherited genes encoded in the 15q11-13 chromosomal region. Reduced expression of Snord116, a small nucleolar RNA highly expressed in hypothalamus. This may be an important cause of defective hypothalamic function in this disorder.
- **Bardet–Biedl syndrome (BBS):** It is a genetically heterogeneous disorder characterized by obesity, mental retardation, retinitis pigmentosa, diabetes, renal and cardiac malformations.
- **Laurence–Moon–Biedl syndrome:** It is an autosomal recessive disorder associated with generalized obesity of early onset (1–2 years), first degree hypogonadism and polydactyly.

Other specific acquired syndromes may be associated with obesity. These include Cushing's syndrome, hypothyroidism, insulinoma, craniopharyngioma and other disorders involving the hypothalamus.

Genetic effects appear to be related to both intake and expenditure of energy. Genes influence the susceptibility to obesity in response to specific diets and availability of nutrition. Cultural factors are also important. These cultural factors relate to both availability and composition of the diet and the level of physical activity. In underdeveloped nations, high economic group females are more often obese. In children, obesity correlates to some degree with time spent watching television. High-fat diets consumed along with simple, rapidly absorbed carbohydrates, promote obesity. Sleep deprivation also leads to increased obesity. Changes in gut microbiome with capacity to alter energy balance may have a possible role for obesogenic viral infections.

Constitutional Influences on Obesity

Many environmental influences can result in long-term, gene-like effects on body weight regulation and have the tendency to susceptible to obesity-related health problems. These modifications of gene expression without modification of the DNA are termed epigenetic effects (refer pages 433–440). These epigenetic changes are due to processes such as DNA methylation and chromatin remodeling.

Effect of environmental influences during intrauterine and perinatal period: The intrauterine environment and the perinatal period have effect on the subsequent weight and health.

- **Undernutrition during the last trimester of pregnancy and in the early postnatal period: This reduces the risk of adult obesity**. However, low birth weight associated with undernutrition (or smoking) in late pregnancy increases the risk of other diseases. These include adulthood hypertension, abnormal glucose tolerance, and CVD.
- **Undernutrition limited to first two trimesters of pregnancy:** In contrast to undernutrition during last trimester, if undernutrition is only limited to the first two trimesters of pregnancy, it is associated with an increased probability of adult obesity.
- **Diabetic mother:** The infants of diabetic mothers tend to be fatter than those of nondiabetic mothers. The children of diabetic mothers also have a greater prevalence of obesity when they are 5–19 years old. This is independent of their mother's obesity status. Intrauterine exposure to the diabetic environment also increases the risk of diabetes mellitus and obesity in the offspring.

Environmental Contributors to Human Obesity

Dramatic changes are observed in the environment over the past 50 years. These changes have resulted in reduced physical activity and reduced expenditure of energy. Also, alterations in the food supply have either increased or failed to decrease in energy intake in comparison with reduced energy expenditure.

Food

Many environmental factors can influence food intake. Dietary factors that promote obesity are as follows: -

Energy density of foods: Consuming energy-dense foods results in greater energy intake. Many high-fat foods are energy dense and consumption of energy dense high fat diet is associated with excess body weight.

Larger food portion size: Larger portions of food and beverage can contribute toward obesity. Food variety can also affect energy intake.

Increased variety of entrees, sweets, snacks, and carbohydrates in the diet: It is associated with an increase in body fat and food intake. On the contrary, there is no associated risk of increased body fat if there is increase in variety of vegetables, because it is not result in an increased energy intake.

Increased palatability and availability, the reduced costs of food and consumption of caloric beverages such as soft drinks and fruit juices is not accompanied by decrease in food intake and these are associated with the extra energy intake.

Physical activity

Physical activity can be divided into three types. These are: (1) Exercise (fitness and sports-related activities), (2) Work-related physical activity, and (3) Nonexercise, nonemployment (spontaneous) activity. Exercise (fitness and sports-related activities) is the main component of physical activity thermogenesis (the process of heat production). To expend a large amount of energy, it is necessary to exercise at high levels or for a sufficient duration. Focusing only on "exercise" as the main component of physical activity will not be useful for energy balance. The benefits and energy spent during nonexercise activity can be greater than the usual amount of exercise. Nonexercise activity thermogenesis (NEAT) is the caloric expense during the performance of all activities other than exercise. These include employment-related and spontaneous activity.

Reduced physical activity is contributing factor of obesity. Increased sedentary behavior (e.g., watching television, computer), decreased work-related (employment) physical activity, and decreased activities of daily living (e.g., these include labor-saving activities such as use of escalators, remote controls, e-mail, online shopping) promotes obesity. The amount of time spent in sedentary activities is an independent predictor of metabolic abnormalities associated with obesity.

Main Components of the Afferent System of the Neurohumoral Mechanisms

Three important components of the afferent system of the neurohumoral mechanisms that regulate energy balance are leptin, adiponectin and gut hormones. They are discussed here.

Leptin

Q. Write a short essay on leptin in obesity.

Leptin is a protein (peptide) and is the product of the *ob* gene. The name leptin is derived from the Greek root *leptos*, meaning thin.

Source: Leptin is from the cytokine family and secreted almost exclusively by adipocytes (adipose cells/fat cells) and acts mainly through the hypothalamus.

Regulation of energy balance by leptins (Fig. 41): Discovery of leptin was the first confirmation that adipose tissue can secrete hormones that have CNS effects on food intake. Leptins output is regulated by the adequacy of fat stores. BMI and body fat stores are directly related to secretion of leptin.

- **Regulation of food intake:** In individuals of stable weight, the activities of the below mentioned pathways are balanced.
    - **Abundant adipose tissue stimulates leptin secretion:** When there is abundant adipose tissue, secretion of leptin is stimulated and it crosses the blood–brain barrier and travels to the hypothalamus. In the hypothalamus it **reduces food intake by stimulating**

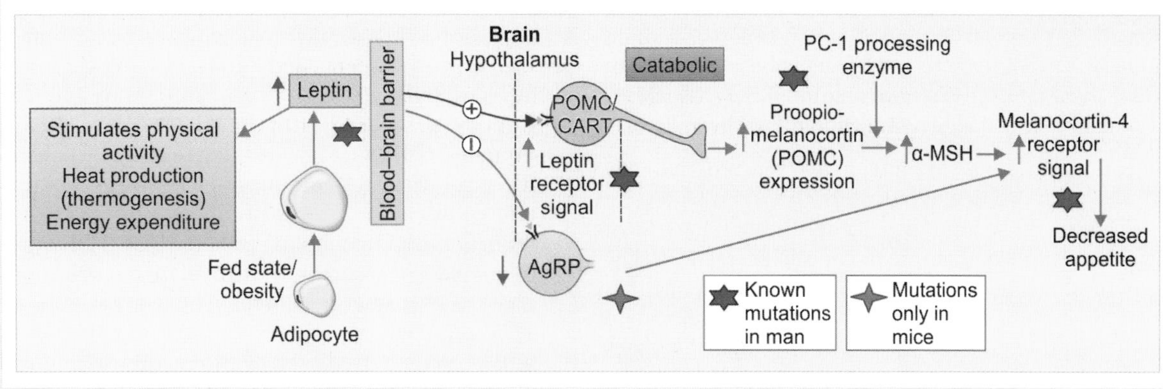

FIG. 41: Central pathway of leptin regulating appetite and body weight. Normally, when adipocytes are in fed state/obesity, produce leptins. These leptin signals are generated when leptin binds to its receptor. It activates proopiomelanocortin (POMC) neurons in the hypothalamus and induces increased production of α-melanocyte-stimulating hormone (α-MSH). This process needs the processing enzyme prohormone convertase 1 (PC-1). α-MSH gives rise to melanocortin-4 receptors. They in turn inhibit appetite. The neuropeptide agouti-related protein (AgRP) acts as an antagonist of melanocortin-4 receptor. Mutations that cause obesity in humans are indicated by the red stars and can lead to obesity. Mutation of AgRp favors stimulation of melanocortin-4 receptor and is found only in mice.

POMC/CART neurons and inhibiting NPY/AgRP neurons. Increased leptin secretion reduces appetite (anorexigenic).

- **Inadequate stores of body fat reduce secretion of leptin:** When there are inadequate stores of body fat, the opposite sequence of events occurs. It causes diminished secretion of leptin and **increases intake of food**.

- **Regulation of energy expenditure:** Leptin not only regulates intake of food but also expenditure of energy through a distinct set of pathways. Thus, an abundance of leptin stimulates physical activity, heat production, and energy expenditure. The neurohumoral mediators of leptin-induced energy expenditure are not clearly known.
  - **Thermogenesis:** Production of heat is called thermogenesis and is an important catabolic effect mediated by leptin. Heat production is controlled in part by hypothalamic signals. These signals increase the release of norepinephrine from sympathetic nerve endings in adipose tissue.

Central role of leptin in energy homeostasis: Study of mutations affecting components of the leptin pathway in mice and in humans and revealed the importance of leptin in energy homeostasis.

- **Mutations in leptin or its receptor gene:** Mice with mutations that disable the leptin gene or its receptor fail to sense the adequacy of fat stores. These mice behave as if they are undernourished, consume large amount of food and become massively obese. In humans, mutations of the leptin gene or receptor are rare. In humans as in mice, the mutations of the leptin gene or receptor cause massive obesity.
- **Mutations in the melanocortin receptor 4 gene:** It is more common and is found in 4–5% of patients with massive obesity.

The above monogenic traits confirm the importance of leptin signaling in the control of body weight. Apart from this, there may be other genetic or acquired defects in the leptin pathway that may play a role in the more common forms of obesity.

Leptin resistance: Normally, leptin produces anorexigenic (causing anorexia/loss of appetite) response. This anorexigenic response of leptin is blunted in states of obesity despite the presence of high levels of circulating leptin. This is called leptin resistance. Also, injections of leptin in obese humans fail to affect food intake and energy expenditure. Hence, initial enthusiasm of leptin therapy for obesity is fruitful.

Insulin exerts anorexigenic responses similar to leptin: Though above discussion is focused on the actions of leptin, there is increasing evidence that like leptin, insulin also exerts anorexigenic responses. Insulin receptors are expressed in both POMC/CART and NPY/AgRP neurons. Though insulin can mimic the actions of leptin, most of the evidence suggests the primacy of leptin in the regulation of energy homeostasis.

Adiponectin

- Fat-burning molecule that **causes oxidation of fatty acid:** Adiponectin is produced in the adipose tissue. In muscle, adiponectin increases glucose transport and increases fatty acid oxidation, partially through the activation of AMP kinase. Adiponectin is called a "fat-burning molecule," because it stimulates oxidation of fatty acid in skeletal muscle and reduces the levels of fatty acid. Excess fatty acids can cross the blood–brain barrier and enter the hypothalamus. In the hypothalamus, fatty acids are sensed by microglial cells. In response to this, the microglial cells releasing inflammatory factors. These factors act on hypothalamic neurons to cause leptin resistance. This in turn blunts its antiadiposity signals. Because adiponectin reduces the fatty acids by promoting their oxidation, adiponectin is called the "guardian angel against obesity".
- **Reduces production of glucose in the liver and increases insulin sensitivity:** In the liver, adiponectin inhibits the expression of gluconeogenic enzymes and the rate of glucose production. It also increases insulin sensitivity. These actions of adiponectin protect against the metabolic syndrome.
- **Other actions:** Adiponectin is an anti-inflammatory cytokine produced exclusively by adipocytes and inhibits many steps in the inflammatory process. Adiponectin has

antiatherogenic, antiproliferative, and cardioprotective effects.

Serum levels of adiponectin are lower in obese than in lean individuals. These effects are responsible for obesity associated insulin resistance, T2DM, and non-alcoholic fatty liver disease.

Mode of action: Adiponectin binds to two receptors namely AdipoR1 and AdipoR2. These receptors are found in several tissues, including the brain. AdipoR1 and AdipoR2 are most highly expressed in skeletal muscle and liver, respectively. Binding of adiponectin to its receptors triggers signals that activate cyclic adenosine monophosphate (cAMP)-dependent protein kinase (protein kinase A). This in turn phosphorylates and inactivates acetyl coenzyme A carboxylase. This is the main enzyme needed for synthesis of fatty acid.

Gut hormones (peptides)

Gut peptides can act as short-term meal initiators and terminators. Examples of gut hormones include ghrelin, PYY (peptide YY), and GLP-1 (glucagon-like peptide-1).

Ghrelin: It is produced by the oxyntic cells of the fundus of the stomach. Ghrelin is the only known gut hormone that increases food intake (orexigenic effect/appetite stimulant/ stimulates feeding). Its injection in experimental rodents produces great increase in crave for feeding, even after repeated administration. Long-term injections produce gain of weight by increasing caloric intake and reducing energy utilization. Ghrelin acts centrally by activating orexigenic NPY/ AgRP neurons. Normally, ghrelin levels rise before meals and fall after 1–2 hours. This fall is reduced in obese individuals. In obese persons ghrelin levels are lower when compared with normal-weight individuals. Ghrelin levels increase with a reduction in obesity. The rise in levels of ghrelin is much reduced in persons who undergo gastric bypass surgery for the treatment of obesity. This suggests that the beneficial effects of such surgery may be partly due to a reduced surface of gastric mucosa that is exposed to food. Other metabolic effects resulting from bypassing the foregut include altered responses of GLP-1, PYY3-36, and oxyntomodulin.

PYY and GLP-1: These are secreted from endocrine (L cells) cells in the ileum and colon. During fasting, the plasma levels of PYY and GLP-1 are low and their level increase shortly after intake of food. Both PYY and GLP-1 act centrally through NPY/AgRP neurons in the hypothalamus. This in turn causes a reduction in food intake. Because of the anorexigenic effect of GLP-1, agonists of GLP-1 receptor are used for treatment of obesity and T2DM. Apart from reducing food intake, GLP-1 increases glucose-dependent insulin secretion.

Adipocyte and Adipose Tissue

Q. Write short essay on endocrine function of adipose tissue

The excess energy consumed by adults is usually stored as TGs in adipocytes. Adipose tissue is composed of the lipid-storing adipose cell (adipocytes) and a stromal/vascular compartment. In the stroma, preadipocytes and macrophages also present.

Types of adipose tissue: There are two types of adipose tissues: white adipose tissue (WAT) and brown adipose tissue (BAT).

Brown adipose tissue: BAT is abundant especially in newborns. It is mainly located in interscapular and supraclavicular areas. Lesser amounts are present around kidneys, aorta, heart, pancreas, and trachea. Some BAT is preserved in adolescents and adults. Physiologic role of BAT is not yet established.

- **Energy produced into heat:** BAT has the unique property of disbursing (spending) energy by nonshivering thermogenesis. BAT produces energy from energy storage and converts the energy produced into heat. In BAT, a mitochondrial uncoupling protein (UCP-1) dissipates the hydrogen ion gradient in the oxidative respiration chain and releases energy as heat. The sympathetic nervous system heavily innervates BAT. The metabolic activity of BAT is increased by a central action of leptin, acting through this sympathetic nervous system. In experimental rodents, BAT deficiency causes obesity and diabetes. In these rodents, development of diabetes and obesity can be protected by stimulation of BAT with a specific adrenergic agonist (β_3 agonist).

White adipose tissue: WAT is used to store energy in the form of lipids. There will be continuous recruitment of new adipocytes (fat cells) from a large preadipocyte pool, to replace dying adipocytes. Primarily, increase of WAT mass occurs by increased (enlarged) size of adipose cells (adipocyte hypertrophy), through deposition of lipid. This process of adipocyte hypertrophy can only store a limited amount of fat. If sufficient fat is deposited, eventually there will be a net increase in number of adipocytes as more new adipocytes (adipocyte hyperplasia) are created than needed to replace dying cells. Weight is gained more from adipocyte hyperplasia than from hypertrophy. In obese adipose tissue, there is also increase inflammatory response (greater numbers of infiltrating macrophages and other immune cells). Adipocytes are derived from mesenchymal preadipocyte and this process involves several differentiation steps mediated by a different specific transcription factor. One of the main transcription factors is peroxisome proliferator-activated receptor γ (PPARγ).

- **Factors released by white adipocytes (Fig. 42):** Generally, white adipocyte is considered as a storage depot for fat. But it is also an endocrine cell that releases numerous molecules in a regulated fashion. These include the energy balance–regulating hormone (e.g., leptin, adiponectin), cytokines, e.g., TNF-α, interleukin

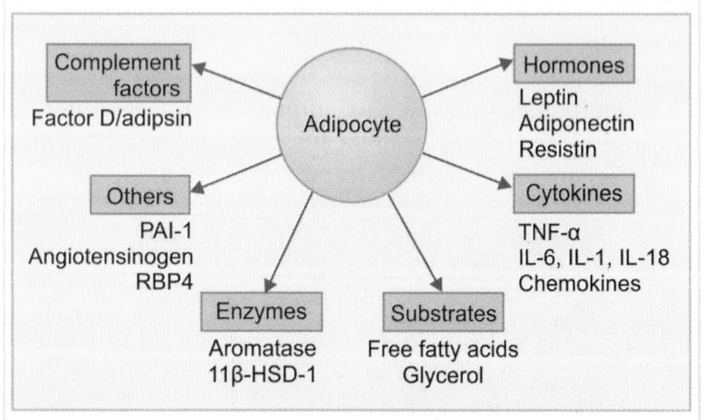

(HSD: hydroxysteroid dehydrogenase, IL: interleukin; PAI: plasminogen activator inhibitor; RBP4: retinol binding protein 4; TNF: tumor necrosis factor)

FIG. 42: Factors released by the adipocyte. These can affect peripheral tissues.

(IL)-6, IL-1, IL-18, chemokines, complement factors (e.g., factor D also known as adipsin), prothrombotic agents (e.g., plasminogen activator inhibitor I), and a component of the blood pressure-regulating system (e.g., angiotensinogen), retinol binding protein 4 (RBP4). and steroid hormones.

- Adiponectin is an abundant adipose-derived protein. Its levels are reduced in obesity. It enhances insulin sensitivity and lipid oxidation and has vascular-protective effects.
- Retinol binding protein 4: It is secreted by fat cells. RBP4 levels are increased in obesity. Its actions counteract with those of insulin and it may induce insulin resistance. Raised levels of RBP4 found in T2DM.
- In obese patients, there is increased production of cytokines and chemokines by adipose tissue. This creates a chronic proinflammatory state and accompanied by high levels of circulating CRP. This suggests that immune cells, particularly tissue macrophages, have important roles in regulating function of adipocyte.

Adipose tissue participates in the control of energy balance and energy metabolism. It functions as a link between lipid metabolism, nutrition, and inflammatory responses.

Recently described adipocytes called beige fat cells resemble BAT cells in expressing UCP-1. They are scattered through WAT. However, their thermogenic potential is uncertain.

In obesity, there is increased fat storage in tissues such as muscle and liver. This ectopic lipid has been linked to metabolic disturbances. These factors along with others unknown factors, play a role in the physiology of lipid homeostasis, insulin sensitivity, blood pressure control, coagulation, and vascular health. These are likely to contribute to obesity-related pathologies.

Endocannabinoids: These are endogenous lipids. They bind to cannabinoid receptors 1 and 2 (CB1 and CB2). CB1 receptors are found in hypothalamic nuclei and are involved in control of energy balance and weight. They are also found in adipose tissue and the GI tract. Activated CB1 receptor stimulates food intake. Thus, these may be involved in the development and maintenance of obesity. Rimonabant is a synthetic blocker of the CB1 receptor. It suppresses appetite and reduces weight in obese individuals. But because of its major side effect of depression, it is not used in the treatment of obesity.

Role of the Gut Microbiome

The microbiome is the genetic material of all the microbes—bacteria, fungi, protozoa and viruses—that live on and inside the human body. Gut microbiome or flora affects body weight. Observations in mice indicated that the gut microbiome may be involved in the development of obesity. It was found that the gut microbiota between genetically obese mice and lean is different. The microbiome of genetically obese mice can generate more energy from food than lean mice. Germ-free mice are protected from diet-induced obesity. If gut of a germ-free mice is colonized by microbiota (intestinal flora) from obese mice (but not microbiota from lean mice), it increases the body weight of germ-free mice. Distal gut flora from obese humans contains different microbes from the flora of lean individuals. Probably, gut bacteria from obese individuals may more efficiently extract calories from complex components of the diet than microbiota from their lean counterparts. However, modern foods of high-caloric density are composed of mostly simple carbohydrates and oils. These are easily absorbed without the assistance microbial flora. However, their role in human obesity is not clear.

Major orexigenic (that promote weight gain) and anorexigenic (that promote weight loss) factors are presented in **Figure 43**.

Psychosocial Aspects of Obesity

These include sexual, physical, and emotional abuse. This can result in long-term adverse consequences such as obesity especially in women. The effects are more severe if abuse occurs in childhood and adolescence. These women may be severely obese and may have chronic depression.

Figure 44 shows physical appearance of a patient with morbid obesity.

Pathologic Consequences of Obesity (Complications of Obesity)

Q. Write short essay on medical complications of obesity.

Morbidity and mortality: Obesity has many adverse effects on health and is associated with an increase in mortality and morbidity. Obese individuals especially those with central obesity are at risk of early death, mainly from T2DM, coronary heart disease cerebrovascular disease and cancer.

Metabolic Complications

Q. Write short essay on metabolic syndrome.

A central or upper body obesity, more than that total fat mass, is predictive of the metabolic complications of obesity. These

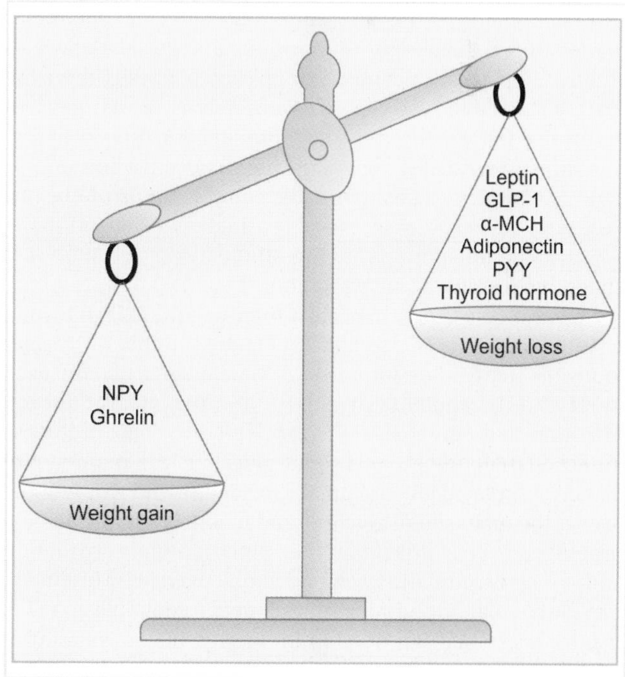

(α-MSH: α-melanocyte-stimulating hormone; GLP-1: glucagon-like peptide-1; NPY: neuropeptide Y; PYY: peptide YY).

FIG. 43: Important chemical mediators that promote fat accumulation (weight gain) and those that promote fat loss (weight loss).

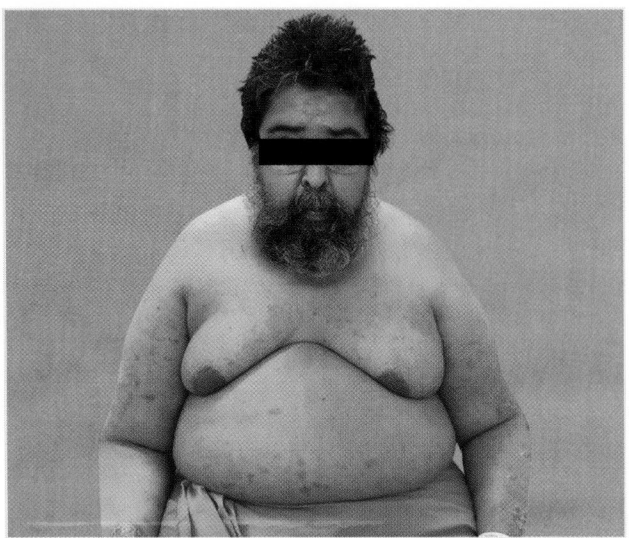

FIG. 44: Appearance of a patient with morbid obesity.

are known as the metabolic syndrome. Metabolic syndrome (syndrome X, insulin resistance syndrome) is characterized by metabolic abnormalities of glucose and lipid metabolism as well as associated with hypertension and evidence of a systemic proinflammatory state. There is increased risk of CVD (cardiovascular disease) and diabetes mellitus. The major features of the metabolic syndrome include central obesity, hypertriglyceridemia, low levels of HDL cholesterol, hyperglycemia, and hypertension.

Normally, lipolysis of adipose tissue releases free fatty acids (FFAs) and glycerol into the circulation. It provides 50–100% of daily energy requirement. Adipose tissue lipolysis is regulated mainly by insulin (inhibition) and catecholamines (stimulation), though growth hormone and cortisol may also stimulate lipolysis. In central or upper body obesity there are many abnormalities of adipose tissue lipolysis, most important being the increased concentrations of FFA due to excess release postprandially. Abnormally high concentrations of FFA can contribute to many metabolic complications of obesity. Free fatty acids and excess levels of lipids in cells and tissue activates the inflammasome. This stimulates secretion of IL-1 and induces systemic inflammation.

Insulin resistance, hyperinsulinemia and T2DM: Insulin resistance is the decrease/failure of target (peripheral) tissues to insulin action. The term insulin resistance is usually used to refer to the ability of insulin to promote glucose uptake, oxidation, and storage as well as to inhibit the release of glucose into the circulation. The skeletal muscle is the main site of insulin stimulated glucose uptake, oxidation and storage. The liver is the main site of glucose production. Normally, insulin promotes glucose utilization (i.e., glucose uptake, oxidation and storage in muscle) as well as to inhibit the release of glucose into the circulation and suppresses concentrations plasma FFA. Insulin resistance can develop in obesity. Insulin resistance initially leads to hyperinsulinemia and may eventually produce T2DM. Central/upper body/visceral obesity associated with insulin resistance and hyperinsulinemia is found in >80% of patients with T2DM. Major factors for insulin resistance include: (1) Insulin itself, by causing downregulation of its receptor, (2) Impairment of insulin action by increased free fatty acids, (3) Intracellular accumulation of lipid, and (4) Modification of insulin action by many circulating peptides secreted by adipocytes (e.g., cytokines TNF-α and IL-6, RBP4, and the "adipokine" adiponectin).

Inflammation induced by IL-1 and excess insulin may play a role in the retention of sodium, increase of blood volume, excess production of norepinephrine, and proliferation of smooth muscle that are the hallmarks of hypertension. Risk of hypertension increases proportionately with weight.

Hypertriglyceridemia and low HDL cholesterol levels: Upper body obesity and T2DM are associated with an atherogenic lipid profile. These include increased TGs (hypertriglyceridemia), increased LDL cholesterol and very-low density lipoprotein (VLDL) cholesterol and decreased HDL cholesterol, and decreased levels of the vascular protective adipokine adiponectin. These alterations increase the risk of cardiovascular diseases (atherosclerosis, coronary heart disease, cardiomyopathy) in the metabolic syndrome. The risk is increased due to the existence of comorbid conditions including diabetes, hypertension, and dyslipidemia.

Pathophysiology of the metabolic syndrome (Fig. 45): Excess of FFAs are released from an increased adipose tissue mass in obesity.

- In the liver, FFAs causes increased production of glucose and TGs and secretion of VLDLs. This is associated with lipid/lipoprotein abnormalities and includes decreased HDL and an increase of LDL.
- In the muscle, FFAs reduce insulin sensitivity by preventing insulin-mediated uptake of glucose. This is associated with reduced conversion of glucose to glycogen and increased accumulation of TG.
- The increased levels of circulating glucose, and to some extent FFAs (free fatty acids), increases insulin secretion by pancreas producing hyperinsulinemia.
- Hyperinsulinemia may increase reabsorption sodium in the kidney. This along with increased levels of circulating FFAs contribute to hypertension.
- Excessive FFAs also produces proinflammatory state and contribute to the insulin resistance. There is increased secretion of IL-6 and TNF-α by adipocytes and monocyte-derived macrophages. This results in more insulin resistance and lipolysis of adipose tissue leading to increased levels of circulating FFAs. IL-6 and other cytokines also increase glucose and VLDL production by liver and insulin resistance in muscle. Insulin resistance also increases accumulation of TG in the liver.
- Cytokines and FFAs also increase production of fibrinogen by liver and production of plasminogen activator inhibitor 1 (PAI-1) by adipocyte. This produces a prothrombotic state. Increased levels of circulating cytokines stimulate production of CRP by liver. There is also reduced production of the anti-inflammatory and insulin-sensitizing cytokine adiponectin is in the metabolic syndrome.

Mechanisms of insulin action and its impairment in metabolic syndrome are presented in **Figures 46A to C**.

Cardiovascular Complications

Hypertension: Obesity is associated with a high risk of hypertension and is associated with increased sympathetic activity. High insulin levels in obese patients with insulin resistance act on pathway not related to glucose metabolism.

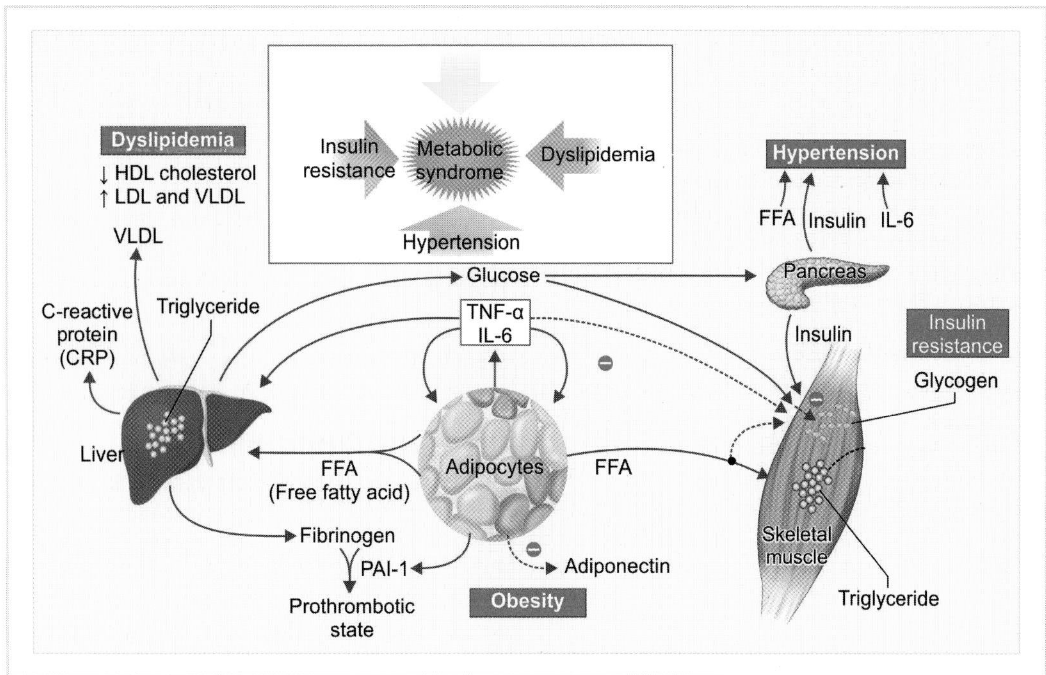

FIG. 45: Pathophysiology of the metabolic syndrome. In obesity, excess of free fatty acids (FFAs) are released from an increased adipose tissue mass. In the liver, FFAs causes increased production of glucose and triglycerides (TGs) and secretion of VLDLs. This leads to lipid/lipoprotein abnormalities such as decreased HDL and an increase of LDL. In the muscle, FFAs reduce insulin sensitivity by preventing insulin-mediated uptake of glucose. This is associated with reduced conversion of glucose to glycogen and increased accumulation of TG. The increased circulating glucose increases insulin secretion by pancreas producing hyperinsulinemia. Hyperinsulinemia may increase reabsorption sodium in the kidney and with increased levels of circulating FFAs, it may contribute to hypertension. Excessive FFAs also produces proinflammatory state and contribute to the insulin resistance. Cytokines and FFAs also increase production of fibrinogen by liver and production of plasminogen activator inhibitor 1 (PAI-1) by adipocyte. This produces a prothrombotic state.

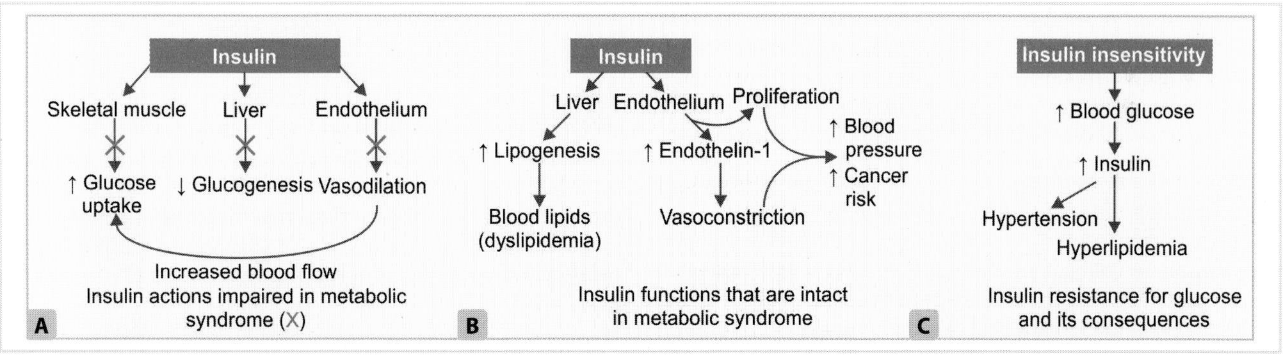

FIGS. 46A TO C: Mechanisms of insulin action and its impairment in metabolic syndrome. (A) Insulin actions that are impaired. (B). Insulin functions that are intact. (C) Insulin resistance for glucose and its consequences in metabolic syndrome.

These include increased renal reabsorption of sodium, which contributes to hypertension, and stimulate production of the vasoconstrictor endothelin-1 by endothelial cells. Adipose tissue in obese individuals also secretes substances such as angiotensin II and its precursors that directly cause vasoconstriction and increase blood pressure. Even a small reduction in weight may decrease blood pressure.

Coronary heart disease: Dyslipoproteinemia and hypertension are major risk factors for atherosclerotic cardiovascular disease linked to obesity.

Congestive heart failure: Obesity is associated with increased risk of heart failure due to eccentric dilatation of heart. Also, the combination of obesity and hypertension leads to thickening of ventricular wall and larger heart volume. Obese individuals are also prone to increased risk of atrial fibrillation and atrial flutter.

Thromboembolic disease: Deep venous thromboses and pulmonary embolism are more common in obese individuals.

Thromboembolic disease of the lower extremities may be due to increased abdominal pressure, impaired fibrinolysis and increased circulating cytokines in abdominal obesity

Hepatobiliary Disease

Non-alcoholic fatty liver disease: Obesity and T2DM is frequently associated with non-alcoholic fatty liver disease (NAFLD). The hepatic steatosis of NAFLD may progresses to inflammatory non-alcoholic steatohepatitis (NASH) and more rarely to cirrhosis and hepatocellular carcinoma. Steatosis usually improves following weight loss, secondary to diet or bariatric surgery.

Cholelithiasis (gallstones): Obesity is associated with increase in total body cholesterol. It causes increased turnover of cholesterol and leads to increased biliary secretion of cholesterol, supersaturation of bile, and a higher incidence of cholesterol-rich gallstones. Gall stones are six times more common in obese than in lean individuals.

Bone, Joint, and Cutaneous Disease

Osteoarthritis: Excessive body weight in obesity predisposes to degenerative joint disease (osteoarthritis) and also gout. Osteoarthritis usually appears in older individuals. It is mainly due to the cumulative effects of wear and tear on joints and activation of inflammatory pathways that promote synovial pathology. More the body burdens of fat, the greater the trauma to joints with the passage of time.

Venous stasis/varicose veins

Acanthosis nigricans: It manifests as darkening and thickening of the skin-folds on the neck, elbows and dorsal interphalangeal spaces. It reflects the severity of underlying insulin resistance.

Increased friability of skin: Especially in skin-folds, thereby increasing the risk of fungal and yeast infections. Excessive hair growth (hirsutism) can occur due to increases in circulating androgens in susceptible women.

Pulmonary Disease

Pulmonary abnormalities associated with obesity include reduced chest wall compliance, increased work of breathing, increased minute ventilation due to increased metabolic rate, and decreased functional residual capacity and expiratory reserve volume. In severe obesity, there may be obstructive sleep apnea and the "obesity hypoventilation syndrome." Sleep apnea may be obstructive (most common), central, or mixed.

Obstructive sleep apnea: Obstructive cessation of breathing (apnea) is common in severely obese individuals. Sleep apnea is most likely due to enlargement of upper airways soft tissue. This results in collapse of the upper airways with inspiration during sleep. The obstruction leads to apnea, with hypoxemia, hypercarbia, and high levels of catecholamine and endothelin. The quality of sleep quality of sleep will be poor due to frequent arousals to restore breathing. Sleep apnea is associated with an increased risk of hypertension. If sleep apnea is severe, consequently it can lead to right-sided heart failure and sudden death. Features suggestive of obstructive sleep apnea include a history of daytime hypersomnolence, loud snoring, restless sleep, or morning headaches.

Obesity hypoventilation syndrome (OHS) (Pickwickian syndrome): Hypoventilation syndrome is respiratory abnormalities in very obese individuals and consists of the triad of obesity, sleep disordered breathing, and chronic hypercapnia during wakefulness in the absence of other known causes of hypercapnia. In Charles Dickens' novel namely "The Pickwick Papers" a young, jovial, generous, fat (plump) boy was constantly falling asleep. Hence, it was called as Pickwickian syndrome.

Hypersomnolence: Hypersomnolence is a condition where an individual experiences significant episode of sleepiness, even after having 7 hours or more of quality sleep. In obese individuals it may develop both at night and during the day. It is often associated with apneic pauses during sleep (sleep apnea), polycythemia and right-sided heart failure (cor pulmonale).

Endocrine Manifestations

Women: Polycystic ovarian syndrome (PCOS) and menstrual abnormalities.

Men: Reduced plasma testosterone and sex hormone–binding globulin (SHBG), increased estrogen levels and gynecomastia.

Obesity and Cancer (Fig . 47)

Obesity is associated with increased risk of certain cancer types and are somewhat more in women than in men. Also, obesity can lead to poorer treatment outcomes and increased cancer mortality. These include cancers of the esophagus, colon, rectum, pancreas, liver, prostate thyroid, and kidney in men and cancers of the gallbladder, bile ducts, breasts, esophagus, endometrium, cervix, ovaries, and kidney in women. Obesity and related cancers are listed in **Table 19**. The mechanisms of development of cancer in obese individuals are unknown and are more likely to be multiple.

Raised levels of insulin: Insulin resistance leads to hyper-insulinemia. This may have multiple effects and may directly or indirectly contribute to cancer development. For example, hyperinsulinemia causes increased levels of free insulin-like growth factor 1 (IGF-1). IGF-1 is a mitogen, and its receptor, IGFR-1, is highly expressed in many human cancers. IGFR-1 activates the RAS and PI3K/AKT signaling pathways. This results in increased growth of both normal and neoplastic cells and inhibits apoptosis.

Steroid hormones: Obesity has effects on steroid hormones that regulate cell growth and differentiation in the breast, uterus, and other tissues. Obesity is associated with increased production of estrogen from androgen precursors in adipose tissue, increases synthesis of androgen in ovaries and adrenals, and enhances the availability of estrogen by inhibiting the production of sex hormone-binding globulin (SHBG) in the liver.

Adiponectin: In obese individuals, secretion of adiponectin from adipose tissue is reduced. Adiponectin suppresses proliferation of cells and increases apoptosis. This anti-neoplastic action of adiponectin is partly achieved by promoting the actions of p53 and p21. In obese individuals, these antineoplastic actions of adiponectin may be compromised.

Proinflammatory state: It is associated with obesity and may be carcinogenic.

Others

These include gastroesophageal reflux disease, urinary incontinence and increased risk of ischemic stroke.

Markers of Inflammation

These include systemic biomarker CRP and proinflammatory cytokines such as IL-1, 6, and 18, resistin and TNF-α. They

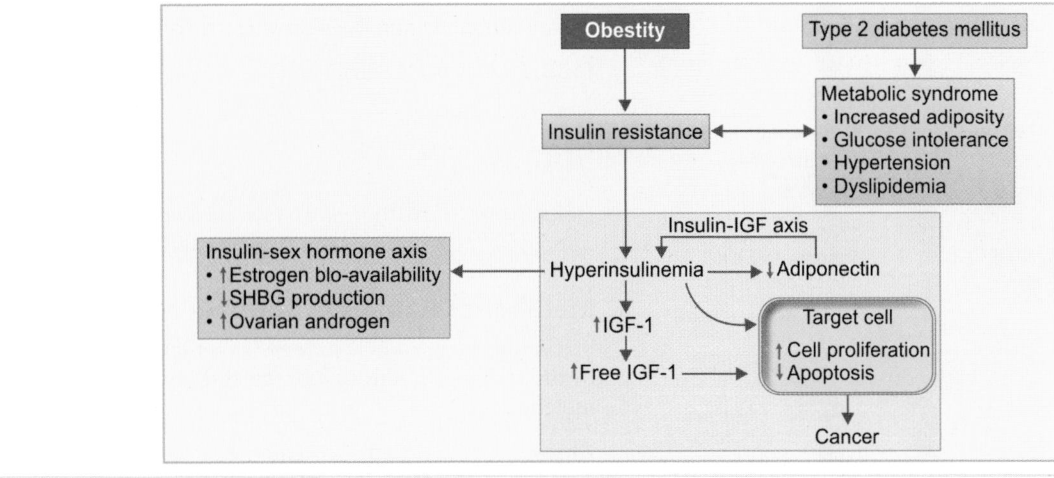

FIG. 47: Obesity, metabolic syndrome, and cancer. Obesity is the precursors of the metabolic syndrome. Metabolic syndrome is associated with insulin resistance, type 2 diabetes mellitus, and hormonal changes. In obesity, there is increase in insulin. Hyperinsulinemia causes increased levels of free insulin-like growth factor 1 (IGF-1). IGF-1 is a mitogen, and its receptor, IGFR-1, is highly expressed in many human cancers. IGFR-1 activates the RAS and PI3K/AKT signaling pathways. This results in increased cell proliferation of both normal and neoplastic cells and inhibits apoptosis. This may contribute to development of cancer. In obesity, there is increased synthesis of androgen in ovaries and adrenals. Hyperinsulinemia also increases availability of estrogen by inhibiting the production of sex hormone-binding globulin (SHBG) in the liver. Obesity is associated with increased production of estrogen from androgen precursors in adipose tissue,

Table 19: Obesity and related cancers.

Males	***Females***
Esophagus	Gallbladder
Colon	Bile ducts
Rectum	Breasts
Pancreas	Esophagus
Liver	Colon
Prostate	Endometrium
Thyroid	Cervix
Kidney	Ovaries

are overproduced by the expanded adipose tissue mass and are often raised in obese persons, in particularly in individuals with central obesity. These may be elevated due to a direct proinflammatory effect of excess circulating lipids and increased release of cytokines from fat-laden adipocytes. Adipose tissue–derived macrophages may be the main source of proinflammatory cytokines locally and in the systemic circulation. Chronic inflammation may be responsible for many of the complications of obesity such as insulin resistance, metabolic abnormalities, thrombosis, cardiovascular disease, and cancer.

Complications of obesity are mentioned in **Figure 48**.

Diet and Cancer

Q. Write short essay on obesity and cancer

Few specific types of cancer are linked to diets. Carcinogenesis may be due to three major aspects of the diet. These are: (1) The presence of exogenous carcinogens, (2) The endogenous production of carcinogens from dietary components, and (3) Absence of protective factors in the diet.

Exogenous carcinogens in diet: One of the exogenous carcinogens in the diet is aflatoxin. It is involved in the development of hepatocellular carcinomas usually in association with hepatitis B virus. Aflatoxin in the diet causes a specific mutation in codon 249 of the *TP53* gene. In hepatocellular carcinomas, this mutation serves as a molecular signature for aflatoxin exposure. It is not clear regarding the carcinogenicity of food additives, artificial sweeteners, and diets contaminated with pesticides.

Endogenous production of carcinogens from dietary components: Main example is gastric carcinomas due to endogenous production of carcinogenic agents from dietary components. These are related to the presence of nitrosamines and nitrosamides in the diet. They induce gastric cancer in animals. These compounds can be formed in the GIT from nitrites and amines or amides in the digested proteins. Nitrites such as sodium nitrite is added to foods as a preservative. Nitrates are present in common vegetables and are reduced in the gut by bacterial flora. However, so far, no particular diet has been well documented to cause or prevent cancer.

Absence of protective factors in the diet: Examples are as follows:

- **High intake of animal fat combined with low fiber intake:** It has been involved in the causation of colon cancer. Increasing average level of total fiber content in the food decreases the risk of colon cancer. Probably, high intake of fat increases the bile acids level in the gut. This may modify the intestinal flora and favor the growth of microaerophilic bacteria. Bile acid metabolites produced by these bacteria may function as carcinogens. The protective effect of a high-fiber diet may be due to the following effects:

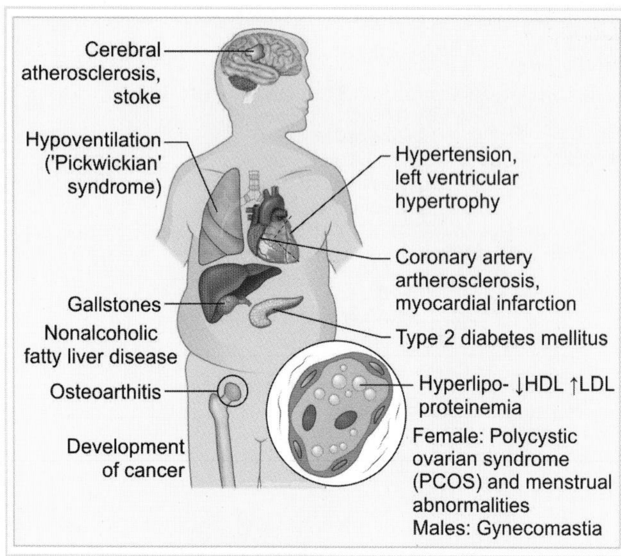

FIG. 48: Complications of obesity.

  - It increases bulk of stool and reduces the transit time of intestinal content. This reduces the exposure of mucosa to probable carcinogen in the diet.
  - Certain fibers are capable of binding to the carcinogens in the diet and thereby protect the intestinal mucosa against exposure to carcinogens in diet.
- **Vitamins C and E, β-carotene, and selenium:** They are believed to have anticarcinogenic effects because of their antioxidant properties. However, there is no convincing evidence that they act as chemopreventive agents.
- Retinoids are effective agents in the therapy of acute promyelocytic leukemia.
- Low levels of vitamin D may be associated with cancer of the colon, prostate, and breast
- Obesity is associated with cancer development. Prevention of obesity by consuming a healthy diet is a best way to preserving good health.

Diet and Systemic Diseases

Composition of the diet even with adequate nutrients may contribute to the causation and progression of a number of diseases. A few examples are mentioned below:

Diet and atherosclerosis: One of the most important and controversial issues is the contribution of diet to atherogenesis. Primary prevention of atherosclerosis is by dietary modification. This specifically consists of reduced consumption of foods rich in cholesterol and saturated animal fats (e.g., eggs, butter, beef). The aim is to reduce serum cholesterol levels and prevents or slows the development of atherosclerosis (mainly coronary heart disease) in individuals without any previous episode of cardiovascular disease. However, its beneficial effect is not clear.

Restricting sodium intake: It reduces hypertension.

Dietary fiber or roughage: It increases the bulk of stool and may be a preventive effect against diverticulosis of the colon.

Caloric restriction: This has been proved to increase lifespan in experimental animals, including monkeys.

Garlic: It may protect against heart disease.

STARVATION

Definition: Starvation is a state of overall deprivation of nutrients. Causes of starvation are listed in **Box 8**.

Metabolic Changes in Starvation

Starvation is a gradual process in which there is decrease in the metabolic rate as storage carbohydrate reserves are metabolized.

Glucose: Normal body has glucose stores that are sufficient only for one day's metabolic needs. During fasting, insulin independent tissues, such as the brain, blood cells and renal medulla continue to utilize glucose. However, insulin-dependent tissues like muscle do not utilize glucose. To maintain normal blood glucose level, there will be release of glycogen stores from the liver. When the liver glycogen stores are depleted (within a few days), the supply of glucose released into the blood decreases. Subsequently, hepatic gluconeogenesis from other sources, such as breakdown of proteins takes place.

Proteins: Protein stores and the TGs of adipose tissue have enough energy for about 3 months. In starvation, the proteins are broken down to release amino acids and these amino acids are utilized as fuel for hepatic gluconeogenesis. Protein is used for energy by means of gluconeogenesis because certain tissues prefer glucose as an energy source. The use of protein for gluconeogenesis produces a negative nitrogen balance.

Fats: When insulin levels decline during fasting, triglycerides of adipose tissue are broken down to form glycerol and free fatty acids. The fatty acids are converted into ketone bodies in the liver and they are used for energy use in place of glucose by most organs including brain. As starvation continues, overall needs for energy are reduced by slowing metabolism. The tissues that usually need glucose for energy adapt by using ketone bodies produced from fat. Eventually lipolysis of stored fat provides the source of required energy, and the use of protein as an energy source decreases. Through this adaptive response the body strives to conserve lean body mass. Overall, there will be reduction and depletion of the body's protein. Fasting (voluntary starving) is not associated with a high mortality unless it is prolonged. Starvation can continue till a stage when all the body fat stores are exhausted. After the exhaustion of fat stores death will occur.

Manifestations: Starved patient has lax, dry skin, wasted muscles and atrophy of internal organs. In chronic starvation the patient is susceptible to infections (**Box 9**).

Laboratory findings: Characteristic findings in starvation include decreased serum glucose levels and urinary nitrogen excretion, along with elevation in the levels of ketone bodies (with ketonuria) and free fatty acids.

Box 8: Causes of starvation.

- Deliberate fasting (religious or political)
- Famine conditions (country or community)
- Secondary undernutrition: Due to chronic wasting illness/ diseases (e.g., infections, inflammatory conditions, liver disease), cancer*

*Cancer cachexia is defined as progressive weight loss accompanied by severe weakness, anorexia and anemia developing in patients with cancer. Its mechanism is poorly understood and may be due to TNF and other cytokines, such as IL-1, interferon-γ, and leukemia inhibitory factor. They may be produced by macrophages in the tumor or by the tumor cells themselves.

Box 9: Infections associated with starvation.

- Gastroenteritis and gram-negative sepsis
- Respiratory infections, e.g., bronchopneumonia
- Viral diseases, e.g., measles, herpes simplex
- Tuberculosis
- Streptococcal and staphylococcal skin infections
- Helminthic infestations

BIBLIOGRAPHY

1. Abdelhamid AS, Brown TJ, Brainard JS, et al. Omega-3 fatty acids for the primary and secondary prevention of cardiovascular disease. *Cochrane Database Syst Rev*. 2018;(7):CD003177.
2. Aune D, Sen A, Prasad M, et al. BMI and all-cause mortality: systematic review and non-linear dose-response meta-analysis of 230 cohort studies with 3.74million deaths among 30.3 million participants, *BMJ*. 2016;353:i2156.
3. Beelen R, Raaschau-Nielsen O, Massimo S, et al. Effects of long-term exposure to air pollution on natural-cause mortality: an analysis of 22 European cohorts within the multicenter ESCAPE project. *Lancet*. 2014;383:785.
4. Berthoud H-R, Munzberg H, Morrison CD. Blaming the brain for obesity: integration of hedonic and homeostatic mechanisms. *Gastroenterology*. 2017;152:1728.
5. Bouter KE, van Raalte DH, Groen AK, et al. Role of gut microbiome in the pathogenesis of obesity and obesity-related metabolic dysfunction. *Gastroenterology*. 2017;152:1671.
6. Cao Y, Willet WC, Rimm EB, et al. Light to moderate intake of alcohol, drinking patterns, and risk of cancer: results from two prospective US cohort studies. *BMJ*. 2015;351:h4238.
7. Chechi K, Nedergaard J, Richard D. Brown adipose tissue as an antiobesity tissue in humans. *Obes Rev*. 2014;15:92.
8. Chen Y, Copeland WK, Vedanthan R, et al. Association between body mass index and cardiovascular disease mortality in east Asians and south Asians: pooled analysis of prospective data from the Asia Cohort Consortium. *BMJ*. 2013;347:f5446.
9. Gialeraki A, Valsami S, Pittaras T et al: Oral contraceptives and HRT risk of thrombosis. *Clin Appl Thromb Hemost*. 2018;24:217.
10. Gonzalez-Muniesa P, Martinez-Gonzalez M-A, Hu FB, et al. Obesity. *Nat Rev Dis Primers*. 2017;3:1.
11. Guy GP Jr, Zhang K, Schieber LZ, et al. County-level opioid prescribing in the United States, 2015 and 2017. JAMA Internal Medicine published online February 11, 2019.
12. Haines A, Ebi K. The imperative for climate action to protect health. *N Engl J Med*. 2019;380:263.
13. Hanna-Attisha M, LaChance J, Sadler RC, et al. Elevated blood lead levels in children associated with the Flint drinking water crisis: a spatial analysis of risk and public health response. *Am J Public Health*. 2016;106:283.
14. Hariz A, Hamdi MS, Boukhris I, et al. Gelatinous transformation of bone marrow in a patient with anorexia nervosa: an uncommon but reversible etiology. *Am J Case Rep*. 2018;19:1449.
15. Hon KL, Fung CK, Leung AKC. Childhood lead poisoning: an overview. *Hong Kong Med J*. 2017;23:616.
16. Jameson JL, Fausi AS, Kasper DL, et al. Harrison's principles of internal medicine (2 vols), 20th edition. New York: McGraw-Hill Medical Publishing. Division; 2018.
17. Kumar V, Abbas AK, Aster JC. Robbins basic pathology, 10th edition. Philadelphia: Saunders Elsevier; 2018
18. Kumar V, Abbas AK, Fausto N, et al. Robbins and Cotran pathologic basis of disease, 10th edition. Philadelphia: WB Saunders; 2021.
19. Kumar V, Abbas AK, Aster JC, Deyrup AT. Robbins essential pathology, 1st edition. Philadelphia: Elsevier; 2021.
20. Maddatu J, Anderson-Baucum E, Evans-Molina C. Smoking and the risk of type 2 diabetes. *Trans Res*. 2017;184:101.
21. Matthew JD, Forsythe AV, Brady Z, et al. Cancer risk in 680,000 people exposed to computed tomography scans in childhood or adolescence: data linkage study of 11 million Australians. *BMJ*. 2013;346:f2360.
22. Million M, Diallo A, Raoult R. Review. Gut microbiota and malnutrition. *Microb Pathog*. 2017;106:127.
23. National Institute on Drug Abuse (NIDA). https://www.drugabuse.gov updated in June 2019.
24. Padayatty SJ, Levine M. Vitamin C: the known and unknown and Goldilocks. *Oral Dis*. 2016;22:463.
25. Ralston SH, Penman ID, Strachan MWJ, et al. Davidson's principles and practice of medicine, 23rd edition. Edinburgh: Churchill Livingstone; 2018.
26. Rautiainen S, Manson J, Lichtenstein AH. Dietary supplements and disease prevention—a global review. *Nat Rev Endocrinol*. 2016;12:407.
27. Rehman K, Fatima F, Waheed I, et al. Prevalence of exposure of heavy metals and their impact on health consequences. *J Cell Biochem*. 2018;119:157.
28. Rigotti NA. Balancing the benefits and harms of e-cigarettes: a national academies of science, engineering, and medicine report. *Ann Intern Med*. 2018;168:666.
29. Sarri JC. Vitamin A metabolism in rod and cone visual cycles. *Annu Rev Nutr*. 2012;32:125.
30. Steele CB, Thomas CC, Henley SJ, et al. Vital signs: trends in incidence of cancers associated with overweight and obesity—United States, 2005-2014. *MMWR Morb Mortal Wkly Rep*. 2017;66(39):1052.
31. Strayer DS, Saffitz JE. Rubin's Pathology: Mechanism of Human Disease, 8th edition. Philadelphia: Wolters Kluwer; 2020.
32. Teng J, Pourmand A, Mazer-Amirshahi M. Vitamin C: the next step in sepsis management? *J Crit Care*. 2018;43:230.
33. Timper K, Bruning JC. Hypothalamic circuits regulating appetite and energy homeostasis: pathways to obesity. *Dis Model Mech*. 2017;10:679.
34. Zhao VW, Scherer PE. Adiponectin, the past two decades. *J Mol Cell Biol*. 2016;8:93.

SECTION

3

IMMUNOPATHOLOGY

CHAPTER 15

Normal Immune Response and Hypersensitivity

CHAPTER OUTLINE

NORMAL IMMUNE RESPONSE

Introduction

Immunity: This term is derived from the Latin word immunitas, which was referred to the protection against legal prosecution offered to Roman senators during their tenures in office. Historically, immunity means protection from disease and, more specifically, infectious disease. However, immunity in its broader sense includes host reactions against cancers (tumor immunity), tissue transplants, and even self-antigens (autoimmunity).

Definition: Immunity is resistance (defense mechanism) by host against invasion by any foreign antigen, including microorganisms.

Immune system and response: The cells and molecules involved in immunity constitute the immune system. The collective and coordinated response of the immune system to the introduction of foreign substances is called the immune response. The foreign agents include microorganisms, viruses, multicellular parasites, toxins, chemicals, drugs, and transplanted foreign tissues.

Importance of normal immune system: The normal immune system is vital for survival because it protects individuals from infectious pathogens that are present in the environment and also from the development of cancer. Predictably, immune deficiencies render the individuals easy prey to infections and increase the incidence of certain cancers.

Double-edged sword: Though normal immune system is protective in most of the situations, it is like a double-edged sword. Sometimes, the immune system is itself capable of causing tissue injury and disease. Examples of disorders caused by immune responses include reactions to environmental substances that cause allergies and reactions against an individual's own tissues and cells (autoimmunity).

Mechanism of immunity (Fig. 1): Defense against microbes is mediated by sequential and coordinated immune responses. These mechanisms of immunity can be divided into two broad categories namely—(1) innate and (2) adaptive immunity.

1. **Innate immunity:** It is also known as natural, or native immunity. It refers to intrinsic mechanisms that react immediately and forms the first line of defense. It is mediated by cells and molecules that recognize products of microbes and dead cells. It produces rapid protective host reactions.
2. **Adaptive immunity:** It is also called acquired, or specific immunity. Its mechanisms are stimulated by ("adapt to") exposure to microbes and other foreign substances. It occurs more slowly than innate immunity. But it is more powerful in fighting against infections. Conventionally, the term immune response is usually used to adaptive immunity.

Innate (Natural/Native) Immunity

Q. Write short essay on innate immunity.

General Features

- Innate immunity is the first line of defense present by birth. It is necessary for defending against microbes in the first few hours or days after infection, before there is development of adaptive immune responses.

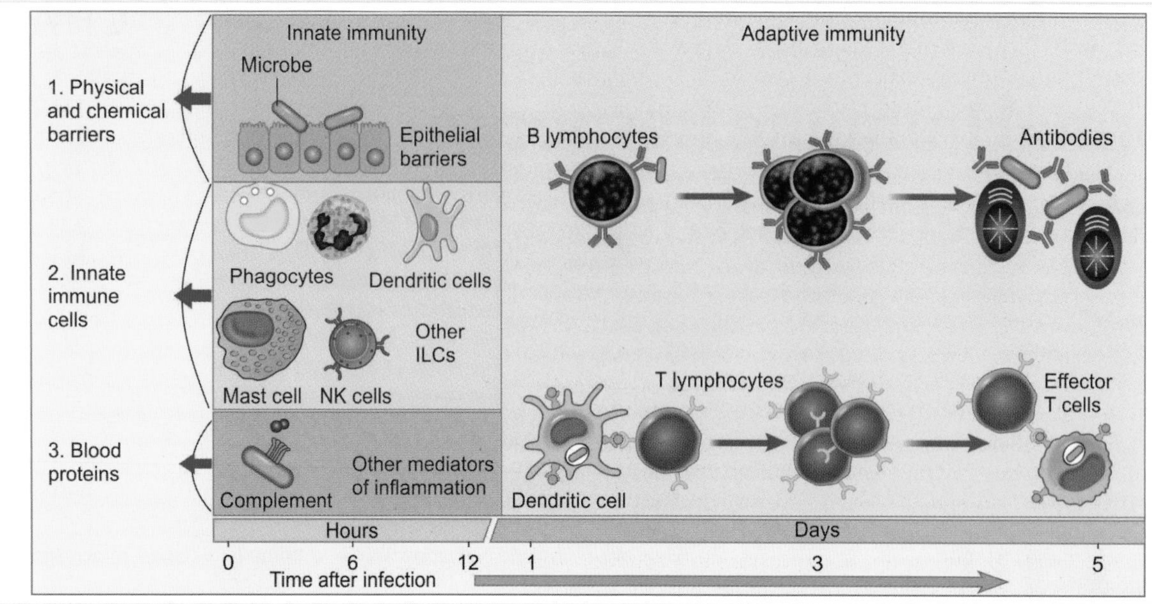

(ILC: innate lymphoid cell; NK: natural killer)

FIG. 1: Main components and mechanism of innate and adaptive immunity. Initial innate immunity provides the defense against infections. Adaptive immune responses develop later and need the activation of lymphocytes.

- It provides immediate, initial protective response against an invading pathogen (microbes) and to remove damaged cells. These purposes are served by evolution of receptors and other components of innate immunity.
- Innate immunity is mediated by mechanisms that are present in an individual even before the occurrence of an infection (hence innate=inherent /inborn).
- It does not depend on the prior contact with foreign antigen or microbes.
- It lacks specificity but is highly effective. No memory and no self/nonself recognition.
- It triggers the adaptive immune response.
- No memory is seen.

Components of Innate Immunity

The main components of innate immunity (**Fig. 1**) are:
- **Physical and chemical barriers**
- **Innate immune cells**
- **Plasma/Blood proteins**

Physical (anatomical) and chemical barriers

These include epithelia (block entry of microbes) and antimicrobial chemicals produced at epithelial surfaces.

Epithelia The epithelia include those lining of skin, gastrointestinal, and respiratory tracts. They are **mechanical barriers** that prevent the entry of microbes from the external environment.

Secretion of antimicrobial chemicals Epithelial cells also produce antimicrobial molecules such as **defensins** at these sites. If microbes breach epithelial boundaries, other defense mechanisms come into play.

Innate immune cells

These include phagocytic cells (mainly neutrophils, macrophages), dendritic cells (DCs), mast cells, natural killer cells (NK cells), and other innate lymphoid cells (ILCs). Many innate immune cells (e.g., macrophages, DCs, mast cells) are always present in most tissues. They keep watch for invading microbes.

Phagocytic cells

Neutrophils and macrophages Most important phagocytic cells are monocytes (macrophages in tissue) and neutrophils in the blood. They can be rapidly recruited to any site of infection. Monocytes from blood enter the tissues and mature. These are called macrophages. Some tissue-resident macrophages (Kupffer cells in the liver, microglia in the brain, and alveolar macrophages in the lungs) develop from the yolk sac or fetal liver early in life and are found in various tissues. Phagocytes sense the presence of microbes and other offending agents. They ingest (phagocytose) these invaders and destroy them. Macrophages are the dominant cells of chronic inflammation (discussed in detail in on pages 306–311).

Dendritic cells These are specialized cells and are present in epithelia, lymphoid organs, and most tissues (see page 16).
- **Functions of DCs:** (1) These cells function as antigen-presenting cells (APCs) to T cells. DCs capture protein antigens and display peptides for recognition by T lymphocytes. (2) DCs have numerous receptors that sense microbes and cell damage. The activated receptors stimulate the secretion of cytokines. These cytokines are mediators that play critical roles in inflammation and antiviral defense. They produce type I interferons (IFNs)

(e.g., IFN-α), which inhibit viral infection and replication. Thus, DCs serve as sentinels and detect danger and initiate innate immune responses. However, in contrast to macrophages, they do not play main role in the destruction of microbes and other offending agents.

Innate lymphoid cells ILCs are **tissue-resident lymphocytes** (especially mucosal tissues such as the lung and intestines) that do not have T-cell antigen receptors **and cannot respond to antigens**. But they are **activated by cytokines** and other mediators produced at sites of tissue damage. Probably, ILCs are sources of inflammatory cytokines during early phases of immune reactions. These **cytokine-secreting ILCs have similar effector functions as CD4+ helper T cells**. ILCs are classified into **three major groups** depending on the predominant cytokines they secrete—groups 1, 2, and 3. These ILCs produce many of the same cytokines as Th1, Th2, and Th17 subsets of CD4+ helper T cells. ILCs are rare in the blood. The common lymphoid progenitor in the bone marrow that gives rise to T and B lymphocytes also gives rise to a common precursor of both NK cells and cytokine secreting ILCs. Both NK cells and ILCs share expression of several lineage-specific markers and transcription factors. A type of ILC called lymphoid tissue-inducer cells secretes the cytokines lymphotoxin (LT) and tumor necrosis factor (TNF) and these are needed for the formation of organized secondary lymphoid tissues.

NK cells: These are one type of ILCs. They provide early protection against many viruses and intracellular bacteria. They are discussed in detail on pages 1044 and 1045.

Other types of cells Many other types of cells can sense and react to microbes. These include mast cells (produce many mediators of inflammation) and epithelial and endothelial cells.

Plasma/Blood proteins

These include components of the complement system and other mediators of inflammation.

Apart from the cells, several soluble proteins also play important roles in innate immunity.

Complement system: The complement system (described in detail on pages 257–263) consists of plasma proteins. These are activated by microbes. In innate immune responses, complements may be activated through the alternative and lectin pathways. In adaptive immune responses, they may be activated through the classical pathway, which involves antibody–antigen complexes.

Other circulating proteins of innate immunity These include mannose-binding lectin and C-reactive protein. Both these proteins coat microbes and aid phagocytosis. In the lung, surfactant is a component of innate immunity and protects against inhaled microbes.

Cellular Receptors in Innate Immunity

The cellular receptors in innate immunity include those for microbes, products of damaged cells, and foreign substances.

Molecular patterns

There are two types of molecular patterns namely, pathogen-associated molecular patterns (PAMPs) and damage-associated molecular patterns (DAMPs). These are derived from microbes, damaged cells or foreign substances.

1. **Pathogen-associated molecular patterns:** Phagocytic cells involved in innate immunity are capable of recognizing certain components of microbes. These components (structures) are shared among related microbes and that are generally essential for the infectivity of these pathogens. These components of microbes are highly conserved common molecular structures shared by entire classes of pathogens. They cannot be mutated to allow the microbes to evade the defense mechanisms. These microbial components (structures) are called PAMPs. These are biochemical moieties expressed by microbes but not by human cells and thus are recognized as nonself. Examples of PAMPs are presented in **Table 1** (refer Table 4 of chapter 8).
2. **Damage-associated molecular patterns:** Leukocytes also recognize molecules released by injured and necrotic cells. These molecules are called as DAMPs. Examples of DAMPs are presented in Table 5 and Box 3 of Chapter 8.

Pattern recognition receptors

PRRs are located in all cellular compartments where microbes may be present. These pattern recognition receptors (PRRs) are as follows:

- **Plasma membrane receptors:** They detect extracellular microbes.
- **Endosomal receptors:** They detect ingested microbes.
- **Cytosolic receptors:** They detect microbes in the cytoplasm.

There are several classes of PRRs. Examples for PRRs are discussed next.

Toll-like receptors These are the best-known PRRs. They are present in the plasma membrane and endosomal vesicles (Figs. 2 and 3 of Chapter 8). About 10 types of human toll-like receptors (TLRs) have been identified. Each receptor recognizes a unique set of microbial patterns. For example, TLR2 recognizes various ligands (e.g., lipoteichoic acid) expressed by gram-positive bacteria, TLR4 recognizes lipopolysaccharides (LPS) of gram-negative bacteria.

Signaling: All TLRs signal by a common pathway. These signals activate two sets of transcription factors.

Table 1: Examples of pathogen-associated molecular patterns (PAMPs).

Nature	*Type of molecule*	*Type of microbe*
Cell wall lipids	Lipopolysaccharide (LPS)	Gram-negative bacteria
	Lipoteichoic acid	Gram-positive bacteria
Cell wall carbohydrates	Mannans	Fungi, bacteria
	Glucans	Fungi
Cell wall (surface) proteins	Flagellin, Pilin	Bacteria
Microbial nucleic acids	ssRNA	Viruses
	dsRNA	Viruses
	CpG sequences	Viruses, bacteria

(CpG: cytidine-guanidine-rich dinucleotide; dsRNA: double-stranded RNA; ssRNA: single-stranded RNA)

1. **NF-κB:** It stimulates the synthesis and secretion of cytokines and the expression of adhesion molecules. Both of them are necessary for the recruitment and activation of leukocytes.
2. **Interferon regulatory factors (IRFs):** They stimulate the production of the antiviral cytokines, type I IFN.

Inherited loss-of-function mutations can involve TLRs and their signaling pathways. Though they are rare, they produce serious immunodeficiency syndromes (refer page 1120).

NOD-like receptors and the inflammasome Nucleotide-binding oligomerization domain (NOD)-like receptors (NLRs) are cytosolic receptors.

Molecules recognized: NOD-like receptors recognize a wide variety of substances. These include products released from necrotic or damaged cells [e.g., uric acid and adenosine triphosphate (ATP)], loss of intracellular K^+ ions, and some microbial products.

Mode of action: Several of the NLRs signal through a cytosolic multiprotein complex called the inflammasome (for details refer pages 224–226). Inflammasome activates an enzyme (caspase-1) that cleaves a precursor form of the cytokine interleukin-1 (IL-1) and produce the biologically active form (Fig. 5 of Chapter 8). IL-1 is a mediator of inflammation and recruits leukocytes and produces fever.

Consequences of mutations in NLRs: Gain-of-function mutations may occur in NLRs and related proteins, and loss-of-function mutations can occur in regulators of the inflammasome. These mutations cause a periodic fever syndrome called **autoinflammatory syndromes**. This syndrome should be distinguished from autoimmune diseases that develop due to T and B lymphocyte reactions against self-antigens. The autoinflammatory syndromes respond very well to treatment with IL-1 antagonists.

Other functions of NLRs: Inflammasome pathway may also be involved in many common disorders. Examples are as follows:

- **Detection of urate crystal:** In gout, urate crystals are recognized by a class of NLRs and are responsible for the inflammation associated with gout.
- **Detection of lipids and cholesterol crystals:** NLRs can also detect lipids and cholesterol crystals deposited in abnormally large amounts in tissues. The resulting inflammation may contribute to obesity-associated type 2 diabetes mellitus and atherosclerosis, respectively.

Other cellular receptors for microbial products

C-type lectin receptors (CLRs) They are expressed on the plasma membrane of macrophages and DCs. They detect fungal glycans and elicit inflammatory reactions to fungi.

RIG-like receptors (RLRs): They are named so after the founding member RIG-I (retinoic acid-inducible gene-I). They are present in the cytosol of most cell types. These receptors detect nucleic acids of viruses that replicate in the cytoplasm of infected cells. RLRs stimulate the production of antiviral cytokines.

Cytosolic receptors for microbial DNA: The receptors activate a pathway called STING (for stimulator of *IFN* genes). This leads to the generation of the antiviral cytokine IFN-α. If STING pathways are excessively activated, they cause systemic inflammatory disorders collectively called interferonopathies.

Plasma membrane G protein-coupled receptors: These receptors are present on neutrophils, macrophages, and most other types of leukocytes. They recognize short bacterial peptides containing N-formylmethionyl residues. All bacterial proteins and few mammalian proteins (only those synthesized within mitochondria) are initiated by N-formylmethionine. Hence, RLR enables neutrophils to detect bacterial proteins and move toward their source (chemotaxis).

Mannose receptors: They recognize microbial sugars (containing terminal mannose residues, unlike mammalian glycoproteins) and induce phagocytosis of the microbes.

Natural Killer Cells

Q. Write short essay on NK cell.

Natural killer cells are first known **ILCs** (refer page 1043). They are cytotoxic cells and play important roles in innate immune responses, mainly against viruses and intracellular bacteria.

Term NK: The term killer was given because their major function is killing infected cells, similar to the killer cells of adaptive immune system namely, the cytotoxic T lymphocytes (CTLs). The term natural was given because, once they develop, they are ready to kill infected cell, without further differentiation. Hence its designation "natural killer." NK cells also secrete IFN-γ and are sometimes called as type of ILC1.

Localization of NK cells: NK cells circulate in the blood and comprise about 5–15% of peripheral blood mononuclear cells. They are also present in various lymphoid tissues. In contrast, the cytokine-producing ILCs are found in peripheral tissues and are rare in the blood and lymphoid organs.

Appearance of NK cells: In the peripheral blood, NK cells appear as large lymphocytes with numerous cytoplasmic granules.

Markers: NK cells do not express diverse, clonally distributed antigen receptors expressed by B or T cells. NK cells can be identified in the blood by expression of **CD56** and there is absence of the T-cell marker CD3. Most blood NK cells also express **CD16**. CD16 is a receptor for IgG Fc tails. It is responsible for antibody-dependent cellular cytotoxicity (ADCC) by NK cells.

Functions of NK cells

Natural killer cells have cytotoxic effector functions similar to CD8+ CTLs. NK cells recognize and **destroy severely stressed or abnormal cells**. The cells destroyed by NK cells include virus-infected (intracellular pathogen) cells and tumor cells (antitumor activity). NK cells produce IFN-γ, which **activates macrophages to destroy phagocytosed microbes**.

Mechanism of NK cell-mediated cytotoxicity Mechanism of killing by NK cells is **similar to that of CD8+ CTLs**. Like CTLs, **NK cells have granules containing proteins** that mediate killing of target cells. When NK cells are activated, exocytosis of granule releases these proteins adjacent to the target cells. One NK cell granule protein is called **perforin**. It facilitates the entry of other granule proteins, called **granzymes**, into the cytosol of target cells. The granzymes are proteolytic enzymes.

They initiate a sequence of signaling events that lead to death of the target cells by apoptosis. Since NK cells kill cells infected by viruses and intracellular bacteria, they remove reservoirs of infection. Killing by NK cells is achieved without prior exposure to or activation by the microbes or tumors. Because of this ability, NK cells act as an early line of defense against viral infections and few tumors.

Activating and inhibitory receptors of NK cells: NK cells distinguish infected and stressed cells from healthy cells. NK cells have a variety of surface receptors and these can be mainly categorized into—(1) activating and (2) inhibitory receptors. Thus, **killing of target cells** by NK cells **is regulated by a balance between signals that are generated from activating and inhibitory receptors**. These receptors on NK cells recognize molecules on the surface of other (target) cells and generate activating or inhibitory signals that promote or inhibit NK responses. The activating receptors stimulate protein kinases that phosphorylate downstream signaling substrates, whereas inhibitory receptors stimulate phosphatases that counteract the kinases.

Ligands for receptors: These are as follows—

- **Ligands for activating receptors:** These include ligands (surface molecules) on infected (microbes), injured (undergone stress, DNA damage) or neoplastic cells.
- **Ligands for inhibitory receptors:** These include ligands [self-class I major histocompatibility complex (MHC) molecules] which are expressed on all healthy normal cells.

Consequences: The function of NK cells is regulated by a balance between signals from these activating and inhibitory receptors. Its consequences depend on the receptors involved.

- **Inhibitory receptors (Fig. 2A):** Engagement of inhibitory receptors block activity of NK cell and prevents killing. MHC class I molecules are normally expressed on healthy/ normal nucleated host cells. NK cell inhibitory receptors recognize self-class I MHC molecules, which are expressed on all normal healthy host cells (MHC class I positive). They prevent NK cells from killing normal host cells by inhibiting the death pathway.
- **Activating receptors (Fig. 2B):** Engagement of activating receptors by ligands on target cell stimulates the killing activity of the NK cells. This leads to destruction of stressed or infected cells. Virus infection or neoplastic transformation usually increases the expression of ligands for activating receptors and at the same time reduces the expression of class I MHC molecules. Thus, when activating receptors of NK cells are engaged by these abnormal cells, the balance is tilted toward activation, and the infected or tumor cell is killed.

***Killing of microbes through activation of macrophages* (Fig. 2C)** NK cells also secrete cytokines such as interferon-γ (IFN-γ). NK cell-derived IFN-γ activates macrophages and increases the capacity of macrophages to kill phagocytosed (ingested) microbes. Thus, NK cells provide an early defense against intracellular microbial infections. The activity of NK cells is regulated by many cytokines. These include the interleukins IL-2, IL-15, and IL-12. IL-2 and IL-15 stimulate proliferation of NK cells, whereas IL-12 activates the killing of target cells and the secretion of IFN-γ.

Antibody-dependent cellular cytotoxicity NK cells bear (CD16) immunoglobulin receptors (FcR) and recognize antibody-coated (IgG-coated) target cells (refer page 1077 and Fig. 31 of Chapter 15). They bind antibody-coated targets leading to lysis of these target cells. This phenomenon is called as antibody-dependent cell-mediated cytotoxicity (type IV).

Functions and Reactions of Innate Immunity

Innate immunity protects the individual against microbes and tissue injury.

Functions of innate immunity: General features of functions of innate immune responses are as follows:

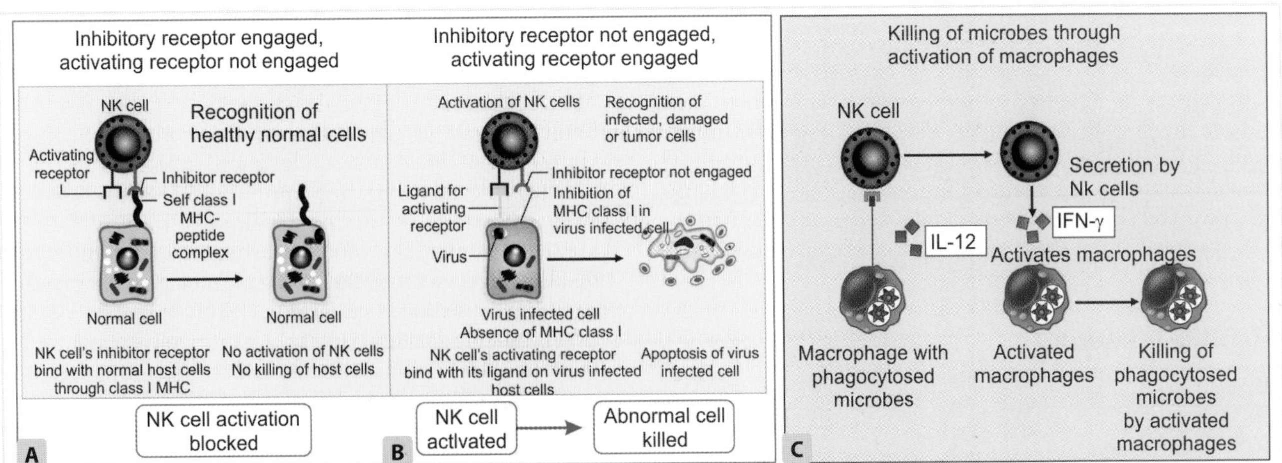

FIGS. 2A TO C: Mechanism of function of natural killer (NK) cells. (A and B) Functions of activating and inhibitory receptors of NK cells. Receptors of NK cells recognize ligands on target cells. (A) Normal cells express self-class I major histocompatibility complex (MHC) molecules. These molecules are recognized by inhibitory receptors of NK cells that bind them and prevent from killing normal cells. However, it is to be noted that healthy cells may express ligands for activating receptors (not shown in figure) or may not express such ligands (as shown in figure). They do not activate NK cells because they engage the inhibitory receptors. (B) In infected and stressed cells, class I MHC expression is reduced so that the inhibitory receptors of NK cells are not engaged. There is expression of ligands for activating receptors. This results in activation of NK cells and killing of infected cells/stressed cells and cytokine secretion. (C) NK cells respond to interleukin-12 (IL-12) produced by macrophages and secrete interferon-γ (IFN-γ). This activates the macrophages to kill phagocytosed microbes.

- **Block the entry of microbia:** The innate immune system blocks the entry of microbia by maintaining physical and chemical defenses at epithelial barriers such as the skin and lining of the gastrointestinal and respiratory tracts. If these barriers are damaged or microbes can cross epithelia, then only microbes can colonize tissues.
- **Prevent, control, or eliminate microbial infection:** This can be achieved by the initial innate immune responses.
- **Elimination of damaged cells and initiation of the process of tissue repair.**
- **Stimulation of adaptive immune responses and make them optimally effective against different types of microbes.** Innate immunity produces the danger signals that stimulate the subsequent more powerful adaptive immune response.

Protective reactions: There are two main types of protective host defense reactions of the innate immune system. These are—(1) inflammation and (2) antiviral defense.

- **Inflammation:** Cytokines, products of complement activation, and other mediators are produced during innate immune reactions. They trigger the vascular and cellular components of inflammation. Inflammation is the process by which circulating leukocytes and plasma proteins are brought into sites of infection in the tissues. They destroy and eliminate the offending agents. Inflammation also occurs as the main reaction to damaged or dead cells and to accumulation of abnormal substances in cells and tissues. The recruited leukocytes in inflammation destroy microbes and ingest and eliminate damaged cells. Also, innate immune response triggers the repair of damaged tissues. Various aspects of inflammation are discussed in detail in Chapter 8.
- **Antiviral defense:** Antiviral defense mechanisms prevent virus replication and promote killing of infected cells. Type I IFNs are produced in response to viral infections. They act on infected and uninfected cells. Type I IFNs activate enzymes that degrade viral nucleic acids and block viral replication. This produces antiviral state. NK cells recognize virus-infected cells and destroy them and thus eliminating reservoirs of viral infection without an inflammatory reaction.

In contrast to adaptive immunity, innate immunity does not have memory or fine antigen specificity. Probably innate immunity uses about 100 different receptors to recognize 1,000 molecular patterns. In adaptive immunity, there are mainly two types of receptors [antibodies and T-cell receptors (TCRs)], and each have millions of variations, to recognize millions of antigens.

Adaptive Immunity

If the innate immune system fails to provide effective protection against invading microbes, the adaptive immune system is activated.

Lymphocytes and their products: The adaptive immune response is mediated by cells called lymphocytes and their products (including antibodies). Lymphocytes of adaptive immunity express highly diverse receptors. These receptors can recognize a vast number of antigens (foreign substances).

Types of lymphocytes: There are **two major types of lymphocytes namely, B lymphocytes and T lymphocytes**. They mediate different types of adaptive immune responses. Both types of lymphocytes express highly specific receptors for a wide variety of substances, which are called antigens.

Types of adaptive immunity: There are two types of adaptive immunity namely (i) humoral and (ii) cell-mediated immunity.

1. **Humoral immunity:** It is mediated by B (bone marrow-derived) lymphocytes and their secreted products, antibodies (also called immunoglobulins, Ig). Antibody is capable of reacting with the specific antigens responsible for its production. It protects against extracellular microbes and their toxins. Antibodies recognize microbial antigens, neutralize the infectivity of the microbes, and these microbes are targeted for elimination by phagocytes and the complement system. Humoral immunity is the main defense mechanism against microbes and their toxins located outside cells (e.g., in the lumens of the gastrointestinal and respiratory tracts and in the blood). This is achieved by attachment of secreted antibodies to the microbes and toxins, and their neutralization and assisting their elimination. The term affinity means binding strength at a single antibody variable region and antigen epitope (part of an antigen molecule to which an antibody attaches) and avidity means, the overall strength of an interaction between an antibody and antigen. Terminologies used in antibodies are:
   i. **Isotype:** Antibodies that differ by constant regions (i.e., IgG, IgA, IgM, IgE, IgD).
   ii. **Idiotype:** Antibodies that differ by hypervariable region. Hypervariable region is the region with three sequences of amino acids with profound variability. They are located within the variable regions of both heavy and light chains. They are responsible for the specificity of antibodies.
   iii. **Allotype:** Antibodies that differ among individuals due to polymorphisms (more than two alleles) in heavy and light chains.
2. **Cell-mediated (or cellular) immunity:** It is localized reaction to organism, usually intracellular pathogens. It is mediated by T (thymus-derived) lymphocytes, macrophages, and their soluble products called cytokines. Many microbes are ingested and survive within phagocytes. Some microbes, such as viruses, infect and replicate in various host cells. In these locations, the microbes are inaccessible to circulating antibodies. Defense against such infections is by cell-mediated immunity. Cell-mediated immunity promotes the destruction of microbes inside phagocytes and the killing of infected cells thereby eliminates reservoirs of infection. Cell-mediated immunity is responsible for defense against intracellular microbes (causes lysis of virus infected cells), immunity against cancers, and rejection of allograft. Active versus passive immunity (**Fig. 3**)—protective immunity against a microbe may be provided by two means. One is by the host's response to the microbe and another is by the transfer of antibodies that defend against the microbe.
   i. **Active immunity (Fig. 3A):** This is induced by exposure to a foreign antigen. It is called active immunity because the immunized individual plays an active role in responding to the antigen. Individuals and lymphocytes that have not come across a particular antigen are said to be naïve. This means that

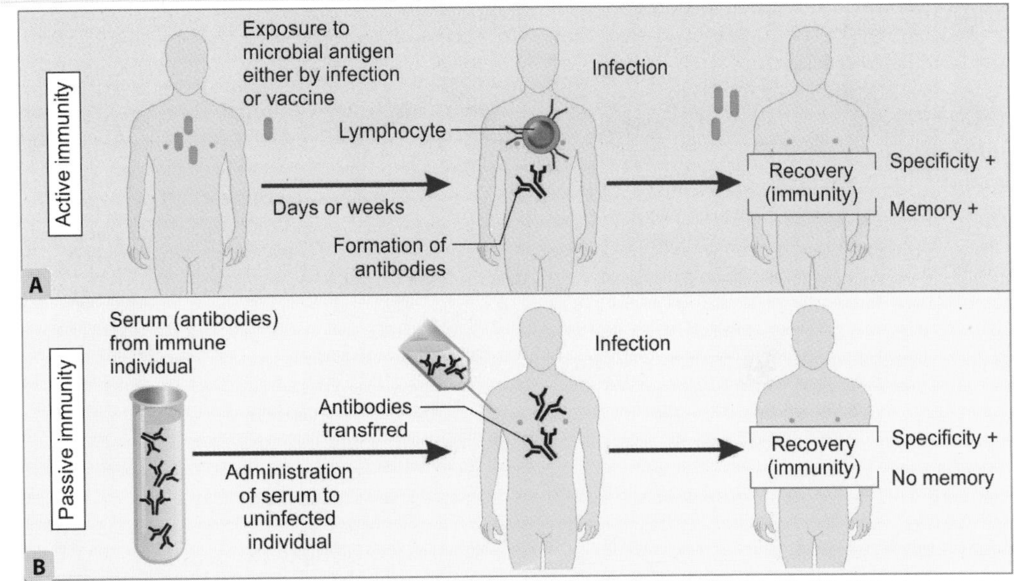

FIGS. 3A AND B: Active and passive immunity. Active immunity develops when a normal individual is exposed to a microbe or microbial antigen (e.g., vaccine). Passive immunity is achieved by transfer of antibodies or T lymphocytes specific for the microbe from an immune individual to an uninfected individual. Both forms of immunity provide resistance to infection and are specific for microbial antigens. However, only active immune responses have immunologic memory. Routinely therapeutic passive transfer of antibodies is performed and not lymphocytes. Physiologically passive immunity occurs during pregnancy from mother to fetus.

they are immunologically inexperienced. Individuals who have been exposed and responded to a microbial antigen are protected from subsequent exposures to that microbe. They are said to be immune. It has both specificity and memory.

ii. **Passive immunity (Fig. 3B):** An individual who has been exposed to an antigen develops antibodies and individual is said to be immunized. Immunity can be conferred on an individual who has not encountered the antigen by transferring antibodies from these immunized individuals. The recipient of such a transfer becomes immune to the particular antigen even though he had no exposure to that antigen. Hence, this form of immunity is called passive immunity. Example for physiologically important passive immunity is the transfer of maternal antibodies through the placenta to the fetus. This passive immunity protects the newborns against infections for several months before they develop the ability to produce antibodies themselves. Passive immunization is also a useful method for conferring resistance rapidly, without having to wait for an active immune response to develop. It has specificity but no memory.

Cardinal Features of Adaptive Immunity

- Second line of defense acquired during life.
- Capable of recognizing both microbial and nonmicrobial substances.
- Takes more time to develop and is more powerful than innate immunity.
- Longlasting protection.
- Prior exposure to antigen is present.
- Three characteristic features are—(1) specificity, (2) diversity, and (3) memory.

Cells of the Adaptive Immune System

T and B lymphocytes and their subsets morphologically appear almost similar to one another. However, they are heterogeneous and specialized in molecular properties and functions. **Figure 4** illustrates major classes of lymphocytes and their functions in adaptive immunity.

Circulation of lymphocytes: In most of the organs, the body cells are fixed to the site. But lymphocytes and other cells involved in immune responses are not fixed in particular tissues. Lymphocytes continuously circulate, moving through the blood, lymphatic vessels, secondary lymphoid organs, and nonlymphoid tissues. This characteristic helps in immune surveillance throughout the body and allows lymphocytes to reach to any site of infection. In lymphoid organs, different classes of lymphocytes are anatomically segregated. But, when they encounter antigens and other stimuli, they can interact with one another.

- **Naïve lymphocytes:** These are mature lymphocytes that have not encountered the antigen for which they are specific. These naïve lymphocytes are immunologically inexperienced.
- **Effector cells:** When naïve lymphocytes encounter and recognize antigens and other signals, they become activated and these lymphocytes differentiate into effector cells. These effector cells perform the function of eliminating microbes.
- **Memory cells:** These lymphocytes live in a state of heightened awareness. In case, microbes infect again, memory cells are able to react rapidly and strongly to combat the microbe.

Lymphocyte specificity and diversity

Specificity (Fig. 5)

Clonal selection: Immune responses are specific for distinct antigens and usually for different portions of a single complex

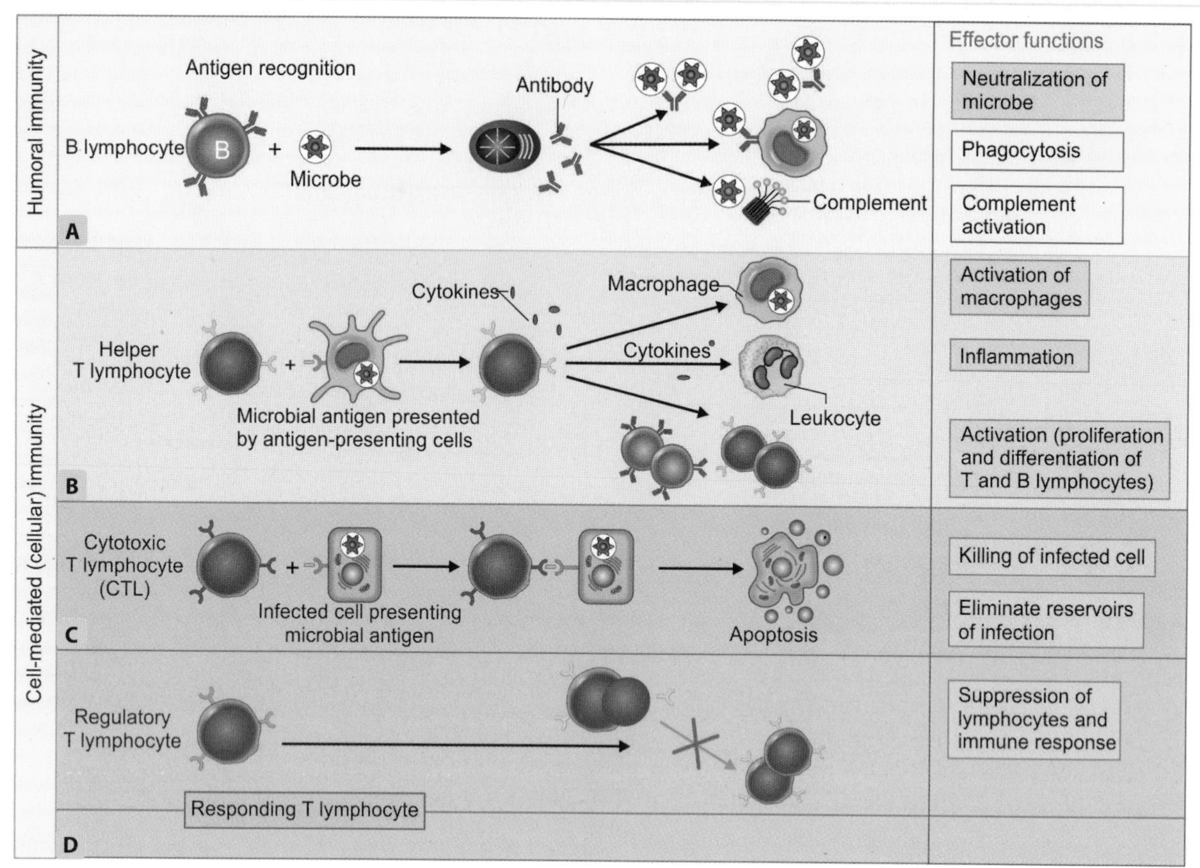

FIGS. 4A TO D: Main classes of lymphocytes and their functions. B and T lymphocytes are the cells of adaptive immunity. (A) B lymphocytes recognize many different types of antigens and develop into antibody-secreting cells. These plasma cells produce antibodies that can neutralize microbe, aid phagocytosis, and activate complement system. (B) Helper T lymphocytes recognize antigens on the surfaces of antigen-presenting cells (APCs) and secrete cytokines. These cytokines stimulate different mechanisms of immunity. They activate macrophages, stimulate inflammation, and activate (proliferation and differentiation) of T and B lymphocytes. (C) Cytotoxic T lymphocytes recognize antigens on infected cells and kill these cells by apoptosis. (D) Regulatory T cells suppress immune responses (e.g., to self-antigens).

protein, polysaccharide, or other macromolecule (**Fig. 5**). The **parts of complex antigens that are specifically recognized by lymphocytes** are termed as determinants or **epitopes**. This fine specificity is because individual lymphocytes express membrane receptors that can distinguish minute differences in structure between distinct epitopes. Clones of lymphocytes with different specificities for a large number of antigens are present in unimmunized individuals (before exposure to antigen). These clones are able to recognize and respond to foreign antigens (**Fig. 6**). When an antigen appears, these clones selectively activate the antigen-specific cells. This fundamental concept is called clonal selection. Lymphocytes of the same specificity are said to constitute a clone. All members of one clone express identical antigen receptors, which are different from the receptors in all other clones.

Clonal expansion: As already mentioned above, antigen-specific clones of lymphocytes develop before and independent of exposure to antigen. An introduced antigen binds to (selects) the lymphocyte of the pre-existing antigen-specific clone and activates these lymphocytes of particular clone. This results in proliferation of lymphocytes specific for the antigen and produces thousands of progeny of lymphocytes with the same specificity. This process is called clonal expansion.

Diversity

Lymphocyte repertoire: It is the total number of antigenic specificities of the lymphocytes in an individual. Lymphocyte repertoire is extremely large. In a healthy adult, there are about 10^{12} lymphocytes, and there are 10^7–10^9 clones with distinct antigenic determinants (each express receptor specific for a different antigen). This **ability of the lymphocyte repertoire to recognize a very large number of antigens is called diversity**.

There are many different clones of lymphocytes. Each clone of lymphocytes has a unique antigen receptor and therefore, a singular antigen specificity. The immune system is capable of producing so many receptors. This is responsible for a total repertoire that is extremely diverse. Thus, diversity is due to the variability in the structures of the antigen-binding sites of lymphocyte receptors for antigens. For the immune system to defend individuals against the many potential pathogens in the environment, diversity is essential.

Mechanism of antigen receptor diversity: Antigen receptor diversity is produced by somatic recombination of the genes that encode antigen receptors. All cells, including lymphocyte progenitors, contain antigen receptor genes in the germline (inherited) configuration. These genes encoding these receptors consist of spatially separated segments. These genes cannot be expressed as mRNAs.

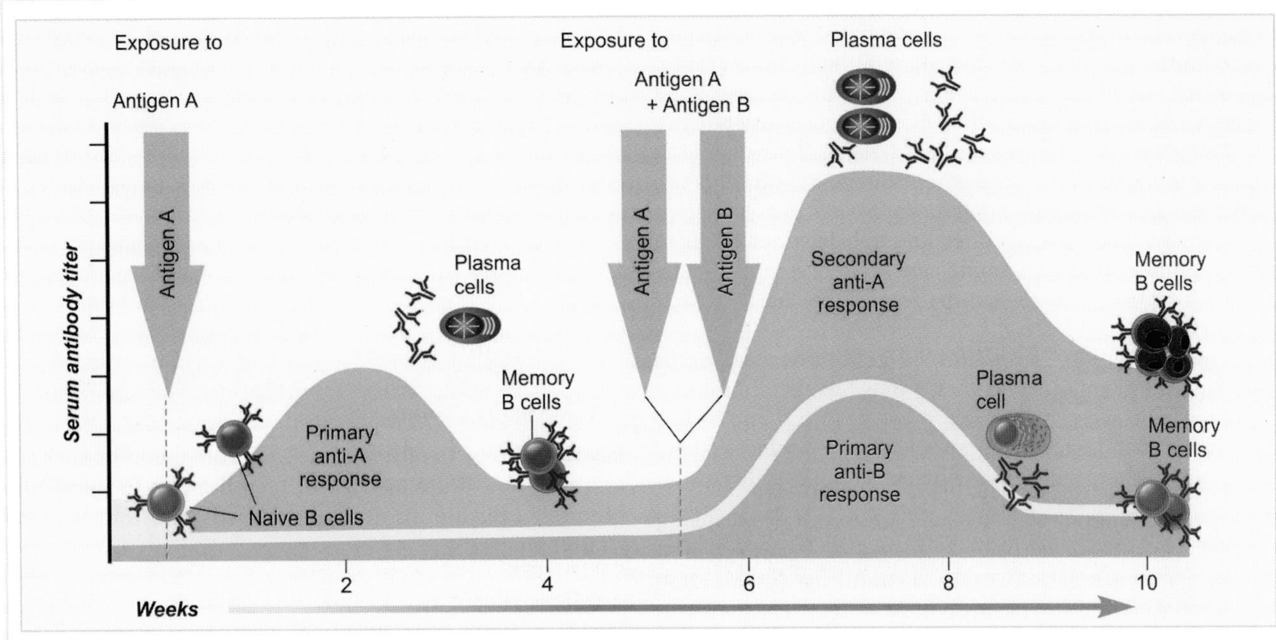

FIG. 5: Specificity, memory, and contraction of adaptive immune responses. In humoral immune response, antigens A and B induce the production of different antibodies (specificity). The secondary response to antigen A is more rapid and larger than the primary response (memory). Antibody levels decline with time after each immunization (contraction, this maintains homeostasis). The same features are also observed in T cell-mediated immune responses.

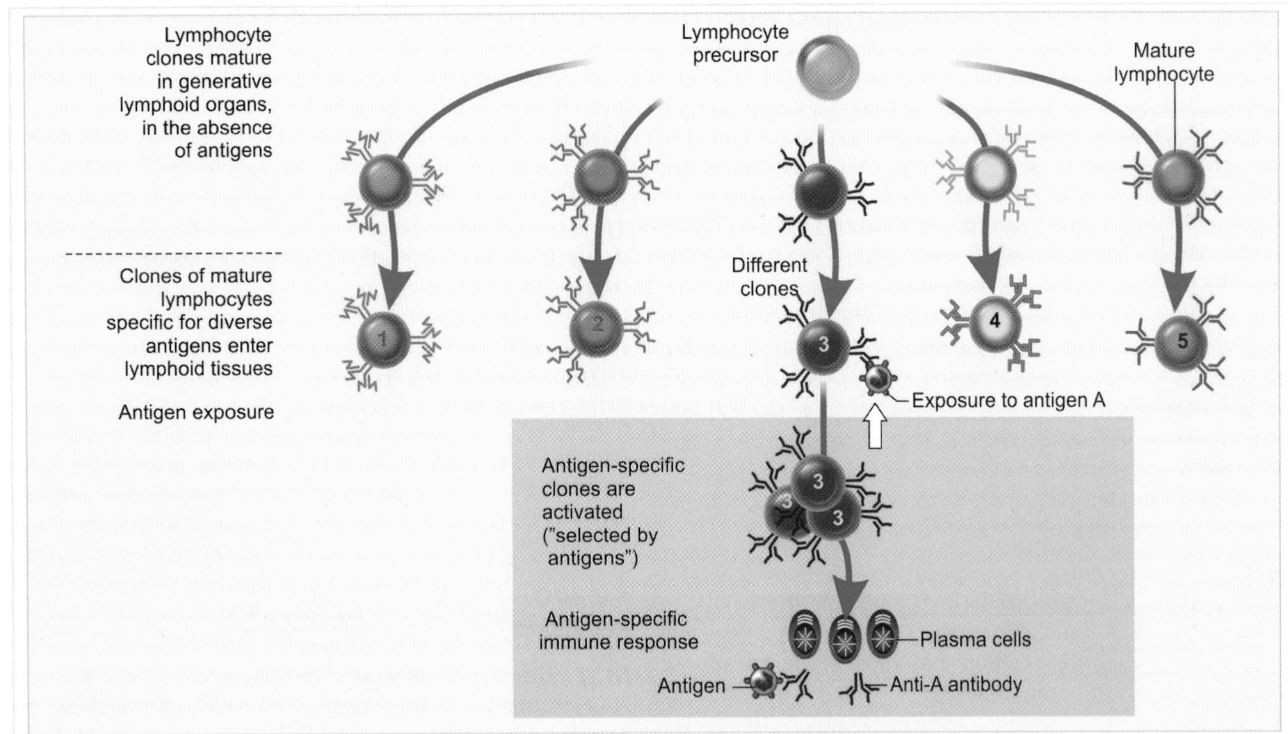

FIG. 6: Clonal selection. Each antigen (A) selects a pre-existing clone of specific lymphocytes. The antigenic exposures stimulate the proliferation and differentiation of that particular clone. In the figure, five pre-existing clones of specific lymphocytes (1 to 5) are shown and only clone 3 B lymphocytes exposed to particular antigen (A) gives rise to antibody-secreting effector cells. The same principle applies to T lymphocytes.

- **Recombination:** Recombination is a process in which pieces of DNA are broken and recombined to produce new combinations of alleles. During lymphocyte maturation (in the thymus for T cells and the bone marrow for B cells), the gene segments that encode antigen receptor are assembled by recombination, and DNA sequence variation is introduced at the sites where the gene segments are joined. This recombination process creates many different genes that can be transcribed and translated into antigen receptors with diverse amino acid sequences. This mainly involves gene in the regions of the receptors that recognize and bind antigen.
- **Products of *RAG-1 and RAG-2* gene:** The enzyme in developing lymphocytes that brings out recombination of the gene segments is the product of RAG-1 and RAG-2 (recombination-activating genes). Inherited defects in RAG proteins lead to failure to produce mature lymphocytes.

Detection of recombined genes by molecular analysis: All cells in the body contain germline antigen receptor genes. But **only T and B cells contain recombined (also called rearranged) antigen receptor genes, i.e.,** *TCR* genes in T cells and *Ig* genes in B cells. Molecular analysis is a marker of T- or B-lineage cells. Hence, the presence of recombined *TCR* or *Ig* genes can be demonstrated by molecular analysis. Each T or B cell and its clonal progeny have a unique DNA rearrangement and hence they have a unique antigen receptor. Lymphocyte proliferations can be polyclonal (nonneoplastic) or monoclonal (neoplastic in lymphoid tumor). It is possible to distinguish polyclonal lymphocyte proliferations from monoclonal lymphoid tumors by assessing the diversity of antigen receptor rearrangements within a population of lymphocytes. Thus, assays that **determine the clonality of antigen receptor gene rearrangements are useful in diagnosing lymphoid neoplasms.**

Memory

Primary or first immune response: When an a foreign antigen is exposed for the first time, the immune response is called primary response. This is due to naïve lymphocytes specific for the antigen present at the time of initial antigen exposure.

Secondary immune response: When the immune system is again exposed to the same antigen, it increases its ability to respond to that antigen. These responses to second and subsequent exposures to the same antigen are called secondary immune responses. These responses are usually more rapid, of greater magnitude, and usually qualitatively different from the first, or primary, immune response to that antigen (**Fig. 5**).

Immunologic memory: Each exposure to an antigen generates long-lived memory cells specific for the antigen. These cells are responsible for immunologic memory. It occurs because of two reasons for the stronger response in the secondary response than the primary immune response:

- Memory cells accumulate and become more numerous during secondary immune response than naïve lymphocytes during primary immune response.
- Memory cells react more rapidly and vigorously to antigen challenge than do naïve lymphocytes.

Memory permits the immune system to escalate heightened responses to persistent or recurring exposure to the same antigen. This helps to fight against infections by microbes that are encountered repeatedly.

T lymphocytes

T lymphocytes consist of three major population (**Figs. 4B** to **D**) having distinct functions. These are—(1) helper T lymphocytes, (2) cytotoxic (killer) T lymphocytes, and (3) regulatory T lymphocytes.

1. **Helper T lymphocytes:** They stimulate B lymphocytes to produce antibodies and activate other leukocytes (e.g., phagocytes) to destroy microbes.
2. **Cytotoxic (killer) T lymphocytes:** They kill infected cells.
3. **Regulatory T lymphocytes:** They limit or regulate immune responses and prevent reactions against self-antigens.

Development: T lymphocytes are derived from precursors that arise from hematopoietic stem cells (HSCs). These T cells **develop in the thymus**.

Distribution of T cells: Mature T cells are found in the blood and they constitute **60–70% of lymphocytes in peripheral blood**. T cells are also found in T-cell zones of secondary lymphoid organs.

T-cell receptor

Q. Write short essay on TCR.

Each T-cell recognizes a specific cell-bound antigen by means of an antigen-specific TCR.

The αβ TCR: In about 95% of T cells, the TCR is composed of a disulfide-linked heterodimer made up of an **α and a β polypeptide chain** (**Fig. 7**). Each polypeptide chain has a variable (antigen binding) region and a constant region. The αβ TCR recognizes peptide antigens that are bound to and presented by MHC molecules on the surfaces of APCs. Thus, this TCR limits the specificity of T cells for peptides displayed by cell surface MHC molecules. It is called MHC restriction. The immune system ensures that T cells see only cell-associated antigens (e.g., those derived from microbes in cells or from proteins ingested by cells).

TCR complex (Fig. 7): Each TCR is noncovalently linked to CD3 complex (composed of polypeptide chains) and the ζ chain dimer (**Fig. 7**). Both CD3 complex and ζ chain proteins are invariant (i.e., identical) in all T cells. When antigen binds to the TCR, these are involved in the transduction of signals into the T cell. Together with the TCR, these proteins form the TCR complex.

The γδ TCR: A small subset of mature T cells expresses another type of TCR composed of γ and δ polypeptide chains. The γδ TCR recognizes peptides, lipids, and small molecules. They do not require display by MHC proteins. γδ T cells form aggregates at epithelial surfaces, such as the skin and mucosa of the gastrointestinal and urogenital tracts. These cells are sentinels that protect against microbes that try to enter through epithelia. Exact functions of γδ T cells are not known.

NK-T cells: Few T cells express markers that are also found on NK cells. These T cells are called NK-T cells. NK-T cells express a very limited diversity of TCRs. They recognize glycolipids that are displayed by the MHC-like molecule CD1. The functions of NK-T cells are also not known.

Other proteins expressed by T cells: Apart from CD3 and ζ proteins, T cells also express many other proteins that help in the functioning of the TCR complex. These include CD4, CD8, CD28, and integrins. CD4 and CD8 are expressed on two mutually exclusive subsets of αβ T cells.

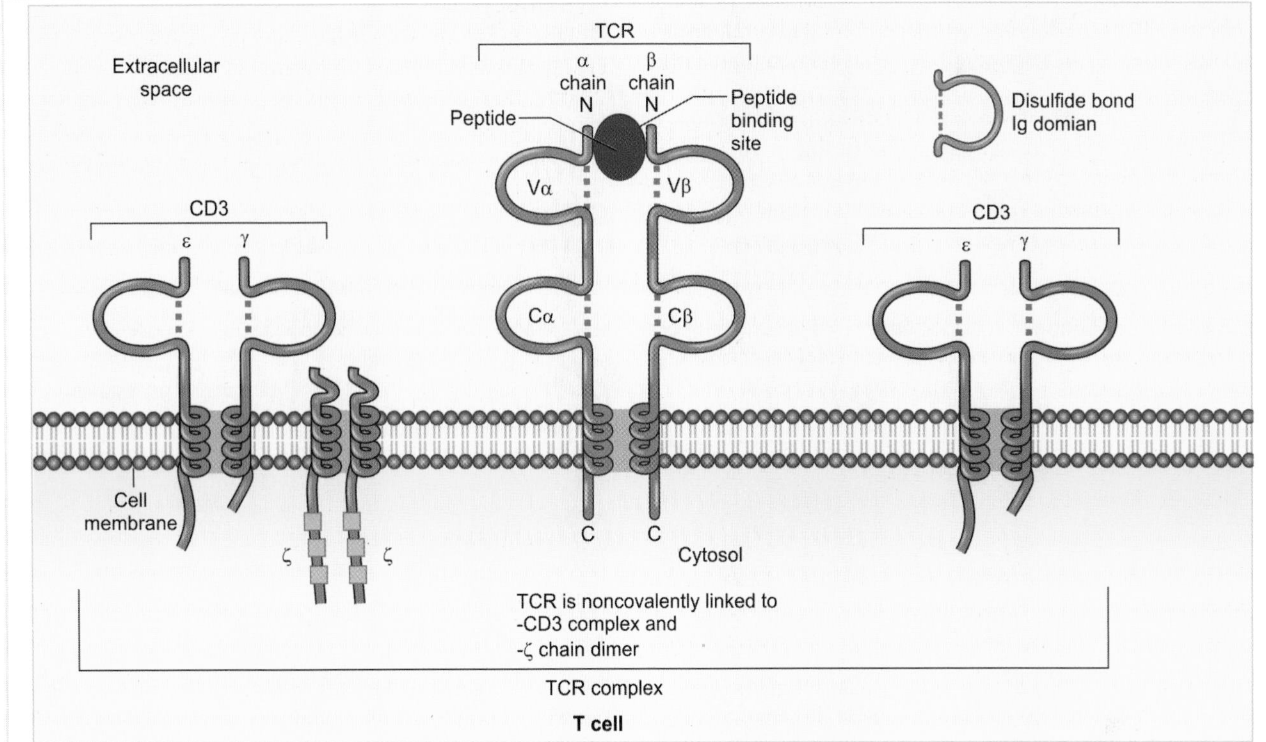

(C: constant region; Ig: immunoglobulin; MHC: major histocompatibility complex; V: variable region)

FIG. 7: Components of the T-cell receptor (TCR) complex (not to scale) in about 95% of T cells. The TCR complex of MHC-restricted T cells consists of the αβ TCR noncovalently linked to the CD3 complex and ζ proteins. In the center is αβ TCR. This is a heterodimer, consisting of an α and a β chain, showing the domains of a typical TCR specific for a peptide-MHC complex. The antigen-binding portion of the TCR is formed by the Vα and Vβ domains. Some T cells express CD8 and not CD4; these molecules serve analogous roles.

CD4+ and CD8+ T cells: Normally, about 60% of mature T cells are CD4+, and 30% are CD8+. Most CD4+ T cells function as cytokine-secreting helper cells. They assist macrophages and B lymphocytes to fight against infections. Most CD8+ cells function as CTLs and kill host cells containing microbes. **Both CD4 and CD8 function as coreceptors in T-cell activation**.

T-cell activation (Fig. 8): During antigen recognition by T cells, CD4 molecules attach to class II MHC molecules that are displaying antigen whereas CD8 molecules attach to class I MHC molecules. CD4 or CD8 coreceptor initiates signals that are required for activation of the T cells. For T-cell activation, these coreceptors are required. Coreceptors, **CD4+ helper T cells can recognize and respond to antigen in association with class II MHC molecules,** whereas **CD8+ cytotoxic T cells recognize cell bound antigens only in association with class I MHC molecules**. This is called MHC restriction. Integrins are adhesion molecules which assist in the attachment of T cells to APCs.

T cells recognize antigen–MHC complexes and also receive additional signals provided by APCs. CD28 plays an important role in this process.

Superantigens

Q. Write short essay on superantigens.

Conventional antigens: T cells can recognize antigen bound to MHC molecules. Conventional (typical) microbial T-cell antigens are processed by APCs and are composed of a peptide bound to the peptide-binding groove (cleft) of an MHC molecule on the APCs. In any individual, these conventional antigens are recognized by a very small fraction of T cells. Conventional antigens bound to class II MHC interact with TCRs of small fraction of T cells and only these T cells are activated (stimulated) to become effector T cells. These effector cells protect the individual against the microbe.

Superantigens: These are antigens (proteins) that bind and activate (stimulates) all of the T cells in an individual that express a particular set (type) or family of TCR Vβ chain. Because they activate many more clones of T cells than do conventional peptide antigens, they are termed as superantigens. Superantigens are special class of T-cell activators and another kind of polyclonal stimulus.

Binding of superantigens to T cells (Fig. 9): Superantigens, like the typical (conventional) antigens, bind to class II MHC molecules of APCs. Superantigens bind to nonpolymorphic regions of class II MHC molecules on APCs and not to the peptide-binding grooves/clefts (conventional antigens bind only to the peptide-binding clefts). Many T cells express a TCR β chain from a particular Vβ family. Superantigens bind to class II MHC molecules outside the peptide-binding groove of APCs and simultaneously interact with the conserved variable (V) region of many different TCR β chains (of TCRs), regardless of the peptide specificity of the TCR. Thus, superantigens bind to T cells in an antigen-nonspecific manner.

Consequences: Superantigens can activate a large number of T cells (activate many more clones of T cells than do

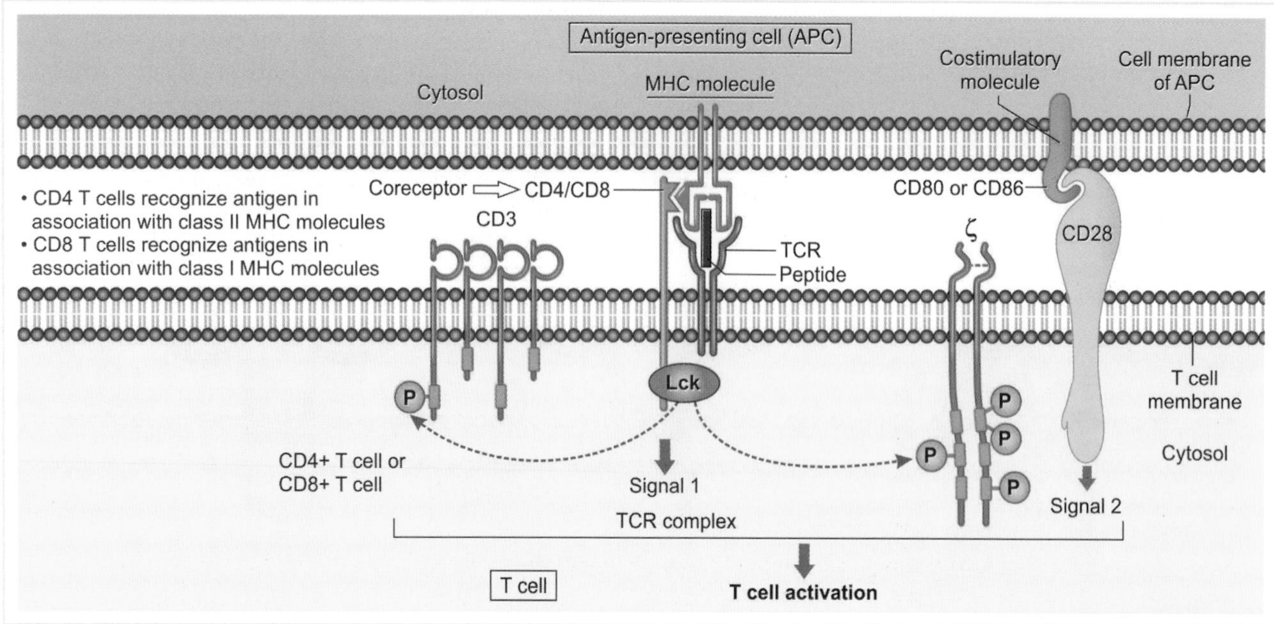

(MHC: major histocompatibility complex)

FIG. 8: T-cell activation (not to scale). When an antigen is presented by antigen presenting cells (APCs), it is recognized by T-cell receptor (TCR) complex. During this recognition, there is clustering of TCR complexes with coreceptors (CD4 in this figure or CD8). CD4 and CD28 are also involved in T-cell activation. CD4-associated Lck (SRC family kinase) becomes active and phosphorylates tyrosines of CD3 and ζ chains. (Note that some T cells express CD8 and not CD4; these molecules serve analogous roles.)

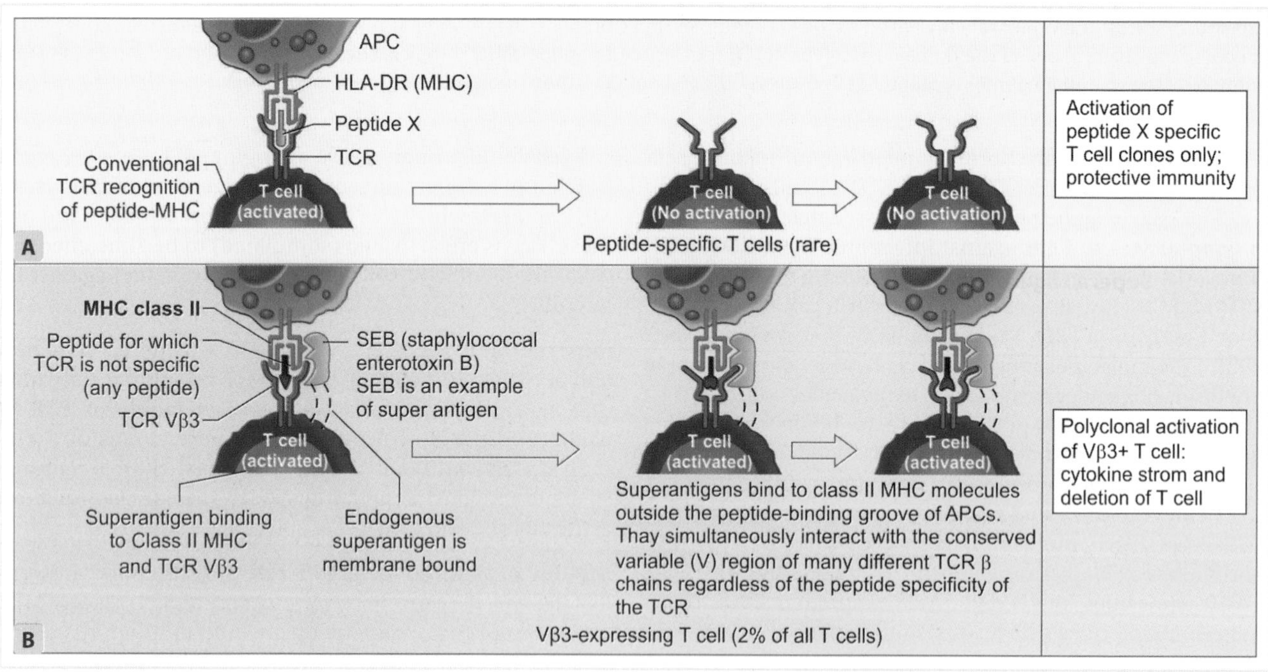

(APC: antigen-presenting cell; HLA: human leukocyte antigen; MHC: major histocompatibility complex; TCR: T-cell receptor)

FIGS. 9A AND B: Superantigen-mediated cross-linkage of T-cell receptor and MHC class II molecules (diagrammatic). (A) Conventional microbial T-cell antigens are composed of a peptide bound to the peptide-binding groove of an MHC molecule. In any individual, conventional T-cell antigens are recognized by a very small fraction of T cells. Only these T cells are activated and form effector T cells that protect against the microbe. (B) In contrast, a superantigen binds to class II MHC molecules outside the peptide-binding groove. A superantigen binds to all TCRs bearing a particular V sequence regardless of their antigen specificity. Superantigens simultaneously bind to the variable region of many different TCR β chains, irrespective of the peptide specificity of the TCR. Different superantigens bind to TCRs of different Vβ families. Many T cells express a TCR β chain from a particular Vβ family. Hence, superantigens can activate a large number of T cells. Exogenous superantigens are soluble secreted bacterial proteins, including various exotoxins. In this example, the superantigen staphylococcal enterotoxin B (SEB) binds to HLA-DR and the V regions of TCRs belonging to the Vβ3 family. Endogenous superantigens are membrane-embedded proteins produced by certain viruses.

conventional peptide antigens). Because superantigens bind outside the TCR antigen-binding cleft/grooves, any T cell expressing that particular V sequence will be activated by a corresponding superantigen. Hence, the activation is polyclonal. Thus, superantigens can cause massive T-cell activation with the subsequent production of large amounts of T-cell cytokines. Overproduction of cytokines can cause systemic toxicity and produce a systemic inflammatory syndrome that is similar to septic shock.

Vβ regions of TCR are encoded by over 65 different genes in humans. Superantigen binding need for costimulation and professional APCs are still required for full T-cell activation by superantigens.

Types of superantigens: It may be endogenous superantigens or exogenous superantigens.

- **Exogenous superantigens:** These are soluble proteins secreted by bacteria. These include a variety of exotoxins secreted by gram-positive bacteria, such as staphylococcal enterotoxins, toxic shock syndrome toxin, and exfoliative dermatitis toxin. Each of these exogenous superantigens binds particular V sequences in TCRs and cross-links the TCR to an MHC class II molecule.
- **Endogenous superantigens:** These are cell-membrane proteins produced by specific viral genes that have integrated into human genomes.

Superantigen-induced cytokine overproduction: Two examples of disorders caused by superantigen-induced cytokine overproduction are—(1) food poisoning induced by staphylococcal enterotoxins and (2) toxic shock induced by toxic shock syndrome toxin. Superantigens in various infections are listed in **Box 1**.

Differences between conventional and superantigens are listed in **Table 2**.

Box 1: Superantigens in various diseases.

Associated with bacterial infection

Pyrogenic bacteria

- Toxic shock syndrome
- Staphylococcal enterotoxin, A, B, C, D, E, F, and H
- Staphylococcal exfoliative toxin
- Streptococcal pyrogenic toxin A, B, C
- Streptococcal scarlet fever toxin

Nonpyrogenic bacteria

- Mycoplasma arthritis mitogen I
- *Yersinia enterocolitica*
- *Y. pseudotuberculosis* superantigen

Associated with viral infection

- Murine mammary tumor virus
- Rabies nucleocapsid protein
- EBV-associated superantigen
- CMV-associated superantigen
- HIV-encoded superantigen

Associated with fungal infection

- *Malassezia furfur*

(CMV: cytomegalovirus; EBV: Epstein–Barr virus; HIV: human immunodeficiency virus)

B lymphocytes

B lymphocytes are the only cells that can produce antibodies. These antibodies are the mediators of humoral immunity. B lymphocytes develop from precursors in the bone marrow.

Distribution of B cells: B cells are distributed as follows—

- Peripheral blood: Mature B cells constitute 10–20% of lymphocytes in the peripheral blood.
- Peripheral lymphoid tissues: B cells are also present in peripheral lymphoid tissues. These include lymph nodes (cortex), spleen (white pulp), and mucosa-associated lymphoid tissues {MALT [pharyngeal tonsils and Peyer's patches of gastrointestinal tract (GIT)]}.

B-cell antigen receptor complex (Fig. 10): B cells recognize antigen through the B-cell antigen receptor complex.

- **Antibodies of the IgM and IgD isotypes:** All mature, naïve B cells have membrane-bound antibodies of the

Table 2: Differences between conventional and superantigens.

Features	*Conventional antigen*	*Superantigen*
Processing of antigen into peptides	Required	Not required
TCR chains involved in recognition of antigen	TCR α and β chains	Only TCR β chains
MHC class involved	Recognition restricted by an MHC class I or II molecule	Bind to almost any MHC class II molecule
Types of protein antigens	Almost all proteins can be conventional antigens	Very few antigens are superantigens

(MHC: major histocompatibility complex; TCR: T-cell receptor)

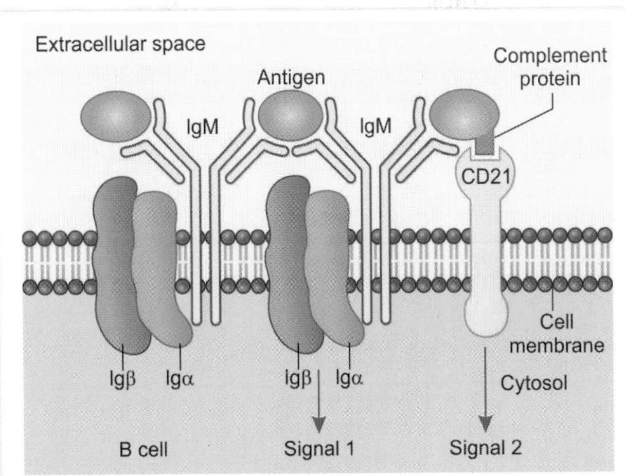

FIG. 10: Structure of antibodies and the B-cell antigen receptor (BCR) complex (not to scale). The BCR complex is composed of membrane immunoglobulin M (IgM; or IgD, not shown) on the surface of mature B cells. They are associated with the invariant Igβ and Igα molecules. BCR recognizes antigens in association with signaling proteins Igα and Igβ. CD21 is a receptor for a complement component that also promotes B-cell activation. Note the similarity of BCR complex to the T-cell receptor (TCR) complex.

IgM and IgD isotypes on their surface. They constitute the antigen-binding component of the B-cell receptor (BCR) complex (**Fig. 10**). After stimulation by antigen and other signals, B cells mature into plasma cells as well as long-lived memory cells. Plasma cells produce antibodies, and a single plasma cell can secrete hundreds to thousands of antibody molecules per second. This indicates the remarkable capacity of the immune response for fighting against pathogens. Salient features of various antibodies are presented in **Table 3**.

- **Igα and Igβ:** Apart from membrane Ig, the B-cell antigen receptor complex contains a heterodimer of two invariant (never changing) proteins namely, Igα and Igβ. Igα (CD79a) and Igβ (CD79b) are essential for signal transduction in response to antigen recognition. Thus, they are similar to the CD3 and ζ proteins of the TCR complex (see **Fig. 7**).
- **Other molecules:** B cells also express many other molecules needed for their responses. These include the type 2 complement receptor (CR2, or CD21) and CD40. CR2 (CD21) recognizes complement products produced during innate immune responses to microbes. CR2 is also used by Epstein–Barr virus (EBV) as a receptor to enter and infect B cells. CD40 receives signals from helper T cells.

Dendritic cells

Dendritic cells are named so because they have numerous fine cytoplasmic processes that resemble dendrites. DCs (sometimes called interdigitating DCs) are the most important APCs for initiating T-cell responses against protein antigens. They have a unique position in the immune system and are involved in both innate and adaptive immunity. They sense the presence of microbes and initiate innate immune defense reactions and capture microbial proteins for display to T cells to initiate adaptive immune responses. Thus, they serve as sentinels of infection that begin the rapid innate response and also link innate responses with the development of adaptive immune responses.

Important features

- **Expression of many receptors:** DCs express many receptors for recognizing, capturing, and responding to microbial molecules (and other antigens). These receptors include TLRs and lectins.
- **Location:** DCs are located at the right places to capture antigens. These places include—(1) **under epithelia** and (2) **interstitia of all tissues**. Under epithelial is the common site of entry of microbes and foreign antigens, and in the interstitium is the site where antigens may be produced. DCs are widely distributed in lymphoid tissues, mucosal epithelium, and organ parenchyma. **Immature DCs within the epidermis are called Langerhans cells** (**Figs. 11A** and **B**).
- **Recruitment to the T-cell zones of lymphoid organs:** In response to microbes, DCs are recruited to the T-cell zones of lymphoid organs. This is the ideal site of their location to present antigens to naïve T cells.
- **Express high levels of MHC and other molecules:** DCs express high levels of MHC and other molecules that are

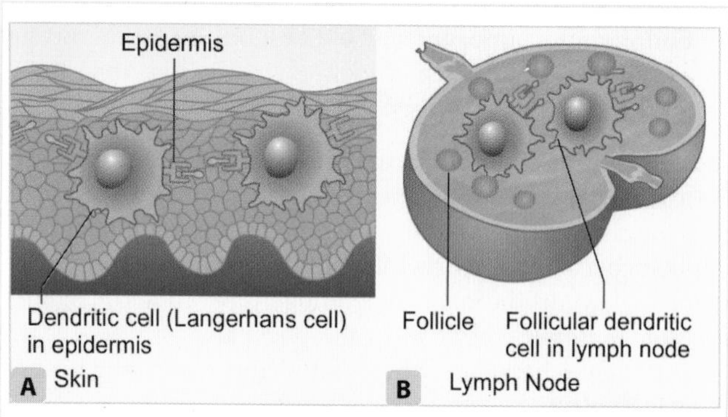

FIGS. 11A AND B: (A) Dendritic cell in epidermis of skin and (B) Follicular dendritic cell (FDC) in lymph node.

Table 3: Salient features of antibodies (immunoglobulins).

Features	*IgM (millionaire's antibody)*	*IgG (subtypes: IgG1, IgG2, IgG3, IgG4)*	*IgA*	*IgE (reaginic/ homocytotropic antibody)*	*IgD*
Approximate % of total Ig	5%	80% (maximum)	15%	Trace	Trace
Molecular weight	900,000 (maximum)	150,000	150,000–300,000	190,000	180,000
Type of heavy chain	μ	γ	α	ϵ	δ
Structure	Pentamer (maximum size)	Monomer	Dimer (in glandular secretions), monomer (in serum)	Monomer	Monomer
Complement activation	Yes (classical pathway)	Yes (classical pathway)	Activates alternate complement pathway	No	No
Transport across placenta	No	Yes	No	No	No
Half-life (days)	5	21	6	2	3
Main function	Primary immune response	• Secondary immune response • Functions as B-cell receptor	• Mucosal immunity • Highly effective at neutralizing toxins	Allergic diseases, defense against parasite infection and anaphylactic reaction	Unknown

required for antigen presentation and T-cell activation. All DCs express both class I and class II MHC molecules, which are needed for presentation of antigens to CD8+ and CD4+ T cells, respectively.

- **Secretion of cytokines:** DCs respond to microbes by secreting cytokines that recruit and activate innate cells at the site of infection.
- **Extremely efficient APCs:** DCs have long membranous projections and phagocytic capacity. DCs are most efficient at capturing protein antigens of microbes, degrading these antigens, and displaying portions of these antigens for recognition by T cells. The innate immune response enhances this antigen-presenting capacity of DCs. This is an important mechanism by which innate immunity promotes adaptive immune responses.

Development of DCs: Most DCs are part of the myeloid lineage of hematopoietic cells. They originate from a precursor that can also differentiate into monocytes. Langerhans cells (type of DC present in the epithelial layer of skin) develop from embryonic precursors in the yolk sac or fetal liver, early during the development.

Follicular dendritic cells (FDCs): These cells have a dendritic morphology but are not related to the DCs. FDCs are **present in the germinal centers of lymphoid follicles in the spleen and lymph nodes**. They are not derived from bone marrow precursors and do not present protein antigens to T cells. But they are involved in B cell activation in lymphoid organs. These cells have Fc receptors for IgG and receptors for C3b and can trap antigen bound to antibodies or complement proteins. Thus, they play a role in humoral immune responses by presenting antigens to B cells in the germinal center.

Macrophages

Macrophages are a part of the mononuclear phagocyte system. They are discussed in detail on pages 306-311. Important functions of macrophages in the induction and effector phases of adaptive immune responses are as follows:

- **Antigen presenting cells (APCs):** Macrophage can phagocytose microbes and antigen. They process the protein antigens and present peptide fragments to T cells. Thus, macrophages function as APCs involved in T-cell activation.
- **Effector cells in cell mediated immunity:** Macrophages can be main effector cells in certain types of cell-mediated immunity. By this, they can eliminate intracellular microbes. In this type of response, T cells can activate macrophages and enhance their ability to kill ingested microbes.
- **Humoral immunity:** Macrophages are also involved in the effector phase of humoral immunity. Macrophages can efficiently phagocytose and destroy microbes that are opsonized (coated) by IgG or C3b through its corresponding receptors.

Tissues of the Immune System

The tissues of the immune system can be divided into—(1) the primary (also called generative, or central) lymphoid organs and (2) the secondary (or peripheral) lymphoid organs.

Primary lymphoid organs

Main primary lymphoid organs are—(1) the **thymus** (where T cells develop) and (2) the **bone marrow** (the site of production of all other blood cells, including naïve B cells). In primary lymphoid organs, T and B lymphocytes mature and become competent to respond to antigens.

Secondary lymphoid organs

The secondary lymphoid organs include **lymph nodes, spleen, and the mucosal and cutaneous lymphoid tissues**. These are the tissues where adaptive immune responses occur.

Lymph nodes Lymph nodes are encapsulated (**Fig. 12**), vascularized secondary lymphoid organs consisting of nodular aggregates of lymphoid tissues present along lymphatic channels throughout the body. Therefore, lymph nodes have access to antigens encountered at epithelia and originating in most tissues, which are drained by lymphatics. There are about 500 lymph nodes in the body. Afferent lymphatics carry lymph to the subcapsular (marginal) sinus followed by substance of the lymph node. Efferent lymphatics drain the lymph out of the lymph node.

Anatomic features of lymph node favor the initiation of adaptive immune responses to antigens carried from tissues by lymphatics. Most foreign antigens (e.g., microbial antigens) enter the body through epithelia or are produced in tissues. Antigen derived from microbes or other sources are recognized, taken up, and transported by APCs present in the location (e.g., entry through epithelia into tissues) as well as DCs. These APCs and DCs enter the lymph. As lymph slowly permeates via afferent lymphatic vessels, these APCs and DCs reach the subscapular sinus of lymph nodes. Thus, the antigens of microbes that enter through epithelia or colonize tissues become concentrated in draining lymph nodes. Macrophages in the subscapular sinus are important phagocytic cells that remove infectious organisms from lymph. Lymph nodes are the main site of generation of the majority of adaptive immune responses.

Spleen The spleen is a highly vascularized, abdominal secondary lymphoid organ. Major functions of spleen are—(1) to remove aging and damaged blood cells and particles (such

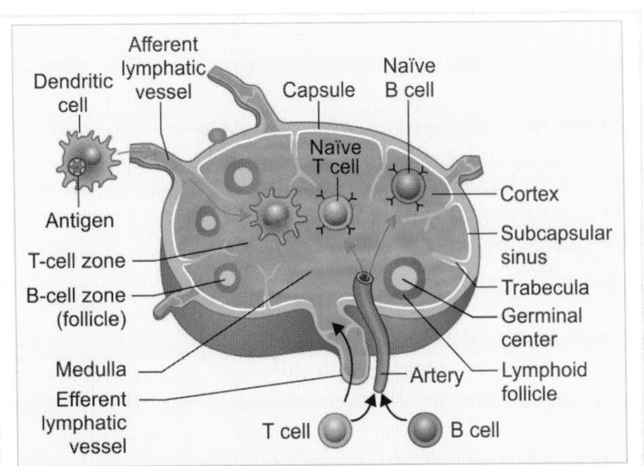

FIG. 12: Diagrammatic illustration of lymph node. B cells and T cells are segregated in different regions of the lymph node (T-cell-rich and B-cell-rich zones). The routes of entry of lymphocytes and antigen are also shown. Antigen presenting cells including dendritic cells carry the antigen from its site of entry through afferent lymphatic vessels into the regional lymph nodes. These cells migrate to the T-cell-rich areas of the node. The naïve lymphocytes enter the node through an artery. The naïve T and B lymphocytes migrate to different areas of a lymph node.

as immune complexes and opsonized microbes) from the circulation and (2) to initiate adaptive immune responses to bloodborne antigens. It has the same role in immune responses to bloodborne antigens as the lymph nodes do in responses to lymph-borne antigens. Sinusoids in the spleen are lined by macrophages and DCs. Blood entering the spleen flows through these networks of sinusoids. Bloodborne antigens are trapped in the spleen by macrophages and DCs lining sinusoids. This can then initiate adaptive immune responses to these antigens.

Cutaneous and mucosal lymphoid systems All major epithelial barriers of the body have their own system of lymph nodes, nonencapsulated lymphoid structures, and diffusely distributed immune cells. These lymphoid systems work in coordinated ways and respond to antigens that enter through breaches in the epithelium. The epithelial barriers include the **skin, gastrointestinal mucosa, and bronchial mucosa** and lymphoid tissue are located under the epithelia at these sites. Thus, skin has cutaneous lymphoid system where MALT is present at GIT and respiratory system. Two anatomically defined mucosal lymphoid tissues are—(1) pharyngeal tonsils and (2) Peyer patches of the intestine. Large fraction of the body's lymphocytes is present in the mucosal tissues, and many of these lymphocytes are memory cells. Thus, the skin and MALT contain a large proportion of the cells of the innate and adaptive immune systems.

Distribution of T and B cells in secondary lymphoid organs: In the secondary lymphoid organs, naïve T and B lymphocytes are separated into different regions.

- **Lymph nodes (Fig. 12):** In lymph nodes, B and T cells are distributed as follows—
    - **Follicles: B cells** are concentrated in discrete structures called **follicles**. The periphery, or cortex of lymph node, contains these lymphoid follicles. After exposure to an antigen, the B cells in a follicle respond and produce pale central region called a germinal center. The follicles contain the FDCs that are involved in the activation of B cells.
    - **Paracortex: T lymphocytes are concentrated in the paracortex** of the lymph node, adjacent to the follicles. The paracortex contains the DCs that present antigens to T lymphocytes.
- **Spleen:** In the spleen, **T lymphocytes** are concentrated **in periarteriolar lymphoid sheaths** surrounding small arterioles. **B cells are present in follicles** similar to those found in lymph nodes (splenic white pulp).

Lymphocyte classes in adaptive immunity are listed in **Box 2**.

Lymphocyte recirculation

Lymphocyte homing refers to adhesion of the circulating lymphocytes in blood to specialized endothelial cells within lymphoid organs. There is constant recirculation of lymphocytes between tissues and they home to particular sites.

Recirculation of T-cell versus B-cell: The process of lymphocyte recirculation is most important for T cells. This is because naïve T cells have to circulate through the secondary lymphoid organs where antigens are concentrated. The effector T cells have to migrate to sites of infection to eliminate microbes. In contrast, B lymphocytes which differentiate into plasma cells remain in lymphoid organs and the bone marrow. They need not circulate to sites of infection. This is because plasma cells secrete antibodies that are carried through the blood to distant tissues.

Box 2: Lymphocyte classes in adaptive immunity.

T Lymphocytes

αβ T lymphocytes
- CD4+ helper T lymphocytes
- CD8+ cytotoxic T lymphocytes
- Regulatory T cells
- Natural killer T (NKT) cells

γδ T lymphocytes

Mucosa-associated invariant T (MAIT) cells

B Lymphocytes
- Follicular B cells
- Marginal zone B cells
- B-1 cells

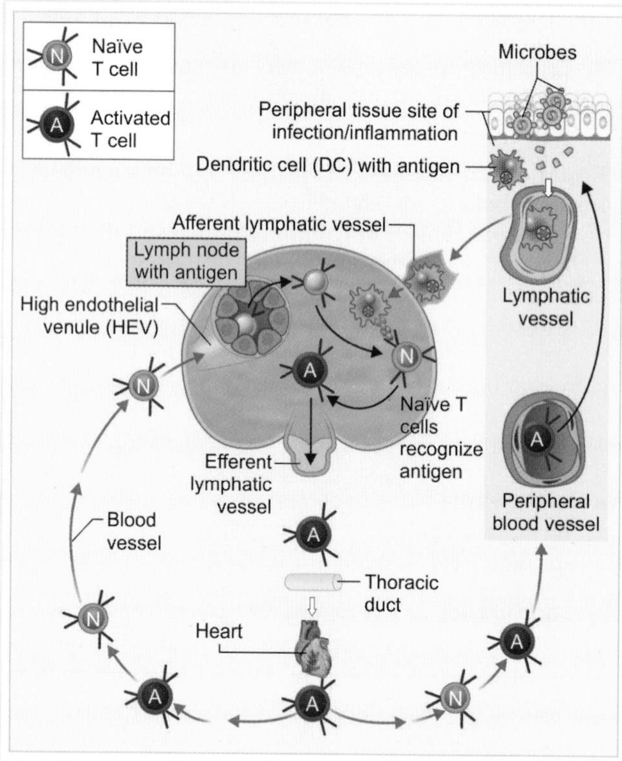

FIG. 13: Pathways of T lymphocyte recirculation. Naïve T cells leave the blood and enter lymph nodes across the high endothelial venules (HEVs). Dendritic cells (DCs) bearing antigen enter the lymph nodes through afferent lymphatic vessels. If the naïve T cells recognize antigen in the lymph node, they become activated. These activated T cells return to the circulation through the efferent lymphatics and the thoracic duct, which empties into the superior vena cava, then into the heart, and ultimately into the arterial circulation. Effector and memory T cells preferentially leave the blood and enter peripheral tissues through venules at sites of inflammation. T cell recirculation through only lymph nodes is shown.

T lymphocyte recirculation (Fig. 13): Naïve lymphocytes traverse the secondary lymphoid organs where immune responses are initiated. The effector lymphocytes migrate to sites of infection and inflammation. This recirculation depends on mechanisms that control entry of naïve T cells from the blood into lymph nodes, as well as molecular signals that control the exit of naïve T cells from the nodes. The homing mechanisms that bring naïve T cells into lymph nodes are very efficient. Specialized postcapillary high endothelial venules (HEV) are located in the T-cell zones.

- **Migration of naïve T cells into lymph nodes:** Homing of naïve T cells into lymph nodes and MALT occurs through HEV. Naïve T lymphocytes are carried to secondary lymphoid tissues through arterial blood flow. In the lymphoid organs, naïve T lymphocytes leave the blood circulation and migrate out of the blood. They enter into the parenchyma of the lymph node through these HEVs. The endothelial cells of HEVs display certain adhesion molecules (e.g., L-selectin and LFA-1) and chemokines (e.g., chemokine receptor CCR7) on their surfaces. This helps in selective homing of only certain population of lymphocytes.
- **Movement of T cells within secondary lymphoid organs:** After entering lymph nodes or mucosal lymphoid tissues, T lymphocytes and DCs actively move in the lymph node in such a way to maximize the chances of interaction between these two cell types.
- **Exit of T cells from lymph nodes:** If naïve T cells that have homed into lymph nodes are not able to recognize antigen presented by DCs, they do not undergo activation. These T cells will eventually return to the bloodstream. The major route of re-entry into the blood is through the efferent lymphatics, then through the lymphatic vasculature to the thoracic duct, which drains into the superior vena cava, and finally into the right subclavian vein. This return of naïve T cells to the blood completes one T cell recirculation loop. These returned naïve T cells have another chance to enter secondary lymphoid organs and search for the antigens they can recognize.

Migration of effector T lymphocytes to sites of infection

Generation of effector T cells: If naïve T cells that have homed into lymph nodes are able to recognize antigen presented by DCs, they undergo activation. Antigen-induced activation of naive T cells generates effector T cells.

Exit of effector T cells from secondary lymphoid organs: The effector T cells leave secondary lymphoid organs through lymphatic drainage and return to the blood.

Migration and homing of effector T cells to site of infection: Circulating effector T cells preferably migrate and home to peripheral tissue sites of infection rather than lymphoid organs. This is because of changes in adhesion molecule and chemokine receptor expression in these effector cells. This migration of effector T cells into infected tissues is antigen independent. However, the effector T cells that encounter antigen in the affected tissue are preferentially retained at the infected site. Thus, effector cells of various specificities can enter tissue sites of infection. This maximizes the chance of T cells finding the antigen for which they are specific.

Subsets of effector cells: There are different subsets of effector T cells and each subset has distinct functions. Effector T cells include CD8+ CTLs and CD4+ helper T cells. Helper T cells have further subsets namely, Th1, Th2, and Th17. Each of these subsets of helper T cells expresses different types of cytokines and protects against different types of microbes. Though these subsets are different, they often have overlapping patterns of migration.

Differences between innate and adaptive immunity are shown in **Table 4**.

Terms used with regard to cells involved in adaptive immunity are presented in **Box 3**.

Major Histocompatibility Complex Molecules

Q. Write short essay on human leukocyte antigen (HLA) (MHC).

All human cells have a series of molecules on their surfaces that are recognized by other individuals as foreign antigens. MHC molecules were discovered as products of genes that evoke rejection of transplanted organs. The name MHC is derived because of their role in determining tissue compatibility between individuals.

Box 3: Terms used with regard to cells involved in adaptive immunity.

Naïve lymphocytes: These are mature lymphocytes which have not encountered the antigen (immunologically inexperienced)
Effector cells: They perform the function of eliminating microbes
Memory cells: They live in a state of heightened awareness and are better able to combat the microbe in case it infects again

Table 4: Differences between innate and adaptive immunity.

	Innate immunity	*Adaptive immunity*
Components		
Cellular and chemical barriers	Skin, mucosal epithelia; antimicrobial molecules	Lymphocytes in epithelia; antibodies secreted at epithelial surfaces
Blood proteins	Complement, various lectins, and agglutinins	Antibodies
Cells	Phagocytes (macrophages, neutrophils), dendritic cells, natural killer cells, mast cells, innate lymphoid cells (ILC)	Lymphocytes
Characteristics		
Specificity	For molecules shared by groups of related microbes and molecules produced by injure or damaged host cells	For microbial and nonmicrobial antigens
Diversity	Limited	Very large
Memory	None or limited	Present

MHC and HLA: The **human MHC is commonly called the HLA complex.** HLAs are also known as histocompatibility antigens. The term human because it was observed in humans; leukocyte because initially the antibodies were detected on leukocytes by the binding of antibodies from other individuals; and antigens because the molecules were recognized by antibodies. Hence the term HLA.

Function of MHC: Physiologic function of **MHC molecules is to display peptide fragments of proteins for recognition by antigen-specific T cells**. They organize many cell-cell interactions fundamental to immune responses. Since MHC molecules are necessary for antigen recognition by T cells, they are linked to many autoimmune diseases. These HLA antigens are major immunogens and thus targets in transplant rejection.

MHC Genes

The MHC molecules are products of *MHC* genes. The genes encoding HLA molecules are densely packed (clustered) on a small segment on chromosome 6 (6p21.3). *MHC* gene occupies about 3,500 kilobases (kb). The best known of these *MHC* genes are the HLA class I and class II genes. Their products are important for immunologic specificity and transplantation histocompatibility. Class I and class II *MHC* genes are the most polymorphic genes in the genome. *MHC* genes are codominantly expressed in each individual. Thus, for a given *MHC* gene, each individual expresses the alleles that are inherited from both parents.

Polymorphism of *MHC* gene

Polymorphism refers to variations in a gene among individuals in a population. The HLA system is highly polymorphic. Polymorphism means that there are many alleles of each *MHC* gene resulting in extreme (high degree) variation in the MHC in human population (genetic diversity). There are thousands of distinct *MHC* gene alleles in humans. Each person inherits one set of these alleles that is different from the alleles in most other persons in the population. The possibility of two different individuals having the same combination of MHC molecules is very remote. Therefore, grafts exchanged between individuals are recognized as foreign and attacked by the immune system. Polymorphism is an important barrier in organ transplantation.

HLA haplotype: It is the combination of HLA alleles in each individual. Each individual inherits one set of *HLA* genes from each parent and thus typically expresses two different molecules for every locus.

Importance of MHC: MHC is the peptide display system of adaptive immunity and is important—(1) in organ/tissue transplantation and (2) HLA is linked to many autoimmune diseases.

Classification of MHC

The *MHC* gene product is classified based on their structure, cellular distribution, and function into two major classes (**Fig. 14**) and one minor class. MHC class I and class II gene products are critical for immunologic specificity and transplantation histocompatibility, and they play a major role in susceptibility to a number of autoimmune diseases.

Structure of MHC Molecules

General properties of MHC molecules

All MHC molecules have certain structural characteristics that are important for their role in peptide display and antigen recognition by T lymphocytes. Each MHC molecule is composed of an—(1) extracellular peptide-binding cleft, followed by an (2) Ig-like domain, and (3) transmembrane and (4) cytoplasmic domains.

Extracellular peptide-binding cleft: The polymorphic amino acid residues of MHC molecules are located in and adjacent to the extracellular peptide-binding cleft (groove).

Immunoglobulin-like domain: The nonpolymorphic Ig-like domains of class I and class II MHC molecules contain binding sites for the T-cell molecules CD8 and CD4, respectively. CD4 and CD8 are expressed on distinct subpopulations of mature T lymphocytes. In the recognition of antigen, both CD4 and CD8 participate together with antigen receptors. Hence, they are called T-cell coreceptors. CD4 binds selectively to class II MHC molecules, and CD8 binds to class I molecules. CD4+ helper T cells recognize class II MHC molecules displaying peptides and CD8+ T cells recognize class I MHC molecules with bound peptides. In other words, CD4+ T cells are class II MHC restricted and CD8+ T cells are class I MHC restricted.

Class I MHC molecules

Expression of Class I MHC: They are the products of MHC class I genes and are constitutively expressed on **all nucleated cells and platelets** (except erythrocytes and trophoblasts).

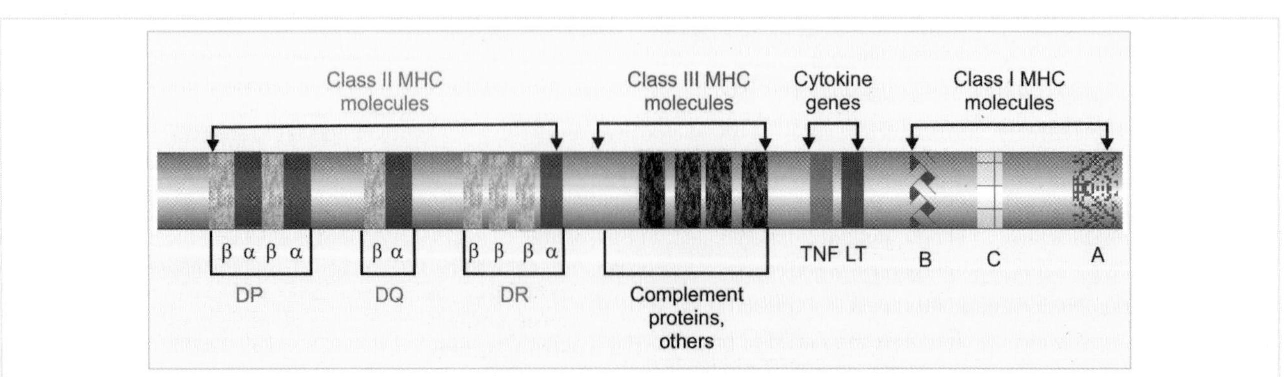

(LT: lymphotoxin; TNF: tumor necrosis factor)

FIG. 14: Major histocompatibility complex (MHC) (human leukocyte antigen complex) showing location of genes.

Their expression is increased by the type I IFNs, IFN-α, and IFN-β, which are produced during the early innate immune response to many viruses.

The *HLA class I genes*: They are **located at the telomeric end of the HLA region.** There are three class I *MHC* genes called *HLA-A, HLA-B,* and *HLA-C,* which encode three types of class I MHC molecules with the same names. They are polymorphic in the population and most highly polymorphic segment known within the human genome. More than 3,400 alleles at HLA-A, 4,300 alleles at HLA-B, and 3,100 alleles at HLA-C have been identified.

Structure of class I MHC molecules (Fig. 15) Class I MHC molecules are heterodimers (a protein composed of two polypeptide chains differing in composition, number, or amino acid residues) and consist of two noncovalently bound polypeptide chains. One chain is an MHC-encoded 44–47 kD polymorphic, transmembrane glycoprotein called α chain (or heavy chain) and other is a non-MHC-encoded 12 kD subunit called β_2-microglobulin. β_2-microglobulin lacks a membrane component. One polypeptide chain (α) encoded in the MHC on chromosome 6 and a second, non-MHC-encoded chain (β_2-microglobulin) on chromosome 15.

α chains: These are encoded by three genes, namely, *HLA-A, HLA-B,* and *HLA-C.* These three genes lie close to one another in the MHC locus. About three quarters of the α chain polypeptide is extracellular; a short hydrophobic segment in the plasma membrane, and the carboxy-terminal residues are located in the cytoplasm.

- **Extracellular region of the α chain:** It is divided into three domains—α_1, α_2, and α_3. The α_1 and α_2 domains form a cleft, or groove (peptide-binding cleft/groove) of class I molecules. The peptides bind to this groove. The polymorphic amino acid residues line the sides and the base of the peptide-binding groove and are confined to this region. This is the reason for the different class I alleles to bind different peptides. The α_3 segment of the α chain folds into an Ig domain. The amino acid sequence of Ig domain is conserved among all class I MHC molecules. This α_3 segment contains most of the binding site for CD8. But β_2-microglobulin and a small portion of the nonpolymorphic C-terminal portion of the α_2 domain also contribute.
- **Transmembrane and cytoplasmic region of the α chain:** At the carboxy-terminal end of the α_3 segment traverses the lipid bilayer of the plasma membrane and in the cytoplasm.

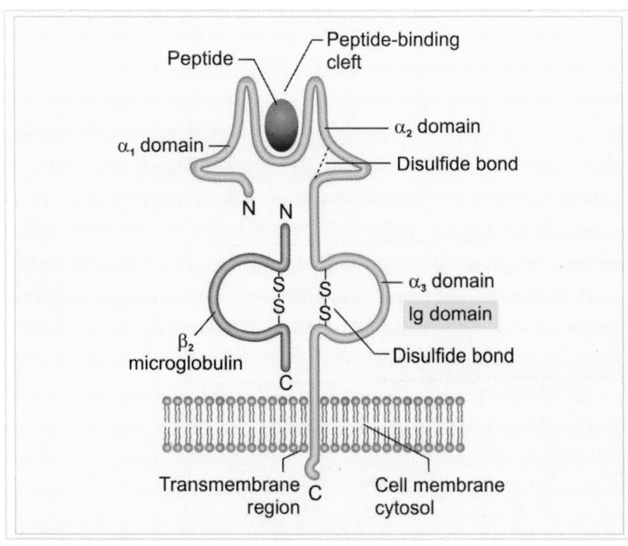

(C: carboxy-terminal; N: amino-terminal; S: sulfide)

FIG. 15: Structure of a class I major histocompatibility complex (MHC) molecule. The diagrammatic appearance of the different regions of the MHC molecule (not to be scaled). Class I MHC molecule consists of a polymorphic α chain noncovalently attached to the nonpolymorphic β_2-microglobulin (β_2m).

β_2-microglobulin: It is the light chain of class I molecules. It is encoded by a gene outside the MHC on chromosome 15. It is named so because of its electrophoretic mobility (β_2), size (micro), and solubility (globulin). It is noncovalently bound to the α_3 domain of the α chain. Similar to the α_3 segment, β_2-microglobulin is structurally homologous to an Ig domain and is conserved among all class I MHC molecules.

Designation of *HLA* genes and their products: It is based on a World Health Organization (WHO) nomenclature. The alleles are given a single designation that indicates locus, allotype, and sequence-based subtype. For example, HLA-A*02:01 designation indicates subtype 1 of a group of alleles that encode HLA-A2 molecules. Subtypes that differ from each other at the nucleotide but not the amino acid sequence level are designated by an extra numeral (e.g., *HLA-B*07:02:01* and *HLA-B*07:02:02* are two variants of *HLA-B*07:02,* both encoding the same HLA-B7 molecule).

Functions Products of *MHC* class I gene are integral participants in the immune response to intracellular infections, tumors, and allografts. Class I molecules interact with CD8+ T lymphocytes during antigen presentation and are involved in cytotoxic reactions. CD8+ T lymphocytes recognize antigens only in the context of self-class I molecules, they are referred to as class I MHC-restricted.

Peptide antigen presentation (Fig. 16): Various sequence of events in antigen presentation on class I MHC molecules APCs are as follows—

- **Sources of protein antigens:** Class I MHC molecules display peptides that are derived from cytoplasmic proteins. These include normal proteins and virus- and tumor-specific antigens. These are all recognized bound to class I MHC molecules by CD8+ T cells.
- **Degradation of proteins in the proteasomes:** Cytoplasmic proteins are degraded in proteasomes and it generates peptides that are able to bind class I MHC molecules.
- **Transport of peptides from the cytosol to the endoplasmic reticulum (ER):** Peptides are transported into the ER by a specialized transporter called transporter associated with antigen processing (TAP). Newly synthesized class I MHC molecules are available to bind the peptides in the ER.
- **Assembly of peptide–class I MHC complexes in the ER:** Peptides translocated into the ER bind to newly synthesized class I MHC molecules. Peptide-loaded MHC molecules then associate with β2-microglobulin to form a structurally stable complex.
- **Surface expression of peptide–class I MHC complexes:** Class I MHC molecules with bound peptides are transported to the cell surface and are expressed on the cell surface.

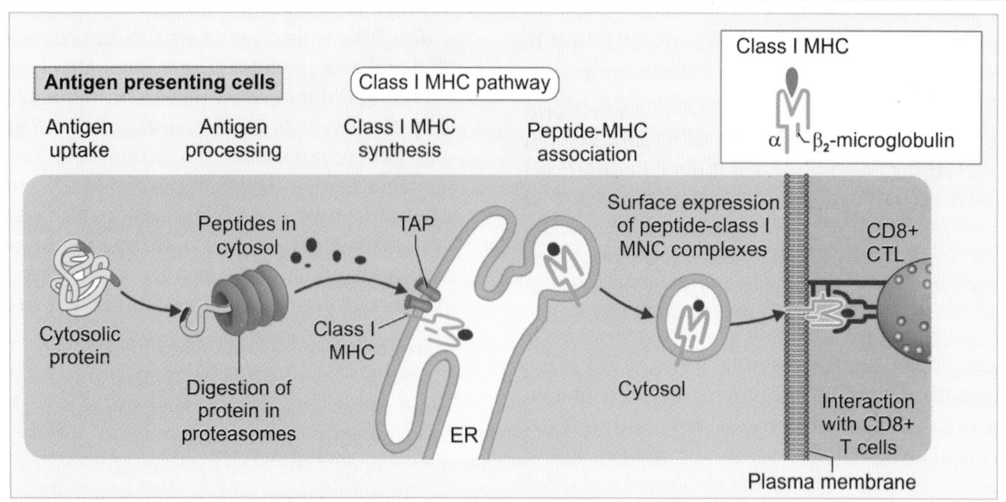

(ER: endoplasmic reticulum; MHC: major histocompatibility complex; TAP: transporter associated with antigen processing)

Fig. 16: Pathways of antigen processing and presentation in the class I MHC pathway. Protein antigens in the cytosol are processed by proteasomes. The proteins in antigens are digested in the proteasomes and peptides are released into the cytosol. These peptides are then transported into the ER. In ER, peptides bind to class I MHC molecules and are transported to the surface of antigen presenting cell (APC). These are recognized by CD8+ T cells.

- **Interaction with CD8+ T cells:** The nonpolymorphic α_3 domain of class I MHC molecules has a binding site for CD8. Hence, the peptide-class I complexes expressed on the cell surface are recognized by CD8+ T cells, which function as CTLs. In this interaction, the TCR of CD8+ T cells recognizes the MHC-peptide complex. The CD8 molecule of CD8+ T cells acts as a coreceptor and binds to the class I heavy chain.
- **CD8+ T cells are class I MHC-restricted:** CD8+ T cells recognize peptides only if presented as a complex with class I MHC molecules. Therefore, CD8+ T cells are said to be class I MHC-restricted.
- **Important functions of CD8+ CTLs:** These include the elimination of viruses (which may infect any nucleated cell) and killing of tumor cells (which may arise from any nucleated cell). Thus, all nucleated cells express class I MHC molecules and can be surveyed by CD8+ T cells.

Class II MHC molecules

They are encoded in a region called HLA-D, which has three su-regions—HLA-DP, HLA-DQ, and HLA-DR.

Cells expressing class II MHC: Class II antigens (HLA-D and -DR, D-related) are expressed only on **professional APCs** (B lymphocytes, monocytes/macrophages, Langerhans cells, and DCs).

Structure of class II MHC molecules (Fig. 17) Class II MHC molecules are heterodimers consisting of two noncovalently associated polypeptide chains namely, α chain (32–34 kD) and β chain (29–32 kD). Unlike class I molecules, the genes encoding both polypeptide chains of class II molecules are polymorphic and located in the MHC locus.

Extracellular portions: Both α and β chains have extracellular portions composing of two domains designated α_1 and α_2 and β_1 and β_2. The amino-terminal α_1 and β_1 segments of the class II chains interact to form the peptide-binding cleft that faces outward. It is in this portion that most class II alleles differ. Thus, similar to class I molecules, polymorphism of class II molecules is associated with differential binding of antigenic peptides. Like class I α_3 and β_2-microglobulin, the α_2 and β_2 segments of class II MHC molecules are folded into Ig domains. These Ig domains are nonpolymorphic (i.e., they do not vary among alleles of a particular class II gene). Both the α_2 and β_2 domains of class II molecules contribute to a concavity that accommodates a protrusion of the CD4 protein, thus allowing binding to occur.

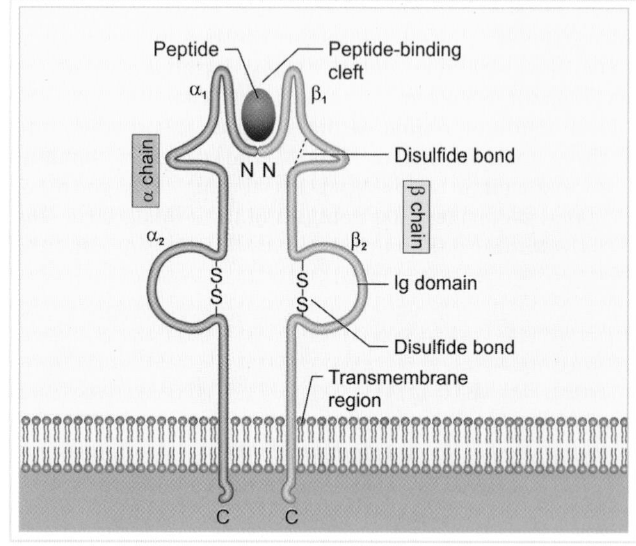

(C: carboxy-terminal; N: amino-terminal; S: sulfide)

FIG. 17: Structure of a class II major histocompatibility complex (MHC) molecule. The diagrammatic appearance of the different regions of the MHC molecule (not to be scaled). Class II MHC molecules consist of a polymorphic α chain noncovalently attached to the polymorphic β chain.

Transmembrane and cytoplasmic region: The carboxy-terminal ends of the α_2 and β_2 segments continue as hydrophobic transmembrane residues, followed by short hydrophilic cytoplasmic tails.

Function This locus contains genes that encode many proteins involved in antigen processing and presentation. The class II-peptide complex is recognized by CD4+ T-cells (function as helper cells) and these CD4 molecules act as the co-receptor.

Peptide antigen presentation (Fig. 18): Class II MHC molecules present antigens derived from extracellular microbes. Various sequences of events in antigen presentation APCs on class I MHC molecules are as follows—

- **Targeting of protein antigens to lysosomes:** The antigens from the extracellular environment are ingested and sequestered in vesicles. Following their internalization, the antigens are proteolytically degraded in lysosomes (or late endosomes).
- **Proteolytic digestion of antigens in lysosomes:** Internalized proteins are degraded enzymatically in late endosomes and lysosomes to produce peptides. These peptides are able to bind to the peptide-binding clefts of class II MHC molecules. Thus, the site of proteolysis mainly determines the class of MHC molecules to which the generated peptides will bind (whether class I or class II).
- **Biosynthesis and transport of class II MHC molecules to endosomes:** In the ER, class II MHC molecules are newly synthesized, and these are transported to endosomes with an associated protein, the invariant chain (I***i***). Invariant chain occupies the peptide-binding clefts of the newly synthesized class II MHC molecules.
- **Association of processed peptides with class II MHC molecules in vesicles:** Within the endosomal vesicles, the I***i*** dissociates from class II MHC molecules. This is achieved by the combined action of proteolytic enzymes and the HLA-DM molecule. HLA-DM molecule is encoded within the MHC and structurally similar to that of class II MHC molecules. The peptides derived from protein antigens are now able to bind to the available peptide-binding clefts of the class II heterodimer molecules. These peptides associate with class II molecules.
- **Expression of peptide–class II MHC complexes on the cell surface:** Class II MHC molecules are stabilized by the bound peptides. The stable peptide–class II complexes are transported from the vesicle to the surface of the APC. In the APC, they are displayed for recognition by CD4+ T cells.
- **Recognition by CD4+ T cells:** The class II β2 domain has a binding site for CD4. So, the class II-peptide complex is recognized by CD4+ T cells. These cells function as helper cells. CD4+ T cells can recognize antigens only in the context of self-class II molecules. Hence, they are referred to as class II MHC restricted. In contrast to class I molecules, class II molecules are mainly expressed on cells that present ingested antigens and respond to T-cell help (macrophages, B lymphocytes, and DCs).

Features of class I and class II MHC molecules are presented in **Table 5**.

Differences in antigen processing and presentation between class I and class II MHC pathways are presented in **Table 6**.

Class III MHC molecules (Fig. 15)

Their genes encode components of the complement system, cytokines, TNF, LT, and some proteins without apparent role in the immune system.

Minor histocompatibility (mH) antigens

Q. Write short essay on minor histocompatibility antigens.

Minor histocompatibility (mH) antigens are non-MHC-encoded cell surface processed peptides. mH antigens are diverse, short segments of normal proteins (peptides). They are polymorphic in a given population These antigens in

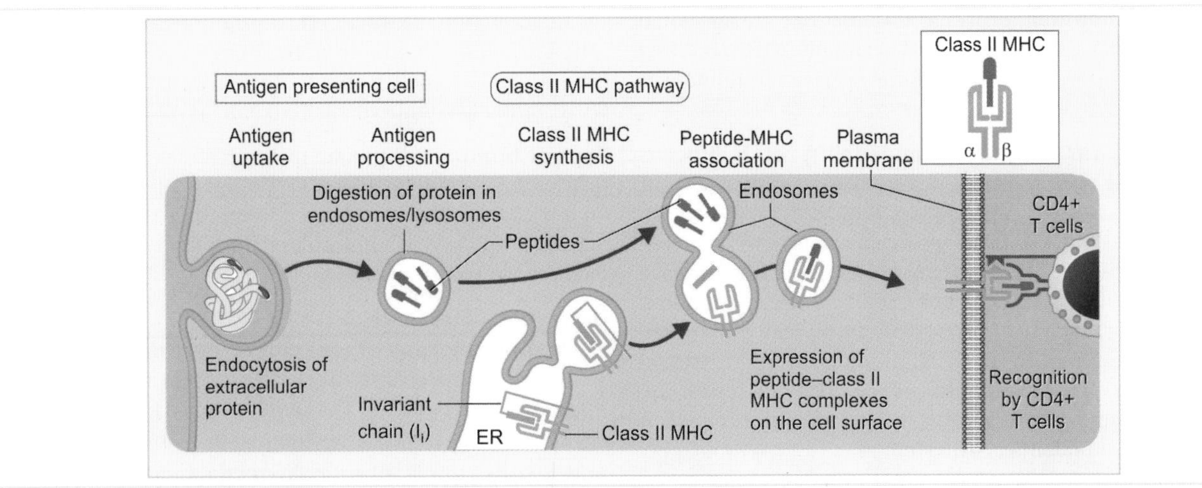

(ER: endoplasmic reticulum; Ii: invariant chain; MHC: major histocompatibility complex)

FIG. 18 Pathways of antigen processing and presentation in the class II MHC pathway. Protein antigens derived from extracellular sources (e.g., microbes). The protein antigen is degraded in lysosomes or late endosomes. In the ER, class II MHC molecules are newly synthesized, and these are transported to endosomes with an associated protein, the invariant chain (Ii). Invariant chain occupies the peptide-binding clefts of the newly synthesized class II MHC molecules. Newly synthesized class II MHC molecules are transported to endosomes. In the endosomes, invariant chain dissociates from class II MHC molecule and allows class II molecule to bind to peptides. The peptides bound to class II MHC molecules are then transported to the surface of antigen presenting cell (APC). These are recognized by CD4+ T cells.

Table 5: Features of class I and class II MHC molecules.

Characteristics	*Class I MHC*	*Class II MHC*
Type of polypeptide chains	α and β_2-microglobulin	α and β
Locations of polymorphic residues	α_1 and α_2 domains	α_1 and β_1 domains
Binding site for T cell coreceptor	CD8 mainly binds to the α_3 domain	CD4 binds to a pocket created by parts of α_2 and β_2 domains
Size of peptide-binding cleft	Peptides of 8–11 residues*	Peptides of 10–30 residues * or more
Nomenclature	HLA-A, HLA-B, HLA-C	HLA-DR, HLA-DQ, HLA-DP

*A series of amino acids joined by peptide bonds form a polypeptide chain, and each amino acid unit in a polypeptide is called a residue.

(HLA: human leukocyte antigen; MHC: major histocompatibility complex)

Table 6: Differences in antigen processing and presentation between class I and class II MHC pathways.

Characteristics	*Class I MHC pathway*	*Class II MHC pathway*
Source of antigens	Cytosolic proteins (usually synthesized in the cell but may enter cytosol from phagosomes); nuclear and membrane proteins	Endosomal and lysosomal proteins (internalized from extracellular environment)
Types of APCs involved in processing and presentation of antigen	All nucleated cells	Dendritic cells, mononuclear phagocytes, B lymphocytes, endothelial cells, thymic epithelium
Site of degradation of antigen	Proteasome	Late endosomes and lysosomes
Enzymes responsible for degradation of protein	Proteasomes (e.g., β_1, β_2, and β_5 subunits)	Endosomal and lysosomal proteases (e.g., cathepsins)
Site of peptide loading of MHC	Endoplasmic reticulum (ER)	Late endosomes/lysosomes
Molecules involved in transport of peptides and loading of MHC molecules	TAP (transporter associated with antigen processing) in ER	Invariant chain (Ii) in ER, Golgi; HLA-DM (has a structure similar to that of class II MHC molecules)
Composition of stable peptide-MHC complex	Polymorphic α chain, β_2-microglobulin	Polymorphic α and β chains peptide
Responsive T cells	CD8+ T cells	CD4+ T cells

(APCs: antigen-presenting cells; MHC: major histocompatibility complex)

association with both the MHC class I and class II proteins. They contribute to graft rejection. Usually, these rejections are less severe than due to MHC disparity. mH antigens are encoded by a large number of chromosomes and are presented only as peptides in the context of recipient MHC (indirect allorecognition). Exact number of mH antigens in humans is not known.

Significance of mH antigens **Incompatibility of mH antigens between donor and recipient**—even when a transplant donor and recipient are identical with regard to *MHC* genes, amino acid differences in these minor proteins can lead to rejection. Thus, there is a risk of developing graft-versus-host disease (GVHD) or graft failure after bone marrow transplantation. This can develop both in HLA phenotypically matched unrelated donors and also in HLA genotypically identical sibling donors. These minor antigens are responsible for the need for immunosuppression even after donation between HLA-matched nonidentical twin siblings.

Antigen types: Most mH antigens are expressed ubiquitously, including on epithelial tissues. They may have **either broad tissue expression or expression restricted to hematopoietic cells** (e.g., HA-1, HA-2, HB-1, and CD19). One of the classical mH antigens is Male or H-Y antigen.

- **Male or H-Y antigens:** These antigens are encoded on the Y chromosome. Females of the species may mount an immune response against these antigens. Alloresponses to this antigen are responsible for reduced long-term graft survival observed in male-to-female donations.

Recognition of such mH antigens by donor T cells following HSC (hematopoietic stem cell) transplantation (hematopoietic cell transplantation or HCT) can lead to GVHD and also, graft-versus-leukemia (GVL).

Type of immune response: mH antigen evokes only MHC-restricted CTL and proliferative T helper cell responses. They do not elicit antibody-mediated immunity. This is in contrast to polymorphic MHC molecules, which evoke even antibody-mediated immune response.

Other roles of mH antigen: These include—

- **Immunotherapy of leukemia:** Some mH antigens can be used as therapeutic T cell targets to augment the GVL effect. In this, CTLs specific for mH antigen peptide are used to prevent or manage leukemia relapse after HCT.
- **Corneal allograft rejection:** mH antigen acts as major barriers and the MHC incompatibility plays a minor role.
- **Secondary recurrent miscarriage:** Immunization of mothers against male-specific minor histocompatibility (H-Y) antigens may have a pathogenic role in secondary recurrent miscarriage (i.e., recurrent abortions in pregnancies succeeding a previous live birth).

HLA Haplotype and its Significance

Q. Write short essay on role of MHC in disease.

Q. Write short essay on HLA and disease.

Q. Write short essay on HLA B27.

Every individual inherits one set of HLA genes from each parent and generally expresses two different HLA molecules for every locus. The combination of HLA alleles in each individual is called the HLA haplotype.

Polymorphism of HLA and its significance: *HLA* genes are highly polymorphic. There are innumerable combinations of HLA molecules in the population and each individual expresses an MHC profile on their cell surface that is different from the haplotypes of most other individuals. Due to polymorphism, it is unlikely to express the same MHC molecules by any two individuals (other than identical twins) in a population, Therefore, the immune system recognizes grafts exchanged between these individuals as foreign and mounts immune attack. Each HLA haplotype is inherited as a block. Because each individual receives two sets of genes from each parent, the chance that siblings will have the same MHC is 1 in 4. For this reason, whenever a kidney or HSC transplant is needed, siblings are first screened as potential donors for patients.

Role of MHC molecule in regulating T-cell-mediated immune responses: MHC molecules play many main roles in regulation of T-cell-mediated immune responses.

- Different antigenic peptides bind to different MHC molecules. An individual can elicit an immune response against a protein antigen only if the individual inherits an MHC variant that can bind peptides derived from the antigen and present it to T cells.
- Peptides are processed by different mechanisms in class I and class II MHC. By this difference, MHC molecules ensure that the correct immune response is mounted against different microbes.
  - CTL-mediated killing of cells harboring cytoplasmic microbes and tumor antigens
  - Helper T-cell-mediated antibody production and macrophage activation to combat extracellular and phagocytosed microbes.

HLA and Disease Association (Table 7)

Many autoimmune and other diseases are associated with the inheritance of particular HLA alleles. These diseases can be broadly grouped into:

- Inflammatory diseases (e.g., ankylosing spondylitis most strikingly associated with HLA-B27).
- Autoimmune diseases (e.g., autoimmune endocrinopathies associated with alleles at the DR locus).
- Inherited errors of metabolism [e.g., 21-hydroxylase deficiency (HLA-BW47) and hereditary hemochromatosis (HLA-A)].

Significance of HLA antigens: (1) Organ transplantation, (2) Play major role in recognition of foreign antigen and immunity, (3) Transfusion medicine and (4) Its association with diseases.

Tests for detection of HLA: (1)Lymphocytotoxicity test (MHC class I), (2) Mixed lymphocyte culture/reaction (MHC class II), (3) Primed lymphocyte typing, and (4) DNA analysis.

Table 7: Association of HLA alleles with diseases.

Disease	*HLA allele*
Class I MHC molecules	
• Ankylosing spondylitis	B27
• Post-gonococcal arthritis	
• Acute anterior uveitis	
• Beçhet's syndrome	B51
• 21-hydroxylase deficiency	HLA-BW47
• Hereditary hemochromatosis	HLA-A
Class II MHC molecules	
• Chronic active hepatitis	DR3
• Primary Sjögren syndrome	
• Rheumatoid arthritis	DR4
• Ulcerative colitis	DR103
• Type 1 diabetes mellitus	DR3/DR4
• Primary biliary cirrhosis	DR8
• Graves' disease and myasthenia gravis	DR3

(HLA: human leukocyte antigen; MHC: major histocompatibility complex)

Cytokines: Messenger Molecules of the Immune System

Immune responses involve multiple interactions among many cells. These cells include lymphocytes, DCs (dendritic cells), macrophages, other inflammatory cells (e.g., neutrophils), and endothelial cells. Some of these interactions are cell-to-cell contact. However, many interactions and effector functions of leukocytes are mediated by **short-acting, soluble, small, secreted proteins called cytokines. Molecularly cytokines are called interleukins**. The term interleukin (IL) was used because cytokines mediate communications between leukocytes. However, many cytokines also act on cells other than leukocytes. These cytokines represent the messenger (specialized regulatory) molecules of the immune system and contribute to different types of immune responses. ILs are a group of cytokines that regulate the immune and inflammatory responses. Most cytokines have a spectrum of effects. Some cytokines are produced by many different types of cells. The majority of cytokines act on the cells that produce them (autocrine actions) or on neighboring cells (paracrine) and rarely at a distance (endocrine).

Role of Cytokine in Immunity

Cytokines of innate immunity

- **Source:** In innate immune responses, cytokines are produced by cells immediately after the encounter with microbes and other stimuli. Main sources are macrophages, DCs, ILCs (innate lymphoid cells), and NK (natural killer) cells. They can also be produced by endothelial and epithelial cells.
- **Function:** These cytokines produce inflammation and inhibit virus replication (antiviral defense).
- **Cytokines involved in innate immunity:** These include TNF, IL-1, IL-12, type I IFNs (interferons), IFN-γ, and chemokines.

Cytokines of adaptive immune responses

- **Source:** These cytokines are produced mainly by CD4+ T lymphocytes in response to antigen and other signals.
- **Function:** They promote lymphocyte proliferation and differentiation and activate effector cells.
- **Cytokines involved in adaptive immunity:** This category includes IL-2, IL-4, IL-5, IL-17, and IFN-γ. Some cytokines limit and terminate immune responses (e.g., TGF-β, IL-10).

Colony-stimulating factors

- **Source:** They are produced by marrow stromal cells, T lymphocytes, macrophages, and other cells. These cytokines stimulate hematopoiesis. They are assayed by their ability to stimulate formation of blood cell colonies from bone marrow progenitors. Examples include granulocyte-macrophage colony-stimulating factor (GM-CSF) and other CSFs (colony-stimulating factors) and IL-3.
- **Function:** They increase the production of leukocyte, thereby increasing their numbers during immune and inflammatory responses. They also replace leukocytes that undergo death (by apoptosis) during such responses.

Therapeutic applications of cytokines: Cytokines have a role in practical therapeutic applications.

- **Inhibiting cytokine production or actions:** This approach is used for controlling the harmful effects of inflammation and tissue-damaging immune reactions. For example, dramatic responses to molecularly targeted therapy with TNF (tumor necrosis factor) antagonists in rheumatoid arthritis. Many other cytokine antagonists are found to be useful for the treatment of various inflammatory disorders.
- **Administration of cytokines to boost reactions:** Cytokines can be used to boost reactions that are normally dependent on these proteins. Cytokines can be used to boost hematopoiesis and defense against some viruses. For example, in stem cell transplantation, cytokines are used to mobilize HSCs from bone marrow to peripheral blood. From peripheral blood, they are collected and used for stem cell transplantation.
  Cytokines are discussed in detail on pages 291–304.

Overview of Lymphocyte Activation and Immune Responses

All adaptive immune responses have many steps and are listed in **Box 4**.

Box 4: Various steps in adaptive immune response.

- Antigen display and recognition
- Activation of specific lymphocytes
- Proliferation and differentiation of activated lymphocytes into effector and memory cells
- Elimination of the antigen
- Decline of the immune response
- Survival of long-lived memory cells

Display and Recognition of Antigens

Recognition of antigen by T cells

Microbes and other foreign antigens can enter the body anywhere. It is not possible for lymphocytes to effectively monitor every possible portal of antigen entry. This is because there are no sufficient antigen-specific lymphocytes to constantly cover all this field. This problem is overcome by capturing microbes and their protein antigens by DCs (one of the APCs) residing in epithelia and tissues. These antigens are carried and concentrated to draining in the lymph nodes. The naïve lymphocytes circulate through lymph nodes (and other secondary lymphoid organs) and increase the likelihood of these naïve lymphocytes to find and recognize the antigens. In the lymph node, the antigens are processed and displayed complexed with MHC molecules on the cell surface. The processed antigens are recognized by T cells.

Recognition of antigen by B cells

B lymphocytes recognize antigens of many different chemical types (including proteins, polysaccharides, and lipids) through their antigen receptors (membrane bound antibody molecules).

Innate immune response

When body comes across the antigens, first innate immune system is activated. This occurs even before the antigens of a microbe are recognized by T and B lymphocytes.

Pattern recognition receptors The microbe elicits an innate immune response through PRRs expressed on innate immune cells. This is the first line of defense and this also activates adaptive immunity.

Costimulators In immunization with a protein antigen, microbial mimics, called adjuvants, are also given along with the antigen. These adjuvants stimulate innate immune responses. During the innate immune response, the microbe or adjuvant activates APCs. These activated APCs express molecules called costimulators and secrete cytokines that stimulate the proliferation and differentiation of T lymphocytes. The main costimulators for T cells are the B7 proteins (CD80 and CD86). These are expressed on APCs and are recognized by the CD28 receptor on naïve T cells (**Fig. 8**). Thus, antigen ("signal 1") and costimulatory molecules produced during innate immune responses to microbes ("signal 2") function together and activate antigen-specific lymphocytes (**Fig. 8**). The requirement for microbe-triggered signal 2 makes sure that the adaptive immune response is induced by microbes and not by harmless substances. In immune responses against tumors and transplants, "signal 2" may be produced by molecules liberated from necrotic cells (the "DAMPs").

Activation of Lymphocytes and Elimination of Microbes

In an immune response, both T and B lymphocytes may be activated concurrently, but their reactions to antigens and functions differ in several ways.

Activation of T lymphocytes in cell-mediated immunity

Presentation of antigen to naïve T lymphocytes: Normally, naïve T lymphocytes pass through and circulate in secondary (peripheral) lymphoid organs. The initial activation of these naïve T lymphocytes occurs mainly in these secondary (peripheral) lymphoid organs. The mature DCs may present antigen to naïve T lymphocytes in secondary lymphoid organs.

Activation and differentiation of naïve T lymphocytes: In secondary (peripheral) lymphoid organs, naïve T lymphocytes are activated by antigens and costimulators. These activated naïve T lymphocytes proliferate and differentiate into effector T cells. The process of differentiation from naïve to effector cells gives these effector cells the capacity to perform specialized functions and the ability to migrate to any site of infection or inflammation. The effector T cells migrate to the site where microbial antigens are present (i.e., sites of infection) (**Fig. 19**). At the site of infection, the effector T cells are again activated by antigens and perform their various functions (e.g., activation of macrophages). The effector T cells may also remain in the lymphoid organs to help B lymphocytes.

Effector T cells of the CD4+ lineage (Fig. 20) One of the earliest responses of CD4+ helper T cells (effector cells) is secretion of the cytokine IL-2 and expression of high-affinity receptors for IL-2 on their surface. This triggers an autocrine loop wherein IL-2 acts as a growth factor that stimulates T-cell proliferation. This leads to an increase in the number of antigen-specific lymphocytes. The functions of CD4+ helper T cells are mediated by the combined actions of CD40-ligand (CD40L) and cytokines. When CD4+ helper T cells recognize antigens displayed by macrophages or B lymphocytes, the T cells express CD40L. This engages CD40 on the macrophages or B cells and activates CD4+ helper T cells. Sequence of events in T cell responses is depicted in **Figure 20**.

Subsets of effector CD4+ T cells: Some of the activated CD4+ T cells can differentiate into different subsets of effector cells. These subsets secrete distinct sets of cytokines and perform different functions (refer Fig. 48 of Chapter 8). The CD4+ T cells subsets are Th1, Th2, Th17, and Tfh.

- **Th1 cell subset:** These cells secrete the cytokine IFN-γ that is a potent macrophage activator. Th1 cells activate macrophages by contact-mediated signals delivered by CD40L-CD40 interactions and by IFN-γ. The combination of CD40- and IFN-γ-mediated activation causes "classical" macrophage activation (refer pages 309 and 310). This leads to the production of microbicidal substances in macrophages and they destroy ingested microbes.
- **Th2 cell subset:** These cells produce IL-4 and IL-5. IL-4 stimulates B cells to differentiate into IgE-secreting plasma cells whereas IL-5 stimulates the production of eosinophils in the marrow and activates eosinophils at sites of immune responses. Eosinophils and mast cells can bind to IgE-coated microbes such as helminthic parasites. Hence, they play a role in the elimination of helminths. Th2 cells also induce the "alternative" pathway of macrophage activation, which is involved in tissue repair and fibrosis.
- **Th17 cell subset:** These cells are named so because the cytokine secreted by these cells is IL-17. This cytokine recruits neutrophils and monocytes, which destroy extracellular bacteria and fungi. They are also involved in some inflammatory diseases such as autoimmune diseases.
- **Tfh cell subset [follicular helper T cells/T follicular helper (Tfh) cells]:** These cells migrate into the follicle and are required for germinal center formation in lymph node.

Effector T cells of the CD8+ lineage (Fig. 20) Activated CD8+ T lymphocytes differentiate into CTLs (cytotoxic T cells). These cells kill cells having ingested microbes in the cytoplasm. By killing the infected cells by CTLs, the reservoir of infection is eliminated. CTLs can also kill tumor cells by recognizing tumor-specific antigens displayed by tumor cells. These tumor antigens may be derived from mutated or abnormal cytoplasmic proteins.

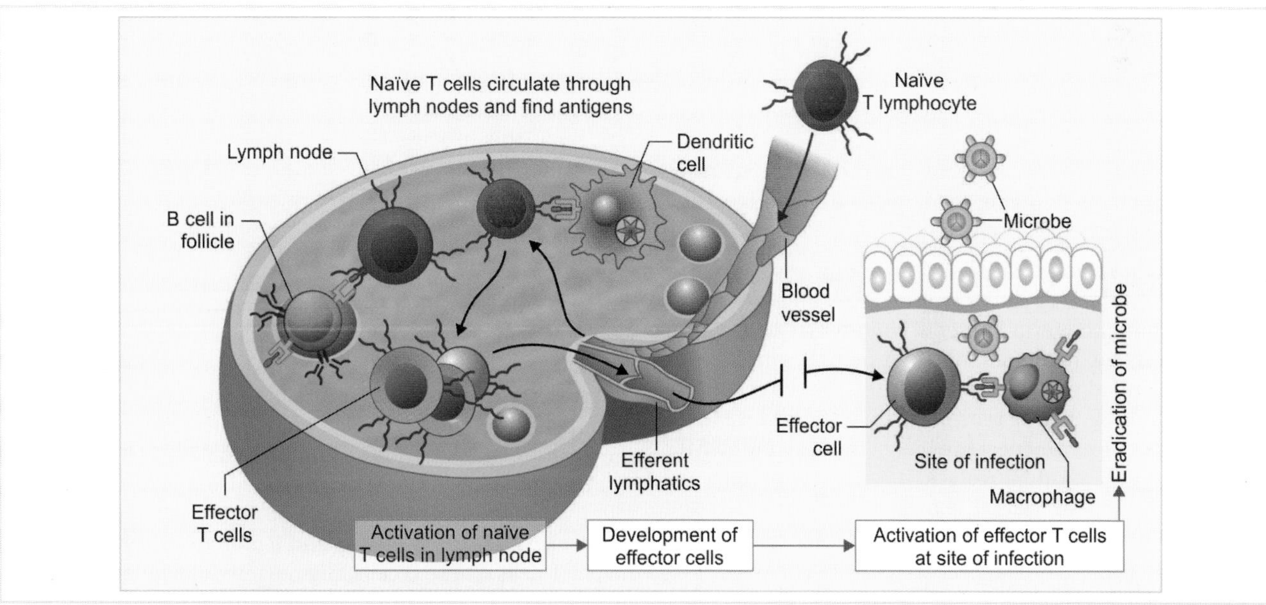

(MHC: major histocompatibility complex)

FIG. 19: Cell-mediated immunity: Activation of naïve and effector T cells by antigen. Dendritic cells capture microbial antigens from epithelia and tissues and transport the antigens to lymph nodes. During this process, the dendritic cells mature, and express high levels of MHC molecules and costimulators. In the lymph node, naïve T cells recognize MHC-associated peptide antigens displayed on dendritic cells. The naïve T cells are activated to proliferate and to differentiate into effector and memory T cells. These effector T cells may remain in the lymphoid organs to help B lymphocytes or migrate to sites of infection. At the site of infection, the effector T cells are again activated by antigens and perform their various functions in cell-mediated immunity (e.g., activation of macrophages).

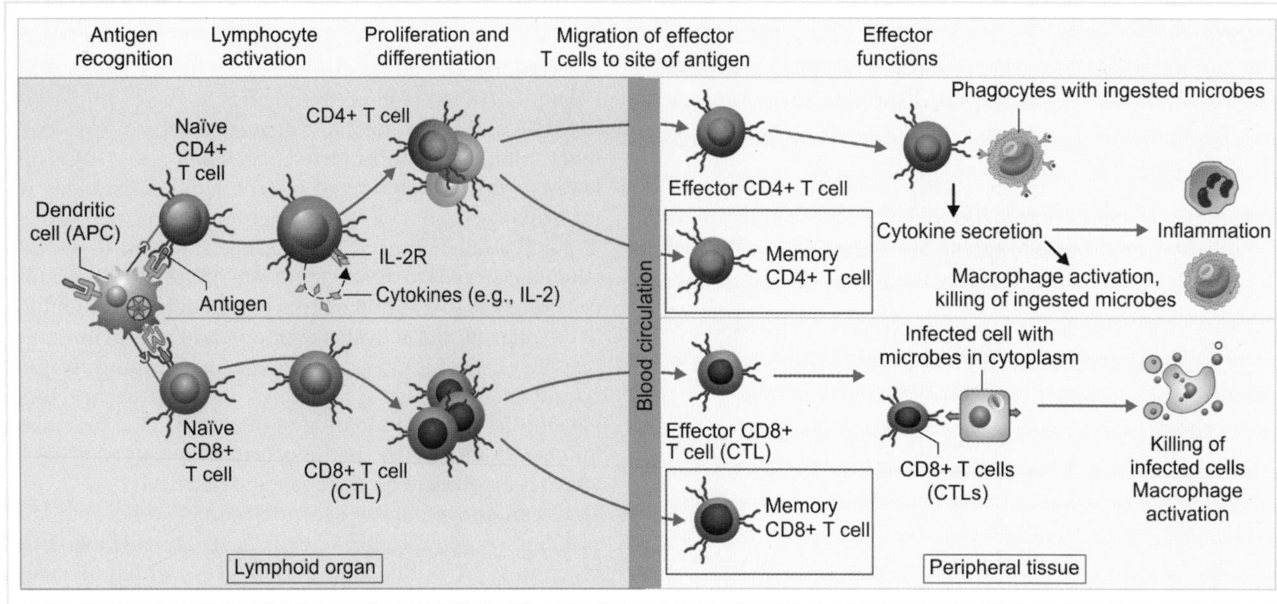

(APC: antigen-presenting cell)

FIG. 20: Sequence of events in T-cell responses. Dendritic cells present antigens to T cells. Antigen recognition by T cells induces cytokine (e.g., IL-2) secretion, particularly in CD4+ T cells. This will produce clonal expansion as a result of T-cell proliferation, and differentiation of the T cells into effector cells or memory cells. The effector CD4+ T cells respond to antigen by producing cytokines that have several actions. CD4+ effector T cells of the Th1 subset recognize the antigens of microbes ingested by phagocytes and activate the phagocytes to kill the microbes. Other subsets of effector cells recruit and activate leukocytes and stimulate different types of immune responses such as inflammation. Cytotoxic T lymphocytes (CTLs) are the effector cells of the CD8+ lineage. Effector CD8+ CTLs kill infected cells containing microbes in the cytoplasm and tumor cells and also secrete inflammatory cytokines that activate macrophages and induce inflammation. Some activated T cells remain in the lymphoid organs and help B cells to differentiate into antibody-secreting plasma cells, and some T cells differentiate into long-lived memory cells.

Activation of B lymphocytes in humoral immunity

In humoral immune responses, recognition of antigen is initiated by specific B lymphocytes in secondary lymphoid organs. The activation of B lymphocytes results in proliferation and differentiation B lymphocytes into antibody-secreting plasma cells and memory cells. Plasma cells secrete different classes of antibodies with distinct functions.

Antibody responses to antigens may be T-dependent or T-independent, depending on the nature of the antigen and the involvement of helper T cells.

T-dependent antibody response Antibody responses to most protein antigens need the help of T cell and are said to be T-dependent. The term helper T lymphocyte came from the realization that T cells stimulate, or help, B lymphocytes to produce antibodies. In these responses, B cells recognize protein antigens by their Ig receptors. They endocytose these antigens into vesicles and degrade them. Then B lymphocytes display peptides bound to class II MHC molecules for recognition by helper T cells. The helper T cells are activated and express CD40L and secrete cytokines. The activated helper T cells together with CD40L and secreted cytokine stimulate the B cells (lymphocytes).

Each plasma cell is derived from an antigen-stimulated B cell. These plasma cells secrete antibodies that recognize the same antigen that was bound by the BCR to initiate the response.

Isotype (class) switching (Fig. 21): In T-independent response to polysaccharides and lipids (described below) secretion by plasma cells is mainly low-affinity IgM antibody. In T-dependent responses to protein antigens, there is involvement of CD40L- and cytokine-mediated helper T-cell actions. In T-dependent responses, some of the progeny of activated IgM- and IgD-expressing B cells are induced to produce antibodies of different classes, or isotypes (IgG, IgA, IgE). This process is called heavy chain isotype (class) switching. This process leads to production of antibodies with heavy chains of different classes, such as γ, α, and ε. Thus, some activated B lymphocytes begin to produce antibodies other than IgM.

Affinity maturation (Fig. 22): As the immune response progresses, helper T cells also stimulate activated B cells to produce antibodies that bind to antigens with high (increasing) affinity. Progressively these B cells dominate the immune response. This process, called affinity maturation, improves the quality of the humoral immune response.

The above two processes (namely isotope switching and affinity maturation) are initiated during responses to protein antigens by activated B cells and simultaneous signals from helper T cells. These B cells migrate into follicles and begin to proliferate to form germinal centers. These **germinal centers of follicles are the major sites of isotype switching and affinity maturation**. The **helper T cells that stimulate these two processes in B lymphocytes also migrate to and reside in the germinal centers**. This type of T helper cells is called T **follicular helper (TFH/Tfh) cells**. Various phases of the humoral immune response are depicted in **Figure 23**.

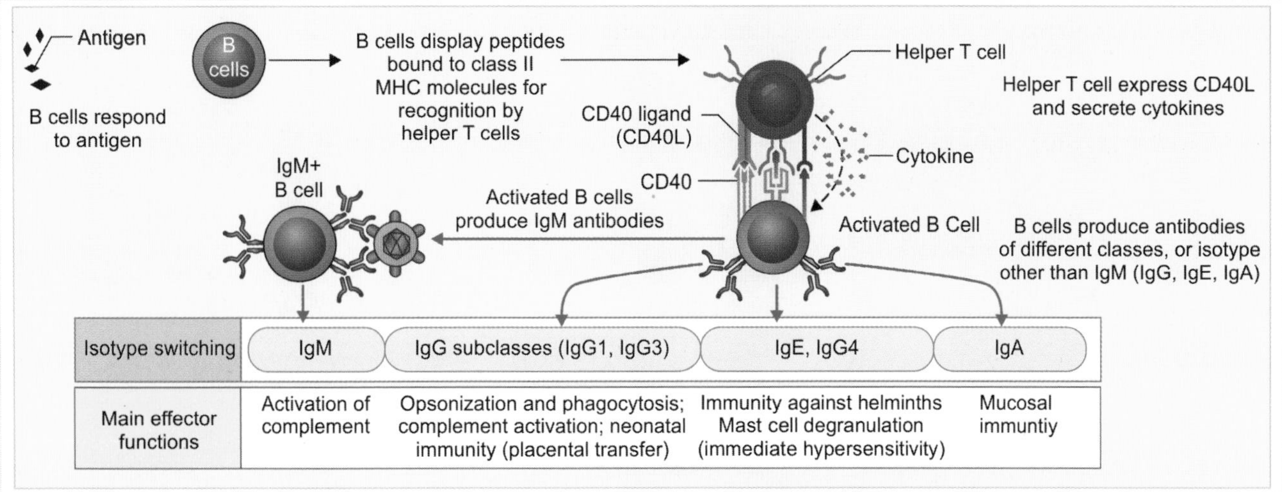

FIG. 21: Immunoglobulin (Ig) heavy chain isotype switching in T-dependent responses to antigens. B cells activated by helper T cell signals (CD40L, cytokines) undergo switching to different Ig isotypes. These different isotypes mediate distinct effector functions.

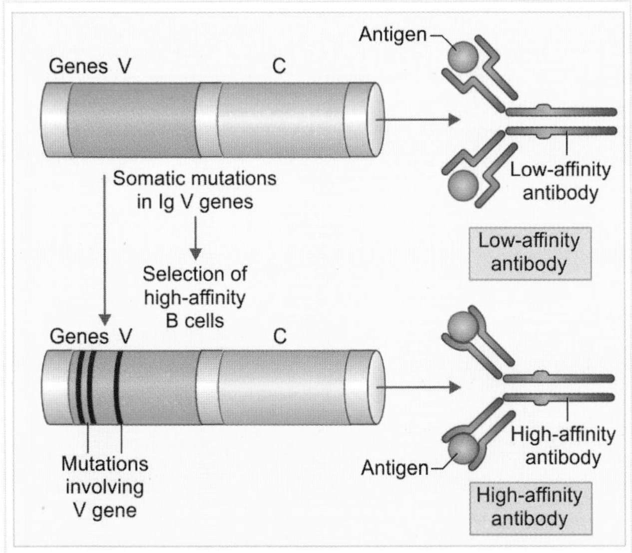

FIG. 22: Affinity maturation. During early immune response, there is production of low-affinity antibodies. During germinal center reaction, somatic mutation of Ig V genes [two genes namely V (variable region of Ig) and C (constant region of Ig)] and selection of B cells with high-affinity antigen receptors lead to the production of antibodies with high affinity for antigen.

Apart from isotype switching and affinity maturation, helper T cells also stimulate the production of long-lived plasma cells and generate memory B cells.

T-independent antibody response: Multivalent antigens with repeating determinants cannot be recognized by T cells. This is because they cannot bind to MHC molecules. But they have multiple identical antigenic determinants (epitopes) that can engage many antigen receptor molecules on each B cell and initiate the process of B-cell activation. This activation of B cells is without T cell help; hence these responses are said to be T-independent. Examples of these include many polysaccharide and lipid antigens. T-independent responses are rapid but relatively simple, consisting mostly of low-affinity IgM antibodies. But T-dependent responses show features such as Ig isotype switching and affinity maturation (described above) and require T cell help. T-dependent responses are slower to develop but are more potent, more varied, and effective.

Functions of antibodies in humoral response: Antibodies are produced by plasma cells in peripheral (secondary) lymphoid organs, inflamed tissues, and bone marrow. These antibodies exert their effector functions at sites distant from their production. The humoral immune response combats microbes in many ways (**Fig. 23**).

- **Neutralization of microbes and toxins:** Antibodies bind to microbes and toxins and neutralize them. This prevents them from infecting or injuring cells.
- **Opsonization and phagocytosis:** IgG antibodies coat (opsonize) microbes and favor them for phagocytosis. Phagocytes such as neutrophils and macrophages express receptors for the Fc fraction of immunoglobulin G (IgG). Phagocytosed microbes are destroyed within the phagocytes.
- **Antibody-dependent cellular cytotoxicity:** Antibodies can mediate cell destruction by antibody-dependent cell-mediated cytotoxicity.
- **Activation of complement:** IgG and IgM activate the complement system by the classical pathway. Products of the complement aid in phagocytosis and destruction of microbes. Activation of complement also leads to inflammation.
- **Special roles of some antibodies:** Some antibodies have special roles at particular anatomic sites.
    - **IgA in mucosa:** It is secreted from mucosal epithelia and they neutralize microbes in the lumens of the respiratory and gastrointestinal tracts. It is also secreted in other mucosal tissues.
    - **IgG transport through placenta:** IgG is actively transported across the placenta into the fetus. It protects the newborn till the immune system becomes mature.

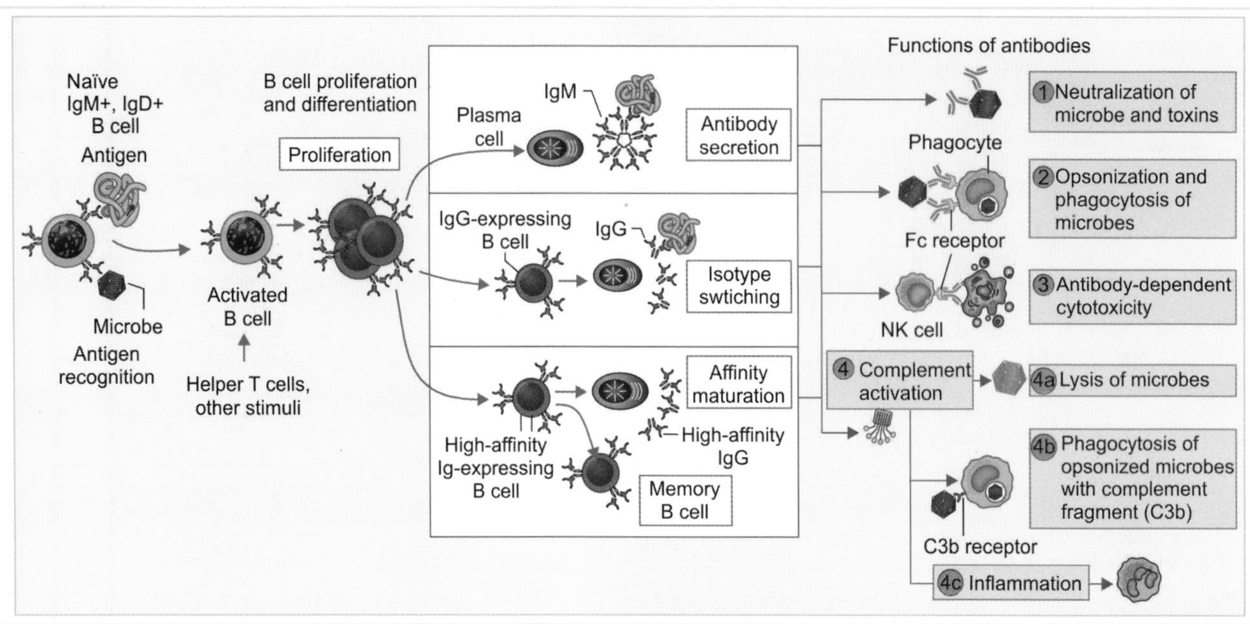

FIG. 23: Phases of the humoral immune response. B-cell activation is initiated by specific recognition of antigens by the surface Ig receptors of the B lymphocytes. Antigen and other stimuli, including helper T cells, stimulate the proliferation and differentiation of the specific B-cell clone. This clone may differentiate into antibody-secreting (IgM type) plasma cells. Some of the activated B cells undergo heavy-chain class switching (other Ig isotypes such as IgG), or may undergo affinity maturation, and some may become long-lived memory cells. These memory cells also usually undergo class switching and affinity maturation. Antibodies of different antibody isotypes (heavy-chain classes) perform different effector functions. Antibodies produced against microbes (and their toxins) neutralize these agents (1), opsonize them for phagocytosis (2), sensitize them for antibody-dependent cellular cytotoxicity (3), and activate the complement system. (4) Activated complement system may cause lysis of microbes (4a), phagocytosis of opsonized microbes (4b), and inflammation (4c).

- **IgE and eosinophils:** They together kill parasites. This is mainly achieved by the release contents present in cytoplasmic granules of eosinophil which are toxic to the worms. Cytokines secreted by Th2 stimulate the production of IgE and activate eosinophils, thereby assisting in killing of worms.

The half-lives of most circulating IgG antibodies are about 3 weeks. Some antibody-secreting plasma cells, especially those produced in germinal centers, migrate to the bone marrow and stay there for months to years. They continuously produce antibodies during this period.

Decline of Immune Responses and Immunologic Memory

After the **elimination of microbe, most of the effector lymphocytes,** induced by an infectious pathogen, **undergo death by apoptosis**. The immune system returns to its resting state.

Memory lymphocytes

Long-lived cells: The activation of lymphocytes by adaptive immunity during infections also produces long-lived memory cells. These memory cells may survive in a functionally quiescent or slowly cycling state for months or years after the elimination of microbial infection.

Frequency of memory cells: Memory cells constitute an expanded pool of antigen-specific lymphocytes. They are more in number than the naïve cells specific for any antigen that are present before encounter with that antigen. As age increases, the frequency of memory cells increases. This is because individuals are continually exposed to environmental microbes. Memory T cells constitute <5% of peripheral blood T cells in a newborn but 50% or more in an adult (**Fig. 24**).

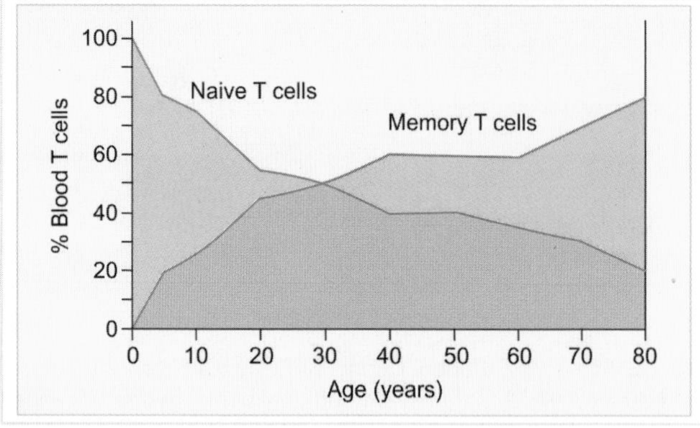

FIG. 24: Change in proportions of naïve and memory T cells in relation to age.

Response to re-exposed antigen: When re-exposed to the antigen, memory cells respond faster and more effectively than do naïve cells.

Subsets of memory cells: Memory cells are heterogeneous. There are subsets that differ in their location and migratory properties.

- **Memory T cells:** Immune responses against an antigen by T cells usually generate memory T cells specific for that antigen. These cells may persist for years, even a lifetime. Memory cells are able to survive in a quiescent state after antigen is eliminated. They mount larger and more rapid responses to antigens than naïve cells. Memory cells express increased levels of antiapoptotic proteins and may be responsible for their prolonged survival.

- **Memory B cells:** These are produced during the germinal center reaction. They cause rapid responses to subsequent introduction of antigen. Since memory B cells are produced mainly in germinal centers, they are seen in T-dependent immune responses.

Production of memory cells is the basis of the effectiveness of vaccination.

HYPERSENSITIVITY: IMMUNOLOGICALLY MEDIATED TISSUE INJURY

Q. Write short essay on concept of hypersensitivity disorders.

Immune response is usually the important function of host defense and is a protective process. But sometimes it is also capable of causing tissue injury and disease. Disorders caused by immune responses are called hypersensitivity diseases. According to the clinical definition, immunity is considered as sensitivity. When an individual who has been exposed to an antigen shows a detectable reaction, or is sensitive, to subsequent contact with the same antigen. Hence the term sensitivity, and individual is said to be sensitized. Normally, immune responses get rid of infectious pathogens without causing any serious injury to host tissues. Hypersensitivity means that the body responds to a particular antigen in an exaggerated fashion, where it does not happen in normal circumstances. Thus, **hypersensitivity is** considered as **an immune response that is inadequately controlled, inappropriately triggered, excessive, or produces undesirable effects on the body**.

Definition: Hypersensitivity reaction is a **pathological, excessive, and injurious immune response to antigen, leading to tissue injury or disease**. Sometimes hypersensitivity can cause death in a sensitized individual. The resulting diseases are named as hypersensitivity diseases.

General Features of Hypersensitivity Disorders

Nature of Antigens

Specific antigens that cause hypersensitivity diseases may be derived from different sources. It may be exogenous antigens or endogenous self-antigens.

Exogenous environmental antigens

These can be microbial and nonmicrobial.

- **Nonmicrobial environmental antigens:** Most healthy individuals do not react against common, generally harmless environmental substances. Some individuals abnormally respond to one or more of these substances. These substances include dust, pollen, food, drugs, and various chemicals. The hypersensitivity reactions against such exogenous antigens may show wide range. For example, in type I hypersensitivity, it may range from mild annoying (irritating) with minor discomforts (e.g., itching of the skin) to potentially fatal diseases (e.g., anaphylaxis). Some of the most common group of diseases known as allergy, are due to reactions against environmental antigens.
- **Microbial environmental antigens:** Immune responses against microbial antigens may cause disease if the reactions are excessive or the microbes are unusually persistent.
    - **Excessive reactions:** Antibodies are usually produced against microbial antigens. These antibodies may bind to the antigens to produce immune complexes. These immune complexes may be deposited in tissues and cause inflammation. For example, immune complex (type III) hypersensitivity.
    - **Unusually persistent microbes:** For example, T-cell responses against persistent microbes such as *Mycobacterium tuberculosis* may cause severe inflammation with formation of granulomas (type IV hypersensitivity). This is the cause of tissue injury in tuberculosis.

Endogenous self-antigens: Immune responses against self, or autologous, antigens, produce autoimmune diseases. By convention, the term hypersensitivity refers to harmful immune responses against exogenous/foreign antigens (environmental antigens, drugs, microbes). It is not used for tissue injury in autoimmune diseases.

Imbalance between the Effector Mechanisms and the Control Mechanisms

In normal immune response, there is a balance between the effector mechanisms and the control mechanisms. This balance regulates and limits the immune responses. Hypersensitivity usually results from an imbalance between the effector mechanisms and the control mechanisms of immune response. Many hypersensitivity diseases are probably due to failure of this normal regulation. This is clearly evident in autoimmunity.

Genetic Susceptibility

Often the development of hypersensitivity diseases (both allergic and autoimmune) is associated with the inheritance of particular susceptibility genes. This includes involvement of both *HLA* genes and *non-HLA* genes in different diseases.

Mechanisms of tissue injury in hypersensitivity reactions In hypersensitivity, the mechanisms of tissue injury are the same as the effector mechanisms of normal defense against infectious pathogens. But, in hypersensitivity, these effector mechanisms are poorly controlled, excessive, or misdirected (e.g., against normally harmless environmental and self-antigens).

Classification of Hypersensitivity Reactions (Table 8)

Hypersensitivity reactions are classified depending on the type of immune response and the effector mechanism responsible for cell and tissue injury (**Table 7**). This classification distinguishes the manner in which an immune response causes tissue injury and disease, and also pathologic and clinical manifestations. These mechanisms include some that are predominantly dependent on antibodies and others predominantly dependent on T cells. However, it is to be noted that both humoral and cell-mediated immunity may be operative in many hypersensitivity diseases.

Table 8: Classification of hypersensitivity reaction according to the effector immune mechanism.

Types	*Mechanism of injury*
Antibody mediated	
1. Immediate hypersensitivity reaction (type I hypersensitivity)	Production of IgE antibody. Immediate release of vasoactive amines and other mediators from mast cells and later recruitment of leukocytes
2. Antibody-mediated disorders (type II hypersensitivity)	IgG and IgM antibodies that bind to fixed tissue or target cell surface antigens; phagocytosis or lysis of target cell by activated complement or Fc receptors; recruitment of leukocytes
3. Immune complex-mediated disorders (type III hypersensitivity)	Deposition of antigen–antibody complexes leads to activation of complement; recruitment of leukocytes by complement products and Fc receptors; Release of enzymes and other toxic molecules
Cell mediated	
4. Cell-mediated immune disorders (type IV hypersensitivity)	Activated T lymphocytes lead to—(1) release of cytokines, inflammation, and activation of macrophage and (2) T-cell-mediated cytotoxicity

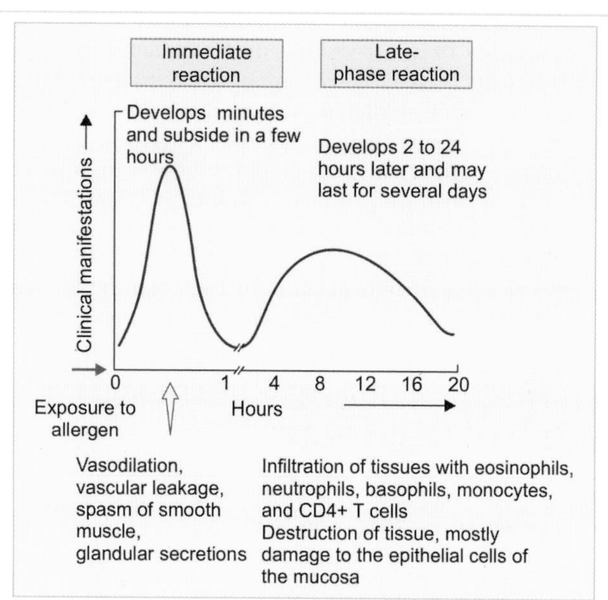

FIG. 25: Two phases of immediate (type I) hypersensitivity reactions consist of immediate and late-phase reactions.

Immediate hypersensitivity (type I hypersensitivity): In this type, the tissue injury is caused by Th2 cells, IgE antibodies, and mast cells and other leukocytes. Mediators released from mast cells act on vessels and smooth muscle. The proinflammatory cytokines released from mast cells also recruit inflammatory cells.

Antibody-mediated disorders (type II hypersensitivity): This type is caused by IgG and IgM antibodies and can produce disease by two mechanisms:

1. Antibodies injure cells by promoting their phagocytosis or lysis and injure tissues by producing inflammation.
2. Antibodies can interfere with cellular functions and cause disease without any tissue injury.

Immune complex-mediated disorders (type III hypersensitivity): IgG and IgM antibodies bind antigens usually in the circulation, and form antigen-antibody complexes deposit. These immune complexes get deposited in tissues and produce inflammation. The leukocytes recruited (neutrophils and monocytes) at the site of deposition produce tissue damage by release of lysosomal enzymes and producing toxic free radicals.

Cell-mediated immune disorders (type IV hypersensitivity): In this type, T lymphocytes (Th1 and Th17 cells and CD8+ CTLs) are the cause of the tissue injury.

Immediate (Type I) Hypersensitivity Reactions

Q. Write short note on type I hypersensitivity reactions and its pathogenesis.

Definition: Immediate, or type I, hypersensitivity reaction is a rapid immunologic reaction occurring in a previously sensitized individual. It is triggered by the binding of an antigen to IgE antibody on the surface of mast cells.

Usually type I hypersensitivity reactions are called as allergy. The exogenous (environmental) antigens that bring out these reactions are known as allergens. It may occur as a local reaction or as a systemic reaction.

- **Local reactions:** They are varied depending on the portal of entry of the allergen. Examples include localized cutaneous rash or blisters (skin allergy, hives), nasal and conjunctival discharge (allergic rhinitis and conjunctivitis), hay fever, bronchial asthma, or allergic gastroenteritis (food allergy).
- **Systemic reaction:** They usually follow injection of an antigen into a sensitized individual (e.g., by a bee sting). However, they can also follow ingestion of antigen (e.g., peanut allergens). Sometimes, the patient goes into a state of shock within minutes and this may be fatal.

Phases of local type I hypersensitivity: Many of the local type I hypersensitivity reactions consist of two well-defined phases—immediate and late reactions (**Fig. 25**).

- **Immediate reaction:** It is characterized by vasodilation and vascular leakage. There is also spasm of smooth muscle or glandular secretions depending on the tissue involved. These changes generally develop within minutes after exposure to an allergen and likely to subside in a few hours.
- **Late-phase reaction:** In many occasions (e.g., allergic rhinitis and bronchial asthma), a second, late-phase reaction occurs in 2–24 hours later without additional exposure to antigen. This may last for several days. This is characterized by infiltration of tissues with eosinophils, neutrophils, basophils, monocytes, and CD4+ T cells. There is also destruction of tissue, mostly damage to the epithelial cells of the mucosa.

Characteristics

Immediate reaction occurring within minutes (5–10 minutes). Hence, type I hypersensitivity is also known as immediate hypersensitivity.

Th2 cells: Most are caused by excessive Th2 responses. Th2 cells play a main role by stimulating IgE production and promoting inflammation.

Exposure to allergens: Reaction develops after the interaction of an environmental antigen (allergens) with IgE antibodies bound to mast cells.

Genetic susceptibility: Occurs in genetically susceptible individuals previously sensitized to the antigen. There is a strong genetic or hereditary linkage regarding the IgE response to antigens (allergens). This genetic component involves both the ability to respond to an allergen and the general ability to produce an IgE antibody response.

Antigens (allergens): Many allergens (e.g., house dust mite, pollens, animal danders or molds) in the environment are harmless for majority of individuals. Allergens elicit significant IgE reactions only in genetically predisposed individuals, who are said to be atopic.

Pathogenesis

Th2-mediated immediate (type I) hypersensitivity reactions (disorders) show a characteristic sequence of events (**Fig. 26**) and are as follows:

Initial exposure to sensitizing antigen: Initial exposure to antigen is called as sensitization. Individuals are exposed to environmental allergens. They may be introduced by—(1) inhalation, (2) ingestion or (3) injection.

Activation of Th2 cells and production of IgE antibody

Probably **DCs capture the antigen** (allergen) from its site of entry and **present it to naïve T cell**. The antigen and other stimuli include cytokines such as IL-4 produced at the local site. This leads to **differentiation of T cells into Th2 cells**. For obscure reasons, only some environmental antigens elicit strong Th2 responses and thus act as allergens. On subsequent exposure to the same antigen, the newly formed Th2 cells produce many cytokines. Main cytokines are IL-4, IL-5, and IL-13.

- **IL-5:** Eosinophils are important effector cells of type I hypersensitivity. IL-5 is involved in the development and activation of eosinophils.
- **IL-13:** It increases production of IgE and acts on epithelial cells to stimulate mucus secretion.
- **IL-4:** It acts on B cells and stimulates class switching to IgE and promotes the development of additional Th2 cells.

Th2 cells (also mast cells and epithelial cells) also produce chemokines. These attract more Th2 cells, as well as other leukocytes, to the reaction site.

- **Th2-high and Th2-low atopic diseases:** Patients with chronic atopic diseases (e.g., asthma, atopic dermatitis) may be classified into Th2-high and Th2-low. This is based on biomarkers that indicate the intensity of the pathologic T-cell response in patients. This may be important for therapy, because antagonists of Th2 cytokines (IL-4, IL-5) are probably most effective in patients belonging to Th2-high group.

Initial response by type 2 ILCs (innate lymphoid cells): Before the development of Th2 responses, type 2 ILCs present in tissues may respond to cytokines produced by damaged epithelia. These ILCs secrete IL-5 and IL-13 and these can produce the same tissue reactions that are induced by the classical Th2 cells. Over time, the Th2 cells become the predominant contributor to the local cytokine response.

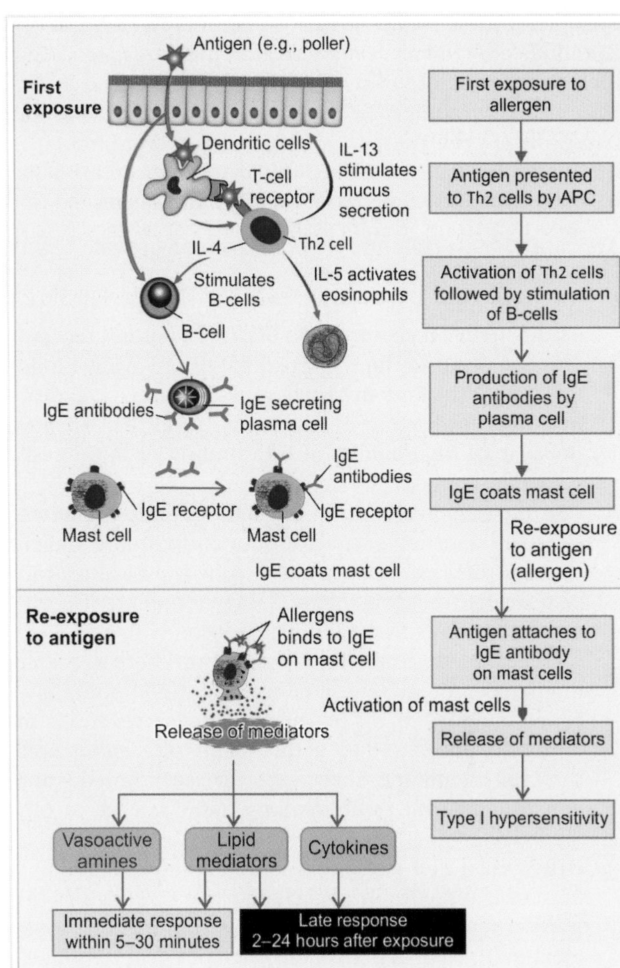

FIG. 26: Sequence of events in immediate (type I) hypersensitivity. It is initiated by the exposure to an allergen. Antigens are taken up by the antigen presenting cell (APC) and presents and stimulate Th2 responses and IgE production, in genetically susceptible individuals. IgE binds to mast cells. On re-exposure to the allergen, antigen binds to IgE on the mast cells and activates it to secrete the mediators. These mediators produce the manifestations of immediate (type I) hypersensitivity.

Production of IgE antibody: IL-4 secreted by Th2 cells acts on B cells and stimulates class switching to IgE. These IgE antibodies are cytotropic.

Sensitization and activation of mast cells

Mast cells and basophils

Mast cells: They play main role in immediate hypersensitivity. These are derived from bone marrow and are widely distributed in the tissues. They are abundant near small blood vessels and nerves and in subepithelial tissues. This is the reason for occurrence of local immediate hypersensitivity reactions usually at these sites. Mast cells contain membrane-bound granules in the cytoplasm and they contain a variety of biologically active mediators (refer page 273).

Basophils: These are the circulating counterpart of mast cells. Basophils are similar to mast cells in many respects. These include the presence of cell surface IgE Fc receptors and the cytoplasmic granules. In contrast to mast cells, normally basophils are not present in tissues but rather circulate in the blood in small numbers. Similar to other granulocytes, basophils can also be recruited to inflammatory sites.

Activators: Mast cells and basophils can be activated by IgE antibodies and nonantibodies.

- **IgE antibody:** Mast cells and basophils express a high-affinity IgE Fc receptor called FcεRI (Fc epsilon receptor). This is specific for the Fc portion of IgE and avidly binds to IgE antibodies. Both mast cells and basophils are activated by the cross-linking of high-affinity IgE Fc receptors. Because of high avidity of IgE binding, it is termed as cytophilic antibody.
- **C5a and C3a:** In addition, mast cells may also be activated by several other stimuli. Some individuals develop urticaria after exposure to an ice cube (physical urticaria) or pressure (dermographism). The complement-derived anaphylatoxins such as complement components C5a and C3a can directly stimulate mast cells by a different receptor-mediated process. These complement components are called anaphylatoxins because they elicit reactions that mimic anaphylaxis. Both of them bind to receptors on the mast cell membrane. They trigger release of stored granule constituents and rapid synthesis and release of other mediators.
- **Other mast cell activators:** Some compounds activate mast cells directly. These include some chemokines (e.g., IL-8), drugs such as codeine and morphine, adenosine, melittin (present in bee venom), and physical stimuli (e.g., heat, cold, sunlight).

Sensitization of mast cells by IgE antibody IgE antibodies produced by B cells attach to the IgE Fc receptors on the mast cells. These IgE antibody bearing mast cells are said to be sensitized because they are activated by subsequent exposure with antigen. IgE bound to Fcε receptors on mast cells and basophils can persist for years.

Activation of mast cells during re-exposure

Activation of mast cells by re-exposure to antigen

Activation of mast cell: In sensitized individual, the mast cell bears IgE antibodies previously produced in response to an antigen. When these mast cells are exposed to the same antigen (specific allergen), the antigen binds to the IgE antibodies on the surface of mast cell. It activates these mast cells. To activate the mast cell, antigen must cross-link at least two adjacent IgE antibody molecules (refer **Fig. 27**).

Release of mediators from mast cells

When multivalent (having several sites for attachment) antigens bind to and cross-link adjacent IgE antibodies, it brings the underlying Fcε receptors together. In the mast cells, this activates signal transduction pathways from the cytoplasmic portion of the receptors. This leads to the release of preformed mediators and de novo (newly synthesized) production of mediators.

Regardless of mast cell activator (IgE antibody or non-antibody), mast cell activations are associated with raised levels of cytosolic free calcium in mast cells. This triggers an increase in cyclic adenosine monophosphate (cAMP) and activates several metabolic pathways within the mast cell. Activated mast cells secrete both preformed and newly synthesized products. These mediators are responsible for the initial, sometimes explosive, symptoms of immediate hypersensitivity. This also set into motion the events that lead to the late-phase reaction. Thus, IgE triggered reactions can be divided into two phases—immediate response and late-phase reaction.

Mediators of Immediate Hypersensitivity

During the effector phase of immediate hypersensitivity reactions, mast cells and eosinophils are activated to rapidly release mediators. They cause increased vascular permeability, vasodilation, and bronchial and visceral smooth muscle contraction. This vascular reaction is called **immediate hypersensitivity** because it begins rapidly, within minutes of antigen challenge in a previously sensitized individual (immediate). Following the immediate response, there is a more slowly developing inflammatory component called the **late-phase reaction**. This is characterized by the accumulation of neutrophils, eosinophils, and macrophages. The term immediate hypersensitivity is usually used to describe the combined immediate and late-phase reactions. Clinically, immediate (type I) hypersensitivity reactions are called **allergy or atopy**, and the associated diseases are called **allergic, atopic, or immediate hypersensitivity diseases.**

Mast cell activation first leads to degranulation with release of preformed (primary), stored mediators in their granules. They are stored in mast cell granules. There is also de novo synthesis (newly synthesized) and release of additional mediators. Two important mediators that are synthesized de novo are lipid products and cytokines.

Granule contents First the mediators contained within mast cell granules are released and these can be divided into three categories:

1. **Vasoactive amines:** Histamine is the most important vasoactive amine released from mast cell granules. Histamine causes severe contraction of both vascular and nonvascular smooth muscle, microvascular dilation, increases vascular permeability, and stimulates mucus secretion by nasal, bronchial, and gastric glands. These effects are mainly mediated through H1 histamine receptors. Gastric acid secretion is mediated through H2 histamine receptors. In the lungs, it causes bronchospasm, vascular congestion, and edema.
2. **Enzymes:** The matrix of mast cell granule contains enzymes. These include neutral proteases (chymase, tryptase, carboxypeptidase) and several acid hydrolases. These enzymes produce damage to the tissue as well as act on the precursor proteins and generate kinins (kinin system) and activated components of complement (complement system) by acting on their precursor proteins. Most important complement component is C3a.
3. **Proteoglycans:** The proteoglycans present in mast cell granules pack and store the vasoactive amines in the granules. These proteoglycans include heparin (anticoagulant) and chondroitin sulfate.

Lipid mediators

- **Arachidonic acid metabolites:** The most important lipid mediators are the products derived from arachidonic acid (refer Fig. 18 and pages 251–254). Mast cell activation is associated with activation of an enzyme called phospholipase A_2. This enzyme converts membrane phospholipids to arachidonic acid. The 5-lipoxygenase and the cyclooxygenase pathways of arachidonic acid produce two main compounds namely, leukotrienes and prostaglandins, respectively.

- **Leukotrienes:** Leukotrienes C_4 and D_4 are the most powerful vasoactive and spasmogenic agents produced through lipoxygenase pathway of arachidonic acid. They are several thousand times more active than histamine. They increase vascular permeability and cause contraction of bronchial smooth muscle. Leukotriene B_4 is also powerful chemotactic mediator for neutrophils, eosinophils, and monocytes.
- **Prostaglandin D_2:** This is the most abundant mediator in mast cells generated by the cyclooxygenase pathway of arachidonic acid. It causes severe bronchospasm and increases mucus secretion.

- **Platelet-activating factor (PAF):** PAF (refer page 254) is a lipid mediator that is not derived from arachidonic acid. It is a mediator derived from membrane phospholipids and is produced by some population of mast cell. It causes platelet aggregation, histamine release, bronchospasm, increased vascular permeability, and vasodilation. However, its role in immediate hypersensitivity reactions is not well established.

Cytokines These are derived from mast cells as well as inflammatory cells recruited to the site during late-phase reaction.

- **Mast cell derived:** Mast cells synthesize and secrete many cytokines. These cytokines may play an important role at several stages of immediate hypersensitivity reactions. The cytokines include TNF (tumor necrosis factor), IL-1, and chemokines, which attract leukocyte (recruitment) to the site (is characteristic of the late-phase reaction); IL-4, which amplifies the Th2 response; and many others.
- **Inflammatory cell derived:** The inflammatory cells that are recruited by mast cell–derived TNF and chemokines are also the sources of cytokines.

Actions of mediators of immediate hypersensitivity (Fig. 27)
Most of the manifestations of immediate hypersensitivity reactions are brought out by the mediators produced by mast cells.

- **Immediate response:** Some mediators such as histamine and leukotrienes are released rapidly from sensitized mast cells. They produce the intense immediate reactions (response) characterized by edema (due to vascular leakage), mucus secretion, and smooth muscle spasm.
- **Late-phase response:** Cytokines, including chemokines, recruit additional leukocytes (inflammatory cells) to the site of hypersensitivity reaction and set the stage for the late-phase response. These inflammatory cells release additional mediators (including cytokines) as well as they cause damage to the epithelial cells. These epithelial cells can also produce soluble mediators, such as chemokines.

Late-phase Reaction

Leukocytes are recruited in the late-phase reaction. These leukocytes amplify and sustain the inflammatory response without additional exposure to the triggering antigen (allergen).

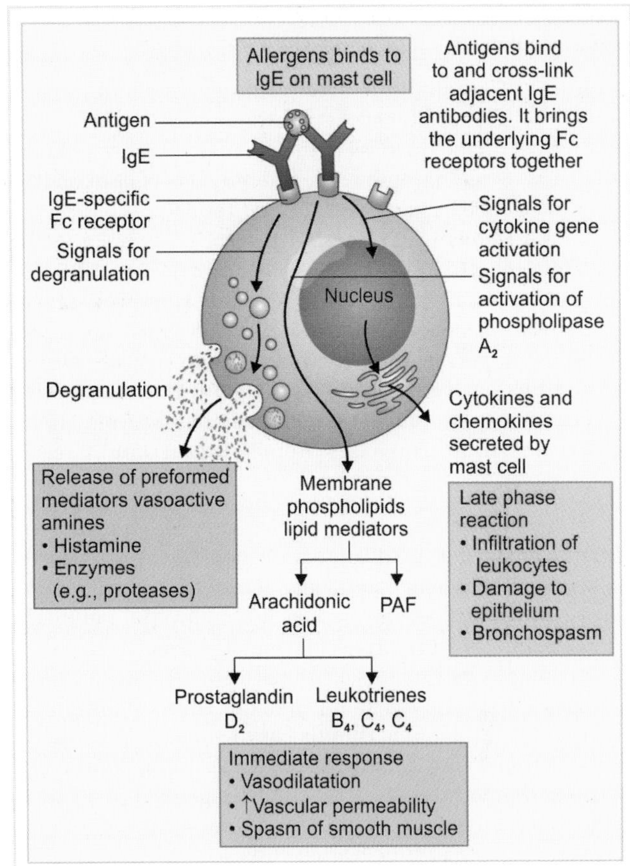

(PAF: platelet-activating factor)

FIG. 27: Mast cell mediators involved in type I hypersensitivity. Activated mast cells release various classes of mediators. These are responsible for the immediate and late-phase reactions.

Eosinophils Eosinophils are the leukocytes that are usually plenty in type I hypersensitivity reactions.

Chemotactic factors that recruit eosinophils: Eosinophils are recruited to sites of immediate hypersensitivity by chemokines, such as eotaxin, and others. These mediators may be produced by epithelial cells, Th2 cells, and mast cells.

- IL-5: IL-5 derived from Th2 is the most potent eosinophil activating cytokine.
- Upon activation, eosinophils release proteolytic enzymes as well as two unique proteins which damage tissues. These proteins are—(1) major basic protein and (2) eosinophil cationic protein.
- **Charcot–Leyden crystals:** Eosinophils contain crystals called as Charcot–Leyden crystals. They are composed of the protein galectin-10. Sometimes, Charcot–Leyden crystals are released into the extracellular space and can be found in the sputum of patients with asthma. These crystals promote inflammation and increase Th2 responses. Thus, they may contribute to allergic reactions.

Secondary (newly synthesized) mediators

Cytokines: Inflammatory infiltrate is mediated by many cytokines. For example, TNF, IL-1, and chemokines promote leukocyte recruitment during the late-phase reaction. Lipid mediators: They are synthesized and secreted by mast cells, include leukotrienes and prostaglandins.

Products of arachidonic acid pathway: Arachidonic acid derivatives are produced by a variety of cell types. Their products of cyclooxygenase pathways include prostaglandins D_2, E_2, and F_2 and thromboxane and products of lipoxygenase pathway include leukotrienes B_4, C_4, D_4, and E_4.

- **Leukotrienes C_4, D_4, and E_4,** are previously known as "slow-reacting substances of anaphylaxis" (SRS-As). Leukotrienes C_4 and D_4 are the most powerful (several thousand times than histamine) and cause increased vascular permeability and bronchial smooth muscle contraction. Leukotriene B_4 is a powerful chemotactic factor for neutrophils, eosinophils, and monocytes.
- **Prostaglandin D_2** causes bronchospasm and increased mucus secretion.

Platelet-activating factor: It is a lipid derived from membrane phospholipids. It is an inflammatory mediator synthesized by mast cells. PAF is a potent inducer of platelet aggregation and release of vasoactive amines. It is also a powerful neutrophil chemotaxin. PAF can activate all types of phagocytic cells.

In some type I hypersensitivity disorders (e.g., allergic asthma), late-phase reaction is a major cause of symptoms. For example, in allergic rhinitis (hay fever) which is due to immediate reaction, antihistamine drugs are beneficial. But diseases due to late-phase reactions (e.g., allergic asthma) require broad-spectrum anti-inflammatory drugs, such as steroids, rather than antihistamine drugs.

Development of Allergies

The development of allergies is the result of **gene–environment interactions**. These interactions are complex and poorly understood.

Genetic predisposition

Susceptibility to and development of immediate hypersensitivity reactions is genetically determined. The role of genetic predisposition for the development of allergies is well known and many susceptibility genes have been identified. There is higher concordance (co-occurrence) of allergies in identical twins than in nonidentical twins. Relatives of individuals with allergy are more likely to have allergies than unrelated individuals, even when they are exposed to different environments.

Atopy: Tendency to develop immediate hypersensitivity reactions is called atopy. In atopy, there is a familial predisposition to produce an exaggerated localized immediate hypersensitivity (IgE-mediated) reaction to inhaled and ingested environmental substances (allergens) that are otherwise harmless. Atopic individuals usually have higher serum levels of IgE, and more IL-4 producing Th2 cells than normal individuals. In 50% of atopic individuals, there is a positive family history of allergy. Though the basis of familial predisposition is not known, in patients with asthma polymorphisms in several genes (in the locus for atopy on chromosome 5q) encoding cytokines with important roles in allergic reactions have been observed. These include the genes for the cytokines IL-3, IL-4, IL-5, IL-9, IL-13, and GM-CSF13 and the IL-4 receptor. Polymorphisms within the *HLA* genes located on chromosome 6 have also been observed.

Environmental factors

Environmental factors (influences) are also important in the development of allergic diseases. They synergize with genetic risk factors.

Atopic allergy Environmental influences include exposure to environmental pollutants (allergens), to infectious organisms, and other factors that impact mucosal barrier function, such as air pollution. It appears that the time of life when exposure to these environmental factors occurs may be important (especially early-life exposure).

Hygiene hypothesis: According to this hypothesis, exposure to some pathogens (microbes) during infancy and childhood benefits individuals and may reduce the risk for developing allergies. Early childhood and even prenatal exposure to microbial antigens "educates" the immune system. On subsequent exposure, this educated immune system prevents pathologic responses against common environmental allergens. If there is improved hygiene in early childhood, there will not be exposure to microbial antigens and immune system is not trained to handle these antigens. Hence, they are more likely to develop allergies later in life.

Nonatopic allergy In about 20–30% of individuals with immediate hypersensitivity reactions, the stimuli are nonantigenic such as extremes of temperature and exercise. They neither involve Th2 cells nor IgE. Such reactions are sometimes called nonatopic allergy. Probably, in these individuals, mast cells are abnormally sensitive to activation by various nonimmune stimuli.

Allergic Diseases in Humans

Clinical manifestations and pathologic features of allergic reactions (diseases) depend on the tissues (point of contact with the allergen) involved, anatomic site of the reaction, and the chronicity of the resulting inflammatory process.

- **Point of contact:** The point of contact with the allergen can determine the organs or tissues where mast cells and Th2 cells are activated. For example, inhaled antigens cause rhinitis or asthma, ingested antigens usually produce vomiting and diarrhea (but if larger doses are ingested, it can also produce skin and respiratory symptoms), and injected antigens cause systemic effects on the circulation.
- **Concentration of mast cells:** The concentration of mast cells varies in different tissues and its concentration in the involved organ influences the severity of responses. Mast cells are particularly abundant in the skin and the mucosa of the respiratory and gastrointestinal tracts. Hence, these tissues generally suffer the most injury in immediate hypersensitivity reactions.
- **Phenotype of mast cells:** The local mast cell phenotype may influence the characteristics of the immediate hypersensitivity reaction. For example, connective tissue mast cells secrete abundant histamine and are responsible for wheal-and-flare reactions in the skin.

Systemic Anaphylaxis

Systemic anaphylaxis is an acute, potentially fatal form of immediate hypersensitivity. It is known as anaphylaxis (ana = without, phylaxis = protection) and is characterized by widespread edema (edema in many tissues) and reduced blood pressure secondary to vasodilation and increased vascular permeability, shock, and difficulty in breathing.

Causes: Usually follows injection of an antigen into a sensitized individual. It may develop in hospital settings after administration of foreign proteins (e.g., antisera), drugs (e.g., antibiotic penicillin), hormones, enzymes, and polysaccharides. It may also be following exposure to food allergens (e.g., proteins in peanuts, tree nuts, fish, shellfish, milk, eggs) or insect toxins (e.g., those in bee venom).

Dose: Systemic anaphylaxis may be triggered by extremely small doses of antigen. For example, very small amounts used in skin testing for allergies.

Clinical features: Within minutes after exposure to allergens, the individual develops itching, hives and skin erythema. It is shortly followed by difficulty in breathing and respiratory distress due to contraction of respiratory bronchioles. May cause shock and death. Laryngeal edema produces hoarseness and laryngeal obstruction, which further aggravates respiratory difficulty. Vomiting, abdominal cramps, and diarrhea may follow. The patient may go into shock and even die within the hour.

The risk of systemic anaphylaxis should be borne in mind when administering certain therapeutic agents. Though patients who had a previous history of some form of allergy are at risk, the absence of such a history does not exclude the possibility of an anaphylactic reaction.

Local Immediate Hypersensitivity Reactions

About 10–20% of the individuals suffer from allergies. This consists of localized reactions to common environmental allergens, such as pollen, animal dander, house dust, foods, and others. Examples of specific diseases include urticaria, allergic rhinitis (hay fever), bronchial asthma, atopic dermatitis, and food allergies.

Protective roles of IgE- and mast cell-mediated immune reactions

immediate hypersensitivity reactions may protect against helminthic infections by promoting IgE- and eosinophil-mediated antibody-dependent cell-mediated cytotoxicity and gut peristalsis. Mast cells may also play a role in innate immune responses to bacterial infections and venoms.

Diagnosis of type I hypersensitivity

- Typical clinical history and examination.
- Skin-prick testing.
- Measuring specific IgE in the serum.

Examples of type I hypersensitivity reactions are listed in **Table 9**.

Table 9: Examples of type I hypersensitivity reactions.

Localized type I hypersensitivity	*Systemic type I hypersensitivity*
• Bronchial asthma (extrinsic) • Hay fever/allergic rhinitis • Allergic conjunctivitis • Urticaria • Atopic dermatitis/eczema • Angioedema • Allergic gastroenteritis (food allergy)	Anaphylaxis due to: • Antibiotics (Most commonly penicillin) • Bee stings • Insect bite • Foreign proteins (e.g., antisera) • Foods (peanuts, fish, and shellfish) • Food additives

Antibody-mediated (Type II) Hypersensitivity Reactions

Definition: Antibody-mediated (type II) hypersensitivity disorders are caused by antibodies (IgG/IgM) which react with target antigens present on the surface of specific cells or fixed in the extracellular matrix (tissues). These antibodies destroy these cells, triggering inflammation, or interfering with normal functions.

Type of antigen: It may be endogenous or exogenous. Endogenous antigens may be normal molecules intrinsic to the cell membrane or extracellular matrix (e.g., autoimmune diseases). Exogenous antigens may be chemical or microbial proteins that may get adsorbed on a cell surface or extracellular matrix. This may cause altered surface antigen (e.g., drug metabolite).

Type of antibodies: IgG (usually) and IgM (rarely) type of antibodies mediate type II reactions. The antibodies may be specific for normal cell or tissue antigens (autoantibodies) or for exogenous antigens as described above (e.g., chemical or microbial proteins). These antibodies bind to a cell surface or tissue matrix (**Fig. 28**).

Mechanism of Injury by Antibodies Against Fixed Cell and Tissue Antigens

Antibodies against fixed cell and tissue antigens in antibody-mediated (type II) hypersensitivity reactions cause disease by three distinct mechanisms. These are as follows:

1. **Opsonization and phagocytosis:** Antibody bound to a target cell can serve as an opsonin. This allows phagocytic cells with Fc receptors or (after complement has been activated by the bound antibodies) receptors for complement fragments such as C3b to bind and phagocytose the antibody-coated cell.

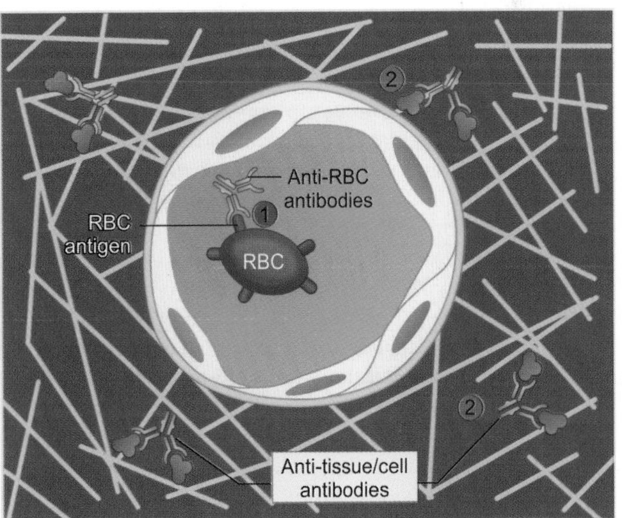

(RBC: red blood cell)

FIG. 28: Different forms of antibodies that may cause disease in antibody-mediated (type II) hypersensitivity. Antibodies to cells may bind to cells [e.g., circulating red cells (1)] and promote destruction of these cells. Anti-tissue antibodies may bind specifically to extracellular tissue antigens (2) and recruit leukocytes leading to tissue injury.

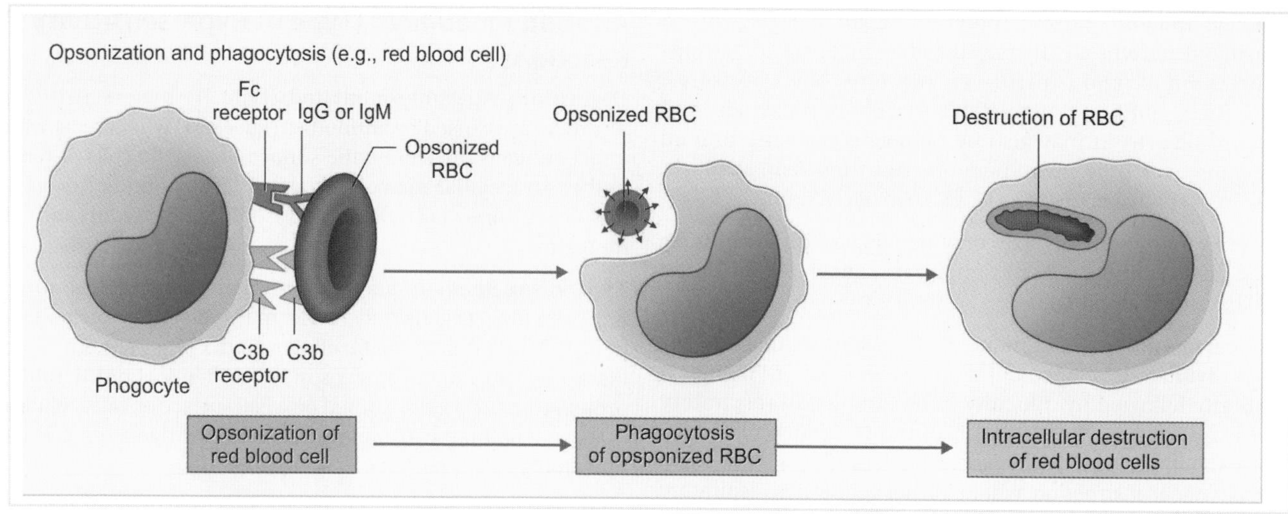

FIG. 29: Antibody-mediated (type II) hypersensitivity reaction by opsonization and phagocytosis. In this example, the red blood cell (RBC) is coated by antibodies and complement components (C3b). The opsonized RBC is phagocytosed followed by their lysis inside the phagocytes (e.g., macrophage in the spleen).

2. **Lysis of target cells through membrane attack complex (MAC):** Certain immunoglobulin subclasses can activate the complement system. This creates pores in the membrane of a foreign cell.
3. **Antibody-dependent cellular cytotoxicity:** Antibodies can mediate cell destruction by antibody-dependent cell-mediated cytotoxicity. In this, cytotoxic cells bearing Fc receptors bind to the Fc region of antibodies on target cells and promote killing of the cells.

Opsonization and phagocytosis (Fig. 29)

- **Opsonization of cell surface antigens:** It may occur directly or opsonization following activation of complement system. In direct opsonization, antibodies bind to target coated cell surface antigens through immunoglobulin Fc receptors on phagocytes thereby opsonizing the cells. Another method of opsonization is activation of the complement system that generates complement proteins and the C3b complement component binds to C3b receptors on target cells and opsonize these cells.
- **Phagocytosis of cells:** Many phagocytic cells, including neutrophils and macrophages, express cell membrane receptors for both Fc and C3b. By binding to these receptors, Ig or C3b enhance the phagocytosis of target and subsequent intracellular destruction of the antibody- or complement-coated cell. Phagocytosis is mainly responsible for depletion of cells coated with antibodies.
    - **Direct opsonization (complement independent):** Cells opsonized by IgG antibodies are recognized by phagocyte Fc receptors, which are specific for the Fc portions of some IgG antibodies. Since this does not need complement, this is a complement-independent opsonization.
    - **Through complement activation (complement-dependent):** Complement and antibody molecules can destroy target cells by opsonization, and this is a complement-dependent opsonization. When IgM or IgG antibodies are deposited on the surfaces of cells, they may activate the complement system by the classical pathway. Complement activation produces cleavage products of C3, mainly C3b. This C3b gets deposited on the surfaces of the cells. C3b is an opsonin and is recognized by phagocytes that express receptors for these complement proteins. These receptors for complement proteins bind to complement component and lead to phagocytosis of the cells.
- **Destruction of cells inside phagocytes:** After phagocytosis, ingested cells inside the phagocytes are destroyed. These are the main mechanisms of cell destruction of red blood cells (RBCs) in autoimmune hemolytic anemia and platelets in autoimmune thrombocytopenia. The antibodies specific for the cells (RBCs or platelets) lead to the opsonization and removal of these cells from the circulation. The same mechanism is responsible for hemolysis in transfusion reactions.

Lysis of target cells through MAC (Fig. 30)

Complement activation through classical pathway on cells also leads to the formation of the MAC (membrane attack complex), also called as C5b-9 complexes. This destroys membrane integrity by forming holes on target cells through the lipid bilayer of the cell. This leads to osmotic lysis of the target cells. Probably destruction through MAC is effective in destroying only cells and microbes with thin cell walls (**Fig. 30**). Example for this type of cell lysis is certain autoimmune hemolytic anemias resulting from antibodies against RBC blood group antigens. In some transfusion reactions that result from major blood group incompatibilities, intravascular hemolysis occurs through activation of complement.

Examples of clinical conditions associated with antibody-mediated cell destruction and phagocytosis are as follows:

- **Transfusion reactions:** These occur when red cells from a blood group mismatched (incompatible) donor react with and are opsonized by preformed antibody in the recipient.
- **Hemolytic disease of the fetus and newborn (erythroblastosis fetalis):** It develops when there is an antigenic difference between the mother and the fetus. IgG anti-RBC antibodies from the mother cross the placenta and cause destruction of fetal RBCs.

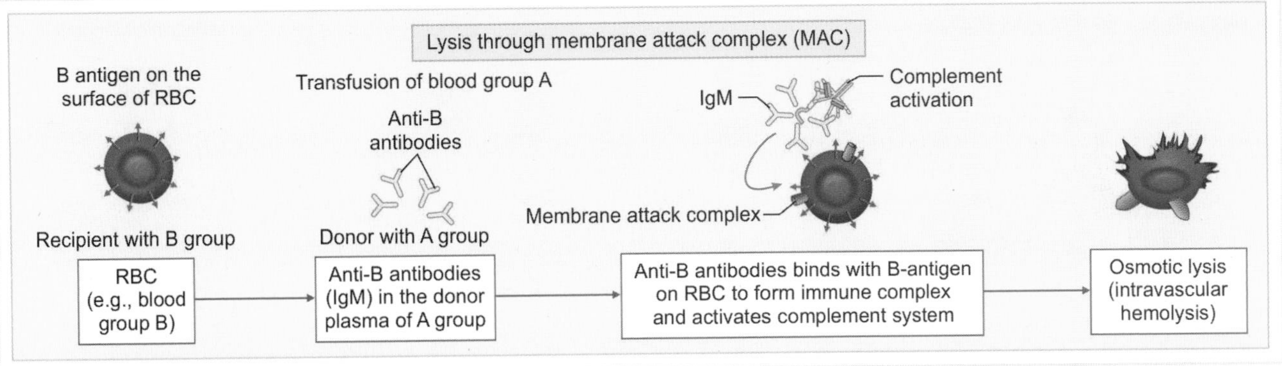

FIG. 30: Antibody-mediated (type II) hypersensitivity reaction causing cell lysis through membrane attack complex (MAC). In this example, individual with blood group B is transfused with blood group A and this leads to transfusion reactions. Binding of IgG or IgM antibody to an antigen promotes complement fixation. Activation of complement leads to formation of MAC which causes cell lysis.

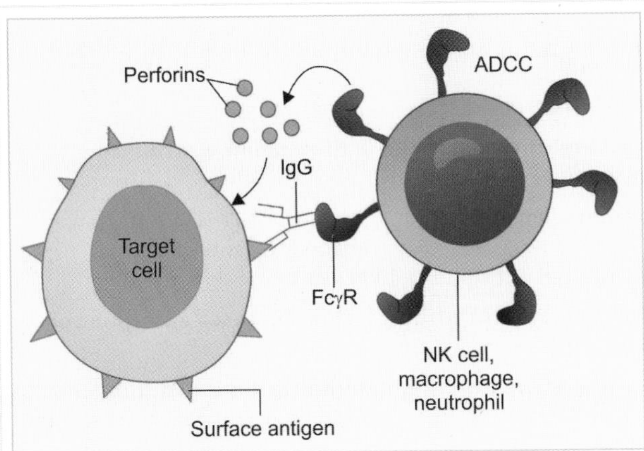

FIG. 31: Antibody-dependent cellular (cell-mediated) cytotoxicity (ADCC). Target cell surface antigens coated with IgG antibody can be killed by mainly natural killer (NK) cells and macrophages. NK cells and macrophages bind to the target cell by their receptors (FcγR) for the Fc fragment of IgG, and lysis of cell occurs without phagocytosis. Effector cells synthesize homologs of terminal complement proteins (e.g., perforins), which participate in cytotoxic events.

- **Autoimmune hemolytic anemia, agranulocytosis, and thrombocytopenia:** They occur when individuals produce antibodies to their own blood cells. These cells are then destroyed.
- **Certain drug reactions:** Use of certain drugs produces drug induced antibody-mediated destruction of blood cells. In certain cases, the offending drug binds to plasma membrane proteins on host cells and forms drug-protein complex. Antibodies are produced against these drug-protein complex. In other cases, the offending drug modifies the conformation of an antigen and generates new antigenic epitopes against which the individual reacts.

Antibody-dependent cellular (cell-mediated) cytotoxicity (Fig. 31)

Antibody-mediated destruction of cells can also occur by another mechanism called ADCC. This mechanism does not require complement, but rather involves cytolytic leukocytes that attack antibody-coated target cells after binding via Fc receptors. Cells coated with IgG antibody can be killed by effector cells, mainly NK cells and macrophages; NK cells and macrophages bind to the target cell by their receptors for the Fc fragment of IgG, and lysis of cell occurs without phagocytosis. Effector cells synthesize homologs of terminal complement proteins (e.g., perforins), which participate in cytotoxic events. Only rarely is antibody alone directly cytotoxic. ADCC is involved in the pathogenesis of some autoimmune diseases (e.g., autoimmune thyroiditis).

Tissue Injury by Inflammation (Fig. 32)

When circulating antibodies get deposited in fixed tissues (e.g., basement membranes, extracellular connective matrix), they bind intrinsic connective tissue antigens. This brings out the destructive local inflammatory responses and injures the fixed tissue due to inflammation. The antibodies deposited in fixed tissue activate complement. Activated complement system produces cleavage products. These complement products include chemotactic agents (mainly C5a), which cause migration of granulocytes and monocytes; and anaphylatoxins (C3a and C5a), which increase vascular permeability (**Fig. 32B**). The leukocytes are activated by engagement of their C3b (with complement C3b) and Fc receptors (Fc portion of antibodies). Activated leukocytes release substances that damage tissues. These include lysosomal enzymes, including proteases capable of digesting basement membrane, collagen, elastin, and cartilage. There is also production of damaging reactive oxygen species.

Examples of antibody-mediated inflammation (**Table 10**) causing tissue injury include some forms of glomerulonephritis (e.g., Goodpasture syndrome), vascular rejection in organ grafts, bullous skin diseases pemphigus and pemphigoid, and numerous other disorders. Goodpasture syndrome is a classic example in which anti-glomerular basement membrane antibody binds to noncollagenous domain of type IV collagen, which is a major structural component of pulmonary and glomerular basement membranes. This activates the complement system and results in neutrophil chemotaxis and activation. The inflammatory cells damage the basement membrane and produce pulmonary hemorrhage and glomerulonephritis. Direct complement-mediated damage to glomerular and alveolar basement membranes through MACs may also be involved.

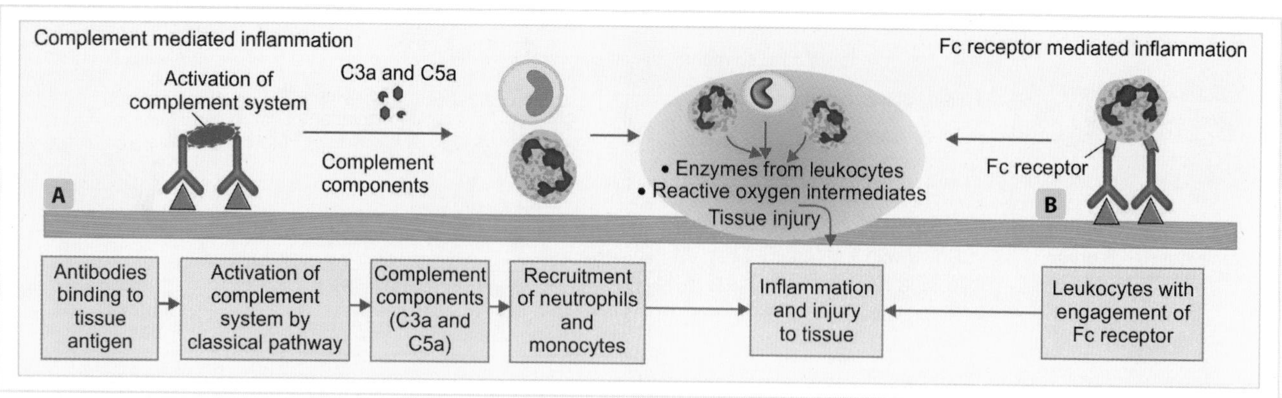

FIGS. 32A AND B: Antibody-mediated (type II) hypersensitivity reaction—complement and Fc receptor mediated inflammation. (A) Antibody binds to a surface antigen, activates the complement system, and leads to the recruitment of tissue-damaging inflammatory cells. Several complement-derived peptides (e.g., C5a) are potent chemotactic factors; (B) Inflammation may also be induced by antibody binding to Fc receptors of leukocytes.

Table 10: Examples of type II hypersensitivity (antibody-mediated) diseases.

Mechanism and disease	*Target antigen*
Opsonization and phagocytosis (IgG-mediated)	
• Autoimmune hemolytic anemia	Cell-surface antigens (Rh blood group antigens, I antigen)
• Autoimmune thrombocytopenic purpura	Platelet membrane glycoprotein IIb: IIIa integrin
Lysis by membrane attack complex (MAC) of the complement system	
Transfusion reactions	The cells from an incompatible donor react with and are opsonized by preformed antibody in the recipient
Neutrophil degranulation and Inflammation	
Vasculitis caused by ANCA	Neutrophil granule proteins, presumably released from activated neutrophils
Complement and Fc receptor-mediated inflammation (IgG-mediated)	
Goodpasture syndrome	Antibody against matrix antigens (basement membrane noncollagenous protein of kidney glomeruli and lung alveoli)
Antibody-mediated activation of proteases and disruption of intercellular adhesions	
Pemphigus vulgaris	Proteins in intercellular junctions of epidermal cells (desmogleins)
Antibody-mediated (complement-independent) cellular dysfunction	
• Graves' disease (hyperthyroidism)	Antibody against receptors: Thyroid-stimulating hormone (TSH) receptor (agonistic antibodies)
• Myasthenia gravis	Antibody against receptors: Acetylcholine receptor (antagonistic antibodies)

Continued

Continued

Mechanism and disease	*Target antigen*
Cross-reactive antibodies (inflammation, macrophage activation)	
Acute rheumatic fever	Streptococcal cell wall antigen; antibody cross-reacts with myocardial antigen
Neutralization of intrinsic factor, decreased absorption of vitamin B_{12}	
Pernicious anemia	Intrinsic factor of gastric parietal cells

(ANCA: antineutrophil cytoplasmic antibodies)

Cellular Dysfunction

It is characterized by deposition of antibodies directed against cell surface receptors. In some antibody mediated (type II) reactions, antibody binds to a specific target cell receptor. They may impair or change the function of the target cell without causing cell death/injury or inflammation (**Fig. 33**). Examples are as follows:

- **Antibody-mediated stimulation of cell function (Fig. 33):** In Graves' disease, there are autoantibodies against the thyroid-stimulating hormone (TSH) receptor on surface of thyroid epithelial cells. These antibodies stimulate the follicular cells of thyroid to produce thyroxin. This leads to hyperthyroidism (thyrotoxicosis).
- **Antibody-mediated inhibition of cell function:** In myasthenia gravis (**Fig. 34**), there are autoantibodies directed against acetylcholine receptors (postsynaptic neurotransmitter receptors) in the motor end plates of skeletal muscles. These antibodies react with acetylcholine receptors and block acetylcholine binding and/or mediate internalization or destruction of receptors. This prevents effective synaptic neuromuscular transmission. This leads to muscle fatigue (weakness of muscles).

Cross-reactive antibodies: Usually, antibodies that cause cell- or tissue-specific diseases are autoantibodies. Less commonly, the antibodies may be produced against a foreign (e.g.,

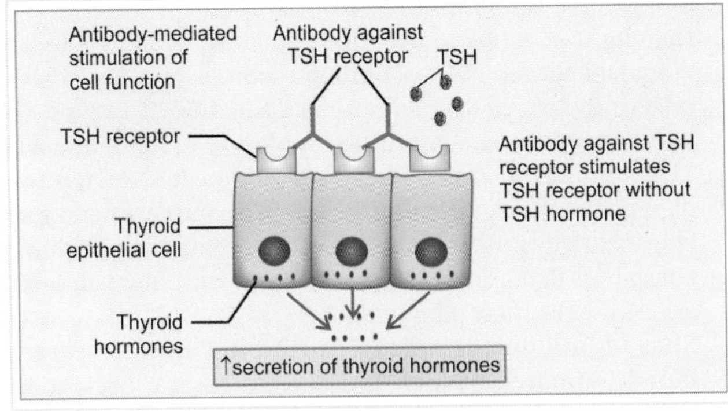

FIG. 33: Antibody-mediated (type II) hypersensitivity reaction: Antibody-mediated stimulation of cell function. Autoantibodies bind against the thyroid-stimulating hormone (TSH) receptor and activate thyroid cells to produce excessive production of hormones and causing hyperthyroidism in Graves' disease.

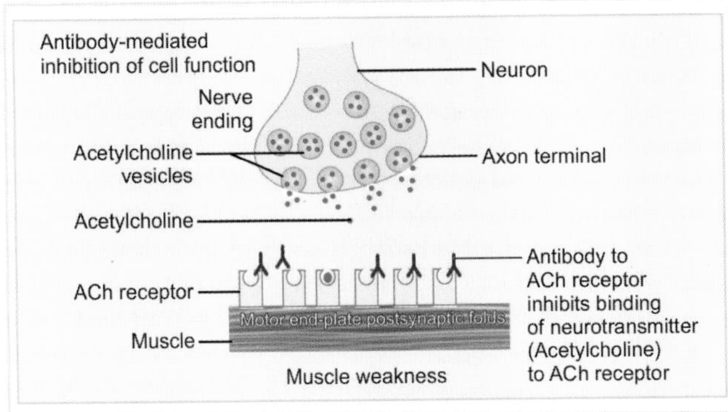

FIG. 34: Antibody-mediated (type II) hypersensitivity reaction: Antibody-mediated inhibition of cell function. Anti-receptor antibodies may inhibit/disturb the normal function of receptors. Example—autoantibodies to the acetylcholine (ACh) receptor on skeletal muscle cells in myasthenia gravis produce disease by blocking neuromuscular transmission and causing progressive muscle weakness.

microbial) antigen. These antibodies are immunologically cross-reactive with a component of self-tissues. For example, in rheumatic fever, antibodies produced against streptococcal antigens. These antibodies cross-react with antigens in the heart, get deposited in this organ, and cause inflammation and tissue damage.

In summary, antibody-mediated (type II) hypersensitivity reactions are directly or indirectly cytotoxic through action of antibodies against antigens on cell surfaces or in connective tissues. Complement system is involved in many of these events. It may—(1) directly cause lysis, or (2) act indirectly by opsonization and phagocytosis or (3) chemotactic attraction of phagocytic cells, which produce a variety of tissue-damaging products. Complement-independent reactions, such as ADCC, also play a role in antibody-mediated (type II) hypersensitivity. **Figure 35** shows summary of mechanism of antibody-mediated (type II) hypersensitivity reaction reactions. Examples of type II hypersensitivity diseases are presented in **Table 10**.

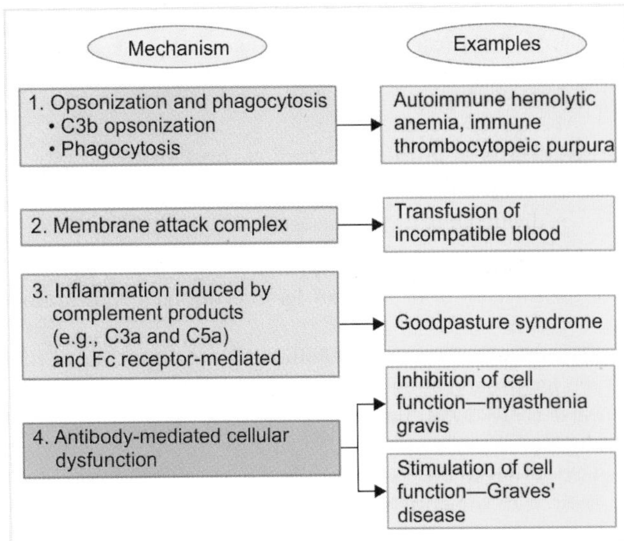

FIG. 35: Summary of mechanism of antibody-mediated (type II) hypersensitivity reaction reactions.

Immune Complex-mediated (Type III) Hypersensitivity Reactions

Q. Write short essay on type III hypersensitivity reactions.

Q. Discuss immune complex disease in humans.

Definition: Immune complex-mediated (type III) hypersensitivity reactions are characterized by formation of immune (antigen and antibody) complexes in the circulation. They may get deposited in blood vessels, leading to complement activation and a subsequent self-sustaining acute inflammation. The inflammatory cells recruited (neutrophils and monocytes) release lysosomal enzymes and generate toxic free radicals leading to tissue damage at the sites of deposition of immune complexes.

Less commonly, the immune complexes may be formed at sites where antigen has been "planted" previously (in situ immune complexes).

Antibodies: These include complement-fixing antibodies namely, **IgG, IgM**, and occasionally IgA.

Antigens: The antigens that form immune complexes may be exogenous or endogenous.

- **Exogenous:** Various foreign proteins such as foreign serum protein injected (e.g., diphtheria antitoxin, horse anti-thymocyte globulin) or produced by an infectious microbe.
- **Endogenous:** Antibody against self-components (autoimmunity), e.g., nucleoproteins.

Immune complex-mediated diseases are usually systemic. The common sites of immune complex deposition are kidney (glomerulonephritis), joints (arthritis), and small blood vessels (vasculitis).

Systemic Immune Complex Disease

Serum sickness is the classical example of systemic immune complex disease. It was once a frequent sequela to the administration of large amounts of foreign serum (e.g., serum from immunized horses used for protection against diphtheria). In present times, the disease is rare and may be seen in individuals who receive antibodies from other individuals or species.

Pathogenesis of immune complex-mediated diseases (Fig. 36)

It can be divided into three phases.

1. ***Formation of immune complexes:***
   Introduction of protein antigen: It initiates an immune response.
   Formation of antibody: Following the injection of the foreign protein antigen, antibodies are usually formed in a week (7–12 days). The antibodies formed are secreted into the blood.
   Formation of immune complex: In the blood, antibodies react with the antigen still present in the circulation and form antigen–antibody complexes.
2. ***Deposition of immune complexes:*** In this phase, the circulating antigen–antibody complexes are deposited in vessels. The exact factors that determine whether immune complex formation will lead to tissue deposition and disease are not fully known. Probably it depends on the characteristics of the immune complexes and local vascular alterations. Most immune complexes are removed effectively before they can cause tissue injury. In type III hypersensitivity, the immune complexes are not removed. The amount of immune complex deposited in tissues depends on the nature of the immune complexes and the characteristics of the blood vessels. Generally, immune complexes that are of medium size, and with slight antigen excess are the most pathogenic.
   Sites of immune complex deposition: Organs in which blood is filtered at high pressure to form other fluids include urine and synovial fluid. These are sites in which immune complexes become concentrated and likely to deposit. Thus, immune complex disease usually affects renal glomeruli (causes glomerulonephritis) and joints (causes arthritis).
3. ***Inflammation and tissue injury:*** Once immune complexes are deposited in the tissues, immune complexes cause local activation of complement and form C5a, which is a potent neutrophil chemoattractant. Other neutrophil chemotactic mediators include leukotriene B_4 and IL-8 are also formed. This leads to development of acute inflammatory reaction at the site of immune complex deposit. This phase occurs about 10 days after antigen administration. During this period, it clinically manifests with fever, urticaria, joint pain, lymph node enlargement, and proteinuria on urine examination.
   Cause of tissue damage: Wherever immune complexes are deposited, inflammation and tissue injury occur. It is mediated through the **antibody-mediated mechanisms** (type II hypersensitivity). **Complement plays an important role in the pathogenesis** of the tissue injury. Supporting evidence for this are as follows:
   Complement proteins can be detected at the site of injury.
   - During the active phase of the disease, consumption of complement leads to a decrease in serum levels of C3. In some cases, estimation of serum C3 levels can be used to monitor activity of the disease.

Recruited neutrophils at the site of immune complex deposition are activated through contact with, and ingestion of, immune complexes. Activated neutrophils release inflammatory mediators, including proteases, reactive oxygen intermediates, and arachidonic acid products. These collectively produce tissue injury.

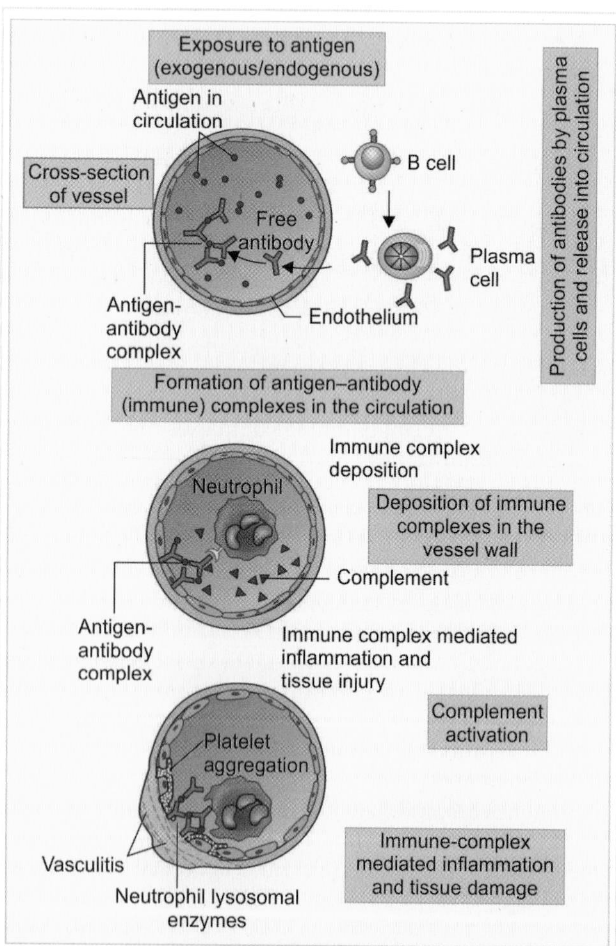

FIG. 36: Pathogenesis of systemic immune complex-mediated disease (type III hypersensitivity). Immune complexes are deposited in tissue activate complement system and recruit tissue-damaging inflammatory cells. The pathogenic ability of immune complexes to mediate tissue injury depends on size, solubility, net charge, and ability to fix complement.

MORPHOLOGY

Main morphologic features of immune complex injury are seen in blood vessels and glomerulus of kidney.

Acute vasculitis: It is associated with necrosis of the vessel wall and severe neutrophilic infiltration. The necrotic tissue and deposits of immune complexes, complement, and plasma protein give a smudgy eosinophilic appearance to the site of tissue destruction. This appearance is termed as **fibrinoid necrosis** (refer page 140 and Fig. 11 of Chapter 7).

Glomerulus: Immune complex deposits in the kidney appear as a **granular lumpy deposit of immunoglobulin** and complement on immunofluorescence microscopy. On electron microscopy, it produces **electron-dense deposits along the glomerular basement membrane**.

Acute serum sickness: It is caused by a single exposure to a large amount of antigen. The lesions usually resolve as a result of catabolism of the immune complexes.

Chronic serum sickness: It results from repeated or prolonged exposure to an antigen and includes several diseases. For example, systemic lupus erythematosus (SLE) is associated with persistent antibody responses to autoantigens. In many immune complex-mediated diseases, the morphologic changes and other findings suggest immune complex deposition, but the causative antigens are unknown. Diseases under this category include membranous glomerulonephritis and several types of vasculitides.

Local Immune Complex Disease

The Arthus reaction is a localized form of experimental immune complex-mediated vasculitis. It is produced by subcutaneous (intracutaneous) injection of an antigen into a previously immunized animal (contains circulating antibodies against that antigen) or an animal that has been given an intravenous injection of antibody specific for the antigen. Circulating antibodies rapidly bind to the injected antigen and form large immune complexes. These immune complexes are deposited in the walls of small blood vessels at the injection site. This immune complex deposition produces local cutaneous vasculitis, with thrombosis of the affected vessels. This leads to fibrinoid necrosis in the tissue. Superimposed thrombosis worsens the ischemic injury.

Examples of immune complex disorders are listed in **Table 11.**

T-cell-mediated (Type IV) Hypersensitivity

Q. Write short essay on T cell-mediated (type IV) hypersensitivity reactions.

Cell-mediated hypersensitivity is the only hypersensitivity reaction that is purely cell mediated (T cell-mediated disease) rather than antibody mediated.

Types (Fig. 37): T lymphocytes can injure tissues either indirectly by producing cytokines that produce inflammation or by directly killing target cells.

Table 11: Examples of immune complex-mediated diseases.

Disease	*Antigen*	*Manifestations*
Exogenous antigen		
Poststreptococcal glomerulonephritis	Streptococcal cell wall antigen(s); may be "planted" in glomerular basement membrane	Glomerulonephritis
Polyarteritis nodosa	Hepatitis B virus antigens in some cases	Systemic vasculitis
Serum sickness	Various proteins, e.g., foreign serum protein (horse anti-thymocyte globulin)	Arthritis, vasculitis, nephritis
Arthus reaction	Various foreign proteins	Cutaneous vasculitis
Endogenous antigen		
Systemic lupus erythematosus (SLE)	Nuclear antigens	Glomerulonephritis, skin lesions, arthritis, others

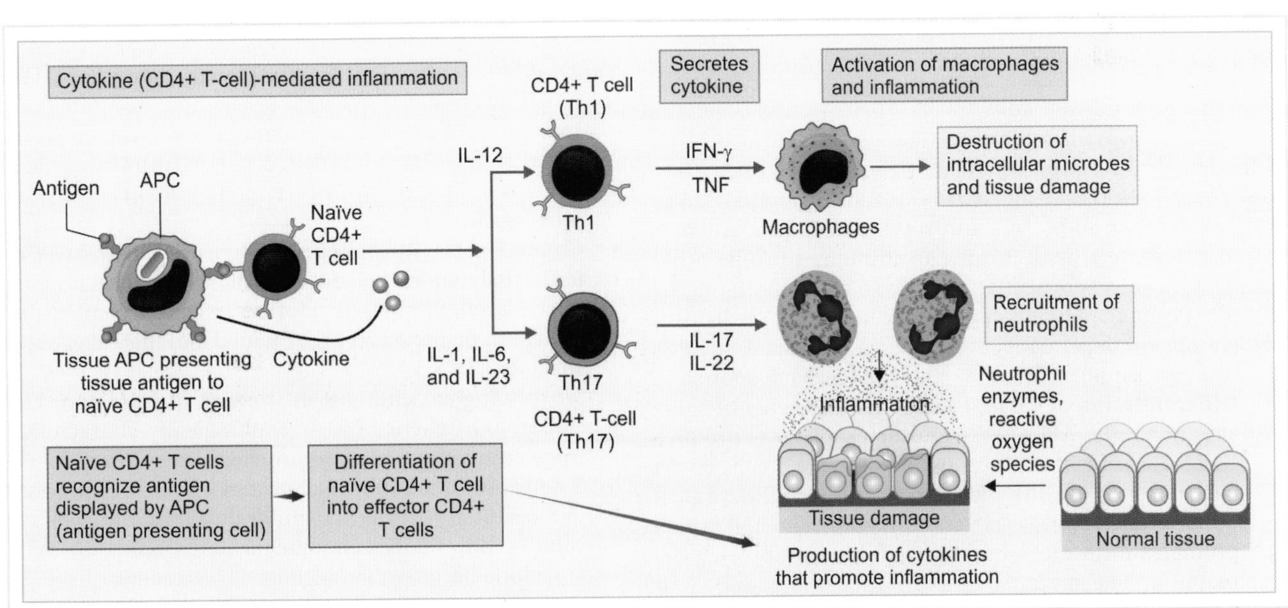

(IFN: interferon; IL: interleukin; TNF: tumor necrosis factor)

FIG. 37: Mechanisms of CD4+ T-cell (cytokine) mediated (type IV) hypersensitivity reactions. In delayed-type hypersensitivity reactions, antigens are presented to naïve T-cells by antigen presenting cell (APC). Depending on the cytokines produced by APC, naïve T-cells may differentiate into CD4+ Th1 or CD4+ Th17. CD4+ Th1 cells secrete cytokines that activate macrophage leading to tissue injury. CD4+ Th17 cells produce cytokines that produce inflammation by recruiting neutrophils. Both mechanisms produce tissue damage.

- **Cytokine-mediated inflammation:** In this type, CD4+ T cells produce cytokines and mainly these cytokines cause inflammation. CD4+ T cell–mediated hypersensitivity may be induced by environmental and self-antigens. It is responsible for many autoimmune and other chronic inflammatory diseases.
- **Direct cell toxicity mediated by CD8+ T cells:** Cell killing by CD8+ cells may also be involved in some autoimmune diseases. It may be the main mechanism of tissue injury in certain reactions, especially those that follow viral infections.

CD4+ T-cell-mediated (Cytokine-mediated) Inflammation

In CD4+ T-cell-mediated hypersensitivity reactions (**Fig. 37**), cytokines produced by T cells produce inflammation. This inflammation may be chronic and destructive.

Q. Write short essay on delayed hypersensitivity reactions.

Delayed-type hypersensitivity (DTH): Classical example of T-cell-mediated inflammation is DTH. DTH is a tissue reaction to antigens given to immune individuals. In DTH reaction, an antigen is administered into the skin of a previously immunized individual. This leads to a detectable cutaneous reaction within 24–48 hours. Since the **reaction is delayed by 24–48 hours**, it is termed delayed, in contrast to immediate hypersensitivity (which occurs immediately).

Inflammatory reactions are prominent aspect of the pathology and are elicited mainly by CD4+ T cells of the Th1 and Th17 subsets. Both Th1 and Th17 subsets of CD4+ T cells contribute to organ-specific diseases. The **inflammatory reaction associated with Th1 cells is dominated by activated macrophages**, whereas that triggered by **Th17 cells has predominantly neutrophils**. The sequential stages of the inflammatory reactions stimulated by CD4+ T cells are described below.

Activation of CD4+ T cells

When the foreign protein antigen is introduced, DCs (dendritic cells) process the antigen and display these antigenic peptides. Naïve CD4+ T cells recognize these peptides displayed by DCs and secrete IL-2. This IL-2 acts as an autocrine growth factor and stimulates proliferation of the antigen-responsive T cells. These antigen-stimulated T cells subsequently differentiate into Th1 or Th17 cells. This differentiation depends on the cytokines produced by APCs (antigen presenting cells) at the time of T-cell activation.

- **Differentiation of CD4+ T cells into Th1 cells:** In some situations, the APCs (DCs and macrophages) produce IL-12. This induces differentiation of CD4+ T cells to the Th1 subset. These Th1 effector cells produce IFN-γ (most powerful macrophage activating cytokine) and TNF which promotes further Th1 development, thus amplifying the reaction. The macrophages produce substances that destroy intracellular microbes and damage tissues.
- **Differentiation of CD4+ T cells into Th17 cells:** If the APCs produce the inflammatory cytokines IL-1, IL-6, and IL-23 (which is closely related to IL-12), the T cells are induced to differentiate to the Th17 subset. Th17 cells produce IL-17, IL-22, chemokines, and other cytokines that promote inflammation by recruiting more neutrophils and monocytes to the site of reaction.

Some of the differentiated effector T cells enter the circulation. They join the pool of memory T cells and persist for long periods (sometimes years).

Responses of differentiated effector T-cells

On re-exposure to an antigen, Th1 cells secrete cytokines, mainly IFN-γ. These cytokines are responsible for many of the manifestations of DTH.

Activation of macrophages: IFN-γ activates macrophages. These IFN-γ-activated ("classically activated") macrophages are altered in several ways:

- Ability of macrophages to phagocytose and kill microorganisms is markedly increased.
- Activated macrophages express more class II MHC molecules on the surface. This increases antigen presentation by these cells.
- Activated macrophages secrete TNF, IL-1, and chemokines, which promote inflammation.
- Activated macrophages produce more IL-12 and amplify the Th1 response.

Sustained activation of macrophages: Activated macrophages try to eliminate the offending antigen. If the activation of macrophages is sustained, it leads to continued inflammation and tissue injury. Activated Th17 cells secrete IL-17, IL-22, chemokines, and several other cytokines. These cytokines recruit neutrophils and monocytes to the reaction and promote inflammation.

Clinical examples of CD4+ T-cell-mediated inflammatory reactions

Four examples of CD4+ T-cell-mediated inflammatory reactions are discussed below. These are—(1) tuberculin reaction, (2) granulomatous inflammation, (3) contact dermatitis, and (4) drug reactions.

Tuberculin reaction (Fig. 38) The classic example of DTH is the tuberculin reaction (Mantoux test).

- **Injection of PPD:** In tuberculin reaction, purified protein derivative (PPD, also called tuberculin), a protein-containing antigen of the tubercle bacillus is injected intracutaneously.
- **Changes at the site of injection:** In a previously sensitized individual, reddening and induration appear at the site of injection of PPD, in 8–12 hours. It reaches a peak (usually 1–2 cm in diameter) in 24–72 hours, and thereafter slowly subside.
- **Morphological changes at the site of injection:** DTH (tuberculin reaction) is morphologically characterized by accumulation of mononuclear cells, mainly CD4+ T cells and macrophages, around venules. It produces perivascular "cuffing". In fully developed lesions, the venules show marked endothelial hypertrophy. This is due to endothelial activation mediated by cytokines.

Granulomatous inflammation Prolonged DTH reaction against certain persistent microbes (e.g., tubercle bacilli deposited in the lungs or other tissues) or other nondegradable antigens (e.g., foreign bodies) injurious agent may produce a special type of microscopic reaction known as granulomatous inflammation.

Mechanisms of granuloma formation (Fig. 39): Different steps involved in granuloma formation are as follows—

- **Exposure to antigen:** APCs present the antigen to naïve CD4+ T cells. These CD4+ T cells undergo differentiation and proliferation into Th1 cells.

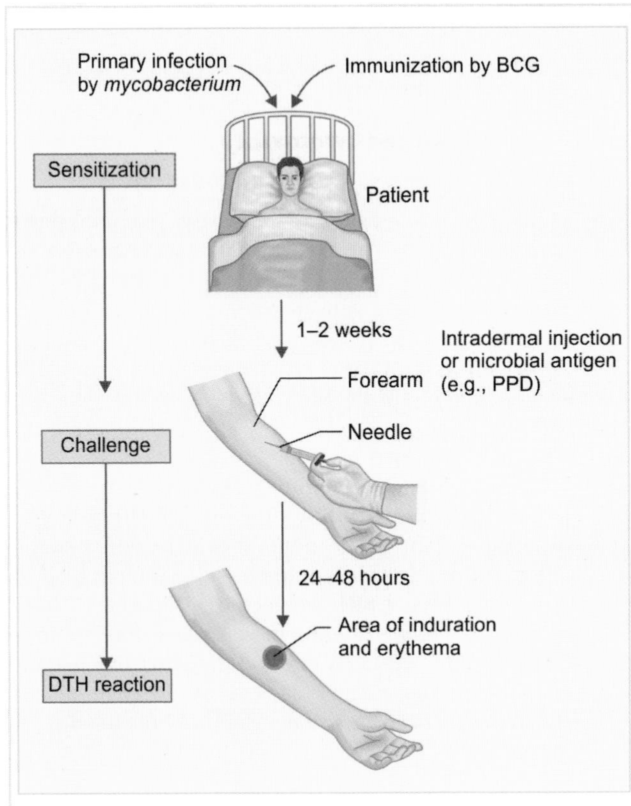

(PPD: purified protein derivative)

FIG. 38: Tuberculin reaction. It is an example for delayed-type hypersensitivity (DTH) reaction. Infection or immunization (vaccination) sensitizes an individual. Subsequent challenge with the same antigen from the infectious agent elicits a DTH reaction. The reaction produces induration with redness and swelling at the site of the intradermal injection of microbial antigen. This reaction peaks at 24–48 hours.

- **Macrophage infiltration: Th1** cells are replaced by activated macrophages and the inflammatory infiltrate predominantly consists of macrophages over a period of 2 or 3 weeks.
- **Transformation of macrophages into epithelioid cells:** TNF secreted by activated macrophages causes recruitment of monocytes from circulation. With sustained antigen activation, activated macrophages usually undergo a morphologic transformation into epithelioid cells. These transformed epithelioid cells are large flat, eosinophilic, and epithelium-like cells with abundant cytoplasm and morphologically resemble the squamous epithelial cells. The cytokines (e.g., IFN-γ) may cause fusion of epithelioid cells to form multinucleated giant cells (e.g., Langhans giant cell).
- **Formation of granuloma:** Aggregates of epithelioid cells are usually surrounded by lymphocytes and form grossly visible small nodules called granulomas (**Fig. 40**). This pattern of chronic inflammation is called granulomatous inflammation. This is commonly found in association with strong Th1 cell activation and production of cytokines such as IFN-γ. It can also be caused by indigestible foreign bodies, which activate macrophages without producing an adaptive immune response. Thus, granuloma is a microscopic aggregate of epithelioid cells (**Fig. 40**), surrounded by a rim of lymphocytes. Older granulomas are enclosed by rim of fibroblasts and connective tissue.

Helminthic infections: In some helminthic infections, such as schistosomiasis, the worms lay eggs in the tissues. These eggs elicit granulomatous reactions. These reactions usually show numerous eosinophils and are elicited by strong Th2 responses. This Th2 response and presence of many eosinophils in tissue is characteristic of many helminthic infections.

Contact dermatitis Contact dermatitis is an example for tissue injury resulting from DTH reactions. Contact with various environmental antigens (e.g., poison ivy, metals such as nickel and chromium, chemicals such as hair dyes, cosmetics, and soaps) may evoke inflammation with blisters in the skin at the site of contact known as contact dermatitis. Urushiol is the antigenic component of poison ivy or poison oak. Contact with poison ivy may be evoked DTH reaction and clinically presents with itchy, vesicular (blistering) dermatitis.

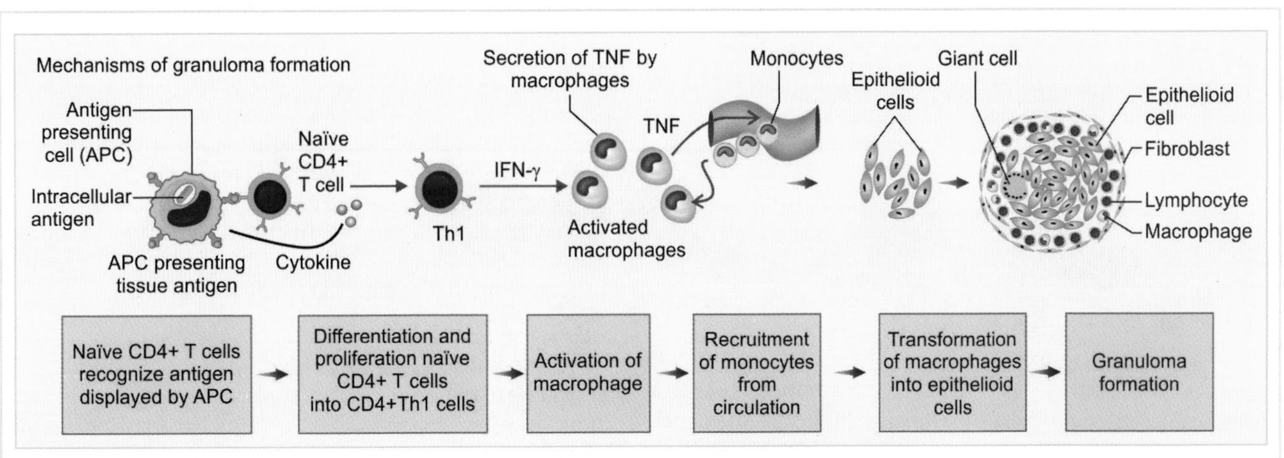

FIG. 39: Mechanisms of granuloma formation in cell-mediated (type IV) hypersensitivity reactions.

Mechanism: Probably, the environmental chemical binds to and structurally modifies self-proteins. The peptides derived from these modified self-proteins are recognized by T cells and elicit the DTH reaction. Chemicals may also modify HLA molecules and make them appear as foreign to T cells.

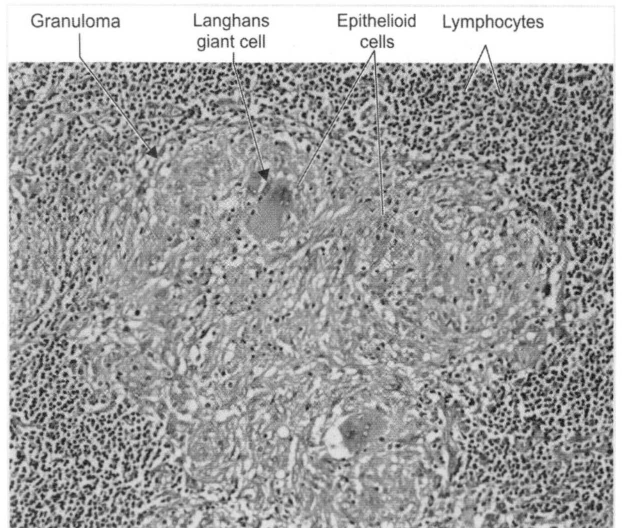

FIG. 40: Granulomatous inflammation. Section of a lymph node with granuloma. It consists of an aggregate of epithelioid cells surrounded by lymphocytes. The granuloma shows several multinucleate giant cells.

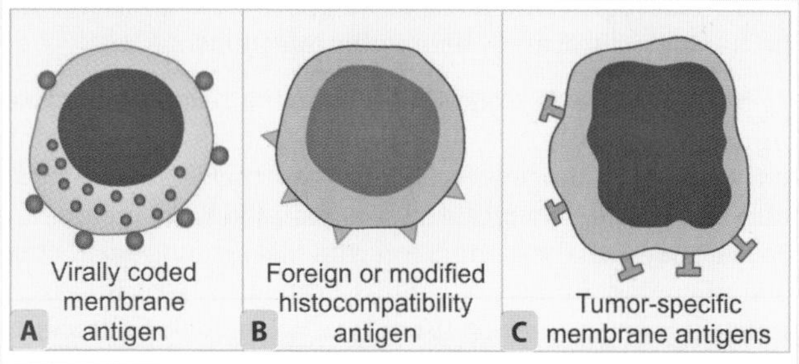

FIG. 41: Potential target cells and antigens in CD8+ T-cell-mediated cytotoxicity. These include—(A) virus-infected host cells; (B) foreign (histoincompatible transplanted); and (C) malignant host cells.

Drug reactions Drug reaction is the most common immunologic reactions in humans. These usually manifest as skin rashes. The mechanism of drug reaction is similar to those for contact dermatitis.

Other examples Other examples of tissue injury (diseases) caused due to CD4+ T cell-mediated inflammation include many organ-specific and systemic autoimmune diseases. Examples are rheumatoid arthritis and multiple sclerosis. Inflammatory bowel disease is linked to uncontrolled reactions to bacterial commensals in the lumen of intestine.

CD8+ T-cell–mediated Cytotoxicity

Q. Write short essay on T-cell mediated cytotoxicity.

It is a type of T-cell mediated tissue injury (reaction) due to CD8+ T lymphocytes. These CD8+ T lymphocytes are also called as CTLs (CD8+ CTLs). In this type, **CD8+ CTLs kill antigen-expressing** (antigen-bearing) **target cells**. Potential target cells and antigens in CD8+ T-cell-mediated cytotoxicity include virus-infected host cells, foreign (histoincompatible transplanted) and malignant host cells (**Fig. 41**).

Destruction of tissues by CTLs may play an important role in some T cell-mediated diseases. Examples include **type 1 diabetes mellitus, graft rejection** (CTLs are directed against cell surface histocompatibility antigens), **killing of virus infected cells** (e.g., in viral hepatitis), and some tumor cells.

- **Viral infection:** In a virus-infected cell, viral peptides are displayed by class I MHC molecules. These class I MHC molecules are recognized by the TCR (T cell receptor) of CD8+ T lymphocytes and they kill the virus-infected cell. The killing of infected cells leads to the elimination of the infection. However, in some cases, it is responsible for cell damage that accompanies the infection (e.g., in viral hepatitis).
- **CTLs against tumor antigens:** In tumors, the tumor antigens are presented on the surface of tumor cells. CTLs are involved in the host response to these transformed tumors cells (for details refer pages 492–495 and Fig. 73 of Chapter 10).

Mechanism of T-cell-mediated killing of targets (Fig. 42)

Perforins and granzymes: Main mechanism of T-cell-mediated killing of targets involves perforins (facilitates the entry of other granule proteins) and granzymes. These are

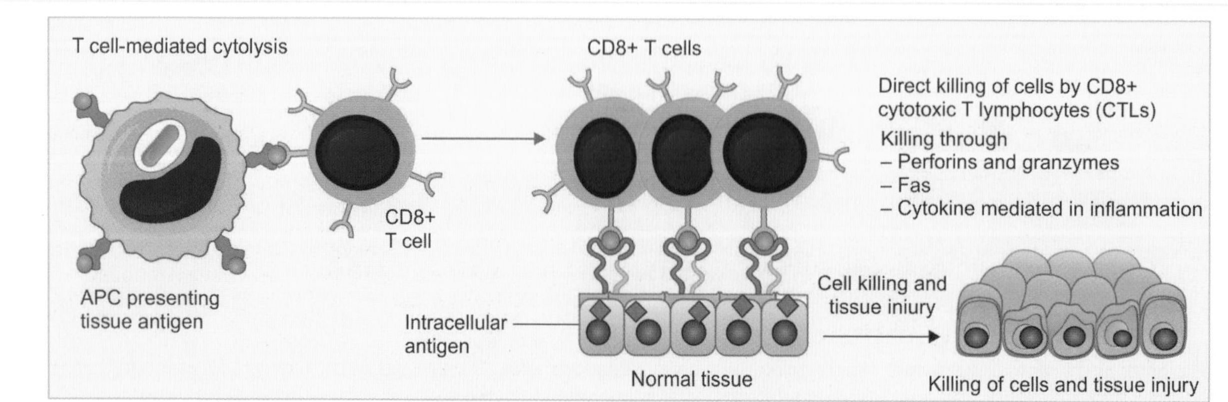

FIG. 42: Mechanisms of T-cell mediated (type IV) hypersensitivity reactions by direct cell toxicity mediated by CD8+ cytotoxic T lymphocytes.

preformed mediators present in the lysosome-like granules of CTLs.

Entry of mediators from CTLs into target cells: CTLs recognize the target cells and secrete a complex consisting of perforin, granzymes, and other proteins. These mediators enter the target cells by endocytosis.

Release and action of the granzymes: In the cytoplasm of target cell, perforin facilitates the release of the granzymes from the complex. Granzymes are proteases that cleave and activate caspases. Activated caspases induce apoptosis of the target cells.

Other mechanisms: These include—

- **Through Fas:** Activated CTLs also express Fas ligand, a molecule with homology to TNF. Fas can produce apoptosis by binding and activating Fas receptor expressed on target cells.
- **Through cytokines:** CD8+ T cells also produce cytokines, especially IFN-γ. These cytokines are involved in inflammatory reactions and resemble DTH. This occurs mainly following infections by viruses and exposure to some contact sensitizing agents.

Examples of T-cell mediated (type IV) hypersensitivity are shown in **Table 12**.

Salient features and differences between hypersensitivity reactions are presented in **Table 13**.

Table 12: Examples of T-cell mediated (type IV) hypersensitivity.

Disease	*Specificity of pathogenic T cells*	*Mechanism*	*Manifestations*
Diseases caused by cytokine-mediated inflammation			
Rheumatoid arthritis	?Collagen; citrullinated self-protein	Inflammation mediated by Th17 (and Th1) cytokines	Chronic arthritis, inflammatory destruction of articular cartilage and bone
Multiple sclerosis	Protein antigens present in myelin (e.g., myelin basic protein)	Inflammation mediated by Th1 and Th17 cytokines; destruction of myelin by activated macrophages	Demyelination in CNS with inflammation; paralysis, optic neuritis
Type 1 diabetes mellitus*	Antigens of pancreatic islet β cells (e.g., insulin, glutamic acid decarboxylase)	T-cell-mediated inflammation (CD4+T) and destruction of islet cells by CTLs	Insulitis (chronic inflammation in islets), destruction of β cells; diabetes mellitus
Inflammatory bowel disease	Enteric bacteria, self-antigen	Inflammation mediated by Th1 and Th17 cytokines	Chronic inflammation of intestine, ulceration, obstruction
Psoriasis	Unknown skin antigens	Inflammation mediated mainly by Th17 cytokines	Plaques in the skin
Hashimoto thyroiditis*	Thyroglobulin and other thyroid proteins	Destruction of thyroid cells by infiltrating cytotoxic T cells, locally released cytokines, or antibody-dependent cytotoxicity	Hypothyroidism
Contact sensitivity (dermatitis)	Environmental chemicals (e.g., urushiol from poison ivy or poison oak)	Inflammation mediated by Th1 (and Th17) cytokines	Necrosis of epidermis, inflammation of dermis; produces skin rash and blisters
Diseases caused by CTLs			
Viral infection	Viral antigen	Destruction of viral infected host cells by CD8+ T lymphocytes	Depends on the virus
Immune response against tumor	Tumor antigen: mutated self-protein, overexpressed or aberrantly expressed self-protein or oncogenic virus	Destruction of tumor cells by CD8+ T lymphocytes	Varies depending on tumor and the response
Rejection of transplant	Foreign (histoincompatible transplanted) cells	Direct killing of graft cells by CD8+ T lymphocytes, inflammation	Transplant rejection

*Involves both CD4+T lymphocytes and CD8+ cytotoxic T lymphocytes.

(CTL: cytotoxic T lymphocyte; CNS: central nervous system)

Table 13: Salient features and differences between hypersensitivity reactions.

Features	*Type I*	*Type II*	*Type III*	*Type IV*
Antigens	Exogenous allergens include: pollen, molds, mites, drugs, food, etc.	Cell surface or tissue bound	Soluble exogenous (viruses, bacteria, fungi, parasites) or endogenous autoantigens	Cell/tissue bound
Antibody involved	IgE	IgG and IgM	IgG, IgM, IgA	None

Continued

Continued

Features	***Type I***	***Type II***	***Type III***	***Type IV***
Mediators	From mast cells	Opsonization and phagocytosis by direct or complement mediated mechanism; membrane attack complex and antibody-mediated cellular dysfunction	Complement	T lymphocytes, activated macrophages
Time taken for reaction to develop	5–10 minutes	6–36 hours	4–12 hours	48–72 hours
Immunopathology	Edema, vasodilatation, mast cell degranulation, eosinophils	Antibody-mediated damage to target cells/tissue	Acute inflammatory reaction, neutrophils, vasculitis	Perivascular inflammation, mononuclear cells, fibrin, granulomas, caseation and necrosis in tuberculosis
Examples of diseases and conditions produced	• Asthma (extrinsic) • Urticaria/edema • Allergic rhinitis • Food allergies • Systemic anaphylaxis	• Autoimmune hemolytic anemia • Transfusion reactions • Hemolytic disease of fetus and newborn • Goodpasture syndrome • Acute rheumatic fever • Pernicious anemia • Graves' disease • Myasthenia gravis	• Autoimmune, e.g., SLE • Glomerulonephritis • Rheumatoid arthritis • Farmer's lung disease • Hypersensitivity pneumonitis • Arthus reaction (localized)	• CD4+ T cell-cytokine-mediated inflammation: e.g., pulmonary tuberculosis, contact dermatitis, tuberculin test, leprosy • Direct cell toxicity mediated by CD8+ T cells: e.g., graft-versus-host

(SLE: systemic lupus erythematosus)

BIBLIOGRAPHY

1. Abbas AK, Lichtman AH, Pillai S. Cellular and Molecular Immunology, 9th edition. Philadelphia: Elsevier; 2018.
2. Actor JA. Introductory Immunology, 2nd edition. United Kingdom: Elsevier; 2019.
3. Broz P, Dixit V. Inflammasomes: mechanisms of assembly, regulation and signaling. *Nat Rev Immunol*. 2016;16:407-20.
4. Brubaker SW, Bonham KS, Zanoni I, et al. Innate immune pattern recognition: a cell biological perspective. *Ann Rev Immunol*. 2015;33:257-90.
5. Crotty S. T follicular helper cell biology: a decade of discovery and diseases. *Immunity*. 2019;50:1132-48.
6. Galli SJ, Tsai M. IgE and mast cells in allergic disease. *Nat Med*. 2012;18:693-704.
7. Goodnow CC, Vinuesa CG, Randall KL, et al. Control systems and decision making for antibody production. *Nat Immunol*. 2010;11:681-8.
8. Goubau D, Deddouche S, Reis E, et al. Cytosolic sensing of viruses. *Immunity*. 2013;38:855-69.
9. Jancar S, Sanchez Crespo M. Immune complex–mediated tissue injury: a multistep paradigm, *Trends Immunol*. 2005;26:48-55.
10. Kauffmann F, Demenais F. Gene-environment interactions in asthma and allergic diseases: challenges and perspectives. *J Allergy Clin Immunol*. 2012;130:1229-40.
11. Klimov VV. From Basic to Clinical Immunology. Switzerland: Springer Nature; 2019.
12. Kumar V, Abbas AK, Aster JC. Robbins basic pathology, 10th edition. Philadelphia: Saunders Elsevier; 2018.
13. Kumar V, Abbas AK, Fausto N, et al. Robbins and Cotran pathologic basis of disease, 10th edition. Philadelphia: WB Saunders; 2021.
14. Kumar V, Abbas AK, Aster JC, Deyrup AT. Robbins essential pathology, 1st edition. Philadelphia: Elsevier;2021.
15. Lakhani SR. Dilly SA, Finlayson CJ, Gandhi M. Basic Pathology-An introduction to the mechanisms of disease,5th edition. Boca Raton: CRC Press; 2016.
16. Lambrecht BN, Hammad H. The immunology of asthma. *Nat Immunol*. 2015;16:45-56.
17. Manthiram K, Zhou Q, Aksentijevich I, et al. The monogenic autoinflammatory diseases define new pathways in human innate immunity and inflammation. *Nat Immunol*. 2017;18:832-42.
18. O'Shea JJ, Paul WE. Mechanisms underlying lineage commitment and plasticity of helper CD4+ T cells. *Science*. 2010;327: 1098-1102.
19. Pandey S, Kawai T, Akira S. Microbial sensing by Toll-like receptors and intracellular nucleic acid sensors. *Cold Spring Harb Persp Biol*. 2014;7:a016246.
20. Portelli MA, Hodge E, Sayers I. Genetic risk factors for the development of allergic disease identified by genome-wide association. *Clin Exp Allergy*. 2015;45:21-31.
21. Punt J, Stranford SA, Jones PP, Owen JA. Kuby Immunology, 8th edition. New York: Macmilan learning; 2019.
22. Raphael I, Nalawade S, Eagar TN, et al. T cell subsets and their signature cytokines in autoimmune and inflammatory diseases. *Cytokine*. 2015;74:5-17.
23. Strayer DS, Saffitz JE. Rubin's Pathology: Mechanism of Human Disease, 8th edition. Philadelphia: Wolters Kluwer; 2020.
24. Sturfelt G, Truedsson L. Complement in the immunopathogenesis of rheumatic disease. *Nat Rev Rheumatol*. 2012;8:458-68.
25. Weaver CT, Elson CO, Fouser LA, et al. The Th17 pathway and inflammatory diseases of the intestines, lungs, and skin. *Annu Rev Pathol Mech Dis*. 2013;8:477-512.

CHAPTER 16

Autoimmune Diseases and Rejection of Tissue Transplants

CHAPTER OUTLINE

AUTOIMMUNE DISEASES

One of the main features of the immune system is its ability to mount an inflammatory response to potentially harmful foreign substances while avoiding damage to self-tissues. Usually, the development of potentially harmful immune responses to self-antigens is prohibited.

Autoimmune disease: Main feature of an autoimmune disease is that tissue injury is caused by the immunologic (humoral and/or T cell–mediated) reaction against its own tissues.

Autoimmunity: It refers merely to the presence of antibodies (humoral) or T lymphocytes (cellular) that react with self-antigens. This does not necessarily signify that the self-reactivity has pathogenic consequences. Autoimmunity is present in all individuals and increases with age. Autoantibodies in the serum can be found in apparently normal individuals. Autoantibody is particularly observed in older age groups. Moreover, sometimes autoantibodies that are not harmful are produced after damage to tissues. These autoantibodies may serve a physiologic process that helps regulate the immune system and also play a role in the removal of tissue breakdown products. For example, recognition of self plays an important role in clearing apoptotic and other tissue debris from sites throughout the body.

In autoimmune disease, the individual may have numerous autoantibodies. Only some or even none of which may be pathogenic. For example, patients with systemic sclerosis (SSc) may have a wide range of antinuclear antibodies (ANAs) but are not clearly pathogenic; in contrast, patients with pemphigus may also have a wide range of autoantibodies, one of which (antibody to desmoglein 1 and 3) is pathogenic.

Autoimmunity versus autoimmune disease: Mere presence of autoantibodies does not indicate the presence of autoimmune disease. When immune reactions against self-antigens produce disease, it is called autoimmune disease. Autoimmunity is an important cause of certain diseases in humans.

Definition: Autoimmunity is defined as immune reactions in which **body produces autoantibodies and immunologically competent T lymphocytes against self-antigens.**

Requirements to categorized disorder as due to autoimmunity are listed in **Box 1**. Sometimes, some disorders with prominent chronic inflammation are grouped under immune-mediated inflammatory diseases. These may be autoimmune, or the immune response may be directed against normally harmless microbes such as gut commensal bacteria (e.g., Crohn disease).

General Features of Autoimmune Diseases

Diseases produce due to by autoimmunity have some important general features.

Chronic progressive disease: Autoimmune diseases tend to be chronic, often progressive, and self-perpetuating (continue indefinitely). Sometimes it may be with relapses

Box 1: Basic requirements to categorize a disorder as due to autoimmunity.

- Presence of an immune reaction specific for some self-antigen or self-tissue
- Evidence to indicate that such a reaction is primary pathogenic significance and not secondary to tissue damage
- Absence of another well-defined cause of the disease

and remissions. The reasons for these features of autoimmune diseases are that the self-antigens that trigger autoimmune reactions are persistent.

- Once an immune response starts, many intrinsic amplification mechanisms are activated that maintain the response.
- When the immune response is inappropriately directed against self-tissues, the same amplification mechanisms worsen and prolong the injury.
- Immune response initiated against one-self antigen that injures tissues and may release other tissue antigens. This in turn activates lymphocytes specific for these other antigens (newly encountered epitopes), and worsen the disease. This phenomenon is termed as epitope spreading. This is the reason for autoimmune disease to become prolonged and self-perpetuating.

Clinical and pathologic manifestations: These are determined by the nature of the underlying immune response.

- **Autoantibodies:** Some are caused by autoantibodies and they may be associated with dysregulated germinal center reactions.
- **Abnormal and excessive Th1 and Th17 responses:** Most autoimmune chronic inflammatory diseases are caused by abnormal and excessive Th1 and Th17 responses. Examples for these diseases include psoriasis, multiple sclerosis, and some types of inflammatory bowel disease.
- **Both antibody and cell-mediated responses:** Some autoimmune diseases involve both antibodies and T cell-mediated inflammation (e.g., rheumatoid arthritis).

Systemic or organ specific: The clinical manifestations of autoimmune disorders are extremely varied. Autoimmune diseases may be systemic or organ specific. It depends on the distribution of the autoantigens.

- **Organ-specific disease:** This develops when the self-antigens with restricted tissue distribution. When the autoimmune responses (autoantibody or T cell responses) are directed against a single organ or tissue, it results in organ-specific disease. Examples of organ-specific autoimmune diseases are type 1 diabetes mellitus (T1DM), multiple sclerosis and myasthenia gravis. In T1DM, the autoreactive T cells and antibodies are specifically against β cells of the pancreatic islets. In multiple sclerosis, the autoreactive T cells react against central nervous system (CNS) myelin.
- **Systemic disease:** When the autoimmune reactions are against widespread antigens, it results in systemic disease. For example, if there is formation of circulating immune complexes (composed of self-antigens and specific antibodies), it usually produces systemic diseases. One of the classical examples for systemic autoimmune disease is systemic lupus erythematosus (SLE). In SLE, diverse antibodies are directed against DNA, platelets, red cells, and protein-phospholipid complexes. This result in widespread lesions throughout the body. The **systemic diseases tend to involve blood vessels and connective tissues.** Therefore, they are **often called collagen vascular diseases or connective tissue diseases.**
- **Involving more than one organ:** In the middle of the spectrum of organ specific and systemic there are very few diseases. For example, Goodpasture syndrome. In this disorder, the antibody acts against the basement membranes of both lung and kidney and produces lesions in both of them.

Autoimmunity results from the loss or breakdown of natural self-tolerance (loss of tolerance to self-antigens). Thus, autoimmune disease occurs only in those individuals in whom the breakdown of one or more of the basic mechanisms regulating immune tolerance. This results in self-reactivity and can produce damage to tissue. Examples of autoimmune diseases are presented in **Table 1**.

Immunologic Tolerance

Q. Write short essay on immunologic tolerance.

Definition: Immunologic tolerance is defined as **unresponsiveness to an antigen that is induced by previous exposure of lymphocytes to that antigen.**

In immunological tolerance, there is no **immune response to specific (usually self) antigens**. It is the result of exposure of lymphocytes to that specific antigen. The term tolerance was used after the experimental observation in animals. Animals that had encountered an antigen under particular conditions would not respond to, i.e., would tolerate, subsequent exposures to the same antigen. When specific lymphocytes encounter antigens, the lymphocytes may be either activated (leading to immune responses), or they may be inactivated or eliminated, leading to tolerance. **Antigens that induce tolerance are called tolerogens, or tolerogenic antigens**, to distinguish them from immunogens, which generate immunity.

Table 1: Examples of autoimmune diseases.

Organ-specific	*Systemic*
Diseases mediated by antibodies	
• Autoimmune hemolytic anemia	• Systemic lupus erythematosus
• Autoimmune thrombocytopenia	
• Autoimmune atrophic gastritis of pernicious anemia	
• Goodpasture syndrome	
• Graves disease	
• Myasthenia gravis	
Diseases mediated by T-cells	
• Type 1 diabetes mellitus	• Rheumatoid arthritis
• Multiple sclerosis	• Systemic sclerosis (scleroderma)
• Hashimoto thyroiditis	• Sjögren's syndrome
Diseases postulated to be autoimmune	
• Inflammatory bowel diseases (Crohn disease, ulcerative colitis)	• Polyarteritis nodosa
• Primary biliary cirrhosis	• Inflammatory myopathies
• Autoimmune (chronic active) hepatitis	

Self-tolerance: Tolerance to self-antigens is also called self-tolerance. Thus, in self-tolerance, there is **absence of immune response to an individual's own antigens**. Self-tolerance is a fundamental property of the normal immune system and it underlies our ability to live in harmony with our cells and tissues. The term tolerance applies to many protections provided by the immune system to prevent the reaction of its cells and antibodies against host components. In other words, individuals should tolerate—or not respond aggressively against—their own antigens (self-antigens).

Mechanism of Self-tolerance

Tolerance to self-antigens is an active process and requires contact between self-antigens and immune cells. In fetal life, tolerance develops to antigens that trigger vigorous immune responses in adults. There are several characteristics of tolerance in T and B lymphocyte populations. Some of the important general principles of tolerance are as follows:

Elimination of lymphocytes that express high-affinity receptors for self-antigens: Numerous different antigen receptors are produced in the developing T and B lymphocytes. These receptors are capable of recognizing self-antigens. These lymphocytes have to be eliminated or inactivated as soon as they recognize the self-antigens, to prevent immune reaction against own antigens. The mechanisms of tolerance eliminate and inactivate these lymphocytes. All individuals inherit fundamentally the same antigen receptor gene segments. These gene segments recombine and are expressed in lymphocytes as these lymphocytes arise from their precursor cells. The specificities of the receptors encoded by the recombined genes are random. They are not determined by natures of antigen as either foreign or self. During this process of producing, some developing T and B cells may express receptors capable of recognizing self-antigens. Therefore, there is a risk for lymphocytes to react against individual's own cells and tissues, causing disease. The mechanisms of immunologic tolerance prevent such reactions.

Tolerance is antigen specific: This results from the recognition of antigens by individual clones of lymphocytes. In contrast, during therapeutic immunosuppression, it affects lymphocytes of many specificities.

Two mechanism of self-tolerance: Several mechanisms induce and maintain tolerance, actively and continuously. Tolerance constantly blocks or aborts potentially harmful immune responses. The mechanisms of self-tolerance can be classified into two groups: (1) central tolerance and (2) peripheral tolerance. Self-tolerance may be induced in immature self-reactive lymphocytes in the generative lymphoid organs (central tolerance) or in mature lymphocytes in peripheral sites (peripheral tolerance) (**Figs. 1A** and **B**).

Central tolerance (Fig. 1A)

In central tolerance, self-reactive immature T and B lymphocytes are "deleted" or changed during their maturation in the "central" lymphoid organs namely thymus and bone marrow, respectively. Central tolerance makes sure that the mature naïve lymphocytes becomes incapable of responding to self-antigens that are expressed in the generative lymphoid organs (also called as central lymphoid organs). The generative lymphoid organs are the thymus for T cells and the bone marrow for B lymphocytes. In the generative (central) lymphoid organs, **both the B and T cells are immature cells**. In central tolerance process, immature self-reactive T and B lymphocytes clones that recognize self-antigens are deleted (killed) or rendered harmless. This process occurs during the maturation of lymphocytes in the central (primary or generative) lymphoid

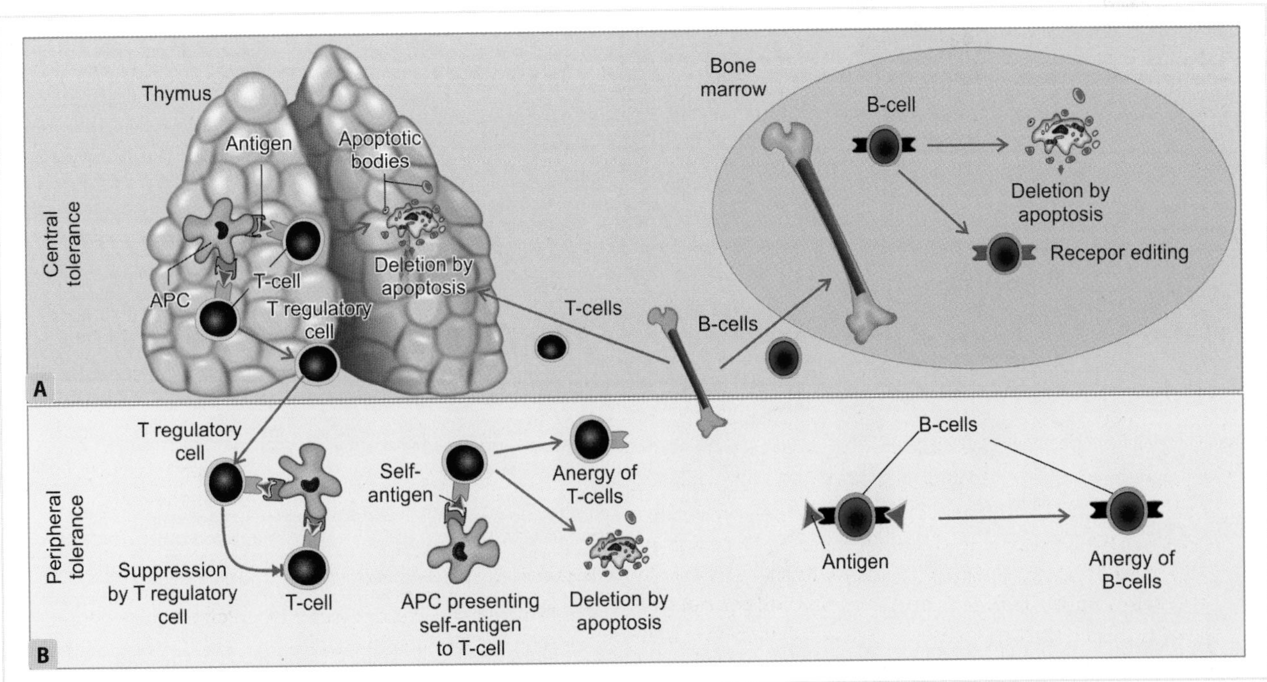

(APC: antigen-presenting cell)

FIGS. 1A AND B: Main mechanisms of central and peripheral immunological self-tolerance.

organs. During the maturation in developing lymphocytes, random somatic antigen receptor gene rearrangements take place. It produces numerous diverse antigen receptors, many of which by chance may have high affinity for self-antigens. The mechanisms of central tolerance completely remove these likely dangerous lymphocytes. As lymphocytes are maturing in the generative lymphoid organs, immature cells may come across antigens in these organs. The antigens that are present in these organs are mostly self and not foreign. This is because foreign (e.g., microbial) antigens that enter from the external environment are usually captured and taken to peripheral lymphoid organs (e.g., lymph nodes, spleen, and mucosal lymphoid tissues), and are not concentrated in the thymus or bone marrow.

Central T cell tolerance **Negative selection or clonal deletion:** During their maturation in the thymus, when **immature T cells expressing T-cell receptors (TCRs) specific for self-antigens come across self-antigens**, signals are produced that **result in killing of the cells by apoptosis**. Thus, **many immature T cells that recognize antigens with high avidity die** by **apoptosis**. This process of death of immature T cells as a result of recognition of antigens in the thymus is known as clonal deletion, or negative selection.

The antigens present in the thymus include: (1) many circulating and (2) cell-associated proteins that are widely distributed in tissues. The thymus also has a special mechanism for expressing many protein antigens that are expressed in different peripheral tissues. These **peripheral tissue antigens** are produced in medullary thymic epithelial cells (MTECs) **under the control of a protein called autoimmune regulator (AIRE) protein**. AIRE stimulates expression of some peripheral tissue–restricted self-antigens in the thymus. Thus, AIRE is thus vital for deletion of immature T cells specific for these antigens. Germline loss-of-function mutations in the *AIRE* gene, produces a multiorgan autoimmune disorder called autoimmune polyendocrine syndrome type 1 (APS1). This group of diseases is characterized by antibody- and lymphocyte-mediated destruction of multiple endocrine organs (e.g., parathyroids, adrenals, and pancreatic islets).

Many autologous protein antigens (including antigens probably restricted to peripheral tissues) are processed and presented by thymic antigen-presenting cells (APCs) in association with self major histocompatibility complex (MHC) molecules. Therefore, these antigens can be recognized by potentially self-reactive T cells.

Regulatory T cells: During maturation immature T cells in the thymus, some of the surviving cells that see self-antigens in the CD4+ lineage do not die but may differentiate and develop into regulatory T-cells (Tregs) (**Figs. 2A** and **B**). The regulatory T cells leave the thymus and inhibit responses against self-antigens in the periphery.

Central B cell tolerance In the bone marrow, immature B cells that recognize self-antigens with high affinity change their specificity or are deleted.

Receptor editing (Fig. 3A): When developing immature B cells strongly recognize self-antigens (that are present at high concentration) in the bone marrow, many of these B cells can reset antigen receptor gene rearrangement. This antigen receptor gene rearrangement causes expression of new antigen receptors, not specific for self-antigens. This process is called "receptor editing". Thus, **receptor editing is a process by which some self-reactive B-cells undergo genes rearrangement of antigen receptor and express new antigen receptors on the B cells.** These new antigen receptors expressed on reprogrammed B cells are no longer self-reactive and thus do not recognize self. Receptor editing is an important mechanism for eliminating self-reactivity. Probably one-fourth to one-half of all B cells in the body may undergone receptor editing during their maturation.

Apoptosis/Deletion (Fig. 3A): If receptor editing does not occur, the self-reactive immature B-cells that recognize self-antigens may undergo apoptosis in the bone marrow.

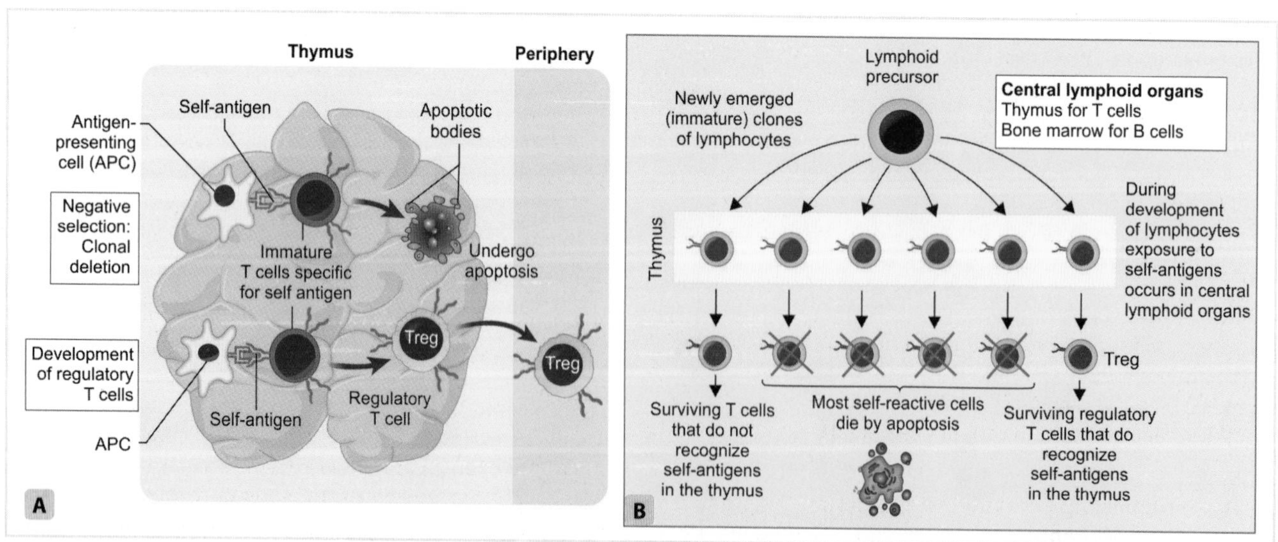

FIGS. 2A AND B: Central T-cell tolerance. (A) Recognition of self-antigens by immature T cells in the thymus leads to the apoptosis of the cells (negative selection, or clonal deletion) or to the development of regulatory T cells (Tregs). Tregs enter peripheral tissues. (B) Central tolerance is established by deletion of lymphocytes in central lymphoid organs (thymus for T cells and bone marrow for B cells) if they possess receptors that can react with self-antigens, or by the emergence of regulatory T cells (Treg) that can inhibit self-reactive cells.

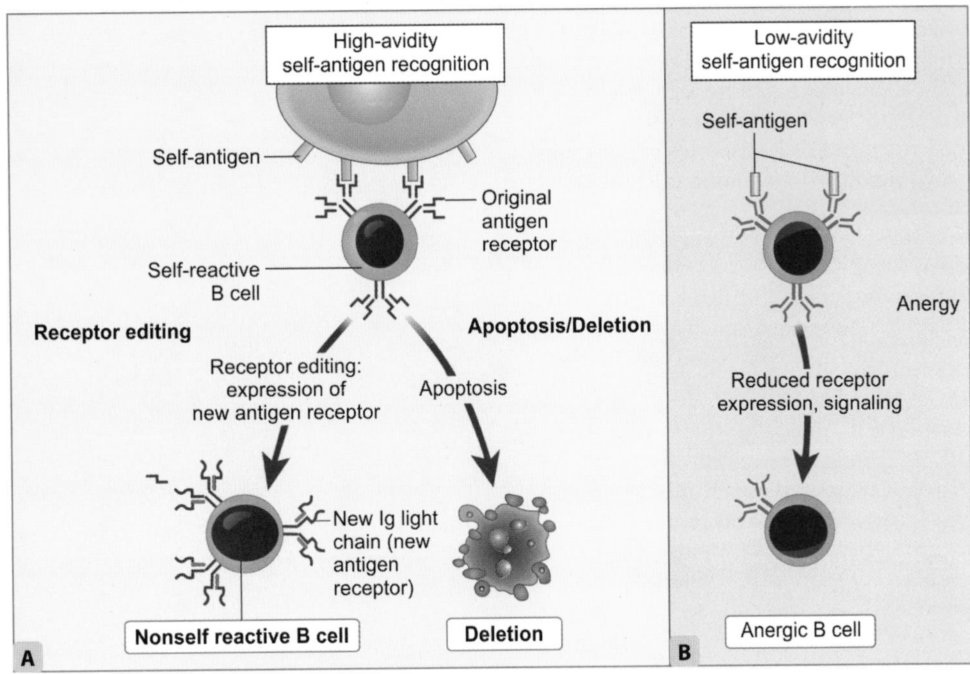

FIGS. 3A AND B: Central tolerance in B cells. (A) Immature developing B cells that recognize self-antigens in the bone marrow with high avidity, change the specificity of their antigen receptors (receptor editing, which involves light chains and in figure shown as change of antigen-binding region of the receptor) or if receptor editing does not occur, they undergo death by apoptosis. (B) Weak recognition of self-antigens in the bone marrow may lead to anergy (functional inactivation) of the B cells.

Thus, potentially dangerous lymphocytes are deleted from the mature B cell.

Anergy (Fig. 3B): A phenomenon that renders lymphocytes to recognize self-antigens to a functionally unresponsive form is called anergy. If developing B cells recognize self-antigens weakly, B cells may become functionally unresponsive (anergic) and exit the bone marrow in this unresponsive state. Weak self-antigens may be because antigen is soluble and does not cross-link many antigen receptors or if the B cell receptors (BCRs) recognize the antigen with low affinity. Anergy is due to downregulation of expression of antigen receptor and a block in antigen receptor signaling.

However, central tolerance is not perfect. Not all self-antigens may be present in the thymus and bone marrow. Many self-reactive lymphocytes (with receptors for autoantigens) complete their maturation escape into the periphery. Therefore, the mechanisms of peripheral tolerance are needed to prevent activation of these potentially dangerous lymphocytes.

Peripheral tolerance

In the periphery, both the B and T cells are mature cells. Silencing of potentially autoreactive T and B cells in peripheral tissues is called as peripheral tolerance. Several mechanisms silence autoreactive T and B cells in peripheral tissues.

Peripheral T cell tolerance (Fig. 4) Peripheral tolerance is important in regulating T cells that escape intrathymic negative selection. Three mechanisms of peripheral T cell tolerance are: (1) anergy (functional unresponsiveness), (2) suppression by Tregs, and (3) deletion (cell death by apoptosis). These three mechanisms may be responsible for peripheral T cell tolerance to tissue-specific self-antigens. This is especially for those self-antigens that are not abundant in the thymus.

Anergy (functional unresponsiveness): If lymphocytes that recognize self-antigens are rendered functionally unresponsive, this phenomenon is called anergy. Normal activation of antigen-specific T cells needs two signals: (1) **recognition of peptide antigen in association with self MHC molecules** on the surface of APCs such as dendritic cell (DC) and (2) set of **costimulatory signals** ("second signals") from APCs (**Fig. 4A**). These second signals are normally provided by some T cell-associated molecules such as CD80/B7-1 and CD86/B7-2 on the APC and CD28 on the T cell. They bind to their ligands (the costimulators B7-1 and B7-2) on APCs.

If the antigen is presented to T cells without adequate costimulatory signals, the T cells become anergic. In normal tissues, the resting DCs do not express or weakly express costimulatory molecules. Downstream T-cell inactivation/unresponsiveness (anergy) can be mediated mainly by two mechanisms.

- **Absence of costimulation (second signal):** When autoreactive T cells bind to specific self-antigens presented by DCs (one of the APCs) in the **absence of the "second signal"**, it may lead to anergy (**Fig. 4B**). Exposure of mature T cells to an antigen in the absence of costimulation may make the cells incapable of responding to that antigen. T cells that recognize self-antigens may receive an inhibitory signal from receptors that are structurally similar to CD28 but serve the opposite functions. Two of these inhibitory receptors are CTLA-4 and PD-1. These inhibitory receptors are sometimes called coinhibitors, because

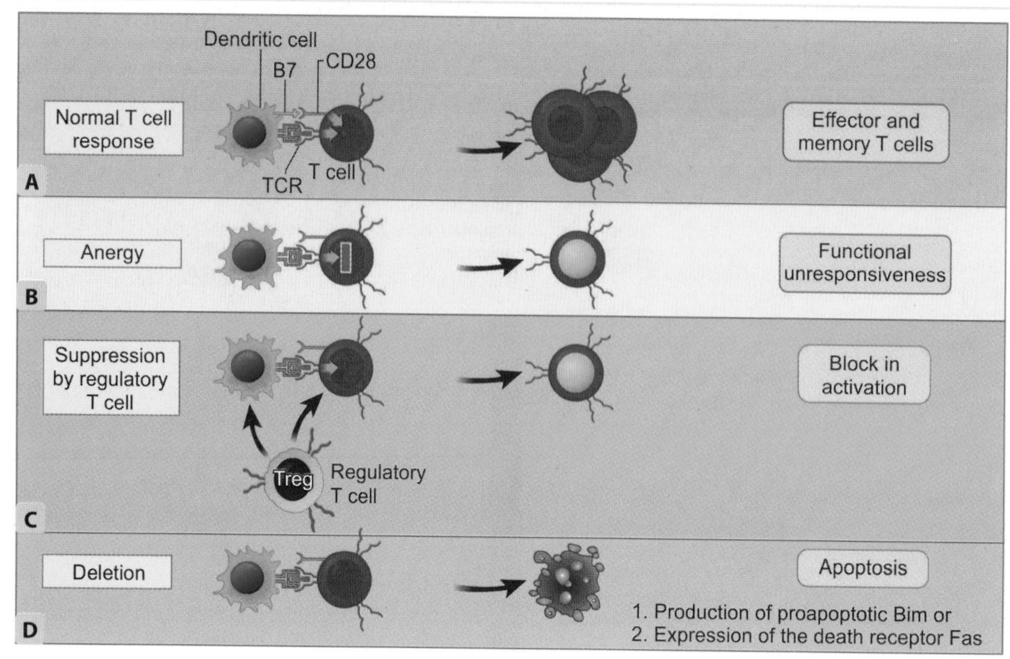

FIGS. 4A TO D: Mechanisms of peripheral T cell tolerance. (A) Signals involved in a normal T cell immune response. One of the antigens presenting cell namely dendritic cell is shown in figure. Three major mechanisms of peripheral T cell tolerance—(B) Anergy; (C) Suppression, and (D) Deletion/apoptosis.

in contrast to those of costimulators, they inhibit T cell activation. CTLA-4 (like CD28) binds to B7 molecules, and PD-1, binds to two ligands, PD-L1 and PD-L2, that are expressed on a different type of cells. This is discussed in detail on pages 498–501 (See Fig. 77 of Chapter 10). Anergy also affects mature B cells in peripheral tissues.

Suppression by regulatory T cells (Tregs) (Fig. 4C): One population of T cells called regulatory T cells that prevent immune reactions against self-antigens. Mainly regulatory T cells develop in the thymus, as a result of recognition of self-antigens, but they may also develop in peripheral lymphoid tissues. Regulatory T cells (Tregs) are a subset of CD4+ T cells suppress immune responses generated in response to exposure to self-antigens and maintain self-tolerance. These Tregs are CD4+, and constitutively expresses high levels of CD25, (the α-chain of the high-affinity IL-2 receptor), and FOXP3 (a transcription factor of the forkhead family).

Both IL-2 and FOXP3 are needed for the development and maintenance of functional CD4+ regulatory T cells. Mutations and polymorphisms affecting CD25, IL-2 or FOXP3 result in autoimmune disorders. Mutations in FOXP3 produce severe autoimmunity and cause a systemic autoimmune disease called IPEX (an acronym for ***i***mmune dysregulation, ***p***olyendocrinopathy, ***e***nteropathy, ***X***-linked). IL-2 is essential for the maintenance of regulatory T cells. Mutation of the gene encoding IL-2 or the IL-2 receptor α or β chain also causes a rare multiorgan autoimmune disease. Polymorphisms in the promoter of the *CD25* gene are associated with T1DM, multiple sclerosis, and other autoimmune diseases.

Suppression of immune responses by regulatory T cells may occur by different mechanisms. They secrete immunosuppressive cytokines (e.g., IL-10, TGF-β), which inhibit lymphocyte activation and effector functions. Regulatory T cells not only suppress immune responses not only against self-antigens but also against the fetus and commensal microbes. Developing fetus expresses paternal antigens (inherited from the father) that are foreign to the mother yet have to be tolerated. Probably regulatory T cells prevent immune reactions against these fetal antigens inherited from the father. Regulatory T cells may play a role in in human pregnancy and probably defects in these Treg cells may be responsible for recurrent spontaneous abortions.

Deletion of T cells by apoptosis (Fig. 4D): T cells that recognize self-antigens may receive signals that promote their death by apoptosis. Depletion of T cells occurs both in the thymus and in the periphery. Deletion of mature T cells in the periphery may occur by two mechanisms.

1. **Production of proapoptotic Bim:** If T cells recognize self-antigens, they may express a proapoptotic member of the Bcl family, called Bim. These T cells do not produce antiapoptotic members of the family like Bcl-2 and Bcl-x. Unopposed pro-apoptotic Bim triggers **apoptosis by the mitochondrial (intrinsic) pathway**.
2. Expression of the death receptor Fas (CD95): This mechanism involves the Fas-Fas ligand system. Upon recognition of self-antigens, T lymphocytes express the death receptor Fas (CD95). Fas is a member of the tumor necrosis factor (TNF)-receptor family. Fas ligand (FasL) is a membrane protein that is structurally similar to the cytokine TNF. FasL is expressed mainly on activated T lymphocytes. The engagement of Fas by FasL induces **apoptosis by the death receptor (extrinsic) pathway**. If self-antigens engage antigen receptors of self-reactive T cells, Fas and FasL are coexpressed. This causes death of

the cells via Fas-mediated apoptosis. Self-reactive B cells may also be deleted by FasL on T cells engaging Fas on the B cells. Mutations in Fas or FasL produce an autoimmune disease reminiscent of SLE called the autoimmune lymphoproliferative syndrome (ALPS).

Sequestered antigens: Some antigens are hidden (sequestered) from the immune system. This is because the tissues in which these antigens are present do not communicate with the blood and lymph. These self-antigens do not elicit immune responses and are ignored by the immune system. The tissues in which the antigens are hidden include the testis, eye, and brain. These sites are called immune-privileged sites, because antigens introduced into these sites tend to elicit weak or no immune responses. If the antigens of these immune-privileged tissues are released (e.g., due to trauma, infection), the resulting immune response may lead to prolonged tissue inflammation and injury. Probably this mechanism involved in the pathogenesis of post-traumatic orchitis and uveitis.

Peripheral B cell tolerance Mechanism of peripheral B cell tolerance is less known than for T cells. In peripheral tissues, mature B lymphocytes that recognize **self-antigens** in the absence of specific helper T cells may be rendered functionally **inactive** (unresponsive) **or die by apoptosis** (**Fig. 5**).

Anergy and deletion by apoptosis: Some self-reactive B cells may be repeatedly stimulated by self-antigens. These B cells become unresponsive to further activation. These anergic B cells need more than normal levels of the growth factor BAFF [B-cell activating factor, also called BLys (B lymphocyte stimulator)] for survival. The anergic B cells cannot compete with normal naïve B cells for BAFF. Because of this, the anergic B cells that have encountered self-antigens have a shortened life span. They are deleted more quickly than B cells that have not recognized self-antigens. In the periphery, mature B cells that bind with high avidity to self-antigens may also undergo apoptotic death by the mitochondrial (intrinsic) pathway.

In peripheral tissues, if B cells encounter self-antigen, especially in the absence of specific helper T cells, the B cells cannot respond to subsequent antigenic stimulation. These B cells may be excluded from lymphoid follicles, resulting in their death by apoptosis.

Signaling by inhibitory receptors: In the periphery, B cells that recognize self-antigens may be prevented from activation by the engagement of various inhibitory receptors.

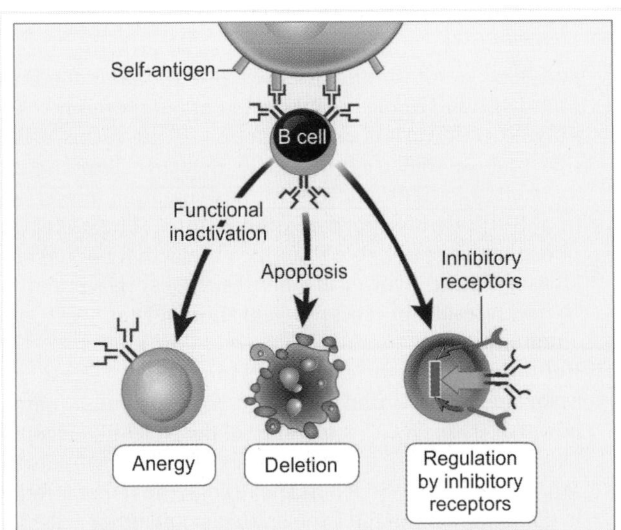

FIG. 5: Peripheral tolerance in B cells. When mature B cells encounter self-antigens in peripheral tissues, they may become functionally inactive by anergy or undergo death by apoptosis. In some B cells, recognition of self-antigens may trigger inhibitory receptors that prevent B cell activation.

Mechanisms of Autoimmunity

Q. Write short essay on mechanism/pathogenesis of autoimmunity.

Normally, the immune system exists in an equilibrium in which there is balance between lymphocyte activation (needed for defense against pathogens), and the mechanisms of tolerance (prevent reactions against self-antigens). Loss (failure) of tolerance allows immune responses to develop against self-antigens and lead to autoimmunity and is the cause of autoimmune diseases.

Major mechanisms that prevent autoimmunity are listed in **Box 2**.

Two main factors that contribute to the development of autoimmunity are: (1) **genetic susceptibility** and (2) **environmental triggers**, such as infections and local tissue injury/damage. Mechanism of autoimmunity may be the result of combination of these two main factors. The inheritance of susceptibility genes may contribute to the breakdown of self-tolerance, and environmental triggers, (e.g., infections and tissue damage) promote the activation of self-reactive lymphocytes (**Fig. 6**). General abnormalities that may to contribute to development of autoimmunity are as follows:

Defective immune tolerance or regulation: Breakdown of self-tolerance may lead to autoimmunity. But, the exact mechanism by which self-tolerance fails is not known in the majority of common autoimmune diseases.

Abnormalities in display of self-antigens: These abnormalities may include

- Increased expression and persistence of self-antigens that are normally cleared.
- Structural changes in the self-antigens resulting from post-translational enzymatic modifications.

Box 2: Major mechanisms that prevent autoimmunity.

- **Sequestration of self-antigens** renders them inaccessible to the immune system
- **Generation and maintenance of tolerance:** Specific unresponsiveness (tolerance or anergy) of relevant T or B cells
  - Central deletion of autoreactive lymphocytes
  - Peripheral anergy of autoreactive lymphocytes
  - Receptor replacement in autoreactive lymphocytes
- **Regulatory mechanisms:** Limitation of potential reactivity by regulatory mechanisms
  - Regulatory T cells (Tregs)
  - Regulatory B cells

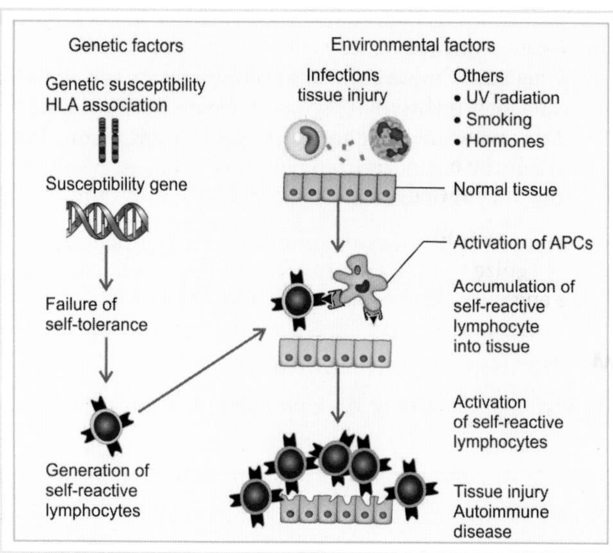

FIG. 6: Pathogenesis of autoimmunity. Various genetic loci may predispose susceptibility to autoimmunity, partly by influencing the maintenance of self-tolerance. Environmental triggers, such as infections and other inflammatory stimuli, promote the accumulation of lymphocytes into tissues and activate self-reactive lymphocytes leading to tissue injury.

- Cellular stress or injury.

Abnormalities in self-antigens lead to the display of "neoantigens" (new epitopes that are not expressed normally). The immune system may not be tolerant to these new epitopes, and immune system may develop antiself-responses.

Inflammation or an initial innate immune response: The innate immune response is a strong stimulus for the subsequent activation of lymphocytes and the production of adaptive immune responses. Microbes or cell injury may bring about local inflammatory reactions and these may trigger subsequent autoimmunity.

Genetic Factors

Role of susceptibility genes

Autoimmunity has a genetic component. Most of autoimmune diseases are complex multigenic disorders in which affected individuals inherit multiple genetic polymorphisms that contribute to disease susceptibility. These genes act with environmental factors to cause the diseases. The proof for genetics contribution is increased incidence of many autoimmune diseases in twins of affected individuals than in the general population, and incidence is greater in monozygotic than in dizygotic twins. Susceptibility genes may disrupt self-tolerance mechanisms and produce autoimmune diseases. Some of these polymorphisms in gene are associated with several autoimmune diseases. This suggests that these causative genes influence general mechanisms of immune regulation and self-tolerance. Other genetic loci are associated with particular diseases, suggesting that they may affect organ damage or autoreactive lymphocytes of particular specificities.

***Association of human leukocyte antigen alleles with autoimmune disease*:** Among the genes that are associated with autoimmunity, the strongest associations are with *MHC (HLA) genes*. *HLA genes* are known to be associated with

Table 2: Examples of non–HLA genes associated with autoimmune diseases.

Presumed gene involved	*Diseases*
Genes involved in immune regulation	
PTPN22	Rheumatoid arthritis, type 1 diabetes mellitus, inflammatory bowel disease
IL23R	Inflammatory bowel disease, psoriasis, ankylosing spondylitis
CTLA4	Type 1 diabetes mellitus, rheumatoid arthritis
IL2RA	Multiple sclerosis, Type 1 diabetes mellitus
Genes involved in immune responses to microbes	
NOD2 and *ATG16*	Inflammatory bowel disease
IRF5 and *IFIH1*	Systemic lupus erythematosus (SLE)

autoimmunity. Examples for autoimmune diseases associated with increased HLA association include rheumatoid arthritis, T1DM, multiple sclerosis, SLE, ankylosing spondylitis, and Celiac disease. There are most striking associations between ankylosing spondylitis and *HLA-B27*; individuals who inherit *HLA-B27* have a 100- to 200-fold greater chance of developing the disease compared with those who do not carry *HLA-B27*.

***Association of non-MHC genes with autoimmune diseases*:** Polymorphisms in many non-MHC (non-HLA) genes are associated with different autoimmune diseases (**Table 2**). Some of these genes are disease-specific, but many of the non-MHC genes are seen in multiple disorders. These observations suggest that the products of these genes affect general mechanisms of immune regulation and self-tolerance. Three genes associations with autoimmunity are briefly discussed here:

1. **Polymorphisms in a gene *PTPN22*:** This gene encodes a protein tyrosine phosphatase. Polymorphisms in a gene *PTPN22* is fairly high with rheumatoid arthritis, T1DM, and other autoimmune diseases. It is probably the most frequent non-HLA gene implicated in autoimmunity. The polymorphic variants of the gene encode forms of the phosphatase that are functionally defective. The disease-associated variant causes complex signaling alterations in multiple immune cell populations. The defective phosphatase is not able to reduce the activity of tyrosine kinases that are involved in many responses of lymphocytes. Hence, it results in excessive activation of lymphocyte and autoimmunity.
2. **Polymorphisms in the gene for *NOD2*:** These are associated with Crohn disease, a form of inflammatory bowel disease. *NOD2*, a member of the NOD-like receptor (NLR) family (see Fig. 2 of chapter 8). It is a cytoplasmic sensor of microbes (bacterial peptidoglycans) that is found in epithelial cells of intestine epithelial and other cells. The disease-associated NOD2 variant reduces the function of NOD2 and is unable to sensing gut microbes, including commensal bacteria. This cannot provide effective defense against certain intestinal microbes. This leads to entry of these bacteria (microbes) into the intestinal epithelium. This initiates a chronic inflammatory reaction in the intestinal

wall against these normally well-tolerated organisms. Crohn disease is believed to be an unregulated response to commensal microbes and not a true autoimmune disease.

3. **Polymorphisms in the gene encoding the IL-2 receptor (CD25):** These are associated with multiple sclerosis and other autoimmune diseases. These variants of gene encoding the IL-2 receptor may influence the expression and activity of IL key receptor. This in turn affect the balance between regulatory and effector T cells.

Inherited single-gene (Mendelian) abnormalities: Sporadic mutations of individual genes may result in autoimmunity, but diseases caused by these single-gene mutations are rare. The individual genes associated with autoimmune diseases include AIRE, CTLA4, PD1, FAS, FASL, and IL2 and its receptor CD25. B cells express an Fc receptor that recognizes IgG antibodies bound to antigens and switches off further antibody production (a normal negative-feedback mechanism). If the mutation affects FC receptor, it can produce autoimmunity, probably because these B cells can no longer be controlled and switches on the production of antibody.

Environmental Factors

Role of Infections

Infections by virus and bacteria may contribute to the development and exacerbation of autoimmunity. Infections by variety of microbes may trigger autoimmune reactions.

Two mechanisms by infections contribute to autoimmunity (**Fig. 7**) are discussed here.

Induction of costimulators on APCs Normally, when a mature self-reactive T cell encounter with a self-antigen presented by a costimulator-deficient resting tissue APC, it results in peripheral tolerance by anergy (**Fig. 7A**).

- Infections by microbes may activate the APCs to express costimulator (**Fig. 7B**). Infections of particular tissues may induce local innate immune responses. This causes recruitment of leukocytes into the tissues and also activates tissue APCs. These APCs begin to express costimulators. When APCs present self-antigens along with costimulators, it results in the breakdown of peripheral T cell self-tolerance by breakdown of anergy. The activated T cells specific for the self-antigens leads to the development of autoimmune disease. This type of response is called bystander activation.

Molecular mimicry (**Fig. 7C**): Some microbes may contain antigens that have the same amino acid sequences as in self-antigens. Immune responses against these microbial antigens may result in the activation of self-reactive lymphocytes. This phenomenon is known as molecular mimicry because the **antigens of the microbe cross-react with, or mimic, self-antigens**. For example, rheumatic heart disease in which anti-streptococcal antibodies formed against streptococcal bacterial proteins cross-react with myocardial proteins. These antibodies are deposited in the heart and cause myocarditis. DNA sequencing has shown many short stretches of homologies between myocardial proteins and streptococcal proteins.

Other abnormalities

- **Polyclonal B-cell activation:** Infections by microbes may produce other abnormalities that promote autoimmune reactions. Some viruses [e.g., Epstein-Barr virus (EBV), human immunodeficiency virus (HIV)], cause polyclonal B-cell activation and may produce autoantibodies.
- **Creation of neoantigens:** Infections produce tissue injury and may release and structurally modify self-antigens. This creates neoantigens (new antigens) that can activate T cells.
- **Cytokine production:** Infections may induce the production of cytokines that recruit lymphocytes to sites of self-antigens. These lymphocytes may be potentially self-reactive lymphocytes.

Infections may protect against autoimmune diseases: Some infections may protect against the development of some autoimmune diseases. Epidemiologic data suggest infections greatly reduce the incidence of disease and reducing infections increases the incidence of T1DM and multiple sclerosis. The mechanisms are not known. Probably, infections promote

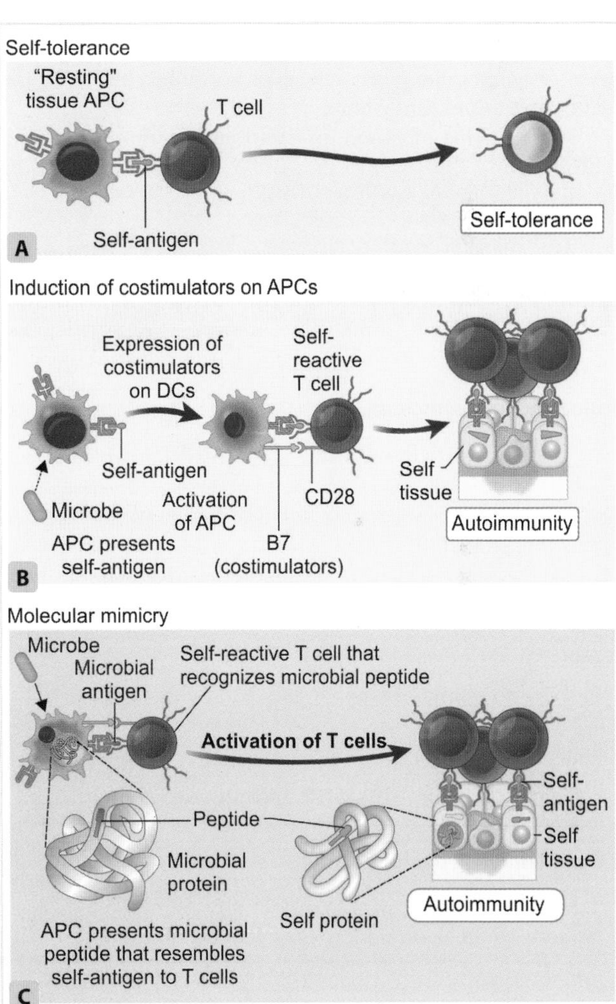

FIGS. 7A TO C: Role of infections in the development of autoimmunity. (A) Normally, when a mature self-reactive T cell encounter with a self-antigen presented by a costimulator-deficient resting tissue antigen presenting cell (APC), it results in peripheral tolerance by anergy. (B) Infections by microbes may activate the APCs to express costimulators (B7). When these APCs present self-antigens, the self-reactive T cells are activated and cause autoimmunity. (C) Some microbial antigens may mimic self-antigens and activate self-reactive lymphocytes. These reactive lymphocytes may cross-react with self-antigens (molecular mimicry).

low-level IL-2 production. IL-2 is essential for maintaining regulatory T cells.

Other environmental factors

Apart from infections, the display of tissue antigens also may be changed by a variety of environmental factors.

Ultraviolet (UV) radiation causes cell death and may lead to the exposure of nuclear antigens. This may trigger pathologic immune responses in systemic lupus erythematosus. This mechanism is the probably responsible for the association for the development of lupus flares with exposure to sunlight.

Smoking is a risk factor for rheumatoid arthritis. Possibly smoking leads to chemical modification of self-antigens.

Local tissue injury due to any cause (e.g., inflammation, ischemic injury, trauma) may release of self-antigens that are normally concealed from the immune system.

Hormones: Autoimmunity has a strong gender bias. Autoimmune diseases are more common in women than in men. This may due to the effects of hormones and unknown genes on the X chromosome.

Mechanisms of tissue injury in autoantibody mediated autoimmune disease are presented in **Table 3** and those mediated by T cells are listed in **Table 4**.

Table 3: Mechanisms of tissue injury in autoantibody mediated autoimmune disease.

Target	*Disease*
Blocking or inactivation	
α chain of the nicotinic acetylcholine receptor	Myasthenia gravis
Phospholipid–β_2-glycoprotein I complex	Antiphospholipid syndrome
Insulin receptor	Insulin-resistant diabetes mellitus
Intrinsic factor	Pernicious anemia
Stimulation	
TSH receptor (LATS)	Graves disease
Proteinase-3 (ANCA)	Granulomatosis with polyangiitis
Epidermal cadherin Desmoglein 3	Pemphigus vulgaris
Complement activation	
α_3 chain of collagen IV	Goodpasture syndrome
Immune complex formation (type III hypersensitivity)	
Double-stranded DNA	Systemic lupus erythematosus
Immunoglobulin	Rheumatoid arthritis
Opsonization	
Platelet GpIIb: IIIa	Autoimmune thrombocytopenic purpura
Rh antigens, I antigen	Autoimmune hemolytic anemia
Antibody-dependent cellular cytotoxicity	
Thyroid peroxidase, thyroglobulin	Hashimoto thyroiditis

(ANCA: antineutrophil cytoplasmic antibodies; DNA: deoxyribonucleic acid; Gp: glycoprotein; LATS: long-acting thyroid stimulator)

Systemic Lupus Erythematosus

Definition: SLE is an autoimmune disease involving multiple organs, characterized by a variety of autoantibodies [particularly ANAs], in which organs and cells damage is initially mediated by tissue-binding autoantibodies and immune complexes.

Systemic lupus erythematosus may be acute or insidious in its onset, and is typically a chronic, remitting and relapsing. Though it can affect almost any organ in the body, **most prominent injury is to the skin, joints, kidney, and serosal membranes**. Thus, SLE is very heterogeneous disease, and any patient may present with any number of clinical features.

Revised criteria for classification of SLE by the American College of Rheumatology are presented in **Table 5**.

A patient is classified as having SLE if four of the clinical and immunologic criteria are present at any time (not necessarily concurrently), including at least one clinical and one immunologic criterion.

Systemic lupus erythematosus is a fairly common disease and predominantly affects women with a female-to-male ratio of 9:1 and affects women of childbearing (reproductive) age of 17–55 years. The female-to-male ratio is only 2:1 for SLE disease developing during childhood or after 65 years of age. Though it usually presents between 20 and 30-year age group, it may manifest at any age, including early childhood.

Autoantibodies in Systemic Lupus Erythematosus

Q. Write short essay on antibodies in SLE.

Q. Write short essay on significance of antineutrophil cytoplasmic antibodies/ANAs.

Systemic lupus erythematosus is characterized by the production of several diverse autoantibodies. The hallmark of SLE is the presence of autoantibodies and includes antibodies to double-stranded DNA (anti-dsDNA) and the so-called Smith (Sm) antigen. These autoantibodies are virtually diagnostic of SLE. Some antibodies are against different nuclear and cytoplasmic components of the cell that are not organ specific. Other antibodies are directed against specific cell surface antigens of blood cells.

Significance: The autoantibodies are pathogenic and produce damage by either forming immune complexes or by attacking their target cells. The levels of these autoantibodies in the blood also help in the diagnosis and management of patients with SLE.

Antinuclear autoantibodies

These autoantibodies are directed against nuclear antigens. They can be grouped into four categories depending on their specificity for: (1) DNA, (2) histones, (3) nonhistone proteins bound to RNA, and (4) nucleolar antigens. Various autoantibodies and their clinical utility in SLE are presented in **Table 6**.

Table 4: Mechanisms of tissue injury in T cell-mediated autoimmune disease.

Mechanism	*Disease*
Cytokine production	Rheumatoid arthritis, multiple sclerosis, type 1 diabetes mellitus
Cellular cytotoxicity	Type 1 diabetes mellitus

Table 5: Revised criteria for classification of systemic lupus erythematosus (American College of Rheumatology Criteria).

Criterion	*Description*
Clinical criteria	
Acute cutaneous lupus	Malar rash (fixed erythema, flat or raised, over the malar eminences tending to spare the nasolabial folds), photosensitivity
Chronic cutaneous lupus	Discoid rash: Erythematous raised patches with adherent keratotic scaling and follicular plugging
Nonscarring alopecia	Diffuse thinning or hair fragility in the absence of other causes
Oral or nasal ulcers	Oral or nasopharyngeal ulceration, usually painless, observed by physician
Joint disease	Nonerosive arthritis involving two or more peripheral joints, joints, characterized by tenderness, swelling, or effusion
Serositis	Pleuritis (pleuritic pain or rub or evidence of pleural effusion), pericarditis
Renal disorder	Persistent proteinuria >0.5 g/day or red cell casts
Neurologic disorder	Seizures, psychosis, myelitis or neuropathy, in the absence of offending drugs or other known causes
Hemolytic anemia	Hemolytic anemia
Leukopenia or lymphopenia	Leukopenia: $<4.0 \times 10^9$ cells/L ($<4{,}000/mm^3$) total on two or more occasions or lymphopenia: $<1.5 \times 10^9$ cells/L ($<1{,}500/mm^3$) on two or more occasions
Thrombocytopenia	Thrombocytopenia: $<100 \times 10^9$ cells/L ($<100{,}000/mm^3$) in the absence of offending drugs and other conditions
Immunologic criteria	
Antinuclear antibody	Abnormal titer of antinuclear antibody by immunofluorescence
Anti-dsDNA antibody	Abnormal titer
Anti-Sm antibody	Presence of antibody to Sm nuclear antigen
Antiphospholipid antibody	Positive finding of antiphospholipid antibody based on: (1) an abnormal serum level of IgG or IgM anti-cardiolipin antibodies, (2) a positive test for lupus anticoagulant using a standard test, or (3) a false-positive serologic test for syphilis known to be positive for at least 6 months and confirmed by negative *Treponema pallidum* immobilization or fluorescent treponemal antibody absorption test
Low complement	Low C3, C4, or CH50
Direct Coombs test	Assay for anti-red cell antibody, in the absence of clinically evident hemolytic anemia

Table 6: Various autoantibodies and their clinical utility in systemic lupus erythematosus (SLE).

Type of antibody (% positivity)	*Antigen recognized*	*Clinical utility*
Antinuclear antibodies		
Antinuclear antibodies (antibodies to DNA) (95–100)	Multiple nuclear	Best screening test; if repeated test is negative SLE unlikely
Anti-dsDNA* (40–70)	DNA (double-stranded)	High titers of IgG antibodies are SLE-specific (but not to single-stranded DNA)
Anti-Sm* (20–30)	Smith (Sm) antigen (core protein of small RNP particles): Protein complexed to 6 species of nuclear U1 RNA	Specific for SLE; do not usually correlate with disease activity or clinical manifestations; most patients also have anti-RNP
Antihistone antibodies (70)	Histones associated with DNA (in nucleosome, chromatin)	More frequent in drug-induced lupus than in SLE
Anti-Ro (SS-A)# (30–50)	Protein complexed to hY RNA	Not specific for SLE; predictive value indicates increased risk for neonatal lupus and Sicca syndrome
Anti-RNP (40)	Protein complexed to U1 RNA	Not specific for SLE; high titers associated with syndromes that have overlap features of several rheumatic syndromes including SLE
Anti-PL# (antiphospholipid) (30–50)	Phospholipid-protein complexes	Antiphospholipid syndrome (in ~10% of SLE patients)
Anti-La (SS-B) (10–20)	47-kDa protein complexed to hY RNA	Usually associated with anti-Ro; associated with decreased risk for nephritis
Other antibodies		
Antierythrocyte (60)	RBC membrane	Measured as direct Coombs test; a small proportion develops overt hemolysis
Antiplatelet (30)	Surface and altered cytoplasmic antigens on platelets	Associated with thrombocytopenia, but neither good sensitivity or specificity; not a useful clinical test
Antineuronal: includes antiglutamate receptor 2 (60)	Neuronal and lymphocyte surface antigens	Positive test in CSF may correlate with active CNS lupus
Antiribosomal P (20)	Protein in ribosomes	Positive test in serum may correlate with depression or psychosis due to CNS lupus

[CNS: central nervous system; CSF: cerebrospinal fluid; U1 RNA: small nuclear ribonucleoprotein (snRNP also known as U1-RNP)]

* Antibodies specific to SLE.

Females with child-bearing potential and SLE should be screened for aPL and anti-Ro.

Method of detection: The most commonly used method for detecting ANAs is indirect immunofluorescence. Immunofluorescence can detect antibodies that bind to a various nuclear antigen, including DNA, RNA, and proteins (collectively called generic ANAs). The pattern of nuclear fluorescence under immunofluorescence suggests the type of antibody present in the patient's serum. Five basic patterns of nuclear fluorescence are as follows (**Table 7**):

1. **Homogeneous or diffuse nuclear staining:** It usually suggest antibodies to chromatin, nucleosomes, histones, and, occasionally, double-stranded DNA. It is common in SLE.
2. **Rim or peripheral staining patterns:** They are usually produced by antibodies to double-stranded DNA and sometimes to nuclear envelope proteins.
3. **Speckled pattern:** It is characterized by the presence of uniform or variable-sized speckles. Though it is one of the most common patterns of fluorescence observed, it is the least specific. It reflects the presence of antibodies to non-DNA nuclear constituents such as Sm antigen, ribonucleoprotein, and SS-A and SS-B reactive antigens.
4. **Nucleolar pattern:** This pattern is characterized by the presence of a few discrete spots of fluorescence within the nucleus. It is typical of antibodies to RNA. This pattern is detected mostly in patients with systemic sclerosis.
5. **Centromeric pattern:** This pattern indicates antibodies specific for centromeres. It is seen in patients with systemic sclerosis.

The immunofluorescence patterns are not absolutely specific for the type of antibody. In a patient with SLE many autoantibodies may be present and combinations of patterns are frequent. However, the immunostaining pattern is still considered as a diagnostic tool.

Other autoantibodies

In addition to ANAs, many other autoantibodies may be found in SLE patients.

***Autoantibodies against blood cells*:** Some antibodies are directed against blood cells. These include antibodies against: (1) red cells, (2) platelets, and (3) lymphocytes.

Q. Write short essay on antiphospholipid antibody.

***Antiphospholipid (aPL) antibodies*:** These are present in 30–40% of SLE patients but they are not specific for SLE.

- The term **antiphospholipid antibody is misleading,** because these **antibodies react with proteins in complex with phospholipids rather than directly with phospholipids** (**Fig. 8**). They are actually specific for epitopes of plasma proteins. These proteins are in complex

Table 7: Pattern of antinuclear antibody staining.

Pattern of staining	*Diagrammatic appearance*	*Staining pattern due to*	*Associated conditions*
Homogeneous or diffuse staining of the entire nucleus with or without apparent masking of the nucleoli		Antibodies to nucleosomes (anti-DNP), histones (anti-histone) and occasionally double-stranded DNA (anti-dsDNA)	Rheumatoid arthritis, systemic lupus erythematosus (SLE), and miscellaneous disorders (anti-ssDNA)
Rim or peripheral staining		Antibodies to double-stranded DNA (anti-DNA) and sometimes to nuclear envelope proteins. Not seen on HEp-2	SLE
Speckled (may be coarse or fine) pattern-the presence of uniform or variable-sized speckles throughout the nucleus. Most common pattern and is least specific		Antibodies to non-DNA nuclear constituents such as Sm antigen (anti-Sm), ribonucleoprotein (anti-RNP), and SS-A (anti-SS-A) and SS-B reactive antigens (anti-SS-B)	SLE, systemic sclerosis (SSc), polymyositis (PM)/ dermatomyositis (DM)
Nucleolar pattern-presence of a few discrete spots within the nucleus-stains nucleoli within the nucleus, sharply separated from the unstained nucleoplasm		Antibodies to RNA (anti-nucleolar)	Most often seen in systemic sclerosis
Centromeric pattern-discrete uniform speckles throughout the nucleus. The number of speckles corresponds to a multiple of the normal chromosome number		Antibodies specific for centromeres (anti-centromere)	Systemic sclerosis, Sjögren syndrome, and other diseases

(ds: double stranded; ss; single stranded).

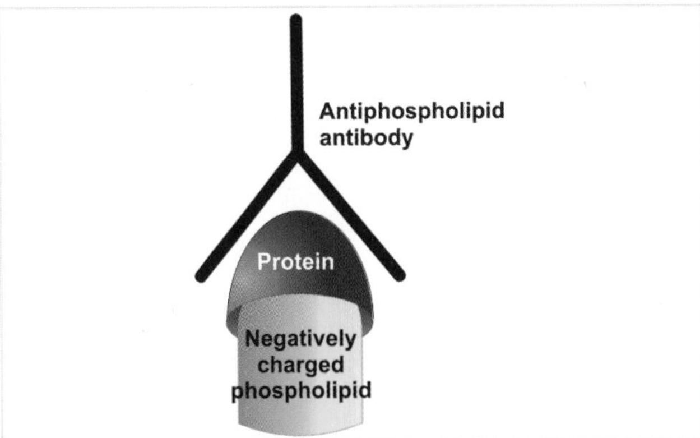

FIG. 8: Antiphospholipid antibody against plasma proteins bound to phospholipids.

with phospholipids. These **proteins include prothrombin, annexin V, β_2-glycoprotein I, protein S, and protein C.**

- **Antibodies against the phospholipid-β_2-glycoprotein** complex also bind to cardiolipin antigen. Since cardiolipin antigen is used in the serological test for syphilis, SLE patients **may give a false-positive serological reaction for syphilis.**
- Some of these antiphospholipid **antibodies interfere with in vitro clotting tests** (e.g., partial thromboplastin time). Therefore, these antibodies are sometimes called to as **lupus anticoagulant**. Though they delay clotting in vitro, these patients with antiphospholipid antibodies may develop complications due to excessive clotting (a hypercoagulable state). For example, they **may develop thrombus.**
- **Complications:** These autoantibodies can lead to **increased venous and arterial thrombosis** and **thrombocytopenia.** They are prone to develop **recurrent spontaneous miscarriages** and **focal cerebral or ocular ischemia.** The antiphospholipid antibody syndrome is discussed on pages 373–374 and 1102.
- Diagnosis: Two tests that measure different antibodies (anticardiolipin and the lupus anticoagulant): (1) ELISA for anticardiolipin, and (2) a sensitive phospholipid-based activated prothrombin time, such as the dilute Russell viper venom test.

In addition to SLE, autoantibodies are found in many diseases. Few examples of systemic autoimmune diseases with corresponding autoantibodies are presented in **Table 8**.

Table 8: Autoantibodies in systemic autoimmune diseases other than SLE.
Sjögren syndrome
• Ro/SS-A • La/SS-B
Systemic sclerosis
• DNA topoisomerase 1 • Centromeric proteins (CENPs) A, B, C • RNA polymerase III
Autoimmune myositis
• Histidyl aminoacyl-tRNA synthetase, Jo1 • Mi-2 nuclear antigen • MDA5 (cytoplasmic receptor for viral RNA) • TIF1γ nuclear protein
Rheumatoid arthritis
• Cyclic citrullinated peptides (CCP); various citrullinated proteins (specific for rheumatoid arthritis) • Rheumatoid factor (not specific)

(DNA: deoxyribonucleic acid; RNA: ribonucleic acid; SLE: systemic lupus erythematosus)

Etiology

Q. Discuss the etiology and pathogenesis of SLE.

Systemic lupus erythematosus is an autoimmune disease in which fundamental defect is failure of the mechanisms that maintains self-tolerance. It leads to production of many autoantibodies that damage the tissue either directly or indirectly by depositing immune complex deposits. As in most of the autoimmune diseases, a combination of genetic and environmental factors plays a role in the pathogenesis of SLE.

Genetic factors

Systemic lupus erythematosus is a genetically complex multigenic disease with contributions from both MHC (HLA) and multiple non-MHC (non-HLA) genes. Many evidences support genetic predisposition and these are as follows:

- **Family members of SLE** patients have an increased risk of developing SLE. Also, about 20% of unaffected first-degree relatives of SLE patients may show autoantibodies and other immune abnormalities.
- **High rate of concordance** (>20%) in monozygotic twins when compared with dizygotic twins (1–3%).
- **HLA associations:** It was observed that *MHC* genes regulate production of particular autoantibodies. Specific alleles of the HLA-DQ locus are linked to the production of anti-double-stranded DNA, anti-Sm, and antiphospholipid antibodies.
- **Inherited deficiencies of early complement components:** This is found in some SLE patients. These deficient early complement components include C2, C4, or C1q. Deficiency of complement may diminish the removal of circulating immune complexes by the mononuclear phagocyte system. This in turn may favor the deposition of immune complexes in the tissue. Probably deficiency of C1q leads to defective phagocytic clearance of apoptotic cells. Normally, many cells undergo apoptosis and are cleared. Deficiency of C1q may lead to defective apoptosis. The nuclear components released from these apoptotic cells may elicit immune responses.
- Studies have identified many genetic loci that may be associated with the SLE. Many of these loci encode proteins involved in lymphocyte signaling and interferon responses. Both these responses may play a role in lupus pathogenesis. But the relative risk for each locus is small, and even if all loci are considered together these loci account for 20% or less of the predisposition to SLE.

Immunologic factors

Several immunological abnormalities of both innate and adaptive immune system have been observed in SLE. These abnormalities collectively may result in the persistence and uncontrolled activation of self-reactive lymphocytes.

Failure of self-tolerance in B-cells: Failure of mechanism of immunologic tolerance against self-reactive B cells. It may occur either in the bone marrow or in peripheral tolerance mechanisms. This leads to failure to remove these self-reactive B cells with accumulation of autoreactive B-cells.

Activation of CD4+ helper T cells: The CD4+ helper T cells specific for nucleosomal antigens that escape tolerance may be activated in SLE. This will help B cells to generate high-affinity pathogenic autoantibodies.

Engagement of toll-like receptor (TLR) by nuclear DNA and RNA present in immune complexes: Normally, the function of TLRs present in B lymphocytes is to sense microbial products, including nucleic acids.

- In SLE, TLR of B cells may be engaged by nuclear DNA and RNA contained in immune complexes. This may activate B lymphocytes. These activated B cells specific for nuclear antigens may get second signals from TLRs. This leads to further activation of B cells and increased production of antinuclear autoantibodies.

Type I interferons: These are antiviral cytokines normally produced by B-cells during innate immune responses to nucleic acid of viruses. Large amounts of type I interferons produced play a role in lymphocyte activation in SLE. Probably, nucleic acids engage TLRs on DCs (dendritic cells) and stimulate the production of interferons, i.e., self-nucleic acids mimic their microbial counterparts. Type I interferons may activate DCs and B cells and promote Th1 responses. All these responses may stimulate the production of pathogenic autoantibodies and produce inflammation.

Environmental factors

Environmental factors may also be involved in the pathogenesis of SLE.

UV radiation: Exposure to UV (ultraviolet) light in the sunlight intensify the lesions of the disease in many patients.

- **Mechanism:** UV irradiation increases apoptosis of host cells (e.g., skin cells). This may alter the DNA and intracellular proteins to make them antigenic. These altered DNA are increasingly recognized by TLRs. Also, UV light may modulate the immune response. For example, UV light stimulates keratinocytes to produce IL-1. IL-1 is a cytokine known to promote inflammation.

Cigarette smoking: It is associated with development of SLE.

Sex hormones: SLE is 10 times greater during the reproductive period (17–55 years) in women than in men. SLE shows exacerbation during normal menses and pregnancy. The gender bias of SLE is partly due to the actions of sex hormones and partly related to unknown genes on the X chromosome, independent of effects of hormone.

Drugs: Examples include **hydralazine, procainamide, isoniazid and D-penicillamine** can produce SLE-like disease. The disease remits after withdrawal of the drug.

Epstein–Barr virus (EBV): It may be one infectious agent that can trigger SLE in susceptible individuals.

Others: Prolonged occupational exposure to crystalline silica (e.g., inhalation of soap powder dust or soil in farming activities) may increase the risk. Drinking alcohol (two glasses of wine a week or ½ of an alcoholic drink daily) reduces the risk of SLE.

Pathogenesis of systemic lupus erythematosus

Q. Write short essay on pathogenesis of systemic lupus erythematosus.

Immunologic abnormalities in SLE are varied and complex. Autoimmunity in SLE results from interplay between genetic susceptibility, environment, gender, race, and abnormal immune responses. The proposed pathogenic mechanisms of SLE (**Fig. 9**) are as follows:

- **Increased apoptosis triggered by environmental agents:** UV irradiation and other environmental agents (insults) may cause death of cells by apoptosis.

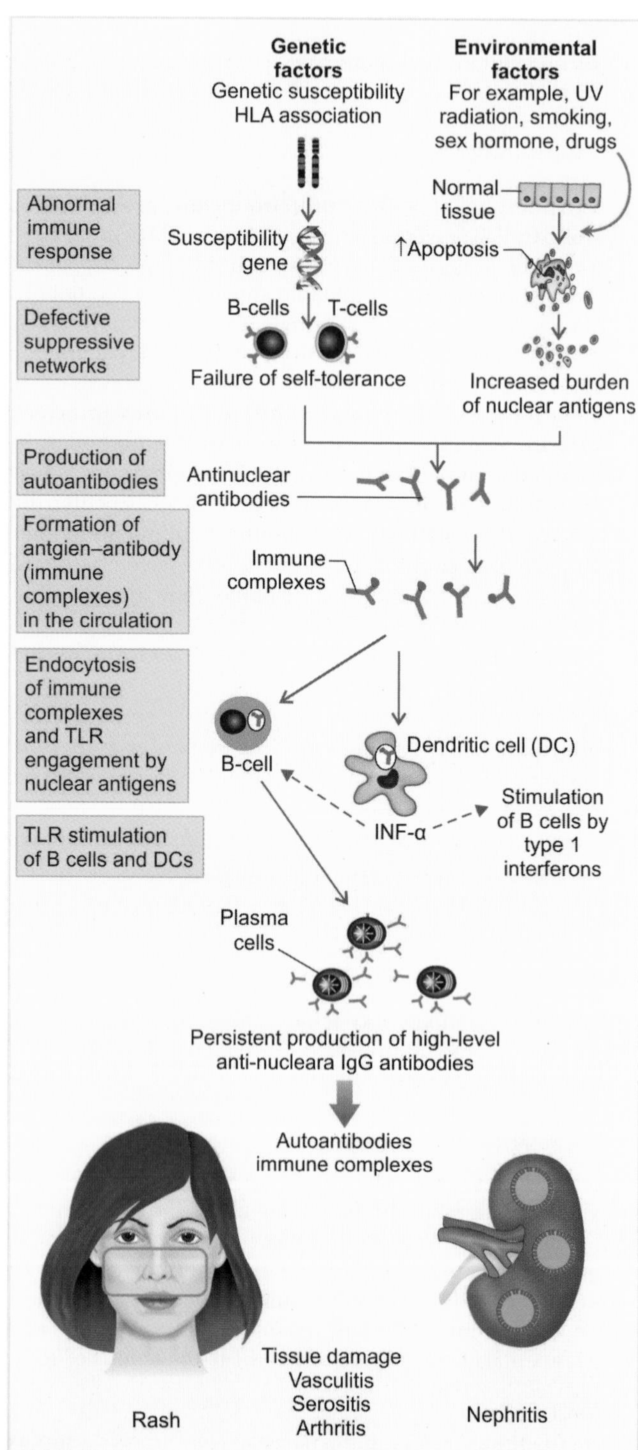

FIG. 9: Pathogenesis of systemic lupus erythematosus.

- **Inadequate clearance of apoptotic bodies:** Inadequate clearance of the nuclei of these apoptotic cells due to abnormal immune responses leads to production of increased quantities and immunogenic forms of nucleic acids, their accompanying proteins, and other self-antigens. Hence, increased amounts of nuclear antigens accumulate.
- **Susceptibility genes with failure of self-tolerance:** Genetic abnormality in B and T lymphocytes is responsible for defect in self-tolerance. Immunogenic forms of nucleic acids and other self-antigens, drive autoimmune-inducing activation of innate immunity, autoantibodies, and T cell. Due to defective self-tolerance, the self-reactive lymphocytes (reactive against self-antigens) survive and remain functional.
- **Production of antibodies and formation of immune complexes:** The self-reactive B lymphocytes are stimulated by nuclear self-antigens, and antibodies are produced against the antigens. They form antigen-antibody (immune) complexes in the circulation.
- **Endocytosis of immune complexes:** The antibody portion of immune complexes bind to Fc receptors on B-cells and DCs (dendritic cells) and the immune complexes may be internalized by endocytosis.
- **Engagement of toll-like receptors by nuclear antigens:** The process of abnormal immune response may begin with autoimmunity-inducing activation of innate immunity. TLRs recognize molecular microbial structures and constitute an important group of pattern recognition receptors of the innate immune system. TLR ligands that bind TLRs are usually exogenous such as lipopolysaccharide, lipopeptides, bacterial DNA and viral RNA and DNA. These ligands are powerful activators of DCs, macrophages and other APCs. However, in SLE, circulating DNA/histone and RNA/protein complexes from apoptotic debris can become endogenous ligands, especially when complexed with autoantibodies. TLRs in B-cells and DCs partly bind endogenous ligands present in nucleic acid components (DNA/RNA/proteins) of immune complexes.
- **TLR induced stimulation of B-cells and DCs:** The binding of endogenous ligands present in nucleic acid components to TLR has following effects:
    - Stimulate B-cells to produce more autoantibodies.
    - Stimulate and activate DCs to produce large amounts interferons and other cytokines. They further amplify immune response and cause more apoptosis. There are two major types of IFNs: type I (IFN-α, IFN-β) and type II (IFN-γ, which is secreted only by T cells). IFN-α strongly stimulates both innate and adaptive immune responses. In SLE, circulating DNA/histone and RNA/protein complexes from apoptotic debris chronically stimulate its production. Most lupus patients have increased circulating levels of IFN-α. Levels of expression of many genes that are upregulated by IFN-α are higher in patients with SLE than in normal patients.
- **Persistent production of autoantibodies:** Thus, a cycle of antigen release and immune activation results in the persistent production of high-affinity IgG autoantibodies.
- **Tissue damage:** Tissue damage begins with deposition of autoantibodies and/or immune complexes. This is followed by destruction brought out through complement activation and release of cytokines/chemokines. Nonimmune tissue-fixed cells (e.g., basal cells of the dermis, synovial fibroblasts, renal mesangial cells, podocytes and tubular epithelium, and endothelial cells throughout the body) are then activated to produce more inflammation and damage.

Mechanisms of Tissue Injury

Q. Write short essay on immune mechanism in SLE.

Different autoantibodies and the immune complexes formed are the causes of most of the lesions of SLE.

Type III hypersensitivity

Most of the systemic lesions are caused by the deposition of **immune complexes** (type III hypersensitivity). It is the **most common cause of tissue injury** and **visceral lesions.** In animal models, DNA-anti-DNA complexes can be detected in the glomeruli and small blood vessels. Serum complement levels are low secondary to consumption of complement proteins. Granular deposits of complement and immunoglobulins are found in the glomeruli. All these findings support the role of immune complex deposition in the pathogenesis.

T-cell: Infiltrates of T lymphocytes are also frequently found in the kidneys and may be involved in damage to tissue.

Q. Write short essay on lupus erythematosus (LE) cells and LE bodies.

Binding of ANAs to nuclei of damaged cells: ANAs present in blood and immune complexes cannot penetrate intact cells. However, if nuclei of the cell are exposed, the ANAs can react and bind to these nuclei.

- **LE bodies or hematoxylin bodies in tissues:** Nuclei released from damaged cells react with ANAs. These nuclei after binding of ANAs lose their chromatin pattern, and appear homogeneous. They produce so-called LE bodies or hematoxylin bodies in tissue.
- **LE cells (Figs. 10A to C):** It is related to phenomenon of LE bodies and can be readily seen when blood is agitated in vitro. To demonstrate LE cells in blood sample, blood is agitated to damage the nucleated cells and it releases the nuclei. The nuclei of damaged cells react with ANAs to form a homogenous denatured nuclear material. The LE cell is any phagocytic leukocyte (blood neutrophil or macrophage) that has engulfed this denatured nucleus of an injured cell. In the past, the demonstration of LE cells in vitro was used as a test for the diagnosis of SLE. With the advent of new techniques for detection of ANAs, this test is of only historical interest. Sometimes, LE cells can be demonstrated in body fluid such as pericardial or pleural effusions in SLE patients. LE cell is positive in about 70% of SLE. It may also be positive in conditions such as rheumatoid arthritis, lupoid hepatitis, penicillin sensitivity, etc.

Type II hypersensitivity

Autoantibodies against cell surface antigens specific for red blood cells (RBCs), white cells and platelets can opsonize

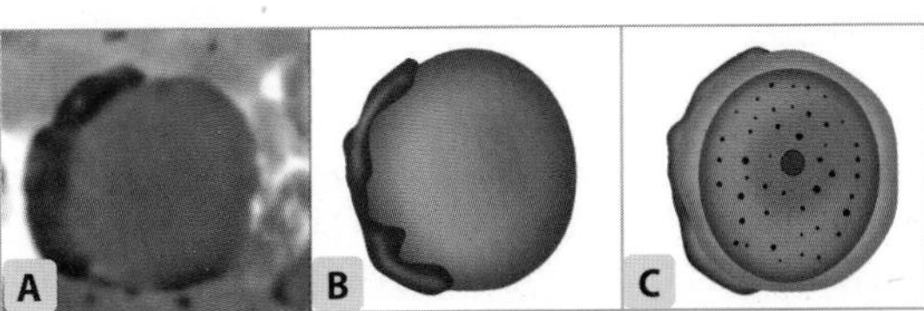

FIGS. 10A TO C: Appearance of lupus erythematosus (LE) cell and tart cells; (A) LE cell with Leishman stain, (B) Diagrammatic presentation of LE cell, (C) Tart cell.

these cells. Opsonization favors their phagocytosis and lysis. Resulting destruction of these blood cells produces cytopenias. These are due to antibody-mediated (type II) hypersensitivity reactions. The most common disorder due to this type of autoantibody is immune thrombocytopenic purpura (ITP). ITP develops in up to 10% of patients with SLE. Most commonly, ITP is due to binding of autoantibodies to the glycoproteins present on membrane of platelet. These autoantibody coated platelets are removed by macrophages, mainly in splenic sinusoids.

Antiphospholipid antibody syndrome

Q. Write short essay on antiphospholipid syndrome (APS).

Antiphospholipid antibody syndrome (APS) is an **autoantibody-mediated acquired thrombophilia** characterized by recurrent arterial or venous thrombosis and/or pregnancy morbidity. This syndrome is associated with recurrent spontaneous miscarriages and focal cerebral or ocular ischemia. It affects mainly females. APS may occur alone (primary) or in association with other autoimmune diseases (secondary). Thus, in **primary antiphospholipid antibody syndrome,** the patient develops autoantibodies and the clinical manifestation **without associated SLE.** Catastrophic APS (CAPS) is characterized by a life-threatening rapidly progressive thromboembolic disease and simultaneously involves three or more organs.

Main autoimmune disease associated with APS that cause **secondary antiphospholipid antibody syndrome** is SLE. These SLE patients with antiphospholipid antibodies (discussed on pages 373–374) show variety of clinical features of APS. These patients are prone to develop **venous and arterial thromboses**. Probably thrombosis develops due to antibodies against clotting factors, platelets, and endothelial cells.

Neuropsychiatric manifestations of SLE: They are probably due to autoantibodies that cross the blood-brain barrier. These antibodies may react with neurons or receptors for various neurotransmitters. Other immune factors (e.g., cytokines), may also be responsible for the cognitive dysfunction and CNS abnormalities associated with SLE.

Q. Write short essay on pathology of SLE.
Q. Write short essay on lupus nephritis.

MORPHOLOGY

Systemic lupus erythematosus is a systemic autoimmune disease and morphologic changes in SLE are **extremely variable**. The most characteristic lesions of SLE are due to deposition of immune complexes in **blood vessels, kidneys, connective tissue, and skin**. The frequency of individual organ involved is listed in **Box 3**.

Blood Vessels

Acute necrotizing vasculitis: It involves **capillaries, small arteries and arterioles**. Acute necrotizing vasculitis may be observed in blood vessels of any involved tissue. Microscopically, vasculitis/arteritis is characterized by **fibrinoid necrosis** in the vessel walls. In **chronic stages**, vessels undergo **fibrous thickening of wall and narrowing of the lumen**.

Continued

Box 3: Common pathologic manifestations of systemic lupus erythematosus.

Pathologic manifestation (prevalence in %)
- Hematologic (100)
- Arthritis, arthralgia or myalgia (80–90)
- Skin (85)
- Renal (50–70)
- Pleuritis (45)
- Pericarditis (25)
- Gastrointestinal (20)

Continued

Kidney

Clinically, significant involvement of kidney may be found in **about 50% of SLE** patients. It is mainly in the form of glomerulonephritis and tubulointerstitial nephritis. It and is one of the **most important organs involved.**

Pathogenesis of glomerulonephritis: The lesions in glomeruli are the result of **deposition of immune complexes**. Immune complexes consist of DNA and anti-DNA antibodies. These immune complex deposits may be on the glomerular basement membrane, in the mesangium, and sometimes throughout the glomerulus. These deposits produce inflammation and proliferation of cells (endothelial, mesangial and/or epithelial) in the glomeruli.

Morphologic classification of lupus nephritis: Six classes (patterns) of glomerular disease are seen in SLE are recognized. There may be some overlap between these classes and over the time lesions may evolve from one pattern to another. Class I is the least common and class IV is the most common pattern.

1. **Minimal mesangial lupus nephritis (Class I):** It is characterized by deposition of immune complex in the mesangium. It is identified by immunofluorescence and by electron microscopy as granular deposits of immunoglobulin and complement. There are no recognizable structural changes by light microscopy. It is very uncommon pattern.
2. **Mesangial proliferative lupus nephritis (Class II):** It is characterized by immune complex deposition in the mesangium. Microscopically, it shows mild-to-moderate increase in mesangial cells (mesangial cell proliferation) and often accompanied by accumulation of mesangial matrix. Immunofluorescent microscopy shows granular mesangial deposits of immunoglobulin and complement component deposition. There is no involvement of glomerular capillaries.
3. **Focal lupus nephritis (class III):** In this glomerulonephritis, there is involvement of ≤50% of all glomeruli. It is seen in 20–35% of patients. The lesions may be segmental (affecting only a portion of the glomerulus) or global (involving the entire glomerulus). Microscopically, involved glomeruli may show swelling and proliferation of endothelial and mesangial cells, leukocyte infiltration, capillary necrosis, and hyaline thrombi (eosinophilic deposits or intracapillary).

Continued

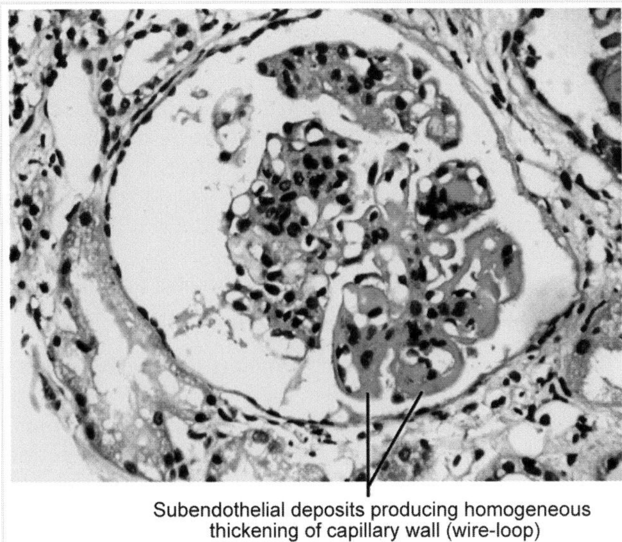

Fig. 11: Diffuse lupus nephritis (class IV) showing glomerulus with "wire-loop" lesions due to extensive subendothelial deposition of immune complexes. It may be seen in class III pattern of systemic lupus erythematosus (SLE).

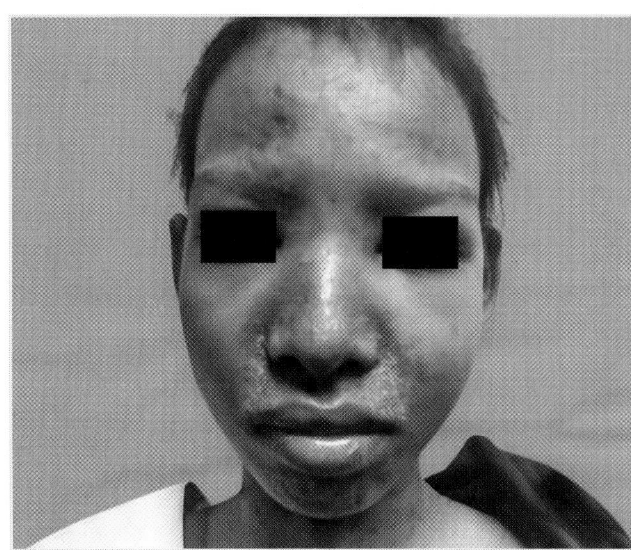

FIG. 12: Systemic lupus erythematosus with malar rash and alopecia.

Continued

There is also often extracapillary proliferation associated with focal fibrinoid necrosis and crescent formation (proliferation parietal epithelial cells of glomerulus). Clinical manifestation may range from mild hematuria and proteinuria to acute renal Insufficiency. Urine shows red blood cell casts when the disease is active. Some patients may progress to diffuse glomerulonephritis. The active (or proliferative) inflammatory lesions may completely heal or progress to chronic global or segmental glomerular scarring.

4. **Diffuse lupus nephritis (Class IV):** It is **most common and severe form of lupus nephritis**. It occurs in 35–60% of patients. The lesions are similar to those in class III, but differ in extent. Typically, in class IV glomerulonephritis ≥50% of all glomeruli (half or more of the glomeruli) involved. Lesions may be **segmental or global**. Depending on this basis, class IV can be subclassified as Class IV segmental (IV-S) or Class IV global (IV-G). Microscopically, involved glomeruli show **proliferation of endothelial, mesangial, and epithelial cells**. The proliferation of parietal epithelial cells may produce cellular crescents that may fill Bowman's space. Prominent, subendothelial immune complex deposits may cause circumferential homogeneous thickening of the capillary wall. On light microscopy this appears to form "**wire-loop "structure** (**Fig. 11**). These wire loops may be seen in both focal and diffuse proliferative (class III or IV) lupus nephritis. Immune complexes can be detected by electron microscopy and immunofluorescence. The glomerular lesions may progress and produce scarring of glomeruli. These patients are usually symptomatic. Urine shows hematuria and proteinuria. Hypertension and mild to severe renal insufficiency are also commonly found.
5. **Membranous lupus nephritis (Class V):** It is seen in 10–15% of patients. It is characterized by **diffuse thickening of the capillary walls**. It shows **subepithelial**

Continued

Continued

immune complexes, similar to idiopathic membranous nephropathy. The immune complex deposits are usually associated with increased production of basement membrane-like material. Class V lesion typically causes severe **proteinuria or nephrotic syndrome**. Class V lesion may occur concurrently with focal (class III) or diffuse (class IV) lupus nephritis.
6. **Advanced sclerosing lupus nephritis (Class VI):** It shows **sclerosis of more than 90% glomeruli**. It represents **end-stage renal disease**.

Interstitium and tubules: Changes in the interstitium and tubules are frequent but are usually not dominant abnormality. Rarely, tubulointerstitial lesions may be the dominant feature. In many lupus nephritis patients, immune complexes similar to those in glomeruli are observed. These are seen in the tubular or peritubular capillary basement membranes. Occasionally, the interstitium may show well-organized B-cell follicles with plasma cells. These plasma cells may be the sources of autoantibodies.

Skin

Skin involvement is common in SLE. Characteristic skin lesion is erythematous rash and affects sun-exposed sites mainly on the face (**Fig. 12**) along the bridge of the nose and cheeks (the malar **"butterfly" rash**). It is seen in about 50% of patients. Similar rash may also develop on the extremities and trunk. Urticaria, bullae, maculopapular lesions, and ulcerations may also occur. Exposure to sunlight triggers or makes the erythema prominent.

Microscopy: The involved skin shows **vacuolar degeneration of the basal layer of the epidermis**. Dermis shows variable edema and perivascular inflammation. Vasculitis with fibrinoid necrosis may be prominent.

Immunofluorescence microscopy: Shows **deposition of immunoglobulin and complement along the dermoepidermal junction ("lupus band")**. It may also be

Continued

Continued

observed in uninvolved skin. This finding is not diagnostic of SLE and is sometimes observed in scleroderma or dermatomyositis.

Joints

Joint involvement is the most common (over 90% of cases) manifestation of SLE. It is typically a **nonerosive synovitis with little deformity**. This is in contrasts with rheumatoid arthritis which shows joint destruction.

Pleuritis, pericarditis and other serosal cavity

Serous membranes are commonly involved. Inflammation of the serosal lining membranes may be acute, subacute or chronic. During the acute phases, the mesothelial surfaces of serosal membrane may be covered with fibrinous exudate. Later serosa become thickened, opaque, and coated with a shaggy fibrous tissue. This may lead to partial or total obliteration of the serosal cavity. More than one-third of patients develop pleuritis and pleural effusions. Pericarditis and peritonitis occur, but are less frequent.

Central Nervous System

It can manifest as psychiatric disease or vasculitis. No clear morphologic abnormalities are characteristics for the neuropsychiatric symptoms of SLE. Sometimes noninflammatory occlusion of small vessels by intimal proliferation is observed. This may be the result of endothelial damage by autoantibodies or immune complexes. Vasculitis can lead to hemorrhage and infarction of the brain and may be life threatening.

Cardiovascular System

SLE can damage any layer of the heart. Various manifestations are as follows:

- **Pericardium:** Symptomatic or asymptomatic pericardial involvement is the most common finding. It can be observed in up to 50% of patients.
- **Myocardium:** Myocarditis, or mononuclear cell infiltration of the myocardium is less common. It may cause resting tachycardia and electrocardiographic abnormalities.
- **Endocardium:** Valvular abnormalities mainly involve the mitral and aortic valves. It manifests as diffuse thickening of valve leaflet that may be associated with valvular dysfunction (stenosis and/or regurgitation). Valvular endocarditis (called **Libman–Sacks endocarditis**) was more common before the widespread use of steroids. Libman–Sacks endocarditis is a nonbacterial verrucous endocarditis and is usually not clinically significant. It is characterized by small nonbacterial vegetations on valve leaflets. The vegetations may be single or multiple and measure 1- to 3-mm and appear as warty deposits on any heart valve. They are distinctively **found on either surface of the leaflets** (**Fig. 13A**). These lesions should be differentiated from vegetations of infective endocarditis and rheumatic heart disease. The vegetations in infective endocarditis (**Fig. 13B**) are considerably larger and bulkier. In rheumatic heart disease, vegetations are smaller and found along the lines of closure of the valve leaflets (**Fig. 13C**).

Coronary artery disease: SLE patients may have coronary artery disease (angina, myocardial infarction) resulting from **coronary atherosclerosis**. This complication is more common in young patients with long-standing disease, and especially prevalent in patients treated with corticosteroids. The pathogenesis of accelerated coronary atherosclerosis is probably multifactorial. Risk factors for atherosclerosis, including hypertension, obesity, and hyperlipidemia, are more common in SLE patients. Also, immune complexes and antiphospholipid antibodies may damage endothelium and promote atherosclerosis.

Lungs

Pleuritis and pleural effusions are observed in almost 50% of patients. Apart from this, some patients may have chronic progressive interstitial fibrosis and increased incidence of secondary pulmonary hypertension. None of these changes is specific for SLE.

Spleen

In SLE there is commonly splenomegaly, capsular thickening, and follicular hyperplasia of spleen. Central penicilliary arteries may show concentric intimal and smooth muscle cell hyperplasia. This produces onion-skin lesions in the vessels.

Lymph nodes

They may be enlarged due to the hyperplastic germinal centers, or may show necrotizing lymphadenitis. It is usually associated with the presence of activated cytotoxic T-cells (CTLs) and macrophages. In some cases, the activated T cells may be so prominent as to mimic certain features of T-cell lymphoma. But these are polyclonal and reactive in nature compared to monoclonal in lymphoma.

Other Organs and Tissues

Presence of LE, or hematoxylin, bodies in the bone marrow or other organs are strongly indicative of SLE.

Continued

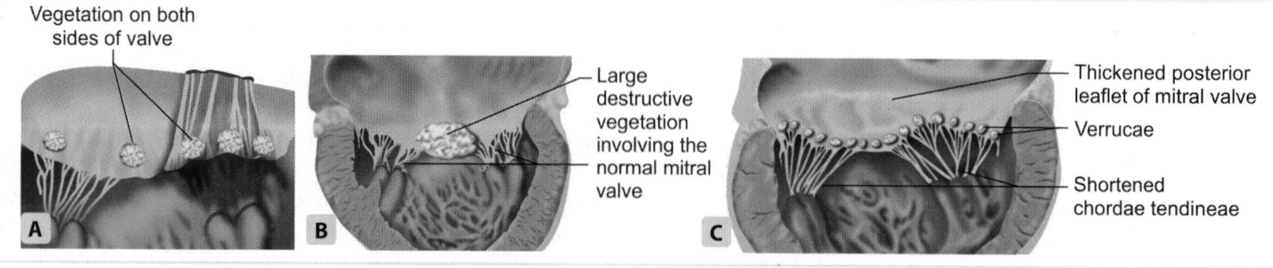

FIGS. 13A TO C: Diagrammatic appearance of vegetations in: (A) Libman–Sacks endocarditis (LSE), (B) Acute bacterial endocarditis, (C) Rheumatic heart disease.

Clinical Features

Systemic lupus erythematosus is a **multisystem disease** with **highly variable clinical presentation**.

- **Age:** It usually occurs in **young woman between 20 and 30 years**, but may manifest at any age.
- **Sex:** It **predominantly affects women**, with female-to-male ratio of 9:1.
- **Onset: Acute or insidious with fever**.

Typical presentation: Butterfly rash over the face, fever, pain in one or more peripheral joints (feet, ankles, knees, hips, fingers, wrists, elbows, shoulders) **without deformity, pleuritic chest pain and photosensitivity**. SLE patients are susceptible to infections, because of immune dysfunction and treatment with immunosuppressive drugs. However, in many patients, it is subtle and may present as a febrile illness of unknown origin, abnormal urinary findings, or joint disease masquerading as rheumatoid arthritis or rheumatic fever.

Musculoskeletal manifestations: Arthralgia and nonerosive arthritis are most common (>85%). Commonly involves proximal interphalangeal and metacarpophalangeal joints of the hand, along with the knees and wrists. In about 10% of patients, deformities result from damage to periarticular tissue, a condition termed Jaccoud's arthropathy.

Cutaneous manifestations: Classic malar rash consists of erythematous (flat or raised) facial rash with a butterfly distribution across the malar and nasal prominences and sparing of the nasolabial folds (see **Fig. 12**) and is seen in 30–60% of patients. Butterfly rash is often triggered by sun exposure. Lupus dermatitis can be classified as acute, subacute, or chronic. Chronic discoid lupus erythematosus (DLE) is the most common chronic dermatitis in lupus (discussed later). SLE patients may have generalized photosensitivity (skin rash on exposure to sunlight) and develop alopecia,

Mucous membrane manifestations: Recurrent crops of small, painful ulcerations on the oral or nasal mucosa. Dryness secondary to Sjögren's syndrome.

Hematologic manifestations: Antibodies that target each of the cellular blood elements are responsible for hematological changes.

- **RBC:** Normocytic normochromic anemia, reflecting chronic illness. In hemolytic anemia, Coombs test is positive or it may be due to microangiopathic hemolysis.
- **WBC:** Leukopenia, particularly lymphopenia
- **Platelets:** Idiopathic/ITP induced by antiplatelet antibodies.
- Antibodies to clotting factors can contribute to impaired clot formation and hemorrhage.
- Laboratory investigations may show evidence of some hematologic abnormality in almost all cases. In some patients presenting manifestation as well as the dominant clinical features are those due to anemia or thrombocytopenia.

Renal manifestations: Many clinical findings may suggest renal involvement. These include hematuria, red cell casts and proteinuria. Some patients may present with the classic nephrotic syndrome.

Some SLE patients may develop mental aberrations, including psychosis or convulsions, or show clinical features of coronary artery disease.

Diagnosis depends on a collective information of clinical, serologic, and morphologic changes (see **Table 5**).

Laboratory findings

Q. Write short essay on laboratory diagnosis of SLE.

Purpose: (1) To establish or rule out the diagnosis, (2) follow the course of disease, and (3) to identify adverse effects of therapies.

Tests for autoantibodies: ANAs are found in almost all patients, but it is not specific. Various methods of detecting antibodies include:

- **Indirect immunofluorescence assay (IFA):** They can identify ANAs. They are discussed on page 1096 (refer Table 7). Significance of IFA assay are:
  - Extremely sensitive (positive in more than 95%)
  - Limited specificity because it is positive in patients with other autoimmune diseases, chronic infections and cancer
- **Multiplex flow cytometry immunoassay**
- **ELISA (for Smith antigen)**

Standard tests for diagnosis: These include complete blood count, platelet count, ESR (raised) and urinalysis.

Tests for following disease course: These tests indicate the status of organ involvement known to be present during SLE flares.

- **Renal involvement:** Urinalysis may show hematuria, red cell casts, proteinuria, or nephrotic syndrome.
- **Hematologic changes:** Hemoglobin levels (anemia) or platelet counts (thrombocytopenia) and ESR.
- Serum levels of creatinine or albumin.
- Decreased complement component levels in serum such as C3 and C4 are often indicators of enhanced consumption and increased disease activity.

Course of the disease

It is variable and unpredictable. Rarely, death may occur within weeks to months. Usually with appropriate therapy, the disease follows a relapsing and remitting course. This may span over a period of years or even decades. During acute exacerbation, there is increased formation of immune complexes and activates complement. This is usually accompanied by hypocomplemententemia. Exacerbations are usually treated with corticosteroids or other immunosuppressive drugs. In some patients, even without therapy, the disease runs an indolent course. They may have relatively mild features, such as skin changes and mild hematuria, for years. Patients treated with steroids and immunosuppressive drugs develop usual risks associated with such therapy.

Cause of death: The most common causes are renal failure, intercurrent infections and coronary artery disease.

Chronic Discoid Lupus Erythematosus

Chronic DLE (discoid lupus erythematosus) is a disease characterized by the presence of skin manifestations (disease remains confined to the skin) that may mimic SLE, but systemic manifestations are rare. In 5–10% of patients with DLE develop multisystem manifestations after many years.

Skin manifestations: It presents with skin plaques (slightly raised patches) showing varying degrees of edema, erythema, adherent keratotic scaliness, follicular plugging, and skin atrophy surrounded by an elevated erythematous border. This rash is primarily seen on the face and scalp. Immunofluorescence studies of skin biopsy show deposition of immunoglobulin and C3 at the dermoepidermal junction. It is similar to that seen in SLE. However, unlike SLE, uninvolved skin contains no immune deposits. In approximately 35% of patients, generic ANAs are positive, but antibodies to double-stranded DNA are rarely present.

Subacute Cutaneous Lupus Erythematosus

A group of patients show subacute cutaneous lupus erythematosus in which the features intermediate between SLE and chronic DLE. This presents with predominant involvement of skin and is distinguished from chronic DLE by following criteria.

- Skin rash tends to be widespread, superficial, and nonscarring (though exceptions occur).
- Most of the patients have mild systemic symptoms consistent with SLE.
- Strong association with antibodies to the SS-A antigen (Ro antigen) (ribonucleoprotein complex) and with the HLA-DR3 genotype are characteristic.

Drug-induced Lupus Erythematosus

An SLE-like syndrome may develop in patients during therapy with certain medications.

Etiology: Variety of drugs that can produce drug-induced lupus erythematosus are as follows:

- **Drugs:** Antiarrhythmics (e.g., procainamide), antihypertensive (e.g., hydralazine), methyl dopa), D-penicillamine, antipsychotics (e.g., chlorpromazine), anticonvulsants (e.g. carbamazepine and phenytoin), antibiotics (e.g., isoniazid), antirheumatic (e.g., sulfasalazine), diuretic (e.g., hydrochlorothiazide) and antihyperlipidemics (e.g., lovastatin).
- **Biologic agents:** Interferons and TNF inhibitors (anti-TNF therapy effective in rheumatoid arthritis and other autoimmune diseases).

Many of these drug-induced lupus erythematosus are positive for ANAs, but most patients do not develop symptoms of SLE. For example, majority (about 80% of patients) on procainamide therapy develop positive test for ANAs, but only one-third of them manifest clinical symptoms (e.g., arthralgias, fever, and serositis). Although it can affect multiple organs, it is distinctly uncommon to find involvement of renal and CNS. Symptoms usually resolve after discontinuation of the offending drug. Antibodies specific for double-stranded DNA are rare, but the positivity of antibodies specific for histones are very high.

Sjögren Syndrome

Definition: Sjögren syndrome is a chronic, slowly progressing, autoimmune **disease** characterized by **immunologically mediated destruction** and **marked lymphocytic infiltration of exocrine glands**, primarily **salivary and lacrimal glands**. It results in dry eyes (keratoconjunctivitis sicca or xerophthalmia) and dry mouth (xerostomia).

Types: It may present as primary or secondary.

- **Primary Sjögren syndrome:** It occurs as an isolated primary disorder (as a single entity) in the absence of any underlying autoimmune disorder. It is also known as the **Sicca syndrome**.
- **Secondary Sjögren syndrome:** It occurs in association with another autoimmune disease. Examples of other associated autoimmune diseases include rheumatoid arthritis (most common), SLE, polymyositis, scleroderma, vasculitis, mixed connective tissue disease, (MCTD) primary biliary cirrhosis, autoimmune thyroiditis, chronic active hepatitis. Secondary form is more common than primary.

Pathogenesis

Lymphocyte infiltration in exocrine glands: Sjögren syndrome is clinically characterized by decrease in tears and saliva (Sicca syndrome). It is the result of dense lymphocytic infiltration, B lymphocyte hyperreactivity and fibrosis of the lacrimal and salivary glands. The infiltrate is predominantly composed of activated CD4+ helper T cells and some B cells, along with plasma cells.

Autoantibodies: Various autoantibodies are as follows:

- **Rheumatoid factor:** About 75% of patients with Sjögren syndrome have rheumatoid factor (an antibody reactive with self IgG) irrespective of whether or not there is coexisting rheumatoid arthritis.
- **ANAs (antinuclear antibodies):** They are found in 50–80% of patients and are assessed by immunofluorescence assay.
- **Autoantibodies to SS-A (Ro) and SS-B (La) antigens:** Many other organ-specific and nonorgan-specific antibodies also can be detected. Most important are antibodies against two cytoplasmic ribonucleoprotein associated antigens namely SS-A (Ro) and SS-B (La). These can be found in as many as 90% of patients by sensitive techniques and are **considered as the serologic markers of the disease**. These autoantibodies are not entirely specific for Sjögren syndrome, because they are also found in few patients with SLE.

HLA association: Similar to other autoimmune diseases, Sjögren syndrome is associated (weakly) with certain HLA alleles. It is highly associated with the HLA DQA1*0501 allele. **Exact pathogenesis** of Sjögren syndrome is **not known**. Following features are important in its pathogenesis.

- **Aberrant activation of both T-cell and B-cell** are probably involved in its pathogenesis.
- **Initial trigger may be a viral infection** of the salivary glands. This causes local death of cell and release tissue self-antigens.
- In **genetically susceptible individuals, CD4+ T cells and B cells specific for these self-antigens may escape tolerance** and react with tissue.
- Produces inflammation, damage to tissue and, eventually, fibrosis.
- Sjögren syndrome–like disease develops in some patients with infections by human T-lymphotropic virus (HTLV), HIV, and hepatitis C virus. However, the exact relationship between these viruses and the autoimmune disorder is not clear.

MORPHOLOGY

Exocrine glands

Lacrimal and salivary glands are the major sites of the disease. Other exocrine glands that may be involved include those lining the respiratory and gastrointestinal tracts (GITs) and the vagina.

Microscopy of salivary glands

- **Lymphocytic infiltration (Fig. 14)**: Initially, the involved glands show periductal and perivascular **lymphocytic infiltration**. Later, there is dense/extensive infiltration by lymphocytes and they **may form lymphoid follicles with germinal centers.**
- **Atrophy of gland in later stages**: The epithelial cells lining the duct may show hyperplasia and obstruct the ducts. Later, atrophy of the acini, fibrosis, and hyalinization occurs. In later stages of the disease process, there may be atrophy of the involved gland and replacement of parenchyma with fat.

Lymphoma: In some patients, the extensive lymphoid infiltrate may give the appearance of a lymphoma. Of course, these patients have a high risk for development of B-cell lymphomas which may destroy acini and ducts. As the disease progresses, the affected glands show atrophy and may be replaced by hyalinized fibrotic tissue.

Cornea

Absence of tears leads to **drying of the corneal epithelium**. This may lead to inflammation, erosion and ulceration of cornea.

Mucosa

Oral mucosa may show atrophy, with inflammatory fissuring and ulceration. **Nose becomes dry and shows crusting**. It may lead to ulcerations and even perforation of the nasal septum.

Clinical Features

Gender and age: Sjögren syndrome is the most common in females between 50 and 60 years of age.

Symptoms

These are the consequences of inflammatory destruction of the exocrine glands and mainly due to lack of tears and saliva.

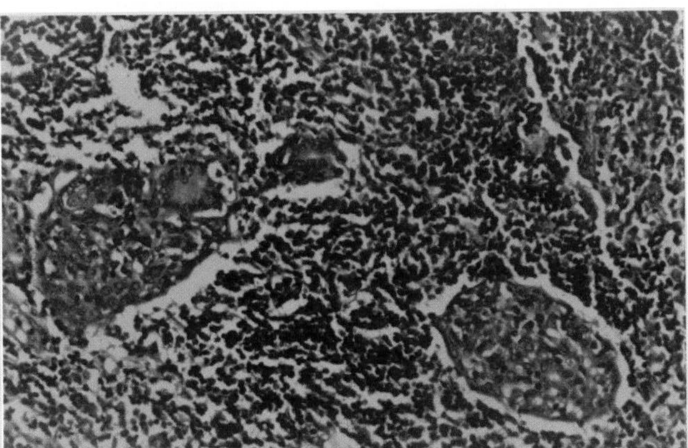

FIG. 14: Parotid gland showing dense lymphocytic and plasma cell infiltration. The duct lining show epithelial hyperplasia.

- **Eye:** Keratoconjunctivitis produces eye discomfort, blurred vision, burning, and itching. There may be accumulation of thick secretions in the conjunctival sac. May develop infections and ulcer of the cornea and conjunctivae.
- **Salivary gland:** Xerostomia produces dry mouth (dryness of the buccal mucosa), difficulty in swallowing solid foods, decrease in taste, cracks, and fissures in the mouth. Parotid gland may be enlarged in 50% of patients. Dry mouth is sometimes accompanied by increased dental caries and by thrush or other mouth infections.
- **Respiratory system:** These symptoms include dryness of the nasal mucosa, epistaxis, recurrent bronchitis, and pneumonitis.
- **Extraglandular disease:** It may develop in one-third of patients. These include synovitis, diffuse pulmonary fibrosis, and peripheral neuropathy. They are more commonly observed in patients having high titers of antibodies specific for SS-A. In Sjögren syndrome, glomerular lesions are extremely rare. However, there may be defects of tubular function (e.g., renal tubular acidosis, uricosuria, and phosphaturia) with tubulointerstitial nephritis. In about 60% of patients there may be another autoimmune disorder (e.g., rheumatoid arthritis).

Mikulicz syndrome: In the past, the combination of lacrimal and salivary gland inflammation was called as Mikulicz disease. Now, this name has been replaced by Mikulicz syndrome. This syndrome includes all the causes that produce **enlargement of both lacrimal and salivary gland**. These include sarcoidosis, IgG4-related disease, lymphoma, and other tumors.

Marginal zone lymphoma: The involved glands show intense inflammatory infiltrates. During the early stages of the disease, this immune inflammatory infiltrate is composed of a mixture of polyclonal T and B cells. However, if the inflammation persists, over time the individual clones within the population of B cells have a strong tendency to gain a growth advantage, probably due to the acquisition of somatic mutations. This dominant B-cell clone may develop into a marginal zone lymphoma. This is a specific type of B-cell malignancy that often arises in the setting of chronic lymphocytic inflammation. About 5% of Sjögren patients develop lymphoma which is 40-fold greater than normal. Certain other autoimmune disorders (e.g., Hashimoto thyroiditis) are also associated with a high risk of marginal zone lymphoma. They arise within the organ or tissue with autoimmune inflammation.

Systemic Sclerosis (Scleroderma)

Definition: Systemic sclerosis (SSc) is a systemic disease characterized by: (1) **chronic inflammation (thought to be the result of autoimmunity)**, (2) **widespread damage to small blood vessels**, and (3) **progressive interstitial and perivascular fibrosis** in the skin and multiple internal organs. It is chronic and frequently has a progressive course, with significant disability, disfigurement and mortality.

Skin is most commonly affected and, in some patients, the disease may remain confined to the skin for many years. For this reason, the term scleroderma is commonly used in clinical medicine. It is better named systemic sclerosis because it is characterized by excessive fibrosis throughout the body and not restricted to skin. **Almost every organ can be affected**, and frequently affect skin, GIT, skeletal muscles, lungs, kidneys, heart, and other tissues. Though in some patients, the initial involvement may be restricted to skin, it progresses to visceral involvement with death from renal failure, cardiac failure, pulmonary insufficiency, or intestinal malabsorption.

Q. Write short essay on CREST syndrome.

Classification: Systemic sclerosis is clinically a heterogeneous disease. Based on its course, systemic sclerosis is classified into two major categories:

1. **Diffuse scleroderma:** At the onset of disease, it is characterized by widespread involvement of skin, with rapid progression and early visceral involvement.
2. **Limited scleroderma:** In this category, the skin involvement is often confined to fingers, forearms, and face. Involvement of the viscera occurs late and it usually follows a benign course. Some patents with the limited disease develop a combination of **C**alcinosis, **R**aynaud phenomenon, **E**sophageal dysmotility, **S**clerodactyly, and **T**elangiectasia. This is called CREST syndrome. Many other variants and related conditions are less frequent (e.g., eosinophilic fasciitis).

Pathogenesis (Fig. 15)

The causes and the pathogenesis of systemic sclerosis are not well understood. The clinical and pathologic manifestations of systemic sclerosis results from three interrelated processes namely: (1) **inflammation and autoimmune responses** (humoral and cellular immunity), (2) **vascular damage** (diffuse microangiopathy characterized by fibroproliferative vascular lesions of small arteries and arterioles), and (3) **excessive and often progressive deposition of collagen**.

Inflammation and autoimmunity

Probably, CD4+ T cells respond to an as yet-unidentified antigen and accumulate in the skin. The CD4+ T cells release cytokines (e.g., IL-13) and growth factor (e.g., TGF-β), that activate inflammatory cells and fibroblasts. Inflammatory infiltrates are usually sparse in the skin of patients with systemic sclerosis. However, activated CD4+ T cells and Th2 cells have been isolated from the skin. Several cytokines released from these T cells (including TGF-β and IL-13), can stimulate the transcription of genes encoding collagen and other extracellular matrix proteins (e.g., fibronectin) in fibroblasts. Other cytokines recruit leukocytes and produce chronic inflammation. There is usually improper activation of humoral immunity. Detection of various autoantibodies, especially ANAs, is helpful for both diagnosis and prognosis. Although the role of these ANAs in the pathogenesis of the disease is not known, probably some of these antibodies may stimulate fibrosis.

Vascular damage

Microvascular disease is common in systemic sclerosis.

- **Microvascular disease** is observed early in the course of systemic sclerosis and may be the initial lesion. **Proliferation of intimal cells** in the digital arteries, **dilatation of capillary dilation with leakage and destruction** are common. **Capillary loops in the nailfold**

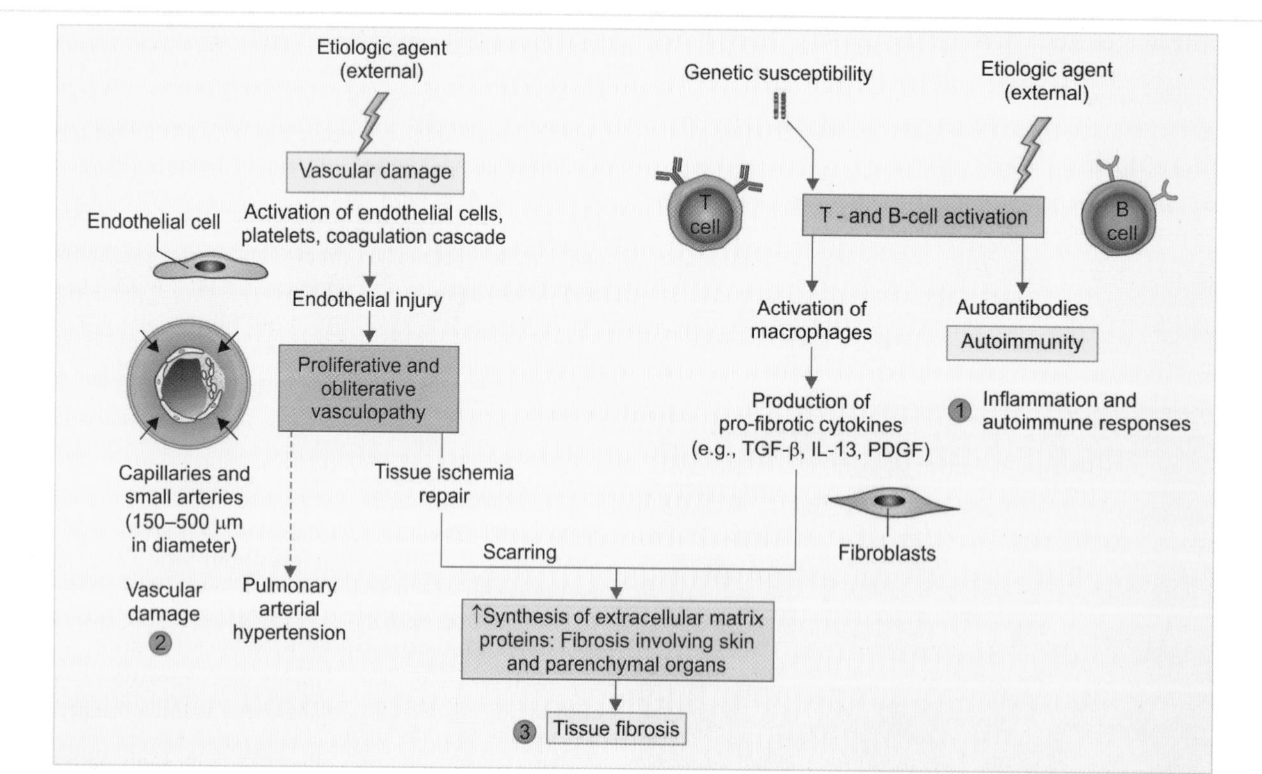

FIG. 15: Pathogenesis of systemic sclerosis. Systemic sclerosis results from three interrelated processes namely: (1) inflammation and autoimmune responses, (2) vascular damage (diffuse microangiopathy characterized by fibroproliferative vascular lesions of small arteries and arterioles), and (3) fibrosis (excessive deposition of collagen).

are distorted during the early course of disease, and later they disappear. Features of endothelial activation and injury (e.g., increased levels of von Willebrand factor) and increased platelet activation (increased circulating platelet aggregates) are also observed.

- **Cause of vascular injury:** Etiological agent that causes damage to the vessel is not known. Vascular injury may be either the initiating event or the result of chronic inflammation. The chemical mediators released by inflammatory cells may produce damage to the microvascular endothelium.
    - **Repeated cycles of endothelial injury** followed by platelet aggregation lead to release of platelet and endothelial factors (e.g., PDGF, TGF-β). These in turn stimulate **perivascular fibrosis**.
    - Smooth muscle cells of vessels also show abnormalities, such as increased expression of adrenergic receptors.
    - **Widespread narrowing of the microvasculature** leads to **ischemic injury and scarring**.

Fibrosis (excessive deposition of collagen)

The progressive fibrosis is characteristic of systemic sclerosis. Fibrosis may be the end result of multiple abnormalities and these include:

- Accumulation of alternatively activated macrophages.
- Actions of fibrogenic cytokines produced by infiltrating leukocytes.
- Hyper-responsiveness of fibroblasts to these fibrogenic cytokines.
- Scarring that follows ischemic damage caused by the vascular lesions.

Fibroblasts in systemic sclerosis may have an intrinsic abnormality that causes them to produce excessive amounts of collagen.

MORPHOLOGY

Sites involved: Systemic sclerosis may affect almost all organs. Most prominently involved are the skin, alimentary tract, musculoskeletal system, and kidney. The lesions are also often present in the blood vessels, heart, lungs, and peripheral nerves.

Skin

Majority of patients develop diffuse, sclerotic atrophy of the skin. It usually starts in the fingers and distal regions of the upper extremities. Then it extends proximally to involve the upper arms, shoulders, neck, and face.

Microscopy: Following are the microscopic features:

- Skin shows edema and perivascular infiltrates by CD4+ T cells. This is accompanied by **swelling and degeneration of collagen fibers** which appear eosinophilic.
- **Capillaries and small arteries** (150–500 µm in diameter): They may show **thickening of the basal lamina, endothelial cell damage, and partial occlusion.**
- **Dermis:** As the disease progresses increased fibrosis occurs in the dermis and the fibrous tissue becomes tightly bound to the subcutaneous structures. With progression of the disease, there is increasing fibrosis of the dermis. With marked increase of compact collagen in the dermis, there is thinning of epidermis, loss of rete pegs, atrophy of the dermal appendages, and hyaline thickening of the walls of dermal arterioles and capillaries.

Continued

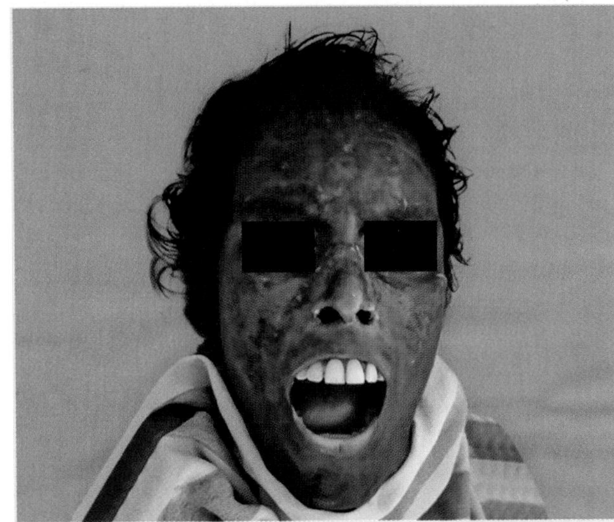

FIG. 16: Systemic sclerosis. Clinical picture shows mask like face with decreased oral aperture in the advanced stage of disease.

Continued

- **Calcification:** Focal and sometimes diffuse subcutaneous calcifications may occur, especially in patients with the CREST syndrome.
- **Advanced stages:** The fingers appear tapered with claw-like appearance, movement of joint is limited, and the face appears like a drawn mask (**Fig. 16**). Loss of blood supply may lead to ulceration of skin and to atrophic changes in the terminal phalanges. Loss of blood supply may produce ulcerations and atrophic changes or autoamputation of the terminal phalanges.

Alimentary tract

It is the most commonly (in about 90% of patients) involved internal organ system. It is characterized by progressive atrophy and fibrous replacement of the muscularis at any level of the gut.

- **Esophagus:** Esophageal involvement is almost universal and most severe. The lower two-thirds of the esophagus may develop a rubber-hose-like inflexibility giving rise to symptoms of gastroesophageal reflux and its complications (e.g., strictures, Barrett esophagus). The mucosa becomes thinned and may ulcerate. The lamina propria and submucosa shows excessive collagenization.
- **Small intestine:** It may show loss of villi and bacterial overgrowth may lead to secondary malabsorption syndrome.

Musculoskeletal system

Musculoskeletal symptoms may be the first manifestations of the disease. Severity may vary. Inflammation of the synovium (synovitis) is common in the early stages and is associated with synovial hypertrophy and hyperplasia. Fibrosis occurs in later stages. These changes appear similar to rheumatoid arthritis, but there is no destruction of joint in systemic sclerosis. In few patients (approximately 10%), inflammatory myositis may develop.

Kidneys and blood vessels

Renal involvement may be found in two-thirds of patients.

- **Thickening of intima:** Most prominent are the vascular lesions characterized by thickening of intima due to

Continued

Continued

deposition of mucinous or finely collagenous material in the interlobular arteries. These intimal deposits stain histochemically for glycoprotein and acid mucopolysaccharides.

- **Proliferation of intimal cells:** Concentric proliferation of intimal cells may resemble those seen in malignant hypertension. But in scleroderma these alterations are seen only in vessels measuring 150–500 µm in diameter and are not always associated with hypertension. However, in 30% of patients with scleroderma have hypertension, and in 20% it follows a rapid, downhill course (malignant hypertension). In hypertension, vascular changes are more prominent and are often associated with fibrinoid necrosis of arterioles, thrombosis, and infarction. Such patients usually die due to renal failure and it accounts for about 50% of deaths from systemic sclerosis. There are no specific changes in the glomerulus.

Lungs

It may be affected in >50% of patients and may manifest as pulmonary hypertension, and interstitial fibrosis. Pulmonary vasospasm, secondary to pulmonary vascular endothelial dysfunction, is involved in the pathogenesis of pulmonary hypertension. Pulmonary fibrosis cannot be distinguished from idiopathic pulmonary fibrosis.

Heart

It may be involved in one-third of patients. It may manifest as pericarditis with effusion, myocardial fibrosis, and thickening of intramyocardial arterioles. The changes in the lung may lead to right ventricular hypertrophy and failure (cor pulmonale). However, clinical impairment due to involvement of myocardium is not common.

Clinical Features

Age and gender: Peak age of presentation is between 50 and 60 years of age. More frequent in females with a female-to-male ratio of 3:1.

Striking cutaneous changes: The distinctive feature of systemic sclerosis is the striking cutaneous changes notably skin fibrosis.

Raynaud phenomenon: It clinically manifests as numbness and tingling of the fingers and toes caused by episodic vasoconstriction of arteries and arterioles. It is seen in almost all patients and in 70% of cases, Raynaud phenomenon precedes other symptoms.

Internal organs

GIT: Dysphagia due to esophageal fibrosis and associated hypomotility are seen in >50% of patients. In later stages, destruction of the esophageal wall leads to atony and dilation, especially at its lower end. Abdominal pain, intestinal obstruction, or malabsorption syndrome can occur due to involvement of the small intestine. Weight loss and anemia due to nutritional deficiencies are observed when there is involvement of the small intestine.

Respiratory system: The pulmonary fibrosis may produce severe respiratory difficulties and is the most common cause of death. It may lead to right-sided cardiac dysfunction.

Heart: Myocardial fibrosis may produce chest pain, arrhythmias and cardiac failure.

Renal system: Mild proteinuria may be found in about 30% of patients and usually does not produce nephrotic syndrome. The most serious manifestation is the development of malignant hypertension leading to renal failure. If there is no hypertension, it progresses slowly. Because of current advances in treatment of the renal crises, pulmonary disease has become the major cause of death in systemic sclerosis.

Autoantibodies: Almost all patients have ANAs that react with a variety of nuclear antigens. Two ANAs strongly associated with systemic sclerosis are:

- **Anti-Scl 70:** Antibody against DNA topoisomerase I (anti-Scl 70) is highly specific and is associated with pulmonary fibrosis and peripheral vascular disease.
- **Anticentromere antibody:** It is associated with CREST syndrome. In patients with this syndrome there is relatively limited involvement of skin, usually confined to fingers, forearms, and face, and calcification of the subcutaneous tissues.

Prognosis: Most of the patients, it steadily follows downhill course over the span of many years.

Inflammatory Myopathies

Definition: Inflammatory myopathies are uncommon, probably immunologically mediated, heterogeneous group of disorders. They are characterized by injury and inflammation of mainly the skeletal muscles.

Depending on clinical, morphologic, and immunologic features, three disorders have been described namely: (1) polymyositis, (2) dermatomyositis, and (3) inclusion body myositis.

Mixed Connective Tissue Disease

Definition: As the name suggests, mixed connective tissue disease (MCTD) is used to describe a disease with clinical features that overlap with those of SLE, systemic sclerosis, and polymyositis.

Pathogenesis of MCTD: It is poorly understood. Patients usually have evidence of B-cell activation with hypergammaglobulinemia and rheumatoid factor. MCTD is associated with HLA-DR4 and HLA-DR2 genotypes, suggesting a role for T cells in autoantibody production.

Laboratory findings: Serologically, MCTD is characterized by a most distinctive ANA directed against an extractable nuclear antigen. These patients have high titers of antibodies to U1 (uridine-rich) ribonucleoprotein (anti-U1-RNP antibody). Most diagnostic criteria for MCTD include high-titer anti-U1-RNP ANA. Anti-RNP antibodies may be also found in SLE, but its titer is much lower than in MCTD. However, their role in the development of any of the characteristic lesions of MCTD is not clear.

Clinical features: It is more common in female and most are adults (mean age, 37 years).

Clinical features of MCTD are shared with other autoimmune diseases. Usually, it presents with synovitis of the fingers, Raynaud phenomenon, mild myositis rash, and renal involvement. They respond favorably to corticosteroids, at least in the short term. There is controversy whether MCTD is a truly separate disease or if different patients with nonclassical presentations of SLE, scleroderma or polymyositis. For example, in some patients, over time, MCTD may evolve into classic SLE, systemic sclerosis or rheumatoid arthritis. However, patients with the mixture of features are maintained over time, and disease remains undifferentiated. Therapeutic beneficial response to steroids is not universal. This suggests that there is a form of MCTD that is distinct from other autoimmune diseases.

Complications: These include pulmonary hypertension, interstitial lung disease, and renal disease.

Polyarteritis Nodosa and Other Vasculitides

Definition: Polyarteritis nodosa is an immunologic disease that belongs to a group of disorders characterized by necrotizing inflammation of the walls of blood vessels. It can involve any type of vessel (arteries, arterioles, veins, or capillaries).

IgG4-related Disease

Q. Write short essay on IgG4-related disease.

Definition: IgG4-related disease (IgG4-RD) is fibroinflammatory disorder characterized by a tendency to form tumor-like (tumefactive) lesions.

Characteristic features: These are as follows:

- Lymphoplasmacytic infiltrate with a high percentage of IgG4-positive (antibody-producing) plasma cells in the tissues. The inflammatory infiltrate is composed of an admixture of both B and T lymphocytes. B cells are usually organized in germinal centers.
- Characteristic pattern of fibrosis termed "storiform" (from the Latin storea, for "woven mat").
- Tendency to target blood vessels, particularly veins, through an obliterative process ("obliterative phlebitis").
- Mild-to-moderate tissue eosinophilia.

Though microscopic appearance of IgG4-RD, is highly characteristic, it requires immunohistochemical confirmation of the diagnosis with IgG4 immunostaining.

Organs involved: IgG4-RD constitutes many conditions previously regarded as separate, organ-specific entities. Initially recognized when extrapancreatic manifestations were identified in patients with autoimmune pancreatitis (AIP). Presently this form of sclerosing pancreatitis is now termed type 1 (IgG4-related) AIP. It is now known that IgG4-related disease can be developed in almost every organ system.

- **Commonly affected organs** include the biliary tree, major salivary glands, periorbital tissues, lymph nodes, kidneys, lungs, and retroperitoneum.
- **Less commonly affected:** It can also involve meninges, aorta, prostate, thyroid, breast, pericardium, and skin.
- **Rarely affected:** Rarely, it can affect the brain parenchyma, the joints, the bone marrow, and the bowel mucosa.

IgG4-RD spectrum: Many other lesions thought as confined to single organs are found to be part of the IgG4-RD spectrum. Examples include some forms of Mikulicz syndrome (enlargement and fibrosis of salivary and lacrimal glands), Riedel thyroiditis, idiopathic retroperitoneal fibrosis, AIP, and inflammatory pseudotumors of the orbit, lungs, and kidneys.

Pathogenesis: Not known, Hallmark of this disease is production of IgG4 in lesions. However, it is not known whether this antibody type contributes to the pathology. Role of B cells is supported by initial clinical trials in which depletion of B cells with anti-B cell reagents (e.g., rituximab) produced clinical benefit. It is not clear whether the disease is really an autoimmune, and no target autoantigens have been so far identified.

Age group and gender: Usually affects middle-aged and older men.

Diagnostic features: Increased numbers of IgG4-producing plasma cells in tissue are required for the diagnosis of this disorder. Though this disorder is often associated with elevated serum IgG4 concentrations, it need not be present in all cases.

REJECTION OF TISSUE TRANSPLANTS

Q. Discuss basic principles of organ transplantation and opportunistic infections.

Q. Write short essay on hematopoietic stem cells (HSCs) transplantation.

Q. Classify rejection reactions and describe pathology of acute rejection.

Q. Write short essay on complications in transplant.

- Transplantation is a procedure for replacement of irreparably damaged tissue or organ to restore their lost function. In transplantation, organs or tissues from one individual is grafted to another.
- Tissue or organ transplanted is called as transplant or graft.
- Individual from which transplant is obtained is known as donor and the individual who receives it is called recipient.
- **Allograft is the term used for a graft exchanged from individual of the same species**. These are usual graft. Grafts from one species to another are called xenografts. They are still an experimental stage.
- A major barrier for transplantation is the process known as rejection. In rejection, the recipient's immune system recognizes the graft as a foreign and attacks it by mounts the immunological reactions against it.

Mechanisms of Recognition and Rejection of Allografts

In transplantation, donor MHC-encoded antigens are immunogenic and can stimulate rejection of transplanted tissues. Rejection is a complex process in which both T lymphocytes and antibodies produced against graft antigens. They react against and destroy the tissue grafts.

Recognition of Graft Alloantigens by T and B Lymphocytes

Optimal survival of graft occurs when recipient and donor are closely matched for histocompatibility antigens. But an exact HLA match is not possible, except between monozygotic twins.

Because *HLA* genes are highly polymorphic, there will be always some differences between individuals. Exception being HLA match in identical twins. The major **antigenic differences between a donor and recipient that cause transplant rejection are mainly due to differences in HLA alleles**. Thus, after organ transplantation, immunosuppressive therapy and vigilant monitoring of graft function are necessary. Present therapeutic advances have greatly improved transplant success rates, even when there is a degree of histoincompatibility. Both cell-mediated immunity and circulating antibodies play a role in transplant rejection. The antigens in the allograft are termed as allogeneic antigens or alloantigens.

Pathways of recognition of graft alloantigens: Following transplantation, the recipient's T cells recognize donor alloantigens from the graft by two pathways namely direct and indirect pathways of recognition of alloantigens.

1. **Direct pathway:** In this pathway, the graft antigens are presented directly to recipient T cells by APCs present in the graft. This pathway may be most important for CTL-mediated acute rejection.
2. **Indirect pathways:** In this pathway, the graft antigens are taken up by host APCs, processed (similar to any other foreign antigen), and presented to host T cells. Indirect pathway may play a greater role in chronic rejection.

Both pathways (direct and indirect) activate CD8+ T cells. They develop into CTLs and CD4+ T cells. CD4+ T cells become cytokine-producing effector cells, mainly Th1 cells.

Stronger immune response by T cells against allograft than against microbes: It is to be noted that the frequency of T cells that can recognize the foreign antigens in a graft is much higher than the frequency of T cells that recognize any microbe. This is responsible for stronger immune responses to allografts than responses to pathogens. These strong immune reactions to allograft can destroy grafts rapidly. Hence, their control needs powerful immunosuppressive agents.

B cell response needs T cell help: B lymphocytes also recognize antigens in the allograft. These include HLA and other antigens that differ between donor and recipient. The activation of these B cells usually needs help of T cells.

Patterns and Mechanisms of Graft Rejection

Classification of rejection reaction

Depending on the clinical and pathologic features, the graft rejection is classified as: (1) hyperacute, (2) acute and (3) chronic. This is the historical classification was based on rejection of kidney allografts. Kidneys were the first solid organs to be transplanted and are most commonly transplanted organ. Hence, the morphologic changes are discussed mainly limited to renal allografts. However, similar changes are observed in other organ transplants.

Hyperacute rejection

- **Mediated by preformed antibodies:** This type of rejection occurs if the host has preformed antibodies specific for antigens on graft endothelial cells in the circulation before transplantation.
- **Causes of preformed antibodies:** These preformed antibodies in the recipient may be natural or acquired. The natural are IgM antibodies specific for blood group antigens. The acquired antibodies may be antibodies specific for allogeneic MHC molecules. These antibodies might have developed by prior exposure of the organ recipient to allogeneic cells. This may occur through following:
  - **Multiparous women**, who develop anti-HLA antibodies against paternal antigens that is shed from the fetus.
  - **Prior blood transfusions**, because platelets and white blood cells are rich in HLA antigens.
  - **Host has previously transplantation of another organ**.

Mechanism: Immediately after the graft is transplanted and blood flow is restored, the alloantibodies bind to antigens on the endothelium of graft vessel. This activates the complement system and causes injury to endothelial cells, produces vascular thrombosis, and ischemic necrosis of the graft (**Fig. 17**). Presently, hyperacute rejection is rare because every donor and recipients are matched for blood type, and recipients are tested for antibodies against the cells of the donor by performing a test called cross-match.

MORPHOLOGY

Gross

In hyperacute rejection, the affected kidney graft rapidly becomes cyanotic, mottled, and flaccid. The recipient may excrete a few drops of bloody urine (i.e., anuria).

Later, cortex undergoes necrosis (infarction), and kidney becomes nonfunctional.

Microscopy

Almost all arterioles and arteries show acute fibrinoid necrosis of their walls. They undergo narrowing or complete occlusion of their lumens by thrombi. Neutrophils accumulate rapidly within arterioles, glomeruli, and peritubular capillaries. As these changes become severe and become diffuse, thrombotic occlusion of the glomerular capillaries occurs. The kidney cortex undergoes severe coagulative necrosis (infarction). The affected kidneys become nonfunctional and have to be removed.

Acute rejection Acute rejection is brought out by recipient **T cells and antibodies** that are **activated by alloantigens in the graft**. It develops within days or weeks after transplantation in the nonimmunosuppressed. It is the main cause of early graft failure. It may also develop suddenly much later after transplantation if immunosuppression is tapered or terminated.

Types: Depending on the role of T cells or antibodies, acute rejection is divided into two types namely: acute cellular and acute antibody-mediated rejection. In most graft rejections, both types are present.

Acute cellular (T cell-mediated) rejection (Fig. 18): It is mediated by **activated recipient T (CD4+ and CD8+) lymphocytes**. CD8+ CTLs may directly destroy graft cells whereas CD4+ T cells secrete cytokines and induce inflammation. The inflammatory reaction injures/damages the graft and results in deterioration in graft function. Recipient **T cells may also react against graft vessels** and produces damage to vessels of the graft. Current immunosuppressive therapy is aimed mainly to prevent and reduce acute rejection by blocking the activation of alloreactive T cells.

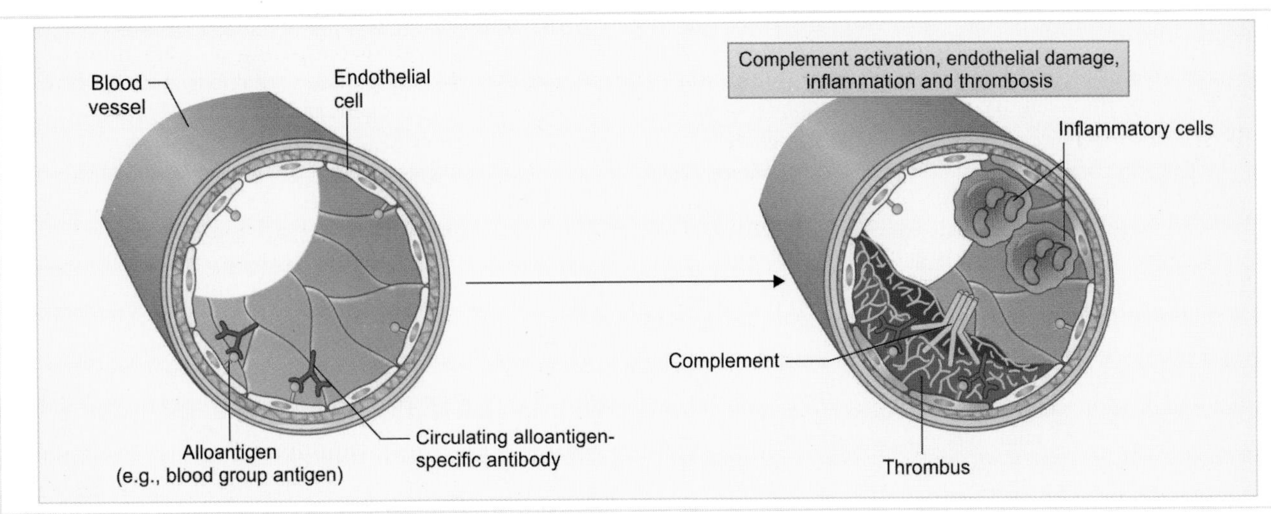

FIG. 17: Hyperacute rejection. Immediately after transplantation, preformed allogenic-specific antibody from recipient of graft, gets deposited on alloantigens on endothelium of graft blood vessels. This activates complement system causes injury to endothelial cells, produces vascular thrombosis, and ischemic necrosis of the graft.

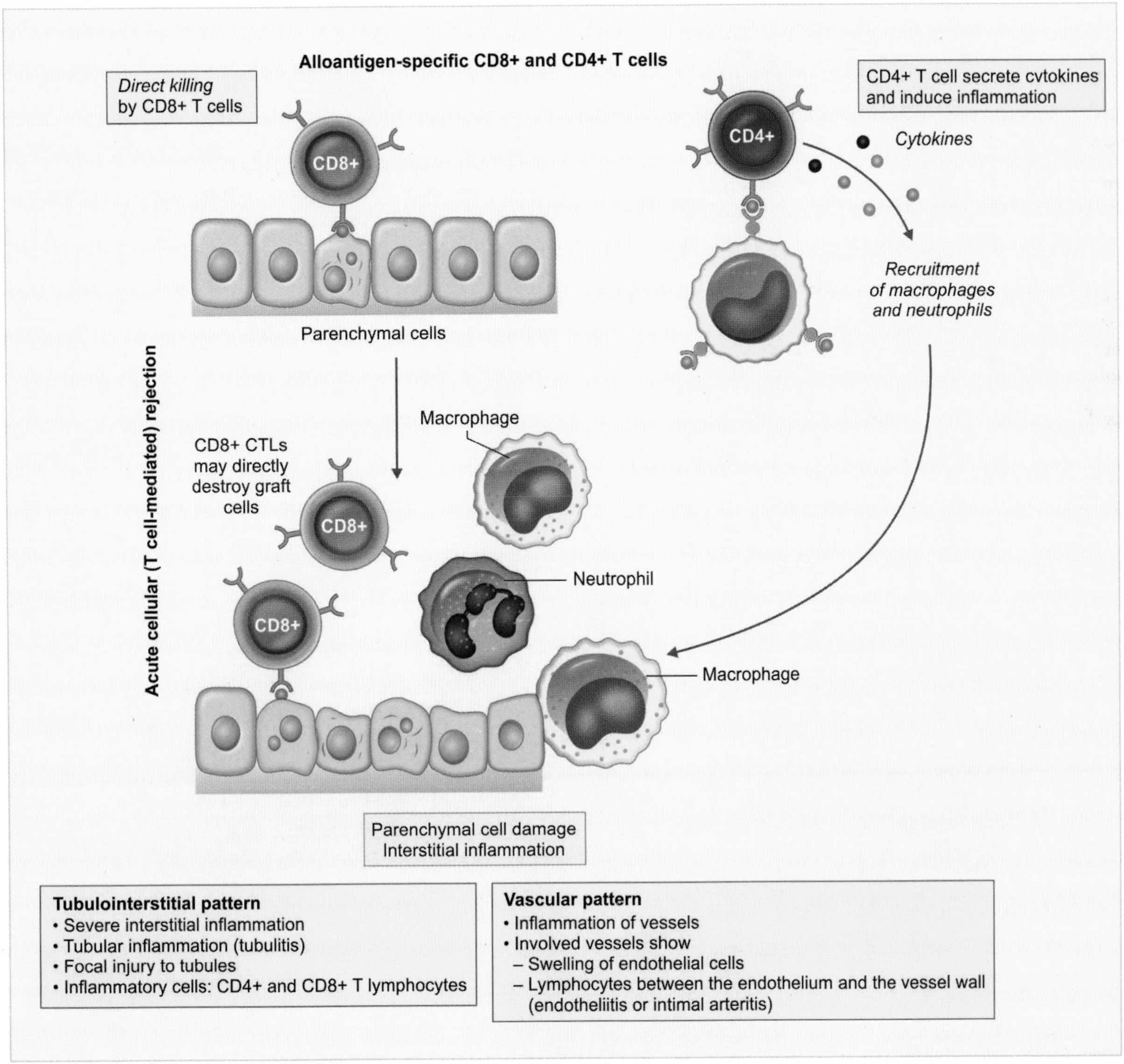

Acute cellular (T cell-mediated) rejection

Alloantigen-specific CD8+ and CD4+ T cells

Direct killing by CD8+ T cells

CD8+

Parenchymal cells

CD4+ T cell secrete cvtokines and induce inflammation

CD4+

Cytokines

Recruitment of macrophages and neutrophils

CD8+ CTLs may directly destroy graft cells

CD8+

CD8+

Macrophage

Neutrophil

Macrophage

Parenchymal cell damage
Interstitial inflammation

Tubulointerstitial pattern
- Severe interstitial inflammation
- Tubular inflammation (tubulitis)
- Focal injury to tubules
- Inflammatory cells: CD4+ and CD8+ T lymphocytes

Vascular pattern
- Inflammation of vessels
- Involved vessels show
  - Swelling of endothelial cells
  - Lymphocytes between the endothelium and the vessel wall (endotheliitis or intimal arteritis)

FIG. 18: Acute cellular rejection. Destruction of graft cells by CD4+ and CD8+ T lymphocytes. CD8+ CTLs directly kill the graft cells whereas by CD4+T cells secrete cytokine and induce inflammation and damages the graft cells.

MORPHOLOGY

Acute cellular (T cell-mediated) rejection may produce two different patterns of injury namely: (1) tubulointerstitial pattern (type I), and (2) vascular pattern (type II and III).

1. **Tubulointerstitial pattern** (sometimes called type I): This is characterized by extensive interstitial inflammation and tubular inflammation (tubulitis). There may be associated focal injury to tubules. The inflammatory infiltrates consist of both activated CD4+ and CD8+ T lymphocytes.
2. **Vascular pattern:** It shows inflammation of vessels (type II) and sometimes accompanied by necrosis of vessel walls (type III). The affected vessels show swelling of endothelial cells, and lymphocytes between the endothelium and the vessel wall. This is termed as **endotheliitis or intimal arteritis.**

The recognition of acute cellular rejection is important because, if not accompanied by acute humoral rejection, most patients respond well to immunosuppressive therapy.

Acute antibody-mediated rejection: In acute antibody-mediated (vascular or humoral) rejection, antibodies bind to alloantigens present in the endothelium of the vessels of the graft. This activates complement via the classical pathway (**Fig. 19**). This induces inflammation and causes endothelial damage. This leads to failure of the graft.

MORPHOLOGY

Acute antibody-mediated rejection: It is characterized by damage to glomeruli and small blood vessels. Activation of the complement system by the antibody-dependent classical pathway induces inflammation of glomeruli and peritubular capillaries. Small vessels may also show focal thrombosis.

Chronic rejection

Chronic rejection is an indolent form of graft damage. It develops over months or years, leading to progressive loss of graft function.

- **T cells:** Chronic rejection is characterized by interstitial fibrosis and gradual narrowing of graft blood vessels (graft arteriosclerosis). Both are due to reaction of T cells against graft alloantigens and secretion of cytokines. These cytokines stimulate the proliferation and activities of fibroblasts and vascular smooth muscle cells in the graft (**Fig. 20**).
- **Alloantibodies:** They also contribute to chronic rejection.

Current methods prevent or reduce acute rejection and have better 1-year survival of transplants. However, chronic rejection is refractory to most therapies and is becoming the main cause of graft failure.

MORPHOLOGY

Chronic rejection: Dominant feature is vascular changes. They show thickening of intima and occlusion of vascular lumen. Chronically rejecting kidney grafts show glomerulopathy, with duplication of the basement membrane. This is probably secondary to chronic endothelial injury. It also shows peritubular capillaritis and multilayering of peritubular capillary basement membranes. Other features include interstitial fibrosis and tubular atrophy with loss of renal parenchyma secondary to the vascular lesions. However, typically the interstitial mononuclear cell infiltrates are sparse.

Differences between hyperacute and acute transplant rejection are presented in **Table 9**.

In addition to the kidney, other organs, such as the liver, heart, lungs, and pancreas, are also transplanted.

Methods of Increasing Graft Survival

HLA matching: The importance of HLA matching between donor and recipient varies according to the solid-organ transplants.

- **Renal transplants:** HLA matching has significant benefit if all the polymorphic HLA alleles are matched (both inherited alleles of HLA-A, -B, and DR).
- **Other solid-organ transplant:** HLA matching is usually not done for transplants of liver, heart, and lungs. This

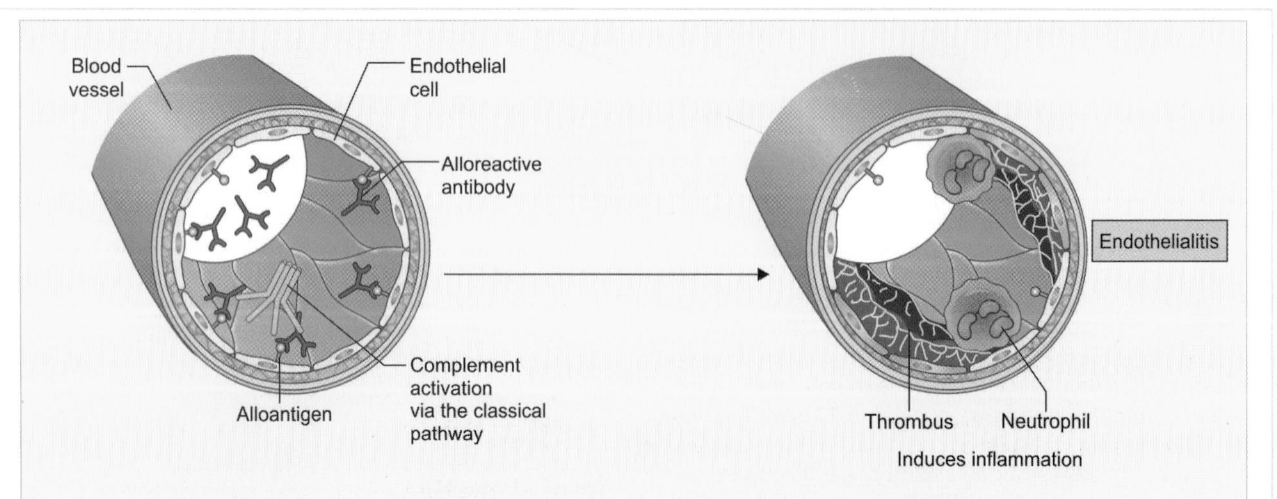

FIG. 19: Acute antibody-mediated (humoral) rejection. Graft damage is caused by antibody deposition in vessels which activates complement system via the classical pathway. This induces inflammation and causes endothelial damage. This leads to failure of the graft. Vessels may also show focal thrombosis.

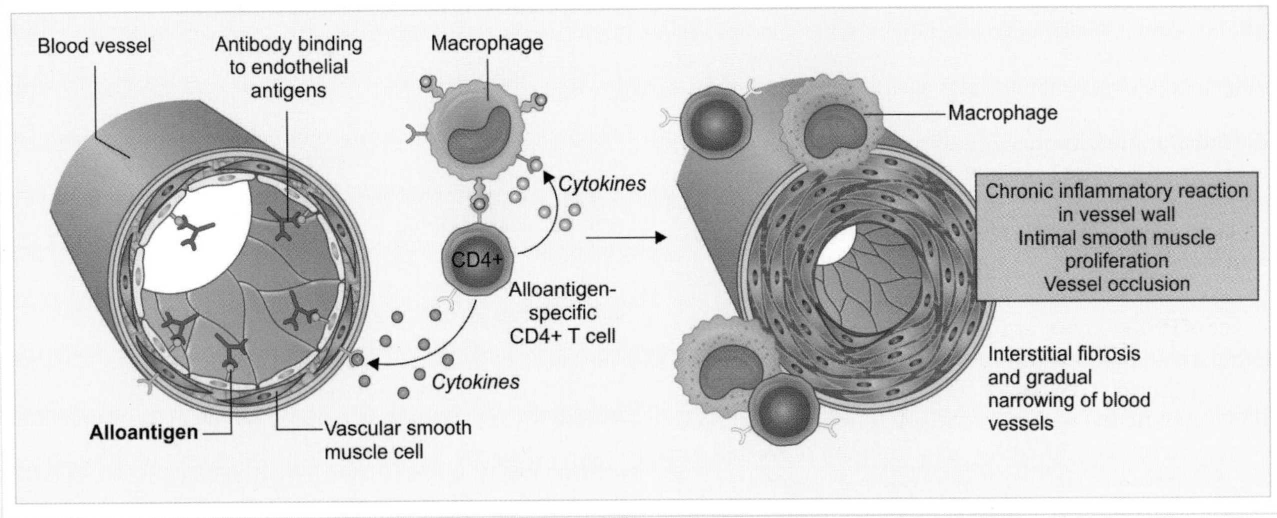

FIG. 20: Chronic rejection. Narrowing of graft blood vessels by T-cell cytokines and antibody deposition.

Table 9: Differences between hyperacute and acute transplant rejection.

Type	*Time of development*	*Mechanism*	*Pathological findings*
Hyperacute rejection	Minutes to hours	Preformed antibody and complement activation (type II hypersensitivity)	Arteritis, thrombosis, and necrosis
Acute cellular rejection	5 days to weeks	Activated T lymphocytes: CD4+ and CD8+ T-cells (type IV hypersensitivity)	Extensive interstitial mononuclear cell infiltration (CD4+ and CD8+), edema and endotheliitis
Acute humoral rejection		Antibody and complement activation	Neutrophilic infiltration and thrombosis
Chronic rejection	Months to years	Immune and nonimmune mechanisms	Fibrosis, scarring

is because other considerations override the potential benefits of HLA matching. These include anatomic compatibility, severity of the underlying illness, and the need to minimize the time of organ storage.

Immunosuppressive therapy: It is essential in all donor-recipient combinations (except for identical twins). Currently used immunosuppressive drugs include steroids (which reduce inflammation), mycophenolate mofetil (which inhibits lymphocyte proliferation), and tacrolimus (FK506). Tacrolimus is an inhibitor of the phosphatase calcineurin. The phosphatase calcineurin is necessary for activation of a transcription factor called nuclear factor of activated T cells (NFATs). NFAT stimulates transcription of cytokine genes (particularly the gene that encodes the growth factor IL-2). Thus, tacrolimus inhibits T cell responses.

Drugs used to treat rejection: These include T cell- and B cell-depleting antibodies, and pooled intravenous IgG (IVIG). IVIG suppresses inflammation by unknown mechanisms.

- **Plasmapheresis:** It is used when there is severe antibody-mediated rejection.
- **Preventing costimulatory signals from DCs:** T cells get activated when these receive both antigen and costimulatory signals. More recent strategy for reducing antigraft immune responses is to prevent host T cells from receiving costimulatory signals. This costimulatory signals from DCs is prevented during the initial phase of sensitization. This can be achieved by preventing the interaction between the B7 molecules on the DCs of the graft donor with the CD28 receptors on host T cells. For example, by administration of proteins that binds to B7 costimulators.

Untoward effects of immunosuppression: Immunosuppression prolongs graft survival. However, it has certain risks. Patients on immunosuppressive drugs are **increasingly susceptible to opportunistic infections.** Most frequent is reactivation of **polyoma virus**. In healthy individuals, the virus establishes latent infection of epithelial cells in the lower genitourinary tract. On immunosuppression, it becomes reactivated and infects renal tubules, and may even produce failure of graft. Patients on immunosuppressive drugs are also at increased risk for **developing EBV-induced lymphomas, human papillomavirus-induced squamous cell carcinomas, and Kaposi sarcoma (KS)**. They are probably due to reactivation of latent viral infections because of diminished host defenses.

These untoward effects of immunosuppression can be overcome by inducing donor-specific tolerance in graft recipients. This may be achieved by injecting regulatory T cells and blocking the costimulatory signals that are required for lymphocyte activation.

Transplantation of Hematopoietic Stem Cells

Hemoglobinopathy such as sickle cell anemia, thalassemia, and immunodeficiency states are progressively increasing each year. Transplantation of genetically "re-engineered" hematopoietic stem cells (HSCs) obtained from affected patients may be used for somatic cell gene therapy. It is also being evaluated in some immunodeficiencies and hemoglobinopathies.

Definition: HSC transplantation is a procedure which involves eliminating an individual's hematopoietic and immune system by chemotherapy and/or radiotherapy and replacing with stem cells either from another individual or with individual's own HSCs.

Source of HSCs: Bone marrow transplantation was the original term used to describe the collection and transplantation of HSCs. Historically, HSCs were obtained from the bone marrow and it is the richest source of HSCs. HSC transplantation is a preferred term. This is because now they are harvested from **peripheral blood and umbilical cord blood**. In the peripheral blood they are obtained after they are mobilized from the bone marrow by administration of hematopoietic growth factors. Umbilical cord blood of new born infants is easily available and also a rich source of HSCs.

Types of HSC transplant: These are as follows:

- Autologous ("from self"): Own HSCs removed, cryopreserved and reinfused.
- Allogeneic ("from different genes"): HSCs obtained from another individual.
- Syngeneic ("from same genes"): HSCs obtained from an identical twin.

Indications for HSC transplantation are listed in **Box 4**.

In most of the conditions in which HSC transplantation is indicated, the recipient is irradiated or treated with high doses of chemotherapy. This destroys the immune system (and sometimes, cancer cells) and opens up niches in the microenvironment of the marrow that nurture HSCs. Thus, it helps the transplanted HSCs to engraft.

Box 4: Indications for hematopoietic stem cell transplantation.

Red blood cell disorders

- Severe aplastic anemia
- Thalassemia major
- Fanconi anemia
- Sickle cell disease
- Pure red cell aplasia

WBC disorders

- Leukemia
  - Acute lymphoblastic leukemia—relapse after initial chemotherapy induced remission
  - Chronic myeloid leukemia, acute myeloid leukemia
- Myelodysplastic syndromes, myelofibrosis
- Lymphomas: Hodgkin lymphoma, non-Hodgkin lymphoma
- Multiple myeloma

Solid tumors: Germ cell tumors, neuroblastoma

Immunological disorders

- Severe autoimmune disorders: Scleroderma, lupus erythematosus
- Immune deficiency syndromes

Complications of HSC Transplantation

Autologous HSC transplants have fewer immunologic complications but have higher rates of relapse of the disease after transplant. Allogeneic HSC transplants have lower rates of relapse but have more immunologic complications, and graft-versus-host disease (GVHD), which can be fatal. HSC transplants differ from solid-organ transplants in several aspects. Two problems unique to HSC transplantation are GVHD and immunodeficiency.

Graft-versus-host disease

Q. Write short essay on GVHD.

It is the major complication that follows allogeneic HSC transplant. Rarely, it may develop following transplantation of solid organs rich in lymphoid cells (e.g., the liver) or transfusion of un-irradiated blood. **GVHD develops when immunologically competent cells or their precursors are transplanted into immunologically compromised recipients. The transferred donor cells recognize alloantigens in the host and attack host tissues.** This is due to infused donor T lymphocytes (CD4+ and CD8+ T-cells) reacting against the recipient's tissues/organs. Three conditions are necessary for the development of GVHD:

1. An immunocompetent graft (i.e., one containing T-cells).
2. HLA mismatch (minor or major) between donor and recipient.
3. An immunosuppressed recipient who cannot mount an immune response to the graft.

When immunosuppressed recipients receive HSCs from allogeneic donors, the immunocompetent T-cells present in the donor HSCs recognize the recipient's HLA antigens as foreign and react against them. GVHD can be minimized by transplanting HSCs between donor and recipient who are HLA-matched using precise DNA sequencing-based methods for molecular typing of HLA alleles.

Acute GVHD It occurs within days to weeks after allogeneic HSC transplantation. Any organ may be affected in acute GVHD. But major clinical manifestations result from involvement of the immune system and three primary target organs namely epithelia of the skin, liver, and intestines.

- **Skin:** It manifests as a generalized rash that may desquamate in severe cases.
- **Liver:** It causes destruction of small bile ducts and gives rise to jaundice.
- **GIT:** It produces ulceration of mucosa of the gut resulting in bloody diarrhea.

Though injury to tissue may be severe, the affected tissues are not usually heavily infiltrated by lymphocytes. Tissue damage is due to direct cytotoxicity by CD8+ T cells as well as cytokines released by the sensitized donor T cells.

Chronic GVHD

Skin: Chronic GVHD may either follow the acute syndrome or may occur insidiously. It is manifested with extensive cutaneous injury. It shows destruction of skin appendages and fibrosis of the dermis. Skin changes may resemble systemic sclerosis.

Liver: Chronic liver disease may cause cholestatic jaundice.

GIT: Damage to the GI tract may produce esophageal strictures.

Immune system: It produces involution of the thymus and depletion of lymphocytes in the lymph nodes.

Other symptoms: Patients develop recurrent and life-threatening infections. Patients may develop autoimmunity, probably to result from the grafted CD4+ helper T cells reacting with host B cells. These stimulated B cells may produce autoantibodies.

Depleting donor T cells before transplantation: GVHD is mediated by T lymphocytes present in the transplanted donor tissue. Depletion of donor T cells before transfusion almost avoids GVHD. However, this protocol is a mixed blessing: prevents GVHD, but tumor recurs in leukemic patients, increased incidence of graft failures and EBV-related B-cell lymphoma. Multifaceted T cells though mediate GVHD but are also needed for engraftment of the transplanted HSCs, suppression of EBV-infected B-cell clones, and control of leukemia cells (graft-versus-leukemia effect). The induction graft-versus-leukemia effect can be achieved by infusion of allogeneic T cells and is used to treat chronic myeloid leukemia that has relapsed after HSC transplantation.

Immunodeficiency: It is a frequent complication of HSC transplantation. The immunodeficiency may be due to prior treatment (e.g., for leukemia), preparation for the graft (myeloablation prior to HSC transplantation), a delay in repopulation of the recipient's immune system, and attack on the host's immune cells by grafted lymphocytes. Immunodeficiency predisposes to infections, particularly infection with cytomegalovirus. This is usually due to activation of latent infection. Cytomegalovirus-induced pneumonitis can be a fatal complication of HSC transplantation.

BIBLIOGRAPHY

1. Abbas AK, Lichtman AH, Pillai S. Cellular and Molecular Immunology, 9th edition. Philadelphia: Elsevier; 2018.
2. Actor JA. Introductory Immunology, 2nd edition. United Kingdom: Elsevier; 2019.
3. Bach JF. The hygiene hypothesis in autoimmunity: the role of pathogens and commensals. *Nat Rev Immunol*. 2018;18:105-120.
4. Cheng M, Anderson MS. Thymic tolerance as a key brake on autoimmunity. *Nat Immunol*. 2018;19:659-64.
5. Cheng MH, Anderson MS. Monogenic autoimmunity. *Annu Rev Immunol*. 2012;30:393-427.
6. Crow MK, Olferiev M, Kirou K. Type I interferons in autoimmune disease. *Ann Rev Pathol Mech Dis*. 2019;14:369-93.
7. Dendrou CA, Petersen J, Rossjohn J, et al. HLA variation and disease. *Nat Rev Immunol*. 2018;18:325-39.
8. Dominguez-Villar M, Hafler DA. Regulatory T cells in autoimmune disease. *Nat Immunol*. 2018;19:665-73.
9. Goodnow CC. Multistep pathogenesis of autoimmune disease. *Cell*. 2007;130:25.
10. Inshaw JRJ, Cutler AJ, Burren OS, et al. Approaches and advances in the genetic causes of autoimmunity and their implications. *Nat Immunol*. 2018;19:674-684.
11. Jennette JC, Falk RJ, Hu P, et al. Pathogenesis of antineutrophil cytoplasmic autoantibody-associated small-vessel vasculitis. *Annu Rev Pathol*. 2013;8:139-60.
12. Katsumoto TR, Whitfield ML, Connolly MK. The pathogenesis of systemic sclerosis. *Annu Rev Pathol Mech Dis*. 2011;6:509-537.
13. Kaul A, Gordon C, Crow MK, et al. Systemic lupus erythematosus. *Nat Rev Dis Primer.s* 2016;2:16039.
14. Klimov VV. From Basic to Clinical Immunology. Switzerland: Springer Nature; 2019.
15. Kumar V, Abbas AK, Aster JC, Deyrup AT. Robbins essential pathology, 1st edition. Philadelphia: Elsevier; 2021.
16. Kumar V, Abbas AK, Aster JC. Robbins basic pathology, 10th edition. Philadelphia: Saunders Elsevier; 2018.
17. Kumar V, Abbas AK, Fausto N, et al. Robbins and Cotran pathologic basis of disease, 10th edition. Philadelphia: WB Saunders; 2021.
18. Lenardo M, Lo B, Lucas CL. Genomics of immune diseases and new therapies. *Ann Rev Immunol* 2016;34:121-49.
19. Mahajan VS, Mattoo H, Deshpande V, et al. IgG4-related disease. *Annu Rev Pathol Mech Dis* 2014;9:315-47.
20. Maria NI, Davidson A. Emerging areas for therapeutic discovery in SLE. *Curr Opin Immunol* 2018;55:1-8.
21. Marson A, Housley WJ, Hafler DA: Genetic basis of autoimmunity. *J Clin Invest*. 2015;125:2234-41.
22. Mathis D, Benoist C. Microbiota and autoimmune disease: the hosted self. *Cell Host Microbe*. 2011;10:297-301.
23. Mavragani CP. Mechanisms and new strategies for primary Sjogren's Syndrome. *Annu Rev Med*. 2017;68:331-43.
24. Mitchell RN. Graft vascular disease: immune response meets the vessel wall. *Annu Rev Pathol Mech Dis*. 2009;4:19-47.
25. Mueller DL. Mechanisms maintaining peripheral tolerance. *Nat Immunol*. 2010;11:21-7.
26. Nagy ZA. Alloreactivity: an old puzzle revisited. *Scand J Immunol*. 2012;75:463-70.
27. Nankivell BJ, Alexander SI. Rejection of the kidney allograft. *N Engl J Med*. 2010;363:1451.
28. Ohkura N, Kitagawa Y, Sakaguchi S. Development and maintenance of regulatory T cells. *Immunity*. 2013;38:414-23.
29. Pattanaik D, Brown M, Postlethwaite BC, et al. Pathogenesis of systemic sclerosis. *Front Immunol*. 2015;6:272.
30. Punt J, Stranford SA, Jones PP, Owen JA. Kuby Immunology, 8th edition. New York: Macmilan learning; 2019.
31. Schildberg FA, Klein SR, Freeman GJ, et al. Coinhibitory pathways in the B7-CD28 ligand-receptor family. *Immunity*. 2016;44: 955-72.
32. Schwartz RH. Historical overview of immunological tolerance. *Cold Spring Harb Perspect Biol*. 2012;4:a006908.
33. Strayer DS, Saffitz JE. Rubin's Pathology: Mechanism of Human Disease, 8th edition. Philadelphia: Wolters Kluwer; 2020.
34. Theofilopoulos A, Kono DH, Baccala R. The multiple pathways to autoimmunity. *Nat Immunol*. 2017;18:716-24.
35. Valenzuela NM, Reed EF. Antibody-mediated rejection across solid organ transplants: manifestations, mechanisms, and therapies. *J Clin Invest* 2017;127:2492-504.
36. Wood KJ, Goto R. Mechanisms of rejection: current perspectives. *Transplantation*. 2012;93:1-10.

CHAPTER 17

Immunodeficiency Diseases and Amyloidosis

CHAPTER OUTLINE

- Immunodeficiency diseases
  - Classification
  - Principal consequence of immunodeficiency
  - Primary immunodeficiencies
  - Secondary (acquired) immunodeficiencies
- Acquired immunodeficiency syndrome
  - Etiology
  - Route of transmission
  - Pathogenesis of HIV infection and AIDS
  - Natural history of HIV infection
  - Clinical features of AIDS
  - Effect of antiretroviral drug therapy
  - Laboratory diagnosis of HIV infection and AIDS
  - Prevention of HIV in healthcare facilities
- Amyloidosis
  - Properties of amyloid proteins
  - Pathogenesis of amyloidosis
  - Pathological effects of amyloid deposits
  - Classification of amyloidosis
  - Clinical features

IMMUNODEFICIENCY DISEASES

Immunity is intrinsic to life and integrity of the immune system is essential for defense against pathogenic microorganisms and their toxic products. Immune system can be divided into two major components—the innate immune system and the adaptive immune system. Defects in one or more components of the immune system can lead to serious and often fatal disorders. These are collectively called immunodeficiency diseases.

Definition: Immunodeficiency is a state in which the ability of the immune system to protect the host against pathogens (disease-causing agents) is reduced due to decreased or complete failure of immune response.

Classification

Immunodeficiency diseases are classified as primary (congenital) or secondary (acquired), and by defective host defense system (innate or adaptive).

- **Primary (hereditary/innate/congenital) immunodeficiency** disorders (PID) are due to an intrinsic defect in the immune system and are genetically determined (i.e., caused by gene mutations).
- **Secondary (or acquired) immunodeficiency** states are not inherited. These occur due to the influence of harmful environmental and endogenous factors. They may arise as complications of an underlying condition. The underlying conditions include cancers, infections, malnutrition, or side effects of immunosuppression, irradiation, or chemotherapy for cancer and other diseases.

Principal Consequence of Immunodeficiency

Susceptibility to infections: Clinically, immunodeficiencies manifest as increased susceptibility to infections. These infections may be either newly acquired or a reactivation of latent infection. The nature of the infection depends mainly on the component of the immune system that is defective (**Table 1**). In combined immunodeficiencies (defect in both humoral and cell-mediated immunity), patients are susceptible to infection by all classes of microorganisms. Immunodeficient patients, especially those with defects in cellular immunity, often present with opportunistic infections. Opportunistic infections are infections by microbes that are commonly encountered but effectively eliminated by healthy individuals.

Susceptible to certain types of cancer: Patients with immunodeficiency are susceptible to cancers. Many of these cancers in patients with immunodeficiency are caused by oncogenic viruses. Examples of oncogenic viruses include Epstein–Barr virus (EBV) and human papilloma viruses (HPVs). T cells play an important role in surveillance against cancer. Hence, an increased incidence of cancer is most often seen in T-cell immunodeficiencies.

Increased incidence of autoimmunity: Paradoxically, some immunodeficiency diseases are associated with an auto-immunity.

Defects in lymphocyte development or activation or in the effector mechanisms of innate and adaptive immunity: Immunodeficiency diseases form a heterogeneous group that are different clinically and pathologically. This is partly because

Table 1: Features of immunodeficiencies affecting T or B lymphocytes.

Feature	*Deficiency of B lymphocytes*	*Deficiency of T lymphocytes*
Deficient immunity	Defects in humoral immunity	Defects in cell-mediated immunity
Susceptibility and type of infection produced	Encapsulated, pus-forming (pyogenic) bacteria (otitis, pneumonia, meningitis, osteomyelitis), enteric bacteria and viruses, some parasites	Intracellular microbes, *Pneumocystis jirovecii*, many viruses, atypical mycobacteria, fungi, reactivation of latent infections
Serum immunoglobulin (Ig) levels	Decreased	Normal or decreased
Delayed-type hypersensitivity (DTH) reactions to common antigens	Normal	Reduced
Morphology findings in lymphoid tissues	Absent or reduced follicles and germinal centers (B cell zones)	Usually normal follicles; May show reduced parafollicular cortical regions (T-cell zones)

different diseases involve different components of the immune system. Abnormalities in lymphocyte development may be caused by mutations in genes encoding enzymes, adaptors, transport proteins, and transcription factors.

Primary Immunodeficiencies

Q. Discuss various primary immunodeficiency disorders.

Primary immunodeficiency diseases are caused by genetic (inherited) defects. These defects may affect the defense mechanisms of innate or adaptive immunity.

- **Innate immunity:** This may involve components of innate immunity such as phagocytes, NK cells, or complement system.
- **Adaptive immunity:** This may involve the humoral and/or cellular arms of adaptive immunity. Humoral immunity is mediated by B lymphocytes and cellular immunity is mediated by T lymphocytes.

Most of the primary immunodeficiency diseases manifest and are detected during infancy, between 6 months and 2 years of age. They are susceptible to recurrent infections.

Defects in Innate Immunity

Innate immunity is the first line of defense against infectious organisms. Two important components of innate immunity are phagocytes and complement system. Therefore, congenital disorders of phagocytes and the complement system are associated with recurrent infections.

Classification of primary immune deficiency diseases due to deficiencies of the innate immune system is presented in **Box 1**. Deficiencies in innate immunity include defects of phagocyte function, innate immune receptors, and complement system. Inherited immune defects in the early innate immune response usually affect leukocyte functions or the complement system (**Table 2**, also see Tables 14 and 21 of Chapter 8). These patients have increased susceptibility to infections.

Box 1: Classification of primary immune deficiency diseases due to deficiencies of the innate immune system.

Defects in leukocyte (phagocytic cells)
- Impaired production: Severe congenital neutropenia (SCN)
- Asplenia
- Impaired adhesion: Leukocyte adhesion deficiency (LAD)
- Impaired formation of phagolysosome: Chédiak–Higashi syndrome
- Impaired killing: Chronic granulomatous disease (CGD)

Innate immunity receptors and signal transduction
- Defects in toll-like receptor (TLR) signaling
- Mendelian susceptibility to mycobacterial disease

Complement deficiencies
- Classical, alternative, and lectin pathways
- Lytic phase

Deficiencies of complement regulatory proteins

Defects in leukocyte function

Few examples are discussed below:

Inherited defects in leukocyte adhesion: It is due to inherited defects in adhesion molecules. It impairs leukocyte recruitment to sites of infection and is characterized by recurrent bacterial infections.

- **Leukocyte adhesion deficiency type 1 (LAD-1):** LAD-1 is caused by defects in biosynthesis of the β_2 chain that is shared by the integrins LFA-1 and Mac-1.
- **Leukocyte adhesion deficiency type 2 (LAD-2):** LAD-2 is caused by the absence of sialyl-Lewis X, the fucose-containing ligand for E- and P-selectins. It is due to a defect in a fucosyl transferase, an enzyme that attaches fucose moieties to protein backbones.

Both conditions result in a failure of leukocyte adhesion to endothelium, preventing the cells from migrating into tissues and making patients prone to bacterial infections, which are often recurrent and frequently life-threatening.

Inherited defects in phagolysosome function: One of the examples is Chédiak–Higashi syndrome. It is an autosomal recessive condition in which there is defective fusion of phagosomes and lysosomes. This results in defective phagocyte function and susceptibility to infections. The gene associated with this disorder encodes a large cytosolic protein called LYST. This LYST regulates lysosomal trafficking. Main leukocyte abnormalities include neutropenia (decreased neutrophils), defective degranulation, and delayed microbial killing. In **peripheral blood smears, the affected leukocytes show giant granules**, which are probably the result from aberrant phagolysosome fusion. Other abnormalities include

Table 2: Examples of inherited defects in innate immunity affecting phagocytic leukocytes and the complement system.

Disease	*Defect*
Defects in leukocyte function	
Leukocyte adhesion deficiency 1	Defective leukocyte adhesion because of mutations in the β chain of CD11/CD18 integrins. There is defective β_2-integrin expression or function
Leukocyte adhesion deficiency 2	Defective leukocyte adhesion because of mutations in fucosyl transferase required for synthesis of sialylated oligosaccharide (receptor for selectins). There is defective fucosylation and selectin binding
Chédiak–Higashi syndrome	• Decreased leukocyte functions due to mutations affecting protein involved in lysosomal membrane traffic (defective lysosomal granules) • Poor chemotaxis
Chronic granulomatous disease	Decreased oxidative burst. Deficient NADPH oxidase, with no production of H_2O_2
X-linked	Defect in phagocyte oxidase (membrane component)
Autosomal recessive	Defect in phagocyte oxidase (cytoplasmic components)
Myeloperoxidase deficiency	Decreased microbial killing because of defective MPO-H_2O_2 system. There is deficient production of $HOCl^-/OCl_2^-$
Defects in the complement system	
C2, C4 deficiency	Defective activation of classical pathway. Results in reduced resistance to infection and reduced clearance of immune complexes
C3 deficiency	Defects in all complement functions, immune-complex syndromes, pyogenic infections
Deficiency of complement regulatory proteins	Excessive activation of complement. It includes angioedema, paroxysmal hemoglobinuria

abnormalities in melanocytes (leading to albinism), cells of the nervous system (associated with nerve defects), and platelets (causing bleeding disorders).

Inherited defects in microbicidal activity: One of the examples of the disease characterized by defect in oxygen-dependent bacterial killing is group of congenital disorders called chronic granulomatous disease of childhood. It is discussed on page 304.

Innate immunity receptors and signal transduction

Defects in TLR signaling: These are rare in which defect is in toll-like receptors (TLRs) and their signaling molecules. For example, defects in TLR3 (a receptor for viral RNA) are associated with recurrent herpes simplex encephalitis and defects in MyD88 (the adaptor protein downstream of multiple TLRs) are associated with destructive bacterial infections of lung producing pneumonias.

Deficiencies affecting the complement system

Hereditary deficiencies can occur with almost all components of the complement system and their regulators (refer page 261–265). One disease, namely paroxysmal nocturnal hemoglobinuria, is due to an acquired deficiency of complement regulatory factors.

Deficiency of C2 or C4: These are early components of the classical pathway. Deficiency of C2 is the most common hereditary complement protein deficiency. A deficiency of C2 or C4 is associated with increased infections by bacteria or virus. However, many patients may not have any clinical manifestation. This may be probably because the alternative complement pathway is adequate for the control of most infections. Surprisingly, some of these patients, as well as in patients with C1q deficiency, may produce systemic lupus erythematosus (SLE)-like manifestation of autoimmune disease.

Deficiency of components of the alternative pathway (properdin and factor D): It is rare and is associated with recurrent pyogenic infections (refer page 261).

Deficiency of C3: The C3 component of complement is needed for both the classical and alternative pathways. Hence, C3 deficiency is associated with susceptibility to serious and recurrent pyogenic infections. It is also associated with an increased incidence of immune complex-mediated glomerulonephritis. Complement is necessary for the removal of immune complexes. Hence, during its absence, inflammation is probably caused by Fc receptor-dependent leukocyte activation.

Deficiency of terminal complement components: The terminal components of complement consist of C5, 6, 7, 8, and 9. They are needed for the formation of the membrane attack complex (MAC) involved in the lysis of organisms. Deficiency of these late-acting components is associated with increased susceptibility to recurrent *Neisseria* (gonococcal and meningococcal) infections. *Neisseria* bacteria have thin cell walls, and they are destroyed by the lytic actions of complement. Absence of lytic component, namely MAC, leads to its susceptibility to infections.

Inheritance of defective form of mannose-binding lectin: This is a plasma protein that activates the lectin pathway of complement. These patients also have increased susceptibility to infections.

Deficiencies of complement regulatory proteins

Deficiency of C1 inhibitor (C1 INH): It gives rise to hereditary angioedema and is discussed in detail on pages 263 and 264.

Others: Examples of deficiencies of other complement regulatory proteins include paroxysmal nocturnal hemoglobinuria, chronic forms of hemolytic uremic syndrome, and age-related macular degeneration.

Defects in Adaptive Immunity

Inherited defects in adaptive immunity can be subclassified depending on the primary component involved (i.e., B cells or T cells or combined) (**Table 3**). However, the distinctions between them are not clear-cut. For example, T-cell defects always lead to impaired synthesis of antibody. Hence, isolated deficiencies of T cells are usually clinically indistinguishable from combined deficiencies of T and B cells. Immunodeficiencies due to the defects in adaptive immunity result from abnormalities in lymphocyte development (maturation), or impaired function (activation). Immunodeficiency may be caused by defects in B- and T-cell maturation (impaired development) or defects in B- and T-cell activation (impaired survival, migration, function). The mutations responsible for many of these immunodeficiency diseases are well known. Main pathways of lymphocyte development and various primary immune deficiency diseases are presented in **Fig. 1**.

Severe combined immunodeficiency

Severe combined immunodeficiency (SCID) consists of over 20 genetically distinct syndromes. All of them are characterized by common defects in both humoral and cell-mediated immune responses. This is due to deficiencies in T-cell and B-cell development and function.

Table 3: Classifications and examples of inherited defects in adaptive immune system.

Combined T and B lymphocytes	
• Impaired development	Severe combined immunodeficiencies (SCIDs)*
• Impaired survival, migration, function	Combined immunodeficiencies
B lymphocytes	
• Impaired development	XL [e.g., Bruton X-linked agammaglobulinemia (XLA)*] and AR agammaglobulinemia
• Impaired function	• Hyper-IgM syndrome* • Common variable immunodeficiency (CVID)* • IgA deficiency*
T lymphocytes	
• Impaired development	DiGeorge's syndrome*
• Impaired survival, migration, function	• Hyper-IgE syndrome (autosomal dominant) • Wiskott–Aldrich syndrome* • Ataxia-telangiectasia* and other DNA repair deficiencies

* These are discussed in detail.

Clinical presentation: Affected infants present in the first few months of life with prominent thrush (oral candidiasis), extensive diaper rash, diarrhea, and failure to thrive. Some infants may develop a scaly skin eruption (morbilliform/rash that looks like measles) rash shortly after birth. This is due to the transfer of maternal T cells across the placenta and these maternal T-cell engraftments attack the fetus, causing graft-versus-host disease (GVHD). Individuals with SCID are extremely susceptible to recurrent, severe infections by a wide range of pathogens. These include *Candida albicans*, *Pneumocystis jirovecii*, *Pseudomonas*, cytomegalovirus (CMV), varicella, and others. SCID is usually fatal and death occurs within the first year of life unless an immune system can be provided by hematopoietic stem cell (HSC) transplantation. Though the clinical features of SCID are common, the underlying genetic defects are varied, and, in many cases, they are not known. Usually, the defect in SCID is in the T-cell with a secondary impairment of humoral immunity.

X-linked SCID It is the most common form of SCID and is responsible for 40–60% of cases. It is X-linked, and hence this type of SCID is more common in boys than in girls.

Molecular basis: The genetic defect is due to mutation in the common γ-chain (γc) subunit of cytokine receptors. This receptor is a transmembrane protein shared by several cytokine receptors (the IL-2, 4, 7, 9, 11, 15, and 21 receptors). IL-7 is needed for the survival and proliferation of lymphoid progenitors, particularly T-cell precursors. As a result of defective IL-7 receptor signaling, there is a severe block in the earliest stages of lymphocyte development, especially T-cell development (**Fig. 1**). T-cell numbers are markedly reduced. Though B cells may be normal in number, because of lack of T-cell help, there is impaired synthesis of antibody. IL-15 is required for the maturation and proliferation of NK cells. Because the common γc is a component of the receptor for IL-15, these patients usually also have deficiency of NK cells.

Autosomal recessive SCID The remaining, about 40%, forms of SCID are autosomal recessive disorders.

Molecular basis: The most common cause of autosomal recessive SCID is a deficiency of the enzyme adenosine deaminase (ADA). Probably ADA deficiency leads to accumulation of deoxyadenosine and its derivatives (e.g., deoxy-ATP). These are toxic to rapidly dividing immature lymphocytes, especially T-cell lineage. Hence there may be a more decrease in the number of T lymphocytes than of B lymphocytes. Other less common causes of autosomal recessive SCID are as follows:

- Mutations in recombinase-activating genes (RAG) or other components of the antigen receptor gene recombination machinery. These mutations prevent the somatic gene rearrangements that are needed for the assembly of TCR and Ig genes. This prevents the development of T and B cells.
- Signal transduction through cytokine receptors containing the common γc (which is mutated in X-linked SCID) requires an intracellular kinase called JAK3. Hence,

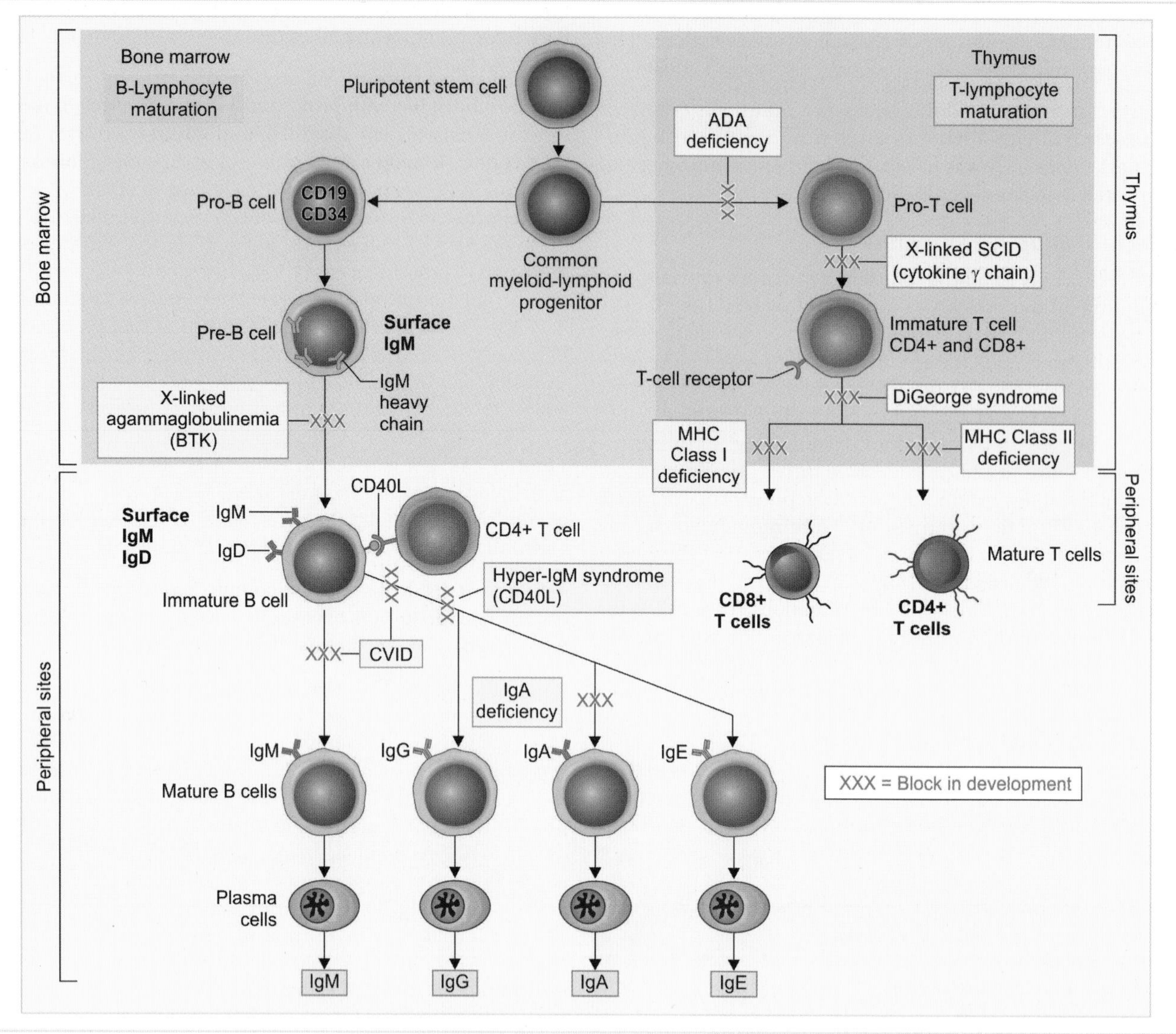

[ADA: adenosine deaminase; BTK: Bruton tyrosine kinase; CD40L: CD40 ligand (also known as CD154); CVID: common variable immunodeficiency; Ig: immunoglobulin; MHC: major histocompatibility complex; SCID: severe combined immunodeficiency]

FIG. 1: Main pathways of lymphocyte development and various primary immune deficiency diseases. Pluripotent stem cells give rise to common myeloid-lymphoid progenitor cells. These cells populate either the bone marrow or thymus. **B cell differentiation**: Common lymphoid progenitors give rise to pre-B cells. The B cell differentiation pathway goes through the pre–B cell stage (expression of surface IgM), and the mature B cell stage (expression of surface IgM and IgD). B cells can differentiate into plasma cells and produce IgM. These B cells produce antibodies of various isotypes. **T-cell differentiation**: In this, common lymphoid progenitors give rise to the T cell precursors that migrate to the thymus. They differentiate into immature T cells with T-cell receptor (TCR). They further develop into CD4+ and CD8+ T cells. More than 100 primary immunodeficiency disorders occur at the genetic and/or molecular levels. Several immunodeficiency disorders result from a discrete molecular defect in the form of "maturational arrest" in the development of fully differentiated and functional lymphocytes. Blocks in these pathways in few primary immune deficiency diseases are depicted in the figure. In some of the disorders, the affected genes are indicated in brackets. The identification of specific molecular lesions helped in the diagnosis and understanding of these diseases.

mutations of JAK3 have the same effects as mutations in the γc.

- Many other mutations may involve signaling molecules, such as kinases associated with the T-cell antigen receptor and components of calcium channels that are needed for the entry of calcium and activation of many signaling pathways.

MORPHOLOGY

Microscopy

It depends on the underlying defect. In the two most common forms (γc mutation and ADA deficiency) of SCID, the thymus is small and there are no lymphoid cells.

Continued

Continued

- **X-linked SCID:** Thymus shows lobules of undifferentiated epithelial cells resembling fetal thymus.
- **SCID caused by ADA deficiency:** It shows remnants of Hassall's corpuscles.

In both types of SCID, other lymphoid tissues are also hypoplastic. There is marked depletion of T-cell areas and in some cases, both T-cell and B-cell zones.

Treatment Currently, the treatment of choice is HSC transplantation.

- **X-linked SCID:** It was the first human disease in which gene therapy has been successful. In this type of SCID ex vivo gene therapy, a normal γc gene is expressed using a viral vector in HSCs taken from patients. These cells are then transplanted back into the patients. The number of cases treated with gene therapy is small to comment on its effect. Some patients have shown improvement for over 10 years after therapy. Unfortunately, about 20% of patients developed T-cell lymphoblastic leukemia. This is one of the dangers of gene therapy. The uncontrolled T-cell proliferation causing leukemia was triggered by the activation of oncogenes by the integrated virus.
- **Patients with ADA deficiency:** They were treated with HSC transplantation. Recently, administration of the enzyme or gene therapy involves the introduction of a normal ADA gene into T-cell precursors.

X-linked agammaglobulinemia (Bruton's agammaglobulinemia)

Bruton's X-linked agammaglobulinemia (XLA) is one of the more common primary immunodeficiency diseases. XLA is characterized by the defect in B-cell development. There is failure of B-cell precursors (pro–B cells and pre–B cells) to develop into mature B cells.

Molecular basis of Ig production by B cells and its maturation in bone marrow: During normal maturation of B-cell in the bone marrow, the Ig heavy-chain genes are rearranged first in pre–B cells. These form a complex with a "surrogate" light chain on the cell surface called the pre–B-cell receptor (pre-BCR). This complex delivers signals that induce rearrangement of the Ig light-chain genes and further maturation. This need for Ig-initiated signals is a quality-control mechanism. It makes sure that maturation will only proceed if functional Ig proteins are expressed.

Molecular basis of XLA: Bruton's XLA is characterized by mutations in a cytoplasmic tyrosine kinase, called Bruton tyrosine kinase (BTK). Gene that encodes BTK is present on the long arm of the X chromosome at Xq21.22. BTK gene product is a protein tyrosine kinase that participates in pre-BCR signaling (**Fig. 1**). It is associated with the pre-BCR and with the BCR complexes present on mature B cells. It is required for maturation of pre–B-cell to B-cell stage. Mutation of *BTK* gene (with defective kinase) blocks B-cell maturation at pre-B-cell stage. The pre-BCR cannot deliver the signals that are needed for light chain rearrangement, and maturation is arrested. There is no production of light chains and it leads to reduced production of immunoglobulin (Ig). BTK is also a transducer of BCR signals. This transduction stimulates growth and increases cell survival in benign and malignant mature B cells. Inhibitors of BTK can be used as effective therapeutic agents for the treatment of several B-cell malignancies. T-cell mediated immunity is intact.

Clinical manifestations Being an X-linked disease, it is seen almost exclusively in males, but sporadic cases can occur in females, probably due to mutations in other genes that function in the same pathway. The disease usually does not manifest until about 6 months of age due to protective maternal antibody (Ig). It presents when the levels of the maternal antibodies become depleted.

Susceptible to infections: These infections include the following:

- **Bacterial infections:** In most cases, patient presents with recurrent bacterial infections of the mucosal surfaces of the respiratory tract. These include acute and chronic pharyngitis, sinusitis, otitis media, bronchitis, and pneumonia. They may develop pyoderma, meningitis, and septicemia. Almost always the infections are caused by *Haemophilus influenzae, Streptococcus pneumoniae,* or *Staphylococcus aureus*. Normally, these organisms are opsonized by antibodies and destroyed by phagocytosis. In the absence of antibodies, these are not effectively cleared.
- **Viral infections:** Antibodies are important for neutralizing infectious viruses. Hence, these patients are also susceptible to certain viral infections. These include enteroviruses, such as echovirus, poliovirus, and coxsackievirus. These enteroviruses infect the gastrointestinal tract (GIT), and they can disseminate from GIT to the nervous system through the blood. Thus, immunization with live attenuated poliovirus can lead to paralytic poliomyelitis, and echovirus can cause fatal encephalitis.
- **Protozoal infections:** *Giardia lamblia* is an intestinal protozoan that is normally destroyed by IgA secreted in the intestine. In XLA patients, it can cause persistent infections. Usually, most fungal, protozoal, and intracellular viral infections are controlled by the intact T-cell-mediated immunity.

Increased susceptibility to autoimmune diseases: Paradoxically, autoimmune diseases (e.g., arthritis and dermatomyositis) develop in as many as 30% of patients. Probably these autoimmune disorders are caused by a breakdown of self-tolerance resulting in autoimmunity. Chronic recurrent infections associated with the immune deficiency may also be responsible for inducing the inflammatory reactions.

Characteristics of a classical form of Bruton's XLA is presented in **Box 2**.

Box 2: Characteristics of a classic form of Bruton's XLA.

- Absent or markedly decreased B lymphocytes in the circulation (peripheral blood)
- Serum levels of all classes of Igs are reduced
- Bone marrow shows normal numbers of pre-B cells. They express the B-lineage marker CD19 but not membrane Ig
- Underdeveloped or poorly developed germinal centers in the lymph nodes, Peyer patches, the appendix, and tonsils
- Absence of plasma cells throughout the body
- Normal T-cell-mediated reactions

Treatment: It is by replacement therapy with Igs. Prophylactic intravenous immunoglobulin (IVIG) therapy will be useful for most patients.

DiGeorge syndrome (thymic hypoplasia)

Q. Write short essay on DiGeorge syndrome.

DiGeorge syndrome is a T-cell immunodeficiency disorder. It is characterized by failure of development of T cells in the thymus and there is absence of cell-mediated immunity due to low numbers of T lymphocytes in the blood and lymphoid tissues.

Etiology

- Normally, the third and fourth pharyngeal pouches give rise to the thymus, the parathyroids, some of the C cells of the thyroid, and the ultimobranchial body, and influence conotruncal cardiac development.
- In DiGeorge syndrome, there is **defective embryologic development** (i.e., congenital malformation) **of the third and fourth pharyngeal pouches**.
    - **Defective development of the thymus:** Thymus shows either hypoplasia or there is complete agenesis/absence of the thymus. This leads to selective T-cell deficiency with deficient T-cell maturation causing variable loss of T-cell-mediated immunity (immunodeficiency). In the absence of a thymus, T-cell maturation is interrupted at the pre–T-cell stage (**Fig. 1**). Most affected patients have "partial" DiGeorge syndrome in which a small remnant of thymus is present.
    - **Absent parathyroid glands:** This causes tetany characterized by abnormal calcium homeostasis and muscle twitching.
    - **Congenital defects (abnormal development) of the heart and great vessels:** These are due to defective conotruncal cardiac development.
    - **Abnormalities in other structures** that develop from the third and fourth pharyngeal pouches during fetal life (e.g., facial deformities such as abnormal appearance of the mouth, ears, and facies).

Molecular genetics: Most (90%) of the DiGeorge syndrome is caused by a small germline deletion that maps to chromosome 22q11. Hence, currently DiGeorge syndrome is considered a component of the 22q11 deletion syndrome (refer page 862). *TBX1* gene lies within the same chromosomal region of chromosome 22q11. *TBX1* gene codes for a transcription factor called T-box 1 (TBX1) and this is required for development of the branchial arch and the great vessels. In a few patients of DiGeorge syndrome without chromosome 22q11 deletions, there are loss-of-function mutations involving *TBX1*.

MORPHOLOGY

Thymus: Hypoplasia or complete agenesis/absence of the thymus
Parathyroid glands: Absent
Congenital defects of the heart and great vessels
Reduced T lymphocytes: Absence of cell-mediated immunity is caused due to decreased numbers of T lymphocytes in the peripheral blood and lymphoid tissues. There is poor defense against certain fungal and viral infections.
Depletion of T-cell zones: In the lymphoid organs, there are reduced T-cell regions. There is depletion of paracortical areas of the lymph nodes as well as the periarteriolar sheaths of the spleen.
Immunoglobulin (Ig): Antibody levels in the serum may be normal or reduced, depending on the severity of the T-cell deficiency.

Clinical manifestations: Usually presents during infancy with conotruncal congenital heart defects and severe hypocalcemia (due to hypoparathyroidism). Infants are prone to recurrent or chronic viral, bacterial, fungal, and protozoal infections. DiGeorge syndrome can be corrected by fetal thymic transplantation or by bone marrow transplantation. However, they are usually not needed, because T-cell function tends to improve with age in many patients and is often normal by 5 years. This improvement is probably either due to presence of some residual thymic tissue or yet undefined extrathymic sites that assume the function of T-cell maturation. With time, it is also possible that thymus tissue may develop at ectopic sites (i.e., other than the normal location). Some patients with 22q11 mutations only show conotruncal cardiac defects.

Other defects in lymphocyte maturation

Several other rare immunodeficiencies can occur due to defect during lymphocyte maturation. In T-lymphocyte development, single-positive CD4+ and CD8+ T cells are produced from double-positive (CD4+ and CD8+) immature T cells. This generation depends on positive selection and lineage commitment events. Specific inherited mutations in genes that regulate the process of positive selection abolish the development of CD4+ T cells or of CD8+ T cells.

Bare lymphocyte syndrome (MHC Class II deficiency): It is a rare heterogeneous group of autosomal recessive diseases. It is usually caused by mutations in transcription factors that are required for class II major histocompatibility complex (*MHC*) gene expression. Deficiency or absence of class II MHC prevents the development of CD4+ T cells (**Fig. 1**). These CD4+ T cells are involved in cellular immunity and provide help to B cells. Hence, class II MHC deficiency results in combined immunodeficiency. These patients express little or no HLA-DP, HLA-DQ, or HLA-DR on B lymphocytes, macrophages, and dendritic cells (DCs). They express normal or only slightly reduced levels of class I MHC molecules.

MHC class I deficiency (Fig. 1): It is an autosomal recessive disorder characterized by decreased CD8+ T-cell numbers and function.

Other defects may be due to mutations in antigen receptor chains or signaling molecules involved in T- or B-cell maturation.

Hyper-IgM syndrome

Hyper-IgM (HIM) syndrome is an Ig production disorder in which the affected patients have IgM antibodies. But there is a deficiency of IgG, IgA, and IgE antibodies.

Molecular basis: Many of the functions of CD4+ helper T cells require the engagement of CD40 on B cells, macrophages, and

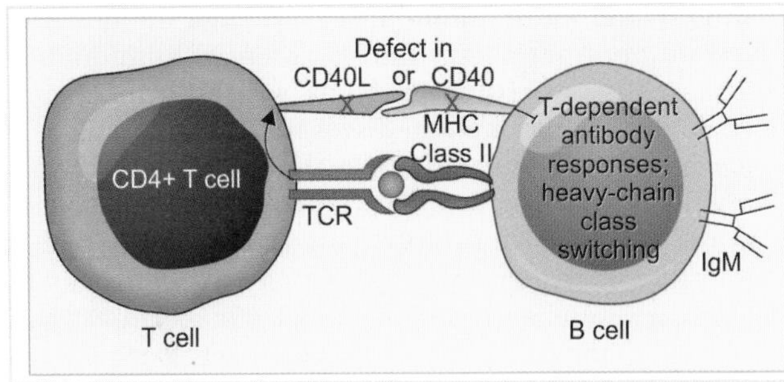

(MHC: major histocompatibility complex; TCR: T-cell receptor).

FIG. 2: Hyper-IgM syndrome. Normally, binding of the CD40L protein on T cells to CD40 on B cells is induced when T cells are activated through their TCR binding to MHC class II molecules on B cells. This interaction results in antibody responses to T-dependent antigens and heavy-chain class switching. Hyper-IgM syndrome can occur due to defects in CD40L on T lymphocytes (cells) or CD40 on B lymphocytes (cells). A defect in either CD40 or CD40L (indicated by red X's) results in a deficiency in T-cell-dependent antibody responses and heavy-chain class switching. This produces raised levels of IgM and the absence or low levels of IgG, IgA, and IgE.

DCs by CD40 ligand (CD40L; also called CD154) expressed on antigen activated T cells. This interaction of CD40 with CD40L (CD40 ligand) triggers Ig class switching and affinity maturation in B cells (**Fig. 2**) and also stimulates the microbicidal functions of macrophages.

In HIM syndrome, mature B cells are present. The circulating B cells bear only IgM and IgD. The "switch" to other heavy-chain isotypes from IgD/IgM is defective. Interaction of CD40 receptor on B-cell membranes with CD40L is required for isotype switching. In the absence of interaction of CD40 with CD40L, B cells are not capable of Ig class switching and affinity maturation. This is either because of a defect in CD4+ helper T cells (absence of CD40L) or an intrinsic B-cell defect (absence of CD40).

- **X-linked hyper-IgM syndrome:** About 70% of patients with HIM syndrome have the X-linked form of the disease. It is caused by mutations in the gene encoding the T-cell effector molecule CD40L/CD154 located on Xq26. This mutation interferes with function of CD4+ helper T-cell.
- **Autosomal recessive disease:** In the remaining patients, the HIM syndrome is inherited in an autosomal recessive pattern. Most of these patients have genetic defects with loss-of-function mutations involving either CD40 or in the enzyme activation-induced cytidine deaminase (AID). AID is a DNA-editing enzyme expressed in B cells that is required for Ig class (heavy chain isotype) switching and affinity maturation.

Laboratory findings: The serum of patients with HIM syndrome shows normal or raised levels of IgM but no IgA or IgE and extremely low levels of IgG. The B and T cells in the blood are normal in number.

Clinical presentation: Patients present with recurrent pyogenic infections. This is because of the low level of opsonizing IgG antibodies and also impaired affinity maturation. Impaired affinity maturation is a process required for production of high-affinity antibodies.

- **CD40L mutations:** These patients are also susceptible to pneumonia caused by the intracellular organism *Pneumocystis jirovecii* (formerly *Pneumocystis carinii*). This is because of defective CD40L-mediated macrophage activation which is a main event in cell-mediated immunity.
- **Autoimmune destruction of blood cells:** Occasionally, the IgM antibodies may react with blood cells and produce autoimmune diseases involving the formed elements of blood, especially autoimmune hemolytic anemia, thrombocytopenic purpura, and recurrent, severe neutropenia. In older patients, there may be a proliferation of IgM-producing plasma cells. These plasma cells infiltrate the mucosa of the GIT.

Common variable immunodeficiency

Common variable immunodeficiency (CVID) is a relatively frequent disorder associated with defects in B-cell differentiation. CVID is a group of **heterogeneous disorders in which the common features are reduced levels of serum Ig** (hypogammaglobulinemia). Usually, it affects all the antibody classes but sometimes only IgG. They are also associated with impaired antibody responses to infection, and increased incidence of infections.

Patterns of disease: It can occur both as familial/inherited and sporadic forms. As the name common variable immunodeficiency implies, the presentation and pathogenesis are highly variable.

- **Familial inherited forms:** There is no single pattern of inheritance. Relatives of patients with familial forms have a high incidence of selective IgA deficiency. This suggests that in some cases, both selective IgA deficiency (see page 1126) and CVID represent different expressions of a common genetic defect in antibody synthesis.
- **Sporadic forms:** Most patients have normal or near-normal numbers of B cells in the blood and lymphoid tissues. However, these B cells can not differentiate into plasma cells.

Etiology: Antibody deficiency may be due to intrinsic defects of B-cell and abnormalities in helper T-cell-mediated activation of B cells. In familial form, mutations in approximately 25 different genes have been identified. Few of them are described below. However, monogenic causes of the known mutations are observed in <10% of all cases of CVID.

- **Abnormalities BAFF-receptor:** BAFF-receptor (BAFF-R) is a receptor for a cytokine and is one of the main pro-survival receptors in B cells. This promotes the survival and differentiation of B cells. Its abnormality may be responsible for CVID.
- **Mutation in ICOS (inducible T-cell costimulator):** ICOS is a molecule homologous to CD28. This CD28 is one of the proteins expressed on T cells that provide co-stimulatory signals required for T-cell activation and survival. ICOS is involved in T-cell activation and is required for T follicular helper cell generation and in interactions between T and B cells.
- **Others** include mutations in *TACI* gene and *CD19* gene.

MORPHOLOGY

Microscopy

The germinal centers in lymphoid tissues (i.e., lymph nodes, spleen, and gut) show hyperplasia. This is due to the proliferation of B cells in response to antigen but are defective in further maturation in some respect.

Clinical manifestations: These are caused by deficiency of antibody. Hence, they resemble those of X-linked agammaglobulinemia (XLA). Both sexes are equally affected, and the onset of symptoms is later than in XLA in childhood or adolescence.

- **Infections:** Usually patients present with recurrent sinopulmonary pyogenic infections. About 20% of patients may develop recurrent herpesvirus infections. Serious enterovirus infections may cause meningoencephalitis. Persistent diarrhea caused by *G. lamblia* may develop. Ig deficiency and associated pyogenic infections with *H. influenzae* and *S. pneumoniae* are major features.
- **Autoimmune diseases:** As in XLA, patients of CVID have a high frequency of autoimmune diseases (about 20%). These include pernicious anemia, hemolytic anemia, inflammatory bowel disease, and rheumatoid arthritis.
- **Malignant tumors:** A high incidence of **lymphomas** and **gastric cancer** has also been reported in association with CVID.

Diagnosis: Serum shows very low IgG levels and decreased IgM and/or IgA. The diagnosis of CVID is usually one of exclusion by ruling out other well-defined primary immunodeficiency causes of decreased antibody production.

Isolated IgA deficiency

Many immunodeficiencies may selectively involve one or a few Ig isotypes. The most common is selective IgA deficiency. Isolated IgA deficiency is a common immunodeficiency. It is caused by impaired differentiation of naïve B lymphocytes to IgA-producing plasma cells. It is characterized by **normal serum levels of IgM and IgG** and **extremely low levels of both serum** (<7 mg/dL) **and secretory IgA**. Normal serum level of IgA is 80–350 mg/dL.

Molecular basis: The defect in isolated IgA deficiency is a block in the differentiation of B cells to IgA antibody-secreting plasma cells. In most patients, the molecular basis of this disease is not known. In few patients, defects in a receptor for a B cell-activating cytokine, BAFF (B cell-activating factor), have been described. Mutations have been also described in TACI (transmembrane activator and calcium modulator and cyclophilin ligand interactor), and APRIL (a proliferation-inducing ligand). BAFF and APRIL are required to stimulate B-cell survival and proliferation.

Clinical presentation: Most individuals are asymptomatic.

- **Infections of mucosal surfaces: IgA is the major antibody in mucosal secretions** and IgA deficiency weakens the mucosal defenses. Infections occur in the respiratory, gastrointestinal, and urogenital tracts. Symptomatic patients commonly present with recurrent sinopulmonary infections and diarrhea.
- **Allergy and autoimmune diseases:** High frequency of respiratory tract allergy and a variety of autoimmune diseases may occur in patients with IgA deficiency. Examples of autoimmune diseases developing in these patients include **SLE and rheumatoid arthritis**. The basis of these diseases in patients with isolated IgA deficiency is not known. When blood containing normal IgA is transfused to patients with IgA deficiency, some patients develop severe, even fatal, anaphylactic reactions. This is because the IgA in the donor blood acts like a foreign antigen.

X-linked lymphoproliferative disease

X-linked lymphoproliferative (XLP) disease is an autosomal recessive disorder of young boys who have a normal response to childhood infections. But they **develop fatal lymphoproliferative disorders after infection with EBV**. Thus, XLP disease is characterized by an **inability to eliminate EBV**. It ultimately leads to **fulminant infectious mononucleosis (IM) and the development of B-cell lymphoma**. Most of the patients die of acute IM.

Molecular pathogenesis: These are as follows—

- **Mutations in the gene encoding SAP:** In approximately 80% of patients, the protein associated is SAP (SLAM-associated protein). The disease is due to **mutations in the gene encoding this SAP**. SAP is an adaptor molecule called signaling lymphocyte activation molecule (SLAM)-associated protein. SAP binds to a family of cell surface molecules involved in the activation of NK cells and T and B lymphocytes. This includes SLAM. Defects in SAP reduces the activation of NK and T-cell. This leads to increased susceptibility to viral infections. SAP is also needed for the development of T follicular helper cells. Because of this defect, in XLP disease, there is neither formation of germinal centers in lymphoid tissues nor production of high-affinity antibodies (hypogammaglobulinemia). These additional abnormalities further contribute to susceptibility to viral infection. These patients develop severe EBV infection, including severe and often fatal IM. However, they do not develop other viral infections and the reasons for this are not clearly known.
- **Mutations in gene coding XIAP:** In about 20% of patients of XLP, the genetic defect is not in the SAP. It is mutation in the gene encoding X-linked inhibitor of apoptosis (XIAP). This mutation results in increased apoptosis of T cells and NK T cells. This in turn leads to a marked depletion of both these cell types. Most commonly, this immunodeficiency is manifested by severe opportunistic EBV infections.

Other defects in lymphocyte activation

Many rare cases of lymphocyte activation defects can also occur. They may affect antigen receptor signaling and various biochemical pathways.

Mendelian susceptibility to mycobacterial disease (MSMD): Environmental *Mycobacterium* species (often called atypical mycobacteria) include *Mycobacterium avium, Mycobacterium kansasii,* and *Mycobacterium fortuitum*. These are weakly virulent mycobacteria and do not cause disease in healthy individuals. In MSMD disorders, the patients are predisposed to severe diseases caused by these weakly virulent mycobacteria, as well as other intracellular pathogens including various bacterial, fungal, and viral species. In MSMD, there are mutations affecting Th1 responses.

Chronic mucocutaneous candidiasis and bacterial infections of the skin: It is a disorder called Job syndrome and is due to inherited defects in Th17 responses.

Immunodeficiencies Associated with Systemic Diseases

Certain inherited (congenital) systemic disorders are characterized by a prominent immune deficiency. These are associated with variable degrees of T- and B-cell immunodeficiency with a wide spectrum of abnormalities involving multiple organ systems. Examples include Wiskott-Aldrich syndrome and ataxia telangiectasia.

Wiskott–aldrich syndrome

Wiskott-Aldrich syndrome is an **X-linked disease**. It is characterized by **thrombocytopenia** (reduced blood platelets), **eczema, and a marked susceptibility to bacterial infection**. These infections are recurrent and can result in **early death**.

Molecular pathogenesis

- **X-linked disease:** Wiskott-Aldrich syndrome is caused by **mutations in the gene located at Xp11.23**. This gene encodes a cytoplasmic protein called **Wiskott-Aldrich syndrome protein (WASP)**. WASP is expressed exclusively in bone marrow-derived cells. *WASP* gene mutations affect not only T lymphocytes but also the other lymphocyte subsets, DCs, and platelets. WASP belongs to a family of proteins that link membrane receptors, such as antigen receptors, to cytoskeletal elements. WASP may be involved in cytoskeleton-dependent responses, including cell migration and signal transduction. There is defective formation of immune synapses between T cells and antigen-presenting cells. This results in poor activation of the lymphocytes and impaired mobility of all leukocytes.
- **Autosomal recessive disease:** This resembles Wiskott-Aldrich syndrome and is caused by **mutations in the gene encoding WIP** (WASP-interacting protein). WIP is a protein that binds to WASP and stabilizes it.

MORPHOLOGY

The thymus is morphologically normal and lymphocyte numbers are normal, at least in the initial stages of the disease. With increasing age, there is a progressive loss of T lymphocytes in the peripheral blood as well as T-cell zones (paracortical areas) of the lymph nodes, with variable defects in cellular immunity. The lymphocytes (and platelets) are smaller than normal.

Clinical features: Main defect is an inability to produce antibodies in response to T-cell-independent polysaccharide antigens, and the response to protein antigens is poor. Because of this, patients are particularly susceptible to infections with encapsulated bacteria. Serum levels of IgM are low, but levels of IgG are usually normal. Paradoxically the levels of IgA and IgE are often raised. Patients may also develop B-cell lymphomas. Treatment is by HSC transplantation.

Ataxia telangiectasia

Ataxia telangiectasia is an autosomal recessive disorder. Its characteristic features are—(1) abnormal gait (ataxia), (2) vascular malformations (telangiectases), (3) neurologic deficits, (4) increased incidence of tumors, and (5) immunodeficiency.

Molecular pathogenesis: The gene responsible for ataxia telangiectasia is located on chromosome 11. It encodes a protein kinase called ATM (ataxia telangiectasia mutated). ATM is related structurally to PI3-kinase. Normally, if there is DNA damage (double-strand breaks), ATM activates p53 by phosphorylation. p53 can activate cell cycle checkpoints and apoptosis in cells with damaged DNA. ATM also contributes to the stability of DNA double strand break complexes during V(D)J recombination. Ataxia telangiectasia is caused by **mutations in a gene that encodes an ATM** and leads to deficiency of ATM. This in turn leads to abnormalities in DNA repair and may generate abnormal antigen receptors. ATM also contributes to DNA stability when double-stranded DNA breaks (DSBs) are generated in the course of Ig class switch recombination. Mutations in ATM result in defective class switching and reduced levels of IgG, IgA, and IgE.

Immunologic defects: They are of variable severity. They may affect both B and T cells. The most important humoral immune abnormalities are defective production of isotype-switched antibodies. This mainly involves IgA and IgG_2 and results in their deficiency. The T-cell defects are usually less prominent and are associated with hypoplasia of thymus. Patients develop bacterial infections of upper and lower respiratory tract, multiple autoimmune abnormalities, and have markedly increased incidence of lymphoma with advancing age.

Secondary (Acquired) Immunodeficiencies

Deficiencies of the immune system can develop due to abnormalities that are not genetic but acquired during life. In fact, acquired immunodeficiency diseases are more common than congenital (primary or genetic) immunodeficiencies. They are caused by different pathogenic mechanisms (**Table 4**). Most serious secondary immunodeficiency is acquired immunodeficiency syndrome (AIDS).

ACQUIRED IMMUNODEFICIENCY SYNDROME

Acquired immunodeficiency syndrome is caused by the **retrovirus human immunodeficiency virus (HIV)**. HIV epidemic was first identified only in the 1980s. It is reported from more than 190 countries around the world. The degree of morbidity and mortality caused by HIV and the worldwide impact of this infection on healthcare resources and economics are enormous and continue to grow. Currently, there is no vaccine or permanent cure for AIDS, but quite effective antiretroviral drugs are capable of controlling the infection. India has the third largest HIV epidemic in the world. Overall, India's HIV epidemic is slowing down.

Characteristic features of AIDS: These include—(1) HIV primarily infects cells of the immune system including CD4+ helper T cells, macrophages, and DCs and **infection of CD4+ T lymphocytes leads to their depletion** and (2)

Table 4: Causes and mechanism of secondary (acquired) immunodeficiencies.

Cause	*Mechanism*
Infections that target cells of the immune system	
Human immunodeficiency virus infection	Depletion of CD4+ helper T cells
Measles virus and human T cell lymphotropic virus 1 (HTLV-1, like HIV, it is a retrovirus)	Infect lymphocytes, HTLV-1 has tropism for CD4+ T cells and transforms them and produces adult T-cell leukemia/lymphoma
Iatrogenic immunodeficiencies as complications of therapy for other diseases	
Irradiation and chemotherapy treatments for cancer	Reduction of bone marrow precursors for all leukocytes with defective lymphocyte maturation
Immunosuppression for transplants (drugs to prevent graft rejection), or to treat autoimmune diseases	Killing or functionally inactivating lymphocyte, cytokine blockade, impaired **leukocyte trafficking**
Complication of another disease processes	
Involvement of bone marrow by cancers (metastases, leukemias)	Reduced site of leukocyte development with defective lymphocyte maturation
Protein–calorie malnutrition	Metabolic derangements inhibit lymphocyte maturation and function, inadequate Ig synthesis
Loss of the spleen due to trauma, sickle cell disease, or removal by surgery (after trauma, as a treatment for autoimmune hemolytic anemia and thrombocytopenia)	Decreased phagocytosis of blood-borne microbes
Diabetes, chronic infection (*Mycobacterium tuberculosis* and various fungi, chronic malarial infections), drugs, and other metabolic diseases	• Variable; lymphocyte depletion (from drugs or severe infections) • Chronic infections result in anergy to many antigens

severe immunosuppression that leads to opportunistic infections, secondary neoplasms, wasting, and neurologic manifestations (nervous system degeneration).

Etiology

Q. Discuss pathogenesis of AIDS with a note on various opportunistic infections.

HIV was discovered independently by *Dr Luc Montagnier, Dr Anthony Gallo, and Dr Jay Levy* in 1983–84.

Properties of HIV

AIDS is caused by human immunodeficiency virus (HIV), which is a nontransforming human retrovirus. It belongs to the lentivirus family. Lentivirus family includes feline immunodeficiency virus, simian immunodeficiency virus (SIV), visna virus of sheep, bovine immunodeficiency virus, and the equine infectious anemia virus. The name for lentivirus came from the Latin word lentus, meaning "slow," because infection develops gradually. **Retroviruses are single-stranded RNA (ssRNA) viruses** having an enzyme called reverse transcriptase, which prepares a DNA copy of the RNA genome of the virus in host cell.

Genetic forms: HIV occurs in **two genetically different** but related main forms namely, **HIV-1 and HIV-2.** They have been isolated from patients with AIDS. Both are similar in structure and function, but are **differentiated from each other by their envelope glycoproteins, point of origin, and latency periods.** Many subspecies or strains of HIV also exist because of the rapid rate of HIV virion mutation.

HIV-1 HIV-1 viruses likely came from chimpanzees and/or gorillas. It is most common in the United States, Europe, and Central Africa. About 10 subtypes of HIV-1 have been identified—group N (YBF30), group O, and group M with 8 subtypes (A, B, C, D, E, F, G, and H). The most common cause of AIDS in India is HIV-1 group M subtype C. Four major groups of HIV-1 are:

1. Group M ("major", 98% of infections worldwide): Group M subtypes exhibit a high degree of diversity and consist of 9 subtypes: A–D, F–H, J, and K (subtypes E and I were subsequently shown to be recombinants of other subtypes).
    c. Subtype C (Africa and India) accounts for half of the strains and is more readily transmitted.
    b. Subtype B predominates in Western Europe, North America, and Australia.
    c. Subtypes A and D are associated with slower and faster disease progression, respectively.
2. Group O ("outlier") subtypes are highly divergent from group M and are largely confined to small numbers centered on Cameroon.
3. Group N (new-"non-major and non-outlier") is mostly restricted to West Central Africa (e.g., Gabon).
4. Group P related to gorilla strains of SIV has been identified from a patient from Cameroon.

HIV-2 HIV-2 viruses likely came from different nonhuman source namely, sooty mangabeys [old World monkey found in forests from Senegal (a country in Africa)]. It is common in West Africa and confined to western and southern India (found near Goa). HIV-2 is differentiated from HIV-1 by a longer clinical latency period from the onset of infection to the development of symptoms. It is possible to have coinfection with both HIV-1 and HIV-2. HIV-2 is morphologically similar to HIV-1. The immunodeficiency state associated with HIV-2 infection is indistinguishable from AIDS caused by HIV-1. The risk factors also appear to be similar. However, HIV-2 is probably more difficult to transmit than HIV-1. Individuals infected with HIV-2 tend to progress to AIDS more slowly than those infected with HIV-1.

Specific tests are available for HIV-2. Blood collected for transfusion is routinely screened for both HIV-1 and HIV-2 seropositivity. The following discussion is mainly on HIV-1 and diseases caused by it, but it is generally applicable to HIV-2 as well.

Structure of HIV (Fig. 3)

HIV-1 is **spherical enveloped virus** which is about 90–120 nm in diameter. It consists of **electron-dense, cone-shaped viral core surrounded by lipoprotein envelope**. This lipid envelope is derived from the host cell membrane. The structure is similar to most retroviruses.

1. **Viral core:** It contains:
   i. **Major capsid protein p24:** The nucleocapsid or viral core is composed of a nucleocapsid protein called p24. This protein p24 is a viral antigen and is most abundant. This antigen and the antibodies against this are used for the diagnosis of HIV infection in enzyme-linked immunosorbent assay (ELISA). ELISA is widely used to diagnose HIV infection.
   ii. **Two identical strands (copies) of ssRNA (single-stranded RNA) viral genome.** The RNA genome of HIV is approximately 9.2 kb long. It has the basic arrangement of nucleic acid sequences, characteristic of all known retroviruses.
   iii. **Three viral enzymes:** These enzymes are very important because they facilitate the conversion of RNA to DNA. (1) Protease (p10) works as a "molecular scissors" and splits the other viral components and activates the virions; (2) reverse transcriptase (p64), which also has ribonuclease H activity, and it is an RNA-dependent DNA polymerase which allows the virus to copy RNA into DNA; and (3) integrase (p32). When the virus infects a cell, viral RNA is not translated, instead transcribed by reverse transcriptase into DNA. The DNA form of the retroviral genome is called a provirus which can be integrated into the chromosome of host cell. There are multiple molecules of each of these three enzymes (for simplicity only one copy is shown in **Figure 3**). The viral core is surrounded by a matrix protein called p17, which lies underneath the virion envelope.
   iv. **Nucleocapsid protein p7/p9**
2. **Matrix protein p17:** Between the lipid envelope and viral core (nucleocapsid), there is a protein layer called p17.
3. **Lipid envelope:** The virus contains a lipoprotein envelope (phospholipid bilayer envelope), which consists of lipid derived from the host cell and about 14 (only 7 shown in **Fig. 3**) glycoprotein projections. Each projection consists of two viral glycoproteins. These glycoproteins are—(1) gp120, projects as knob-like spikes (looks like a studded ball) on the surface and is associated with gp41; and (2) gp41, a transmembrane molecule that crosses the lipid bilayer of the viral envelope and forms the anchoring transmembrane pedicle for gp120 and covers the viral particle surface. gp120 is the most external and distal part of each "stud/knob-like," whereas gp41 is the bridge that holds it onto the virion surface. These glycoproteins are essential for HIV infection of cells. The transmembrane gp41 subunit and an external, noncovalently associated, gp120 subunit form viral envelope glycoprotein complex, called Env. These subunits (gp120 and gp41) are produced by proteolytic cleavage of a gp160 precursor. The Env complex is expressed as a trimeric structure of three gp120/gp41 pairs. This Env complex mediates a multistep process of bind and fusion of the virion envelope to the target receptor (CD4) and coreceptor (CXCR4 or CCR5) present on the membrane of the target cell.

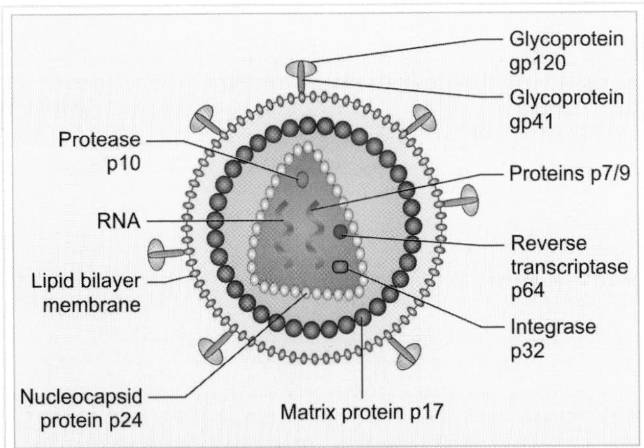

FIG. 3: Cross-sectional diagrammatic representation of structure of the human immunodeficiency virus (HIV)-1 virion. Each virion is covered by a lipid bilayer derived from the host cell and contains about 14 (only 7 shown in Figure) glycoprotein projections, each composed of viral glycoproteins gp41 and gp120. The gp41 is a transmembrane molecule that crosses the lipid bilayer of the viral envelope, and gp120 is associated with gp41. These proteins are encoded by the env gene. Their function is to bind to the target receptor (CD4) and coreceptor (CXCR4 or CCR5) on host cells and initiate infection. Inside the viral capsid, there are two copies of the HIV genome composed of single-stranded RNA (ssRNA), along with multiple molecules of each of three enzymes: reverse transcriptase (p64), which also has ribonuclease H activity, a protease (p10), and an integrase (p32). These enzymes are products of the *pol* gene.

HIV Genome (Fig. 4 and Table 5)

The HIV-1 RNA genome is approximately 9.2 kb long. It has the basic arrangement of nucleic acid sequences characteristic of all known retroviruses. Long terminal repeats (LTRs) are present at each end of the genome. They regulate viral gene expression, viral integration into the host genome, and viral replication. The genome contains two main groups of genes and their products act as antigens. Its RNA encodes for nine genes, i.e., three standard genes and six accessory genes (**Fig. 4**).

1. **Standard genes:** HIV-1 RNA genome contains three standard retroviral genes, which are typical of retroviruses. These include ***gag, pol***, and ***env*** genes. Initially, the protein products of the *gag* and *pol* genes are translated into large precursor proteins and are later cleaved by the viral enzyme protease to form mature proteins. The *gag* gene encodes the core antigen proteins that form the virus particle. The *pol* gene encodes reverse transcriptase proteins. The *env* gene encodes the viral envelope protein, glycoprotein gp160, which is split into two fragments, gp120 and gp41, by cellular protease.

Accessory genes: HIV contains six accessory genes namely, *tat, rev, vif, nef, vpr,* and *vpu.* They regulate the synthesis (regulatory genes) and assembly of infectious viral particles and the pathogenicity of the virus. For example, the product of the *tat* (transactivator) gene causes a 1,000-fold increase in the transcription of viral genes. It is important for replication of virus.

The functions of all viral genes are summarized in **Table 5.**

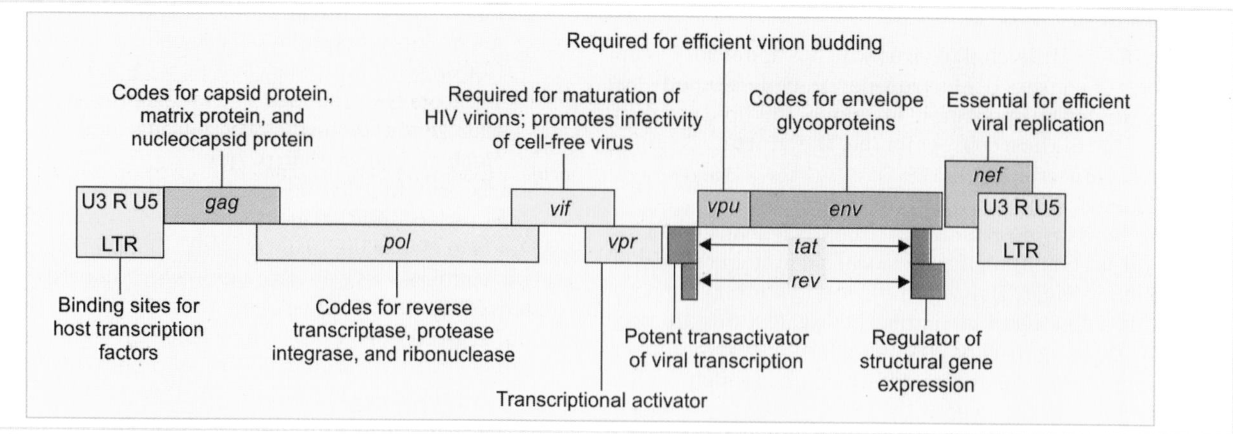

(LTR: long terminal repeat; gag: group-specific antigen; env: envelope; nef: negative effector; pol: polymerase; rev: regulator of viral gene expression; tat: transcriptional activator; vif: viral infectivity factor; vpr: viral protein R; vpu: viral protein u)

FIG. 4: Human immunodeficiency virus-1 (HIV-1) genome. The genes along the linear genome are indicated by different colored blocks. Some genes use some of the same sequences as other genes and these are shown by overlapping blocks. But these are read differently by host cell RNA polymerase. The coding sequences of the *tat* and *rev* genes are separated in the genome into noncontiguous pieces. These gene segments need RNA splicing to produce functional mRNA.

Table 5: Various genes in the HIV-1 genome and their function.

Gene	*Function*
LTRs (Long terminal repeats) are present at each end of the genome	• Required for the initiation of transcription of viral genome • Contain control regions/sites that bind host transcription factors (NF-κB, NFAT, Sp1, TBP) • Required for integration of viral DNA into host cell genome • Contain RNA trans-acting response element (TAR) that binds Tat
Standard genes	
gag (group-specific antigen -Pr55gag)	Nucleocapsid core and matrix proteins Polyprotein processed by PR MA, matrix (p17) • Undergoes myristylation that helps target Gag polyprotein to lipid rafts, promoting virus assembly at cell surface Capsid (CA) protein (p24): • Binds cyclophilin A and CPSF6 • Target of TRIM5 Nucleocapsid protein (p7): • Zn finger, RNA binding protein p6: • Regulates the terminal steps in virion budding through interactions with TSG101 and ALIX 1 • Incorporates Vpr into viral particles
pol (polymerase)	Encodes a variety of viral enzymes, including protease (PR) (p10), reverse transcriptase (RT) and RNAse H (p66/51), integrase (p32), ribonuclease, and all processed by protease (PR). These enzymes are required for viral replication
env (gp160 envelope protein)	Viral coat proteins (gp120 and gp41) • gp160 is cleaved in endoplasmic reticulum to gp120 (SU) and gp41 (TM). gp120 and gp41 are noncovalently associated with each other • gp120 mediates CD4 and chemokine receptor binding, while gp41 mediates fusion • Contains RNA response element (RRE) that binds Rev
Accessory genes	
vif [viral infectivity factor (p23)]	Overcomes inhibitory effect of host cell enzyme (APOBEC3G) preventing hypermutation and viral DNA degradation; promotes viral replication
vpr [viral protein R (p15)]	Increases viral replication; especially promotes HIV infection of macrophages; blocks cell cycle progression by promoting G_2 cell-cycle arrest

Continued

Continued

Gene	**Function**
tat [transcriptional activator (p14)]	Required for elongation of viral transcripts; binds TAR in presence of host cyclin T1 and CDK9 enhances RNA Pol II–mediated elongation of integrated viral DNA (on the viral DNA template)
rev [regulator of viral gene expression (p19)]	Inhibits viral RNA splicing and promotes nuclear export of partially (incompletely) spliced viral RNAs; Binds RRE (Rev response element)
vpu (viral protein u)	Promotes CD4 degradation; enhances release of virions from cells; overcomes inhibitory effects of tetherin
nef [negative effector (p27)]	• Downregulates host cell surface CD4 and class I MHC expression; modulates intracellular signaling to facilitate viral replication; blocks apoptosis; and enhances virion activity • Progression to disease slowed significantly in **absence of Nef**

Route of Transmission

HIV-1 and HIV-2 are relatively weak viruses outside of the body. HIV is found in every bodily fluid and is broadly disseminated in the body. Since it is present in very low titers in saliva, tears, cerebrospinal fluid, amniotic fluid, and feces, it is not transmitted through these body fluids. Transmission of HIV occurs when there is an exchange of blood or body fluids containing the virus or virus-infected cells. The three major routes of transmission are:

1. **Sexual transmission:** It is the main route of infection in >75% of cases of HIV.
   i. **Homosexual or bisexual men or heterosexual contacts:** It may be male-to-male, or male-to-female or female-to-male transmission. HIV infections are less in circumcised men. This may be because the foreskin is less well keratinized than other parts of the penis and has a higher concentration of cutaneous DCs (Langerhans cells).
   ii. **HIV is present in genital fluids** such as vaginal secretions and cervical secretions/cells (in women) and semen (in men). The virus is carried in the semen from men. Virus enters the recipient's body through abrasions in rectal or oral mucosa or by direct contact with mucosal lining cells.
   iii. **Coexisting sexually transmitted diseases:** Risk of sexual transmission of HIV is increased when there is coexisting sexually transmitted diseases, especially those associated with genital ulceration (e.g., syphilis, chancroid, and herpes). Other sexually transmitted diseases (e.g., gonorrhea, chlamydia) are also cofactors for transmission of HIV. This may be because in these genital inflammatory conditions, there are increased numbers of inflammatory cells in the semen. This leads to greater concentration of the virus and virus-containing cells in genital fluids.
   iv. **Viral transmission** can occur in two ways:
      a. Direct inoculation of virus or infected cells into the blood vessels at the site of breach caused by trauma, and
      b. Infection of the mucosal DCs **or CD4+ cells within the mucosa.**
2. **Parenteral transmission:** It occurs via blood, blood products, or blood-contaminated needles or syringes. Three groups of individuals are at risk.
   i. **Intravenous drug abusers:** Transmission occurs by sharing of needles and syringes contaminated with HIV-containing blood.
   ii. **Hemophiliacs:** Mainly those who received large amounts of factor VIII and factor IX concentrates before 1985. Now increasing use of recombinant clotting factors has eliminated this mode of transmission.
   iii. **Transfusion of HIV-infected whole blood or blood component:** Transfusion of whole blood or blood component (e.g., platelets, plasma) is one of the modes of HIV transmission. Three public health measures greatly reduce the risk of this mode of transmission. These are—(1) screening of blood and plasma for antibody to HIV, (2) stringent purity criteria for factor VIII and factor IX preparations, and (3) screening of donors on the basis of history. Because recently infected individuals may be antibody-negative (seronegative), there is a small risk of acquiring AIDS through transfusion of seronegative blood.
   iv. **Organs from HIV-infected donors can also transmit AIDS.**
3. **Perinatal transmission (mother-to-infant transmission):** This is the **major mode of transmission of AIDS in children** (pediatric AIDS). Transmission of infection from infected mothers to their offspring can occur by three routes:
   i. **In utero:** It is transmitted by transplacental spread.
   ii. **Perinatal spread:** During normal vaginal delivery or childbirth (intrapartum) through an infected birth canal and in the immediate period (peripartum)
   iii. **After birth:** It is transmitted by ingestion of breastmilk or from the genital secretions.

   Of the above three, perinatal transmission, i.e., during birth (intrapartum) and in the immediate period thereafter (peripartum), is the most common mode. Risk of transmission is higher when the maternal viral load is high, low CD4+ T-cell counts, and presence of chorioamnionitis in mother.

Routes by which HIV infection is not transmitted are listed in **Box 3**. There is an extremely small risk of transmission to healthcare professional, after accidental needlestick injury or exposure of nonintact skin to infected blood in laboratory accidents. After needlestick accidents, the risk of serocon-

Box 3: Routes by which HIV is not transmitted.

- Nonsexual close/casual personal contact (including kissing, hugging) with infected people
- Sharing of utensils and insect bites
- Household contact
- Contact at workplace, or school, swimming pool, etc.
- Insect bites

version may be about 0.3%. If postexposure antiretroviral prophylaxis is given within 24–48 hours of a needlestick, it can reduce the risk of infection 8-fold.

Pathogenesis of HIV Infection and AIDS

Q. Write short essay on pathogenesis of HIV infection and AIDS.

Infection is transmitted when the virus enters the blood or tissues of an individual.

Major targets: HIV can infect many tissues, but two major targets of HIV infection are (i) immune system and (ii) central nervous system.

1. **Immune system:** HIV is an RNA retrovirus that causes a severe immune deficiency, primarily involving the cell-mediated immunity. It may progress to AIDS. Mainly, there is infection and subsequent death of CD4+ T cells. There is also an impairment in the function of surviving helper T cells. But infection of macrophages and DCs also contributes to its pathogenesis of HIV infection.
2. **Central nervous system** (CNS) is discussed on page 1146.

Life Cycle of HIV

Life cycle of HIV consists of three main steps, namely—(1) infection of cells by HIV, (2) integration of the provirus into the host cell genome, and (3) activation of viral replication with production and release of infectious virus.

Infection of cells by HIV

At the time of exposure to the HIV, HIV enters the body of new individual through mucosal tissues and blood. Infection occurs when the virus moves across the epithelium or mucosal membrane of the body.

Cell tropism **CD4 molecule as receptors for HIV infection:** Once inside the body, HIV has selective affinity for host cells with surface CD4 molecule receptor and various chemokine receptors as coreceptors. The cells with such receptors include **CD4+ T cells** and other CD4+ cells such as **monocytes/macrophages and DCs**. The infection becomes established in lymphoid tissues. The HIV envelope contains two glycoproteins, surface gp120 (expressed in all HIV strains) noncovalently attached to a transmembrane protein and gp41.

Binding of HIV to Host Cell (Fig. 5A)

First step in HIV infection is the binding of envelope protein gp120 to CD4 molecule receptor on the host cell in the mucosal or other tissue at or near the site of exposure.

Coreceptor molecules: Binding to CD4 molecule alone is not enough for infection (for fusion of the virion and host cell) and requires participation of another surface molecules namely coreceptor molecules. These coreceptors on the target cells are necessary for the virus to gain entry into cells. These coreceptors are chemokine receptors. More than seven chemokine receptors can serve as coreceptors for HIV entry into host cells. Most important of these chemokine receptors for HIV are CCR5 (must be present for the HIV particles to bind to the CD4+ cells, especially in early infection) and/or CXCR4 (present in later infection). Chemokines (chemoattractant cytokines that regulate leukocyte trafficking to sites of inflammation) play a significant role in the pathogenesis of HIV disease. New recognition site on gp120 of HIV binds to chemokine receptors, i.e., CCR5 and CXCR4. Chemokine receptors play a role in viral cell entry.

Tropism of HIV to coreceptors: All HIV strains can infect and replicate in freshly isolated human CD4+ T cells that are activated in vitro. In contrast, some HIV strains have selective binding. HIV isolates can be distinguished by their use of these receptors:

- **Macrophage-tropic (M-tropic) virus:** HIV variants are described as R5 for CCR5 binding. R5 strains use CCR5 as coreceptor. They preferentially infect cells of the monocyte/macrophage lineage and are thus referred to as M-tropic.
- **T-tropic virus:** HIV variants are described as X4 for CXCR4 binding. X4 strains use CXCR4 as coreceptor. They preferentially infect T cells and are referred to as T-tropic.
- **Dual-tropic virus:** HIV variants are described as R5X4 for the ability to bind to both chemokine receptors. Some strains (R5X4) use both T-cell lines and macrophages.

In majority (about 90%) of HIV-infected cases, early in the disease (acutely infected individuals), there is production of virus that uses CCR5 and is predominantly macrophage-tropic and is T-tropic late in the disease. However, over the course of infection, there is a change from the M-tropic to virus that binds to CXCR4 (T-tropic viruses). These T-tropic viral strains tend to be more virulent because they can infect many T cells including T-cell precursors in thymus. Thus, they produce greater depletion and impairment of T cells more than M-tropic strains.

Importance of coreceptors: The requirement of binding of HIV to coreceptors on host cell may be important for the pathogenesis of AIDS. Individuals who do not express this CCR5 coreceptor on their cell surface due to an inherited homozygous deletion in the CCR5 gene have been found resistant to HIV infection. Chemokines (chemokine is a cytokine with chemotactic properties, produced by lymphocytes and macrophages) that block these chemokine coreceptors can prevent HIV infection of cells in culture. Therefore, the efficiency of viral infection may depend on the level of chemokines in the tissues. Susceptibility to HIV infection may be influenced by the polymorphisms in the gene encoding CCR5. Those who inherit two mutant copies of the *CCR5* gene are found to be resistant to infection and the development of AIDS associated with R5 HIV isolates. Individuals who are heterozygous for this protective CCR5 allele are not protected from AIDS, but the onset of their disease after infection may be delayed.

The understanding of molecular details of binding between HIV glycoproteins and their cell surface receptors on host cell is important because they may provide the basis for additional anti-HIV therapies.

Conformational change (Fig. 6)

- **Conformational change in gp120 (Fig. 5B):** First gp120 envelope glycoprotein of HIV binds to CD4 molecule on host cell. This leads to a conformational change (change in shape by refolding) in the gp120. This promotes the formation of a new (secondary) recognition site on gp120 for the coreceptors CCR5 or CXCR4. Thus, gp120 binds to chemokine receptor.
- **Conformational change in gp41 (Fig. 5C):** Binding of gp120 to the coreceptor (CCR5 or CXCR4) in the target cell induces a conformational change in gp41. This exposes a hydrophobic region in gp41 called the fusion peptide at the tip of gp41. This peptide in turn inserts into the cell membrane (**Fig. 5D**) of the target/host cells (e.g., CD4+ T cells or macrophages).

Penetration of host cell membrane by gp41

- **Membrane fusion:** After the binding of HIV particle to both the CD4 receptor and the chemokine receptor on the host cell, fusion peptide at the tip of gp41 implants itself in the cell membrane. By this event, the target cell allows the viral membrane to fuse with the target (host CD4+ T cells or macrophages) cell membrane.
- **Entry of viral genome into cytoplasm of host cell:** Membrane fusion allows the virus core containing the HIV genome to enter into the cytoplasm of host cell. Once internalized, the infection is produced.

Integration of the proviral DNA into the genome of the host cell (Fig. 6)

- **Synthesis of double-stranded complementary DNA (cDNA;** proviral DNA): After the membrane fusion, HIV virion enters into the cytoplasm of host cell. The enzymes within the nucleoprotein complex of HIV become active and begin the viral reproductive cycle. The nucleoprotein core of the virus becomes disrupted. The viral core consists of two strands of ssRNA. The RNA genome of HIV is reverse transcribed into a double-stranded DNA by viral reverse transcriptase. First, the enzyme reverse transcriptase synthesizes a single-stranded DNA from a ss RNA. Using this single-stranded DNA as a template, DNA polymerase copies it to make a second (complementary) DNA strand and destroys the original RNA strands. Thus, it produces double-stranded DNA. This **double-stranded complementary DNA is called as cDNA or proviral DNA or preintegration complex (PIC).** The accuracy of DNA transcription is poor, with mutations occurring frequently. This tendency to mutate makes HIV resistant to antiviral medications.
- **Episomal form:** In quiescent T cells, HIV cDNA may remain as a linear episomal form in the cytoplasm of infected cell.
- **Integration of the cDNA (proviral DNA) into the host genome:** In dividing T cells, the cDNA (viral DNA) forms a circular group, migrates to the nucleus of host cell. The viral integrase also enters the nucleus and catalyzes the integration of viral DNA into the host cell genome in the nucleus. The integrated HIV DNA is called the provirus.

Activation of viral replication with production and release of infectious virus (Fig. 6)

The integrated HIV DNA may follow one of the paths mentioned below:

Latent infection After integration into host genome, the provirus may remain transcriptionally inactive (silent) for months or years. There is little or no production of new viral proteins or virions. In this manner, HIV infection of an individual cell can be latent.

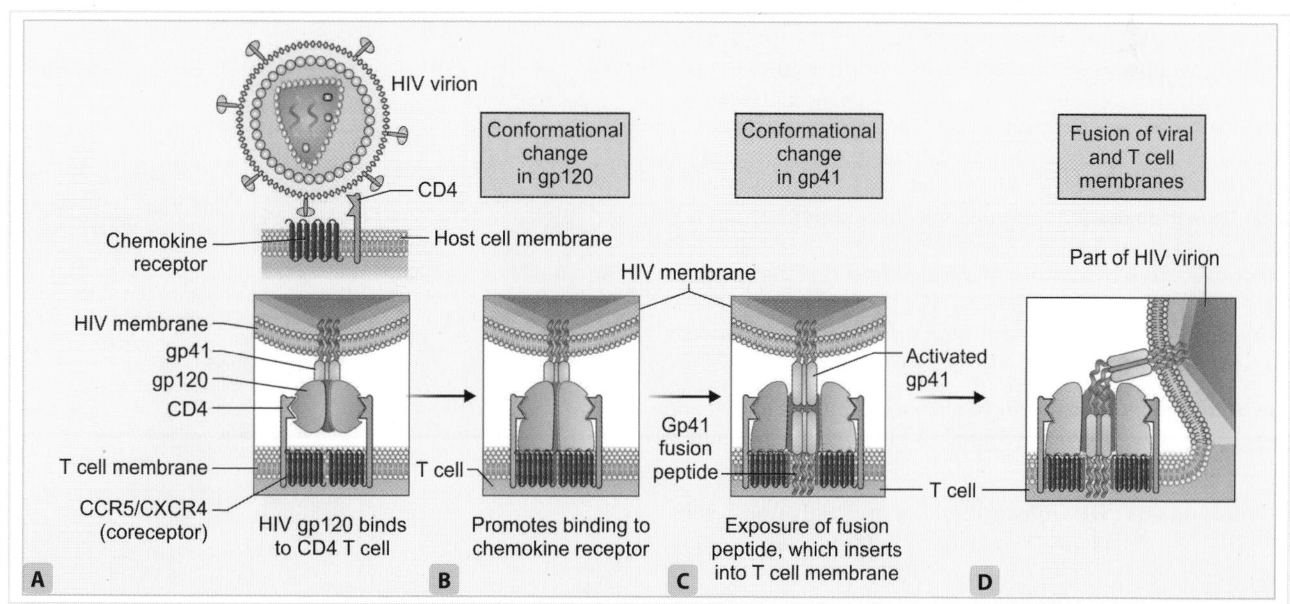

FIGS. 5A TO D: Diagrammatic representation of mechanism of HIV entry into the host cell (e.g., CD4+ T cells). (A) First gp120 envelope glycoprotein of HIV binds to CD4 molecule on host cell. (B) The binding leads to a conformational change (change in shape by refolding) in the gp120. This promotes the formation of a new (secondary) recognition site on gp120 for the coreceptors CCR5/ CXCR4. Thus, gp120 binds to chemokine receptor. (C) Binding of gp120 to the coreceptor (CCR5 or CXCR4) in the target cell induces a conformational change in gp41. These changes expose a hydrophobic region in gp41 called the fusion peptide at the tip of gp41. (D) The fusion peptide inserts into the cell membrane of the target/host cells (e.g., CD4+ T cells or macrophages). The fusion of the HIV-1 and host cell membranes occurs.

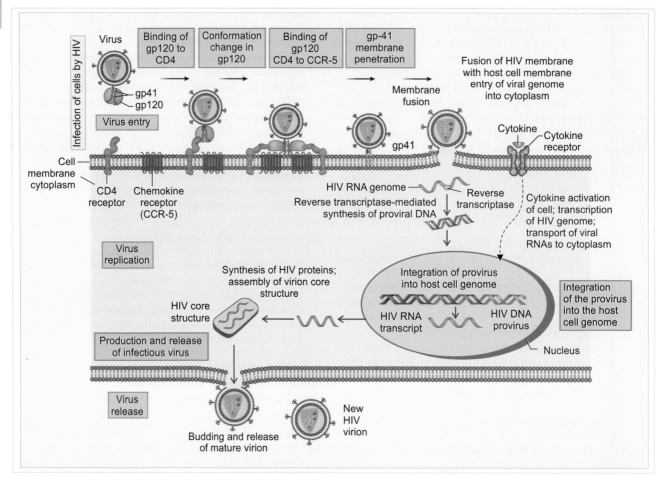

FIG. 6: Various molecular steps involved in the life cycle of HIV.

Productive infection (Fig. 7) Alternatively, provirus may be transcribed and produce complete viral particles and is called productive infection. After the virus completes its life cycle in the infected cell, the complete virus particles (free viral particles) are formed. These new infectious virus particles bud from the host cell membrane and are released from the infected cell (**Fig. 7A**). These new virus particles bind to an uninfected cell, thus propagating the infection. In addition, gp120 and gp41 are expressed on the plasma membrane of infected cells before virus is released. These infected host cells can mediate cell–cell fusion with an uninfected cell that expresses CD4 and coreceptors. HIV genomes can be directly passed between these fused host cells (**Fig. 7B**).

Death of infected host cell: When such productive infection is associated with extensive viral budding, it causes death of infected cells.

T cells and HIV: HIV infects memory and activated T cells. But HIV is not efficient at productively infecting naïve (resting) T cells.

- **Naïve T cells:** They contain an active form of an enzyme that can produce mutations in the HIV genome. This enzyme is a cytidine deaminase and is called as APOBEC3G (for apolipoprotein B mRNA-editing, enzyme-catalytic, polypeptide-like 3G). This enzyme produces cytosine-to-uracil mutations in the viral DNA by reverse transcription. These mutations inhibit further replication of viral DNA.

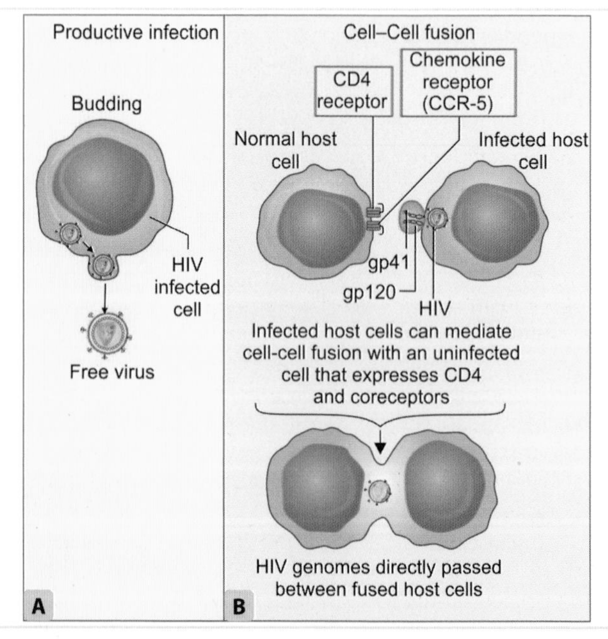

FIGS. 7A AND B: Productive infection of HIV. (A) By budding. (B) Cell-to-cell fusion. Infected cells express gp120 and gp41 on the plasma membrane before virus is released. These infected host cells can mediate cell–cell fusion with an uninfected cell that expresses CD4 and coreceptors. HIV genomes can be directly passed between these fused host cells.

- **Activated T cells:** Activation of T cells converts APOBEC3G into an inactive, high molecular mass complex. This allows replication of the previously activated (e.g., memory) T cells.
- **Evolution of HIV:** HIV has evolved a method to counteract this cellular defense mechanism which prevents their production. This is achieved by binding of viral protein Vif to APOBEC3G. This causes degradation of APOBEC3G by cellular proteases.

Activation of infection in latent infection The virus infection remains latent for long periods in lymphoid tissues. In latently infected cells, **completion of the life cycle of HIV occurs only after activation of infected host cell (e.g., CD4+ T cells).** In most of the cases of CD4+ T cells, viral replication and its shedding result in lysis of the infected cells.

Resting T cells: In resting T cells, one of transcription factors called NF-κB is in inactive form in the cytoplasm by forming a complex with the IκB (inhibitor of κB) protein.

Activation of T cells: T cells can be activated by antigens or cytokines.

- **Mechanism of T-cell activation:** Antigens or cytokines upregulate several transcription factors, including NF-κB. In turn, NF-κB stimulates transcription of genes encoding cytokines such as IL-2 and its receptor. Stimulation of T cells by antigen or cytokines activates cytoplasmic kinases. These kinases phosphorylate inhibitor of κB namely IκB and are enzymatically degraded. This releases transcription factor NF-κB and allows it to translocate to the nucleus. In the nucleus, NF-κB binds to the regulatory sequences of several genes. This includes even those cytokines that are expressed in activated T cells.
- **NF-κB binding sites in HIV:** The LTR sequences that are present at the two ends of the HIV genome also contain NF-κB binding sites. This can also drive the expression of viral RNA.
- **Activation of T cells by environmental antigen:** When a latently infected CD4+ T cell encounters an environmental antigen, it upregulates NF-κB in such a cell. It is a physiologic response. This upregulates NF-κB that binds to NF-κB–binding sites in HIV and also activates the expression of HIV genes. This is a pathologic outcome. Thus, there is production of virions, leading to lysis of CD4+ T cells.
- **TNF and other cytokines** produced by activated macrophages also stimulate NF-κB activity in T cells.

Thus, HIV thrives when the host T cells and macrophages are physiologically activated. Such activation may be due to antigenic stimulation by HIV itself or by other infecting microorganisms. Patients with HIV are prone to other infections, which cause lymphocyte activation and production of proinflammatory cytokines. These, in turn, stimulate production of more HIV, more infection, and loss of additional CD4+ T cells. Active viral replication is associated with more infection of cells and progression to AIDS.

Mechanisms of immunodeficiency (T-cell depletion) caused by HIV infection

Direct cytopathic effects of the replicating virus: HIV infects CD4+ T cells. A major cause of loss of infected CD4+ T cells in HIV-infected individuals is the direct cytopathic effects of the replicating HIV virus. In infected individuals, every day about 10,000 crores of new viral particles are produced, and about 100–200 crores of CD4+ T cells die each day.

- **Site of death:** Frequency of infected cells in the circulation is very low, and many infected cells are within tissues (e.g., secondary lymphoid organs and mucosal sites). Death of cells within tissues is a major cause of severe loss of cells.
- **Replacement by new T cells:** Immune system can replace the dying T cells especially in the early (acute) phase of the infection. Hence, the rate of T-cell loss may appear low in the beginning of the disease. But as the disease progresses, renewal of CD4+ T cells cannot compensate for the loss. Also, apart from direct killing of cells by the virus, other mechanisms may also cause loss of T cells.

Other mechanisms of T-cell destruction: These include the following—

Apoptosis of uninfected T cells: Uninfected T cells may be chronically activated as a response to HIV infection itself or to infections that are common in patients with AIDS. These activated uninfected cells undergo apoptosis by the process of activation-induced cell death. Thus, the numbers of death of uninfected CD4+ T cells may be considerably more than the numbers of death of infected cells. The molecular mechanism is unknown. Viral production can interfere with cellular protein synthesis and thereby lead to cell death.

Pyroptosis: Noncytopathic (abortive) HIV infection activates the inflammasome pathway. This produces a form of cell death known as pyroptosis (refer pages 151 and 152). Pyroptosis releases inflammatory cytokines and cellular contents. They cause recruitment of new cells and increasing the numbers of cells that can be infected. Pyroptosis may also play a role in spread of the infection.

Destruction of the architecture of secondary lymphoid organs: HIV infects cells in secondary lymphoid organs such as spleen, lymph nodes, and tonsils. This may produce progressive destruction of architecture of these organs as well as cellular composition of lymphoid tissues.

Loss of immature precursors of CD4+ T cells: This may be either due to direct infection of progenitor cells in the thymus or by infection of accessory cells that secrete cytokines needed for maturation of CD4+ T-cell.

Fusion of infected and uninfected cells: This may lead to formation of syncytia (giant cells). In tissue culture, it was found that the gp120 expressed on productively infected cells binds to CD4 molecules on uninfected T cells (**Fig. 7B**). This leads to cell fusion. The process of HIV-induced syncytia formation can be lethal to both HIV-infected T cells and uninfected CD4+ T cells that fuse to the infected cells. These fused cells usually die within a few hours. This syncytia formation is usually seen only in T-tropic X4 type of HIV-1. So this type of HIV virus is often called as syncytia-inducing (SI) virus, in contrast to the R5 virus. However, this phenomenon was observed in vitro, and syncytia are rarely seen in the tissues of patients with AIDS.

CD8+ cytotoxic T cells: Destruction of infected CD4+ T cells may occur by antigen-specific CD8+ cytotoxic T cells.

Qualitative defects in T cells: Marked reduction in CD4+ T cells is hallmark of AIDS. It accounts for most of the immunodeficiency late in the course of HIV infection. However, qualitative defects in T cells can be found even in asymptomatic HIV infected individuals. These qualitative defects include reduced antigen-induced T-cell proliferation, decreased Th1-type responses, and defects in intracellular signaling. The loss of Th1 responses results in severe deficiency of cell-mediated immunity. This leads to increased susceptibility to infections by viruses and other intracellular microbes. Early in the course of disease, there is also a selective loss of the memory subset of CD4+ helper T cells.

Low level chronic or latent infection of T cells is an important feature of HIV infection. The integrated provirus, without viral gene expression (latent infection), can remain in the cells for months to years. Potent antiviral therapy can sterilize the peripheral blood from virus, but latent virus remains hidden within the CD4+ cells (both T cells and macrophages) in the lymph nodes. In the lymph nodes, about 0.05% of CD4+ T cells are latently infected. Most of these CD4+ T cells are memory cells. Hence, they are long-lived and remain for months to years. This is a persistent reservoir of virus.

CD4+ T cells play a critical role in regulating both cellular and humoral immune responses. Therefore, destruction of CD4+ T cells by HIV-1 affects every component of the immune system and can disable the entire immune system (**Box 4**). Thus, in a typical patient with AIDS, all elements of the immune system are eventually crippled. These include T cells, B cells, NK cells, the monocyte/macrophage lineage of cells, and Ig production.

HIV infection of non-T cells

Apart from infection and destructive loss of CD4+ T cells, HIV may infect or injure macrophages, DCs, and follicular dendritic cells (FDCs). Their abnormalities are also important in the pathogenesis of HIV infection and progression of immunodeficiency.

Infection of macrophages Similar to CD4+ T cells, the number of macrophages infected by HIV in the tissues is much more than the number of infected monocytes in the peripheral blood. In some tissues (e.g., lungs, brain), 10–50% of macrophages may be infected. General features of HIV infection of macrophages are as follows:

HIV can infect terminally differentiated nondividing macrophages: Most retroviruses require cell division for their nuclear entry and replication. However, HIV-1 can infect and multiply in terminally differentiated nondividing macrophages. This is because of the viral *vpr* gene of HIV-1. The Vpr protein (the product of *vpr* gene) allows nuclear entry through the nuclear pore.

Macrophages are relatively resistant to cytopathic effects of HIV: Infected macrophages bud relatively small number of virus from their cell surface. But these macrophages contain numerous virus particles, often located in intracellular vesicles. Though macrophages allow replication of HIV virus, these macrophages are resistant to killing by HIV. This is in contrast to CD4+ T cells which are highly susceptible to cytolysis. Thus, in late stages of HIV infection, **when numbers of CD4+ T-cell markedly reduced, macrophages may be an important site of continued replication of HIV virus**. They also **form a reservoir for persistence of virus in the patient**. In fact, the quantity of macrophage-associated HIV exceeds T-cell-associated virus in most tissues from patients with AIDS (e.g., brain and lung).

Macrophages may act as portals of infection: This is because in >90% of cases, acute HIV infection is by M-tropic strains, which has affinity for macrophages. Macrophages express much lower levels of CD4 molecules than CD4+ T lymphocytes. But they express CCR5 coreceptors and are susceptible to HIV infection.

Functional defects in uninfected monocytes: Uninfected monocytes may have unexplained functional defects. These defects include decreased chemotaxis and phagocytosis, impaired microbicidal activity, decreased secretion of IL-1, inappropriate secretion of TNF, and poor capacity to present antigens to T cells. Infected monocytes may carry HIV from the blood to various parts of the body. This is especially in the nervous system, where infiltrating infected monocytes may be a source of the virus that infects resident microglial cells.

Infection of dendritic cells In addition to macrophages, there are two types of DCs that are also important targets for the initiation and maintenance of HIV infection. These are mucosal and follicular DCs.

Mucosal DCs: Mucosal DCs are infected by the virus and may transport HIV to regional lymph nodes. In the lymph nodes, the virus is transmitted to CD4+ T cells. DCs also express a lectin-like receptor that binds HIV. These DCs display HIV in intact, infectious form to T cells, thus promoting infection of the T cells.

Follicular dendritic cells: FDCs are present in the germinal centers of lymph nodes and the spleen. They are potential

Box 4: Important abnormalities of immune system in AIDS.

Lymphopenia
- Mainly due to death of the CD4+ helper T-cell subset

Decreased T-cell function in vivo
- Loss of activated and memory T cells
- Decreased delayed-type hypersensitivity
- Susceptibility to opportunistic infections and neoplasms

Altered T-cell function in vitro: Following are decreased—
- Proliferative response to mitogens, alloantigens, and soluble antigens
- Cytotoxicity
- Helper function for B-cell antibody production
- Production of interleukin-2 (IL-2) and interferon-γ(IFN-γ)

Polyclonal activation of B-cell
- Hypergammaglobulinemia and circulating immune complexes
- No de novo antibody response to new antigens
- Poor responses to normal B-cell activation signals in vitro

Altered functions of monocyte/macrophage: Following are decreased—
- Chemotaxis and phagocytosis
- Microbicidal activity
- Expression of class II human leukocyte antigen (HLA)
- Capacity to present antigen to T cells
- Secretion of interleukin-1 (IL-1), tumor necrosis factor (TNF)

reservoirs of HIV. Though some of the FDCs may be susceptible to HIV infection, they trap large amounts of HIV on their surfaces, Thus, most HIV particles are found on the surface of their dendritic processes and not inside the DCs. FDCs have receptors for the Fc portion of Igs. FDCs can also trap anti-HIV antibodies coated HIV virions through Fc receptor-mediated binding. The antibody-coated virions localized to FDCs retain the capability to infect CD4+ T cells as they traverse the intricate meshwork formed by the dendritic processes of the FDCs. Infected T follicular helper cells present in the germinal centers also act as reservoirs of HIV. Since cytotoxic T cells (CTLs) are largely excluded from germinal centers, these viral reservoirs (FDCs) cannot be destroyed by the host immune response. FDCs contribute to the pathogenesis of HIV-associated immunodeficiency in at least two ways:

1. FDC surface is a reservoir for HIV. They can infect macrophages and CD4+ T cells in the lymph nodes.
2. In HIV infection, normal functions of FDCs in immune responses are impaired. They may eventually be destroyed by the virus by unknown mechanism. The net result of their destruction is loss of the FDC network in the lymph nodes and spleen. This causes dissolution of the architecture of the peripheral lymphoid system.

B-cell function in HIV infection

HIV infects T cells, macrophages, and DCs. But individuals with AIDS also show severe abnormalities of B-cell function. Surprisingly, during early course of the disease, there is polyclonal activation of B cells. This produces germinal center B-cell hyperplasia and may be associated with autoimmune phenomena (e.g., immune thrombocytopenic purpura).

Mechanisms of B-cell activation: B-cell activation may be due to different mechanisms:

- Reactivation of or reinfection with EBV: EBV is a polyclonal activator of B-cell.
- Viral gp41: This can promote B-cell growth and differentiation.
- Increased production of IL-6: This stimulates proliferation of B cells by HIV infected macrophages.

B-cell activation is also accompanied by increase in number of plasma cells. This leads to hypergammaglobulinemia and bone marrow plasmacytosis.

Defective antibody response (humoral immunity): Though there is B-cell activation and risk of autoimmunity in patients with AIDS, these patients are not able to mount effective antibody responses to newly encountered pathogens. This may be partly due to lack of T-cell help, but there is also suppression of antibody responses against T-independent antigens. Hence, there may be also intrinsic defects in B cells. Because of impaired humoral immunity, these patients are susceptible to disseminated infections caused by encapsulated bacteria. These include *S. pneumoniae* and *H. influenzae*, both of which require antibodies for effective opsonization and clearance of these microbes.

NK cell: Its activity is also severely decreased in AIDS. NK cells kill both virus-infected cells and tumor cells. Their defect may contribute to the malignant tumors and viral infections in these patients. Reduced activity of NK cell is due to both, a decrease in number of NK cells as well reduced levels of IL-2 owing to a loss of CD4+ T cells.

Pathogenesis of central nervous system involvement

In addition to the lymphoid system, the nervous system is also involved in HIV infection. The term HIV-associated neurocognitive disorder (HAND) is used for clinical syndrome of CNS abnormalities in HIV.

Cells infected: Microglial cells in the CNS belong to the macrophage lineage. In the brain, microglial cells are the main type of cell types that are infected with HIV. Probably infected T cells or monocytes carry the HIV into the brain.

Mechanism of damage: The mechanism of HIV-induced damage of the brain is not clearly known. HIV does not infect the neurons. In HIV patients, in comparison to the severity of neurologic symptoms, the extent of neuropathologic changes is less than expected.

- **Indirect damage:** Probably, the neurologic damage is indirect rather than direct HIV infection. The indirect damage may be brought out by viral products and soluble factors produced by infected microglia. Examples of the soluble factors are IL-1, TNF, and IL-6. Also, nitric oxide induced in neuronal cells by gp41 may also cause indirect damage.
- **Direct neuronal damage:** It may be caused by soluble HIV gp120.

Natural History of HIV Infection (Fig. 8)

The virus enters the new host through mucosal epithelia and the subsequent pathologic changes and clinical manifestations of the HIV infection can be divided into mainly three phases—(1) an acute retroviral syndrome; (2) a middle, chronic phase (in this phase most are asymptomatic); and (3) clinical AIDS.

Acute Infection and Acute Retroviral Syndrome (Fig. 8)

Primary mucosal infection

HIV disease begins with acute infection. Infection develops following exposure to virus through mainly sexual contact. The virus usually enters through mucosal epithelia.

Infection of memory CD4+ T cells: Acute (early) **infection involves memory CD4+ T cells** (which express CCR5) present in the lymphoid tissues of mucosa and produces death of many infected cells. Mucosal tissues are the largest reservoir of memory T cells in the body. Hence, infection of memory T cells by HIV produces considerable **local loss due to death and leads to depletion of these lymphocytes**. There is also death of abortively infected bystander CD4+ T cells. Indeed, within 2 weeks of infection, there may be destruction of large number of CD4+ T cells. Few infected memory CD4+ T cells are detectable in the blood and other tissues. Mucosal infection is usually associated with damage to the mucosal epithelium, defects in mucosal barrier functions, and translocation of other microbes across the epithelium.

Virus dissemination

Capture of HIV by DCs in the mucosa: Mucosal infection is followed by dissemination of the virus. This causes **development of immune responses by infected host**. At sites of virus entry, DCs present in mucosal epithelia capture the virus.

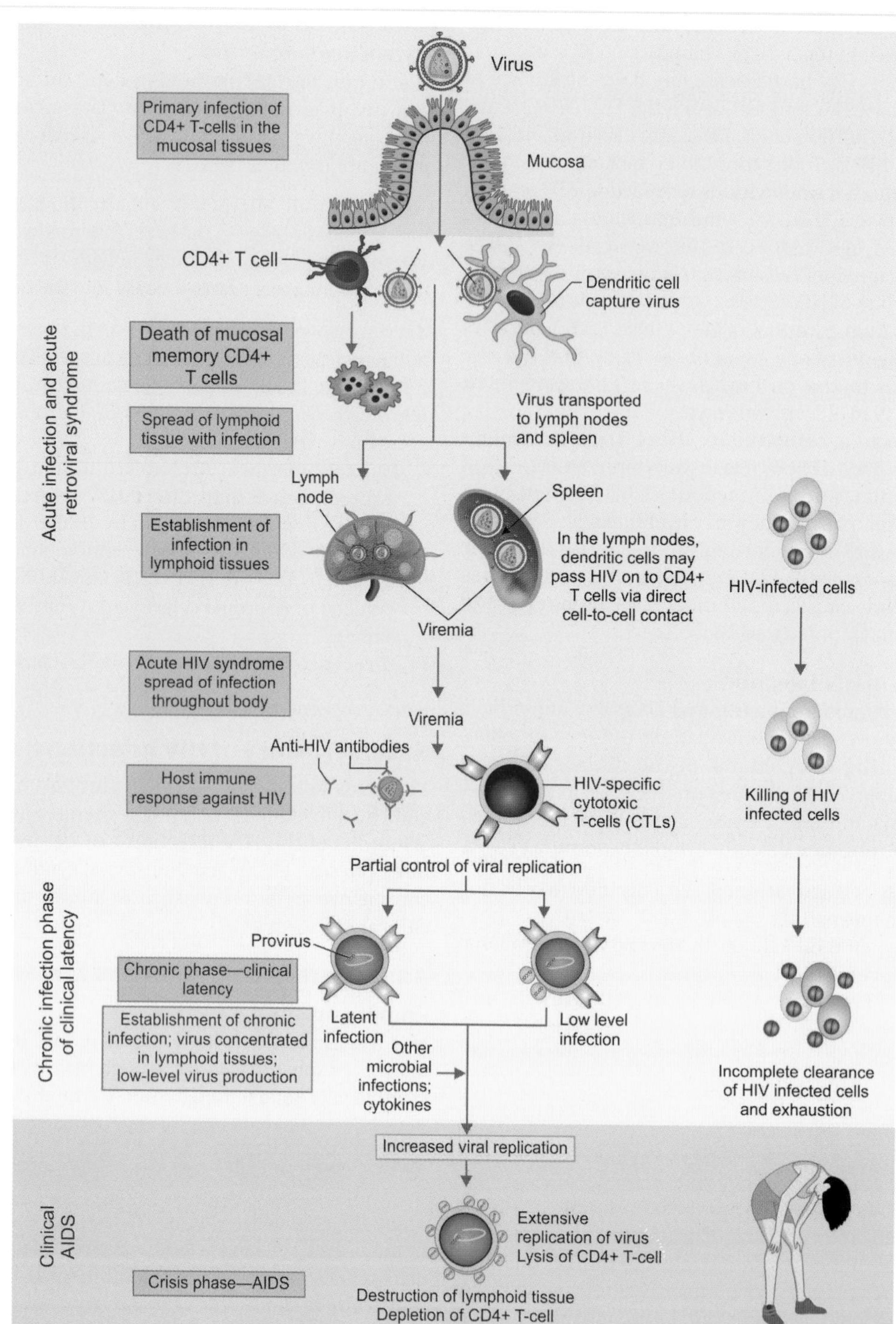

FIG. 8: Pathogenesis and progression of HIV infection. HIV initially infects mucosal tissues, involving mainly memory CD4+ T cells and dendritic cells, and spreads to lymphoid tissues throughout the body (lymph nodes and spleen). Viral replication in lymph node leads to viremia and widespread seeding of lymphoid tissue. This phase corresponds to the early acute phase of HIV infection. The viremia is temporarily controlled by the immune response of host and the disease enters a phase of clinical latency. Immune response of the host does not prevent the establishment of chronic infection of cells in lymphoid tissues. During this phase, viral replication continues both in T cells and macrophages. Ultimately, there is progressive decrease of CD4+ T cells and patient develops clinical symptoms of full-blown AIDS entering the crisis phase. Cytokine stimuli induced by other microbes serve to enhance HIV production and progression to AIDS.

Migration to lymph nodes: DCs with captured viruses migrate to the regional lymph nodes. DCs express a protein with a mannose-binding lectin domain, called DC-SIGN. This may be involved in binding the HIV envelope and transporting the virus.

Pass HIV on to CD4+ T cells: In the lymphoid tissues, DCs may pass HIV on to CD4+ T cells via direct cell-to-cell contact.

Viral replications and dissemination: Within days after the first exposure to HIV, virus replicates in the lymph nodes and this leads to viremia. During viremia, large numbers of HIV particles are present in the patient's blood.

Infection of other cells: The virus disseminates throughout the body and infects helper T cells, macrophages, and DCs in peripheral lymphoid tissues.

Development of immune responses by infected host: As the HIV infection spreads, the infected individual mounts **antiviral humoral and cell-mediated immune responses** (directed at viral antigens). These immune responses **lead to seroconversion** (usually within 3-7 weeks after exposure) and the **production of virus-specific CD8+ cytotoxic T cells**. HIV-specific CD8+ T cells are detected in the blood at about the time when viral titers begin to fall. Probably HIV-specific CD8+ T cells are responsible for the initial control of HIV infection. These **immune responses partially control the HIV infection as well as viral production**. This is observed as a drop in viremia to low but detectable levels by about 12 weeks after the primary exposure.

Acute retroviral syndrome

Acute retroviral (HIV) syndrome represents the clinical presentation of the initial spread of the virus and the response of host. About 40–90% of individuals who acquire a primary infection develop this syndrome. It usually occurs 3–6 weeks after infection and resolves spontaneously in 2–4 weeks.

Presenting features: Acute retroviral (HIV) syndrome presents with a variety of **nonspecific,** self-limited, acute illness with flu-like symptoms. These signs and symptoms are typical of many viral infections and they are nonspecific. These symptoms include sore throat, myalgias, fever, weight loss, and fatigue. Sometimes patient may develop rash, cervical adenopathy, diarrhea, and vomiting. Neurological symptoms are common, including myelopathy, neuropathy, headache, and photophobia. The illness lasts up to 3 weeks and followed by complete recovery.

Viral load: Viral load refers to the amount of virus in an infected person's blood. The viral load in HIV infection is assessed by estimating the level of HIV-1 RNA in the blood. It is a **useful marker of HIV disease progression** and is **useful in the management of patients** with HIV infection. The viral load at the end of the acute phase reflects the equilibrium reached between the virus and the host response. It may remain fairly stable for several years. This level of steady-state viremia is termed viral set point. It is a predictor of the rate of decline of CD4+ T cells and, therefore, progression of HIV disease. If the viral load is less, progression to clinical AIDS is slower than with a higher viral load.

Standard HIV-1 enzyme immunoassay (EIA) and Western blot testing, which depend on the presence of anti-HIV-1 *gag* antibodies, are negative during the initial stage of the infection.

Categories of HIV infection depending on CD4+ cell counts: Centers for Disease Control and Prevention (CDC) classifies HIV infection into three categories based on age-specific CD4+ T lymphocyte count or CD4+ T lymphocyte percentage of total lymphocytes (**Table 6**). Perhaps, for clinical management, CD4+ T-cell count in the blood is the most reliable short-term indicator of disease progression. Hence, the CD4+ cell count (rather than viral load) is mainly used to determine when to start antiretroviral therapy (ART).

Table 6: Centers for Disease Control and Prevention (CDC) HIV infection stages 1–3 based on age-specific CD4+ T lymphocyte count or CD4+ T lymphocyte percentage of total lymphocytes.

*Stage**	*Age on date of CD4+ T-lymphocyte test*					
	<1 year		1–5 years		≥6 years	
	Cells/µL	%	Cells/µL	%	Cells/µL	%
1	≥1,500	≥34	≥1,000	≥30	≥500	≥26
2	750–1,499	26–33	500–999	22–29	200–499	14–25
3	<750	<26	<500	<22	<200	<14

*The stage is based primarily on the CD4+ T-lymphocyte count; the CD4+ T-lymphocyte count takes precedence over the CD4 T-lymphocyte percentage, and the percentage is considered only if the count is missing. There are three situations in which the stage is not based on this table: (1) if the criteria for stage 0 are met, the stage is 0 regardless of criteria for other stages (CD4 T-lymphocyte test results and opportunistic illness diagnoses); (2) if the criteria for stage 0 are not met and a stage-3-defining opportunistic illness has been diagnosed, then the stage is 3 regardless of CD4 T-lymphocyte test results; or (3) if the criteria for stage 0 are not met and information on the above criteria for other stages is missing, then the stage is classified as unknown.

Chronic Infection: Phase of Clinical Latency (Fig. 8)

Following acute phase, HIV disease progresses to next phase namely chronic phase.

Minimal or no clinical manifestations: During this chronic phase, virus continuously replicates in the lymph nodes and spleen and there is associated cell destruction (**Fig. 8**). During this period, there are few or no clinical manifestations of the HIV infection. Minimal symptoms may be due to minor opportunistic infections, such as oral candidiasis (thrush), vaginal candidiasis, herpes zoster, and perhaps tuberculosis. Autoimmune thrombocytopenia may also develop. However, the immune system remains competent at handling most infections. Hence, this phase of HIV disease is called the clinical latency period.

Persistent generalized lymphadenopathy: A subgroup of patients may develop persistent generalized lymphadenopathy (PGL). PGL is defined as lymphadenopathy (>1 cm) at two or more extrainguinal sites for >3 months in the absence of causes other than HIV infection. Biopsy reveals nonspecific lymphoid hyperplasia. The lymph nodes are usually symmetrical, firm, mobile, and nontender. Nodes may disappear as the disease progresses.

Progressive decrease of CD4+ T cells: Majority of peripheral blood T cells do not contain the virus during this phase, but they are present in secondary lymphoid organs. Normally, >90% of the body's (about 10^{11}) T cells are found in peripheral and mucosal lymphoid tissues and secondary lymphoid organs. During chronic phase, there is continuous destruction of CD4+ T cells in these lymphoid tissues. Probably, HIV destroys up to 2×10^9 CD4+ T cells each day. This is accompanied by a steady decrease in number of CD4+ T cells in the peripheral blood. During the early course of disease, the loss of CD4+ T cells can be replaced by new T cells almost as quickly as they are destroyed. During initial period of this stage, up to 10% of CD4+ T cells in lymphoid organs may be infected and the infected CD4+ T cells in the blood may be <0.1% of the total circulating CD4+ T cells. However, over a period of years, the slow increase in virus infection, death of T-cell, and new infection lead to a steady decrease in the number of CD4+ T cells, both in the lymphoid tissue and in circulation. Accompanying this loss of CD4+ T cells, host defenses diminish. The ratio of the surviving CD4+ cells to infected with HIV increases and also there is increase in the viral burden per CD4+ cell.

Increase in HIV RNA levels: Not unexpectedly, levels of HIV RNA increase as the host begins to lose the battle with the virus. The mechanism of escape of HIV from immune control is not clearly known. These mechanisms may include destruction of the CD4+ T cells that are important for effective immunity, antigenic variation, and down-modulation of class I MHC molecules on infected cells so that viral antigens are not recognized by CD8+ CTLs.

Evolve and switching of coreceptors: During chronic phase, the virus may evolve and switch from depending solely on coreceptor CCR5 for their entry into target cells to relying on either CXCR4 or both CCR5 and CXCR4. This coreceptor switch is associated with more rapid reduction in CD4+ T-cell counts, probably due to infection of large number of T cells.

Clinical AIDS (Fig. 9)

In most of the untreated patients (not all), HIV disease progresses to the final and almost invariably lethal phase, called AIDS.

Characteristics: It is characterized by a failure of host defense, a striking increase in viral load (viremia may be accelerated unchecked in reservoirs other than T cells), the blood CD4+ T-cell count drops below 200 cells/mm^3, and severe, life-threatening clinical disease.

Patterns of HIV progression

Typical progressors: Typically, it presents with long-lasting fever (>1 month), fatigue, weight loss, diarrhea, and generalized lymphadenopathy. After a variable period, patient develops serious multiple opportunistic infections, secondary neoplasms, or clinical neurologic disease and the patient is said to have developed AIDS. Most of untreated (but not all) patients with HIV infection progress to AIDS after a chronic phase lasting from 7 to 10 years. Exceptions to this typical course of HIV are as follows:

- **Rapid progressors:** In these patients, the middle, chronic phase is shortened to 2–3 years after primary infection and they rapidly progress to AIDS.
- **Long-term nonprogressors:** These are untreated HIV-1-infected patients who are asymptomatic for 10 years or more, with stable CD4+ T-cell counts and low levels of plasma viremia (usually <500 viral RNA copies per milliliter). They form about 5–15% of infected individuals.
- **Slow progressors:** They have a CD4 decline that is very slow compared to the typical progressors.
- **Elite controllers:** About 1% of patients have undetectable plasma virus (<50–75 RNA copies/mL) and are called elite controllers. This group is heterogeneous with respect to the variables that influence the course of the disease and all have a vigorous anti-HIV immune response. Some patients have high levels of HIV-specific CD4+ and CD8+ T-cell responses during the course of infection. The

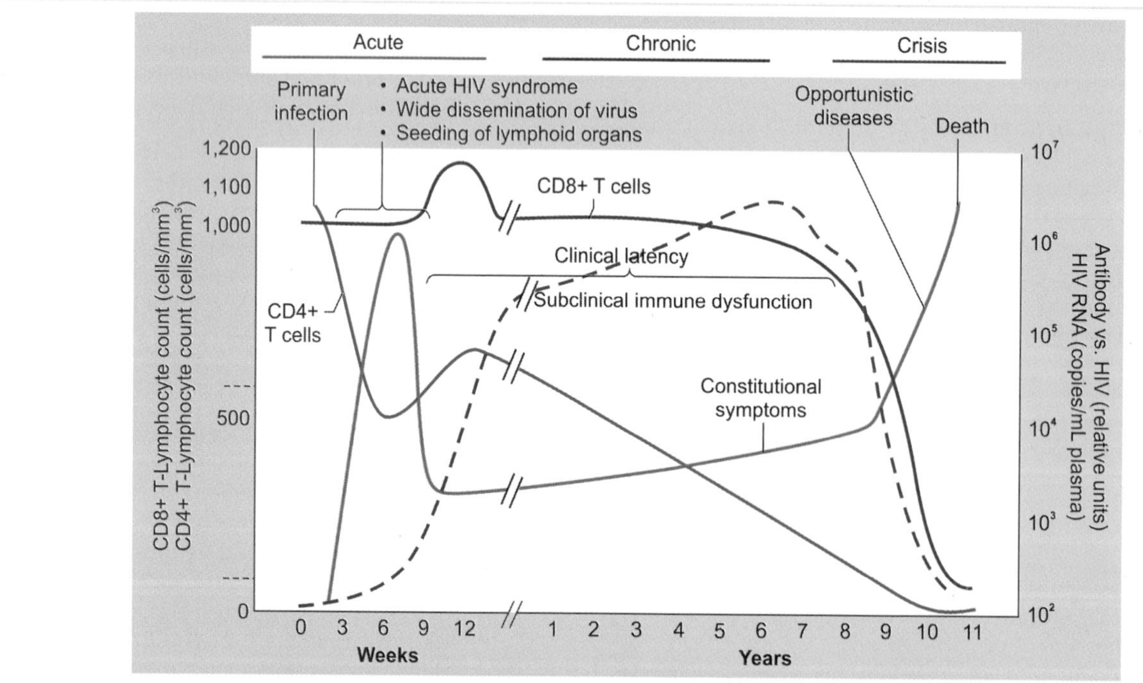

FIG. 9: Generalized time course of human immunodeficiency virus-1 (HIV-1) infection. After primary HIV infection, during the early period, the virus disseminates and there is development of a host immune response to HIV. This often causes an acute viral syndrome. During the period of clinical latency, replication of virus continues in lymphoid organs and the CD4+ T-cell count gradually decreases. When CD4+ T cells reach a critical level, it is associated with considerable risk of AIDS-associated diseases. Clinical syndrome, virus loads, and CD8+ lymphocyte population dynamics are also shown over time.

inheritance of particular HLA alleles may be responsible for the resistance against progression of disease.

HIV disease progression with CD+ T cell level and viral load in different phases of HIV infection are presented in **Figure 9**. Immune response by host to HIV infection is presented in **Figure 10**.

Clinical Features of AIDS

Clinical manifestations and type of opportunistic infections associated with AIDS vary in different parts of the world. Currently available antiretroviral therapies have considerably modified the course of the disease as well many destructive complications. These complications were common before the presently available antiretroviral therapies and are presently infrequent.

The adult patient with AIDS usually presents with fever, weight loss, diarrhea, generalized lymphadenopathy, multiple opportunistic infections, neurologic disease, and secondary neoplasms. AIDS-defining opportunistic infections and neoplasms found in patients with HIV infection are presented in **Table 7**.

Opportunistic Infections

Q. Write short essay on opportunistic infections in AIDS.

Centers for Disease Control and Prevention has listed diagnostic criteria for AIDS with regards to any HIV-related illness. CDC has classified certain serious and life-threatening diseases that are directly associated with advanced HIV infection, called "AIDS-defining" illnesses. When an individual has any one of these illnesses, the individual is diagnosed with the advanced stage of HIV infection known as AIDS. While some of these diseases can occur in individual without HIV, they are only considered AIDS-defining in the presence of an HIV infection, AIDS-defining conditions (**Box 5**) include opportunistic infections and cancers that are life-threatening in a person with HIV. Pattern of opportunistic infections associated with declining CD4+ T cell counts is shown in **Figure 11**.

Opportunistic infections are responsible for the majority of deaths in untreated patients with AIDS. Most of these infections represent reactivation of latent infections. Normally, these infections are controlled by the immune system but are not completely eradicated. This is because the infectious agents coexist with their hosts. The frequency of these

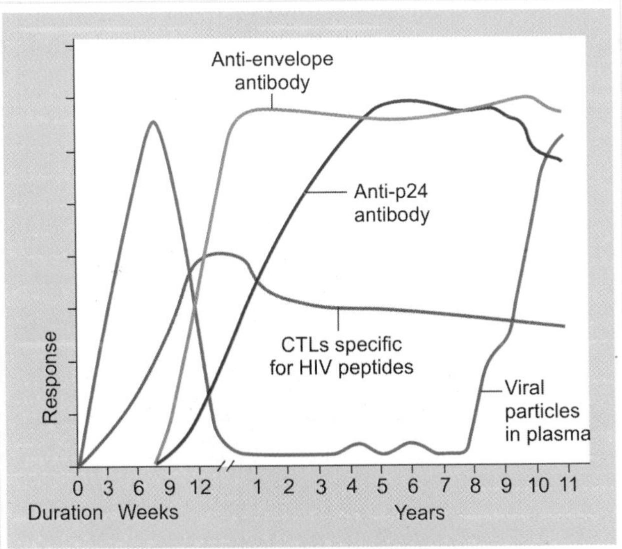

FIG. 10: Immune response to HIV infection. A cytotoxic T lymphocyte (CTL) response to HIV is observed by 2–3 weeks after the initial HIV infection and it peaks by 9–12 weeks. The humoral immune response (anti-envelope antibody and anti-p24 antibody) of host to HIV peaks at about 12 weeks. Viral particles in plasma peak during acute phase (6 weeks) and decline during chronic phase. It spurts during terminal phase of AIDS.

Table 7: AIDS-defining opportunistic infections and neoplasms found in patients with HIV infection.

Opportunistic infections	*Organ or site involved or type of damage*
Protozoal and helminthic infections	
Cryptosporidium or *Cystoisospora*	Enteritis
Toxoplasma	Pneumonia or central nervous system (CNS) infection
Fungal infections	
Candida	Esophageal, tracheal, or pulmonary
Pneumocystis	Pneumonia or disseminated infection
Cryptococcus	Infection of central nervous system
Coccidioides	Disseminated
Histoplasma	Disseminated
Bacterial infections	
Mycobacterium	
Mycobacterium atypical, e.g., *Mycobacterium avium-intracellulare*	Disseminated or extrapulmonary
Mycobacterium tuberculosis	Pulmonary or extrapulmonary
Nocardia	Pneumonia, meningitis, disseminated
Salmonella infections	Disseminated
Viral infections	
Cytomegalovirus	Pulmonary, intestinal, retinitis, or CNS infections
Herpes simplex virus	Localized or disseminated
Varicella-zoster virus	Localized or disseminated
Progressive multifocal leukoencephalopathy	Central nervous system
Neoplasms	**Cause**
Kaposi sarcoma (KS)	Kaposi sarcoma herpes virus (KSHV) also called human herpesvirus 8 (HHV8)
Primary lymphoma of brain	Epstein–Barr virus (EBV)
Invasive cancer of the uterine cervix	Human papillomavirus (HPV)
Anal carcinoma	HPV

Box 5: AIDS-defining conditions (CDC).

- Bacterial infections, multiple or recurrent
- Candidiasis of bronchi, trachea, or lungs
- Candidiasis of esophagus
- Cervical cancer, invasive
- Coccidioidomycosis, disseminated or extrapulmonary
- Cryptococcosis, extrapulmonary
- Cryptosporidiosis, chronic intestinal (>1 month's duration)
- Cytomegalovirus disease (other than liver, spleen, or nodes), onset at age >1 month
- Cytomegalovirus retinitis (with loss of vision)
- Encephalopathy, HIV related
- Herpes simplex: chronic ulcers (>1 month's duration) or bronchitis, pneumonitis, or esophagitis (onset at age >1 month)
- Histoplasmosis, disseminated or extrapulmonary
- Isosporiasis, chronic intestinal (>1 month's duration)
- Kaposi's sarcoma
- Lymphoid interstitial pneumonia or pulmonary lymphoid hyperplasia complex
- Lymphoma, Burkitt (or equivalent term)
- Lymphoma, immunoblastic (or equivalent term)
- Lymphoma, primary, of brain
- *Mycobacterium avium* complex or *Mycobacterium kansasii*, disseminated, or extrapulmonary
- *Mycobacterium tuberculosis* of any site, pulmonary, disseminated or extrapulmonary
- *Mycobacterium*, other species or unidentified species, disseminated or extrapulmonary
- *Pneumocystis jirovecii* pneumonia
- Pneumonia, recurrent
- Progressive multifocal leukoencephalopathy
- *Salmonella* septicemia, recurrent
- Toxoplasmosis of brain, onset at age >1 month
- Wasting syndrome attributed to HIV

opportunistic infections varies in different regions of the world. Currently available combinations of three or four drugs by ART (antiretroviral therapy) block different steps of the HIV life cycle. They have markedly reduced these infections. Salient features of some infections in AIDS are discussed briefly.

- **Pneumonia due to *Pneumocystis jirovecii*:** The majority of patients with HIV-1/AIDS suffer from opportunistic pulmonary infections. This has been greatly reduced by the use of prophylactic antibiotics. About 15–30% of untreated HIV patients develop pneumonia during the course of the disease caused by the fungus *Pneumocystis jirovecii* (formerly called *P. carinii*). This is usually reactivation of a prior latent infection. Before the advent of ART, this was the presenting feature in about 20% of cases. Currently, the incidence is much less.
- **Other opportunistic infections:** Many patients develop other opportunistic infections. Most common include *Candida*, CMV, atypical and typical mycobacteria, *Cryptococcus neoformans, Toxoplasma gondii, Cryptosporidium*, herpes simplex virus, papovaviruses, and *Histoplasma capsulatum.*
- ***Candidiasis*:** It is the most common fungal infection in patients with AIDS. Most common clinical manifestations are those involving the oral cavity (see Fig. 62 Chapter 11), vagina, and esophagus (**Fig. 12**). In asymptomatic HIV-infected individuals, oral candidiasis is a sign of immunologic decompensation. It often indicates the transition to AIDS. However, invasive candidiasis is infrequent in patients with AIDS. If it occurs, it is usually when there is drug-induced neutropenia or with the use of indwelling catheters.
- ***Cytomegalovirus*:** It may cause disseminated disease or may be localized (e.g., eye, GIT). The incidence of CMV chorioretinitis was high (in about 25% of patients), but it has dramatically reduced due to ART. CMV retinitis almost exclusively occurs in patients with CD4+ T cell counts of <50/μL. Gastrointestinal disease (5–10% of cases) manifests as esophagitis and colitis (associated with multiple mucosal ulcerations).

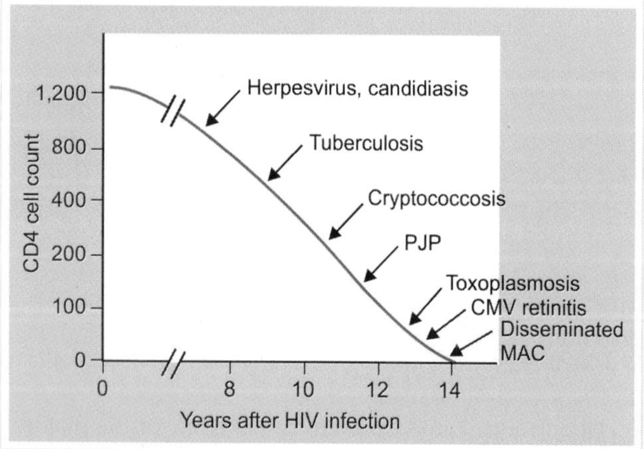

(CMV: cytomegalovirus; HIV: human immunodeficiency virus; MAC: *Mycobacterium avium* complex; PJP: *Pneumocystis jirovecii* pneumonia)

FIG. 11: Pattern of opportunistic infections associated with declining CD4+ T-cell counts.

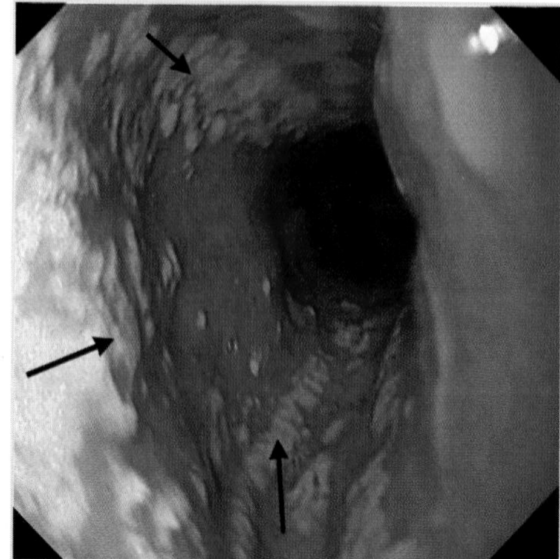

FIG. 12: Esophageal candidiasis.

- **Disseminated infection with atypical mycobacteria:** Disseminated bacterial infection with atypical mycobacteria (mainly *Mycobacterium avium-intracellulare*) develops late when there is severe immunosuppression. After AIDS epidemic, the incidence of tuberculosis has dramatically raised. Worldwide, about one-third of all deaths in AIDS patients are due to tuberculosis. Patients with AIDS have an increased risk for reactivation of latent pulmonary disease as well as primary infection. In contrast to infection with atypical mycobacteria, *M. tuberculosis* infection develops early in the course of AIDS. Tuberculosis may be restricted to lungs or may involve multiple organs. The extent of infection depends on the degree of immunosuppression; dissemination occurs more commonly when the CD4+ T-cell count is very low. Most warning are the growing number of cases that are resistant to multiple available antimycobacterial drugs.
- **Infections of the CNS:** A variety of opportunistic infections affect the CNS. *Cryptococcosis* is observed in about 10% of AIDS patients and mainly presents as devastating meningitis. *Toxoplasma gondii* causes encephalitis and is responsible for 50% of all mass lesions in the CNS. *JC virus* is a human papovavirus, another important cause of CNS infection that produces progressive multifocal leukoencephalopathy.
- **Other infections:** They may involve the GIT and genitalia. *Herpes simplex virus* infection presents as mucocutaneous ulcerations involving the mouth, esophagus, external genitalia, and perianal region. Persistent diarrhea is common in untreated patients with advanced AIDS. It is usually caused by infections with protozoans such as *Cryptosporidium, Isospora belli*, or microsporidia. These patients present with chronic, profuse, watery diarrhea with massive loss of fluid. Diarrhea may also be due to infection with enteric bacteria, such as *Salmonella* and *Shigella*, as well as *M. avium-intracellulare.*
- **Skin disease:** Almost all patients with AIDS develop some form of skin disease and infections are the most prominent. Most commonly, *Staphylococcus aureus* causes bullous impetigo, deeper purulent lesions (ecthyma), and folliculitis. Chronic mucocutaneous herpes simplex (**Fig. 13**) infection is characteristic of AIDS and it is considered an index infection in establishing the diagnosis of AIDS. Other skin lesions include those due to *Molluscum contagiosum* (**Fig. 14A**) and genital warts (**Fig. 14B**) by HPV, scabies, and infections with *Candida* species. A varicella zoster eruption (herpes zoster) (**Fig. 14C**) developing below the age of 50 should raise the suspicion of a possible occult HIV-1 infection.

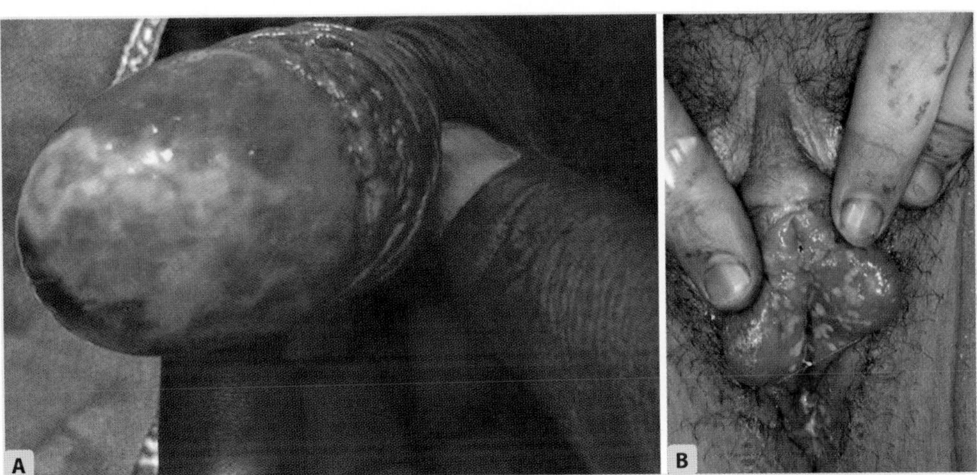

FIGS. 13A AND B: Genital herpes simplex involving external genitalia. (A) Male and (B) Female.

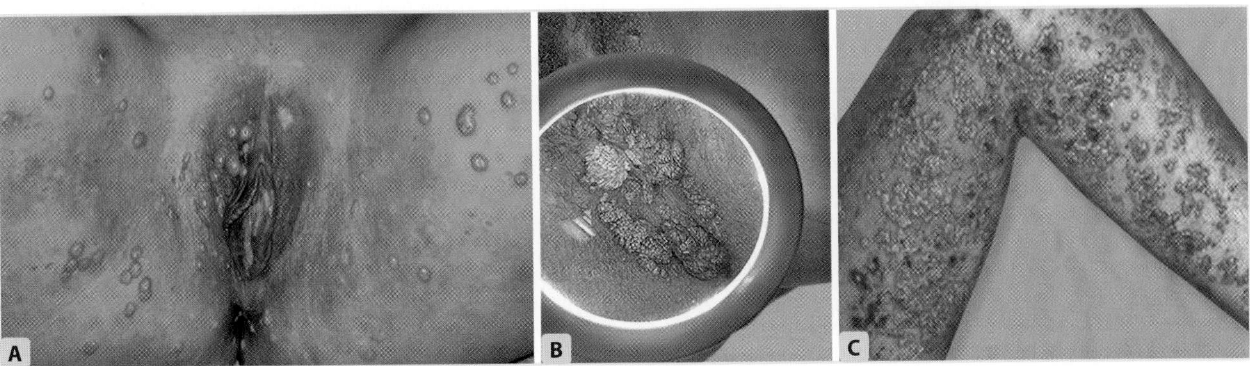

FIGS. 14A TO C: (A) Molluscum contagiosum; (B) Genital warts; and (C) Herpes zoster hand.

Tumors

Q. Write short essay on AIDS-related neoplasms.

High incidence of certain tumors is observed in patients with AIDS. These include Kaposi sarcoma (KS), B-cell lymphoma, cervical cancer in women, and anal cancer in men. About 25–40% of untreated HIV-infected individuals may develop a malignancy. A common feature of these tumors in HIV is that they are caused by oncogenic DNA viruses. These are human herpesvirus-8 (HHV8; causing KS), EBV (causing B-cell lymphoma), and HPV (causing cervical and anal carcinoma). These oncogenic DNA viruses may produce latent infections even in healthy individuals, but a competent immune system usually keeps them in check. Thus, the risk of malignancy in AIDS patients is because of failure to control the infections and decreased immunity against the tumors.

Kaposi sarcoma (Fig. 15)

Kaposi sarcoma (KS) is a **vascular tumor** and is the most common neoplasm in patients with AIDS especially in untreated patients. In recent years, due to the use of ART, their incidence has been dramatically reduced. KS can also occur in patients not infected with HIV (sporadic form) and here only features relevant to AIDS-related form of KS are discussed.

Microscopically, KS shows **proliferation of spindle-shaped cells**. These cells express **markers of both endothelial cells** (vascular or lymphatic) **and smooth muscle cells**. They also show **numerous slit-like vascular spaces**. This suggests that they may arise from primitive mesenchymal precursors of vascular channels. Also, KS lesions show chronic inflammatory cell infiltrates.

Nature of KS: Despite its name sarcoma, many of the features of KS suggest that it is not a malignant tumor. For example, spindle cells in many of the lesions of KS are polyclonal or oligoclonal and not monoclonal. However, occasionally more advanced lesions show monoclonality.

Etiology and pathogenesis: KS is caused by HHV8, also called as KS herpesvirus (KSHV). HHV8 virus has been detected in both spindle cells and endothelial cells of KS. The presence of HHV8 in the blood strongly predicts later development of KS. About 75% of HIV-infected people with HHV8 in the blood developed KS within 5 years. It is thought that HHV8 is sexually transmitted.

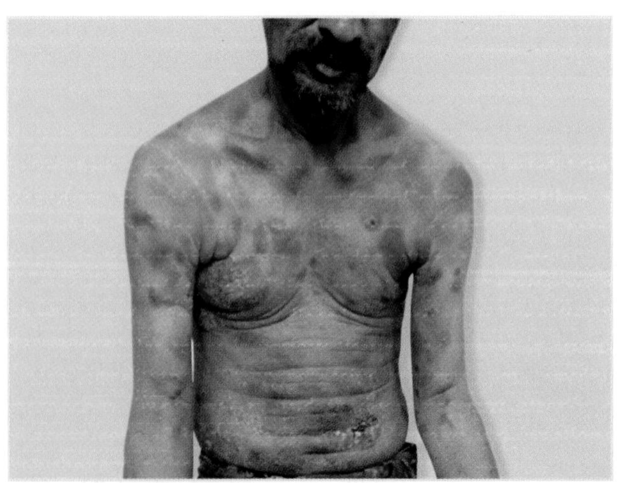

FIG. 15: Kaposi sarcoma.

Exact mechanism of production of KS by HHV8 infection is not known. Like other herpesviruses, HHV8 establishes latent infection. During this period, several proteins are produced. These stimulate proliferation of spindle cells and prevent apoptosis. These proteins include a viral homolog of cyclin D and several inhibitors of p53. However, though HHV8 infection is necessary for development of KS, it is not sufficient to produce KS. It requires additional cofactors. In the AIDS-related KS, this cofactor is clearly HIV, whereas the relevant cofactors for HIV negative KS are not known. HIV-mediated immune suppression may assist in widespread dissemination of HHV8 in the host.

Probably the proliferated spindle cells produce proinflammatory and angiogenic factors. They mobilize the inflammatory and neovascular components of the lesion, respectively. The neovascular components provide signals that help in survival and growth of spindle cell.

HHV8 virus and its associated tumors: It is related phylogenetically (evolutionary development) to the lymphotropic subfamily of herpesviruses (γ-herpesvirus). HHV8 infection is not limited to only endothelial cells. The genome of HHV8 virus is found in B cells of infected individuals. Thus, HHV8 infection may also be associated with peculiar, rare B-cell lymphomas in AIDS patients. This is called **primary effusion lymphoma**. Apart from neoplasms, HHV8 may cause **AIDS-associated multicentric Castleman disease** (B-cell lymphoproliferative disorder).

AIDS-associated KS versus sporadic form of KS: Clinically, AIDS-associated KS is totally different from the sporadic form. In HIV-infected individuals, KS is usually widespread, affecting the skin (**Fig. 15**), mucous membranes, GIT, lymph nodes, and lungs. These KS are also more aggressive than classic sporadic form of KS.

Lymphomas

In patient with AIDS, about 5% of them present with lymphoma and about another 5% develop lymphoma during the subsequent course of the disease. Lymphoma is one of the several AIDS-defining conditions. Almost all lymphomas arise from transformed B cells. Though currently available effective ART has substantially reduced the incidence of lymphoma in some HIV-infected populations, it occurs in HIV-infected individuals more than the population average.

Pathogenies of B-cell lymphoma in AIDS (Fig. 16) The association of B-cell lymphoma and HIV infection is maybe partly due to T-cell immunodeficiency. Two mechanisms may be responsible for the increased risk of B-cell tumors in HIV-infected individuals:

1. **Uncontrolled proliferation of B cells:** In AIDS patients, there is **severe depletion of T cells**. This may lead to uncontrolled **proliferation of B cells infected with oncogenic herpesviruses**. To prevent the proliferation of B cells infected with oncogenic viruses (e.g., EBV and HHV8), it needs control by T-cell immunity. In the late course of HIV infection, due to severe depletion of T cells, this control is lost. So, AIDS patients have a high risk of developing aggressive B-cell lymphomas. These B-cell lymphomas are

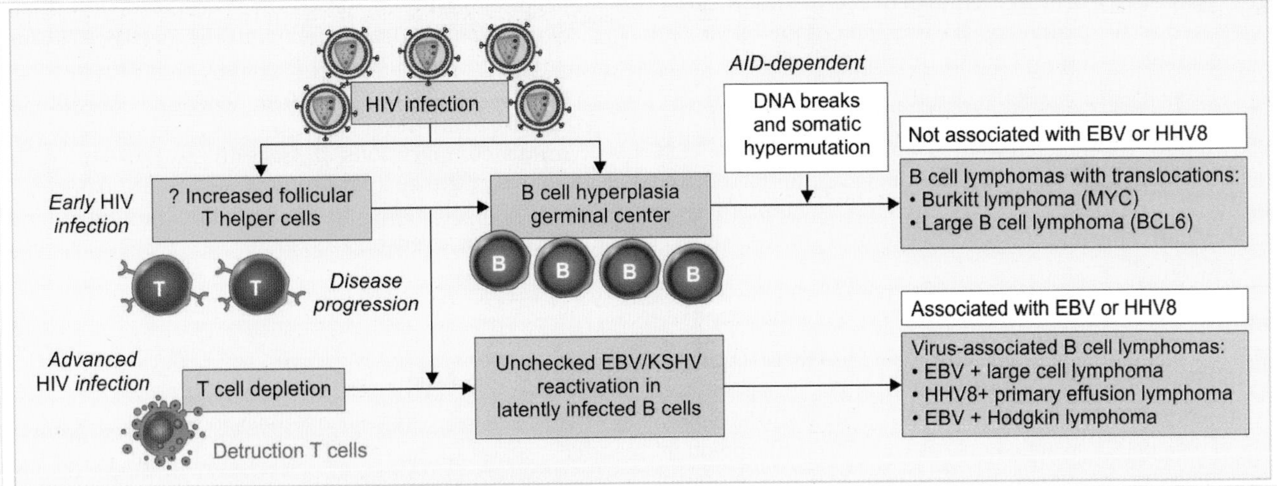

FIG. 16: Probable pathogenesis of B-cell lymphomas in HIV infection. The mechanism of lymphoma in early HIV infections is due to B-cell hyperplasia in germinal center followed by DNA breaks and somatic hypermutation which depend on HIV infection. In advanced HIV infection (AIDS), T-cell depletion is associated with unchecked proliferation of latently infected (by EBV or KSHV/HHV8) B cells. An increase in T follicular helper cells early in the course of the disease may also be involved in both early and advanced HIV infection.

composed of tumor cells infected by oncogenic viruses, particularly EBV.

Most normal individuals get infected with EBV by the time they become adults. With normal immunity, **EBV persists as a latent infection** in about 1 in 100,000 B cells. Most of these B cells have a memory B-cell phenotype. When these memory **B cells are activated by antigen or by cytokines,** there is emergence of an EBV-encoded program of gene expression. This leads to proliferation of B cells. **AIDS patients have high levels of several cytokines** and some of them (e.g., IL-6) are growth factors for B cells. AIDS patients are also chronically infected with many pathogens and this may also stimulate proliferation of B cells. In AIDS patients, due to severe depletion of T-cell immunity, these EBV-infected clones proliferate and may acquire additional somatic mutations. This leads to their uncontrolled proliferation forming full-blown EBV-positive B-cell lymphomas.

B-cell lymphomas in AIDS: The tumors usually develop in the **extranodal sites, such as the CNS, GIT, orbit, lungs, and bone marrow**. The **primary effusion lymphomas** present as malignant effusions, and the tumor cells are typically coinfected by both EBV and HHV8. This is an unusual example of cooperativity and mutual friendship between two oncogenic viruses to harm the host harboring it.

2. **B-cell hyperplasia in germinal center: During early HIV infection, the germinal center shows hyperplasia of B cells.** B-cell hyperplasia is usually manifested as generalized lymphadenopathy. Even with effective ART currently available, there is overall high rate of B-cell lymphoma in the HIV-infected population. This is true even in patients with normal CD4+ T-cell counts. **Majority of the lymphomas that develop in patients with normal CD4+ T-cell counts are not associated with EBV or HHV8.** Though the exact pathogenesis is not known, probably it may be due to severe B-cell hyperplasia in the germinal center that is observed early in HIV infection. **In germinal centers, B cells** undergo two processes namely, **class switching and somatic hypermutation in their *Ig* genes.** Both these processes **produce breaks in DNA, and they are error prone.** Sometimes this may lead to translocation of oncogenes.

B-cell lymphomas in early HIV infections: B-cell tumors that occur early in HIV infections (before the development of full-blown AIDS) include **Burkitt lymphoma and diffuse large B-cell lymphoma.** These are often associated with translocations of oncogenes into *Ig* gene loci. Thus, the marked B-cell hyperplasia in germinal center that occurs early in HIV infection may contribute to production of lymphoma. This may partly be due to increasing number of B cells that are prone for acquiring lymphoma-initiating events.

Other EBV-related proliferations in HIV Several other EBV-related proliferations also occur in HIV patients. These are as follows:

- **Hodgkin lymphoma:** Hodgkin lymphoma is an unusual B-cell tumor with a marked tissue inflammatory response with characteristic tumor cells namely Reed–Sternberg cells that constitute 1–3%. Hodgkin lymphoma also occurs at an increased frequency in HIV-infected individuals. In almost all cases of HIV-associated Hodgkin lymphoma, the characteristic Reed–Sternberg cells are infected with EBV. Low CD4+ counts are observed in many (but not all) HIV-associated Hodgkin lymphoma patients at the time of presentation.
- **Oral hairy leukoplakia:** It develops in immunocompromised individuals including AIDS. Oral hairy leukoplakia appears as white projections on the tongue, EBV infection is responsible for it. It results from EBV-driven squamous cell proliferation of the oral mucosa.

Other tumors

In addition to KS and lymphoma, AIDS patients have increased risk for other tumors. These include **HPV-associated carcinomas of the uterine, cervix, and the anus.**

HPV-associated SIL and carcinoma of cervix: HPV is closely associated with squamous cell carcinoma of the cervix and its precursor namely squamous intraepithelial lesion (SIL). HPV-associated SIL is almost 10 times more common in HIV-infected women when compared to uninfected women. It is restricted to HIV-infected women with CD4+ counts of <500 cells/μL. Thus, the increased risk may be due to reduced immune surveillance. In HIV-infected women, there is acceleration of the rate of progression from SIL to overt cervical carcinoma.

Central Nervous System Disease

CNS involvement is common (**Box 6**) and produces important manifestations of AIDS. Clinically apparent neurologic dysfunction is found in 40–60% of HIV patients. At autopsy, 90% of patients show some form of neurologic involvement. In some patients, neurologic manifestations may be the only or earliest presenting feature of HIV infection. CNS involvement includes the following:

- **Opportunistic infections and neoplasms**
- **HIV-related neuropathologic changes:** These include a self-limited meningoencephalitis (occurs at the time of seroconversion), aseptic meningitis, vacuolar myelopathy, peripheral neuropathies, and **progressive encephalopathy**. The progressive encephalopathy is most common and is designated clinically as HIV-associated neurocognitive disorder. Probably, it results due to a combination of HIV infection of microglia and an immune response in the CNS.

Various complications of AIDS due to HIV-1-mediated destruction of the cellular immune system are depicted in **Figure 17**. The infectious and neoplastic complications of AIDS can affect almost every organ system.

Box 6: CNS lesions in AIDS.

- Non-Hodgkin B-cell lymphoma—primary lymphoma of the brain
- Self-limited meningoencephalitis
- AIDS dementia complex
- Progressive multifocal leukoencephalopathy
- Meningoencephalitis (tuberculous, cryptococcal)
- Aseptic meningitis
- Peripheral neuropathy
- Demyelinating lesions of the spinal cord (vacuolar myelopathy)

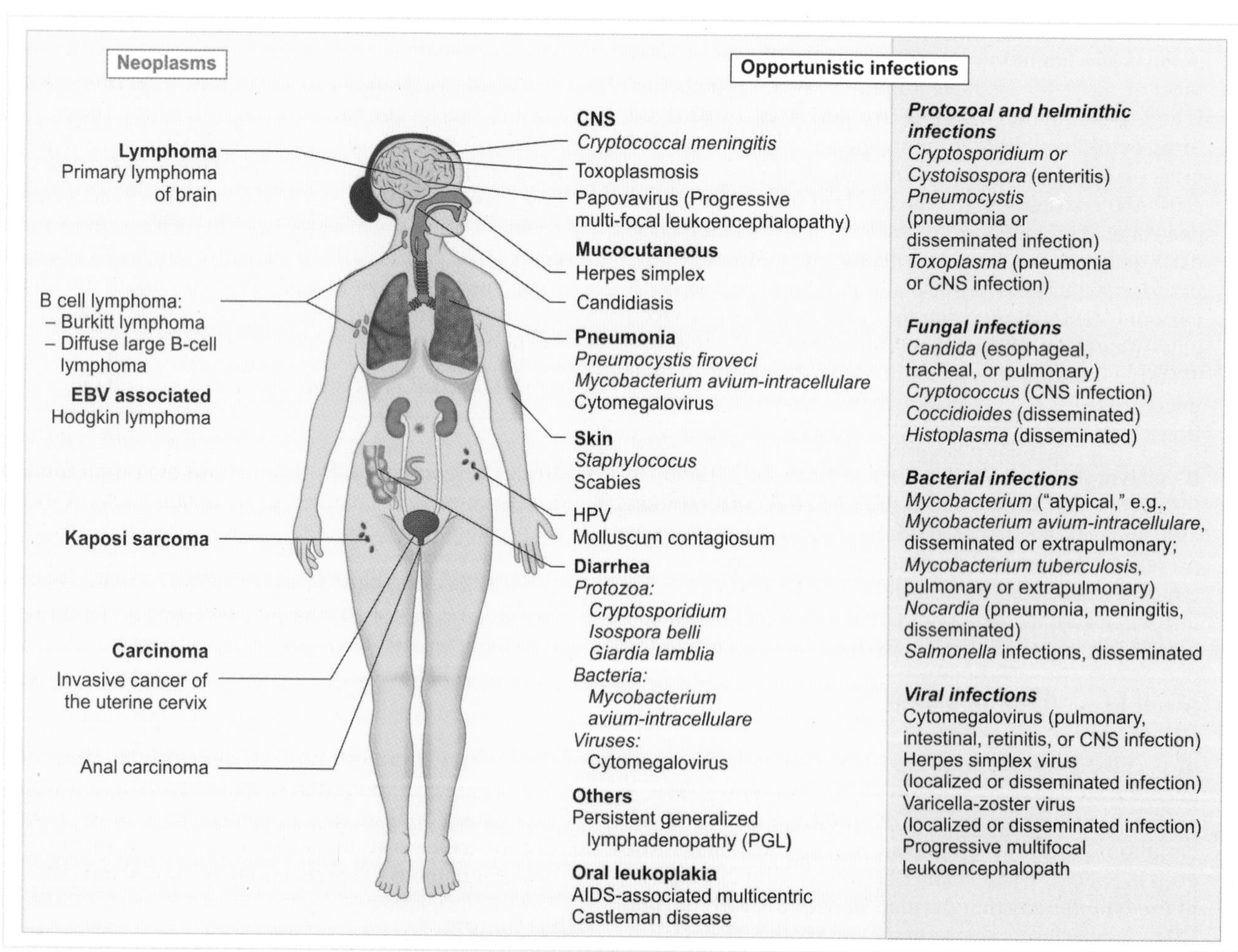

(CNS: central nervous system; HPV: human papilloma virus)

FIG. 17: Various complications of AIDS due to human immunodeficiency virus-1 (HIV-1)-mediated destruction of the cellular immune system.

Effect of Antiretroviral Drug Therapy

Q. Write short essay on effect of antiretroviral drug therapy (ART) in HIV.

Initial agents used for the treatment of HIV were designed to inhibit the function of HIV reverse transcriptase and protease.

Antiretroviral drug therapy (ART): New strategies or medications of ART are developed to treat patients with HIV/AIDS. ART (**Box 7**) consists of drugs that target the viral reverse transcriptase, protease, integrase, and coreceptor CCR5. They have dramatically changed the clinical course of HIV infection. ART reduced AIDS-related mortality and increased all indices of health in HIV-1-infected patients. HIV virus mutates much more than most other viruses. To reduce the emergence of drug-resistant mutants, ART drugs are given in combination. Currently, more than 25 antiretroviral drugs from six distinct drug classes are available for the management of HIV infection.

Effect of ART: When a combination of at least three effective drugs is used, HIV viral load is reduced to below the level of detection (<50 copies RNA/mL). This level remains indefinitely as long as the patient takes the therapy. Even if the virus develops drug resistance, there are several second- and third-line drugs available to fight against these drug-resistant viruses.

- **CD4+ T cells:** Once the virus is suppressed by ART, the progressive loss of CD4+ T cells is prevented. The CD4+ T-cell count in peripheral blood slowly increases and over a period of several years, often returns to normal. HIV patients with even undetectable viral loads for years on ART develop active infection if they stop drug treatment.
- **Decreased death rate:** With the use of ART, the death rate from AIDS has decreased.
- **Reduced AIDS-associated disorders:** Many AIDS-associated disorders (e.g., *P. jirovecii* infection, KS) are very uncommon after the ART.
- **Reduced transmission of the virus:** ART has also reduced the transmission of the virus. This is especially from infected mothers to newborns. Due to the reduced mortality, more individuals are living with HIV.

ART less effective against HIV in CNS and macrophages: ART drugs do not satisfactorily cross the blood–brain barrier. They are less effective in inhibiting HIV-1 persistence in macrophages. Thus, the CNS and other organs, especially mononuclear phagocytes in other organs such as the GIT and lung, may be a safe place for the virus.

Consequences of ART

The introduction of effective ART has led to many unanticipated new complications and consequences.

Box 7: Distinct classes of antiretroviral medicines.

- Nucleoside reverse transcriptase inhibitors
- Non-nucleoside reverse transcriptase inhibitors
- Protease inhibitors
- Integrase inhibitors
- Fusion inhibitors
- Entry inhibitors

Immune reconstitution inflammatory syndrome

In some patients with advanced disease and on ART, even after the recovery of immune system, the clinical condition paradoxically deteriorated. This occurs in spite of increased CD4+ T-cell counts and decreased viral load. This disorder is called immune reconstitution inflammatory syndrome. This syndrome affects about one-sixth of HIV patients and usually develops shortly after ART begins. The mechanism is not known. Probably it is due to a poorly regulated host response to the high antigenic burden of persistent microbes.

Adverse effects of ART

Important complication of long-term ART is due to adverse side effects of the ART drugs. These include lipoatrophy (loss of facial fat), lipoaccumulation (excess fat deposition centrally), raised levels of lipids, insulin resistance, and peripheral neuropathy. Drugs can also damage cardiovascular, renal, and hepatic function. In long-term ART-treated patients, the CD4+ T-cell counts are normalized. Hence, non-AIDS morbidity is far more common than classic AIDS-related morbidity in patients on long-term ART. These morbidities include cancer and increased rate of cardiovascular, kidney, and liver diseases. The exact mechanism for these non-AIDS-related complications is not known. Probably it may be due to persistent inflammation and immune dysfunction.

MORPHOLOGY

Morphological changes in the tissues are neither specific nor diagnostic of HIV infection. Common pathologic features of AIDS include opportunistic infections, KS, and B-cell lymphomas.

Lymph nodes: Though changes in lymph nodes are not specific, they have certain strange features.

- In the **early stages** of HIV infection, they show marked hyperplasia of B-cell follicles. The **germinal follicles are enlarged** and usually assume an **unusual serpiginous shape**. There is **attenuation of mantle zones** that surrounds these germinal follicles. The **germinal centers encroach on interfollicular T-cell areas**. The germinal hyperplasia of B cells reflects the polyclonal B-cell activation that is observed in HIV-infected individuals.
- **With disease progression**, the uncontrolled proliferation of B-cell subsides and produces **severe shrinkage of lymphoid tissue**. There is depletion of lymphocytes and disruption of the organized network of follicular dendritic cells (FDCs). There may be even **hyalinization of germinal centers**. The lymph node becomes small, atrophic, and "burnt-out." These lymph nodes **may show numerous opportunistic pathogens**, often within macrophages. Due to severe immunosuppression, there may be minimal or atypical inflammatory responses to infections, both in the lymph nodes and at extranodal sites. For example, mycobacteria may not produce granuloma because of deficiency of CD4+ T cells. In the empty-looking lymph nodes and in other organs, without special stains, the presence of infectious agents may not be readily identified.

Spleen and thymus: Apart from lymph nodes, **shrinkage of lymphoid tissue** is also found in the spleen and thymus in later stages of AIDS. They are almost devoid of lymphocytes.

Pathogenesis of Long-term Complications

Exact pathogenesis of long-term complications of HIV-1 infection following ART is not completely known. Probable pathogenesis is depicted in **Figure 18**.

With the advent of ART, the mortality rate has declined in HIV, but treated patients still carry viral DNA in their lymphoid tissues, and a cure remains difficult to achieve. To develop a vaccine, there are many hurdles. So far, it was not successful to have a vaccine-based prophylaxis for HIV. Molecular analyses have shown a worrying degree of variation in viral isolates from patients. This makes the task of producing a vaccine extremely difficult. Presently, the mainstays in the fight against AIDS are public health measures and antiretroviral drugs.

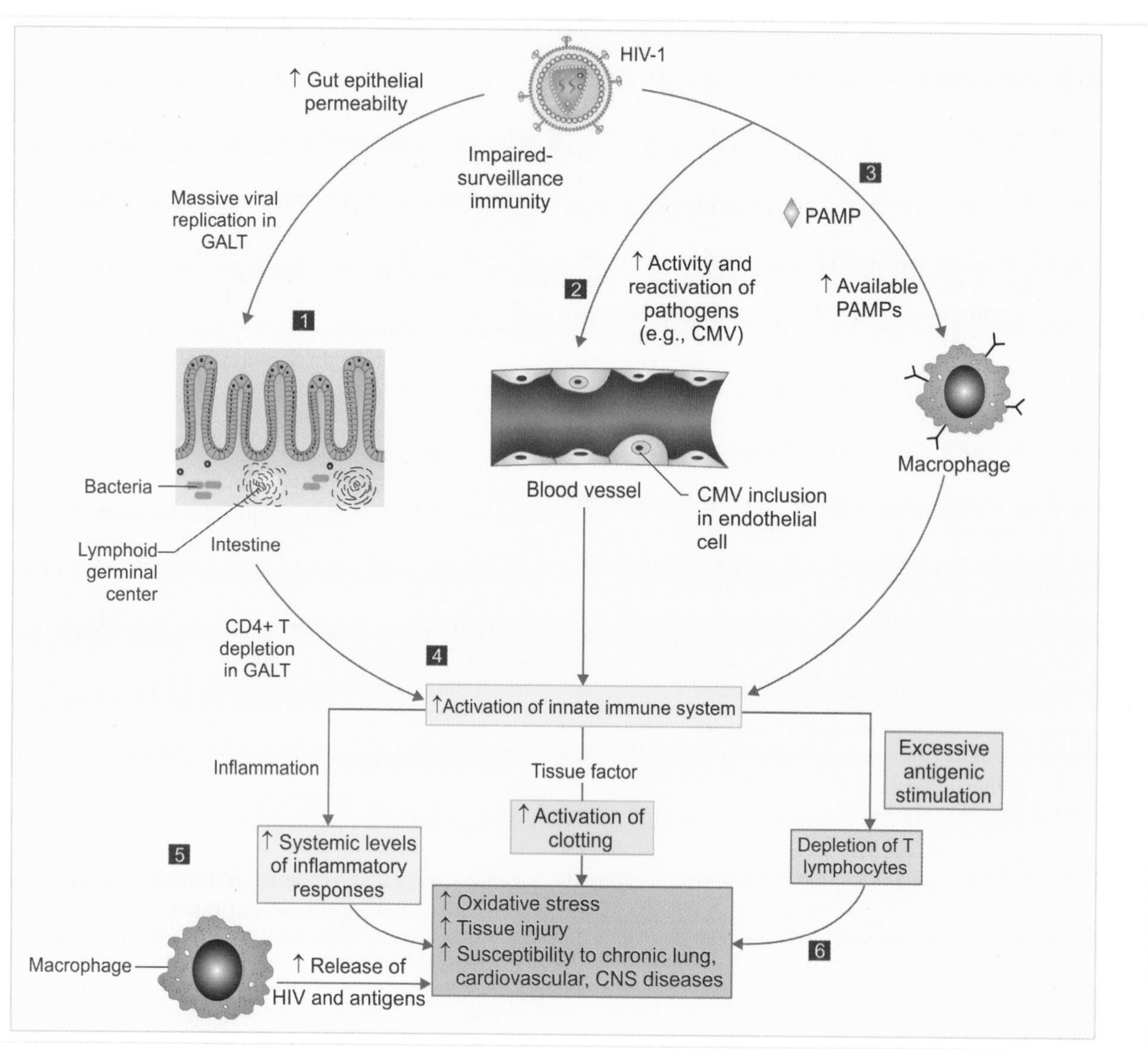

(GALT: gut-associated lymphoid tissue)

FIG. 18: Probable pathogenesis of long-term complications of human immunodeficiency virus-1 (HIV-1) infection following antiretroviral therapy (ART). 1. Chronic antigenic stimulation: HIV-1 infection impairs the barrier function of the gut epithelium. This leads to chronic antigenic stimulation by bacteria and other microbes in the gastrointestinal lumen. 2. Reactivation of pathogens: Impaired surveillance immunity against latent resident pathogens leads to reactivation of pathogens. For example, cytomegalovirus (CMV) within vasculature. 3. Excessive pathogen-associated molecular patterns (PAMPs): Antigens present macrophages and other cells of the innate immune system circulating in the blood. These increased circulating microbial antigens are associated with excessive levels of PAMPs. They stimulate their corresponding receptors (PRRs) on these cells. 4. Excessive activation of the innate immune system: The above three factors, all combined together, excessively activate the innate immune system. 5. Activated innate immune system in turn contributes to tissue injury by the following: (i) increases the systemic levels of inflammatory responses, (ii) tissue factor triggers clotting, and (iii) excessive antigenic stimulation with depletion of T-cell compartment. 6. Persistent HIV-1 infection of macrophage produces continuing production of HIV-1 antigens and virus particles. Along with this, combination of the three factors (mentioned under 5) leads to increased oxidative stress, depleting antioxidant reserves, and increased tissue injury, especially of cardiovascular, lung, and CNS.

Laboratory Diagnosis of HIV Infection and AIDS

Q. Write short essay on laboratory diagnosis of HIV infection and AIDS.

The diagnosis of HIV infection depends on three main types of tests—(1) the demonstration of antibodies to HIV (antibody tests), (2) the direct detection of HIV or one of its components (HIV RNA, i.e., viral load tests), and (3) a combination test that detects both antibodies and viral protein called p24 (antibody-antigen test, or HIV Ab-Ag test).

Demonstration of Antibodies to HIV

Antibodies to HIV usually appear in the circulation 3–12 weeks following infection. The standard blood screening tests for HIV infection depend on the detection of antibodies to HIV. It is detected by ELISA, also referred to as an EIA. Most diagnostic laboratories use kits that contain antigens from both HIV-1 and HIV-2, and they can detect antibodies to either. In fourth-generation EIA tests, the antibodies to HIV as well as the p24 antigen of HIV can be detected. EIA tests are generally reported as positive (highly reactive), negative (nonreactive), or indeterminate (partially reactive).

False-positive EIA tests: It may be seen when there are antibodies to class II antigens (e.g., following pregnancy, blood transfusion, or transplantation), autoantibodies, hepatic disease, recent influenza vaccination, and acute viral infections. Hence, in individuals suspected of having HIV infection based on a positive or inconclusive fourth-generation EIA result, it should be confirmed by a more specific assay such as an HIV-1- or HIV-2-specific antibody immunoassay, a western blot, or a plasma HIV RNA level.

Western blot assay: Multiple HIV antigens of different molecular weights can produce specific antibodies. In western blot assay, these antigens can be separated on the basis of molecular weight, and antibodies to each component can be detected. Though the western blot is an excellent confirmatory test for HIV infection in patients with a positive or indeterminate EIA, it is a poor screening test.

Point-of-care tests: Many point-of-care tests can give results in 1–60 minutes. They can be performed on blood, plasma, or saliva. The sensitivity and specificity of this test are approximately 99% when performed using whole blood.

Direct Detection of HIV or One of its Components

Many laboratory tests are available for the direct detection of HIV or its components (**Table 8**). These tests may be useful in making a diagnosis of HIV infection when the antibody determination assays or western blot results are indeterminate. Also, the tests for detecting the levels of HIV RNA can be used to determine prognosis and to assess the response to antiretroviral therapies.

Table 8: Characteristics of tests for direct detection of HIV.

Test	*Technique*
Immune complex–dissociated p24 antigen capture assay	Measurement of levels of HIV-1 core protein in an enzyme immunoassay (EIA)-based format. This is done following dissociation of antigen–antibody complexes by using weak acid treatment
HIV RNA by polymerase chain reaction (PCR)	Target amplification of HIV-1 RNA via reverse transcription followed by PCR
HIV RNA by branched DNA (bDNA)	Measurement of levels of particle-associated HIV RNA in a nucleic acid capture assay using signal amplification
HIV RNA by transcription-mediated amplification (TMA)	Target amplification of HIV-1 RNA through reverse transcription followed by T7 RNA polymerase
HIV RNA by nucleic acid sequence-based amplification (NASBA)	Isothermal nucleic acid amplification with internal controls

Immune complex-dissociated p24 antigen capture assay: It is the **simplest and economical test** for the direct detection. This is an EIA-type assay in which the solid phase consists of antibodies to the p24 antigen of HIV. It detects the viral protein p24 in the blood of HIV-infected individuals which may be present either as free antigen or complexed to anti-p24 antibodies. When blood samples are treated with a weak acid to dissociate antigen-antibody complexes, it gives increased positivity (in ~50% of infected patients). Throughout the course of HIV infection, there is usually an equilibrium between p24 antigen and anti-p24 antibodies. During first few weeks of HIV infection, before there is an immune response, the p24 antigen levels are markedly raised. These levels decrease after the development of anti-p24 antibodies. The p24 antigen capture assay is very useful as a screening test for HIV infection in patients suspected of having the acute HIV syndrome. This is because high levels of p24 antigen are present before the development of antibodies. Currently, its use as a routine blood donor screening for HIV infection has been replaced by nucleic acid test (NAT) or "fourth-generation" assays that combine antigen and antibody testing.

Measurement of HIV RNA levels in the plasma: Measuring and monitoring the levels of HIV RNA in the plasma of patients with HIV infection have helped in understanding of the pathogenesis of HIV infection and in monitoring the response to combination antiretroviral therapy (cART). Mainly four assays are used for measurement of HIV RNA in the plasma. They are—(1) reverse transcriptase PCR (RT-PCR); (2) branched DNA (bDNA); (3) transcription-mediated amplification (TMA); and (4) nucleic acid sequence-based amplification (NASBA). These tests are useful for the diagnosis of HIV infection, in establishing initial prognosis, and in monitoring the effects of therapy.

A **positive EIA with a confirmatory western blot or HIV RNA assay remains the "gold standard" for a diagnosis of HIV infection**. Culture of virus from the monocytes and CD4+ T cells can also be performed.

Prevention of HIV in Healthcare Facilities

Q. Write short essay on prevention of HIV in healthcare facilities.

It is to be borne in mind that there is a small but definite occupational risk of HIV transmission. This includes healthcare workers, laboratory personnel, and others who work with HIV-containing materials, particularly when sharp objects are used.

Potentially Infectious Source of HIV

Primary source of HIV infection: Healthcare workers are usually exposed while handling blood or body fluids in direct contact with an open wound, or by needle or sharp stick; also, during obstetric procedures, labor and delivery, and immediate care of the infant with HIV.

It is mainly transmitted through **blood and blood products**. Apart from blood, others such as **bloody body fluids, semen, and vaginal secretions** also are considered potentially infectious. However, they are usually not involved in occupational transmission from patients to healthcare workers.

- **Potentially infectious:** The fluids that are considered potentially infectious are cerebrospinal fluid, synovial fluid, pleural fluid, peritoneal fluid, pericardial fluid, and amniotic fluid. The risk for transmission after exposure to fluids or tissues other than HIV-infected blood is probably lower than the risk after blood exposures.
- **Not potentially infectious:** These include feces, nasal secretions, saliva, sputum, sweat, tears, urine, and vomitus. These are not considered potentially infectious for HIV unless they are visibly bloody.
- **Human bite:** Rare cases of HIV transmission via human bites may occur but not due to occupational exposure.

Mode of transmission: There is documented evidence for transmission of HIV through intact skin. The potential risks of HIV infection in healthcare worker are percutaneous injuries (e.g., a needle pricks or cut with a sharp object) or contact of mucous membrane or nonintact skin (e.g., skin with crack, abrasion, or dermatitis) with **blood, tissue, or other potentially infectious body fluids**.

- **Percutaneous transmission:** An increased risk for HIV infection following percutaneous exposures to HIV-infected blood is associated with exposures to relatively large amount of blood. For example, in case of a device visibly contaminated with the patient's blood, a procedure where a hollow-bore needle is placed directly in a vein or artery, or a deep injury.
- **Mucocutaneous transmission:** Factors that may lead to mucocutaneous transmission of HIV include exposure to an unusually large volume of blood and prolonged contact. In addition, the risk increases for exposures to blood from untreated patients with high levels of HIV in the blood.

Frequency of risk: The risk of HIV transmission following skin puncture from a needle or a sharp object that was contaminated with blood from an individual with documented HIV infection is approximately 0.23% and after a mucous membrane exposure, it is 0.09%. This risk is if the injured and/or exposed individual is not treated within 24 hours with antiretroviral drugs.

Prevention of HIV Transmission

It is necessary to prevent transmission from patient to healthcare worker or healthcare worker to patient or from patient to another patient. The basic preventive measures include:

Follow universal precautions: Universal precautions is an approach in infection control to treat all human blood and certain human body fluids as if they were known to be infectious for HIV, HBV, and other bloodborne pathogens. It is applied "universally" in caring for all patients, regardless of the diagnosis in order to minimize or avoid exposure to infection.

CDC guidelines for universal precautions are as follows:

- **Use of protective barriers [Personal protective equipment (PPE)]:** Use appropriate barrier precautions to prevent skin and mucous membrane exposure during contact with blood or other body fluids of any patient. Gloves should be worn while handling blood and body fluids, mucous membranes, or nonintact skin of all patients, for handling items or surfaces soiled with blood or body fluids, and for performing venipuncture and other vascular access procedures. Gloves should be changed after contact with each patient. Masks and protective eyewear or face shields should be worn during procedures that are likely to generate droplets of blood or other body fluids to prevent exposure of mucous membranes of the mouth, nose, and eyes. Gowns or aprons should be worn during procedures that are likely to generate splashes of blood or other body fluids.
- **Hands and other skin surfaces should be washed** immediately and thoroughly if contaminated with blood or other body fluids. Hands should be washed immediately after gloves are removed.
- **Use and dispose needles and sharps safely:** Should take precautions to prevent injuries caused by needles, scalpels, and other sharp instruments or devices during procedures; when cleaning used instruments; during disposal of used needles; and when handling sharp instruments after procedures. To prevent needlestick injuries, needles should not be recapped, purposely bent or broken by hand, removed from disposable syringes, or otherwise manipulated by hand.
- **Safe handling/disposal of contaminated material:** After their use, disposable syringes and needles, scalpel blades, and other sharp items should be placed in puncture-resistant containers for disposal; the puncture-resistant containers should be located as close as practical to the use area. Large-bore reusable needles should be placed in a puncture-resistant container for transport to the reprocessing area.
- Though saliva may not transmit HIV transmission, to **minimize the need for emergency mouth-to-mouth resuscitation, mouth pieces**, resuscitation bags, or other ventilation devices should be available for use in areas in which the need for resuscitation is predictable.
- **Healthcare workers having exudative lesions or weeping dermatitis should refrain from all direct patient care** and from handling patient-care equipment until the condition resolves.
- **Pregnant healthcare workers should be familiar with and strictly adhere** to precautions to minimize the risk of HIV transmission.

Other measures include:

- Decontamination of equipment and devices
- Cleaning of contaminated surfaces and prompt cleaning up of blood and body fluid spills
- Precautions during invasive procedures
- Precautions for dentistry
- Precautions for autopsies

- Precautions for dialysis
- Precautions for laboratories

To prevent transmission from patient to patient: Sterilize all contaminated equipment and devices.

Management of Exposures

Postexposure prophylaxis: Currently almost all puncture wounds and mucous membrane exposures in healthcare workers involving blood from a patient with documented HIV infection are treated prophylactically with combination antiretroviral therapy (cART). This practice is called as **postexposure prophylaxis or PEP**. This has dramatically reduced the occurrence of puncture-related transmissions of HIV to healthcare workers.

Laboratory Monitoring of Patients with HIV Infection

Q. Write short essay on laboratory monitoring in a patient on ART.

The laboratory tests play a key role in assessing HIV infection in an individual before ART is initiated and also for monitoring their treatment response and possible toxicity of antiretroviral drugs. There is a close relationship between clinical manifestations of HIV infection and CD4+ T cell count. Hence, measurement of CD4+ T cell numbers is routinely done for the evaluation of HIV-infected individuals. Another test for monitoring is by assessing the plasma levels of HIV RNA in the blood. Determination of peripheral blood CD4+ T-cell counts and measurement of the plasma levels of HIV RNA are powerful tools for determining prognosis and monitoring response to therapy.

CD4+ T-cell counts

CD4+ T-cell count is the laboratory test which is the best indicator of the immediate state of immunologic competence of the patient with HIV infection.

Direct CD4+ T-cell count or as percentage of total lymphocytes: This measurement can be done directly or calculated as the percentage of CD4+ T cells and the total lymphocyte count. The CD4+ T cells percentage is determined by counting the CD4+ T cells by flow cytometry and total lymphocyte count determined by the white blood cell (WBC) count multiplied by the lymphocyte differential percentage. A CD4+ T-cell percentage of 15 is comparable to a CD4+ T-cell count of 200/μL.

CD4+ T-cell count and possible infection: The CD4+ T-cell count correlates very well with the level of immunologic competence. When the **CD4+ T-cell counts <200/μL**, patients are at a high risk of infection by ***P. jirovecii***, whereas when the CD4+ T cell counts <50/μL, the patients are also at higher risk of infection from ***CMV*, mycobacteria of the *M. avium complex* (MAC), and/or *T. gondii***.

Monitoring of CD4+ T-cell count: In patients with HIV infection, CD4+ T-cell measurements should be done **first at the time of diagnosis and every 3–6 months thereafter**. More frequent measurements are necessary if there is a declining trend. For patients who have been on cART for at least 2 years with HIV RNA levels persistently <50 copies/mL and CD4 counts >500/μL, the monitoring of the CD4 count may be optional.

Clinical situations in which the CD4+ T-cell count may be misleading: These include—

- **Co-infection:** If patients have HTLV-1/HIV coinfection, elevated CD4+ T-cell counts do not accurately reflect their degree of immune competence.
- **CD4+ T-cell percentage:** CD4+ T-cell percentage may be a more reliable indication of immune function than the CD4+ T-cell count in certain situations. These include patients with hypersplenism or with splenectomy, and in patients receiving medications that suppress the bone marrow (e.g., IFN-α).

HIV RNA determinations

Measurement of serum or plasma levels of HIV RNA is an essential component in the monitoring of patients with HIV infection. Most common technique used to measure HIV RNA is the RT-PCR (reverse transcriptase PCR) assay. By this assay, number of copies of HIV RNA per milliliter of serum or plasma can be reliably detected with as few as 40 copies of HIV RNA per milliliter of plasma. More sensitive assay is by nested PCR techniques. Thus, it is possible to study tissue levels of virus as well as plasma levels of HIV RNA in patient with HIV infection.

Precautions: HIV RNA measurements are influenced by the state of activation of the immune system. It may fluctuate greatly when there is secondary infection or immunization. Hence, decisions based on HIV RNA levels should never be made on a single determination.

Monitoring: It should be as follows—

- Measurement of plasma HIV RNA levels should be performed **at the time of HIV diagnosis and every 3–6 months thereafter in the untreated patient**.
- **After the initiation of therapy or any change in therapy**, plasma HIV RNA levels should be monitored **every 4 weeks until the effectiveness of the therapeutic regimen** is determined. The effectiveness is indicated by the development of a new steady-state level of HIV RNA. With most effective ART, the plasma level of HIV RNA will drop to <50 copies/mL within 6 months of the initiation of treatment.
- **During therapy**, levels of HIV RNA should be monitored **every 3–6 months** to evaluate the continuing effectiveness of therapy.

HIV resistance testing

Presently many antiretroviral drugs are available for treatment. It is possible to measure the sensitivity of an individual' HIV to different antiretroviral agents.

Types of testing: HIV resistance testing can be done through either genotypic or phenotypic measurements.

- **Genotypic assays:** In this, sequence analyses of the HIV genomes obtained from patients is done. They are compared with sequences of viruses with known antiretroviral resistance profiles.
- **Phenotypic assays:** In this, the in vivo growth of viral isolates obtained from the patient. This is compared with the growth of reference strains of the virus in the presence or absence of different antiretroviral drugs. A modification of this phenotypic approach is available. In this technique, the enzymatic activities of the reverse transcriptase, protease, or integrase genes obtained by molecular

cloning of patients' isolates are performed. These are then compared with the enzymatic activities of genes obtained from reference strains of HIV in the presence or absence of different drugs targeted to these genes.

Indications for drug resistance testing: These are as follows—

- Recommended at the time of **initial diagnosis** and, if therapy is not started at that time of initial diagnosis, it should be done at **the time of initiation of cART**.
- **If there is virologic failure**, it should be performed while the patient is still on the failing regimen. This is because HIV may rapidly revert to wild-type in the absence of the selective pressures of cART. It helps in the selection of new drugs in patients with virologic failure.

Co-receptor tropism assays

Following the use of first CCR5 antagonist for the treatment of HIV infection, it became necessary to determine whether a patient's virus was likely to respond to this treatment.

Type of co-receptor: Early in the course of infection, patients tend to have CCR5-tropic virus and later in disease, they trend toward CXCR4 viruses.

Other tests

Other measurements are markers of disease activity and they help to increase our understanding of the pathogenesis of HIV disease. However, currently, they do not play a major role in the monitoring of patients with HIV infection. These include:

- Quantitative culture of replication-competent HIV from plasma, peripheral blood mononuclear cells, or resting memory CD4+ T cells.
- Circulating levels of β_2-microglobulin, soluble IL-2 receptor, IgA, acid-labile endogenous IFN, or TNF-α.
- Presence or absence of activation markers such as CD38, HLA-DR, and PD-1 on CD4+ or CD8+ T cells.
- Nonspecific serologic markers of inflammation and/or coagulation such as IL-6, d-dimer, and sCD14: These have been a high correlation with all-cause mortality.

Table 9 summarizes the recommended laboratory tests for HIV screening and monitoring. This also includes approaches to screen for coinfections and noncommunicable diseases.

Table 9: Summary of recommended laboratory tests for HIV screening and monitoring.

Recommended	***Desirable (If feasible)***
HIV diagnosis	
• HIV serology • CD4+ T-cell count • Screening for tuberculosis • Plasma HIV RNA levels (viral load)	• *Cryptococcus* antigen if CD4+ T-cell count ≤100 cells/mm^2 • Screening for sexually infections • Assessment for major noncommunicable chronic diseases and comorbidities • HBV (HBsAg) and HCV serology
Follow-up before ART	
• CD4+ T-cell count (every 6–12 months) • HIV resistance testing (before initiation of therapy)	
ART initiation	
• CD4+ T-cell count • Plasma HIV RNA levels (viral load)	• Pregnancy test • Measurement of blood pressure • Urine for glycosuria and estimated glomerular filtration rate (eGFR) • Depending the drug used: Serum creatinine, alanine aminotransferase
Receiving ART	
• CD4+ T-cell count (every 6 months) • Plasma HIV RNA levels (viral load at 6 months after initiating ART and every 12 months thereafter)	• Urine for glycosuria • Serum creatinine (depends on the drug used)
Virologic (treatment) failure	
• CD4+ T-cell count • Plasma HIV RNA levels (viral load) • HIV resistance testing	HBV (HBsAg) serology (before switching ART regimen if this testing was not done or if the result is negative at baseline)

AMYLOIDOSIS

Q. Discuss classification, chemical nature, pathogenesis, and clinical syndrome of amyloidosis. Enumerate the special stains for amyloid.

Definition: Amyloidosis is a **group of protein misfolding disorders in which there is extracellular deposition of insoluble fibrillar proteins** (that form insoluble β-pleated sheets) **in tissues and organs**. The deposit is called amyloid.

It is a pathologic condition associated with a number of inherited and inflammatory disorders. Amyloid is deposited in the extracellular space in various tissues and organs in several clinical conditions. With progressive accumulation, amyloid encroaches (impinges) on and produces pressure atrophy of adjacent cells. This can cause tissue damage and functional disturbances in the involved organ or tissue.

Aggregation of misfolded proteins: Proteins in their normal folded configuration are soluble. In amyloidosis, these are abnormal fibrils which are produced by the aggregation of misfolded proteins. These misfolded proteins are folded into an incorrect three-dimensional shape. They are usually nonfunctional. They are often resistant to breakdown and are not soluble. The fibrillary deposits bind a variety of proteoglycans and glycosaminoglycans present in the extracellular space. These include heparan sulfate and dermatan sulfate, and plasma proteins (especially serum amyloid P).

Contain charged sugar groups: The adsorbed proteins in these extracellular deposits contain abundant charged sugar groups. These sugar groups give the deposits staining characteristics that were thought to resemble starch (amylose, meaning crystallizable form starch). The term amyloid was coined around 1854 by the pathologist Rudolf Virchow. He thought that these deposits resembled starch (Latin *amylum*) under the microscope. This term amyloidosis is firmly established and unlikely to change despite being aware of fact that these deposits are unrelated to starch.

Amyloid deposition usually occurs gradually and sometimes difficult to explain (mysterious). Its clinical recognition basically depends on morphologic identification of this distinctive substance in appropriate biopsy specimens. Under the **light microscope and hematoxylin and eosin stains, amyloid appears as an amorphous, eosinophilic, hyaline, extracellular substance**. To differentiate amyloid from other hyaline materials (e.g., collagen, fibrin), many histochemical techniques are used. Most widely used is the Congo red stain. Under ordinary light, **Congo red** imparts a pink or red color to tissue deposits. But far more impressive and specific is the **green birefringence of the stained amyloid when viewed by polarizing microscopy**.

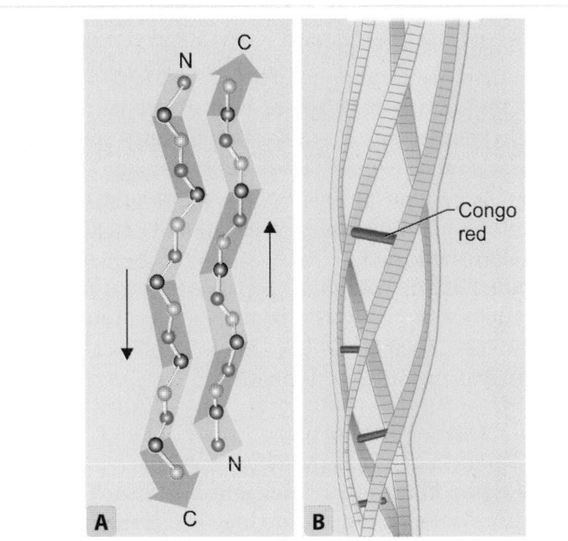

FIGS. 19A AND B: Schematic diagram of structure of amyloid fiber. β-pleated sheet contains extended stretches of polypeptide chain (sheets). Strands have a zig-zag shape. (A) Showing two fibrils arranged in antiparallel fashion. N represents amino terminal and C represents carboxy terminal (B) Showing four fibrils (there can be as many as six in each fiber) wound around one another with regularly spaced binding of the Congo red dye.

Properties of Amyloid Proteins

Microscopically, all amyloid deposits appear similar. But amyloid is not a single chemical entity. About more than 20 different proteins can aggregate to form amyloid. There are **three major and several minor biochemical forms**. These are deposited by different pathogenic mechanisms. So, amyloidosis is not a single disease. It is a group of diseases having in common the deposition of similar-appearing proteins in the extracellular space.

Physical Nature of Amyloid

Under electron microscopy, all types of amyloid, irrespective of clinical setting or chemical composition, are composed of **continuous, nonbranching fibrils**. These fibrils have **7.5–10 nm diameter.** X-ray crystallography (determines the atomic and molecular structure of a crystal, in which the crystalline structure causes a beam of incident X-rays to diffract into many specific directions) and infrared spectroscopy (deals with the infrared region of the electromagnetic spectrum, that is light with a longer wavelength and lower frequency than visible light) of **amyloid shows a characteristic cross-β-pleated sheet conformation (Fig. 19)**. This arrangement is responsible for the peculiar Congo red staining and green birefringence of amyloid when viewed by polarizing microscopy.

Chemical Nature of Amyloid

About **95% of the amyloid consists of fibril proteins** and remaining **5% consists of the P component and other glycoproteins**. The standard nomenclature is AX, where A indicates amyloidosis and X represents the protein present in the fibril. Amyloid consists of three major distinct proteins and more than 20 minor forms (**Box 8**). The two most common forms of amyloid are as follows:

Box 8: Chemical Forms of Amyloid

Major forms
- Amyloid light chain (AL) protein (λ and κ)
- Amyloid-associated (AA) protein
- β-amyloid (Aβ) protein

Minor types
- Transthyretin (TTR)
- β_2-microglobulin (β_2M)
- Leukocyte chemotactic factor-2 (LECT2) amyloid
- Apolipoprotein A and C variants: Apolipoprotein AI (AApoAI), apolipoprotein AII (AApoAII), apolipoprotein AIV (AApoAIV), apolipoprotein CII (AApoCII) and apolipoprotein CIII (AApoCIII).
- Gelsolin (AGel) amyloid
- Lysozyme (ALys) amyloid
- Fibrinogen Aα (AFib)
- Heavy chain (AH) amyloid
- Atrial natriuretic factor (AANF)
- Procalcitonin (ACal)
- Islet amyloid polypeptide/amylin (AIAPP)
- Amyloid precursor protein (APP) (Aβ)

1. **Major forms:** Three major forms are as follows—
   i. **Amyloid light chain (AL) protein:** Consists of complete Ig light chains or the amino-terminal fragments of light chains, or both.
      - Most of the AL proteins are composed of λ light chains or their fragments. In some cases, it may be κ chains.
      - The amyloid fibril protein of the AL type is produced from free Ig light chains secreted by a monoclonal population of plasma cells. AL is associated with certain plasma cell tumors.

   ii. **Amyloid-associated (AA) protein:** This amyloid is derived from a unique non-immunoglobulin (non-Ig) protein synthesized by the liver.
      - The AA protein found in the fibrils is derived from the proteolysis of a larger precursor in the serum called serum amyloid-associated (SAA) protein.

SAA protein is synthesized by the liver and circulates in the blood bound to high-density lipoproteins.

- Increased synthesis of SAA protein occurs in inflammatory states as part of the acute phase response. It occurs under the influence of cytokines (e.g., IL-6 and IL-1) during inflammation.
- This form of amyloidosis is associated with chronic inflammation and is usually called as secondary amyloidosis.

iii. **β-amyloid (Aβ) protein:** It is seen in the core of cerebral plaques and also the amyloid deposited in walls of cerebral blood vessels in patients with Alzheimer disease.

- Derived by proteolysis from a much larger transmembrane glycoprotein called amyloid precursor protein (APP).

2. **Minor types:** Many other biochemically distinct proteins can also be deposited as amyloid in different clinical conditions. Most often among these rare forms of amyloid are as follows:

i. **Transthyretin (TTR):** It is a normal tetrameric serum protein that binds and transports thyroxine and retinol. This protein is on chromosome 18. TTR can fold into beta sheets and is synthesized and secreted into the blood by the liver. Transthyretin amyloid (ATTR) is found in 13–17% of amyloid cases owing to its prevalence in the heart and lung. It is divided into hereditary disease associated with genetic mutations (ATTRm) and acquired disease associated with the wild-type protein (ATTRwt). Most patients are heterozygotes and have a mix of mutant and wild-type subunits.

a. **Hereditary mutated TTR:** It is caused by inherited TTR mutations. Different mutations in gene encoding TTR (and its fragments) can alter its structure and lead to misfolds. They constitute a group of genetically determined disorders called as familial amyloid polyneuropathies.

b. **Acquired disease associated unmutated TTR:** It may be deposited as amyloid in the heart of aged individuals and is called as senile systemic amyloidosis.

ii. **β_2-microglobulin (β_2M):** It is a normal serum protein and a component of MHC class I molecules and is present on all cells. It is normally cleared by glomerular filtration and later reabsorbed and catabolized in proximal tubules. It forms a major component (subunit) of a form of amyloid ($A\beta_2m$) that gets deposited in or around the joints or soft tissues of patients on long-term hemodialysis.

iii. **Leukocyte chemotactic factor-2 (LECT2) amyloid:** Initially, LECT2 was thought to result from only the wild-type protein without associated genetic abnormalities. However, recently it was found to be associated with genetic abnormality. LECT2 amyloid (ALECT2) can be found in renal amyloidosis, hepatic amyloidosis, and can also involve the spleen, pulmonary alveoli and septa, and adrenal gland.

iv. **Other minor types:** These include—

a. Apolipoprotein (AApo) A and C variants **amyloid:** It is caused by deposition of one of the apolipoprotein family of proteins, which are encoded on chromosome 11. It includes apolipoprotein AI (AApoAI), apolipoprotein AII (AApoAII), apolipoprotein AIV (AApoAIV), apolipoprotein CII (AApoCII) and apolipoprotein CIII (AApoCIII).

b. **Gelsolin (AGel) amyloid:** It is found in a systemic and hereditary amyloidosis. It typically presenting as an autosomal dominant polyneuropathy syndrome.

c. **Lysozyme (ALys) amyloid:** It is a consequence of mutation in the lysozyme enzyme and may be found in many organ systems but is predominantly nephropathic or involves the GI tract.

d. **Fibrinogen Aα (AFib):** It is found in an autosomal dominant systemic amyloidosis caused by mutations in the fibrinogen Aα-chain gene on chromosome 4.

e. **Heavy chain (AH) amyloid:** It is rare and may occur with or without accompanying AL amyloidosis, and usually involves IgG or IgA.

f. In a minority of patients of prion disease in the CNS, the misfolded prion proteins aggregate in the extracellular space. This acquires the structural and staining characteristics of amyloid.

Pathogenesis of Amyloidosis (Fig. 20)

Q. Write short essay on amyloidogenesis.

Amyloidosis results from **abnormal folding (misfolding) of proteins**. Misfolded proteins are normally degraded by quality control mechanisms. Thus, they are degraded intracellularly in proteasomes, or extracellularly by macrophages. In amyloidosis, these quality control mechanisms fail, and misfolded abnormal proteins accumulate outside cells. These **abnormal proteins become insoluble, aggregate, and deposit as fibrils in extracellular tissues**.

Two categories of proteins: The proteins that form amyloid belong to two general categories (**Fig. 20**):

1. **Production of abnormal amounts of normal protein:** Normal proteins may have an inherent tendency to fold improperly, associate, and form fibrils. A healthy cellular machinery is normally present in the body to chaperone (to look after or supervise) proteins during the process of synthesis and secretion. This makes sure that there is correct tertiary conformation and function, and to eliminate proteins that misfold. Improper folding occurs when the proteins are produced in increased amounts that exceeds the capacity for degradation. These proteins have an inherent tendency to fold improperly or undergo misfolding, associate, and form fibrils. For example, during inflammation, SAA is synthesized by the liver cells under the influence of cytokines such as IL-6 and IL-1 secreted by activated macrophages and is degraded by monocyte-derived enzymes. In individuals prone to amyloidosis, there may be defect in the monocyte-derived enzymes, incomplete breakdown of SAA, and formation of insoluble AA molecules. Genetically defective SAA may also be responsible for resistant degradation by macrophages. The amyloid fibril protein of the AL type is produced from

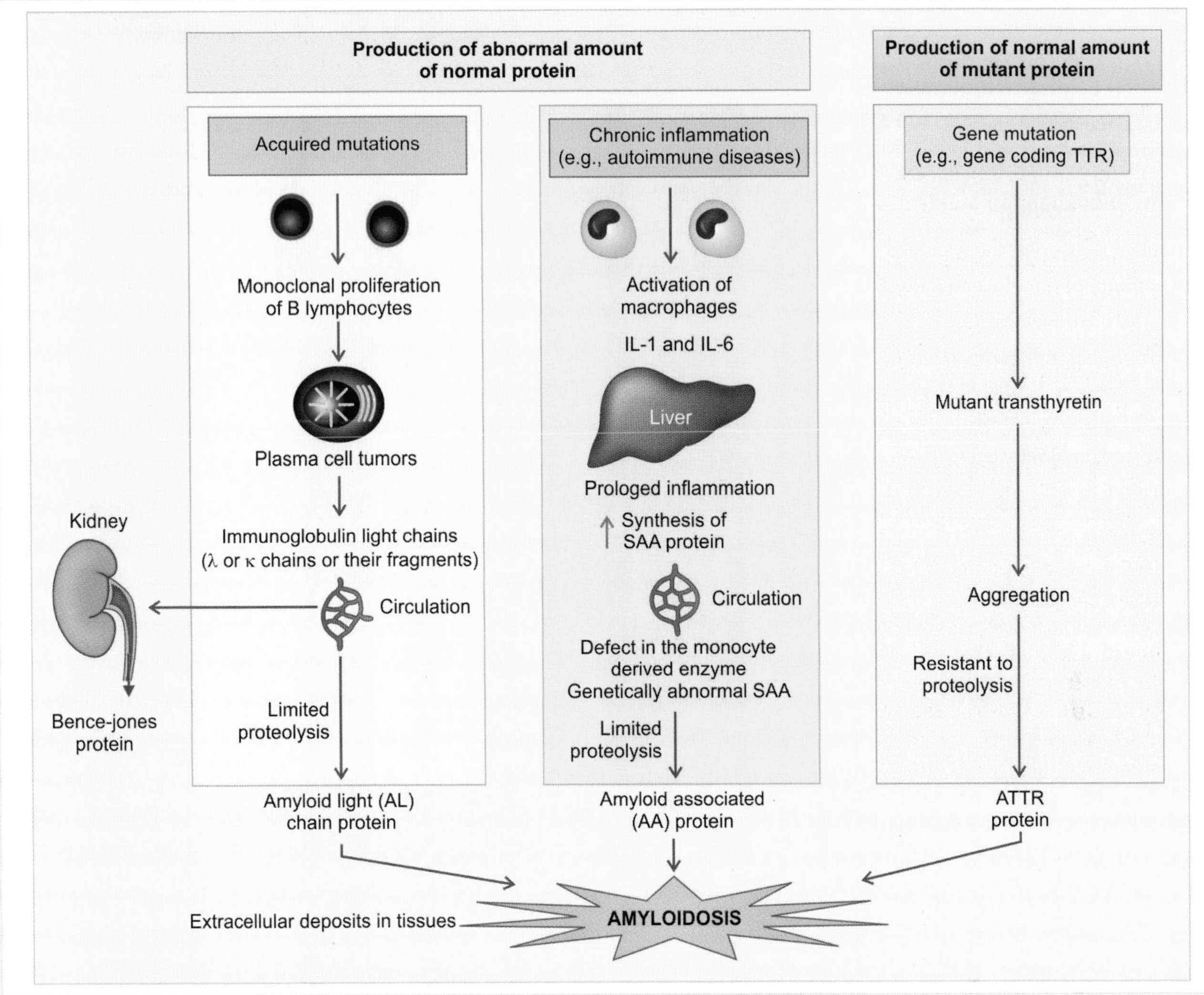

(AL: amyloid light chain; ATTR: amyloid transthyretin; IL: interleukin; SAA: serum amyloid-associated; TTR: transthyretin)

FIG. 20: Pathogenesis of amyloidosis. AL protein is seen in association with B lymphocyte and plasma cell proliferation (e.g., multiple myeloma) which secrete immunoglobulin light chains that are amyloidogenic. AA protein is seen in variety of diseases associated with the activation of macrophages, which, in turn, leads to the synthesis and release of SAA. The SAA is converted to AA protein. ATTR protein is due to mutant proteins which aggregate and deposit as amyloid.

free Ig light chains secreted by a monoclonal population of plasma cells and is associated with plasma cell tumors (e.g., multiple myeloma).

2. **Production of normal amount of mutant protein:** These proteins are liable to undergo misfolding and subsequent aggregation to form amyloid. For example, in familial amyloidosis, mutation of gene encoding TTR leads to alterations in structure of serum protein TTRs. These proteins are prone to misfolding, aggregate, and are resistant to proteolysis.

Pathological Effects of Amyloid Deposits

- Pressure on adjacent normal cells leads to atrophy of cells.
- Deposition in the blood vessel wall causes:
  - Narrowing of the lumen leading to ischemic damage
  - Increased permeability of vessels and escape of protein out of vessel

Classification of Amyloidosis

A given biochemical form of amyloid (e.g., AA) may be associated with amyloid deposition in different clinical conditions. Hence, a combined biochemical-clinical classification is more appropriate (**Table 10**).

- Depending on the distribution of amyloid, it may be classified as **systemic (generalized),** involving several organ systems, or **localized** to a single organ (e.g., heart).
- On clinical grounds, the systemic, or generalized, pattern is subclassified into:
  - Primary amyloidosis, associated with clonal plasma cell proliferations.
  - Secondary amyloidosis occurs as a complication of an underlying chronic inflammatory process.
  - Hereditary or familial amyloidosis constitutes a separate, but a heterogeneous group, with several distinctive patterns of organ involvement.

Table 10: Classification of amyloidosis.

Type	*Precursor protein*	*Fibril protein*	*Associated disease/s*
A. Systemic (generalized) amyloidosis			
Immunoglobulin light chain amyloidosis (primary amyloidosis)	Immunoglobulin light chains (mainly λ)	AL	Multiple myeloma, other monoclonal plasma cell proliferations
Reactive systemic amyloidosis (secondary amyloidosis)	Serum amyloid associated (SAA)	AA	Chronic inflammatory process
Hemodialysis-associated amyloidosis	β_2-microglobulin	$A\beta_2m$	Chronic renal failure
B. Hereditary or familial amyloidosis			
Familial Mediterranean fever	SAA	AA	
Familial amyloidotic neuropathies (several types)	Transthyretin	ATTR	
Systemic senile amyloidosis	Transthyretin	ATTR	
C. Localized amyloidosis			
• Senile cerebral	Amyloid precursor protein (APP)	Aβ	Alzheimer disease
• Endocrine			
○ Thyroid	(Pro)calcitonin	A Cal	Medullary carcinoma
○ Islets of Langerhans	Islet amyloid peptide (amylin) (IAPP)	AIAPP	Type 2 diabetes mellitus
○ Isolated atrial amyloidosis	Atrial natriuretic factor (ANF)	AANF	

(AA: amyloid associated; AL: amyloid light chain; ATTR: amyloid transthyretin; Cal: calcitonin; IL: interleukin; SAA: serum amyloid-associated; TTR: transthyretin)

Primary Amyloidosis: Plasma Cell Disorders Associated with Amyloidosis

Systemic and AL type: This category of amyloidosis is the most common form of amyloidosis. It is usually **systemic in distribution** and is of the **AL type**.

AL with plasma cell disorders: This type of amyloidosis is systemic, AL type, and is associated with plasma cell disorders. Plasma cell is derived from B cells. Plasma cell disorders are caused due to clonal proliferation of plasma cells that **synthesize an Ig (immunoglobulin) light chain**. These light chains are prone to form amyloid due to its intrinsic physiochemical properties. One of the well-defined diseases causing this type of systemic amyloidosis is **multiple myeloma**.

- **Multiple myeloma:** It is a malignant plasma cell tumor characterized by multiple osteolytic lesions throughout the skeletal system. The malignant plasma cells produce abnormal amounts of a single Ig. This produces an M (myeloma) protein "spike" on serum electrophoresis. Apart from the production of whole Ig molecules, the malignant plasma cells usually secrete **free, unpaired κ or λ light chains**. These light chains are called as **Bence-Jones protein**. Bence-Jones proteins have small molecular size and are often found in the serum and are excreted and concentrated in the urine. In primary amyloidosis, the free light chains are present in serum, urine, and are also deposited in tissues as amyloid. It should be noted that majority of myeloma patients who have free light chains in serum and urine do not develop amyloidosis. **Primary amyloidosis occurs in 5–15% of patients with myeloma.** It indicates that not all free light chains are equally likely to produce amyloid. The amyloidogenic property of any particular light chain is probably determined by its specific amino acid sequence.

AL without overt B cell neoplasm: Most individuals with AL amyloid are without any classic multiple myeloma or any other overt (apparent) B cell neoplasm. These are **classified as primary amyloidosis.** This is because their clinical features are due to the effects of amyloid deposition **without any other associated disease**.

- **Ig or free light chains:** Almost all these individuals **have monoclonal Igs or free light chains, or both**. These can be found in the serum or urine.
- **Monoclonal gammopathy:** Most of these patients also have a moderate increase in the number of plasma cells in the bone marrow. Probably, these plasma cells secrete the precursors of AL protein. Thus, these patients have an underlying monoclonal proliferation of Ig-producing cells (monoclonal gammopathy). In this category, plasma cell disorder with production of an abnormal protein is the dominant manifestation rather than presence of tumor masses.

Reactive Systemic (Secondary) Amyloidosis

Systemic and AA type: In this type of amyloidosis, deposits are systemic in distribution and biochemically are composed of AA proteins.

Develops as a complication of chronic inflammatory conditions: It develops as a complication of (secondary to) chronic inflammatory condition or tissue-destructive process. Hence, was previously termed as secondary amyloidosis. Complicates or occurs in association with diseases, such as:

- **Chronic infections:** At one time, it used to develop as a complication of chronic inflammatory conditions such as tuberculosis, leprosy, bronchiectasis, and chronic osteomyelitis. Because of presently available effective antibiotic therapy, the importance of these conditions has reduced as a cause of reactive systemic amyloidosis.

- **Autoimmune states:** Now, more commonly reactive systemic amyloidosis develops as **complications of rheumatoid arthritis** (most frequent), other connective tissue disorders such as **ankylosing spondylitis, SLE, and inflammatory bowel disease** (Crohn's disease and ulcerative colitis). About 3% of patients with rheumatoid arthritis develop amyloidosis and one-half of these produces clinically significant disease.
- **Heroin abusers:** Heroin users who inject the drug subcutaneously have a high rate of development of generalized AA amyloidosis. These patients develop chronic skin infections or abscesses due to subcutaneous self-administration of narcotics.
- **Solid tumors:** Reactive systemic amyloidosis may also develop in association with certain solid tumors. Most common examples include **renal cell carcinoma and Hodgkin lymphoma**.

Mechanism of amyloid deposition: In reactive systemic amyloidosis, production of SAA by hepatocytes is stimulated by cytokines. These cytokines include IL-6 and IL-1. These are produced during inflammation. When the inflammation is chronic and prolonged, there is sustained elevation of SAA levels. However, only just increased synthesis of SAA itself is not sufficient for the deposition of amyloid. This may occur by two possible mechanisms:

1. **Defect in the monocyte derived enzyme:** Normally, SAA is degraded to soluble end products by the action of enzyme derived from monocytes. Individuals who develop amyloidosis have an enzyme defect and this leads to improper or incomplete breakdown of SAA. This produces insoluble AA molecules.
2. **Genetically abnormal SAA:** Genetical structural abnormality in the SAA molecule may make it resistant to degradation by macrophages.

Hemodialysis-associated Amyloidosis

Chemical nature of amyloid: Patients with chronic or end-stage kidney disease who are on long-term hemodialysis can develop amyloidosis due to deposition of β_2-microglobulin. This β_2-microglobulin is present in high concentrations in the serum of individuals with chronic renal disease. This is because β_2-microglobulin cannot be filtered through dialysis membranes and gets deposited as amyloid.

Sites of amyloid deposits: In these patients, β_2-microglobulin gets deposited in joints, muscle, tendons, or ligaments. Patients usually present with local symptoms related to these deposits. One of the relatively common presentations is **carpal tunnel syndrome**. The incidence of hemodialysis related amyloidosis has substantially decreased with the increased use of new high-flux dialysis membranes.

Hereditary or Familial (Heredofamilial) Amyloidosis

It is a heterogeneous group consisting of variety of familial forms of amyloidosis. Most of them are rare and occur in certain geographic areas.

Familial mediterranean fever

- It is an autosomal recessive disorder and sometimes associated with widespread amyloidosis.
- It is an autoinflammatory syndrome in which there is excessive production of the cytokine IL-1 in response to inflammatory stimuli.
- It is clinically characterized by recurrent attacks of fever accompanied by inflammation of serosal surfaces (peritoneum, pleura, and synovial membrane).
- The gene for familial Mediterranean fever encodes a protein called pyrin. This is called so because of its relation to fever. Pyrin is one of the complex of proteins that regulate inflammatory reactions through activation of the inflammasome (refer pages 224–226).
- **Chemical nature of amyloid:** The amyloid fibril proteins are of AA type derived from SAA. SAA is produced in excessive amount in response to excessive IL-1 secretion. Increased IL-1 is observed during recurrent bouts of inflammation.

Familial amyloidotic neuropathies

- It is a group of autosomal dominant familial disorders characterized by deposition of amyloid mainly in peripheral and autonomic nerves.
- **Chemical nature of amyloid:** In this group of genetic disorders, the fibrils are composed of **mutant TTRs**. These genetically determined alterations of TTR structure render mutant TTR prone to misfolding and aggregation and resistant to proteolysis. The mutant TTR is deposited as amyloid fibrils.

Localized Amyloidosis

- Sometimes amyloid deposits are limited to a single organ (e.g., heart) or tissue. There is no involvement of any other site in the body as observed in generalized amyloidosis.
- The deposits may produce either grossly visible nodular masses or detected only by microscopic examination.
- **Sites:** Common sites of nodular deposits of amyloid are lung, larynx, skin, urinary bladder, tongue, and the region around the eye.
- **Microscopy:** Amyloid deposits may be surrounded by lymphocytes and plasma cells.
- **Chemical nature of amyloid:** In some cases, the amyloid consists of AL protein. Therefore, they may be localized form of plasma cell–derived amyloid.

Endocrine amyloid

- Endocrine tumors such as **medullary carcinoma of the thyroid, islet tumors of the pancreas**, and **pheochromocytomas** may show microscopic deposits of localized amyloid.
- Localized amyloid deposits may be observed in **islets of Langerhans in type 2 diabetes mellitus** (T2DM).

Chemical nature of amyloid: The amyloid proteins are probably derived either from polypeptide hormones (e.g., medullary carcinoma) or from unique proteins (e.g., islet amyloid polypeptide). The presence of amyloid in medullary carcinoma of the thyroid is a helpful diagnostic feature.

Amyloid of Aging

Q. Write short essay on senile amyloid.

Many well-documented forms of amyloid deposition are found with aging. Senile systemic amyloidosis is characterized by the systemic deposition of amyloid in elderly patients. The age of patients is usually between 70 and 80 years. Its dominant involvement produces dysfunction of the heart. Hence, this was previously called as senile cardiac amyloidosis. Those who are symptomatic present with the symptoms related to restrictive cardiomyopathy and arrhythmias. Usually this from is sporadic senile systemic amyloidosis, but rarely due to mutation of gene encoding TTR.

Chemical nature of amyloid: The amyloid in amyloid of aging is derived from the normal TTR molecule. Rarely a mutant form of TTR may predominantly affect the heart. In this mutant form of TTR, cardiomyopathy develops in both homozygous and heterozygous patients.

MORPHOLOGY

Main Organs Involved

In any categories of amyloidosis, there are **no consistent or distinctive patterns of organ or tissue distribution of amyloid deposits**. However, a few general features are as follows:

Immunoglobulin light chain amyloidosis: Amyloidosis associated with plasma cell proliferations **more often involves the heart, GIT, respiratory tract, peripheral nerves, skin, and tongue**.

Reactive systemic amyloidosis: In amyloidosis secondary to chronic inflammatory disorders, usually involved organs are **kidneys, liver, spleen, lymph nodes, adrenals, and thyroid**.

Hereditary amyloidosis: The amyloid deposits in the hereditary syndromes vary. In familial Mediterranean fever, the amyloidosis may be widespread and may involve the **kidneys, blood vessels, spleen, respiratory tract**, and (rarely) liver. The localization of amyloid in the remaining hereditary syndromes depends on the designation of these entities. For example, in familial amyloidotic neuropathies, deposition of amyloid is mainly in peripheral and autonomic nerves.

Gross

In any clinical disorder associated with amyloidosis, the deposits of amyloid may or may not be apparent grossly (macroscopically). If there is accumulation of large amount amyloid, affected organs are usually enlarged. The tissue appears gray with a waxy (**Fig. 21A**) appearance and firm in consistency.

Cut surface: If the amyloid deposits are large, painting the cut surface with iodine gives a yellow color, which is transformed to blue violet after application of sulfuric acid (which acidifies iodine). This method was used for demonstrating cellulose or starch. This staining property was responsible for the coining of the term amyloid (starch-like). But amyloid is neither starch nor cellulose.

Microscopy

Hematoxylin and eosin stain

- Amyloid deposits are **always extracellular** (**Fig. 21B**). The deposits begin between the cells (intercellular space) and often closely adjacent to basement membranes. In AL form associated with plasma cell proliferation, it is common to find deposits in the **perivascular region and in the vessel wall**.

Continued

Continued

- Progressive accumulation of amyloid encroaches on the cells. **Later it produces pressure atrophy of adjacent cells** and destroys them.
- **Appears as an amorphous, acellular, pale, eosinophilic** (**Fig. 22A**), **hyaline, glassy, extracellular substance** (material)
- Many other substances (e.g., collagen, fibrin) also stain eosinophilic with hematoxylin and eosin. Hence, it is **necessary to differentiate amyloid from these other hyaline deposits by using special stains**. The microscopic diagnosis of amyloid depends almost entirely on its staining characteristics.

Staining (tinctorial) properties of amyloid

1. **Congo red stain:** Staining technique using the dye Congo red is the **most common special stain used for the diagnosis of amyloidosis. Amyloid stains pink or red with the Congo red dye** under ordinary light under light microscope (**Fig. 22B**). But more specific when viewed **under polarizing microscope; amyloid gives so-called apple-green birefringence** (**refer Fig. 23**). This reaction with Congo red is seen in all forms of amyloid. This **staining reaction is due to the cross-β-pleated configuration of amyloid fibrils**. The fibrillar deposits organized in one plane exhibit one color, and those opposite to that plane appear the other color. Other regular protein structures (e.g., collagen) appear white under these conditions. The 10-nm-diameter amorphous nonoriented thin fibrils can also be seen by electron microscopy of paraformaldehyde-fixed tissue and are confirmatory for the diagnosis of amyloid.
2. **Van Gieson stain:** Amyloid takes up khaki color.
3. **Alcian blue:** Amyloid imparts blue color to glycosaminoglycans in amyloid.
4. **Periodic acid–Schiff (PAS) reaction:** Amyloid stains pink.
5. **Methyl violet and cresyl violet:** These metachromatic stains (belong to rosaniline group of basic dyes) give magenta or rose pink color to the amyloid deposits whereas surrounding tissue is colored blue.
6. **Iodine solution** produces a **dark, mahogany brown color** when poured over the cut surface of the organ involved by amyloidosis. It is **transformed to blue violet after application of sulfuric acid**.
7. **Thioflavin T:** It is not specific and may be less sensitive for amyloid, but amyloid fluoresce when viewed in ultraviolet light. Thioflavin T highlights amyloid with enhanced fluorescence emission at 480 nm, when excited at 450 nm. There are few reports of Congo red-negative amyloid requiring thioflavin T or crystal violet for diagnosis.
8. **Immunohistochemical staining:** Specific immunohistochemical staining can distinguish AA, AL, and ATTR types.

Morphology of Major Organs Involved

The pattern of organ involvement in different clinical forms of amyloidosis varies. Morphology of major organs involved in primary and/or secondary amyloidosis is discussed below.

Continued

Continued

Kidney

Kidney involvement is the **most common and the most serious form** of organ involvement.

Gross (Fig. 21A): It may be of normal size and color during early stages. In advanced stages, it may be shrunken due to ischemia. Ischemia is due to vascular narrowing induced by amyloid deposits within arterial and arteriolar walls.

Microscopy: Most commonly renal amyloid is of light-chain (AL in primary amyloidosis) or AA (in secondary amyloidosis type).

- **Glomeruli:** It is the main site of amyloid deposition (**Fig. 21B**).
    - First, focal deposits within mesangial matrix and produces subtle or minimal thickenings of the mesangial matrix. This is accompanied by diffuse or nodular uneven thickening/widening of the glomerular basement membranes.
    - Later, both the mesangial and basement membranes deposits cause narrowing of capillaries and distortion of the glomerular vascular tuft. Progressive accumulation of amyloid results in obliteration of the capillary lumen and the obsolescent glomerulus shows broad ribbons of amyloid.
- Amyloid may also be deposited in the peritubular interstitial tissue, arteries, and arterioles.
- **Congo red stain:** Histological sections when stained by dye Congo red, amyloid appears pink or red under light microscope, But it gives so-called apple-green birefringence when same is viewed under polarizing microscope (**Fig. 23**).

Spleen

Gross: It may be normal in size or may cause moderate to marked splenomegaly (200–800 g). For completely strange reasons, it may show one of the two patterns of deposition:

1. **Sago spleen:** Amyloid deposits are **mainly limited to the splenic follicles**. Grossly it appears like tapioca/sago granule; hence known as sago spleen. Microscopically, the **amyloid is deposited in the wall of arterioles in the white pulp**.
2. **Lardaceous spleen:** Amyloid is **deposited in the walls of the splenic sinuses and connective tissue framework in the red pulp**. This may result in moderate to marked enlargement of spleen. Fusion of the early deposits gives rise to large, map-like areas of reddish color on cut surface. This resembles pig fat (lardaceous) and hence called as lardaceous spleen. Microscopically, it shows **amyloid deposits in the wall of the sinuses**.

Light microscopy: These deposits appear homogenous pink, which when stained with Congo red and viewed under polarizing microscope, give rise to characteristic green birefringence.

Liver

Gross: The amyloid deposits may be inapparent grossly or may cause moderate to marked enlargement of liver (hepatomegaly). In advance stages, it appears pale, gray, and waxy.

Continued

Continued

Microscopy

- Amyloid first deposits in the space of Disse and then progressively encroaches on adjacent hepatic parenchymal cells and sinusoids.
- Progressive accumulation leads to deformity, pressure atrophy, and disappearance of liver cells. This can cause total replacement of large areas of liver parenchyma. Vascular involvement is frequent. Even with extensive involvement of liver, its function is usually preserved.

Heart

Q. Write short essay on cardiac amyloidosis.

It may be involved in any form of systemic amyloidosis (AL type). It is the major organ involved in senile systemic amyloidosis.

Gross: Heart may be enlarged and firm. But often it does not show any significant changes on gross examination. The amyloid deposits first begin in the subendocardial region and may appear as gray-pink like dew drop.

Microscopy: First, amyloid deposits are seen in the subendocardial region. Later, amyloid is deposited between the muscle fibers (**Fig. 24**). Their progressive accumulation causes pressure atrophy of myocardial fibers.

Clinical significance: When the amyloid deposits are subendocardial, they may damage the conduction system. This may be responsible for the electrocardiographic abnormalities observed in some individuals.

Other Organs

Tongue: Nodular deposits of amyloid in the tongue may cause macroglossia. This gives rise to the designation tumor-forming amyloid of the tongue.

Respiratory tract: It may be involved focally or diffusely from the larynx down to the smallest bronchioles.

Brain: A distinct form of amyloid is seen in the brains of patients with Alzheimer disease. It may form so-called plaques or get deposited in the blood vessels.

Peripheral and autonomic nerves: Amyloidosis of peripheral and autonomic nerves is a feature of many familial amyloidotic neuropathies.

Wrist: Depositions of amyloid can occur in patients on long-term hemodialysis. It involves most prominently the carpal ligament of the wrist and causes compression of the median nerve (carpal tunnel syndrome). There may also be extensive deposits of amyloid in the joints.

Medullary carcinoma of thyroid: Acellular amyloid deposits in the stroma is often found in medullary carcinoma of thyroid (**Figs. 22** and **23**).

Common chemical types of amyloid in different organ systems are presented in **Table 11**.

Clinical Features

Clinical presentation of amyloidosis is variable. No single set of symptoms points unequivocally to amyloidosis as a diagnosis. Amyloidosis may not produce any clinical manifestations, or it may produce symptoms related to the sites or organs affected. Amyloidosis may be diagnosed unexpectedly in the course of evaluation for something unrelated, with no clinical manifestations referable to the amyloidosis itself. It may cause serious clinical illness and even death. Clinical manifestations initially may be nonspecific (e.g., weakness, weight loss, lightheadedness, syncope) and be detected as an unsuspected anatomic change. The symptoms depend on the underlying disease, the quantity of amyloid deposited, and the sites or organs affected. However, organ dysfunction differs greatly between individuals and between different organs. Specific symptoms appear later and are related to renal, cardiac, and gastrointestinal involvement.

Renal involvement: Kidney involvement may cause proteinuria. Sometimes, proteinuria is so massive to produce nephrotic syndrome. In advanced cases, the obliteration of glomeruli by amyloid deposits may lead to renal failure and uremia. Renal failure is a common cause of death in amyloidosis with renal involvement.

Cardiac amyloidosis: Involvement of heart may gradually and slowly produce congestive heart failure. Most serious consequences of cardiac amyloidosis are conduction disturbances and arrhythmias, which may prove fatal. Occasionally, it may lead to a restrictive pattern of cardiomyopathy and clinically resemble features of chronic constrictive pericarditis. Short of biopsy, two-dimensional echocardiography and Doppler studies are helpful in suggesting the diagnosis of cardiac amyloidosis. Cardiac magnetic resonance imaging with late gadolinium enhancement may also be useful. Serum cardiac troponin and N-terminal pro-brain natriuretic peptide concentrations are powerful predictors of cardiac involvement and prognosis.

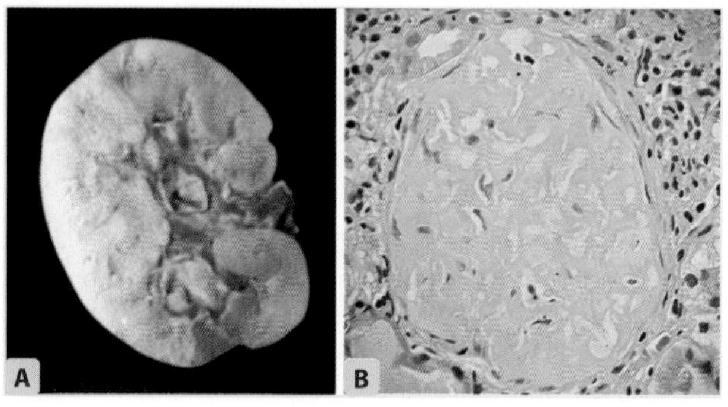

FIGS. 21A AND B: Amyloid kidney. (A) Cut section of an amyloid kidney showing waxy appearance; (B) Microscopic appearance of amyloidosis of kidney showing pink, amorphous extracellular amyloid deposits in the entire glomerulus (H&E stain).

Gastrointestinal amyloidosis: Amyloid may involve the ganglia, smooth muscle, vasculature, and submucosa of the GIT. Deposits in these locations can alter gastrointestinal motility and absorption. Usually, GIT involvement is clinically silent or entirely asymptomatic. If symptomatic, it may present in a variety of ways:

- Amyloidosis of the tongue may cause **marked enlargement of tongue (macroglossia)**. Enlarged tongue (**Fig. 25A**) is pathognomonic of AL amyloidosis that may be found in about 10% of patients. **The inelasticity of tongue may restrict the speech and swallowing.**
- Amyloid depositions in the **stomach and intestine** may lead to malabsorption, diarrhea, and digestive disturbances.

Vascular amyloidosis. Deposits of amyloid in the vessel (capillaries) cause vascular fragility and may lead to easy bruising and bleeding. Sometimes, it may be massive and can occur spontaneously or following mild or insignificant trauma. In some patients, AL amyloid binds and inactivates factor X (important coagulation factor). This can lead to a life-threatening bleeding disorder. Cutaneous ecchymosis especially around the eyes and can produce "raccoon-eye" (dark circles around the eyes) sign (**Fig. 25B**).

Neuropathies: Autonomic dysfunction with gastrointestinal motility disturbances (diarrhea, constipation) and peripheral sensory neuropathies are relatively common. Carpal tunnel syndrome with weakness and paresthesia of the hands may be an early presenting feature.

Diagnosis of Amyloidosis

Diagnosis depends on the microscopic demonstration of amyloid deposits in tissues.

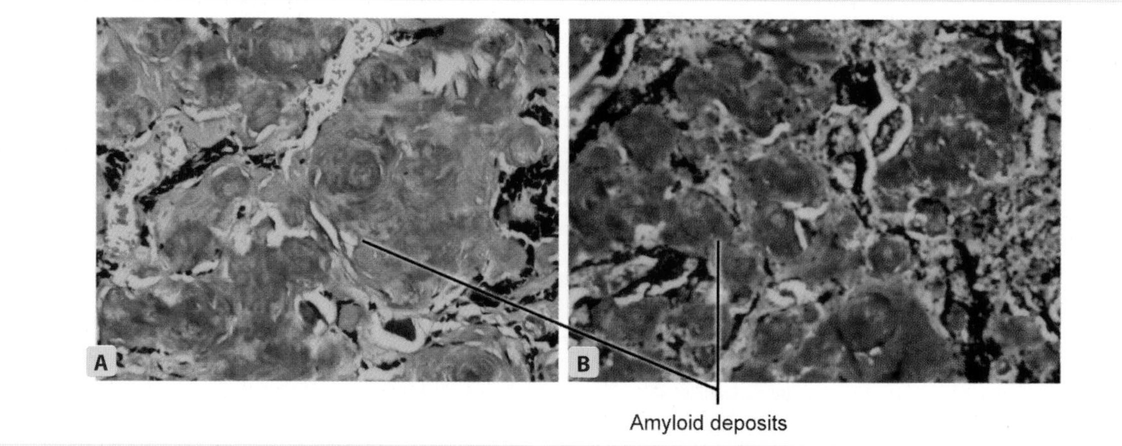

FIGS. 22A AND B: Amyloid deposits in medullary carcinoma of thyroid. (A) Amyloid appears as extracellular, amorphous, eosinophilic substance under H and E stain; (B) Congo red stain gives red color to the amyloid deposits.

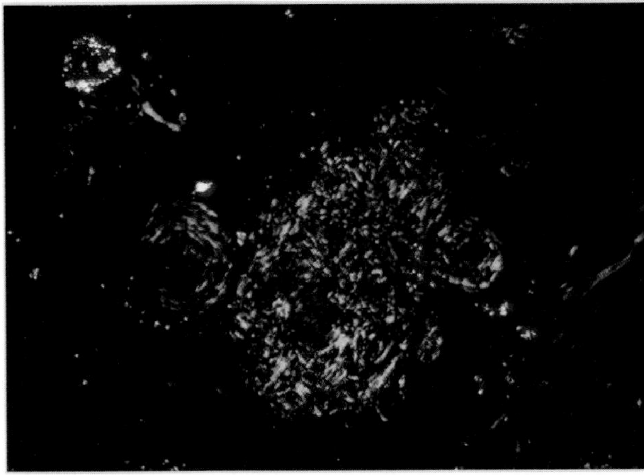

FIG. 23: Medullary carcinoma of thyroid. Congo red stain viewed under polarizing microscope gives apple-green birefringence to amyloid deposits.

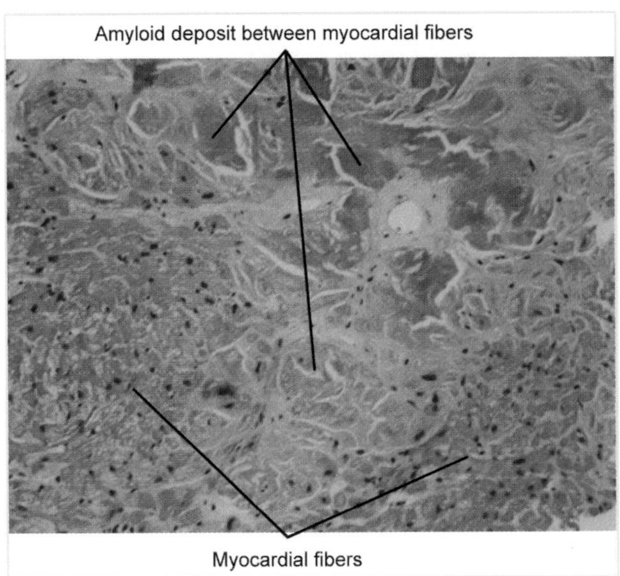

FIG. 24: Amyloid deposits between cardiac muscle fibers.

Table 11: Common chemical types of amyloid in different organ systems.

Organ system	*Common amyloid types*
Heart	AL, ATTR
Kidney	AL, AA, ALECT2
Gastrointestinal tract	AL, AA, ATTR
Liver	AL, ATTR, ALECT2
Lung	AL, ATTR, AA
Peripheral nervous system	AL, ATTR
Carpal tunnel, joints	AL, Aβ_2M (if on dialysis)

(AA: serum amyloid A; Aβ_2M: β_2-microglobulin; AL: light chain; ALECT2: leukocyte chemotactic factor-2; ATTR: transthyretin)

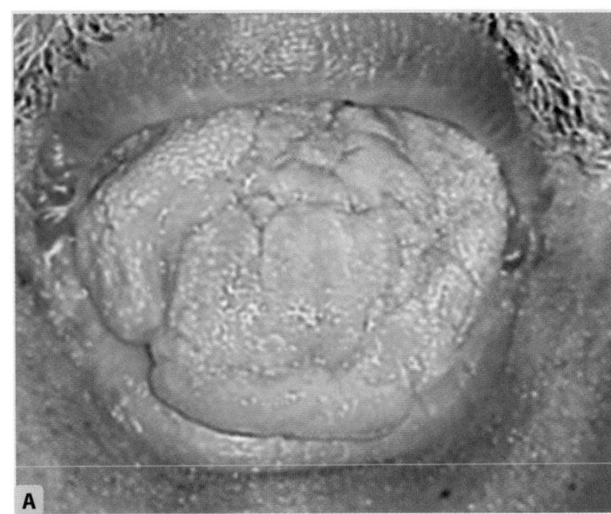

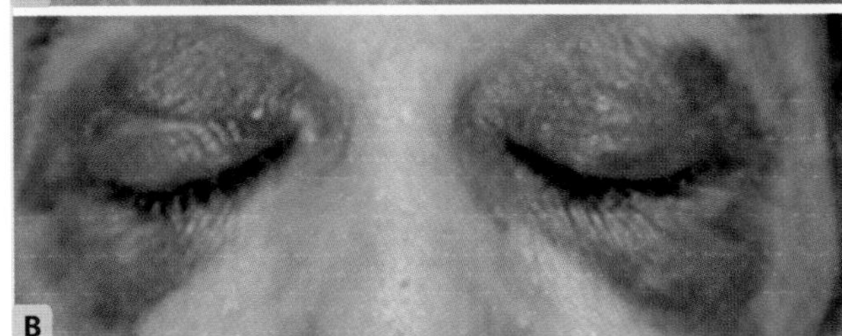

FIGS. 25A AND B: Amyloidosis. (A) Macroglossia; (B) Periorbital ecchymoses producing dark circles around the eyes.

- **Biopsy:** The most common sites of biopsy are the kidneys when there are renal manifestations. Biopsy of rectum or gingival tissues is the most common site of biopsy in patients having suspicion of systemic amyloidosis.
- **Examination of abdominal fat aspirates stained with Congo red** can also be for the diagnosis of systemic amyloidosis. It is **quite specific but has low sensitivity**. For obtaining fat aspirate, local anesthesia is given to the abdominal region and abdominal fat aspirated with a 16-gauge needle. Fat globules expelled onto a glass slide can be stained with Congo red stain. This procedure avoids a surgical procedure. If this material is negative, more invasive biopsies of the kidney, heart, liver, or GIT can be considered in patients in whom amyloidosis is suspected.
- **In suspected cases of AL amyloidosis** (in plasma cell disorders associated with amyloidosis), **serum and urine protein electrophoresis** and immunoelectrophoresis should be done. Bone marrow aspirates may show monoclonal plasmacytosis, even in the absence of multiple myeloma.
- **Scintigraphy with radiolabeled serum amyloid P (SAP) component** is a **rapid, noninvasive, and specific test**. Radiolabeled human SAP is a quantitative in vivo tracer for amyloid deposits. SAP binds to the amyloid deposits and reveals their presence. It is also helpful for measuring the extent of amyloidosis and can be used to follow patients undergoing treatment.

- **Determine the precursor protein type:** Once amyloid is found on microscopy; the precursor protein type must be determined. It may be done **by using immunohistochemistry, immunoelectron microscopy, or extraction and biochemical analysis** employing mass spectrometry; gene sequencing is used to identify mutants causing hereditary amyloidosis.

Prognosis

For generalized amyloidosis, prognosis is poor. In AL amyloidosis, overall median survival is 2 years after diagnosis. Prognosis is even poorer in patients with myeloma-associated AL amyloidosis. Prognosis of reactive systemic amyloidosis is somewhat better. It depends to some extent on the control of the underlying primary condition.

BIBLIOGRAPHY

1. Abbas AK, Lichtman AH, Pillai S. Cellular and Molecular Immunology, 9th edition. Philadelphia: Elsevier; 2018.
2. Actor JA. Introductory Immunology, 2nd edition. United Kingdom: Elsevier; 2019.
3. Buxbaum JN, Linke RP. A molecular history of the amyloidosis. *J Mol Biol*. 2012;421:142-59.
4. Casanova JL, Abel L. Human genetics of infectious diseases: unique insights into immunological redundancy. *Semin Immunol*. 2018;36:1-12.
5. Cohen MS, Shaw GM, McMichael AJ, et al. 1 infection. *N Engl J Med*. 2011;364:1943-54.
6. Dogan A. Amyloidosis: insights from proteomics. *Annu Rev Pathol Mech Dis*. 2017;12:277-304.
7. Douek DC, Roederer M, Koup RA. Emerging concepts in the immunopathogenesis of AIDS. *Annu Rev Med*. 2009;60:471.
8. Durandy A, Kracker S, Fischer A. Primary antibody deficiencies. *Nat Rev Immunol*. 2013;13:519-33.
9. Fischer A, Notarangelo LD, Neven B, et al. Severe combined immunodeficiencies and related disorders. *Nat Rev Dis Primers*. 2015;1:15061.
10. Giannini G, Nast CC. An Organ System–Based Approach to Differential Diagnosis of Amyloid Type in Surgical Pathology. *Arch Pathol Lab Med*. 2020;144:379.
11. Jameson JL, Fausi AS, Kasper DL, et al. Harrison's principles of internal medicine (2 vols), 20th edition. New York: McGraw-Hill Medical Publishing. Division; 2018.
12. Klimov VV. From Basic to Clinical Immunology. Switzerland: Springer Nature; 2019.
13. Kumar V, Abbas AK, Aster JC, Deyrup AT. Robbins essential pathology, 1st edition. Philadelphia: Elsevier; 2021.
14. Kumar V, Abbas AK, Aster JC. Robbins basic pathology, 10th edition. Philadelphia: Saunders Elsevier; 2018.
15. Kumar V, Abbas AK, Fausto N, et al. Robbins and Cotran pathologic basis of disease, 10th edition. Philadelphia: WB Saunders; 2021.
16. Merlini G, Dispenzieri A, Sanchorawala V, et al. Systemic immunoglobulin light chain amyloidosis. *Nat Rev Dis Primers*. 2018;4:38.
17. Moir S, Chun TW, Fauci AS. Pathogenic mechanisms of HIV disease. *Annu Rev Pathol Mech Dis*. 2011;6:223-48.
18. Parvaneh N, Casanova JL, Notarangelo LD et al. Primary immunodeficiencies: a rapidly evolving story. *J Allergy Clin Immunol*. 2013;131:314-23.
19. Punt J, Stranford SA, Jones PP, Owen JA. Kuby Immunology, 8th edition. New York: Macmilan learning; 2019.
20. Ralston SH, Penman ID, Strachan MWJ, et al. Davidson's principles and practice of medicine, 23rd edition. Edinburgh: Churchill Livingstone; 2018.
21. Strayer DS, Saffitz JE. Rubin's Pathology: Mechanism of Human Disease, 8th edition. Philadelphia: Wolters Kluwer; 2020.
22. Westermark GT, Fandrich M, Westermark P: AA amyloidosis: pathogenesis and targeted therapies. *Ann Rev Pathol Mech Dis*. 2015;10:321.

INDEX

Page numbers followed by *b* refer to box, *f* refer to figure, *fc* refer to flowchart, and *t* refer to table.

B

C

D

E

F

G

H

I

J

K

L

M

O

P

Q

R

S

T

U

V

W

X

Y

Z